10TH EDITION

TOPLEY & WILSON'S

MICROBIOLOGY & MICROBIAL INFECTIONS

IMMUNOLOGY

10TH EDITION

TOPLEY & WILSON'S

MICROBIOLOGY & MICROBIAL INFECTIONS

Topley & Wilson's Microbiology and Microbial Infections has grown from one to eight volumes since first published in 1929, reflecting the ever-increasing breadth and depth of knowledge in each of the areas covered. This tenth edition continues the tradition of providing the most comprehensive reference to microorganisms and the resulting infectious diseases currently available. It forms a unique resource, with each volume including examples of the best writing and research in the fields of virology, bacteriology, medical mycology, parasitology, and immunology from around the globe.

www.topleyandwilson.com

VIROLOGY Volumes 1 and 2

Edited by Brian W.J. Mahy and Volker ter Meulen
Volume 1 ISBN 0 340 88561 0; Volume 2 ISBN 0 340 88562 9; 2 volume set ISBN 0 340 88563 7

BACTERIOLOGY Volumes 1 and 2

Edited by S. Peter Borriello, Patrick R Murray, and Guido Funke
Volume 1 ISBN 0 340 88564 5; Volume 2 ISBN 0 340 88565 3; 2 volume set ISBN 0 340 88566 1

MEDICAL MYCOLOGY

Edited by William G. Merz and Roderick J. Hay
ISBN 0 340 88567 X

PARASITOLOGY

Edited by F.E.G. Cox, Derek Wakelin, Stephen H. Gillespie, and Dickson D. Despommier
ISBN 0 340 88568 8

IMMUNOLOGY

Edited by Stephan H.E. Kaufmann and Michael W. Steward
ISBN 0 340 88569 6

Cumulative index

ISBN 0 340 88570 X

8 volume set plus CD-ROM

ISBN 0 340 80912 4

CD-ROM only

ISBN 0 340 88560 2

For a full list of contents, please see the *Complete table of contents* on page 1027

10TH EDITION

TOPLEY & WILSON'S
MICROBIOLOGY & MICROBIAL INFECTIONS

IMMUNOLOGY

EDITED BY

Stefan H.E. Kaufmann PHD
Director, Department of Immunology
Max-Planck-Institute for Infection Biology, Berlin, Germany

Michael W. Steward BSC PHD DSC
Emeritus Professor of Immunology
London School of Hygiene and Tropical Medicine, London, UK

Hodder Arnold
A MEMBER OF THE HODDER HEADLINE GROUP

ASM PRESS

First published in Great Britain in 1929
Second edition 1936
Third edition 1946
Fourth edition 1955
Fifth edition 1964
Sixth edition 1975
Seventh edition 1983 and 1984
Eight edition 1990
Ninth edition 1998
This tenth edition published in 2005 by
Hodder Arnold, an imprint of Hodder Education and a member of the Hodder Headline Group,
338 Euston Road, London NW1 3BH

http://www.hoddereducation.com

Distributed in the United States of America by ASM Press, the book publishing division of the American Society for Microbiology, 1752 N Street, N.W. Washington, D.C. 20036, USA

British Library Cataloguing in Publication Data
A catalogue record for this book is available from the British Library

Library of Congress Cataloging-in-Publication Data
A catalog record for this book is available from the Library of Congress

This volume only ISBN-10 0 340 885 696 ISBN-13 978 0 340 885 697
Complete set and CD-ROM ISBN-10 0 340 80912 4 ISBN-13 978 0 340 80912 9
Indian edition ISBN-10 0 340 88559 9 ISBN-13 978 0 340 88559 8

1 2 3 4 5 6 7 8 9 10

Commissioning Editor: Serena Bureau / Joanna Koster
Development Editor: Layla Vandenberg
Project Editor: Zelah Pengilley
Production Controller: Deborah Smith
Index: Merrall-Ross International Ltd.
Cover Designer: Sarah Rees

Cover image: Coloured SEM of macrophage engulfing protozoan / Science Photo Library

Typeset in 9/11 Times New Roman by Lucid Digital, Salisbury, UK
Printed and bound in Italy

What do you think about this book? Or any other Hodder Arnold title? Please send your comments to www.hoddereducation.com

Contents

Contributors

Rafi Ahmed
Emory Vaccine Center; and
Department of Microbiology and Immunology
Emory University School of Medicine
Atlanta, GA, USA

Antonio Alcami PHFD
Department of Medicine
University of Cambridge
Addenbrooke's Hospital
Cambridge, UK; and
Senior Research Assistant
Centro Nacional de Biotecnologia (CSIC)
Campus Universidad Autonoma
Madrid, Spain

Brigitte A. Askonas
Department of Biological Sciences
Imperial College London
London, UK

Richard J. Aspinall
Reader in Immunology
Division of Investigative Science and Medicine
Imperial College London
London, UK

Michel Aurrand-Lions PHD
Senior Scientist
Department of Pathology and Immunology
Centre Medical Universitaire
Geneva, Switzerland

Marco Baggiolini MD
Professor
University of Lugano (USI)
Lugano, Switzerland

Marc Bonneville
Research Director, CNRS
INSERM U601
Institute of Biology
Nantes, France

Gillian Borland PHD
Division of Biochemistry & Molecular Biology
Institute of Biomedical & Life Sciences
University of Glasgow, UK

Frances Bowe
Centre for Molecular Microbiology and Infection
Department of Biological Sciences
Imperial College London
London, UK

Prosper N. Boyaka
Department of Microbiology
The University of Alabama at Birmingham
Birmingham, AL, USA

Aoife P. Boyd BA(Mod) PHD
Lecturer, Department of Microbiology
National University of Ireland
Galway, Ireland

Gordon D. Brown PHD
Institute of Infectious Disease and Molecular Medicine
Faculty of Health Sciences, CLS
University of Cape Town
Cape Town, South Africa

Shane Crotty PHD
Assistant Member
Division of Vaccine Discovery
La Jolla Institute for Allergy & Immunology (LIAI)
San Diego, CA, USA

Helena Crowley
Department of Pathology
Tufts University School of Medicine
Boston, MA, USA

William Cushley PHD
Division of Biochemistry & Molecular Biology
Institute of Biomedical & Life Sciences
University of Glasgow, UK

Anthony L. DeFranco
Department of Microbiology and Immunology
University of California
San Francisco, CA, USA

Giuseppe Del Giudice MD
IRIS Research Center, Chiron SrI
Siena, Italy

Gordon Dougan
Professor and Director
Centre for Molecular Microbiology and Infection
Department of Biological Sciences
Imperial College London
London, UK

Stefan Ehlers MD
Professor, Division of Molecular Infection Biology
Research Center Borstel
Borstel, Germany

Antonio Ferrante FRCPATH PHD
Director of Department of Immunopathology
Women's and Children's Hospital
South Australia; and
Professor, Department of Paediatrics
University of Adelaide; and
Professor of Immunopharmacology
School of Pharmacy and Medical Sciences
University of South Australia
Adelaide, Australia

Alain Fischer
Inserm U429
Necker University Hospital
Paris, France

Bernhard Fleischer
Bernhard Nocht Institute for Tropical Medicine
and Institute for Immunology
University Hospital Eppendorf
Hamburg, Germany

Kohtaro Fujihashi
Department of Pediatric Dentistry
Immnunobiology Vaccine Center
School of Dentistry
University of Alabama at Birmingham
Birmingham, AL, USA

Antoine Galmiche MD PHD
Department of Cellular Microbiology
Max Planck Institute fur Ifektions Biologie
Berlin, Germany

Tomas Ganz PHD MD
Departments of Medicine and Pathology
David Geffen School of Medicine at UCLA
Los Angeles, CA, USA

Paul Garside PHD
Professor of Immunobiology
Division of Immunology, Infection and Inflammation
University of Glasgow, Western Infirmary
Glasgow, UK

Andrew J.T. George MA PHD FRCPATH
Professor of Molecular Immunology
Department of Immunology
Division of Medicine
Imperial College London
Hammersmith Hospital
London, UK

Siamon Gordon MB CHB FAMS PHD
Glaxo Wellcome Professor of Cellular Pathology
Sir William Dunn School of Pathology
University of Oxford
Oxford, UK

Adrian Hayday BA MA PHD
Head of Division of Immunology, Infection
and Inflammatory Diseases
Kay Glendinning Professor, and Chair
The Peter Gorer Department of Immunobiology
Guy's, King's, and St Thomas' Medical School
King's College London
London, UK

Ann B. Hill MB BS FRACP PHD
Associate Professor
Department of Molecular Microbiology
and Immunology
Oregon Health and Science University
Portland, OR, USA

Christoph Hölscher PHD
Junior Professor, Junior Research Group
Molecular Infection Biology
Research Center Borstel
Borstel, Germany

Shiou-Chih Hsu (Stephen) PHD
Postdoctoral Research Scientist
Institute of Animal Health
Compton, Berkshire, UK

Brigitte T. Huber PHD
Department of Pathology
Tufts University School of Medicine
Boston, MA, USA

Ralf Ignatius
Department of Medical Microbiology and Infection Immunology
Charité University Medicine Berlin
Berlin, Germany

Beat A. Imhof PHD
Professor and Chairman
Department of Pathology and Immunology
Centre Medical Universitaire
Geneva, Switzerland

Elizabeth R. Jarman PHD
Wellcome Trust Research Laboratories
Malawi-Liverpool School of Tropical Medicine
Blantyre, Malawi

Klas Kärre
Microbiology and Tumorbiology Center (MTC)
Karolinska Institute
Stockholm, Sweden

Linda S. Klavinskis BSC PHD
Senior Lecturer
Peter Gorer Department of Immunobiology
Guys, Kings' and St. Thomas' School of Medicine
Guys Hospital, London, UK

Ulrich H. Koszinowski
Chair of Virology
Max von Pettenkofer-Institut
München, Germany

Jonathan R. Lamb DSC FRCPATH FMEDSCI FRSE
GlaxoSmithKline Immunology Group
Translational Medicine and Technology
Clinical Pharmacology and Discovery Medicine
Greenford, UK

Robert I. Lehrer MD
Department of Medicine
UCLA School of Medicine
Los Angeles, CA, USA

Myron M. Levine MD DTPH
Professor and Director
Center for Vaccine Development
University of Maryland School of Medicine
Baltimore, MD, USA

Pius Loetscher PD PHD
Novartis Institutes of Biomedical Research
Novartis Pharma AG
Basel, Switzerland

Richard Lucius
Full Professor, Department of Molecular Parasitology
Institute of Biology
Humboldt-University Berlin
Berlin, Germany

Daniela N. Männel
Department of Immunology
University of Regensburg
Germany

Jerry R. McGhee
Department of Microbiology
The University of Alabama at Birmingham
Birmingham, AL, USA

Graham F. Medley BSC PHD
Professor of Infectious Disease Epidemiology
Department of Biological Sciences
University of Warwick
Coventry, UK

Kingston H.G. Mills BA(Mod) PHD
Professor of Experimental Immunology
Department of Biochemistry
Trinity College Dublin
Ireland

Edward E.S. Mitre MD
Clinical Associate
Laboratory of Parasitic Diseases
National Institute of Allergy and Infectious Diseases
National Institutes of Health
Bethesda, MD, USA

B. Paul Morgan FRCPATH MRCP PHD
Department of Medical Biochemistry and Immunology
University of Wales College of Medicine
Cardiff, UK

Anne Marie Moulin MD PHD
Directeur de Recherche
Centre National de la Recherche Scientifique, CEDEJ
Le Caire, Egypte

Allan M. Mowat BSC(Hons) MBCHB PHD FRCPATH
Division of Immunology, Infection and Inflammation
University of Glasgow, Western Infirmary
Glasgow, UK

Claude P. Muller
Professor of Immunology
University of Trier, Trier, Germany; and
Institute of Immunology, LNS; and
Director, WHO Collaborating Center for Measles and
European Reference Laboratory for Measles
and Rubella
Luxembourg, Grand-Duchy of Luxembourg

James P. Nataro MD PHD
Professor of Pediatrics and Medicine
Center for Vaccine Development; and
Associate Chair for Research
Department of Pediatrics
University of Maryland School of Medicine
Baltimore, MD, USA

D. James Nokes BSC PHD
Senior Lecturer, Ecology and Epidemiology Group
Department of Biological Sciences
University of Warwick, Coventry, UK; and
Senior Research Officer
Centre for Geographic Medicine Research (Coast)
Kenya Medical Research Institute
Kilifi, Kenya

Thomas B. Nutman MD
Head, Helminth Immunology Section, and
Head, Clinical Parasitology Unit
Laboratory of Parasitic Diseases
National Institute of Allergy and
Infectious Diseases
National Institutes of Health
Bethesda, MD, USA

Charles W. Parker
Emeritus Professor of Medicine Microbiology/
Immunology
Washington University School of Medicine
St. Louis, MO, USA

Charalambos D. Partidos DVM MSc PHD
Senior Research Scientist
UPR 9021, CNRS
Immunologie et Chimie Thérapeutiques
Institut de Biologie Moléculaire et Cellulaire
Strasbourg, France

Sidney Pestka MD
Professor and Chairman
Department of Molecular Genetics,
Microbiology and Immunology
University of Medicine and Dentistry
Robert Wood Johnson Medical School
Pistcataway NJ, USA; and
Program Director
Cancer Institute of New Jersey
New Brunswick, NJ, USA; and
Chief Scientific Officer
PBL Biomedical Laborateries
Piscataway, NJ, USA

Liljana Petrovska DVM MSC PHD
Centre for Molecular Microbiology and Infection
Department of Biological Sciences
Imperial College London
London, UK

Eckhard R. Podack
Professor and Chairman
Department of Microbiology
and Immunology
University of Miami School of Medicine
Miami, FL, USA

Mike M. Putz MENG PHD
Department of Virology
Faculty of Medicine, Imperial College London
London, UK

Rino Rappuoli PHD
IRIS Research Center, Chiron Srl
Siena, Italy

John G. Raynes BSC PHD
Senior Lecturer
London School of Hygiene and Tropical Medicine
London, UK

Sergio Romagnani
Department of Internal Medicine
University of Florence, Italy

Thomas Schneider
Gastroenterologie, Infektiologie, Rheumatologie
Charité, Campus Benjamin Franklin
Universitätsmedizin
Berlin, Germany

Nicolas W.J. Schröder MD
Institute for Microbiology and Hygiene
'Charité' University Medical Center
Medical Faculty of The Humboldt-University
Berlin, Germany

Ralf R. Schumann MD PHD
Professor of Medicine and Microbiolobgy
Institute for Microbiology and Hygiene
'Charité' University Medical Center
Medical Faculty of The Humboldt-University
Berlin, Germany

Marie-Anne Shaw BSc PhD
Senior Lecturer in Human Genetics
School of Biology
University of Leeds
Leeds, UK

Werner Solbach MD
Professor and Chair
Institute for Medical Microbiology and Hygiene
University Luebeck
Luebeck, Germany

Carrie Steele BA MSc PhD
The Peter Gorer Department of Immunology
Guy's, King's, and St Thomas' Medical School
King's College London
London, UK

Emil R. Unanue MD
Professor and Chair
Department of Pathology and Immunology
Washington University School of Medicine
St Louis, MO, USA

Jonathan W. Yewdell
Laboratory of Viral Diseases
National Institute of Allergy and
Infectious Diseases
Bethesda, MD, USA

Jens Zerrahn PhD
Max-Planck-Institute for Infection Biology
Department of Immunology
Berlin, Germany

Arturo Zychlinsky
Max Planck Institut fur Infektions Biologie
Department of Cellular Microbiology
Berlin, Germany

Preface

Since its first publication in 1929, Topley and Wilson has focused on microbiology and microbial infections. The Tenth edition not only covers virus infection and all types of pathogen, but for the first time also includes one specific volume on immunology. Microbiology and immunology both emerged from infectious disease research which experienced its golden age in the second half of the 19th century. At that time, microbiology - in Paris under the direction of Louis Pasteur and in Berlin under the leadership of Robert Koch - not only led to the discovery of the major pathogens but also to the elucidation of the principal host defense mechanisms effected by the immune system. Elias Metchnikoff in Paris, and Emil von Behring and Paul Ehrlich in Berlin can be considered as the pioneers of immunology of those days. These researchers strongly emphasized the immune response as a defense mechanism against infectious agents. Subsequently however, medical microbiology and immunology developed in their separate ways. A large part of immunology became integrated into pathology, transplantation, and internal medicine. Whilst this broad diversification of immunology illustrates the importance of the immune system in all aspects of life, no doubt exists that the immune system developed first of all as a defense mechanism against infection. We therefore consider it a wise decision of the editorial board of Topley and Wilson to dedicate a full volume to immunology in its Tenth edition.

Infectious disease is best understood as the outcome of the cross-talk between the microbial pathogen and the host immune response. Therefore the understanding of infectious disease cannot be complete if one of these aspects is underrepresented. Previous editions of Topley and Wilson covered several aspects of host immunity to infectious agents. These chapters were, however, divided in volumes discussing the different classes of microbial pathogens. This allowed for direct reference to the relevant immune mechanisms in the same volume. However, the basic immune mechanisms of host defense against pathogens are independent of the type of pathogen being counteracted. Therefore, by covering specific immune responses to distinct types of pathogens, some overlap was unavoidable. This also led to the omission of both general basic aspects and specific topics of immunology not directly related to infectious disease. These obstacles are now overcome by including a single volume on immunology in Topley and Wilson which allows us to cover the whole spectrum of immunology ranging from basic mechanisms to medical application.

This volume comprises 46 chapters subsumed under the following topics: innate immunity and inflammation, soluble mediators, acquired immunity, infection and immunity, immunopathology and immunodeficiency, and vaccines. This structure allows the reader to both identify the specific topics related to infectious diseases and find sufficient information on basic mechanisms underlying immunity. Moreover, the reader is provided with information on clinical issues of immunology as they relate to immunopathology and immunodeficiency. Finally, seven chapters are dedicated to the different aspects of vaccination and vaccine development. Vaccinology represents the most direct application of immunology and although the first vaccine against smallpox was developed by Edward Jenner without knowledge of immunological mechanisms, immunology has subsequently proved to be vital for the rational design of new vaccines. Vaccination remains the most cost-efficient measure in medicine and, in the future, it is likely to provide us with powerful means for combating infectious diseases, and hopefully for controlling autoimmunity and cancer.

Based on our conviction that infectious disease is the outcome of cross-talk between microbial pathogen and host immune response, we are pleased that the discipline of immunology now has been given a whole volume of Topley and Wilson. In many infectious diseases prevalent today, immunopathology is equally important for disease outbreak and progression as are microbial virulence factors. This is perhaps most impressively illustrated by AIDS (Acquired Immune Deficiency Syndrome). The responsible pathogen, HIV (Human Immunodeficiency Virus), directly attacks CD4 helper T cells, the central coordinators of the immune response, in this way causing immunodeficiency and immunopathology. In fact, numerous microbial pathogens are now being implicated as being directly or indirectly involved in the development of autoimmune diseases and immunodeficiences.

We are proud to have attracted an internationally-recognized panel of experts to share their insights into the different aspects of immunology. We wish to thank all these authors for their contributions which make this volume an invaluable asset for all those interested in how the immune system works. We would also like to take the opportunity of expressing our thanks to the editorial team at Hodder and to Yvonne Bennett, for their immense input and efforts. Last but not least, we would like to thank our wives for their understanding that we spent so much time with this book rather than with our families.

Stefan H. E. Kaufmann
Michael W. Steward
Berlin and London
May 2005

Abbreviations

AA arachidonic acid
AAE acquired angioedema
Ab antibodies
ABMT autologous bone marrow transplantation
AC-Hly adenylyl cyclase hemolysin toxin
AC accessory chain
α_1-ACT α_1-antichymotrypsin
ACTH adrenocorticotropic hormone
ADA adenosine deaminase deficiency
ADCC antibody-dependent cell-mediated cytotoxicity; or antibody-dependent cellular cytotoxicity
ADP adenosine diphosphate
AEC airway epithelial cell
AF-1 accessory factor-1
Ag antigen
AGP acid glycoprotein
AHR airway hyperresponsiveness
AICD activation-induced cell death; or antigen induced cell death
AID activation-induced cytokine deaminase
AIDS acquired immune deficiency syndrome
ALPS autoimmune lymphoproliferative syndrome
AND anaphylactic degranulation
ANT adenine nucleotide translocator
anti-GST anti-glutathione *S*-transferase
AP antiproliferative activity
Apaf-1 apoptosis protease-activating factor-1
APC antigen-presenting cells
APECED autoimmune polyendocrinopathy–candidiasis–ectodermal dystrophy
APP acute phase proteins; or amyloid precursor protein
APR acute phase response
APRF acute phase response factor
APS-1 autoimmune polyendocrine syndrome type 1
ARDS adult respiratory distress syndrome
ASC antibody-secreting cell
ASM airway smooth muscle mass
ASP acylation stimulating protein
AT ataxia telangiectasia
ATL adult T-cell leukemia/lymphoma
ATP adenosine triphosphate
ATPase adenosine triphosphatase
AV antiviral activity
AVP arginine vasopressin

BAL bronchoalveolar lavage
BALT bronchus-associated lymphoepithelial tissue
BB biobreeding
BCA-1 B-cell-attracting chemokine
BCG Bacillus Calmette–Guérin
BCR B-cell receptor
BcR B-cell antigen receptor complex
BGH bovine growth hormone
BH Bcl-2 homology
bHLH basic-loop-helix
BIR baculoviral IAP repeat
BLS bare lymphocyte syndrome
BPI bactericidal/permeability-increasing protein
BCR B-cell receptors
BSA bovine serum albumin
BSAP early B cell factor
Btk Bruton's tyrosine kinase

C3NeF C3 nephritic factors
C4NeF C4 nephritic factors
C complement
CAB-2 C activation blocker-2
CAM cell adhesion molecule
cAMP cyclic adenosine monophosphate
CARD caspase-recruitment domain
Cbp Csk-binding protein
cDNA complementary DNAs
CDR complementarity determining regions
CDT cytolethal distending toxins
CDV canine distemper virus
CEA carcinoembryonic antigen
CETP cholesterol ester-transfer protein
CF cystic fibrosis
CFA complete Freund's adjuvant
CGD chronic granulomatous disease
cGMP cyclic guanosine monophosphate
CHH cartilage hair hypoplasia
CHO Chinese hamster ovary
CHS Chédiak–Higashi syndrome
CIITA class II transactivator
CL cutaneous leishmaniasis
CLA cutaneous lymphocyte-associated antigen
CLC Charcot–Leyden crystal
CLIP class II-associated invariant chain peptide
CLP common lymphoid progenitor cells

CLR collagen-like region
CMC carboxymethylcellulose
CMI cell-mediated immunity
CMIS common mucosal immune system
CML chronic myelogenous leukemia
CMP common myeloid progenitor cells
CMV cytomegalovirus
CNS central nervous system
CNTF ciliary neurotropic factor
Con A concanavalin A
COP-1 coat protein 1
COX-2 cyclooxygenase 2
CpG cytidine phosphate-guanosine dinucleotide
CR complement receptor
CR2 complement receptor 2
CRAMP cathelin-related antimicrobial peptide
CRF corticotropin-releasing factor
CRM crossreacting material
CrmA cytokine response modifier A
CRP C-reactive protein
CRS congenital rubella syndrome
CS-1 corticostatin-1
CSF cerebrospinal fluid
CSF colony-stimulating factor
CSP circum sporozoite protein
CSR class switch recombination
CT cholera toxin; or cholera enterotoxin
CTACK cutaneous T-cell attracting chemokine
CTAPIII connective tissue-activating peptide III
CT-B cholera toxin B
CTL cytotoxic T-lymphocyte
CV cowpox virus
CVF cobra venom factor
CVID common variable immunodeficiency

dAb domain antibodies
DAF decay accelerating factor
DAG diacylglygerol
DARC Duffy antigen receptor for chemokines
DBM diazobenzyloxymethyl
DC-SIGN cell-specific ICAM-grabbing nonintegrin
DC dendritic cells
DD death domain
DED death effector domains
DETC dendritic epidermal T cells
DIC disseminated intravascular coagulation
DISC death-inducing signal complex
DISC death-inducing signaling complex
DN dominant negative; or double negative
DNA-PK DNA-dependent protein kinase
DRD2 dopamine receptor D2
DRiP defective ribosomal products
dsDNA double-stranded DNA
dsRNA double-stranded RNA
DT diphtheria toxin or toxid
DTH delayed type hypersensitivity
DTP diphtheria/tetanus/pertussis

EAE experimental autoimmune encephalomyelitis
EBA erythrocyte-binding antigen
EBF terminal deoxynucleotidyl transferase
EBV Epstein–Barr virus
ECM extracellular matrix
ECP eosinophil cationic protein
ECSIT evolutionarily conserved signaling intermediate in Toll pathways
EDF eosinophil differentiating factor
EDN eosinophil derived neurotoxin
EGF epidermal growth factor
ELAM endothelial leukocyte adhesion molecule 1
ELC Epstein–Barr virus-induced receptor ligand chemokine
eIF-2α translation initiation factor 2α
ELISA enzyme-linked immunosorbent assay
EPEC enteropathogenic *Escherichia coli*
EPO erythropoietin; or eosinophil peroxidase
EpoR erythropoietin receptor
ER endoplasmic reticulum
ERAD endoplasmic reticulum-associated degradation
ERGIC endoplasmic reticulum–Golgi intermediate compartment
ERK extracellular regulated kinase; or extracellular signal-regulated kinase
ES excretory/secretory
ESR erythrocyte sedimentation rate
ETEC enterotoxigenic *E. coli*
EV ectromelia virus
EV epidermodysplasia verruciformis

FACS fluorescence activated cell sorter
FAD flavin adenine dinucleotide
FAE follicle-associated epithelium
FAK focal adhesion kinase
FasL Fas ligand
FcαRI Fcα receptor
FcγR Fcγ receptor
FDA Food and Drug Administration (USA)
FDC follicular dendritic cells
FGF fibroblast growth factor
FHA filamentous hemagglutinin
FHL familial hemophagocytic lymphohistiocytosis
fHL-1 fH-like-1
FLIP FLICE-inhibitory proteins
FLK2 fetal liver kinase 2
FMDV foot-and-mouth disease virus
fMLP formyl-methionine-leucine-phenylalanine
FPLV feline panleukopenia virus

Gab1 Grb-2-associated binding protein 1
G6PD glucose-6-phosphatase dehydrogenase
GAD glutamic acid decarboxylase
GAG glycosaminoglycans
GALT gut-associated lymphoepithelial tissues
GBS Guillain–Barré syndrome
GC germinal center

GCP-2	granulocyte chemoattractant protein 2
G-CSF	granulocyte colony-stimulating factor
gG	glycoprotein G
GH	growth hormone
GI	gastrointestinal
GIT	GI tract
GM-CSF	granulocyte–monocyte colony-stimulating factor
GnRH	gonadotropin-releasing hormone
GPCR	G-protein-coupled receptors
GPI	glycosyl-phosphatidy-linositol; or glucose-6-phosphate isomerase
GRO	growth-related oncogene
GROα/β	growth-related gene product α/β
GST	glutathione *S*-transferases
GTPase	guanosine triphosphatase
HA	hemagglutinin
HAART	highly active antiretroviral therapy
HAE	hereditary angioedema
HAM/TSP	HTLV-1-associated myelopathy/tropical spastic paraparesis
HAMA	human anti-mouse (or rat) antibody
HAV	hepatitis A virus
HBD	human β-defensin
HBD-1	human β-defensin-1
HbS	hemoglobin S
HBV	hepatitis B virus
HBeAg	hepatitis Be antigen
HBsAG	hepatitis B virus surface antigen
HCMV	human cytomegalovirus
HCG	human chorionic gonadotropin
HCV	hepatitis C virus
HD	human intestinal defensins
HDL	high-density lipoprotein
5-HETE	5-Hydroxyeicosatetraenoic acid
5-HPETE	5-hydroperoxide eicosatetraenoate
HEL	hen egg white lysozyme
HEV	high endothelial venules
HGF	hemopoietic growth factors
Hh	hemopoietic histocompatibility
HHT	12-hydroxy-5, 8, 10-heptadecatraenoic acid
HHV-6	Human herpesvirus 6
HHV-8	human herpesvirus 8
Hib	*Haemophilus influenzae* b
HIES	hyper-IgE syndrome
HIV	human immunodeficiency virus
HIVA	HIV-1 clade A
HIgM	hyper-IgM syndrome
HLA	human leukocyte antigen
hLPO	human lactoperoxidase
HlyA	α-haemolysin
HMGB1	high mobility group 1 protein
HNE	hemagglutinin noose epitope
HNP	human neutrophil peptide
HPLC	high-performance liquid chromatography
HPRT	hypoxanthine–guanine phosphoribosyl transferase
HPS	hemophagocytic syndrome
HPV	human papilloma virus
HRF	histamine-releasing factor
HRR	haplotype relative risk
HSC	hemopoietic stem cell
HSK	herpetic stromal keratitis
HSP	heat shock protein
hSPO	human salivary peroxidase
HSV	herpes simplex virus
HTLV	human T-cell lymphotropic virus
HU	HTLV-1 uveitis
HUS	hemolytic uremic syndrome
HUVS	hypocomplementemic urticarial vasculitis
HV4	hypervariable region 4
HVEM	herpesvirus entry mediator
HVR1	hypervariable region 1
HVS	herpesvirus Saimiri
IAP	inhibitor of apoptosis
IAVI	International AIDS Vaccine Initiative
IBD	identical by descent
IBD	inflammatory bowel disease
IBS	identical by state
ICAM-1	intercellular adhesion molecule 1
ICE	IL-1β-converting enzyme
iCOS	inducible co-stimulatory molecule
iDC	immature dendritic cell
IE	immediate early
IEC	intestinal epithelial cell
IEL	intraepithelial lymphocyte
IFA	incomplete Freund's adjuvant
IFN-γ	interferon-γ
IFN	interferon
IFNGR1	interferon γ receptor β_1 subunit
Ig	immunoglobulin
IGF-1	insulin-like growth factor 1
IL	interleukin
IL-1	interleukin-1
IL-1β	interleukin-1β
IL-2	interleukin-2
IL-10	interleukin-10
IL-12	interleukin-12
IL-1R	interleukin-1 receptor
IL-1Ra	IL-1 receptor antagonist
ILF	isolated lymphocyte follicle
iNOS	inducible nitric oxide synthase
IP10	interferon-inducible protein 10
IP_3	inositol triphosphate
IPV	inactivated polio vaccine
IRF	IFN-regulatory factor
IRF-1	IFN-regulatory factor-1
ISCAR	immunostimulatory carriers
ISCOM	immunostimulating complex
ISS	immunostimulatory sequences
I-TAC	interferon-inducible T-cell α-chemoattractant
ITAM	immunoreceptor tyrosine based activation motif

ITIM	immunoreceptor tyrosine-inhibition motif
JAK	Janus kinase
Jaks	Janus-family kinase
JI	jet injectors
JNK	c-Jun NH_2-terminal kinase
KIR	killer cell Ig-like receptors
KL	kit ligand
KLH	keyhole limpet hemocyanin
KO	knock-out
KSHV	Kaposi's sarcoma-associated herpesvirus
L-OasA	lipidated outer surface protein A
LAB	linker for activation of B cells
LAD	leukocyte adhesion deficiency
LAK	lymphokine-activated killer
LAM	lipoarabinomannan
LAP	latency-associated protein
LAT	linker for activation of T cells
LBP	lipopolysaccharide-binding protein
LC	Langerhans' cell
LCMV	lymphocytic choriomeningitis virus
LDH	lactate dehydrogenase
LDL	low-density lipoprotein
LDLR	low-density lipoprotein receptor
LFA-1	lymphocyte function-associated antigen 1
LFA-1α	leukocyte function antigen-1α
LGL	large granular lymphocyte
LHR	late phase response
LHRH	luteinizing hormone-releasing hormone
LIF	leukemia inhibitory factor
LIR-1	leukocyte immunoglobulin-like receptor 1
LLO	cytolysin listeriolysin O
LMP	low-molecular-weight protein
LOS	lipooligosaccharide
LP	lamina propria
LPG	lipophosphoglycan
LPL	lamina propria lymphocytes
LPS	lipopolysaccharide
LRC	leukocyte receptor cluster
LRR	leucin-rich repeat
LSA-1	liver stage-specific antigen 1
LSA-3	liver stage antigen 3
LSC	lymphoid stem cells
LT	lymphotoxin; or leukotrienes; or heat-labile enterotoxin
LT-α	lymphotoxin α
LTA	lipoteichoic acid
LT-B	heat-labile enterotoxin B subunit
LTB_4	leukotriene B_4
LTC_4	leukotriene C_4
LTD_3	leukotriene D_3
LTNP	long-term non-progressing
LTR	long terminal repeat
M	microfold
Mϕ	macrophage
mAb	monoclonal antibodies
MAC	membrane attack complexes
MAC	multiple antigen constructs
MACPF	membrane attack complex/perforin
MadCAM-1	mucosal addressin-cell adhesion molecule-1
MAF	macrophage activating factor
MAGUK	phospholipase
MALP	mycoplasma lipopeptide-2
MALT	mucosa-associated lymphoepithelial tissue
MAM	*M. arthritidis* mitogen
MAP	mitogen-activated protein
MAPK	mitogen-activated protein kinase
MAS	*M. arthritidis* superantigen
MASP	mannose-binding protein-associated serine protease
MBL	mannan-binding lectin
MBP	major basic protein; or mannan-binding protein
McAbs	monoclonal antibodies
MCGF	mast cell growth factor
MCL	mucocutaneous lesions
MCMV	murine cytomegalovirus
MCP	membrane co-factor protein; or monocyte chemoattractant protein
MCP-1	monocyte chemoattractant protein-1
MCP-2	monocyte chemoattractant protein-2
MCP-3	monocytic chemoattractant protein-3
mCT	mutant cholera toxin
MCV	molluscum contagiosum virus
MDC	monocyte-derived chemokine
mDC	myeloid dendritic cells
MDP	muramyl dipeptide
MenA	*Neisseria meningitidis* group A
MenB	*Neisseria meningitidis* group B
MenC	*Neisseria meningitidis* group C
MenW135	*Neisseria meningitidis* group W135
MenY	*Neisseria meningitidis* group Y
MF	mitogenic factor
MHC	major histocompatibility complex
MHC I	major histocompatibility complex class I
MHCII	major histocompatibility complex class II
MHV-68	murine γ-herpesvirus 68
MI	myocardial infarction
MIF	migration inhibiting factor
Mig	monokine induced by interferon γ
mIg	membrane immunoglobulin
MIP	macrophage inflammatory protein
MIP-1α	macrophage infectivity potentiator 1α
MIP-α/β	macrophage inflammatory protein 1-α/β
MLN	mesenteric lymph nodes
Mls	minor lymphocyte-stimulating antigens
mLT	mutant labile toxin
MMP	matrix metalloproteases
MMR	macrophage mannose receptor
MMR	measles, mumps, and rubella
MMTV	mouse mammary tumor virus
MOF	Multiple organ failure

MOG myelin oligodendrocyte glycoprotein
MOM mitochondrial outer membrane
MPL monophosphoryl lipid A
MPL-TDM monophosphoryl lipid A/trehalose dicorynomycolate
MPO myeloperoxidase
MPT mitochondria-permeability transition
MRI magnetic resonance imaging
mRNA messenger RNA
MS multiple sclerosis
αMSH α-melanocyte-stimulating hormone
MSP merozoite surface proteins
MSP-1 major merozoite surface protein-1
MTOC microtubule-organizing center
MULT-1 mouse ULBP-like transcript-a
MV myxoma virus
MVA modified vaccinia virus Ankara

N-CAM neuronal cell adhesion molecule
NA neuraminidase
NADPH nicotinamide adenine dinucleotide phosphate
NALT nasopharyngeal-associated lymphoepithelial tissue
NAP-2 neutrophil-activating protein 2
NBS nigmegen breakage syndrome
NBT nitroblue tetrazolium
NE neutralizing epitope
NF-κB nuclear factor κB
NFAT nuclear factor-activated T cell
NGF nerve growth factor
NHEJ nonhomologous end-joining
NK natural killer
NLS nuclear localization sequences
NMR nuclear magnetic resonance
NO Nitric oxide
2NOS-2 nitric oxide synthase
NOD non-obese diabetic
NOD nucleotide-binding oligomerization domain
NPL nonparametric linkage
Nramp-1 natural resistance-associated macrophage protein-1
nS nanosiemens
NspA neisserial surface protein A
NTAL non-T cell activation linker
NV Norwalk virus
NVCP Norwalk virus capsid protein
NZB New Zealand black
NZW New Zealand white

2′,5′-OAS 2′,5′-oligoadenylate system
OAT ornithine aminotransferase
ODC ornithine carbamoyltransferase
ODN oligodeoxynucleotide
OMP outer membrane protein
OMV outer membrane vesicle
OPN osteopontin
OPV oral polio vaccine
orf open reading frame
Osp outer surface protein
OspA outer surface protein A
OVA ovalbumin

P3C tripalmitoyl-*S*-glyceryl-cysteinylserylserine
PA phosphatidic acid
PAF platelet-activating factor
PAI-1 plasminogen activator inhibitor type I
PAI pathogenicity island
PAMP pathogen-associated microbial patterns
PARP poly-ADP-ribose-polymerase
PBMC peripheral blood mononuclear cells
PC phosphorylcholine
PCR polymerase chain reaction
pDC plasmacytoid dendritic cells
PDGF platelet-derived growth factor
PECAM-1 platelet endothelial cell adhesion molecule-1
PET positron emission tomography
PET pyrogenic exotoxins
PG prostaglandin
PGD_2 prostaglandin D_2
PGE_2 prostaglandin E_2
PGN peptidoglycan
PHA phytohemagglutinin
PHI primary HIV-1 infection
PI-9 protease inhibitor 9
PI3K phosphatidylinositol 3-kinase
PI phosphatidyl inositol
PIC polymorphism information content
pIgA polymeric IgA
pIgR polymeric immunoglobulin receptor
PIP_2 phosphatidylinositol biphosphate
PIP_3 phosphatidylinositol 3,4,5-triphosphate
PKC protein kinase C
PKDL post kala-azar dermal leishmaniasis
PKH paroxysmal cold hemoglobinuria
PKR protein kinase
PLA_2 phospholipase A_2
PLC-β-1 phosphatidylinositol 4,5,-bisphosphate
PLCγ1 phospholipase Cγ1
PLCγ2 phospholipase Cγ2
PLG poly(lactide-co-glycolide)
PLP proteolipid protein
PLSP polymeric lamellar substrate particles
PLTP phospholipid-transfer protein
PMA phorbol myristate acetate
PMD piecemeal degranulation
PMN polymorphonucleated neutrophilic granulocytes
PNG Papua New Guinea; or polymorphonuclear granulocytes
PNH paroxysmal nocturnal hemoglobinuria
PNP Purine nucleoside phosphorylase
POPG palmitoyloleoylphosphatidylglycerol
PP Peyer's patches
PPARα peroxisome proliferator receptor α
PPD purified protein derivative

PR	peptide-receptive
pro-IL-1β	proinflammatory cytokine IL-1β
PrP	prion protein
PRR	pattern recognition receptors
PT	pertussis toxin
Ptd Ins (3,4,5) P3	phosphatidylinositol 3,4,5-trisphosphate
PtdSer	phosphatidylserine
PTHrP	parathyroid hormone-related protein
PTK	protein tyrosine kinase
PTX3	long pentraxin
PVM	pneumonia virus of mice
PYD	pyrin domain
PfEMP1	P. falciparum erythrocyte membrane protein 1
RA	rheumatoid arthritis
RAE	retinoic acid early inducibles
r-Ad	recombinant adenoviruses
RAG	recombinant-activating genes
RaLPS	detoxified lipopolysaccharide
rBCG	recombinant BCG
RBL-1	rat basophilic leukemia cells
RCA	regulators of C activation
RESA	ring-infected erythrocyte surface antigen
RFLP	restriction fragment length polymorphism
RID	receptor internalization
RNI	reactive nitrogen intermediates
ROI	reactive oxygen intermediates
ROS	reactive oxygen species
RSS	recombination signal sequences
RSV	respiratory syncytial virus
RT-PCR	Reverse transcription-polymerase chain reaction
RTD	rhesus theta (θ) defensins
RTX	repeat-in-toxin
SAA	serum amyloid A
SAGE	serial analysis of gene expression
SALT	skin-associated lymphoid tissue
SAP	SLAM-associated protein; or serum amyloid P
SARS	severe acute respiratory syndrome
SAg	superantigens
SC	secretory component; or stratum corneum
SCF	stem cell factor
SCID	severe combined immunodeficiency
SCN	severe congenital neutropenia
SCR	short consensus repeat
sCR1	soluble form of the C receptor CR1
SDF-1	stromal cell-derived factor 1
SDF-1α	Stromal cell-derived factor 1α
SDS	sodium dodecylsulfate
SDS-PAGE	sodium dodecylsulfate–polyacrylamide gel electrophoresis
SE	staphylococcal enterotoxins
SEB	staphylococcal enterotoxin B
SEC	serpin enzyme complex
SED	subepithelial dome
serpin	serine protease inhibitor
SF	splicing factor; or steel factor
SHIV	simian–human immunodeficiency virus
SHM	somatic hypermutations
SHP-1	-SH2-domain-containing tyrosine phosphatase
sICAM	soluble intercellular adhesion molecule
s-IgA	secretory IgA
SIR	susceptible, infectious, resistant
SIRPα	signal regulatory protein alpha
SIRS	systemic inflammatory response syndrome
SIV	simian immunodeficiency virus
SLAM	signaling lymphocyte activation molecule
SLC	secondary lymphoid tissue chemokine
SLE	systemic lupus erythematosus
SLN	solitary lymph nodes
SLPI	secretory leukocyte protease inhibitor
SMAC	supramolecular activation clusters
SMEZ	streptococcal mitogenic exotoxin Z
SNP	single nucleotide polymorphisms
SOCS	suppressors of cytokine synthesis
SPDP	*N*-succinimidyl-3-(2-pyridyldithio) propionate
SPE	streptococcal pyrogenic exotoxins
SPEB	streptococcal erythrogenic toxin B
SPECT	single photon emission computed tomography
SRBC	sheep erythrocytes
SRE	serum response element
SRS	slow-reacting substance
STAT	signal transducer and activator of transcription
STAT6	signal transducer and activator of transcription 6
STI	sexually transmitted infection
sTNFR2	TNF receptor 2
svCAM	soluble vascular cell adhesion molecule
T3	triiodothyronine
T4	thyroxine
TAA	tumor-associated antigens
TAO	Thyroid-associated ophthalmopathy
TAP	transporter associated with antigen presentation or processing
TB	tuberculosis
TbpB	transferrin-binding protein B
Tc	cytotoxic T cells
TCC	terminal C complex
TCGF	T-cell growth factor
TCI	transcutaneous immunization
T_{CM}	central memory T cells
TCR	T cell receptor
TCRβ	T cell receptor β
TCR^+	T cell receptor positive
TDA	thymus-dependent areas
TDT	transmission disequilibrium test
TdT	X-linked agammaglobulinemia; or terminal deoxynucleotidyl transferase
TE	toxoplasmic encephalitis
TEA	T-early α
TEC	thymic medullary epithelial cells
TECK	thymus-expressed chemokine
T_{EM}	effector memory T cells

TF tissue factor
T_{FH} follicular B-helper T
TGF transforming growth factor
TGF-β transforming growth factor β
TGF-β1 transforming growth factor-β1
TGN trans Golgi network
Th T-helper
Th1 T-helper type 1
Th2 T-helper type 2
ThCE T-helper cell epitope
TI B-cell stimulatory/activatory protein
TIMP tissue inhibitors of metalloproteases
TIR Toll/IL-1R receptor
TL thymus leukemia
TLR Toll-like receptor
TLR 2 Toll-like receptor 2
TLR 4 Toll-like receptor 4
TLR 9 Toll-like receptor 9
TNF tumor necrosis factor
TNF-α tumor necrosis factor-α
TNF-β tumor necrosis factor-β
TPD transdermal powder delivery
TPI triose phosphate isomerase
TPO thrombopoietin
TPPII tripeptidyl peptidase
Tr regulatory T
Tr1 T-regulatory 1
Treg T-regulatory
TRAF-6 tumor necrosis factor receptor-associated factor 6
TRAIL tumor necrosis factor-related, apoptosis-inducing ligand
TRAP thrombospondin-related adhesive protein
TREC T-cell receptor excition circles
TRH thyrotropin-releasing hormone
TRLA treatment-resistant Lyme arthritis
TSH thyroid-stimulating hormone
TSP tropical spastic paraparesis
TSS toxic shock syndrome
TSST-1 toxic shock syndrome toxin-1
TT tetanus toxoid
TTSS type III secretion system
TxA_2 thromboxane A_2
TxB_2 thromboxane B_2

ULBP UL16-binding proteins
URT upper respiratory tract
USF-1 upstream stimulatory factor-1

VCAM vascular cell adhesion molecule
VCAM-1 vascular cell adhesion molecule 1
vCKBP viral chemokine-binding proteins
VCP viral complement control protein
VEGF vascular endothelial growth factor
vFLIPs viral FLICE inhibitor proteins
VGF vaccinia growth factor
vhs viral host protein shut off
vIFN-γR viral IFN-γ receptor
vIL-6 IL-6 homolog
vIL-10 IL-10 homolog
vIL-17 IL-17 homolog
vIL-18BP IL-18 binding protein
vIL-1βR viral IL-1β receptor
VIPR vasoactive intestinal peptite receptor
VL visceral leishmaniasis
VLA-4 very late activated antigen-4
VLDL very-low-density lipoprotein
VLP virus-like particles
VNTR variable number tandem repeat
vSag viral superantigens
vSEMA semaphorin homologue
VSG variant surface glycoprotein
VSP variable small protein
vTNFR viral TNF receptor
VV vaccinia virus
VZV varicella-zoster virus

WAS Wiskott–Aldrich syndrome
WASP Wiscott–Aldrich syndrome protein
WHO World Health Organization
XLA X-linked agammaglobulinemia
XLAAD X-linked autoimmunity-allergic disregulation syndrome

XLP X-linked lymphoproliferative
XLPS X-linked lymphoproliferative syndrome

YAC monoclonal antibodies
YPM Y. pseudotuberculosis mitogen

ZAP ζ-associated protein

PART I

INTRODUCTION

1

Introduction

BRIGITTE A. ASKONAS

The publication of this immunology volume as a separate entity in *Topley & Wilson's Microbiology and Microbial Infections* is a welcome innovation and a reflection of extensive progress in our understanding of the immune system in recent decades. Nevertheless there are still enormous gaps in our knowledge that need to be investigated before we will be able to manipulate immune responses predictably to our advantage. Recent advances are widely distributed in numerous different journals and publications, and this makes it difficult to keep up with so much new information relating to the complex and now vast field of immunology. Present knowledge relied on a whole range of interdisciplinary research activities such as molecular and cellular biology, protein chemistry, proliferation and differentiation signals, regulation of gene expression, membrane biology, etc. Hence this well-referenced book will be most useful to many investigators.

The editors have collected 46 chapters written by different experts and have assembled much basic knowledge to update us on both innate and adaptive (or acquired) immune responsiveness. The innate cellular responses provide the first line of defense against invading microbes. By production of mediators when activated they set the scene for the activation of the adaptive responses with specificity for the challenging antigen(s). Type I interferons are produced very rapidly in many infections (see Chapter 14); natural killer (NK) cells and their subsets (see Chapters 6 and 14), γ/δ cells (see Chapter 23), complement components (see Chapter 9), phagocytes and granulocytes (i.e. macrophages and neutrophils; see Chapters 3 and 4) are of central importance in innate responsiveness by formation of various chemokines and cytokines (interleukins). Pattern recognition receptors (such as Toll-like receptors (TLR)) are expressed by certain cell types. They recognize particular groups of microbes or their components and play a major role in early cell signaling events (see Chapter 7). Although the innate immune responses do exert some control over the pathogen load early in infection, they are rarely sufficient to totally clear intracellular microbial infections, be they caused by viruses or parasites.

Adaptive immunity depends on a highly complex and intricate network of interactions between different cell types and their subpopulations, regulated by their production of mediators, i.e. cytokines, chemokines, interferons type I and II (see Chapters 13, 14, and 15). The adaptive immune responses are driven to a large extent by antigenic challenge resulting in the clonal expansion, differentiation, and maturation of diverse clones of antigen-specific B cells to form circulating antibodies (humoral immunity) and of antigen-specific cell-mediated responses by thymus-derived T cells. These vary in phenotype, cytokine formation, and effector function. In this brief introduction it is impossible to do justice to all the main players in this amazingly multifaceted system. However, this volume contains detailed articles on the many cell types involved, the lymphocytes and their subpopulations differing in phenotype and function, their lifestyle, and their antigen recognition receptors and patterns (see Chapters 16, 17, 19–25, 27 and 29). In addition the main antigen-presenting cells (APC), i.e. dendritic cells and macrophages, are essential to activate B and T cells from their resting and naive state (see Chapters 19 and 21).

The T cells are divided into two major subpopulations according to their phenotype, the expression of the CD4 and CD8 surface markers, as well as their functional differences (see Chapters 20 and 22). Chapters 19 and 21 convey the antigen-processing pathways and the assembly of the major histocompatibility complexes (MHC) with antigen-derived fragments for recognition by the T-cell receptors. $CD4^+$ T cells recognize antigen-derived fragments in conjunction with MHC class II molecules on the cell surface while $CD8^+$ cytotoxic

T cells (CTL) see antigen-derived peptides in association with MHC class I. The MHC gene complex is of course highly polymorphic and the binding of diverse antigen fragments to the polymorphic MHC molecules varies in different haplotypes in the population. Both T and B cells are the source of many cytokines and chemokines when they recognize antigen. Nonantigen-specific B and T cells are also recruited by chemokines into infected or damaged areas, and become activated by bystander cytokines in the environment of lymphoid organs to further enhance inflammation.

Excessive levels of certain immune responses and resulting cytokines can cause serious immunopathology as seen, for example, in certain infections, autoimmune disorders, allergic reactions, or hypersensitivity reactions (see Chapters 34–37). Thus it is not sufficient to activate and induce immune responses, but, to prevent lymphoproliferative disorders and overactivation of cells in the lymphoid tissues or infected organs, it is also essential that the immune cells can be down-regulated. Regulatory T cells and their formation of inhibitory cytokines (such as the interleukin (IL)-10 and transforming growth factor (TGF)-β) or apoptotic signals (see Chapters 8 and 15) fulfill this need.

Chapters 40–46 are devoted to recent approaches used in efforts to develop new vaccines. There are no effective vaccines as yet against serious health threats caused by some extensively studied and fully characterized pathogens, as well as by newly emerging infectious agents. However, this is an area that still requires intensive research and study. Each infectious microbe is a law unto itself and differs in tissue tropism; it is endowed with different mechanisms to evade immune control (see Chapters 31, 32, and 33), varies in its host–pathogen relationship, lifestyle, and the effects of host genetic influences (see Chapter 30). Therefore each microbial infection has to be examined as such and there are no obvious shortcuts. Not all immune responses are beneficial and deleterious reactivities have to be avoided. Clearly, there is a need to define appropriate protective responses against intracellular infections. We would like to be left also with immune memory (i.e. antigen-specific lymphoid cells that respond more rapidly and are present at a higher frequency than found in naive hosts) for defense against subsequent challenges with the same microbes (see Chapter 26). The induction of antibodies alone is not necessarily the answer to all our prayers. Chapter 18 addresses the therapeutic application of monoclonal antibodies.

This *Immunology* volume provides basic information on broad aspects of immunology that must be taken into consideration when dealing with infectious diseases and so many clinical problems and disorders involving lymphoid cells and pathological inflammatory responses. This volume will be invaluable to students and postdoctoral investigators, as well as experts, microbiologists, immunologists, basic or clinical scientists, and clinicians in many fields.

2

History

ANNE MARIE MOULIN

IMMUNOLOGY WITH AN EMPHASIS ON INFECTIOUS DISEASES: A RETROSPECTIVE

The modern science of immunology stemmed from the germ theory of diseases at the end of the nineteenth century and then developed in close connection to it. At that time, immunology was decisively empowered by the early successes of rabies vaccine and anti-diphtheria serotherapy and contributed to establish bacteriology as one of the pillars of modern medicine.

In the twentieth century, immunology acquired a growing autonomy and distanced itself from the domain of infectious diseases. Immunology dealt with a growing number of affections with no infectious agent identified, or even hypothesized. The enlargement of the definition of antigenicity, addressing a whole array of molecules (Landsteiner 1936), helped to emancipate immunology from its historical origins.

Immunology as the 'science of the immune system' acquired connections with other systems in the body such as the endocrine or the nervous apparatus. The immune system played a major role in the selection of species and individuals and the present ontogeny reflected these developments. Immunology, the 'latest language of medicine' as tentatively named (Moulin 1991), could claim to be becoming the science of the 'system of systems', because the immune system was increasingly shown interacting with other vital functions and regulating them.

The dream of the eradication of microbes was nurtured by the success over smallpox and infectious diseases, and the observation of the world's spectacular demographic expansion. Yet, in the immunology of the last quarter of the twentieth century, the share of research linked to infectious diseases declined. Some scientists, focusing on idiotypic–anti-idiotypic relations, went so far as to discard the primacy of infections in the understanding of immune responses, and set forth the distinction between a so-called peripheral system dealing with external pathogens, corresponding more or less to the infection-oriented immunological tradition, and a central part, or immunological core, described as a self-centered network (Coutinho et al. 1984).

These last years have been marked by a revived interest in infectious diseases. In sharp contrast with the previous period, the last decade of the twentieth century has witnessed a growing anxiety over the so-called return of infectious diseases, and disenchantment over the perspectives of a rapid and complete eradication. The fight against ancient and new plagues has been resumed with accrued vigor and traditional tools have been refurbished with the help of all-powerful molecular biology.

Inflammation, an antiquated concept taking us back to Celsius and Roman times, is again finding a central place in immunology. Inflammation associated to infection is a crossroad phenomenon that includes secretion of multiple factors. A whole network of molecules, entertaining complex relationships with each other, thus contributes to the permanent homeostatic control of the body and adjustment essential to life (Canguilhem 1966).

The immunology of infectious diseases has been rehabilitated in a new guise, most notably expressed in a molecular language. Immunology, once described as a science attached to the ideal of specificity, or the 'science of boundaries' trespassed only in rare cases (Moulin 1997), is by now deeply concerned with the exchange of biological material across the species barrier. The trends of innate and acquired immunity, dubbed natural and adaptive immunity, go intertwined through recent immunological literature, opening a flow of speculations over evolution, selection, and survival.

THE 'RETURN' OF INFECTIOUS DISEASES

With the development of microbiology at the end of the nineteenth century, the initiative seemed to be in the medical camp for ever, and a definitive advantage given to the doctors' side. The isolation and cultivation of germs made plausible the hope of destroying them.

The eradication goal was immediately perceived as at hand not only by journalists but also by scientists (Gradman 2000). Louis Pasteur set the tone by predicting the demise of tuberculosis, rabies, plague, and cholera. Although Pasteur admitted that new plagues were to come, he was confident that, as they would show up, fresh science would take over. This fighting adopted almost mystical tones. Scientists crusaded to relieve humankind from the original sin lurking in the body in the guise of germs. Not that the physicians of the past had ignored any ontology of disease. On the contrary, they had all the time been familiar with the general idea of the 'seeds of the disease' (Nutton 1983). But so long as this theory was of little practical value for curing patients, this had been a mere speculative luxury.

Operating in the wake of World War II, the World Health Organization (WHO) decided to give a decisive impulse to the eradication of infectious diseases. Its officers launched the campaign against smallpox which led to the announcement of its eradication in 1979 and provided the model, to be followed by tuberculosis, malaria, poliomyelitis, and other diseases.

Although immunology provided a whole line of vaccines, antibiotics, by alleviating the burden of infections, reduced the pressure on immunologists to explore the inadequacies of the immune response. Immunologists interacted more closely with biological research in embryology, neurology, cognitive sciences, cancer studies, and pharmacology, and provided tools and concepts to other disciplines.

Between the 1980s and the present time, the period under scrutiny in this chapter, immunology faced events that boosted and remodeled its activity in the domain of infections.

Today, in Africa and Asia, countries still bear an enormous infectious burden and AIDS has shortened by many years the gain in life expectancy, which immunization and modern medicine had helped to procure. In contrast, in industrialized countries, less than 10 percent of mortality is attributed to infectious diseases, and even AIDS has only globally induced a rise of about 1 percent. Yet, infectious diseases have stepped again to the forefront for many reasons:

- As a result of the neglect of immunization and political unrest, some ancient plagues have burst out again in Africa. Yellow fever erupted in Brazil, in urban settings, in 1998. A threat weighs over Asia, historically free from yellow fever without demonstrable immunity to it, in spite of the presence of other flaviviruses. Hemorrhagic dengue is now expanding in South America and the Caribbean.
- The microbial world has displayed a previously unheard of diversity, including new classes of pathogens, among which bacteria such as legionellae, viruses such as the bunyaviruses, the parvoviruses, the arenaviruses to which belong the viruses of hemorrhagic fevers (Machupo, Junin, Lassa, Sabia), the filoviruses (Ebola, Marburg), and above all the retroviruses.

Systematic investigation in birds and rodents around the world has detected thousands of viruses that have no ascertained pathogenic role. Field studies represent at best a glimpse into the diversity of viruses circulating among rodents, vectors, and mammals – a potential reservoir of pests for the rest of the living world.

Defying the dogmas of molecular biology, unconventional particles of poorly defined status, such as prion proteins, have been involved in the genesis of neurological disorders (Gajdusek 1977). With the demonstration of the transmissibility of the bovine encephalitis to humans, natural order was challenged, because the species barrier is no longer an absolute protection. Inasmuch as the tomato spotted wild virus, a bunyavirus akin to the Rift Valley fever virus, is adapted to plants, plant viruses could grow on vertebrate cells.

Laboratories and hospitals are no longer sanctuaries. Hospitals, considered once as hotbeds of infection, a threat to neighborhoods, reappear as dangerous places. Nosocomial infections are scaled up to 10 percent of the registered infections, even in Africa, although with germs differing from those in the West. It is in a hospital, in 1976, that the Ebola epidemic burst out, as well as a few months later, in Yambuku in Zaire, and in 1995 again in Zaire.

In the laboratories of the industrialized world, accidents may happen. The Marburg virus, close to the Ebola virus, draws its name from the city where it made its way from monkey cells used for vaccine production in 1967. Until recently, there have been reported cases of infected people among the staff handling the Rift Valley fever virus, identified in 1983 and extremely contagious. The creation of high security laboratories (P4) illustrates the difficulty of manipulating ultra-virulent and unidentified infectious material. But there are no P4 laboratories close to the infection foci in Africa. Moreover, growing resistance of microbes to antibiotics instilled the idea that no defense line would soon remain available. In a pre-vision of this therapeutic collapse, the mechanisms of immunity should be revisited, and immunologically inspired treatments investigated more carefully.

The return of infectious diseases, at the beginning of the new millennium, has roused an anxiety aggravated by the recent threat of bacteriological warfare. Mass media currently discuss germ pulverization in the atmosphere; they evoke the mad scientist working for terrorists, flooding germs and toxins in water pipes, inventing genetically modified microorganisms, resuscitating the smallpox virus in populations deprived of immunity.

The 'Conquest of Diseases' (Winslow 1943) has been replaced by the idea of a 'victory à la Pyrrhus' (Ameisen 1999, p. 158), with nobody vanquishing or being vanquished. Epiloguing on this 'return', which typically reveals postmodern distress in a 'global' world, we have to admit that the notion of 'new virus' actually reflects our previous ignorance and witnesses the extension of our inventory of the living world. It is as much the vanishing of an illusion, thanks to the improvement of our detection tools, as the awareness of a grim reality. It is not only the immune system that has been taken off guard; many systems of surveillance in the world have been dismantled, in the former Soviet Union, for example, or in Africa.

This so-called return, be it the emergence of radically new plagues, or the re-emergence of previously tamed epidemics, confronts long-term germ evolution with the quickening step of human history (Moulin 1996b). The relationship between humans and the environment has been transformed, some say perverted, by human activity, and a debate bears on the necessity of rethinking a new alliance or even a 'new contract' (Serres 1990) between 'Man' and 'Nature', which he possesses far less than he is possessed by it.

The AIDS epidemics has provided an unmatched opportunity for dissecting the immune mechanisms. The virus, when dormant in the cells of the immune system, is relatively unobnoxious for most human tissues, with perhaps an exception for the nervous system, but it is deleterious to the immune system and transforms the body into a 'city without walls' (Epicurus) ready for 'opportunistic' attacks. Our present pessimism is rooted in our failure to produce a vaccine rapidly, in spite of the unprecedented research effort. We still miss a satisfactory animal model and an anchorage in the natural history of the disease, documenting spontaneous cure. Virus lines developed in the laboratory swiftly behave like 'circus strains', to use a phrase coined by French biologist Charles Nicolle, too obedient to the dompter's whistles and falling rapidly apart from wild viruses. After the introduction of active tritherapy, much is expected from the manipulation of the immune system, giving it a chance to take over when specific therapy is discontinued.

THE NEW AGE OF INFECTION AND IMMUNITY

The development of monoclonal antibody technique has followed a paper published by Cesar Milstein and Georges Köhler in 1975 in *Nature* and crowned by the Nobel prize. This technique, initially conceived by Milstein to explore the immunoglobulin genes and the diversity of antibody formation, turned out to be available for all kinds of studies. Hybridoma technology (the name appeared 2 years later) has resulted in immortal cell lines producing, at will, any human or murine antibody of chosen specificity, a wonderful tool for genetics and immunogenetics. The T4 count (CD4 cells still rank among the major indicators of the risk for opportunistic infections) was defined with the help of monoclonal antibodies (Cambrosio and Keating 1995). Flux cytometry uses monoclonal antibodies to mark cells and the cell sorter has turned into a quantitating machine (Cambrosio and Keating 1994). Novel ligands for cell-surface molecules can be identified using high-avidity recombinant reagents displayed on fluorescent beads. These reagents allow description of interactions between cells and molecular analogs of receptors or targets (Wedderburn and Dianda 2000).

Genetics had at first been little concerned with infectious diseases, being absorbed in the model of 'innate errors of metabolism' (Garrod 1909) and research on diseases recognized for a long time as being hereditary, based on family pedigrees and aiming at genetic counseling. Innovations included karyotyping techniques and the selection of new animal models that mimic human pathologies. Standard mice were produced between the two world wars by the Jackson Laboratory, established by the geneticist Little (Löwy and Gaudillière 1998). The center has become the world leader in the study and production of inbred, genetically homologous strains of mice.

'Knock-out' (KO), with artificially defective genomes, have provided exquisite tools for the analysis of the immune system (Mak et al. 2001). Studies have shown that the immune system finds a new balance when it loses some component. The deletion of a gene coding for an important molecule of immunity may have consequences in a remote sector of physiological life, e.g. mice missing the *PrP* gene, which are insensitive to prion infection, display anomalies in systems other than the immune system. But genetic manipulations do not necessarily result in gross alterations in development and survival. The block that occurs to some pathways through genetic defects does not necessarily compromise the formation of innate or even acquired immunity, suggesting flexibility and redundancy as major features of the immune system, which is critical for survival.

In the two last decades, the actors of the immune system, studied with new tools, have multiplied. The immunological band once cartooned by Gershon in the 1970s has by now expanded to the dimensions of a symphonic orchestra (Gershon 1980).

In the mouse, two functionally different CD4 populations were described in 1989: T-helper 1 (Th1) and T-helper 2 (Th2) (Mosmann and Coffmann 1989). The T-/B-cell dichotomy, corresponding more or less to the historical split between the cellular and humoral response, has mirrored itself in a new subdivision in the T-cell population between Th1 and Th2 subsets, key tuned to different classes of pathogens, extra- and intracellular. Characteristically, this division was based on different patterns of lymphocyte secretions. The observation was soon extended to the human case (Romagnani 1996).

Another new subset of cells has been dendritic cells. When they were described by Paul Langerhans in the dermis (Langerhans 1868), they had nothing to do with immunity. Langerhans called them dendritic because of their aspect, which was reminiscent of nerve cells, and hypothesized that they belonged to the nervous system. The French dermatologist Darier later noticed their frequency in inflammatory lesions (Darier 1900). Dendritic cells are scattered throughout the body, close to the main portals of microbe entry. Although the phenomenon called crosspriming or crosspresentation was described in 1976 (Bevan Cross 1976), their role was diversely interpreted before being viewed as essential to the onset and modulation of the immune response. In lymph nodes, they are sufficiently 'professionalized' (Amigorena 1999, p. 932) to instruct naïve lymphocytes and present antigens from infected cells, in association with class I molecules, to T-cytotoxic lymphocytes. In AIDS, they are among the first cells to capture the virus in contaminated fluids. This strategic position makes them appear as good targets for potential vaccines at an early stage of primoinfection.

Dendritic cells identify pathogen agents via toll-like receptors, so called because of an analogy with proteic receptors in *Drosophila*, which are mediators of embryogenesis. Toll receptors recognize molecular patterns shared by numerous pathogens of the gram-negative families (Rock et al. 1998). The activation of these receptors in mammals leads to the production of antimicrobial peptides such as cecropin and defensin.

The genetic diversity of B lymphocytes results primarily from the recombination of the many genes harvested in our body libraries. To build the receptors that display specific targets on their shields, lymphocytes make use of enzymes under the dependence of two genes called recombinant-activating genes (RAG). These genes, shared by all species endowed with T lymphocytes such as mammals, birds, and some fish, probably derive from a very primitive microorganism, a transposon, that was integrated into the human genome millions of years ago.

In 'the golden age of genetics and the dark age of infectious diseases' (Tibayrenc 2001), how did immunology evolve? The biologist Paul Ewald sharply subtitled his popular book *Plague Time* (Ewald 2002) *The new germ theory of disease*. Post-modern immunology features:

- a new definition of pathogens and pathogenicity
- a focus on infection currently redefined
- a genetic agenda for the assessment of the germ/host relationship.

The nature of the pathogen has diversified. RNA viruses are particularly proteiform, because they mutate rapidly when they multiply in the host cells and because their polymerase, an enzyme essential in the synthesis of nucleic acids, does not entail any mechanism for repairing errors. RNA viruses, numerous in plants and animals, are good candidates for the etiology of many chronic affections such as multiple sclerosis or Parkinson's disease.

Genetic recombinations frequently happen between two subpopulations of one microbial species, in a vector or a host, with unpredictable consequences for pathogenicity.

The nature of pathogens has become elusive. It is not excluded that viroides, small monocatenary pieces of RNA involved in transmissible diseases in plants, play a role in humans and animals. In the cerebral tissue of patients suffering from Creutzfeldt–Jakob dementia, the PrP protein results from the alteration of a normal protein. Although the modalities of infection by prions remain far from understood in their entirety, the infectious role of proteins is now well established.

Some pathogens had been known about for a long time in the animal kingdom, but damaged immunity in humans (whatever the cause, and they are many in the modern world, such as chemotherapy, transplantation, severe congenital defects) procures them new opportunities. These 'opportunist infections' are best illustrated in the case of microsporidia.

Microsporidia are unicellular parasites that are widespread in the animal kingdom. The German zoologist Naegeli described corpuscles, which he called *Noema bombyci*, under the skin of the silkworms in rearings. Babiani suggested, in 1882, the name microsporidia because of their tiny dimensions. Their position in taxonomy is still controversial. The absence of mitochondria favors a 'regressive evolution', with loss of important organelles. With the help of the high-resolution electronic microscope, it became possible to investigate the pathogenic power of this supposedly benign parasite. The first human case described was in a patient stricken with AIDS (Desportes et al. 1985). The story of this patient, whom the author came to know personally, was most unfortunate because for a long time there was a failure to attribute the disease correctly to a transfusion in Haiti. Many cases have been reported since in AIDS and immunosuppressed patients. In athymic or severe combined immunodeficient (SCID) mice, parasites invade the whole organism and infections of microsporidia are lethal.

The very notion of infection has lost its clear outlook (Evans 1993). Medical interest has moved from canonical descriptions of infections, almost in Hippocratic format, to the search for all possible symptoms. Computer technology has played a crucial role in this shift from clinical to bibliographic knowledge. Primoinfection linked to a given pathogen is shown to generate a broad spectrum of situations, from the healthy carrier to acute and severe forms, and to chronic diseases pursuing their course in the absence of a detectable pathogen. Murine models, in the case of leishmania infections, for example, illustrate the clinical diversity of human forms, from the benign oriental sore to deadly kala-azar.

The opposition between infection and hereditary disease is no longer clear cut. The transmissible spongiform encephalitis such as that of Creutzfeldt–Jakob disease exists under two forms: the infectious one, including cases that result from treatment using growth hormone extracted from patients who died with dementia, and the hereditary one.

Since the late 1980s, the role of chronic infections as facilitators of more severe diseases has been discussed: they would weaken the immune system by overstraining or overstimulating its capacity to respond. In 1989, in order to explain HIV diffusion, Luc Montagnier suggested such a role for mycoplasma infections. Later, sexually transmitted diseases associated with *Chlamydia* have been incriminated. The general idea of an infection ecosystem in unstable equilibrium in populations, or 'pathocenosis', as put forward by the late historian Mirko Grmek (1969), has led to the global incrimination of chain reactions in the immune system without assigning the first signal.

New immunology addresses the question why an epidemic intervenes in the course of the silent co-evolution of germs and their potential hosts. Closer articulation of the innate response, allegedly more primitive, and the adaptive response, claimed to be the privilege of the most recent species, has reinforced the link between our sophisticated organisms and the rest of the living world, and restored a more balanced view of the respective advantages and disadvantages among species. Already sobered by moral considerations on the cyclic return of the 'brute beast' in humans (Nicolle 1933), our positivist optimism has been dampened by the discovery of the highly innovative capacity of germs and their ability to exploit molecular niches in the intimacy of the body.

To address these challenges, immunology operates within the framework of the selective theory (Silverstein 1989), which still prevails, even though it has lost its original simplicity since Burnet offered the idea that the antigen selects the corresponding clone, which subsequently expands T cells to identify the molecules of the self carried by the histocompatibility complex on antigen-presenting cells. As far as immunity is concerned, the differences in repertoires between individuals account for both the havoc caused by epidemics and the survival of a few. Differences between high and low responders were suggested by Ludwig Hirschfeld in his seminal book, *Konstitutionserologie* (Hirschfeld 1928). Biological individuality is considered alternately as an obstacle to general strategies of immunization, leading some authors to recommend immunization 'à la carte', and as a providential reservoir of biodiversity, illustrating the leibnizian principle of 'multiple splendor' in 'Creation' (Moulin 2001) and the maximization of good.

The history of primoinfection is one of mounting a powerful immune response that involves all known components of immunity, from the old crones, antibodies and cells, to the creatures of novel immunology, cytotoxic cells, Th1 and Th2, from Metchnikoff's phagocytes to dendritic cellules and natural killers, from Jules Bordet's complement to cytokines and lymphokines.

Today, knowledge about HIV infections illustrates the general development of such knowledge about the immune system, the vulnerability of which was thus exposed. The way HIV infection proceeds fatally toward a chronic form by escape from the immune system is extreme and cannot constitute the general model of all kinds of primoinfection. Yet it has reshaped our understanding of the encounter between germs and organisms that may shelter them.

Transmission of germs and genes, now more integrated than in the past, constitutes a general and unifying perspective. A century and half after the beginning of bacteriology, there is space for multicausal explication. With the emergence of notions such as genetic pattern or pathogenicity islets in the genome, which mean more than constitution, terrain, soil, natural immunity, predisposition, etc., immunogenic knowledge and epidemiological data point to the inequality of bodies, without denying the role played by lifestyle.

THE MOLECULARIZATION OF IMMUNOLOGY

Immunology has entered the modern era by exploring the genetic aspects of the immune response and by adopting molecularization. Molecular immunology is convenient shorthand for the study of the molecules of the immunological orchestra and their interactions (Moulin and Silverstein 1990), with the tools of molecular biology. This abbreviation refers to both an ideal and an enterprise in the making.

The molecularization of immunology raises the question of the changing position of immunology among other biological disciplines. Did it significantly help it to solve physiological issues and open new diagnostic and therapeutic vistas in diseases (Panem 1984)? In the 1980s, cancer was the main target of the 'immunological revolution' (Fridman 2000): molecularized immunology was expected to open a 'fourth line' of therapies, after radiotherapy, chemotherapy, and surgery (Löwy 1997). In the 1990s, infectious diseases were reconsidered as possible beneficiaries of advances in the field, from a curative and also a preventive viewpoint (vaccines).

The breaking of the genetic code and the identification of the nucleic acids as the support of heredity have been presented as *The Eighth Day of Creation* (Judson 1979). But it was only the beginning of an era that saw biologists manipulating gene segments and expressing them in vectors. The colossal enterprise of the Human Genome Project, in contrast to the medical programs for eradicating diseases, has been regularly ahead of its deadlines. Mapping the human genome has become the totem of the new molecular biology, in a planetary vision (Jordan 1995).

If the development of restriction enzymes from the 1975s onwards marked an important milestone of molecular genetics, the 1975 hybridoma paper by Köhler and Milstein (1975), ending with a few lines on the applications for the production of antibodies of medical interest, is considered as a similarly crucial step in the molecularization of immunology, in terms of phenomenological analysis, and production of tools and therapies. Either ancillary to molecular biology or bringing its own recipes, immunology has come into the scientific mainstream. Immunologists can pursue the historical mission that its pioneers had assigned themselves. The goal of specificity, a major tenet of early immunology (Mazumdar 1995), is alleged to be reached thanks to elegant techniques allowing the dissection of the immune response into all its components and the identification of all relevant pathways. Since the 1980s, molecular biology has allowed the localization of genes for capsules, toxins, adherence factors, invasion and survival cell factors on plasmids, bacteriophages, and even on chromosomes, leading to a description of 'pathogenicity islets' and the identification of a whole array of molecules involved in infection and immunity.

Interferons were first described by Isaacs and Lindenmann in 1957, referring to the phenomenon of viral interference. They were used as antitumoral agents only some 30 years later. They are today considered as both constitutive and induced immunity factors.

David (1966) and Bloom and Bennett (1966), independently hypothesized that a substance, formed by lymphoid cell–antigen interaction, inhibits macrophage migration. Bloom called this factor migration inhibiting factor (MIF). In 1969, Dumonde et al. suggested the term 'lymphokines' for substances different from classic antibodies, generated by antigen-activated lymphocytes.

In 1975, while investigating a viral etiology of leukemia in Gallo's laboratory, Morgan and Ruscetti noted that media from phytohemagglutinin (PHA)-stimulated lymphocytes were capable of prolonging the growth of cells from leukemic cells in continuous cultures. The new molecule (called T-cell growth factor (TCGF)), and not the antigen, allowed cultured normal lymphocytes to maintain their functions. In 1978, a murine cytotoxic cell line was used as a bioassay for testing this lymphokine. An assembly of immunologists recognized the identity of thymocyte mitogenic factor, killed helper factor, and lymphocyte mitogenic factor, which have previously been described, and co-chromatograph with TCGF. The subsequent cloning and purification of interleukin (IL) 2 by Taniguchi et al. in 1983 confirmed that all these activities were ascribed to a single molecule. IL-2 is presently one of the best-known molecules. B-cell-stimulating lymphokines, such as IL-4, IL-5 (also active on eosinophils), and IL-6, were successively defined. Human lymphokines were thought to be similar to their mouse homologs, although most experiments needed to prove it were impossible for obvious ethical reasons.

The availability of a variety of hemopoietic growth factors has allowed the development of in vitro approaches to the differentiation of hemopoietic lineages. These factors regulate genes that are required for the maintenance of viability during proliferation and differentiation. With the advances in modern biotechnology, many of them have become available in sufficient amounts and purity to study their effects in vitro and in vivo. It was expected that knowledge gained from these studies would lead to new approaches to the treatment of human disease.

As more factors were identified and cloned, the complexity of their effects and interactions was perceived. 'Cytokines', immunologically active proteins that bind to specific receptors on target cells, can be produced by a wide variety of cells, e.g. IL-1, stimulated by lipopolysaccharide (LPS) and a component of Gram-negative bacteria, is secreted by monocytes; many other cells can, however, make IL-1. Among many bacterial products, the ubiquitous LPS (Besredka 1906) has been characterized as a potent stimulus of both immunity and inflammation (Cavaillon and Le Garrec 1998).

As growth factors, cytokines have been particularly useful for facilitating the culture of cells reputed to be difficult to grow in vitro. With further recognition of the numerous cell subsets involved in immunity, additional ingredients were poured into the 'cauldron'. How these molecules are classified has currently depended on whether an endocrinologist, immunologist, or hematologist described them first. Later, their protean properties have somewhat bewildered researchers, who are always eager to advertise them as potential immunostimulants or more generally immunomodulators, but embarrassed for classifying them and putting them into a hierarchy. The availability of purified recombinant factors, the development of radioligand assays, and the production of monoclonal antibodies to surface determinants have permitted quantitative study of the chemistry of ligand–receptor interactions. The information contained within the structure of the factor is received by the receptor and rapidly translated into a limited repertoire of chemical internal signals that affect cellular functions.

Cytokines characteristically act at a site distant from the cells that produce them, witnessing the potential of the immune response to reach target organs far from the microbial entry. However, a regulation is required to provide balances and checks of cytokine production. Cytokines are now viewed as the key to the understanding of the inflammatory reaction and the regulation of the immune response. Anti-inflammatory cytokines, such as the 'quintet' of IL-4, IL-10, IL-13, interferon-α and the transforming growth factor (TGF) would have the capacity to repress proinflammatory cytokines elaborated by activated macrophages.

Chemokines, described in 1992, are a family of small proteins that recruit circulating cells and play an important role during inflammatory reactions. Their function is chemotaxis or attraction exerted on cells. Chemokines play also a role in angiogenesis, collagen production, and proliferation of hemopoietic cells. This family includes numerous members, among which is IL-8, and has raised a considerable interest, because of its potential therapeutic action in AIDS.

In contrast to the ideal of narrow specificity, the system is redundant. Chemokines are promiscuous in receptor usage – several cells produce several chemokines with an overlapping sector of action. The robustness of biochemical pathways renders their output relatively insensitive to change. The natural polymorphism occurring in an outbred cell population does not usually affect the immune response for this reason. No chemokine is uniquely active on one leukocyte, and usually a given leukocyte population has receptors for and responds to different molecules. Most known receptors interact with multiple ligands, and most ligands interact with more than one receptor.

Generally speaking, it is impossible to discriminate between 'good' and 'evil' cells and molecules. Infection is a drama with successive steps where immediate destruction of viruses by specific cytotoxic cells may be associated with negative indirect effects on non-infected cells. Antigen–antibody complexes can protect viruses hidden in lymph nodes. Although chemokines can stick to ligands, preventing infection of the cells by viruses, cytokines can diminish the regeneration of cell lines, and trigger destruction in neighboring cells.

The molecular biologist Jean-Pierre Changeux has characterized the immune system as an allosteric orchestra, to emphasize the role of allostery or alternate changes in chemical structure, which induces functional diversity, as illustrated by hemoglobin in the Wyman–Changeux–Monod model. Shared signals, structural analogies in receptors forming families that overlap the species barrier, manifest the unity of the molecular language in which infection and immunity are described today.

AN EMPIRICAL VIEW OF THE IMMUNE SYSTEM

In 1990, the author wrote, with Silverstein in a book dedicated to 'The role of cells and cytokines in immunity and inflammation, that "the past decade has been marked more by technologic than by conceptual developments"' (Moulin and Silverstein 1990, p. 3).

A tentative model of disease has been based on dysfunctional production of and responsiveness to cytokines. The administration of LPS reproduces some of the disease events by inducing an outburst of cytokines. Coordinated reactions, facing danger, involve a reorganization of self-perception and behavior. Anorexia, sleepiness and drowsiness bordering on comatose states, onirism, and retreating from the world had been described for a long time by patients themselves. Infectious disease has been one of the most studied human behaviors. A masterpiece of Elizabethan literature in the Renaissance is John Donne's *Reflections upon Emergent Occasions*. Donne wrote, during a typhus epidemic, his detailed personal account of the events accompanying disease, fever, and delirium, and the effects of consulting the physician and the priest.

The cold/hot opposition was among the basic tenets of the humoral theory that for centuries shaped medical thinking. Fever has remained the clinical hallmark of inflammation, and is narrowly associated with disease, trauma, or infection. The physiology of fever is better understood in the context of recent immunology: cytokines are responsible for fever induction and the behavioral changes during the acute phase of infection.

In response to a stimulus such as LPS, the body's thermostatic control center within the hypothalamus increases its set-point temperature. The body then increases its core temperature to match the new level. Physiological (vasoconstriction, reduced sweating) and also behavioral modifications (drinking warm liquids, putting on warmer clothes) drive up the body's temperature. When the fever breaks, the body temperature again is too high relative to the new set-point, and physiological and behavioral modifications result in a lowering of core temperature, increased blood flow in the skin, sweating, and the desire to drink cold liquids. Fever is a central episode of immunity and infection. Clinical considerations on the onset and rhythm of fever paroxysms remain a decisive component of the biomedical enterprise in the era of the cytokine orchestra.

At the onset of the disease, inflammation is a nonspecific restorative response of tissues to soluble chemical mediators produced after injury. If the harmful agent is not removed or the disequilibrium persists, a pathological state of chronic inflammation ensues. If the inflammatory cycle is broken, the host is restored to its preinflammatory state of physiological equilibrium, but, as the French philosopher of medicine Georges Canguilhem stated in many of his writings, there is no return to cellular innocence.

IN SEARCH OF A MECHANISM UNIFYING IMMUNOLOGY

The tantalizing identification of multiple factors in constant interaction has resulted in a 'balkanization' of research, i.e. division of research into small separate sections. It has blurred the primitive simplicity of the immune response with its two arms – the informative and the effective – once gracefully linked in a kind of reflexive arc.

The distinction between self and nonself is still very much there, even if many doubts are expressed about its pertinence. Frank Mcfarlane Burnet had long ago envisioned the possibility of accounting for the nature of the self in precise molecular terms, before retreating to use of the phrase in a metaphorical sense. Zinkernagel and Doherty's (1979) demonstration that the T-lymphocyte receptor reacts with a polypeptide attached to a major histocompatibility complex (MHC) molecule reinforced the notion of the recognition of nonself in the context of self. At the onset of molecular immunology, there were attempts to describe more precisely the self as the 'peptidic self' (Kourilsky and Claverie 1988).

Generally speaking, however, the self/nonself distinction functions more as a general background than as an effective theoretical construct (Moulin 1994), an indication that, although many questions remain to be clarified, most immunological reactivity is oriented for the sake of survival of the organism. It does not radically differ from expressions such as 'genes' or 'immunity', the meaning of which is constantly fluctuating. Although it has been said that 'The self is constantly defined anew, which is another way of saying it doesn't really exist at all' (Richardson 1996), the reference to self and nonself ensures communication between generations of scientists and between scientists and their public.

The last few decades have seen an outburst of data where it is difficult to single out unambiguous signals. Epistemologists insist on the dependence of scientists, more than theory, on the experimental systems that they handle on a daily basis (Rheinberger 1997). It had been suggested for a long time that tolerance can be induced by small as well as overwhelming doses of antigen, but never has it been made clearer that the self/nonself distinction is made empirically, case by case, and the meaning of immunological phenomena is practically determined. For Zinkernagel (2000), there is nothing absolute: immunity is, in his own words, a matter of dose, space, and time. Philippe Kourilsky (1998), inaugurating the first chair of 'molecular immunology' in France in 1998, stated the same idea:

> Specificity in the immune system, more than on the complementarity of structures, is founded on the dynamic of cellular activations: some defence mechanisms are deprived of specificity and acquire it only by operating at the right time, at the right place.

This perspective is not as empirical as it appears at first sight. It simply moves the emphasis to the importance of microenvironment and local determinism. Cells and factors are not identical because, following a 'leibnizian' doctrine of individuality, they are always located in space and time. Obviously, we miss an all-encompassing and simultaneous view of all compatible phenomena in the realm of immunity – the vision of GOD (for Generator Of Diversity), to recall Melvin Cohn's jocular and unmistakably serious address. Any activation can result in overreaction and destruction of antigen-stimulated cells. The recognition of autoreactivity as a physiological phenomenon resulting in autoimmunity has illustrated this empirical turn.

The identification of autoreactive cells within the lymphocyte repertoire recalls the interpretation of these cells playing a role in body homeostasis, such as immunocircuits controlling the antibody level, e.g. through idiotypic interactions. Autoimmunity became pathogenic only when effector cells penetrated organs, favored by microchanges in the environment.

It is currently being suggested (and has been suggested for decades) that infections may cause autoimmune diseases. The molecular basis still remains to be established in many cases, but it is a fascinating hypothesis, also available for many idiopathic diseases. The scenario would be the following: molecular mimicry between a pathogen-derived antigen and a host antigen would set off subliminal autoimmunity.

T-cell receptor recognition of antigen looks highly degenerate. In experimental models, myelin basic protein, involved in multiple sclerosis, may display similarities with peptides presented by MHC structures. Mimicry of human sphingolipids by lipopolysaccharides from *Haemophilus influenzae* may provoke the Guillain–Barré syndrome or Lewis-like polysaccharide antigens from *Helicobacter pylori* lead to atrophic gastritis in humans. The analogy can go beyond primary amino acid sequence homology and includes shapes in space (e.g. between arrangements of a three-domain coil of HIV-1 glycoproteins and contact areas of IL-2 with the α, β, and γ chains of the IL-2 receptor), considerably extending the possibilities of chain reactions, even if one does not know to what extent in vitro studies can be extrapolated to autoimmunity in humans: 'Molecular mimicry is round every corner' (Regner and Lambert 2001, p. 185). The production of proinflammatory cytokines would play a decisive role. A genetic component might determine susceptibility to autoimmune diseases, and environmental factors play a role. Everything is possible if the worst does not necessarily happen. In the empirical frame of mind presented above, it has been suggested that autoimmunity can benefit self-maintenance and even be 'a cause of health' (Schwartz and Cohen 2000).

As autoimmune diseases involve stimulation against certain antigens in the individual, no wonder some concerns have arisen about the flirtation with infection called immunization or vaccination, which might also contribute to an autoimmune effect (Shoenfeld and Aron-Maor 2000). Vaccination does not differ substantially from casual immunization through infection, in that it stimulates various pathways depending on both the antigen and the host, and irreversible disorder may be created. The examples of hepatitis B and multiple sclerosis have recently been scrutinized, and the impact of immunization programs on the repertoire of the immune responses in populations taken seriously. The multiplication of vaccines has raised the iconoclastic question of whether they still offer the best strategy for preventing infections. Unfortunately, most of the time, autoimmune diseases have over the last few years been associated with immunization based almost exclusively on case reports – the weakest of scientific evidence.

Although immunization remains a major tool in the management of public health, the consideration of individual reactions, in conformity with the principle of precaution, is forcibly discussed in industrialized countries, where there is a move in favor of immunization 'à la carte'. These considerations reflect the individual and liberal mood of the last few years, with uncertainty about the consequences of this change, at economic, symbolic, or demographic levels.

In the sound and fury of molecular signaling, immunology remains in search of an innovative theoretical framework that would shelter its empirical work and substantiate its claims for solving medical problems and offering clues to general physiology, beyond the sole study of infectious diseases. Not satisfied with the elusiveness of the self/nonself topic, some immunologists have searched for phenomena that convey a general physiological meaning. These attempts have generated much interest and debate and also some confusion; if they stimulated imagination, they fell short of revolutionizing immunology.

The 'danger theory' brought forth by Polly Matzinger has been a flamboyant and significant episode of this quest for a new unifying trend. Matzinger considers that her 'danger theory' has undermined Burnet's classic view of self/nonself discrimination and the paradigm of clonal selection that ruled immunology for more than 30 years. She suggests that, in place of being sensitive to the discrimination between self and nonself, the immune system is in a state of permanent alarm, detecting cellular lesions, which she labels 'danger', after various events, ranging from exposure to tetanus toxin, to a pollutant interfering with the environment, and consequently reacting. In the nineteenth century, physiologists included, in the definition of inflammation, besides Celsius' triad of 'rubor–dolor–edema' (redness, pain, swollenness), '*functio laesa*' or impaired function. Matzinger aimed to discard teleological explanations and introduce simple mechanisms to account for accumulated data in cellular and molecular immunology. The use of the danger notion remains, however, as contextual and teleological as the self/nonself distinction and, even if it clashes with the almost excessive mystique of the self (Silverstein 1997), it does not induce any revolutionary changes in immunologists' theoretical thinking.

The emphasis on apoptosis has also played a role in bringing together different axes of research. The formation of small fragmented bodies, which contain remnants of nuclei, has been documented for a long time in scattered single cells. They were described for the first time in the liver in yellow fever as 'Councilman's bodies'. The Greek word *apoptosis*, used to describe the dropping of petals from flowers or leaves from the trees in autumn, was applied in 1972 by Kerr and collaborators to controlled cell deletion (Kerr et al. 1972) – a genetically programmed cell death, recognized as a vital biological phenomenon. The structural changes would comprise the formation of apoptotic bodies, and their subsequent degradation and phagocytosis.

Apoptosis appears to play an opposite, but also complementary, role to mitosis in the regulation of cell populations. It is determined by intrinsic clocks that are specific to the cell type involved, and plays an important role in the regulation of cell numbers in a variety of tissues under both physiological and pathological conditions. In 1991, Clem and Fechheimer described, in baculovirus (an insect virus), two proteins that inhibit molecules triggering cellular death. One of them at least would belong to a large molecular family operating throughout species. Most viruses such as the human papilloma virus, responsible in the long term for the occurrence of genital cancers, interfere with gene reparation and apoptosis. Anti-infectious defense, aging, and carcinogenesis seem so closely interrelated that any therapeutic or even preventive strategy is at risk of provoking undesired effects.

Apoptosis bears some analogies with Pasteur's hypothesis of 1882 that bacteria invading the organisms rapidly run short of food, a scorched earth tactic on the part of the organism. This theory was rapidly discarded and replaced by a more positive theory focusing on Metchnikoff's phagocytosis. Cell suicide triggered during primoinfection comes very close to the idea of a mechanism that allows the pathogen to starve to death.

Apoptosis has been put in sharp focus by contemporary studies of the immune system. Immortalized cells may transform into cancer cells and give birth to lymphomas, if the immune system is weakened or strained. Apoptosis offers a clue to the mechanisms that determine whether the immune response will be positive or negative, activation or tolerance. In 1995, Douglas and Thomas Ferguson offered two mirroring images of apoptosis: in sanctuaries such as the eye and brain or the pregnant woman's womb, the cells of the immune system are forced to commit suicide, whereas, in the immune system, it is the infected cells that are forced to commit suicide (Green 1998).

Apoptosis captured the imagination in the scientific race for new ideas. *La Sculpture du Vivant* by Jean-Claude Ameisen, dedicated to apoptosis in immunology, refers to an episode of Odyssey on Ulysses in the Messina Straits (Ulysses attached to the mast in the ship listens to the mermaids' songs and wants to die with them; the sailors who do not hear them go on rowing). The myth illustrates the modern science of biological signals, the contradictory or alternate messages of which determine cell behavior.

With apoptosis as the key concept to the understanding of immunity as interference with cell suicide, we have to pay attention to the merging of two functions that are historically claimed by immunologists: infection control and cancer surveillance. The molecular description of a cycle of gene repressors leading to cellular death enables reconsideration of Burnet's past effort to associate them. The new orientation in anti-infectious strategy is no longer the mere destruction, either chemical or cellular, of the pathogen, but the exploitation of programmed suicide, by sending the cells a signal that is ordinarily repressed. The link between potent life and death metaphors, and the schemes of thought favored by scientists will remain a matter of debate for those who wish to elucidate the mechanisms of discovery and serendipity in research.

THE MOLECULARIZATION OF VACCINOLOGY

If new immunology is still uncertain about its theoretical foundations (is the self more than philosophical platitudes?), can it at least rely on its medical practical successes in the molecular era?

'The 1990s will be remembered as the decade of vaccines', a researcher from Connaught laboratories exclaimed in 1995, in Canada, during a congress on vaccines (Klein 1996, p. 295). And he went on to explain how research would update the classic vaccines and deliver new ones. The vaccine model had unified and stimulated the field of immunity studies and powerfully motivated scientists and governments. But the old models of war against germs appeared inappropriate in a sophisticated era where cognitive modes of thought tended to replace bellicose metaphors (Fox-Keller 1995).

Although the notion of species fixity has always been controversial (Amsterdamska 1987), vaccines were first conceived on the basis of a supposedly stable bacterial order. This order has been shattered. The constant mutations of flu viruses oblige us to invent new vaccines each winter. Bacteria or viruses, we have learnt, contain revertant individuals displaying the virulence of wild strains, or a new virulence, after mutations induced by the environment or through hybridization with other strains in a propitious environment. Reversion to virulence and polio cases that happen after oral immunization are probably the result of recombinations in the gut of the three vaccinal strains, or possibly between vaccinal viruses and other enteroviruses. A genetic drift makes strains of pertussis, the agent of whooping cough, diverge from the vaccinal prototypes, increasing the burden of the vaccinal enterprise.

The whole historical enterprise of immunization, notwithstanding its numerous 'hazards', was rather successful in the long run. Yet, molecularization was expected to fare better still and provide safer vaccines in diseases that were already controlled. Overall, it was advertised as coping with diseases refractory to immunization, such as leprosy or dengue fever, or new plagues such as AIDS.

Molecular vaccinology stands in sharp contrast to the former empirical methods of pathogen attenuation and is celebrated as the achievement of Landsteiner's ideal, with the replacement of crude preparations by molecules of exquisite specificity. Technical advances in gene splitting, gene sequencing, and protein engineering would allow the identification and optimization of new protective antigens against bacterial, viral, and parasitic diseases, on the basis of the most recent knowledge on the immune response pathways.

As vaccines played an important role in the popularity of immunology, although the development of immunology followed rather than caused the advent of early vaccines, molecularization – the shift from mere empiricism to rational design – was considered as the historical opportunity for immunology to produce at last ideal vaccines.

Several pathways offered for molecularization deserve comment:

- The first is the cloning of genes coding for virulence factors, islets grouping all sites involved in cellular invasion, toxin production, for the rational development of knock-out bacterial strains, or their introduction in vectors (Kourilsky 1987). Although BCG, administered soon after birth, avoids meningitis and disseminated infections in infants, it protects imperfectly against pulmonary tuberculosis in adult life. The new BCG projects plan to replace one of the most controversial vaccines by a modern one (Palfy et al. 1999).

- The second pathway is the recombinant subunit vaccines, the prototype for which is the hepatitis B vaccine.
- Genetic immunization is presented as an elegant way of making muscular tissue produce a vaccine.
- Finally, synthetic vaccines would mark the peak of innovation. The computerized invention of vaccinal structures, e.g. polypeptidic antigens, flatters the esthetic taste and comforts the quest for vaccines tailored to each individual's genetic make-up and life-style.

Adenoviruses were the first vectors in favor. They had been used as oral vaccines for respiratory infections since 1969. Then came the poxviruses (Panicali and Paoletti 1982). Cowpox, in use for two centuries, had allowed smallpox eradication. The first recombinant successfully produced as a vaccine was the canarypox rabies vaccine for dogs.

One of the great successes of molecular immunology was the production of recombinant vaccine against hepatitis B (Blumberg 1975). The research was fueled by anxiety linked to the use of hepatitis B carrier plasmas and the threat of transmission of an unknown virus undetected by the tests and undestroyed by inactivation techniques (Muraskin 1995). The recombinant vaccine obtained in vitro by expression of hepatitis B antigen in yeasts was licensed in 1986 (McAleer et al. 1984). Polysaccharidic vaccines protecting against capsular bacteria such as *Neisseria meningitidis* or *Haemophilus infuenzae* were also produced.

The programs have led more to a gathering of an unprecedented amount of information on immunity than to solving the practical issues that they had in mind. In spite of the adoption of current methods of molecular biology, reviews of the processes employed concluded that the choice of various preparations was still empirical. More clinical trials, especially in infants, were necessary to help understand 'conjugate immunology' (Moreau 1996, p. 148).

Expression of the foreign antigen by the carrier is not sufficient to elicit an immune response. The presentation of the antigen to the immune system depends on its physical location on the bacterial surface, and its accessibility is crucial for the magnitude of the immune response. Rather than choosing attenuated pathogens, it has been suggested that commensal microorganisms should be used to deliver vaccine antigens, but they then have to compete with the local flora. Molecular biology forces us to enter a realm always further away, toward an artificially produced environment. This strategy requires surveillance of its short- and long-term consequences, in terms of infection, morbidity, and mortality rates. Are we prepared to sustain this challenge, especially in countries where health services are inadequate or disorganized through internal or external conflicts?

In spite of its proponents' enthusiasm, it appears that the revolution has not yet borne all the expected fruit. Parasitic diseases do not give way, even the leishmaniases that had fostered well-founded hopes, since the early attempts at empirical immunization went back to the eighteenth century in the Middle East. The WHO has recently encouraged clinical trials for a modernized version of this legacy of the past (Mudabber 1989).

Genetic vaccines, although made attractive by their simple, cheap, and easy manufacture, seem to be inefficient and raise numerous queries about the advent of genes into the microenvironment of the body. The old adjuvant, alum, which is still in use, was recently charged as provoking untoward effects. There is an agreement about its replacement by synthetic molecules: this means that research starts again from zero, with clinical trials required for assessing the new adjuvants.

The rational approach paradoxically does not guarantee that the deleted bacterium will produce the desired immunity. Although usually passage of strains through animals leads to attenuation, biological engineering modifies pathogenicity without offering parallel constant immunogenicity. In any case, the new vaccine must be tested in phase I studies, without the benefit of more than one century of experimentation and results in the field of immunity. Molecularization leads to purity that is not synonymous with antigenicity, an event that could be expected, after revisiting early studies on haptens by Karl Landsteiner at the turn of the twentieth century. Landsteiner expressed the necessity of coupling small well-known chemicals, which he labeled as 'haptens', with large molecules playing an elusive role (carriers) in the triggering of the immune response.

The cytoxic lymphocyte (CTL) epitopes, supposed to provide clues for the treatment of cancer and of chronic infectious diseases, are not necessarily potent antigens, and subunit and peptide vaccines often behave as poor antigens.

The unification of vaccines under the banner of molecular immunology has not been completed to date, never mind the economic problems linked to the cost of new technologies and the difficulty of replacing old vaccines by new ones, bearing in mind modern regulations about innovation and their approval.

If molecularization has not resulted in a general program for safe and effective vaccines, is this for structural or historical reasons? The optimists argue that we just have to wait for appropriate tools and molecules, exquisite specificity retaining its long-term promises. The pessimists argue that immunization has reached its historical limits and will fail when confronted with pathogens that have evolved, or rather coevolved, with potent mechanisms for using the organism's cells and the immune system itself to survive and direct the components of the organisms to their profit: incorporation in the cell genome, fixation on receptors, use of chemokines as growth factors or decoys. Failures would occur inexorably and the number of invading viruses (the 'emergence' phenomenon) would rise, to the point where it may be discussed whether we have reached a limit along this pathway in our capacity to deal with infections (Moulin 1996a). Have we not dealt in the first place with the easiest-going pathogens, those secreting a toxin (diphtheria, tetanus)? Does it remain possible to reach those that are more or less integrated into the nuclei of our cells? Killing infected cells may go too far and trigger an array of inflammatory phenomena.

This could change the very meaning of immunization and point to relative rather than absolute prevention, as is actually the case in AIDS trials where vaccine may be administered in the course of infection, to help the organism to cure the disease or reduce its severity. But this change in the biological meaning of vaccines would entail a dramatic revision in both popular and medical perceptions of immunization as a tool of public health, and would probably undermine its current applications.

THE IMMUNE SYSTEM AS A SUBSYSTEM OR A PART OF THE WHOLE

Jerne and others had already described formal analogies between the nervous and the immune systems, and suggested mathematical modeling for the sake of comparison (Lefkovits 1980). Molecularization of immunology, with the emergence of multiple families, has led to the relativization of the frontiers between organs and awareness of the narrow relationships among organs, cell lines, and systems. Compared with the nervous system, its paragon and model, the immune system, is first characterized by the mobility of its elements. Fridman (1992) called it the mobile brain. Cells of the immune system move continuously and this movement is essential for immunosurveillance and clonal selection, 'in the sea of microbes, toxins, parasites and mutagens we call Earth' (Anderson 1990, p. 14).

The immune system shares more than cursory similarities with other systems such as the endocrine or nervous systems. Bidirectional communication between them seems to occur as a result of common hormones and receptors. Revisited in the era of molecular biology, the list is impressive and ever increasing. Not only do neuroendocrine and immune tissues produce, communicate, and regulate a battery of informational molecules, but also there is growing evidence that these systems may use similar, if not identical, molecules to achieve their ends. Receptors for neuroendocrine molecules on immune cells and for lymphokines on neuroendocrine cells provide ample means for the two systems to interact. Cytokines are secreted by immunocompetent and glial cells. Neuroendocrine factors such as corticotropin-releasing hormone or growth hormone could have been qualified as cytokines if they had initially been described by immunologists, and molecules that were seemingly typically immune could have been qualified as neuropeptides if there had been timely identification by neurobiologists.

Receptors for cytokines present in the brain emit information that modulates the reaction to infection by pathogens. There are ligands for norepinephrine (noradrenaline) and other neuropeptides on the surface of macrophages, lymphocytes, and other immunocompetent cells. Immunoblotting has allowed the identification of receptors on immune and neural cells, ascertaining their molecular identity. β-Endorphin, which participates in analgesia during stress, can link with opioid receptors on lymphocytes (Dantzer et al. 1999). The humoral immune response is accompanied by an activation of the hypothalamic–hypophyseal–cortical–adrenocorticotropic axis and the rise of cortiscosterone in blood. A lesion of the hypothalamic–hypophyseal axis by radiofrequency suppresses the cytotoxic activity of natural killer (NK) cells in mice (Blalock 1997). Immune cells behave like a sensorial organ that is able to convey information to the brain.

These data suggest the importance of taking seriously not only the unity of the organism, but also the difficulty of interfering with its inner organization.

IMMUNOLOGY OF INFECTION: A POST-MODERN PERSPECTIVE

The immune system is a biomedical construct, the elaboration of which has proceeded over several periods, during which the understanding of its functions and its composition have been radically modified: after defense against germs, these functions were the self/nonself discrimination, tumor surveillance, participation in homeostasis, etc.

During the second half of the twentieth century, the microbial element lost its importance as the most immediate correlate of immune function, and the immune system appeared more and more able to respond to various stimulations and to interact with other systems that share the bodily space.

As we began to consider the complexity of microorganisms, and their considerable flexibility, resistance, and capacity to escape, disenchantment has set in to match the ingenious nature of parasites and viruses, strategies have become more sophisticated, clever, and costly. This observation opens on human history and evolution of the living world that coexist and collide under our eyes.

How will the new immunology meet the challenge of the dark infectious age agents? Not only had the microbial world accrued diversity, but also the pathways of pathogens into the organism were known to be multiple: how does the immune system deal with pathogens ranging from telluric bacteria, such as the tetanus bacillus secreting a toxin that can be absorbed *per os* without causing the least trouble, to viruses able to invade the genome of the immune system and remain there silent for long periods of time before bursting out?

The return of infectious diseases has prompted the need for fresh knowledge and the urge to deepen both immunological and genetic components of the immune response. Not only did it revive the idea that heredity and immunity, or vertical and horizontal transmission, are two faces of the same coin, it also led to the idea that immunity is strongly integrated into many physiological and pathological responses.

With the new challenges posed by the return of infectious diseases, now that we are aware of the two-edged nature of most of our therapeutic tools and the ambivalence of most drugs, we can start to appreciate how the scientific revolution that is ritually celebrated has so far been incomplete, and to measure the extent of the work that lies ahead of us. There is a huge need for specific studies, but integrated approaches are also badly needed. It is a concern for the author of this chapter that the historical and philosophical approach attempted allows us to cast a critical glance over our accumulated knowledge and the seemingly impressive breakthroughs that deepen our knowledge, but also to move the future targets forward.

There is no such thing in history as a return to a former perspective. Even if the rallying cry of the fight against infectious diseases has sounded over these last few years for immunologists, it is by no means a return to the past. Contemporary immunology, with an emphasis on infectious diseases, can indeed be redefined as an immunity of infection rather than immunology of infections. Although infectious diseases are many, this chapter on the recent past of immunology spells 'infection' in the singular. Infection does not point to a separate chapter on pathology, but is a central episode corresponding not only to traditional infectious diseases but to many other disorders, from poorly understood autoimmune syndromes to diseases once labeled neurological, endocrine, or otherwise, and cancers. The advances made in the understanding of the immune system illuminate some crucial events in the genesis of disease and the fabric of normal life through all kinds of encounters with pathogens both internal and external. The immune system can be assimilated, in a sixth sense, for sensing pathogens, the key organ of interaction between the organism and its environment. The central position of immunology today in medicine echoes the centrality of infection as a crossroads in the economy of the organism.

REFERENCES

Ameisen, J.-C. 1999. *La sculpture du vivant*. Paris: Le Seuil.

Amigorena, S. 1999. Présentation antigénique par les cellules dendritiques. *Méd Sci*, **15**, 932.

Amsterdamska, O. 1987. Medical and biological constraints: early research on variations in bacteriology. *Soc Studies Sci*, **17**, 657–87.

Anderson, A.O. 1990. Structure and organization of the lymphatic system. In: Oppenheim, J.J. and Shevach, E.M. (eds), *Immunophysiology*. Oxford: Oxford University Press, 14.

Besredka, A. 1906. De l'antiendotoxine typhique et des anti-endotoxines en général. *Ann Instit Pasteur Immunol*, **20**, 149.

Bevan Cross, M.J. 1976. Priming for a secondary cytotoxic response to minor antigens with H-2 congenic cells which do not crossreact in the cytotoxic assay. *J Expl Med*, **143**, 1283–8.

Blalock, J.E. (ed.) 1997. *Neuroimmunoendocrinology*. Basel: Karger.

Bloom, B.R. and Bennett, B. 1966. Mechanism of a reaction in vitro associated with delayed-type hypersensitivity. *Science*, **153**, 80–2.

Blumberg, B. 1975. Hepatitis B virus and vaccine. In: Gallagher, R.L., Nossal, G.V., et al. (eds), *Immunology, the making of a modern science*. London: Academic Press, 223–9.

Cambrosio, A. and Keating, P. 1994. 'Ours is an engineering approach': Flow cytometry and the constitution of human T-cell subsets. *J Hist Biol*, **27**, 449–79.

Cambrosio, A. and Keating, P. 1995. *Exquisite specificity. The monoclonal antibody revolution*. Cambridge: Cambridge University Press.

Canguilhem, G. 1966. *Le normal et le pathologique*. New York: Zone Books, (English translation by C.R. Fawcett.).

Cavaillon, J.-M. and Le Garrec, Y. 1998. Alexandre Besredka (1870–1940): a famous endotoxinologist. *Endotoxin Newsletter*, **8**, 4.

Clem, R.J. and Fechheimer, M. 1991. Prevention of apoptosis by a baculovirus gene during infection, of insect cells. *Science*, **254**, 1388–90.

Coutinho, E., Forni, D.I., et al. 1984. From an antigen-centered, clonal perspective of immune responses to an organism-centered network perspective of autonomous activity in a self-referential immune system. *Immunol Rev*, **79**, 151–68.

Dantzer, R., Wollman, E.E. and Yimiya, R. (eds) 1999. *Cytokines, stress and depression*. New York: Plenum.

Darier, P. 1900. Anatomie et physiologie de la peau. In: Besnier, E., Brocq, E. and Jacquet, L. (eds), *La pratique dermatologique*, vol 1. . Paris: Masson, 46–7.

David, J.R. 1966. Delayed hypersensitivity in vitro: its mediation by cell-free substances formed by lymphoid cell-antigen interaction. *Proc Nat Acad Sci*, **56**, 72–7.

Desportes, I., Le Charpentier, Y. and Gelian, A. 1985. Occurrence of a new microsporidian *Enterocytozoon bieneusi* n.g n.sp. in the enterocytes of a human patient with Aids. *J Protozool*, **32**, 250–4.

Dumonde, D.C., Wolsencroft, R.A., et al. 1969. Lymphokines: 'non antibody' mediators of cellular immunity generated by lymphocyte activation. *Nature*, **224**, 38–42.

Evans, A.S. 1993. *Causation and disease*. New York: Plenum Medical Books.

Ewald, P. 2002. *Plague time: The new germ theory of disease*. New York: Anchor Books.

Fox-Keller, E. 1995. *Refiguring life: metaphors of twentieth-century biology*. New York: Columbia University Press.

Fridman, W.H. 1992. *Le cerveau mobile*. Paris: Hermann.

Fridman, W.H. 2000. *La révolution immunologique. Les défenses naturelles contre le cancer*. Paris: Lattès.

Gajdusek, D.C. 1977. Unconventional viruses and the origin and disappearance of kuru. *Science*, **197**, 943–60.

Garrod, A.E. 1909. *The innate errors of metabolism*. London: Frowde.

Gershon, R.K. 1980. Immunoregulation circa 1980: Some comments on the state of the art. *J Allergy Clin Immunol*, **66**, 18–24.

Gradman, C. 2000. Invisible enemies and the language of politics in imperial Germany. *Science in Context*, **130**, 9–30.

Green, D.R. 1998. Apoptotic pathways, the roads to ruin. *Cell*, **94**, 695–8.

Grmek, M.D. 1969. Préliminaires d'une étude historique des maladies. *Annales ESC*, **1**, 1473–83.

Hirschfeld, L. 1928. *Konstitutionserologie und Blutgruppenforschung*. Berlin: Springer.

Isaacs A, Lindenmann J, 1957. Virus interference. I. The Interferon. *Proceedings of the Royal Society, Biology*, vol. 147. London: Royal Society, 258–67.

Jordan, B. 1995. *Voyage au pays des gènes*. Paris: Les Belles Lettres-INSERM.

Judson, H.F. 1979. *The eighth day of creation. Makers of a revolution in biology*. New York: Simon & Schuster.

Kerr, J.B., Wylie, A.H. and Currie, A.R. 1972. Apoptosis: A basic biological phenomenon with wide-ranging implications in tissue kinetics. *Br J Cancer*, **26**, 239–57.

Klein, M. 1996. Future prospects for vaccinology. In: Plotkine, S. and Fantini, B. (eds), *Vaccinia, vaccine, vaccinology*. Paris: Elsevier, 295.

Köhler, G. and Milstein, C. 1975. Continuous cultures of fused cells secreting antibodies of predetermined specificity. *Nature*, **256**, 495–7.

Kourilsky, P. 1987. *Les artisans de l'hérédité*. Paris: Odile Jacob.

Kourilsky, P. 1998. *Conference for the inauguration of the immmunology chair*. Paris: Collège de France, 6.

Kourilsky, P. and Claverie, J.M. 1988. Le modèle du soi peptidique. *Méd Sci*, **4**, 177–83.

Landsteiner, K. 1936. *The specificity of serological reactions*. Springfield: CC Thomas.

Langerhans, P. 1868. Über die Nerven der Menschlichen Haut. *Virchows Arch*, **44**, 325–37.

Lefkovits, I. (ed.) 1980. *The immune system. A festschrift in honor of Niels Kaj Jerne*. Basel: S. Karger.

Löwy, I. 1997. *Between bench and bedside, science, healing and interleukin-2 in a cancer ward*. Cambridge: Harvard University Press.

Löwy, I. and Gaudillière, J.-Pb. 1998. Disciplining cancer. Mice and the practice of genetic purity. In: Löwy, I. and Gaudillière, J.-P. (eds), *The invisible industrialist. Manufacturers and the production of scientific knowledge*. London: Macmillan, 209–49.

McAleer, W.J., Markus, H.Z. and Bailey, J.F. 1984. Human hepatitis B vaccine from recombinant yeast. *Nature*, **1**, 178–80.

Mak, T.W., Penninger, J.M. and Ohashi, P.S. 2001. Knock-out mice, a paradigm shift in modern immunology. *Rev Immunol*, **1**, 11–19.

Mazumdar, P.H. 1995. *Species and specificity. An interpretation in the history of immunology*. Cambridge: Cambridge University Press.

Moreau, M. 1996. Conjugation technologies. In: Plotkin, S. and Fantini, B. (eds), *Vaccinia, vaccination and vaccinology*. Elsevier: Paris,, 148.

Mosmann, T.R. and Coffmann, R.L. 1989. Th1 and Th2 cells: different patterns of lymphokine secretions lead to different functional properties. *Ann Rev Immunol*, **7**, 145–73.

Moulin, A.M. 1991. *Le dernier langage de la médecine, Histoire de l'immunologie, de Pasteur au Sida*. Paris: PUF.

Moulin, A.M. 1994. Les horizons du soi biologique. In: *Rencontres internationales de Genève, Les identités*. Neuchatel: La Baconnnière, 99–145.

Moulin, A.M. (ed.) 1996a. *L'aventure de la vaccination*. Paris: Fayard.

Moulin, A.M. 1996b. L'actualité des maladies infectieuses dans les pays industrialisés: évolution ou histoire? *Rev Epidémiol Santé Publique*, **44**, 519–29.

Moulin, A.M. 1997. A 'science dans le siècle', Immunology or the science of boundaries. In: Krige, J. and Pestre, D. (eds), *Science in the twentieth century*. Amsterdam: Harwood, 479–95.

Moulin, A.M. 2001. Multiple splendor. The one and many versions of the immune system. In: Moulin, A.M. and Cambrosio, A. (eds), *Singular selves, historical debates and contemporary issues in immunology*. Paris: Elsevier, 228–43.

Moulin, A.M. and Silverstein, A.M. 1990. History of immunophysiology. In: Oppenheim, J.J. and Shevach, E.M. (eds), *Immunophysiology: The role of cells and cytokines in immunity and inflammation*. Oxford: Oxford University Press, 3–13.

Mudabber, F. 1989. Experiences with vaccines against cutaneous leishmaniasis of men and mice. *Parasitology*, **98**, 849–60.

Muraskin, W. 1995. *The war against hepatitis B. A history of the International Task Force on hepatitis B immunization*. Philadelphia: University of Pennsylvania Press.

Nicolle, C. 1933. *Le destin des maladies infectieuses*. Paris: Alcan.

Nutton, V. 1983. The seeds of disease: an explanation of contagion and infection from the Greeks to the Renaissance. *Med Hist*, **27**, 1–34.

Palfy, G., Dutour, O., et al. (eds) 1999. *Tuberculosis past and present*. Budapest: Tuberculosis Foundation.

Panem, S. 1984. *The interferon crusade*. Washington DC: Brookings Institution.

Panicali, D. and Paoletti, E. 1982. Construction of poxvirus as cloning vectors: insertion of the thymidine kinase gene from herpes simplex virus into the DNA of infectious vaccinia virus. *Proc Natl Acad Sci USA*, **79**, 4927–31.

Regner, M. and Lambert, P.H. 2001. Autoimmunity through infection or immunization? *Nature Immunol*, **2**, 185–8.

Rheinberger, H.J. 1997. *Toward a history of epistemic things, synthesizing proteins in the test tube*. Stanford: Stanford University Press.

Richardson, S. 1996. The end of the self. *Discovery*, **5**, 17, 80.

Rock, F.L., Hardiman, G. and Timans, J.C. 1998. A family of human receptors structurally related to Drosophila Toll. *Proc Natl Acad Sci USA*, **95**, 588–93.

Romagnani, S. 1996. Th1 and Th2 in human diseases. *Clin Immunol Immunopathol*, **80**, 225–35.

Schwartz, M. and Cohen, I.R. 2000. Autoimmunity can benefit self-maintenance. *Immunol Today*, **265**, 265–7.

Serres, M. 1990. *Le contrat naturel*. Paris: François Bourin.

Shoenfeld, Y. and Aron-Maor, A. 2000. Vaccination and autoimmunity. 'Vaccinosis': a dangerous liaison? *J Autoimmun*, **14**, 1–10.

Silverstein, A.M. 1989. *A history of immunology*. San Diego: Academic Press.

Silverstein, A.M. 1997. On the mystique of the immunological self. *Immunol Rev*, **159**, 197–206.

Taniguchi, T., Matsui, H., et al. 1983. Structure and expression of a cloned cDNA for human interleukin 2. *Nature*, **302**, 305–10.

Tibayrenc, M. 2001. Editorial. Infection. *Genetics and Evolution*, **1**, 1.

Wedderburn, L. and Dianda, L. 2000. T cells at the turn of the twenty-first century. *Immunol Today*, **120**, 120–2.

Winslow, C.E. 1943. *The conquest of epidemic diseases*. Princeton: Princeton University Press.

Zinkernagel, R.M. 2000. Self-nonself revisited. *Semin Immunol*, **12**, 169.

Zinkernagel, R.M. and Doherty, P.C. 1979. MHC-restricted cytotoxic T cells. *Adv Immunol*, **27**, 51–177.

PART II

INNATE IMMUNITY AND INFLAMMATION

3

Phagocytes part 1: Macrophages

GORDON D. BROWN AND SIAMON GORDON

Macrophages (Mϕ) play an essential role in anti-infectious immunity. They are key players in the innate immune system, detecting and responding to microbial invasion, restricting the spread of microbes, and recruiting other immune cells to the site of infection. Mϕs can act as accessory cells in secondary lymphocyte activation and as effector cells in cell-mediated immunity, and participate in humoral immunity by eliminating foreign antigens. The functions of Mϕs are enhanced when these cells are activated; thus activation represents a crucial step in anti-infective immunity and defects in this process result in an increased susceptibility to pathogens. Mϕs produce a number of anti-inflammatory molecules, which contribute to the resolution of inflammatory responses, and are also involved in many essential homeostatic functions, such as the clearance of apoptotic cells.

In this chapter we present an overview of Mϕ functions, as they relate to anti-infectious immunity. We describe the origins and types of Mϕs, the mechanisms they use for microbial recognition, uptake, and killing, as well as describing their interactions with the adaptive immune system through the release of cytokines and other soluble factors, and through the presentation of antigens. We explore Mϕ activation, their role in homeostatic processes, as it relates to infection, and briefly discuss Mϕ-induced pathology. With such an important role in anti-infective immunity, the Mϕ also provides an ideal niche for pathogens able to modify Mϕ functions, and we demonstrate some of the mechanisms that pathogens use to achieve these goals.

ORIGINS OF MACROPHAGES

Macrophages originate from blood monocytes which are generated in the bone marrow from monoblasts and promonocytes. Monocytes enter the bloodstream constitutively throughout life, accounting for 1–6 percent of the total normal adult white blood cell count (Ross and Auger 2002). These cells leave the bloodstream by adhering to endothelial cells through interactions of a variety of surface receptors, including β_1- and β_2-integrins, such as VLA-4 and LFA-1, which interact with immunoglobulin-domain-containing endothelial receptors, such as intercellular adhesion molecule-1 (ICAM-1) and vascular cell adhesion molecule 1 (VCAM-1) (Springer 1994; Yusuf-Makagiansar et al. 2002). Pathogen-derived molecules, such as lipopolysaccharide (LPS), and a number of inflammatory cytokines cause upregulation of these receptors, resulting in increased leukocyte delivery to sites of infection and inflammation (Roebuck and Finnegan 1999). After adherence, monocytes pass between the endothelial cells by diapedesis, involving interactions with other molecules such as CD31 (platelet endothelial cell adhesion molecule-1 (PECAM-1)), and subsequently migrate into tissues where they differentiate into mature macrophages (Muller and Randolph 1999). A diagrammatic repre-

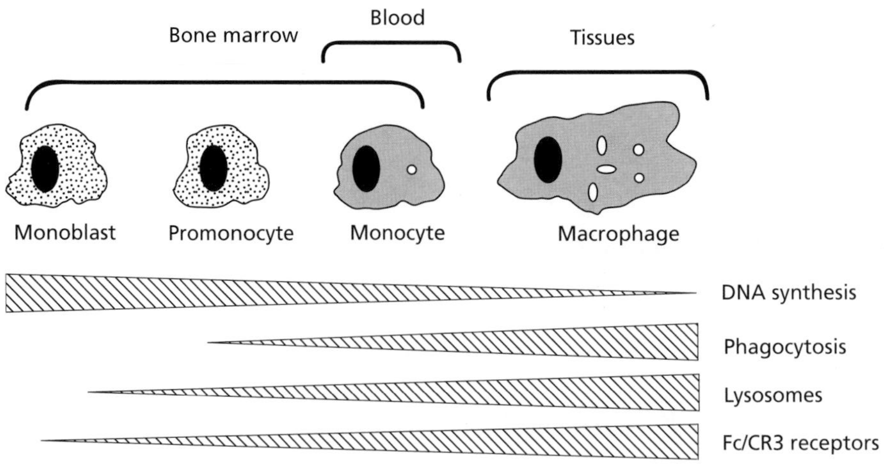

Figure 3.1 *The origins and characteristics of cells giving rise to tissue macrophages. (Adapted with permission from Auger and Ross 1992.)*

sentation of the development of tissue macrophages and some of their characteristics is shown in Figure 3.1.

Tissue macrophages display great functional and morphological heterogeneity, depending on their functional state as well as their interactions with other cells and molecules in the local microenvironment (Gordon 1999, 2001, 2003b). The characterization of these cells has been made possible by the development of tools such as monoclonal antibodies that recognize distinct macrophage proteins (Gordon et al. 1992; Gordon 1999). Resident populations of Mϕs are found at or close to portals of entry (e.g. lung, gut, skin), as sinusoidal cells in liver (Kupffer cells), as stromal cells in bone marrow, and spleen and lymph nodes, and as part of the neural parenchyma (microglia) (Crocker et al. 1991; Perry et al. 1993). They display considerable phenotypic microheterogeneity, e.g. in splenic red pulp, white pulp, and marginal zone, where blood-borne pathogens interact with specialized Mϕ subpopulations and other immune cells (Kraal 1992; Martinez-Pomares and Gordon 1999). An analogous subpopulation of Mϕs is present in the subcapsular region of lymph nodes, encountering potential antigens and dendritic cells in afferent lymph. An example of macrophage heterogeneity in the spleen is shown in Figure 3.2.

Monocytes can also differentiate into dendritic cells (DCs), specialized cells that have the unique ability to migrate out of tissues to secondary lymphoid organs and prime naïve T cells (Mellman and Steinman 2001). These cells are found in most tissues, such as the Langerhans' cells of the skin, and display functional and morphological heterogeneity. They have two distinct functional stages, based on their ability to take up and process antigens (the immature stage) and their ability to migrate to the lymphoid organs and activate antigen-specific T and B cells, directing the generation of the adaptive immune response (the mature stage). Although possessing unique abilities, many of the functions of DCs are similar to those found in macrophages, including their ability to recognize and internalize pathogens and their ability to recruit other immune cells, such as macrophages, neutrophils, natural killer (NK) cells and immature DCs, to the sites of infection. Aspects of this are covered below and in other chapters.

RECOGNITION OF PATHOGENS

During initial infection, the recognition of pathogens by macrophages and other phagocytes is reliant on germline-encoded molecules, termed pattern recognition receptors (PRR) (Janeway 1992). These molecules do not undergo the somatic mutation characteristically required by the adaptive immune response. As the name implies, these receptors recognize conserved microbial structures (the pathogen-associated microbial patterns (PAMP)), such as lipoteichoic acid (LTA) of gram-positive bacteria, LPS of gram-negative bacteria, and β-glucan of fungi. By recognizing these conserved structures, the host can recognize a variety of microbes with a limited set of receptors. Expression of these receptors is varied in different macrophage populations and can also be regulated by cytokines and other immune-modulating agents, including microbial components such as LPS (McKnight and Gordon 1998). In addition to pathogen recognition, the PRRs also determine the mechanism and route of cellular uptake, the response mediated by the Mϕ, and ultimately the immune response generated toward the pathogen.

The PRRs are either found free in the serum, as membrane receptors, or located intracellularly. A list of selected molecules in each of these classes, as well as their microbial ligands, is shown in Table 3.1. The serum-derived PRRs include the collectins, pentraxins, and complement, which coat the microbe (opsonization), allowing recognition and binding by opsonic receptors on host phagocytes. Specific antimicrobial antibodies,

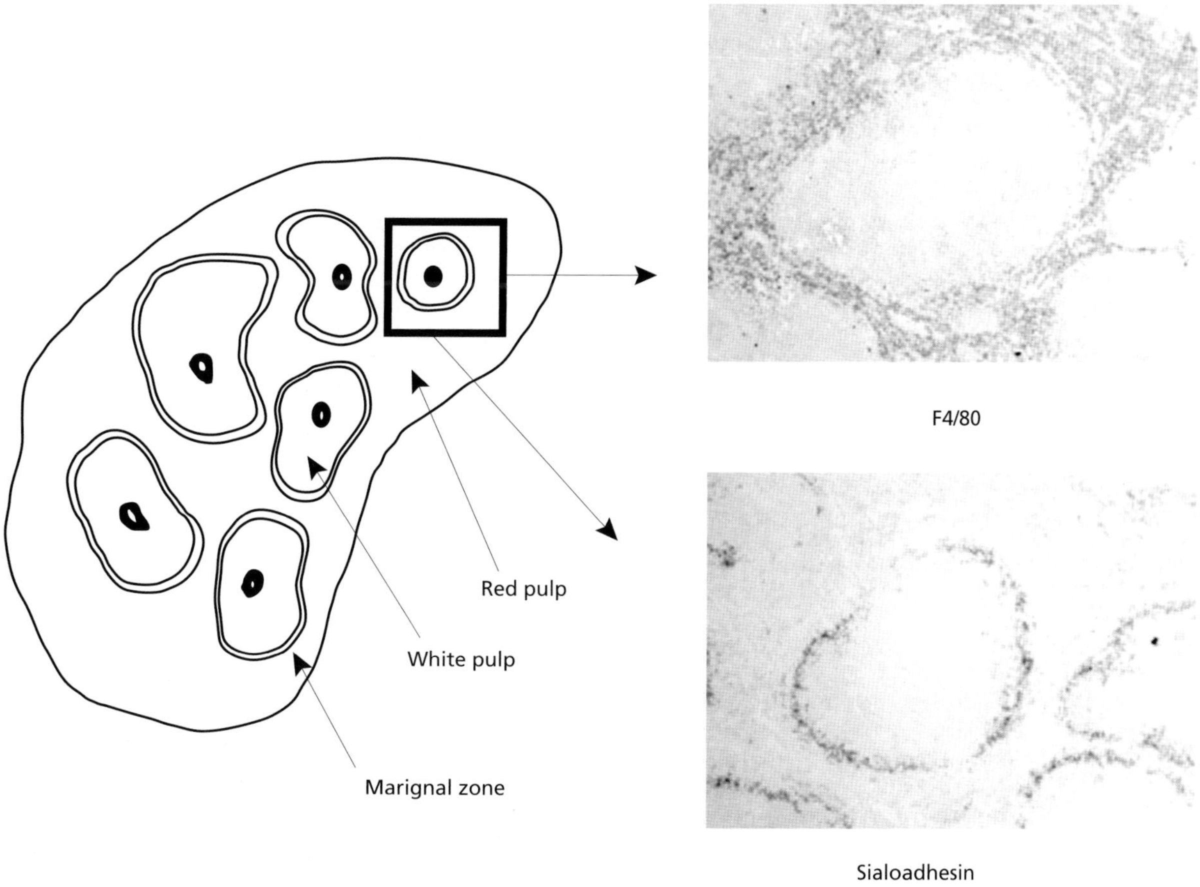

Figure 3.2 *Mouse spleen showing macrophage heterogeneity. Red pulp macrophage (Mϕ) can be detected with F4/80, whereas metallophilic Mϕs (in the marginal zone) can be detected with the anti-sialoadhesin antibody (3D6). (Images courtesy of Dr Luisa Martinez-Pomares, University of Oxford.)*

produced after the induction of acquired immunity, enhance the opsonic recognition of microbes. Although some of the opsonic receptors on host cells have been described, including the complement receptors and those that recognize the Fc portion of antibodies (the so-called Fc receptors) (Ravetch and Clynes 1998), many are still unknown. The nonopsonic or direct recognition and binding of microbes is mediated by a variety of membrane-bound PRRs on phagocytes, including classic and nonclassic C-type lectins, leucine-rich proteins, scavenger receptors, and integrins. Intracellular PRRs include the recently described 'nucleotide-binding oligomerization domain (NOD)' proteins as well as a variety of proteins involved in the recognition of viruses. It should be remembered that the in vivo recognition of microbes probably involves coordinated recognition by many of these receptors, e.g. binding of *Mycobacterium tuberculosis* to macrophages has been shown to involve the complement and mannose receptors, as well as CD14 and the surfactant protein A (collectin) receptor (Ernst 1998).

Although less well characterized, molecules other than the PRRs can also be used by pathogens to bind to and/or enter Mϕs. This is especially true for viruses that make use of cellular molecules, such as the proteoglycans, or other receptors, such as the chemokine receptor CCR5 used by HIV (Miller and Gordon in press). The use of these 'nonimmune' molecules to gain entry into cells enables pathogens to bypass the antimicrobial effects normally generated by the PRRs.

While the binding and internalization of microbes is mediated by various PRRs, generation of the appropriate responses has been ascribed to a recently identified family of receptors, the Toll-like receptors (TLRs). These receptors were originally identified by homology to a receptor in *Drosophila*, and are a family of receptors with homology to the interleukin (IL) 1 (IL-1) receptor (Hoffmann and Reichhart 2002). The various TLR family members can distinguish between various pathogens, often by acting in combinations, and initiate signaling cascades similar to those induced by the IL-1 receptor, via MyD88 and IRAK to activate the factor NFκB, resulting in the production and/or release of proinflammatory mediators and cytokines (Medzhitov 2001; Underhill et al. 1999; Ozinsky et al. 2000). Although a number of TLRs and their ligands have been identified, they all appear to

Table 3.1 *Microbial pattern recognition molecules*

Location	Family	Member(s)	Selected microbial ligand(s)	Reference(s)
Serum	Collectins	SP-A, SP-D	Influenza A virus, herpes simplex virus, *Staphylococcus aureus, Klebsiella pneumoniae, Pseudomonas aeruginosa, Haemophilus influenzae, Escherichia coli, Pneumocystis carinii, C. neoformans, Aspergillus fumigatus*	Crouch (1998); Haagsman (1998)
		Mannose-binding lectin	HIV, influenza A virus, *S. aureus, Neiserria meningitidis, Chlamydia pneumoniae, Candida albicans, Cryptococcus neoformans, A. fumigatus*	Kilpatrick (2002)
	Pentraxins	C-reactive protein, serum amyloid P	*S. aureus, E. coli, Streptococcus pyogenes, N. meningitidis, A. fumigatus, C. albicans, Plasmodium falciparum, influenza A virus*, LPS	Noursadeghi et al. (2000); Szalai (2002)
	Complement	C1q	Antibody-coated microbes, *Listeria monocytogenes, Legionella pneumophila, E. coli*, HIV	Nicholson-Weller and Klickstein (1999); Stoiber et al. (2001)
		C3	Microbial surfaces	Taylor et al. (1998)
	Lipid transferases	LBP	LPS	Jack et al. (1997)
Membrane bound	Classic C-type lectins	Mannose receptor	*Candida albicans, P. carinii, Mycobacterium tuberculosis, K. pneumoniae, Leishmania donovani*, HIV-1, zymosan	East and Isacke (2002)
		DC-SIGN	HIV, Ebola virus, *Leishmania* spp.	Geijtenbeek et al. (2002)
	Non-classic C-type lectins	Dectin-1	β-Glucans, zymosan, *Saccharomyces cerevisiae, C. albicans*	Brown and Gordon (2001)
	Leucine-rich proteins	CD14	*E. coli*, LPS, LTA, peptidoglycan	Landmann et al. (2000)
		Toll-like receptors (1–10)	LPS, LTA, zymosan, bacterial lipoproteins, peptidoglycan, viral proteins, flagellin, bacterial DNA	Medzhitov (2001)
	Scavenger receptors	SR-A (I and II), LOX-1, MARCO	*E. coli, S. aureus, L. monocytogenes, M. tuberculosis, Enterococcus faecalis, N. meningitidis*, LPS, LTA, bacterial DNA	Peiser et al. (2002); Shimaoka et al. (2001); Sankala et al. (2002)
	Integrins	CR3, CR4	Complement-coated microbes, LPS, LPG, *C. albicans, M. tuberculosis, C. neoformans*	Ehlers (2000); Ingalls and Golenbock (1995); Taborda and Casadevall (2002)
Intracellular	NODs	NOD-1, NOD-2	LPS, *S. flexneri*	Inohara et al. (2002)
	Interferon-induced proteins	PKR, OAS, ADAR1	Viral dsRNA	Samuel (2001)
		Mx GTPase	Viral–protein complexes	Ponten et al. (1997)

LPG, lipophosphoglycan; LPS, lipopolysaccharide; LTA, lipotechoic acid; NODs, nucleotide-binding oligomerization domains.

signal via the same pathway and it is therefore not yet understood how specific responses to each pathogen are initiated. There is some evidence that response specificity is mediated by specific intracellular adaptors, such as TIRAP, and also by the PRRs involved in recognition and binding (Engering et al. 2002; Horng et al. 2002).

It should be remembered that Mϕs also possess many other surface receptors that play a role in the response to infection, but are not involved in microbial recognition. These receptors include the cytokine and chemokine receptors, as well as receptors involved in migration, adhesion, and antigen presentation. Some of these aspects are covered in more detail below and in later chapters.

INGESTION OF MICROBES

Macrophages have a prodigious capacity to ingest microbes and are capable of engulfing very large particles. This ability may be the result of their, apparently unique, ability to utilize membrane from the endoplasmic reticulum (ER) for this uptake (Gagnon et al. 2002). Ingestion is initiated by binding of microbes to the Mϕ surface receptors, which triggers the transmembrane activation signals leading to their internalization. For microbes larger than 0.5 μm, internalization occurs through a heterogeneous actin-dependent process called phagocytosis (Aderem and Underhill 1999). Many of the details of these processes are incompletely understood and made more complex by the fact that microbes are recognized by more than one receptor, each of which may be dictating a different mechanism of uptake. The receptors themselves may also interact with other surface receptors, such as CD172a (signal regulatory protein alpha (SIRPα)) (Oldenborg et al. 2001), either stimulating or inhibiting uptake.

The understanding of phagocytosis, first observed by Elie Metchnikoff in the 1890s, is currently based on the study of two receptors, the Fcγ and complement receptors. The Fcγ receptor (FcγR) mediates what is known as the zipper model of phagocytosis, whereby actin-rich pseudopods extend over the particle surface through the sequential binding of cell surface receptors to the microbe, ultimately engulfing the entire particle (Griffin et al. 1975, 1976). This process is initiated by receptor clustering, occurring from interactions with the microbe, and leads to the phosphorylation of tyrosine residues in specific motifs (the immunoglobulin gene family tyrosine activation motifs) of the cytoplasmic tail of the receptor (Daeron 1997). These phosphorylation events are dependent on cytoplasmic enzymes, the src kinases, and result in the sequential recruitment and signaling via a variety of other molecules, including Syk, Cdc42, and Rac, which results in actin assembly, membrane protrusion, pseudopod extension, and finally closure of the phagocytic cup (Caron and Hall 1998; Aderem and Underhill 1999).

Complement receptor (CR)-mediated phagocytosis is less well understood but is known to require an additional stimulus to occur, such as tumor necrosis factor α (TNF-α) or attachment to extracellular matrix proteins. In contrast to the FcγR, the particle is not engulfed by pseudopods but rather appears to sink into the cell, forming a phagosome where the membrane is less adherent, held by point-like contacts to the microbe (Kaplan 1977; Aderem and Underhill 1999). CR-mediated phagocytosis also requires intact microtubules, uses different signaling molecules, such as Rho, and is not blocked by inhibitors of tyrosine kinases (Allen and Aderem 1996; Caron and Hall 1998).

Microbes can be ingested through a variety of other mechanisms, including macropinocytosis, coiling phagocytosis, and endocytosis. Macropinocytosis describes a process whereby membrane ruffles form a large spacious vacuole around the adjacent microbe, leading to subsequent ingestion (Rittig et al. 1999). In coiling phagocytosis, there is an initial extension of a single pseudopod, which wraps around the microbe. Subsequent pseudopods form, giving the characteristic whorl-like appearance, which ultimately fuse to form the phagosome (Rittig et al. 1999). Endocytosis is a heterogeneous group of cellular processes used for the internalization of particles smaller than 0.5 μm, such as viruses, and includes caveolae- and clathrin-mediated endocytosis (Gruenberg 2001; Shin and Abraham 2001; Sieczkarski and Whittaker 2002).

Receptor-mediated endocytosis and phagocytosis are used for homeostatic functions by Mϕ and to clear up the debris released by infection, including necrotic and apoptotic cells. In addition, these mechanisms are used or subverted by a variety of pathogens, the study of which has given many insights into the molecular mechanism underlying these processes.

After internalization, the phagosome matures through a number of sequential steps involving interactions with the endocytic pathway (Desjardins et al. 1994). This consists of extensive vesicle budding and fusion, controlled by a variety of cytoplasmic proteins including the rab guanosine triphosphatases (GTPases) (Aderem and Underhill 1999). During maturation the phagosome moves along the microtubule network from the periphery to a perinuclear location. As it matures, the phagosome acquires hydrolytic enzymes, such as cathepsin-D, and the proton pump adenosine triphosphatase (ATPase), which contributes to a lowering of the phagosomal pH. The late stages of maturation involve fusion with lysosomes generating a low pH phagolysosomal compartment containing a variety of degradative lysosomal hydrolases (Alvarez-Dominguez et al. 1999). The process of maturation therefore generates an increasingly antimicrobial environment in which the ingested microbe is ultimately killed and digested. A simplified schematic diagram of these processes is shown in Figure 3.3.

ANTIMICROBIAL MECHANISMS

Macrophages possess a variety of antimicrobial mechanisms including the use of toxic metabolites, enzymes, and peptides, as well as through physical restraint of the pathogens, by ingestion into phagosomes, or through the formation of a granuloma. Most organisms are killed within the phagosome after phagocytosis, through a number of mechanisms that can work synergistically. The maturing phagosome generates an increasingly antimicrobial environment, achieved through lowering of the phagosomal pH, limitation of nutrients required for microbial growth, and generation of reactive metabolites. After fusion of the phagosome with lysosomes, there is also the acquisition of hydrolytic enzymes, antimicrobial proteins, and peptides, such as the membrane-permeabilizing peptide defensins, which have a broad spectrum of microbial targets, and lysozyme, which attacks the peptidoglycan layer of bacterial cell walls.

The confinement of microbes within the phagosome acts as a physical barrier to the microbe, limiting the availability of essential nutrients required for microbial growth, such as iron. The supply of nutrients to the phagosome is further restricted by active mechanisms within the cells. The transferrin receptor, for example, which transports iron via the endosomal pathway, is downregulated upon infection whereas another molecule, natural resistance-associated macrophage protein-1

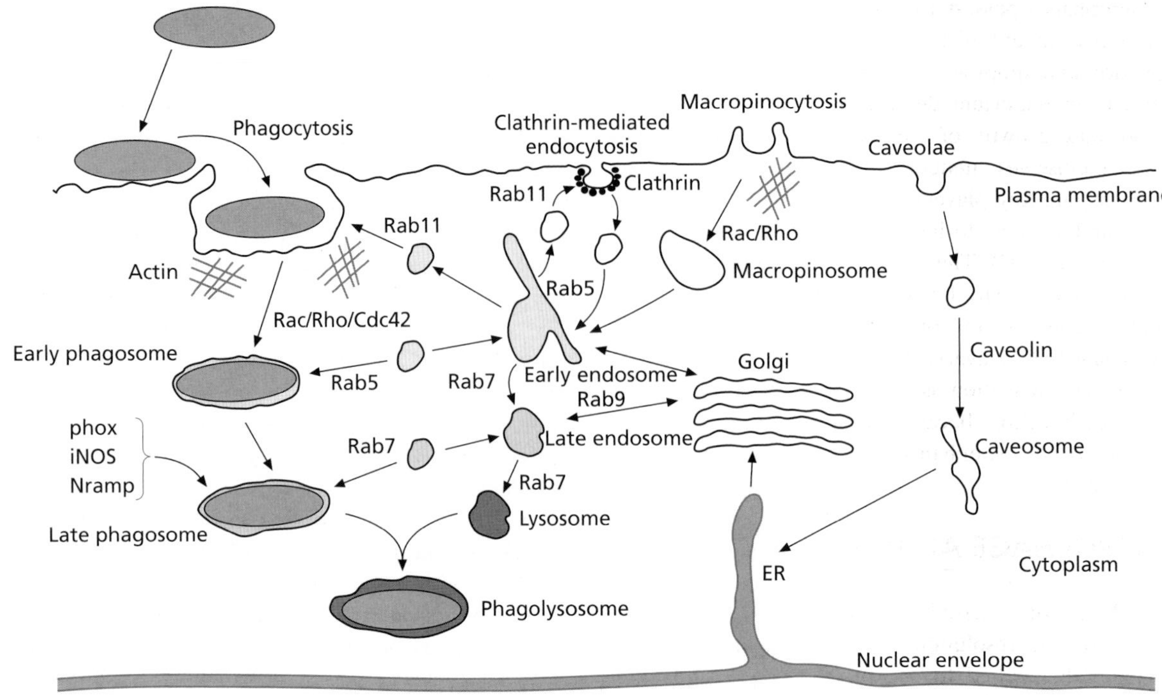

Figure 3.3 *A schematic representation depicting the various routes used by macrophage (Mϕ) to internalize microbes. Some of the molecules associated with this process are also indicated. (Adapted in part from Sieczkarski and Whittaker 2002.)*

(Nramp-1), is recruited to the phagosome, ensuring removal of iron and other essential divalent cations (Gruenheid et al. 1997; Sunder-Plassmann et al. 1999; Forbes and Gros 2001).

The production of reactive oxygen intermediates (ROIs), described as the respiratory burst of Mϕs, is a very efficient antimicrobial defense. Superoxide ion ($O_2^{-\bullet}$) is generated by the activated, membrane-associated, protein complex, the phagocyte reduced nicotinamide adenine dinucleotide phosphate (NADPH) oxidase (phox), which transfers electrons from NADPH to O_2. Toxic oxidants, including hydroxyl radicals and hydrogen peroxide, are then generated in the phagosomal lumen, and kill the internalized organism (Hampton et al. 1998). The phox proteins may also assemble in the plasma membrane, resulting in the generation of extracellular toxic oxidants, which may also contribute to pathology. Superoxide ions can also act as a signal for the activation of granule proteases in neutrophils (Reeves et al. 2002). Activation and localization of the oxidase complex are determined by the cellular receptors involved in recognition of the pathogen, and involve numerous signal transduction cascades that result in phosphorylation of one of the cytosolic phox proteins ($p47^{phox}$) (Karlsson and Dahlgren 2002). Chronic granulomatous disease (CGD) is a disease characterized by recurrent infections with a number of pathogens, and results from mutations in the phox proteins, highlighting the importance of this antimicrobial mechanism for the host (Goldblatt and Thrasher 2000).

Myeloperoxidase (MPO) is a major neutrophil granule protein that is also found in monocytes. MPO generates hypochlorous acid from hydrogen peroxide, one of the most potent antimicrobial agents produced (Winterbourn et al. 2000). Although MPO is not produced in Mϕs, it can be taken up via the macrophage mannose receptor and is known to augment macrophage antimicrobial activity (Shepherd and Hoidal 1990; Marodi et al. 1998).

The inducible nitric oxide synthase (iNOS) of phagocytes is another important enzyme contributing to the antimicrobial actions of Mϕs. Induction of iNOS leads to the production of nitric oxide (NO), through the oxidative deamination of l-arginine, which subsequently reacts with superoxide or thiol groups to produce antimicrobial compounds, such as peroxynitrite and nitrosothiols (Burgner et al. 1999). The production of NO by iNOS requires homodimerization and interaction with many other molecules, including calmodulin, and NADPH. Microbial products, such as LPS, and cytokines, such as TNF-α or interferon γ (IFN-γ), can act either individually or synergistically to induce the production of iNOS (MacMicking et al. 1997). The use of iNOS inhibitors and knockout mice has clearly demonstrated the importance of this antimicrobial mechanism in the control of many infections (Wei et al. 1995).

Macrophages possess two other notable features that play a role in antimicrobial activities, that of cellular activation and apoptosis. Apoptosis, or programmed cell death, is an important defense mechanism limiting the spread and growth of intracellular organisms. Mϕs, which themselves undergo apoptosis during certain infections, are key players in the clearance of apoptotic bodies and are able to induce this process in other cells (Geske et al. 2002). The role of apoptosis in infection is not always so clear, however, because in some cases apoptosis appears to favor the pathogen (Weinrauch and Zychlinsky 1999; Navarre and Zychlinsky 2000). Finally, macrophage activation is extremely important for the control of infection, because activation, via cytokines or microbial products, enhances the antimicrobial activities of these cells.

MACROPHAGE ACTIVATION

The ability of macrophages to become activated is critical for the resolution of infection. This term has been loosely applied to describe the selective, stereotypical responses of Mϕs to different stimuli, mainly of a microbial or immunological nature. Recent gene array studies have started to illustrate the diversity of genes expressed in various infectious and other experimental models. Earlier phenotypic characterization made it possible to discern the following types of cell activation: innate activation, classic immune activation, and alternate activation. Finally, the control of this process, through the deactivation of Mϕs, is critically important to reduce pathology.

Innate activation, induced by microbial products and intact microorganisms, is mediated by specific receptors and signaling pathways described already, and results in altered pro- and anti-inflammatory metabolite secretion, enhanced expression of co-stimulatory molecules, and induction of plasma membrane receptors such as MARCO, a type A scavenger receptor (Gordon 2001). Thus, antimicrobial and immune functions are induced, as well as cell migration and dendritic cell maturation.

Classic immune activation was originally described by Mackaness as enhanced, antigen non-specific, antimicrobial activation of Mϕs during *Listeria monocytogenes* and BCG (mycobacterial) infection (Gordon 1999, 2003b). This can now be ascribed to IFN-γ, acting on specific Mϕ receptors and their signaling pathway (Gordon 1999, 2003b). IFN-γ is produced by natural killer (NK) cells and activated T lymphocytes in response to cytokines produced by antigen-presenting cells (APCs), IL-12, IL-18, and IL-15. Genetic studies in mouse and humans have confirmed the importance of this pathway in cellular immunity to infection by mycobacteria and other selected pathogens. Secondary deficiency contributes to opportunistic infections in AIDS. In addition, IFN-γ induces major histocompatibility complex class II (MHCII) and iNOS expression and primes Mϕs to secrete high levels of mediators in response to microbial stimuli.

Alternate immune activation can be induced by the cytokines IL-4 and IL-13, acting on a common receptor subunit and resulting in a distinct program of gene expression in Mϕs to promote humoral immunity, especially against extracellular parasites (Gordon 2003a). Phenotypic markers include elevated MHCII, enhanced mannose receptor, and, in some situations, giant cell formation. Certain chemokines (MDC and TARC) and a range of other markers are also selectively upregulated. Inducible NOS is downregulated, whereas l-arginine metabolism is switched to favor collagen production by fibroblasts, and repair.

Deactivation is mediated by cytokines such as IL-10 and transforming growth factor β (TGF-β) which profoundly downregulate Mϕ proinflammatory, immunological, and cytotoxic activities (Gordon 2003a). The balance between activation and deactivation is critical in preventing host injury, as illustrated in inflammatory bowel disease and genetic deficiency of the above cytokines. New findings have highlighted the importance of inhibitory receptors on the Mϕ surface, such as SIRPα, which limit activation of Mϕ. Distinct receptor pairs that regulate Mϕ activation include CD200/CD200R – microglia become spontaneously activated in CD200-deficient mice; experimental autoimmune disease is regulated, in part, by this pathway. Important intracellular regulatory systems include the suppressors of cytokine synthesis (SOCS) family and type I interferons. The uptake of apoptotic cells downregulates inflammatory responses of Mϕs.

SECRETION OF SOLUBLE MEDIATORS AND OTHER FACTORS

In addition to the secretion of ROIs, described above, Mϕs produce and secrete a variety of other products either constitutively or after stimulation. These include factors that are involved in homeostasis, such as pro- and antiangiogenic factors controlling vascular supply, or those, such as lysozyme, that are involved in combating infection. Other secretion products include enzymes, such as lysosomal hydrolases, proteases, and lipases, some of which help to maintain extracellular matrix balance, and promote and interact with plasma protein cascades (coagulation, fibrinolysis, complement, kinin generation) in response to injury (Gordon 2003b). Mϕs produce complement components, which opsonize microbes and are major producers of arachidonic acid intermediates (Ross and Auger 2002).

Macropages produce cytokines and chemokines, which recruit other immune cells to the site of infection and which, along with antigen presentation to lymphocytes, help direct the generation and type of the adaptive immune response. Cytokines are central molecules of the immune response, forming a complex network that

Table 3.2 *Selected cytokines produced by or having an effect on macrophages (Mϕs)*

Cytokine	Major producer	Effect
IL-4/IL-13	T cells	Alternate Mϕ activation ↑ MHCII, B7-1, B7-2 ↑ giant cell formation ↓ IL-1, TNF-α, IL-6, IL-12
IL-10	Mϕ DC Activated T and B cells	Mϕ deactivation ↓ IL-1, TNF-α, IL-6, IL-12 ↓ MHCII, B7-1, B7-2
IL-12	Mϕ DC Others	T-cell proliferation $CD4^+$ Th1 differentiation ↑ IFN-γ ↑ CTL activity
IFNγ	T cells NK cells	Mϕ and PMN activation $CD4^+$ Th1 differentiation B-cell isotype switching (IgG2a, IgG3) ↑ NK cell cytolytic activity ↑ vascular adhesion molecules ↑ MHCI and MHCII ↑ TNF-α, IL-1, IL-12, IFN-β ↓ IL-10
IL-18	Mϕ	T-cell proliferation $CD4^+$ Th1 differentiation ↑ IFNγ ↓ IL-10
IFN-α/β	Mϕ Others	Mϕ and NK activation ↑ CTL activity ↑ MHCI
TNF-α	Mϕ Others	Mϕ and PMN activation Inflammatory cell recruitment ↑ vascular adhesion molecules ↑ MHCI ↑ acute phase proteins ↑ T-cell apoptosis
TGF-β	Platelets Mϕ	Monocyte activation Mϕ deactivation ↑ extracellular matrix proteins ↑ selected growth factors

CTL, cytotoxic T lymphocyte; DC, dendritic cell; Th1, T-helper cell 1; IFN, interferon; IgG, immunoglobulin G; IL, interleukin; PMN, polymorphonuclear neutrophil; MHC, major histocompatibility complex; Mϕ, macrophage; NK, natural killer; TGF, transforming growth factor; TNF, tumor necrosis factor.

mediates and regulates many local and systemic immune functions. Cytokines bind to their cognate cell surface receptors and signal through a variety of pathways, including the Janus-family kinase (Jaks) and signal transducer and activator of transcription (Stat) proteins (Imada and Leonard 2000). The properties and characteristics of a few selected cytokines are listed in Table 3.2. Many of those listed are involved in macrophage activation (IL-4, IL-13, IL-12, IL-18, and IFN-γ) or deactivation (IL-10 and TGF-β). Cytokines, such as TGF-β, also play an important role in the suppression and resolution of the immune response (Ashcroft 1999).

Chemokines, or chemotactic cytokines, are small, structurally related peptides that are recognized by seven transmembrane G-protein-coupled receptors on their target cells (Thomson 1998). They are involved in a variety of homeostatic functions, including organogenesis and hemopoiesis, but also function to recruit neutrophils, monocytes, immature dendritic cells, and activated T cells to the sites of infection (Olson and Ley 2002). Chemokines are highly basic proteins and can bind to glycosaminoglycans on extracellular matrix surfaces, generating gradients that attract leukocytes and promote their attachment and diapedesis through vascular endothelium, as described above. Chemokines are divided into four families, based on the number and position of conserved cysteines: C, CC, CXC, and the CX3C chemokines. In general, CXC chemokines, such as IL-8, attract neutrophils, whereas CC and C chemokines, such as monocytic chemotactic peptide 1 (MCP-1) and lymphotactin, attract monocytes and lymphocytes. Chemokines can also induce the release of proinflammatory mediators and stimulate the respiratory burst.

ANTIGEN PRESENTATION

Antigen presentation, along with cytokine production, is a critical component of innate immunity required for the generation of the adaptive immune response and resolution of most infections (Fearon and Locksley 1996). Mϕs present antigens only to primed T cells, whereas DCs have the ability to prime naïve T cells (Mellman and Steinman 2001). Antigen presentation results in the generation of pathogen-specific immunity and specific subsets of T cells. These subsets include the $CD4^+$ T cells, which are involved in the resolution of intracellular (T-helper (Th) 1 cells) and extracellular (Th2 cells) pathogens, and $CD8^+$ T cells, which are involved in killing cells infected with cytosolic pathogens. Both $CD4^+$ and $CD8^+$ T cells can activate the antimicrobial activities of Mϕs, although $CD4^+$ Th2 cells normally mediate Mϕ-independent responses to extracellular parasites, such as helminths.

Antigen presentation requires the noncovalent association of the antigen with MHC molecules. This association occurs via two main routes, through loading of antigens onto MHCII, which have been ingested and degraded in the lysosomes, and loading of antigens onto MHCI, which are derived from the cytosol. This is an oversimplified scheme, however, because lysosomally derived antigens can be loaded on MHCI molecules, although the mechanisms involved are less clear. Antigens loaded onto MHC molecules are normally peptides, but lipids and glycolipids can be presented through MHC-like molecules to T cells. We describe the various cellular mechanisms in antigen loading and presentation to T cells, including a brief description of the co-stimulatory molecules and cytokines involved.

MHCI is expressed by nearly all cells and presents cytosolic peptides to cytotoxic $CD8^+$ T cells (Guermonprez et al. 2002). These peptides are generated by the proteasome and are translocated into the ER by transporter associated with antigen processing (TAP) protein where they associate with the MHCI molecules before transport to the cell surface. As the presented peptides originate from the cytosol, MHCI presentation is important in the control of cytosolic pathogens, such as viruses.

MHCII is expressed by Mϕs, DCs, and B cells and presents exogenously derived peptides to $CD4^+$ T-helper cells (Guermonprez et al. 2002). MHCII is upregulated after activation of Mϕs and on maturation of DCs. Exogenous antigens released from the degradative late endosomal and/or phagosomal compartments are thought to be loaded onto MHCII in the MIIC compartment. MHCII molecules are associated with an invariant chain (Ii), which prevents association with endogenous peptides during synthesis in the ER and Golgi body. Ii is removed by proteolysis and the actions of an auxiliary molecule, HLA-DM, in the MIIC compartment, allowing the binding of foreign peptide and transport to the cell surface. In certain circumstances peptides can be also be loaded onto MHCII in the ER, early endosomes, and at the plasma membrane (Robinson and Delvig 2002). As peptides derived from the endosomal/phagosomal pathway are presented through MHCII, this presentation pathway is, however, critical for the control of intracellular pathogens.

Antigen can also be presented to T cells through two other classes of molecules: MHCIb and CD1 (Porcelli and Modlin 1999; Schaible et al. 1999). MHCIb present short *N*-formylmethionine-containing peptides of bacterial and/or mitochondrial origin to $CD8^+$ T cells. Although MHCIb is structurally similar to MHCIc, the processing and peptide-loading mechanisms are unclear and may be TAP independent. Also structurally related to MHCI is the CD1 family of proteins, consisting of five members, four of which (CD1a, -b, -c, -e) are found only in humans. Most of these proteins, expressed mainly by activated Mϕs, DCs, and B cells, are capable of presenting microbial lipid and glycolipid antigens, such as mycolic acids from mycobacteria, to cytotoxic $CD4^-$ $CD8^-$ T cells and possibly also $CD8^+$ T cells. Antigen loading is TAP independent.

In addition to T-cell receptor (TCR) recognition of antigen presented on MHC molecules, the activation and proliferation of T cells requires a 'second' signal (Guermonprez et al. 2002). This additional signal is mediated by co-stimulatory molecules on the APCs, including CD40, B7-1, and B7-2 which interact with CD40L, CD28, and CTLA4 on the lymphocytes. These interactions activate the APCs and mediate the type of $CD4^+$ T-helper cell (Th1 or Th2) produced.

The differentiation of $CD4^+$ T cells into Th1- or Th2-type cells is also mediated by cytokines. Activation of DCs in the periphery and crosslinking of CD40 during the presentation of antigens induce IL-12 production, which biases the development of naïve T cells to the Th1 type, suppressing the production of Th2-type cells. Conversely, IL-4 stimulates the production of Th2-type cells, while suppressing Th1-type development. The driving factors behind Th2 development are still unknown, leading some investigators to propose that Th2 is the default pathway. The role and generation of Th1 and Th2 T cells in infection are discussed in greater detail in later chapters.

Macrophages and other APCs have the ability to ingest apoptotic or necrotic cells and present the antigens they contain in a process known as cross-presentation, or crosspriming (Heath and Carbone 2001). These antigens can be presented on both MHCI and MHCII molecules by a process that is influenced by several factors in vivo, including antigen dose, age of the host, and tissue type. It should be noted that cross-presentation of cellular antigens can also lead to T-cell tolerance (cross-tolerance).

SUBVERSION OF MACROPHAGE FUNCTION BY PATHOGENS

Although Mϕs are very efficient at recognizing and destroying microbes, pathogens have evolved numerous strategies to avoid or subvert the antimicrobial functions of these leukocytes. Pathogens can evade or promote recognition through specific PRRs, and they can block or modify the phagocytic pathway, the antimicrobial mechanisms, the production of soluble mediators, and the ability of Mϕs to present antigens. Studies of these microbial subversion strategies have, however, greatly aided our understanding of the basic mechanisms underlying the cellular processes in Mϕs and other leukocytes.

Pathogens have developed mechanisms to avoid phagocytosis or to direct phagocytosis through specific receptors. Phagocytosis mediated by FcγR, but not CR3, for example, results in the production of proinflammatory mediators and induces the respiratory burst (Underhill and Ozinsky 2002). Consequently, CRs are commonly used by intracellular pathogens, such as *Mycobacterium tuberculosis*, to gain access to host cells (Ernst 1998). Pathogens may induce entry into macrophages, such as salmonellae, which stimulate macropinocytosis by transferring proteins into the host cytosol using a type III secretion system (Goosney et al. 1999). Other pathogens actively block phagocytosis, such as *Yersinia* which use a type III secretion system to transfer proteins to block the signaling mechanisms that control cytoskeletal rearrangements (Fallman et al. 1995; Cornelis 2002).

Macrophages also provide numerous niches for intracellular pathogens, which have evolved a variety of mechanisms for survival within these cells. Some pathogens interfere with phagosomal maturation, such as *Mycobacterium tuberculosis*, which arrests maturation at an early stage (Armstrong and Hart 1971). Pathogens such as *Legionella*, are able to convert the phagosome to a unique vacuole, whereas others, such as *Shigella* spp., escape the phagosome completely and reside in the host cytosol (Portnoy et al. 1988; High et al. 1992). Some pathogens, such as *Leishmania* and *Coxiella* spp., have even adapted to life within the harsh environment of the phagolysome (Chang and Dwyer 1976; Heinzen et al. 1996; Rabinovitch and Veras 1996).

The antimicrobial mechanisms of Mϕs present other obstacles that have been overcome by pathogens, leading to the development of a number of resistance mechanisms. Pathogens overcome the acidification of the phagosome by excluding the vesicular proton pump ATPase, such as occurs with mycobacteria, or escape into the cytoplasm, as mentioned above (Sturgill-Koszycki et al. 1994). Essential nutrients can be acquired by, for example, secreting siderophores, which bind iron with a higher affinity than host molecules, such as the mycobactins and exochelins of mycobacteria (De Voss et al. 1999). The respiratory burst can be avoided by entry through specific receptors, as discussed, but it can also be suppressed by inhibiting the activation cascades, as occurs with *Yersinia* spp. (Cornelis 2002). Microbes, such as salmonellae and mycobacteria, protect themselves from toxic oxidants and reactive nitrogen intermediates by producing enzymes, such as catalase, glutathione reductase, alkyl hydroperoxide reductase, and superoxide dismutase, which break down these compounds (Storz et al. 1990; Manca et al. 1999).

Pathogens are able to modulate the ability of Mϕs to interact with the rest of the immune system, by affecting their ability to produce cytokines and to present antigens. Pathogens such as the pox and herpes viruses produce virokines and viroceptors, which mimic cytokines and cytokine receptors, whereas pathogens such as mycobacteria can deactivate Mϕs, making them refractory to activating cytokines, and induce the production of the anti-inflammatory cytokine, TGF-β (McFadden et al. 1998; Mosser and Karp 1999). Viruses and bacteria have also been shown to prevent surface expression of both MHCI and MHCII, or they can produce super-antigens that can cause extensive nonspecific T-cell activation (Herman et al. 1991; Schaible et al. 1999; Yewdell and Bennink 1999; Papageorgiou and Acharya 2000). Thus, pathogens have not only evolved mechanisms to subvert Mϕ function, they have also evolved mechanisms to modulate the entire immune response.

ROLE OF MACROPHAGES IN HOMEOSTASIS

Macrophages, as a system, display features consistent with a major role in tissue homeostasis. They are constitutively dispersed throughout the body, in the absence of inflammation, and can be recruited in increased numbers to sites of local injury and infection. They are relatively long-lived cells, remaining biosynthetically active, display a range of plasma membrane receptors for recognition of endogenous and exogenous ligands, and are able to secrete a wide variety of products in response to stimulation. Through these activities they regulate the activity of many cell types in their local microenvironment, as well as systemically. Here we touch briefly on selected aspects to illustrate diverse homeostatic aspects of Mϕ function particularly relevant to infection.

As discussed above, resident tissue Mϕs show great variation, the functions of which are not well understood, but can be broadly interpreted as homeostatic. In bone marrow, for example, stromal Mϕs play a tropic role in hemopoiesis by interacting with developing myeloid and erythroid cells (as well as removing erythrocyte nuclei) (Crocker et al. 1991). In lung, alveolar Mϕs contribute to surfactant metabolism as well as host defense. In the central nervous system, microglia persist throughout adult life, closely associated with neurons and astrocytes, possibly contributing to neurotransmitter catabolism (Perry et al. 1993).

Macrophages play a major role in the uptake and destruction of apoptotic, senescent, and necrotic cells, through a range of scavenger and other receptors (Fadok et al. 2001; Peiser et al. 2002). Apart from their phagocytic and surface immune interaction molecules such as MHC and co-stimulatory antigens, Mϕs are well placed to remove a wide range of ligands from the circulation, or extravascular tissue fluids by phagocytosis and endocytosis. Examples include classic reticuloendothelial cell clearance functions of Kupffer cells, often shared with liver sinusoidal, true endothelial cells. Thus many lysosomal hydrolases express a terminal saccharide recognized by the Mϕ mannosyl/fucosyl receptor (East and Isacke 2002). Other important host-protective endocytic clearance systems include CD91 (α_2-macroglobulin–protease complexes) and CD163 (haptoglobin–hemoglobin complexes) (Binder et al. 2001; Kristiansen et al. 2001). The products of activated neutrophils can also be removed by several of the above receptors.

Macrophages express a variety of constitutive and inducible metabolic activities that help to catabolize substrates such as hemoglobin, and inactivate chemical compounds including drugs. Mϕs contribute to bile pigment formation through hemoxygenase and other enzymes, and can express high levels of cytochrome P450. They contribute to iron homeostasis through a variety of pathways.

MACROPHAGE-INDUCED PATHOLOGY

Many of the properties of Mϕs, described above, can be readily extrapolated to pathological responses to infection and metabolic diseases in which Mϕs play a central role, with or without contributions from other cells (Gordon 1999, 2001, 2003b). We illustrate the range of diseases by selected examples, in which Mϕs are overactive or deficient in function. These include chronic infections and/or inflammatory diseases, such as tuberculosis and rheumatoid arthritis in which Th1 responses and TNF-α production predominate, and a range of storage diseases, such as atherosclerosis.

Granuloma development is a characteristic of mycobacterial infection. Persistence of a microbial stimulus, in Mϕs themselves, can result in the focal accumulation of newly recruited monocytes and their differentiation into Mϕs (epithelioid and Langhans' giant cells), together with T lymphocytes, other myeloid cells, and fibroblasts. The granuloma Mϕs express a range of cell activation markers including lysozyme and proinflammatory cytokines (TNF-α, IL-1β, IL-6), as well as IL-10. TNF-α is essential for granuloma formation, as shown in antibody and genetic depletion studies. The type 3 complement receptor is also important in mobilization of monocytes to form granulomas. A granuloma stained with F4/80 is shown in Figure 3.4.

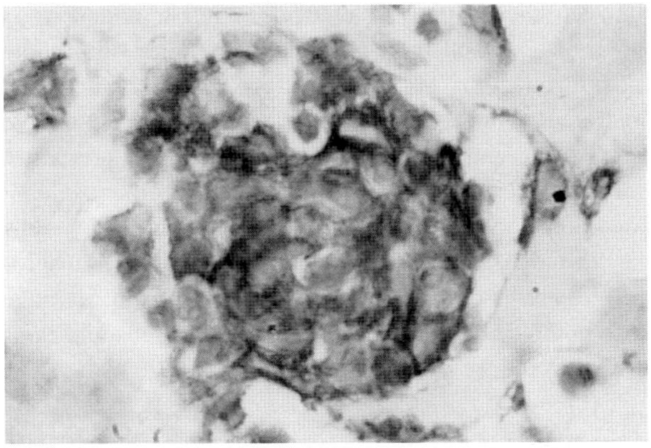

Figure 3.4 C. parvum-*induced granuloma in the liver stained with F4/80. The majority of the cells in the granuloma stain positive for F4/80, as do some adjacent Kupffer cells.*

The immunologically primed host is exquisitely sensitive to LPS or microbial stimuli, which readily precipitate a septic shock syndrome, mediated through CD14 and TLR pathways, with diffuse intravascular coagulation and vascular collapse, mainly through the actions of cytokines such as TNF-α and IL-1β on the endothelium. Infection by a range of other intracellular pathogens mentioned above can give rise to widespread local and systemic inflammatory sequelae, including wasting, fibrosis, and secondary amyloidosis, as well as immunosuppression.

Other types of modified chronic inflammation in which Mϕs are prominent include atherosclerosis and, perhaps, Alzheimer's disease. Accumulation of intra- or extracellular lipoprotein or fibrillar deposits in large arteries or brain, respectively, results in persistent Mϕ secretion of tropic and destructive products. Classic Mϕ storage diseases include lysosomal storage of macromolecules caused by genetic enzyme deficiency and iron overload. Such Mϕs can become potent secretory sources of enzymes that serve as markers (e.g. chitotriosidase in Gaucher's disease), or mediators of tissue injury (elastase, collagenase).

Deficiencies of Mϕ function include failure to clear apoptotic cells, which may contribute to autoantigen formation in diseases such as systemic lupus erythematosus, and the inability to destroy opportunistic pathogens in AIDS. Rare inherited deficiencies of respiratory burst components result in inefficient killing of a range of microorganisms, in chronic granulomatous disease.

CONCLUSION

We have briefly highlighted the various roles that Mϕs play in anti-infectious immunity and have shown that, through their ability to recognize, ingest, and destroy microbes, as well as recruit other immune cells to the sites of infection, Mϕs are key cells in innate immunity. We have demonstrated that Mϕs play an essential role in specific immunity by modulating this response through the release of cytokines, and other soluble mediators, and acting as effector cells and accessory cells in secondary lymphocyte activation. Although macrophages are essential for the control of infection, we have also noted some of their homeostatic functions and their ability to induce pathology.

ACKNOWLEDGMENTS

We thank the Wellcome Trust and Medical Research Council for funding, and Dr Philip Taylor for critically reading this manuscript.

REFERENCES

Aderem, A. and Underhill, D.M. 1999. Mechanisms of phagocytosis in macrophages. *Annu Rev Immunol*, **17**, 593–623.

Allen, L.A. and Aderem, A. 1996. Molecular definition of distinct cytoskeletal structures involved in complement- and Fc receptor-mediated phagocytosis in macrophages. *J Exp Med*, **184**, 627–37.

Alvarez-Dominguez, C., Mayorga, L. and Stahl, P.D. 1999. Sequential maturation of phagosomes provides unique targets for pathogens. In: Gordon, S. (ed.), *Phagocytosis: The host*. Stamford, CT: JAI Press, Inc, 285–97.

Armstrong, J. and Hart, P. 1971. Response of cultured macrophages to *Mycobacterium tuberculosis* with observations on fusion of lysosomes with phagosomes. *J Exp Med*, **134**, 713–40.

Ashcroft, G.S. 1999. Bidirectional regulation of macrophage function by TGF-beta. *Microbes Infect*, **1**, 1275–82.

Auger, M.J. and Ross, J.A. 1992. The biology of the macrophage. In: Lewis, C.E. and McGee, J.O.'D. (eds), *The macrophage*. New York: Oxford University Press.

Binder, R.J., Karimeddini, D. and Srivastava, P.K. 2001. Adjuvanticity of alpha 2-macroglobulin, an independent ligand for the heat shock protein receptor CD91. *J Immunol*, **166**, 4968–72.

Brown, G.D. and Gordon, S. 2001. Immune recognition: A new receptor for beta-glucans. *Nature*, **413**, 36–7.

Burgner, D., Rockett, K. and Kwiatkowski, D. 1999. Nitric oxide and infectious diseases. *Arch Dis Child*, **81**, 185–8.

Caron, E. and Hall, A. 1998. Identification of two distinct mechanisms of phagocytosis controlled by different Rho GTPases. *Science*, **282**, 1717–21.

Chang, K.P. and Dwyer, D.M. 1976. Multiplication of a human parasite (*Leishmania donovani*) in phagolysosomes of hamster macrophages in vitro. *Science*, **193**, 678–80.

Cornelis, G.R. 2002. Yersinia type III secretion: send in the effectors. *J Cell Biol*, **158**, 401–8.

Crocker, P.R., Morris, L. and Gordon, S. 1991. Adhesion receptors involved in the erythroblastic island. *Blood Cells*, **17**, 83–91, discussion 91-6.

Crouch, E.C. 1998. Structure, biologic properties, and expression of surfactant protein D (SP-D). *Biochim Biophys Acta*, **1408**, 278–89.

Daeron, M. 1997. Fc receptor biology. *Annu Rev Immunol*, **15**, 203–34.

De Voss, J.J., Rutter, K., et al. 1999. Iron acquisition and metabolism by mycobacteria. *J Bacteriol*, **181**, 4443–51.

Desjardins, M., Huber, L.A., et al. 1994. Biogenesis of phagolysosomes proceeds through a sequential series of interactions with the endocytic apparatus. *J Cell Biol*, **124**, 677–88.

East, L. and Isacke, C. 2002. The mannose receptor family. *Biochim Biophys Acta*, **1572**, 364.

Ehlers, M.R. 2000. CR3: a general purpose adhesion-recognition receptor essential for innate immunity. *Microbes Infect*, **2**, 289–94.

Engering, A., Geijtenbeek, T.B. and van Kooyk, Y. 2002. Immune escape through C-type lectins on dendritic cells. *Trends Immunol*, **23**, 480–5.

Ernst, J.D. 1998. Macrophage receptors for *Mycobacterium tuberculosis*. *Infect Immun*, **66**, 1277–81.

Fadok, V.A., Bratton, D.L. and Henson, P.M. 2001. Phagocyte receptors for apoptotic cells: recognition, uptake, and consequences. *J Clin Invest*, **108**, 957–62.

Fallman, M., Andersson, K., et al. 1995. Yersinia pseudotuberculosis inhibits Fc receptor-mediated phagocytosis in J774 cells. *Infect Immun*, **63**, 3117–24.

Fearon, D.T. and Locksley, R.M. 1996. The instructive role of innate immunity in the acquired immune response. *Science*, **272**, 50–3.

Forbes, J.R. and Gros, P. 2001. Divalent-metal transport by NRAMP proteins at the interface of host-pathogen interactions. *Trends Microbiol*, **9**, 397–403.

Gagnon, E., Duclos, S., et al. 2002. Endoplasmic reticulum-mediated phagocytosis is a mechanism of entry into macrophages. *Cell*, **110**, 119–31.

Geijtenbeek, T.B., Engering, A. and Van Kooyk, Y. 2002. DC-SIGN, a C-type lectin on dendritic cells that unveils many aspects of dendritic cell biology. *J Leukoc Biol*, **71**, 921–31.

Geske, F.J., Monks, J., et al. 2002. The role of the macrophage in apoptosis: hunter, gatherer, and regulator. *Int J Hematol*, **76**, 16–26.

Goldblatt, D. and Thrasher, A.J. 2000. Chronic granulomatous disease. *Clin Exp Immunol*, **122**, 1–9.

Goosney, D.L., Knoechel, D.G. and Finlay, B.B. 1999. Enteropathogenic E. coli, Salmonella and Shigella: masters of host cell cytoskeletal exploitation. *Emerg Infect Dis*, **5**, 216–23.

Gordon, S. 1999. Macrophages and the immune response. In: Paul, W.E. (ed.), *Fundamental immunology*. Philadelphia: Lippincott-Raven Publishers, 533–45.

Gordon, S. 2001. Mononuclear phagocytes in immune defence. In: Roitt, I., Brostoff, B. and Male, D. (eds), *Immunology*. Edinburgh: Mosby, 147–62.

Gordon, S. 2003a. Alternative macrophage activation. *Nat Rev Immunol*, **3**, 23–35.

Gordon, S. 2003b. Macrophages and the immune response. In: Paul, W.E. (ed.), *Fundamental immunology*. Philadelphia: Lippincott-Raven Publishers.

Gordon, S., Lawson, L., et al. 1992. Antigen markers of macrophage differentiation in murine tissues. In: Russell, S. and Gordon, S. (eds), *Macrophage biology and activation*, vol. 181. . Berlin: Springer-Verlag, 1–37.

Griffin, F.M. Jr, Griffin, J.A., et al. 1975. Studies on the mechanism of phagocytosis. I. Requirements for circumferential attachment of particle-bound ligands to specific receptors on the macrophage plasma membrane. *J Exp Med*, **142**, 1263–82.

Griffin, F.M. Jr, Griffin, J.A. and Silverstein, S.C. 1976. Studies on the mechanism of phagocytosis. II. The interaction of macrophages with anti-immunoglobulin IgG-coated bone marrow-derived lymphocytes. *J Exp Med*, **144**, 788–809.

Gruenberg, J. 2001. The endocytic pathway: a mosaic of domains. *Nat Rev Mol Cell Biol*, **2**, 721–30.

Gruenheid, S., Pinner, E., et al. 1997. Natural resistance to infection with intracellular pathogens: the Nramp1 protein is recruited to the membrane of the phagosome. *J Exp Med*, **185**, 717–30.

Guermonprez, P., Valladeau, J., et al. 2002. Antigen presentation and T cell stimulation by dendritic cells. *Annu Rev Immunol*, **20**, 621–67.

Haagsman, H.P. 1998. Interactions of surfactant protein A with pathogens. *Biochim Biophys Acta*, **1408**, 264–77.

Hampton, M.B., Kettle, A.J. and Winterbourn, C.C. 1998. Inside the neutrophil phagosome: oxidants, myeloperoxidase, and bacterial killing. *Blood*, **92**, 3007–17.

Heath, W.R. and Carbone, F.R. 2001. Cross-presentation, dendritic cells, tolerance and immunity. *Annu Rev Immunol*, **19**, 47–64.

Heinzen, R.A., Scidmore, M.A., et al. 1996. Differential interaction with endocytic and exocytic pathways distinguish parasitophorous vacuoles of *Coxiella burnetii* and *Chlamydia trachomatis*. *Infect Immun*, **64**, 796–809.

Herman, A., Kappler, J.W., et al. 1991. Superantigens: mechanism of T-cell stimulation and role in immune responses. *Annu Rev Immunol*, **9**, 745–72.

High, N., Mounier, J., et al. 1992. IpaB of *Shigella flexneri* causes entry into epithelial cells and escape from the phagocytic vacuole. *EMBO J*, **11**, 1991–9.

Hoffmann, J.A. and Reichhart, J.M. 2002. Drosophila innate immunity: an evolutionary perspective. *Nat Immunol*, **3**, 121–6.

Horng, T., Barton, G.M., et al. 2002. The adaptor molecule TIRAP provides signalling specificity for Toll-like receptors. *Nature*, **420**, 329–33.

Imada, K. and Leonard, W.J. 2000. The Jak-STAT pathway. *Mol Immunol*, **37**, 1–11.

Ingalls, R.R. and Golenbock, D.T. 1995. CD11c/CD18, a transmembrane signaling receptor for lipopolysaccharide. *J Exp Med*, **181**, 1473–9.

Inohara, N., Ogura, Y. and Nunez, G. 2002. Nods: a family of cytosolic proteins that regulate the host response to pathogens. *Curr Opin Microbiol*, **5**, 76–80.

Jack, R.S., Fan, X., et al. 1997. Lipopolysaccharide-binding protein is required to combat a murine gram-negative bacterial infection. *Nature*, **389**, 742–5.

Janeway, C.A. Jr 1992. The immune system evolved to discriminate infectious nonself from noninfectious self. *Immunol Today*, **13**, 11–16.

Kaplan, G. 1977. Differences in the mode of phagocytosis with Fc and C3 receptors in macrophages. *Scand J Immunol*, **6**, 797–807.

Karlsson, A. and Dahlgren, C. 2002. Assembly and activation of the neutrophil NADPH oxidase in granule membranes. *Antioxid Redox Signal*, **4**, 49–60.

Kilpatrick, D. 2002. Mannan-binding lectin: clinical significance and applications. *Biochim Biophys Acta*, **1572**, 401.

Kraal, G. 1992. Cells in the marginal zone of the spleen. *Int Rev Cytol*, **132**, 31–74.

Kristiansen, M., Graversen, J.H., et al. 2001. Identification of the haemoglobin scavenger receptor. *Nature*, **409**, 198–201.

Landmann, R., Muller, B. and Zimmerli, W. 2000. CD14, new aspects of ligand and signal diversity. *Microbes Infect*, **2**, 295–304.

McFadden, G., Lalani, A., Everett, H., Nash, P. and Xu, X. 1998. Virus-encoded receptors for cytokines and chemokines. *Semin Cell Dev Biol*, **9**, 359–68.

McKnight, A.J. and Gordon, S. 1998. Membrane molecules as differentiation antigens of murine macrophages. *Adv Immunol*, **68**, 271–314.

MacMicking, J., Xie, Q.W. and Nathan, C. 1997. Nitric oxide and macrophage function. *Annu Rev Immunol*, **15**, 323–50.

Manca, C., Paul, S., et al. 1999. Mycobacterium tuberculosis catalase and peroxidase activities and resistance to oxidative killing in human monocytes in vitro. *Infect Immun*, **67**, 74–9.

Marodi, L., Tournay, C., et al. 1998. Augmentation of human macrophage candidacidal capacity by recombinant human myeloperoxidase and granulocyte-macrophage colony-stimulating factor. *Infect Immun*, **66**, 2750–4.

Martinez-Pomares, L. and Gordon, S. 1999. The mannose receptor and its role in antigen presentation. *Immunologist*, **7**, 119–23.

Medzhitov, R. 2001. Toll-like receptors and innate immunity. *Nat Rev Immunol*, **1**, 135–45.

Mellman, I. and Steinman, R.M. 2001. Dendritic cells: specialized and regulated antigen processing machines. *Cell*, **106**, 255–8.

Miller, J.L. and Gordon, S. in presss. Innate recognition of viruses by macrophage and related receptors. In: Gordon, S. (ed.), *Pharmacology of macrophages*. Heidelberg: Springer-Verlag.

Mosser, D.M. and Karp, C.L. 1999. Receptor mediated subversion of macrophage cytokine production by intracellular pathogens. *Curr Opin Immunol*, **11**, 406–11.

Muller, W.A. and Randolph, G.J. 1999. Migration of leukocytes across endothelium and beyond: molecules involved in the transmigration and fate of monocytes. *J Leukoc Biol*, **66**, 698–704.

Navarre, W.W. and Zychlinsky, A. 2000. Pathogen-induced apoptosis of macrophages: a common end for different pathogenic strategies. *Cell Microbiol*, **2**, 265–73.

Nicholson-Weller, A. and Klickstein, L.B. 1999. C1q-binding proteins and C1q receptors. *Curr Opin Immunol*, **11**, 42–6.

Noursadeghi, M., Bickerstaff, M.C., et al. 2000. Role of serum amyloid P component in bacterial infection: protection of the host or protection of the pathogen. *Proc Natl Acad Sci USA*, **97**, 14584–9.

Oldenborg, P.A., Gresham, H.D. and Lindberg, F.P. 2001. CD47-signal regulatory protein alpha (SIRPalpha) regulates Fcgamma and complement receptor-mediated phagocytosis. *J Exp Med*, **193**, 855–62.

Olson, T.S. and Ley, K. 2002. Chemokines and chemokine receptors in leukocyte trafficking. *Am J Physiol Regul Integr Comp Physiol*, **283**, R7–28.

Ozinsky, A., Underhill, D.M., et al. 2000. The repertoire for pattern recognition of pathogens by the innate immune system is defined by cooperation between toll-like receptors. *Proc Natl Acad Sci USA*, **97**, 13766–71.

Papageorgiou, A.C. and Acharya, K.R. 2000. Microbial superantigens: from structure to function. *Trends Microbiol*, **8**, 369–75.

Peiser, L., Mukhopadhyay, S. and Gordon, S. 2002. Scavenger receptors in innate immunity. *Curr Opin Immunol*, **14**, 123–8.

Perry, V.H., Andersson, P.B. and Gordon, S. 1993. Macrophages and inflammation in the central nervous system. *Trends Neurosci*, **16**, 268–73.

Ponten, A., Sick, C., et al. 1997. Dominant-negative mutants of human MxA protein: domains in the carboxy-terminal moiety are important for oligomerization and antiviral activity. *J Virol*, **71**, 2591–9.

Porcelli, S.A. and Modlin, R.L. 1999. The CD1 system: antigen-presenting molecules for T cell recognition of lipids and glycolipids. *Annu Rev Immunol*, **17**, 297–329.

Portnoy, D.A., Jacks, P.S. and Hinrichs, D.J. 1988. Role of hemolysin for the intracellular growth of *Listeria monocytogenes*. *J Exp Med*, **167**, 1459–71.

Rabinovitch, M. and Veras, P.S. 1996. Cohabitation of *Leishmania amazonensis* and *Coxiella burnetii*. *Trends Microbiol*, **4**, 158–61.

Ravetch, J.V. and Clynes, R.A. 1998. Divergent roles for Fc receptors and complement in vivo. *Annu Rev Immunol*, **16**, 421–32.

Reeves, E.P., Lu, H., et al. 2002. Killing activity of neutrophils is mediated through activation of proteases by K^+ flux. *Nature*, **416**, 291–7.

Rittig, M.G., Wilske, B. and Krause, A. 1999. Phagocytosis of microorganisms by means of overshooting pseudopods: where do we stand? *Microbes Infect*, **1**, 727–35.

Robinson, J.H. and Delvig, A.A. 2002. Diversity in MHC class II antigen presentation. *Immunology*, **105**, 252–62.

Roebuck, K.A. and Finnegan, A. 1999. Regulation of intercellular adhesion molecule-1 (CD54) gene expression. *J Leukoc Biol*, **66**, 876–88.

Ross, J.A. and Auger, M.J. 2002. The biology of the macrophage. In: Burke, B. and Lewis, C.E. (eds), *The macrophage*. Oxford: Oxford University Press, 1–72.

Samuel, C.E. 2001. Antiviral actions of interferons. *Clin Microbiol Rev*, **14**, 778–809, table of contents.

Sankala, M., Brannstrom, A., et al. 2002. Characterization of recombinant soluble macrophage scavenger receptor MARCO. *J Biol Chem*, **277**, 33378–85.

Schaible, U.E., Collins, H.L. and Kaufmann, S.H. 1999. Confrontation between intracellular bacteria and the immune system. *Adv Immunol*, **71**, 267–377.

Shepherd, V.L. and Hoidal, J.R. 1990. Clearance of neutrophil-derived myeloperoxidase by the macrophage mannose receptor. *Am J Respir Cell Mol Biol*, **2**, 335–40.

Shimaoka, T., Kume, N., et al. 2001. LOX-1 supports adhesion of Gram-positive and Gram-negative bacteria. *J Immunol*, **166**, 5108–14.

Shin, J.S. and Abraham, S.N. 2001. Caveolae as portals of entry for microbes. *Microbes Infect*, **3**, 755–61.

Sieczkarski, S.B. and Whittaker, G.R. 2002. Dissecting virus entry via endocytosis. *J Gen Virol*, **83**, 1535–45.

Springer, T.A. 1994. Traffic signals for lymphocyte recirculation and leukocyte emigration: the multistep paradigm. *Cell*, **76**, 301–14.

Stoiber, H., Kacani, L., et al. 2001. The supportive role of complement in HIV pathogenesis. *Immunol Rev*, **180**, 168–76.

Storz, G., Tartaglia, L.A. and Ames, B.N. 1990. The OxyR regulon. *Antonie Van Leeuwenhoek*, **58**, 157–61.

Sturgill-Koszycki, S., Schlesinger, P.H., et al. 1994. Lack of acidification in Mycobacterium phagosomes produced by exclusion of the vesicular proton-ATPase. *Science*, **263**, 678–81.

Sunder-Plassmann, G., Patruta, S.I. and Horl, W.H. 1999. Pathobiology of the role of iron in infection. *Am J Kidney Dis*, **34**, S25–9.

Szalai, A.J. 2002. The antimicrobial activity of C-reactive protein. *Microbes Infect*, **4**, 201–5.

Taborda, C.P. and Casadevall, A. 2002. CR3 (CD11b/CD18) and CR4 (CD11c/CD18) are involved in complement-independent antibody-mediated phagocytosis of *Cryptococcus neoformans*. *Immunity*, **16**, 791–802.

Taylor, P., Botto, M. and Walport, M. 1998. The complement system. *Curr Biol*, **8**, R259–261.

Thomson, A. 1998. *The cytokine handbook*. San Diego, CA: Academic Press.

Underhill, D.M. and Ozinsky, A. 2002. Phagocytosis of microbes: complexity in action. *Annu Rev Immunol*, **20**, 825–52.

Underhill, D.M., Ozinsky, A., et al. 1999. The Toll-like receptor 2 is recruited to macrophage phagosomes and discriminates between pathogens. *Nature*, **401**, 811–15.

Wei, X.Q., Charles, I.G., et al. 1995. Altered immune responses in mice lacking inducible nitric oxide synthase. *Nature*, **375**, 408–11.

Weinrauch, Y. and Zychlinsky, A. 1999. The induction of apoptosis by bacterial pathogens. *Annu Rev Microbiol*, **53**, 155–87.

Winterbourn, C.C., Vissers, M.C. and Kettle, A.J. 2000. Myeloperoxidase. *Curr Opin Hematol*, **7**, 53–8.

Yewdell, J.W. and Bennink, J.R. 1999. Mechanisms of viral interference with MHC class I antigen processing and presentation. *Annu Rev Cell Dev Biol*, **15**, 579–606.

Yusuf-Makagiansar, H., Anderson, M.E., et al. 2002. Inhibition of LFA-1/ICAM-1 and VLA-4/VCAM-1 as a therapeutic approach to inflammation and autoimmune diseases. *Med Res Rev*, **22**, 146–67.

4

Phagocytes part 2: Neutrophils

ANTONIO FERRANTE

INTRODUCTION

The importance of neutrophils in host defense is best demonstrated in hereditary and acquired neutropenias, conditions that place an individual at risk of life-threatening infections. Neutrophils devote their activity mainly to producing oxygen-reactive species, which combine with granule constituents to form very potent microbicidal systems. This was first appreciated in the late 1950s when it was discovered that respiration was not dependent on mitochondria. Through the combined efforts of a number of independent investigators, not only was the identification of the release of hydrogen peroxide and superoxide discovered as a major feature of the cell (Paul and Sbarra 1968; Babior et al. 1973), but also the special location of the unassembled and assembled components of the oxidase were described (reviewed by Heyworth et al. 1999). A much more comprehensive understanding of the biochemistry of the oxidase came through the efforts of Segal and colleagues (1978), who identified a *b*-type cytochrome which formed a key component of the oxidase system of the cell and which was found to be the defect in some patients who had chronic granulomatous disease (CGD) whose cells failed to generate oxygen radicals and kill some bacteria. Subsequently, the complexity of the oxidase became evident with the identification of several different components that exist in a dormant form until phosphorylated and assembled at the phagosome membrane. The understanding of the generation of antimicrobial substances by neutrophils was further extended by the work of Klebanoff (1968), who demonstrated the reaction of the azurophilic granule enzyme, myeloperoxidase (MPO), with H_2O_2 and chloride to yield hypochlorous acid.

During this time, excitement about the characteristics of the respiratory burst of neutrophils overshadowed many other important discoveries such as the identification of antimicrobial cationic proteins in granules by Zeya and Spitznagel (1966), and it was not until the 1990s, when Lehrer and Ganz (1990) purified these as defensins, that major interest developed.

The discovery in the late 1970s and early 1980s of the role of specific colony-stimulating factors (CSFs) in the regulation of neutrophil hemopoiesis through the efforts of Metcalf and colleagues (Metcalf 1989) opened new vistas in granulocyte biology with potential therapeutic applications in neutrophil disorders.

In the 1980s, the author's group and others discovered more intriguing properties of this cell, that of priming. In this process, the neutrophil interacts with cytokines such as tumor necrosis factor (TNF) and gains significantly greater antimicrobial powers (Ferrante and Mocatta 1984; Klebanoff et al. 1986). Thus it became evident for the first time that the neutrophil can be educated by factors released by tissues, endothelial cells,

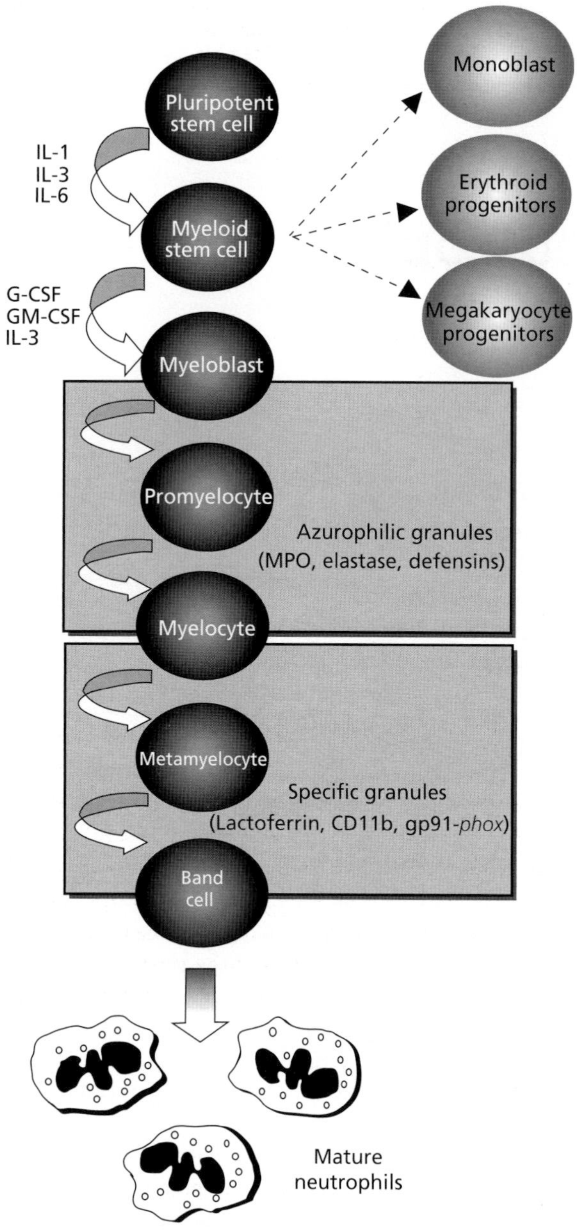

Figure 4.1 *Scheme showing the different stages of neutrophil development in the bone marrow from stem cells. Cytokines that promote granulocyte development are outlined. Note the initial appearance of azurophilic granules and later expression of specific granules. Some of the markers specific for the different granules are also shown.*

lymphocytes and monocytes in the way that macrophages were shown to be activated by interferon-γ in the 1970s.

When Tiku et al. (1986) reported that zymosan-stimulated neutrophils released interleukin (IL) 1 (IL-1), it was appreciated that neutrophils were able to promote the immunological response through the release of cytokines that regulate macrophage and lymphocyte function.

The ability of neutrophils to migrate rapidly into tissue at infection sites, release oxygen reactive species, and degranulate in order to kill bacteria needs to be regulated because of their tissue-damaging properties. The discovery that neutrophils die by programmed cell death (apoptosis), which protects against tissue damage mediated by this cell, has contributed significantly to our understanding of the mechanism of regulation of the inflammatory reaction.

The concept of neutrophil emigration from blood to tissues under a gradient of molecules had already been put in place in the mid- to late 1800s by the founding fathers, such as Metchnikoff (1893). Since then, substantial complexity has been added to this concept. This includes the array of the chemotactic factors generated during inflammation, the mechanisms of cell movement, and the interactions required between neutrophils and the endothelium for emigration into tissues.

Although the neutrophil has always been considered the 'poor cousin' of the mononuclear phagocyte because of its short life and inability to be educated to perform many of the intricate functions of the macrophage necessary to develop a strong immunological defense system, it is evident that singular properties of the neutrophil are becoming apparent. This chapter covers the properties of neutrophils in general and attempts not only to describe properties that are considered classic from the times of Elie Metchnikoff, but also to illustrate those properties that have only recently been appreciated.

NEUTROPHIL DEVELOPMENT

The bone marrow is involved in the production of neutrophils. This is the site for proliferation of neutrophil precursors and maturation to the mature stage (Figure 4.1) (Bainton 1999). Once cells evolve from pluripotent stem cells to progenitor cells, they can no longer differentiate into any type of blood cell and will differentiate into the mature cells. Hemopoiesis is regulated by a number of cytokines. Four of these, the CSFs, IL-3 (multi-CSF), macrophage (M)-CSF, granulocyte–macrophage (GM)-CSF, and G-CSF regulate development of leukocytes (Metcalf 1989). The granulocyte lineages come under the control of G-CSF, GM-CSF, and IL-3. These factors regulate the production of neutrophils.

During neutrophil development in the bone marrow, at different stages the cell acquires functional properties necessary for optimal antimicrobial activity (Figure 4.1) (Borregaard and Cowland 1997). As constituents of granules such as MPO and eventually lactoferrin are synthesized, they are packaged in their respective granules. Components of the oxidase, such as the gp91^{phox} and functional surface receptors (CD18, CD11b) which ligate complement-opsonized bacteria, also become expressed at the plasma membrane of these cells as the cells differentiate toward the mature neutrophil. The granules to appear first are the azurophilic (primary) granules containing MPO and elastase, morphologically

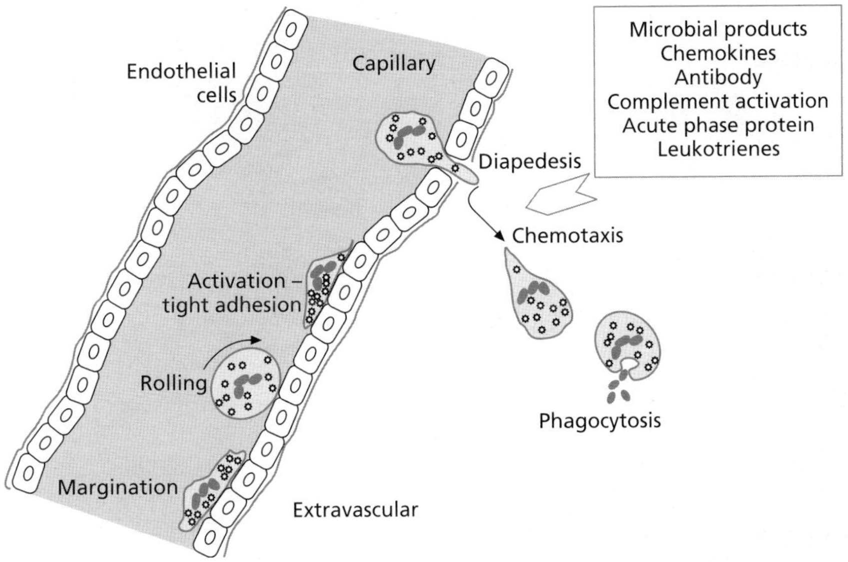

Figure 4.2 *Diagrammatic representation of early events in the recruitment of neutrophils to inflammatory sites. Stimulation of both neutrophils and the endothelium will promote the process of rolling, attachment, and transendothelial cell migration. The nature of the inflammatory response and mediators produced dictates a preference for selective recruitment of neutrophils at the level of neutrophil receptors for promoting adhesion and chemotaxis and, also, endothelial cell activation.*

seen at the promyelocyte stage. The secondary granules (specific) characterize the myelocyte stage. Once the cell lineages reach the metamyelocyte stage, the cells cease to divide.

MOBILIZATION TO SITES OF INFECTION AND DAMAGED TISSUES

Accumulation of neutrophils at infection foci and sites of tissue damage begins with margination, whereby the neutrophils attach to the capillary wall and have the potential to migrate out of the blood vessel (Gallin and Snyderman 1999) (Figure 4.2). This is followed by diapedesis, a step in which the cells squeeze through gaps in the endothelial cell layer. Their chemotactic properties enable the cells to migrate preferentially towards the source of infection and local tissue damage, and may experience migration inhibition to enable retention of cells at the infection site.

To achieve cell accumulation in tissues, a number of complex interactions occur between receptors on neutrophil surfaces and various soluble or cell surface ligands, which stimulate the cells to respond (Gallin and Snyderman 1999). Bacterial infiltration of tissues leads to the release of microbial products (e.g. lipopolysaccharide (LPS)), which can promote neutrophil accumulation in tissues themselves, via their ability to activate the endothelium and/or act as chemotactic factors. These microbial products and structures can also promote the generation of chemotactic active peptides of complement such as C5a and stimulate tissues to produce chemokines (cytokines such as IL-8) and the leukotriene, LTB_4, a chemotactic factor produced during the metabolism of arachidonic acid via the lipoxygenase pathway. Some cytokines such as TNF can also cause migration inhibition, especially at concentrations likely to be generated at inflammatory sites (Ferrante 1992).

Although many of the properties of the mediator effects on cells are reasonably well understood, how the network of interactions coordinately brings about a physiological response and when this response becomes uncontrolled to give rise to pathophysiology are far from clear and continue to be an area of research interest.

The cell cytoskeleton

The intracellular components are embedded in a supporting frame, the cytoskeleton, which consists of microfilaments, microtubules, intermediate filaments, and the microtrabecular lattice. Second messengers link the surface ligand-binding receptor to the cytoskeleton. Changes in this cytoskeleton then form the basis for cell movement, phagocytosis, granule movement, receptor recycling, and activation of the reduced nicotinamide adenine dinucleotide phosphate (NADPH) oxidase (Edwards 1994; Stossel 1999).

Microfilaments found predominantly beneath the plasma membrane are considered to be the most dynamic of the components of the cytoskeleton. Microfilaments are composed of actin molecules that exist as monomers (G-actin), which can reversibly assemble into actin filament (F-actin). Actin polymerization is initiated by the activation of actin monomers by divalent cations. A range of actin-binding proteins is involved in maintaining actin in an unpolymerized state in cells and promoting rapid assembly during cell activation. Microtubules consist of α- and β-tubulin subunits arranged in a

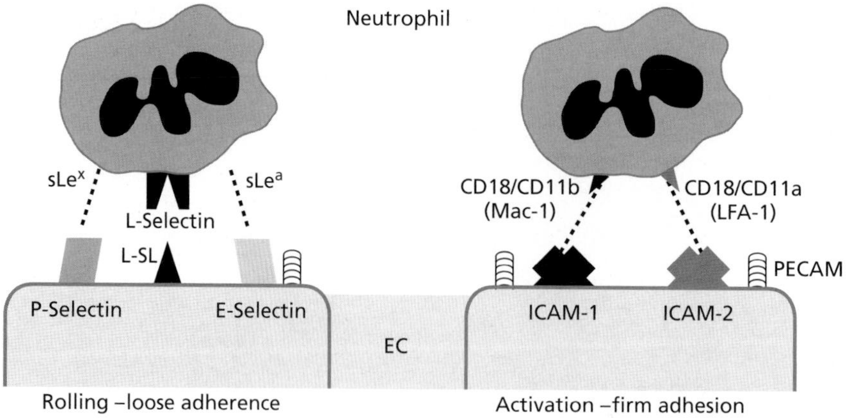

Figure 4.3 *The receptor ligand involved in the interaction of neutrophils with endothelial cells. Interaction of the tetrasaccharides sialyl Lewis^a (sLe^a), sLe^x, L-selectin with the counter-receptor/ligand, E-selectin, P-selectin, and L-selectin ligand (L-SL) promotes loose adherence and enables the neutrophils to roll. Endothelial cell (EC) activation induces/upregulates expression of cell adhesion molecules, ICAM-1/-2 enabling interactions with β_2-integrins and promoting firm adhesion of the cell to the endothelial surface. PECAM then facilitates transendothelial cell migration.*

helical structure. Assembly of these is increased during cell activation. Assembly is upregulated by cyclic guanosine monophosphate (cGMP) and decreased by cyclic adenosine monophosphate (cAMP) and Ca^{2+}. Neutrophils also have intermediate filaments, which consist of vimentin molecules that can be rapidly polymerized. Their function is not clearly known but they may be involved in connecting the peripheral region of the cell to the central regions. The microtrabecular lattice, an intricate network of fine strands, is also part of the cytoskeleton. Actin is the major polypeptide of this lattice. Cytoplasmic granules can be found associated within this lattice.

Neutrophil–endothelial cell interactions

Recruitment of neutrophils to sites of inflammation requires a series of events involving rolling, activation, adhesion, and transendothelial cell migration, which are depicted in Figures 4.2 and 4.3. The type of inflammation may dictate the cell types that leave the circulation and migrate into tissues which is in part a reflection of the type of adhesion molecules upregulated, i.e. members of the common cell adhesion molecule (CAM) family, apart from their selection by specific chemokines.

The events seen at inflammatory sites are the emigration of neutrophils from the circulation in the post-capillary venules and their loose and reversible adhesion to the endothelial cells (see Figure 4.2). This interaction, which mainly involves the selectin family and the sialylated Lewis-bearing ligands (see Figure 4.3), enables the cells to roll under the influence of forces of blood flow (Robinson et al. 1999). This interaction leads to neutrophil activation as such and indirectly by mediators released by the endothelial cells. Integrins are upregulated to high-affinity states, rolling ceases, and the cells show tight binding to the endothelium through the counter-receptor, intercellular adhesion molecule (ICAM)-1, and ICAM-2 (members of the immunoglobulin gene superfamily) (see Figure 4.3) (Kishimoto et al. 1999).

The neutrophils advance to crawl/squeeze between the endothelial cell junctions in an amoeboidal manner (Muller 1999). This transendothelial cell migration is highly dependent on platelet endothelial cell adhesion molecule-1 (PECAM-1). Having traversed the intercellular junctions, neutrophils need to migrate across the basal lamina. This again involves recognition molecules such as PECAM-1 and either physical penetration or degradation of the matrix by release of proteases.

Chemotaxis

Neutrophils are quick to respond to a gradient of chemical agents generated at a site of infection and tissue damage. These chemotactic agents bind to receptors on the cell surface to bring about a network of interactions that promotes directional movement of the cell toward the source of the chemical agent (Uhing and Snyderman 1999). This involves the recognition of a concentration gradient spanning the front and rear ends of the cell, and a combination of calcium mobilization, actin, actin-binding proteins, and proteins that regulate the cytoskeleton of the cell.

After the binding of chemotactic agents to neutrophils, the cell undergoes a shape change, characteristically bipolar. The leading edge of the cell orients toward the source of chemotactic factor and forms a pseudopod or lamellapodium that adheres to the substratum. Toward the rear of the cell can be found the nucleus and the contractile uropod exhibiting retraction fibers, which enable the cell to adhere. A repeated sequence of lamellapodia extension towards the chemotactic source and uropod retraction towards the cell body leads to cell migration.

RECOGNITION AND PHAGOCYTOSIS OF MICROBIAL PATHOGENS

Innate immunity in vertebrates expresses primitive forms of recognition system that involve recognition of structures generally based on their charge and special arrangement of chemical groups (Gallin and Snyderman 1999). These possibly evolved from scavenger properties of primitive cells such as amoebae. Thus carbohydrate residues on the surface of a pathogen may be recognized by receptors that perform scavenger functions. These types of recognition system may play an important role at sites in which complement and antibody levels are very low or absent.

Neutrophils display a wide range of receptors on their surface, which enable a highly regulated attack on microorganisms, although such receptors will also direct the neutrophil attack toward damaged tissue. Several well-characterized receptors are outlined in Table 4.1. These receptors are set into operation when bacteria are opsonized with antibody and/or complement components (Greenberg 1999), enabling neutrophils to attach to the bacteria via the Fc portion of the immunoglobulin molecule involving FcγR or FcαR. Deposition of complement components on the surface of bacteria leads to binding of neutrophils to bacteria via the complement receptors, CR1, CR3, and CR4. The ligation of these receptors promotes the phagocytosis of the microorganisms and their killing by stimulating the neutrophil respiratory burst and degranulation.

The binding of antibody to the surface antigens of microbial pathogens leads to the exposure of a region in the Fc domain of the immunoglobulin molecule, which can be recognized by the Fc receptors (FcRs) on the neutrophil. There are three types of FcγR on neutrophils recognized to date: FcγRI (CD64), FcγRIIA (CD32), and FcγRIIIB (CD16). The function of these is to recognize the Fc domain of IgG, but their ability to do this is dependent on various physiological and pathophysiological conditions. The FcγRI is a glycosylated 72-kDa transmembrane protein which is absent in blood neutrophils but is upregulated and detected following pre-exposure to interferon-γ (IFN-γ) which involves transcription. This contrasts with the regulation of FcγRIIIB, which can be upregulated by release from granules and downregulated by shedding. The FcγRI, in comparison to FcγRIIA and FcγRIIIB binds monomeric IgG with high affinity.

Table 4.1 *Functional receptors mediating phagocytosis of opsonized particles and activation in neutrophils*

Receptor type	Ligand
FcγRI (CD64)[a]	Fc domain of IgG
FcγRIIA (CD32)	Fc domain of IgG
FcγRIII B (CD16)	Fc domain of IgG
FcαR (CD89)	Fc domain of IgA
CR1 (CD35)	C3b
CR3 (CD11b/CD18)	C3bi
CR4 (CD11c/CD18)	C3bi

a) CD classification of Fcγ and CR on neutrophils.

The significance of FcγRI on neutrophils is not clear because it is expressed by neutrophils only after long-term exposure to IFN-γ. However, this may argue for an important role for neutrophil activation and priming in a similar manner to mononuclear phagocytes (Ferrante 1992). Similarly, the role of FcγRIIIB in neutrophils is not clear because it lacks a transmembrane or cytoplasmic domain, suggesting that it is not involved in intracellular signaling for a respiratory burst and/or degranulation. But, because it is expressed in abundance on neutrophils, its main function may be the binding and removal of immune complexes. Presumably FcγRIIIB promotes the binding of bacteria but it needs to cooperate with FcγRIIA to stimulate the relevant intracellular signals.

FcαR which recognizes the Fc domain of IgA is also expressed by neutrophils. IgA in high concentration opsonizes and facilitates microbial phagocytosis and activation of the neutrophil respiratory burst through this receptor. This is likely to be an important defense mechanism in mucosal surfaces where the complement concentration is likely to be too low to promote phagocytosis.

During inflammation, whether induced by microbial pathogens or altered tissues, complement is activated in a cascade manner to generate components that are recognized by neutrophils, some of which act as opsonins to promote phagocytosis. The component C3 is of vital importance because it generates fragments, C3b and C3bi, which when deposited on bacteria facilitate recognition by neutrophils usually through the receptors CR1, CR3, and CR4 (Greenberg 1999) (see Chapter 9, Complement). Whether particles are coated with C3b or C3bi is dependent on whether complement is activated via the classic or the alternate pathway. CR1 (LAF-1) binds C3b primarily and has very weak affinity for C3bi. In contrast CR3 (Mac-1) binds to C3bi deposited on bacteria with very high affinity. CR4 also probably recognizes C3bi. Neutrophils can recognize microbial surfaces in the absence of antibody and complement by an opsonin-independent system that may involve CR3 receptors recognizing other residues.

Appropriate recognition and adherence of neutrophils to bacteria and fungi lead to the engulfment of these microbes, thereby confining and limiting their harmful effects. This involves the formation of a pseudopod, which extends around the surface of the bacteria in a 'zipper hypothesis' manner to confine the organisms within a vacuole. The cell is then able to deal with the engulfed bacteria by a combination of pH changes in the

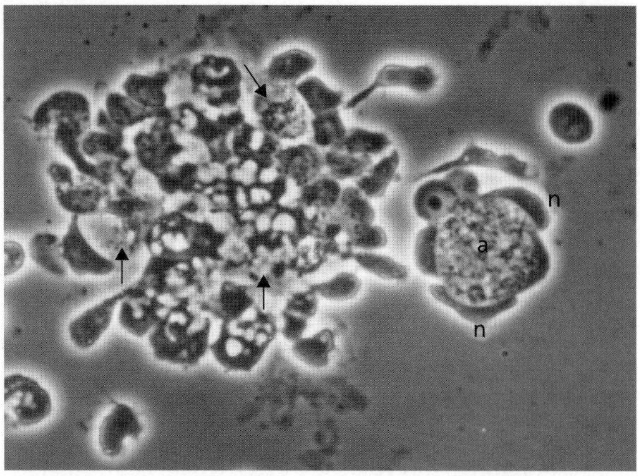

Figure 4.4 *The interaction of neutrophils with pathogenic free-living amoebae in the peritoneal cavity of mice immune to* Naegleria fowleri. *Mice were injected intraperitoneally with living amoebae and, after 8 h, the peritoneal content harvested and examined. A motile amoeba* **(a)** *is seen with attached neutrophils* **(n)**. *Several amoebae are seen highly vacuolated or lysed (→) because these are attacked by neutrophils.*

phagocytic vacuole and the release of toxic oxygen intermediates and granule constituents, some of which have enzymatic properties. A unique interaction between neutrophils and parasites has been described in which the neutrophil extracts *Plasmodium falciparum* from within an erythrocyte without lysis of the erythrocyte (Kumaratilake et al. 1994).

Frustrated phagocytosis has been found to occur when a particle is too large to be engulfed by the neutrophil. This may occur with some large unicellular protozoan parasites such as amoebae (Figure 4.4) and in the case of multicellular parasites and hyphae of *Candida albicans*. Interaction with altered tissues may also lead to an event of frustrated phagocytosis. In these situations, a 'partial vacuole' is formed in which the environment seen in a complete phagocytic vacuole is created. The reactive oxygen species and granule constituents are released and able to damage and lyse the cells. Usually a number of neutrophils will attack one multicellular parasite and presumably it is the net effect of surface parasite damage induced by several neutrophils that leads to parasite death. In autoimmune diseases such as glomerulonephritis and rheumatoid arthritis, the antigen–antibody complexes deposited on the membranes and their ability to activate complement promote this neutrophil-mediated cellular cytotoxicity.

ANTIMICROBIAL ARMORY OF THE NEUTROPHIL

Once neutrophils localize at an infection site and come into contact with bacteria, the cells are stimulated to produce an array of microbicidal substances within seconds and minutes. The neutrophil microbicidal systems can be divided into the nonoxidative and oxidative components. Depending on the type of bacteria or parasite, either one of these components may be effective or, in other cases, both systems are seen to operate synergistically.

Nonoxidative antimicrobial systems

Neutrophils contain two major granules, specific and azurophilic granules which can be distinguished by the presence of different constituents (Table 4.2). The constituents present in the azurophilic granules have primarily an antimicrobial function. The ability of these constituents to kill microbial pathogens contrasts with a mechanism by which organisms can be killed in their absence, simply by being confined in a phagocytic vacuole and destroyed by the microbe's own products. Evidence for a role of nonoxidative mechanisms in neutrophil-mediated microbial killing is seen from experiments where neutrophils from patients with CGD, lacking NADPH oxidase activity, while unable to kill some bacteria can still kill others. In addition, others have found that crude fractions of neutrophils were able to kill gram-negative bacteria (Borregaard and Cowland 1997). Granule constituents play various roles in nonoxidative killing of microorganisms. These mechanisms are continuing to be an area of major research interest. Some of the granule enzyme components show direct antimicrobial activities and in purified forms can kill bacteria. Others, although not directly microbicidal, are involved in the digestion of the bacteria. Nonenzymatic granule proteins have also been shown to be highly antimicrobial. The following azurophilic granule constituents are of interest in relation to nonoxidative killing of microbial pathogens:

- Defensins, cationic peptides of 3.5–4.5 kDa, have a broad-spectrum antimicrobial activity (Lehrer and Ganz 1990). Both α- and β-defensins have been found

Table 4.2 *An abridged summary of the two major neutrophil granule constituents*[a]

Azurophilic/primary granules	Specific/secondary granules
Myeloperoxidase	Lysozyme
β-Glucuronidase	Lactoferrin
Elastase	Vitamin B_{12}-binding protein
Cathepsin G	Receptors – CR3, fMLP receptor
Defensins	Components of NADPH oxidase
BPI	
Lysozyme	

fMLP, formyl–methionine–leucine–phenylalanine or f-Met-Leu-Phe; BPI, bactericidal permeability-increasing protein.
a) Note that these two granules need to be considered along with a tertiary granule (gelatinase granules) and secretory vesicles.

in these neutrophil granules. The peptides show cytotoxic activity towards fungi, parasites, and gram-negative bacteria. They are released into the phagocytic vacuole during phagocytosis of bacteria.

- Serprocidins such as elastase, azurocidin, and cathepsin G, which have microbicidal activity, are also contained in azurophilic granules (Edwards 1994). This microbicidal activity is independent of proteolytic action.
- Cathepsin G is active against a range of gram-positive and gram-negative bacteria, particularly against *Neisseria gonorrheae* and fungi.
- A highly cationic protein (bactericidal/permeability – increasing protein) with marked bactericidal activity, particularly towards gram-negative bacteria, is also found in azurophilic granules (Elsbach and Weiss 1983). The molecule inserts into bacterial outer membranes causing increased permeability.

Oxidative systems

THE OXYGEN-DEPENDENT RESPIRATORY BURST

When phagocytes adhere to bacteria, one of the most dramatic responses seen is the oxygen-dependent respiratory burst and the generation of a spectrum of reactive oxygen intermediates (ROIs) which are either directly or indirectly microbicidal. The enzyme responsible for this is NADPH oxidase, which consists of several different components that assemble on the phagosome membrane (Heyworth et al. 1999). When neutrophils are stimulated most of the glucose is oxidized via the hexose monophosphate shunt which is closely linked to the reduction of oxygen by the NADPH oxidase. The initial product of the respiratory burst is the production of superoxide ($O_2^{\bar{}}$).

It was only a few decades ago that the unique characteristics of the neutrophil respiratory burst were first described. It was shown that bacterial killing still occurred in the presence of cyanide, suggesting that mitochondria and the citrate cycle were not involved, consistent with the finding of very few active mitochondria in neutrophils. The ATP generation comes mainly from glycolysis, which does not require oxygen, and this is considered as an advantage because neutrophils need to kill microorganisms in oxygen-depleted tissue sites. Later, it became evident that the majority of the oxygen consumed by the neutrophil was converted to $O_2^{\bar{}}$ (Barbior et al. 1973; Fridovich 1978). Thus, during a respiratory burst, glucose is oxidized via the hexose monophosphate shunt, generating NADPH which together with oxygen provides the source of electrons to produce superoxide anion. From $O_2^{\bar{}}$ several ROIs are formed in the phagocytic vacuole. These are shown below.

$$\underset{\text{(Superoxide)}}{O_2^{\bar{}} + O_2^{\bar{}}} + 2H + \xrightarrow[\text{Dismutase}]{\text{Superoxide}} \underset{\text{(Hydrogen Peroxide)}}{O_2 + H_2O_2}$$

Haber–Weiss reaction:

$$O_2^{\bar{}} + Fe^{3+} \rightarrow O_2 + Fe^{2+}$$

$$Fe^{2+} + H_2O_2 \rightarrow Fe^{3+} + \underset{\text{(Hydroxyl radical)}}{OH^{\cdot}} + \underset{\text{(Hydroxyl ion)}}{OH^-}$$

The activation of the respiratory burst oxidase can be demonstrated in the reduction of nitroblue tetrazolium (NBT) by the cells which causes the dye to change from a yellow, soluble compound to a blue–black, formazan-insoluble substance in the cell (Figure 4.5).

COMPONENTS AND ASSEMBLY OF NADPH OXIDASE

NADPH is essentially dormant and becomes rapidly activated after the stimulation of appropriate intracellular signals by agonists ligating the cell surface receptors on neutrophils (Heyworth et al. 1999). Activation occurs once the various components become rapidly assembled at the plasma membrane (vacuole membrane), involving both membrane and cytosolic components of this system (Figure 4.6). Within the membrane is a unique cytochrome b_{245} (Segal and Jones 1978), a heterodimer of two subunits, $gp91^{phox}$ and $p22^{phox}$, suggested to contain two different types of redox centers. There is one flavin adenine dinucleotide (FAD) domain and at least two heme prosthetic groups (Babior and Kipnes 1977; Segal et al. 1992). The three cytosolic proteins are believed to be necessary to associate with the cytochrome at the membrane, $p40^{phox}$, $p47^{phox}$, and $p67^{phox}$, forming the active enzyme system (Wientjes et al. 1993; Heyworth et al. 1999). Other constituents such as the small GTP-binding proteins are also involved (Heyworth et al. 1999). The oxidase is strategically located to generate ROIs in the vacuole containing the ingested bacteria. Consequently, the binding site for the substrate, NADPH, is on the cytoplasmic side and superoxide is formed at the phagosome membrane side (Figure 4.6).

MYELOPEROXIDASE–H_2O_2–HALIDE SYSTEM

Myeloperoxidase is present in very high amounts in neutrophil azurophilic granules. During phagocytosis, activation of the respiratory burst is accompanied by degranulation, resulting in release of H_2O_2 and MPO into the phagosome. Interestingly, some of the bacteria phagocytosed can also be a source of H_2O_2. Chloride is then oxidized to hypochlorite (HOCl) by the MPO and H_2O_2. The system produces other toxic agents, including chloramines, hydroxyl radicals, and singlet oxygen.

$$H_2O_2 + 2Cl^- \xrightarrow{\text{MPO}} 2HOCl$$

This system causes destruction of microorganisms in phagocytic vacuoles in two main ways: by halogenation and by oxidation (Klebanoff 1968, 1999); it has been

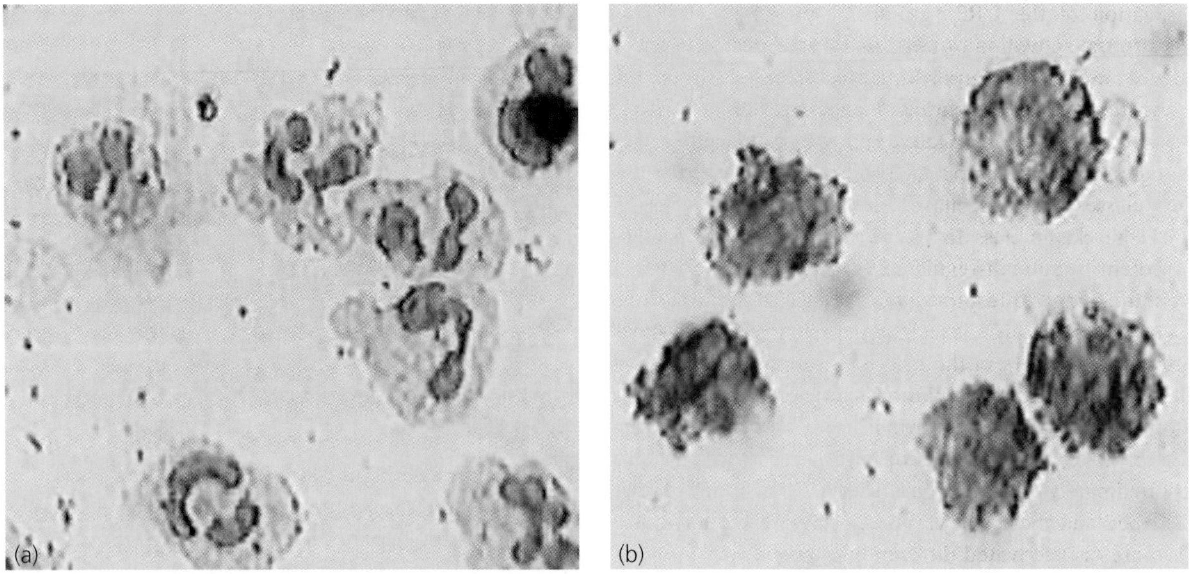

Figure 4.5 *Oxidative burst activity in stimulated neutrophils shown by the nitroblue tetrazolium (NBT) reduction assay.* **(a)** *Non-stimulated neutrophils lacking positive NBT staining compared with phorbol myristate acetate (PMA)-activated neutrophils* **(b)**, *which show the blue–black formazan deposits.*

shown to damage/kill a wide range of microorganisms, including bacteria, protozoan parasites and metazoan parasites (Klebanoff 1999), as well as tumor tissues during inflammation (Klebanoff 1999). Bacterial toxins are also inactivated by the MPO–H_2O_2–halide system.

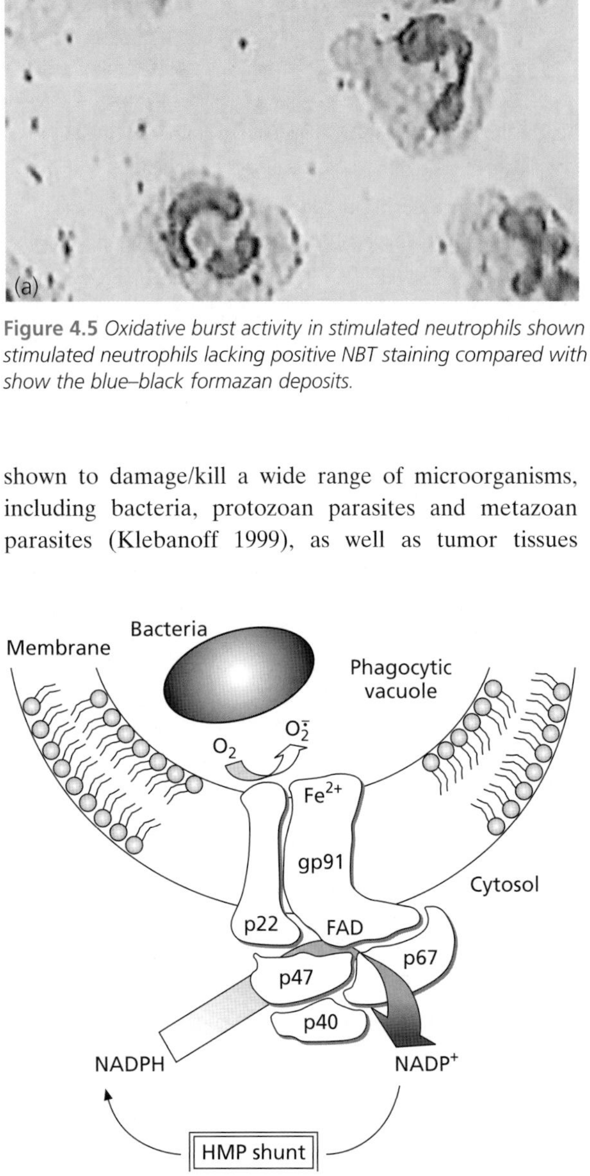

Figure 4.6 *The positioning of the activated oxidase in the membrane of the phagocytic vacuole and the link between the oxidation of NADPH and the generation and release of superoxide into the bacteria-containing phagocytic vacuole. The components of the NADPH oxidase are also depicted. The cytochrome b gp91^{phox} and p22^{phox} are localized in the membrane and require the recruitment of at least three cytosolic components, p40^{phox}, p47^{phox}, and p67^{phox} for the complex to act as the oxidase. The substrate for oxidase is generated when glucose is oxidized via the hexose monophosphate (HMP) shunt. In this reaction two electrons are transferred from the NADPH to FAD, followed by the reduction of Fe^{3+} to Fe^{2+} and direct binding of the reduced hemes to oxygen molecules to form superoxide.*

INTRACELLULAR SIGNALING AND NEUTROPHIL FUNCTIONS

The chemoattractant coupling of the surface receptor is coupled to the intracellular second messengers by the heterotrimeric G-proteins (guanine nucleotide-binding proteins). The second messengers, inositol triphosphate (IP_3), Ca^{2+} mobilization, phosphatidic acid (PA), arachidonic acid (AA), and cyclic nucleotides, have all been shown to participate in cell movement. Antibody- and/or complement-opsonized microorganisms ligate the FcγR and CR3 receptors and induce signal transduction mechanisms, involving G-proteins, protein kinases, and phospholipids, which control phagocytosis, activation of NADPH oxidase, and degranulation.

Nonstimulated neutrophils express a transmembrane FcγRIIA and FcγRIIIB, which is the GDP-dissociation inhibitory factor GPI linked to the membrane. Ligation and crosslinking of these receptors stimulates tyrosine phosphorylation as well as phospholipase Cγ. This then leads to the activation of protein kinase C (PKC), Ca^{2+} mobilization, and activation of phosphotidylinositol-3-kinase (PI3-K) signaling pathways. These molecules are then responsible for activating downstream signals such as the mitogen-activated protein (MAP) kinases, leading to a network interaction to stimulate functional responses including phagocytosis, activation of the respiratory burst, and degranulation. The complement receptors such as CR1 and CR2 are likely to associate with the Fcγ receptors to promote these responses.

Ligation of the CR3 (CD18/CD11b) on neutrophils leads to the activation of upstream signals including PI3-K. A number of intracellular molecules have been shown to regulate the various neutrophil functions. The PI3-K, a family of kinases, phosphorylates inositol-containing phospholipids to form phosphatidyl inositol. Two classes of PI3-K have been identified in neutrophils: the classic class Ia (p85/p110) heterodimer and a G-protein βγ subunit-regulated PI3-K. PI3-K is required for stimulating the respiratory burst and degranulation.

Protein kinase C is a family of serine/threonine kinases that resides in the cytoplasm and translocates to the particulate fraction (plasma membrane and cytoskeleton associated) after neutrophil stimulation. Translocation of PKC is closely associated with its activation. Approximately 12 different PKC isozymes have been described and these will vary from cell type to cell type. They are also activated differently by individual agonists and various isozymes may be responsible for different cellular functions. In neutrophils the expression of PKCα, β1, β11, δ, and ξ has been reported. Evidence has been presented that PKC is required for the neutrophil functions of chemotaxis, respiratory burst, and phagocytosis.

There are three distinct families of MAP kinases recognized: the extracellular signal-regulated kinase (ERK), c-Jun NH_2-terminal kinase (JNK), and p38. The role of JNK in neutrophil function has not been identified because various agonists fail to activate JNK, unless special conditions are met such as pre-adherence of cells and addition of protease inhibitors (Avdi et al. 2001).

ERK1 and ERK2, which can be activated via various receptors including FcγR, have been shown to play a role in the activation of the oxidase by phosphorylating $p47^{phox}$, a cytosolic component of the oxidase. More recent studies have, however, demonstrated that the ERK cascade plays a major role in chemokinesis and a lesser role in bacterial and fungal killing by neutrophils (Hii et al. 1999).

Of the four recognized isoforms of p38, neutrophils express the α and δ isoforms. Activation of p38 can be achieved by both G-protein-coupled receptors as well as non-G-protein-coupled receptors. In terms of neutrophil functions, p38 plays a role in chemotaxis, respiratory burst, degranulation, and apoptosis.

NEUTROPHIL PRIMING

There is now overwhelming evidence that neutrophils can be educated for increased performance in their antimicrobial activity (Coffey 1992). A variety of exogenous and endogenous mediators has been shown to prime neutrophils for increased antimicrobial function but perhaps the most interesting have been the cytokines (Ferrante 1992). Priming of neutrophils requires short-term exposure to cytokines and in most cases is optimal with a 30-min pre-treatment time (Ferrante et al. 1993b). Cytokine-primed neutrophils are then able to respond more effectively to a challenging agonist, be it soluble or particulate, including microbial pathogens. This has been shown as an increased expression of functional surface receptors (CR3, FcγR), increased particle adhesion and phagocytosis, increased release of ROIs and degranulation, and increase in microbial killing or tissue damage (Klebanoff et al. 1986; Ferrante et al. 1987; Ferrante 1989).

Many cytokines have been shown to alter neutrophil responses, in terms of priming. These include TNF-α, TNF-β, GM-CSF, G-CSF, IL-1, IFN-γ, IFN-β, IL-2, and IL-8 (Coffey 1992). Receptors for many of these cytokines have been described on neutrophils. Treatment of neutrophils with some of these cytokines alone produces little response, fulfilling the role as primers and enabling the cell to undergo rapid stimulation upon engagement of microbial pathogens (Ferrante 1992). Increases in formyl-methionine-leucine-phenylalanine (fMLP) receptor, CR3, and FcγR expression have been described during the priming phase (Klebanoff et al. 1986; Kumaratilake et al. 1995). Priming of neutrophils can also be achieved by exposing the cells to cytokine-rich supernatants from stimulated T cells or macrophages, or from purified cytokine from these cells (Kumaratilake et al. 1991; Ferrante 1992) and even after direct contact with activated T lymphocytes (Zhang et al. 1992). Peripheral blood mononuclear cells stimulated with heat-killed *Staphylococcus aureus* produce high amounts of TNF-α and IL-1. These supernatants were found to prime neutrophils for increased killing of opsonized *S. aureus* and this property was primarily caused by TNF-α (Ferrante 1992). Table 4.3 outlines the properties of TNF-α more extensively.

An examination of the various models of microbial killing by cytokine-primed neutrophils shows that, in models such as the killing of opsonized, pathogenic, free-living amoebae, e.g. *Naegeria fowleri*, unprimed neutrophils have little effect and only attain amoebicidal properties once primed with cytokines (Ferrante and Mocatta 1984). In other cases, the neutrophils kill the bacteria, such as *S. aureus*, but this killing can be markedly improved by priming the neutrophils (Ferrante et al. 1993b). Interestingly, Kowanko et al. (1996) showed that such priming for killing of *S. aureus* was oxygen-dependent, but oxygen-independent for killing of intraerythrocytic asexual blood stages of *Plasmodium falciparum*. In the case of blood stages of *P. falciparum*, the merozoite and asexual intraerythrocytic stages, TNF-primed neutrophils will also show enhanced killing in the absence of opsonins, although it is much more marked when the parasites have been opsonized with antibody and complement (Kumaratilake et al. 1991, 1992; Ferrante et al. 1993a). This suggests that priming may also enhance killing when recognition is via a pattern-recognition system.

Table 4.3 *Properties of TNF-primed neutrophils*

Increased expression of CR3, FcγR, fMLPR
Inhibited migration
Increased agonist-induced respiratory burst in response to:
fMLP
opsonized bacteria
opsonized yeast/fungi
opsonized parasites
Increased agonist-induced degranulation in response to:
fMLP
opsonized bacteria
opsonized yeast/fungi
opsonized parasites
Increased microbial killing, e.g. for
Staphylococcus aureus
Streptococcus pneumoniae
Candida albicans
Plasmodium falciparum merozoites and intraerythrocytic asexual blood stage
pathogenic free-living amoebae
Increased tissue damage:
articular cartilage

fMLP, formyl–methionine–lysine–phenylalanine or f-Met-Lys-Phe; fMLPR, fMLP receptor; TNF, tumor necrosis factor.

Neutrophil priming by other exogenous and endogenous inflammatory mediators, apart from cytokines, also occurs, e.g. fMLP, a microbial peptide, is a poor neutrophil stimulator of respiratory burst and degranulation but a strong chemotactic agent and a strong neutrophil priming agent for the former two responses. This thus enables cells to arrive at inflammatory sites relatively controlled and primed to respond to bacteria. Products of the cyclooxygenase pathway, in particular LTB_4 and 5-oxo-6,8,11,14-eicosatetraenoic acid (5-oxo-ETE), will also act as neutrophil priming agents to increase neutrophil adhesion, superoxide production, and degranulation (Powell et al. 1997; Ferrante et al. 1999).

ROLE OF NEUTROPHILS IN MICROBIAL DEFENSE

The importance of neutrophils in immunity to bacterial and fungal infections has been appreciated for over a century and their role in immunity to protozoan and metazoan parasites has been more recently recognized. The first line of evidence for a role of neutrophils in resistance against infection is demonstrated by the susceptibility of microbial pathogens to various products of neutrophils. Second, provided that the relevant opsonic factors are present, neutrophils have been shown to engulf bacteria such as *S. aureus*, *Pseudomonas aeruginosa*, *Streptococcus pneumoniae*, and *Haemophilus influenzae* and also fungi such as *Candida albicans*. Asexual intraerythrocytic blood stages of *P. falciparum* are readily engulfed and destroyed by neutrophils (Ferrante et al. 1993a). Larger unicellular (amoebae) and multicellular (such as nematodes, microfilaria, etc.) parasites are, however, killed by an extracellular mechanism.

There is an overwhelming demonstration of the accumulation of neutrophils at sites of microbial pathogens in the tissues. These include numerous types of bacteria, fungi, and parasites. It is not uncommon to find neutrophils with engulfed bacteria at these sites. Furthermore, a range of microbial products promotes neutrophil accumulation at inflammatory sites.

Experiments of nature demonstrate an important role of neutrophils in resistance against infection. Neutropenia, whether hereditary or drug induced, leads to increased risk of infection and death from overwhelming infection. Neutropenic patients are in particular susceptible to both bacterial and fungal infections. Several neutrophil functional defects also predispose children to severe/recurrent life-threatening infection.

In experimental animal models of infection, the role of the neutrophil has also been established. Experimentally induced neutropenia makes animals highly susceptible to bacterial, fungal, and parasitic infections. In some cases, such as infections with nematodes and pathogenic free-living amoebae, depletion of neutrophils from immune mice renders them highly susceptible to these infections (Penttila et al. 1985; Ferrante 1992).

Primed neutrophils show increase antimicrobial activity. In vitro there is evidence that neutrophil-mediated killing of microbial pathogens can be increased dramatically by priming with cytokines such as TNF, GM-CSF, IL-1, LTs, and IFN-γ (Coffey 1992; Tan et al. 1995). In some cases neutrophils fail to show any significant killing of the microorganism unless the cells have been primed with these agents (Ferrante 1992). It is interesting that human peripheral blood mononuclear cells stimulated with heat-killed *S. aureus* generate supernatants that are very effective neutrophil-priming agents, and this activity can be ablated by treatment with anti-TNF antibodies (Ferrante 1992). The role of TNF-primed neutrophils in microbial killing has been extended to several bacteria, including *H. influenzae* and *Legionella pneumophila* (Blanchard 1992; Tan et al. 1995).

Interestingly, neutrophils recovered from immune mice can kill microbial pathogens at significantly greater rates (Ferrante 1992; Penttila et al. 1984). In other studies with experimental infection models, it has been shown that infusion of cytokines increases the resistance against bacterial, fungal, and parasitic infection. Furthermore, immunized mice resistant to microbial pathogens can be severely compromised by treatment with anti-TNF or anti-GM-CSF antibodies (Coffey 1992; Ferrante 1992).

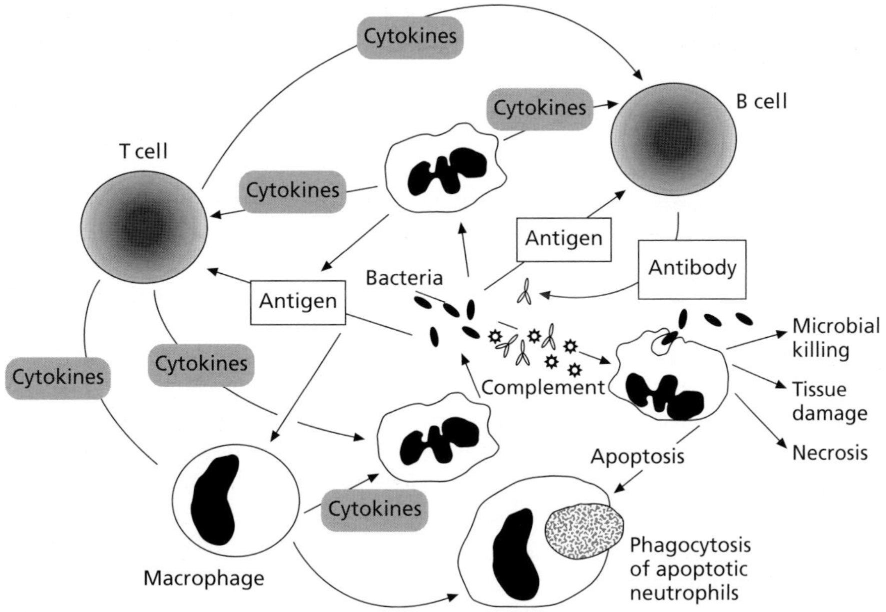

Figure 4.7 *An abridged version of the intricate interrelationship of neutrophils, lymphocytes, and mononuclear phagocytes. The main function of the neutrophil is to phagocytose microbial pathogens. Phagocytosis is promoted by coating of the bacteria with antibody and complement. Neutrophil recognition of particles, phagocytosis, and killing is greatly accelerated by priming neutrophils with cytokines released by T lymphocytes and macrophages. Downregulation of tissue damage by activated neutrophils is achieved through the stimulation of apoptosis in neutrophils and engulfment by macrophages. The likely contribution of neutrophils to T- and B-lymphocyte responses is also demonstrated in this scheme.*

APOPTOSIS

Activation of a cell-intrinsic suicide program results in programmed cell death or apoptosis, which can be distinguished from degenerative cell death or necrosis. The dying cell is characterized by several properties such as shrinkage, crenation, condensed chromatin, and DNA fragmentation. Apoptosis is controlled by many types of endogenous and exogenous mediators. Neutrophil apoptosis is considered a host tissue-protective property because these cells lose their functional receptors and ability to produce toxic products, and are eventually engulfed and removed by macrophages (Fanning et al. 1999). This aging fate of neutrophils was first indicated by Metchnikoff (1893).

Neutrophils reaching inflammatory sites engulf and kill microbial pathogens and die at these sites. Death via necrosis leads to the release of tissue-damaging products. Thus, the physiological response, besides initiating events that lead to microbial killing, also ensures the subsequent initiation of apoptotic signals to downregulate the powerful oxidative and nonoxidative responses of the neutrophils and finally leads to the clearance of neutrophils from these sites (Newman et al. 1982). Inflammatory leukocytes, such as activated neutrophils, express Fas, a death factor receptor. Ligation of this receptor transduces the intracellular signals for apoptotic death (French and Tschopp 1997). Apoptotic signals in neutrophils lead to a loss in their ability to respond to inflammatory mediators because their cell surface receptors are downregulated. There is also a major loss in chemotactic, phagocytic, degranulation, and respiratory burst function. Further isolation from their toxic products results from the engulfment of the apoptotic neutrophils by macrophages. Essentially, this is a means of limiting tissue injury as demonstrated in Figure 4.7. It is believed that apoptotic neutrophils are recognized by either the exposure of phosphatidylserine on their surface and/or expression of a thrombospondin-binding moiety that recognizes thrombospondin and allows binding to the vitronectin (CD16) receptor on macrophages (Fadok et al. 1992).

Inflammatory fluids contain many different factors some of which protect against apoptosis. The cytokines G-CSF, GM-CSF and IL-2, as well as LPS and glucocorticoids, inhibit neutrophil apoptosis. However, conflicting data have been presented for TNF and fMLP.

PRODUCTION OF INFLAMMATORY MEDIATORS

Neutrophils play a central role in the inflammatory response in contributing to the inflammatory mediator network by releasing a range of mediators, including oxygen radicals, enzymes such as MPO, LTs, and prostaglandins (PGs) as well as a range of cytokines (Table 4.4). In this manner, neutrophils could have a significant influence on the acute and chronic inflammatory responses, as well as the immune response, by regulating T lymphocyte, macrophage, and antigen-presenting cell functions (Figure 4.8).

Table 4.4 *Products of stimulated neutrophils which may regulate inflammation and immune responses*

Class of mediator	Mediator
Lipids	PAF, AA, LTB4, PGE2, lipoxins, TXA4, 5-oxo-ETE
Cytokines	IL-1, TNF-α, IFN-α, IL-8, IL-6, TGF-β, IL-12, IL-10, IL-3, G-CSF, M-CSF, MCP-1, MIP-2, IL-1α

AA, arachidonic acid; CSF, colony-stimulating factor; G-CSF, granulocyte CSF; M-CSF, macrophage CSF; IFN, interferon; IL, interleukin; LT, leukotriene; MCP, monocytic chemotactic peptide; MIP, macrophage inflammatory protein; PAF, platelet-activating factor; PG, prostaglandin; 5-oxo-ETE, 5-oxo-6,8,11,14-eicosatetraenoic acid; TGF, transforming growth factor; TNF, tumor necrosis factor; Tx, thromboxane.

Lipid inflammatory mediators

Through the action of a number of cellular enzymes, such as phospholipase (PLA_2), cyclooxygenases, and lipoxygenases, neutrophils release a range of mediators (see Table 4.4). Several mediators produced are known for their marked effects on inflammation and immune responses (Haeggstrom and Serhan 1999). These include arachidonic acid (AA), LTB_4, PGE_2, and platelet-activating factor (PAF), all of which regulate neutrophil, eosinophil, basophil, T-lymphocyte, macrophage, and endothelial cell function.

Platelet-activating factor plays a role in both acute and chronic inflammation. It stimulates a range of neutrophil activities including chemotaxis, aggregation, adherence, respiratory burst, and degranulation. LTs have diverse effects and may promote the pathophysiological process during infection by stimulating endothelial cell function, upregulating macrophage, and lymphocyte functions. This contrasts with their role in promoting pathophysiology in rheumatoid arthritis, airway diseases such as asthma and adult respiratory distress syndrome, allergic inflammation, and cystic fibrosis (Penrose et al. 1999).

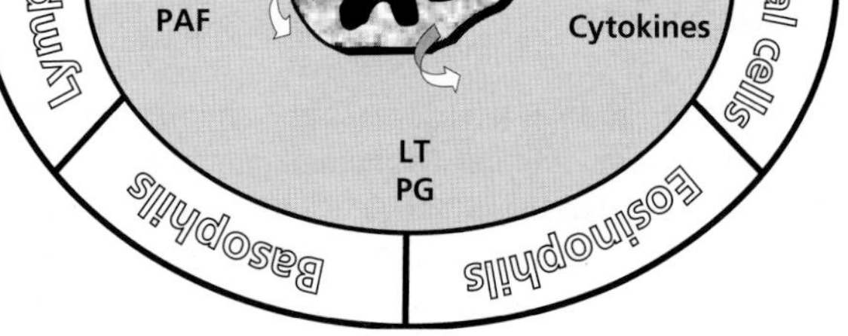

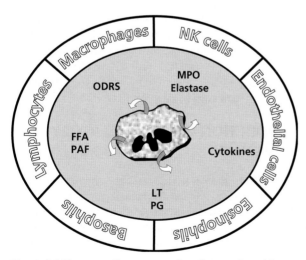

Figure 4.8 *Diagrammatic summary of mediators released by stimulated neutrophils and the cells that these may regulate. FFA, free fatty acid; LT, leukotriene; MPO, myeloperoxidase; NK, natural killer; PAF, platelet-activating factor; PG, prostaglandin.*

Prostaglandins, produced during the oxidation of AA via the cyclooxygenase pathway, have a wide range of effects and play a role in both physiological and pathophysiological responses (Griffith 1999). These regulate pain, edema, fever, and granulocyte, macrophage and lymphocyte function. PGE_2 suppresses neutrophil functions, chemotaxis, and respiratory burst. It also inhibits the activation of mononuclear phagocytes, depressing TNF synthesis. Inhibition of T-cell function, lymphoproliferation, and cytokine production are also inhibited by PGE_2, in particular the Th1 cytokines.

Cytokines

Although mature neutrophils have been considered as end cells not capable of RNA and protein synthesis, more recent evidence suggests that they can be induced to synthesize new proteins (Cassatella 1999). Most interesting has been the discovery that neutrophils can produce a wide range of cytokines (see Table 4.4). In this manner, the cells can regulate immune reactions. Although these cytokines are produced in very low amounts by neutrophils compared with macrophages, with a predominance of neutrophils in some inflammatory sites, it is possible that neutrophils release effective amounts of these cytokines to control other cells of the inflammatory response. Through the ability to release the spectrum of cytokines outlined in Table 4.4, neutrophils have the potential to control migration of mononuclear cells into tissues as well as to promote their activation. Thus, T lymphocytes as well as B lymphocytes may be under neutrophil control through the release of cytokines such as IL-1, IL-6, IL-10, IL-3, etc. Similarly, these and others will influence the function of mononuclear phagocytes and APCs. In this manner neutrophils that arrive early in inflammatory sites and antigen injection sites are likely to have some influence on the inflammatory response. The examination of the spectrum of cytokines produced by neutrophils shows that these may be of either Th1 or Th2 type, suggesting that the neutrophil could influence the type of immune response elicited by microbial antigens. Similarly, there are cytokines that regulate macrophage functions.

Interestingly, apart from a wide range of compounds able to stimulate cytokine production by neutrophils, there is also evidence that different stimulators may cause the production of different types of cytokines and that both extrinsic and intrinsic stimulators can induce cytokine production in these cells (Cassatella 1999). Extrinsic agents include bacteria, fungi, and viruses and fMLP. Intrinsic stimulators include LTB_4, PAF, C5a and of course the cytokines themselves. The ability to produce IL-1 receptor antagonist (IL-1ra) enables the neutrophil to regulate the activity of the pyrogenic cytokine, IL-1.

Neutrophils, through the release of IL-8 (a CXC chemokine), can regulate the migration of other neutrophils and stimulate these cells for antimicrobial functions. As IL-8 is also chemotactic for T lymphocytes and basophils, neutrophils could be involved in exerting influence on these cell types during inflammation. Other CXC chemokines produced by neutrophils that have effects similar to IL-8 on neutrophils are growth-related gene product α/β (GROα/β) and IFN-γ-inducible protein (IP-10) which are mainly chemotactic for natural killer (NK) cells, and may therefore be important in the recruitment of these cells, as well as T cells and monocytes. Neutrophils can also secrete CC chemokines, such as macrophage inflammatory protein 1-α/β (MIP-α/β), which have potent chemotactic properties for monocytes and T lymphocytes.

The three cytokines that are classically referred to as the pyrogenic cytokines, TNF-α, IL-1, and IL-6, can also be produced by neutrophils. Thus, there is the potential for neutrophils to mediate pathogenesis by releasing these cytokines. Both TNF-α and IL-1 are also known to prime neutrophils for increased antimicrobial activity and it is possible that neutrophils may autoregulate their antimicrobial functions in this manner. The ability of these cytokines to regulate lymphocyte activation and differentiation enables neutrophils also to influence this property of the immunological system. The expression of the CD30 ligand (CD30L), a member of the nerve growth factor (NGF)/TNF receptor super family) on neutrophils suggests that neutrophils could interact via CD30 on T lymphocytes to promote activation of these cells. Neutrophils can also produce IL-1ra, which controls the effects of IL-1. This represents another level of regulation of inflammation and pathogenesis by neutrophils. A variety of agents is also capable of inducing the production of IL-1ra in neutrophils. The influence that stimulated the effects that neutrophils may have on the development of the Th1 versus the Th2 response can be extrapolated from their reported ability to produce and release IL-12, which induces IFN-γ production from NK cells and T lymphocytes, and a cytokine that facilitates Th1 lymphocyte responses and thereby suppresses IgE formation.

Although the amount of cytokine produced by neutrophils compared with macrophages is very small, in a number of inflammatory conditions neutrophils are present in substantial numbers and may contribute to immunoregulation through the release of selective cytokine patterns. Important consideration needs, however, to be given in specific situations, e.g. the ability of neutrophils to produce IFN-α in similar levels to that produced by monocytes when infected with Sendai virus suggests an important role for neutrophils in defense against viruses.

NEUTROPHIL IMMUNODEFICIENCY DISEASES

Congenital defects

The spectrum of primary neutrophil disorders is listed in Table 4.5. These range from disorders in which the numbers of neutrophils are too low to cope with infections to others that show functional defects of chemotaxis, adhesion, respiratory burst, and degranulation (Quile et al. 1996).

NEUTROPENIA

Leukocyte counts of below 1500 cells/mm^2 will increase the risk of infection in a progressive manner as the numbers continue to decrease below this level. A dramatic increase in incidence of infection is seen once the levels are below 500 cells/mm^2. Hereditary neutropenia occurs, ranging from severe, as seen in infantile genetic agranulocytosis, to moderate, as in familial neutropenia. The former disorder is a result of maturation arrest that is inherited in an autosomal recessive manner. Patients with hereditary neutropenia experience severe infection and death in infancy. Another neutropenia characterized by the periodic disappearance of neutrophils from the blood is cyclic neutropenia, an autosomal dominant disorder. During the period of low neutrophil counts, the patient can present with cutaneous infections and associated fever and malaise. Overcoming the neutropenic oscillations can be achieved with G-CSF or prednisolone treatment.

LEUKOCYTE ADHESION DEFICIENCY

Two types of leukocyte adhesion deficiency (LAD) have been described. In type 1 there is a defect in the integrin molecule. This is the result of an abnormal β-chain synthesis presenting as a spectrum of mutations in the β gene. Although the α chain is produced in normal amounts, the assembly of the α and β chains is poor and is poorly transported to the cell surface. The neutrophils have impaired adherence, chemotaxis, and respiratory burst in response to complement- but not antibody-coated particles. Although cells from these individuals display normal rolling adhesion, they cannot bind firmly to venule walls and hence are unable to migrate out of the blood vessels. This is an autosomal recessive disease after a history of consanguinity. Patients are likely to present with prolonged, as well as recurrent, infections with *Pseudomonas* and *Staphylococcus* spp. during

Table 4.5 *Summary of primary immunodeficiencies of neutrophils*

Disease	Function affected
Neutropenia	
Infantile genetic agranulocytosis	
Familial neutropenia	
Cyclic neutropenia	
Leukocyte adhesion deficiency	
Type 1 (CR3 deficiency)	Adhesion, chemotaxis, aggregation, spreading
Type 2 (sialyl Lewis deficiency)	Selectin ligation, rolling, adhesion
Chronic granulomatosis disease	
Membrane defects of	Oxidase (lack of production of oxygen reactive species)
$gp91^{phox}$	
$p22^{phox}$	
Cytosol defects of	
$p47^{phox}$	
$p67^{phox}$	
Chédiak–Higashi syndrome	Granules (giant lysosomal granules): decreased chemotaxis, degranulation and bactericidal activity, increased H_2O_2 production, deficient elastase and cathepsin G
Specific granule deficiency	Specific granules are absent; decreased chemotaxis, O_2^- production, bactericidal activity
Myeloperoxidase (MPO) deficiency	Absent or low MPO
Hyper-IgE (Job's) syndrome	Chemotactic defect

infancy. Poor wound healing can also occur which can manifest in delayed umbilical cord separation. Infection sites include the intestinal tract, soft tissues, and mucosal surfaces. Those individuals who survive infancy are likely to develop acute gingivitis and eventually gingival hypertrophy. Patients with the moderate phenotype may survive to adulthood. It has been estimated that two-fifths of patients with type 1 LAD die before 2 years of age.

In LAD type 2, the defect is an absence of expression of the primary selectin ligand sLe^x on the neutrophils. This is an autosomal recessive disorder in which poor random mobility and chemotactic responses by neutrophils are exhibited. However, the respiratory burst response to opsonized particles does lie within a normal range. The neutrophils fail to adhere to stimulated venules and lack rolling adhesion. As the integrin expression is normal the neutrophils still adhere to blood vessel walls. Patients present from early childhood with recurrent bacterial infections.

CHRONIC GRANULOMATOUS DISEASE

Chronic granulomatous disease is a group of disorders of phagocyte oxidative respiratory burst which can be inherited either in an X-linked or an autosomal recessive manner. The basis of this deficiency is the result of a defect in one of several components that make up the oxidase. Abnormalities in the membrane-bound component $gp91^{phox}$ of cytochrome b_{558} give rise to the most common form of CGD (55–60 percent). Defects of the light chain of the membrane cytochrome, $gp22^{phox}$ have also been described with an approximate frequency of 5 percent. Defects in the cytosolic components $p47^{phox}$ and $p67^{phox}$ account for 30–35 and 5 percent of the CGD, respectively.

Chronic granulomatous disease is manifested clinically by the development of serious infections in early childhood. Pneumonia, skin and soft tissue infections, lung abscesses, osteomyelitis, and hepatic abscesses may be common. The majority of the infections can be accounted for by *S. aureus* and *Serratia burkholderia* and, less commonly, by infection with *Aspergillus* and *Nocardia* spp. Management of patients with CGD primarily involves aggressive antibiotic cover, surgical drainage, and even white cell transfusion. Prophylactic IFN-γ has recently been employed which has reduced the occurrence of these life-threatening infections. It is recommended that IFN-γ be used in conjunction with trimethoprim–sulfamethoxazole. Efforts are being made at present to use gene therapy to correct the defect in CGD, with some early success with retroviral-mediated gene therapy for $p47^{phox}$ deficiency.

CHÉDIAK–HIGASHI SYNDROME

Neutrophils from patients with Chédiak–Higashi syndrome (CHS) show abnormal (large) granules as a result of fusion of two granules. Although the cells can phagocytose particles, chemotaxis and microbial killing are abnormal. The respiratory burst and its ability to produce oxygen-reactive species is normal but the release of MPO is delayed. The neutrophils show deficiency in cathepsin G and elastase. There is abnormal fusion of granules, possibly as a result of defects in membrane fluidity and the microtubules. The bactericidal activity of the cell is greatly diminished as a consequence of a delay in the delivery of granule constituents to the phagocytic vacuole. Apart from neutrophils, defective functions of other cells of the immune system occur, impaired NK cell activity, and antibody-dependent, cell-mediated cytotoxicity. Cytotoxic T-cell activity is also affected. Decreased neutrophil and monocyte migration and reduced bactericidal activity are likely to explain the delayed inflammatory response and the increased susceptibility to infections expressed by patients with CHS, who usually die from infections at an early age.

SPECIFIC GRANULE DEFICIENCY

Patients with an absence of specific granules have been described. Their neutrophils lack specific granule constituents such as lactoferrin and vitamin B_{12}-binding protein. However, it has also been found that the cells are devoid of defensins, which are major components of the azurophilic granule. Thus, there is likely to be a more general defect. As a result of the lack of specific granules, upregulation of functional surface receptors is compromised. It is not surprising to find that neutrophils have chemotactic defects. Patients present with recurrent infections.

MYELOPEROXIDASE DEFICIENCY

This is the most common of the neutrophil disorders. This deficiency may go unnoticed because, in many individuals, the susceptibility to infection is not easily recognized and only a few cases have been reported with serious infections, mainly candidiasis. Killing of microorganisms is delayed because of the absence of MPO. Other functions such as chemotaxis, phagocytosis, respiratory burst, and degranulation are normal. Superoxide levels may be increased because of the lack of MPO and this may compensate for the lack of killing of bacteria via the MPO–H_2O_2–halide system.

HYPER-IgE SYNDROME (JOB'S SYNDROME)

Patients with extremely high levels of IgE have depressed neutrophil chemotaxis and depressed acute inflammation. One of the suggested causes of this is the release of histamine. These patients present with recurrent cutaneous and sinopulmonary infections. Characteristically, the infections are caused by *S. aureus*, but in some cases *H. influenzae* causes pulmonary infections. T lymphocytes from these patients have also been reported to be deficient in IFN-γ production and it has been suggested that an imbalance between IL-4 and IFN-γ production leads to downstream switching of immunoglobulin genes, giving rise to elevated IgE. Although some sporadic cases have been described, hyper-IgE syndrome is an autosomal dominant disease.

Acquired immunodeficiencies of neutrophils

Secondary immunodeficiency of neutrophils, as with primary immunodeficiency, spans a wide range, but will usually occur in combinations because of the nonspecific nature of the causative agent. This includes malnutrition, cancer and chemotherapy, infection, immaturity of the immune system in neonates, and deterioration as a result of age. The hallmark of these diseases is the increased severity and recurrence of infection, as for primary immunodeficiencies, although it is considered not to be as severe.

Drug therapy is responsible for acquired neutropenias, seen in patients undergoing chemotherapy for immunological and neoplastic disorders. Idiosyncratic reaction may occur when drugs such as penicillin, cephalosporins, vancomycin, sulfonamides, and phenothiazines are used. With antibody-mediated neutrophil damage or hypersplenism, neutropenia is experienced because of sequestration of the neutrophils in splenic tissue (Palmblad et al. 2001).

Diseases in which circulating immune complexes occur, including rheumatoid arthritis, systemic lupus erythematosus, etc., can show a high rate of oxidative respiratory burst and granule release, and decrease in chemotactic responses. Other forms of serum chemotactic inhibitors have been found. Bactericidal products may cause neutrophil chemotactic abnormalities as seen, for example, in some patients with gingival infections with *Bacterioides ochraceus* (Clark et al. 1977).

Treatment of these infections restores chemotactic responsiveness. IgG antineutrophil antibodies have also been implicated with neutrophil chemotactic responsiveness seen in patients with recurrent skin infections. Other agents that can cause decreased chemotactic responsiveness include the drugs amphotericin B and tetracyclines, and alcohol. Other causes of acquired chemotactic immunodeficiencies include malnutrition, physiological immaturity of the neonate, viral infections, sepsis, and thermal injury. In leukemia, thermal injury, various autoimmune conditions, sepsis, and viral infections, the neutrophil microbicidal activity can also be significantly reduced. Viral infections can lead to decreased neutrophil functions and associated risk of bacterial infections (Faden and Ogra 1986). Thus, during epidemics of influenza, deaths have been associated with bacterial pneumonia. Viruses have been shown to depress neutrophil chemotaxis, phagocytosis, and respiratory burst/intracellular killing.

A range of bacteria as well as fungi and parasites cause depressed neutrophil chemotaxis, phagocytosis, and oxidative burst. The pneumococcal toxin, pneumolysin was found to cause marked inhibition of neutrophil-mediated killing of *S. pneumonia* and the respiratory burst of the cell (Paton and Ferrante 1983).

Therapies for neutrophil disorders

Marked neutropenia and severe neutrophil function defects lead to life-threatening infections (Walsh et al. 1994). Antibiotic prophylaxis is used in most cases, although the development of antibiotic-resistant organisms presents another problem. Other forms of therapies include neutrophil transfusion, bone marrow transplantation, and cytokine infusions.

Neutrophil transfusion is of possible benefit to neutropenic patients with infections, although the results from some of the clinical trials have questioned whether the patients actually benefit. Nevertheless, benefits can be achieved if a careful approach is taken (Strauss 1999). There are various explanations for the inconsistencies in results with this type of therapy, including the severity of the infection and the various antibiotics used. Thus transfusions should be used in combination with the various therapies, antibiotics, immunoglobulin, and recombinant growth factors. The decision to proceed with neutrophil infusion should be guided by ensuring that relevant preparation methods are used and effective doses are given to patients. Neutrophils prepared from donors who have received G-CSF seem to give a more favorable response.

Bone marrow transplantation has been used successfully in LAD and CGD and more recently hemopoietic progenitor cell transfusions have become an attractive option. The treatment of patients with recombinant hemopoietic growth factors such as G-CSF is very attractive; it has proved useful to enhance bone marrow recovery as a consequence of chemotherapy and was beneficial in protecting against infection in these patients. According to reported information, low-dose G-CSF in patients with cyclic and idiopathic neutropenia is effective in elevating circulating neutrophil numbers and decreasing the episodes of fever and infections. In congenital neutropenia high doses of G-CSF are needed.

Trials have also been conducted on the use of G-CSF in non-neutropenic patients with pneumonia. These patients experienced an increase in neutrophil levels as well as clinical improvement. In addition, cytokine therapy has been used in CGD. The incidence of life-threatening infection in CGD patients can be markedly reduced with prophylactic IFN-γ. Both the number and the severity of infections are dramatically reduced (Quie et al. 1996). The action is most likely through a multiple effect, including restoration of some functional oxidase activity, macrophage granule stimulation, and increased expression of functional receptors such as FcγR. This cytokine is recommended in conjunction with antimicrobial agents as a prophylactic for CGD.

Laboratory diagnosis of neutrophil deficiencies

The various neutrophil immunodeficiency syndromes can be easily diagnosed by a series of laboratory tests (Metcalf, Gallin et al. 1986; Kuijpers et al. 1999; Virella 1999). These tests can range from very simple procedures to those requiring much more sophistication. Although some tests will measure a specific pathway, others measure the activity of several pathways culminating in a final event. When the defect in neutrophil function is severe, patients will usually present with recurrent and life-threatening infections. An outline of the tests used to assess the competence of neutrophils in a patient is summarized in Table 4.6. Usually evaluations would proceed to this group of tests when recurrent bacterial and fungal infections in patients cannot be explained by neutropenia, defects of antibody or complement, and T-cell abnormalities.

Leukocyte adhesion deficiency can be diagnosed by functional and flow cytometric analysis and the two forms, LAD1 and LAD2, should be differentiated. In LAD1 there is deficient expression of the α and β chains

Table 4.6 *Neutrophil functional tests for diagnosis of primary immunodeficiency*

Function	**Tests**
LAD1	Adhesion of neutrophils
	Flow cytometry
LAD2	Flow cytometry
Chemotaxis	Migration under agarose
	Boyden chamber
	Modified/commercial Boyden chamber
Phagocytosis	Uptake of yeast particles/by microscopy
	Uptake of particles by flow cytometry
	Radiometric assay
	Erythrocyte lysis assay
NADPH oxidase	NBT assay
	Chemiluminescence (lucigenin)
	O_2^{-} or H_2O_2 assays
	HMP shunt
MPO	Quantitative leukocyte iodination assay
	MPO enzyme assay
	Histochemical assay
Microbicidal activity	Bactericidal assay
	Fungicidal assay

HMP, hexose monophosphate; LAD, leukocyte adhesion deficiency; MPO, myeloperoxidase; NADPH, reduced nicotinamide adenine dinucleotide phosphate; NBT, nitroblue tetrazolium.

of the integrins, and hence antibodies to these surface molecules can be used in conjunction with flow cytometry to diagnose this deficiency. Similarly the detection of the surface expression of sLe^x is a diagnostic tool for LAD2. The ability for neutrophils from these patients to adhere to plasma-coated surfaces in microtiter plates can be measured when these cells are either treated or not treated with agonists such as TNF or fMLP. The ability to respond to complement-coated particles that are ligated to neutrophils via the CR3 receptor can also be diagnostic for LAD1. Because these cells are unable to adhere to substrates they will also show a deficiency of chemotaxis.

Chemotactic assays have now been relatively standardized and defects of chemotaxis can be identified by these assay methods. The two methods that are usually used are the technique of migration under agarose and in chemotactic chambers, developed by Boyden and referred to as the Boyden chamber (Boyden 1962), and modifications thereof (Rot 1999). In the former assay, wells are cut into agarose into which cells and a chemotactic agent such as fMLP can be applied. As the fMLP diffuses through the agarose, a chemotactic gradient is set up which attracts the cells and the distance migrated can be measured microscopically.

The Boyden chamber and related chambers consist of two compartments separated by a filter that contains pores to enable neutrophils to crawl through from one chamber toward the chemotactic agent in the other chamber. The distance moved or number of cells moved into the filter is measured to ascertain the chemotactic response. Once again fMLP is used most commonly as the chemotactic agent but others include LTB_4 and complement, e.g. C5a, IL-8.

Measurement of the phagocytic activity of the cell can be quite difficult because it is difficult to distinguish between adhered and engulfed particles. Some techniques can be rather subjective when microscopic counting of internalized particles is conducted. The particles used include zymosan (yeast), *C. albicans*, and erythrocytes. These are opsonized for promoting recognition by neutrophils. One means of distinguishing between adhered and ingested particles is to use radiolabeled *S. aureus* and then eliminate those that have not been ingested by treating with lysostaphin. A radiometric technique has also been described that takes into consideration that there is little RNA synthesis in neutrophils. In this assay, after an incubation period to allow phagocytosis to take place, $[^3H]$uridine, which is readily taken up by non-engulfed bacteria or fungi, is added to the cultures. The amount of inhibition of uridine uptake measures an index of phagocytic power. Other systems make use of erythrocytes and hypotonic lysis of nonphagocytosed erythrocytes. A flow cytometry method has also been developed which makes use of fungi or bacteria with fluorescent labels and quenching of any nonengulfed bacteria with trypan blue.

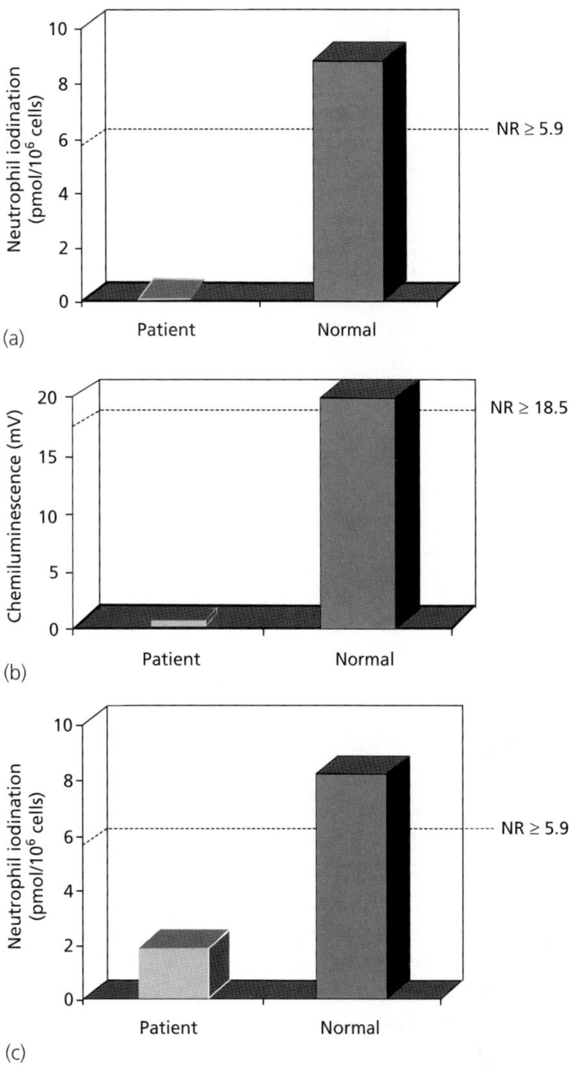

Figure 4.9 *The neutrophil iodination reaction in chronic granulomatous disease (CGD) and myeloperoxidase (MPO)-deficient neutrophils.* **(a)** *Lack of chemiluminescence response in neutrophils from patients with chronic granulomatous disease stimulated with formyl-methionine–leucine–phenylalanine (fMLP).* **(b)** *Poor leukocyte iodination reaction in the same cells stimulated with opsonized zymosan.* **(c)** *Depressed leukocyte iodination reaction in neutrophils from an MPO-deficient patient. NR, normal range.*

Defects in the oxidase can be assessed by a range of assays. The cells fail to undergo respiratory burst activity and hence do not produce oxygen-derived reaction species. Various assays are available for measuring O_2^- and H_2O_2. A standard assay for O_2^- is the superoxide dismutase-inhibitable cytochrome *c* reduction assay, which measures a color change that is read spectrophotometrically (Figure 4.9). In another system, a lucigenin-dependent chemiluminescence assay is used for measuring the superoxide produced by cells. This assay is facilitated by the used of a luminometer which dark-adapts the cells and is able to inject various components into the assay mixture.

The classic test for GGD and a detective oxidase system is the nitroblue tetrazolium (NBT) dye reduction. This is readily performed on cells adherent to microscope slides. A stimulus is used to activate the oxidase. In this reaction, the pale-yellow NBT is reduced to form a blue formazan. The cells positive for this reaction are scored microscopically. Normal cells will have more than 98 percent of the cell staining positively for NBT reduction while neutrophils from CGD patients lack staining. As a defect of the oxidase is being sought, phorbol myristate acetate (PMA) is the preferred stimulus which bypasses the surface receptor and stimulates the assembly of the oxidase by activating PKC. This excludes other possible defects such as β_2-integrin deficiencies, which can give rise to lack of activation of the oxidase because of particle adhesion defects. Then, by using opsonized zymosan in combination with PMA, defects of adhesion and ingestion can be diagnosed by the same testing system.

Flow cytometers are now readily available and a fluorescence assay that is based on the oxidation of an intracellular 2′,7′-dichlorofluorescein diacetate to the highly fluorescent 2′,7′-dichlorofluorescein can also be used to detect oxidase activity in stimulated neutrophils. Other fluorescence indicators include dihydrorhodamine 123. Both PMA and opsonized zymosan can be used to stimulate the respiratory burst.

Myeloperoxidase deficiency is the most common neutrophil disorder and various methods can be used to detect the presence or absence of MPO as well as to quantify MPO levels. This includes histochemical staining of the enzyme in cells or examining a leukocyte extract for the enzyme. A convenient method is the quantitative leukocyte iodination reaction (see Figure 4.9). This takes into consideration both the release of MPO and the production of H_2O_2 (i.e. oxidase activity). Thus, in conjunction with a measurement of the oxidase assay such as NBT or chemiluminescence, the assay can be a first-line screen for MPO deficiency (see Figure 4.9).

Neutrophil microbial killing assays are important because these represent the net effect of all the cellular components and, if the appropriate opsonin and microorganisms are chosen, this will detect most of the neutrophil defects such as LAD, MPO deficiency, NADPH oxidase defects, degranulation deficiency, and phagocytosis defects. The particles used will usually be complement-opsonized bacteria or fungi. Samples taken over the period of 1 hour for bacteria and 2 hours for fungi can be used to determine both the amount and the rate of killing, e.g. with MPO deficiency, neutrophils will show a delay in killing of *C. albicans*. For killing of bacteria, *S. aureus* is usually chosen. As this bacterium can produce H_2O_2, the lack of NADPH oxidase activity can be overcome. Thus, it is essential that the *S. aureus* used is catalase positive.

REFERENCES

Avdi, N.J., Nick, J.A., et al. 2001. Tumor necrosis factor-alpha activation of the c-Jun N-terminal kinase pathway in human neutrophils. Integrin involvement in a pathway leading from cytoplasmic tyrosine kinases apoptosis. *J Biol Chem*, **276**, 2189–99.

Bainton, D.F. 1999. Developmental biology of neutrophils and eosinophils. In: Gallin, J.I. and Snyderman, R. (eds), *Inflammation: basic principles and clinical correlates*. Philadelphia: Lippincott Williams & Wilkins, 13–34.

Babior, B.M. and Kipnes, R.S. 1977. Superoxide-forming enzyme from human neutrophils evidence for a flavin requirement. *Blood*, **50**, 517–24.

Babior, B.M., Kipnes, R.S. and Curnutte, J.T. 1973. Biological defence mechanisms: The production of leukocytes of superoxide, a potential bactericidal agent. *J Clin Invest*, **52**, 741–4.

Blanchard, D.K. 1992. TNF in Legionella infection. In: Beutler, B. (ed.), *Tumor necrosis factor: The molecules and their emerging role in medicine*. New York: Raven Press Ltd, 293–302.

Borregaard, N. and Cowland, J.B. 1997. Granule of the human neutrophilic polymorphonuclear leukocyte. *Blood*, **89**, 3503–21.

Boyden, S. 1962. The chemotactic effect of mixtures of antibody and antigen on polymorphonuclear leukocytes. *J Exp Med*, **115**, 453–66.

Cassatella, M.A. 1999. Production of cytokines by polymorphonuclear neutrophils. In: Gabrilovich, D. (ed.), *The neutrophils: new outlook for old cells*. London: Imperial College Press, 151–229.

Clark, R.A., Page, R.C. and Wilde, G. 1977. Defective neutrophil chemotaxis in juvenile periodontitis. *Infect Immun*, **18**, 694–700.

Coffey, R.G. (ed.) 1992. *Granulocyte responses to cytokines: basic and clinical research*. New York: Marcel Dekker Inc.

Edwards, S.W. 1994. *Biochemistry and physiology of the neutrophil*. New York: Cambridge University Press.

Elsbach, P. and Weiss, J. 1983. A re-evaluation of the roles of the O_2-dependent and O_2-independent microbicidal systems of phagocytes. *Rev Infect Dis*, **5**, 843–53.

Faden, H. and Ogra, P. 1986. Neutrophil and antiviral defence. *Pediatr Infect Dis J*, **5**, 86–92.

Fadok, V.A., Savill, J.S., et al. 1992. Different populations of macrophage use either the vitronectin receptor or the phosphatidylserine receptor to recognise and remove apoptotic cells. *J Immunol*, **149**, 4029–35.

Fanning, N.F., Redmond, H.P. and Bouchier-Hayes, D. 1999. Neutrophil apoptosis. In: Gabrilovich, D.I. (ed.), *The neutrophils: New outlook for old cells*. London: Imperial College Press, 231–42.

Ferrante, A. 1989. Tumour necrosis factor alpha potentiates neutrophil antimicrobial activity: increased fungicidal activity against *Torulopsis glabrata/Candida albicans* and associated increases in oxygen radical production and lysosomal enzyme release. *Infect Immun*, **57**, 2115–22.

Ferrante, A. 1992. Activation of neutrophils by interleukins-1 and 2 and tumor necrosis factors. In: Coffey, R.G. (ed.), *Granulocyte responses to cytokines, basic and clinical research*. Tampa, FL: Marcel Dekker Inc, 417–36.

Ferrante, A. and Mocatta, T. 1984. Human neutrophils require activation by mononuclear leukocyte conditioned medium to kill the pathogenic free-living amoeba, *Naegeria fowleri*. *Clin Exp Immunol*, **56**, 556–9.

Ferrante, A., Hill, N.L., et al. 1987. A role for myeloperoxidase in the killing of *Naegleria fowleri* by lymphokine-altered human neutrophils. *Infect Immun*, **55**, 1047–50.

Ferrante, A., Kumaratilake, L.M. and Rathjen, D.A. 1993a. Cytokine regulation of phagocytic cells in immunity to malaria. In: Good, M. and Saul, A. (eds), *Molecular immunological consideration in malaria vaccine development*. Boca Raton, CA: CRC Press, 47–95.

Ferrante, A., Martin, A.J., et al. 1993b. Killing of *Staphylococcus aureus* by tumor necrosis factor α-activated neutrophils: the role of serum opsonins integrin receptors, respiratory burst and degranulation. *J Immunol*, **151**, 4821–8.

Ferrante, A., Hii, C.S.T., et al. 1999. Regulation of neutrophil function by fatty acids. In: Gabrilovich, D. (ed.), *The neutrophils: New outlook for the old cells*, Vol. 4. . London: Imperial College Press, 79–150.

French, L.E. and Tschopp, J. 1997. Thyroiditis and hepatitis: Fas on the road to disease. *Nature Med*, **3**, 387–8.

Fridovich, I. 1978. The biology of oxygen radicals: The superoxide radical is an agent of oxygen toxicity, superoxide dismutase provide an impact defence. *Science*, **201**, 875–80.

Gallin, J.I. and Snyderman, R. (eds) 1999. *Inflammation: Basic principles and clinical correlates*. Philadelphia: Lippincott Williams & Wilkins.

Greenberg, S. 1999. Biology of phagocytosis. In: Gallin, J.I. and Snyderman, R. (eds), *Inflammation: Basic principles and clinical correlates*. Philadelphia: Lippincott Williams & Wilkins, 681–701.

Griffith, R.J. 1999. Prostaglandins and inflammation. In: Gallin, J.I. and Snyderman, R. (eds), *Inflammation: Basic principles and clinical correlates*. Philadelphia: Lippincott Williams & Wilkins, 349–60.

Haeggstrom, J.Z. and Serhan, C.N. 1999. Update on arachidonic acid cascade: Leukotrienes and lipoxins in disease models. In: Serhan, C.N. and Ward, P.A. (eds), *Molecular and cellular basis of inflammation*. Totowa, NJ: Human Press Inc, 51–92.

Heyworth, P.G., Curnutte, J.T. and Badwey, J.A. 1999. Structure and regulation of NADPH oxidase of phagocytic leukocytes: insights from chronic granulomatosus disease. In: Serhan, C.N. and Ward, P.A. (eds), *Molecular and cellular basis of inflammation*. Totowa, NJ: Humana Press Inc, 165–91.

Hii, C.S.T., Stacey, K., et al. 1999. Role of extracellular signal-regulated protein kinase cascade in neutrophil killing of *S. aureus and C. albicans* and in migration. *Infect Immun*, **67**, 31297–302.

Kishimoto, T.K., Baldwin, E.T. and Anderson, D.C. 1999. The role of β_2 integrins in inflammation. In: Gallin, J.I. and Snyderman, R. (eds), *Inflammation: Basic principles and clinical correlates*. Philadelphia: Lippincott Williams & Wilkins, 537–70.

Klebanoff, S.J. 1968. Myeloperoxidase-halide-hydrogen peroxide antibacterial systems. *J Bacteriol*, **95**, 2131–8.

Klebanoff, S.J. 1999. Oxygen metabolites from phagocytes. In: Gallin, J.I. and Snyderman, R. (eds), *Inflammation: Basic principles and clinical correlates*. Philadelphia: Lippincott Williams & Wilkins, 721–768.

Klebanoff, S.J., Vadas, M.A., et al. 1986. Stimulation of neutrophils by tumor necrosis factor. *J Immunol*, **136**, 4220–5.

Kowanko, I.C., Ferrante, A., et al. 1996. Tumor necrosis factor primes neutrophils to kill *Staphylococcus aureus* by an oxygen-dependent mechanism and *Plasmodium falciparum* by an oxygen-independent mechanism. *Infect Immunity*, **64**, 3435–7.

Kuijpers, T.W., Weening, R.S. and Roos, D. 1999. Clinical and laboratory work-up patients with neutrophil shortage and dysfunction. *J Immunol Methods*, **232**, 211–29.

Kumaratilake, L.M., Ferrante, A. and Rzepczyk, C.M. 1991. The role of T lymphocytes in immunity to *Plasmodium falciparum:* enhancement of neutrophil-mediated parasite killing by lymphotoxin and interferon gamma and comparisons with tumour necrosis factor effects. *J Immunol*, **146**, 762–7.

Kumaratilake, L.M., Ferrante, A., et al. 1992. Effects of cytokines, complement and antibody on the neutrophil respiratory burst and phagocytic response to merozoites of *Plasmodium falciparum. Infect Immun*, **60**, 3731–8.

Kumaratilake, L.M., Ferrante, A., et al. 1994. Focus: Extraction of intraerythrocytic malarial parasites by phagocytic cells. *Parasitol Today*, **10**, 193–6.

Kumaratilake, L.M., Rathjen, D.A., et al. 1995. A synthetic TNFα agonist peptide enhances human PMN-mediated killing of *Plasmodium falciparum* in vitro and suppresses *P. chabaudi* infection in mice. *J Clin Invest*, **95**, 2315–24.

Lehrer, R.I. and Ganz, T. 1990. Antimicrobial polypeptides of human neutrophils. *Blood*, **76**, 2169–81.

Metcalf, D. 1989. The molecular control cell division, differentiation, commitment and maturation in haemopoietic cells. *Nature*, **339**, 27–30.

Metcalf, J.A., Gallin, J.I., et al. (eds). 1986. *Laboratory manual of neutrophil functions*. New York: Raven Press.

Metchnikoff, E. 1893. Lecture VII. In: Starling, F.A. and Starling, E.H. (eds), *Lectures on comparative pathology of inflammation*. London: Keyan, Paul, Trench, Trubner & Co, 107–31, (Republished 1968. London: Dover Publication, 1–218.).

Muller, W.A. 1999. Leukocyte-endothelial cell adhesion molecules in transendothelial migration. In: Gallin, J.I. and Snyderman, R. (eds), *Inflammation: Basic principles and clinical correlates*. Vol. 6. Philadelphia: Lippincott Williams & Wilkins, 585–92.

Newman, S.L., Henson, J.E. and Henson, P.M. 1982. Phagocytosis of senescent neutrophils by human monocyte-derived macrophages and rabbit inflammatory cells. *J Exp Med*, **156**, 430–2.

Palmblad, J., Papadaki, H.A. and Eliopoulos, G. 2001. Acute and chronic neutropenias. What is new? *J Intern Med*, **250**, 476–91.

Paton, J.C. and Ferrante, A. 1983. Inhibition of human polymorphonuclear leukocyte respiratory burst, bactericidal activity. and migration by pneumolysin. *Infect Immun*, **41**, 1212–16.

Paul, B. and Sbarra, A.J. 1968. The role of the phagocyte in host-parasite interactions. 13. The direct quantitative estimation of H_2O_2 in phagocytosing cells. *Biochim Biophys Acta*, **156**, 168–78.

Penrose, J.F., Austen, K.F. and Lam, B.K. 1999. Leukotrienes, biosynthetic pathway, releaseand receptor-mediated actions with relevance to disease states. In: Gallin, J.I. and Synderman, R. (eds), *Basic principles and clinical correlates*. Philadelphia: Lippincott Williams & Wilkins, 361–72.

Penttila, I.A., Ey, P.L. and Jenkin, C.R. 1984. Reduced infectivity of *Nematospiroides dubius* after incubation in vitro with neutrophils or eosinophils from infected mice and lack of effect by neutrophils from normal mice. *Parasite Immunol*, **6**, 295–308.

Penttila, I.A., Ey, P.L., et al. 1985. Suppression of early immunity of *Nematospiroides dubius* in mice by selective depletion of neutrophils with monoclonal antibody. *Aust J Exp Biol Med Sci*, **63**, 531–43.

Powell, W.S., Gravel, S., et al. 1997. Effect of 5-oxo-6,8,11,14-eicosatetraenoic acid on expression of CD11b, actin polymerization and adherence in human neutrophils. *J Immunol*, **159**, 2952–9.

Quie, P.G., Mills, E.L., et al. 1996. Disorders of the polymorphonuclear phagocytic system. In: Stiehm, E.R. (ed.), *Immunologic disorders in infants and children*. Philadelphia: WB Saunders Co, 443–68.

Robinson, L.A., Steeber, D.A. and Tedder, T.F. 1999. The selectins in inflammation. In: Gallin, J.I. and Synderman, R. (eds), *Inflammation: Basic principles and clinical correlates*. Philadelphia: Lippincott Williams & Wilkins, 571–84.

Rot, A. 1999. Neutrophil migration and methods for its in vitro study. In: Gabrilovich, D.I. (ed.), *The neutrophils: New outlook for old cells*. London: Imperial College Press, 243–74.

Segal, A.W. and Jones, O.T.G. 1978. Novel cytochrome b system in phagocytic vacuoles of human granulocytes. *Nature*, **276**, 515–17.

Segal, A.W., Jones, O.T.G., et al. 1978. Absence of a newly described cytochome b from neutrophils of patients with CGD. *Lancet*, **ii**, 446–9.

Segal, A.W., West, I., et al. 1992. Cytochrome b_{245} is a flavocytochrome containing FAD and the NADPH-binding site of the microbial oxidase of phagocytes. *Biochem J*, **284**, 781–8.

Stossel, T.P. 1999. Mechanical responses of white blood cells. In: Gallin, J.I. and Synderman, R. (eds), *Inflammation: Basic principles and clinical correlates*. Philadelphia: Lippincott Williams & Wilkins, 661–79.

Strauss, R.G. 1999. Neutrophil transfusion therapy. In: Gabrilovich, D.I. (ed.), *The neutrophils: New outlook for old cells*. London: Imperial College Press, 345–62.

Tan, A.-M., Ferrante, A., et al. 1995. Activation of the neutrophil bactericidal activity for non-typable *Haemophilus influenzae* by tumor necrosis factor and lymphotoxin. *Pediatr Res*, **37**, 155–9.

Tiku, K., Tiku, M.L. and Skosey, J.L. 1986. Interleukin, 1 production by human polymorphonuclear neutrophils. *J Immunol*, **136**, 3677–85.

Uhing, R.J. and Snyderman, R. 1999. Chemoattractant – response coupling. In: Gallin, J.I. and Synderman, R. (eds), *Inflammation: Basic principles and clinical correlates*. Philadelphia: Lippincott Williams & Wilkins, 607–26.

Virella, G. 1999. Diagnostic evaluation of neutrophil function. In: Gabrilovich, G.I. (ed.), *The neutrophils: New outlook for old cells*. London: Imperial College Press, 275–97.

Walsh, T.J., De Panw, B., et al. 1994. Recent advances in the epidemiology, prevention and treatment of invasive fungal infections in neutropenic patients. *J Med Vet Myc*, **32**, suppl 1, 33–51.

Wientjes, F.B., Hsuan, J.J., et al. 1993. P40^{phox}, a third cytosolic component of the activation complex of the NADPH oxidase to contain src homology, 3 domains. *Biochem J*, **296**, 557–61.

Zeya, H. and Spitznagel, J.K. 1966. Cationic proteins of polymorphonuclear lysosomes, I. Resolution of antibacterial and enzymatic activities. *J Bacteriol*, **91**, 750–4.

Zhang, J.-H., Ferrante, A., et al. 1992. Neutrophil stimulation by activated T lymphocytes. *J Immunol*, **148**, 177–92.

5

Basophils and eosinophils

EDWARD E.S. MITRE AND THOMAS B. NUTMAN

Basophils and eosinophils are leukocytes with large cytoplasmic granules that originate from $CD34^+$ progenitor cells. Although both are present at tissue sites of inflammation in allergic and helminthic disease, basophils reside predominantly in the circulation, whereas the majority of eosinophils are found in the tissues. Both cell types have lifespans of a few days, which can be prolonged through the actions of the interleukins IL-3, IL-5, and other growth factors; there is a large overlap in the mediators that cause them to traffic from the circulation to sites of inflammation. Both cell types release multiple inflammatory mediators, with histamine being the primary effector molecule of basophils and granule proteins being the primary effector molecules of eosinophils. Basophils typically degranulate through an IgE-dependent pathway, whereas eosinophils are most often activated by cytokine–cytokine receptor interaction. Although both cells are classically considered part of the innate immune system, they also modify the adaptive immune system through the release of cytokines and chemokines. In addition, histamine released from basophils has multiple immunomodulatory effects, and eosinophils have the ability to process and present antigen. Finally, basophils and eosinophils are clearly involved in the immune response to helminth infections and play a role in HIV and respiratory virus infections.

BASIC BIOLOGY

Basophils

MORPHOLOGY

Basophils are the least common white blood cell, making up 0.5–1 percent of the circulating peripheral blood cell population and accounting for 0.33 percent of the nucleated cells in the marrow (Juhlin 1963). They have lobulated nuclei of various forms and contain multiple prominent amorphous granules that stain purple to red with blue aniline dyes (Figures 5.1a and 5.2a). This staining pattern is the result of the presence within the granules of highly sulfated proteoglycans which are often complexed to proteases, histamine, and cytokines.

GROWTH AND DIFFERENTIATION

Basophils, as well as eosinophils, mast cells, monocytes, and neutrophils, originate from pluripotential $CD34^+$ progenitor cells found in cord blood, peripheral blood, and bone marrow (Kirshenbaum et al. 1991; Metcalf 1989). Basophils and eosinophils are believed to derive from a subset of $CD34^+$ cells that are also interleukin (IL) IL-3Rα^+ and IL-5R$^+$ (Boyce et al. 1995). The existence of a common progenitor cell for eosinophils and basophils is supported by the finding of granulocytes with hybrid eosinophil/basophil phenotype in vivo in patients with chronic myelogenous leukemia (Weil and Hrisinko 1987) and in vitro in cultures of peripheral blood and bone marrow from normal human donors (Leary and Ogawa 1984; Denburg et al. 1985). There is also evidence that basophils share a common progenitor with mast cells. Traditionally, basophils have been thought to arise from a separate cell lineage than mast cells, the progenitor cells of which are $CD34^+/CD38^+$ (Kempuraj et al. 1999) or $CD34^+$/c-kit$^+$/$CD13^+$ (Kirshenbaum et al. 1999). Recently, however, a new monoclonal antibody (97A6 – which targets ectonucleotide pyropho-

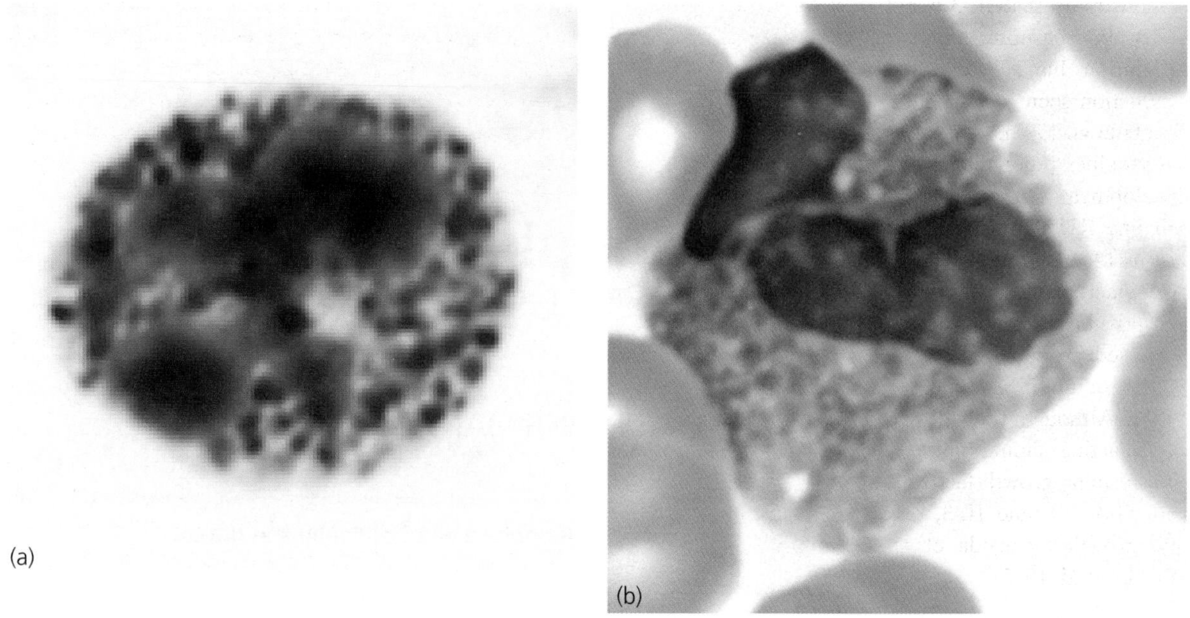

Figure 5.1 (a) *May–Grünwald stain of a human peripheral blood basophil at 1000 × magnification with typical multilobulated nucleus and multiple large purple-staining granules of variable size.* (b) *Wright–Giemsa stain of a human peripheral blood eosinophil viewed at 1000 × demonstrating the characteristic bilobed nucleus and red-staining granules.*

sphatase/phosphodiesterase 3) has been described that is specific for mast cells, basophils, and their precursors (Buhring et al. 1999, 2001), suggesting that mast cells and basophils arise from a similar lineage.

The principal cytokine required for basophil growth and differentiation is IL-3 (Valent 1995); 9.5–50 percent of cord blood and bone marrow cells differentiated in the presence of IL-3 becomes basophils, with the remaining cells consisting of eosinophils, neutrophils, and macrophages (Saito et al. 1988). Growth of chronic myelogenous leukemia basophils, and of the human basophil-like cell line KU 812, is supported by IL-3 through high-affinity binding sites (Valent et al. 1989, 1990); moreover, humans treated with recombinant human IL-3 (rhIL-3) develop basophilia (Ganser et al. 1990). Studies with IL-3 knock-out (KO) mice have

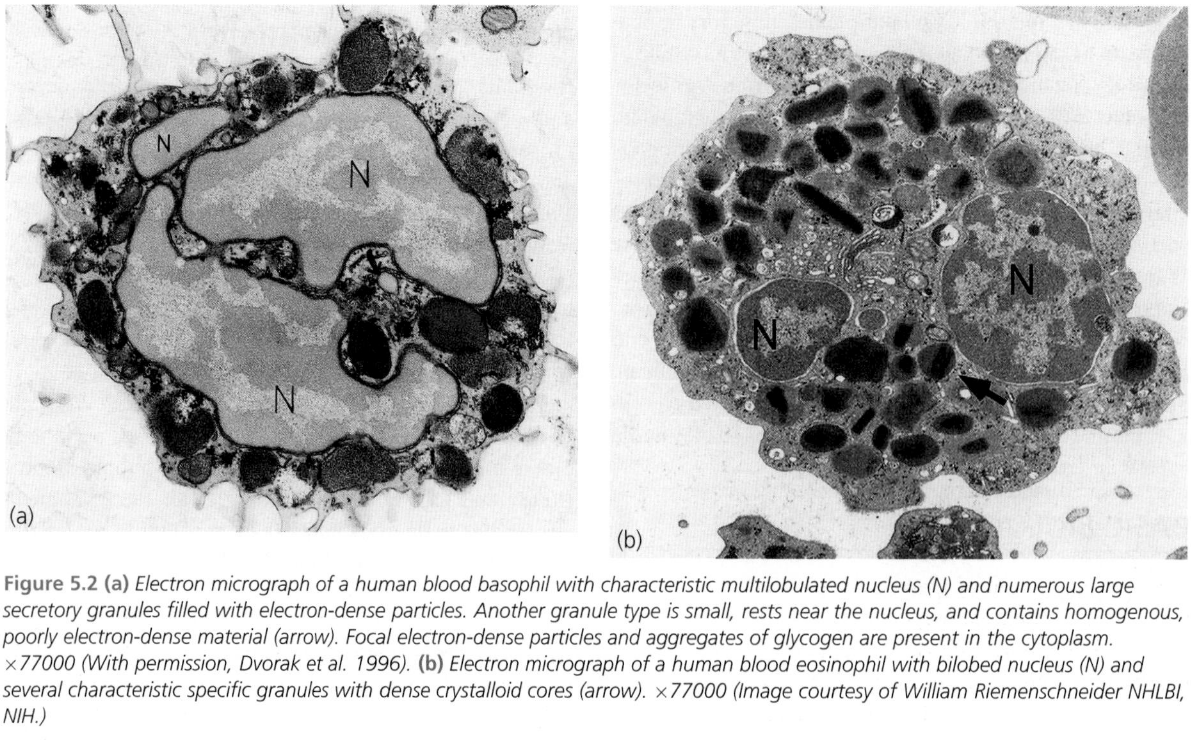

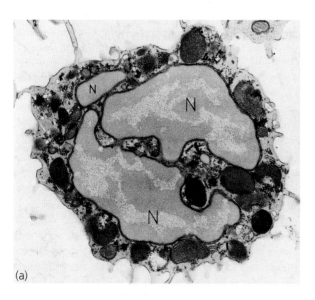

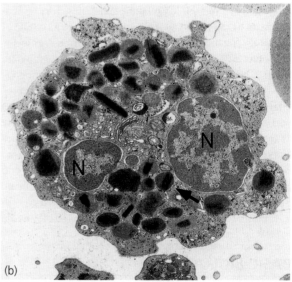

Figure 5.2 (a) *Electron micrograph of a human blood basophil with characteristic multilobulated nucleus (N) and numerous large secretory granules filled with electron-dense particles. Another granule type is small, rests near the nucleus, and contains homogenous, poorly electron-dense material (arrow). Focal electron-dense particles and aggregates of glycogen are present in the cytoplasm. ×77000 (With permission, Dvorak et al. 1996).* (b) *Electron micrograph of a human blood eosinophil with bilobed nucleus (N) and several characteristic specific granules with dense crystalloid cores (arrow). ×77000 (Image courtesy of William Riemenschneider NHLBI, NIH.)*

demonstrated that IL-3 is not required for development of baseline basophil numbers in the bone marrow and circulation, but is necessary for the enhanced basophil production seen in mouse models of helminth infection (Lantz et al. 1998).

Cytokines other than IL-3 also contribute to basophil development. Differentiation of the human basophil-like cell line KU 812 can be promoted by IL-6 and tumor necrosis factor α (TNF-α) (Nilsson et al. 1994); granulocyte–macrophage colony-stimulating factor (GM-CSF) and possibly IL-5 can cause basophil differentiation and increased production from the peripheral blood (Hutt-Taylor et al. 1988; Saito et al. 1988; Denburg et al. 1991). Although they do not have much of an effect when acting alone, nerve growth factor (NGF) and transforming growth factor β (TGF-β) can act in synergy with GM-CSF and IL-3, respectively, to enhance basophil growth (Matsuda et al. 1988; Tsuda et al. 1991; Sillaber et al. 1992).

NATURAL HISTORY

Basophils, which primarily remain in the circulation after maturation in the bone marrow, can infiltrate tissues at sites of active inflammation in parasitic diseases (Cross et al. 1987), asthma (Kepley et al. 2001), and allergy (Mitchell et al. 1982; Guo et al. 1994). The typical basophil has a relatively short lifespan, ranging from a few days to a few weeks. IL-3, IL-5, and NGF all improve the basophil lifespan in culture, with IL-3 improving viability the most (Miura et al. 2001). Whereas basophils cultured in media alone die within 3 days, basophils cultured with IL-3 have $>$ 95 percent viability at 3 days (Miura et al. 2001). The basophil lifespan is also prolonged slightly by GM-CSF but not by IL-4, G-CSF, M-CSF (Yamaguchi et al. 1992), or stem cell factor (Dvorak et al. 1994). Basophils differentiated in vitro appear at about 1 week, peak at 3 weeks, and then decrease in number thereafter (Kirshenbaum et al. 1989). Basophils usually die through apoptosis, which can be induced by glucocorticoids (Yoshimura et al. 2001) and inhibited by IL-3 (although not by IL-5 or GM-CSF) (Zheng et al. 2002).

Eosinophils

MORPHOLOGY

Eosinophils have bilobed nuclei and large cytoplasmic granules that stain with eosin and other acidic dyes (see Figures 5.1b and 5.2b). Specific granules have dense crystalloid cores and store the major secretory effector proteins as well as various enzymes and cytokines. Another population of granules, so-called primary granules, contain Charcot–Leyden crystal protein. Smaller granules contain acid phosphatase and arylsulfatase, and non-membrane-bound organelles called lipid bodies contain arachidonic acid, 5-lipoxygenase, and cyclooxygenase (and are probably the main sites of prostaglandin and leukotriene production in the eosinophil) (Weller and Dvorak 1994). Eosinophils also have vesiculotubular structures that contain cytochrome b_{558}, a component of reduced nicotinamide adenine dinucleotide phosphate (NADPH) oxidase that enables eosinophils to produce superoxide upon activation.

GROWTH AND DIFFERENTIATION

Like basophils, eosinophils develop in the bone marrow from pluripotent $CD34^+$ cells in approximately 1 week. Differentiation into eosinophils is primarily guided by IL-3, IL-5, and GM-CSF. Of these, IL-5 is the most powerful inducer of eosinophilopoiesis, as the usual bone marrow eosinophilia that develops in sensitized mice challenged with allergen is almost completely abrogated by treatment with anti-IL-5, yet hardly diminished by either anti-IL-3 or anti-GM-CSF (Tomaki et al. 2002). Eosinophilopoiesis is not dependent exclusively on these three cytokines, because mice that lack the IL-5 receptor (Foster et al. 1996) or the common receptor β chain for these three cytokines (Nishinakamura et al. 1995) are able to produce eosinophils, although the basal level is lower than normal and the mice are unable to increase their eosinophil counts in response to helminths or allergic challenge. Unlike IL-3 and GM-CSF, which promote the development of multiple lineages, IL-5 acts most specifically on eosinophils. IL-5 is made predominantly by type II $CD4^+$ T cells, but can also be made by natural killer (NK) cells, $CD8^+$ T cells, and eosinophils.

Eosinophilopoiesis can be inhibited by IL-12. Mice lacking IL-12 have higher bone marrow eosinophil counts than control mice (Zhao et al. 2000), and treatment of allergic mice with intrapulmonary IL-12 decreases bone marrow eosinophil counts by up to 45 percent (Rais et al. 2002). IL-12 may inhibit eosinophil production by upregulation of interferon γ (IFN-γ), because IL-12 inhibition of eosinophilopoiesis does not occur in IFN-γ KO mice (Rais et al. 2002).

NATURAL HISTORY

After differentiation, a pool of mature eosinophils remains in the bone marrow and can be rapidly released after IL-5 or eotaxin administration (Palframan et al. 1998a, 1998b). Eosinophils typically circulate for 3–26 hours in the circulation before migration into tissues, where the vast majority of eosinophils exist and where they survive for several days to weeks. In vivo studies of mice infected with *Angiostrongylus cantonensis* show that eosinophils taken from the site of infection have prolonged survival compared with that of peripheral blood eosinophils (Sugaya et al. 2001). The eosinophil lifespan is prolonged by IL-5, IL-3, and GM-CSF, each of which prevents apoptosis of eosinophils in in vitro culture systems (Simon and Blaser 1995). In the absence of stimulating cytokines, eosinophils soon undergo apoptosis (Walsh 1997). Eosinophils survive up to 10 days in the presence of IL-5 but only up to 4 days in its absence (Yamaguchi et al. 1991); 53 percent of eosinophils cultured in vitro with IL-3 are viable at 14 days, whereas only 10 percent are viable in its absence (Rothenberg et al. 1988). After 7 days of culture with GM-CSF, 43 percent of human eosinophils remain alive, whereas most eosinophils cultured in media alone are dead (Owen et al. 1987). IL-5, IL-3, and GM-CSF most probably prolong eosinophil survival by inhibiting apoptosis by signaling through the β subunit of their receptors, which they all share. This β subunit interacts with Lyn and syk tyrosine kinases involved in anti-apoptotic signaling in eosinophils (Yousefi et al. 1996).

Eosinophil survival can also be prolonged by IL-15 (probably through induction of autocrine GM-CSF production by eosinophils) (Hoontrakoon et al. 2002), TNF-α (Valerius et al. 1990), nitric oxide (Beauvais et al. 1995), and engagement of CD40 (Bureau et al. 2002). Although IFN-γ and IFN-α are generally considered capable of prolonging eosinophil survival (Valerius et al. 1990), one study showed that interferons diminished eosinophil survival (Morita et al. 1996).

Eosinophils usually die through apoptosis. This occurs in the absence of activating cytokines and is most probably induced through events mediated by the Fas receptor (CD95) (Matsumoto et al. 1995), which eosinophils express on their surface (Druilhe et al. 1996). Apoptosis of eosinophils can also be induced by glucocorticoids (Meagher et al. 1996), TNF-α (Fujihara et al. 2002), TGF-β_1 (Atsuta et al. 1995), and through ligation of CD69, a type II membrane antigen expressed on cytokine-stimulated eosinophils (Walsh et al. 1996). The recent finding that CD69 expression on eosinophils of patients with asthma increases after stimulation with a specific inhalation challenge suggests that CD69 may play a role in a negative feedback loop in eosinophilia (Pignatti et al. 2002).

Eosinophils that have undergone apoptosis are ingested by macrophages using macrophage surface proteins CD36 and $\alpha_v\beta_3$ (Stern et al. 1996), thus preventing unwanted deleterious release of toxic intracellular products upon eosinophil death.

CELL TRAFFICKING

Trafficking of basophils and eosinophils from the peripheral circulation to sites of inflammation occurs through a multistep process (Springer 1994), with leukocytes rolling on endothelial cells through binding of selectins, firmly adhering to endothelium via integrins, transmigrating through the endothelial cell layer by diapedesis, and finally proceeding to sites of inflammation through the effects of chemotactic agents. The exact mechanisms by which this occurs have been studied in greater detail in eosinophils than in basophils. As a result of the large number of adhesion and chemotaxis factors common to both cell types (Tables 5.1 and 5.2), it is likely that trafficking of basophils and eosinophils is quite similar. The extent of the overlap between the pathways of basophil and eosinophil recruitment and the extent to which these cell types are recruited independently of one another are areas of active investigation (Bochner and Schleimer 2001). Factors that alter expression of adhesion molecules and the relative importance of different chemotactic factors with regard to each cell type are discussed below.

Basophils

BASOPHIL ADHESION

Expression of basophil adhesion molecules is modulated by several factors. Pretreatment with IL-1 and TNF-α (Bochner et al. 1988), as well as FcεR1 aggregation (Bochner et al. 1989), enhances the ability of basophils to bind to endothelial cells, probably by upregulating CD18 on basophils. IL-3 increases basophil adhesiveness to endothelial cells, possibly by increasing CD11b – a molecule that can bind to intercellular adhesion molecule 1 (ICAM-1), fibrinogen, and complement component C3bi (Bochner et al. 1990) – on basophils. In addition to CD11b, basophil activation also increases surface expression of CD11c and αd, two other β integrins (Bochner 2000).

The type 2 cytokines IL-4 and IL-13 increase the ability of basophils and eosinophils to bind to endothelial cells by increasing endothelial cell expression of vascular cell adhesion molecule 1 (VCAM-1), to which basophils and eosinophils, but not neutrophils, can bind (Columbo et al. 1992; Bochner et al. 1995).

CHEMOTAXIS

Multiple factors – including cytokines, chemokines, complement components, and lipid products – serve as basophil chemoattractants. Of the CC chemokines, RANTES and monocytic chemotactic peptide (MCP-3) 3 have the greatest ability to attract basophils, followed by MCP-1 and macrophage infectivity potentiator 1α (MIP-1α) (Dahinden et al. 1994). In terms of the effects of the CC chemokines on basophils, RANTES acts mostly as a chemoattractant, MCP-1 as an inducer of basophil degranulation, and MCP-3 as a combination, serving as both a strong chemoattractant and an inducer of basophil degranulation (Rot et al. 1992; Dahinden et al. 1994). MCP-2, another CC chemokine, is also chemoattractive for basophils (Weber et al. 1995). Stromal cell-derived factor 1α (SDF-1α), a CXC chemokine that is the only known ligand for CXCR4, has been shown to recruit basophils with even greater potency than RANTES and MCP-1 (Jinquan et al. 2000). Of the

Table 5.1 *Basophil and eosinophil adhesion molecules and chemotaxis factors*

		Adhesion molecule expression by	
Adhesion molecules	**Ligands**	**Basophils**	**Eosinophils**
Integrins			
β_1 *(VLA family)*			
$\alpha_4\beta_1$ (CD49d/CD29)	VCAM-1, fibronectin	+	+
$\alpha_5\beta_1$ (CD49e/CD29)	Fibronectin	+	+
$\alpha_6\beta_1$ (CD49f/CD29)	Laminin	–	+
β_2 *family*			
LFA-1 (CD11a/CD18)	ICAM-1, -2, -3	+	+
Mac-1 (CD11b/CD18)	C3bi, ICAM-1, fibronectin	+	+
P150,95 (CD11c/CD18)	C3bi, others	+	+
αd (αd/CD18)	ICAM-3, VCAM-1	+	+
β_7 *family*			
$\alpha_4\beta_7$	MAdCAM-1, VCAM-1, fibronectin	+	+
Ig gene superfamily			
ICAM-1 (CD54)	LFA-1, Mac-1	+	+
ICAM-3 (CD50)	LFA-1	+	+
PECAM-1 (CD31)	CD31	+	+
ICAM-2 (CD102)	LFA-1	+	–
Selectins			
L-Selectin (CD62L)	GlyCAM-1, CD34, MAdCAM-1	+	+
PSGL-1 (CD162)	P-Selectin	+	+
Sialyl Lewis-X (CD15s)	E-Selectin, P-selectin	+	+
Sialyl-dimeric Lewis-X	E-Selectin	+	+
Lewis-X (CD15)	P-Selectin	–	+
Others			
Pgp-1 (CD44)	Hyaluronic acid	+	+
Siglec-8	Sialic acid	+	+

Table 5.2 *Basophil and eosinophil adhesion molecules and chemotaxis factors*

		Recepter expression by	
Chemotaxis factors	**Predominant recepter**	**Basophils**	**Eosinophils**
Chemokines			
MIP-1α, RANTES, MCP-2[a]	CCR1	+	+
Eotaxin, MCP-3, MCP-4, RANTES	CCR3	+	+
SDF-1α	CXCR4	+	+
MCP-1	CCR2	+	–
MIP-3α	CCR6	+	–
Cytokines			
IL-3	IL-3R	+	+
IL-5	IL-5R	+	+
IL-8	CXCR1, CXCR2	?	?
GM-CSF	GM-CSFR	+	+
TNF-α	TNF-αR	–	+
Others			
C3a	C3aR	+	+
C5a	C5aR (CD88)	+	+
fMLP	fMLPR	+	+
PAF	PAFR	+	+
Prostaglandin D_2	CRTH1	+	+
Leukotriene B_4	LTB_4R	?	+

See text for abbreviations.
a) MCP-2 can also use CCR2B and CCR3 as functional receptor.

cytokines, IL-3 and GM-CSF are strong basophil chemoattractants, and IL-5 and IL-8 are weak ones (Tanimoto et al. 1992; Yamaguchi et al. 1992).

Eotaxin, eotaxin-2, and eotaxin-3, which are usually considered primarily as eosinophil chemoattractive proteins, are also potent basophil chemoattractants (Yamada et al. 1997; Dulkys et al. 2001; Menzies-Gow et al. 2002). Other basophil chemoattractants include the complement components C3a and C5a, leukotriene B_4 (LTB_4), and platelet-activating factor (PAF) (Lett-Brown et al. 1976; Tanimoto et al. 1992). Recently, prostaglandin D_2 has been shown to induce migration of basophils and eosinophils through the CRTH2 receptor (Hirai et al. 2001).

The ability of basophils to migrate toward chemoattractants C5a, IL-3, and IL-8 is inhibited by dexamethasone (Yamaguchi et al. 1994).

Eosinophils

ADHESION

Recruitment of eosinophils out of the circulation begins with binding of VLA-4 ($\alpha_4\beta_1$) and selectins on eosinophils to VCAM-1 and E-selectin present on activated endothelial cells (Sriramarao et al. 1994, 2000; Ulfman et al. 1999). The ability to bind to VCAM-1, in particular, allows eosinophils and basophils to be selectively recruited from the circulation, because neutrophils lack VLA-4 (Walsh et al. 1991).

Once tethered, eosinophils can be acted upon by inflammatory mediators to upregulate integrins and other cell adhesion molecules to enable firm adhesion. IL-8, MCP-1, C3a, C5a, and PAF can all induce activation-dependent adhesion of rolling eosinophils, probably through upregulation of β_2-integrins that can bind to ICAM-1 on endothelial cells (Discipio et al. 1999; Gerszten et al. 1999; Ulfman et al. 2001; Broide 2002). Although CD11b–CD18 binding to ICAM-1 is considered important for firm adhesion, it is not necessary for tissue eosinophilia, because patients with CD18 deficiency still have eosinophils present in inflamed tissues (Anderson et al. 1985). After firm adhesion, cells then diapedese across the endothelial wall. In addition to inducing firm adhesion, C5a has been shown to enable eosinophils to migrate across the vascular endothelium (Discipio et al. 1999). Once across, leukocytes migrate through tissues under the guidance of chemoattractants.

Eosinophil-binding molecules are affected by numerous factors. As with basophils, IL-4 increases selective recruitment of eosinophils from the circulation by specifically upregulating expression of VCAM-1 on endothelial cells and enhancing VLA-4/VCAM-1 binding (Moser et al. 1992; Schleimer et al. 1992). IL-4, as well as TNF-α, has also been shown to upregulate VCAM-1 expression by lung fibroblasts (Sabatini et al. 2002). TNF-α also causes lung fibroblasts to increase ICAM-1 expression and to release the eosinophil chemoattractants MCP-1 and eotaxin. IL-4 and IL-13 have been shown in a mouse model of *Onchocerca volvulus* keratitis to recruit eosinophils to the cornea through upregulation of ICAM-1 expression on limbal vascular endothelial cells (Berger et al. 2002).

Other cytokines that can affect eosinophil adhesion include IL-3 and GM-CSF, which were shown to upregulate expression of VLA-4 and VLA-5 on eosinophils in a study of patients infected with *Onchocerca volvulus* (Brattig et al. 1995). This study also found that infective onchocerca larvae had fibronectin deposited on their surface, raising the possibility that eosinophils bind directly to helminths through fibronectin, a known ligand for VLA-4 and VLA-5.

Together, TNF-α and C5a increase eosinophil attachment to human bronchial epithelial cells threefold through upregulation of $\alpha_5\beta_1$ integrin, which appears to bind fibronectin (Burke-Gaffney et al. 2002).

In a sheep model of trichostrongylus infection, eosinophils at sites of helminth infection exhibit increased CD18 expression compared with circulating eosinophils (Stevenson et al. 2001). One agent that has been shown to increase CD18 and CD11b expression on eosinophils is leukotriene D_3 (LTD_3), which probably does so through the cysLT-1 receptor and β_2 integrin (Nagata et al. 2002).

The eotaxin proteins can also affect eosinophil adhesion. Eotaxin-1 has been shown to enhance binding of eosinophils to VCAM-1 (Kitayama et al. 1997). Eotaxin-2 appears to cause eosinophils to shift from VCAM-1 to ICAM-1 adhesion, possibly acting to enable firm adhesion after eosinophils have been tethered (Tachimoto et al. 2002). Eotaxin-2 also plays a role in eosinophil de-adhesion (Tachimoto et al. 2000), whereas eotaxin-3 induces transmigration of eosinophils across the endothelium (Cuvelier and Patel 2001).

CHEMOTAXIS

Eotaxin

Initially isolated from the bronchiolar fluid of sensitized guinea pigs, eotaxin-1 is an 8- to 9-kDa protein with an amino acid sequence very similar to that of the CC chemokines MCP-1, MCP-2, and MCP-3 (Jose et al. 1994). Eotaxin is a powerful and specific eosinophil chemoattractant (Jose et al. 1994; Garcia-Zepeda et al. 1996). It acts by binding to CCR3, which is also the receptor for RANTES, MCP-2, MCP-3, and MCP-4 (Marleau et al. 1996; Alkhatib et al. 1997; Heath et al. 1997), and its production probably occurs via activation of the transcription factor NF-κB (Jedrzkiewicz et al. 2000). The importance of eotaxin and other CC chemokines in eosinophil recruitment is underscored by the finding that CCR3 KO mice fail to recruit eosinophils to the small intestine and skeletal muscle even after infection with *Trichinella spiralis* (Gurish et al. 2002). Eotaxin can be made by pulmonary epithelial cells, because eotaxin mRNA is detectable in human epithelial cell lines after stimulation with TNF-α and IL-1β (Lilly et al. 1997). Production of eotaxin-1 by human airway fibroblasts is increased by TGF-β and IL-13 (Wenzel et al. 2002). IL-4, another type 2 cytokine, has differential effects on the production of eotaxin, upregulating its production by human lung epithelial cells and downregulating its production by peripheral blood mononuclear cells (PBMCs) (Nakamura et al. 2001). This differential effect probably serves to increase eosinophil recruitment out of the peripheral circulation and into the tissues.

Mice lacking the eotoxin gene have lower baseline levels of peripheral blood eosinophils and less eosinophilia in response to antigen challenge than normal mice (Rothenberg et al. 1997; Matthews et al. 1998). The findings that plasma eotaxin levels are significantly elevated in patients with acute asthma compared with age-, sex-, and ethnicity-matched patients with stable asthma (Lilly et al. 1999) and that bronchoalveolar lavage (BAL) levels of eotaxin increase after segmental allergen challenge (Lilly et al. 2001) suggest that eotaxin contributes to the eosinophilia in asthma and allergic diseases of humans. Intradermal injection of eotaxin and eotaxin-2 into atopic and nonatopic human volunteers results in infiltration of eosinophils, basophils, neutrophils, and macrophages, as well as in histological changes consistent with mast cell degranulation (Menzies-Gow et al. 2002).

As discussed in the previous section, eotaxin also mediates eosinophil adhesion. Notably, the ability of eotaxin to upregulate CD11b is three times greater in IL-5 transgenic mice than in normal mice, a finding that suggests synergy between eosinophil-specific cytokines such as IL-5 and chemokines in terms of inducing eosinophil aggregation (Kudlacz et al. 2002). Glucocorticoids, which suppress eosinophilia, have been shown to suppress eotaxin mRNA expression (Lilly et al. 1997).

Eotaxin-2 and eotaxin-3 (so named because of functional, not structural, similarities to eotaxin) are other CC chemokines that mediate their effects through CCR3. They serve as chemoattractants for both eosinophils and basophils and have been shown to have similar efficacy for inducing calcium flux, activating Gi proteins, and inducing superoxide anion generation as eotaxin (Forssmann et al. 1997; Dulkys et al. 2001; Badewa et al. 2002).

Interleukin 5

In addition to supporting differentiation and growth of eosinophils, IL-5 is a strong eosinophil chemoattractant (Lampinen et al. 2001). Although IL-5 does not appear to regulate baseline eosinophil blood counts, as IL-5 KO mice have normal basal peripheral eosinophil counts (Kopf et al. 1996), IL-5 is one of the major factors responsible for recruiting eosinophils into tissues. IL-5 KO mice sensitized to ovalbumin do not develop the eosinophilia, hyperreactivity, and lung damage that normal sensitized mice do after allergen challenge (Foster et al. 1996). Overexpression of IL-5 in transgenic mice results in increased numbers of eosinophils in the gastrointestinal mucosa compared with those in control mice (Mishra et al. 2002), and treatment of patients with asthma with monoclonal anti-IgE antibody results in significant decreases in sputum eosinophils (Fahy et al. 1997).

Although important, IL-5 is not an absolute requirement for the recruitment of eosinophils into tissues, because pulmonary eosinophilia with morphologically normal eosinophils occurs in the lungs of IL-5KO mice infected with pneumonia virus of mice (PVM) to the same degree as in those of control mice (Domachowske et al. 2002).

Other chemotaxis factors

Many other factors have been shown to serve as eosinophil chemoattractants, including the complement components C3a and C5a, the CC chemokines MCP-2, MCP-3, and RANTES, and the cytokines GM-CSF, IL-2, IL-3, and IL-8 (Resnick and Weller 1993; Noso et al. 1994; Schweizer et al. 1994; Weber et al. 1995; Discipio et al. 1999). It has been shown that LTB_4 and PAF can induce eosinophil chemotaxis (Klein et al. 2001; Oliveira et al. 2002), and TNF-α has been show to recruit eosinophils in ulcerative colitis (Lampinen et al. 2001). Ligation of SDF-1α to CXCR4 also induces eosinophil migration (Nagase et al. 2000). Although not directly acting on eosinophils, intranasal delivery of IL-13 into mice causes lung and airway eosinophilia by increasing IL-5 and eotaxin production (Pope et al. 2001). Finally, it has been shown that eosinophils can accumulate at sites of helminth infection even in mice lacking B and T cells, suggesting that eosinophils may be directly recruited by some helminth molecule or some factor released by normal tissue in response to a helminth infection (Shinkai et al. 2002).

CELL FUNCTION

Basophils

As a result of their ability to bind IgE, individual basophils can specifically recognize and be activated by many different antigens. Activation of basophils causes release of preformed and newly synthesized inflammatory mediators that play important roles in vascular reaction, exudation, leukocyte accumulation, and wound healing. In addition, basophils have the ability to produce and release cytokines and to phagocytose particles.

ACTIVATION

IgE-mediated activation

The most important molecules for basophil function are their high-affinity IgE receptors (FcεR1s). These receptors are highly specific for IgE and bind them in a 1:1 ratio, with the Cε3 domain of the Fc portion of the IgE antibody serving as the principal binding site for FcεR1 (Weetall et al. 1990). When a multivalent antigen binds to several IgE molecules, the receptors aggregate and initiate cell activation, stimulating mediator generation and release (Turner and Kinet 1999). Basophil degranulation occurs very quickly, with crosslinking of IgE causing half-maximum histamine release from basophils in 7 minutes (Kuna et al. 1992).

Although maximal histamine response occurs when about 10 percent of the FcεR1 is aggregated, aggregation of as few as 100 receptors is enough to activate a basophil (Menon et al. 1984). As basophils can express well over 200 000 FcεR1s per cell (MacGlashan et al. 1997), a single basophil can theoretically hold enough different IgE molecules to enable that basophil specifically to recognize and be activated by well over 1000 antigens.

FcεR1 upregulation on basophils is mediated by the interaction of IgE with FcεR1 (MacGlashan et al. 1999). As a result of this, the number of FcεR1s expressed on basophils is proportional to the amount of IgE in the serum (MacGlashan et al. 1997). IL-3 and IL-5, but not NGF, also probably induce FcεR1 upregulation, because they have been shown to induce FcεR1β mRNA expression in basophils in culture in vitro (Miura et al. 2001).

Human FcεR1 can be expressed as a tetrameric ($\alpha\beta\gamma_2$) or trimeric ($\alpha\beta_2$) structure (Kinet 1999). There is a large range in the ratio of the FcεR1 α:β subunits in basophils from different human donors (Saini et al. 2001). As the β subunit of FcεR1 amplifies IgE-triggered signaling (Lin et al. 1996; Dombrowicz et al. 1998) and increases surface FcεR1 expression (Donnadieu et al. 2000), the finding of different FcεR1β:FcεR1α ratios suggests that basophil responsiveness is modulated in part by changes in this ratio.

In addition to FcεR1, human basophils also express FcγRIIb, a low-affinity IgG receptor. In vitro studies using human basophils have shown that co-aggregation of FcγRIIb and FcεR1 molecules decreases IgE-dependent activation (Daeron et al. 1995).

Non-IgE activation

Basophils can be activated by a number of substances through IgE-independent mechanisms. These factors, known as histamine-releasing factors, include complement proteins, human histamine-releasing factor (HRF), chemokines, cytokines, substance P, PAF, contrast media, ionophores, opiates, the bacterial peptide formylmethionine-leucine-phenylalanine (f-Met-Leu-Phe or fMLP), and HIV glycoprotein 120.

The complement proteins C3a, C4a, and C5 cause basophil as well as mast cell degranulation (Schulman et al. 1988; Bischoff et al. 1990b). They may have a role in anaphylactoid reactions and are therefore known as anaphylatoxins. It has been suggested that anaphylatoxins may be activated in immune complex-mediated diseases, reactions to iodinated contrast media, and reactions to dialysis tubing. C3a requires the presence of IL-3 or GM-CSF to enable basophils to release histamine (Bischoff et al. 1990b). In addition to histamine release, C5a in the presence of IL-3 can cause long-lasting release of leukotriene C_4 (LTC_4), IL-4, and IL-13 by continuous signaling through the C5a receptor (Eglite et al. 2000).

Histamine-releasing factor (p23) is made by lymphocytes of atopic children and causes histamine and IL-4 release from a subset of basophils in patients with allergy (MacDonald et al. 1995; Schroeder et al. 1996). Initially believed to act through IgE, it has recently been shown to activate basophils in an IgE-independent manner, although its basophil receptor has yet to be identified (Wantke et al. 1999).

Of the CC chemokines, MCP-1 and MCP-3 are the most potent HRFs described (Dahinden et al. 1994). MCP-1 has been shown to be equivalent to IgE and C5a in its ability to cause basophils to degranulate, and it induces histamine release from basophils within 30 seconds (Alam et al. 1992; Kuna et al. 1993). Other CC chemokines that induce basophils to release histamine include MCP-2, RANTES, and MIP-1α (Alam et al. 1994; Dahinden et al. 1994). Of interest, although it is a weak inducer of basophil degranulation, MCP-2 also causes basophils not pretreated with IL-3 to lose their ability to be degranulated by MCP-1 and MCP-3, suggesting that MCP-2 may act as a functional inhibitor of MCP-1 and MCP-3 (Weber et al. 1995). SDF-1α, a CXC chemokine, induces histamine release from basophils as well as MCP-1 does (Jinquan et al. 2000).

Other less potent basophil activators include fibroblast-induced cytokine (Alam et al. 1994), MIP-1α, connective tissue-activating peptide III (CTAPIII), secretory IgA (Iikura et al. 1998), neutrophil-activating peptide-2 (NAP-2) (Kuna et al. 1993), and stem cell factor (Columbo et al. 1992). IL-18, a proinflammatory cytokine that activates NK cells and Th1 responses, induces basophils to release histamine, IL-4, and IL-13 when co-cultured with IL-3 (Yoshimoto et al. 1999). When IL-18 is given with IL-12, however, it inhibits IgE-triggered histamine activation (Yoshimoto et al. 1999).

Degranulation

Basophils release granule contents in two different ways. Anaphylactic degranulation (AND), the typical way in which basophils degranulate after IgE-mediated activation, occurs through granule-to-plasma membrane fusion and allows for very rapid release of large amounts of granule materials (Dvorak et al. 1980). Piecemeal degranulation (PMD), on the other hand, occurs through trafficking of small vesicles from granules to the plasma membrane and results in a slow, piecemeal loss of granule contents (Dvorak et al. 1976). The most effective trigger for AND is anti-IgE (then MCP-1, then recombinant HRF or rHRF), whereas rank orders for PMD and granule-vesicle attachments are MCP-1 > anti-IgE > rHRF (Dvorak et al. 1996). Although morphologically they appear very different, AND and PMD actually represent anatomical extremes of a continuum of basophil degranulation, because, at very high rates of PMD, vesicles form into tubules by vesicle-to-vesicle fusions, allowing for direct granule-to-plasma membrane fusion, leading to the morphological release pattern termed AND (Dvorak et al. 1991).

Activation markers

CD63 has been the most commonly used marker of basophil activation. IgE-dependent activation of basophils is associated with upregulation of CD63, and the kinetics of this upregulation parallel those of histamine release from basophils (Knol et al. 1991). Increased expression of CD63 on basophils as detected by flow cytometry after in vitro allergen challenge correlates strongly with in vitro assays of histamine and LTC_4, release and has been shown to correlate with a history of allergy to both pollen (Paris-Kohler et al. 2000) and hymenoptera venom (Sainte-Laudy et al. 2000). In addition to CD63, activated basophils also upregulate several β_2-integrins (Bochner 2000).

As CD63 and integrins are not specific only for basophils, studies for other markers of activation are being actively pursued. One possible candidate is E-NPP3 (CD203c), a type II transmembrane protein exclusively expressed on basophils, mast cells, and their $CD34^+$ precursor cells (Buhring et al. 1999, 2001). E-NPP3 has recently been shown to be upregulated on peripheral blood basophils from sensitized individuals after exposure to antigen (Hauswirth et al. 2002).

Degranulation potentiators

Major potentiators of basophil degranulation include IL-3, IL-5, GM-CSF, mast cell growth factor (c-kit ligand), and NGF (Bischoff and Dahinden 1992; Kuna et al. 1993). Although none of these by itself induces basophil degranulation, they all potentiate the effects of factors that cause basophil degranulation. IL-5 enables NAP-1 and C3a to cause basophils to degranulate (Bischoff et al. 1990a) and primes basophils for IgE-dependent histamine release (Kuna et al. 1993). The ability of IL-5 to potentiate the basophil response to C5a is unclear, with studies showing both increased degranulation in response to C5a (Bischoff et al. 1990a) and no change (Miura et al. 2001). IL-3 enables IL-8 and RANTES to induce basophil degranulation (Fureder et al. 1995) and enables C5a-induced LTC_4 generation (Miura et al. 2001). Secretory IgA causes degranulation only after basophils have been exposed to IL-3, IL-5, or GM-CSF, suggesting that the intracellular signaling that primes the basophil for degranulation occurs through the shared β chain of these cytokine receptors (Iikura et al. 1998).

Other factors that potentiate IgE-mediated histamine release from basophils include recombinant human stem cell factor, IL-1α, IL-1β, mast cell growth factor (c-kit ligand), and insulin-like growth factor II (Massey et al. 1989; Columbo et al. 1992; Kuna et al. 1993).

IL-8 inhibits CTAPIII- and IL-3-dependent histamine release from basophils, although it does not inhibit anti-IgE- or fMLP-induced basophil degranulation (Kuna et al. 1991).

EFFECTOR MOLECULES

Basophils release both preformed and newly synthesized inflammatory mediators (Table 5.3). Preformed inflammatory mediators include histamine, chondroitin sulfates, neutral protease, elastase, β-glucuronidase, major basic protein, cathepsin G-like enzyme, Charcot–Leyden crystal protein, tryptase, chymase, and carboxypeptidase. Basophils also store basogranulin, the function of which is unknown, and IL-4. Factors that basophils synthesize on activation include LTC_4, PAI-1, IL-4, IL-13, and MIP-1α.

Histamine

Basophils are the predominant source of histamine in human peripheral blood (Porter and Mitchell 1972).

Table 5.3 *Basophil effector molecules*

Basophil effector molecules
Preformed inflammatory mediators
Histamine
Chondroitin sulfates
Neutral protease with bradykinin-generating activity
Elastase
β-Glucuronidase
Major basic protein
Cathepsin G-like enzyme
Charcot–Leyden crystal protein
Tryptase
Chymase
Carboxypeptidase A
Factors produced upon basophil activation
Leukotriene C_4
Plasminogen-activator inhibitor 1
Cytokines
IL-4 (preformed and *de novo* synthesis on activation)
IL-13 (*de novo* synthesis on activation)
Chemokines
MIP-1α (*de novo* synthesis on activation)

Histamine is made from histidine through the action of histidine carboxylase (Bauza and Lagunoff 1981). Circulating basophils have an average concentration of 1 pg histamine per basophil (Schulman et al. 1983; Fox et al. 1985). Histamine binds to the carboxyl groups of proteins and proteoglycans in secretory granules through ionic forces. During degranulation, histamine dissociates from the proteoglycan–protein complex by cation exchange with extracellular sodium at neutral pH. Histamine probably acts close to its site of release, because it is degraded into either methylhistamine or imidazole acetic acid within minutes of release. Histamine affects cells through its interactions with cell-specific H_1-, H_2-, and H_3-receptors (Black et al. 1972; Arrang et al. 1987). H_1-receptors induce vascular permeability, dilate arterioles, and stimulate intestinal and bronchial smooth muscle contraction. H_2-receptors stimulate gastric acid production by parietal cells, increase mucus secretion, cause endothelial cells to release prostacyclin (PGI_2 – a potent inhibitor of platelet aggregation), and modulate the immune response by inhibiting secretion from cytotoxic lymphocytes as well as neutrophils and basophils. H_3-receptors modulate neuroconduction by affecting neurotransmitter release in the central and peripheral nervous systems. Histamine also has specific immunomodulatory effects that are discussed below.

Other effector molecules

The effects of LTC_4 overlap significantly with those of histamine, because it causes smooth muscle contraction, increased vascular permeability, and mucus secretion. As it is not preformed, LTC_4 is released several hours after basophil activation and, thus, is a contributor to the late-phase response seen in allergic reactions. MIP-1α is a potent inflammatory mediator that stimulates further histamine release, causing a positive feedback loop of basophil degranulation (Li et al. 1996b).

C5a stimulation of the basophil cell line KU 812 results in production of plasminogen activator inhibitor-1, suggesting that basophils may play a role in the modulation of fibrinolysis (Wojta et al. 2002). Basogranulin is a recently identified basic protein that appears to be unique to basophils, is located in secretory granules, and is secreted (McEuen et al. 1999, 2001). Its physiological role is as yet undetermined.

Eosinophils

Upon activation, eosinophils migrate towards chemoattractants, release stored granules, and produce reactive oxygen metabolites. Eosinophils can also phagocytose foreign antigens and other materials, but do not do so as efficiently as neutrophils.

ACTIVATION

Non-Ig-mediated activation

Eosinophils are predominantly activated by non-Ig-dependent mechanisms. IL-3, IL-5, and GM-CSF, in addition to prolonging eosinophil survival, can all activate eosinophils (Owen et al. 1987; Rothenberg et al. 1988; Yamaguchi et al. 1988). In addition to its role as an eosinophil chemoattractant, eotaxin also activates eosinophils, causing calcium mobilization, production of reactive oxygen species, and upregulation of CD11b through pertussis-sensitive signaling pathways (Tenscher et al. 1996). SDF-1α, through ligation of CXCR4, also causes intracellular calcium fluxes in eosinophils (Nagase et al. 2000).

Eosinophils have receptors to many other cytokines, including IL-1α, IL-2, IL-4, IL-16, stem cell factor (c-kit), TNF-α, IFN-α, and IFN-γ, although the exact effects of these cytokines on eosinophils are not yet known.

In addition to responding to signals made by other cells, eosinophils may be able to respond directly to pathogens. While eosinophils have been shown to express mRNA for Toll-like receptors 1, 2, 4, 7, 9, and 10 (Plotz et al. 2001; Nagase et al. 2003), the functional significance of these receptors on eosinophils remains unclear. While an initial study found that LPS was able to activate eosinophils (Plotz et al. 2001), two subsequent studies have found no effect of LPS on eosinophils (Sabroe et al. 2002; Nagase et al. 2003). Interestingly, R-848, a ligand of TLR7 and TLR8, has been demonstrated to prolong survival and induced superoxide generation in eosinophils (Nagase et al. 2003). These data suggest that eosinophils have the ability to directly respond to pathogens.

Ig-mediated activation

Eosinophils have both high-affinity FcϵRI and low-affinity FcϵRII IgE receptors on their surface. One study showed that binding of IgE to FcϵRI mediated the release of eosinophil peroxidase (EPO) from activated eosinophils (Khalife et al. 1986). A more recent study, however, showed that eosinophils have almost no surface expression of FcϵRI (Seminario et al. 1999). Rather, eosinophils contain large quantities of FcϵRIα (but no FcϵRIβ) intracellularly and release this into the supernatant (Seminario et al. 1999). As FcϵRIα binds to IgE, extracellular release of FcϵRIα may serve as a way to inhibit IgE-mediated events by binding up free IgE.

Eosinophils express both IgA and IgG receptors on their surface. Of the IgG receptors, eosinophils primarily express FcγRII (CDw32), the low-affinity IgG receptor, although they also express small amounts of FcγRI (CD64), a high-affinity IgG receptor, and can express FcγRIII after exposure to IFN-γ. Crosslinking of either the IgG or IgA receptors stimulates rapid eosinophil degranulation (Abu-Ghazaleh et al. 1989; De Andres et al. 1997; Motegi and Kita 1998), but these processes also cause the eosinophils to die and may not be physiological (Weiler et al. 1996). Thus, the role IgG and IgA receptors play in human eosinophil function remains unknown.

Degranulation

Unlike basophils, the exact mechanisms by which eosinophils undergo degranulation have not yet been elucidated. Electron microscopic analysis suggests that eosinophilic granules release their contents into small vesicles that transport them to and release them at the cell surface, akin to piecemeal degranulation in basophils (Dvorak and Weller 2000; Karawajczyk et al. 2000). In a mouse model of Nippostrongylus infection, it has been shown that, although not necessary for eosinophil accumulation at sites of helminth infection, $CD4^+$ T cells are required to enable eosinophil degranulation (Shinkai et al. 2002). The signal transmitted by $CD4^+$ T cells to cause eosinophil degranulation in this model is not known, but even $CD4^+$ T cells deficient in IL-4, IL-13, and the signal-transducing element Stat6, were able to mediate degranulation (Shinkai et al. 2002).

Once activated, eosinophils take on characteristic morphological changes with generation of cytoplasmic vacuolizations, fewer specific granules, and increased numbers of lipid bodies. Activated eosinophils are less dense and more metabolically active than unstimulated eosinophils. These hypodense eosinophils have been described in both allergic and parasitic diseases and exhibit increased surface expression of several proteins, including CD25, CD69, HLA-DR, ICAM-1, FcγRIII, and β_2-integrins (Mawhorter et al. 1996; Bochner 2000). To date, however, no unique marker of eosinophil activation has been described.

EFFECTOR MOLECULES

Effector molecules that eosinophils release include granule proteins, Charcot–Leyden crystal protein, lipid mediators, and enzymes (see Table 5.4), all of which are released into the extracellular space upon activation via degranulation.

Major granule proteins

Major granule proteins include major basic protein (MBP), EPO, eosinophil-derived neurotoxin (EDN), and ECP. All are located in specific granules, have markedly basic isoelectric points, and have a broad range of direct in vitro toxicity against many organisms (including helminths) and normal cells. MBP, so named because of its predominance in specific granules, is located in the central core of the specific granule, whereas the others are found in the matrix of the granule around the core. Although MBP can be found in low amounts in basophils (and EDN and ECP can be found in neutrophils) (Sur et al. 1998), eosinophils are the primary source of these proteins. In addition to its direct cytotoxic effects, MBP induces histamine release from basophils and mast cells, and superoxide production from neutrophils (Moy et al. 1990).

Eosinophil peroxidase catalyzes conversion of hydrogen peroxide and halides such as bromide and

Table 5.4 *Eosinophil effector molecules*

Eosinophil effector molecules
Major granule proteins
Eosinophil-derived neurotoxin
Eosinophil peroxidase
Major basic protein
Eosinophil cationic protein
Primary granule protein
Charcot–Leyden crystal protein
Lipid mediators
Leukotriene C_4
Lipoxins
5-HETE
5,15- and 8,15-diHETE
15-Oxo-ETE
Platelet-activating factor (PAF)
Prostaglandins E_1 and E_2
Thromboxane B_2
Enzymes
Acid phosphatase
Arylsulfatase
Catalase
Hexoseaminidase
Histaminase
Lysophospholipase
Phospholipase D
Oxidative products
Hydrogen peroxide
Hydroxyl radical
Superoxide anion
Singlet oxygen
Cytokines
GM-CSF
TGF-α
TGF-β_1
TNF-α
IFN-γ
Nerve growth factor (NGF)
Neurotrophin 3
Interleukins IL-1α, IL-2, IL-3, IL-4, IL-5, IL-6, IL-10, IL-12, IL-16
Chemokines
IL-8
MIP-1α
RANTES
MCP-3S
Eotaxin

See text for abbreviations.

chloride to hypohalous acids. EDN and ECP are ribonuclease A superfamily members; however, it is not clear what role their enzymatic ability serves, because the cytotoxic activity of ECP does not require its ribonuclease activity (Rosenberg 1995). EDN, named because of its neuropathic effect on rabbits, has never been shown to be neurotoxic for humans.

Charcot–Leyden crystal protein

Located in primary granules (Dvorak et al. 1988), Charcot–Leyden crystal (CLC) protein makes up 7–10 percent of the eosinophil total protein. CLC is a lysophospholipase, which suggests that eosinophils have a role in lipid and membrane metabolism (Weller et al. 1984). X-ray crystallography of CLC shows a structural similarity to galectins (β-galactoside-binding proteins) (Leonidas et al. 1995). CLC is able to bind specifically to β-galactoside sugars, but a natural ligand for CLC has yet to be found (Dyer and Rosenberg 1996).

Other effector molecules

Eosinophils store esterified arachidonic acid in their lipid bodies. Arachidonic acid metabolism through the 5-lipoxygenase pathway results in production and release of LTC_4, which causes vasoconstriction, bronchoconstriction, and smooth muscle contraction (Lewis and Austen 1984). Arachidonic acid metabolism through 15-lipoxygenase results in lipoxins, and metabolism by cyclooxygenase pathways produces prostaglandin E_2 (PGE_2) and thromboxane B_2. Eosinophils also release several oxidative products (including hydrogen peroxide, superoxide anion, and hydroxyl radical and singlet oxygen) and release PAF (Lee et al. 1984).

IMMUNOMODULATORY CAPABILITIES

Although basophils and eosinophils are typically thought of as cells of the innate immune system, they also serve to modify the adaptive immune system by releasing cytokines. In addition, histamine released by basophils has immunomodulatory effects, and eosinophils have the ability to process and present antigen.

Basophils

CYTOKINE RELEASE

Basophils release both IL-4 and IL-13. IL-4 induces $CD4^+$ T-helper (Th) 0 cells to become Th2 cells, and both cytokines can, in combination with ligation of CD40, cause B cells to switch to IgE isotype. Of all PBMCs, basophils are the only ones with the ability to provide IL-4 early in response to a stimulus (Gibbs et al. 2000), releasing preformed IL-4 within 5–10 minutes of IgE stimulation (Gibbs et al. 1996). After activation, basophils also synthesize IL-4 and IL-13 *de novo*, with time-course experiments showing a second peak of IL-4 release after 4 hours and a first peak of IL-13 release at 24 hours (Gibbs et al. 1996).

IL-4 release is increased in basophils exposed to IL-3 but not to basophils exposed to IL-5, GM-CSF, or NGF (Brunner et al. 1993; Dahinden et al. 1997). IL-13 production is also enhanced by IL-3 (Li et al. 1996a). There are probably some differences in the regulation of IL-4 and IL-13 production by basophils, because only IL-13 is secreted from basophils after stimulation with IL-3 alone and IL-4 production is inhibited by the immunosuppressant FK506, whereas IL-13 production is not (Redrup et al. 1998). Also, 20 hours after activation, the amount of IL-4 released from basophils after stimulation with IL-3 and anti-IgE correlates strongly with the percentage of histamine secreted, whereas the amount of IL-13 released does not (Redrup et al. 1998).

Eotaxin also modulates basophil cytokine production, augmenting antigen-dependent IL-4 production and release from basophils by two- to fourfold and lowering the threshold for basophil activation and IL-4 production by 40-fold (Devouassoux et al. 1999). Other factors that enhance basophil IL-4 production include the chemokines MCP-2, MCP-3, MCP-4, RANTES, and eotaxin-2, all of which act on basophils through CCR-3 (Devouassoux et al. 1999), and the recombinant HRF (rp21) (Schroeder et al. 1997).

As they can express CD40 ligand as well as release IL-4 and IL-13, basophils have the ability to induce B cells to switch to IgE isotype (Gauchat et al. 1993), potentially creating a positive feedback loop whereby IgE-dependent activation of basophils results in the production of more IgE by B cells.

ANTIGEN PRESENTATION

Unlike eosinophils, there is no evidence that basophils can act as antigen-presenting cells (APCs).

IMMUNOMODULATORY PROPERTIES OF HISTAMINE

Basophils can modulate the immune response through secreted histamine. Histamine modulates the expression and action of several cytokines, having been shown to increase production of IL-2, IL-5, IL-6, IL-8, IL-10, IL-11, IL-16, GM-CSF, and RANTES and to downregulate production of IL-2, IL-4, IL-12, IFN-γ, and TNF-α (Igaz et al. 2001).

Signaling through the different histamine receptors mediates different effects on the Th response. Triggering of the H1R on $CD4^+$ T cells enhances Th1-type responses, causing increased IFN-γ production and subsequent downregulation of Th2-type responses, whereas triggering through the H2R downregulates both Th1 and Th2 responses (Elenkov et al. 1998; Jutel et al. 2001). As the Th2-type response is integral to the production of IgE through the actions of IL-4 and IL-13, the downregulation of the Th2 arm of the cellular immune system through H_1- and H_2-receptors may serve as a negative feedback on the response that initially accounted for the production of IgE which led to the basophil degranulation.

It is clear that histamine affects a variety of cell types and modulates the Thl/Th2 balance at several different points. Histamine affects monocytes by decreasing their production of IL-12 (van der Pouw Kraan et al. 1998) and inhibiting ICAM-1 expression induced by IL-18 (Takahashi et al. 2002). Through interaction with the H_2-receptor, histamine causes increased IL-10 and decreased IL-12 production by dendritic cells (Mazzoni et al. 2001). Histamine also increases the release of IL-10 from unstimulated and LPS-stimulated human alveolar macrophages by PGE_2 and nitric oxide (NO) production (Sirois et al. 2000). One study suggests that many of the effects of histamine may be the result of its upregulation of IL-18 production, because addition of anti-IL-18 abolished all cytokine changes caused by histamine in in vitro studies of PBMCs (Kohka et al. 2000).

Eosinophils

CYTOKINE RELEASE

Eosinophils release a multitude of cytokines (see Table 5.2), many of which amplify a type 2 response. Eosinophils produce and release IL-1α, which can work in concert with APCs as a stimulator for Th2 lymphocytes (Del Pozo et al. 1990; Weller et al. 1993). In murine schistome granulomas, eosinophils are the predominant source of IL-4. Eosinophils also release IL-3, IL-5, and GM-CSF (Kita et al. 1991; Moqbel et al. 1991; Broide et al. 1992; Desreumaux et al. 1993), the cytokines most responsible for eosinophilopoeisis in the bone marrow, suggesting that eosinophil degranulation results in increased eosinophil production. In a murine model of Nippostrongylus infection, eosinophils accumulate at sites of helminth infection and express IL-4 even in mice lacking B and T cells, raising the possibility that eosinophils may even have the capacity to initiate a Th2 response (Shinkai et al. 2002).

In addition to contributing to the Th2 response, several cytokines released by eosinophils play a direct role in the inflammatory response. IL-1α and TNF-α, both secreted by eosinophils (Del Pozo et al. 1990; Weller et al. 1993; Finotto et al. 1994), are potent inflammatory agents that can enhance local blood flow, activate macrophages, and induce fibroblast growth. TGF-α and TGF-β, also released by eosinophils, are potent promoters of fibroblast growth and collagen synthesis and may play a role in the tissue fibrosis that occurs in diseases of chronic eosinophilic inflammation (Todd et al. 1991; Finotto et al. 1994).

It has recently been shown that eosinophils synthesize and release NGF and neurotrophin-3 (Kobayashi et al. 2002), factors that are essential for the survival and development of peripheral neurons. Although the physiological relevance of this finding has yet to be determined, it suggests that eosinophils may be involved in processes such as guiding tissue homeostasis and development. Alternatively, as NGF can activate eosinophils (Solomon et al. 1998), release of NGF by eosinophils may serve as a means by which eosinophil activation is amplified in an autocrine fashion.

ANTIGEN PRESENTATION

Eosinophils express MHC class II (HLA-DR) when cultured with GM-CSF in vitro (Lucey et al. 1989). In vivo, eosinophils taken from sites of inflammation in patients with asthma, allergy, and chronic eosinophilic pneumonia also express MHC class II (Hansel et al. 1991; Beninati et al. 1993). Evidence that eosinophils can function as APCs comes from in vitro and mouse models showing that eosinophils can stimulate antigen-specific T-cell proliferation (Del Pozo et al. 1992; Hansel et al. 1992; Weller et al. 1993). The extent to which eosinophils actually present antigen in vivo is unclear, especially as they are not particularly efficient at phagocytosis, often a first step required for antigen presentation.

BASOPHILIA AND EOSINOPHILIA AS DISEASE MARKERS

Eosinophilia, which is usually defined as an eosinophil count > 500 cells/mm^3, is a common finding in helminth infections, allergy, asthma, and several other diseases. Basophilia is a rare finding in all disease processes except for chronic myelogenous leukemia. Tables 5.5 and 5.6 list the infectious and non-infectious diseases in which basophilia and eosinophilia have been reported to occur.

ROLE IN INFECTIOUS DISEASES

The majority of research on eosinophils and basophils has focused on their roles in diseases such as asthma and allergy. In addition to these states, however, it is clear that basophils and eosinophils play large roles in the immunological response to infectious diseases – especially to helminths and possibly to viruses. Despite decades of study, however, the exact function that these cells serve in the response to infection remains unclear.

Helminth infections

BASOPHILS

Several factors suggest that basophils play an important role in the immune response to helminth infections. While a recent retrospective study suggests that basophilia does not occur in helminth infections of humans (Mitre and Nutman 2003), it clearly occurs in animal

Table 5.5 *Diseases associated with basophilia*

Diseases associated with basophilia
Infectious diseases
Helminths (in animal models, not reported in humans)
Tuberculosis
Viruses
Influenza[a]
Smallpox[a]
Varicella-zoster[a]
Non-infectious causes
Allergic reactions to medication or food
Diabetes mellitus
Erythroderma
Estrogen administration
Hodgkin's disease
Hypothyroidism
Iron deficiency
Juvenile rheumatoid arthritis
Myeloproliferative/neoplastic diseases
Chronic myelogenous leukemia
Myelofibrosis
Polycythemia vera
Primary thrombocythemia
Serum sickness
Ulcerative colitis
Urticaria

a) Mentioned in other reviews; primary sources not found.

models of parasitic infection. One of the earliest reports of this phenomenon came from Chan in the 1960s, who showed that bone marrow and circulating basophil counts increase within 48 hours of subcutaneous injection of Ascaris body (Chan 1965) and ova fluid (Chan 1968) into guinea pigs. Since then, several other investigators have reported similar findings in several different animal models of parasitic infection. *Trichostrongylus colubriformis* infection has been shown to increase basophil numbers in the bone marrow, small intestine, and peripheral circulation of guinea pigs (Rothwell and Love 1975). Infection of rats (Ogilvie et al. 1978; Roth and Levy 1980; Kasugai et al. 1993) and gerbils (Okada et al. 1997) with *Nippostrongylus brasiliensis* resulted in up to a 50-fold increase in peripheral basophil counts at 2 weeks. *Trichinella spiralis* infection in rats (Ogilvie et al. 1980) and guinea pigs (Lindor et al. 1983) also results in a marked basophilia that precedes the onset of eosinophilia by approximately 1 week. Fasciola infection of guinea pigs is associated with a chronic peripheral basophilia that is detectable up to 4 months after infection (Conboy and Stromberg 1991), and strongyloides infection of *Erythrocebus patas* monkeys causes peripheral basophilia that is occasionally detectable for more than a month after infection (Harper et al. 1984).

Basophils clearly respond to helminth infections, because basophils from patients infected with *Toxocara*, *Ascaris*, *Onchocerca*, *Wuchereria*, *Strongyloides*, and *Schistosoma* spp. have been shown to release histamine in response to parasite antigen (Ottesen et al. 1979; Genta et al. 1983; Hofstetter et al. 1983; Nielsen et al. 1994; Gonzalez-Munoz et al. 1999). Helminth infections are associated with high levels of IgE (Rossi et al. 1993; Estambale et al. 1995; Ramirez et al. 1996), and the amount of histamine released by basophils in response to toxocara antigen is proportional to the serum concentration of toxocara antigen-specific IgE (Nielsen et al. 1994).

In addition to high levels of IgE, human helminth infections are also associated with increased production of IL-4, the prototypical Th2 cytokine. Basophils from filaria-infected patients have been shown to release IL-4 in response to infective stage (L3) larvae and filarial antigen (King 2001), and basophils from non-infected individuals have been shown to release IL-4 after stimulation with schistosoma egg antigen (Falcone et al. 1996). Although basophils make up only a small percentage of peripheral white blood cells, they have the ability specifically to recognize many different antigens by virtue of binding different IgE antibodies on their surface. Consequently, it is possible that the number of basophils that specifically recognize and are activated by helminth antigen may equal or even exceed the number of antigen-specific T cells responding to helminths. Indeed, results from a recent study showed that the number of basophils producing IL-4 in response to filarial antigen was usually equal to or greater than the number of IL-4-producing T-cells in filaria-infected patients (Mitre et al. 2004). Whereas filarial antigen was only shown to cause basophil activation in filaria-infected patients with filarial-Ag specific IgE, it has been demonstrated that a glycoprotein from *Schistosoma mansoni* eggs can cause basophils to degranulate and release IL-4 by binding and crosslinking non-antigen-specific IgE (Falcone et al. 1996; Haisch et al. 2001), raising the possibility that some helminth antigens may act as a type of 'super-allergen' by being able to bind directly to the nonvariable portion of IgE. This suggests that, in some cases, basophils may serve as the initial source of IL-4, providing the stimulus for T cells to differentiate toward a Th2 phenotype.

Similarly, homologs of mammalian, translationally controlled tumor protein, a calcium-binding protein that directly stimulates histamine release from basophils, have recently been cloned from *Schistosoma mansoni* (Rao et al. 2002) and the filarial parasites *Wuchereria bancrofti* and *Brugia malayi* (Gnanasekar et al. 2002).

EOSINOPHILS

Eosinophilia is a frequent finding in invasive helminth infections; such eosinophilia is probably mediated by IL-5, because treatment of mice with anti-IL-5 results in ablation of helminth-induced eosinophilia (Coffman et al.

Table 5.6 *Diseases associated with eosinophilia*

Infectious diseases		Non-infectious causes	
Bacteria		**Allergic diseases**	
	Resolving scarlet fever		Allergic rhinitis[a]
	Tuberculosis[a]		Asthma[a]
Fungi			Atopic dermatitis[a]
	Allergic bronchopulmonary aspergillosis[a]		Medication allergy[a]
	Coccidioidomycosis		Urticaria/angioedema[a]
Helminths		**Dermatological diseases**	
	Angiostrongyliasis[a]		Atopic dermatitis[a]
	Anisakiasis[a]		Bullous pemphigoid
	Ascariasis[a]		Urticaria/angioedema[a]
	Capillariasis[a]	**Immunodeficiencies**	
	Clonorchiasis[a]		Wiskott–Aldrich syndrome
	Coenurosis[a]		Hyper-IgE (Job's) syndrome
	Cysticercosis		Autoimmune lymphoproliferative syndrome (ALPS)
	Dicrocoeliasis[a]	**Rheumatological diseases**	
	Echinococcosis[a]		Eosinophilic fasciitis[a]
	Echinostomiasis[a]		Hypersensitivity vasculitis
	Enterobiasis		Rheumatoid arthritis
	Fascioliasis[a]	**Myeloproliferative/neoplastic diseases**	
	Filariasis[a]		Eosinophilic leukemia[a]
	Gnathostomiasis[a]		Hodgkin's disease
	Heterophyiasis[a]		Idiopathic hypereosinophilic syndrome
	Hookworm[a]		Kimura disease
	Hymenolepsiasis[a]		Lymphomas
	Metagoniamiasis[a]		Myeloid leukemia
	Opisthorciasis[a]		Solid tumors
	Paragonomiasis[a]	**Gastrointestinal diseases**	
	Schistosomiasis[a]		Celiac sprue
	Sparganosis[a]		Eosinophilic gastroenteritis[a]
	Strongyloidiasis[a]		Inflammatory bowel disease
	Trichinosis[a]	**Respiratory diseases**	
	Trichuriasis[a]		Asthma[a]
	Visceral larva migrans[a]		Allergic rhinitis[a]
Protozoa			Churg–Strauss syndrome
	Isosporiasis		Eosinophilic pneumonia
Viruses		**Miscellaneous**	
	HIV		Eosinophilic myalgia syndrome
	Respiratory syncytial virus		Graft-versus-host disease
			GM-CSF therapy
			Histiocytosis
			Hypereosinophilic syndrome
			IL-2 therapy
			Toxic oil syndrome

a) Disease in which eosinophilia commonly occurs.

1989; Sher et al. 1990). After treatment of human patients infected with onchocerciasis or lymphatic filariasis, serum IL-5 levels increase and circulating eosinophil levels decrease, suggesting that eosinophils are recruited out of the circulation and into the tissues by IL-5 in response to dying helminths (Limaye et al. 1991, 1993; Cooper et al. 1999). In addition to increased production and recruitment of eosinophils by IL-5, eosinophilia in response to helminth infections may be the result of a prolonged eosinophil lifespan, because eosinophils from splenic granulomas of *Schistosoma mansoni*-infected mice have been shown to be resistant to apoptosis in vivo and protected from Fas–FasL-mediated apoptosis by the absence of Fas ligand expression (Rumbley et al. 2001).

Studies in mice and in vitro clearly show that eosinophils are toxic to helminths. Culture of freshly isolated human eosinophils with antibody-coated *Schistosoma mansoni* larvae results in death of 14 percent of the parasites. After addition of IL-3, the eosinophils kill over 50 percent of the *S. mansoni* larvae (Rothenberg et al. 1988). IL-5 can also enhance the toxicity of eosinophils against *S. mansoni* (Mazza et al. 1991).

Binding of CD11b and VLA-4 on the eosinophil surface to C3a and plasma fibronectin deposited on the cuticular surface of *Nippostrongylus brasiliesis* larvae after experimental infection of transgenic IL-5 mice allows eosinophils to adhere directly to the larvae (Shin et al. 2001). Electron microscopy reveals that the cuticular surface of *N. brasiliensis* larvae in this model becomes damaged from electron-dense materials released from the eosinophils. Indeed, purifed eosinophil granule proteins have been shown to have direct toxicity on various helminths, including *Trichinella spiralis* (Hamann et al. 1987), *S. mansoni* (Ackerman et al. 1985), *Brugia malayi* (Hamann et al. 1990), and *Trypanosoma cruzi* (Molina et al. 1988). Eosinophil toxicity of helminths has been shown to occur via antibody-dependent (Butterworth et al. 1974) and antibody-independent (Shin et al. 2001) mechanisms.

Whether eosinophils actively protect against helminth infections remains controversial. Several studies using rabbit anti-mouse eosinophil serum, which depletes mice of circulating eosinophils, showed that eosinophils probably have a protective effect against Schistoma, Trichinella, and Trichostrongylus infections (Mahmoud et al. 1975; Grove et al. 1977; Gleich et al. 1979).

In contrast to these findings, more recent studies using anti-IL-5 antibodies to deplete circulating eosinophils in experimental helminth infections have shown mixed results in terms of the importance of eosinophils in mediating helminth protection. Mouse models of Schistosoma, Trichinella, and Trichuris infections found no differences in parasite burden in eosinophil-depleted mice compared with control mice (Sher et al. 1990; Herndon and Kayes 1992; Betts and Else 1999). On the other hand, elimination of eosinophils using IL-5-neutralizing antibodies, although not affecting the number of tissue-migrating larvae recovered from the lungs in primary infection with *Strongyloides venezuelensis*, does result in greater numbers of adult Strongyloides worms in the intestine, suggesting that eosinophils are important in the control of infection, although perhaps not during the initial establishment of infection (Korenaga et al. 1994). Also, anti-IL-5-treated mice become susceptible to re-infection with *Onchocerca lienalis*, a helminth to which mice are usually resistant (Folkard et al. 1996).

Other approaches to ascertain the role of eosinophils in response to helminth infection also come to different conclusions. Mice deficient in IL-5 cannot develop circulating or tissue eosinophilia. These IL-5 KO mice have been shown to have similar susceptibility to *Mesocestoides corti*, *Hymenolepis diminuta*, and *Fasciola hepatica* as control mice (Kopf et al. 1996; Ovington and Behm 1997). *Toxocara canis*, *Strongyloides ratti*, and *Heligmosomoides polygyrias* infections, however, appear to be more severe and cause greater tissue damage in IL-5-deficient mice than in control mice (Ovington and Behm 1997). In one study, IL-5 transgenic mice, which have high baseline peripheral blood eosinophil levels, were shown to have the same susceptibility to infection with *Schistosoma mansoni* as control mice (Freeman et al. 1995). Another study, however, demonstrated that IL-5 transgenic mice have greater resistance against helminths, with a sevenfold decrease in the worm recovery rate 60 days after infection with *Litomosoides sigmodontis* compared with control mice (Martin et al. 2000). In an ex vivo gut loop experimental infection of *Fasciola hepatica*, protection correlated strongly with the frequency of eosinophils in the gut (Van Milligen et al. 1999). CCR3 KO mice, which are unable to recruit eosinophils to the small intestine and skeletal muscle after infection with *Trichinella spiralis*, exhibit normal rejection rates of adult worms from the small intestine but have greater total numbers of cysts in the skeletal muscle and these cysts exhibit less necrosis than those of normal mice (Gurish et al. 2002).

There are several possible explanations for the discrepant results of studies of eosinophils and helminth infections. It may be that eosinophils play different roles in different animal species. Moreover, there are significant differences between human and mouse eosinophils: murine eosinophils lack Fcε receptors (de Andres et al. 1997), and there are large differences between the amino acid sequences of mouse EDN and ECP compared with human EDN and ECP (Larson et al. 1996; Nittoh et al. 1997). Also, eosinophils may be efficacious against some helminth infections (or some stages of the infections) but not all. To date, one of the major barriers to studying the role of eosinophils in helminth infections has been the lack of a specific method for selective depletion of eosinophils. A monoclonal antibody to CCR3 has recently been developed and been shown selectively to deplete eosinophils in mice (Grimaldi et al. 1999). Studies using this antibody are currently under way and will, it is hoped, better elucidate the role of eosinophils in the immune response to helminths.

Viral infections

BASOPHILS

Although the role, if any, that basophils play in host defense against HIV is unknown, it is clear that basophils may be an important reservoir for HIV infection. Basophils express CD4 as well as the HIV co-receptors CCR3 and CXCR4, can be infected with M-tropic HIV in vitro, and have been shown to be infected with HIV in many patients with AIDS (Li et al. 2001). HIV-1 Tat protein upregulates CCR3 expression on basophils, increasing the likelihood that the virus successfully infects the cells (Marone et al. 2001). IL-16, which can bind to CD4, makes basophils less susceptible to infection with M-tropic HIV (Qi et al. 2002). Notably, HIV-1 gp120 can act as a 'super-allergen' by interacting with the heavy chain variable 3 (V[H]3) region of IgE to induce cytokine and histamine release from $Fc\epsilon R1^+$ cells (Marone et al. 2001). The physiological significance of this phenomenon is unknown.

Basophils also interact with respiratory viruses. In vitro, infection of human PBMCs with respiratory viruses results in enhanced IgE-mediated histamine release from basophils (Chonmaitree et al. 1988), and experimental infection of allergic rhinitis patients with rhinovirus 16 results in increased plasma histamine levels (Calhoun et al. 1991). Rhinovirus infection of the basophil cell line KU 812 augments anti-IgE-induced histamine release and increases maximal IL-4 and IL-6 production by basophils (Hosoda et al. 2002). These results suggest that some respiratory viruses may trigger asthma attacks by causing release of histamine and type 2 cytokines from basophils. The effect that the basophils have in terms of host defense in these infections is not known.

EOSINOPHILS

Asymptomatic eosinophilia occurs in 18 percent of patients with HIV (Caterino-de-Araujo 1994), and occurrence of eosinophilia in HIV correlates with low $CD4^+$ cell counts (Smith et al. 1994; Tietz et al. 1997). Eosinophilia in HIV patients, however, is neither a useful clinical marker for eosinophil-related diseases nor a predictive factor for the future course of HIV infection. In a study of blood counts in HIV patients over a 4-year period, no etiological agent could be found in patients with eosinophilia (Cohen and Steigbigel 1996). Other than a moderate increase in the prevalence of rash, a case–control study of HIV patients with and without eosinophilia found no significant clinical correlation between eosinophilia and other diseases such as parasitic infection, allergic reaction, or malignancy (Skiest and Keiser 1997).

Like basophils, eosinophils express CD4 and CCR3 and can be infected by macrophage-tropic strains of HIV (Weller et al. 1995; Alkhatib et al. 1997). Eotaxin, which binds to CCR3, diminishes HIV entry into eosinophils (Alkhatib et al. 1997).

Some in vitro data suggest that eosinophils may aid in eliminating HIV. EPO has been shown to have marked antiviral activity against HIV-1 (Klebanoff and Coombs 1996), and eosinophils have been shown to inhibit cellular transduction by a mouse retrovirus through a mechanism dependent on eosinophil ribonucleases (Domachowske and Rosenberg 1997); however, subcutaneous injection of IL-3 into humans with HIV, which resulted in a 17-fold increase in absolute eosinophil counts, caused no significant quantitative changes in viral load, suggesting that IL-3 and corresponding eosinophilia do not enhance HIV elimination in humans (Scadden et al. 1995).

Eosinophils may also play a role in the pathogenesis of respiratory syncytial virus (RSV) infection. Eosinophils are often found in nasal washes of children with RSV (Zhao et al. 2002), and are occasionally found in increased numbers in the peripheral circulation as well (Ehlenfield et al. 2000). Whether eosinophils serve a protective role against RSV has not yet been completely determined, although such a role has been postulated (Rosenberg and Domachowske 2001). The tissue eosinophilia induced by RSV infection may, however, exacerbate asthma. The degree of eosinophilia in nasopharyngeal secretions correlates with the degree of asthma exacerbation in children with asthma who are infected with RSV, but not influenza (Zhao et al. 2002). In addition, higher peripheral blood eosinophil counts at the time of RSV bronchiolitis are associated with an increased risk of developing childhood asthma (Ehlenfield et al. 2000).

REFERENCES

Abu-Ghazaleh, R.I., Fujisawa, T., et al. 1989. IgA-induced eosinophil degranulation. *J Immunol*, **142**, 2393–400.

Ackerman, S.J., Gleich, G.J., et al. 1985. Comparative toxicity of purified human eosinophil granule cationic proteins for schistosomula of *Schistosoma mansoni*. *Am J Trop Med Hyg*, **34**, 735–45.

Alam, R., Lett-Brown, M.A., et al. 1992. Monocyte chemotactic and activating factor is a potent histamine-releasing factor for basophils. *J Clin Invest*, **89**, 723–8.

Alam, R., Forsythe, P., et al. 1994. Monocyte chemotactic protein-2, monocyte chemotactic protein-3, and fibroblast-induced cytokine. Three new chemokines induce chemotaxis and activation of basophils. *J Immunol*, **153**, 3155–9.

Alkhatib, G., Berger, E.A., et al. 1997. Determinants of HIV-1 coreceptor function on CC chemokine receptor 3. Importance of both extracellular and transmembrane/cytoplasmic regions. *J Biol Chem*, **272**, 20420–6.

Anderson, D.C., Schmalsteig, F.C., et al. 1985. The severe and moderate phenotypes of heritable Mac-1, LFA-1 deficiency: their quantitative definition and relation to leukocyte dysfunction and clinical features. *J Infect Dis*, **152**, 668–89.

Arrang, J.M., Garbarg, M., et al. 1987. Highly potent and selective ligands for histamine H3 receptors. *Nature*, **327**, 117–23.

Atsuta, J., Fujisawa, T., et al. 1995. Inhibitory effect of transforming growth factor β 1 on cytokine-enhanced eosinophil survival and degranulation. *Int Arch Allergy Immunol*, **108**, 31–5.

Badewa, A.P., Hudson, C.E. and Heiman, A.S. 2002. Regulatory effects of eotaxin, eotaxin-2, and eotaxin-3 on eosinophil degranulation and superoxide anion generation. *Exp Biol Med (Maywood)*, **227**, 645–51.

Bauza, M.T. and Lagunoff, D. 1981. Histidine transport by isolated rat peritoneal mast cells. *Biochem Pharmacol*, **30**, 1271–6.

Beauvais, F., Michel, L. and Dubertret, L. 1995. The nitric oxide donors, azide and hydroxylamine, inhibit the programmed cell death of cytokine-deprived human eosinophils. *FEBS Lett*, **361**, 229–32.

Beninati, W., Derdak, S., et al. 1993. Pulmonary eosinophils express HLA-DR in chronic eosinophilic pneumonia. *J Allergy Clin Immunol*, **92**, 442–9.

Berger, R.B., Blackwell, N.M., et al. 2002. IL-4 and IL-13 regulation of ICAM-1 expression and eosinophil recruitment in *Onchocerca volvulus* keratitis. *Invest Ophthalmol Vis Sci*, **43**, 2992–7.

Betts, C.J. and Else, K.J. 1999. Mast cells, eosinophils and antibody-mediated cellular cytotoxicity are not critical in resistance to *Trichuris muris*. *Parasite Immunol*, **21**, 45–52.

Bischoff, S.C. and Dahinden, C.A. 1992. Effect of nerve growth factor on the release of inflammatory mediators by mature human basophils. *Blood*, **79**, 2662–9.

Bischoff, S.C., Brunner, T., De Weck, A.L. and Dahinden, C.A. 1990a. Interleukin 5 modifies histamine release and leukotriene generation by human basophils in response to diverse agonists. *J Exp Med*, **172**, 1577–82.

Bischoff, S.C., De Weck, A.L. and Dahinden, C.A. 1990b. Interleukin 3 and granulocyte macrophage colony-stimulating factor render human basophils responsive to low concentrations of complement component C3a. *Proc Natl Acad Sci USA*, **87**, 6813–17.

Black, J.W., Duncan, W.A., et al. 1972. Definition and antagonism of histamine H 2 receptors. *Nature*, **236**, 385–90.

Bochner, B.S. 2000. Systemic activation of basophils and eosinophils: markers and consequences. *J Allergy Clin Immunol*, **106**, S292–302.

Bochner, B.S. and Schleimer, R.P. 2001. Mast cells, basophils, and eosinophils: distinct but overlapping pathways for recruitment. *Immunol Rev*, **179**, 5–15.

Bochner, B.S., Peachell, P.T., et al. 1988. Adherence of human basophils to cultured umbilical vein endothelial cells. *J Clin Invest*, **81**, 1355–64.

Bochner, B.S., MacGlashan, D.W. Jr, et al. 1989. IgE-dependent regulation of human basophil adherence to vascular endothelium. *J Immunol*, **142**, 3180–6.

Bochner, B.S., McKelvey, A.A., et al. 1990. IL-3 augments adhesiveness for endothelium and CD11b expression in human basophils but not neutrophils. *J Immunol*, **145**, 1832–7.

Bochner, B.S., Klunk, D.A., et al. 1995. IL-13 selectively induces vascular cell adhesion molecule-1 expression in human endothelial cells. *J Immunol*, **154**, 799–803.

Boyce, J.A., Friend, D., et al. 1995. Differentiation in vitro of hybrid eosinophil/basophil granulocytes: autocrine function of an eosinophil developmental intermediate. *J Exp Med*, **182**, 49–57.

Brattig, N.W., Abakar, A.Z., et al. 1995. Cell-adhesion molecules expressed by activated eosinophils in *Onchocerca volvulus* infection. *Parasitol Res*, **81**, 398–402.

Broide, D. 2002. Fast flowing eosinophils: signals for stopping and stepping out of blood vessels. *Am J Respir Cell Mol Biol*, **26**, 637–40.

Broide, D.H., Paine, M.M. and Firestein, G.S. 1992. Eosinophils express interleukin 5 and granulocyte macrophage colony-stimulating factor mRNA at sites of allergic inflammation in asthmatics. *J Clin Invest*, **90**, 1414–24.

Brunner, T., Heusser, C.H. and Dahinden, C.A. 1993. Human peripheral blood basophils primed by interleukin 3 (IL-3) produce IL-4 in response to immunoglobulin E receptor stimulation. *J Exp Med*, **177**, 605–11.

Buhring, H.J., Simmons, P.J., et al. 1999. The monoclonal antibody 97A6 defines a novel surface antigen expressed on human basophils and their multipotent and unipotent progenitors. *Blood*, **94**, 2343–56.

Buhring, H.J., Seiffert, M., et al. 2001. The basophil activation marker defined by antibody 97A6 is identical to the ectonucleotide pyrophosphatase/phosphodiesterase 3. *Blood*, **97**, 3303–5.

Bureau, F., Seumois, G., et al. 2002. CD40 engagement enhances eosinophil survival through induction of cellular inhibitor of apoptosis protein 2 expression: possible involvement in allergic inflammation. *J Allergy Clin Immunol*, **110**, 443–9.

Burke-Gaffney, A., Blease, K., et al. 2002. TNF-α potentiates C5a-stimulated eosinophil adhesion to human bronchial epithelial cells: a role for α5β1 integrin. *J Immunol*, **168**, 1380–8.

Butterworth, A.E., Sturrock, R.F., et al. 1974. Antibody-dependent cell-mediated damage to schistosomula in vitro. *Nature*, **252**, 503–5.

Calhoun, W.J., Swenson, C.A., et al. 1991. Experimental rhinovirus 16 infection potentiates histamine release after antigen bronchoprovocation in allergic subjects. *Am Rev Respir Dis*, **144**, 1267–73.

Caterino-De-Araujo, A. 1994. HIV-1 infection and eosinophilia. *Immunol Today*, **15**, 498–9.

Chan, B.S. 1965. Quantitative changes in the basophil cells of guinea-pig bone marrow following the administration of Ascaris body fluid. *Immunology*, **8**, 566–77.

Chan, B.S. 1968. Quantitative changes in the basophil cells of guinea-pig bone marrow following the administration of desiccated Ascaris ova. *Immunology*, **14**, 99–106.

Chonmaitree, T., Lett-Brown, M.A., et al. 1988. Role of interferon in leukocyte histamine release caused by common respiratory viruses. *J Infect Dis*, **157**, 127–32.

Coffman, R.L., Seymour, B.W., et al. 1989. Antibody to interleukin-5 inhibits helminth-induced eosinophilia in mice. *Science*, **245**, 308–10.

Cohen, A.J. and Steigbigel, R.T. 1996. Eosinophilia in patients infected with human immunodeficiency virus. *J Infect Dis*, **174**, 615–18.

Columbo, M., Horowitz, E.M., et al. 1992. The human recombinant c-kit receptor ligand, rhSCF, induces mediator release from human cutaneous mast cells and enhances IgE-dependent mediator release from both skin mast cells and peripheral blood basophils. *J Immunol*, **149**, 599–608.

Conboy, G.A. and Stromberg, B.E. 1991. Hematology and clinical pathology of experimental *Fascioloides magna* infection in cattle and guinea pigs. *Vet Parasitol*, **40**, 241–55.

Cooper, P.J., Awadzi, K., et al. 1999. Eosinophil sequestration and activation are associated with the onset and severity of systemic adverse reactions following the treatment of onchocerciasis with ivermectin. *J Infect Dis*, **179**, 738–42.

Cross, D.A., Klesius, P.H., et al. 1987. Dermal cellular responses of helminth-free and *Ostertagia ostertagi*-infected calves to intradermal injections of soluble extracts from *O ostertagi* L3 larvae. *Vet Parasitol*, **23**, 257–64.

Cuvelier, S.L. and Patel, K.D. 2001. Shear-dependent eosinophil transmigration on interleukin 4-stimulated endothelial cells: a role for endothelium-associated eotaxin-3. *J Exp Med*, **194**, 1699–709.

Daeron, M., Latour, S., et al. 1995. The same tyrosine-based inhibition motif, in the intracytoplasmic domain of FcγRIIB, regulates negatively BCR-, TCR- and FcR-dependent cell activation. *Immunity*, **3**, 635–46.

Dahinden, C.A., Geiser, T., et al. 1994. Monocyte chemotactic protein 3 is a most effective basophil- and eosinophil-activating chemokine. *J Exp Med*, **179**, 751–6.

Dahinden, C.A., Rihs, S. and Ochsensberger, B. 1997. Regulation of cytokine expression by human blood basophils. *Int Arch Allergy Immunol*, **113**, 134–7.

de Andres, B., Rakasz, E., et al. 1997. Lack of Fcε receptors on murine eosinophils: implications for the functional significance of elevated IgE and eosinophils in parasitic infections. *Blood*, **89**, 3826–36.

Del Pozo, V., De Andres, B., et al. 1990. Murine eosinophils and IL-1: αIL-1 mRNA detection by *in situ* hybridization. Production and release of IL-1 from peritoneal eosinophils. *J Immunol*, **144**, 3117–22.

Del Pozo, V., De Andres, B., et al. 1992. Eosinophil as antigen-presenting cell: activation of T cell clones and T cell hybridoma by eosinophils after antigen processing. *Eur J Immunol*, **22**, 1919–25.

Denburg, J.A., Telizyn, S., et al. 1985. Heterogeneity of human peripheral blood eosinophil-type colonies: evidence for a common basophil-eosinophil progenitor. *Blood*, **66**, 312–18.

Denburg, J.A., Silver, J.E. and Abrams, J.S. 1991. Interleukin-5 is a human basophilopoietin: induction of histamine content and basophilic differentiation of HL-60 cells and of peripheral blood basophil-eosinophil progenitors. *Blood*, **77**, 1462–8.

Desreumaux, P., Janin, A., et al. 1993. Synthesis of interleukin-5 by activated eosinophils in patients with eosinophilic heart diseases. *Blood*, **82**, 1553–60.

Devouassoux, G., Metcalfe, D.D. and Prussin, C. 1999. Eotaxin potentiates antigen-dependent basophil IL-4 production. *J Immunol*, **163**, 2877–82.

Discipio, R.G., Daffern, P.J., et al. 1999. A comparison of C3a and C5a-mediated stable adhesion of rolling eosinophils in postcapillary venules and transendothelial migration in vitro and in vivo. *J Immunol*, **162**, 1127–36.

Domachowske, J.B. and Rosenberg, H.F. 1997. Eosinophils inhibit retroviral transduction of human target cells by a ribonuclease-dependent mechanism. *J Leukoc Biol*, **62**, 363–8.

Domachowske, J.B., Bonville, C.A., et al. 2002. Pulmonary eosinophilia in mice devoid of interleukin-5. *J Leukoc Biol*, **71**, 966–72.

Dombrowicz, D., Lin, S., et al. 1998. Allergy-associated FcRβ is a molecular amplifier of IgE- and IgG-mediated in vivo responses. *Immunity*, **8**, 517–29.

Donnadieu, E., Jouvin, M.H. and Kinet, J.P. 2000. A second amplifier function for the allergy-associated FcεRI-β subunit. *Immunity*, **12**, 515–23.

Druilhe, A., Cai, Z., et al. 1996. Fas-mediated apoptosis in cultured human eosinophils. *Blood*, **87**, 2822–30.

Dulkys, Y., Schramm, G., et al. 2001. Detection of mRNA for eotaxin-2 and eotaxin-3 in human dermal fibroblasts and their distinct activation profile on human eosinophils. *J Invest Dermatol*, **116**, 498–505.

Dvorak, A.M. and Weller, P.F. 2000. Ultrastructural analysis of human eosinophils. *Chem Immunol*, **76**, 1–28.

Dvorak, A.M., Mihm, M.C. Jr and Dvorak, H.F. 1976. Degranulation of basophilic leukocytes in allergic contact dermatitis reactions in man. *J Immunol*, **116**, 687–95.

Dvorak, A.M., Newball, H.H., et al. 1980. Antigen-induced IgE-mediated degranulation of human basophils. *Lab Invest*, **43**, 126–39.

Dvorak, A.M., Letourneau, L., et al. 1988. Ultrastructural localization of the Charcot-Leyden crystal protein (lysophospholipase) to a distinct crystalloid-free granule population in mature human eosinophils. *Blood*, **72**, 150–8.

Dvorak, A.M., Warner, J.A., et al. 1991. F-met peptide-induced degranulation of human basophils. *Lab Invest*, **64**, 234–53.

Dvorak, A.M., Seder, R.A., et al. 1994. Effects of interleukin-3 with or without the c-kit ligand, stem cell factor, on the survival and cytoplasmic granule formation of mouse basophils and mast cells in vitro. *Am J Pathol*, **144**, 160–70.

Dvorak, A.M., Schroeder, J.T., et al. 1996. Comparative ultrastructural morphology of human basophils stimulated to release histamine by anti-IgE, recombinant IgE-dependent histamine-releasing factor, or monocyte chemotactic protein-1. *J Allergy Clin Immunol*, **98**, 355–70.

Dyer, K.D. and Rosenberg, H.F. 1996. Eosinophil Charcot-Leyden crystal protein binds to β-galactoside sugars. *Life Sci*, **58**, 2073–82.

Eglite, S., Pluss, K. and Dahinden, C.A. 2000. Requirements for C5a receptor-mediated IL-4 and IL-13 production and leukotriene C4 generation in human basophils. *J Immunol*, **165**, 2183–9.

Ehlenfield, D.R., Cameron, K. and Welliver, R.C. 2000. Eosinophilia at the time of respiratory syncytial virus bronchiolitis predicts childhood reactive airway disease. *Pediatrics*, **105**, 79–83.

Elenkov, I.J., Webster, E., et al. 1998. Histamine potently suppresses human IL-12 and stimulates IL-10 production via H2 receptors. *J Immunol*, **161**, 2586–93.

Estambale, B.B., Simonsen, P.E., et al. 1995. Bancroftian filariasis in Kwale District of Kenya. III. Quantification of the IgE response in selected individuals from an endemic community. *Ann Trop Med Parasitol*, **89**, 287–95.

Fahy, J.V., Fleming, H.E., et al. 1997. The effect of an anti-IgE monoclonal antibody on the early- and late-phase responses to allergen inhalation in asthmatic subjects. *Am J Respir Crit Care Med*, **155**, 1828–34.

Falcone, F.H., Dahinden, C.A., et al. 1996. Human basophils release interleukin-4 after stimulation with *Schistosoma mansoni* egg antigen. *Eur J Immunol*, **26**, 1147–55.

Finotto, S., Ohno, I., et al. 1994. TNF-α production by eosinophils in upper airways inflammation (nasal polyposis). *J Immunol*, **153**, 2278–89.

Folkard, S.G., Hogarth, P.J., et al. 1996. Eosinophils are the major effector cells of immunity to microfilariae in a mouse model of onchocerciasis. *Parasitology*, **112**, 323–9.

Forssmann, U., Uguccioni, M., et al. 1997. Eotaxin-2, a novel CC chemokine that is selective for the chemokine receptor CCR3, and acts like eotaxin on human eosinophil and basophil leukocytes. *J Exp Med*, **185**, 2171–6.

Foster, P.S., Hogan, S.P., et al. 1996. Interleukin 5 deficiency abolishes eosinophilia, airways hyperreactivity, and lung damage in a mouse asthma model. *J Exp Med*, **183**, 195–201.

Fox, C.C., Dvorak, A.M., et al. 1985. Isolation and characterization of human intestinal mucosal mast cells. *J Immunol*, **135**, 483–91.

Freeman, G.L. Jr, Tominaga, A., et al. 1995. Elevated innate peripheral blood eosinophilia fails to augment irradiated cercarial vaccine-induced resistance to *Schistosoma mansoni* in IL-5 transgenic mice. *J Parasitol*, **81**, 1010–11.

Fujihara, S., Ward, C., et al. 2002. Inhibition of nuclear factor-κB activation un-masks the ability of TNF-α to induce human eosinophil apoptosis. *Eur J Immunol*, **32**, 457–66.

Fureder, W., Agis, H., et al. 1995. Differential response of human basophils and mast cells to recombinant chemokines. *Ann Hematol*, **70**, 251–8.

Ganser, A., Lindemann, A., et al. 1990. Effects of recombinant human interleukin-3 in patients with normal hematopoiesis and in patients with bone marrow failure. *Blood*, **76**, 666–76.

Garcia-Zepeda, E.A., Rothenberg, M.E., et al. 1996. Human eotaxin is a specific chemoattractant for eosinophil cells and provides a new mechanism to explain tissue eosinophilia. *Nature Med*, **2**, 449–56.

Gauchat, J.F., Henchoz, S., et al. 1993. Induction of human IgE synthesis in B cells by mast cells and basophils. *Nature*, **365**, 340–3.

Genta, R.M., Ottesen, E.A., et al. 1983. Specific allergic sensitization to Strongyloides antigens in human strongyloidiasis. *Lab Invest*, **48**, 633–8.

Gerszten, R.E., Garcia-Zepeda, E.A., et al. 1999. MCP-1 and IL-8 trigger firm adhesion of monocytes to vascular endothelium under flow conditions. *Nature*, **398**, 718–23.

Gibbs, B.F., Haas, H., et al. 1996. Purified human peripheral blood basophils release interleukin-13 and preformed interleukin-4 following immunological activation. *Eur J Immunol*, **26**, 2493–8.

Gibbs, B.F., Haas, H., et al. 2000. Early IgE-dependent release of IL-4 and IL-13 from leukocytes is restricted to basophils: a comparison with other granulocytes and mononuclear cells. *Inflamm Res*, **49**, suppl 1, S9–10.

Gleich, G.J., Olson, G.M. and Herlich, H. 1979. The effect of antiserum to eosinophils and susceptibility and acquired immunity of the guinea pig to *Trichostronglyus colubriformis*. *Immunology*, **37**, 873–80.

Gnanasekar, M., Rao, K.V., et al. 2002. Molecular characterization of a calcium binding translationally controlled tumor protein homologue from the filarial parasites *Brugia malayi* and *Wuchereria bancrofti*. *Mol Biochem Parasitol*, **121**, 107–18.

Gonzalez-Munoz, M., Garate, T., et al. 1999. Induction of histamine release in parasitized individuals by somatic and cuticular antigens from *Onchocerca volvulus*. *Am J Trop Med Hyg*, **60**, 974–9.

Grimaldi, J.C., Yu, N.X., et al. 1999. Depletion of eosinophils in mice through the use of antibodies specific for C-C chemokine receptor 3 (CCR3). *J Leukoc Biol*, **65**, 846–53.

Grove, D.I., Mahmoud, A.A. and Warren, K.S. 1977. Eosinophils and resistance to *Trichinella spiralis*. *J Exp Med*, **145**, 755–9.

Guo, C.B., Liu, M.C., et al. 1994. Identification of IgE-bearing cells in the late-phase response to antigen in the lung as basophils. *Am J Respir Cell Mol Biol*, **10**, 384–90.

Gurish, M.F., Humbles, A., et al. 2002. CCR3 is required for tissue eosinophilia and larval cytotoxicity after infection with *Trichinella spiralis*. *J Immunol*, **168**, 5730–6.

Haisch, K., Schramm, G., et al. 2001. A glycoprotein from *Schistosoma mansoni* eggs binds non-antigen-specific immunoglobulin E and releases interleukin-4 from human basophils. *Parasite Immunol*, **23**, 427–34.

Hamann, K.J., Barker, R.L., et al. 1987. Comparative toxicity of purified human eosinophil granule proteins for newborn larvae of *Trichinella spiralis*. *J Parasitol*, **73**, 523–9.

Hamann, K.J., Gleich, G.J., et al. 1990. In vitro killing of microfilariae of Brugia pahangi and Brugia malayi by eosinophil granule proteins. *J Immunol*, **144**, 3166–73.

Hansel, T.T., Braunstein, J.B., et al. 1991. Sputum eosinophils from asthmatics express ICAM-1 and HLA-DR. *Clin Exp Immunol*, **86**, 271–7.

Hansel, T.T., De Vries, I.J., et al. 1992. Induction and function of eosinophil intercellular adhesion molecule-1 and HLA-DR. *J Immunol*, **149**, 2130–6.

Harper III, J.S., Genta, R.M., et al. 1984. Experimental disseminated strongyloidiasis in *Erythrocebus patas*. I. Pathology. *Am J Trop Med Hyg*, **33**, 431–43.

Hauswirth, A.W., Natter, S., et al. 2002. Recombinant allergens promote expression of CD203c on basophils in sensitized individuals. *J Allergy Clin Immunol*, **110**, 102–9.

Heath, H., Qin, S., et al. 1997. Chemokine receptor usage by human eosinophils. The importance of CCR3 demonstrated using an antagonistic monoclonal antibody. *J Clin Invest*, **99**, 178–84.

Herndon, F.J. and Kayes, S.G. 1992. Depletion of eosinophils by anti-IL-5 monoclonal antibody treatment of mice infected with *Trichinella spiralis* does not alter parasite burden or immunologic resistance to reinfection. *J Immunol*, **149**, 3642–7.

Hirai, H., Tanaka, K., et al. 2001. Prostaglandin D2 selectively induces chemotaxis in T helper type 2 cells, eosinophils, and basophils via seven transmembrane receptor CRTH2. *J Exp Med*, **193**, 255–61.

Hofstetter, M., Fasano, M.B. and Ottesen, E.A. 1983. Modulation of the host response in human schistosomiasis. IV. Parasite antigen induces release of histamine that inhibits lymphocyte responsiveness *in vitro*. *J Immunol*, **130**, 1376–80.

Hoontrakoon, R., Chu, H.W., et al. 2002. Interleukin-15 inhibits spontaneous apoptosis in human eosinophils via autocrine production of granulocyte macrophage-colony stimulating factor and nuclear factor-κB activation. *Am J Respir Cell Mol Biol*, **26**, 404–12.

Hosoda, M., Yamaya, M., et al. 2002. Effects of rhinovirus infection on histamine and cytokine production by cell lines from human mast cells and basophils. *J Immunol*, **169**, 1482–91.

Hutt-Taylor, S.R., Harnish, D., et al. 1988. Sodium butyrate and a T lymphocyte cell line-derived differentiation factor induce basophilic differentiation of the human promyelocytic leukemia cell line HL-60. *Blood*, **71**, 209–15.

Igaz, P., Novak, I., et al. 2001. Bidirectional communication between histamine and cytokines. *Inflamm Res*, **50**, 123–8.

Iikura, M., Yamaguchi, M., et al. 1998. Secretory IgA induces degranulation of IL-3-primed basophils. *J Immunol*, **161**, 1510–15.

Jedrzkiewicz, S., Nakamura, H., et al. 2000. IL-1β induces eotaxin gene transcription in A549 airway epithelial cells through NF-κB. *Am J Physiol Lung Cell Mol Physiol*, **279**, L1058–1065.

Jinquan, T., Jacobi, H.H., et al. 2000. Chemokine stromal cell-derived factor 1α activates basophils by means of CXCR4. *J Allergy Clin Immunol*, **106**, 313–20.

Jose, P.J., Griffiths-Johnson, D.A., et al. 1994. Eotaxin: a potent eosinophil chemoattractant cytokine detected in a guinea pig model of allergic airways inflammation. *J Exp Med*, **179**, 881–7.

Juhlin, L. 1963. Basophil leukocyte differential in blood and bone marrow. *Acta Haematol*, **29**, 89–95.

Jutel, M., Watanabe, T., et al. 2001. Histamine regulates T cell and antibody responses by differential expression of H1 and H2 receptors. *Nature*, **413**, 420–5.

Karawajczyk, M., Seveus, L., et al. 2000. Piecemeal degranulation of peripheral blood eosinophils: a study of allergic subjects during and out of the pollen season. *Am J Respir Cell Mol Biol*, **23**, 521–9.

Kasugai, T., Okada, M., et al. 1993. Infection of *Nippostrongylus brasiliensis* induces normal increase of basophils in mast cell-deficient Ws/Ws rats with a small deletion at the kinase domain of c-kit. *Blood*, **81**, 2521–9.

Kempuraj, D., Saito, H., et al. 1999. Characterization of mast cell-committed progenitors present in human umbilical cord blood. *Blood*, **93**, 3338–46.

Kepley, C.L., McFeeley, P.J., et al. 2001. Immunohistochemical detection of human basophils in postmortem cases of fatal asthma. *Am J Respir Crit Care Med*, **164**, 1053–8.

Khalife, J., Capron, M., et al. 1986. Role of specific IgE antibodies in peroxidase (EPO) release from human eosinophils. *J Immunol*, **137**, 1659–64.

Kinet, J.P. 1999. The high-affinity IgE receptor (FcεRI): from physiology to pathology. *Annu Rev Immunol*, **17**, 931–72.

King, C.L. 2001. Transmission intensity and human immune responses to lymphatic filariasis. *Parasite Immunol*, **23**, 363–71.

Kirshenbaum, A.S., Goff, J.P., et al. 1989. IL-3-dependent growth of basophil-like cells and mastlike cells from human bone marrow. *J Immunol*, **142**, 2424–9.

Kirshenbaum, A.S., Kessler, S.W., et al. 1991. Demonstration of the origin of human mast cells from CD34+ bone marrow progenitor cells. *J Immunol*, **146**, 1410–15.

Kirshenbaum, A.S., Goff, J.P., et al. 1999. Demonstration that human mast cells arise from a progenitor cell population that is CD34+, c-kit+, and expresses aminopeptidase N (CD13). *Blood*, **94**, 2333–42.

Kita, H., Ohnishi, T., et al. 1991. Granulocyte/macrophage colony-stimulating factor and interleukin 3 release from human peripheral blood eosinophils and neutrophils. *J Exp Med*, **174**, 745–8.

Kitayama, J., Fuhlbrigge, R.C., et al. 1997. P-selectin, L-selectin, and α4 integrin have distinct roles in eosinophil tethering and arrest on vascular endothelial cells under physiological flow conditions. *J Immunol*, **159**, 3929–39.

Klebanoff, S.J. and Coombs, R.W. 1996. Virucidal effect of stimulated eosinophils on human immunodefciency virus type 1. *AIDS Res Hum Retroviruses*, **12**, 25–9.

Klein, A., Talvani, A., et al. 2001. Stem cell factor-induced leukotriene B4 production cooperates with eotaxin to mediate the recruitment of eosinophils during allergic pleurisy in mice. *J Immunol*, **167**, 524–31.

Knol, E.F., Mul, F.P., et al. 1991. Monitoring human basophil activation via CD63 monoclonal antibody 435. *J Allergy Clin Immunol*, **88**, 328–38.

Kobayashi, H., Gleich, G.J., et al. 2002. Human eosinophils produce neurotrophins and secrete nerve growth factor on immunologic stimuli. *Blood*, **99**, 2214–20.

Kohka, H., Nishibori, M., et al. 2000. Histamine is a potent inducer of IL-18 and IFN-γ in human peripheral blood mononuclear cells. *J Immunol*, **164**, 6640–6.

Kopf, M., Brombacher, F., et al. 1996. IL-5-deficient mice have a developmental defect in CD5+ B-1 cells and lack eosinophilia but have normal antibody and cytotoxic T cell responses. *Immunity*, **4**, 15–24.

Korenaga, M., Hitoshi, Y., et al. 1994. Regulatory effect of anti-interleukin-5 monoclonal antibody on intestinal worm burden in a primary infection with *Strongyloides venezuelensis* in mice. *Int J Parasitol*, **24**, 951–7.

Kudlacz, E., Whitney, C., et al. 2002. Functional effects of eotaxin are selectively upregulated on IL-5 transgenic mouse eosinophils. *Inflammation*, **26**, 111–19.

Kuna, P., Reddigari, S.R., et al. 1991. IL-8 inhibits histamine release from human basophils induced by histamine-releasing factors, connective tissue activating peptide III and IL-3. *J Immunol*, **147**, 1920–4.

Kuna, P., Reddigari, S.R., et al. 1992. Monocyte chemotactic and activating factor is a potent histamine-releasing factor for human basophils. *J Exp Med*, **175**, 489–93.

Kuna, P., Reddigari, S.R., et al. 1993. Characterization of the human basophil response to cytokines, growth factors, and histamine releasing factors of the intercrine/chemokine family. *J Immunol*, **150**, 1932–43.

Lampinen, M., Carlson, M., et al. 2001. IL-5 and TNF-α participate in recruitment of eosinophils to intestinal mucosa in ulcerative colitis. *Dig Dis Sci*, **46**, 2004–9.

Lantz, C.S., Boesiger, J., et al. 1998. Role for interleukin-3 in mast cell and basophil development and in immunity to parasites. *Nature*, **392**, 90–3.

Larson, K.A., Olson, E.V., et al. 1996. Two highly homologous ribonuclease genes expressed in mouse eosinophils identify a larger subgroup of the mammalian ribonuclease superfamily. *Proc Natl Acad Sci USA*, **93**, 12370–5.

Leary, A.G. and Ogawa, M. 1984. Identification of pure and mixed basophil colonies in culture of human peripheral blood and marrow cells. *Blood*, **64**, 78–83.

Lee, T., Lenihan, D.J., et al. 1984. Increased biosynthesis of platelet-activating factor in activated human eosinophils. *J Biol Chem*, **259**, 5526–30.

Leonidas, D.D., Elbert, B.L., et al. 1995. Crystal structure of human Charcot-Leyden crystal protein, an eosinophil lysophospholipase, identifies it as a new member of the carbohydrate-binding family of galectins. *Structure*, **3**, 1379–93.

Lett-Brown, M.A., Boetcher, D.A. and Leonard, E.J. 1976. Chemotactic responses of normal human basophils to C5a and to lymphocyte-derived chemotactic factor. *J Immunol*, **117**, 246–52.

Lewis, R.A. and Austen, K.F. 1984. The biologically active leukotrienes. Biosynthesis, metabolism, receptors, functions, and pharmacology. *J Clin Invest*, **73**, 889–97.

Li, H., Sim, T.C. and Alam, R. 1996a. IL-13 released by and localized in human basophils. *J Immunol*, **156**, 4833–8.

Li, H., Sim, T.C., et al. 1996b. The production of macrophage inflammatory protein-1α by human basophils. *J Immunol*, **157**, 1207–12.

Li, Y., Li, L., et al. 2001. Mast cells/basophils in the peripheral blood of allergic individuals who are HIV-1 susceptible due to their surface expression of CD4 and the chemokine receptors CCR3, CCR5 and CXCR4. *Blood*, **97**, 3484–90.

Lilly, C.M., Nakamura, H., et al. 1997. Expression of eotaxin by human lung epithelial cells: induction by cytokines and inhibition by glucocorticoids. *J Clin Invest*, **99**, 1767–73.

Lilly, C.M., Woodruff, P.G., et al. 1999. Elevated plasma eotaxin levels in patients with acute asthma. *J Allergy Clin Immunol*, **104**, 786–90.

Lilly, C.M., Nakamura, H., et al. 2001. Eotaxin expression after segmental allergen challenge in subjects with atopic asthma. *Am J Respir Crit Care Med*, **163**, 1669–75.

Limaye, A.P., Abrams, J.S., et al. 1991. Interleukin-5 and the posttreatment eosinophilia in patients with onchocerciasis. *J Clin Invest*, **88**, 1418–21.

Limaye, A.P., Ottesen, E.A., et al. 1993. Kinetics of serum and cellular interleukin-5 in posttreatment eosinophilia of patients with lymphatic filariasis. *J Infect Dis*, **167**, 1396–400.

Lin, S., Cicala, C., et al. 1996. The FcεRI β subunit functions as an amplifier of FcεRIβ-mediated cell activation signals. *Cell*, **85**, 985–95.

Lindor, L.J., Wassom, D.L. and Gleich, G.J. 1983. Effects of trichinellosis on levels of eosinophils, eosinophil major basic protein, creatine kinase and basophils in the guinea pig. *Parasite Immunol*, **5**, 13–24.

Lucey, D.R., Nicholson-Weller, A. and Weller, P.F. 1989. Mature human eosinophils have the capacity to express HLA-DR. *Proc Natl Acad Sci USA*, **86**, 1348–51.

MacDonald, S.M., Rafnar, T., et al. 1995. Molecular identification of an IgE-dependent histamine-releasing factor. *Science*, **269**, 688–90.

McEuen, A.R., Buckley, M.G., et al. 1999. Development and characterization of a monoclonal antibody specific for human basophils and the identification of a unique secretory product of basophil activation. *Lab Invest*, **79**, 27–38.

McEuen, A.R., Calafat, J., et al. 2001. Mass, charge, and subcellular localization of a unique secretory product identified by the basophil-specific antibody BB1. *J Allergy Clin Immunol*, **107**, 842–8.

MacGlashan, D. Jr, Lichtenstein, L.M., et al. 1999. Upregulation of FcεRI on human basophils by IgE antibody is mediated by interaction of IgE with FcεRI. *J Allergy Clin Immunol*, **104**, 492–8.

MacGlashan, D.W., et al. 1997. Down-regulation of FcεRI expression on human basophils during in vivo treatment of atopic patients with anti-IgE antibody. *J Immunol*, **158**, 1438–45.

Mahmoud, A.A., Warren, K.S. and Peters, P.A. 1975. A role for the eosinophil in acquired resistance to *Schistosoma mansoni* infection as determined by antieosinophil serum. *J Exp Med*, **142**, 805–13.

Marleau, S., Griffiths-Johnson, D.A., et al. 1996. Human RANTES acts as a receptor antagonist for guinea pig eotaxin *in vitro* and in vivo. *J Immunol*, **157**, 4141–6.

Marone, G., Florio, G., et al. 2001. Human mast cells and basophils in HIV-1 infection. *Trends Immunol*, **22**, 229–32.

Martin, C., Le Goff, L., et al. 2000. Drastic reduction of a filarial infection in eosinophilic interleukin-5 transgenic mice. *Infect Immun*, **68**, 3651–6.

Massey, W.A., Randall, T.C., et al. 1989. Recombinant human IL-1α and -1β potentiate IgE-mediated histamine release from human basophils. *J Immunol*, **143**, 1875–80.

Matsuda, H., Coughlin, M.D., et al. 1988. Nerve growth factor promotes human hemopoietic colony growth and differentiation. *Proc Natl Acad Sci USA*, **85**, 6508–12.

Matsumoto, K., Schleimer, R.P., et al. 1995. Induction of apoptosis in human eosinophils by anti-Fas antibody treatment *in vitro*. *Blood*, **86**, 1437–43.

Matthews, A.N., Friend, D.S., et al. 1998. Eotaxin is required for the baseline level of tissue eosinophils. *Proc Natl Acad Sci USA*, **95**, 6273–8.

Mawhorter, S.D., Stephany, D.A., et al. 1996. Identification of surface molecules associated with physiologic activation of eosinophils. Application of whole-blood flow cytometry to eosinophils. *J Immunol*, **156**, 4851–8.

Mazza, G., Thorne, K.J., et al. 1991. The presence of eosinophil-activating mediators in sera from individuals with *Schistosoma mansoni* infections. *Eur J Immunol*, **21**, 901–5.

Mazzoni, A., Young, H.A., et al. 2001. Histamine regulates cytokine production in maturing dendritic cells, resulting in altered T cell polarization. *J Clin Invest*, **108**, 1865–73.

Meagher, L.C., Cousin, J.M., et al. 1996. Opposing effects of glucocorticoids on the rate of apoptosis in neutrophilic and eosinophilic granulocytes. *J Immunol*, **156**, 4422–8.

Menon, A.K., Holowka, D. and Baird, B. 1984. Small oligomers of immunoglobulin E (IgE) cause large-scale clustering of IgE receptors on the surface of rat basophilic leukemia cells. *J Cell Biol*, **98**, 577–83.

Menzies-Gow, A., Ying, S., et al. 2002. Eotaxin (CCL11) and eotaxin-2 (CCL24) induce recruitment of eosinophils, basophils, neutrophils, and macrophages as well as features of early- and late-phase allergic reactions following cutaneous injection in human atopic and nonatopic volunteers. *J Immunol*, **169**, 2712–18.

Metcalf, D. 1989. The molecular control of cell division, differentiation commitment and maturation in haemopoietic cells. *Nature*, **339**, 27–30.

Mishra, A., Hogan, S.P., et al. 2002. Enterocyte expression of the eotaxin and interleukin-5 transgenes induces compartmentalized dysregulation of eosinophil trafficking. *J Biol Chem*, **277**, 4406–12.

Mitchell, E.B., Crow, J., et al. 1982. Basophils in allergen-induced patch test sites in atopic dermatitis. *Lancet*, **i**, 127–30.

Mitre, E. and Nutman, T.B. 2003. Lack of basophilia in human parasitic infections. *Am J Trop Med Hyg*, **69**, 87–91.

Mitre, E., Taylor, R.T., et al. 2004. Parasite antigen-driven basophils are a major source of IL-4 in human filarial infections. *J Immunol*, **172**, 2439–5.

Miura, K., Saini, S.S., et al. 2001. Differences in functional consequences and signal transduction induced by IL-3, IL-5, and nerve growth factor in human basophils. *J Immunol*, **167**, 2282–91.

Molina, H.A., Kierszenbaum, F., et al. 1988. Toxic effects produced or mediated by human eosinophil granule components on *Trypanosoma cruzi*. *Am J Trop Med Hyg*, **38**, 327–34.

Moqbel, R., Hamid, Q., et al. 1991. Expression of mRNA and immunoreactivity for the granulocyte/macrophage colony-stimulating factor in activated human eosinophils. *J Exp Med*, **174**, 749–52.

Morita, M., Lamkhioued, B., et al. 1996. Induction by interferons of human eosinophil apoptosis and regulation by interleukin-3, granulocyte/macrophage-colony stimulating factor and interleukin-5. *Eur Cytokine Netw*, **7**, 725–32.

Moser, R., Fehr, J. and Bruijnzeel, P.L. 1992. IL-4 controls the selective endothelium-driven transmigration of eosinophils from allergic individuals. *J Immunol*, **149**, 1432–8.

Motegi, Y. and Kita, H. 1998. Interaction with secretory component stimulates effector functions of human eosinophils but not of neutrophils. *J Immunol*, **161**, 4340–6.

Moy, J.N., Gleich, G.J. and Thomas, L.L. 1990. Noncytotoxic activation of neutrophils by eosinophil granule major basic protein. Effect on superoxide anion generation and lysosomal enzyme release. *J Immunol*, **145**, 2626–32.

Nagase, H., Miyamasu, M., et al. 2000. Expression of CXCR4 in eosinophils: functional analyses and cytokine-mediated regulation. *J Immunol*, **164**, 5935–43.

Nagase, H., Okugawa, S., et al. 2003. Expression and function of Toll-like receptors in eosinophils: activation by Toll-like receptor 7 ligand. *J Immunol*, **171**, 3977–82.

Nagata, M., Saito, K., et al. 2002. Leukotriene D4 upregulates eosinophil adhesion via the cysteinyl leukotriene 1 receptor. *J Allergy Clin Immunol*, **109**, 676–80.

Nakamura, H., Luster, A.D., et al. 2001. IL-4 differentially regulates eotaxin and MCP-4 in lung epithelium and circulating mononuclear cells. *Am J Physiol Lung Cell Mol Physiol*, **281**, L1288–1302.

Nielsen, B.W., Lind, P., et al. 1994. Immune responses to nematode exoantigens: sensitizing antibodies and basophil histamine release. *Allergy*, **49**, 427–35.

Nilsson, G., Carlsson, M., et al. 1994. TNF-α and IL-6 induce differentiation in the human basophilic leukaemia cell line KU 812. *Immunology*, **81**, 73–8.

Nishinakamura, R., Nakayama, N., et al. 1995. Mice deficient for the IL-3/GM-CSF/IL-5 βc receptor exhibit lung pathology and impaired immune response, while β IL3 receptor-deficient mice are normal. *Immunity*, **2**, 211–22.

Nittoh, T., Hirakata, M., et al. 1997. Identification of cDNA encoding rat eosinophil cationic protein/eosinophil-associated ribonuclease. *Biochim Biophys Acta*, **1351**, 42–6.

Noso, N., Proost, P., et al. 1994. Human monocyte chemotactic proteins-2 and -3 (MCP-2 and MCP-3) attract human eosinophils and desensitize the chemotactic responses towards RANTES. *Biochem Biophys Res Commun*, **200**, 1470–6.

Ogilvie, B.M., Hesketh, P.M. and Rose, M.E. 1978. Nippostrongylus brasiliensis: peripheral blood leucocyte response of rats, with special reference to basophils. *Exp Parasitol*, **46**, 20–30.

Ogilvie, B.M., Askenase, P.W. and Rose, M.E. 1980. Basophils and eosinophils in three strains of rats and in athymic (nude) rats following infection with the nematodes *Nippostrongylus brasiliensis* or *Trichinella spiralis*. *Immunology*, **39**, 385–9.

Okada, M., Nawa, Y., et al. 1997. Development of basophils in Mongolian gerbils: formation of basophilic cell clusters in the bone marrow after *Nippostrongylus brasiliensis* infection. *Lab Invest*, **76**, 89–97.

Oliveira, S.H., Costa, C.H., et al. 2002. Sephadex induces eosinophil migration to the rat and mouse peritoneal cavity: involvement of mast cells, LTB4, TNF-α, IL-8 and PAF. *Inflamm Res*, **51**, 144–53.

Ottesen, E.A., Neva, F.A., et al. 1979. Specific allergic sensitsation to filarial antigens in tropical eosinophilia syndrome. *Lancet*, **i**, 1158–61.

Ovington, K.S. and Behm, C.A. 1997. The enigmatic eosinophil: investigation of the biological role of eosinophils in parasitic helminth infection. *Mem Inst Oswaldo Cruz*, **92**, 93–104.

Owen, W.F. Jr, Rothenberg, M.E., et al. 1987. Regulation of human eosinophil viability, density, and function by granulocyte/macrophage colony-stimulating factor in the presence of 3T3 fibroblasts. *J Exp Med*, **166**, 129–41.

Palframan, R.T., Collins, P.D., et al. 1998a. Eotaxin induces a rapid release of eosinophils and their progenitors from the bone marrow. *Blood*, **91**, 2240–8.

Palframan, R.T., Collins, P.D., et al. 1998b. Mechanisms of acute eosinophil mobilization from the bone marrow stimulated by interleukin 5: the role of specific adhesion molecules and phosphatidylinositol 3-kinase. *J Exp Med*, **188**, 1621–32.

Paris-Kohler, A., Demoly, P., et al. 2000. In vitro diagnosis of cypress pollen allergy by using cytofluorimetric analysis of basophils (Basotest). *J Allergy Clin Immunol*, **105**, 339–45.

Pignatti, P., Perfetti, L., et al. 2002. Increased CD69 expression on peripheral blood eosinophils after specific inhalation challenge. *Allergy*, **57**, 411–16.

Plotz, S.G., Lentschat, A., et al. 2001. The interaction of human peripheral blood eosinophils with bacterial lipopolysaccharide is CD14 dependent. *Blood*, **97**, 235–41.

Pope, S.M., Brandt, E.B., et al. 2001. IL-13 induces eosinophil recruitment into the lung by an IL-5- and eotaxin-dependent mechanism. *J Allergy Clin Immunol*, **108**, 594–601.

Porter, J.F. and Mitchell, R.G. 1972. Distribution of histamine in human blood. *Physiol Rev*, **52**, 361–81.

Qi, J.C., Stevens, R.L., et al. 2002. IL-16 regulation of human mast cells/basophils and their susceptibility to HIV-1. *J Immunol*, **168**, 4127–34.

Rais, M., Wild, J.S., et al. 2002. Interleukin-12 inhibits eosinophil differentiation from bone marrow stem cells in an interferon-γ-dependent manner in a mouse model of asthma. *Clin Exp Allergy*, **32**, 627–32.

Ramirez, R.M., Ceballos, E., et al. 1996. The immunopathology of human schistosomiasis. III. Immunoglobulin isotype profiles and response to praziquantel. *Mem Inst Oswaldo Cruz*, **91**, 593–9.

Rao, K.V., Chen, L., et al. 2002. Cloning and characterization of a calcium-binding, histamine-releasing protein from *Schistosoma mansoni*. *J Biol Chem*, **277**, 31207–13.

Redrup, A.C., Howard, B.P., et al. 1998. Differential regulation of IL-4 and IL-13 secretion by human basophils: their relationship to histamine release in mixed leukocyte cultures. *J Immunol*, **160**, 1957–64.

Resnick, M.B. and Weller, P.F. 1993. Mechanisms of eosinophil recruitment. *Am J Respir Cell Mol Biol*, **8**, 349–55.

Rosenberg, H.F. 1995. Recombinant human eosinophil cationic protein. Ribonuclease activity is not essential for cytotoxicity. *J Biol Chem*, **270**, 7876–81.

Rosenberg, H.F. and Domachowske, J.B. 2001. Eosinophils, eosinophil ribonucleases, and their role in host defense against respiratory virus pathogens. *J Leukoc Biol*, **70**, 691–8.

Rossi, C.L., Takahashi, E.E., et al. 1993. Total serum IgE and parasite-specific IgG and IgA antibodies in human strongyloidiasis. *Rev Inst Med Trop São Paulo*, **35**, 361–5.

Rot, A., Krieger, M., et al. 1992. RANTES and macrophage inflammatory protein 1α induce the migration and activation of normal human eosinophil granulocytes. *J Exp Med*, **176**, 1489–95.

Roth, R.L. and Levy, D.A. 1980. Nippostrongylus brasiliensis: peripheral leukocyte responses and correlation of basophils with blood histamine concentration during infection in rats. *Exp Parasitol*, **50**, 331–41.

Rothenberg, M.E., Owen, W.F. Jr, et al. 1988. Human eosinophils have prolonged survival, enhanced functional properties, and become hypodense when exposed to human interleukin 3. *J Clin Invest*, **81**, 1986–92.

Rothenberg, M.E., MacLean, J.A., et al. 1997. Targeted disruption of the chemokine eotaxin partially reduces antigen-induced tissue eosinophilia. *J Exp Med*, **185**, 785–90.

Rothwell, T.L. and Love, R.J. 1975. Studies of the responses of basophil and eosinophil leucocytes and mast cells to the nematode *Trichostrongylus colubriformis*. II. Changes in cell numbers following infection of thymectomised and adoptively or passively immunised guinea pigs. *J Pathol*, **116**, 183–94.

Rumbley, C.A., Sugaya, H., et al. 2001. Elimination of lymphocytes, but not eosinophils, by Fas-mediated apoptosis in murine schistosomiasis. *Am J Trop Med Hyg*, **65**, 442–9.

Sabatini, F., Silvestri, M., et al. 2002. Fibroblast-eosinophil interaction. Modulation of adhesion molecules expression and chemokine release by human fetal lung fibroblasts in response to IL-4 and TNF-α. *Immunol Lett*, **84**, 173–8.

Sabroe, I., Jones, E., et al. 2002. Toll-like receptor (TLR) 2 and TLR4 in human peripheral blood granulocytes: a critical role for monocytes in leukocyte lipopolysaccharide responses. *J Immunol*, **168**, 4701–10.

Saini, S.S., Richardson, J.J., et al. 2001. Expression and modulation of FcεRIα and FcεRIβ in human blood basophils. *J Allergy Clin Immunol*, **107**, 832–41.

Sainte-Laudy, J., Sabbah, A., et al. 2000. Diagnosis of venom allergy by flow cytometry. Correlation with clinical history, skin tests, specific IgE, histamine and leukotriene C4 release. *Clin Exp Allergy*, **30**, 1166–71.

Saito, H., Hatake, K., et al. 1988. Selective differentiation and proliferation of hematopoietic cells induced by recombinant human interleukins. *Proc Natl Acad Sci USA*, **85**, 2288–92.

Scadden, D.T., Levine, J.D., et al. 1995. In vivo effects of interleukin 3 in HIV type 1-infected patients with cytopenia. *AIDS Res Hum Retroviruses*, **11**, 731–40.

Schleimer, R.P., Sterbinsky, S.A., et al. 1992. IL-4 induces adherence of human eosinophils and basophils but not neutrophils to endothelium. Association with expression of VCAM-1. *J Immunol*, **148**, 1086–92.

Schroeder, J.T., Lichtenstein, L.M. and MacDonald, S.M. 1996. An immunoglobulin E-dependent recombinant histamine-releasing factor induces interleukin-4 secretion from human basophils. *J Exp Med*, **183**, 1265–70.

Schroeder, J.T., Lichtenstein, L.M. and MacDonald, S.M. 1997. Recombinant histamine-releasing factor enhances IgE-dependent IL-4 and IL-13 secretion by human basophils. *J Immunol*, **159**, 447–52.

Schulman, E.S., Post, T.J., et al. 1988. Differential effects of the complement peptides, C5a and C5a des Arg on human basophil and lung mast cell histamine release. *J Clin Invest*, **81**, 918–23.

Schulman, E.S., Kagey-Sobotka, A., et al. 1983. Heterogeneity of human mast cells. *J Immunol*, **131**, 1936–41.

Schweizer, R.C., Welmers, B.A., et al. 1994. RANTES- and interleukin-8-induced responses in normal human eosinophils: effects of priming with interleukin-5. *Blood*, **83**, 3697–704.

Seminario, M.C., Saini, S.S., et al. 1999. Intracellular expression and release of FcαRIα by human eosinophils. *J Immunol*, **162**, 6893–900.

Sher, A., Coffman, R.L., et al. 1990. Ablation of eosinophil and IgE responses with anti-IL-5 or anti-IL-4 antibodies fails to affect immunity against *Schistosoma mansoni* in the mouse. *J Immunol*, **145**, 3911–16.

Shin, E.H., Osada, Y., et al. 2001. Involvement of complement and fibronectin in eosinophil-mediated damage to *Nippostrongylus brasiliensis* larvae. *Parasite Immunol*, **23**, 27–37.

Shinkai, K., Mohrs, M. and Locksley, R.M. 2002. Helper T cells regulate type-2 innate immunity *in vivo*. *Nature*, **420**, 825–9.

Sillaber, C., Geissler, K., et al. 1992. Type β transforming growth factors promote interleukin-3 (IL-3)-dependent differentiation of human basophils but inhibit IL-3-dependent differentiation of human eosinophils. *Blood*, **80**, 634–41.

Simon, H.U. and Blaser, K. 1995. Inhibition of programmed eosinophil death: a key pathogenic event for eosinophilia? *Immunol Today*, **16**, 53–5.

Sirois, J., Menard, G., et al. 2000. Importance of histamine in the cytokine network in the lung through H2 and H3 receptors: stimulation of IL-10 production. *J Immunol*, **164**, 2964–70.

Skiest, D.J. and Keiser, P. 1997. Clinical significance of eosinophilia in HIV-infected individuals. *Am J Med*, **102**, 449–53.

Smith, K.J., Skelton, H.G., et al. 1994. Hypereosinophilia secondary to immunodysregulation in patients with HIV-1 disease. *Arch Dermatol*, **130**, 119–21.

Solomon, A., Aloe, L., et al. 1998. Nerve growth factor is preformed in and activates human peripheral blood eosinophils. *J Allergy Clin Immunol*, **102**, 454–60.

Springer, T.A. 1994. Traffic signals for lymphocyte recirculation and leukocyte emigration: the multistep paradigm. *Cell*, **76**, 301–14.

Sriramarao, P., Von Andrian, U.H., et al. 1994. L-selectin and very late antigen-4 integrin promote eosinophil rolling at physiological shear rates *in vivo*. *J Immunol*, **153**, 4238–46.

Sriramarao, P., Discipio, R.G., et al. 2000. VCAM-1 is more effective than MAdCAM-1 in supporting eosinophil rolling under conditions of shear flow. *Blood*, **95**, 592–601.

Stern, M., Savill, J. and Haslett, C. 1996. Human monocyte-derived macrophage phagocytosis of senescent eosinophils undergoing apoptosis. Mediation by αvβ 3/CD36/thrombospondin recognition mechanism and lack of phlogistic response. *Am J Pathol*, **149**, 911–21.

Stevenson, L.M., Colditz, I.G. and Lejambre, L.F. 2001. Expression of cell surface adhesion molecules by peripheral blood eosinophils during *Trichostrongylus colubriformis* infection in sheep. *Immunol Cell Biol*, **79**, 240–4.

Sugaya, H., Abe, T. and Yoshimura, K. 2001. Eosinophils in the cerebrospinal fluid of mice infected with *Angiostrongylus cantonensis* are resistant to apoptosis. *Int J Parasitol*, **31**, 1649–58.

Sur, S., Glitz, D.G., et al. 1998. Localization of eosinophil-derived neurotoxin and eosinophil cationic protein in neutrophilic leukocytes. *J Leukoc Biol*, **63**, 715–22.

Tachimoto, H., Burdick, M.M., et al. 2000. CCR3-active chemokines promote rapid detachment of eosinophils from VCAM-1 *in vitro*. *J Immunol*, **165**, 2748–54.

Tachimoto, H., Kikuchi, M., et al. 2002. Eotaxin-2 alters eosinophil integrin function via mitogen-activated protein kinases. *Am J Respir Cell Mol Biol*, **26**, 645–9.

Takahashi, H.K., Yoshida, A., et al. 2002. Histamine regulation of interleukin-18-initiating cytokine cascade is associated with down-regulation of intercellular adhesion molecule-1 expression in human peripheral blood mononuclear cells. *J Pharmacol Exp Ther*, **300**, 227–35.

Tanimoto, Y., Takahashi, K. and Kimura, I. 1992. Effects of cytokines on human basophil chemotaxis. *Clin Exp Allergy*, **22**, 1020–5.

Tenscher, K., Metzner, B., et al. 1996. Recombinant human eotaxin induces oxygen radical production, Ca^{2+} mobilization, actin reorganization and CD11b upregulation in human eosinophils via a pertussis toxin-sensitive heterotrimeric guanine nucleotide-binding protein. *Blood*, **88**, 3195–9.

Tietz, A., Sponagel, L., et al. 1997. Eosinophilia in patients infected with the human immunodeficiency virus. *Eur J Clin Microbiol Infect Dis*, **16**, 675–7.

Todd, R., Donoff, B.R., et al. 1991. The eosinophil as a cellular source of transforming growth factor α in healing cutaneous wounds. *Am J Pathol*, **138**, 1307–13.

Tomaki, M., Zhao, L.L., et al. 2002. Comparison of effects of anti-IL-3, IL-5 and GM-CSF treatments on eosinophilopoiesis and airway eosinophilia induced by allergen. *Pulm Pharmacol Ther*, **15**, 161–8.

Tsuda, T., Wong, D., et al. 1991. Synergistic effects of nerve growth factor and granulocyte-macrophage colony-stimulating factor on human basophilic cell differentiation. *Blood*, **77**, 971–9.

Turner, H. and Kinet, J.P. 1999. Signalling through the high-affinity IgE receptor FcεRI. *Nature*, **402**, B24–30.

Ulfman, L.H., Kuijper, P.H., et al. 1999. Characterization of eosinophil adhesion to TNF-α-activated endothelium under flow conditions: α4 integrins mediate initial attachment and E-selectin mediates rolling. *J Immunol*, **163**, 343–50.

Ulfman, L.H., Joosten, D.P., et al. 2001. IL-8 induces a transient arrest of rolling eosinophils on human endothelial cells. *J Immunol*, **166**, 588–95.

Valent, P. 1995. Cytokines involved in growth and differentiation of human basophils and mast cells. *Exp Dermatol*, **4**, 255–9.

Valent, P., Besemer, J., et al. 1989. Interleukin 3 activates human blood basophils via high-affinity binding sites. *Proc Natl Acad Sci USA*, **86**, 5542–6.

Valent, P., Besemer, J., et al. 1990. IL-3 promotes basophilic differentiation of KU 812 cells through high affinity binding sites. *J Immunol*, **145**, 1885–9.

Valerius, T., Repp, R., et al. 1990. Effects of IFN on human eosinophils in comparison with other cytokines. A novel class of eosinophil activators with delayed onset of action. *J Immunol*, **145**, 2950–8.

van der Pouw Kraan, T.C., Snijders, A., et al. 1998. Histamine inhibits the production of interleukin-12 through interaction with H2 receptors. *J Clin Invest*, **102**, 1866–73.

Van Milligen, F.J., Cornelissen, J.B. and Bokhout, B.A. 1999. Protection against *Fasciola hepatica* in the intestine is highly correlated with eosinophil and immunoglobulin G1 responses against newly excysted juveniles. *Parasite Immunol*, **21**, 243–51.

Walsh, G.M. 1997. Mechanisms of human eosinophil survival and apoptosis. *Clin Exp Allergy*, **27**, 482–7.

Walsh, G.M., Mermod, J.J., et al. 1991. Human eosinophil, but not neutrophil, adherence to IL-1-stimulated human umbilical vascular endothelial cells is α4β1 (very late antigen-4) dependent. *J Immunol*, **146**, 3419–23.

Walsh, G.M., Williamson, M.L., et al. 1996. Ligation of CD69 induces apoptosis and cell death in human eosinophils cultured with granulocyte-macrophage colony-stimulating factor. *Blood*, **87**, 2815–21.

Wantke, F., MacGlashan, D.W., et al. 1999. The human recombinant histamine releasing factor: functional evidence that it does not bind to the IgE molecule. *J Allergy Clin Immunol*, **103**, 642–8.

Weber, M., Uguccioni, M., et al. 1995. Monocyte chemotactic protein MCP-2 activates human basophil and eosinophil leukocytes similar to MCP-3. *J Immunol*, **154**, 4166–72.

Weetall, M., Shopes, B., et al. 1990. Mapping the site of interaction between murine IgE and its high affinity receptor with chimeric Ig. *J Immunol*, **145**, 3849–54.

Weil, S.C. and Hrisinko, M.A. 1987. A hybrid eosinophilic-basophilic granulocyte in chronic granulocytic leukemia. *Am J Clin Pathol*, **87**, 66–70.

Weiler, C.R., Kita, H., et al. 1996. Eosinophil viability during immunoglobulin-induced degranulation. *J Leukoc Biol*, **60**, 493–501.

Weller, P.F. and Dvorak, A.M. 1994. Lipid bodies: intracellular sites for eicosanoid formation. *J Allergy Clin Immunol*, **94**, 1151–6.

Weller, P.F., Bach, D.S. and Austen, K.F. 1984. Biochemical characterization of human eosinophil Charcot-Leyden crystal protein (lysophospholipase). *J Biol Chem*, **259**, 15100–5.

Weller, P.F., Rand, T.H., et al. 1993. Accessory cell function of human eosinophils. HLA-DR-dependent, MHC-restricted antigen-presentation and IL-1α expression. *J Immunol*, **150**, 2554–62.

Weller, P.F., Marshall, W.L., et al. 1995. Infection, apoptosis, and killing of mature human eosinophils by human immunodeficiency virus-1. *Am J Respir Cell Mol Biol*, **13**, 610–20.

Wenzel, S.E., Trudeau, J.B., et al. 2002. TGFβ- and IL-13 synergistically increase eotaxin-1 production in human airway fibroblasts. *J Immunol*, **169**, 4613–19.

Wojta, J., Kaun, C., Smith, X.X. and Smith, X.X. 2002. C5a stimulates production of plasminogen activator inhibitor-1 in human mast cells and basophils. *Blood*, **100**, 517–23.

Yamada, H., Hirai, K., et al. 1997. Eotaxin is a potent chemotaxin for human basophils. *Biochem Biophys Res Commun*, **231**, 365–8.

Yamaguchi, M., Hirai, K., et al. 1992. Haemopoietic growth factors induce human basophil migration *in vitro*. *Clin Exp Allergy*, **22**, 379–83.

Yamaguchi, M., Hirai, K., et al. 1994. Dexamethasone inhibits basophil migration. *Allergy*, **49**, 371–5.

Yamaguchi, Y., Hayashi, Y., et al. 1988. Highly purified murine interleukin 5 (IL-5) stimulates eosinophil function and prolongs *in vitro* survival. IL-5 as an eosinophil chemotactic factor. *J Exp Med*, **167**, 1737–42.

Yamaguchi, Y., Suda, T., et al. 1991. Analysis of the survival of mature human eosinophils: interleukin-5 prevents apoptosis in mature human eosinophils. *Blood*, **78**, 2542–7.

Yoshimoto, T., Tsutsui, H., et al. 1999. IL-18, although antiallergic when administered with IL-12, stimulates IL-4 and histamine release by basophils. *Proc Natl Acad Sci USA*, **96**, 13962–6.

Yoshimura, C., Miyamasu, M., et al. 2001. Glucocorticoids induce basophil apoptosis. *J Allergy Clin Immunol*, **108**, 215–20.

Yousefi, S., Hoessli, D.C., et al. 1996. Requirement of Lyn and Syk tyrosine kinases for the prevention of apoptosis by cytokines in human eosinophils. *J Exp Med*, **183**, 1407–14.

Zhao, J., Takamura, M., et al. 2002. Altered eosinophil levels as a result of viral infection in asthma exacerbation in childhood. *Pediatr Allergy Immunol*, **13**, 47–50.

Zhao, L.L., Linden, A., et al. 2000. IL-12 regulates bone marrow eosinophilia and airway eotaxin levels induced by airway allergen exposure. *Allergy*, **55**, 749–56.

Zheng, X., Karsan, A., et al. 2002. Interleukin-3, but not granulocyte-macrophage-stimulating factor and interleukin-5, inhibits apoptosis of human basophils through phosphatidylinositol 3-kinase: requirement of NF-κB-dependent and -independent pathways. *Immunology*, **107**, 306–15.

6

Natural killer cells

KLAS KÄRRE AND JENS ZERRAHN

DEFINITION AND GENERAL CHARACTERISTICS OF NATURAL KILLER CELLS

Historical perspective

Natural killer cells were discovered in the early 1970s, through their capacity to kill certain tumor cells in cytotoxicity assays in vitro. In the search for evidence of a specific immune response in patients or experimental animals with tumors, several groups observed a cytotoxic activity by lymphocytes isolated from the blood or the spleen. It was soon realized that this activity occurred also in healthy individuals, and had nothing to do with a specific tumor response. Although some considered this activity as 'nonspecific background', others went on to analyze the phenomenon in more detail. This research soon provided evidence that the cytotoxicity was mediated by a previously undescribed, lymphocyte-like cell with unique characteristics, and the term natural killer (NK) cell was then coined (Herberman et al. 1975a, b; Kiessling et al. 1975a, b). Equally important, it became clear that the activity observed in vitro correlated with natural resistance to transplantable tumors in vivo in animals (Kiessling et al. 1975c). The NK cells were soon also identified as the effector cell responsible for a peculiar form of bone marrow transplant rejection that had puzzled immunologists for a decade (Kiessling et al. 1977). The notion of one novel cell type with in vivo relevance triggered further research, mainly in tumor immunology, but eventually also in infection immunology. Evidence for a role of NK cells in the early defense against viral infections soon emerged. Other researchers also observed effects mediated by NK cells in bacterial and parasite infections. The microbiology-oriented NK cell research has been particularly important for defining additional effector functions of NK cells. Their capacity to secrete cytokines such as interferon (IFN)-γ is in many situations more important than the killer function that forms the basis of their name.

It took a relatively long time before NK cell recognition could be defined in molecular terms. Research on inhibitory, major histocompatibility complex (MHC) class I-recognizing receptors, as postulated in the 'missing self' model, provided a platform for identification of the first NK cell receptors (Kärre 1985, 2002; Ljunggren and Kärre 1990). Intensive research during the 1990s has defined a large number of activating and inhibiting receptors (Moretta et al. 1993, 2001; Yokoyama and Plougastel 2003). A challenge for the current and coming years of research is to transform the reductionist study of individual receptors into a comprehensive view of how these molecules interact in decision processes created by different challenges, especially different microbial agents.

Identification and isolation of NK cells – cell surface markers

There is no single cell surface molecule or other feature that can be used to identify all NK cells, and nothing but NK cells. Any efforts to define or isolate these cells must therefore rely on a combination of characteristics. NK cells are of lymphoid lineage and are often associated with a special morphology, that of the large granular lymphocyte (LGL) (Figure 6.1) (Timonen and Saksela 1980). In the normal blood of healthy individuals, there is a good correlation between NK cells and this morphological phenotype. However, not all NK cells are LGLs, and not all LGLs are NK cells.

Natural killer cells are usually defined through a combination of cell surface markers – in the human as $CD56^{+}CD16^{+}CD3^{-}$ immunoglobulin (Ig) cells with the morphology of lymphocytes (Moretta et al. 1994; Carson and Caligiuri 1996). CD56 is the neuronal cell adhesion molecule (N-CAM), but it is unclear whether and how this marker relates to the function of NK cells. In the mouse, the allotypic marker NK1.1 is used instead of CD56, although the two markers are completely unrelated (Yokoyama 1999). NK cells express a number of additional adhesion molecules, cytokine receptors, and cognate recognition molecules (Tables 6.1 and 6.2), many of which are discussed further later in the chapter in relation to the functional aspects.

The NK cells represent about 5–15 percent of the lymphocytes in the blood, and about 1 percent of the lymphocytes in the spleen. These are the two usual sources for isolation of NK cells in the human and mouse, respectively. An enriched or purified population requires cell sorting by flow cytometry or immunomagnetic beads, based on the combinations of surface marker characteristics discussed above. NK cells can also be isolated from the thymus, liver, and lymph nodes, although they are rare in these tissues.

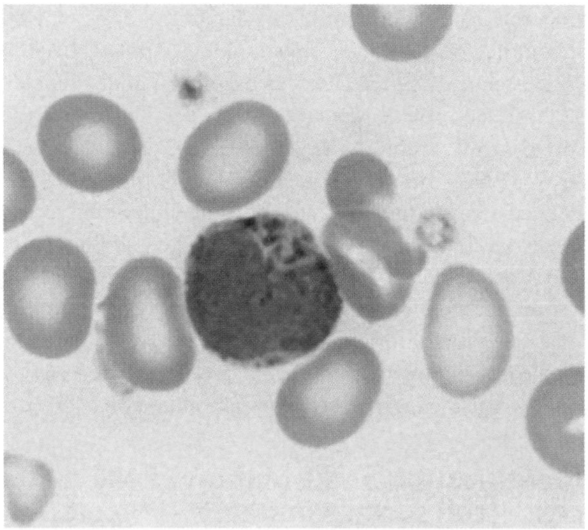

Figure 6.1 *A large granular lymphocyte. Blood smear – large granular lymphocyte. (Photograph kindly provided by Dr V. Krenn, Charité, Berlin.)*

Table 6.1 *Cell surface molecules expressed by natural killer (NK) cells*

Antigen	Ligand
CD2	CD58, CD48
CD11a/LFA-1	ICAM-1, ICAM-2
CD11b/Mac1	ICAM-1, ICAM-2, complement
CD16	IgG
CD27	CD70
CD28	B7–1, B7–2
CD40L	CD40
CD44	Hyaluronic acid
CD45/B220	
CD49b/DX5	
CD49e	Collagen, laminin
CD56 (human)	
CD62L	
CD69	–
CD94	
IFN-$\alpha\beta$R	IFN-α, IFN-β
IL-2Rβ	IL-2, IL-15
IL-12R	IL-12
IL-18R	IL-18
Asialo-GM1 (rodent)	

ICAM, intercellular adhesion molecule; IFN, interferon; Ig, immunoglobulin; IL, interleukin.

NK cells do not display the typical clonal receptor distribution seen in T and B cells, and they do not rely on rearrangement of gene segments in a germline repertoire for generation of receptors. Hence, their development is not disturbed in severe combined immunodeficient (SCID) or RAG gene-deficient mice (Yokoyama 1999). However, NK cells are heterogeneous in their receptor repertoire, in the sense that different cells express different combinations of activating and inhibitory receptors. In addition, a functional heterogeneity is emerging, at least in the human. The majority of blood NK cells express moderate levels of CD56 in combination with various molecules of the killer cell immunoglobulin receptor (KIR) family (Cooper et al. 2001). This population also expresses high levels of perforin, a pore-forming protein secreted on triggering of the killer machinery. In addition, there is a small subpopulation of blood NK cells that expresses high levels of CD56 in combination with the inhibitory receptor NKG2A, and no receptors of the KIR family. This subset has low perforin levels and seems to be specialized for high cytokine secretion rather than direct killing. The latter subset may be the only NK cells present in the lymph nodes, an organ that was initially thought to be completely devoid of NK cells (Ferlazzo et al. 2004). NK cells are also observed in the capillary beds of the lungs and liver, and they can evidently deliver effector functions in the skin as well as in the peritoneal cavity.

Table 6.2 *Mouse strains useful for studies of natural killer (NK) cells*

Mutation	Development	Comment
Beige	Normal	Defect in natural killing
Tgϵ26	Compromised	Lack NK and T cells (transgenic for human CD3e
Ly49A#7-tg	Compromised	NK-cell deficiency (accidentally)
IL-15	Compromised	Development and homeostasis
$\gamma c^{-/-}$	Compromised	Reduced cytotoxicity and cytokine production
Ikaros$^{-/-}$	Compromised	Reduced cytotoxicity
Ets1$^{-/-}$	Compromised	Reduce cytotoxicity and cytokine production
PU.1$^{-/-}$	Compromised	Normal cytotoxicity
IRF1$^{-/-}$	Compromised	Reduced cytotoxicity
ID2$^{-/-}$	Compromised	compromised cytotoxicity
MITF$^{-/-}$	Normal	Reduced cytotoxicity and cytokine production
CEBP$\gamma^{-/-}$	Normal	Reduced cytotoxicity and cytokine production
CD3e$^{-/-}$ FcϵRIg$^{-/-}$	Normal	Compromised specific killing
Syk$^{-/-}$ ZAP70$^{-/-}$	Normal	Compromised specific killing
DAP12$^{-/-}$	Normal	Cytotoxicity and cytokine production compromised
Fyn$^{-/-}$	Normal	Non-MHC receptor-mediated cytotoxicity compromised
STAT-1$^{-/-}$	Normal	Impaired rejection of tumors
dnSHP1-tg	Normal	Non-MHC receptor-mediated cytotoxicity compromised
Perforin$^{-/-}$	Normal	Perforin-independent cytotoxicity (Fas-L, TRAIL)

γc, common cytokine receptor γ chain; CEBP, CCAAT/enhancer binding protein; Ets1, E26 avian leukemia oncogene 1; Fas-L, Fas ligand; ID2, inhibitor of DNA binding 2; IRF1, interferon regulatory factor 1; MITF, microphthalmia-associated transcription factor; ZAP70, ζ-chain associated protein 70 kDa; DAP12/KARAP, killer cell activating receptor associated protein; STAT, signal transducer and activator of transcription; dnSHP1, dominant-negative SH_2-domain-containing protein tyrosine phosphatase; TRAIL, tumor necrosis factor (TNF)-related, apoptosis-inducing ligand. For further information see (Colucci et al. 2003).

Effector functions

As indicated by their name, the ability to kill various target cells is a central functional feature of NK cells. They possess several different mechanisms to do this, most of which they share with cytotoxic T lymphocytes. The most important one is perforin-dependent killing (Young and Cohn 1986). Perforin is a pore-forming protein, which is stored in the secretory granules of NK cells. When killing is triggered, the secretory apparatus is oriented toward the interface with the target cell, and the granule contents are released in the 'immune synapse' between the two cells (Davis et al. 1999; Henkart 1999; Lieberman 2003). The granules contain additional proteins, such as the serine proteases granzyme A, B, and C. These are introduced into the target cell via the pores formed by perforin, and subsequently activate apoptotic pathways. These, as well as osmotic effects created by the perforin-induced pores, eventually lead to target cell death. The process involves considerable temporospatial specificity – one NK cell can bind and initiate a 'synapse' with several cells simultaneously, and still kills only those that present the appropriate triggering signals; the others are left intact (Eriksson et al. 1999).

This rapid and efficient killer mechanism, allowing elimination of numerous target cells within minutes to hours, is defective in perforin-deficient mice. The NK cells from such mice can still kill many target cells, although this usually requires longer observation times (12–24 h) (Wallin et al. 2003). This killing is dependent on membrane-bound death receptors such as Fas ligand (Fas-L or CD178) and tumor necrosis factor (TNF)-related, apoptosis-inducing ligand-dependent receptors (Arase et al. 1995; Kayagaki et al. 1999). These interact in a cognate fashion with Fas and tumor necrosis factor-related, apoptosis-inducing ligand (TRAIL) and can thereby activate apoptosis in target cells expressing these molecules. Such mechanisms may dominate in certain situations, even when the NK cells express perforin.

Natural killer cells can also secrete cytokines, particularly IFN-γ and TNF-α (Trinchieri et al. 1984; Degliantoni et al. 1985). These cytokines may be directly cytotoxic in certain situations, but they are mainly viewed as regulators of other cellular functions. In this way NK cells may contribute to host defense by influencing infected cells and other white blood cells as well as noninfected cells outside the immune system, but which nevertheless are important for the inflammatory response (e.g. endothelial cells) (Trinchieri 1995; Biron et al. 1999). For example, IFN-γ induces increased expression of a number of cell surface molecules, including MHC class I and II products and intracellular proteins involved in antigen processing. IFN-γ can also induce intracellular pathways that limit the replication or even lead to the direct elimination of microorganisms. It can influence the profile of the ensuing specific adaptive response, deviating the T cells toward a T-helper (Th) type 1 response. Other cytokines that can be secreted by NK cells include the interleukin (IL)-10, IL-13, and granulocyte–macrophage colony-stimulating factor (GM-CSF).

The soluble effectors expressed by NK cells also include molecules with antimicrobial activity. The peptide granulysin is one of the granule components, allowing NK cells to exert direct bactericidal effects (Krensky 2000). Finally, a relatively recently discovered effector function involves cognate receptors that can stimulate T cells directly. The cell surface molecule 2B4 and its ligand CD48 appear to play a central role here (Lee et al. 2003).

Many stimuli can induce several parallel effector functions, e.g. the recognition of target cells via activating and inhibitory receptors will in many cases lead to cytotoxicity as well as IFN-γ secretion. Other stimuli, such as cytokine receptors, may elicit more restricted action.

Methods to study NK cell function in vitro and in vivo

Natural killer cell activity is often measured with the type of cytotoxicity assays that allowed their discovery (Kiessling et al. 1975a, b; Herberman et al. 1975a, b). These are usually based on assessing the proportion of target cells that releases an intracellular marker as a sign of cell damage or death after incubation with a cellular preparation containing NK cells. The target cells are usually 'labeled' with the marker before the assay, e.g. with the isotope ^{51}Cr that binds to intracellular proteins and is therefore minimally released during 4–8 h used for the assay, unless the target cells are killed.

Some target cells, e.g. normal resting cells, label poorly or are difficult to prepare to give minimal 'spontaneous release' of the isotope in the absence of killer cells. An alternative in such cases in experimental animal research is a type of assay based on 'in vivo elimination'. Target cells labeled with isotope or fluorescent dyes are inoculated into mice, usually intravenously, and the numbers of surviving cells are measured by sacrificing the animals and counting radioactivity or fluorescent cells in different organs (Riccardi et al. 1979). These assays have the advantage of demonstrating killer activity directly in vivo, which is usually more efficient than the in vitro activity. When used with tumor cells, the most efficient NK cell-mediated elimination is usually observed in the lungs, where many tumor cells are initially trapped in the capillary bed (Smyth et al. 2002). This type of assay has so far been used only to a limited extent in microbiological NK research.

A more complex, but of course highly relevant, way to study NK cells is to assess their influence on the incidence or outcome of disease or a treatment. This has been done extensively in relation to infectious agents as well as tumors. In such studies, it is of course vital to have parallel control animals in which NK cells are defective in some way or totally depleted. Measuring the survival or replication of the microorganism, and/or signs of disease and ultimately death of the infected animal, can then follow infection. Some examples on the role of NK cells in infections are discussed further below. In cancer research, the outcome can be measured by complete rejection or outgrowth of a subcutaneously inoculated tumor (Kiessling et al. 1975c). This requires the use of titrated, low doses of tumor inocula, but gives the advantage of demonstrating that NK cells can 'finish the job' and eradicate the last tumor cells (Kärre et al. 1986). Alternately, higher tumor doses can be used, and the outcome assessed by measuring the tumor size or number of metastases at given time points. NK cells are particularly efficient at preventing hematogenous metastases to the lungs (Smyth et al. 2002), which may reflect their efficient activity in the blood and the capillary beds. NK cells have been studied extensively in experimental bone marrow transplantation in lethally irradiated mice (Kiessling et al. 1977; Bennett et al. 1995; Barao and Murphy 2003). The outcome is then evaluated about a week after the transplantation, and based on assessing the spleen colonization by transplanted cells. This is done either by counting colonies or by measuring how an injected isotope is taken up specifically by proliferating hematopoietic cells.

Controls used to assure that effects are caused by NK cells are usually based on removal of the NK cells from the cell population or the animal. In this case, most investigators use treatment with a monoclonal antibody or antiserum directed against a cell surface marker of NK cells, such as DX5, NK1.1, or asialo GM1 (Ehl et al. 1996). As these reagents are not entirely specific for NK cells, additional controls may be required, e.g. NK 1.1 is expressed on a subpopulation of T cells, the so-called NK-T cells, and it may therefore be appropriate to perform the experiment also in mice lacking such cells. There is, to date, no natural mutant or intentionally constructed gene knock-out mouse with a complete and selective lack of NK cells. However, an experiment aimed at producing a transgenic strain unexpectedly led to a complete NK cell defect in one founder, presumably as a result of the insertion site of the transgene (Kim et al. 2000). The strain derived from this founder is a useful tool to study development of NK cells, but can also be used as a negative control for NK cell effects in vivo, particularly in long-term experiments where it is difficult to maintain absence of NK activity by repeated injections of antibodies (Table 6.3). Several genetically manipulated mouse strains with an approximately normal size of the NK cell population, but with defects in single receptors or signal transduction pathways affecting NK cell functions, have been established (Colucci et al. 2003). These strains will be useful to dissect the importance of different NK functions in

Table 6.3 *Activating and inhibiting receptors of natural killer (NK) cells and expression on T cells*

Receptor	mu	hu	Ligand	References	T cells
Inhibiting					
Ly49	+	–	MHCI	Anderson et al. (2001); Kane et al. (2001)	+ ($CD8^-$ effector/memory subset)
Ly49A			D^d, D^k, (D^b)	Karlhofer et al. (1992)	
Ly49C			K^b, (K^d, D^d, D^k, D^b)		
Ly49G			D^d, L^d		
Ly49I			K^d, MCMV m157	Arase et al. (2002); Smith et al. (2002)	
Ly49O			D^b, D^d, D^{dk}, L^d		
Ly49V			H-2^b, H-2^d, H-2^k		
Ly49B, -E, -F, -J, -Q, -S, -T			Specificity n.d.		
KIR	–	+	HLA cl.I	Lanier (1998); Natarajan et al. (2002)	+ ($CD8^-$ effector/memory subset)
2DL2, 2DL3			HLA-C group 1[a]		
2DL1			HLA-C group 2[a]		
3DL1			HLA-Bw4		
3DL2			HLA-A3, -A11		
2DL5, 3DL7					
CD94/NKG2A/B	+	+	Qa-1, HLA-E, HLA-E/UL40	Braud et al. (1998); Tomasec et al. (2000)	+ ($CD8^-$ subset, all activated)
KLRG1/MAFA	+	+			+ ($CD8^-$ effector/memory subset)
LIR1/ILT2	+		HCMV UL18	Reyburn et al. (1997)	+ ($CD8^-$ subset)
NKR-P1D	+	+	Clr-b	Iizuka et al. (2003)	
Activating					
Ly-49[b]	+	–		Anderson et al. (2001); Kane et al. (2001)	
Ly-49D			H-$2D^d$, ligand on CHO cells	Idris et al. (1999)	–
Ly-49H			MCMV m157	Arase et al. (2002); Smith et al. (2002)	
Ly-49P			D^d		
Ly-49R			D^d, D^k, L^d		
Ly-49W			H-2^d, H-2^k		
Ly-49L, -M, -U			Specificity n.d.		

(*Continued over*)

Table 6.3 *Activating and inhibiting receptors of natural killer (NK) cells and expression on T cells (Continued)*

Receptor	mu	hu	Ligand	References	T cells
KIR	–	+	HLA cl.I	Lanier (1998); Natarajan et al. (2002)	+ ($CD8^-$ memory subset)
2DS2			HLA-C group 1		
2DS1			HLA-C group 2		
2DL4			HLA-G		
2DS4			HLA-C		
2DS3, 2DS5, 3DS1					
CD94/NKG2C	+	+	Qa-1, HLA-E	Braud et al. (1998); Vance et al. (1999)	+ ($CD8^-$ subset)
CD94/NKG2E/H	+	+	Qa-1	Vance et al. (1999)	+ ($CD8^-$ subset)
NKG2D	+	+	Rae-1, H60; MIC-A/B, ULBP	Raulet (2003)	+ ($CD8^-$ subset; hu-all, mu-effectors)
NKp30	+	+	Ligand on iDCs	Moretta (2002)	–
NKp44	–	+	Influenza HA		–
NKp46	+	+	Influenza HA	Mandelboim et al. (2001)	–
NKR-P1A	+	+			
NKR-P1C/NK1.1	+	–			+ ($CD8^+$ effector/memory subset)
Co-receptors					
NKp80		+		Moretta et al. (2001)	+ subset
2B4	+	+	CD48	Moretta et al. (2001)	+
DNAM-1		+	Nectins		+
NTB-A		+			

Further inhibiting receptors: P75/AIRM, IRp60, LAIR-1, gp49B1.

CHO, Chinese hamster ovary; CMV, human cytomegalovirus; HA, hemagglutinin; iDCs, immature dendritic cells; ITIM, immunoreceptor tyrosine-based inhibitory motif; KIR, killer cell immunoglobulin-like receptors; MCMV, murine cytomegalovirus; n.d., not defined yet.

Low-affinity ligands are indicated in parenthesis.

a) HLA-C: group 1 – Ser-77, Asn-80 in Cw1, Cw3, Cw7, Cw8; group 2 – Asn-77, Lys-80 in Cw2, Cw4, Cw5, Cw6.

b) As 'activating' have been designated Ly49 receptors (1) for which stimulatory activity has been revealed or (2) that have no ITIMs and a positively charged residue in the transmembrane segment (Anderson et al. 2001; Kane et al. 2001).

complex in vivo scenarios, e.g. in infectious diseases. Similarly, mice defective in genes critical for various effector functions can be used to study exactly how NK cells contribute to a complex response or development of disease.

There are mice with a profound immune deficiency that involves NK cells as well as other cells, e.g. mice deficient for the common γ chain of cytokine receptors (γc) (Table 6.3). Despite such a broad defect, these mice can be used for the study of NK cells by adoptive transfer of isolated NK cells. Cytokine-stimulated NK cells can also be used in adoptive transfer to improve the resistance to tumor cells in normal mice.

Ontogeny and regulation

Like other white blood cells, NK cells are derived from hematopoietic stem cells in the bone marrow. In the fetus, NK cells and other lineages also develop in the yolk sac, liver, and aorta–gonad–mesonephros region. Studies in mice indicate that generation of NK cells may be critically dependent on the microenvironment of the bone marrow during adult life. Mice treated with the marrow-ablating agents ^{89}Sr and estradiol, in which other pathways of myelo- and lymphopoiesis are taken over by the spleen, show severely impaired NK cell development (Colucci et al. 2003). Stroma cells of the marrow appear to have a critical role, providing cytokines as well as cognate interactions required for NK cell development.

Through the use of well-defined culture conditions, it is possible to generate NK cells from hematopoietic cells from different sources in the mouse as well as in the human (Mrozek et al. 1996; Williams et al. 1997; Colucci et al. 2003). Multiple intermediate stages have been proposed. Although these differ between species, source of stem cells, and culture conditions, a general pathway emerges that is remarkably similar in the human and the mouse. This simplified scheme has three phases.

The first phase leads to NK cell precursors, via initial commitment to the lymphoid lineage and subsequently to the NK cell lineage. The NK precursors in the human as well as in the mouse express the IL-2 receptor IL-2Rβ, but lack many of the typical NK cell markers. The second phase leads to immature NK cells, during which the NK precursors gradually acquire surface markers and several functions of NK cells. NKRP-1 and CD2 molecules appear early, followed by DX5 (mouse) or CD56 (human), in parallel with the development of the cytolytic potential. The MHC receptors are acquired late; those of the NKG2 family precede those of the Ly49 (mouse) and KIR (human) families. In the third and final phase NK cells are exported to the periphery. Phase 1 and at least part of phase 2 can be achieved in culture by the correct cytokine combinations, without the need for stromal cells. The cytokines stem cell factor (SCF) (also known as c-KIT ligand), fetal liver kinase 2 (FLK2) ligand (also known as FMS-like tyrosine kinase 3 ligand or FLT3L), and IL-7 can drive the cells through phase 1, although none of these is essential by itself for NK development in vivo (Williams et al. 1997). IL-15 is critical in phase 2 (Mrozek et al. 1996). The latter requirement may explain the block in NK cell development in mice with common cytokine receptor γ-chain deficiency – this chain is an essential part of the IL-15 and IL-2 receptor. Although high doses of IL-2 can substitute for IL-15 in vitro, there is overwhelming evidence that in vivo development is critically dependent on IL-15, and not at all on IL-2. Under the influence of IL-15 in vitro, NK cells acquire cytotoxic capacity, but they still lack several characteristics of mature NK cells, such as receptors of the Ly49 or KIR families. Complete maturation requires interaction of NK cell precursors with MHC and possibly other molecules on bone marrow stromal cells, in order to develop and fine-tune the receptor repertoire (Roth et al. 2000; Raulet et al. 2001). The latter aspect is discussed separately.

Developmental processes are regulated by transcription factors, some of which can act as crucial master switches in hematopoietic lineage commitment (Colucci et al. 2003). Mice deficient in the Ikaros gene show a block in lymphoid development, including T, B, and NK cells, whereas myelopoiesis is unaffected (see Table 6.3). NOTCH-1 and PAX5 act as master switches for the development of T cells and B cells, respectively. Mutations in these genes do not affect NK cell development. There is evidence that ID molecules (inhibitors of DNA-binding proteins), which negatively regulate the basic-loop-helix (bHLH) family of DNA-binding proteins, are important to favor the NK over the T- and B-cell lineage (Yokota et al. 1999). Deficiency in several other transcription factors can partially impair NK cell development, or skew the receptor repertoire (Colucci et al. 2003).

Natural killer cell precursors can be isolated from the thymus. It is, however, not clear whether this signifies a closer relationship to the T-cell lineage. In any case, the thymus plays no critical role in NK cell development; athymic patients (di George syndrome) and mice (nu/nu genotype) have normal if not increased NK cell numbers and activity (Yokoyama 1999).

Once mature, NK cells have a lifespan of at least several weeks. They circulate in the blood and can enter mucosae as well as parenchymatous organs. A special subset is detected in the placenta (Moffett-King 2002). During local infection or inflammation, NK cells may infiltrate the site by attraction through chemokines and the use of integrins such as very late antigen 4 (VLA-4) (or CD49d/CD29) (see Table 6.1). The homeostatic survival may, like NK development, depend critically on IL-15. Adoptive transfer experiments suggest that mature NK cells are blocked from dividing under normal conditions, but homeostatic proliferation can take place if the number of NK cells is low (Prlic et al. 2003). There is a vast proliferation on overproduction of the cytokine IL-15 in vivo and NK cells may become dominant in the spleen (Fehniger and Caligiuri 2001). In vitro, NK cells can be induced to proliferate by IL-2. As a result of the constitutive expression of IL-2Rβ, they are the major responding cell population when normal blood or spleen cells are exposed to high doses of IL-2, in what has been termed lymphokine-activated killer (LAK) cultures (Rosenberg 1988; Yokoyama 1999). Hence, they are the major effector cells in the antitumoral responses observed after adoptive transfer of LAK cells in experimental and clinical situations (Smyth et al. 2002). The physiological role of IL-2 in NK cell regulation and proliferation is unclear, but it is not a critical factor for development or proliferation of NK cells in vivo (Colucci et al. 2003). There is evidence for nonspecific, cytokine-driven, as well as specific, cognate, recognition-driven proliferation of NK cells during viral infection (Biron et al. 1999).

Many cytokines, chemokines and other mediators can increase the cytotoxic activity of NK cells. Type I IFNs secreted in response to virus infection or artificial stimuli, such as poly(I:C) and tilorone, are frequently used to optimize NK activity in murine experimental models (Biron et al. 1999; Yokoyama 1999). IL-12, IL-18, IL-21, as well as several chemokines can all act to increase NK cytotoxic function (Trinchieri 2003b). Combinations of one or more of these factors often show potentiating effects. Some pathways of regulation have a more profound influence on certain NK cell functions. There is, for example, dichotomy in murine cytomegalovirus (CMV) infection where IL-12 appears more important for NK cell-derived IFN-γ, whereas type I IFNs induce the cytotoxic function. NK cytotoxicity can be down-regulated by IL-10 and transforming growth factor β (TGF-β) (Biron et al. 2002).

Various conditions, diseases, diets, and activities – from high yogurt consumption to laughter and space trips – have been investigated with respect to their influence on NK activity. It is difficult to discern any specific patterns or regulatory pathways from the literature. In general, NK activity may vary considerably and appears relatively easy to modulate on a short-term basis. The functional impact of such spontaneous or induced alterations is unclear.

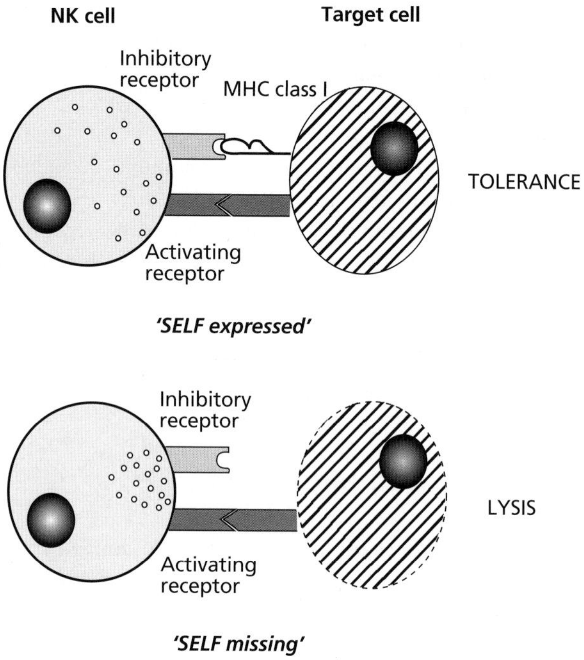

Figure 6.2 *The 'missing self' model. The expression of major histocompatibility complex class I (MHC class I) (*SELF expressed*) on a potential target cell can be sensed by inhibitory natural killer (NK) cell receptors. Tolerance is caused by dominance of inhibitory signals over NK cell triggering signals exerted by activating receptors engaging ligands on the potential target cell. Reduced or no MHCI expression (*SELF missing*) leads to a reduced or lack of inhibitory signals. Consequently activating signals dominate and killing of the target cell is triggered (Kärre 1985; Ljunggren and Kärre 1990).*

SPECIFICITY OF NK CELLS – A BALANCE BETWEEN ACTIVATING AND INHIBITORY RECEPTORS

The 'missing self' model

It is now clear that the specificity of NK cells depend on the integration of different recognition events mediated by activating as well as inhibitory receptors. This basic paradigm was first formulated within the 'missing self' model for NK cell recognition (Figure 6.2) (Kärre 1985, 1997, 2002; Ljunggren and Kärre 1990). Briefly, this model proposed that one (but not the only) function of NK cells is to recognize and act on information that is missing in the target and present in the host rather than the opposite, which is how T cells work. More specifically, the information in question would be host MHC class I molecules. An immune mechanism eliminating cells without, or with too few, MHC class I molecules could have evolved as an alternative, as well as a necessary complement to T cells: an alternative because aberrant cells do not always express novel epitopes – loss of gene products might represent an early or even unique change in infected or transformed cells; complementary, because without MHC class I molecules, no antigens would be presented to CD8 T cells, which open for microbial escape mechanisms targeting this pathway. The postulated recognition strategy would also eliminate cells from other individuals, as a result of lack of host MHC molecules. Exposure to such cells occurs frequently in certain invertebrates, for which it has long been recognized that they possess graft rejection mechanisms based on self-recognition (Kärre 2002). Transfer of cells between individuals can also occur in mammals, e.g. during intimate contacts or pregnancy, and this could represent a way for spreading infections. It can thus be argued that mechanisms in 'primitive' defense systems may have evolved further and adapted to the MHC system of mammals in the form of missing self-recognition.

This model provided a number of testable predictions (Kärre 2002), many of which are alluded to in the sections on cancer and transplantation in this chapter. A key prediction related to the main mechanistic model for missing self-recognition, depicted in Figure 6.2, is based on the idea that NK cells depend on two (sets of) receptors, one activating and one inhibiting. The activating receptor(s) were postulated to recognize ubiquitously expressed ligands, present on most normal cells. This would allow NK cells to bind most cells in the body and receive a preliminary triggering signal. The ultimate decision would then be taken by the inhibitory receptors, recognizing one or more self MHC class I ligands of the host. This would inhibit the triggering signal. If critical class I molecules were missing or too few in number, the inhibitory signal would be insufficient, and lysis of the target cell would proceed by default. This predicted the existence of MHC class I allele-specific receptors on NK cells, and that antibodies prepared against such receptors should induce lysis (by blocking of the inhibitory recognition) rather than block it. This experimental prediction was confirmed with the identification of two different inhibitory receptor families in the human and mouse, respectively (Karlhofer et al. 1992; Moretta et al. 1993, 1994; Yokoyama 1999). The use of antibodies against such receptors allowed a further dissection of specificity and eventually the identification of activating receptors. Although the basic platform provided by the missing self model has turned out to be correct, it is now clear that the picture is immensely more complex, with a variety of activating and inhibitory receptors balancing each other. The decision does not always lie with the inhibitory receptors – some of the activating receptors recognize ligands expressed only by infected or stressed cells, and they can induce NK effector functions even if the target cell expresses self MHC class I molecules (Moretta et al. 2001; Raulet 2003; Yokoyama and Plougastel 2003). Most of the known NK receptors are summarized in Table 6.4; the most important ones are discussed in more detail below.

Inhibitory receptors

Natural killer cells express inhibitory receptors that recognize MHC class I molecules with varying degrees of allele specificity. Interestingly, these receptors are encoded by two entirely different gene families in the human and in the mouse – the KIR and the Ly49 receptors (Ly49R) in the lectin-like superfamily, respectively (Moretta et al. 2001; Yokoyama and Plougastel 2003). Even though the proteins are in two different structural groups, the receptor systems in the two species show remarkable similarities at the functional level. Both types of receptor recognize a subgroup of MHC class I alleles. Both deliver inhibitory signals by immunotyrosine inhibitory motifs (ITIM) (with the sequence V/I–x–Y–x–x–L/V) in the cytoplasmic tail, which on phosphorylation can recruit phosphatases acting on substrates in the signaling pathways initiated by activating receptors (Lanier 2003). Both are encoded in complex gene families showing considerable polymorphism between individuals, and also include activating receptors of similar specificity and structure, except for the ITIM in the cytoplasmic tail (Trowsdale et al. 2001; Yokoyama and Plougastel 2003).

Table 6.4 *Key features of signal transduction in natural killer (NK) cells*

Receptor	Module/adaptor	Downstream elements
$Ly49_{inhibiting}$	ITIM	SHP1
$Ly49_{activating}$	+TM/DAP12	SYK, ZAP70
$KIR_{inhibiting}$	ITIM	SHP1
$KIR_{activating}$	+TM/DAP12	SYK, ZAP70 – PLCγ1, ERK1/2
CD94/NKG2A	ITIM	SHP1
CD94/NKG2C, -E	+TM/DAP12	SYK, ZAP70
NKG2D	$+TM/DAP10_{(YINM)}$[a], $+TM/DAP12_{(ITAM)}$[b]	SLP-76, PI3K, Grb2 – Vav, PLCγ2, SYK, ZAP70
2B4	SAP or SHP1; LAT	PI3K
NKp30	FcεRIγ, CD3ζ	SYK, ZAP70
NKp44	+TM/DAP12	SYK, ZAP70
NKp46	FcεRIγ, CD3ζ	SYK, ZAP70
Nkrp-1c	FcεRIγ, CD3ζ	SYK, ZAP70
CD16	FcεRIγ, CD3ζ	SYK, ZAP70 – PI3K, PLCγ2, Vav

ITAM, immunoreceptor tyrosine-based activation motif; ITIM, immunoreceptor tyrosine-based inhibitory motif; KIR, killer cell immunoglobulin receptor; LAT, linker for activation of T cells; PI3K, phosphatidylinositol 3-kinase; PLCγ1, phospholipase C γ1, SAP, SLAM-associated protein; SHP1, SH_2-domain-containing protein tyrosine phosphatase; +TM, positively charged residues in the transmembrane portion; ZAP70 – ζ chain-associated protein 70 kDa. More detailed information is provided in Colucci et al. (2002), Lanier (2003), and Trinchieri (2003a).

a) Resting and activated NK cells.

b) Activated NK cells.

Both types of receptor are expressed in complex patterns within one individual, yielding NK cells or clones or subpopulations with different but partly overlapping combinations of receptors (Raulet et al. 2001; Parham and McQueen 2003). Most importantly, both types of receptor allow the NK cells to distinguish between cells with normal or insufficient self MHC class I expression, by inhibiting effector function in response to the former but not to the latter. In the following, the mouse and human receptors are discussed separately, with emphasis on the features that distinguish them. It is nevertheless clear that the unifying functional aspects dominate. It is a conundrum why evolution has selected two different complex receptor systems with such similar functions in different species.

HLA CLASS I RECOGNIZING KIR RECEPTORS

As evident from their name, the KIR belong to the immunoglobulin superfamily of genes. The KIR genes are located within a larger gene complex termed the leukocyte receptor cluster (LRC) on chromosome 19q13.4 (Trowsdale et al. 2001). Fourteen different expressed KIRs have been described so far (Lanier 1998; Parham and McQueen 2003). The inhibitory receptors have two or three Ig-like folds, and the commonly used terminology is partly based on this feature (e.g. KIR2DL1 means KIR of 2 Ig-like domains, with long cytoplasmic tail including ITIM). As summarized in Table 6.2, the 2D KIRs distinguish two major subgroups of HLA-C alleles on the basis of a dimorphism involving residues 77 and 80. The KIRs bind on top of the MHC class I molecule, interacting with both α helices and the peptide (Boyington and Sun 2002; Natarajan et al. 2002) (Figure 6.3). This explains why the peptide bound by the MHC molecule can influence the KIR recognition, although there is no generalized difference between self and nonself (e.g. microbe-derived) peptides. The KIR3DL1 receptor recognizes a subgroup of HLA-B molecules with the Bw4 serological motif determined by residues 77–83, in a manner that can also be influenced by the bound peptide.

A given NK clone can express between 0 and 3 inhibitory KIRs. This expression pattern appears stable within each clone (Lanier 1998). The composition and expression pattern of the KIR-gene complex differ among individuals (Vilches and Parham 2002). The expression pattern is genetically determined; it is stable within one individual and similar in monozygotic twins but, surprisingly, it is not strongly influenced by the HLA type of the individual. The issue of receptor repertoires in rela-

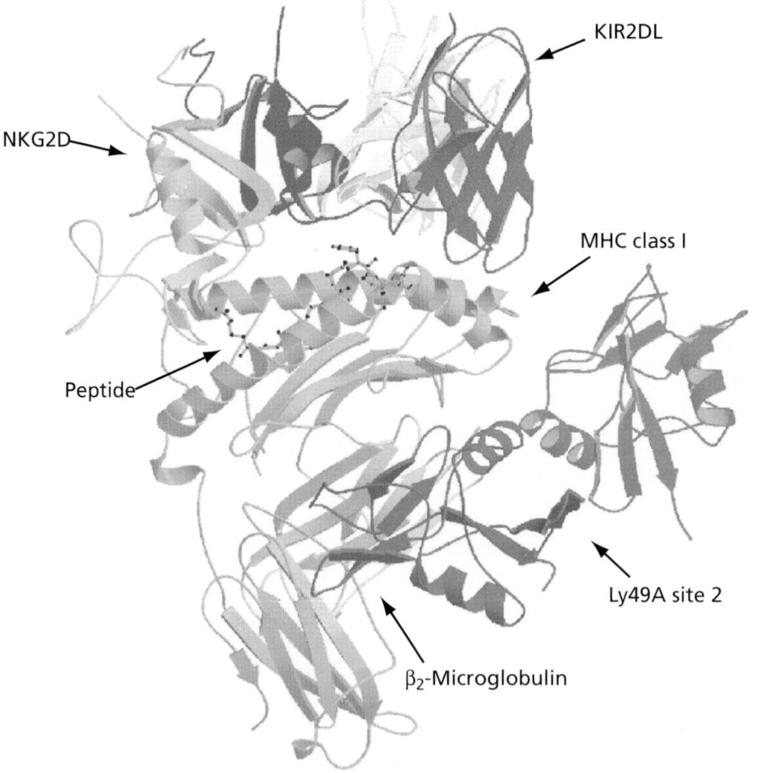

Figure 6.3 *Structural aspects of major histocompatibility complex class I (MHC class I) recognition by three natural killer (NK) receptors. Binding sites for Ly49A, KIR2DL, and NKG2D on MHC class I (shown is H-2DS^d). Ly49A interacting at site 2 is depicted in cyan/light blue, KIR2DL in magenta, and NKG2D in green/pink. (Figure reproduced with permission from Natarajan et al. (2002) © 2004 Annual Reviews. For detailed discussions see Boyington and Sun (2002); Natarajan et al. (2002), and Dam et al. (2003).)*

tion to tolerance and disease susceptibility is discussed in more detail below.

In addition, the LRC contains the *LIR/ILT* gene family, which includes inhibiting as well as activating receptors (Borges and Cosman 2000; Colonna et al. 2000; Trowsdale et al. 2001). They differ from KIRs in the expression pattern, and are found mainly on other cells in the immune system (Natarajan et al. 2002), e.g. LIR-1/ILT-2 is expressed by B cells, macrophages, and dendritic cells, and only on a smaller fraction of NK cells. This receptor can recognize several different MHC class I molecules but, interestingly, its affinity for the human cytomegalovirus (HCMV) protein UL 18 is 1000-fold higher (Chapman et al. 1999). LIR-2/ILT-4 also bind to MHC class I molecules, whereas the specificity of other members of this family is elusive.

H-2 CLASS I RECOGNIZING LY49 RECEPTORS

The *Ly49* genes are encoded within the NK gene complex (NKC) of distal chromosome 6 in the mouse, together with several other genes that also belong to the lectin superfamily (Yokoyama and Plougastel 2003). There are, however, structural features of Ly49 molecules that argue against a true lectin function, i.e. carbohydrate recognition. A total of 16 full-length Ly49 genes have been identified; the number of genes varies between different mouse strains (Kane et al. 2001). They are expressed as homodimers with type II membrane orientation on the cell surface (Lanier 1998). Like the KIR family, the Ly49 family also includes genes that encode activating receptors.

The Ly49 receptors bind mouse MHC class I molecules with varying degree of allele specificity (see Table 6.4) (Kane et al. 2001). The Ly49A receptor, co-crystallized with its ligand, surprisingly revealed two sites of interaction: 'site 1' at the top of the groove near the N terminus of the peptide, and 'site 2' below the antigen-binding groove, with several contact residues in the $\alpha 3$ domain and β_2-microglobulin (Kane et al. 2001; Natarajan et al. 2002). Although 'site 1' was initially believed to represent the physiological binding, multiple lines of evidence now argue in favor of 'site 2' being the important recognition zone (Dam et al. 2003). This puts the issue of allelic specificity in focus, because many contact residues at 'site 2' are nonpolymorphic. The most likely explanation is that alterations in polymorphic residues distant from the contact zone can nevertheless affect it by structural changes transmitted through the molecule, ultimately affecting the orientation of nonpolymorphic contact residues. Even polymorphic residues in the floor of the antigen-binding groove can influence allele specificity, which may explain why certain Ly49 receptors are influenced by the nature of the peptide bound to the groove. Perhaps the opposing ways by which KIR and Ly49 molecules bind and distinguish different MHC class I molecules may explain why the two species have evolved different types of receptors.

Each NK cell expresses between 0 and 6 Ly49 receptors, the average estimated as being 2.6 different ones per cell (Kubota et al. 1999; Raulet et al. 2001). The development of the inhibitory receptor repertoire is discussed below.

HLA-E/QA-1 RECOGNIZING NKG2A RECEPTORS

NKG2A receptors are also encoded in the NKC, but, in contrast to the Ly49 family, they and the family of genes they belong to are encoded in the syntenic human chromosome 12p13 (Yokoyama and Plougastel 2003). NKG2A, with two intracytoplasmic ITIMs, is expressed as a heterodimer together with CD94, also encoded within the NKC (Carretero et al. 1997; Lanier 1998). NKG2A recognizes the nonclassic conserved MHC class I molecule HLA-E or its homolog Qa-1 in the mouse. These ligands are not transported from the endoplasmic reticulum (ER) to the cell surface unless they bind peptides with specific anchor motifs, present mainly in leader sequences of polymorphic MHC class I molecules (Braud et al. 1998). Paradoxically, the loading of such leader sequences in HLA-E/Qa-1 molecules requires the ER membrane-bound peptide transporter associated with antigen presentation (TAP). The NKG2A receptor will thus allow the scanning for expression of MHC class I molecules and/or TAP on potential target cells. Reduced production of such molecules will indirectly lead to insufficient HLA-E/Qa-1 expression, which is required to inhibit via the NKG2A receptor (Leibson 1998).

The division of labor between NKG2A and KIR/Ly49 receptors is not clear. Perhaps they are used as complementary tools to sense intact antigen-processing/MHC class I machinery. NKG2A can be expressed together with one or several KIRs, but they can also be expressed in the absence of KIR.

INHIBITING RECEPTORS WITH OTHER SPECIFICITIES

The inhibiting receptors in the mouse also include NKR-P1B and -D. The latter recognizes a lectin expressed by dendritic cells. Interestingly, the gene for this inhibitory ligand is closely linked to the receptor, suggesting that tolerance in this system evolved by linked inheritance of receptor and ligand (Iizuka et al. 2003). In the human, an Ig-like molecule termed p75/AIRM has been identified as an ITIM containing inhibitory NK receptors. It is a member of the sialoadhesin family in the LRC, and it is also expressed by myeloid cells. It mediates sialic acid-dependent recognition but the functional specificity is unknown (Vitale et al. 2001).

The existence of inhibitory receptors with specificities other than MHC class I suggests that the 'missing self' concept may be extended to include situations where target cells need to be protected from NK cells, although MHC class I expression is suboptimal. One obvious example is the red blood cell. It is not known how erythrocytes escape NK lysis. So far, unknown inhibitory receptor–ligand pairs represent one possibility, but it is also possible that red blood cells do not express adhesion molecules and activating ligands for initial binding and triggering of NK cells.

Activating receptors

ACTIVATING RECEPTORS IN THE KIR AND LIR FAMILIES

Several of the inhibitory KIRs have closely related homologs, which, however, differ in that they only have a short cytoplasmic tail, without ITIMs. These receptors are designated with an S (for short cytoplasmic tail) instead of a D, e.g. KIR2DS1. They possess a charged amino acid in the intramembrane-spanning domain (Lanier 1998), allowing the association with the adaptor molecule KARAP/DAP-12 that couples to activating signal transduction pathways through immunoreceptor tyrosine-based activation motifs (ITAM) in their cytoplasmic tail (Tomasello et al. 2000; Lanier 2003). These are based on the semiconserved peptide sequence YxxL(I)x_{6-8}YxxL(I) (Lanier and Bakker 2000). Cross-linking of the activating KIRs thus leads to triggering of NK cells, although the role for this type of recognition for overall NK cell function is not clear. It could represent one of several activating recognition systems for ligands expressed by most cells, and necessary for NK cells to mediate surveillance for the missing self. A more popular idea is that the activating KIRs directly recognize ligands preferentially expressed by infected or stressed cells – either 'altered self' in the form of MHC class I/peptide combinations, or pathogen-encoded, MHC class I-like molecules. There is evidence that activating KIRs may have lower affinity for MHC class I ligands than inhibitory KIRs, and that they are mostly expressed together with the inhibitory homolog (Khakoo and Brooks 2003). These aspects could be important to avoid autoreactivity. As discussed below, the activating KIRs appear to undergo rapid evolution, in line with the idea of an evolutionary pressure created by pathogens.

Some receptors in the LIR/ILT family, such as LIR-6a/b and LIR7/ILT1, share the features of activating KIRs, i.e. a short cytoplasmic tail with a charged amino acid in the membrane-spanning region (Borges and Cosman 2000; Colonna et al. 2000). The function of activating LIRs is not known.

ACTIVATING RECEPTORS IN THE LY49 FAMILY

The Ly49 family also includes activating receptors. Ly49H and Ly49D are the most well characterized (Nakamura et al. 1999; Yokoyama and Plougastel 2003). Like the activating KIRs, they lack ITIMs (despite a long cytoplasmic tail) and instead harbor a charged amino acid in the membrane-spanning region. Similar to activating KIRs, this allows them to signal through the adaptor molecule KARAP/DAP-12 (Lanier and Bakker 2000). Ly49H recognizes a murine cytomegalovirus (MCMV)-encoded ligand, and this receptor is indeed the product of a CMV resistance gene studied for a long time in the mouse strain C57BL, as discussed below (Scalzo et al. 2003). Ly49D, also associating with DAP-12, can bind to the murine MHC class I molecule H-$2D^d$. Ly49D$^+$ NK cells from mice lacking H-$2D^d$ can use the receptor to kill cells that express this MHC allele (Nakamura et al. 1999). An appealing hypothesis that integrates these seemingly disparate specificities of Ly49H and Ly49D, addressing the function and evolution of activating of MHC class I-recognizing receptors in general, is discussed below.

NKG2D: AN ACTIVATING RECEPTOR RECOGNIZING LIGANDS INDUCED IN STRESSED, INFECTED, AND TRANSFORMED CELLS

NKG2D is closely linked genetically to NKG2A and -C, but only distantly related to them with respect to sequence homology (28 percent). Furthermore, it is expressed as a homodimer rather than complexing with CD94. It is expressed by T cells (all in the human and by subsets of $\gamma\delta$T and activated $\alpha\beta$T cells in the mouse) and by activated macrophages (Raulet 2003). Through a charged amino acid in the membrane-spanning region, it can associate and induce activating signals through the adaptor molecule DAP10 in T cells, which enables it to work as a co-receptor for T-cell receptor (TCR) triggering. In NK cells it can act as an activating receptor on its own. This is the result of two splice variants, allowing association with KARAP/DAP12 as well as DAP10 (Lanier 2003). NKG2D can recognize a large variety of ligands distantly related to MHC class I, expressed mainly on certain stressed, infected, or transformed cells. The ligands for human NKG2D include MICA and MICB, expressed on stressed epithelial cells, and the CMV-encoded proteins ULBP1–3. Murine NKG2D binds to Rae-1 and HL-60 expressed by stressed cells and certain tumor cells, and a recently identified ligand termed mouse ULBP-like transcript-a (MULT-1) (Raulet 2003). The last appears to be constitutively expressed in many tissues. Structural studies of NKG2D co-crystallizing with its ligands have provided an explanation of how this receptor can bind to different ligands (see Figure 6.3) (Natarajan et al. 2002). NKG2D was initially thought to be completely independent of inhibitory signals; it now appears that these signals can inhibit activation of NKG2D, but less efficiently than other activating receptors (Pende et al. 2001). Stressed normal cells can therefore be killed through recognition by NKG2D even if they express considerable levels of MHC class I molecules. NKG2D and its ligands provide many exciting lines of research in infection and tumor immunology, discussed further in the specialized sections below.

ACTIVATING RECEPTORS WITH UNKNOWN SPECIFICITY, INCLUDING RECEPTORS RECOGNIZING NON-MHC MOLECULES ON NORMAL CELLS

The 'missing self' model postulates that the activating NK cell receptors recognize ligands on most normal cells. There is strong evidence that NK cells can indeed kill normal cells, which lack MHC class I, and which also lack the stress-induced ligands for NKG2D discussed previously. Thus, there must be other activating receptors. Some of the receptors discussed here play a role in the surveillance of normal cells, but it must be emphasized that the exact (combination of) receptors used in different situations remain to be clarified. One of the reasons for this may be that NK cells use several receptors in a parallel and redundant fashion, which makes it difficult to prove the role of one by targeting it genetically or in antibody blockade experiments. It is therefore interesting that several activating receptors were identified in an experimental approach with xenogeneic effector target cell combinations, in order to minimize the number of receptor–ligand pairs involved. Using this approach, antibodies binding to the three so-called NCRs, NKp30, NK p44, and NKp46, were identified (Moretta et al. 2001). All NK cells, in humans as well as in mice, express NKp30 and NKp46. The former is the main activating receptor in NK cell interactions with dendritic cells (Moretta 2002). NKp46 is involved in recognition of normal as well as many tumor cells, and there is also evidence that it can recognize influenza virus-infected cells via sialic residues of the hemagglutinin (Mandelboim et al. 2001). The level of NKp46 varies between NK cells, and this correlates with their cytotoxic potential. Only human activated NK cells express NKp44 (Moretta et al. 2001). Its ligands are unknown.

There is intensive ongoing research on the specificity and expression patterns of these activating receptors, as well as their role in recognition of various target cells. A frequently used strategy to define the specificity of receptors is to produce multimeric, soluble proteins to identify ligands in different types of cells. This is not always as straightforward as it sounds – the geometry and affinity of these constructs may not always allow ligand-specific binding above background levels. The final answer as to which activating receptors NK cells use in different situations must be based on methods allowing the direct measurement of ligands on target cells, as well as antibody cocktails combining different antibodies to completely block the critical interactions (Moretta et al. 2001).

Transduction and integration of signals after NK cell recognition

The ligation of activating and inhibitory receptors must be transduced to intracellular signals, and these must be integrated and read out to activate different NK cell programs. This is an intensive area of research, and only a fragmentary picture is currently available (Colucci et al. 2002; Lanier 2003). Upon ligation of inhibitory receptors, the phosphorylated ITIMs in their cytoplasmic tails recruit -SH2-domain-containing tyrosine phosphatase (SHP-1) and other phosphatases. These are thought to act on substrates that have been phosphorylated in the proximal part of activating pathways. There are multiple, parallel, proximal signaling pathways for activating receptors, which generally signal through noncovalently associated adaptor molecules. This association commonly involves an aspartic acid residue in the transmembrane region of the adaptor molecule, interacting with a positively charged amino acid in corresponding domain of the ligand-binding receptor. Some of the adaptor molecules, such as CD3ζ, FcεRIγ, and KARAP/DAP-12, contain ITAMs in their cytoplasmic tails. Ligation of an NK receptor linked to an ITAM-containing adaptor initiate proximal signaling events in a protein tyrosine kinase (PTK) cascade similar to ITAM-dependent mechanisms in T- and B-cell activation. It involves activation of PTK in the Src family, leading to activation of ZAP70 and Syk in the Syk PTK family (Colucci et al. 2002). DAP10, one of the adaptor molecules associating with NKG2D, lacks ITAMs (Lanier 2003). Its cytoplasmic tail instead contains the motif YINM, which can bind and activate phosphatidylinositol 3-kinase (PI3K) (Trinchieri 2003a).

Further downstream, additional intracellular adaptor molecules are activated, e.g. linker for activation of T cells (LAT), SLP 76, phospholipase Cγ (PLCγ1), PI3K, and Vav family members of guanine nucleotide exchange factors. Examples of receptors interacting with ITAM-containing molecules are CD16, NKp46, and NKp30, as well as the activating KIRs and Ly49Rs (Yokoyama 1999; Moretta et al. 2001; Colucci et al. 2003).

Table 6.4 summarizes the pathways known so far, including examples of interacting receptors, adaptor molecules, and some information on downstream signaling. The multiple pathways may just represent redundancy as a result of evolutionary tinkering, but it is also possible that they are needed to preserve hierarchies of interactions and specific consequences of certain interactions. As a result of these multiple, partly parallel pathways, specific defects caused by gene deletion or pharmacological intervention may in many cases have few if any consequences for overall NK function, whereas T- and B-cell function and even development may be severely affected. The highly NK-sensitive target cell YAC-1 is, for example, killed efficiently by mice with defects in Syk, ZAP70, or both (Colucci et al. 2002). One may speculate that this and other 'prototype' NK targets were once chosen initially as highly reliable for NK assays, just because they express multiple activating ligands, although that was of course not known at the time. Some NK functions appear to rely critically on one pathway, e.g. Ly49H–KARAP/DAP-12, relevant for mouse CMV infection (Yokoyama and Plougastel 2003). Cytokines and adhesion molecules can also trigger or modulate NK function; this is regulated by pathways common to many white blood cells.

As more is learned about activating and inhibiting receptors, tools must be developed to dissect the complexity created by multiple inputs. Can all pathways interact and, if so, are the signals simply additive or subtractive? Are some activating receptors specialized in the sense that they are less (or not at all) influenced by inhibitory receptors, or activate only some effector function? This analysis will require imaging techniques to assess intracellular clustering of receptors and signaling molecules, as well as mathematical models for prediction and interpretation of the final outcome in effector function in response to different inputs. A few studies on inhibitory and activating immune synapses between NK cells and target cells have been published (Davis 2002). Although this field is just starting, it is clear that inhibitory receptors and their MHC class I ligands cluster in the center of the synapse in many situations.

Expression of NK receptors on T cells

Many of the NK receptors discussed above can also be expressed by subpopulations of T cells under certain conditions (Mingari et al. 2000; McMahon and Raulet 2001; Young and Uhrberg 2002; Trinchieri 2003a). One may indeed question the term NK receptors, which is usually based on the notion that the given receptor was first identified on NK cells. A detailed discussion is beyond the scope of this chapter, but an overview is integrated into Table 6.2. Suffice it to say that the function of these receptors is not clear; it has been proposed that these receptors can be used to fine-tune the action of T cells with respect to effector function, proliferation, survival, or homeostasis. A common theme is that they appear to act exclusively as co-receptors for activation or inhibition; they can thus act only by superimposing signals on those triggered via TCR recognition.

Polymorphism and complexity: implications for receptor repertoires, tolerance, and disease associations

As evident from the discussion of each NK receptor type, there are several levels of polymorphisms and complexity in this system. There are multiple genes encoding activating and inhibiting receptors within one individual. Some of these genes are present in all individuals and are conserved; some are present in all individuals, but with different alleles; some are expressed only in some individuals (Vilches and Parham 2002; Parham and McQueen 2003). Furthermore, within one individual, different NK cells express different combinations of receptors (Raulet et al. 2001; Hsu et al. 2002; Vilches and Parham 2002). Most of the mechanisms behind these patterns, as well as the functional implications, are unknown. In the following, the first section reviews a number of solid observations about NK repertoires. The next two sections deal with interpretations and hypotheses about this complexity, first in relation to tolerance development and then in relation to resistance against disease associations and evolutionary pressures.

DEVELOPMENT OF RECEPTOR REPERTOIRES

Natural killer cells acquire their MHC class I-specific receptors relatively late during ontogeny. The development of the receptor repertoire has been studied mainly in mice (Raulet et al. 2001). Some key observations from such studies are described below, with reference to human studies whenever there are similar or different data available.

The patterns with different combinations of receptors expressed by each NK cells arise from the basic notion that each receptor gene is either on or off in a given cell. This 'variegated' pattern of Ly49Rs and KIRs is determined at the gene expression level in a partly stochastic process. Some transcription factors influencing this process have been identified, but the detailed regulation remains unclear (Held et al. 1999). The receptor genes are usually, but not always, expressed in a monoallelic fashion, indicating that the stochastic mechanisms determining whether a particular gene is on or off apply to different loci as well as to different alleles at one locus. As a result, the proportion of cells in an individual that express a given receptor can vary between 5 and 80 percent. Expression of multiple different receptors on one cell follows the 'product rule'. This means that the probability for simultaneous expression of two different Ly49Rs (as well as the KIRs) can be calculated by multiplying the proportion of cells that express each single receptor (Raulet et al. 2001).

The NK cells in a newborn mouse or human cord blood initially express NKG2A/CD94, but not Ly49Rs or KIRs. The Ly49Rs then appear sequentially in certain patterns, Ly49A usually preceding Ly49C and Ly49G2, but this order is not absolute. Interaction with MHC class I molecules on stromal cells influence this process (Roth et al. 2000), in a manner that is not well understood, but which reduces the number of cells expressing several receptors of the same specificity. After 3–4 weeks, the Ly49R expression has developed to the adult pattern, which means that each NK cell expresses at least one and often several receptors (Raulet et al. 2001).

Concurrently, the proportion of NKG2A-positive cells falls to approximately 50 percent in the mouse, whereas the majority of human NK cells express this receptor throughout life. Once established, the receptor expression of each cell appears stable. Long-term follow-up of human NK clones in vitro shows a similar pattern.

NK CELL REPERTOIRE IN RELATION TO AUTOLOGOUS MHC MOLECULES

Most NK cells have the potential to kill according to the 'missing self' model, i.e. their interactions with most normal cells are ultimately controlled by the inhibitory MHC class I receptors. As the latter, at least the ones in the KIR and Ly49R families, are allospecific, there is a risk for autoreactivity. How can 'tolerance' be ascertained in the system, given the complexity described above? Not only do receptors differ between individuals, and between NK cells within the individual, but in addition, the MHC class I ligands are extremely polymorphic and not genetically linked to the receptor genes. The ability to be triggered by activating ligands expressed by most cells must thus somehow be matched somatically with the expression of inhibitory receptors independently recognizing segregating ligands on autologous cells. How this is achieved has so far remained an enigma.

There are several theoretical possibilities. A simple positive selection model is based on stochastic expression of different receptor combinations in each NK cell, followed by a selection step in which only those receptors recognizing that at least one self MHC class I molecule during development receives a survival signal. Models based on this principle predict that the presence of a given MHC class I gene product should select for increased numbers of NK cells with this specificity. However, there is little or no influence at all of HLA on the KIR repertoire; in the mouse, H-2 has a minor influence on the frequency of NK cells with given Ly49 receptors, but in the opposite direction: the number of cells expressing a given receptor are marginally, but reproducibly, fewer if their ligands are present in the host. MHC class I-deficient mice therefore have somewhat more cells expressing any given Ly49R than normal mice (Raulet et al. 2001).

A second possibility, 'the sequential receptor expression' model, postulates that developing NK cells express and test receptors against the environment in sequential and cumulative order, in a process that is terminated as soon as one receptor detects self-ligands in the environment. This predicts a reduced probability for expression of multiple different receptors, which can recognize the same ligand in each NK cell. There is supporting evidence for this in normal mice as well as in transgenic mice where one receptor is forced on the whole NK cell population. The mechanisms limiting expression of several receptors for the same self-ligand appear to act late in differentiation in an interaction between NK cells and stromal cells. It may represent a way to render NK cells as 'useful' as possible, because limited inhibitory receptor expression specific for any MHC product would lead to more sensitive detection of cells in which this particular product is partly down-regulated (Raulet et al. 2001; Salmon-Divon et al. 2003).

Despite these observations, the complete available data do not fit the simplest form of the sequential receptor expression model, which would predict that all NK cells in MHC class I-deficient mice or humans should express all inhibitory receptors (and this should still not be sufficient for tolerance). However, these individuals have normal numbers of NK cells, which display the usual variegated expression pattern of Ly49Rs and KIRs, and which are tolerant to autologous cells (Raulet et al. 2001). They retain other cytotoxic NK functions against certain tumor cells and antibody-coated target cells in antibody-dependent cell-mediated cytotoxicity (ADCC) assays.

It must thus be questioned whether tolerance is based solely on inhibitory, MHC class I-recognizing receptors. In the human, complete analysis of in vitro cultured NK clones from a few individuals indicate that each NK cell expresses at least one self-receptor (Valiante et al. 1997). To be conclusive as to whether inhibitory receptors can account for tolerance, corresponding studies must be done on freshly derived cells. These have so far been performed only in mice, and always reveal a fraction of cells where no known self-receptor is expressed (Raulet et al. 2001). However, it can be argued that this observation is also inconclusive until there is a complete panel of receptors identified (and the corresponding reagents).

The currently most accepted, modified model is based on the idea that the sequential receptor expression of inhibitory receptors is only one of several contributing to tolerance, and that it acts only during a limited time window in differentiation. It would therefore not allow expression of all receptors in one NK cell. Additional mechanisms to consider in conjunction with this model, or independently, are those that do not rely on inhibitory MHC class I-specific receptors. Some NK cells could thus acquire tolerance by expression of another type of inhibitory receptor(s), or by down-regulating the receptors or critical links in signal transduction pathways that are responsible for the initial activation in missing self-recognition (Held et al. 2003).

It should be possible to identify these mechanisms by comparative transcriptomic or proteomic profiles on NK cells from mice that differ only in one MHC class I allele (and, hence, NK cell tolerance to cells that lack this allele). The most dramatic influence of MHC type on NK receptors observed so far is a down-regulation of Ly49R (by 30–90 percent) when their high-affinity ligands are present in the host (Olsson et al. 1995; Raulet et al. 2001). This appears to result partly from a direct, post-translational response to interaction with the ligand, most probably leading to internalization or shedding of the receptor. It has not been observed with the KIR in humans. Although this down-regulation leads to enhanced sensitivity to detect impaired expression of the corresponding allele, potentially making the NK cell more 'useful', the functional significance of this phenomenon is unclear. Finally, there is evidence that the receptor levels of NK cells are influenced by the ligand expression of the NK cell itself (Kase et al. 1998; Doucey et al. 2004). This has led to speculations that Ly49Rs can interact with their ligands in '*cis*', and that this may be involved in regulation or tolerance (Held et al. 2003).

Whether tolerance is based on alteration of activating or inhibitory pathways, one must finally consider whether it is irreversible, or whether mature NK cells can alter their specificity once they are mature. In mice with mosaic MHC class I expression where a part of the cells lacked one self-allele out of three expressed by the remaining cells, NK cells were nonreactive to both MHC class I phenotypes but retained the ability to kill cells lacking all MHC class I alleles (Johansson et al. 1997). When NK cells of the two MHC phenotypes were separated and cultured in IL-2 in vitro, the ones with complete expression of three alleles acquired the ability to kill the cells expressing only two alleles. Although this demonstrates that some tolerant cells are preserved and not deleted, it remains to be investigated whether tolerance is actually reversible in vivo.

In summary, it seems plausible that NK cells acquire tolerance by a combination of mechanisms influencing activating as well as inhibiting mechanisms. This can be manifested at the level of gene expression, but post-translational mechanisms, where the cellular distribution and even membrane topology for receptor expression patterns influence the specificity, are not excluded. Further research is required to understand the general principles behind the development of receptor repertoires and tolerance in the NK system.

NK RECEPTOR GENES: EVOLUTIONARY ASPECTS AND IMPLICATIONS FOR DISEASE ASSOCIATIONS

Figure 6.4 provides a schematic overview of the two major families. The activating and the inhibiting receptors in the NKG2 family have been largely conserved. The mouse has four genes in the Nkrp1 family, the human only one (Yokoyama and Plougastel 2003). There are several other more or less related genes encoded in the NKC, such as CD69, an early activation marker for lymphocytes, including NK cells. The NK cells in these two species, as well as in the rat, are thus similar in many respects. However, there is a dramatic difference in the expansion of the Ly49 family in the mouse and rat. The Ly49L gene in humans does not encode a functional product, and this gene family therefore plays no role in humans.

The human genome instead contains the gene families in the LRC on chromosome 19 (Figure 6.4) (Trowsdale et al. 2001). For both KIR and Ly49R families, there is considerable polymorphism and evidence that they undergo rapid evolution – the KIRs may even be evolving at a higher pace than human MHC genes (Kane et al. 2001; Hsu et al. 2002; Vilches and Parham 2002). It is believed that infectious agents drive this evolution, although the mechanisms are not well understood. One key to the problem may lie in the function of the MHC class I-specific activating receptors in each family, which, at least in humans, are the genes that show the highest diversity. It has been proposed that their specificity goes beyond MHC class I molecules, and that they may recognize pathogen-encoded ligands, either in association with MHC molecules or by themselves. The latter is certainly the case for the activating Ly49H receptor in the mouse, as discussed in the section on CMV.

The considerable polymorphism and dynamic evolution of the KIR genes in the human population opens the possibility for studies of disease associations. Individuals differ in the number of loci as well as the alleles carried by these loci. Certain typical 'haplotypes' (combinations of loci and their respective alleles) are now being defined, and observed to be present in different frequencies in different ethnic groups (Hsu et al. 2002; Parham and McQueen 2003). Do different genes or haplotypes affect the incidence or course of infectious, malignant, or autoimmune diseases and is there an impact on the outcome of transplantation? Some associations, open for different mechanistic interpretations, have been reported (Table 6.5) and more are probably waiting in the wings in this intensive research field.

NK CELLS IN INFECTIONS

Virus infections

CLINICAL OBSERVATIONS

The picture emerging from the study of natural infections and their correlation with impaired NK activity in patients suggests that NK cells may be particularly important for the defense against viruses in the herpes family (Biron et al. 1989; Cerwenka and Lanier 2001; Orange et al. 2002). These have in common that they remain latent with no or little viral replication after the primary infection; they may be reactivated and cause opportunistic infections under conditions where the immune system is compromised, e.g. in malignant or infectious diseases and transplantation. This group includes, among others, varicella-zoster virus (VZV), herpes simplex type 1 virus (HSV-1), Epstein–Barr virus (EBV), and HCMV. The evidence is often anecdotal and sometimes difficult to interpret, because impaired

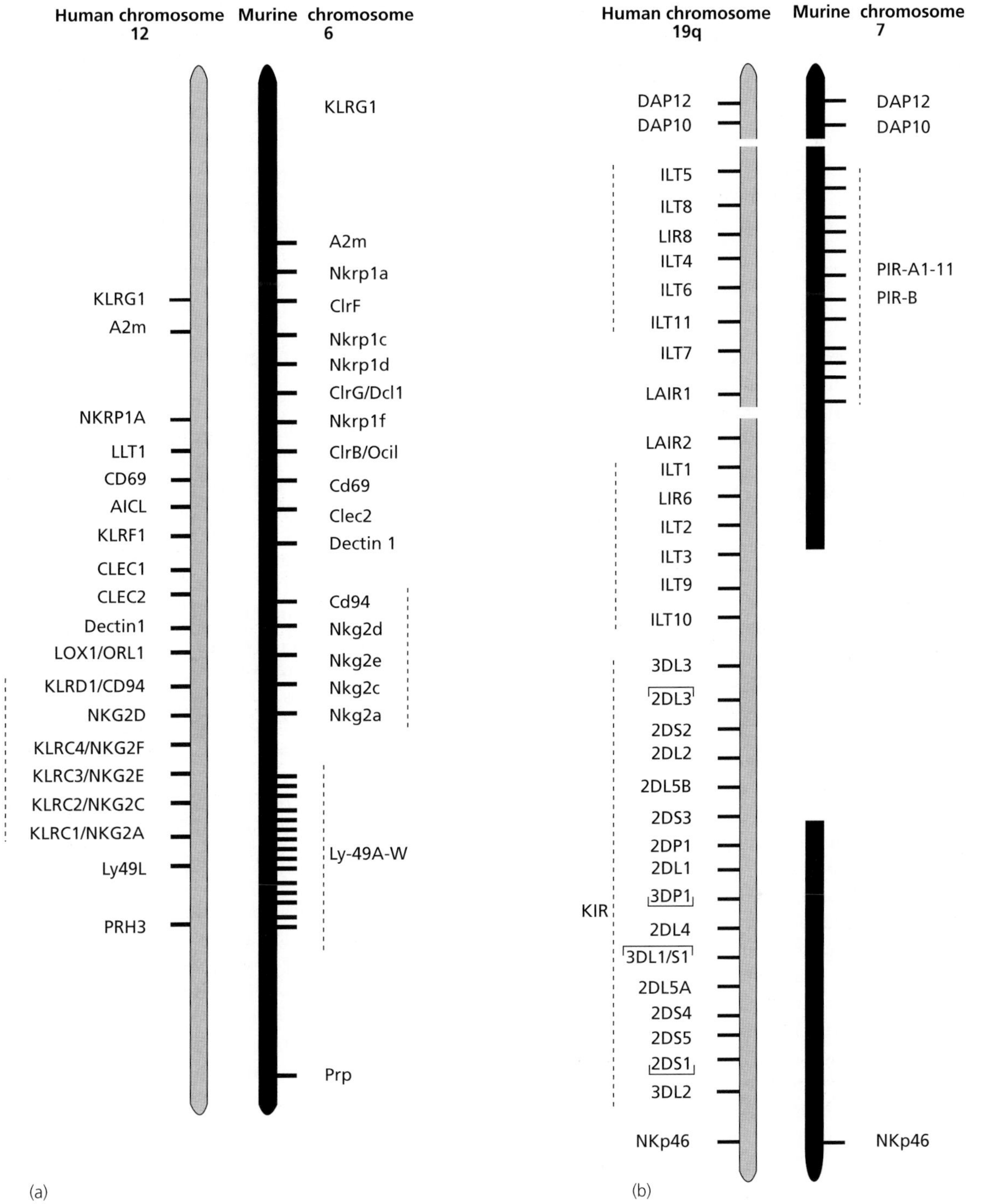

Figure 6.4 **(a)** *The natural killer (NK) gene complex (NKC) and* **(b)** *the leukocyte receptor cluster (LRC). The NKC is present on human chromosome 12p13.1 and mouse distal chromosome 6 whereas the LRC is on human chromosome 19q13 and mouse chromosome 7 (Trowsdale et al. 2001; Hsu et al. 2002; Yokoyama and Plougastel 2003). Dashed vertical lines denote the NKG2/CD94-, the Ly49-, the LIR/ILT-, the PIR-, and the KIR-gene families. The brackets comprise the variable KIR gene regions, opposed to the three conserved framework genes* 3DL3, 3DL2, *and* 2DL4 *(Vilches and Parham 2002). Positions of genes are not drawn to scale.*

NK cell function may be the nonspecific consequence of infectious disease rather than its specific cause. Furthermore, NK deficiency is usually relative rather than absolute, and often associated with other immune defects. A typical example is the X-linked lymphoproliferative syndrome (Moretta et al. 2001), resulting from defective control of EBV, which is associated with perturbed function of NK cells as well as of T cells as a result of a defect in the signaling lymphocyte activation molecule-associated protein (SAP), involved in regulation of the signaling lymphocyte activation molecule (SLAM) pathway.

Table 6.5 *Killer cell immunoglobulin receptor (KIR) polymorphisms and disease associations*

KIR	Disease association
KIR3DS1	HLA-Bw-80Ile^{+} HIV-1-infected individuals – delayed progression to AIDS In case of HLA-Bw-80Ile absence KIR3DS1 is associated with more rapid progression (Martin et al. 2002a)
KIR2DS2	Development of rheumatoid vasculitis associated with 2DS2^{+} CD4^{+} CD28^{null} T cells (Namekawa et al. 2000)
KIR2DS1, KIR2DS2	Associated with psoriatic arthritis, but only when the HLA ligands for their homologous inhibitory receptors were absent (Martin et al. 2002b)
KIR2DS2	Susceptibility to develop type 1 diabetes when present with group 1 HLA-C ligands (van der Silk et al. 2003)

There is an often cited example of an NK-deficient patient that is particularly informative (Biron et al. 1989). A 13-year-old girl presented with an unusually severe chickenpox (varicella) infection. She was found to have a complete and selective lack of NK cells. Other cells of the innate immune system were normal, and so were T- and B-cell responses, which eventually resolved the infection. Within 5 years, she developed first a severe HCMV infection and then a disseminated HSV-1 infection. Siblings and relatives showed normal NK cell development and function, and the mechanism behind this immune defect remains a mystery. Such total and selective NK cell deficiency is apparently extremely rare, and one may ask why. It may be that it is usually lethal in the intrauterine or early postnatal period. Another possibility is simply that it requires a combination of genetic defects for which the probability is extremely low. For future research it may be important to identify patients with more discrete effects, e.g. patients who retain a normal or close to normal NK cell number that, however, lacks one or more receptor or effector functions.

Patients with human immunodeficiency (HIV) infection and/or acquired immune deficiency syndrome (AIDS) represent one of the most well-studied patient categories in clinical immunology laboratories. A consistent pattern in these patients is that NK cell activity is reduced (Scott-Algara and Paul 2002). This can occur relatively early in infection, and often without diminished NK cell numbers in the blood. The functional defect appears more prominent for the direct NK cytotoxicity than the ADCC activity mediated through a FcγRIII receptor. There may be an association with reduced expression levels of the activating receptors NKp30 and NKp46 (De Maria et al. 2003; Mavilio et al. 2003). NK cells may contribute to various defense mechanisms, including production of chemokines blocking co-receptors for viral infection; NK cells may also be important for control of human herpesvirus 8 (HHV-8) and Kaposi's sarcoma (Cerwenka and Lanier 2001). The Nef gene product of the virus down-regulates HLA-A and -B expression, but does not affect HLA-C and -E molecules, ligands for the inhibitory NK receptors KIR2D and NKG2A (Cohen et al. 1999; Cerwenka and Lanier 2001; Mavilio et al. 2003).

EXPERIMENTAL STUDIES

The role of NK cells has been studied in a variety of animal models, mainly in mice, and usually by depleting the NK cells before injection of a relatively high dose of pathogenic virus. Normal mice respond with increased NK cell activity, locally and systemically, to most if not all viruses 2–4 days after infection (Tay et al. 1998; Biron et al. 1999). Early cytokines, particularly type I interferons and IL-12, are important factors for this rapid augmentation of NK activity. In some virus infections, such as MCMV, Pichinde virus, HSV-1, influenza virus, Coxsackie virus, vaccinia virus, ectromelia virus, encephalomyocarditis virus, and Theiler's virus, the early NK defense is crucial. NK cell-depleted mice show dramatically increased viral replication locally or systemically (Biron et al. 1999). Depending on the infection dose and the virus, the NK cell-depleted mice may die within one week, whereas normal mice limit the replication and survive until the adaptive T- and B-cell response reaches effective activity and clears the infection. As discussed in more detail in relation to MCMV, NK cells contribute to early defense by direct killing of infected cells, as well as by secretion of chemokines and cytokines, particularly IFN-γ (Biron et al. 1999).

With other viruses, NK cell depletion has no effect on the course of the infection, even though there may be strong initial augmentation of NK cell activity. A typical example in this category is lymphocytic choriomeningitis virus (LCMV), which otherwise is extremely sensitive to immune mechanisms and cytotoxic T cells (Tay et al. 1998; Biron et al. 1999). The reasons why certain viruses are 'NK insensitive' are not known. It may relate to whether NK cells can specifically target the virus-infected cells. Antiviral NK cell-mediated defense through cytotoxicity implies that NK cells should be able to recognize the infected cells and specifically eliminate them. In many cases, virus-infected human or murine cells are more NK susceptible than non-infected controls, but this is not a general rule. For certain viruses, infected cells may even become more resistant. Viruses may affect NK sensitivity by a variety of molecular mechanisms, including reduced MHC class I expression, leading to killing by recognition of 'missing self'. There is good evidence for this in the case of HSV-1- and vaccinia virus-infected cells (Orange et al. 2002). The pattern with HCMV and MCMV, known to possess multiple mechanisms for interference with the MHC class I pathway, is more complex, as discussed in detail below.

NK CELLS IN CMV INFECTION: MOLECULAR ASPECTS OF RECOGNITION, EFFECTOR FUNCTION, AND ESCAPE

MCMV and HCMV are the most well-studied infections with respect to NK cells, and several interesting molecular mechanisms have been revealed. These closely related viruses are therefore discussed in more detail, as an example of the complex pattern that may emerge in co-evolution of host and virus. HCMV and MCMV establish latent infections, and their large DNA-based genomes encode many proteins that are not required for replication in host cells in vitro, but act instead to modulate and interfere with host immune responses, including NK cells.

Mice with NK cell deficiency caused by low age, experimental depletion, or gene defects are highly sensitive to experimental infection with MCMV (Tay et al. 1998; Lee et al. 2002). Adoptive transfer of NK cells can restore resistance. NK cells appear to mediate their effect by at least two mechanisms: perforin-dependent cytotoxicity, which is the more important mechanism in the spleen, and IFN-γ secretion, which is crucial to limit viral replication in the liver (Biron et al. 1999; Lee et al. 2002). The cytotoxic response depends on type I interferons acting through the STAT-1 signaling pathway in NK cells, whereas the cytokine response depends on IL-12 produced by macrophages and acting through STAT-4 (Biron et al. 2002). IFN-γ can exert its effect directly on hepatocytes to limit viral replication, but may also act by stimulating macrophages for inducible nitric oxide synthase. There is thus an important crosstalk between NK cells and macrophages in the liver, emphasized also by a crucial role of the macrophage-secreted chemokine macrophage inflammatory protein 1-α (MIP-1α) for NK cell migration into the liver during infection (Lee et al. 2002).

How can NK cells target CMV-infected cells? Given that both HCMV and MCMV possess several different genes for interference with the MHC class I pathway, NK cells are important innate effector cells against infection in both species, and the particularly strong CMV resistance in the mouse strain C57Black has for a long time been shown to map to a locus within or close to the Ly49 family (CMV1), it has been speculated whether 'missing self' recognition plays an important role (Lee et al. 2002). However, C57Black mice deficient for MHC class I molecules, the NK cells of which cannot perform missing self-recognition, show a strong NK-mediated resistance to the infections. Research in recent years has instead identified the activating Ly49H receptor as the product of the CMVR1 locus (Yokoyama and Scalzo 2002). Resistance is impaired in mice treated with Ly49H antibodies, and in mice deficient in the adaptor molecule crucial for Ly49H signaling, KARAP/DAP12 (Sjolin et al. 2002; Yokoyama and Plougastel 2003). The Ly49 receptor acts by recognizing the virus-encoded, GPI membrane-attached molecule m157 on infected cells (Arase et al. 2002; Smith et al. 2002). This viral gene, which shows distant homology to MHC class I genes, is not required for virus replication in vitro, and one may wonder why and how the virus has evolved it, because it acts to limit spread of the virus. An attractive model proposes that m157 evolved as a ligand to target the inhibitory MHC class I-recognizing receptor Ly49I (Yokoyama and Scalzo 2002), thereby allowing the virus to escape missing self-recognition in spite of its interference with host cell MHC class I molecules. The Ly49H receptor would represent the evolutionary countermove of the host, resulting in the selection of a receptor gene where recombination and other mechanisms would have maintained recognition of m157, but not of host MHC class I molecules, and switched the intramembrane/cytoplasmic domains to convey activating rather than inhibiting signals.

This scenario may be difficult if not impossible to test, but it has profound implications for our understanding of infections as an evolutionary pressure for the NK cell system. MCMV carries at least half a dozen additional genes encoding distant MHC class I homologs (Yokoyama and Scalzo 2002), the function of which remain to be determined. Similarly, mice as well as humans have a number of activating MHC class I receptors in the Ly49 and KIR families with poorly understood function (see Table 6.2). It may be that the inhibitory MHC class I-specific receptors provide a platform for development of viral escape strategies that can easily be turned into counter-weapons in the next host, or in the next evolutionary step. The intensive research on activating KIRs, and their possible association with diseases (Martin et al. 2002a, b; Namekawa et al. 2000; van der Slik et al. 2003) (Table 6.5), may give important clues in this research field.

One may still ask why CMV interference with MHC class I recognition is not sufficient to induce NK cell susceptibility. This is probably a result of a variety of parallel viral mechanisms that interfere with NK cell recognition and triggering (Figure 6.5). MCMV and HCMV both possess genes, *UL16* and *m152* respectively, the products of which bind to and prevent cell surface expression of ligands for the activating NKG2D receptor, such as MIC, ULBP1 and -2 in humans, and Rae-1 and H-60 in mice (Cerwenka and Lanier 2001; Krmpotic et al. 2002; Orange et al. 2002; Dunn et al. 2003; Lodoen et al. 2003; Rolle et al. 2003). Even if the NKG2D receptor is not believed to be the primary activating receptor for 'missing self' surveillance of normal cells, there is evidence that the activating ligands of this

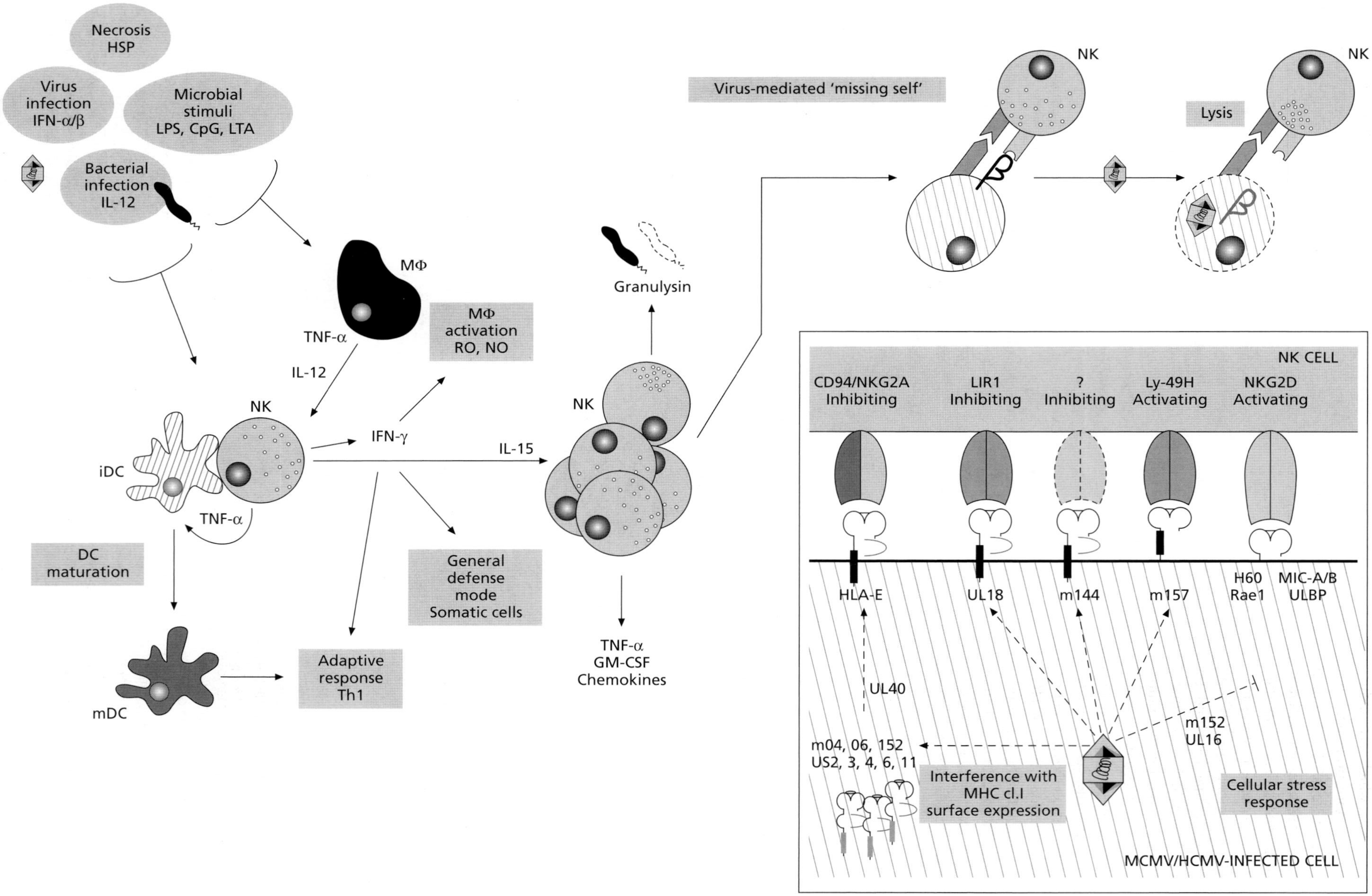

Necrosis
HSP
Virus
infection
IFN-α/β
Microbial
stimuli
LPS, CpG, LTA
Bacterial
infection
IL-12
MΦ
TNF-α
IL-12
MΦ
activation
RO, NO
NK
iDC
TNF-α
IFN-γ
IL-15
DC
maturation
mDC
Adaptive
response
Th1
General
defense
mode
Somatic cells
NK
Granulysin
TNF-α
GM-CSF
Chemokines
Virus-mediated 'missing self'
NK
NK
Lysis
NK CELL
CD94/NKG2A
Inhibiting
LIR1
Inhibiting
?
Inhibiting
Ly-49H
Activating
NKG2D
Activating
HLA-E
UL18
m144
m157
H60
Rae1
MIC-A/B
ULBP
UL40
m152
UL16
m04, 06, 152
US2, 3, 4, 6, 11
Interference with
MHC cl.I
surface expression
Cellular stress
response
MCMV/HCMV-INFECTED CELL

receptor, which are induced during HCMV infection, play a more prominent role for NK cell recognition of infected cells. This implies that the virus in parallel down-regulates the activating ligands that are important in normal cells, but, as these are not completely known, this hypothesis remains to be tested.

Furthermore, the HCMV gene *UL40* provides a signal sequence that can bind to and promote expression of HLA-E, which may counteract the reduced expression of this ligand for the inhibitory NKG2A receptor caused by HCMV products that interfere with TAP function (Braud et al. 2002; Orange et al. 2002). HCMV also contains the gene *UL18*, which binds to the LIR-1 receptor on NK, B and dendritic cells with 1000-fold higher affinity than MHC class I molecules (Chapman et al. 1999). The UL18 protein has been proposed to act as a decoy ligand that inhibits NK cells (Reyburn et al. 1997), but this is controversial and the pathophysiological role of this viral product is not clear (Orange et al. 2002).

The overall picture emerging in the case of CMV is that the NK cell defense is important, because the virus has evolved different mechanisms to avoid it. The recognition strategy of NK cells with multiple activating and inhibitory receptors has probably emerged in dynamic co-evolution with CMV and other infectious agents, and it continues to provide a complex platform for ongoing evolution where activating and inhibitory receptors and their ligands interact.

Bacterial infections

Several effector functions of NK cells contribute to antibacterial responses. Granulysin, a membrane-perturbing peptide component of human (but not mouse) NK cell granules, is directly active against gram-positive and gram-negative bacteria, including *Mycobacterium tuberculosis* (Krensky 2000). NK cells can also lyse target cells infected with bacteria, e.g. *Shigella*, *Listeria*, *Salmonella*, *Legionella*, and *Mycobacterium* spp. (Bancroft 1993; Yokoyama 1999). Finally, by secretion of IFN-γ, they can activate macrophages and induce more efficient intracellular and extracellular elimination of bacteria, e.g. through reactive oxygen metabolites and reactive nitrogen intermediates. As IFN-γ can also deviate the ensuing adaptive response toward a Th1 type, NK cells cannot contribute only to early innate resistance; they also provide a link to adaptive responses against bacteria. In this context, one may also note that NK cells interact efficiently with dendritic cells (DC) (Moretta 2002; Zitvogel 2002). Upon infection with *M. tuberculosis*, DCs develop the capacity to activate NK cells, but they also become resistant to NK cell attack. The activated NK cells can, however, kill uninfected, immature DCs. This process, which involves altered expression levels of DC ligands for the NKp30-activating receptor and NKG2A-inhibiting receptor, may be important for optimal antigen presentation to T cells.

Although depletion of NK cells in experimental infection in mice led to enhanced growth of *Mycobacterium avium* (Florido et al. 2003), there is so far no model where NK cells have an absolutely critical role in immunocompetent animals. This is presumably because numerous partly overlapping mechanisms cooperate in antibacterial resistance. In several infections, the contribution of NK cells is most clearly recognized in the absence of one or more other immune components. A well-studied example is resistance to *Listeria monocytogenes* in SCID mice (Bancroft 1993). NK cells are critical for the early limitation of bacterial spread. Under the influence of IL-12 and other cytokines produced by infected macrophages, NK cells are induced to secrete IFN-γ, which in turn activates the macrophages. Their induced antibacterial pathways can limit the spread of bacteria, but T cells are required ultimately to resolve the infection. Similar schemes can be drawn for several other intracellular bacteria, e.g. *M. tuberculosis*.

It is also uncertain whether there is a particularly prominent role for NK cells in any disease in the clinical panorama. Bacterial infections, particularly in the respiratory tract, have been reported in certain patients with defects of dysregulation of NK cells, but it cannot be excluded that these reflect secondary infections

Figure 6.5 *A consensus model for the role of natural killer (NK) cells in infections. During infection NK cells can be activated either directly by recognition of microbial components or indirectly by cytokines (interferon IFN-αβ, interleukin IL-12) produced from infected cells or activated macrophages (Mϕ) (Biron et al. 1999; Trinchieri 2003b). The interaction with immature dendritic cells (iDC) encountering antigens or pathogens leads to reciprocal activation, driving, on the one hand, maturation of DCs, which is crucial for induction of the adaptive immune response, and, on the other, NK cell activation (Moretta 2002). This is accompanied by strong NK cell-derived IFN-γ production, most probably IL-15-driven NK cell proliferation and ordered NK cell recruitment to the site of infection, which is orchestrated by chemokines. Although IFN-γ is crucial for induction of a variety of defense programs exerted by macrophages and also somatic cells, NK cells contribute to pathogen destruction by cytotoxic mechanisms. Missing or altered self as a consequence of pathogen invasion can be recognized by NK cells and induces killing of the infected cell. The elaborate interplay between NK cells and murine or human cytomegalovirus (MCMV and HCMV) is illustrated (Cerwenka and Lanier 2001; Braud et al. 2002; Orange et al. 2002). The virus interferes with MHCI surface expression (m04, -06, -152; US2, -3, -4, -6, -11), expresses MHCI-like surrogates (m144, m157, UL18), and interferes with surface expression (m152, UL16) of cellular 'stress'-indicative molecules (H60, Rae-1, MIC-A/B, ULBP). The viral MHCI-like m144 protein binds to an unknown inhibitory receptor, whereas the viral m157 protein is recognized by the activating Ly49H receptor, which significantly contributes to resistance against MCMV in certain mouse strains (Arase et al. 2002; Smith et al. 2002). Cells expressing 'stress'-indicative molecules (altered SELF) are recognized via the activating receptor NKG2D (Raulet 2003).*

complicating an initial viral disease (Orange et al. 2002). The lack of evidence for an essential role of NK cells or any other innate component in an infection does not mean that these are unimportant. There are large individual variations in the severity of initial disease developing before the sterilizing adaptive responses step in. Future research in bacterial diseases will address this if such patterns can be correlated to selective defects of, for example, NK receptor pathways.

Upon bacterial infection, NK cells may not only become activated indirectly via cytokines secreted by macrophages and DCs. Cognate interactions involving the sensing of reduced MHC class I expression of infected macrophages may occur with *Salmonella*, *Yersinia*, and *Chlamydia* spp. (Kirveskari et al. 1999). Through the Toll-like receptor 9, NK cells can be directly activated by unmethylated CpG sequences in bacterial DNA (Ashkar and Rosenthal 2002). There is also evidence that human NK cells can use the activating NKp46 receptor to directly recognize and kill *M. tuberculosis*-infected monocytes, without concurrent down-regulation of MHC class I molecules (Vankayalapati et al. 2002). The future research on NK cells may well identify several direct molecular recognition pathways for bacteria or bacteria-infected cells.

PARASITE INFECTIONS

The parasites represent a very heterogeneous group of organisms. Nevertheless, common patterns emerge with respect to the role of NK cells in infections, some resembling those seen with NK responses to intracellular bacteria (Figure 6.5). Infected human or murine hosts often show an early augmentation of NK cell activity, e.g. in toxoplasma, leishmania, and trypanosoma infection (Scott and Trinchieri 1995). This activation is partly indirect via cytokines such as IL-12 and TNF-α secreted by infected macrophages. In addition, there is evidence for direct recognition of parasites, their products or infected cells. Human NK cells can be stimulated by the leishmania lipophosphoglycan via Toll-like receptor 2 (Becker et al. 2003), and they can also recognize *Plasmodium falciparum*-infected erythrocytes by a so far unknown receptor (Artavanis-Tsakonas and Riley 2002). Apart from activation, there may also be local recruitment of NK cells; these represent the second wave of infiltrating cells (after granulocytes) at the site of leishmania infection in mice.

As a consequence of activation, NK cells can secrete cytokines to stimulate macrophage-mediated elimination of intracellular and extracellular parasites. Leishmania antigens can also induce a proliferative response of NK cells in vitro. Furthermore, activated NK cells can destroy infected host cells as well as extracellular parasites, e.g. tachyzoites of *Toxoplasma gondii* and trypomastigotes in Chagas' disease. As with many intracellular bacteria, IFN-γ appears to be a key cytokine (Cardillo et al. 1996), even if clear evidence for the in vivo role of NK cells may require models where other components are defective. Infection of mice with *T. gondii* may serve as an example. In β_2-microglobulin-deficient mice, with defective T-cell responses, there is a strong proliferative response of NK cells (Denkers et al. 1993). These eventually become the dominating cell population in the spleen and secrete high levels of IFN-γ, acting to limit the infection. IL-15 may play a role for this expansion of the NK cell population. In immunocompetent mice, NK cells contribute to the IFN-γ response, as do $CD8^+$ T cells, which are required to clear the infection.

As with other microorganisms, one focus of future research will be the identification of parasite structures that can be directly recognized by activating (or inhibiting) receptors of NK cells. Parasites represent a particular challenge in such studies, given their complex life cycles, with extracellular and intracellular stages, and in several cases also mechanisms for antigenic variation.

NK CELLS IN CANCER

Natural killer cells were discovered by virtue of their capacity to kill cancer cells. Furthermore, it was the correlation between strong NK activity and resistance to tumor transplants in mice that stimulated further interest in the field, at the early stage when this cytotoxic activity was frequently questioned as an in vitro artifact. There is now overwhelming evidence from animal models that NK cells can reject transplantable tumors of various histological types (Smyth et al. 2002). As expected from an innate nonadaptive mechanism, NK cell effects operate early, within hours to days of tumor inoculation, and they can be overruled by increasing the dose of transplanted tumor cells (Riccardi et al. 1979; Kärre et al. 1986; Smyth et al. 2002).

In some situations, the NK resistance is particularly efficient. These include host tumor combinations allowing 'missing self' recognition of the tumor, e.g. a F1 hybrid or transgenic host expressing MHC class I molecules that are not present in the tumor (Kiessling et al. 1975c) (discussed further below), or grafts of tumor cells with impaired MHC class I expression (Kärre et al. 1986; Smyth et al. 2002). However, efficient rejection can take place with, as well as without, alterations of the MHC phenotype of the tumor, e.g. the murine lymphoma RMA is not efficiently rejected by NK cells in the autologous C57Black strain. Strong rejection is, however, seen with sublines of the lymphoma such as RMA-S, selected for reduced MHC class I expression, as well as with sublines with normal MHC class I expression, but transfected with Rae-1, the ligand for the activating NKG2D receptor (Kärre et al. 1986; Raulet 2003). Other tumor lines are rejected because they express Rae-1 constitutively. Furthermore, NK-mediated resistance is most efficient in models assessing hematogenous metastasis, usually to the lungs (Hanna 1982; Smyth et al. 2002). This correlates with the rapid NK cell-mediated elimination that can be observed in the lungs in short-term in vivo assays with isotope- or fluorescence-labeled tumor cells. Rapid, perforin-dependent cytotoxicity is thus a major, but not the only, mechanism in tumor cell rejection by NK cells. In its absence, Fas ligand-dependent killing can be observed, even though it is slower and appears less efficient in terms of the number of tumor cells that can be cleared (Screpanti et al. 2001; Wallin et al. 2003). It has also been proposed that NK cells can interact in concert with adaptive response mechanisms in tumor immunity. One obvious example is ADCC. NK cells can exert antitumor effects via this mechanism, at least in situations where monoclonal antibodies are used for treatment (Ravetch and Bolland 2001; Smyth et al. 2002). Another possibility is that early NK cell killing of tumor cells can promote antigen uptake and presentation by DCs, which will lead to more efficient T-cell responses.

There is limited information on the capacity of NK cells to eliminate primary tumor cells in the autochthonous host, as a result of the lack of good experimental models. Transgenic mice developing certain types of tumors at high frequency may become a useful tool here. It is clear that normal NK cell-defective mice to not develop spontaneous tumors in dramatic excess, arguing against classic immunosurveillance as the major function of NK cells. This does not exclude that they may be exploited for cancer therapy. Clinical studies may provide more answers in this context. The NK activity of cancer patients is often weakened. This observation is, however, difficult to interpret – it may simply reflect a consequence of advanced disease.

Adoptive transfer of NK cells was an inherent part of clinical trials with LAK cells performed during the 1980s. These were based on activation and expansion of lymphocytes from cancer patients in vitro, in medium containing relatively high doses of IL-2 (Rosenberg 1988; Smyth et al. 2002). Reinfusion of the cells led to documented shrinkage of tumor deposits in a minor part of the patients, and anecdotal dramatic responses. The available evidence suggests that NK cells were the dominant effector cells in the heterogeneous LAK cell populations, in the human as well as in the murine models providing the platform for this therapy (Whiteside et al. 1998; Wu and Lanier 2003). The therapy was abandoned as a result of limited efficacy, considerable safety problems with severe side effects often requiring intensive care, and development of novel cytokine modalities. However, these efforts demonstrated that activated, expanded, and reinfused NK cells could exert some antitumoral effects in a clinical setting, an important milestone. This has led to several protocols to activate and/or transfer NK cells for cancer therapy. In today's perspective, it is clear that many protocols are based on quite nonspecific stimulation of the NK system, with little attention being paid to specificity and tumor phenotype. In the future, it is reasonable to expect new modalities based on advances in understanding the molecular aspects of NK recognition, e.g. it has recently been reported that colon cancer cells may not only express the NKG2D ligand MICA, but may also shed this molecule in the circulation, where it can block recognition as well as down-modulate the activating NKG2D receptors (Salih et al. 2002). In future studies it may be more critical to assess that the tumor and NK cells in trials express the correct receptor–ligand pair, and take action to diagnose and remove soluble blocking factors. Another example where (mis)matching for missing self-recognition can be used to obtain antitumor effects is discussed below.

NK CELLS IN TRANSPLANTATION

The first thorough studies of an in vivo phenomenon associated with NK cells, at least with respect to genetics, was initiated more than 10 years before the discovery of the NK cells themselves. In the 1960s, it was recognized that lethally irradiated mice, whose adaptive T- and B-cell responses had been abrogated, could still reject MHC-mismatched bone marrow grafts. The mismatch combinations included not only completely allogeneic grafts (A/A rejecting B/B) but also parental grafts into F1 hybrid hosts (A/B rejecting B/B). The latter combination should not lead to T-cell-mediated rejection according to the classic transplantation laws, and this type of rejection was coined as 'hybrid resistance' (Cudkowicz and Bennett 1971). It was also demonstrated against tumor grafts and, in the rat, against grafts of normal lymphocytes. On the discovery of NK cells, it was soon demonstrated that they are the effector cells behind this peculiar type of rejection (Kiessling et al. 1977; Barao and Murphy 2003).

Natural killer cell-mediated rejection of allogeneic and parental grafts is controlled by the MHC region, but it was initially believed that MHC class I molecules were not involved. One major model proposed a new type of recessive, MHC-linked hemopoietic histocompatibility (Hh) locus (Yu et al. 1992). Today, the phenomena are interpreted within the paradigm of MHC class I receptors on NK cells, and missing self-recognition in particular: a graft of MHC type B/B lacks A alleles expressed by an allogeneic A/A as well as an F1 A/B host. NK cells with an inhibitory receptor for A may therefore not be inhibited by the B/B graft, leading to rejection (Kärre 1985; Kärre et al. 1986; Barao and Murphy 2003). Strong evidence for this has been provided by studies of mice made transgenic for a new MHC class I allele (the NK cells of which reject bone marrow from wild-type cells) and mice with deficient MHC class I expression (the bone marrow of which is rejected by NK cells from wild-type mice) (Ohlen et al. 1989; Bix et al. 1991). However, missing self-recognition does not dominate in all combinations; NK cells can also use activating MHC class I-recognizing receptors to recognize an allogeneic graft, and this is the dominant mechanism in certain combinations (Nakamura et al. 1999; Smyth et al. 2002). The role of NK cells in rejection of organ grafts, where rejection is observed only in allogeneic, and not F1 anti-parental, combinations is less clear. They can infiltrate transplanted kidneys and hearts, and it has been proposed that they may attack allogeneic cells; alternatively they may regulate the T-cell responses that are initiated.

It is not clear whether recipient NK cells can affect the outcome of hematopoietic transplantation in the human. However, the role of NK cells in the grafted marrow or stem cells is now the focus of intensive studies. This started with a retrospective analysis of the outcome of so-called haploidentical transplantations between siblings or between parents and children, where one MHC haplotype is shared and the other not (A/B to B/C). One set of HLA-B- and -C-encoded ligands for inhibiting KIRs are thus matched, but the remaining ones may result in a combination where the graft carries an inhibitory KIR ligand that is absent from the host. The murine studies predict that this should lead to NK recognition in the graft-versus-host direction. A subgroup of transplantations representing this combination did indeed show fewer relapses of myeloid leukemia (compared with groups with complete match or KIR ligands present in the recipients but absent from the donor) (Farag et al. 2002; Ruggeri et al. 2002). Parallel studies of human NK cells in vitro or transferred to mice with human leukemia supported the role of an NK-mediated graft-versus-leukemia effect. Surprisingly, there was a reduced incidence of graft-versus-host disease in the same combinations. Experimental studies indicate that this may have been caused by efficient NK cell removal of host DCs, which initiate graft-versus-host reactivity. Follow-up studies, where the same type of mismatches occur in transplantations between unrelated individuals, have given divergent results, possibly as a result of the different recipient conditioning and graft T-cell depletion protocols involved (Davies et al. 2002; Giebel et al. 2003). The role of allogeneic, and particularly KIR-ligand-mismatched, NK cells will undoubtedly be addressed in many different clinical settings in the future, including the use of allogeneic donor lymphocyte infusions and minitransplantations for the treatment of solid tumors (Farag et al. 2002).

NK CELLS IN PREGNANCY

In immunological terms, the fetus can be regarded as an allograft. One of its HLA haplotypes is from the father, and thus foreign to the mother's immune system. The fetal–maternal interface in the decidua must provide tolerance and allow trophoblast invasion, but not beyond certain limits; defense against infections must also be provided. Cells of the NK lineage are the dominating lymphocytes in the decidua, and they may play an important role in one or several of these processes (Moffett-King 2002). The uterine NK (uNK) cells are of a particular phenotype, resembling the minor CD56^{bright} subset in the blood. Their number in the endometrium starts to increase already during the post-ovulatory, secretory phase of the menstrual cycle. The uNK cells normally die as menstruation starts but, if an implantation occurs, they continue to expand and dominate the deciduas until midgestation, when placentation is complete. They then gradually disappear. The expansion of the population may be driven by IL-15 and prolactin, produced by stromal cells under the influence of the pregnancy hormone progesterone (Moffett-King et al. 2002). There are very few T cells in the decidua and no B cells.

The functional role of uNK cells is not clear. It is, however, intriguing that the MHC class I molecules expressed by the extravillous trophoblast in the decidua are HLA-E, HLA-G, and HLA-C, all of which can be recognized by different NK receptors (Moffett-King 2002). The uNK cells all express the inhibitory receptor NKG2A (recognizing HLA-E), like the CD56^{bright} cells in the blood. However, the uNK cells differ from the latter in that a high proportion also expresses KIR, especially the ones recognizing HLA-C alleles. It has been proposed that inhibitory receptors prevent uNK cell lysis of trophoblast, but antibody-blocking studies in vitro do not support this. An alternate possibility is that the receptors regulate cytokine production. The uNK cells can produce the same cytokines as blood NK cells, and the invading trophoblast cells have receptors for many of these (e.g. IFN-γ, CSF1, and TNF). In addition, uNK cells produce several factors involved in angiogenesis and vascular stability. One hypothesis is that NK cells regulate trophoblast invasion and a process intimately connected to this, the transformation of maternal blood vessels in the decidua (Moffett-King 2002; Moffett-King et al. 2002). This is required for adequate fetal blood supply. Dysregulation of this process may lead to the condition preeclampsia, with risk for growth retardation of the fetus or still birth.

There are major differences in the anatomy of placentation between species, and it is therefore difficult to extrapolate observations from murine models to humans. There are some common factors and some intriguing observations from studies in mice (Croy et al. 2003). NK cells also represent the dominating lymphocyte in the mouse decidua, and they appear to be recruited from secondary lymphoid tissues during pregnancy. Mice lacking NK (and uNK) cells breed, and these cells are therefore not essential for implantation, decidualization, and completion of pregnancy. However, in the absence of uNK cells, pregnant mice show several decidual abnormalities at midgestation, such as thick-walled decidual spiral arteries with narrow lumen diameters and a dramatic acellularity of the decidua (Moffett-King 2002; Croy et al. 2003). Studies of gene defective mice have shown that uNK cell-produced IFN-γ may be a central cytokine for vascular modifications (dilatation, elongation, and branching) of spiral arteries.

In conclusion, studies from humans and mice indicate that uNK cells play a role in regulating the trophoblast invasion and vascular transformation in the decidua. Although they are not absolutely required under normal conditions, they may be critical in pregnancies complicated by other factors.

NK CELLS IN AUTOIMMUNE DISEASES

Natural killer cell numbers and functions are often altered in patients with autoimmune disease. As in cancer and infection, such findings are not easy to interpret, because they may represent secondary alterations resulting from, for example, metabolic or other disturbances in the disease. Infiltration of autoimmune target organs by NK cells has been observed in, for example, pancreatic islets in diabetes and the synovial fluid in rheumatoid arthritis (French and Yokoyama 2004). In the latter case, all the infiltrating NK cells are of the $CD56^{bright}CD16^{low}$ cytokine-producing phenotype, which is rare in the blood. Their role in the pathogenesis of rheumatoid arthritis is unclear.

There are two rare clinical conditions where a role for 'missing self' recognition by NK cells has been proposed as responsible for autoreactivity. In the 'bare lymphocyte syndrome', there is complete lack or severely impaired MHC class I expression on cells. This can be caused by different gene defects, one of which affects the so-called TAP. When TAP expression is impaired, the HLA molecules become unstable as a result of deficient loading of peptides in the ER. A subgroup of patients with TAP deficiency suffers from necrotizing granulomatous lesions in skin and lungs, characterized by infiltration of NK cells and T cells, and leading to clinical manifestations in these organs (Zimmer et al. 1998; Moins-Teisserenc et al. 1999). There is indirect evidence that these lesions are caused by autodestructive NK cells that can recognize the 'missing self' phenotype of cells in the target tissue. There must be additional factors required for triggering of this condition, because it does not develop in all patients with the bare lymphocyte syndrome; even patient's siblings who have inherited the TAP deficiency may not develop this pattern. Most MHC class I-deficient patients thus acquire NK cell tolerance toward their own cells, just as mice with the corresponding defects. One possibility is that certain infectious agents can break this tolerance, which could explain why only certain TAP-deficient individuals are affected.

It has also been proposed that the red cell aplasia associated with benign or malignant LGL expansions may be caused by 'missing self' recognition of erythroblasts (with poor MHC class I expression) by the KIRs expressing LGLs (Lamy and Loughran 2003). Such LGL expansions may consist of T cells ($\alpha\beta$or $\gamma\delta$) or NK cells, but both populations can express KIRs.

Several experimental studies have addressed the role of NK cells in animal models of autoimmunity by depleting them just before the induction or during progression of disease. Although corresponding studies in cancer, infection, and transplantation in most cases show impaired reactivity against the target or in some cases no effect, but never evidence for increased reactivity, any of the three outcomes can be observed in autoimmune models (Baxter and Smyth 2002; Flodstrom et al. 2002; French and Yokoyama 2004). There is as yet no clear-cut pattern with respect to type or localization of disease – opposite effects of NK cell depletion have even been reported in different studies of the same disease model (experimental allergic encephalomyelitis). These divergent observations are not surprising, given the complexity in the responses leading to autoimmune manifestations. The effect may thus depend on whether NK cells have a role early in induction or deviation of adaptive responses, or late as effector cells in target tissues, e.g. in a model of myasthenia gravis, NK cells promoted disease by cytokines, which skewed the response toward Th1 and production of autoantibodies to the acetylcholine receptor (Shi et al. 2000).The most consistent results have been observed in diabetes models, where NK cells in three of three cases seemed to promote disease (Flodstrom et al. 2002). The mechanisms behind this are not known, although there is evidence that NK cells can kill pancreatic β cells in vitro, suggesting a direct role as effector cells. NK cells can kill several additional normal cell types in vitro, e.g. oligodendrocytes and neurons.

In conclusion, NK cells may contribute to or prevent autoimmune disease at several levels, including cytokine-mediated stimulation, suppression or deviation of adaptive responses, and cytokine- or perforin-dependent destruction of cells in target organs. One important focus of future research is to reveal the receptors and ligands involved.

REFERENCES

Anderson, S.K., Ortaldo, J.R. and McVicar, D.W. 2001. The ever-expanding Ly49 gene family. Repertoire and signaling. *Immunol Rev*, **181**, 79–89.

Arase, H., Arase, N. and Saito, T. 1995. Fas-mediated cytotoxicity by freshly isolated natural killer cells. *J Exp Med*, **181**, 1235–8.

Arase, H., Mocarski, E.S., et al. 2002. Direct recognition of cytomegalovirus by activating and inhibitory NK cell receptors. *Science*, **296**, 1323–6.

Artavanis-Tsakonas, K. and Riley, E.M. 2002. Innate immune response to malaria. Rapid induction of IFN-gamma from human NK cells by live *Plasmodium falciparum*-infected erythrocytes. *J Immunol*, **169**, 2956–63.

Ashkar, A.A. and Rosenthal, K.L. 2002. Toll-like receptor 9, CpG DNA and innate immunity. *Curr Mol Med*, **2**, 545–56.

Bancroft, G.J. 1993. The role of natural killer cells in innate resistance to infection. *Curr Opin Immunol*, **5**, 503–10.

Barao, I. and Murphy, W.J. 2003. The immunobiology of natural killer cells and bone marrow allograft rejection. *Biol Blood Marrow Transplant*, **9**, 727–41.

Baxter, A.G. and Smyth, M.J. 2002. The role of NK cells in autoimmune disease. *Autoimmunity*, **35**, 1–14.

Becker, I., Salaiza, N., et al. 2003. *Leishmania* lipophosphoglycan (LPG) activates NK cells through toll-like receptor-2. *Mol Biochem Parasitol*, **130**, 65–74.

Bennett, M., Yu, Y.Y., et al. 1995. Hybrid resistance. 'Negative' and 'positive' signaling of murine natural killer cells. *Semin Immunol*, **7**, 121–7.

Biron, C.A., Byron, K.S. and Sullivan, J.L. 1989. Severe herpesvirus infections in an adolescent without natural killer cells. *N Engl J Med*, **320**, 1731–5.

Biron, C.A., Nguyen, K.B., et al. 1999. Natural killer cells in antiviral defense. Function and regulation by innate cytokines. *Annu Rev Immunol*, **17**, 189–220.

Biron, C.A., Nguyen, K.B. and Pien, G.C. 2002. Innate immune responses to LCMV infections. Natural killer cells and cytokines. *Curr Top Microbiol Immunol*, **263**, 7–27.

Bix, M., Liao, N.S., et al. 1991. Rejection of class I MHC-deficient haemopoietic cells by irradiated MHC-matched mice. *Nature*, **349**, 329–31.

Borges, L. and Cosman, D. 2000. LIRs/ILTs/MIRs, inhibitory and stimulatory Ig-superfamily receptors expressed in myeloid and lymphoid cells. *Cytokine Growth Factor Rev*, **11**, 209–17.

Boyington, J.C. and Sun, P.D. 2002. A structural perspective on MHC class I recognition by killer cell immunoglobulin-like receptors. *Mol Immunol*, **38**, 1007–21.

Braud, V.M., Allan, D.S., et al. 1998. HLA-E binds to natural killer cell receptors CD94/NKG2A, B and C. *Nature*, **391**, 795–9.

Braud, V.M., Tomasec, P. and Wilkinson, G.W. 2002. Viral evasion of natural killer cells during human cytomegalovirus infection. *Curr Top Microbiol Immunol*, **269**, 117–29.

Cardillo, F., Voltarelli, J.C., et al. 1996. Regulation of *Trypanosoma cruzi* infection in mice by gamma interferon and interleukin, 10. Role of NK cells. *Infect Immun*, **64**, 128–34.

Carretero, M., Cantoni, C., et al. 1997. The CD94 and NKG2-A C-type lectins covalently assemble to form a natural killer cell inhibitory receptor for HLA class I molecules. *Eur J Immunol*, **27**, 563–7.

Carson, W. and Caligiuri, M. 1996. Natural killer cell subsets and development. *METHODS*, **9**, 327–43.

Cerwenka, A. and Lanier, L.L. 2001. Natural killer cells, viruses and cancer. *Nat Rev Immunol*, **1**, 41–9.

Chapman, T.L., Heikeman, A.P. and Bjorkman, P.J. 1999. The inhibitory receptor LIR-1 uses a common binding interaction to recognize class I MHC molecules and the viral homolog UL18. *Immunity*, **11**, 603–13.

Cohen, G.B., Gandhi, R.T., et al. 1999. The selective downregulation of class I major histocompatibility complex proteins by HIV-1 protects HIV-infected cells from NK cells. *Immunity*, **10**, 661–71.

Colonna, M., Nakajima, H. and Cella, M. 2000. A family of inhibitory and activating Ig-like receptors that modulate function of lymphoid and myeloid cells. *Semin Immunol*, **12**, 121–7.

Colucci, F., Di Santo, J.P. and Leibson, P.J. 2002. Natural killer cell activation in mice and men. Different triggers for similar weapons? *Nat Immunol*, **3**, 807–13.

Colucci, F., Caligiuri, M.A. and Di Santo, J.P. 2003. What does it take to make a natural killer? *Nat Rev Immunol*, **3**, 413–25.

Cooper, M.A., Fehniger, T.A. and Caligiuri, M.A. 2001. The biology of human natural killer-cell subsets. *Trends Immunol*, **22**, 633–40.

Croy, B.A., He, H., et al. 2003. Uterine natural killer cells. Insights into their cellular and molecular biology from mouse modelling. *Reproduction*, **126**, 149–60.

Cudkowicz, G. and Bennett, M. 1971. Peculiar immunobiology of bone marrow allografts. II. Rejection of parental grafts by resistant F 1 hybrid mice. *J Exp Med*, **134**, 1513–28.

Dam, J., Guan, R., et al. 2003. Variable MHC class I engagement by Ly49 natural killer cell receptors demonstrated by the crystal structure of Ly49C bound to H-2K(b). *Nat Immunol*, **4**, 1213–22.

Davies, S.M., Ruggieri, L., et al. 2002. Evaluation of KIR ligand incompatibility in mismatched unrelated donor hematopoietic transplants. Killer immunoglobulin-like receptor. *Blood*, **100**, 3825–7.

Davis, D.M. 2002. Assembly of the immunological synapse for T cells and NK cells. *Trends Immunol*, **23**, 356–63.

Davis, D.M., Chiu, I., et al. 1999. The human natural killer cell immune synapse. *Proc Natl Acad Sci USA*, **96**, 15062–7.

De Maria, A., Fogli, M., et al. 2003. The impaired NK cell cytolytic function in viremic HIV-1 infection is associated with a reduced surface expression of natural cytotoxicity receptors (NKp46, NKp30 and NKp44). *Eur J Immunol*, **33**, 2410–18.

Degliantoni, G., Murphy, M., et al. 1985. Natural killer (NK) cell-derived hematopoietic colony-inhibiting activity and NK cytotoxic factor. Relationship with tumor necrosis factor and synergism with immune interferon. *J Exp Med*, **162**, 1512–30.

Denkers, E.Y., Gazzinelli, R.T., et al. 1993. Emergence of NK1.1+ cells as effectors of IFN-gamma dependent immunity to *Toxoplasma gondii* in MHC class I-deficient mice. *J Exp Med*, **178**, 1465–72.

Doucey, M.A., Scarpellino, L., et al. 2004. Cis association of Ly49A with MHC class I restricts natural killer cell inhibition. *Nat Immunol*, **5**, 328–36.

Dunn, C., Chalupny, N.J., et al. 2003. Human cytomegalovirus glycoprotein UL16 causes intracellular sequestration of NKG2D ligands, protecting against natural killer cell cytotoxicity. *J Exp Med*, **197**, 1427–39.

Ehl, S., Nuesch, R., et al. 1996. A comparison of efficacy and specificity of three NK depleting antibodies. *J Immunol Methods*, **199**, 149–53.

Eriksson, M., Leitz, G., et al. 1999. Inhibitory receptors alter natural killer cell interactions with target cells yet allow simultaneous killing of susceptible targets. *J Exp Med*, **190**, 1005–12.

Farag, S.S., Fehniger, T.A., et al. 2002. Natural killer cell receptors. New biology and insights into the graft-versus-leukemia effect. *Blood*, **100**, 1935–47.

Fehniger, T.A. and Caligiuri, M.A. 2001. Interleukin 15. Biology and relevance to human disease. *Blood*, **97**, 14–32.

Ferlazzo, G., Thomas, D., et al. 2004. The abundant NK cells in human secondary lymphoid tissues require activation to express killer cell Ig-like receptors and become cytolytic. *J Immunol*, **172**, 1455–62.

Flodstrom, M., Shi, F., et al. 2002. The natural killer cell – friend or foe in autoimmune disease? *Scand J Immunol*, **55**, 432–41.

Florido, M., Correia-Neves, M., et al. 2003. The cytolytic activity of natural killer cells is not involved in the restriction of *Mycobacterium avium* growth. *Int Immunol*, **15**, 895–901.

French, A.R. and Yokoyama, W.M. 2004. Natural killer cells and autoimmunity. *Arthritis Res Ther*, **6**, 8–14.

Giebel, S., Locatelli, F., et al. 2003. Survival advantage with KIR ligand incompatibility in hematopoietic stem cell transplantation from unrelated donors. *Blood*, **102**, 814–19.

Hanna, N. 1982. Role of natural killer cells in control of cancer metastasis. *Cancer Metastasis Rev*, **1**, 45–64.

Held, W., Kunz, B., et al. 1999. Clonal acquisition of the Ly49A NK cell receptor is dependent on the trans-acting factor TCF-1. *Immunity*, **11**, 433–42.

Held, W., Coudert, J.D. and Zimmer, J. 2003. The NK cell receptor repertoire. Formation, adaptation and exploitation. *Curr Opin Immunol*, **15**, 233–7.

Henkart, P.A. 1999. Cytotoxic T lymphocytes. In: Paul, W.E. (ed.), *Fundamental immunology*. New York: Lippincott-Raven, 1021–49.

Herberman, R.B., Nunn, M.E., et al. 1975a. Natural cytotoxic reactivity of mouse lymphoid cells against syngeneic and allogeneic tumors. II. Characterization of effector cells. *Int J Cancer*, **16**, 230–9.

Herberman, R.B., Nunn, M.E. and Lavrin, D.H. 1975b. Natural cytotoxic reactivity of mouse lymphoid cells against syngeneic acid allogeneic tumors. I. Distribution of reactivity and specificity. *Int J Cancer*, **16**, 216–29.

Hsu, K.C., Chida, S., et al. 2002. The killer cell immunoglobulin-like receptor (KIR) genomic region. Gene-order, haplotypes and allelic polymorphism. *Immunol Rev*, **190**, 40–52.

Idris, A.H., Smith, H.R., et al. 1999. The natural killer gene complex genetic locus Chok encodes Ly-49D, a target recognition receptor that activates natural killing. *Proc Natl Acad Sci USA*, **96**, 6330–5.

Iizuka, K., Naidenko, O.V., et al. 2003. Genetically linked C-type lectin-related ligands for the NKRP1 family of natural killer cell receptors. *Nat Immunol*, **4**, 801–7.

Johansson, M.H., Bieberich, C., et al. 1997. Natural killer cell tolerance in mice with mosaic expression of major histocompatibility complex class I transgene. *J Exp Med*, **186**, 353–64.

Kane, K.P., Silver, E.T. and Hazes, B. 2001. Specificity and function of activating Ly-49 receptors. *Immunol Rev*, **181**, 104–14.

Karlhofer, F.M., Ribaudo, R.K. and Yokoyama, W.M. 1992. MHC class I alloantigen specificity of Ly-49+ IL-2-activated natural killer cells. *Nature*, **358**, 66–70.

Kärre, K. 1985. Role of target histocompatibility antigens in regulation of natural killer activity. A reevaluation and a hypothesis. In: Callewaert, D. and Herberman, R.B. (eds), *Mechanisms of cytotoxicity by NK cells*. London: Academic Press, 81–91.

Kärre, K. 1997. How to recognize a foreign submarine. *Immunol Rev*, **155**, 5–9.

Kärre, K. 2002. NK cells, MHC class I molecules and the missing self. *Scand J Immunol*, **55**, 221–8.

Kärre, K., Ljunggren, H.G., et al. 1986. Selective rejection of H-2-deficient lymphoma variants suggests alternative immune defence strategy. *Nature*, **319**, 675–8.

Kase, A., Johansson, M.H., et al. 1998. External and internal calibration of the MHC class I-specific receptor Ly49A on murine natural killer cells. *J Immunol*, **161**, 6133–8.

Kayagaki, N., Yamaguchi, N., et al. 1999. Expression and function of TNF-related apoptosis-inducing ligand on murine activated NK cells. *J Immunol*, **163**, 1906–13.

Khakoo, S.I. and Brooks, C.R. 2003. MHC class I receptors on natural killer cells. On with the old and in with the new. *Clin Sci (Lond)*, **105**, 127–40.

Kiessling, R., Klein, E., et al. 1975a. 'Natural' killer cells in the mouse. II. Cytotoxic cells with specificity for mouse Moloney leukemia cells. Characteristics of the killer cell. *Eur J Immunol*, **5**, 117–21.

Kiessling, R., Klein, E. and Wigzell, H. 1975b. 'Natural' killer cells in the mouse. I. Cytotoxic cells with specificity for mouse Moloney leukemia cells. Specificity and distribution according to genotype. *Eur J Immunol*, **5**, 112–17.

Kiessling, R., Petranyi, G., et al. 1975c. Genetic variation of in vitro cytolytic activity and in vivo rejection potential of non-immunized semi-syngeneic mice against a mouse lymphoma line. *Int J Cancer*, **15**, 933–40.

Kiessling, R., Hochman, P.S., et al. 1977. Evidence for a similar or common mechanism for natural killer cell activity and resistance to hemopoietic grafts. *Eur J Immunol*, **7**, 655–63.

Kim, S., Iizuka, K., et al. 2000. In vivo natural killer cell activities revealed by natural killer cell-deficient mice. *Proc Natl Acad Sci USA*, **97**, 2731–6.

Kirveskari, J., He, Q., et al. 1999. Enterobacterial infection modulates major histocompatibility complex class I expression on mononuclear cells. *Immunology*, **97**, 420–8.

Krensky, A.M. 2000. Granulysin. a novel antimicrobial peptide of cytolytic T lymphocytes and natural killer cells. *Biochem Pharmacol*, **59**, 317–20.

Krmpotic, A., Busch, D.H., et al. 2002. MCMV glycoprotein gp40 confers virus resistance to CD8+ T cells and NK cells in vivo. *Nat Immunol*, **3**, 529–35.

Kubota, A., Kubota, S., et al. 1999. Diversity of NK cell receptor repertoire in adult and neonatal mice. *J Immunol*, **163**, 212–16.

Lamy, T. and Loughran, T.P. Jr. 2003. Clinical features of large granular lymphocyte leukemia. *Semin Hematol*, **40**, 185–95.

Lanier, L.L. 1998. NK cell receptors. *Annu Rev Immunol*, **16**, 359–93.

Lanier, L.L. 2003. Natural killer cell receptor signaling. *Curr Opin Immunol*, **15**, 308–14.

Lanier, L.L. and Bakker, A.B. 2000. The ITAM-bearing transmembrane adaptor DAP12 in lymphoid and myeloid cell function. *Immunol Today*, **21**, 611–14.

Lee, K.M., Bhawan, S., et al. 2003. Cutting edge. The NK cell receptor, 2B4 augments antigen-specific T cell cytotoxicity through CD48 ligation on neighboring T cells. *J Immunol*, **170**, 4881–5.

Lee, S.H., Webb, J.R. and Vidal, S.M. 2002. Innate immunity to cytomegalovirus. The Cmv1 locus and its role in natural killer cell function. *Microbes Infect*, **4**, 1491–503.

Leibson, P.J. 1998. Cytotoxic lymphocyte recognition of HLA-E. utilizing a nonclassical window to peer into classical MHC. *Immunity*, **9**, 289–94.

Lieberman, J. 2003. The ABCs of granule-mediated cytotoxicity. New weapons in the arsenal. *Nat Rev Immunol*, **3**, 361–70.

Ljunggren, H.G. and Kärre, K. 1990. In search of the 'missing self'. MHC molecules and NK cell recognition. *Immunol Today*, **11**, 237–44.

Lodoen, M., Ogasawara, K., et al. 2003. NKG2D-mediated natural killer cell protection against cytomegalovirus is impaired by viral gp40 modulation of retinoic acid early inducible, 1 gene molecules. *J Exp Med*, **197**, 1245–53.

McMahon, C.W. and Raulet, D.H. 2001. Expression and function of NK cell receptors in CD8+ T cells. *Curr Opin Immunol*, **13**, 465–70.

Mandelboim, O., Lieberman, N., et al. 2001. Recognition of haemagglutinins on virus-infected cells by NKp46 activates lysis by human NK cells. *Nature*, **409**, 1055–60.

Martin, M.P., Gao, X., et al. 2002a. Epistatic interaction between KIR3DS1 and HLA-B delays the progression to AIDS. *Nat Genet*, **31**, 429–34.

Martin, M.P., Nelson, G., et al. 2002b. Cutting edge. Susceptibility to psoriatic arthritis. Influence of activating killer Ig-like receptor genes in the absence of specific HLA-C alleles. *J Immunol*, **169**, 2818–22.

Mavilio, D., Benjamin, J., et al. 2003. Natural killer cells in HIV-1 infection. Dichotomous effects of viremia on inhibitory and activating receptors and their functional correlates. *Proc Natl Acad Sci USA*, **100**, 15011–16.

Mingari, M.C., Ponte, M., et al. 2000. Expression of HLA class I-specific inhibitory receptors in human cytolytic T lymphocytes. A regulated mechanism that controls T-cell activation and function. *Hum Immunol*, **61**, 44–50.

Moffett-King, A. 2002. Natural killer cells and pregnancy. *Nat Rev Immunol*, **2**, 656–63.

Moffett-King, A., Entrican, G., et al. 2002. Natural killer cells and reproduction. *Trends Immunol*, **23**, 332–3.

Moins-Teisserenc, H.T., Gadola, S.D., et al. 1999. Association of a syndrome resembling Wegener's granulomatosis with low surface expression of HLA class-I molecules. *Lancet*, **354**, 1598–603.

Moretta, A. 2002. Natural killer cells and dendritic cells. Rendezvous in abused tissues. *Nat Rev Immunol*, **2**, 957–64.

Moretta, A., Vitale, M., et al. 1993. P58 molecules as putative receptors for major histocompatibility complex (MHC) class I molecules in human natural killer (NK) cells. Anti-p58 antibodies reconstitute lysis of MHC class I-protected cells in NK clones displaying different specificities. *J Exp Med*, **178**, 597–604.

Moretta, A., Bottino, C., et al. 2001. Activating receptors and coreceptors involved in human natural killer cell-mediated cytolysis. *Annu Rev Immunol*, **19**, 197–223.

Moretta, L., Ciccone, E., et al. 1994. Human natural killer cells. Origin, clonality, specificity, and receptors. *Adv Immunol*, **55**, 341–80.

Mrozek, E., Anderson, P. and Caligiuri, M.A. 1996. Role of interleukin-15 in the development of human CD56+ natural killer cells from CD34+ hematopoietic progenitor cells. *Blood*, **87**, 2632–2640.

Nakamura, M.C., Linnemeyer, P.A., et al. 1999. Mouse Ly-49D recognizes H-2Dd and activates natural killer cell cytotoxicity. *J Exp Med*, **189**, 493–500.

Namekawa, T., Snyder, M.R., et al. 2000. Killer cell activating receptors function as costimulatory molecules on CD4+CD28null T cells clonally expanded in rheumatoid arthritis. *J Immunol*, **165**, 1138–45.

Natarajan, K., Dimasi, N., et al. 2002. Structure and function of natural killer cell receptors. Multiple molecular solutions to self, nonself discrimination. *Annu Rev Immunol*, **20**, 853–85.

Ohlen, C., Kling, G., et al. 1989. Prevention of allogeneic bone marrow graft rejection by H-2 transgene in donor mice. *Science*, **246**, 666–8.

Olsson, M.Y., Karre, K. and Sentman, C.L. 1995. Altered phenotype and function of natural killer cells expressing the major histocompatibility complex receptor Ly-49 in mice transgenic for its ligand. *Proc Natl Acad Sci USA*, **92**, 1649–53.

Orange, J.S., Fassett, M.S., et al. 2002. Viral evasion of natural killer cells. *Nat Immunol*, **3**, 1006–12.

Parham, P. and McQueen, K.L. 2003. Alloreactive killer cells. Hindrance and help for haematopoietic transplants. *Nat Rev Immunol*, **3**, 108–22.

Pende, D., Cantoni, C., et al. 2001. Role of NKG2D in tumor cell lysis mediated by human NK cells. Cooperation with natural cytotoxicity receptors and capability of recognizing tumors of nonepithelial origin. *Eur J Immunol*, **31**, 1076–86.

Prlic, M., Blazar, B., et al. 2003. In vivo survival and homeostatic proliferation of natural killer cells. *J Exp Med*, **197**, 967–76.

Raulet, D.H. 2003. Roles of the NKG2D immunoreceptor and its ligands. *Nat Rev Immunol*, **3**, 781–90.

Raulet, D.H., Vance, R.E. and McMahon, C.W. 2001. Regulation of the natural killer cell receptor repertoire. *Annu Rev Immunol*, **19**, 291–330.

Ravetch, J.V. and Bolland, S. 2001. IgG Fc receptors. *Annu Rev Immunol*, **19**, 275–90.

Reyburn, H.T., Mandelboim, O., et al. 1997. The class I MHC homologue of human cytomegalovirus inhibits attack by natural killer cells. *Nature*, **386**, 514–17.

Riccardi, C., Puccetti, P., et al. 1979. Rapid in vivo assay of mouse natural killer cell activity. *J Natl Cancer Instit*, **63**, 1041–5.

Rolle, A., Mousavi-Jazi, M., et al. 2003. Effects of human cytomegalovirus infection on ligands for the activating NKG2D receptor of NK cells. Up-regulation of UL16-binding protein (ULBP)1 and ULBP2 is counteracted by the viral UL16 protein. *J Immunol*, **171**, 902–8.

Rosenberg, S.A. 1988. Immunotherapy of patients with advanced cancer using interleukin-2 alone or in combination with lymphokine activated killer cells. *Important Adv Oncol*, **Review**, 217–57.

Roth, C., Carlyle, J.R., et al. 2000. Clonal acquisition of inhibitory Ly49 receptors on developing NK cells is successively restricted and regulated by stromal class I MHC. *Immunity*, **13**, 143–53.

Ruggeri, L., Capanni, M., et al. 2002. Effectiveness of donor natural killer cell alloreactivity in mismatched hematopoietic transplants. *Science*, **295**, 2097–100.

Salih, H.R., Rammensee, H.G. and Steinle, A. 2002. Cutting edge. Down-regulation of MICA on human tumors by proteolytic shedding. *J Immunol*, **169**, 4098–102.

Salmon-Divon, M., Hoglund, P. and Mehr, R. 2003. Models for natural killer cell repertoire formation. *Clin Dev Immunol*, **10**, 183–92.

Scalzo, A.A., Wheat, R., et al. 2003. Molecular genetic characterization of the distal NKC recombination hotspot and putative murine CMV resistance control locus. *Immunogenetics*, **55**, 370–8.

Scott, P. and Trinchieri, G. 1995. The role of natural killer cells in host–parasite interactions. *Curr Opin Immunol*, **7**, 34–40.

Scott-Algara, D. and Paul, P. 2002. NK cells and HIV infection. Lessons from other viruses. *Curr Mol Med*, **2**, 757–68.

Screpanti, V., Wallin, R.P., et al. 2001. A central role for death receptor-mediated apoptosis in the rejection of tumors by NK cells. *J Immunol*, **167**, 2068–73.

Shi, F.D., Wang, H.B., et al. 2000. Natural killer cells determine the outcome of B cell-mediated autoimmunity. *Nat Immunol*, **1**, 245–51.

Sjolin, H., Tomasello, E., et al. 2002. Pivotal role of KARAP/DAP12 adaptor molecule in the natural killer cell-mediated resistance to murine cytomegalovirus infection. *J Exp Med*, **195**, 825–34.

Smith, H.R., Heusel, J.W., et al. 2002. Recognition of a virus-encoded ligand by a natural killer cell activation receptor. *Proc Natl Acad Sci USA*, **99**, 8826–31.

Smyth, M.J., Hayakawa, Y., et al. 2002. New aspects of natural-killer-cell surveillance and therapy of cancer. *Nat Rev Cancer*, **2**, 850–61.

Tay, C.H., Szomolanyi-Tsuda, E. and Welsh, R.M. 1998. Control of infections by NK cells. *Curr Top Microbiol Immunol*, **230**, 193–220.

Timonen, T. and Saksela, E. 1980. Isolation of human NK cells by density gradient centrifugation. *J Immunol Methods*, **36**, 285–91.

Tomasec, P., Braud, V.M., et al. 2000. Surface expression of HLA-E, an inhibitor of natural killer cells, enhanced by human cytomegalovirus gpUL40. *Science*, **287**, 1031.

Tomasello, E., Blery, M., et al. 2000. Signaling pathways engaged by NK cell receptors. Double concerto for activating receptors, inhibitory receptors and NK cells. *Semin Immunol*, **12**, 139–47.

Trinchieri, G. 1995. Natural killer cells wear different hats. Effector cells of innate resistance and regulatory cells of adaptive immunity and of hematopoiesis. *Semin Immunol*, **7**, 83–8.

Trinchieri, G. 2003a. The choices of a natural killer. *Nat Immunol*, **4**, 509–10.

Trinchieri, G. 2003b. Interleukin-12 and the regulation of innate resistance and adaptive immunity. *Nat Rev Immunol*, **3**, 133–46.

Trinchieri, G., Matsumoto-Kobayashi, M., et al. 1984. Response of resting human peripheral blood natural killer cells to interleukin, 2. *J Exp Med*, **160**, 1147–69.

Trowsdale, J., Barten, R., et al. 2001. The genomic context of natural killer receptor extended gene families. *Immunol Rev*, **181**, 20–38.

Valiante, N.M., Uhrberg, M., et al. 1997. Functionally and structurally distinct NK cell receptor repertoires in the peripheral blood of two human donors. *Immunity*, **7**, 739–51.

van der Slik, A.R., Koeleman, B.P., et al. 2003. KIR in type I diabetes. disparate distribution of activating and inhibitory natural killer cell receptors in patients versus HLA-matched control subjects. *Diabetes*, **52**, 2639–42.

Vance, R.E., Jamieson, A.M. and Raulet, D.H. 1999. Recognition of the class Ib molecule Qa-1(b) by putative activating receptors CD94/NKG2C and CD94/NKG2E on mouse natural killer cells. *J Exp Med*, **190**, 1801–12.

Vankayalapati, R., Wizel, B., et al. 2002. The NKp46 receptor contributes to NK cell lysis of mononuclear phagocytes infected with an intracellular bacterium. *J Immunol*, **168**, 3451–37.

Vilches, C. and Parham, P. 2002. KIR. Diverse, rapidly evolving receptors of innate and adaptive immunity. *Annu Rev Immunol*, **20**, 217–51.

Vitale, C., Romagnani, C., et al. 2001. Surface expression and function of p75/AIRM-1 or CD33 in acute myeloid leukemias. engagement of CD33 induces apoptosis of leukemic cells. *Proc Natl Acad Sci USA*, **98**, 5764–9.

Wallin, R.P., Screpanti, V., et al. 2003. Regulation of perforin-independent NK cell-mediated cytotoxicity. *Eur J Immunol*, **33**, 2727–35.

Whiteside, T.L., Vujanovic, N.L. and Herberman, R.B. 1998. Natural killer cells and tumor therapy. *Curr Top Microbiol Immunol*, **230**, 221–44.

Williams, N.S., Moore, T.A., et al. 1997. Generation of lytic natural killer, 1.1+, Ly-49- cells from multipotential murine bone marrow progenitors in a stroma-free culture. definition of cytokine requirements and developmental intermediates. *J Exp Med*, **186**, 1609–14.

Wu, J. and Lanier, L.L. 2003. Natural killer cells and cancer. *Adv Cancer Res*, **90**, 127–56.

Yokota, Y., Mansouri, A.S., et al. 1999. Development of peripheral lymphoid organs and natural killer cells depends on the helix-loop-helix inhibitor Id2. *Nature*, **397**, 702–6.

Yokoyama, W.M. 1999. Natural killer cells. In: Paul, W.E. (ed.), *Fundamental immunology*, 4th edn. New York: Lippincott-Raven, 575–603.

Yokoyama, W.M. and Plougastel, B.F. 2003. Immune functions encoded by the natural killer gene complex. *Nat Rev Immunol*, **3**, 304–16.

Yokoyama, W.M. and Scalzo, A.A. 2002. Natural killer cell activation receptors in innate immunity to infection. *Microbes Infect*, **4**, 1513–21.

Young, J.D. and Cohn, I.Z.A. 1986. Cell-mediated killing. A common mechanism? *Cell*, **46**, 641–2.

Young, N.T. and Uhrberg, M. 2002. KIR expression shapes cytotoxic repertoires. A developmental program of survival. *Trends Immunol*, **23**, 71–5.

Yu, Y.Y., Kumar, V. and Bennett, M. 1992. Murine natural killer cells and marrow graft rejection. *Annu Rev Immunol*, **10**, 189–213.

Zimmer, J., Donato, L., et al. 1998. Activity and phenotype of natural killer cells in peptide transporter (TAP)-deficient patients (type I bare lymphocyte syndrome). *J Exp Med*, **187**, 117–22.

Zitvogel, L. 2002. Dendritic and natural killer cells cooperate in the control/switch of innate immunity. *J Exp Med*, **195**, F9–14.

7

Pattern recognition

NICOLAS W.J. SCHRÖDER AND RALF R. SCHUMANN

BRIEF HISTORIC INTRODUCTION

'Putrid poison', 'sepsin', and the birth of microbiology

After a long time of devastating infectious diseases, limiting the average life-time expectancy of the population worldwide until the late nineteenth century, several key findings by research pioneers in Europe not more than 120 years ago led the way to the understanding of basic principles of infection, and to the development of successful prevention and treatment strategies over the last decade. Even before the discovery of living microorganisms as the cause of infectious diseases inaugurating the discipline of microbiology, it was postulated by Panum that a 'putrid poison' was responsible for the lethal outcome of an infection (Panum 1874). Ernst von Bergmann of the Charité, Berlin in the late nineteenth century believed that a chemically defined substance was responsible for fatal infections, which he termed 'sepsin' (Bergmann and Schmiedeberg 1868).

Of course it was Louis Pasteur and Robert Koch in their ground-breaking discoveries who revealed that microorganisms are the cause of infectious diseases and they founded the new discipline of microbiology (reviewed in: Dubos 1995; Brock 1999). Although especially Koch in Berlin isolated several important bacteria presenting proof that they were the cause of disease, it still for a long time remained unclear how a given pathogen would cause a specific disease and it took a long time to define both the 'toxic' elements of microorganisms and the host's reaction patterns involved in the disease (reviewed in Beutler and Rietschel 2003).

Host–pathogen interaction as cause of many diseases of importance

Introduction of hygiene measures preventing spread of infectious diseases and the development of powerful antibiotics during the twentieth century reduced the lethality of infectious diseases in the industrial world dramatically. However, even today, certain diseases caused by microorganisms remain a clinical problem despite the highest hygiene standards and broad-spectrum antibiotics: sepsis and septic shock caused by microorganisms are still a major threat in intensive care units and statistically sepsis is a major killer in the western world (Hotchkiss and Karl 2003). Apparently, here the host reacts early to pathogens and induces a response, unfortunately not leading to limitation of the disease but to a critical state.

On the other hand, chronic inflammatory reactions account for a large number of diseases that are also particularly difficult to treat, and that lead to major financial healthcare burdens. It is very likely that microorganisms persisting within the host account for many of these diseases, although they are not directly treatable by antibiotics (Relman 2002). Other important clinical syndromes characterized by a distinct host reaction include different forms of toxic shock syndrome, chronic parasitic diseases, or virally caused cancers, to name just a few.

Molecular mechanisms of pathogen recognition

The two reaction patterns as examples mentioned above of septic shock, on the one hand, and of chronic inflammation, on the other, depict the wide spectrum of host–pathogen interactions that can take place during an infection, and for a long time the following questions were asked:

- How is this interaction of the pathogen and the host determined?
- What molecules are involved on both sides?
- Can this reaction pattern be influenced?
- Could this be the basis for a therapy for infectious or inflammatory diseases?

Only recently, key molecular elements of the host detection system of innate immune cells were discovered with the family of Toll-like receptors (TLR), which are discussed in detail in this chapter. Furthermore, soluble molecules with the ability to detect pathogens and intracellular molecular elements of the innate immune system have been discovered, which are also outlined.

Microorganisms and their hosts – the 'battle of the genomes'

The last 120 years of microbiology since Koch have also led to the discovery of a large multitude of microorganisms displaying a wide variety of genomic organization and phenotypic appearance. Even though just a small portion of the existing microorganisms is pathogenic for humans, there is still an extremely wide variety of potentially pathogenic microorganisms. The human host, on the other hand, possesses a much larger genome compared with the microbes; however, as was revealed recently, it is smaller than expected with limited variation even between humans and other mammals. As a consequence any host organism must be overwhelmed by the task of recognizing the huge variety of potentially pathogenic microorganisms.

It has thus been postulated, and confirmed by research, lately, that the host's recognition system searches for molecular *patterns* present on distinct families of pathogens. The host apparently has sensors for these 'pathogen-associated molecular patterns (PAMP)' described in the next section and this interaction is a key step in pathogenesis of related diseases. The following section describes how the host, with the help of soluble and cellular recognition molecules, senses foreign material or dangerous situations in order to mount an appropriate response.

MICROBIAL TOXINS

Lipopolysaccharide as paradigm for pathogen-associated molecular patterns

It took several more years until the first theories on 'toxins', postulated in the pre-microbiological era by Panum and von Bergmann, were substantiated by direct evidence for the existence of a microbial substance causing the host's immune response. It was Pfeiffer who, for the first time, showed that even in the absence of live bacteria a toxic potential was present originating from bacteria and not being a protein (reviewed in Rietschel and Cavaillon 2002). This work later led to the discovery of endotoxin or lipopolysaccharide (LPS), now viewed as a classic PAMP inducing a strong activation of the innate immune system via defined molecular structures as outlined in detail below (Rietschel et al. 1996; Raetz and Whitfield 2002).

Lipopolysaccharide has a long history of excellent, thorough chemical analysis, and synthetic LPS was shown to elicit similar responses to isolated bacterial LPS in host cells. With the discovery of lipopolysaccharide-binding protein (LBP) and CD14, two of the first 'pattern-recognition receptors (PRR)' were discovered, 20 years ago, and functionally characterized in 1990 (Schumann et al. 1990; Wright et al. 1990). Further biomedical research on LPS also recently led to the discovery and functional analysis of the important PRR family of TLRs (reviewed in Beutler 2003).

A large variety of PAMPs on pathogenic microorganisms

Meanwhile, numerous pathogenic bacteria have been studied extensively, and have been analyzed chemically and genetically. Both secreted toxins, and elements of their cell walls have been well characterized and shown to bear the potential to induce innate immune responses. In addition, it has been shown that bacterial and viral nucleic acids, i.e. GC-rich oligonucleotides, can be sensed by the host's innate immune system leading to cellular activation (reviewed in Wagner 2002). These bacterial elements have furthermore been shown to be important co-stimulatory factors for inducing the adaptive immune responses, and thus are key elements as adjuvants for immunization.

MOLECULAR PATTERNS OF PATHOGENS

Are the patterns really known?

Until now it is still quite puzzling that, although certain patterns, such as LPS, present in all gram-negative bacteria, are characterized and well defined, other potentially immunostimulatory ligands of microbial source with the ability to activate immune cells are quite diverse, and seem to include such structurally distinct molecules as proteins, nucleic acids, and simple carbohydrates. Although this is still the focus of research, some molecular patterns, such as lipid structures, have been identified and are discussed at the end of this chapter.

The process of pattern recognition may also be very likely to change over time when microorganisms and the host live in symbiosis. Furthermore, selective pressure caused by antimicrobial agents may lead to rapid changes in the gene expression pattern of the pathogens and, as a consequence, to a shift in PAMP expression. Evasion and escape mechanisms of the microorganisms may lead to additional variations in patterns expressed on the surface, yet the host, in order to survive, still has to retain the ability to detect them. Novel gene array techniques may aid in analyzing this delicate balance of genetic adaptation between host and pathogen (Whitney et al. 2003). Furthermore, it has become clear that redundant pattern-recognition systems exist in order to ensure survival of the host in a changing environment.

Is pattern recognition part of the problem or part of the solution?

Despite the large success of recent research regarding both the host's and the pathogen's molecular 'arsenal', it is still not clear whether PAMPs are elements that are instrumental for the microbe to attack the host and improve survival of the pathogen, or whether the host's detection of these molecules is a key defense mechanism helping to fight off the microbes. Inflammation may be part of a successful defense reaction, and at the same time also contribute to the pathophysiology of disease. Recent results with LBP knock-out mice point in the direction that pattern recognition by the host is needed in order to combat live pathogens successfully (Jack et al. 1997; Wurfel et al. 1997; Heinrich et al. 2001; Fierer et al. 2002). Mice lacking certain PRRs were found to be unresponsive to isolated PAMPs and exhibited a worsened outcome when inoculated with whole bacteria (summarized in Werling and Jungi 2003).

Lately, studies investigating frequent single nucleotide polymorphisms (SNP) in genes encoding for TLRs in humans have been helpful for analyzing the role of these PRRs in health and disease (Lazarus et al. 2002). Analyses on the correlation of these SNPs with susceptibility to infectious diseases, discussed in detail in the final section of this chapter, are, however, controversial: although some reports show increased disease susceptibility when a PRR is genetically defective, one recent study revealed a protective effect of a TLR-4 SNP; these results were, however, obtained not for an acute infectious disease, but for an inflammatory disease, atherosclerosis (Kiechl et al. 2002).

Commensals, pathogens, and chronic inflammation

Recent research has focused on questions about the potentially beneficial role of commensal bacteria and the role of their host interaction – or lack thereof – for health and disease. Every human carries in the epigastrium more bacterial than human cells and this physiological flora clearly has important physiological functions. Why these commensals, despite carrying many of the known PAMPs, do not induce inflammatory responses is currently not known, but may be caused by a different arsenal or expression pattern of PRRs in the epigastrium (Melmed et al. 2003).

An overreaction to harmless commensals, on the other hand, has been suggested to be pathogenic in certain chronic inflammatory diseases of the gastrointestinal tract. The delicate balance between a strong defense reaction followed by the elimination of microorganisms and a 'silent symbiosis', based on the lack of early detection and interaction, most probably plays a key role in chronic inflammatory diseases in general (Kanai et al. 2002). These questions are not discussed in detail in this chapter because of a lack of space. They are closely related to topics of 'molecular mimicry' of microorganisms and the subject of autoimmune diseases, which are broadly covered in other chapters of this volume.

INNATE IMMUNITY

Adaptive and innate immunity

The discovery of the complex cellular system of the adaptive immune system during the twentieth century led to the broad application of one of the most important and successful concepts in modern medicine – immunization. The adaptive defense system, which is extensively covered in other parts of this volume, as we now know, needs repeated encounters of the host with the pathogen, and it cannot account for the rapid and potentially dramatic early reactions seen during acute infectious diseases.

In 1884, almost simultaneous with the groundbreaking discoveries of Koch and Pasteur described above, Metschnikoff discovered and described the phenomenon that certain cells within the host, which he called 'phagocytes', are able to detect and destroy foreign structures (Metschnikoff 1844). He also recognized that phagocytes of animals immunized against *Bacillus anthracis* were able to clear bacteria faster compared with their non-immune counterparts.

With these observations, Metschnikoff founded the basic principle of innate immunity, a defense system within the host that rapidly detects foreign microorganisms, kills them, and, if necessary, evokes further adaptive mechanisms against them. Meanwhile we know that, in addition to macrophages, granulocytes and dendritic cells (DC) also contribute to this part of the immune system, as discussed in detail below.

Self, nonself, and danger

To recognize invading organisms, innate immune cells need receptors that are able to distinguish self from nonself. These receptors should be germ-line encoded in order to allow for a rapid response, i.e. within hours, in contrast to the more time-consuming processes of adaptive immunity. Furthermore, these receptors should recognize common patterns not present within the host, which are vital for the invading organisms, and therefore cannot easily be switched off. The innate immune system then activates and controls the adaptive immunity bridging these two systems (Medzhitov and Janeway 1997).

As mentioned above, these patterns are now commonly referred to as PAMPs, but it should be noted that they are expressed not only by pathogens, but also by commensals. The so-called PRRs are able to recognize a wide array of different PAMPs, including proteins, polysaccharides, glycolipids, lipids, and nucleic acid, as discussed below. Notably, some PRRs also detect endogenous ligands. These findings may be explained by the recently proposed 'danger model' (Matzinger 2002), which, in contrast to the 'self–nonself' model explained before, states that PRRs not only recognize structures of invading organisms, but also recognize molecules associated with dangerous circumstances in common, including, for example, breakdown products of necrotic cells (Figure 7.1). Recent studies confirm this hypothesis by showing that only structures released by necrotic (or 'attacked') cells, but not apoptotic (or 'selfinduced death') cells, share this feature (Sauter et al. 2000).

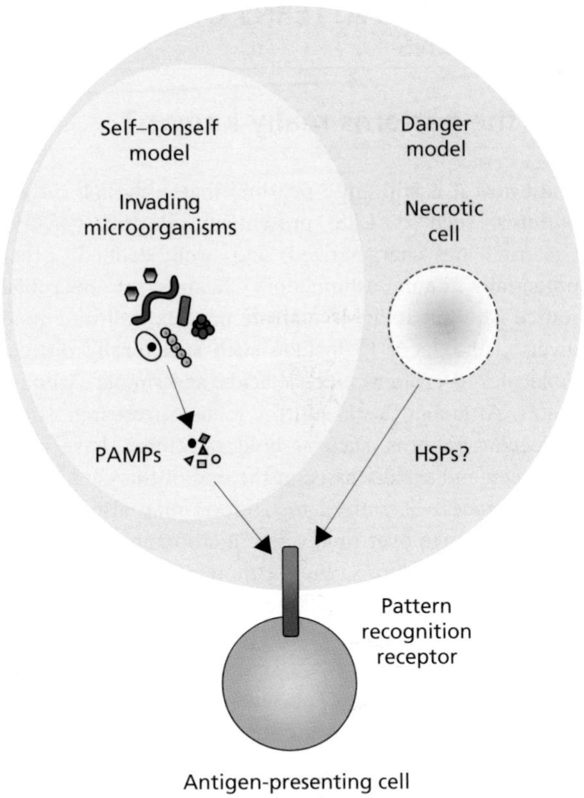

Figure 7.1 *General principles of pattern recognition by antigen-presenting cells (APC). APCs such as macrophages or dendritic cells (DC) play a key role in early innate immunity. They recognize molecular patterns associated with infection or danger via pattern recognition receptors (PRR). According to the self–nonself model, PRRs exclusively recognize pathogen-associated molecular patterns (PAMP), followed by the initiation of immune responses. The proposed danger model suggests that, in addition to PAMPs, endogenous molecular patterns associated with infection or trauma, e.g. partial structures of necrotic cells or released heat shock proteins (HSP), bind to PRRs, initiating an immune response.*

CELLS OF THE INNATE IMMUNE SYSTEM

Antigen-presenting cells

Cells participating in innate immune recognition share the ability of detecting invading microorganisms via PRRs, followed by phagocytosis and digestion. Next, partial structures are shuttled to the outside of the cell in order to present them to other immune cells via major histocompatibility complex (MHC) class I and II molecules (Thery and Amigorena 2001). The complex process of antigen presentation is described in detail in other chapters of this volume. Immune cells sharing this feature are commonly referred to as antigen-presenting cells (APC).

Antigen-presenting cells include granulocytes, monocytes, and macrophages, as well as DCs (Underhill et al. 1999a). As a result of their capacity to present antigen and thus to orchestrate the induction of the adaptive immune response, DCs are currently studied extensively in almost all fields of immunology, including tumor immunology (Banchereau and Steinman 1998). To give an overview of these cells centrally involved in pattern recognition and innate immunity, Figure 7.2 shows how hemopoietic stem cells differentiate early on into common myeloid progenitor cells (CMP) and common lymphoid progenitor cells (CLP).

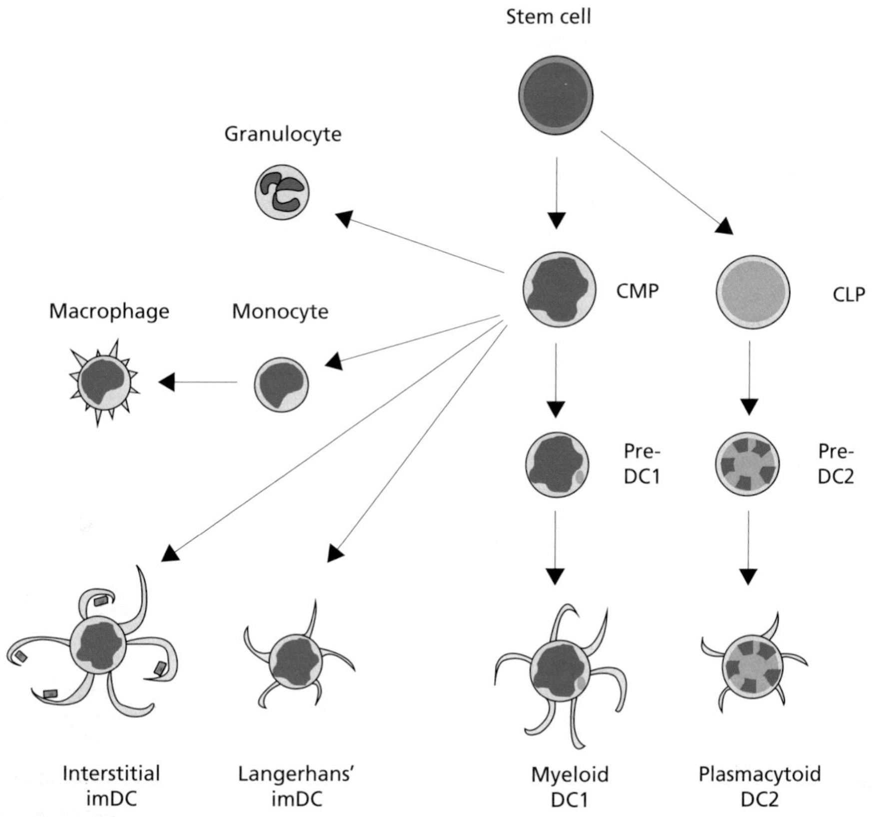

Figure 7.2 *Overview on the hemopoiesis of antigen-presenting cells. Hemopoietic stem cells differentiate into common myeloid progenitor cells (CMP) and common lymphoid progenitor cells (CLP). CMPs give rise to granulocytes and monocytes, which are able to differentiate into tissue macrophages. CMPs can also differentiate into immature dendritic cells (imDC). The imDCs found in the skin are referred to as Langerhans' imDCs, whereas those migrating to the dermis and other tissues are called interstitial imDCs. These are, in contrast to the Langerhans' cells, capable of large-scale phagocytosis and produce interleukin 10 (IL-10), leading to activation of T and B lymphocytes. CMPs are furthermore progenitors of the so-called premature myeloid or DC type 1 cells (pre-DC1), which, similar to their immature interstitial counterparts, are capable of phagocytosis. Premature plasmacytoid or DC type 2 (pre-DC2) cells, in contrast, are unable to phagocytose microorganisms; instead they are producers of the type 1 interferons, i.e. interferon-α and -β.*

Hemopoiesis of dendritic cells

Different classes of DCs have been described and are found in specific tissues of the host: CMPs differentiate into granulocytes, monocytes, and $CD34^+$ late progenitor cells. The last include two subsets: CLA^+ and CLA^- cells. CLA^+ cells differentiate into $CD11c^+CD1a^+$ Langerhans' cell precursors, which migrate into the skin and develop into Langerhans' immature DCs (imDC). CLA^- cells differentiate into $CD11c^+CD1a^-$ interstitial DC precursors, which travel to the dermis, becoming interstitial dendtritic cells. This subset of imDCs is capable of ingesting large quantities of microbial material and initiating IgM production by B cells. CMPs also differentiate into pre-DCs type 1 or monocytic pre-DCs, whereas CLPs differentiate into pre-DCs type 2 or plasmacytoid DCs. Pre-DCs type 1 express antigens related to monocytes, including CD14, CD11, CD13, and CD33 (Liu et al. 2001), whereas pre-DCs type 2 bear markers related to lymphocytes, such as pre-T-antigen and Spi-B (Spits et al. 2000; Bendriss-Vermare et al. 2001). In general, pre-DCs type 1 are capable of phagocytosis of microorganisms, whereas pre-DCs type 2 synthesize large amounts of class 1 interferons, with implications for immune responses to viral infections, as discussed in detail below (Kadowaki and Liu 2002).

PATTERN RECOGNITION RECEPTORS

Basic characteristics

A growing number of PRRs have been identified and are summarized in Table 7.1. Generally two classes can be distinguished: one binds microbial structures leading to detoxification and inhibition of cellular responses. The other group is involved in the induction of signal transduction and the stimulation of responses of the innate immune system. Cellular PRRs are generally found within the membrane of any host cell; however, they are predominantly found in APCs. Furthermore, intracellular forms of PRRs have been described with the function of binding microbial structures after phagocytosis of microorganisms. Finally, soluble PRRs, with

Table 7.1 *Overview on pattern recognition receptors*

Receptor	Origin	Ligands	Function
Cell surface			
Type 3 complement receptor	Monocytes/macrophages	Complement opsonized particles	Phagocytosis
Scavenger receptors	Macrophages	Anionic polymers	Clearance/phagocytosis
C-type lectins	Macrophages	Carbohydrates with mannose residues	Phagocytosis
CD14	Monocytes/macrophages	LPS, LTA, lipoproteins, peptidoglycan	Cytokine induction
Toll-like receptors	Various, including monocytes/ macrophages, dendritic cells, endothelia	Various, including compounds derived from bacteria, virus, fungi, and protozoa	Cytokine induction
Intracellular			
BPI	Neutrophilic granulocytes	LPS	Killing of engulfed gram-negative bacteria
nod1/nod2	Various, including monocytes/ macrophages and epithelia	Peptidoglycan	Innate immune responses
Soluble			
LPS-binding protein	Acute phase protein synthesized in the liver	LPS, LTA	Cytokine induction
CRP	Acute phase protein synthesized in the liver	Phosphorylcholine	Activation of the classic complement pathway
Soluble CD14	Monocytes/macrophages	LPS, LTA, lipoproteins Peptidoglycan	Cytokine induction

According to Medzhitov et al. (1997), PRRs can be classified regarding their distribution in cell-surface, intracellular and soluble PRRs. This table gives an overview on some PRRs, their origin and their function. Note that, in some cases, origin and function are currently still the subject of controversial discussion.
BPI, bactericidal/permeability increasing protein; CRP, C-reactive protein; LBP, LPS-binding protein; LPS, lipopolysaccharide; LTA, lipoteichoic acid.

the function of binding and presenting the microbial target to cellular receptor or enabling phagocytosis (opsonic function), have also been described. A common feature of all PRRs is that they recognize common structures of invading microorganisms, followed by the initiation of immune responses. PRRs can be distinguished into cell-surface, intracellular, and secreted PRRs (Medzhitov 2001) (Table 7.1).

Cell-surface PRRs

Besides the TLR family, which is discussed in detail later, other cellular receptors for microbial ligands have been described, and three examples are given here. A membrane-bound PRR is the type 3 complement receptor, a β_2-integrin also known as CD18/CD11b. It is present on macrophages, enabling phagocytosis of complement-opsonized particles or whole pathogens (Ross 2000). CD18/CD11b has been proposed as being involved in LPS-mediated signal transduction in cooperation with CD14; however, these results are still not conclusive (Flo et al. 2000). Furthermore, the large family of scavenger receptors is expressed not only by macrophages but also by certain endothelial cells. They bind to a wide array of polyanionic ligands, including exogenous molecules such as LPS of gram-negative bacteria or endogenous compounds, i.e. low-density lipoprotein (LDL) (Krieger and Stern 2001). Interaction of bacterial ligands with members of the scavenger receptor family does not induce signal transduction, but leads to detoxification of the ligands.

Another group of cell surface PRRs is the C-type lectins, including mannose receptors and dendritic cell-specific ICAM-grabbing nonintegrin (DC-SIGN). Mannose receptors are expressed by macrophages, DCs, and some endothelial cells, whereas DC-SIGN is restricted to DCs (Geijtenbeek et al. 2002). They bind mannosyl/fucosyl as well as glucosamine residues (East and Isacke 2002), which are commonly found on the bacterial surface. The interaction of mannose receptors with pathogens, affecting intracellular signaling, is not fully elucidated by now, however, there is evidence that virulent strains of *Mycobacterium tuberculosis* are phagocytosed via a pathway involving mannose receptors, whereas their avirulent counterparts are not (Kang and Schlesinger 1998).

Intracellular PRRs

BACTERICIDAL/PERMEABILITY INCREASING PROTEIN

Bactericidal/permeability-increasing protein (BPI) is a predominantly intracellular protein with the ability to bind LPS with high affinity (Weiss et al. 1978). It can therefore be referred to as an intracellular PRR. BPI is found within the primary granules of polymorphonuclear neutrophils (PMN), has bactericidal properties toward gram-negative bacteria, and apparently binds whole bacteria or LPS within the phagocytic compartment of the cell in order to kill engulfed bacteria. BPI is one of the first PRRs that entered clinical trials (Neuprex) in order to modulate the innate immune response brought about by LPS during sepsis, which is discussed in the final chapters (Elsbach and Weiss 1998).

Recently, intracellular PRRs termed 'NOD1' and 'NOD2' were described with the ability to participate in the induction of programmed cell death. It has been suggested that NODs, which share structural similarity with TLRs, are involved in intracellular recognition of LPS and other bacterial partial structures; however, these results still have to be confirmed (Inohara and Nunez 2001). The next section covers some of the results from basic science on NOD2 and the final section of this chapter summarizes the findings of the relationship between NOD2 polymorphisms and Crohn's disease. TLR-9 is another intracellular PRR that recognizes bacterial DNA, which is discussed separately later under Recognition of bacterial DNA by TLR-9.

PRR ROLE FOR NOD2/CARD 15?

A member of a recently discovered, growing family of proteins containing a so-called caspase-recruitment domain (CARD) involved in apoptosis regulation, originally termed 'nucleotide-binding oligomerization domain (NOD)', has recently been postulated to recognize LPS and bacterial muramyldipeptide (MDP) intracellularly (Girardin et al. 2003; Inohara et al. 2003). NOD proteins are related to the family of membrane-bound R-proteins of plants involved in plant host defense (Dangl and Jones 2001). Several NOD proteins in humans have been identified and NOD1 (also called CARD 4) has been implicated with LPS recognition, whereas NOD2 (also called CARD 15), although previously suggested also to recognize LPS, has recently been shown to be involved in MDP recognition (Inohara and Nunez 2001; Inohara et al. 2003).

The NOD proteins all contain leucin-rich repeat (LRR) domains and share homology with the apoptosis regulator apoptotic protease-activating factor-1 (Apaf-1) (Bertin et al. 1999). NOD2/CARD 15 is expressed only by monocytes and recently has gained attention because of a correlation of SNPs with the incidence of Crohn's disease and a rare disease called Blau syndrome (arthritis, uveitis, and skin rash) in humans (see details later under The NOD2/*CARD15* SNPs). A frameshift mutation here leads to a truncated protein that is apparently unable to respond to LPS or MDP (Ogura et al. 2001b; Girardin et al. 2003; Inohara et al. 2003).

The CARD-containing proteins and certain TLRs signal via a CARD-containing serine/threonine kinase termed 'RICK/Rip2/CARDIAK', leading to NF-κB translocation (Kobayashi et al. 2002). The family of CARD/NOD proteins, in summary, are related to TLRs and CD14 with regard to their structure of LRRs, and may serve as intracellular sensors for PAMPs.

Soluble PRRs

SOLUBLE CD14

CD14 is a PRR present on monocytes, macrophages, granulocytes, and DCs, attached to the cell via a phosphatidylinositol (PI) anchor that is unable to transduce signals into the cell (Goyert et al. 1988; Pugin et al. 1994). Cellular CD14 has been shown to be part of a lipid raft allowing for clustering of several PRRs upon ligand stimulation (Pfeiffer et al. 2001). This may serve the function of concentrating bacterial ligands locally in order to be presented to a signal-transducing receptor such as members of the TLR family (Schmitz and Orso 2002).

A second, slightly smaller, form of CD14 termed 'soluble CD14' (sCD14) is released into serum, and both forms play a crucial role in pattern recognition (Schumann and Latz 2000). CD14 has been shown to bind to LPS, a glycolipid present in the outer membranes of gram-negative bacteria (Wright et al. 1990; Rietschel et al. 1996; Alexander and Rietschel 2001). CD14 is also involved in recognition of other bacteria and in initiation of phagocytosis. It leads to an accumulation of PAMPs, enabling recognition by the signal-transducing molecules of the TLR family (Schumann et al. 1994; Landmann et al. 2000). CD14 contains LRRs, a structural characteristic typical of many PRRs including the TLRs addressed in detail below under The family of Toll-like receptors (Ziegler-Heitbrock and Ulevitch 1993).

LIPOPOLYSACCHARIDE-BINDING PROTEIN

During cell growth and death, gram-negative microorganisms release LPS (Brandtzaeg et al. 1989), and in serum it is primarily recognized and bound by LPS-binding protein (LBP), (Figure 7.3), another soluble PRR. LBP is mainly synthesized in the liver, catalyzing the transfer of LPS to CD14 (Schumann et al. 1990) and enabling the cells to respond with, for example, cytokine release (Figure 7.3 and Table 7.1) (Alexander and Rietschel 2001). LBP is a typical acute phase protein that is induced upon stimulation during the acute phase response via interleukin 1 (IL-1), IL-6, and dexamethasone (Schumann et al. 1996). It belongs to a family of proteins that share the ability to bind lipid-like structures including another LBP called BPI, cholesterol ester-transfer protein (CETP), and phospholipid-transfer protein (PLTP) (Kirschning et al. 1997).

Epithelial cells both of intestinal origin and from the respiratory tract have been found to be sources of LBP as well (Vreugdenhil et al. 1999; Dentener et al. 2000). Both CD14 and LBP have been found to be involved in

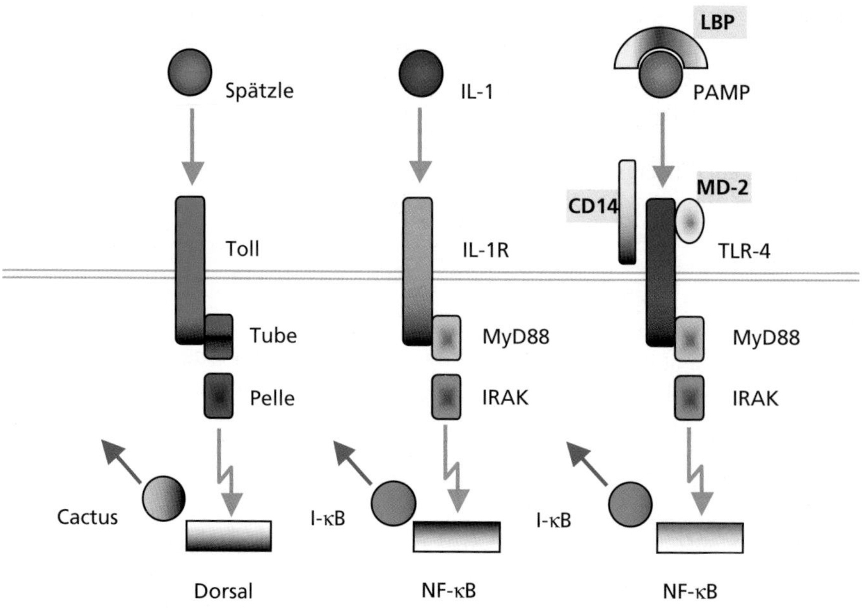

Figure 7.3 *Comparison of signal transduction via drosophila Toll-like receptors (TLR), interleukin 1 receptor (IL-1R), and TLR-4. In* Drosophila, *signal transduction via Toll is initiated by the cleavage of the endogenous ligand* spätzle, *which binds to Toll, initiating a signal transduction cascade involving the adapter molecule* tube *and the kinase* pelle. *After the inhibitory factor* cactus *has dissociated, the transcription factor dorsal translocates into the nucleus, initiating certain transcriptional events. This pathway – because of the sequence homologies – shares striking similarities with the known IL-1R, as well as with the recently identified TLR-4 signaling pathway (almost similar among all other members of the TLR family). After the receptor has recognized its ligand (IL-1 or lipopolysaccharide (LPS)), signaling in both cases involves the adapter molecule MyD88 and the kinase IRAK. The inhibitory factor IF-κB dissociates and the transcription factor NF-κB translocates to the nucleus inducing immune responses. An equivalent of the protease cascade, leading to release of the endogenous ligand* spätzle *in the IL-1/TLR pathway has not yet been found. Instead, for recognition of LPS, several soluble pattern recognition receptors (PRR) are involved with LPS-binding protein (LBP), transferring LPS to the receptor complex, which in addition to TLR-4 also involves CD14 and MD-2.*

recognition of other bacterial structures, such as spirochetal glycolipids, pneumococcal peptidoglycan, lipoteichoic acid (LTA), and others (Perera et al. 1997; Kurt-Jones et al. 2000; Schroder et al. 2000, 2003).

Recently LBP was found to serve a dual role during infection, depending on the local concentration in relation to the concentration of the bacterial ligand. Although small concentrations of LBP enable host cell responses to LPS, high concentrations of LBP, as present in human serum, inhibited cellular LPS-induced signaling (Lamping et al. 1998; Hamann et al. 2000; Zweigner et al. 2001). The soluble PRR LBP may serve both of the functions of innate immunity mentioned above. Early detection of pathogens and induction of the immune response, and fighting off the bacteria and inhibiting its host effects, depend on its concentration, which is tightly regulated during the acute phase.

THE FAMILY OF TOLL-LIKE RECEPTORS

General characteristics of TLRs

BASIC LESSONS LEARNED FROM FLIES

Drosophila Toll was discovered in the early 1980s during a mutagenesis screen by Anderson and Nüsslein-Vollhard (1984). It was further characterized as a factor crucial for dorsoventral axis formation within the drosophila embryo and includes a total of 12 genes (Hashimoto et al. 1988). It is said that the German researcher and Nobel laureate Christine Nüsslein-Volhard, after discovery of this factor, spontaneously shouted 'Toll!', which in German means 'great!'. Toll activation in *Drosophila* also involves a ligand termed *spätzle*, the adaptor protein *tube*, the protein kinase *pelle*, as well as the transcription factor *dorsal* and its inhibitor *cactus* (Medzhitov and Janeway 1998) (see Figure 7.3).

In the late 1990s it was found that there are striking sequence similarities between all members of this pathway and the mammalian interleukin 1 receptor (IL-1R) signal transduction pathway (Medzhitov et al. 1997). It was postulated that *toll* may also play a role in the innate immunity of *Drosophila*. This was supported by the finding that fruit flies deficient of members of this pathway are highly susceptible to fungal infections, however, immunity against bacteria is not impaired (Lemaitre et al. 1996). Another member of the *toll* family, 18-wheeler, is apparently involved in bacterial recognition (Williams et al. 1997), although the signaling pathways involved are different from *toll* (Medzhitov 2001). A further demonstration of an immune function of *toll* relates to its involvement in the induction of antimicrobial peptides, i.e. Drosomycin and Metchnikowin (reviewed in Imler and Hoffmann 2002, 2003).

FIRST EVIDENCE FOR THE ROLE OF TLRS IN MAMMALS

The previous results, and the fact that IL-1 stimulation of human cells leads to similar effects as compared with stimulation with bacterial ligands, led to studies investigating the potential role of mammalian homologs of *toll*, also called 'Toll-like receptors' in innate immunity (Rock et al. 1998). First reports concluded that human TLR-2 was involved in LPS-mediated signaling (Kirschning et al. 1998; Yang et al. 1998). Later it was found that these studies may have been performed in the presence of lipoproteins, structures now known to be classic TLR-2 agonists. Extensive positional cloning studies that analyzed LPS-hyporesponsive C3H/HeJ mice and the formerly termed LPS gene, leading to hyporesponsiveness to LPS, led to the finding that these mice carried a mutation in the gene encoding for TLR-4. These studies and the development of the TLR-4 knockout mouse revealed that TLR-4 was the long-sought-after LPS gene responsible for detection of LPS (Poltorak et al. 1998; Beutler et al. 2001). It is now agreed that TLR-2 recognizes a wide variety of other bacterial ligands, mainly of gram-positive pathogens (see below under Ligands of the heterodimeric TLR-2–TLR-1–TLR-6 complex, and Table 7.2) and some rare and atypical forms of LPS.

STRUCTURE OF TLRs

All TLRs described by now are type I transmembrane receptors characterized by the presence of LRRs within the extracellular domain (O'Neill and Dinarello 2000). The role of LRRs in TLR function is currently not completely elucidated. However, proteins exhibiting LRRs, e.g. ribonuclease inhibitors (Kobe and Deisenhofer 1995), have been shown to exhibit a 'horseshoe-like' structure (Figure 7.4), with the LRRs being relevant for interaction with a proteinaceous ligand. It should be noted that other PRRs besides the TLRs, such as CD14, the NODs, and RP105, share the LRR architecture (Kirschning and Schumann 2002). It is thus tempting to speculate that this structural feature is involved in pattern recognition brought about by these proteins.

Toll-like receptors all possess an intracellular signaling region exhibiting homologies to IL-1R, also referred to as Toll/IL-1R receptor (TIR) domain (see Figure 7.3). There are a total of 20 proteins with TIR domains so far identified in the human genome, and many TIR-domain-containing proteins have been described in other species including plants (O'Neill 2002). The structure of the TIR domain of TLR-1 and -2 has recently been solved; it contains a crucial region for signaling, as the mutation of the LPS-unresponsive HeJ mouse is located in this region (Xu et al. 2000). Signal transduction events initiated by TLR–ligand interaction are discussed in detail later under Signal transduction cascade induced by TLR-ligand interaction. It may be noteworthy that RP105, a receptor associated with MD-1 and also containing LRRs, lacks a TIR domain. Apparently, most of the TLRs described form heterodimers in order to induce signaling, TLR-4 most probably forming homodimers.

Table 7.2 *Toll-like receptors and their agonists: an overview*

Receptor	Ligand
TLR-1	Diacylated lipoproteins/lipopeptides (TLR-1/2 heterodimers)
TLR-2	Lipoproteins/lipopeptides (various)
	Peptidoglycan (gram-positive bacteria)
	Lipoteichoic acid (gram-positive bacteria)
	Lipoarabinomannan (mycobacteria)
	Spirochetal glycolipids (*Treponema* spp.)
	Zymosan (crude candida particles)
	Atypical lipopolysaccharide (LPS) (*Leptospira interrogans*)
	Atypical LPS (*Porphyromonas gingivalis*)[a]
	Glycoinositolphospholipids (*Trypanosoma cruzi*)
	Neisseria porins
	Heat shock protein (HSP) 70 (host)
TLR-3	Double-stranded RNA
TLR-4	LPS (gram-negative bacteria)[b]
	Respiratory syncytial virus fusion protein
	HSP 60 (*Chlamydia* spp.)
	β-Defensins (host)
	HSP 60 (host)
	HSP 70 (host)[c]
TLR-5	Bacterial flagellin
TLR-6	Triacylated lipoproteins/lipopeptides (TLR-1/6/ heterodimers)
TLR-7	Imidazoquinolines (antiviral compounds)
	Loxoribine (antiviral compounds)
	Single-stranded V-rich RNA (in mice)
TLR-8	See TLR-7
TLR-9	CpG DNA
TLR-11	Uropathogenic *E. coli* (in mice)

Ligands are ordered according to the different members of the TLR family. Note that some reports have been questioned.
a) Synthetic LPS of *P. gingivalis* has been reported to act as a TLR-4 ligand.
b) According to some investigators, LPS is the sole ligand for TLR-4.
c) Human HSP 70 has been reported to be devoid of stimulating capacities in the absence of contaminating LPS.

TLR TISSUE DISTRIBUTION

Toll-like receptors are not equally distributed among APCs, with monocytes as well as monocytoid or type 1 DCs expressing a rather wide variety of TLRs, whereas plasmacytoid or type 2 DCs preferentially express TLR-7 and TLR-9 (Kadowaki et al. 2001) (Table 7.2). Other cells types not exclusively contributing to innate immunity have also been described as expressing different TLRs, e.g. endothelial cells predominantly exhibit TLR-4, whereas TLR-2 is usually weakly expressed (Faure et al. 2000), a pattern that is also found in intestinal epithelial cells (Melmed et al. 2003). TLR-3 expression appears to be restricted to DCs, whereas TLR-9 is

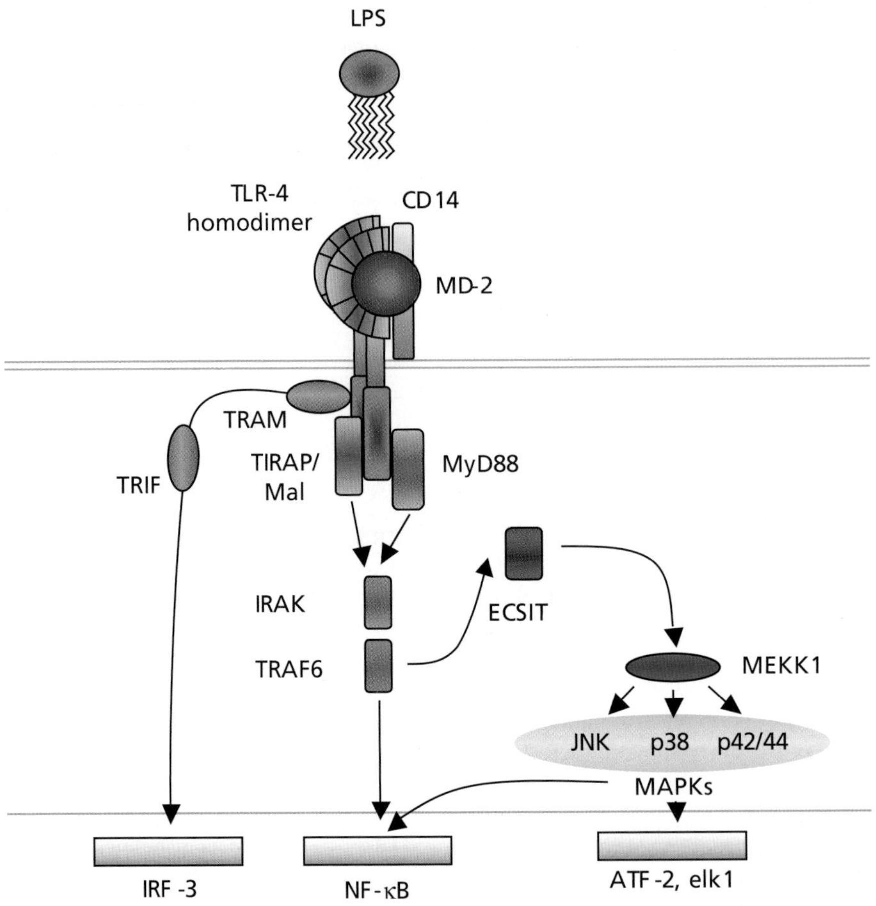

Figure 7.4 *Signaling pathways of Toll-like receptor 4 (TLR-4). Lipopolysaccharide (LPS) interacts with its receptor complex consisting of CD14, MD-2, and a TLR-4 homodimer or multimer. There are several pathways leading to signal transduction into the nucleus, which are discussed in detail later under Signal transduction cascade induced by TLR-ligand interaction. The MyD88-dependent pathway, in addition to MyD88, involves IRAK, TRAF-6, and the transcription factor NF-κB. TRAF6 also interacts with ECSIT, in turn leading to activation of MAP/erk kinase kinase (MEKK1) and subsequently several MAPKs, involving p38, p42/44, and JNK. Diacylated amphiphilic ligands, such as MALP-2 or lipotechoic acid (LTA) interacting with TLR-2/TLR-6 heterodimers, have been shown to activate several other transcription factors, including ATF-2 and elk1. There are at least two MyD88-independent signal transduction pathways: One involves TIRAP/Mal, which activates IRAK and the other downstream elements known from the MyD88-dependent pathway. Furthermore, activation of the TLR-4 receptor complex via recently identified signaling elements TRAM and TRIF leads to activation of Interferon regulatory factor 3 (IRF-3).*

detectable predominantly on B cells and, as mentioned above, type 2 DCs (Muzio et al. 2000). TLR-2 has been shown to be expressed, or upregulated, within the brain (Koedel et al. 2003). The following sections discuss the characteristics of particular TLR subfamilies in detail; a general overview on the agonists found for the given TLRs is given in Table 7.3.

TLR-1, TLR-2, TLR-6, and TLR-10

LIGANDS OF THE HETERODIMERIC TLR-2–TLR-1–TLR-6 COMPLEX

Toll-like receptor 2 was the first member of the TLR family shown to be involved in pattern recognition (Kirschning et al. 1998). Over the last few years TLR-2 has been found to be involved in recognition of microorganisms of almost all types including, for example, peptidoglycan and LTA of gram-positive bacteria (Schwandner et al. 1999; Opitz et al. 2001), bacterial lipopeptides of *Borrelia* and *Mycoplasma* spp. (Lien et al. 1999), lipoarabinomannan of mycobacteria (Means et al. 1999), and zymosan of *Candida* spp. (Underhill et al. 1999b) (reviewed in Kirschning and Schumann 2002). TLR-2 apparently does not interact with MD-2 but, as CD14 has been shown to play a crucial role in cytokine induction by LTA, peptidoglycan, and lipopeptides (Weidemann et al. 1997; Sellati et al. 1998; Hermann et al. 2002), it is very likely that CD14 is also part of the TLR-2 receptor complex. TLR-2, next to its cell surface expression, also appears intracellularly, but only after phagocytic processes (Underhill et al. 1999b).

The high degree of homology among TLR-2, TLR-1, and TLR-6 corresponds to the fact that these receptors are able to form heterodimers (Ozinsky et al. 2000). Apparently, LTA and mycoplasma lipopeptide

Table 7.3 *Ligands of Toll-like receptors classified according to their origins*

Organism	Substance class	Ligand	Receptor
Bacteria	Glycolipid	LPS (gram-negative)	TLR-4
		LPS *L. interrogans*	TLR-2
		LTA (gram-positive) lipoarabinomannan (mycobacteria)	TLR-2
		Spirochetal glycolipids (*Treponema* spp.)	TLR-2
	Lipoprotein/lipopeptide	Lipoprotein (*Borrelia burgdorferi*)	TLR-2/-1
		Mycoplasma spp. (lipopeptide)	TLR-2/-6
	Nucleic acid	CpG	TLR-9
	Protein	Flagellin	TLR-5
		Neisseria porins	TLR-4
		Chlamydia HSP	TLR-2
	?	Uropathogenic *E. coli*	TLR-11
Fungi	Various	Zymosan	TLR-2
Protozoa	Glycolipids	Glycoinositolphospholipids	TLR-2
Virus	Nucleic acid	Double-stranded RNA	TLR-3
		Single-stranded RNA	TLR-7/-8
	Protein	RSV fusion protein	TLR-4
Endogenous	Saccharides	Hyaluronic acid oligomers	TLR-4
		Heparan sulfate	TLR-4
	Proteins	HSP 60 and 70	TLR-4
		HSP 70	TLR-2
		β-Defensins	TLR-4
Others		Paclitaxel	TLR-4
		Antiviral compounds	TLR-7/-8

TLR ligands are classified according to their origin. Ligands derived from bacteria, viruses, fungi, and parasites are listed. Note that there are also reports on endogenous ligands of TLRs derived from the host, not listed here.
HSP, heat shock protein; LPS, lipopolysaccharide; LTA, lipoteichoic acid; RSV, respiratory syncytial virus.

(MALP-2) are recognized by dimers consisting of TLR-2 and TLR-6 (Morr et al. 2002; Takeuchi et al. 2001), whereas borrelia lipoproteins and their synthetic lipopeptide counterparts, respectively, interact with TLR-2/TLR-1 dimers (Takeuchi et al. 2002). Taken together, these data indicate that diacylated amphiphilic molecules (i.e. MALP and LTA) in common are recognized by TLR-2/TLR-6, whereas triacylated molecules (i.e. borrelia lipoproteins) are recognized by TLR-2/TLR-1 (Figure 7.5). Until now, however, no ligand has been described for TLR-10. As this putative receptor exhibits high homology to TLR-1 and TLR-6, it is tempting to speculate that it also forms heterodimers with TLR-2.

IS THERE STILL EVIDENCE FOR TLR-2 BEING AN LPS RECEPTOR?

There have been several reports on 'atypical' LPS molecules interacting with TLR-2 and not with TLR-4. These reports mainly focused on the LPS of *Leptospira interrogans* and *Porphyromonas gingivalis* (Hirschfeld et al. 2001; Werts et al. 2001). In this context, the term 'atypical' describes a lipid A portion of LPS being less phosphorylated and lacking secondary fatty acids compared with the well-characterized Enterobacteriaceae lipid A. However, *Porphyromonas gingivalis* LPS has been described to act as a sole TLR-4 agonist after extensive purification, and synthetic preparations of its lipid A also do not display any interaction with TLR-2 (Ogawa et al. 2002).

Toll-like receptor 3

Toll-like receptor 3 has been shown to recognize double-stranded RNA (dsRNA), which is found during viral infections (Alexopoulou et al. 2001). This evidence was obtained by transfection of a TLR-3-negative cell line, rendering it responsive to dsRNA, as well as studies on TLR-3-deficient mice, which were more susceptible to administered dsRNA in comparison to their wild-type counterparts.

Signal transduction involves MyD88 and NF-κB, or the MyD88-independent TICAM-1 pathway (see later under Signal transduction cascade induced by TLR-ligand interaction). Double-stranded RNA, or its synthetic counterpart, polyinosinic–polycytidylic acid [poly(I):poly(C)] (Alexopoulou et al. 2001) is known to be a potent inducer of type I interferons, such as interferon-α (IFN-α) and IFN-β, which are mainly synthesized by plasmacytoid DCs. However, these cells do not express TLR-3 (Kadowaki et al. 2001). Thus, dsRNA may in addition interact with other receptors. Furthermore, TLR-3, predominantly expressed in monocytoid DCs, may also bind other as yet unidentified ligands. TLR-3 stimulation has recently been

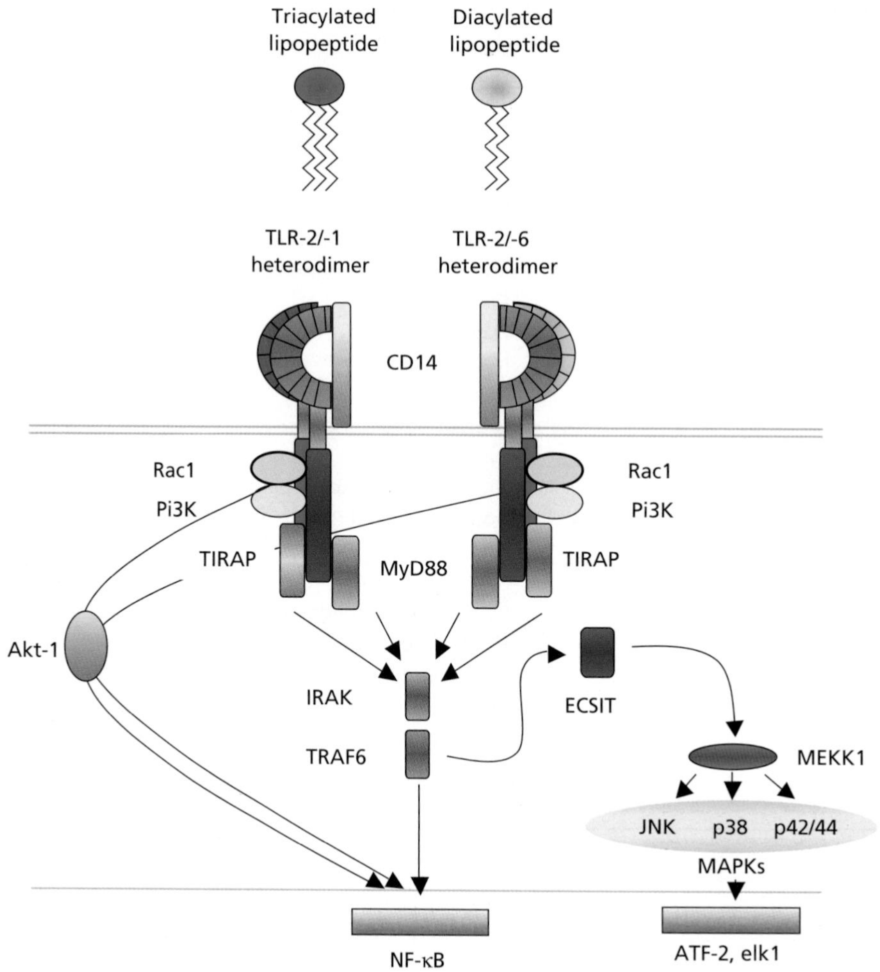

Figure 7.5 *Toll-like receptor 2 (TLR-2)-associated signaling pathways. The TLR-2 receptor complex consists of a heterodimer and apparently involves CD14, as well as TLR-1 or TLR-6. Triacylated amphiphilic molecules, i.e. lipopeptides based on the lipoprotein basic structure of* Borrelia burgdorferi *lipoproteins, interact with TLR-2/TLR-1 heterodimers, whereas diacylated amphiphilic ligands, such as MALP-2 or lipoteichoic acid (LTA), interact with TLR-2/TLR-6 heterodimers. Signal transduction involves the MyD88-dependent pathway or the TIRAP/Mal pathway, largely MyD88 independent (see Figure 7.4). Furthermore, NF-κB translocation is brought about by a signaling cascade involving phosphatidylinositol 3 (PI-3) kinase and Rac1, forming a complex with TLR-2, and AKT. Note that this pathway has also been demonstrated for TLR-4.*

found to induce a complex set of antiviral responses, which are more efficient in fighting viruses compared with stimulation of TLR-4 (Doyle et al. 2003).

Toll-like receptor 4

THE LPS RECEPTOR

With the exception of the LPS–TLR-2 interaction mentioned above, TLR-4 is currently viewed as the sole receptor for bacterial LPS (Beutler et al. 2001). The term 'receptor' appears premature because LPS binding to TLR-4 has not been shown yet; however, binding of LPS to MD-2, a TLR-4 adaptor protein, could be demonstrated (Viriyakosol et al. 2001). It is most likely that TLR-4 forms homodimers or multimers and this receptor complex also involves CD14 and the adaptor molecule MD-2 (da Silva Correia et al. 2001).

Despite the previous finding that TLR-2 is involved in LPS recognition, numerous studies have provided evidence that TLR-4 is the main cellular 'receptor' for LPS (Chow et al. 1999; Heine et al. 1999). TLR-4, therefore, has been found to contain the ability to discriminate LPS types differing in their lipid content within their lipid A moiety, leading to divergent levels of activity (Lien et al. 2000). Transfection of TLR-4 from different species was able to transfer the ability of certain types of LPS to act as active agonist, inactive non-competitive molecule, or antagonist (Poltorak et al. 2000). It has also been shown, by laser scanning microscopy, that the CD14–TLR-4–MD-2 complex specifically travels within the cell to and from the Golgi apparatus transporting LPS, a process that is, however, separate from the induction of signal transduction (Latz et al. 2002).

The crucial role of MD-2 for LPS recognition by TLR-4 could be demonstrated by transfection experiments

(Shimazu et al. 1999), as well as by studies employing MD-2-mutant cell lines (Schromm et al. 2001). Recently, the generation of MD-2-deficient mice clearly showed that MD-2 is absolutely essential for host LPS recognition (Nagai et al. 2002). MD-2 has been shown to form dimers; however, the monomeric form seems to be important for LPS recognition (Re and Strominger 2002). The principle of TLR-4 and MD-2 forming a receptor complex exhibits striking similarities with RP105, the LRR-containing receptor present on B lymphocytes that is associated with an MD-2-related adaptor protein called MD-1 (Miyake and Shimazu 1998). RP105, however, is the only LRR-containing molecule lacking the TIR domain described later, which has been found to be essential for signaling (Miyake 2003).

NON-LPS LIGANDS OF TLR-4

Following the finding that LPS is an agonist for TLR-4, other potential ligands have been proposed to interact with the TLR-4 receptor complex, which are, apart from paclitaxel (Kawasaki et al. 2000), proteins. These include bacterial chlamydia heat shock proteins (HSP) (Costa et al. 2002), viral respiratory syncytial virus (RSV) fusion protein (Kurt-Jones et al. 2000), as well as endogenous compounds, especially host HSPs (Ohashi et al. 2000) (summarized in Table 7.3). It should be noted that studies of interactions of TLR-4 with proteins expressed in gram-negative bacteria, such as *E. coli*, are often hampered by contaminating LPS. Therefore, results obtained with recombinant proteins have to be interpreted carefully, and recent studies came to the conclusion that some of the effects described were mediated by contaminating LPS (Bausinger et al. 2002).

However, RSV-F protein, after protease digestion, exhibited a diminished activity, indicating an interaction of this proteinaceous ligand with TLR-4. For the large and quite diverse family of HSPs, which may be viewed as sensors for necrosis, it has been shown that they also activate innate immune cells (reviewed in Vabulas et al. 2002). For HSPs of both bacterial and mammalian origin, TLR involvement in signaling has been proposed, with human HSP60 and Gp96 being the most prominent ones (Vabulas et al. 2001). The regulation of the host's innate immune response by proteins released by cells may be explained by the above-mentioned 'danger model', with HSPs indicating tissue injury or imbalance of hemostasis. HSPs activate macrophages and DCs and evidence has been obtained that both CD14 and TLR-2, as well as TLR-4, may be involved (Asea et al. 2002).

Toll-like receptor 5

BACTERIAL FLAGELLIN IS THE AGONIST OF TLR-5

Many enteric bacteria possess flagella responsible for motility and directed movement. The flagellum consists of a filament and a hook with the filament being made up of 11 flagellin monomers (reviewed in Smith and Ozinsky 2002). This 55-kDa flagellin protein has been shown to be a potent inducer of inflammation. Flagellin has been recently demonstrated to act as an agonist for another member of the TLR family, TLR-5 (Hayashi et al. 2001). Besides many enteric gram-negative bacteria, gram-positive *Listeria* spp. and spirochetes also contain flagellin, potentially leading to an interaction with TLR-5.

The signal transduction cascade, as has been shown for the other members of the TLR-family, involves MyD88 and NF-κB (Hayashi et al. 2001). Next to mammalians, flagellin is also detected by the immune system of insects and plants. In *Arabidopsis*, a receptor-like kinase termed FLS2 has been identified which interacts with flagellin (Gomez-Gomez and Boller 2000). Interestingly, FLS2 exhibits similarities with TLRs over the presence of LRRs within the extracellular domain. Therefore, recognition of bacterial flagellin appears to be a ubiquitous mechanism of innate immune responses.

POTENTIAL CLINICAL IMPLICATIONS OF TLR-5 FOR GASTROINTESTINAL DISEASES

Intestinal epithelia are only weakly responsive to LPS; however, they react with strong cytokine release on exposure to flagellin (Gewirtz et al. 2001b). TLR-5 appears to be expressed exclusively on the basolateral surface of intestinal cells (Gewirtz et al. 2001a). Therefore, flagellin has to be translocated from the luminal to the basolateral surface in order to elicit immune responses. Pathogenic *Salmonella* spp. translocate into the epithelium, whereas commensal *Escherichia* spp. do not (Gewirtz et al. 2001a). Thus, basolateral expression of TLR-5 might represent a mechanism to distinguish pathogenic from colonizing bacteria. Furthermore bacteria have developed mechanisms to regulate flagellin expression in order to evade TLR-5 recognition, i.e. the human pathogen *Listeria monocytogenes* suppresses flagellin expression at 37°C, whereas the non-pathogenic species *L. innocua* does not (Kathariou et al. 1995).

Toll-like receptors 7, TLR-8, and TLR-9

IMIDAZOQUINOLINES AS LIGANDS FOR TLR-7 AND TLR-8

Toll-like receptors TLR-7, TLR-8, and TLR-9 are closely related. TLR-7 and TLR-8 have been shown to recognize antiviral compounds, the imidazoquinolines, such as imiquimod and R-848 (Hemmi et al. 2002; Jurk et al. 2002), which are commonly used for treatment of anogenital warts caused by human papilloma virus. Recently it has been shown that TLR-7 and -8 recognize single-stranded, V-rich viral RNA (Heil et al. 2004; Diebold et al. 2004; Lund et al. 2004). TLR-9 recognizes bacterial DNA as outlined below. Signal transduction through these receptors, as has been shown for TLR-4 and TLR-2, also involves MyD88 (Hemmi et al. 2000, 2002).

RECOGNITION OF BACTERIAL DNA BY TLR-9

Over the few last years the discovery was made that bacterial DNA differs from eukaryotic DNA in that it exhibits unmethylated CG-rich regions (commonly referred to as 'CpG'). Oligonucleotides containing certain typical nucleotides have been shown to exhibit extensive immunostimulatory capacities (Sparwasser et al. 1997; Krieg 2002). TLR-9 recognizes bacterial DNA, as revealed by studies employing TLR-9-deficient mice that could not be stimulated by CpG oligonucleotides for proinflammatory activation (Hemmi et al. 2000).

TLR-9 is predominantly expressed in plasmacytoid DCs (pre-DC2), and stimulation with CpG-DNA leads to production of high levels of IL-12, initiating a Th1 response. This makes CpG motifs that interact with TLR-9 interesting candidates for immunization strategies (Wagner 2002). In addition, CpG motifs may in the future play a role in gene therapy and cancer immunization strategies (Krieg 1999). It is obvious that, during infections treated by antibiotics, bacterial DNA is released; however, the precise role of CpG-DNA in the pathogenesis of inflammatory diseases or septic shock is still not completely elucidated. In contrast to other TLRs, TLR-9 is not found on the cell surface, but within endosomes (Ahmad-Nejad et al. 2002).

SIGNAL TRANSDUCTION CASCADE INDUCED BY TLR–LIGAND INTERACTION

As mentioned above, there are numerous homologies in the signaling pathways of human TLR activation, drosophila Toll protein, and even plant R-protein signaling (Lemaitre et al. 1996; Kimbrell and Beutler 2001). All systems initially appear to require LRR-containing molecules and, in order to initiate signaling, the presence of TIR domains is essential (Fluhr and Kaplan-Levy 2002). In addition, the human IL-1 signaling pathway displays many similarities to the TLR signaling, which may reflect the ability of the host to amplify certain responses to PAMPs via host molecules such as IL-1, released by immune cells (O'Neill and Dinarello 2000). The homologies among vertebrates, insects, and plants are numerous, and are present basically in every step of signaling. In the following section only the main pathways of TLR signaling in humans are shown.

Myd88-dependent pathways

The signal transduction cascade activated upon interaction of LPS with the TLR-4–CD14–MD-2 receptor complex, as an example for typical and largely similar TLR signaling, is shown in Figure 7.4. MyD88 is an adaptor molecule containing a TIR domain involved in signaling induced by many receptors of the TLR family (Takeuchi and Akira 2002). A difference exists in the additional utilization of the Mal/TIRAP protein mentioned in detail below and termed 'MyD88 independent' (reviewed in O'Neill 2002). Next to the TIR domain, MyD88 also contains a 'death domain' that is found in the downstream signaling molecule IL-1R-associated kinase (IRAK) (Cao et al. 1996). MyD88 activation after interaction of PAMP ligands with its specific TLR and subsequent multimerization is followed by an activation of IRAK and TNF receptor-associated factor 6 (TRAF-6), a member of a family of proteins involved in TNF signaling (Lomaga et al. 1999). Upon this activation, NF-κB dimers are formed involving the NF-κB-inducing kinase (NIK) (Malinin et al. 1997). After inactivation of inhibitory factor I-κB by I-κB kinase (IKK) (DiDonato et al. 1997) NF-κB translocates to the nucleus initiating transcription of genes encoding for, for example, proinflammatory cytokines.

Recruitment of TRAF-6 also leads to activation of 'evolutionarily conserved signaling intermediate in Toll pathways (ECSIT)', which in turn activates mitogen-activated protein (MAP)/extracellular stress-related kinas (eerk) kinase kinase (MEKK1), thus forming a link between Toll-mediated signaling and the MAP kinase pathways (Kopp et al. 1999). These pathways are commonly referred to as 'MyD88-dependent pathways' and seem to be involved in signal transduction by several other TLRs. Furthermore, there is evidence for another signal transduction pathway involving Rac1/PI3K/AKT, leading to the translocation of NF-κB (Arbibe et al. 2000). This pathway has originally described for TLR-2 ligands; however, recent data suggest that it may also play a role in TLR-4-mediated signaling (Ojaniemi et al. 2003).

MyD88-independent

The observation that MyD88-deficient mice at least partially respond to LPS led to the hypothesis of MyD88-independent signal transduction by TLR-4 (Kawai et al. 1999). Meanwhile, a novel TIR-domain-containing adaptor protein (TIRAP) has been described, which has been termed by others 'MyD88 adaptor-like' (Mal) (Horng et al. 2001). As TIRAP/Mal plays no role in IL-1R-mediated signaling, it represents a bifurcation between these pathways. The TIRAP/Mal knock-out mouse confirmed this bifurcation and led to the discovery that TIRAP/Mal is apparently involved in TLR-4, TLR-2, TLR-1, and TLR-6 signaling, but not in signaling brought about by activation of TLR-5, TLR-7, and TLR-9 (Horng et al. 2002; Yamamoto et al. 2002).

Recently, another MyD88-independent pathway has been discovered which leads to the activation of interferon regulatory factor-3 (IRF-3, Kawai et al. 2001). At least three other TIR-domain-containing adaptor proteins exist (reviewed in O'Neill et al. 2003). Two of them, termed TRAM and TRIF have recently been shown to mediate the Myd-88 independent activation of IRF-3.

LINKS TO ADAPTIVE IMMUNITY

Antigen presentation

One major task of the cells of the innate immune system is to screen for pathogen-associated patterns and subsequently detect and kill invading microorganisms as first-line defense. APCs, as mentioned above (Chapter 19, Processing and presentation of the antigen by the class II histocompatibility system; and Chapter 21, MHC class I antigen processing system), also act as a link between innate and adaptive immunity by presenting antigens to lymphocytes, which is extensively covered in other chapters of this volume. This link is in particular represented by immature imDCs (see above under Cells of the innate immune system), with interstitial imDCs being most important. These cells reside within peripheral tissues and scan their environment via endocytosis. After having contact with a wide variety of ligands, mainly via TLRs, they undergo maturation (reviewed in Banchereau and Steinman 1998).

PAMPs recognized by imDCs involve LPS, CpG-DNA, lipoproteins, and peptidoglycan (reviewed in Takeda et al. 2003). Maturation involves the expression of MHC molecules as well as CD80/CD86; furthermore proinflammatory cytokines, such as IL-12, are secreted. Mature DCs travel to lymph NODs and present processed antigen to T lymphocytes, initiating adaptive immune responses.

Type 1 interferons

Another link between innate and adaptive immunity is represented by plasmacytoid or type 1 pre-DCs. These cells, as shown above, express TLR-7 and TLR-9 and secrete type 1 interferons upon stimulation with adequate ligands (Kadowaki and Liu 2002). These cytokines, besides directly inhibiting viral replication and stimulating macrophages and NK cells, also activate T and B lymphocytes. They enhance proliferation of CD8 T lymphocytes, enhance the survival of T cells in general, and elicit antibody production by B lymphocytes. Obviously, type 1 interferons are crucial for immune responses against viral infections; however, they have also been described to act against bacteria and protozoa.

A TWO-STEP MODEL OF PATTERN RECOGNITION

Although the discoveries of the last few years improved understanding of pattern recognition, the general mechanism is far from being completely understood. As outlined in previous chapters, the diversity of microbial ligands is large and there are only first real molecular similarities, which allow for a definition of 'patterns'. Here, a hypothetical two-step model is proposed where, on one the hand, charged molecules are sensed, followed by a fine recognition system focusing on atypical lipids.

As described above, the PRR CD14 is able to bind a variety of ligands, including LPS, LTA, and triacylated lipopeptides. The structure of these ligands is quite different: LPS is a glycolipid with a lipid part and a polymeric part made up of carbohydrates (Raetz and Whitfield 2002). The lipid part of LPS, lipid A, is substituted with up to six fatty acids and exhibits a high degree of polarity as a result of its phosphate content (Figure 7.6). In contrast, LTA of *Staphylococcus aureus* is a glycolipid with a lipid anchor, being composed of glycerol and two fatty acids (diacylglycerol) and fewer phosphate charges. The polymeric region mainly consists of polyglycerophosphate, partially substituted with carbohydrates (Schroder et al. 2003). Lipopeptides are not glycolipids at all, but are amphiphiles bearing diacylglycerol linked to a peptide chain via cysteine. All these molecules are recognized by CD14 and LBP. Therefore, LBP and CD14 may represent a 'first-line' pattern recognition system shuttling amphiphiles to their receptor complexes.

Cellular PRRs such as the TLRs are able to discriminate further these molecular patterns with TLR-4 interacting with LPS, whereas TLR-2/TLR-6 dimers interact with LTA (and diacylated lipopeptides) and TLR-2/-TLR-1 dimers interact with triacylated lipopeptides (Takeuchi et al. 2001). Following this principle, TLRs would be regarded as 'second-line' PRRs initiating a more specific response to different patterns. This is reflected by the fact that the TLR-4-mediated response differs from that initiated by TLR-2 by involving IRF-3. A similar model can be proposed for the TLRs discriminating different types of nucleic acid which are TLR-3, TLR-7, and TLR-9.

CLINICAL IMPLICATIONS AND CONCLUSIONS

Exploitation of pattern recognition for therapy?

As a strong inflammatory reaction is widely viewed as playing a role in the pathology of sepsis and septic shock, interfering with innate immune responses has for many years been the focus of experimental sepsis therapy. Some of these approaches, which all failed to improve sepsis outcome, now show surprising results in the treatment of chronic inflammatory diseases. Interfering with TLR signaling is thus very likely to be the focus of a next generation of novel therapeutic strategies for both types of diseases (Beutler 2003).

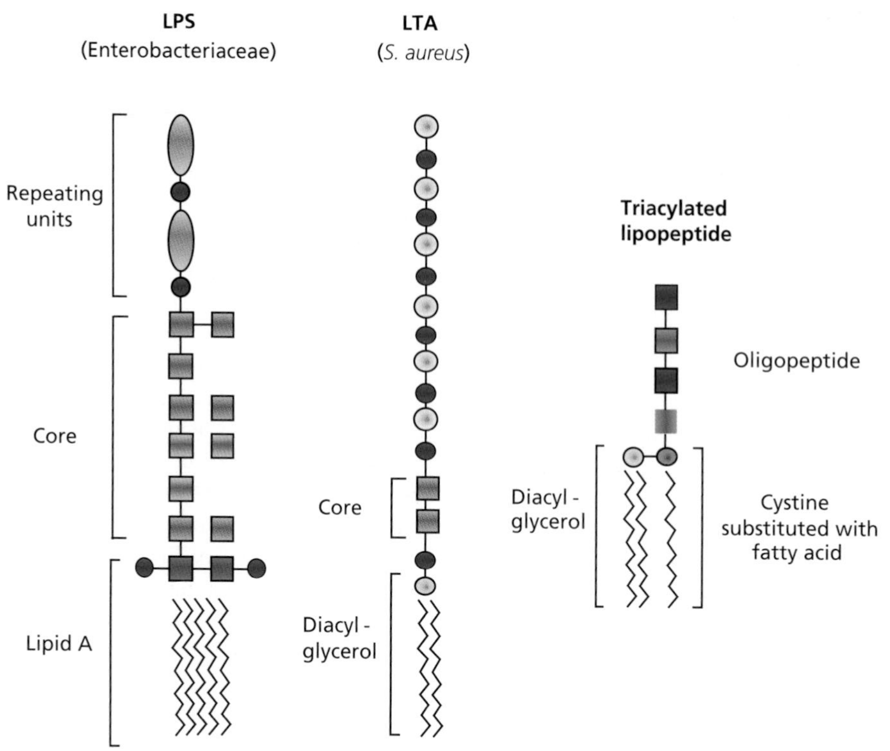

Figure 7.6 *Structural comparison of CD14 ligands. To attempt to define the structural requirements of a pathogen-associated molecular pattern (PAMP), here the simplified structures of lipopolysaccharide (LPS, as found in Enterobacteriaceae), lipoteichoic acid (LTA, from* Staphylococcus aureus*) and triacylated lipopeptide are compared: LPS is a glycolipid composed of a lipid part termed 'lipid A', a carbohydrate core region, and carbohydrate repeating units. Lipid A part contains up to six fatty acids. Major changes in this composition largely reduce the immunostimulatory capacity of LPS. LTA is glycolipid with a simple diacylglycerol lipid anchor, a small core region, and a polymeric backbone of polyglycerophosphate. In contrast, triacylated lipopeptides are diacylglycerols linked to cystine, which is substituted by a third fatty acid and linked to an oligopeptide.*

The LPS-inhibiting PMN protein BPI binds bacterial LPS, and in addition is bactericidal. BPI does not transfer LPS to any other receptor, leading to subsequent signal transduction and cytokine release, and therefore a potential therapeutic effect during infections with gram-negative bacteria was assumed. The recombinant amino-terminal part of BPI (rBPI21) has been applied to children with meningococcemia, which is usually associated with high levels of LPS in the bloodstream. Within the first phase I/II trials positive effects of administration of rBPI21 were observed (Giroir et al. 1997), and a phase III study came to the result that complications were less frequent among children receiving rBPI (Levin et al. 2000).

Although final results are currently not available, the concept of an early blocking of a key PAMP appears to be promising. Application of high concentrations of LBP may be an additional approach for inhibiting LPS-induced inflammatory responses (Lamping et al. 1998; Zweigner et al. 2001). LBP as an acute phase serum protein has a longer half-life compared with BPI and also inhibits effects of LPS and other PAMPs in concentrations found in serum. The host releases large quantities of LBP during the acute phase, apparently to achieve inhibition of inflammation brought about by PAMP–PRR interaction.

Genetic polymorphisms of PRRs and their impact on disease

Genetic polymorphisms, also referred to as 'nucleotide polymorphisms' (SNP), are frequent variations within a gene, which are found at least among 1 percent of individuals within a population. SNPs may have an impact on protein function; however, most SNPs reported so far are 'silent'. The relationship of genetic variations among humans and their susceptibility to disease is currently often investigated in order to identify high-risk populations and subsequently to be able to prevent diseases in these populations by specific prophylaxis.

CD14 AND LBP SNPs

During the past few years, several SNPs of PRRs were reported, including CD14 and LBP. For CD14, two polymorphisms within the promoter were reported, with one (Cys159Thr) being correlated with incidence of septic shock (Gibot et al. 2002), whereas another (Cys260Thr) apparently had no impact on the incidence of sepsis in trauma patients (Heesen et al. 2002). With regard to LBP, two SNPs were identified which were both correlated with a worsened outcome in patients with sepsis (Hubacek et al. 2002).

TOLL-LIKE RECEPTOR SNPS

Shortly after the identification of TLR-4 as the receptor for LPS, SNPs within the TLR-4 gene were described. These polymorphisms, Asp299Thr and Thr399Ile, were initially reported to be associated with decreased asthmatic reactions to inhaled LPS (Arbour et al. 2000). Meanwhile, evidence has been presented that the Asp299Thr SNPs may also be associated with the incidence of sepsis (Lorenz et al. 2002). These SNPs were mainly investigated with regard to a potential increase of susceptibility to infection. However, a decreased incidence of TLR-4 SNPs was found among patients with atherosclerosis (Kiechl et al. 2002), indicating that the limited recognition of pathogens may influence the course of a disease in a beneficial manner. SNPs were also reported for TLR-2 (Lorenz et al. 2000) and TLR-9 (Lazarus et al. 2003); however, their potential impact on human infectious diseases has not been conclusively investigated yet.

THE NOD2/*CARD15* SNPS

A striking correlation between an SNP of a PRR and disease susceptibility has been found for several mutations in the NOD2/*CARD15* gene and the incidence of Crohn's disease, which is a chronic inflammatory disease of the gastrointestinal tract occurring as frequently as 1 per 1000 in western countries (Hugot et al. 2001; Ogura et al. 2001a). Furthermore, the same mutations were found to be associated with 'Blau syndrome', a rare autosomal dominant disease consisting of uveitis, arthritis, and skin rash (Miceli-Richard et al. 2001). As mentioned above, several lines of evidence point in the direction that NOD2/*CARD15* acts as an intracellular PRR recognizing LPS or bacterial MDP (Bonen et al. 2003; Girardin et al. 2003; Inohara et al. 2003).

On the other hand, the NOD proteins similar to many of the related family members contain the caspase recruitment domain centrally involved in apoptosis regulation. It has thus been suggested that disturbance of NOD2 does not change pattern recognition but changes apoptosis regulation (Beutler 2001). This would correspond to the fact that anti-TNF treatment is highly efficient in Crohn's disease patients because TNF is a major apoptosis regulator. Recently, for Crohn's disease another, NOD2-independent genetic linkage has been found; the nature of the gene is, however, currently not known (Hampe et al. 2002).

Studies with different ethnic groups confirmed a role of NOD2/*CARD15* for Crohn's disease, ruling out an involvement in ulcerative colitis (Hampe et al. 2001). Ulcerative colitis, in contrast, was recently found in a small study to be associated with a polymorphism in the CD14 promoter, further supporting the concept of PRR SNPs being responsible for chronic inflammatory diseases of the gastrointestinal tract (Obana et al. 2002). The variation among different ethnic groups is reflected by one study showing the absence, in Japanese Crohn's disease patients, of the NOD2/*CARD15* mutations found in European populations (Kimouchi 2003). A recent study revealed an additional SNP in NOD2/*CARD15* among Ashkenazi Jews which also predisposes to the development of Crohn's disease (Sugimura et al. 2003).

New members of the CARD-containing protein family have recently been identified and several missense mutations have been found to be associated with rare inflammatory diseases, such as Muckle–Wells syndrome, familial cold urticaria, and chronic infantile neurological cutaneous and articular syndrome (McDermott 2002; Albrecht et al. 2003).

Most studies performed so far that investigate the potential effect of SNPs on the course of a particular disease focused on genetic variations of only a few proteins, including cytokines. However, the development and course of a bacterial infection are most probably a multifactorial event. Therefore, future studies investigating several SNPs in parallel and employing high-throughput technologies such as gene arrays may clarify whether SNPs of PRRs really influence the incidence and course of infectious and inflammatory diseases.

CONCLUSION

Pattern recognition is a key feature of the host's repertoire to react early to encounters with pathogens. Innate immunity most probably has an impact on both acute infectious disease complications, such as septic shock, and chronic illnesses caused by microorganisms. Innate immune responses are elicited by microbial compounds released from organisms, and thus cannot be 'treated' successfully by the application of antibiotics. APCs possess the ability to check the environment for these and other danger signals and orchestrate a response bridging innate and adaptive immunity. Major discoveries of the last 5 years include central host receptors of the Toll-like receptor family and their function. These results may lead to novel intervention strategies in acute and chronic infectious diseases that are currently not treatable by antibiotics. Genomic analyses confirm a central role of PRRs for incidence and course of infectious diseases. Intense basic and clinical research, with the help of modern molecular technologies, is, however, needed in order to exploit this growing field of immunology successfully.

REFERENCES

Ahmad-Nejad, P., Hacker, H., et al. 2002. Bacterial CpG-DNA and lipopolysaccharides activate Toll-like receptors at distinct cellular compartments. *Eur J Immunol*, **32**, 1958–68.

Albrecht, M., Domingues, F.S., et al. 2003. Identification of mammalian orthologs associates PYPAF5 with distinct functional roles. *FEBS Lett*, **538**, 173–7.

Alexander, C. and Rietschel, E.T. 2001. Bacterial lipopolysaccharides and innate immunity. *J Endotoxin Res*, **7**, 167–202.

Alexopoulou, L., Holt, A.C., et al. 2001. Recognition of double-stranded RNA and activation of NF-kappaB by Toll-like receptor 3. *Nature*, **413**, 732–8.

Anderson, K.V. and Nüsslein-Volhard, C. 1984. Information for the dorsal-ventral pattern of the Drosophila embryo is stored as maternal mRNA. *Nature*, **311**, 223–7.

Arbibe, L., Mira, J.P., et al. 2000. Toll-like receptor, 2-mediated NF-kappa B activation requires a Rac1-dependent pathway. *Nat Immunol*, **1**, 533–40.

Arbour, N.C., Lorenz, E., et al. 2000. TLR4 mutations are associated with endotoxin hyporesponsiveness in humans. *Nat Genet*, **25**, 187–91.

Asea, A., Rehli, M., et al. 2002. Novel signal transduction pathway utilized by extracellular HSP70: role of Toll-like receptor (TLR) 2 and TLR4. *J Biol Chem*, **277**, 15028–34.

Banchereau, J. and Steinman, R.M. 1998. Dendritic cells and the control of immunity. *Nature*, **392**, 245–52.

Bausinger, H., Lipsker, D., et al. 2002. Endotoxin-free heat-shock protein, 70 fails to induce APC activation. *Eur J Immunol*, **32**, 3708–13.

Bendriss-Vermare, N., Barthelemy, C., et al. 2001. Human thymus contains IFN-alpha-producing CD11c(−), myeloid CD11c(+), and mature interdigitating dendritic cells. *J Clin Invest*, **107**, 835–44.

Bergmann, E. and Schmiedeberg, O. 1868. Über das schwefelsaure Sepsin, das Gift faulender Substanzen (About sulfur-acidic Sepsin, the poison of fowl substances). *Centralbl Med Wissenschaften*, **32**, 497–8.

Bertin, J., Nir, W.J., et al. 1999. Human CARD4 protein is a novel CED-4/Apaf-1 cell death family member that activates NF-kappaB. *J Biol Chem*, **274**, 12955–8.

Beutler, B. 2001. Autoimmunity and apoptosis: the Crohn's connection. *Immunity*, **15**, 5–14.

Beutler, B. 2003. Innate immune responses to microbial poisons: Discovery and function of the Toll-like receptors. *Annu Rev Pharmacol Toxicol*, **43**, 609–28.

Beutler, B. and Rietschel, E.T. 2003. Timeline: Innate immune sensing and its roots: the story of endotoxin. *Nat Rev Immunol*, **3**, 169–76.

Beutler, B., Du, X., et al. 2001. Identification of Toll-like receptor, 4 (Tlr4) as the sole conduit for LPS signal transduction: genetic and evolutionary studies. *J Endotoxin Res*, **7**, 277–80.

Bonen, D.K., Ogura, Y., et al. 2003. Crohn's disease-associated NOD2 variants share a signaling defect in response to lipopolysaccharide and peptidoglycan. *Gastroenterology*, **124**, 140–6.

Brandtzaeg, P., Sandset, P.M., et al. 1989. The quantitative association of plasma endotoxin, antithrombin, protein C, extrinsic pathway inhibitor and fibrinopeptide A in systemic meningococcal disease. *Thromb Res*, **55**, 459–70.

Brock, T. 1999. *Robert Koch – A life in medicine and bacteriology*. Washington DC: ASM Press.

Cao, Z., Henzel, W.J., et al. 1996. IRAK: a kinase associated with the interleukin-1 receptor. *Science*, **271**, 1128–31.

Chow, J.C., Young, D.W., et al. 1999. Toll-like receptor-4 mediates lipopolysaccharide-induced signal transduction. *J Biol Chem*, **274**, 10689–92.

Costa, C.P., Kirschning, C.J., et al. 2002. Role of chlamydial heat shock protein, 60 in the stimulation of innate immune cells by *Chlamydia pneumoniae*. *Eur J Immunol*, **32**, 2460–70.

da Silva Correia, J., Soldau, K., et al. 2001. Lipopolysaccharide is in close proximity to each of the proteins in its membrane receptor complex. transfer from CD14 to TLR4 and MD-2. *J Biol Chem*, **276**, 21129–35.

Dangl, J.L. and Jones, J.D. 2001. Plant pathogens and integrated defence responses to infection. *Nature*, **411**, 826–33.

Dentener, M.A., Vreugdenhil, A.C., et al. 2000. Production of the acute-phase protein lipopolysaccharide-binding protein by respiratory type II epithelial cells: implications for local defense to bacterial endotoxins. *Am J Respir Cell Mol Biol*, **23**, 146–53.

DiDonato, J.A., Hayakawa, M., et al. 1997. A cytokine-responsive IkappaB kinase that activates the transcription factor NF-kappaB. *Nature*, **388**, 548–54.

Diebold, S.S., Kaisho, T., et al. 2004. Innate antiviral responses by means of TLR-7-mediated recognition of single-stranded RNA. *Science*, **303**, 1531–3.

Doyle, S.E., O'Conell, R., et al. 2003. Toll-like receptor, 3 mediates a more potent antiviral response than Toll-like receptor, 4. *J Immunol*, **170**, 3565–71.

Dubos, R. 1995. *Pasteur and modern science*. Madison, WI: Science Tech Publishers.

East, L. and Isacke, C.M. 2002. The mannose receptor family. *Biochim Biophys Acta*, **1572**, 364–86.

Elsbach, P. and Weiss, J. 1998. Role of the bactericidal/permeability-increasing protein in host defence. *Curr Opin Immunol*, **10**, 45–9.

Faure, E., Equils, O., et al. 2000. Bacterial lipopolysaccharide activates NF-kappaB through Toll-like receptor, 4 (TLR-4) in cultured human dermal endothelial cells. Differential expression of TLR-4 and TLR-2 in endothelial cells. *J Biol Chem*, **275**, 11058–63.

Fierer, J., Swancutt, M.A., et al. 2002. The role of lipopolysaccharide binding protein in resistance to Salmonella infections in mice. *J Immunol*, **168**, 6396–403.

Flo, T.H., Ryan, L., et al. 2000. Involvement of CD14 and beta2-integrins in activating cells with soluble and particulate lipopolysaccharides and mannuronic acid polymers. *Infect Immun*, **68**, 6770–6.

Fluhr, R. and Kaplan-Levy, R.N. 2002. Plant disease resistance: commonality and novelty in multicellular innate immunity. *Curr Top Microbiol Immunol*, **270**, 23–46.

Geijtenbeek, T.B., Engering, A. and Van Kooyk, Y. 2002. DC-SIGN, a C-type lectin on dendritic cells that unveils many aspects of dendritic cell biology. *J Leukoc Biol*, **71**, 921–31.

Gewirtz, A.T., Navas, T.A., et al. 2001a. Cutting edge: bacterial flagellin activates basolaterally expressed TLR5 to induce epithelial proinflammatory gene expression. *J Immunol*, **167**, 1882–5.

Gewirtz, A.T., Simon, P.O. Jr, et al. 2001b. *Salmonella typhimurium* translocates flagellin across intestinal epithelia, inducing a proinflammatory response. *J Clin Invest*, **107**, 99–109.

Gibot, S., Cariou, A., et al. 2002. Association between a genomic polymorphism within the CD14 locus and septic shock susceptibility and mortality rate. *Crit Care Med*, **30**, 969–73.

Girardin, S.E., Boneca, I.G., et al. 2003. Nod2 is a general sensor of peptidoglycan through muramyl dipeptide (MDP) detection. *J Biol Chem*, **278**, 8869–72.

Giroir, B.P., Quint, P.A., et al. 1997. Preliminary evaluation of recombinant amino-terminal fragment of human bactericidal/ permeability-increasing protein in children with severe meningococcal sepsis. *Lancet*, **350**, 1439–43.

Gomez-Gomez, L. and Boller, T. 2000. FLS2: an LRR receptor-like kinase involved in the perception of the bacterial elicitor flagellin in Arabidopsis. *Mol Cell*, **5**, 1003–11.

Goyert, S.M., Ferrero, E., et al. 1988. The CD14 monocyte differentiation antigen maps to a region encoding growth factors and receptors. *Science*, **239**, 497–500.

Hamann, L., Schumann, R.R., et al. 2000. Binding of lipopolysaccharide (LPS) to CHO cells does not correlate with LPS-induced NF-kappaB activation. *Eur J Immunol*, **30**, 211–16.

Hampe, J., Cuthbert, A., et al. 2001. Association between insertion mutation in NOD2 gene and Crohn's disease in German and British populations. *Lancet*, **357**, 1925–8.

Hampe, J., Frenzel, H., et al. 2002. Evidence for a NOD2-independent susceptibility locus for inflammatory bowel disease on chromosome, 16p. *Proc Natl Acad Sci USA*, **99**, 321–6.

Hashimoto, C., Hudson, K.L. and Anderson, K.V. 1988. The Toll gene of Drosophila, required for dorsal-ventral embryonic polarity, appears to encode a transmembrane protein. *Cell*, **52**, 269–79.

Hayashi, F., Smith, K.D., et al. 2001. The innate immune response to bacterial flagellin is mediated by Toll-like receptor, 5. *Nature*, **410**, 1099–103.

Heesen, M., Bloemeke, B., et al. 2002. The −260 C→T promoter polymorphism of the lipopolysaccharide receptor CD14 and severe sepsis in trauma patients. *Intens Care Med*, **28**, 1161–3.

Heil, F., Hemmi, H., et al. 2004. Species-specific recognition of single-stranded RNA via Toll-like receptor 7 and 8. *Science*, **303**, 1529–31.

Heine, H., Kirschning, C.J., et al. 1999. Cutting edge: cells that carry A null allele for Toll-like receptor 2 are capable of responding to endotoxin. *J Immunol*, **162**, 6971–65.

Heinrich, J.M., Bernheiden, M., et al. 2001. The essential role of lipopolysaccharide-binding protein in protection of mice against a peritoneal Salmonella infection involves the rapid induction of an inflammatory response. *J Immunol*, **167**, 1624–8.

Hemmi, H., Takeuchi, O., et al. 2000. A Toll-like receptor recognizes bacterial DNA. *Nature*, **408**, 740–5.

Hemmi, H., Kaisho, T., et al. 2002. Small anti-viral compounds activate immune cells via the TLR7 MyD88-dependent signaling pathway. *Nat Immunol*, **3**, 196–200.

Hermann, C., Spreitzer, I., et al. 2002. Cytokine induction by purified lipoteichoic acids from various bacterial species-role of LBP, sCD14, CD14 and failure to induce IL-12 and subsequent IFN-gamma release. *Eur J Immunol*, **32**, 541–51.

Hirschfeld, M., Weis, J.J., et al. 2001. Signaling by Toll-like receptor, 2 and, 4 agonists results in differential gene expression in murine macrophages. *Infect Immun*, **69**, 1477–82.

Horng, T., Barton, G.M. and Medzhitov, R. 2001. TIRAP: an adapter molecule in the Toll signaling pathway. *Nat Immunol*, **2**, 835–41.

Horng, T., Barton, G.M., et al. 2002. The adaptor molecule TIRAP provides signalling specificity for Toll-like receptors. *Nature*, **420**, 329–33.

Hotchkiss, R.S. and Karl, I.E. 2003. The pathophysiology and treatment of sepsis. *N Engl J Med*, **348**, 138–50.

Hubacek, J.A., Pitha, J., et al. 2002. Polymorphisms in the lipopolysaccharide-binding protein and bactericidal/permeability-increasing protein in patients with myocardial infarction. *Clin Chem Lab Med*, **40**, 1097–100.

Hugot, J.P., Chamaillard, M., et al. 2001. Association of NOD2 leucine-rich repeat variants with susceptibility to Crohn's disease. *Nature*, **411**, 599–603.

Imler, J.L. and Hoffmann, J.A. 2002. Toll receptors in *Drosophila*: a family of molecules regulating development and immunity. *Curr Top Microbiol Immunol*, **270**, 63–79.

Imler, J.L. and Hoffmann, J.A. 2003. Toll signaling: the TIReless quest for specificity. *Nat Immunol*, **4**, 105–6.

Inohara, N. and Nunez, G. 2001. The NOD: a signaling module that regulates apoptosis and host defense against pathogens. *Oncogene*, **20**, 6473–81.

Inohara, N., Ogura, Y., et al. 2003. Host recognition of bacterial muramyl dipeptide mediated through NOD2. Implications for Crohn's disease. *J Biol Chem*, **278**, 5509–12.

Jack, R.S., Fan, X., et al. 1997. Lipopolysaccharide-binding protein is required to combat a murine gram-negative bacterial infection. *Nature*, **389**, 742–5.

Jurk, M., Heil, F., et al. 2002. Human TLR7 or TLR8 independently confer responsiveness to the antiviral compound R-848. *Nat Immunol*, **3**, 499.

Kadowaki, N. and Liu, Y.J. 2002. Natural type I interferon-producing cells as a link between innate and adaptive immunity. *Hum Immunol*, **63**, 1126–32.

Kadowaki, N., Ho, S., et al. 2001. Subsets of human dendritic cell precursors express different Toll-like receptors and respond to different microbial antigens. *J Exp Med*, **194**, 863–9.

Kanai, T., Ilyama, R., et al. 2002. Role of the innate immune system in the development of chronic colitis. *J Gastroenterol*, **37**, suppl 14, 38–42.

Kang, B.K. and Schlesinger, L.S. 1998. Characterization of mannose receptor-dependent phagocytosis mediated by Mycobacterium tuberculosis lipoarabinomannan. *Infect Immun*, **66**, 2769–77.

Kathariou, S., Kanenaka, R., et al. 1995. Repression of motility and flagellin production at, 37 degrees C is stronger in *Listeria monocytogenes* than in the nonpathogenic species *Listeria innocua*. *Can J Microbiol*, **41**, 572–7.

Kawai, T., Adachi, O., et al. 1999. Unresponsiveness of MyD88-deficient mice to endotoxin. *Immunity*, **11**, 115–22.

Kawai, T., Takeuchi, O., et al. 2001. Lipopolysaccharide stimulates the MyD88-independent pathway and results in activation of IFN-regulatory factor, 3 and the expression of a subset of lipopolysaccharide-inducible genes. *J Immunol*, **167**, 5887–94.

Kawasaki, K., Akashi, S., et al. 2000. Mouse Toll-like receptor, 4 MD-2 complex mediates lipopolysaccharide-mimetic signal transduction by Taxol. *J Biol Chem*, **275**, 2251–4.

Kiechl, S., Lorenz, E., et al. 2002. Toll-like receptor, 4 polymorphisms and atherogenesis. *N Engl J Med*, **347**, 185–92.

Kimbrell, D.A. and Beutler, B. 2001. The evolution and genetics of innate immunity. *Nat Rev Genet*, **2**, 256–67.

Kimouchi, Y. 2003. CARD15/NOD2 mutational analysis in Japanese patients with Crohn's disease. *Clin Genet*, **63**, 160–2.

Kirschning, C.J. and Schumann, R.R. 2002. TLR2: cellular sensor for microbial and endogenous molecular patterns. *Curr Top Microbiol Immunol*, **270**, 121–44.

Kirschning, C.J., Au-Young, J., et al. 1997. Similar organization of the lipopolysaccharide-binding protein (LBP) and phospholipid transfer protein (PLTP) genes suggests a common gene family of lipid-binding proteins. *Genomics*, **46**, 416–25.

Kirschning, C.J., Wesche, H., et al. 1998. Human Toll-like receptor, 2 confers responsiveness to bacterial lipopolysaccharide. *J Exp Med*, **188**, 2091–7.

Kobayashi, K., Inohara, N., et al. 2002. RICK/Rip2/CARDIAK mediates signalling for receptors of the innate and adaptive immune systems. *Nature*, **416**, 194–9.

Kobe, B. and Deisenhofer, J. 1995. A structural basis of the interactions between leucine-rich repeats and protein ligands. *Nature*, **374**, 183–6.

Koedel, U., Angele, B., et al. 2003. Toll-like receptor, 2 participates in mediation of immune response in experimental pneumococcal meningitis. *J Immunol*, **170**, 438–44.

Kopp, E., Medzhitov, R., et al. 1999. ECSIT is an evolutionarily conserved intermediate in the Toll/IL-1 signal transduction pathway. *Genes Dev*, **13**, 2059–71.

Krieg, A.M. 1999. Mechanisms and applications of immune stimulatory CpG oligodeoxynucleotides. *Biochim Biophys Acta*, **1489**, 107–16.

Krieg, A.M. 2002. CpG motifs in bacterial DNA and their immune effects. *Annu Rev Immunol*, **20**, 709–60.

Krieger, M. and Stern, D.M. 2001. Series introduction: multiligand receptors and human disease. *J Clin Invest*, **108**, 645–7.

Kurt-Jones, E.A. and Popova, L. 2000. Pattern recognition receptors TLR4 and CD14 mediate response to respiratory syncytial virus. *Nat Immunol*, **1**, 398–401.

Lamping, N., Dettmer, R., et al. 1998. LPS-binding protein protects mice from septic shock caused by LPS or gram-negative bacteria. *J Clin Invest*, **101**, 2065–71.

Landmann, R., Muller, B. and Zimmerli, W. 2000. CD14, new aspects of ligand and signal diversity. *Microbes Infect*, **2**, 295–304.

Latz, E., Visintin, A., et al. 2002. Lipopolysaccharide rapidly traffics to and from the Golgi apparatus with the Toll-like receptor, 4-MD-2-CD14 complex in a process that is distinct from the initiation of signal transduction. *J Biol Chem*, **277**, 47834–43.

Lazarus, R., Klimecki, W.T., et al. 2003. Single-nucleotide polymorphisms in the Toll-like receptor, 9 gene (TLR9): frequencies, pairwise linkage disequilibrium, and haplotypes in three U.S. ethnic groups and exploratory case-control disease association studies. *Genomics*, **81**, 85–91.

Lazarus, R., Vercelli, D., et al. 2002. Single nucleotide polymorphisms in innate immunity genes: abundant variation and potential role in complex human disease. *Immunol Rev*, **190**, 9–25.

Lemaitre, B., Nicolas, E., et al. 1996. The dorsoventral regulatory gene cassette spatzle/Toll/cactus controls the potent antifungal response in *Drosophila* adults. *Cell*, **86**, 973–83.

Levin, M., Quint, P.A., et al. 2000. Recombinant bactericidal/permeability-increasing protein (rBPI21) as adjunctive treatment for children with severe meningococcal sepsis: a randomised trial. rBPI21 Meningococcal Sepsis Study Group. *Lancet*, **356**, 961–7.

Lien, E., Sellati, T.J., et al. 1999. Toll-like receptor, 2 functions as a pattern recognition receptor for diverse bacterial products. *J Biol Chem*, **274**, 33419–25.

Lien, E., Means, T.K., et al. 2000. Toll-like receptor, 4 imparts ligand-specific recognition of bacterial lipopolysaccharide. *J Clin Invest*, **105**, 497–504.

Liu, Y.J., Kanzler, H., et al. 2001. Dendritic cell lineage, plasticity and cross-regulation. *Nat Immunol*, **2**, 585–9.

Lomaga, M.A., Yeh, W.C., et al. 1999. TRAF6 deficiency results in osteopetrosis and defective interleukin-1, CD40 and LPS signaling. *Genes Dev*, **13**, 1015–24.

Lorenz, E., Mira, J.P., et al. 2000. A novel polymorphism in the Toll-like receptor, 2 gene and its potential association with staphylococcal infection. *Infect Immun*, **68**, 6398–401.

Lorenz, E., Mira, J.P., et al. 2002. Relevance of mutations in the TLR4 receptor in patients with gram-negative septic shock. *Arch Intern Med*, **162**, 1028–32.

Lund, J.M., Alexopoulou, L., et al. 2004. Recognition of single-stranded RNA viruses by Toll-like receptor 7. *DNAS*, **101**, 5598–603.

McDermott, M.F. 2002. Genetic clues to understanding periodic fevers, and possible therapies. *Trends Mol Med*, **8**, 550–4.

Malinin, N.L., Boldin, M.P., et al. 1997. MAP3K-related kinase involved in NF-kappaB induction by TNF, CD95 and IL-1. *Nature*, **385**, 540–4.

Matzinger, P. 2002. The danger model: a renewed sense of self. *Science*, **296**, 301–5.

Means, T.K., Wang, S., et al. 1999. Human Toll-like receptors mediate cellular activation by Mycobacterium tuberculosis. *J Immunol*, **163**, 3920–7.

Medzhitov, R. 2001. Toll-like receptors and innate immunity. *Nat Rev Immunol*, **1**, 135–45.

Medzhitov, R. and Janeway, C.A. Jr. 1997. Innate immunity: impact on the adaptive immune response. *Curr Opin Immunol*, **9**, 4–9.

Medzhitov, R. and Janeway, C.A. Jr. 1998. Self-defense: the fruit fly style. *Proc Natl Acad Sci USA*, **95**, 429–30.

Medzhitov, R., Preston-Hurlburt, P. and Janeway, C.A. Jr. 1997. A human homologue of the Drosophila Toll protein signals activation of adaptive immunity. *Nature*, **388**, 394–7.

Melmed, G., Thomas, L.S., et al. 2003. Human intestinal epithelial cells are broadly unresponsive to Toll-like receptor, 2-dependent bacterial ligands: implications for host-microbial interactions in the gut. *J Immunol*, **170**, 1406–15.

Metschnikoff, E. 1844. Über eine Sprosspilzkrankheit der Daphnien. Beitrag zur Lehre über den Kampf der Phagocyten gegen Krankheitserreger (A disease of *Daphnia* caused by yeast. A contribution to the theory of phagocytes as agents for attack on disease-causing organisms). *Arch Pathol Anatom Physiol Klin Med (Virchow's Archiv)*, **96**, 177–95.

Miceli-Richard, C., Lesage, S., et al. 2001. CARD15 mutations in Blau syndrome. *Nat Genet*, **29**, 19–20.

Miyake, K. 2003. Innate recognition of lipopolysaccharide by CD14 and Toll-like receptor, 4-MD-2: unique roles for MD-2. *Int Immunopharmacol*, **3**, 119–28.

Miyake, K. and Shimazu, R. 1998. Mouse MD-1, a molecule that is physically associated with RP105 and positively regulates its expression. *J Immunol*, **161**, 1348–55.

Morr, M., Takeuchi, O., et al. 2002. Differential recognition of structural details of bacterial lipopeptides by Toll-like receptors. *Eur J Immunol*, **32**, 3337–47.

Muzio, M., Bosisio, D., et al. 2000. Differential expression and regulation of Toll-like receptors (TLR) in human leukocytes: selective expression of TLR3 in dendritic cells. *J Immunol*, **164**, 5998–6004.

Nagai, Y., Akashi, S., et al. 2002. Essential role of MD-2 in LPS responsiveness and TLR4 distribution. *Nat Immunol*, **3**, 667–72.

O'Neill, L.A. 2002. Signal transduction pathways activated by the IL-1 receptor/ Toll-like receptor superfamily. *Curr Top Microbiol Immunol*, **270**, 47–61.

O'Neill, L.A. and Dinarello, C.A. 2000. The IL-1 receptor/ Toll-like receptor superfamily: crucial receptors for inflammation and host defense. *Immunol Today*, **21**, 206–9.

O'Neill, L.A., Fitzgerald, K.A., et al. 2003. The Toll-IL1 receptor adaptor family grows to five members. *Trends Immunol*, **24**, 286–9.

Obana, N., Takahashi, S., et al. 2002. Ulcerative colitis is associated with a promoter polymorphism of lipopolysaccharide receptor gene, CD14. *Scand J Gastroenterol*, **37**, 699–704.

Ogawa, T., Asai, Y., et al. 2002. Cell activation by *Porphyromonas gingivalis* lipid A molecule through Toll-like receptor, 4- and myeloid differentiation factor, 88-dependent signaling pathway. *Int Immunol*, **14**, 1325–32.

Ogura, Y., Bonen, D.K., et al. 2001a. A frameshift mutation in NOD2 associated with susceptibility to Crohn's disease. *Nature*, **411**, 603–6.

Ogura, Y., Inohara, N., et al. 2001b. Nod2, a Nod1/Apaf-1 family member that is restricted to monocytes and activates NF-kappaB. *J Biol Chem*, **276**, 4812–18.

Ohashi, K., Burkart, V., et al. 2000. Cutting edge: heat shock protein, 60 is a putative endogenous ligand of the Toll-like receptor-4 complex. *J Immunol*, **164**, 558–61.

Ojaniemi, M., Glumoff, V., et al. 2003. Phosphatidylinositol, 3-kinase is involved in Toll-like receptor, 4-mediated cytokine expression in mouse macrophages. *Eur J Immunol*, **33**, 597–605.

Opitz, B., Schroder, N.W., et al. 2001. Toll-like receptor-2 mediates *Treponema* glycolipid and lipoteichoic acid-induced NF-kappaB translocation. *J Biol Chem*, **276**, 22041–7.

Ozinsky, A., Underhill, D.M., et al. 2000. The repertoire for pattern recognition of pathogens by the innate immune system is defined by cooperation between Toll-like receptors. *Proc Natl Acad Sci USA*, **97**, 13766–71.

Panum, P. 1874. Das putride Gift, die Bakterien, die putride infektion oder ntoxikation und die Septikämie (putrid poison, bacteria, putrid infection or intoxication and septicemia). *Arch Pathol Anat Physiol Klin Med (Virchow's Arch)*, **60**, 301–52.

Perera, P.Y., Vogel, S.N., et al. 1997. CD14-dependent and CD14-independent signaling pathways in murine macrophages from normal and CD14 knockout mice stimulated with lipopolysaccharide or Taxol. *J Immunol*, **158**, 4422–49.

Pfeiffer, A., Bottcher, A., et al. 2001. Lipopolysaccharide and ceramide docking to CD14 provokes ligand-specific receptor clustering in rafts. *Eur J Immunol*, **31**, 3153–64.

Poltorak, A., He, X., et al. 1998. Defective LPS signaling in C3H/HeJ and C57BL/10ScCr mice: mutations in Tlr4 gene. *Science*, **282**, 2085–8.

Poltorak, A., Ricciardi-Castagnoli, P., et al. 2000. Physical contact between lipopolysaccharide and Toll-like receptor, 4 revealed by genetic complementation. *Proc Natl Acad Sci USA*, **97**, 2163–7.

Pugin, J., Heumann, I.D., et al. 1994. CD14 is a pattern recognition receptor. *Immunity*, **1**, 509–16.

Raetz, C.R. and Whitfield, C. 2002. Lipopolysaccharide endotoxins. *Annu Rev Biochem*, **71**, 635–700.

Re, F. and Strominger, J.L. 2002. Monomeric recombinant MD-2 binds Toll-like receptor, 4 tightly and confers lipopolysaccharide responsiveness. *J Biol Chem*, **277**, 23427–32.

Relman, D.A. 2002. New technologies, human-microbe interactions, and the search for previously unrecognized pathogens. *J Infect Dis*, **186**, suppl 2, S254–8.

Rietschel, E.T. and Cavaillon, J.M. 2002. Endotoxin and anti-endotoxin. The contribution of the schools of Koch and Pasteur: life, milestone-experiments and concepts of Richard Pfeiffer (Berlin) and Alexandre Besredka (Paris). *J Endotoxin Res*, **8**, 3–16.

Rietschel, E.T., Brade, H., et al. 1996. Bacterial endotoxin: Chemical constitution, biological recognition, host response, and immunological detoxification. *Curr Top Microbiol Immunol*, **216**, 39–81.

Rock, F.L., Hardiman, G., et al. 1998. A family of human receptors structurally related to Drosophila Toll. *Proc Natl Acad Sci USA*, **95**, 588–93.

Ross, G.D. 2000. Regulation of the adhesion versus cytotoxic functions of the Mac-1/CR3/alphaMbeta2-integrin glycoprotein. *Crit Rev Immunol*, **20**, 197–222.

Sauter, B., Albert, M.L., et al. 2000. Consequences of cell death: exposure to necrotic tumor cells, but not primary tissue cells or apoptotic cells, induces the maturation of immunostimulatory dendritic cells. *J Exp Med*, **191**, 423–34.

Schmitz, G. and Orso, E. 2002. CD14 signalling in lipid rafts: new ligands and co-receptors. *Curr Opin Lipidol*, **13**, 513–21.

Schroder, N.W., Opitz, B., et al. 2000. Involvement of lipopolysaccharide binding protein, CD14 and Toll-like receptors in the initiation of innate immune responses by Treponema glycolipids. *J Immunol*, **165**, 2683–93.

Schroder, N.W., Morath, S., et al. 2003. Lipoteichoic acid (LTA) of *S. pneumoniae* and *S. aureus* activates immune cells via Toll-like receptor (TLR)-2, LPS binding protein (LBP) and CD14 while TLR-4 and MD-2 are not involved. *J Biol Chem*, **278**, 15587–94.

Schromm, A.B., Lien, E., et al. 2001. Molecular genetic analysis of an endotoxin nonresponder mutant cell line: a point mutation in a conserved region of MD-2 abolishes endotoxin-induced signaling. *J Exp Med*, **194**, 79–88.

Schumann, R.R. and Latz, E. 2000. Lipopolysaccharide-binding protein. *Chem Immunol*, **74**, 42–60.

Schumann, R.R., Leong, S.R., et al. 1990. Structure and function of lipopolysaccharide binding protein. *Science*, **249**, 1429–31.

Schumann, R.R., Rietschel, E.T. and Loppnow, H. 1994. The role of CD14 and lipopolysaccharide-binding protein (LBP) in the activation of different cell types by endotoxin. *Med Microbiol Immunol (Berl)*, **183**, 279–97.

Schumann, R.R., Kirschning, C.J., et al. 1996. The lipopolysaccharide-binding protein is a secretory class, 1 acute-phase protein whose gene is transcriptionally activated by APRF/STAT/3 and other cytokine-inducible nuclear proteins. *Mol Cell Biol*, **16**, 3490–503.

Schwandner, R., Dziarski, R., et al. 1999. Peptidoglycan- and lipoteichoic acid-induced cell activation is mediated by Toll-like receptor 2. *J Biol Chem*, **274**, 17406–9.

Sellati, T.J., Bouis, D.A., et al. 1998. Treponema pallidum and Borrelia burgdorferi lipoproteins and synthetic lipopeptides activate monocytic cells via a CD14-dependent pathway distinct from that used by lipopolysaccharide. *J Immunol*, **160**, 5455–64.

Shimazu, R., Akashi, S., et al. 1999. MD-2, a molecule that confers lipopolysaccharide responsiveness on Toll-like receptor, 4. *J Exp Med*, **189**, 1777–82.

Smith, K.D. and Ozinsky, A. 2002. Toll-like receptor-5 and the innate immune response to bacterial flagellin. *Curr Top Microbiol Immunol*, **270**, 93–108.

Sparwasser, T., Miethke, T., et al. 1997. Bacterial DNA causes septic shock. *Nature*, **386**, 336–7.

Spits, H., Couwenberg, F., et al. 2000. Id2 and Id3 inhibit development of CD34(+) stem cells into predendritic cell (pre-DC)2 but not into pre-DC1. Evidence for a lymphoid origin of pre-DC2. *J Exp Med*, **192**, 1775–84.

Sugimura, K., Taylor, K.D., et al. 2003. A Novel NOD2/CARD15 Haplotype conferring risk for Crohn disease in Ashkenazi Jews. *Am J Hum Genet*, **72**, 509–18.

Takeda, K., Kaisho, T. and Akira, S. 2003. Toll-Like receptors. *Annu Rev Immunol*, **21**, 335–76.

Takeuchi, O. and Akira, S. 2002. MyD88 as a bottle neck in Toll/IL-1 signaling. *Curr Top Microbiol Immunol*, **270**, 155–67.

Takeuchi, O., Kawai, T., et al. 2001. Discrimination of bacterial lipoproteins by Toll-like receptor, 6. *Int Immunol*, **13**, 933–40.

Takeuchi, O., Sato, S., et al. 2002. Cutting edge: role of Toll-like receptor, 1 in mediating immune response to microbial lipoproteins. *J Immunol*, **169**, 10–14.

Thery, C. and Amigorena, S. 2001. The cell biology of antigen presentation in dendritic cells. *Curr Opin Immunol*, **13**, 45–51.

Underhill, D.M., Bassetti, M., et al. 1999a. Dynamic interactions of macrophages with T cells during antigen presentation. *J Exp Med*, **190**, 1909–14.

Underhill, D.M., Ozinsky, A., et al. 1999b. The Toll-like receptor, 2 is recruited to macrophage phagosomes and discriminates between pathogens. *Nature*, **401**, 811–15.

Vabulas, R.M., Ahmad-Nejad, P., et al. 2001. Endocytosed HSP60s use Toll-like receptor, 2 (TLR2) and TLR4 to activate the Toll/interleukin-1 receptor signaling pathway in innate immune cells. *J Biol Chem*, **276**, 31332–9.

Vabulas, R.M., Wagner, H. and Schild, H. 2002. Heat shock proteins as ligands of Toll-like receptors. *Curr Top Microbiol Immunol*, **270**, 169–84.

Viriyakosol, S., Tobias, P.S., et al. 2001. MD-2 binds to bacterial lipopolysaccharide. *J Biol Chem*, **276**, 38044–51.

Vreugdenhil, A.C., Dentener, M.A., et al. 1999. Lipopolysaccharide binding protein and serum amyloid A secretion by human intestinal epithelial cells during the acute phase response. *J Immunol*, **163**, 2792–8.

Wagner, H. 2002. Interactions between bacterial CpG-DNA and TLR9 bridge innate and adaptive immunity. *Curr Opin Microbiol*, **5**, 62–9.

Weidemann, B., Schletter, J., et al. 1997. Specific binding of soluble peptidoglycan and muramyldipeptide to CD14 on human monocytes. *Infect Immun*, **65**, 858–64.

Weiss, J., Elsbach, P., et al. 1978. Purification and characterization of a potent bactericidal and membrane active protein from the granules of human polymorphonuclear leukocytes. *J Biol Chem*, **253**, 2664–72.

Werling, D. and Jungi, T.W. 2003. TOLL-like receptors linking innate and adaptive immune response. *Vet Immunol Immunopathol*, **91**, 1–12.

Werts, C., Tapping, R.I., et al. 2001. Leptospiral lipopolysaccharide activates cells through a TLR2-dependent mechanism. *Nat Immunol*, **2**, 346–52.

Whitney, A.R., Diehn, M., et al. 2003. Individuality and variation in gene expression patterns in human blood. *Proc Natl Acad Sci USA*, **100**, 1896–901.

Williams, M.J., Rodriguez, A., et al. 1997. The, 18-wheeler mutation reveals complex antibacterial gene regulation in Drosophila host defense. *EMBO J*, **16**, 6120–30.

Wright, S.D., Ramos, R.A., et al. 1990. CD14, a receptor for complexes of lipopolysaccharide (LPS) and LPS binding protein. *Science*, **249**, 1431–3.

Wurfel, M.M., Monks, B.G., et al. 1997. Targeted deletion of the lipopolysaccharide (LPS)-binding protein gene leads to profound suppression of LPS responses ex vivo, whereas in vivo responses remain intact. *J Exp Med*, **186**, 2051–6.

Xu, Y., Tao, X., et al. 2000. Structural basis for signal transduction by the Toll/interleukin-1 receptor domains. *Nature*, **408**, 111–15.

Yamamoto, M., Sato, S., et al. 2002. Essential role for TIRAP in activation of the signalling cascade shared by TLR2 and TLR4. *Nature*, **420**, 324–9.

Yang, R.B., Mark, M.R., et al. 1998. Toll-like receptor-2 mediates lipopolysaccharide-induced cellular signalling. *Nature*, **395**, 284–8.

Ziegler-Heitbrock, H.W. and Ulevitch, R.J. 1993. CD14: cell surface receptor and differentiation marker. *Immunol Today*, **14**, 121–5.

Zweigner, J., Gramm, H.J., et al. 2001. High concentrations of lipopolysaccharide-binding protein in serum of patients with severe sepsis or septic shock inhibit the lipopolysaccharide response in human monocytes. *Blood*, **98**, 3800–8.

8

Apoptosis

ANTOINE GALMICHE AND ARTURO ZYCHLINSKY

INTRODUCTION

In multicellular organisms, cells often die by apoptosis. This form of death occurs as a physiological event in the organism's tissues, where it ensures the elimination of unwanted cells and maintains tissue homeostasis. Apoptosis is an active process, i.e. the cell itself produces the effector proteins that kill it. For this reason, apoptosis is often compared to a cell 'suicide' (Hengartner 2000).

Characteristic morphological alterations accompany apoptosis (Mills et al. 1999; Hengartner 2000). In the nucleus, the chromatin condenses and accumulates at the level of the nuclear membrane. Cytoplasmic shrinkage and plasma membrane blebbing are also evident. Membrane blebs can ultimately pinch off the cell, forming vesicles called apoptotic bodies which contain cell organelles and nuclear material. These morphological alterations are distinct from the ones observed during necrosis, a form of cell death that follows accidental injury. In contrast to necrosis, there is no cytoplasmic swelling, and the integrity of the cell organelles is conserved until the late stages of apoptosis.

During apoptosis, the nuclear DNA is cleaved at the internucleosomal region, generating fragments ranging from 180 to 200 base-pairs. These fragments produce a typical 'ladder' when resolved on agarose gels. The surface of the cell is also modified. Phosphatidylserine, an amino-phospholipid normally restricted to the inner leaflet of the plasma membrane, flips to the outer leaflet. These changes allow phagocytes to recognize and remove apoptotic cells efficiently. Until their latest stages, apoptotic cells, however, display no changes of their plasma membrane integrity. This characteristic, together with the efficient clearance process mediated by phagocytes, ensures that the apoptotic cell does not release its contents.

THE INDUCTION OF APOPTOSIS: EXTRINSIC VERSUS INTRINSIC PATHWAYS

Apoptosis can occur as a consequence of: (1) extracellular stimulation via the engagement of death receptors present at the surface of the cell (e.g. Fas/CD95 or tumor necrosis factor (TNF) receptor), (2) changes in the transcriptional control (glucocorticoids), (3) disruption of organelles or DNA lesions induced, for example, by ionizing radiation or chemotherapy reagents, and (4) absence of trophic factors (reviewed in Hengartner 2000).

These stimuli activate two major cellular pathways controlling the occurrence of apoptosis (Figure 8.1): The extrinsic pathway is activated by extracellular stimuli such as the binding of death receptor ligands to their cognate receptors on the cell surface. In contrast, the intrinsic pathway is initiated as a consequence of many cell stresses (Figure 8.1). Although these two pathways are initiated and controlled in distinct fashions, two systems play a key role in their transduction: (1) mito-

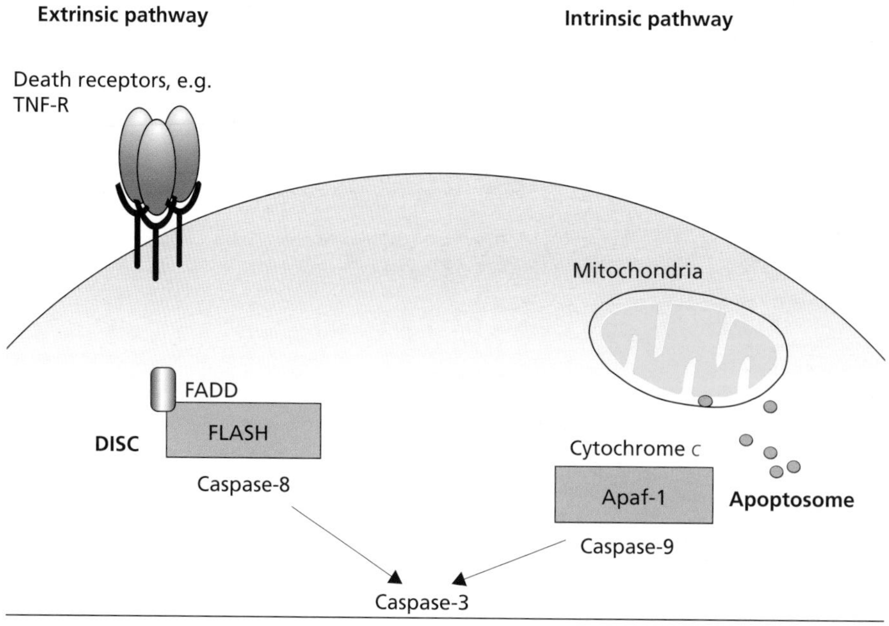

Figure 8.1 *Key components of the apoptotic pathway in mammalian cells. Two major pathways control the occurrence of apoptosis: one, called the intrinsic pathway, is activated by extracellular stimuli, e.g. the binding of death receptor ligands to their cognate receptors on the cell surface. These receptors transduce their death signal via adaptor proteins. These adaptor proteins mediate interactions between participants of the apoptotic cascade, e.g. the adaptor protein FADD is recruited by the activated tumor necrosis factor α (TNF-α) receptor. It in turn recruits and activates the initiator caspase caspase-8. In contrast, the intrinsic pathway is initiated as a consequence of cell stresses. A key role is played by the mitochondrial release of factors such as cytochrome c, activating the formation of a protein complex called apoptosome. The apoptosome contains the initiator caspase caspase-9 complexed with apoptosis protease-activating factor-1 (Apaf-1). Both the intrinsic and the extrinsic pathways activate the common downstream executioner caspase caspase-3. This executioner caspase is ultimately responsible for the cleavage of many cellular substrates.*

chondria and (2) caspases. In the following paragraphs, we summarize what is known about these two systems.

MITOCHONDRIA

Mitochondria are membrane organelles localized in the cytoplasm of most eukaryotic cells. They are formed by two membranes delineating an intermembrane space and the mitochondrial matrix. Mitochondria contain multiple enzyme and protein complexes involved in respiration and energy metabolism, at the level of the inner membrane and in the matrix. They also contain several factors, the release of which into the cytosol contributes to apoptosis: cytochrome *c*, the flavoprotein AIF, Smac/Diablo, HtrA2/Omi, endonuclease G, and some pro-caspases (Kroemer and Reed 2000). Cytochrome *c* is the mitochondrial factor with the best documented contribution to apoptosis induction. Upon its release from the mitochondrial intermembrane space, it serves as a cofactor for the assembly of the apoptosome and the activation of caspase-9 (see later). The mitochondrial outer membrane (MOM) is normally only permeable to solutes of small size, i.e. molecular weight or $M_r < 1.5$ kDa, and not to proteins such as cytochrome *c* (Kroemer and Reed 2000). An increased permeability of the MOM occurs early in the course of apoptosis. How apoptogenic stimuli are converted into changes in the permeability of the MOM is controversial, but different models have been proposed (Kroemer and Reed 2000), implicating either the formation of pores in the MOM or its complete rupture.

The proteins of the Bcl-2 family play a key role in regulating mitochondrial permeability (Cory and Adams 2002). In mammals, there are at least 20 relatives of the protein Bcl-2 (Figure 8.2). These proteins share at least one conserved Bcl-2 homology (BH) domain, BH1–4. Members of the Bcl-2 family can be classified into different subtypes: the most evident classification is based on their opposing functions: (1) the pro-survival family and (2) the pro-apoptotic family.

The pro-survival members of the Bcl-2 family

Bcl-2 and Bcl-XL are the best-characterized members of this family. These proteins share a carboxy-terminal membrane-targeting sequence. Bcl-XL is predominantly located in the MOM, whereas Bcl-2 has a broader membrane distribution, including the endoplasmic reticulum and nuclear envelope (Kaufmann et al. 2003). The pro-survival members of the Bcl-2 family are probably required in every cell of the organism in order to

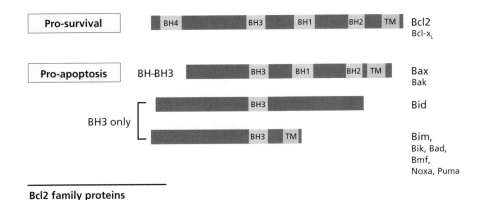

Figure 8.2 *Bcl-2 proteins. Proteins of the Bcl-2 family are often classified into anti- and pro-apoptotic subfamilies. They share some conserved domains (BH1–BH4), and hydrophobic carboxy-terminal membrane-targeting domain. The BH1–BH3 domains allow the members of the Bcl-2 protein family to associate to each other. The BH3 domain is present in all the members of the Bcl-2 family – it is essential for the pro-apoptotic function of the proteins Bax and Bak. The members of the BH3-only subfamily, such as Bad and Bid, function upstream of Bax/Bak. The BH3-only proteins constitute cellular sentinels, being able to activate the Bax/Bak system in response to a variety of death-inducing stimuli. Bcl-2 contains a BH4 domain which allows its interaction with other proteins. A caspase-cleavage site in this region eliminates this domain, thereby converting Bcl-2 into an apoptosis-promoting protein.*

prevent the spontaneous occurrence of apoptosis. Therefore, they play a critical function in tissue homeostasis.

The pro-apoptotic members of the Bcl-2 family

This family can be further separated into a BH3-only subfamily (Bad, Bid, Bim, Bmf, Noxa, Puma), and a BH1–3 subfamily (Bax and Bak) (reviewed in Cory and Adams 2002). The proteins Bax and Bak constitute the BH1–3 subfamily. Genetic evidence supports their role as core components of the apoptotic machinery, because Bax/Bak double knock-out cells are resistant to most apoptotic stimuli (Wei et al. 2001). The members of the BH3-only subfamily function upstream of Bax/Bak (Cheng et al. 2001; Zong et al. 2001). The BH3-only proteins constitute cellular sentinels, able to activate the Bax/Bak system in response to a variety of death-inducing stimuli. In a living cell, they are normally kept in check by different mechanisms, including sequestration at the subcellular level (interaction with the cell cytoskeleton in the case of Bim and Bmf), post-translational modifications (phosphorylation in the case of Bad, proteolytic processing in the case of Bid), or regulation at the transcriptional level (Noxa and Puma) (review in Cory and Adams 2002).

Kuwana et al. (2002) recently reported the use of a cell-free assay using purified components to reconstitute the permeation of the MOM by the protein Bax in vitro. In this system, Bax added to liposomes mimicking the composition of the MOM could permeate them to large-molecular-weight dextran molecules. This process occurred in the absence of any intrinsic mitochondrial proteins, but required the lipid cardiolipin (Kuwana et al. 2002). During apoptosis, protein efflux from mitochondria might be a consequence of local reorganization of the lipids in the MOM, driven by the proapoptotic protein Bax. This lipid reorganization might also cause the mitochondrial fragmentation that occurs during apoptosis (Karbowski et al. 2002).

The members of the pro-survival family of Bcl-2 proteins are able to bind directly and counteract the effect of the pro-apoptotic family members. In addition, they could protect cells from apoptosis independently of their mitochondrial effect (Kaufmann et al. 2003). Although the mechanisms involved are not yet clear, they may directly inhibit caspases (Marsden et al. 2002).

Clearly, many different events take place in the apoptotic mitochondria, and it is not yet possible to establish a causality link between them. Lately, a phenomenon known as the mitochondria-permeability transition (MPT) occurs. It is caused by the opening of a pore formed at the contact of the mitochondrial outer and inner membranes. This pore results in a drop in mitochondrial inner membrane polarity and swelling of the matrix, causing the rupture of the MOM and its non-selective permeabilization (review in Kroemer and Reed 2000).

CASPASES

Caspases (*c*ysteine *as*partyl-specific *prote*ase) are a family of proteases that play a critical role in apoptosis (review in Earnshaw et al. 1999). As their name indicates, they are cysteine proteases that cleave their substrates after an aspartate residue. Caspases are initially produced as inactive zymogens. They share a common structural organization in three domains: an amino-terminal prodomain, and two catalytic domains p20 and p10 (Figure 8.3).

Depending on the level at which they participate in the apoptotic program, caspases are classified as initiator or executioner. Initiator caspases play a role in the early

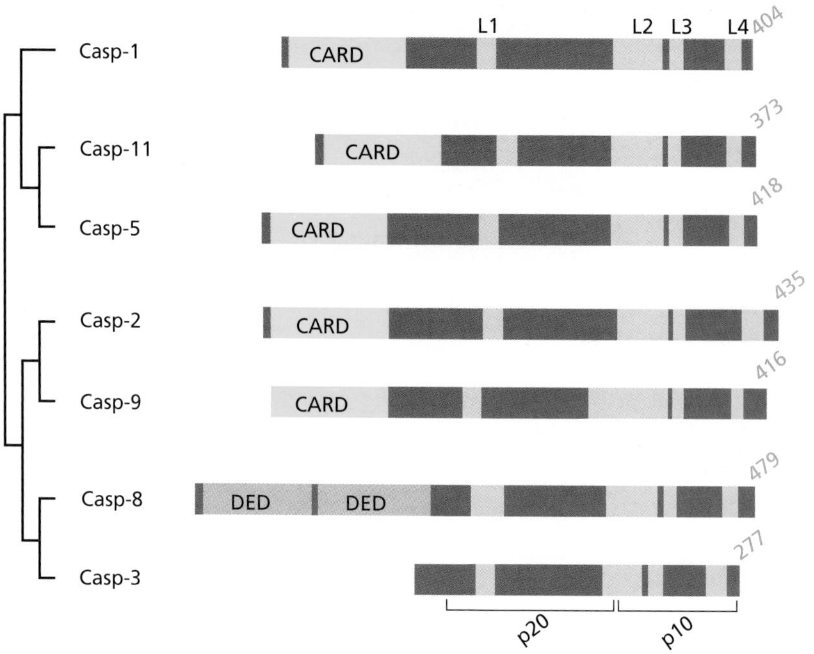

Figure 8.3 *Structure of caspases. Caspases are cysteine proteases that cleave their substrates after an aspartate residue. They are initially produced as inactive zymogens, and share a common structural organization in three domains: an amino-terminal prodomain, and the catalytic domains p20 and p10. Prodomain sequences vary among the members of the caspase family. In contrast to effector caspases such as caspase-3, initiator caspases such as caspase-9 or -1 contain a long amino-terminal prodomain. These prodomains contain one of the protein–protein interaction modules of the death adaptor family – death-effector domain (DED) in the case of caspase-8, caspase activation and recruitment domain (CARD) for other caspases: 1, 2, 9. These domains mediate homotypic interactions between the caspases themselves and with adaptor proteins. They therefore play a critical role in the activation of initiator caspases. (Adapted from Shi 2002.)*

phase of apoptosis, at the time the cell becomes committed to death. In contrast, executioner caspases are activated downstream of initiator caspases, and they are responsible for the morphological alterations that characterize apoptosis. These two types of caspases rely on two important mechanisms for their activation (review in Shi 2002): proteolytic cleavage of their constitutive domains and protein–protein interactions.

Proteolytic cleavage between their constitutive domains

Cleavage can be either autocatalytic or performed by other caspases. Proteolysis is the usual activation mode for the effector caspases, the prototype of which is caspase-3. Activated effector caspases cleave many proteins of the cytoskeleton, nucleus as well as other cellular organelles, thereby resulting in the characteristic hallmarks of apoptosis.

Protein–protein interactions

This activation mode is encountered with initiator caspases, which contain one of the protein–protein interaction modules of the death adaptor family in their prodomain. Members of this family are the death domain (DD), death effect or domain (DED), caspase activation and recruitment domain (CARD), and the newly described pyrin domain (PYD). Although they share no sequence homology, these domains have a common structural organization. Work so far suggests that they mediate homotypic interactions, typically between caspases and adaptor proteins (review in Shi 2002). These homotypic interactions between members of the death effector family are of paramount importance for the assembly of the large protein complexes that activate initiator caspases.

Here, we summarize only the data about the assembly of the death-inducing signaling complex (DISC), a complex that activates caspase-8, and the apoptosome, a complex that activates caspase-9. Other protein complexes contribute to the activation of caspase-1 (Martinon et al. 2002) and caspase-2 (Read et al. 2002), and are not described here.

The DISC is a large protein complex that activates caspase-8. It assembles as a consequence of the interaction between death ligands, such as TNF-α or Fas ligand, and their cognate receptors on the cell surface. TNF receptor family members contain a DD in their cytoplasmic tail, which allows them to recruit the adaptor protein FADD. FADD in turn recruits FLASH, a protein that assembles in a platform that recruits and activates caspase-8 by means of homotypic DED interactions (Imai et al. 1999).

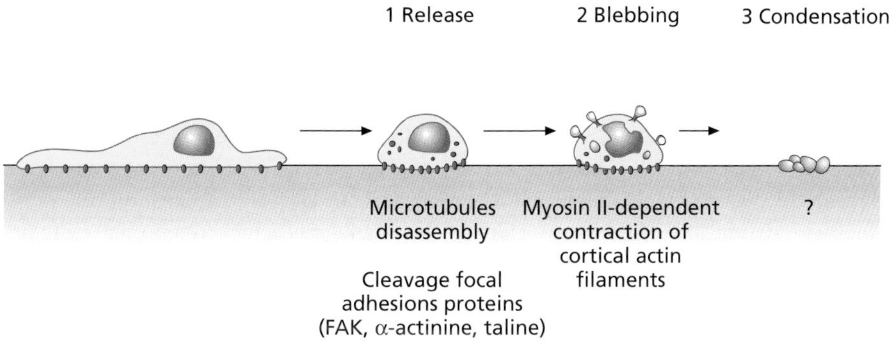

Figure 8.4 *The cytoplasmic execution phase of apoptosis. The cytoplasmic execution phase of apoptosis can be schematically divided into distinct steps: (1) a first step of release of the cell from its environment. The cell loses its attachment to extracellular matrix and to other cells, and thereby adopts a round appearance. The cleavage of some focal adhesion proteins, and a disassembly of the microtubule network, account for these modifications; (2) a step of blebbing, driven by the myosin II-dependent contraction of the cortical actin cytoskeleton; (3) ultimately, blebbing ceases and the cell leaves apoptotic bodies as only remnants. At that time, actin and microtubule cytoskeletons are disassembled or degraded. (Adapted from Mills et al. 1999.)*

The apoptosome is a cytoplasmic complex that assembles as a consequence of the release of cytochrome *c* from mitochondria. The cytoplasmic protein apoptosis protease-activating factor-1 (Apaf-1) is its main component. It recruits caspase-9 after binding cytochrome *c* in the presence of ATP/dATP. Pro-caspase-9 contains a CARD that mediates a specific interaction with the CARD of Apaf-1 (Shiozaki et al. 2002). A first determination of the structure of the apoptosome revealed that the Apaf-1/cytochrome *c* complex is a wheel-shaped oligomer, composed of seven Apaf-1 subunits (Acehan et al. 2002). The multimerized Apaf-1 forms a platform on which caspase-9 can dock and become activated in a CARD-dependent fashion.

Recently, a new potential aspect of caspase regulation has been highlighted: their subcellular compartmentalization. This could be an important determinant in their activation and substrate specificity, e.g. intracellular filaments recruit activated caspase-8 (Siegel et al. 1998). Nuclear import could also play a role in the compartmentalization of caspases. Candidate nuclear localization sequences (NLS) have been identified in the prodomains of caspase-1 (Mao et al. 1998) and caspase-2 (Baliga et al. 2002).

BASIC CELLULAR MECHANISMS AND REGULATION

Although caspase activation and mitochondrial permeabilization are involved in the changes observed in apoptotic cells, it is unclear to what extent these two systems are involved in the initial decision to die, and how much they contribute to reaching the 'point of no return' in the execution of death. Evolutionary considerations point to the importance of mitochondria in phylogenetically ancient organisms (Leist and Jaattela 2001). In mammals, however, this remains a controversial issue, and caspases might play a role upstream of mitochondria as initiators of the stress-induced apoptosis (Lassus et al. 2002). Nevertheless, there is a large consensus to attribute a role in the morphology of the dying cell to caspases.

Living cells normally prevent the spontaneous activation of the apoptotic systems. Among the proteins mediating this inhibitory effect, inhibitors of apoptosis (IAPs) are direct inhibitors of caspases (Shi 2002). All members of this family contain one or more BIR (baculovirus IAP repeat) domains, a domain of about 70 amino acids forming a zinc-coordinating fold. The proteins XIAP, c-IAP1, and c-IAP2 are direct caspase inhibitors: they bind to and inhibit caspases-3, -7, and -9. In addition, XIAP, c-IAP1, and c-IAP2 possess a RING-finger domain at their carboxy-termini. The RING-finger domain endows these proteins with a substrate-specific ubiquityl ligase activity toward caspase-3 and -7 (Jesenberger and Jentsch 2002). Ubiquitinylation is a post-translational modification of proteins consisting of the covalent attachment of ubiquitin, a small protein of 76 amino acids. Ubiquitin often targets proteins for degradation by the proteasome, a large cytoplasmic protease. Therefore, IAPs exert both direct and indirect inhibitory effects on caspases, by regulating their activity and controlling their destruction by the proteasome.

Decoy proteins also prevent the spontaneous activation of the apoptotic machinery in living cells. They exploit the use of protein domains involved in the apoptosis transduction pathway. Decoy proteins containing these domains prevent the spontaneous assembly of the caspase-activating complexes. This strategy is typically illustrated by the FLICE-inhibitory proteins (FLIP), proteins that possess DEDs and compete with caspase-8 for incorporation into the DISC.

Other systems appear to regulate cellular susceptibility to apoptosis although they are not directly part of its core machinery. The transcription factor NF-κB controls the synthesis of many regulators of the apoptotic pathway, such as members of the Bcl-2 or IAP family, and it therefore plays a major regulatory role during apoptosis (Karin and Lin 2002).

Once the initial brakes are relieved, activated caspases mediate the programmed demise of the cell. As more and more caspase substrates are described, we are gaining a better understanding of the key events responsible for the disposal of the cellular contents.

Important events take place in the nucleus. The DNase caspase-activated DNase (CAD) is activated as a consequence of the degradation of ICAD, its associated inhibitory protein, by caspase-3 (Enari et al. 1998; Sakahira et al. 1998). Activation of CAD is responsible for the cleavage of chromosomal DNA at the internuclosomal region, generating the typical DNA fragments visualized as a ladder on an agarose gel. Nuclear lamins, which are components of the nuclear membrane, are also cleaved. Lamin cleavage is probably partly responsible for chromatin condensation during apoptosis (Ruchaud et al. 2002).

The cytoskeleton participates actively in the morphological modifications that characterize apoptosis (Figure 8.4, review in Mills et al. 1999). In fibroblasts committed to apoptosis by death receptor activation, plectin constitutes an early substrate for caspase-8 (Stegh et al. 2000). Plectin, a member of the family of plakins, serves as a link among the three major constituents of the cell cytoskeleton: actin microfilaments, microtubules, and intermediate filaments. The cleavage of plectin is responsible for the early reorganization of the cytoskeleton observed in dying cells (Stegh et al. 2000). In epithelial cells, intermediate filaments (mostly of the cytokeratin family) are an early substrate of effector caspases (review in Oshima 2002). The cleavage of cytokeratins by activated caspases provides an interesting paradigm: in addition to contributing to the programmed dismantling of the cell, it probably provides a positive feedback for further caspase activation (Oshima 2002).

Membrane organelles such as the Golgi apparatus undergo fragmentation during apoptosis. The cleavage of protein p115, a key vesicle tethering protein required for the maintenance of this organelle, contributes to this fragmentation process (Chiu et al. 2002). Here, again, a cleavage product of p115 plays a key role by further amplification of the apoptotic response.

Taken together, the preliminary analysis of the apoptotic dismantling of the cell is consistent with the view that this process is highly organized, its multiple aspects being highly coordinated.

WHAT HAPPENS AFTER DEATH?

Apoptotic cells are efficiently recognized and removed by phagocytes (review in Savill and Fadok 2000). It is widely accepted that dying cells exhibit molecules that signal for their identification and clearance. A large number of cell adhesion molecules could participate in this process, although it is not yet clear which candidates really play a role in vivo.

A change in the distribution of phosphatidylserine (PtdSer), a phospholipid normally restricted to the inner leaflet of the plasma membrane, probably constitutes an important event for the recognition of apoptotic cells. In addition to the appearance of PtdSer on the outer face of the plasma membrane, apoptosis leads to the inappropriate surface localization of molecules that are normally restricted to internal cellular compartments. Many candidate receptors for PtdSer have been identified. The only candidates for which an in vivo contribution has been documented are the product of the proto-oncogene Mer (Scott et al. 2001), and the milk fat globule epidermal growth factor (EGF) 8 (MFG-E8), a secreted glycoprotein that might bridge PtdSer with integrins on macrophages (Hanayama et al. 2002). It is likely that they contribute in a cell- and tissue-specific fashion to the recognition of apoptotic cells.

Interestingly, the report of Brown et al. (2002) recently modulated the classic view that only 'positive' signals are responsible for the clearance of apoptotic cells. These authors showed that viable cells can deactivate macrophage phagocytic ability: a 'repulsive' signal follows the initial contact with the macrophage, and it is mediated by the homophilic interaction of the CD31 molecule present on both the macrophage and its prey. Apoptosis-induced disablement of this signal would promote the engulfment of non-viable cells (Brown et al. 2002).

The interface between the dying cell and the macrophage that attempts to eliminate it is an active one (review in Conradt 2002). The recognition of a dying cell triggers its phagocytosis by means of activation of effectors such as the small GTPase Rac. In return, the recognition of dying cells by macrophages could participate in the completion of the apoptotic program (Conradt 2002). Apoptotic cells signal not only toward macrophages, but also toward their neighbors: early during the apoptotic program, dying epithelial cells provoke their extrusion by an active, Rho GTPase-dependent contraction mechanism performed by their neighbors (Rosenblatt et al. 2001).

Traditionally, the recognition of apoptotic material is considered to have mostly anti-inflammatory and immunosuppressive effects (Savill and Fadok 2000). This view has been challenged recently and more work is clearly needed to determine how apoptosis influences the immune reaction. As the receptors involved in the clearance of apoptotic cells are better characterized, the role of apoptosis in inflammation and immunity will be better understood (Savill et al. 2002).

BACTERIAL-INDUCED APOPTOSIS

Bacterial pathogens induce apoptosis by a variety of mechanisms (Weinrauch and Zychlinsky 1999). One mechanism is the production of bacterial toxins, either pore-forming or with an intracytoplasmic mode of action.

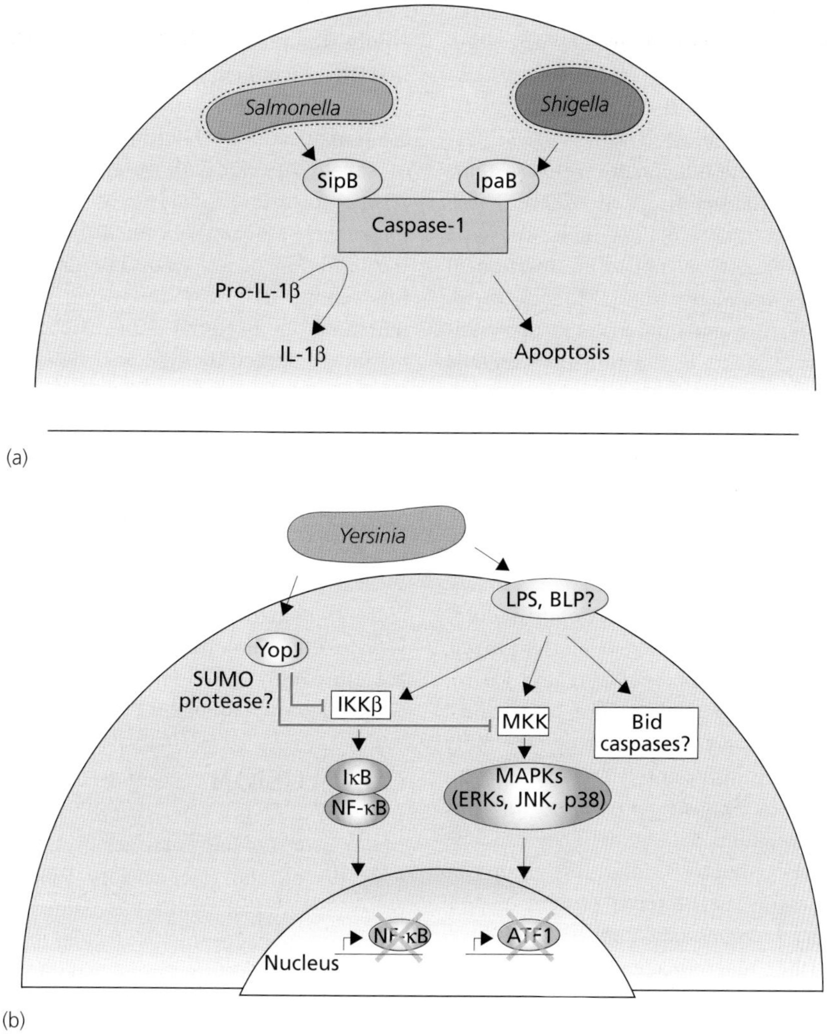

FIG020.5 **Figure 8.5** *Bacterial-induced apoptosis.* **(a)** Salmonella *and* Shigella *spp.-induced apoptosis.* Salmonella *and* Shigella *spp. provoke the death of macrophages by introducing, respectively, the proteins IpaB and SipB into their cytoplasm. The apoptosis that ensues is dependent on caspase-1. It is characterized by the simultaneous production and release of the proinflammatory cytokines interleukin (IL)-1β and IL-18. The molecular detail of the interactions between IpaB or SipB and caspase-1 are still unknown.* **(b)** Yersinia *spp.-induced apoptosis. The factor YopJ accounts for the ability of* Yersinia *spp. to kill its host's macrophages. YopJ has recently been shown to act as a cysteine protease, having the ubiquitin-like molecule SUMO as substrate. YopJ disrupts this post-translational modification. As a consequence, it inhibits the mitogen-activated protein kinase (MAPK) and NF-κB signaling pathways. These two pathways are used by the activated macrophages to produce proinflammatory cytokines, i.e. tumor necrosis factor (TNF)-α. As a result, macrophage death is not accompanied by the production of inflammatory mediators. Other bacterial factors recognized by surface receptors of the Toll-like receptor (TLR) family, such as bacterial lipopolysaccharide or lipoproteins, probably play a cofactor role in macrophage death induced by* Yersinia *spp.*

Other bacterial products can be secreted and translocated into host cells by means of specialized secretion systems, such as type III secretion. We have chosen to discuss here three model microorganisms, *Salmonella*, *Shigella*, and *Yersinia* spp., which induce apoptosis of macrophages as part of their pathogenic strategy.

P020.36 *Shigella* spp are the etiological agent of bacterial dysentery, a diarrheal syndrome. This intestinal infection is an acute, inflammatory disease caused by an acute destruction of the colonic epithelium. In contrast, *Salmonella typhi* disseminates in the immune tissues of its host, causing systemic infections such as typhoid fever in humans. Early during the course of its infection, *Shigella* spp. induce apoptosis of macrophages in the lymphoid follicles of the intestinal mucosa. The bacterial protein IpaB is responsible for macrophage death. IpaB is introduced into the cytoplasm by a type III secretion apparatus. Macrophage apoptosis induced by the bacteria of the genus *Salmonella* is mediated by the bacterial protein SipB, which shares more than 40 percent sequence identity with IpaB (Hersh et al. 1999). Both IpaB and SipB induce macrophage apoptosis by activating caspase-1: macrophages from caspase-1 knock-out mice survive infection by *Shigella* (Hilbi et al. 1998) or *Salmonella* spp. (Hersh et al. 1999). In addition to its role in macrophage death, caspase-1 is also a cytokine processor (it was initially named interleukin 1β (IL-1β)-converting enzyme, or ICE): its activation provokes, together with macrophage death, the release of the proinflammatory cytokines IL-1β and IL-18.

Caspase-1 knock-out mice infected with *Shigella flexneri* do not develop the acute inflammation that is characteristic of shigellosis (Sansonetti et al. 2000). These mice are also much less sensitive than their wild-type counterparts to oral infection, but not to intraperitoneal infection, by virulent *Salmonella* spp. (Monack et al. 2000). Caspase-1 activation and macrophage apoptosis are therefore important events in the course of shigella and salmonella infections. Both these bacteria use macrophage apoptosis as a virulence strategy to initiate an inflammatory response that probably favors their invasion of the intestinal mucosa.

The *Yersinia* genus offers another example of bacterial-induced macrophage programmed cell death. It includes three species that are pathogenic in humans: *Y. pestis*, *Y. enterocolitica*, and *Y. pseudotuberculosis*. Whereas *Y. pestis* is the causative agent of the plague, *Y. enterocolitica* and *Y. pseudotuberculosis* cause gastrointestinal syndromes, lymphadenitis, and septicemia. These symptoms appear as a consequence of the ability of *Yersinia* spp. to survive inside the lymphatic tissue of the host. In contrast to *Shigella* or *Salmonella* spp., *Yersinia* spp. are extracellular pathogens. They are able to induce macrophage apoptosis, and this apoptotic response is dependent on the bacterial protein YopJ/P (YopJ in *Y. pestis* and *Y. pseudotuberculosis*, YopP in *Y. enterocolitica*). In the macrophage cytosol, YopJ/P blocks the activation of the transcription factor NF-κB and the activity of a family of kinases: the MAPKs (Figure 8.5). It probably does so by cleaving the protein SUMO, a ubiquitin-like molecule that is covalently added to numerous regulatory proteins (Orth et al. 2000). NF-κB controls the transcription of genes that promote cell survival and the production of proinflammatory cytokines. In contrast to *Shigella* or *Salmonella* spp., by preventing the activation of NF-κB, *Yersinia* spp. induce macrophage apoptosis without causing inflammation. This response probably represents an adaptation to the extracellular lifestyle of *Yersinia* spp., which renders these bacteria extremely sensitive to inflammatory mediators such as IL-8, interferon-γ (IFN-γ)- or TNF-α. The simultaneous elimination of phagocytic cells and the suppression of proinflammatory cytokine production promote systemic dissemination of *Yersinia* spp. (Monack et al. 1998).

Apoptosis induction is not only induced by bacteria for purposes of pathogenicity, but is also an immune response used by the host against bacteria, in order to limit the extension of the infection. In mammals, this mechanism might particularly operate at the level of epithelia. In a mouse model of *Pseudomonas aeruginosa* pneumonia, Grassme et al. (2000) observed that bronchial cell apoptosis mediated by the cell death receptor CD95 allowed an increased survival of the animals. Apoptosis might contribute to the elimination of cells that are in contact with germs and to the prevention of bacterial dissemination. Apoptosis might therefore serve as an important mechanism preventing the establishment of 'sanctuaries' for pathogens.

Apoptosis is probably not only a mechanism that limits the pathogen's niche. It might also contribute to the initiation of a specific immune response. Following the apoptosis of *Salmonella typhimurium*-infected macrophages, bacterial antigens can be efficiently taken up and presented by bystander dendritic cells (Yrlid and Wick 2000). It is not yet clear how much the processing of antigens obtained from apoptotic macrophages contributes to the activation of antibacterial immune mechanisms. However, during the course of bacterial infection, macrophages could, by committing 'altruistic' suicide, (1) favor the recruitment of potent bactericidal effectors such as polymorphonuclear cells to the site of infection and (2) help deliver antigenic material in an efficient way to other immunocompetent cells. Apoptosis might therefore play a role in the immune response against some bacterial pathogens.

CONCLUSION

Major progress has been achieved in the field of apoptosis during the last decade. While the existence of programmed cell death has gained widespread acceptance, it has been possible to identify some key components of the death pathway. Apoptosis is now acknowledged as an important step in the pathogenicity of many diseases, including bacterial infections.

ACKNOWLEDGMENTS

We would like to thank David Weiss for critical reading of the manuscript and Diane Schad for her help with the figures.

REFERENCES

Acehan, D., Jiang, X., et al. 2002. Three-dimensional structure of the apoptosome: implications for assembly, procaspase-9 binding, and activation. *Mol Cell*, **9**, 423–32.

Baliga, B.C., Colussi, P.A., et al. 2002. Role of prodomain in importin-mediated nuclear localization and activation of caspase-2. *J Biol Chem*, **278**, 4899–905.

Brown, S., Heinisch, I., et al. 2002. Apoptosis disables CD31-mediated cell detachment from phagocytes promoting binding and engulfment. *Nature*, **418**, 200–3.

Cheng, E.H., Wei, M.C., et al. 2001. BCL-2, BCL-XL sequester BH3 domain-only molecules preventing BAX- and BAK-mediated mitochondrial apoptosis. *Mol Cell*, **8**, 705–11.

Chiu, R., Novikov, L., et al. 2002. A caspase cleavage fragment of p115 induces fragmentation of the Golgi apparatus and apoptosis. *J Cell Biol*, **159**, 637–48.

Conradt, B. 2002. With a little help from your friends: cells don't die alone. *Nat Cell Biol*, **4**, E139–143.

Cory, S. and Adams, J.M. 2002. The Bcl2 family: regulators of the cellular life-or-death switch. *Nat Rev Cancer*, **2**, 647–56.

Earnshaw, W.C., Martins, L.M. and Kaufmann, S.H. 1999. Mammalian caspases: structure, activation, substrates, and functions during apoptosis. *Annu Rev Biochem*, **68**, 383–424.

Enari, M., Sakahira, H., et al. 1998. A caspase-activated DNase that degrades DNA during apoptosis, and its inhibitor ICAD. *Nature*, **391**, 43–50.

Grassme, H., Kirschnek, S., et al. 2000. CD95/CD95 ligand interactions on epithelial cells in host defense to *Pseudomonas aeruginosa*. *Science*, **290**, 527–30.

Hanayama, R., Tanaka, M., et al. 2002. Identification of a factor that links apoptotic cells to phagocytes. *Nature*, **417**, 182–7.

Hengartner, M.O. 2000. The biochemistry of apoptosis. *Nature*, **407**, 770–6.

Hersh, D., Monack, D.M., et al. 1999. The *Salmonella* invasin SipB induces macrophage apoptosis by binding to caspase-1. *Proc Natl Acad Sci USA*, **96**, 2396–401.

Hilbi, H., Moss, J.E., et al. 1998. Shigella-induced apoptosis is dependent on caspase-1 which binds to IpaB. *J Biol Chem*, **273**, 32895–900.

Imai, Y., Kimura, T., et al. 1999. The CED-4-homologous protein FLASH is involved in Fas-mediated activation of caspase-8 during apoptosis. *Nature*, **398**, 777–85.

Jesenberger, V. and Jentsch, S. 2002. Deadly encounter: ubiquitin meets apoptosis. *Nat Rev Mol Cell Biol*, **3**, 112–21.

Karbowski, M., Lee, Y.J., et al. 2002. Spatial and temporal association of Bax with mitochondrial fission sites, Drp1 and Mfn2 during apoptosis. *J Cell Biol*, **159**, 9318.

Karin, M. and Lin, A. 2002. NF-kappaB at the crossroads of life and death. *Nat Immunol*, **3**, 221–7.

Kaufmann, T., Schlipf, S., et al. 2003. Characterization of the signal that directs Bcl-xL, but not Bcl-2, to the mitochondrial outer membrane. *J Cell Biol*, **160**, 53–64.

Kroemer, G. and Reed, J.C. 2000. Mitochondrial control of cell death. *Nat Med*, **6**, 513–19.

Kuwana, T., Mackey, M.R., et al. 2002. Bid, Bax, and lipids cooperate to form supramolecular openings in the outer mitochondrial membrane. *Cell*, **111**, 331–42.

Lassus, P., Opitz-Araya, X. and Lazebnik, Y. 2002. Requirement for caspase-2 in stress-induced apoptosis before mitochondrial permeabilization. *Science*, **297**, 1352–4.

Leist, M. and Jaattela, M. 2001. Four deaths and a funeral: from caspases to alternative mechanisms. *Nat Rev Mol Cell Biol*, **2**, 589–98.

Mao, P.L., Jiang, Y., et al. 1998. Activation of caspase-1 in the nucleus requires nuclear translocation of pro-caspase-1 mediated by its prodomain. *J Biol Chem*, **273**, 23621–4.

Marsden, V.S., O'Connor, L., et al. 2002. Apoptosis initiated by Bcl-2-regulated caspase activation independently of the cytochrome c/Apaf-1/caspase-9 apoptosome. *Nature*, **419**, 634–7.

Martinon, F., Burns, K. and Tschopp, J. 2002. The inflammasome: a molecular platform triggering activation of inflammatory caspases and processing of proIL-beta. *Mol Cell*, **10**, 417–26.

Mills, J.C., Stone, N.L. and Pittman, R.N. 1999. Extranuclear apoptosis. The role of the cytoplasm in the execution phase. *J Cell Biol*, **146**, 703–8.

Monack, D.M., Mecsas, J., et al. 1998. Yersinia-induced apoptosis in vivo aids in the establishment of a systemic infection of mice. *J Exp Med*, **188**, 2127–37.

Monack, D.M., Hersh, D., et al. 2000. Salmonella exploits caspase-1 to colonize Peyer's patches in a murine typhoid model. *J Exp Med*, **192**, 249–58.

Orth, K., Xu, Z., et al. 2000. Disruption of signaling by Yersinia effector YopJ, a ubiquitin-like protein protease. *Science*, **290**, 1594–7.

Oshima, R.G. 2002. Apoptosis and keratin intermediate filaments. *Cell Death Differ*, **9**, 486–92.

Read, S.H., Baliga, B.C., et al. 2002. A novel Apaf-1-independent putative caspase-2 activation complex. *J Cell Biol*, **159**, 739–45.

Rosenblatt, J., Raff, M.C. and Cramer, L.P. 2001. An epithelial cell destined for apoptosis signals its neighbors to extrude it by an actin- and myosin-dependent mechanism. *Curr Biol*, **11**, 1847–57.

Ruchaud, S., Korfali, N., et al. 2002. Caspase-6 gene disruption reveals a requirement for lamin A cleavage in apoptotic chromatin condensation. *EMBO J*, **21**, 1967–77.

Sakahira, H., Enari, M. and Nagata, S. 1998. Cleavage of CAD inhibitor in CAD activation and DNA degradation during apoptosis. *Nature*, **391**, 96–9.

Sansonetti, P.J., Phalipon, A., et al. 2000. Caspase-1 activation of IL-1beta and IL-18 are essential for *Shigella flexneri*-induced inflammation. *Immunity*, **12**, 581–90.

Savill, J. and Fadok, V. 2000. Corpse clearance defines the meaning of cell death. *Nature*, **407**, 784–8.

Savill, J., Dransfield, I., et al. 2002. A blast from the past: clearance of apoptotic cells regulates immune responses. *Nat Rev Immunol*, **2**, 965–75.

Scott, R.S., McMahon, E.J., et al. 2001. Phagocytosis and clearance of apoptotic cells is mediated by MER. *Nature*, **411**, 207–11.

Shi, Y. 2002. Mechanisms of caspase activation and inhibition during apoptosis. *Mol Cell*, **9**, 459–70.

Shiozaki, E.N., Chai, J. and Shim, Y. 2002. Oligomerization and activation of caspase-9, induced by Apaf-1 CARD. *Proc Natl Acad Sci USA*, **99**, 4197–202.

Siegel, R.M., Martin, D.A., et al. 1998. Death-effector filaments: novel cytoplasmic structures that recruit caspases and trigger apoptosis. *J Cell Biol*, **141**, 1243–53.

Stegh, A.H., Herrmann, H., et al. 2000. Identification of the cytolinker plectin as a major early in vivo substrate for caspase 8 during CD95- and tumor necrosis factor receptor-mediated apoptosis. *Mol Cell Biol*, **20**, 5665–79.

Wei, M.C., Zong, W.X., et al. 2001. Proapoptotic BAX and BAK: a requisite gateway to mitochondrial dysfunction and death. *Science*, **292**, 727–30.

Weinrauch, Y. and Zychlinsky, A. 1999. The induction of apoptosis by bacterial pathogens. *Annu Rev Microbiol*, **53**, 155–87.

Yrlid, U. and Wick, M.J. 2000. Salmonella-induced apoptosis of infected macrophages results in presentation of a bacteria-encoded antigen after uptake by bystander dendritic cells. *J Exp Med*, **191**, 613–24.

Zong, W.X., Lindsten, T., et al. 2001. BH3-only proteins that bind pro-survival Bcl-2 family members fail to induce apoptosis in the absence of Bax and Bak. *Genes Dev*, **15**, 1481–6.

9

Complement

B. PAUL MORGAN

INTRODUCTION

Complement (C) is a central component of innate immunity, playing important roles in defense against pathogens and the handling of dead and dying cells and cell debris. It also influences adaptive immunity, providing a bridge between these defense systems. The C system has been reviewed and revisited scores of times over the past three decades and it is not my intention in this chapter to rehash the reviews that have gone before. Instead, I will summarize what I believe is essential for an understanding of the system and then focus on more recent developments that have made the study of C exciting again, particularly those of relevance to human disease. Along the way I will, of course, show my own biases and give undue attention to aspects that I find personally fascinating. I hope that these excursions will be excused and perhaps even entertain.

Complement comprises a group of 17 soluble plasma proteins that interact with one another in three distinct enzymatic activation cascades (the classical alternative and lectin pathways) and in the nonenzymatic assembly of a cytolytic complex (the membrane attack pathway) (Figure 9.1 and Table 9.1). It is rigidly controlled by a battery of at least 10 regulatory proteins (CReg) present in plasma and on cell membranes which together prevent damage to self and rapid consumption of C in vivo. In the following sections, the anatomy of the C system, its activation and control, the physiological and pathological roles of C and its activation, the diseases associated with defective C function, and therapies targeting C are described.

HISTORICAL ASPECTS

Complement was discovered during the last decade of the nineteenth century from studies of the capacity of immune sera to kill bacteria and lyse foreign erythrocytes. Two serum factors were required for these bactericidal and hemolytic activities: a heat-stable factor present only in immune serum and a heat-labile factor that was present in both immune and nonimmune sera (Ehrlich and Morgenroth 1899, 1900). The heat-stable factor, termed 'immune body' by Ehrlich, was of course antibody present only in the immune serum. The factor destroyed by warming the serum (a critical cut-off of 56°C was demonstrated later), Bordet and, later, Ehrlich considered 'a complement' to the killing capacity of the immune bodies, coining the name we now all know and love (Bordet 1900). Another important finding from these early studies was the demonstration that C was used up or consumed during lysis of erythrocytes, indicating that it was more than the accessory factor postulated by Ehrlich, and rather an active participant in the lytic reaction, defined by Muir as 'that labile substance of normal serum which is taken up by the combination of an antigen and its antisubstance' (Muir and Browning 1904). The multi-component nature of C was first demonstrated by Ferrata (1907) in the first decade of the twentieth century. He showed that C comprised both water-soluble (euglobulin) and insoluble (pseudoglobulin) components, later termed C′1 and C′2 respectively. Application of other fractionation techniques identified further 'components', termed C′3 and C′4, so

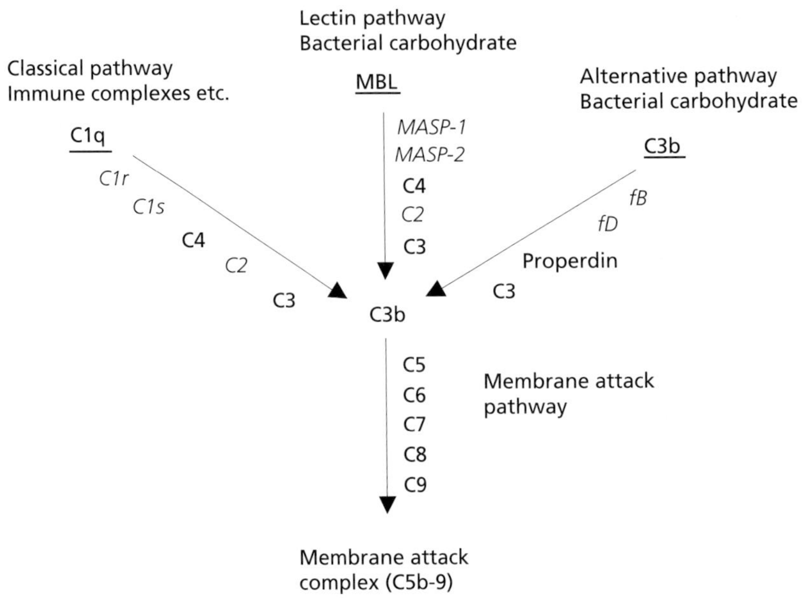

Figure 9.1 *The complement system. The constituent pathways of the C system and the component proteins are shown in sequential order. The initiating component of each pathway is underlined. Components that are enzymes or proenzymes are shown in italics. Abbreviations are as in the text.*

that by the mid-1920s it was clear that C comprised at least four different and separable activities from serum (Whitehead et al. 1925). However, the nature of these activities was unknown. Definitive evidence that at least some of the 'components' were protein in nature was first provided by Pillemer in his seminal work during the 1940s and 1950s, applying the new electrophoretic and ultracentrifugation techniques (Pillemer et al. 1954). These studies also revealed the presence of a second activation pathway, distinct from the antibody-triggered 'classical' pathway of Ehrlich, which was termed the 'alternative' pathway (Pillemer et al. 1954; Blum et al. 1959). Over the next two decades, pioneering use of separation methods by the group of Muller-Eberhard provided further dissection of the C system with the identification of at least nine protein components by the mid-1960s (Muller-Eberhard 1969). Complementary functional analyses, particularly from the groups of Mayer and Lepow, established the enzymatic nature of C activation and the reaction sequences from which the pathways emerged (Mayer 1965).

THE ANATOMY OF THE C SYSTEM

Complement can be activated in several different ways, reflecting the various targets for the system. The hemolytic and bacteriolytic phenomena observed by Bordet and Ehrlich were dependent on antibody that triggers activation of the classical pathway. However, pathogens and other 'foreign' targets activate C in the absence of antibody via two more recently described pathways, the alternative pathway and the lectin pathway.

Activation of the classical pathway

The classical pathway is 'classically' triggered by antibody attached to particulate antigen, although many other substances, including components of damaged cells, bacterial lipopolysaccharide (LPS), C-reactive protein (CRP), and nucleic acids, can also trigger the classical pathway in an antibody-independent manner. Attachment of immunoglobulin (IgG) antibody in sufficient density on the particle surface creates an environment in which the first component of C, C1, can bind. Not all subclasses of IgG antibodies are capable of binding C1; sequence differences in the antibody Fc (Cγ2 domain) regions influence the C1-binding site such that, in humans, IgG1 and IgG3 are strong binders, IgG2 binds weakly, and IgG4 does not bind. Classical pathway-activating capacity correlates precisely with C1 binding (Lucisano Valim and Lachmann 1991). IgM antibody is a strong binder of C1 and, because of its multimeric (pentameric) nature, does not require a high surface density to activate C. Conformational changes occur in the IgM molecule on attachment to antigen, making the Fc (Cμ3 domain) regions available for binding C1 (Perkins et al. 1991). C1 is a large multicomponent complex (molecular weight or M_r about 800 kDa), comprising a single molecule of the recognition unit, C1q, and two molecules each of the enzymatic units, C1r and C1s (Arlaud et al. 1989). The C1q molecule is a member of a growing family of proteins, the collectins, which have both collagen-like and lectin-like domains (Holmskov et al. 1994). Six subunits, each composed of three homologous chains (A, B, and C), associate along an extended collagenous tail and then

Table 9.1 *The component proteins of the C system*

Component	Structure	Sub-component	Plasma concn (mg/l)	(μmol/l)
Classical pathway				
C1	Complicated molecule, composed of three proteins, C1q (460 kDa), C1r (80 kDa), C1s (80 kDa) in a complex (C1qr2s2)	C1q	180	0.40
		C1r	34	0.43
		C1s	31	0.39
C4	Three chains (α, 97 kDa; β, 75 kDa, γ, 33 kDa); from a single precursor		600	2.93
C2	Single chain, 102 kDa		20	0.20
Alternative pathway				
fB	Single chain, 93 kDa		210	2.26
fD	Single chain, 24 kDa		2	0.08
Properdin	Oligomers of identical 53 kDa chains		5	0.09
Lectin pathway				
MBL/MASP	Complicated molecule, composed of three proteins, MBL (about 600 kDa), MASP-1 (93 kDa), MASP-2 (76 kDa) in a complex. Excess of MASP-1 over MBL in plasma	MBL	1[a]	0.002[a]
		MASP-1	6	0.07
		MASP-2	nk	–
Common				
C3	Two chains: α, 110 kDa, β, 75 kDa		1300	7.03
Terminal pathway				
C5	Two chains: 115 kDa, 75 kDa		70	0.39
C6	Single chain, 120 kDa		65	0.54
C7	Single chain, 110 kDa		55	0.50
C8	Three chains: α 65 kDa; β 65 kDa; γ 22 kDa		55	0.36
C9	Single chain, 69 kDa		60	0.89

a) The plasma concentration of MBL varies widely among normal individuals. The proteins that constitute the classical, alternative, and membrane attack pathways are listed. MBL, mannin-binding lectin; MASP, MBL-associated serine proteases; nk, not known. Modified from: Morgan, B.P. and Harris, C.L. 1999: *Complement regulatory proteins*. London: Academic Press.

separate to form the six globular heads, each of which represents a binding site for antibody Fc. Between the heads sits the enzymatic core, the $(C1r{:}C1s)_2$ complex (Figure 9.2). C1r and C1s are homologous single-chain molecules of M_r 80 kDa, which associate with one another and with C1q in a Ca^{2+}-dependent complex (Reid 1986; Reid and Day 1989). Upon binding to antibody through several head groups, conformational changes occur within the C1q molecule which in turn cause conformational alterations in the C1r proenzyme, triggering autocatalytic activation by cleaving a single site (R^{446}–I^{474}) in the molecule. Active C1r cleaves C1s at a single site (R^{422}–I^{423}) to activate the C1s serine protease (Arlaud et al. 1989). C1s in the activated C1 complex will cleave and activate the next component of the classical pathway, C4.

C4 is a large, plasma protein (M_r 200 kDa) containing three disulfide-bonded chains (α, β, and γ) (Schreiber and Muller-Eberhard 1974; Janatova and Tack 1981). C1s cleaves C4 at a single site (R^{737}–A^{738}), near the amino-terminus of the α chain, releasing a small fragment, C4a (M_r about 9 kDa), and exposing a labile, reactive, thioester group in the α chain of the large fragment, C4b. The thioester, formed between residues C^{991} and Q^{994} in the sequence GCGEQT, is key to the way that C acts selectively on targets (Dodds et al. 1996; Law and Dodds 1997). The exposed thioester in C4b forms covalent amide or ester bonds with exposed amino or hydroxyl groups, respectively, on the activating surface, locking the molecule to the surface. The two isotypes of C4, C4A and C4B, although identical apart from four clustered amino acids in the α chain, differ in their

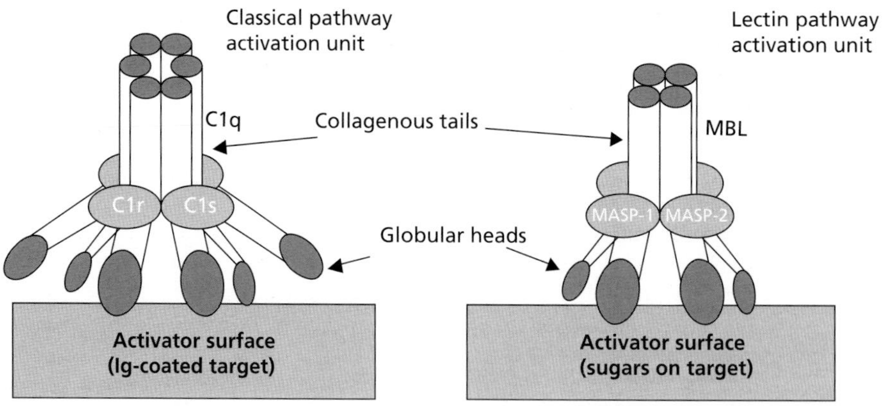

Figure 9.2 *The initiating molecules of the classical and lectin pathways. The activating unit of the classical pathway comprises one molecule of the multimeric C1q (itself made up of six subunits, each composed of three polypeptide chains), together with two molecules each of C1r and C1s arranged as a tetramolecular complex close to the heads of C1q. The activating unit of the lectin pathway has a very similar structure, comprising one molecule of mannan-binding lectin (MBL) (itself made up of between two and six subunits), together with two molecules each of MBL-associated serine proteases (MASP) MASP-1 and MASP-2 arranged as a tetramolecular complex close to the heads of MBL. Each unit binds an activating surface through its globular head groups, thereby triggering activation of the enzymatic components of the complex.*

surface-binding proclivities such that C4A preferentially binds amino groups and forms amide bonds whereas C4B favors hydroxyl groups and forms ester bonds (Tosi et al. 1985). The terminology used for C4 represents one of the many opportunities for confusion in the complement system, the lower case suffixes a and b denoting the fragments generated on cleavage of C4 and the upper case suffixes A and B the isotypes, both of which are cleaved by C1. Attachment of C4b is an inefficient process because the thioester is rapidly inactivated in the fluid phase by hydrolysis, effectively limiting the spread of 'active' C4b to the area surrounding the activating C1. C4b bound close to C1 provides a receptor for the next component of the classical pathway, C2, and presents it for cleavage by C1.

C2 is a single chain plasma protein of molecular weight 102 kDa (Kerr and Porter 1978). In the presence of Mg^{2+} ions, the proenzyme C2 binds membrane-bound C4b and is cleaved by C1s in an adjacent C1 complex at a single site (R^{223}–K^{224}). Cleavage is absolutely dependent on the association of C2 with C4b and fluid-phase C2 is not cleaved by C1. The larger carboxy-terminal fragment, C2a, containing the serine protease domain, remains attached to C4b to form the C4b2a complex, the next enzyme in the classical pathway, whereas C2b is released. Again, terminology is confusing. For most cleavages in C activation, the larger fragment that is required for propagation of activation is termed the 'b' fragment; for historical reasons, C2 does not follow this pattern.

C3, a 185-kDa two-chain molecule, is the most abundant of the C components (1–2 mg/ml in serum) and is essential for activity of all activation pathways (Lambris 1988). C3 attaches loosely to the C4b2a complex and is cleaved at a single site in the α-chain (R^{726}–S^{727}) by the C2a enzyme. Cleavage releases a small, biologically active peptide, C3a (77 amino acids; M_r 9 kDa), from the amino-terminus of the α chain and exposes in the large fragment, C3b, a labile thioester group formed between residues C^{988} and Q^{991} in the sequence GCGEQN. The thioester shares the properties of that in C4b and is similarly susceptible to inactivation by hydrolysis. C3b binds covalently via the thioester either to the activating C4b2a complex or to the adjacent membrane (Kozono et al. 1990; Ebanks et al. 1992). C3b bound to the activating C4b2a complex creates a new enzyme, C4b2a3b, the C5-cleaving enzyme (convertase) of the classical pathway (Kinoshita et al. 1988).

C5 is a two-chain protein of molecular weight 190 kDa, present in plasma at about 75 μg/ml (Tack et al. 1979). C5 is structurally related to C3 and C4 but lacks the thioester so it cannot bind covalently to surfaces. C5 attaches to C3b in the C4b2a3b convertase and is cleaved at a single site in the α chain (R^{733}–L^{734}) by C2a in the complex. A small, glycosylated fragment, C5a (74 amino acids; M_r about 10 kDa), is released from the amino terminus of the α chain, the large fragment, C5b, remaining attached to the convertase.

Activation of the alternative pathway

The alternative pathway provides a rapid, antibody-independent route for activation and amplification of C on foreign surfaces (Figure 9.3). The efficiency of alternative pathway activation results in large part from the fact that it is in a constant state of low-level or 'tickover' activation which targets all exposed surfaces (Lachmann and Hughes-Jones 1984; Law and Dodds 1990). As in the classical pathway, C3 is the central player, but three unique proteins, factor B (fB), factor D (fD), and properdin, are also involved. During tickover, C3 in plasma is hydrolyzed to form a metastable C3(H_2O) molecule which, in the presence of Mg^{2+} ions, binds fB, a single-chain (M_r 90 kDa) protein closely related to C2 and performing, in the alternative pathway, a role analogous to that of C2 in the classical pathway. Once bound to C3(H_2O), fB is cleaved by fD, a highly specific and constitutively active serine protease (M_r 25 kDa) present in plasma at very low concentrations (2 μg/ml). FD cleaves fB in the C3(H_2O) complex at a single site (R^{234}–K^{235}), releasing the smaller fragment Ba (M_r 30 kDa) and exposing in the larger fragment, Bb, a cryptic serine protease domain (Gotze 1986). The fluid-phase C3 convertase thus formed can now cleave plasma C3 at a single site identical to that described for the classical pathway, releasing C3a and exposing the thioester in C3b that allows covalent binding to surfaces. C3b binds indiscriminately to surfaces but further propagation continues only on so-called 'activator' surfaces such as invading bacteria. Healthy self-cells are 'nonactivator' and do not favor propagation. On activator surfaces, covalently bound C3b binds fB, enabling fD cleavage to form a surface C3bBb enzyme that cleaves more C3b, driving amplification and coating of the activating particle with C3b. Self-cells are nonactivators in part because of the expression of membrane C regulators, described below. However, it is now clear that the fluid-phase C regulator factor H (fH) is the main discriminating factor, binding and inhibiting C3bBb enzymes on nonactivators but ignoring those on activator surfaces (Jokiranta et al. 1996). Properdin, a single-chain plasma protein, also contributes to the survival of C3bBb on activator surfaces by binding and stabilizing the clustered complex (Lambris et al. 1984).

A proportion of the nascent C3b formed will attach directly to the C3bBb enzyme, creating in the trimolecular complex, $(C3b)_2Bb$, a binding site for the next component, C5, and simultaneously altering the substrate specificity of the enzyme to a C5 convertase. This enzyme binds and cleaves C5 in precisely the same way as described above for the classical pathway C5 convertase.

The lectin pathway

This newly characterized antibody-independent pathway of C is perhaps better described as a C1 bypass route because, apart from the initiating component, it is identical to the classical pathway (Gadjeva et al. 2001). The role of C1 is played by another complex molecule, structurally related to C1 and comprising a collectin recognition unit and associated serine proteases. The recognition unit, mannan-binding lectin (MBL) is a high-molecular-weight serum lectin, made up of between two and six structural units, each a trimer of a single 32-kDa chain. The subunits associate in a collagenous tail and separate into heads that form the recognition units (see Figure 9.2). MBL binds the simple carbohydrates

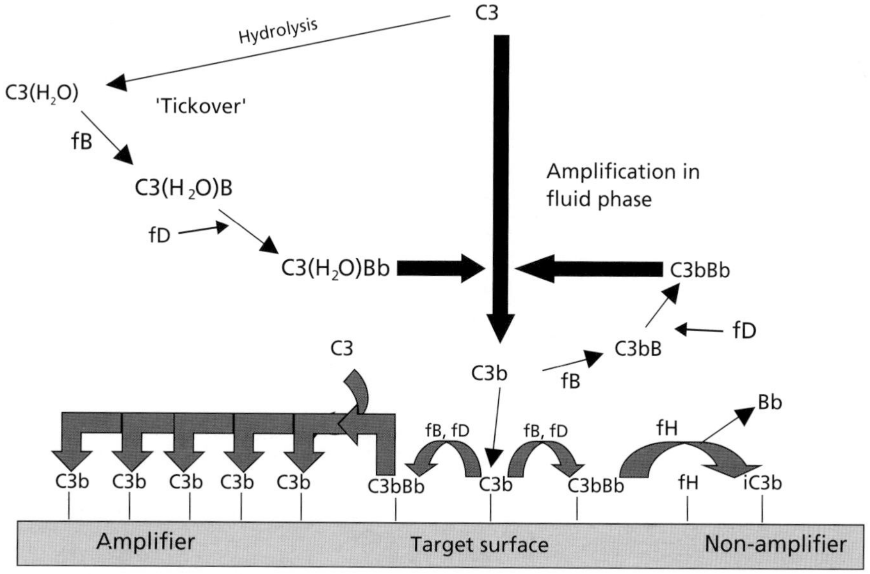

Figure 9.3 The alternative pathway activation loop and the role of fH. Activation begins in the fluid phase with the slow, spontaneous hydrolysis of C3 to form C3(H_2O). Binding of fB to C3(H_2O) and subsequent cleavage by fD generates a fluid-phase convertase, C3(H_2O)Bb, that cleaves C3 to C3b. Some of the C3b formed will bind fB and perpetuate activation in the fluid phase but a proportion will bind surrounding surfaces and form C3 convertases. On nonactivating surfaces (self-cells), fH (present in the fluid phase and on the surface) inactivates the bound convertase and stops further activation. On activator surfaces, amplification proceeds unhindered and the surface rapidly becomes coated with C3b.

mannose and *N*-acetylglucosamine present on the cell walls or envelopes of diverse pathogens, including bacteria, yeast, fungi, and viruses (Holmskov et al. 1994; Reid and Turner 1994). The enzymatic activity resides in MBL-associated serine proteases (MASP) MASP-1 and MASP-2, structural and functional homologues of C1r and C1s. Binding of the MBL–MASP complex to targets causes autolytic cleavage at a single site in MASP-1 and MASP-2 to unmask the serine protease domains. Although the precise roles of the two proteases are unclear, the weight of evidence suggests that MASP-2 in the complex is the C2-cleaving moiety. The activated MBL–MASP complex cleaves C4 and subsequently C2 in a manner identical to that described for C1 in the classical pathway. There is in vitro evidence that MASP-1 directly cleaves C3, bypassing the requirement for C4 and C2. The physiological relevance of this observation is not known. Recent evidence indicates that the ficolins, a family of lectin-like proteins present in plasma, can substitute for MBL and form C-activating complexes with the MASPs (Matsushita and Fujita 2001).

The membrane attack pathway

The membrane attack or terminal pathway involves the noncovalent association of C5b with the four terminal C components, C6, C7, C8, and C9, to form an amphipathic membrane-inserted complex, the membrane attack complex (MAC) (Muller-Eberhard 1986). The four terminal components are homologous molecules that have arisen by gene reduplication during evolution, a fact that is apparent from studies of the primitive C system of sharks (Jensen et al. 1981). Sharks generate a functional MAC from a single terminal component that most closely resembles human C9. The added complexity in mammals probably provides a more efficient targeting system to limit damage to self. The first step in MAC assembly involves the capture by C5b, still attached to the C5 convertase, of C6, a large single chain protein (M_r 120 kDa) present in plasma at about 50 μg/ml (DiScipio and Hugli 1989). A binding site newly exposed in C6 enables the C5b6 complex to capture the next component in the sequence, C7, a single chain protein (M_r 90 kDa; about 90 μg/ml in plasma) (DiScipio et al. 1988; DiScipio 1992a). Capture of C7 triggers release of the trimolecular complex from the convertase, and creates a binding site for the next component (C8), and a labile hydrophobic binding site through which C5b67 can bind tightly to the membrane. As a result of the lability of the membrane-binding site and the presence of plasma inhibitors (described below, under The membrane attack pathway), most of the C5b67 formed does not attach to membrane but 'decays' to an inactive complex that can be detected in plasma as an index of C activation. C5b67 that does bind membrane becomes tightly associated but does not disrupt the bilayer. C8, a large, heterotrimeric plasma protein (150 kDa; 80 μg/ml in plasma), binds C7 in membrane-associated C5b67, causing the tetrameric C5b-8 complex to insert deeper in the membrane and creating binding sites for the final terminal component, C9 (M_r 70 kDa; 60 μg/ml in plasma) (Sodetz 1989). C9 undergoes a major conformational change upon binding C5b-8, from a compact, globular shape to an extended conformation that traverses the membrane. As well as disrupting the integrity of the bilayer, this event exposes C9 binding sites for additional C9 molecules which in turn unfold, insert in the membrane, and recruit more C9 until a rigid ring structure, the classical MAC, has assembled (Podack and Tschopp 1984). The MAC ring, comprising between 12 and 18 C9 molecules, surrounds a pore through which ions and water can pass, causing osmotic lysis of the target. It should be noted that complete rings, the hallmark of the MAC, are not essential for this lytic process; even complexes containing as few as two or three C9 molecules cause considerable bilayer disruption, generating functional pores.

The active products of C

The physiological roles of C are mediated by the products of the pathways described above. In the activation pathways, the small fragments of C3 and C5 shed upon enzymatic cleavage, C3a and C5a, are powerful cell activators whereas the large fragments of C3 and C4 bound to the activating surface, C3b and C4b, direct phagocyte attack. The MAC can cause direct lysis of targets but may also trigger activation events in cells.

The opsonic C fragments

During C activation, pathogens become coated with C3b, C4b, and their breakdown products, a process termed 'opsonization'. These large fragments bind specific C receptors on phagocytes, triggering internalization and destruction of the pathogen. The important phagocyte receptors are C receptor 1 (CR1, CD35), which binds C3b and C4b, and CR3 (CD11b/CD18) and CR4 (CD11c/CD18) which both bind inactivated C3b (iC3b) (Krych et al. 1992). CR1 is a member of the regulators of C activation (RCA) family and, indeed, also functions as a C regulator (see below) (Rey-Campos et al. 1990). CR3 and CR4 are members of the integrin family of cell surface receptors (Myones et al. 1988). C3 fragments iC3b and C3d also bind another receptor, CR2 (CD21), an RCA family member structurally related to CR1 (Krych et al. 1992). CR2, absent on phagocytes but expressed on B cells, some T cells, follicular dendritic cells, and a few other cell types, plays important roles in the response to antigen, described below, under Role of C in the adaptive immune response. CR1 is also expressed on erythrocytes where it plays an important role in the transport of immune complexes (Madi et al. 1991; Pascual and Schifferli 1992). Immune complexes, coated with C3b through classical pathway activation, bind to CR1 on the erythrocyte, effectively removing the immune complex from the circulation – the immune adherence phenomenon. Immune complexes are stripped from erythrocytes passing through the spleen and liver and transferred to fixed macrophages, expressing C receptors and antibody Fc receptors, which endocytose and destroy the complex. The mechanism by which the immune complex is released from erythrocyte CR1 and the fate of CR1 during this process of immune complex stripping are still the subject of debate. Early studies suggested that CR1 was cleaved from the erythrocyte and lost during delivery; indeed, the reduced expression of CR1 on erythrocytes in systemic lupus erythematosus (SLE) was ascribed to this process (Davies et al. 1990, 1992). However, others showed that there was little or no loss of CR1 during passage of immune complex-loaded erythrocytes through the spleen and proposed a dynamic binding model for erythrocyte transport of immune complexes (Schifferli and Peters 1983; Schifferli and Taylor 1989). C3b attached to CR1, a cofactor for fI, is rapidly cleaved to iC3b, thereby releasing the attachment, only for another C3b to take up the attachment. In the spleen, macrophages expressing multiple C receptors and Fc receptors compete to capture the immune complex without loss of erythrocyte CR1. To complicate things still further, more recent elegant studies of immune complex handling in nonhuman primates clearly show that proteolysis of CR1 occurs together with delivery of the immune complex, brought about by specific proteases on the macrophage surface after the immune complex-laden erythrocyte has been captured through macrophage Fc receptors (Nardin et al. 1999).

The anaphylactic and chemotactic C peptides

Several active fragments are released into the fluid phase during C activation. C3a and C5a are structurally similar peptides (77 and 74 amino acids, respectively) released by the convertases of the activation pathways that mediate biological effects through distinct cell receptors, the C3a receptor (C3aR) and C5a receptor (C5aR, CD88) (Hugli 1984; Gerard and Gerard 1994; Ames et al. 1996). These are both members of the large family of seven-transmembrane, G-protein-coupled receptors and signal upon binding their respective ligands. C5a is arguably the most biologically active of the activation products. Binding of C5a to its receptor on neutrophils and other phagocytes triggers cell activation, chemotaxis towards the source, generation of reactive oxygen species, release of toxic cytoplasmic granule contents (enzymes, histamine, leukotrienes, etc.), and upregulation of adhesion properties. The net result is the recruitment of 'angry phagocytes' to the site of complement activation. C5aR is expressed on numerous other cell types, including astrocytes, smooth muscle cells, and endothelia, but the effects of C5a on these cells are still unclear. C3aR is also expressed on phagocytes – in high number on eosinophils and basophils, but in very low number on neutrophils (Zwirner et al. 1999). Binding of C3a activates cells abundantly expressing C3aR, but has little or no role in neutrophil activation. As with C5a, the effects of C3a on the many other cell types that express the receptor are unclear. The effects of C3a and C5a are focally and temporally limited because they are rapidly inactivated by a plasma enzyme termed carboxypeptidase N (anaphylatoxin inactivator). This enzyme cleaves the carboxy-terminal arginine (Arg) to generate the 'desArg' forms (C3a-desArg, C5a-desArg), thereby completely inactivating C3a and reducing the activity of C5a by one or two logs.

An intriguing story has emerged over the last decade linking C3a-desArg with the regulation of fat metabolism (Cianflone et al. 1994). The story began with the identification of a plasma protein, termed acylation stimulating protein (ASP), which stimulated triglyceride synthesis in fibroblasts and adipocytes in vitro. Characterization of purified ASP revealed that it was identical to C3a-desArg! This, together with the demonstration that adipose tissue was a major site of synthesis of fD (originally termed 'adipsin' in this context) and also produced C3 and fB, led to the proposal that a novel pathway involving local alternative pathway activation in adipose tissue to produce C3a-desArg (ASP) was a major homeostatic factor for fat metabolism (Sniderman and Cianflone 1997). In support of this proposal, a putative receptor for C3a-desArg was demonstrated on adipocytes. Doubt has been cast on the central role of this 'adipsin-ASP' pathway in fat metabolism, perhaps most persuasively from those who point out that C3 deficiency in humans and mice is not associated with deficits in lipid metabolism (Kildsgaard et al. 1999).

Of the other fragments and complexes generated during activation, the C4a fragment, although structurally related to C3a and C5a, does not appear to have any biological role in humans. The fragment Ba released during alternative pathway activation has been implicated as an immunosuppressive agent, but the evidence is weak and the mechanisms undefined (Oppermann et al. 1991). The fluid-phase product of terminal pathway activation, SC5b-9 (also called terminal C complex (TCC)), has been shown to activate both neutrophils and endothelia, although no receptor for this complex has yet been identified (Tedesco et al. 1997; Dobrina et al. 2002).

Role of C in the adaptive immune response

The activities described above, opsonization of immune complexes and pathogens, chemotactic attraction and activation of phagocytes, and other cell activation events, can be considered as the 'classical' consequences of C activation, acting to dispose of pathogens and other toxic entities. It is now apparent that there are other, less well-defined but equally important roles of C activation that contribute to homeostasis and the immune response.

A role for C in the adaptive immune response to antigen was first suggested by Pepys in a landmark paper in 1974. Pepys (1974) showed that the antibody response to T-cell-dependent antigens was severely blunted in C-depleted mice, implying a role for C in the immune response to antigen. The mechanism underlying this seminal and controversial finding was not identified until the early 1990s when Tedder, Fearon, and co-workers identified a critical role for CR2 (Tedder et al. 1986; Matsumoto et al. 1991; Fearon 1991). They showed that CR2 expressed on B cells is present in a complex with CD19 and other signaling molecules and plays a key role in the B-cell response to antigen (Figure 9.4). Particulate antigens coated with C3d, the cell-bound end-product of C3b inactivation, will bind both through the B-cell receptor and through CR2, delivering additional stimuli to the B cell and lowering the threshold of cell response to antigen by several orders of magnitude (Tedder et al. 1997; Fearon and Carroll 2000). CR2 on follicular dendritic cells plays a similar, though less well-defined, role and appears to be required for efficient antigen trapping. This key role of C3d in the generation of an efficient immune response is now being exploited in immunization studies where C3d coupled to antigen acts as a molecular adjuvant (Dempsey et al. 1996). C thus provides a strong link between the innate and adaptive immune systems that had previously been considered primarily as discrete, non-interacting systems.

Role of C in apoptosis

Cell death follows one of two pathways: either necrosis involving disruption of the plasma membrane by an external agent and release of intracellular contents, or apoptosis involving the triggering of an endogenous cell death program that leaves the plasma membrane intact and does not release cell contents. Given the lytic capacity of the MAC, a role for C in necrosis is easy to envi-

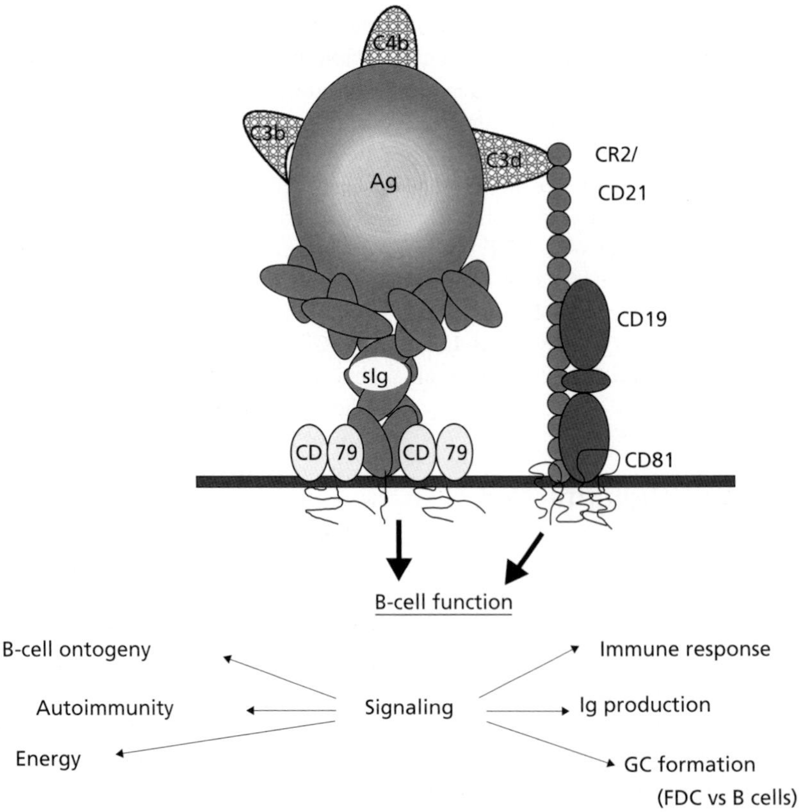

Figure 9.4 *The role of C in the B-cell response to antigen. The antigen (Ag) or immune complex becomes coated with C3b and other C fragments. Enzymatic degradation of C3b leaves C3d fragments, the ligand for CR2, attached to the activating complex. When antigen binds the specific B-cell membrane receptor (sIg), CR2 together with its associated molecules (CD19, CD81) is recruited through binding of C3d. The net result is that signals are transmitted to the B cell both through the B-cell receptor complex and through the CR2/CD19/CD81 complex, thereby lowering the threshold for B-cell response to antigen.*

sage. Indeed, in numerous models of ischemic injury where necrotic cell death is predominant, an important role for C, and specifically the MAC, has been demonstrated (see section on Complement in specific pathologies). Necrotic cell debris triggers further inflammation and C activation, in part through binding of the C activator, CRP, to the cell debris (Griselli et al. 1999). This in turn exacerbates injury in the models. Apoptosis, in contrast, is a 'clean' process that does not involve the release of cell contents and is not proinflammatory. Apoptotic cells will eventually undergo necrotic changes, making efficient removal by phagocytes an essential part of the process. Although C opsonization is an excellent means of targeting phagocytosis, it is somewhat counterintuitive to suggest that the proinflammatory C system might be involved in apoptosis. Indeed, numerous non-C recognition and uptake systems have been identified for the safe removal of apoptotic cells (Savill et al. 1993; Savill and Fadok 2000). Nevertheless, there is abundant evidence from in vitro studies that cells undergoing apoptosis activate C and are opsonized for uptake by phagocytes using the opsonic C receptors described above (Navratil and Ahearn 2001; Mold and Morris 2001). The relevance of opsonization to removal of apoptotic cells in vivo is a continuing source of controversy and the activating triggers a source of debate (Medzhitov and Janeway 2002). Early studies indicated that apoptotic cells activated the alternative pathway (Matsui et al. 1994), whereas later work demonstrated binding of C1q and MBL to sites on the apoptotic blebs, implicating the classical and lectin pathways (Navratil et al. 1999, 2001; Mevorach 2000; Ogden et al. 2001). Whatever the activating pathway, the consequences of C activation will be the same. Opsonization may aid clearance but, if activation were to proceed through to MAC formation, then lysis would ensue with unwanted inflammatory consequences. It has been suggested that activation of the terminal pathway on apoptotic cells is restricted, although no mechanism has yet emerged (Gershov et al. 2000).

Further evidence implicating the classical pathway in apoptotic cell clearance came from analysis of mice deficient in C1q. The mice developed an autoimmune glomerulonephritis with an accumulation of apoptotic cells in the kidney, apparently caused by defective clearance (Botto et al. 1998). These symptoms closely resembled those seen in C-deficient individuals with SLE or lupus-like disease, and provided a new concept of how C deficiency causes SLE, defects in clearance of apoptotic cells rather than immune complexes being key (Taylor et al. 2000). Perhaps the best analogy for the role of C, and specifically the classical pathway, in the prevention of SLE is that suggested by Walport (2001a), the 'waste disposal' hypothesis. This suggests that activation of C on immune complexes, apoptotic cells, and perhaps other debris labels these items as garbage for rapid and efficient clearance by phagocytes. Failure of this system, because of either C deficiencies or a garbage load that exceeds the labeling capacity of the system, will lead to the accumulation of garbage with resultant disease.

C activation products have also been implicated as modulators of apoptosis. C5a has been shown to protect neutrophils from apoptosis (Lee et al. 1993; Perianayagam et al. 2002), but accelerate apoptosis in thymocytes (Guo et al. 2000; Riedemann et al. 2002). In neurons, different studies have reported C5a-induced protection from (Mukherjee and Pasinetti 2001) or induction of (Farkas et al. 1998) apoptosis. The MAC can also influence apoptosis. Using C6-deficient rats in models of renal disease, the MAC was shown to drive apoptosis of mesangial and endothelial cells (Sato et al. 1999; Hughes et al. 2000). In contrast, exposure to nonlethal MAC attack of Schwann cells and oligodendrocytes, the myelin-producing cells of the peripheral and central nervous systems, respectively, protected against apoptosis (Dashiell et al. 2000; Soane et al. 2001). The overall picture is one of confusion, with different cell types responding in dramatically differing ways, the only common thread being that C activation products exert an influence, positive or negative, on the apoptotic process.

REGULATION OF C

It is evident from the above description of the active products that the C system carries with it the potential to harm self, hence the much-repeated adage that C is a 'double-edged sword'. To minimize damage to self, C is tightly controlled at multiple stages in the pathway by regulatory proteins present in plasma and on cell membranes (Table 9.2 and Figure 9.5) (Morgan and Harris 1999).

Regulation in the activation pathways

The first step of the classical pathway is regulated by C1-inhibitor (C1inh), a serine protease inhibitor (serpin), present in plasma at about 150 μg/ml. C1inh binds activated C1 and removes C1r and C1s from the complex (Davis 1988, 1989). C1inh forms a covalent complex comprising two molecules of C1inh and one each of the target proteases C1r and C1s ($C1inh_2C1rC1s$), and is itself cleaved in the process, therefore acting as a suicide pseudosubstrate inhibitor. C1inh is the only plasma inhibitor of activated C1 but also regulates kallikrein in the contact activation system of kinin generation and factors XIa and XIIa in the coagulation system. C1inh may also act to stabilize the proenzymic C1 complex by binding C1 in plasma, thereby reducing the likelihood of activation (Ziccardi 1982).

Although still a matter of debate, the weight of evidence indicates that C1inh also regulates the initial step in the lectin pathway (Matsushita et al. 2000). Regulation by C1inh mirrors that described for C1, acting to remove the proteases MASP-1 and MASP-2

Table 9.2 *The regulatory proteins of the C system*

Regulator	Structure/function	Plasma concn/tissue distribution
Activation pathways		
C1inh	Single chain, two-domain heavily glycosylated, approx. M_r 104 kDa. Suicide inhibitor of activated C1	150 μg/ml (approx. 2 μmol/l)
fH	Single chain, 20 SCRs, approx. M_r 155 kDa; cofactor and decay accelerator for AP convertases	550 μg/ml (approx. 3.5 μmol/l)
fHL-1	Single chain, 7 SCRs, approx. M_r 42 kDa, cofactor and decay accelerator for AP convertases, adhesion	30 μg/ml (approx. 0.7 μmol/l)
C4BP	Oligomer comprising 7 α chains (8 SCRs) and 1 β chain (3 SCRs), approx. M_r 550 kDa. Cofactor and decay accelerator for CP convertases	250 μg/ml (approx. 0.45 μM)
fI	Two-chain from single chain precursor, serine protease, approx. M_r 90 kDa. Cleavage of C3b/C4b in convertases	35 μg/ml (approx. 0.40 μmol/l)
DAF	Single chain, 4 SCRs, GPI tail, approx. M_r kDa. Decay of CP and AP convertases	Broadly distributed, all blood cells, endothelia. Soluble DAF in plasma
MCP	Single chain, 4 SCRs, tm tail, approx. M_r 60 kDa (two major isoforms), cofactor for CP and AP convertases	Broadly distributed, not on human E
Terminal pathway		
S-protein	Single chain, 75 kDa, binds C5b-7 complex and prevents membrane insertion	350 μg/ml (approx. 4.5 μmol/l)
Clusterin	Two chains (α and β each approx. 40 kDa) from single chain precursor. Binds C5b-7 complex and prevents membrane insertion	200 μg/ml (approx. 3 μmol/l)
CD59	Single chain, compact, globular, GPI tail, approx. M_r 20 kDa, heavily glycosylated. Inhibits MAC assemby	Broadly distributed, all blood cells, endothelia, etc.

For references, see the text.
AP, alternative pathway; CP, classical pathway; DAF, decay accelerating factor; GPI, glycosyl phosphatidylinositol; SCRs, short consensus repeats

from the activated MBL–MASP complex. C1inh forms covalent complexes with the MASPs, although the precise stoichiometry of these complexes is uncertain (Petersen et al. 2000). Regulation of MBL–MASP

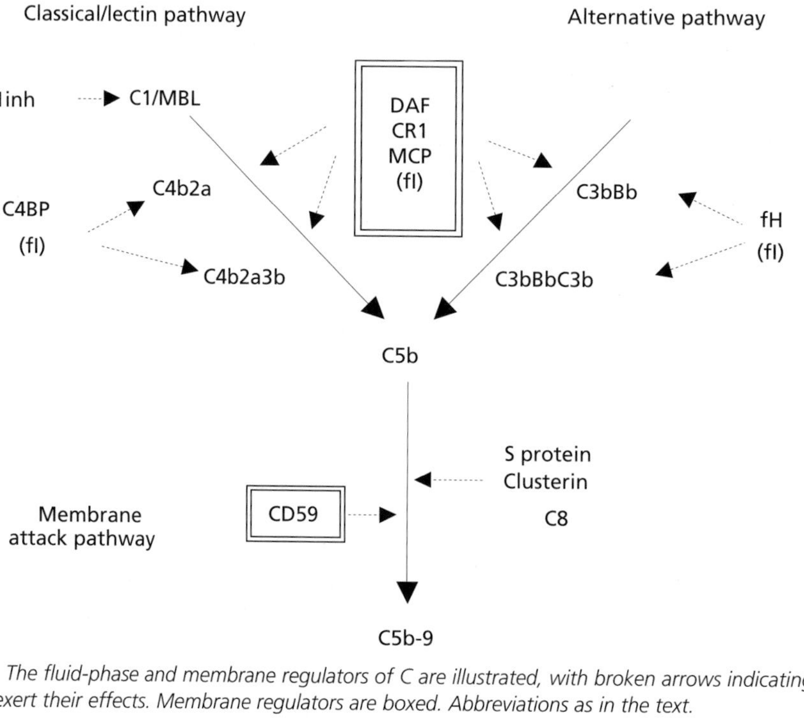

Figure 9.5 *C regulators. The fluid-phase and membrane regulators of C are illustrated, with broken arrows indicating the points in the pathway at which they exert their effects. Membrane regulators are boxed. Abbreviations as in the text.*

activity by α_2-macroglobulin, a plasma protease inhibitor structurally related to C3/C4, has also been reported in vitro, and complexes of MBL–MASP with α_2-macroglobulin have been detected in plasma (Terai et al. 1995). The physiological relevance of this interaction is unknown.

Control of the C3 and C5 convertases is provided by fI, a highly specific serine protease, which, in the presence of essential cofactors, cleaves the α chains of C3b and C4b to inactivate the convertases (DiScipio 1992b). In plasma, two proteins act as cofactors for fI, factor H (fH) in the alternative pathway and C4-binding protein (C4BP) in the classical pathway (Dahlback 1983). Both fH and C4BP also inhibit by accelerating the decay of the convertases. fH is the index member of a large family of structurally related proteins (Zipfel et al. 1999). One of these, fH-like-1 (fHL-1) arises by alternative splicing in the *fH* gene and regulates C. The others, fH-related proteins 1–5 (fHR-1 to fHR-5) are encoded by linked genes in the RCA cluster; their function is still under study.

On the membrane, decay accelerating factor (DAF) (CD55) acts to accelerate the decay of convertases, whereas membrane cofactor protein (MCP, CD46) acts as cofactor for the cleavage of C4b and C3b by fI, irreversibly inactivating the enzyme (Lublin and Atkinson 1990). Both are widely distributed, present on most cell types, although MCP is conspicuously absent from erythrocytes in humans. CR1, a large transmembrane protein mentioned above as a C fragment receptor, is also a regulator of C with both decay accelerating and cofactor activities (Holers et al. 1986). It is expressed on erythrocytes, B cells, polymorphonuclear leukocytes, follicular dendritic cells, and several other cell types. The active sites for C regulation in CR1 are placed a considerable distance from the membrane in the large CR1 molecule, provoking the suggestion that CR1 acts extrinsically to regulate C activation on surrounding cells and surfaces.

With the exception of fI, all of the regulators of C3/C5 convertases and several of the receptors for fragments of C3, C4, and C5 are members of a gene family, called the RCA family, encoded in the RCA locus on chromosome 1q32 (Hourcade et al. 1989). All contain multiple copies of a conserved structural unit, the short consensus repeat (SCR), comprising a compact motif of 60 amino acids with conserved disulfide bridges. Some RCA proteins, such as fH, are made up entirely of SCR units, whereas others contain additional domains performing other roles. The SCR unit is also found in non-RCA molecules that interact with C3, C4, or C5, including the C proteins C1r, C1s, C2, fB, C6, and C7.

Control in the membrane attack pathway

The membrane attack pathway is also regulated by inhibitors present in the fluid phase and on membranes. The fluid-phase C5b-7 complex is the target of S-protein (vitronectin) and clusterin, abundant plasma proteins (each about 0.2–0.5 mg/ml) that, among their many other roles, help regulate C activation by binding the hydrophobic site in C5b-7 and preventing its association with membranes (Podack and Muller-Eberhard 1979; Tschopp and French 1994). Binding of C8 to the fluid-phase C5b-7 complex also blocks attachment to the membrane. On the membrane, CD59, a small, compact, glycolipid-anchored membrane protein unrelated to the RCA-encoded regulators, binds tightly to C8 in the C5b-8 complex and perhaps also to C9 in the C5b-9_1 complex, thereby blocking further incorporation of C9 and assembly of the MAC (Lachmann 1991; Morgan 1999).

COMPLEMENT DEFICIENCIES

Deficiencies of almost every C protein and regulator have been described, giving a wide range of signs and symptoms, depending on the pathways affected by the deficiency (Figure 9.6). These 'experiments of nature' give important information on the physiological roles of C and have pointed the way to some surprising discoveries.

Classical pathway deficiencies

Deficiencies of components of the classical pathway (C1, C4, or C2) are strongly associated with a syndrome clinically indistinguishable from SLE, a consequence of the failure of immune complex solubilization (Walport and Lachmann 1990). The frequency and severity of disease are greatest with deficiencies of one of the subunits of C1 (C1q, C1r, C1s), closely followed by total C4 deficiency (Kolble and Reid 1993). The incidence of SLE is almost 100 percent in C1q deficient subjects, close to 70 percent in those deficient in C1r and/or C1s, and 75 percent in total C4 deficiency. C4 is unusual in that it is encoded by duplicated genes differing in only a few amino acids but yielding proteins (C4A and C4B) that are functionally distinct (Schifferli and Paccaud 1989). As a result of the presence of four loci, complete deficiency of C4 is exceedingly rare, but null alleles at one or more of the four C4 loci are common, giving rise to partial or complete deficiencies of either C4A or C4B. Deficiencies of each isotype have been associated with an increased incidence of lupus-like disease, bacterial infection, and numerous other disorders. Deficiency of C2 is the most common homozygous C deficiency in white people but infrequently causes disease – most C2 deficiencies have been identified by chance in healthy individuals. About 10 percent of C2-deficient individuals present with SLE. The strong association of immune complex disease with classical pathway deficiencies is a consequence of the failure of the 'waste

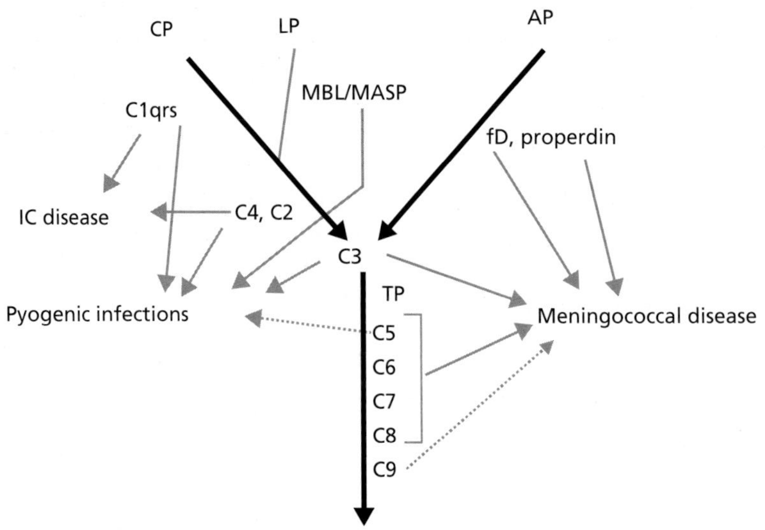

Figure 9.6 *C deficiencies. The clinical sequelae of deficiencies in different parts of the C system are summarized. AP, alternative pathway; CP, clasical pathway; IC, immune complex; LP, lectin pathway; other abbreviations as in the text.*

disposal' role of the classical pathway described in earlier. Bacterial infections are not usually a prominent feature of deficiencies in the classical pathway, illustrating the dominant role of the alternative pathway in dealing with bacteria.

Alternative pathway deficiencies

Deficiencies of alternative pathway components are rare. A few individuals deficient in fD have been described, all of whom have presented with severe and/or recurrent neisseria infections, usually meningococcal meningitis (Biesma et al. 2001). Homozygous deficiency of fB has not been reported, leading to the assumption that the defect was lethal. However, the mild phenotype observed in fB-deficient mice indicates that survival is possible in the absence of fB (Matsumoto et al. 1997).

Deficiency of the positive regulator, properdin, is the most common disorder of the alternative pathway and is also associated with meningococcal infection (Sjoholm et al. 1982). Properdin is encoded on the short arm of the X-chromosome and deficiencies are therefore found only in males. Three distinct forms of the deficiency have been described: type 1, the most common, is associated with complete absence of the protein, type 2 with low levels (1–10 percent) of apparently active protein, and type 3 with normal levels of a functionally impaired protein (Sjoholm et al. 1988a, b; Fijen et al. 1999). Affected individuals usually present with fulminant meningococcal disease that is frequently fatal. Disease onset occurs later than is usual for meningococcal disease (average age of onset 14 years) and is frequently caused by unusual serotypes of the meningococcus. Survivors rarely get recurrence because the antibody response developed during first infection is protective. Screening of male siblings is essential when properdin deficiency is identified because immunization can forestall the risk of a potentially fatal outcome.

Lectin pathway deficiencies

Defects in the lectin pathway are surprisingly common. Indeed, discovery of the pathway followed analyses in a cohort of infants presenting with recurrent bacterial infections. These infants exhibited a reduced capacity of their serum to opsonize yeast particles with C3b, initially ascribed to a defect in the alternative pathway (Soothill and Harvey 1976, 1977). Population screens identified this opsonic defect in up to 5 percent of the population, the large majority of whom had no history of recurrent infections. On closer analysis, no specific alternative pathway deficiency was identified in these individuals. More than a decade later, an association of the opsonic defect with a deficiency of MBL, the C1q-like lectin that is the recognition unit of the lectin pathway, was demonstrated (Super et al. 1989; Turner 1991). About 5 percent of the population in northern Europe have little or no MBL in plasma; in almost all cases, one of three point mutations in the *mbl* gene is present, each causing a single amino acid substitution in the collagen-like domain (Lipscombe et al. 1996; Summerfield et al. 1997). These substitutions interfere with the oligomerization of MBL monomers into the functional protein. Plasma levels in homozygotes are essentially zero, whereas, in heterozygotes, plasma levels vary from about 10 to 50 percent of normal, depending on the polymorphism, although functional activity may be much lower because oligomers containing mutant chains are functionally impaired. Clinical sequelae of MBL deficiency were initially considered to be restricted to infants; however, recent studies have demonstrated that MBL deficiency is also a risk factor for infection in immunodeficient adults and may be associated with increased disease severity in autoimmunity (Sumiya and Summerfield 1996; Petersen et al. 2001).

Inherited and acquired deficiencies of C3

C3 is the lynchpin of the C system, an essential component of all activation pathways and vital for efficient opsonization of bacteria. Deficiency is associated with a marked susceptibility to bacterial infections and, because of the critical role of C3 fragments in responses to antigen, a generalized reduction in immune responsiveness (Botto and Walport 1993). Some C3-deficient individuals also develop glomerulonephritis or lupus-like illness as a result of defects in immune complex handling. Skin rashes are a frequent feature, particularly during infective episodes. The large majority of C3-deficient individuals present with severe, recurrent infections early in life that can be fatal. However, prophylactic antibiotic therapy can now rescue such individuals, enabling survival into adulthood.

Secondary deficiencies of C3 resulting from consumption can also occur. C3 consumption associated with deficiencies of C regulators is discussed below; here, other factors that cause pathological consumption of C3 are introduced. Perhaps the most clinically relevant are autoantibodies, termed C3 nephritic factors (C3NeF), which bind and stabilize the C3 convertase of the alternative pathway, C3bBb (Walport et al. 1994). C3NeFs usually occur in the absence of other features of autoimmunity and the underlying trigger for their production is unknown. Although C3 is consumed systemically and plasma C3 levels can be very low, the dominant clinical consequence is membranoproliferative glomerulonephritis. Less commonly, C3NeFs cause an unusual and distressing syndrome, partial lipodystrophy, in which near-total fat loss occurs, predominantly in the upper body (Mathieson et al. 1993). Adipose tissue is targeted because it is the major site of synthesis of fD in the body. C3bBb complexes can thus form readily in the tissue and, in the presence of a C3NeFs, these complexes are stabilized and cause local activation of C sufficient to kill adipocytes. The gradient of fat loss, with the face and upper extremities most affected, reflects a differential capacity of adipose tissue to produce fD (Mathieson et al. 1993). Rarely, autoantibodies that bind and stabilize the classical pathway convertase C4b2a, C4 nephritic factors (C4NeF), occur; like C3NeFs, these consume C3 and are associated with glomerulonephritis and also lupus-like pathology (Daha et al. 1976).

Terminal pathway deficiencies

Deficiencies of terminal pathway components (C5, C6, C7, C8, or C9) cause susceptibility to infection with organisms of the genus *Neisseria* – meningococcal meningitis and systemic infection with the meningococcus (Wurzner et al. 1992). This reflects the role that the MAC plays in bactericidal activity against this group of organisms. It should, however, be stressed that most individuals with terminal pathway deficiencies remain healthy and are ascertained by chance. Deficiency of C5 causes loss not only of MAC function but also of the potent chemotactic and cell-activating fragment C5a. Despite this, the spectrum of disease in C5-deficient individuals does not differ from that in deficiencies of other terminal components. C6 deficiency is the second most common C deficiency in caucasians; other terminal pathway deficiencies are rare in this group. Deficiency of C9 deserves special mention for three reasons: first, because the link with meningococcal disease, although still present, is weaker, probably because C9-deficient serum kills bacteria, albeit inefficiently (Pramoonjago et al. 1992). Second, because it is extremely common in Japan where 0.1 percent of the population are deficient in C9. Virtually all Japanese C9-deficient individuals carry the same defect, a stop mutation early in the coding region ($D^{95}\rightarrow$Stop) (Horiuchi et al. 1998). Almost 7 percent of the Japanese population are carriers for this mutation. Third, the C9 concentration in neonates is extremely low, reaching adult levels a few months after birth (Lassiter et al. 1992; Hogasen et al. 2000). Neonates are thus likely to have reduced capacity to form MAC and may as a consequence be more susceptible to infection with *Neisseria* spp.

Deficiencies of C regulators

The activation pathways are regulated from the fluid phase by the serpin C1inh and by the enzyme fI, together with its cofactors, fH in the alternative pathway and C4BP in the classical pathway. Deficiency of C1inh deserves particular attention because it causes a syndrome termed hereditary angioedema (HAE), a relatively common, distressing and potentially lethal disorder characterized by episodic painless swelling of areas of the skin or mucosa (Carugati et al. 2001). Involvement of the laryngeal mucosa can cause asphyxia and gut involvement may mimic an acute abdominal emergency. HAE is unusual in that symptoms manifest in individuals heterozygous for defects in the C1inh gene. C1inh is the sole plasma regulator of activated C1 and also regulates activation in the contact and coagulation systems. Because C1inh is a 'suicide inhibitor', consumed when it interacts with its enzyme target, plasma levels reflect a balance between ongoing consumption and biosynthesis. A decreased rate of biosynthesis in the face of sustained consumption will therefore rapidly result in very low plasma levels of C1inh. In heterozygotes, synthesis will be reduced by around 50 percent but plasma levels of C1inh may be 10 percent or less. Attacks often follow minor trauma that initiates activation of the C and contact systems, normally held in check by C1inh. The products of uncontrolled activation, particularly bradykinin and fragments of C2, cause local increased vascular permeability that underlies the tissue edema. HAE affects about 1 in 50 000 people (Davis 1988); more than 20 percent of cases are the result of new mutations and therefore lack a family history of disease (Agostoni and Cicardi 1992). The most common form of HAE, type 1, involves mutations in the C1inh gene that yield little or no protein. Measurement of C1inh protein and function correlate and are both low. In some 15 percent of cases the mutated gene yields an abnormal, functionally compromised protein usually resulting from point mutations that cause amino acid substitutions at or near the active site of the enzyme (Davis et al. 1993). The abnormal protein is detected in antigenic assays, giving normal or elevated serum concentrations and masking the deficiency (type 2 HAE). Functional assays are essential to make the diagnosis. Angioedema indistinguishable from that in HAE may also occur in older individuals, usually in association with lymphoproliferative disease and, occasionally, other malignancies (Cicardi et al. 1996). Here, low level activation of the classical pathway by the large tumor mass and resultant consumption of C1inh causes a secondary deficiency (acquired angioedema (AAE)). Rarely, AAE may occur, in the absence of malignancy, caused by the presence of blocking autoantibodies against C1inh (Mandle et al. 1994).

The factors fI and fH collaborate to control the alternative pathway convertases in the fluid phase and on surfaces. In the absence of either, control fails causing unregulated activation of C and consumption of C3 and other components. Individuals deficient in fI or fH thus have profound secondary deficiency of C3 and the clinical consequences are essentially identical to those described for C3 deficiency. Individuals deficient in fH often have, in addition, renal disease, most commonly membranoproliferative glomerulonephritis or the hemolytic uremic syndrome (HUS). The association of idiopathic (noninfectious) HUS with fH deficiency is of particular interest. Although the link was first noted in patients with low plasma levels of fH, it has now become clear that apparently trivial mutations in the carboxy-terminal region of fH, which have little effect on the plasma level of the protein, can cause HUS, perhaps by interfering with the capacity of fH to bind surfaces (Taylor 2001; Zipfel 2001).

Deficiency of C4BP is rare and the few reports in the literature are lacking in information. Various autoimmune-like symptoms and angioedema have been seen in individuals with complete or partial deficiencies of C4BP but no clear evidence of causative association has emerged.

On membranes, DAF and MCP, the latter as a cofactor for fI, control the activation pathway convertases. No reports of MCP deficiency exist in the literature. DAF deficiency can occur as a global absence of DAF as a result of mutations in the *Daf* gene, or absence from circulating cells in the syndrome paroxysmal nocturnal hemoglobinuria (PNH), secondary to defects in glycosyl phosphatidylinositol (GPI) anchor synthesis. In PNH, erythrocytes and other circulating cells arising from the mutant hemopoietic stem cell clone lack all GPI-anchored proteins on the membranes (Rosse and Ware 1995). The absence of the C regulators DAF and CD59 renders the cells susceptible to C damage in the circulation, causing hemolysis, thrombosis, and leukocyte activation. Erythrocytes are particularly affected because they naturally lack MCP and are thus essentially devoid of protection from C. Several DAF-deficient individuals have been described, recognized because of the absence of the Cromer blood group antigens (the *Inab* phenotype), known to reside within DAF (Merry et al. 1989; Telen and Green 1989). Individuals deficient in DAF were healthy apart from a vague association with intestinal problems in some families. In particular, DAF-deficient individuals did not have intravascular hemolysis or other evidence of C damage to circulating cells.

No reports of complete deficiencies of S-protein (vitronectin) or clusterin, the fluid-phase inhibitors of the terminal pathway, have been published. These proteins have numerous biological roles outside the C system that probably make them indispensable. On the membrane, CD59 regulates the terminal pathway (Davies and Lachmann 1993). As noted above, PNH cells are deficient in CD59 and DAF as a result of defective GPI anchor synthesis and are, as a consequence, susceptible to C damage. A single individual with global absence of CD59 caused by *Cd59* gene mutation has been reported, presenting at a young age with symptoms compatible with PNH (Yamashina et al. 1990). Taken together with the lack of symptoms associated with DAF deficiency, these observations make it clear that CD59 is crucial for survival of cells in the circulation.

COMPLEMENT IN SPECIFIC PATHOLOGIES

Inappropriate activation of C occurs in a large number of inflammatory, iatrogenic, ischemic, and other diseases and, in many, is a major contributor to the initiation or perpetuation of tissue damage (Table 9.3). Pathological effects are mediated by precisely the same mediators that are responsible for the protective roles of C described above. The anaphylactic and chemotactic peptide C5a drives inflammation by recruiting and activating neutrophils, C3a may cause pathological activation of other phagocytes, the MAC may kill or injure cells, and so on. Evidence for a role of C may be sought in humans by looking for the products of C activation either in the tissues or in plasma. In many cases, animal

Table 9.3 *Examples of diseases in which C is implicated*

Disease	Evidence of C involvement
Immune-mediated diseases	
Rheumatoid arthritis (RA)	Consumption of plasma C in acute disease; C activation products in synovial fluid and synovial membrane; C inhibition (various agents) suppresses disease in animal models of rheumatoid arthritis (RA); C deficiency suppresses disease in mouse models of RA
Membranoproliferative glomerulonephritis (MPGN)	Abundant deposits of C activation products, including membrane attack complex (MAC), in glomeruli; C inhibition (various agents) suppresses disease in models of MPGN; intrarenal administration of C regulators suppresses disease in models
Multiple sclerosis (MS)	C activation products in CSF and around areas of demyelination in the CNS; C inhibition (various agents) suppresses disease in animal models of MS; C deficiency suppresses disease in rodent models of MS
Myasthenia gravis (MG)	Abundant C activation products at motor end plate during attacks; C deficiency or depletion abrogates disease in rodent models; C inhibition (CVF; sCR1) suppresses disease in models of MG
Degenerative diseases	
Alzheimer's disease	C activation products in and around plaques in CNS; anti-inflammatory therapy appears to slow progression
Ischaemia–reperfusion injuries	
Myocardial infarct (MI)	Reperfusion associated with C activation in ischemic area; abundant deposits of C activation products in and around infarct; C inhibition at time of reperfusion in models reduces size of infarct
Stroke	Evidence as described above for MI

For references, see the text.

models have proved invaluable in dissecting the roles of C in diseases. Here, no attempt is made to discuss all of these diseases but instead a few examples of disease groups where C plays a part are given.

Complement in SLE and related syndromes

Systemic lupus erythematosus (SLE) is characterized pathologically by the presence of immune complex deposits in affected tissues such as the kidney and skin, which are invariably associated with deposition of C components. Plasma C activity and plasma levels of specific components, particularly C3 and C4, are low in severe disease, reflecting the massive C consumption that occurs in the tissues. These observations have generated the consensus view that C activation drives tissue damage in SLE and related diseases. However, this consensus is difficult to reconcile with the knowledge that disease closely resembling SLE occurs in individuals deficient in components of the classical pathway, where the capacity to generate the toxic products of C activation will be impaired (Navratil et al. 1999). A better explanation for the occurrence of SLE in C-deficient and C-sufficient individuals is provided by Walport's 'waste disposal' hypothesis (Walport 2001b). This suggests that a crucial role of C is the safe disposal of immune complexes and apoptotic cells via binding of C1 and C4 and subsequent engulfment by macrophages. In C deficiency the process fails because of a global lack of these components. In idiopathic SLE it fails because consumption of C causes a localized, secondary deficiency of C1 and C4. In either situation, accumulation of 'garbage' in the tissues is toxic and initiates further tissue damage.

An additional precipitating factor in some individuals with idiopathic SLE is the presence of autoantibodies against the collagen-like region (CLR) of C1q (anti-C1q CLR), which are thought to affect C1 function (Strife et al. 1989; Wener et al. 1989). The presence of anti-C1q CLR antibodies correlates strongly with the severity of renal disease in SLE. These autoantibodies are also found in association with several other pathologies, including membranous glomerulonephritis, rheumatoid vasculitis, and hypocomplementemic urticarial vasculitis (HUVS). Virtually all patients with HUVS have anti-C1q CLR antibodies and the presence of these antibodies has been used as a diagnostic test for this syndrome (Wisnieski and Naff 1989; Wisnieski et al. 1995).

Complement in ischemia–reperfusion injuries

Many common conditions are caused by a transient or permanent loss of blood supply to tissue. Examples include myocardial infarction (MI), ischemic strokes, and malfunction in newly transplanted organs. In transient ischemia, much of the damage is done during reperfusion rather than in the ischemic period. Restoration of blood flow, either spontaneous or achieved through thrombolytic therapy, is accompanied by tissue damage and destruction that often extend far beyond the margins of the ischemic area. One of the major tissue-damaging factors is C activation. Dead and damaged cells are efficient activators of C and local activation during reperfusion of ischemic tissue will cause further tissue damage, propagating the injury into surrounding viable tissue. In MI, the infarct and surrounding 'penumbra' of damaged but viable tissue contains abundant deposits of C activation products, also detectable in plasma for days after the episode (Kilgore et al. 1994). CRP is also deposited in and around the infarct where it binds to damaged cells and triggers further activation of C (Griselli et al. 1999).

Similar evidence is apparent in stroke where the effects of C activation may be magnified because of the remarkable sensitivity of brain cells to C damage (Singhrao et al. 2000). In transplanted organs, the degree of C activation and tissue damage correlate closely with the ischemic interval between organ harvest and implantation. The involvement of C during the brief window of reperfusion in all these injuries presents an ideal opportunity for the use of anti-C agents. Early studies, using the C-depleting agent cobra venom factor (CVF) showed a marked protective effect when given before reperfusion in a baboon model of MI (Crawford et al. 1988). CVF pre-treatment also markedly increased graft survival in rodent models of heart and kidney transplantation (Thomas et al. 1977; Forbes et al. 1978). CVF is a toxic and highly antigenic agent that inactivates C by depleting the system to exhaustion and it is therefore not suitable for use as a therapeutic. Modern C therapies have also been used in ischemia–reperfusion models. A recombinant soluble form of the C receptor CR1 (sCR1), an efficient inhibitor of C in vivo, markedly reduces infarct volume when given at the time of reperfusion in a rat model of MI (Weisman et al. 1990).

Complement in neurological diseases

Complement has been implicated in diverse disorders of the nervous system, including such conditions as stroke, traumatic injury, demyelinating disorders, and neurodegenerative diseases. A summary of the information from the last two groups of diseases follows.

Demyelination in the central nervous system causes multiple sclerosis (MS), a distressing, progressive disease that causes severe disability and even death in sufferers. The underlying cause of MS remains the subject of debate, although it is now broadly accepted that there is an underlying autoimmune component. T cells infiltrating the areas of pathology in the brain are prime suspects. Indeed, in animal models of MS, disease can be transferred by T cells from affected animals to naïve recipients. A role for C in MS was first suggested by demonstrating C consumption and C activation products in plasma and cerebrospinal fluid (CSF) (Morgan et al. 1984; Mollnes et al. 1987). Others showed C deposition in and around plaques in MS brain (Compston et al. 1989) and demonstrated that myelin in vitro directly activated C via the classical pathway (Liu et al. 1983). Recently, detailed clinical and histopathological studies have divided MS into several subgroups, C activation being a major feature in some but not all the groups (Lucchinetti et al. 2000). Decomplementation or therapy with anti-C agents reduced myelin injury in rodent models of MS, further implicating C in myelin loss (Linington et al. 1989; Piddlesden et al. 1994). Demyelination in the peripheral nervous system causes several related pathologies, the most common of which is the Guillain–Barré syndrome (GBS). A role for C was first suggested from demonstrations of the capacity of peripheral nerve myelin to activate C (Koski et al. 1985). C activation products were found in CSF (Sanders et al. 1986) and peripheral nerve (Hafer-Macko et al. 1996) from GBS patients, and decomplementation inhibited disease in the rodent model of GBS (Vriesendorp et al. 1995).

Taken together, these data make a persuasive case for the use of anti-C therapy in at least some forms of demyelinating diseases. The problem is that none of the currently available agents is suitable for long-term therapy, so treatment in MS will probably have to await the development of better drugs. GBS, unlike MS, is a relatively acute disease, most patients making a complete or partial recovery from the demyelinating episode. Anti-C therapy given early in the course of disease might have particularly beneficial effects and could be undertaken with contemporary agents.

To suggest that the innate immune system contributes to degenerative disorders of the nervous system smacks of heresy, yet there is a substantial and growing body of evidence to support the suggestion. Neurodegeneration underlying Alzheimer's disease and related syndromes is, despite an enormous research effort over the past decade, poorly understood. Many mechanisms have been proposed but none has yet proved to be the key to understanding and preventing loss of neurons. The first suggestion of a role of C came from histological studies that showed deposits of C activation products in and around the plaques and tangles that typify the brain in Alzheimer's disease (McGeer et al. 1991, 1994; Eikelenboom et al. 1992). The β-amyloid peptide that is present in plaques activates C in an antibody-independent manner. These findings have led several workers in the field to suggest that Alzheimer's disease is a low-grade inflammatory disease and that anti-inflammatory or anti-C therapy would slow or reverse cognitive decline in Alzheimer's disease (McGeer and McGeer 1999). Trials of anti-inflammatory agents have begun and time will tell whether this approach is likely to be of benefit. Studies in the many animal models of Alzheimer's disease may also help establish whether C plays a significant role in neurodegeneration.

Complement in iatrogenic syndromes

With increasingly sophisticated interventions, iatrogenic or treatment-caused injuries are becoming more frequent. Here, focus is given to one group of injuries where C is known to have a role and anti-C therapies might prove beneficial.

Numerous interventions involve exposure of blood to a foreign surface in an extracorporeal circuit. In renal dialysis, blood is exposed to the dialyzer membrane, usually made of cellulosic materials such as cuprophane, or polymeric materials such as polysulfone. All these materials are, to a greater or lesser extent, bioincompatible and trigger activation of many plasma effector systems, including C. Activation of C and generation of C activation products, particularly C5a, activates neutrophils and other cells in the plasma and can cause fever, neutropenia, and other unwanted effects. The problem can be circumvented to a degree by choosing the least activating surface or by precoating the dialyzer membrane with either albumin or plasma proteins. Membranes that are used several times are always most activating on first use because of this surface-coating phenomenon. C activation can be reduced by pretreating the membrane with heparin, an inhibitor of C activation. C activation may be even more marked in cardiopulmonary bypass circuits, where not only the extensive surfaces of membranes and tubing, but also the plasma-expanding fluids and the gas–liquid interface in the oxygenator, may all activate C (Mollnes et al. 1991; Mollnes 1997). Secondary activation of neutrophils and other blood cells, and generation of inflammatory cytokines, will contribute to the injury and it is not uncommon for patients coming off bypass to be severely compromised for several days, necessitating prolonged intensive care – the post-bypass syndrome. Again, choice of the least activating system and precoating of circuits with protein and/or heparin may reduce activation in the circuit and minimize iatrogenic injury (Svennevig et al. 1993; Fosse et al. 1994). Studies in vitro and in animal models indicate that administration of anti-C agents during the period of bypass may be of great benefit in reducing the risk of unwanted sequelae (Gillinov et al. 1993; Moat et al. 1993; Finn et al. 1996; Lazar et al. 1999).

COMPLEMENT THERAPIES

It should be clear from the previous sections that an ability to manipulate the C system therapeutically might be of considerable benefit in many diseases. Until very recently, no agents suitable for the inhibition of C in humans were available. Crude methods using agents that consumed C (CVF) or, at high doses, expressed a modest anti-C activity (e.g. low-molecular-weight heparins) had been used in animals with some promising results. However, problems of toxicity, antigenicity, or other unwanted effects rendered such agents unusable in humans. The breakthrough came with the demonstration, in the early 1990s, that an engineered recombinant soluble form of a natural C regulator, CR1, was a powerful inhibitor of C activation both in vitro and in vivo (Weisman et al. 1990). Over the last decade, the field of C therapies has exploded and we now have numerous agents on the verge of application in the clinic (Table 9.4).

There are various considerations to be taken into account when developing anti-C therapies. These include the side effects of long-term systemic inhibition of the C system, choice of the most efficient point at which to inhibit C, rapid clearance of reagents in vivo, and the high cost of biological therapies. Inhibition of C will render the recipient less capable of fending off bacterial infections, may predispose to immune complex diseases, and could cause defects in immune tolerance. Although short-term inhibition, as might be used in acute situations, is unlikely to cause many problems, long-term therapy for chronic conditions might well do so. Judicious choice of the stage of inhibition in the C pathway may reduce the risk. Given that so many of the 'physiological' effects of C are mediated by C3 and its fragments, agents that inhibit after C3 cleavage are unlikely to cause significant detrimental effects. Considerations of half-life and cost also relate primarily to long-term uses. A variety of strategies has been proposed to create longer-acting, cheaper anti-C agents for use in chronic conditions.

Recombinant soluble forms of the naturally occurring C regulators

As noted above under Complement therapies, sCR1 (TP10), generated by removing the membrane-anchoring domain from CR1, led the new wave of anti-C agents and has proved efficacious in a large and diverse range of disease models. sCR1 inhibits formation of the C3 and C5 convertase enzymes, preventing C3b opsonization, C5a generation, and MAC formation. It has been awarded 'orphan drug' status from the Food and Drugs Administration (FDA) for therapy of adult respiratory distress syndrome (ARDS) and as a treatment for infants undergoing cardiac surgery (Zimmerman et al. 2000; Rioux 2001). Numerous modifications have been made to sCR1 to alter or improve efficacy in vivo. Removal of the amino-terminal seven SCRs generates a reagent termed sCR1[desLHR-A], an alternative pathway-specific inhibitor which permits continued classical pathway activation for immune complex handling (Murohara et al. 1995; Scesney et al. 1996). Both sCR1 and sCR1[desLHR-A] have been derivatized with the sialyl Lewis^{x} (sLe^{x}) carbohydrate antigen, a ligand for E- and P-selectins (Rittershaus et al. 1999). These agents

Table 9.4 *Current C therapies*

Agent	History and status	Pros	Cons
sCR1 (TP10)	The first of the new generation of anti-C therapies; used in many models; first in clinical trials. Now superseded?	Proof of concept; works across species	Expensive Systemic
SLe^{x}-sCR1 (TP20)	First of the modified sCR1 agents; binds endothelium at sites of inflammation, tested in many models, no clinical trial	May be more 'site specific' than sCR1	Expensive Systemic
APT-070	Truncated, membrane-targeted sCR1 derivative, tested in several models, early stages of clinical trials	'Site specific'?, retained at injection site? Made in bacteria so cheaper?	Unproven Systemic
h5G1.1 and derivatives	Recombinant scFv of anti-C5 monoclonal antibody (mAb); permits opsonization; effective in several models; well advanced in clinical trials	Long half-life compared with sCR1; relatively cheap; nearest to the clinic. The mAb-based therapies well accepted	Systemic
C5aR antagonists	Several agents vying for this niche; attractive drug target; many positive results in models	Small molecule agents (peptides and others); may be inexpensive, may work orally or topically	Unproven
Small molecule antagonists of components	Numerous agents, best explored is the C3 inhibitor Compstatin; good results in models, no trials	May be inexpensive, may be active orally or topically	Unproven

For references to these agents, see the text.

showed enhanced efficacy in murine models of stroke and ischemia–reperfusion injury and rat models of ARDS, probably as a result of the combined activities of localizing C inhibition to the endothelial cell membrane and blockade of leukocyte adhesion to the endothelium (Huang et al. 1999; Mulligan et al. 1999; Schmid et al. 2001).

A truncated form of sCR1, comprising the amino-terminal three SCRs, has been successfully expressed and refolded from *Escherichia coli* and shown to retain activity (Dodd et al. 1995; Mossakowska et al. 1999). Chemical modification of the carboxy-terminus with an 'addressin', comprising a membrane-targeting peptide and a lipophilic acyl chain, myristate, results in a powerful regulator of C activation (Smith and Smith 2001). The 'addressed' reagent, termed APT070, is 100-fold more active than the parent molecule and has proved to be beneficial in various models of disease including arthritis and ischemia–reperfusion (Linton et al. 2000).

Recombinant, soluble forms of MCP and DAF have also been generated and proved effective at inhibiting C in vitro and in various models of C-mediated disease (Moran et al. 1992; Christiansen et al. 1996b). Unlike sCR1, which has both cofactor and decay-accelerating activity, sDAF and sMCP have only one anti-C activity. The sCR1 form is a more effective fluid phase inhibitor than either sDAF or sMCP and mixtures of the two agents are more effective than either alone, illustrating cooperative activities (Christiansen et al. 1996a). A hybrid comprising sMCP fused to the amino terminus of sDAF, termed C activation blocker-2 (CAB-2), is a potent inhibitor both in vitro and in models (Higgins et al. 1997; Kroshus et al. 2000).

The membrane MAC regulator, CD59, has also been generated as a soluble form (sCD59) (Sugita et al. 1994; Quigg et al. 2000). However, sCD59 is a poor inhibitor of C in whole serum, a consequence of its short plasma half-life and tendency to bind plasma lipoproteins.

Antibody-based therapies

Antibodies targeting either C components or C receptors have attracted considerable attention as potential therapies, buoyed by the many other antibody-based agents that have already reached the clinic. Perhaps the most successful of the current anti-C agents is an antibody, h5G1.1, that binds C5 and prevents its enzymatic cleavage (Thomas et al. 1996). This agent does not prevent cleavage of C3, so opsonization of pathogens and immune complexes with C3b can occur, whereas generation of C5a and MAC are prevented. A recombinant, humanized, single-chain Fv of this antibody has been used in clinical trials for treatment of ARDS and ischemia–reperfusion injury, and has been particularly successful in cardiopulmonary bypass at reducing the post-bypass syndrome (Thomas et al. 1996; Fitch et al. 1999). Other antibodies have been generated that target other components of the terminal pathway (Rollins et al. 1995), C fragments such as C3a and C5a (Czermak et al. 1999), or the receptors for these fragments (C3aR, C5aR) (Morgan et al. 1993).

Small molecule inhibitors

A different approach to the generation of anti-C agents has been to seek small molecule inhibitors. Such agents potentially have major advantages over biological agents in terms of cost and ease of administration but are not without problems. Several groups have probed libraries of phage-display random peptides to identify agents. This approach has identified a cyclic 13-residue peptide, termed compstatin, which binds C3 and prevents its cleavage by convertase enzymes (Sahu et al. 1996; Nilsson et al. 1998; Fiane et al. 1999), and peptides that inhibit C1 activation (Roos et al. 2001). Other approaches have identified small molecule serine protease inhibitors specifically targeting C1s and factor D (fD) in the classical pathway and alternative pathway, respectively (Buerke et al. 1995; Kimura et al. 1998; Ueda et al. 2000). Numerous small molecule agents, peptide and non-peptide, targeting the C5aR (C5aR antagonists) have been developed and shown to be effective in models of ischemia–reperfusion injury and shock, and in the reverse passive Arthus reaction (Heller et al. 1999; Short et al. 1999; Riley et al. 2000; Strachan et al. 2001). Therapeutic effects have been demonstrated with some of these C5aR antagonists after oral or topical administration; such agents may be important therapeutic agents for the future.

CONCLUDING REMARKS

Complement, now over 110 years old, has finally come of age. The influence of C in many different areas of immunology and cell biology is now being realized; in fact, one would be hard pressed to identify a more protean part of the immune system. It should be clear from what has gone before that C is core to innate immunity, casts a large influence over adaptive immunity, plays key roles in cell death and clearance of debris, and is a major pathological factor in diverse diseases. The field is now ready to shed its slightly shady past and is prepared to be accepted as a 'respectable' branch of immunology. Welcome it with open arms!

REFERENCES

Agostoni, A. and Cicardi, M. 1992. Hereditary and acquired C1-inhibitor deficiency: biological and clinical characteristics in 235 patients. *Medicine*, **71**, 206–15.

Ames, R.S., Li, Y., et al. 1996. Molecular cloning and characterization of the human anaphylatoxin C3a receptor. *J Biol Chem*, **271**, 20231–4.

Arlaud, G.J., Thielens, N.M. and Aude, C.A. 1989. Structure and function of C1r and C1s: current concepts. *Behring Inst Mitt*, **84**, 56–64.

Biesma, D.H., Hannema, A.J., et al. 2001. A family with complement factor D deficiency. *J Clin Invest*, **108**, 233–40.

Blum, L., Pillemer, L. and Lepow, I.H. 1959. The properdin system and immunity. XIII. Assay and properties of a heat labile serum factor (factor B) in the properdin system. *Z Immunitatsforsch*, **118**, 349–57.

Bordet, J. 1900. Les serums hemolytiques, leurs antitoxines et les theories des serum cytolytiques. *Ann Inst Pasteur*, **15**, 257–70.

Botto, M. and Walport, M.J. 1993. Hereditary deficiency of C3 in animals and humans. *Int Rev Immunol*, **10**, 37–50.

Botto, M., Dell'Agnola, C., et al. 1998. Homozygous C1q deficiency causes glomerulonephritis associated with multiple apoptotic bodies. *Nat Genet*, **19**, 56–9.

Buerke, M., Murohara, T. and Lefer, A.M. 1995. Cardioprotective effects of a C1 esterase inhibitor in myocardial ischemia and reperfusion. *Circulation*, **91**, 393–402.

Carugati, A., Pappalardo, E., et al. 2001. C1-inhibitor deficiency and angioedema. *Mol Immunol*, **38**, 161–73.

Christiansen, D., Milland, J., et al. 1996a. A functional analysis of recombinant soluble CD46 in vivo and a comparison with recombinant soluble forms of CD55 and CD35 in vitro. *Eur J Immunol*, **26**, 578–85.

Christiansen, D., Milland, J., et al. 1996b. Engineering of recombinant soluble CD46: an inhibitor of complement activation. *Immunology*, **87**, 348–54.

Cianflone, K., Roncari, D.A., et al. 1994. Adipsin/acylation stimulating protein system in human adipocytes: regulation of triacylglycerol synthesis. *Biochemistry*, **33**, 9489–95.

Cicardi, M., Beretta, A., et al. 1996. Relevance of lymphoproliferative disorders and of anti-C1 inhibitor autoantibodies in acquired angiooedema. *Clin Exp Immunol*, **106**, 475–80.

Compston, D.A., Morgan, B.P., et al. 1989. Immunocytochemical localization of the terminal complement complex in multiple sclerosis. *Neuropathol Appl Neurobiol*, **15**, 307–16.

Crawford, M.H., Grover, F.L., et al. 1988. Complement and neutrophil activation in the pathogenesis of ischemic myocardial injury. *Circulation*, **78**, 1449–58.

Czermak, B.J., Sarma, V., et al. 1999. Protective effects of C5a blockade in sepsis. *Natural Medicines*, **5**, 788–92.

Daha, M.R., Fearon, D.T. and Austen, K.F. 1976. C3 nephritic factor (C3NeF): stabilization of fluid phase and cell-bound alternative pathway convertase. *J Immunol*, **116**, 1–7.

Dahlback, B. 1983. Purification of human C4b-binding protein and formation of its complex with vitamin K-dependent protein S. *Biochem J*, **209**, 847–56.

Dashiell, S.M., Rus, H. and Koski, C.L. 2000. Terminal complement complexes concomitantly stimulate proliferation and rescue of Schwann cells from apoptosis. *Glia*, **30**, 187–98.

Davies, A. and Lachmann, P.J. 1993. Membrane defence against complement lysis: the structure and biological properties of CD59. *Immunol Res*, **12**, 258–75.

Davies, K.A., Hird, V., et al. 1990. A study of in vivo immune complex formation and clearance in man. *J Immunol*, **144**, 4613–20.

Davies, K.A., Peters, A.M., Beynon, H.L. and Walport, M.J. 1992. Immune complex processing in patients with systemic lupus erythematosus. In vivo imaging and clearance studies. *J Clin Invest*, **90**, 2075–83.

Davis, A.E. 1988. C1 inhibitor and hereditary angioneurotic edema. *Annu Rev Immunol*, **5**, 595–628.

Davis, A.E. 1989. Hereditary and acquired deficiencies of C1 inhibitor. *Immunodef Rev*, **1**, 207–26.

Davis, A.E., Bissler, J.J. and Cicardi, M. 1993. Mutations in the C1 inhibitor gene that result in hereditary angioneurotic edema. *Behring Inst Mitt*, **93**, 313–20.

Dempsey, P.W., Allison, M.E., et al. 1996. C3d of complement as a molecular adjuvant: bridging innate and acquired immunity. *Science*, **271**, 348–50.

DiScipio, R.G. 1992a. Formation and structure of the C5b-7 complex of the lytic pathway of complement. *J Biol Chem*, **267**, 17087–94.

DiScipio, R.G. 1992b. Ultrastructures and interactions of complement factors H and I. *J Immunol*, **149**, 2592–9.

DiScipio, R.G. and Hugli, T.E. 1989. The molecular architecture of human complement component C6. *J Biol Chem*, **264**, 16197–206.

DiScipio, R.G., Chakravarti, D.N., et al. 1988. The structure of human complement component C7 and the C5b-7 complex. *J Biol Chem*, **263**, 549–60.

Dobrina, A., Pausa, M., et al. 2002. Cytolytically inactive terminal complement complex causes transendothelial migration of polymorphonuclear leukocytes in vitro and in vivo. *Blood*, **99**, 185–92.

Dodd, I., Mossakowska, D.E., et al. 1995. Overexpression in *Escherichia coli*, folding, purification, and characterization of the first three short consensus repeat modules of human complement receptor type 1. *Protein Exp Purn*, **6**, 727–36.

Dodds, A.W., Ren, X.D., Willis, A.C. and Law, S.K. 1996. The reaction mechanism of the internal thioester in the human complement component C4. *Nature*, **379**, 177–9.

Ebanks, R.O., Jaikaran, A.S., et al. 1992. A single arginine to tryptophan interchange at beta-chain residue 458 of human complement component C4 accounts for the defect in classical pathway C5 convertase activity of allotype C4A6. Implications for the location of a C5 binding site in C4. *J Immunol*, **148**, 2803–11.

Ehrlich, P. and Morgenroth, J. 1899. Zur theorie der lysinwirkung. *Berlin Klin Wochenchr*, **36**, 6–9.

Ehrlich, P. and Morgenroth, J. 1900. Ueber haemolysin dritte Mitteilung. *Berl Klin Wochenchr*, **37**, 453–85.

Eikelenboom, P., Hack, C.E., et al. 1992. Distribution pattern and functional state of complement proteins and alpha 1-antichymotrypsin in cerebral beta/A4 deposits in Alzheimer's disease. *Res Immunol*, **143**, 617–20.

Farkas, I., Baranyi, L., et al. 1998. A neuronal C5a receptor and an associated apoptotic signal transduction pathway. *J Physiol*, **507**, 679–87.

Fearon, D.T. 1991. Anti-inflammatory and immunosuppressive effects of recombinant soluble complement receptors. *Clin Exp Immunol*, **86**, 43–6.

Fearon, D.T. and Carroll, M.C. 2000. Regulation of B lymphocyte responses to foreign and self-antigens by the CD19/CD21 complex. *Annu Rev Immunol*, **18**, 393–422.

Ferrata, A. 1907. Die univerksamkeit der komplex haeolysise in salzfrein losungen und ihre ursache. *Berlin Klin Wochenschr*, **44**, 366–9.

Fiane, A.E., Mollnes, T.E., et al. 1999. Compstatin, a peptide inhibitor of C3, prolongs survival of ex vivo perfused pig xenografts. *Xenotransplantation*, **6**, 52–65.

Fijen, C.A., van den Bogaard, R., et al. 1999. Properdin deficiency: molecular basis and disease association. *Mol Immunol*, **36**, 863–7.

Finn, A., Morgan, B.P., et al. 1996. Effects of inhibition of complement activation using recombinant soluble complement receptor 1 on neutrophil CD11b/CD18 and L-selectin expression and release of interleukin-8 and elastase in simulated cardiopulmonary bypass. *J Thorac Cardiovasc Surg*, **111**, 451–9.

Fitch, J.C., Rollins, S., et al. 1999. Pharmacology and biological efficacy of a recombinant, humanized, single-chain antibody C5 complement inhibitor in patients undergoing coronary artery bypass graft surgery with cardiopulmonary bypass. *Circulation*, **100**, 2499–506.

Forbes, R.D., Pinto-Blonde, M. and Guttmann, R.D. 1978. The effect of anticomplementary cobra venom factor on hyperacute rat cardiac allograft rejection. *Lab Invest*, **39**, 463–70.

Fosse, E., Moen, O., et al. 1994. Reduced complement and granulocyte activation with heparin-coated cardiopulmonary bypass. *Ann Thorac Surg*, **58**, 472–7.

Gadjeva, M., Thiel, S. and Jensenius, J.C. 2001. The mannan-binding-lectin pathway of the innate immune response. *Curr Opin Immunol*, **13**, 74–8.

Gerard, C. and Gerard, N.P. 1994. C5a anaphylatoxin and its seven transmembrane-segment receptor. *Ann Rev Immunol*, **12**, 775–808.

Gershov, D., Kim, S., et al. 2000. C-Reactive protein binds to apoptotic cells, protects the cells from assembly of the terminal complement components, and sustains an antiinflammatory innate immune response: implications for systemic autoimmunity. *J Exp Med*, **192**, 1353–64.

Gillinov, A.M., DeValeria, P.A., et al. 1993. Complement inhibition with soluble complement receptor type 1 in cardiopulmonary bypass. *Ann Thorac Surg*, **55**, 619–24.

Gotze, O. 1986. C5a anaphylatoxin. In: Rother, K. and Till, G.O. (eds), *The complement system*. Berlin: Springer, 154–68.

Griselli, M., Herbert, J., et al. 1999. C-reactive protein and complement are important mediators of tissue damage in acute myocardial infarction. *J Exp Med*, **190**, 1733–40.

Guo, R.F., Huber-Lang, M., et al. 2000. Protective effects of anti-C5a in sepsis-induced thymocyte apoptosis. *J Clin Invest*, **106**, 1271–80.

Hafer-Macko, C.E., Sheikh, K.A., et al. 1996. Immune attack on the Schwann cell surface in acute inflammatory demyelinating polyneuropathy. *Ann Neurol*, **39**, 625–35.

Heller, T., Hennecke, M., et al. 1999. Selection of a C5a receptor antagonist from phage libraries attenuating the inflammatory response in immune complex disease and ischemia/reperfusion injury. *J Immunol*, **163**, 985–94.

Higgins, P.J., Ko, J.L., et al. 1997. A soluble chimeric complement inhibitory protein that possesses both decay-accelerating and factor I cofactor activities. *J Immunol*, **158**, 2872–81.

Hogasen, A.K., Overlie, I., et al. 2000. The analysis of the complement activation product SC5 b-9 is applicable in neonates in spite of their profound C9 deficiency. *J Perinat Med*, **28**, 39–48.

Holers, V.M., Seya, T., et al. 1986. Structural and functional studies on the human C3b/C4b receptor (CR1) purified by affinity chromatography using a monoclonal antibody. *Complement*, **3**, 63–78.

Holmskov, U., Malhotra, R. and Sim, R.B. 1994. Collectins, collectin receptors and the lectin pathway of complement activation. *Immunol Today*, **15**, 67–74.

Horiuchi, T., Nishizaka, H., et al. 1998. A non-sense mutation at Arg95 is predominant in complement 9 deficiency in Japanese. *J Immunol*, **160**, 1509–13.

Hourcade, D., Holers, V.M. and Atkinson, J.P. 1989. The regulators of complement activation (RCA) gene cluster. *Adv Immunol*, **45**, 381–416.

Huang, J., Kim, L.J., et al. 1999. Neuronal protection in stroke by an sLex-glycosylated complement inhibitory protein. *Science*, **285**, 595–9.

Hughes, J., Nangaku, M., et al. 2000. C5b-9 membrane attack complex mediates endothelial cell apoptosis in experimental glomerulonephritis. *Am J Physiol Renal Physiol*, **278**, F747–57.

Hugli, T.E. 1984. Structure and function of the anaphylatoxins. *Springer Semin Immunopathol*, **7**, 193–219.

Janatova, J. and Tack, B.F. 1981. Fourth component of human complement: studies of an amine-sensitive site comprised of a thiol component. *Biochemistry*, **20**, 2394–402.

Jensen, J.A., Festa, E., Smith, D.S. and Cayer, M. 1981. The complement system of the nurse shark: hemolytic and comparative characteristics. *Science*, **214**, 566–9.

Jokiranta, T.S., Zipfel, P.F., et al. 1996. Analysis of the recognition mechanism of the alternative pathway of complement by monoclonal anti-factor H antibodies: evidence for multiple interactions between H and surface bound C3b. *FEBS Lett*, **393**, 297–302.

Kerr, M.A. and Porter, R.R. 1978. The purification and properties of the second component of human complement. *Biochem J*, **171**, 99–107.

Kildsgaard, J., Zsigmond, E., et al. 1999. A critical evaluation of the putative role of C3adesArg (ASP) in lipid metabolism and hyperapobetalipoproteinemia. *Mol Immunol*, **36**, 869–76.

Kilgore, K.S., Friedrichs, G.S., et al. 1994. The complement system in myocardial ischaemia/reperfusion injury. *Cardiovasc Res*, **28**, 437–44.

Kimura, T., Andoh, A., et al. 1998. A blockade of complement activation prevents rapid intestinal ischaemia-reperfusion injury by modulating mucosal mast cell degranulation in rats. *Clin Exp Immunol*, **111**, 484–90.

Kinoshita, T., Takata, Y., et al. 1988. C5 convertase of the alternative complement pathway: covalent linkage between two C3b molecules within the trimolecular complex enzyme. *J Immunol*, **141**, 3895–901.

Kolble, K. and Reid, K.B. 1993. Genetic deficiencies of the complement system and association with disease-early components. *Int Rev Immunol*, **10**, 17–36.

Koski, C.L., Vanguri, P. and Shin, M.L. 1985. Activation of the alternative pathway of complement by human peripheral nerve myelin. *J Immunol*, **134**, 1810–14.

Kozono, H., Kinoshita, T., et al. 1990. Localization of the covalent C3b-binding site on C4b within the complement classical pathway C5 convertase, C4b2a3b. *J Biol Chem*, **265**, 14444–9.

Kroshus, T.J., Salerno, C.T., et al. 2000. A recombinant soluble chimeric complement inhibitor composed of human CD46 and CD55 reduces acute cardiac tissue injury in models of pig-to-human heart transplantation. *Transplantation*, **69**, 2282–9.

Krych, M., Atkinson, J.P. and Holers, V.M. 1992. Complement receptors. *Current Opin Immunol*, **4**, 8–13.

Lachmann, P.J. 1991. The control of homologous lysis. *Immunol Today*, **12**, 312–15.

Lachmann, P.J. and Hughes-Jones, N.C. 1984. Initiation of complement activation. *Springer Semin Immunopathol*, **7**, 143–62.

Lambris, J.D. 1988. The multifunctional role of C3, the third component of complement. *Immunol Today*, **9**, 387–93.

Lambris, J.D., Alsenz, J., et al. 1984. Mapping of the properdin-binding site in the third component of complement. *Biochem J*, **217**, 323–6.

Lassiter, H.A., Watson, S.W., et al. 1992. Complement factor 9 deficiency in serum of human neonates. *J Infect Dis*, **166**, 53–7.

Law, S.K. and Dodds, A.W. 1990. C3, C4 and C5: the thioester site. *Biochem Soc Trans*, **18**, 1155–9.

Law, S.K. and Dodds, A.W. 1997. The internal thioester and the covalent binding properties of the complement proteins C3 and C4. *Protein Sci*, **6**, 263–74.

Lazar, H.L., Bao, Y., et al. 1999. Total complement inhibition: An effective strategy to limit ischemic injury during coronary revascularization on cardiopulmonary bypass. *Circulation*, **100**, 1438–42.

Lee, A., Whyte, M.K. and Haslett, C. 1993. Inhibition of apoptosis and prolongation of neutrophil functional longevity by inflammatory mediators. *J Leukoc Biol*, **54**, 283–8.

Linington, C., Morgan, B.P., et al. 1989. The role of complement in the pathogenesis of experimental allergic encephalomyelitis. *Brain*, **112**, 895–911.

Linton, S.M., Williams, A.S., et al. 2000. Therapeutic efficacy of a novel membrane-targeted complement regulator in antigen-induced arthritis in the rat. *Arthritis Rheum*, **43**, 2590–7.

Lipscombe, R.J., Beatty, D.W., et al. 1996. Mutations in the human mannose-binding protein gene: Frequencies in several population groups. *Eur J Hum Genet*, **4**, 13–19.

Liu, W.T., Vanguri, P. and Shin, M.L. 1983. Studies on demyelination in vitro: the requirement of membrane attack components of the complement system. *J Immunol*, **131**, 778–82.

Lublin, D.M. and Atkinson, J.P. 1990. Decay-accelerating factor and membrane cofactor protein. *Curr Top Microbiol Immunol*, **153**, 123–45.

Lucchinetti, C., Bruck, W., et al. 2000. Heterogeneity of multiple sclerosis lesions: implications for the pathogenesis of demyelination. *Ann Neurol*, **47**, 707–17.

Lucisano Valim, Y.M. and Lachmann, P.J. 1991. The effect of antibody isotype and antigenic epitope density on the complement-fixing activity of immune complexes: a systematic study using chimaeric anti-NIP antibodies with human Fc regions. *Clin Exp Immunol*, **84**, 1–8.

McGeer, E.G. and McGeer, P.L. 1999. Brain inflammation in Alzheimer disease and the therapeutic implications. *Curr Pharm Des*, **5**, 821–36.

McGeer, P.L., McGeer, E.G., et al. 1991. Reactions of the immune system in chronic degenerative neurological diseases. *Can J Neurol Sci*, **18**, 376–9.

McGeer, P.L., Rogers, J. and McGeer, E.G. 1994. Neuroimmune mechanisms in Alzheimer disease pathogenesis. *Alzheimer Dis Assoc Disord*, **8**, 149–58.

Madi, N., Paccaud, J.P., et al. 1991. Immune complex binding efficiency of erythrocyte complement receptor 1 (CR1). *Clin Exp Immunol*, **84**, 9–15.

Mandle, R., Baron, C., et al. 1994. Acquired C1 inhibitor deficiency as a result of an autoantibody to the reactive center region of C1 inhibitor. *J Immunol*, **152**, 4680–5.

Mathieson, P.W., Wurzner, R., et al. 1993. Complement-mediated adipocyte lysis by nephritic factor sera. *J Exp Med*, **177**, 1827–31.

Matsui, H., Tsuji, S., et al. 1994. Activation of the alternative pathway of complement by apoptotic Jurkat cells. *FEBS Lett*, **351**, 419–22.

Matsumoto, A.K., Kopicky-Burd, J., et al. 1991. Intersection of the complement and immune systems: a signal transduction complex of the B lymphocyte-containing complement receptor type 2 and CD19. *J Exp Med*, **173**, 55–64.

Matsumoto, M., Fukuda, W., et al. 1997. Abrogation of the alternative complement pathway by targeted deletion of murine factor B. *Proc Natl Acad Sci USA*, **94**, 8720–5.

Matsushita, M. and Fujita, T. 2001. Ficolins and the lectin complement pathway. *Immunol Rev*, **180**, 78–85.

Matsushita, M., Thiel, S., et al. 2000. Proteolytic activities of two types of mannose-binding lectin-associated serine protease. *J Immunol*, **165**, 2637–42.

Mayer, M.M. 1965. In: Kabat, E.A. and Mayer, M.M. (eds), *Experimental immunochemistry*. Springfield, IL: Charles C. Thomas, 133–240.

Medzhitov, R. and Janeway, C.A. Jr. 2002. Decoding the patterns of self and nonself by the innate immune system. *Science*, **296**, 298–300.

Merry, A.H., Rawlinson, V.I., et al. 1989. Studies on the sensitivity to complement-mediated lysis of erythrocytes (Inab phenotype) with a deficiency of DAF (decay accelerating factor). *Br J Haematol*, **73**, 248–53.

Mevorach, D. 2000. Opsonization of apoptotic cells. Implications for uptake and autoimmunity. *Ann NY Acad Sci*, **926**, 226–35.

Moat, N.E., Shore, D.F. and Evans, T.W. 1993. Organ dysfunction and cardiopulmonary bypass: the role of complement and complement regulatory proteins. *Eur J Cardio-Thorac Surg*, **7**, 563–73.

Mold, C. and Morris, C.A. 2001. Complement activation by apoptotic endothelial cells following hypoxia/reoxygenation. *Immunology*, **102**, 359–64.

Mollnes, T.E. 1997. Biocompatibility: complement as mediator of tissue damage and as indicator of incompatibility. *Exp Clin Immunogenet*, **14**, 24–9.

Mollnes, T.E., Vandvik, B., et al. 1987. Intrathecal complement activation in neurological diseases evaluated by analysis of the terminal complement complex. *J Neurol Sci*, **78**, 17–28.

Mollnes, T.E., Videm, V., et al. 1991. Complement activation and bioincompatibility. *Clin Exp Immunol*, **86**, suppl 1, 21–6.

Moran, P., Beasley, H., et al. 1992. Human recombinant soluble decay accelerating factor inhibits complement activation in vitro and in vivo. *J Immunol*, **149**, 1736–43.

Morgan, B.P. 1999. Regulation of the complement membrane attack pathway. *Crit Rev Immunol*, **19**, 173–98.

Morgan, B.P. and Harris, C.L. 1999. *Complement regulatory proteins*. London: Academic Press.

Morgan, B.P., Campbell, A.K. and Compston, D.A. 1984. Terminal component of complement (C9) in cerebrospinal fluid of patients with multiple sclerosis. *Lancet*, **ii**, 251–4.

Morgan, E.L., Ember, J.A., et al. 1993. Anti-C5a receptor antibodies. Characterization of neutralizing antibodies specific for a peptide, C5aR-(9-29), derived from the predicted amino-terminal sequence of the human C5a receptor. *J Immunol*, **151**, 377–88.

Mossakowska, D., Dodd, I., Pindar, W. and Smith, R.A. 1999. Structure-activity relationships within the N-terminal short consensus repeats (SCR) of human CR1 (C3b/C4b receptor, CD35): SCR 3 plays a critical role in inhibition of the classical and alternative pathways of complement activation. *Eur J Immunol*, **29**, 1955–65.

Muir, R. and Browning, C.H. 1904. On chemical combination and toxic action as exemplified in haemolytic sera. *Proc R Soc Lond*, **74**, 298–305.

Mukherjee, P. and Pasinetti, G.M. 2001. Complement anaphylatoxin C5a neuroprotects through mitogen-activated protein kinase-dependent inhibition of caspase 3. *J Neurochem*, **77**, 43–9.

Muller-Eberhard, H.J. 1969. Complement. *Annu Rev Biochem*, **38**, 389–414.

Muller-Eberhard, H.J. 1986. The membrane attack complex of complement. *Annu Rev Immunol*, **4**, 503–28.

Mulligan, M.S., Warner, R.L., et al. 1999. Endothelial targeting and enhanced antiinflammatory effects of complement inhibitors possessing sialyl Lewis(x) moieties. *J Immunol*, **162**, 4952–9.

Murohara, T., Guo, J.P., et al. 1995. Cardioprotective effects of selective inhibition of the two complement activation pathways in myocardial ischemia and reperfusion injury. *Met Find Exp Clin Pharmacol*, **17**, 499–507.

Myones, B.L., Dalzell, J.G., et al. 1988. Neutrophil and monocyte cell surface p150,95 has iC3b-receptor (CR4) activity resembling CR3. *J Clin Invest*, **82**, 640–51.

Nardin, A., Lindorfer, M.A. and Taylor, R.P. 1999. How are immune complexes bound to the primate erythrocyte complement receptor transferred to acceptor phagocytic cells? *Mol Immunol*, **36**, 827–35.

Navratil, J.S. and Ahearn, J.M. 2001. Apoptosis, clearance mechanisms, and the development of systemic lupus erythematosus. *Curr Rheumatol Rep*, **3**, 191–8.

Navratil, J.S., Korb, L.C. and Ahearn, J.M. 1999. Systemic lupus erythematosus and complement deficiency: Clues to a novel role for the classical complement pathway in the maintenance of immune tolerance. *Immunopharmacology*, **42**, 47–52.

Navratil, J.S., Watkins, S.C., et al. 2001. The globular heads of C1q specifically recognize surface blebs of apoptotic vascular endothelial cells. *J Immunol*, **166**, 3231–9.

Nilsson, B., Larsson, R., et al. 1998. Compstatin inhibits complement and cellular activation in whole blood in two models of extracorporeal circulation. *Blood*, **92**, 1661–7.

Ogden, C.A., deCathelineau, A., et al. 2001. C1q and mannose binding lectin engagement of cell surface calreticulin and CD91 initiates macropinocytosis and uptake of apoptotic cells. *J Exp Med*, **194**, 781–95.

Oppermann, M., Kurts, C., et al. 1991. Elevated plasma levels of the immunosuppressive complement fragment Ba in renal failure. *Kidney Int*, **40**, 939–47.

Pascual, M. and Schifferli, J.A. 1992. The binding of immune complexes by the erythrocyte complement receptor 1 (CR1). *Immunopharmacology*, **24**, 101–6.

Pepys, M.B. 1974. Role of complement in induction of antibody production in vivo. Effect of cobra venom factor and other C3-reactive agents on thymus-dependent and thymus-independent antibody responses. *J Exp Med*, **140**, 126–45.

Perianayagam, M.C., Balakrishnan, V.S., et al. 2002. C5a delays apoptosis of human neutrophils by a phosphatidylinositol 3-kinase-signaling pathway. *Kidney Int*, **61**, 456–63.

Perkins, S.J., Nealis, A.S., et al. 1991. Solution structure of human and mouse immunoglobulin M by synchrotron X-ray scattering and molecular graphics modelling. A possible mechanism for complement activation. *J Mol Biol*, **221**, 1345–66.

Petersen, S.V., Thiel, S., et al. 2000. Control of the classical and the MBL pathway of complement activation. *Mol Immunol*, **37**, 803–11.

Petersen, S.V., Thiel, S. and Jensenius, J.C. 2001. The mannan-binding lectin pathway of complement activation: biology and disease association. *Mol Immunol*, **38**, 133–49.

Piddlesden, S.J., Storch, M.K., et al. 1994. Soluble recombinant complement receptor 1 inhibits inflammation and demyelination in antibody-mediated demyelinating experimental allergic encephalomyelitis. *J Immunol*, **152**, 5477–84.

Pillemer, L., Blum, L., et al. 1954. The properdin system and immunity: demonstration and isolation of a new serum protein, properdin, and its role in immune phenomena. *Science*, **120**, 279–85.

Podack, E.R. and Muller-Eberhard, H.J. 1979. Isolation of human S-protein, an inhibitor of the membrane attack complex of complement. *J Biol Chem*, **254**, 9808–14.

Podack, E.R. and Tschopp, J. 1984. Membrane attack by complement. *Mol Immunol*, **21**, 589–603.

Pramoonjago, P., Kinoshita, T., et al. 1992. Bactericidal activity of C9-deficient human serum. *J Immunol*, **148**, 837–43.

Quigg, R.J., He, C., et al. 2000. Production and functional analysis of rat CD59 and chimeric CD59-Crry as active soluble proteins in *Pichia pastoris*. *Immunology*, **99**, 46–53.

Reid, K.B. 1986. Activation and control of the complement system. *Essays Biochem*, **22**, 27–68.

Reid, K.B. and Day, A.J. 1989. Structure–function relationships of the complement components. *Immunol Today*, **10**, 177–80.

Reid, K.B. and Turner, M.W. 1994. Mammalian lectins in activation and clearance mechanisms involving the complement system. *Springer Semin Immunopathol*, **15**, 307–26.

Rey-Campos, J., Baeza-Sanz, D. and Rodriguez de Cordoba, S. 1990. Physical linkage of the human genes coding for complement factor H and coagulation factor XIII B subunit. *Genomics*, **7**, 644–6.

Riedemann, N.C., Guo, R.F., et al. 2002. C5a receptor and thymocyte apoptosis in sepsis. *FASEB J*, **16**, 887–8.

Riley, R.D., Sato, H., et al. 2000. Recombinant human complement C5a receptor antagonist reduces infarct size after surgical revascularization. *J Thorac Cardiovasc Surg*, **120**, 350–8.

Rioux, P. 2001. TP-10 (AVANT Immunotherapeutics). *Curr Opin Invest Drugs*, **2**, 364–71.

Rittershaus, C.W., Thomas, L.J., et al. 1999. Recombinant glycoproteins that inhibit complement activation and also bind the selectin adhesion molecules. *J Biol Chem*, **274**, 11237–44.

Rollins, S.A., Matis, L.A., et al. 1995. Monoclonal antibodies directed against human C5 and C8 block complement-mediated damage of xenogeneic cells and organs. *Transplantation*, **60**, 1284–92.

Roos, A., Nauta, A.J., et al. 2001. Specific inhibition of the classical complement pathway by C1q-binding peptides. *J Immunol*, **167**, 7052–9.

Rosse, W.F. and Ware, R.E. 1995. The molecular basis of paroxysmal nocturnal hemoglobinuria. *Blood*, **86**, 3277–86.

Sahu, A., Kay, B.K. and Lambris, J.D. 1996. Inhibition of human complement by a C3-binding peptide isolated from a phage-displayed random peptide library. *J Immunol*, **157**, 884–91.

Sanders, M.E., Koski, C.L., et al. 1986. Activated terminal complement in cerebrospinal fluid in Guillain-Barre syndrome and multiple sclerosis. *J Immunol*, **136**, 4456–9.

Sato, T., Van Dixhoorn, M.G., et al. 1999. The terminal sequence of complement plays an essential role in antibody-mediated renal cell apoptosis. *J Am Soc Nephrol*, **10**, 1242–52.

Savill, J. and Fadok, V. 2000. Corpse clearance defines the meaning of cell death. *Nature*, **407**, 784–8.

Savill, J., Fadok, V., et al. 1993. Phagocyte recognition of cells undergoing apoptosis. *Immunol Today*, **14**, 131–6.

Scesney, S.M., Makrides, S.C., et al. 1996. A soluble deletion mutant of the human complement receptor type 1, which lacks the C4b binding site, is a selective inhibitor of the alternative complement pathway. *Eur J Immunol*, **26**, 1729–35.

Schifferli, J.A. and Paccaud, J.P. 1989. Two isotypes of human C4, C4A and C4B have different structure and function. *Complement Inflamm*, **6**, 19–26.

Schifferli, J.A. and Peters, D.K. 1983. Complement, the immune-complex lattice, and the pathophysiology of complement-deficiency syndromes. *Lancet*, **ii**, 957–9.

Schifferli, J.A. and Taylor, R.P. 1989. Physiological and pathological aspects of circulating immune complexes. *Kidney Int*, **35**, 993–1003.

Schmid, R.A., Hillinger, S., et al. 2001. TP20 is superior to TP10 in reducing ischemia/reperfusion injury in rat lung grafts. *Transplant Proc*, **33**, 948–9.

Schreiber, R.D. and Muller-Eberhard, H.J. 1974. Fourth component of human complement: description of a three polypeptide chain structure. *J Exp Med*, **140**, 1324–35.

Short, A., Wong, A.K., et al. 1999. Effects of a new C5a receptor antagonist on C5a- and endotoxin-induced neutropenia in the rat. *Br J Pharmacol*, **126**, 551–4.

Singhrao, S.K., Neal, J.W., et al. 2000. Spontaneous classical pathway activation and deficiency of membrane regulators render human neurons susceptible to complement lysis. *Am J Pathol*, **157**, 905–18.

Sjoholm, A.G., Braconier, J.H. and Soderstrom, C. 1982. Properdin deficiency in a family with fulminant meningococcal infections. *Clin Exp Immunol*, **50**, 291–7.

Sjoholm, A.G., Kuijper, E.J., et al. 1988a. : Dysfunctional properdin in a Dutch family with meningococcal disease. *N Engl J Med*, **319**, 33–7.

Sjoholm, A.G., Soderstrom, C. and Nilsson, L.A. 1988b. A second variant of properdin deficiency: the detection of properdin at low concentrations in affected males. *Complement*, **5**, 130–40.

Smith, G.P. and Smith, R.A. 2001. Membrane-targeted complement inhibitors. *Mol Immunol*, **38**, 249–55.

Sniderman, A.D. and Cianflone, K. 1997. The adipsin-acylation-stimulating protein pathway and microenvironmental metabolic regulation. *World Rev Nutr Diet*, **80**, 44–81.

Soane, L., Cho, H.J., et al. 2001. C5b-9 terminal complement complex protects oligodendrocytes from death by regulating Bad through phosphatidylinositol 3-kinase/Akt pathway. *J Immunol*, **167**, 2305–11.

Sodetz, J.M. 1989. Structure and function of C8 in the membrane attack sequence of complement. *Curr Top Microbiol Immunol*, **140**, 19–31.

Soothill, J.F. and Harvey, B.A. 1976. Defective opsonization. A common immunity deficiency. *Arch Dis Childhood*, **51**, 91–9.

Soothill, J.F. and Harvey, B.A. 1977. A defect of the alternative pathway of complement. *Clin Exp Immunol*, **27**, 30–3.

Strachan, A.J., Shiels, I.A., et al. 2001. Inhibition of immune-complex mediated dermal inflammation in rats following either oral or topical administration of a small molecule C5a receptor antagonist. *Br J Pharmacol*, **134**, 1778–86.

Strife, C.F., Leahy, A.E. and West, C.D. 1989. Antibody to a cryptic, solid phase C1Q antigen in membranoproliferative nephritis. *Kidney Int*, **35**, 836–42.

Sugita, Y., Ito, K., et al. 1994. Recombinant soluble CD59 inhibits reactive haemolysis with complement. *Immunology*, **82**, 34–41.

Sumiya, M. and Summerfield, J.A. 1996. Mannose-binding protein, genetic variants and the risk of infection. *Q J Med*, **89**, 723–6.

Summerfield, J.A., Sumiya, M., et al. 1997. Association of mutations in mannose binding protein gene with childhood infection in consecutive hospital series. *BMJ*, **314**, 1229–32.

Super, M., Thiel, S., et al. 1989. Association of low levels of mannan-binding protein with a common defect of opsonisation. *Lancet*, **ii**, 1236–9.

Svennevig, J.L., Geiran, O.R., et al. 1993. Complement activation during extracorporeal circulation. In vitro comparison of Duraflo II heparin-coated and uncoated oxygenator circuits. *J Thorac Cardiovasc Surg*, **106**, 466–72.

Tack, B.F., Morris, S.C. and Prahl, J.W. 1979. Fifth component of human complement: purification from plasma and polypeptide chain structure. *Biochemistry*, **18**, 1490–7.

Taylor, C.M. 2001. Complement factor H and the haemolytic uraemic syndrome. *Lancet*, **358**, 1200–2.

Taylor, P.R., Carugati, A., et al. 2000. A hierarchical role for classical pathway complement proteins in the clearance of apoptotic cells in vivo. *J Exp Med*, **192**, 359–66.

Tedder, T.F., Weis, J.J., et al. 1986. The role of receptors for complement in the induction of polyclonal B-cell proliferation and differentiation. *J Clin Immunol*, **6**, 65–73.

Tedder, T.F., Inaoki, M. and Sato, S. 1997. The CD19-CD21 complex regulates signal transduction thresholds governing humoral immunity and autoimmunity. *Immunity*, **6**, 107–18.

Tedesco, F., Pausa, M., et al. 1997. The cytolytically inactive terminal complement complex activates endothelial cells to express adhesion molecules and tissue factor procoagulant activity. *J Exp Med*, **185**, 1619–27.

Telen, M.J. and Green, A.M. 1989. The Inab phenotype: characterization of the membrane protein and complement regulatory defect. *Blood*, **74**, 437–41.

Terai, I., Kobayashi, K., et al. 1995. alpha 2-Macroglobulin binds to and inhibits mannose-binding protein-associated serine protease. *Int Immunol*, **7**, 1579–84.

Thomas, F., Naff, G., et al. 1977. Prevention of hyperacute kidney rejection of decomplementation using purified cobra venom factor. *J Surg Res*, **22**, 189–94.

Thomas, T.C., Rollins, S.A., et al. 1996. Inhibition of complement activity by humanized anti-C5 antibody and single-chain Fv. *Mol Immunol*, **33**, 1389–401.

Tosi, M., Levi-Strauss, M., et al. 1985. Duplications of complement and non-complement genes of the H-2S region: evolutionary aspects of the C4 isotypes and molecular analysis of their expression variants. *Immunol Rev*, **87**, 151–83.

Tschopp, J. and French, L.E. 1994. Clusterin: modulation of complement function. *Clin Exp Immunol*, **97**, 11–14.

Turner, M.W. 1991. Deficiency of mannan binding protein – a new complement deficiency syndrome. *Clin Exp Immunol*, **86**, 53–6.

Ueda, N., Midorikawa, A., et al. 2000. Inhibitory effects of newly synthesized active center-directed trypsin-like serine protease inhibitors on the complement system. *Inflamm Res*, **49**, 42–6.

Vriesendorp, F.J., Flynn, R.E., et al. 1995. Complement depletion affects demyelination and inflammation in experimental allergic neuritis. *J Neuroimmunol*, **58**, 157–65.

Walport, M.J. 2001a. Complement. First of two parts. *N Engl J Med*, **344**, 1058–66.

Walport, M.J. 2001b. Complement. Second of two parts. *N Engl J Med*, **344**, 1140–4.

Walport, M.J. and Lachmann, P.J. 1990. Complement deficiencies and abnormalities of the complement system in systemic lupus erythematosus and related disorders. *Curr Opin Rheumatol*, **2**, 661–3.

Walport, M.J., Davies, K.A., et al. 1994. C3 nephritic factor and SLE: report of four cases and review of the literature. *Q J Med*, **87**, 609–15.

Weisman, H.F., Bartow, T., et al. 1990. Soluble human complement receptor type 1: in vivo inhibitor of complement suppressing post-ischemic myocardial inflammation and necrosis. *Science*, **249**, 146–51.

Wener, M.H., Uwatoko, S. and Mannik, M. 1989. Antibodies to the collagen-like region of C1q in sera of patients with autoimmune rheumatic diseases. *Arthritis Rheum*, **32**, 544–51.

Whitehead, H.R., Gordon, J. and Wormall, A. 1925. The 'third component', a heat-stable factor of complement. *Biochem J*, **19**, 618–25.

Wisnieski, J.J. and Naff, G.B. 1989. Serum IgG antibodies to C1q in hypocomplementemic urticarial vasculitis syndrome. *Arthritis Rheum*, **32**, 1119–27.

Wisnieski, J.J., Baer, A.N., et al. 1995. Hypocomplementemic urticarial vasculitis syndrome. Clinical and serologic findings in 18 patients. *Medicine*, **74**, 24–41.

Wurzner, R., Orren, A. and Lachmann, P.J. 1992. Inherited deficiencies of the terminal components of human complement. *Immunodef Rev*, **3**, 123–47.

Yamashina, M., Ueda, E., et al. 1990. Inherited complete deficiency of 20-kilodalton homologous restriction factor (CD59) as a cause of paroxysmal nocturnal hemoglobinuria. *N Engl J Med*, **323**, 1184–9.

Ziccardi, R.J. 1982. A new role for C-1-inhibitor in homeostasis: control of activation of the first component of human complement. *J Immunol*, **128**, 2505–8.

Zimmerman, J.L., Dellinger, R.P., et al. 2000. Phase I trial of the recombinant soluble complement receptor 1 in acute lung injury and acute respiratory distress syndrome. *Crit Care Med*, **28**, 3149–54.

Zipfel, P.F. 2001. Hemolytic uremic syndrome: how do factor H mutants mediate endothelial damage? *Trends Immunol*, **22**, 345–8.

Zipfel, P.F., Jokiranta, T.S., et al. 1999. The factor H protein family. *Immunopharmacology*, **42**, 53–60.

Zwirner, J., Gotze, O., et al. 1999. Evaluation of C3a receptor expression on human leucocytes by the use of novel monoclonal antibodies. *Immunology*, **97**, 166–72.

10

Antimicrobial peptides: defensins and cathelicidins

ROBERT I. LEHRER AND TOMAS GANZ

Leukocytes, inflammatory exudates, and many secretions exert antimicrobial activity that results from the individual and combined effects of their constituents. The responsible components may include enzymes such as lysozyme, metal-binding proteins such as lactoferrin, highly cationic proteins such as histones or fragments thereof, various lipopolysaccharide (LPS)-binding molecules, and antimicrobial peptides. Surprisingly, there is large interspecies variation in the number and nature of these effector molecules, and considerable cell-to-cell and tissue-to-tissue variation within any given species. This chapter covers two large groups of antimicrobial peptides found in mammals: defensins and cathelicidins.

We define antimicrobial peptides as molecules with fewer than 100 amino acids, which exist in host defense settings, and exhibit antimicrobial activity under locally prevailing conditions. Antimicrobial peptides are ancient weapons of host defense, and many have been found in organisms that antedate mammals. A partial roster of these antimicrobial peptides includes the microhalocins of Archaebacteria (O'Connor and Shand 2002), the bacteriocins (Diep and Nes 2002), and lantibiotics (Pag and Sahl 2002) of Eubacteria, the amoebapores of protozoa (Leippe 1999), the cysteine-rich 'defensins' of plants (Broekaert et al. 1995; Garcia-Olmedo et al. 1998; Thomma et al. 2002), and numerous peptides of insects and other invertebrates (Dimarcq et al. 1998; Bulet et al. 1999). Readers seeking a broader view of antimicrobial peptides should consult the cited references, and the many fascinating studies in *Drosophila* spp. (Hoffmann and Reichhart 2002; Tzou et al. 2002).

Much information about mammalian antimicrobial peptides has come from studying the leukocytes found in blood and their precursors in the bone marrow. In humans, the most abundant blood leukocytes are granulocytes – cells with cytoplasm that contains multiple granules. Those most important for antimicrobial defense are variously called neutrophils, 'polys' – shorthand abbreviation of their more formal (and formidable) name: polymorphonucleated neutrophilic granulocytes (PMN). The several thousand small granules within the cytoplasm of each human PMN are tiny storage organelles that contain a variety of peptides and proteins, many with antimicrobial properties. The PMNs of rabbits and chickens have such an abundance of highly cationic peptides in their granules that they appear eosinophilic after conventional blood staining (Wetzel et al. 1967; Kogut et al. 1994; Stabler et al. 1994). These cells, often called 'heterophils' or pseudo-eosinophils, are the functional equivalent of the human PMN.

The cytoplasmic granules in human PMNs are of several types, and they behave differently after the cell ingests microbes or detects molecular signals (e.g. *N*-formylated peptides, complement-derived chemotaxins, etc.) denoting their presence. The PMN's primary ('azurophil') granules are formed early during its differentiation in the bone marrow, and these granules largely transfer their contents to intracellular phagocytic vacuoles. The secondary ('specific') granules of PMNs form after the azurophil granules and contain a substantially different set of proteins and peptides. Most of the contents of specific granules are secreted outside the PMN; whereas defensins are stored in azurophil granules, cathelicidins are stored in the specific granules. As a result of these storage and delivery patterns, defensins and cathelicidins operate in environments that differ in ionic composition, pH, local peptide concentration, presence or absence of serum proteins, etc. Not surprisingly, they have different structures and properties.

DEFENSINS

Defensins constitute a large and growing family of antimicrobial peptides, the members of which have been identified in mammals, birds, and some reptiles. All defensins have a largely β sheet structure that is stabilized by a tri-disulfide framework formed by six paired cysteines. These peptides were initially called 'lysosomal cationic proteins' and were first noticed in studies of rabbit and guinea-pig granulocytes (Zeya and Spitznagel 1966a, 1966b). Technical advances in peptide purification and characterization allowed more detailed chemical descriptions of the rabbit molecules by the mid-1980s (Lehrer et al. 1983; Selsted et al. 1983, 1984), and homologous peptides were identified soon thereafter in human leukocytes (Ganz et al. 1985; Selsted et al. 1985a). Defensins are also produced by epithelial cells (Ouellette et al. 1989) and may contribute prominently to innate mucosal host defense in the respiratory, reproductive, and gastrointestinal tracts (Huttner and Bevins 1999).

Structural considerations

Cysteine-rich antimicrobial peptides that are also called defensins occur in the hemolymph of insects (Boman and Hultmark 1987; Hoffmann et al. 1996) and in various plant tissues (Broekaert et al. 1995; Garcia-Olmedo et al. 1998). In antifungal plant defensins, the peptide backbone is stabilized by four cystine disulfide bonds, rather than the three intramolecular S-S bonds present in mammalian defensins. At least 13 putative defensin genes have been identified in *Arabidopsis thaliana*, and these genes may encode 11 different defensins. The evolutionary relationship of insect and plant defensins to those of vertebrates is uncertain.

A short α-helical domain is present in several human β defensins (Hoover et al. 2000; Sawai et al. 2001; Schibli et al. 2002), insect defensins (Cornet et al. 1995; Bulet et al. 1999), and some plant defensins (Fant et al. 1998). However, the disulfide connectivity of insect defensins (cysteines 1–4, 2–5, 3–6) differs from that of any mammalian defensin. Structures of several α and β defensins have been solved by two-dimensional nuclear magnetic resonance (NMR) and X-ray crystallography (Selsted et al. 1985a; Bach et al. 1987; Pardi et al. 1988, 1992; Zhang et al. 1992; Zimmermann et al. 1995; Hoover et al. 2000; Sawai et al. 2001; Schibli et al. 2002). Although the cysteine spacing of mammalian α and β defensins differs considerably, and their connectivity differs slightly (Figure 10.1), all contain a triple-stranded β sheet with a distinctive 'defensin fold'. The six cysteines of α defensins are linked in a 1–6, 2–4, 3–5 pattern (Selsted and Harwig 1989), whereas a 1–5, 2–4, 3–6 pattern is found in β defensins (Tang and Selsted 1993). As cysteines 5 and 6 are positioned right next to each other in both α and β defensins, this connectivity difference has little impact on their backbone structure (Zimmermann et al. 1995). Several human β defensins and insect defensins are illustrated in Figure 10.2. Recent forays into the human genome have revealed a large number of β-defensin genes and/or pseudogenes, the integrity and functionality of which remain to be determined (Schutte et al. 2002).

Defensin evolution

The presence of β-defensin-like peptides in snake venom (e.g. growth-arresting peptide and crotamines (Zhao et al. 2001b)) suggests that some of these host defense peptides can be used against targets considerably larger than bacteria, fungi, and viruses. Three members of a structurally unique defensin subfamily were recently identified in leukocytes and bone marrow of the rhesus macaque (Tang et al. 1999; Leonova et al. 2001). Called rhesus theta (θ) defensins (RTD), these molecules are cyclic octadecapeptides with three intramolecular disulfide bonds and a β-sheet structure (Tang et al. 1999). Their production involves post-translational splicing of two nonapeptide segments, each derived from a truncated, α-defensin-like precursor (Figure 10.3). The adjoining chromosomal locations of their genes, and

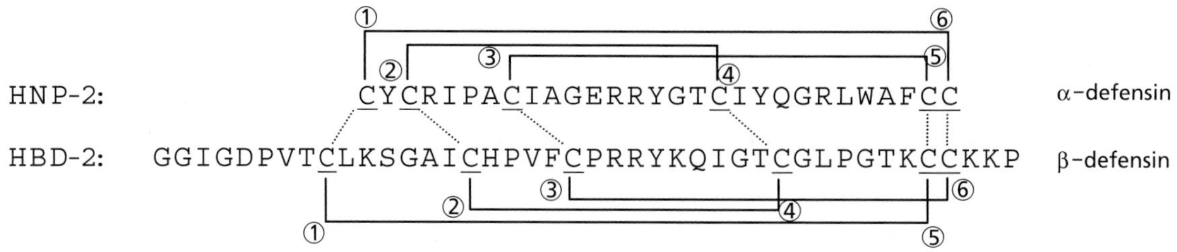

Figure 10.1 *α and β defensins. Human neutrophil peptide-2 (HNP-2), an α-defensin, and human β-defensin-2 (HBD-2) are shown. Both contain six cysteines, that have been numbered from the amino terminus. The cysteines of α and β-defensins have a different pairing pattern, as described in the text, and β defensins are somewhat larger.*

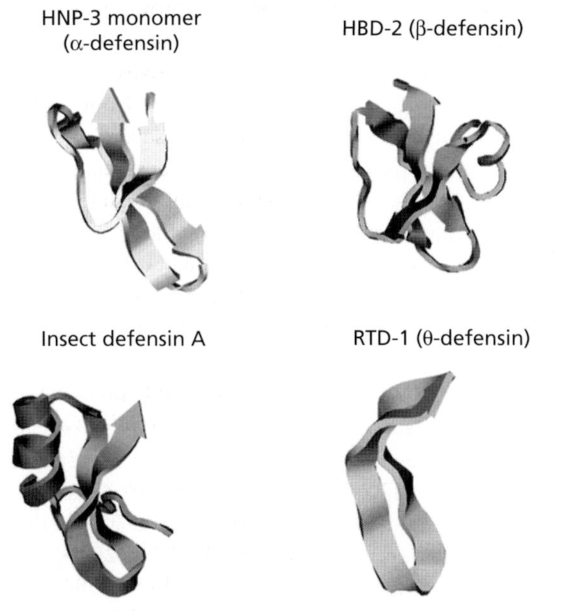

Figure 10.2 *Backbone structures of four different types of defensins. The α-, β-, and θ-defensin peptides expressed by animals arose from a common ancestral gene, the relatedness of which to insect defensin genes is unknown.*

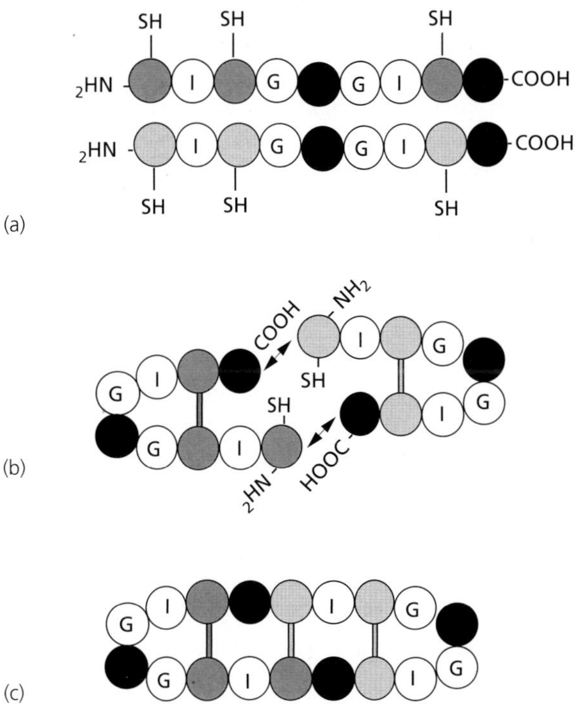

Figure 10.3 *Making a θ defensin. In these cartoons, each circle represents an amino acid residue identified either by single letter code (G, glycine; I, isoleucine) or color (black, arginine; gray, cysteine). The two identical nonapeptides in* **(a)** *correspond to a portion of the retrocyclin-1 precursor described in the text. In* **(b)**, *the double-headed arrows show where these nonapeptides will be spliced to form the cyclic octadecapeptide (θ defensin) shown in* **(c)**. *The events shown in this figure are illustrative – the actual intracellular biochemistry of θ-defensin production remains to be established.*

the structural similarity of their peptides or peptide precursors, make it virtually certain that α, β, and θ defensins arose from a common ancestral gene (Liu et al. 1997).

Just as the existence of β defensins in birds and reptiles identifies them as the oldest vertebrate defensin subfamily, the initial appearance of θ defensins in Old World Monkeys marks them as the youngest subfamily. We have identified intact *DEFT* (θ defensin) genes in several Old World Monkeys, siamangs (a lesser ape), and orangutans. In contrast, we found that the corresponding *DEFT* genes of humans, gorillas, and chimpanzees contained a mutation (a stop codon in the signal sequence) that prevented translation. From phylogenetic considerations, we infer that a hominid ancestor who lived between 7.5 and 10 million years ago sustained the mutation that removed θ defensins from the innate host-defense arsenal of his or her descendants. θ defensins are interesting for many reasons, not the least of which is their ability to inhibit the uptake of HIV-1 by otherwise susceptible $CD4^+$ target cells (Cole et al. 2002).

Variability of expression

Although α- and/or β-defensin peptides probably exist in all mammals and birds, relatively few different species have been studied to date. Defensin expression by neutrophils demonstrates remarkable interspecies variability. Whereas the PMNs of humans, rats (Eisenhauer et al. 1989, 1990), and rabbits contain large amounts of α defensins, the PMNs of cattle (Selsted et al. 1993) and chickens (Harwig et al. 1994) have only β defensins, and murine PMNs contain neither α nor β defensins. Several other mammals, including pigs, sheep, goats, and horses, have PMNs that lack defensins. In some of these animals (e.g. pigs and sheep), the PMNs may compensate by expanding their cathelicidin content. In other species, PMNs may rely more on oxidative microbicidal mechanisms mediated via reduced nicotinamide adenine dinucleotide phosphate (NADPH) oxidase (Wientjes and Segal 1995) and/or inducible nitric oxide synthase (MacMicking et al. 1997; Sethi and Dikshit 2000).

The highest local concentrations of defensins (>10 mg/ml) occur in the storage organelles (granules) of leukocytes (Ganz 1987). When leukocytes ingest microbes and sequester them within phagocytic vacuoles, fusion of the granule and vacuole membranes deposits the defensins and other contents directly on the captured microbe. As little 'empty' space exists in phagocytic vacuoles, ingested microbes are exposed to very high peptide concentrations which, by favoring defensin oligomer/multimer formation, could enhance their efficacy and override any inhibitory effects of the intravacuolar ionic milieu or pH.

Paneth cells are specialized host-defense cells that occupy the base of the crypts in the small intestines of humans and other omnivores. Their prominent secretory granules contain α defensins, and these peptides are secreted into the narrow crypt lumen after bacteria or bacterial LPS enters the intestine. Paneth cell secretion is also stimulated by cholecystokinin or parasympathomimetic agents (Satoh 1988; Satoh et al. 1989). Intestinal crypts are the exclusive sites where the epithelial cells that line intestinal villi arise. Consequently, anticipatory secretion of defensins by Paneth cells may protect this vital cell nursery from adventurous microbes that enter the crypts. Given the crypt lumen's narrow dimensions, its post-secretory defensin concentration may resemble that found in PMN phagocytic vacuoles (Ayabe et al. 2000).

Skin keratinocytes and various epithelia produce β-defensins constitutively (Valore et al. 1998) or in response to infection or inflammation (Harder et al. 2001; Schonwetter et al. 1995). On average, the concentration of defensins in these epithelia ranges from 10 to 100 μg/ml (Harder et al. 1997; Shi et al. 1999), but may be much higher locally if the peptides are unevenly distributed. In the human skin, human β-defensin-2 production is massively induced by interleukin-1 released from myeloid cells, and is secreted by lamellar bodies into the intercellular space between differentiating keratinocytes (Liu et al. 2002, 2003; Oren et al. 2003). Keratinocytes that overexpress human β-defensin-1 (HBD-1) show greater expression of keratin 10, a differentiation marker, suggesting that HBD-1 may enhance cell keratinocyte differentiation (Frye et al. 2001).

Although murine PMNs lack leukocyte defensins and rat PMNs have them in abundance, the Paneth cells of both species express multiple α defensins, and their epithelial tissues express many β defensins. In some cases, defensin expression may be induced by a combination of a specific cell type and local environment. Inflammatory macrophages are leukocytes that arise from circulating blood monocytes which differentiate under the influence of local tissue signals. Rabbit alveolar (lung) macrophages contained two α defensins (NP-1 and NP-2) in amounts approaching their abundance in rabbit neutrophils, but no defensins were present in peritoneal macrophages from the same animals (Ganz et al. 1989). Although defensin expression in monocytes, macrophages, and lymphocytes of some mammals can be detected by highly sensitive techniques (Ryan et al. 1998; Agerberth et al. 2000; Duits et al. 2001), high levels of defensins within macrophages have been documented only in the rabbit alveolar macrophage (Patterson-Delafield et al. 1980, 1981). Some peculiarities in the variable pattern of defensin expression may be driven by evolutionary pressure from species-specific or organ-specific pathogens.

Antimicrobial and antiviral properties

Most defensins display microbicidal activity against bacteria and fungi, especially if tested under low ionic strength conditions or with low concentrations of divalent cations, plasma proteins, or other interfering substances (Selsted et al. 1985b; Lehrer et al. 1988). Under optimal conditions, defensin-mediated antimicrobial activity is evident at peptide concentrations in the low micromolar range. Increasing the medium's salinity inhibits the antimicrobial efficacy of defensins against many organisms, especially gram-negative bacteria. Certain plasma proteins bind defensins, e.g. α_2-macroglobulin (Panyutich and Ganz 1991), and are also inhibitory. In general, metabolically active bacteria are much more sensitive to defensins than bacteria made inactive by nutrient deprivation or metabolic inhibitors. Some bacteria, e.g. *Brucella* and *Burkholderia* spp., are intrinsically resistant to defensins and many other antimicrobial peptides (Martinez et al. 1995; Jones et al. 1996).

Infection by enveloped viruses, such as herpes simplex and vesicular stomatitis virus (Lehrer et al. 1985; Daher et al. 1986), and by adenovirus, a nonenveloped virus (Gropp et al. 1999; Bastian and Schafer 2001), is inhibited by defensins. Human α defensins HNP-1, -2, and-3 suppressed HIV replication (Nakashima et al. 1993). Their production by αβ-$CD8^+$ T cells may promote resistance to developing AIDS (Zhang et al. 2002).

As some defensins are cytotoxic to mammalian cells in vitro (Lichtenstein et al. 1986, 1988; Lichtenstein 1991; Zhang et al. 2001), especially when they are tested at high concentrations or under serum-free conditions, it is possible that defensins may contribute to inflammatory tissue damage in vivo.

ANTIMICROBIAL MECHANISMS

An indicator bacterium (*Escherichia coli* ML-35) (Lehrer et al. 1989) and the K562 mammalian cell line (Lichtenstein 1991) became permeable to small molecules, such as sugars and trypan blue, after being treated with α defensins. In the bacteria, the onset of permeabilization coincided with inhibition of RNA, DNA, and protein synthesis, and decreased bacterial viability as assessed by colony-forming assays. In the K562 cell line, permeabilized cells could be rescued for up to 1 h by removing the defensin. There is evidence that intracellular sites of action also contribute to cell death (Gera and Lichtenstein 1991; Lichtenstein 1991).

In experiments with artificial membranes composed of phosphatidylethanolamine, phosphatidylcholine, and phosphatidylserine in a 2:2:1 ratio, defensins NP-1 (rabbit) and HNP-1 (human) formed voltage-dependent channels, requiring negative potential on the membrane side opposite to where defensins were applied (Kagan et al. 1990). Evidently, insertion of defensin molecules into the membrane is aided when transmembrane electrical forces attract the positively charged defensin molecule. Unlike melittin, a bee-venom peptide that indiscriminately rendered vesicles composed of neutral or anionic phospholipids permeable, defensins were much more active against vesicles containing negatively charged phospholipids (Fujii et al. 1993).

In general, the membranolytic activity of defensins on phospholipid vesicles was diminished by increased salt concentrations, supporting the importance of electrostatic interactions between the cationic (positively charged) defensins and the anionic (negatively charged) head groups of membrane phospholipids. In other experiments, large unilamellar vesicles composed of palmitoyloleoylphosphatidylglycerol (POPG), a negatively charged phospholipid) were permeabilized by human defensin HNP-2 and adding neutral phospholipids to the lipid mix inhibited both defensin binding and permeabilization (Wimley et al. 1994). The importance of anionic phospholipids in defensin–membrane interactions was also shown by calorimetric measurements of phase transitions in membranes (Lohner et al. 1997). In the aggregate, these studies show that both externally applied and local electric fields influence the ability of defensin molecules to insert into a target membrane.

It is less certain what happens once the defensin molecules are in the membrane. The observed leakage of dye markers from liposomes implies the formation of stable or transient transmembrane pores. (We use the term 'pore' to refer to any type of ion or water-permeable structure or lesion within the membrane.) For some defensins, the release of internal markers from each vesicle appeared to occur in an all-or-none fashion (Wimley et al. 1994), suggesting the formation of stable pores with a diameter estimated at 2.5 nm by using markers with different sizes. The authors proposed a model of a defensin pore – a hexamer of dimers that could generate an opening of the observed size. However, stable pore formation is not the only mechanism of defensin interaction with membranes. The more cationic rabbit defensins induced a partial release of markers from individual vesicles, indicating that the pores formed were not stable. Possibly, electrostatic repulsion between the highly cationic rabbit defensin molecules destabilizes the pores.

MICROBIAL RESISTANCE

Specific mechanisms that confer increased bacterial resistance to defensins have been identified by insertional mutagenesis. Disruption of the two-component transcriptional regulator phoP-phoQ increased the sensitivity of *Salmonella* spp. to defensins and other cationic peptides (Groisman et al. 1989, 1992; Miller et al. 1990; Miller 1991). The phoP-phoQ directly regulates multiple genes involved in resistance to cationic peptides and also exerts some of its activity by modulating a second two-component regulator, PmrA-PmrB. The function of the downstream genes includes covalent modification of LPSs that decreases their affinity for cationic peptides (Guo et al. 1998) and expression of membrane proteases that degrade cationic peptides (Guina et al. 2000). In *Neisseria gonorrhoeae*, a bacterium that is naturally resistant to defensins (Qu et al. 1996), the energy-dependent efflux system *mtr* increases the resistance to protegrins, potently antimicrobial β-hairpin peptides originally isolated from pig neutrophils (Shafer et al. 1998). In staphylococci, the disruption of either of two genes, *dlt* or *MprF*, increased sensitivity to defensins (Peschel et al. 1999, 2001). The *dlt* gene is required for covalent modification of cell wall teichoic acid by alanine, and *MprF* is needed for covalent modification of membrane phosphatidylglycerol with l-lysine. By decreasing the negative charge of the cell wall and bacterial membrane, respectively, these mutations diminish their attraction for the cationic defensins. Homologs of these resistance genes exist in many bacterial species, indicating that similar mechanisms may be widespread.

OTHER ACTIVITIES

Various defensins have chemotactic activity for monocytes, T lymphocytes, and dendritic cells (Territo et al. 1989; Chertov et al. 1996; Yang et al. 1999, 2000). Human β defensins-1 and -2 (HBD-2) attract memory T cells and immature dendritic cells, apparently by binding to the chemokine receptor CCR6 (Yang et al. 1999). Although the physiological significance of this interaction is uncertain, the high concentrations of HBD-2 in inflamed skin might allow this defensin to compete effectively with the natural chemokine ligand (variously named CCL20, LARC, or MIP-3α) despite the latter's higher affinity for the CCR6 receptor. Recent structural analysis of CCL20 pointed out remarkable similarities to HBD-2 in the putative receptor-binding region of CCL20. The role of this region in the chemotactic activity of HBD-2 needs to be confirmed by mutating the amino acid residues suspected in its interaction with CCR6. Human neutrophil defensins HNP-1–3 were reported to be chemotactic for monocytes (Territo et al. 1989), naive T cells, and immature dendritic cells (Yang et al. 2000) but a specific receptor remains to be identified. Murine β-defensin-2 acted like an in vivo adjuvant for anti-tumor immunization, and induced dendritic cell maturation by activating Toll-like receptor-4 (TLR4), leading to a type 1 polarized adaptive response in vivo.

Certain defensins, especially rabbit NP-3A, can oppose the action of adrenocorticotropic hormone (ACTH) by binding to ACTH receptor without activating it (Tominaga et al. 1990). NP-3A was called Corticostatin-1 (CS-1) by some investigators (Zhu et al. 1989; Solomon et al. 1991) who failed either to recognize or to acknowledge that their sequences were identical.

By inhibiting production of cortisol (an immunosuppressive hormone) in vivo, this property might enhance the net response to infections. Tominaga et al. (1992) used an antiserum against synthetic rabbit NP-3a (CS-1 in their terminology) to examine the peptide's distribution in several rabbit tissues, including the hypothalamic–pituitary–adrenal axis. Lung and spleen had the highest levels of immunoreactivity, and relatively high levels were also detected in the pituitary, adrenal medulla, and small intestine, although not in the hypothalamus. Plasma levels of NP-3A averaged 7.8 ng/ml, and increased to 185.4 ng/ml with infection. Levels of NP-3A in the adrenal gland, small intestine, and hypothalamus also increased in rabbits with active inflammation. Although these data suggest that NP-3A (CS-1) may affect the hypothalamic–pituitary–adrenal axis in an endocrine or paracrine manner, the physiological role – if any – of corticostatic activity remains to be demonstrated.

Nanomolar concentrations of some defensins activate nifedipine-sensitive calcium channels in mammalian cells (MacLeod et al. 1991; Bateman et al. 1996). Certain mouse Paneth cell defensins (called 'cryptdins' to commemorate their presence in murine small intestinal crypts) activate chloride secretion, most probably by forming channels in the apical membrane of epithelial cells (Lencer et al. 1997; Merlin et al. 2001). This activity is limited to a subset of cryptdins, and its structural basis is not yet known. It is difficult, at present, to reconcile the multiple and varied activities of defensins with any simple receptor–ligand model.

We have recently discovered that certain α and θ defensins interact with various sugars and that this lectin-like property underlies their high-affinity binding to functionally significant glycoproteins and glycolipids. As immunoglobulins, cellular receptors, and viral envelope proteins used to promote cell entry are frequently glycosylated, this property (sugar binding) may affect many activities of defensins, especially their antiviral properties.

Defensin biosynthesis

In humans, multiple genes encoding various α and β defensins are clustered on chromosome 8p23 (Sparkes et al. 1989; Harder et al. 1997; Liu et al. 1997, 1998; Frohlich et al. 2001). Additional defensin-related genes were identified in four other clusters, so that, overall, as many as 30 transcribed defensin genes may exist in 'mice and men' (Schutte et al. 2002). It has been difficult to map the primary defensin locus in 8p23, presumably as a result of its polymorphic nature and because individuals and their chromosomes differ in the number of copies of certain defensin genes (Mars et al. 1995). α defensins are generally encoded as a tripartite pre-propeptide sequence, wherein a 90–100 amino acid precursor contains an amino terminus consisting of a 19 amino signal sequence, an anionic propiece of about 45 amino acids, and a carboxy-terminal mature cationic defensin of about 30 amino acids (Daher et al. 1988) (Figure 10.4). In many cases, the charges of the propiece and the mature defensin approximately balance (Michaelson et al. 1992), and this arrangement may be important for folding and/or to prevent intracellular interactions with membranes (Liu and Ganz 1995; Valore et al. 1996).

α-defensin synthesis by PMNs takes place in the bone marrow, in precursor cells called promyelocytes (Yount et al. 1995; Arnljots et al. 1998; Cowland and Borregaard 1999). Mature neutrophils in blood or inflamed tissues contain large amounts of defensin peptides, but no longer synthesize significant amounts of the peptides or their RNA. In myeloid cell lines, the defensin signal sequence is rapidly removed during synthesis. Subsequent proteolytic processing takes many hours, and is completed in maturing cytoplasmic granules (Valore and Ganz 1992). Defensin processing is a very efficient process, because only small amounts of incompletely processed intermediates are detectable in mature neutrophils (Harwig et al. 1992).

Processing the α-defensins (cryptdins) of murine intestinal Paneth cells requires a metalloprotease called matrilysin (MMP-7), because mice with homozygous disruption of the matrilysin gene fail to process Paneth cell pro-defensins past the removal of the signal sequence. In humans, processing of Paneth cell defensins takes place after secretion and involves Paneth cell trypsin (Ghosh et al. 2002). β-defensin precursors are structurally less complex than α-defensin precursors, having a signal sequence, a short or absent propiece, and a C-terminal mature defensin domain. It is not yet clear why β-defensin precursors can lack an anionic propiece and α-defensin precursors apparently must have one.

Defensin sequences and composition

Except for the conservation of their cystine framework and a few additional residues, the amino acid sequences of mature defensins are highly variable. Clusters of positively charged amino acids are characteristic of most α and β defensins but their specific distribution within the defensin molecule is inconstant (Figure 10.5 and see Figure 10.4).

STORAGE AND DELIVERY

In leukocytes and Paneth cells of the small intestine, defensins are stored in granules. These subcellular storage organelles are rich in negatively charged glycosaminoglycans (Spicer et al. 1967; Olsson 1970; Fromm et al. 1995; Hileman et al. 1998). With the exception of chicken gallinacins, these α and β defensins contain arginine as the predominant cationic amino acid. In contrast, β defensins that are secreted from epithelial cells contain similar amounts of arginine and lysine. The preferential use of arginine in defensins stored in

Rabbit NP-1	MRTLALLAAILLVALQAQA	Signal sequence
Rabbit NP-5	MRTLALLAAILLVTLQAQA	
Rabbit NP-3A	MRTLILLAAILLAALQAQA	
Rat NP-1	MRTLTLLTALLLLALHTQA	
Rat NP-3	MRTLTLLTTLLLLALHTQA	
Rat NP-4	MRTLTLLITLLLLALHTQA	
Human NP-1	MRTLAILAAILLVALQAQA	
Human DEF5	MRTIAILAAILLVALQAQA	
Human NP-4	MRIIALLAAILLVALQVRA	
Guinea pig NP	MRTVPLFAACLLLTLMAQA	
Mouse cryptdin-1	MKKLVLLFALVLLGFQVQA	

(a)

Rabbit NP-1	EHVSVSIDEVVDQQPPQAEDQDVAIYVKEHESSALEALGVKAG	Anionic propiece
Rabbit NP-5	ELHSGMADDGVDQQQPRAQDLDVAVYIKQDETSPLEVLGAKAG	
Rabbit NP-3A	ELFSVNVDEVLDQQQP-GSDQDLVIHLTGEESSALQVPDTK	
Rat NP-1	KSPQGTAEEAPDQEQLVMEDQDISISFGGDKGTALQDADVKAG	
Rat NP-3	ESPQGSTKEAPD------EEQDISVFFGGDKGTALQDAAVKAGVT	
Rat NP-4	ESPQERAKAAPDQD-MVMEDQDIFISFGGYKGTVLQDAVVKAGQ	
Human NP-1	EPLQARADEVAAAPEQIAADIPEVVVSLAWDESLAPKHPGSRKNM	
Human DEF5	ESLQERADE-ATTQKQSGEDNQDLAISFAGNGLSALRTSGSQAR	
Human NP-4	GPLQARGDEAPGQEQRGPEDQDISISFAWDKSSALQVSGSTRGM	
Guinea pig NP	EPLPRAADHSDTKMKGDREDHVAVISFWEEESTSLEDAGAGAG	
Mouse cryptdin-1	DSIQNTDEETKTEEQPGEEDQAVSVSFGDPEGTSLQEES	

(b)

Rabbit NP-1	VV**C**A**C**RRAL**C**LPRERRAGF**C**RIRGRIHPL**CC**RR	95	Mature defensin
Rabbit NP-5	VF**C**T**C**RGFL**C**GSGERASGS**C**TINGVRHTL**CC**RR	95	
Rabbit NP-3A	GI**C**A**C**RRRF**C**PNSERFSGY**C**RVNGARYVR**CC**SRR	93	
Rat NP-1	VT**C**Y**C**RRTR**C**GFRERLSGA**C**GYRGRIYRL**CC**R	94	
Rat NP-3	**C**S**C**RTSS**C**RFGERLSGA**C**RLNGRIYRL**CC**	87	
Rat NP-4	A**C**Y**C**RIGA**C**VSGERLTGA**C**GLNGRIYRL**CC**R	93	
Human NP-1	A**C**Y**C**RIPA**C**IAGERRYGT**C**IYQGRLWAF**CC**	94	
Human DEF5	AT**C**Y**C**RTGR**C**ATRESLSGV**C**EISGRLYRL**CC**R	94	
Human NP-4	V**C**S**C**RLVF**C**RRTELRVGN**C**LIGGVSFTY**CC**TRVD	97	
Guinea pig NP	RR**C**I**C**TTRT**C**RFPYRRLGT**C**IFQNRVYTF**CC**	93	
Mouse cryptdin-1	LRDLV**C**Y**C**RSRG**C**KGRERMNGT**C**RKGHLLYTL**CC**R	93	

(c)

Figure 10.4 *Sequences of α-defensin precursors. Eleven α defensins from four species are shown. Positively charged amino acids, arginine (R) and lysine (K), are red; negatively charged residues, aspartic (D) or glutamic (E) acid, are blue; cysteine (C) is black. Note that:* **(a)** *the signal sequences are highly conserved;* **(b)** *the long propiece has a net negative charge; and* **(c)** *the mature defensin domain contains 29 (human NP-1) to 35 (mouse cryptdin-1) residues, including six conserved cysteines, and has a net positive charge.*

granules may reflect the constraints imposed by packing defensin molecules into the glycosaminoglycan matrix of granules. Alternately, synergistic interactions between defensin and myeloperoxidase, or its downstream products (e.g. HOCl), might have favored the selection of arginines over lysines. Myeloperoxidase is present in mammalian neutrophils but is absent from those of chickens and other fowl (Penniall and Spitznagel 1975; Rausch and Moore 1975).

STRUCTURE–FUNCTION CONSIDERATIONS

At present, no single mechanism explains how defensins kill bacteria, or even if the critical lethal event that defensins inflict is membrane permeabilization. In part, the present uncertainty reflects the diversity in net charge, amino acid sequence, and quaternary structure (monomers versus dimers) found among defensins. It seems likely that these differences evolved to allow defensins to recognize and target bacteria with different cell wall or membrane structures, or different patterns of metabolism or growth. Furthermore, although interactions between defensins with model membranes have been examined (Wimley et al. 1994), they may provide only a first approximation of the events that transpire in more complex biological systems. Further work in this area is needed.

	Signal sequence	Mature peptide
HBD-1	MRTSYLLLFTLCLLLSEMASG	GNFLTGLGHRSDHYN**C**VSSGGQ**C**LYSA**C**PIFTKIQGT**C**YRGKAK**CC**K
MBD-1	MKTHYFLLVMICFLFSQMEPG	VGILTSLGRRTDQYK**C**LQHGGF**C**LRSS**C**PSNTKLQGT**C**KPDKPN**CC**KS
RBD-1	MKTHYFLLVMLFFLFSQMELG	AGILTSLGRRTDQYR**C**LQNGGF**C**LRSS**C**PSHTKLQGT**C**KPDKPN**CC**RS
HBD-2	MRVLYLLFSFLFIFLMPLPGVFG	GIGDPVT**C**LKSGAI**C**HPVF**C**PRRYKQIGT**C**GLPGTK**CC**KKP
HBD-3	MRIHYLLFALLFLFLVPVPGHG	GIINTLQKYY**C**RVRGGR**C**AVLS**C**LPKEEQIGK**C**STRGRK**CC**RRKK
PBD-1	MRLHRLLLVFLLMVLLPVPGLL	KNIGNSVS**C**LRNKGV**C**MPGK**C**APKMKQIGT**C**GMPQVK**CC**KR
TAP	MRLHHLLLALLFLVLSAWSGFTQGVG	NPVS**C**VRNKGI**C**VPIR**C**PGSMKQIGT**C**VGRAVK**CC**RKK
GAL1	MRIVYLLLPFILLLAQGAAGSSQAL	GRKSD**C**FRKSGF**C**AFLK**C**PSLTLISGK**C**S-RFYL**CC**KRIWG
BNBD-4	MRLHHLLLAVLFLVLSAGSGFT	QRVRNPQS**C**RWNMGV**C**IPFL**C**RVGMRQIGT**C**FGPRVP**CC**RR

Figure 10.5 *Sequences of β-defensin precursors. Nine peptides from six species are shown. β-Defensin precursors are considerably shorter than α-defensin precursors, primarily as a result of the presence of a much smaller propiece. Mature β-defensin peptides are positively charged (especially so in HBD-3 or TAP – transporter associated with antigen processing), are longer than α defensins, and the spacing of their six conserved cysteines differs from that seen in α defensins.*

CATHELICIDINS

Cathelicidins are bipartite molecules with a conserved amino-terminal 'cathelin' domain containing about 100 amino acid residues (Zanetti et al. 1995, 2000). The word cathelin is an acronym for cathepsin L inhibitor, and was chosen to commemorate the domain's homology to cystatins, a family of proteins that inhibit cysteine proteases. This inference was supported by later X-ray crystallography and NMR studies (Sanchez et al. 2002a, 2002b). These studies revealed that the cathelin domain and other cystatin family members had similar backbone folds; namely an amino-terminal helix surrounded by a four-stranded β sheet. In addition, the core hydrophobic residues and disulfides of cathelin and cystatins were conserved. Although the function of the cathelin domain remains uncertain, it may protect cathelicidin precursors from premature proteolytic activation during their targeting, packaging, and storage. In many cathelicidins, the carboxy-terminal domain has both antimicrobial and LPS-binding properties. Although the antimicrobial properties of cathelicidins remain latent until the C-terminal peptide is separated from the cathelin domain by limited proteolysis (Zanetti et al. 1993), the LPS-binding properties may not require this activation step (Zarember et al. 2002).

Cathelicidins with short antimicrobial domains

Cathelin-associated antimicrobial peptides vary considerably in size and structure. The smallest are the 12-residue dodecapeptides (also called cyclic 'bactenecins') found in cattle and sheep. The peptides have similar sequences – RLCRIVVIRVCR (bovine) and RICRIIFLRVCR (sheep) – and contain a disulfide bond between their cysteine residues. Bovine indolicidin has 13 residues (ILPWKWPWWPWRR), including 5 tryptophans. Its small size and unusual composition has made it a favorite for analog design and structure–activity studies. NMR studies of indolicidin performed in a membrane-like environment composed of dodecylphosphocholine micelles revealed a well-defined, extended backbone between residues 3 and 11, with half-turns at residues Lys5 and Trp8. The peptide's central hydrophobic core, which is proline and tryptophan rich, was bracketed by positively charged side chains closer to its ends. All but one tryptophan side chain folded flat against the backbone, imparting a wedge shape to the molecule. Indolicidin's preferred location in micelles and lipid bilayers was at the membrane interface. It bound purified LPS with high affinity, and permeabilized the outer and inner membranes of *E. coli* (Falla et al. 1996). When a sufficiently electronegative potential (threshold −70 to −80 mV) was applied to the distal face of a model planar lipid bilayer, the peptide induced transmembrane currents and formed discrete channels with a conductance ranging from 0.05 to 0.15 nanosiemens (nS).

Tritrpticin (VRRFPWWWPFLRR) is a 13-residue antimicrobial peptide with a precursor that is expressed by porcine leukocytes as part of the pro-piece of a 79-residue proline and phenylalanine-rich peptide called prophenin (Harwig et al. 1995). The initial studies of tritrpticin showed activity against *Escherichia coli*, *Pseudomonas aeruginosa*, *Klebsiella pneumoniae*, *Staphyloccus epidermidis*, *Proteus mirabilis*, group D streptococci, and *Aspergillus fumigatus*. The peptide was bactericidal rather than bacteriostatic and its activity was completely inhibited by 2 mmol/l $MgCl_2$ (Lawyer et al. 1996).

In sodium dodecylsulfate micelles, tritrpticin's adjacent turns cluster its hydrophobic residues and separate them from the positively charged arginines, making the peptide amphipathic (Schibli et al. 1999). Spin-label studies showed tritrpticin near the micelle surface, with its aromatic side chains equally partitioned into the hydrophilic–hydrophobic interface and its tryptophan residues inserted. The tryptophan side chains inserted more deeply in vesicles that contained phospholipids with anionic phosphatidylglycerol head groups (Schibli et al. 2002).

Cathelicidins with β-sheet antimicrobial domains

To date, protegrins are the only cathelin-associated antimicrobial peptides with a β-sheet structure. Three protegrin peptides (PG-1,-2, and-3 were purified from porcine leukocytes, and two additional protegrins (PG-4 and-5) were identified by cloning studies. Porcine protegrins contain 16–18 amino acid residues, including four cysteines that form two intramolecular disulfides. These disulfides are essential to preserve optimal broad-spectrum antimicrobial activity in physiological saline. Although protegrins are much smaller than defensins, they show substantial sequence similarity to rabbit defensin, NP-3a. Relatively low concentrations of protegrins (<5 μg/ml) rapidly kill a very wide range of bacteria and fungi, including organisms that are resistant to conventional antibiotics. These properties, in combination with their small size and relatively simple production by direct chemical synthesis, has led to their use in mechanistic studies and as templates for pharmaceutical development (Bellm et al. 2000). Protegrins PG-1 and PG-3 have immunomodulatory properties, because both initiated the processing of pro-interleukin-1β from LPS-stimulated human monocytes, resulting in the efficient release of mature interleukin 1β (IL-1β) (Perregaux et al. 2002).

Cathelicidins with proline-rich antimicrobial domains

The cathelicidins of pigs and ruminants include several with remarkably proline-rich (40–50 percent proline!)

antimicrobial domains (Table 10.1), with either arginine or phenylalanine the next most abundant residue. In bovine bactenecin-7 (Bac7), most prolines are evenly spaced and separated by a single nonproline residue. Bovine Bac5 and porcine PR-39 contain several repeats of a 'PPXX' motif (i.e. two prolines followed by two nonproline residues). The initial 60 residues of prophenins 1 and 2 are repeated proline-rich decamers. Both of these prophenin isoforms were found in porcine lung surfactant preparations prepared by chloroform/methanol extraction (Wang et al. 1999) and contained, in addition to the expected components (98 percent phospholipids and 1–2 percent surfactant-associated proteins B and C), three prophenin-related molecules. These were: full-length prophenin-1; FPPPPPFRPPP FGPPRF – the carboxy-terminal octadecapeptide of prophenin-1; and a variant of prophenin-2 with an amino-terminal pyroglutamic acid extension. These components may have contributed to the antimicrobial properties of the preparation, the commercial equivalent of which (Curosurf) has been given to tens of thousands of pre-term infants with respiratory distress syndrome since its European introduction in 1992.

PR-39, a proline- and arginine-rich cathelicidin peptide found in porcine PMNs, has no known human counterpart. The peptide was initially detected as a result of its antimicrobial properties, but was subsequently reported to modulate proteoglycan production in wounds (Gallo et al. 1994), to promote leukocyte chemotaxis (Huang et al. 1997), to interact with intracellular -SH_3 proteins (Chan and Gallo 1998), and to inhibit superoxide production by PMNs (Shi et al. 1996). Expression of PR-39 and protegrin by porcine bone marrow increased substantially after experimental infection with *Salmonellas typhimurium* or in vivo administration of LPS (Wu et al. 2000). In vitro, expression of PR-39 and protegrin by cultured porcine bone marrow cells increased in response to IL-6 or all-*trans*-retinoic acid. The PR-39 and protegrin genes have upstream binding sites for IL-6 and retinoic acid, as well as potential C/EBP-binding motifs (Wu et al. 2000).

Cathelicidins with α-helical domains

Most cathelin-associated antimicrobial peptides are α helical. Typically, such peptides have 23–37 residues and a net positive charge of +6 or more (see Table 10.1). In addition, many possess an amidated C terminus – a feature that further increases overall cationicity. SMAP-29, an α-helical cathelicidin-derived peptide of sheep, has unusually potent, broad-spectrum antimicrobial activity in vitro (Travis et al. 2000). Brogden and associates induced a *Mannheimia haemolytica* pneumonia in lambs and, 24 h later, administered 0.5 mg SMAP-29 directly to the affected part of the lung (Brogden et al. 2001; Kalfa et al. 2001). Twenty-four hours later, the experimental and control animals were euthanized and their lungs examined. The peptide-treated animals showed reduced inflammation and consolidation, and had lower numbers of bacteria in their bronchoalveolar lavage fluid.

Sites of cathelicidin synthesis and storage

The neutrophils of cattle store cathelicidin peptides in large cytoplasmic granules. The stored peptides remain inactive until their cathelin and antimicrobial domains

Table 10.1 *Sequences of selected cathelicidin peptides*

Structure	Species	Sequence
α Helical		
LL-37	Human	LLGDFFRKSKEKIGKEFKRIVQRIKDFLRNLVPRTES
RL-37	Rhesus	RLGNFFRKVKEKIGGGLKKVGQKIKDFLGNLVPRTAS
CRAMP	Mouse	LLRKGGEKIGEK----LKKIGQKIKNFFQKLVPQPEQ
Proline rich		
Bac-5	Cow	RFRPPIRRPPIRPPFYPPFRPPIRPPIFPPIRPPFRPPLGPFP*
PR-39	Pig	RRRPRPPYLPRPRPPPFFPPRLPPRIPPGFPPRFPPRFP*
Prophenin-1	Pig	AFPPPNVPGPR[FPPPNFPGPR]$_3$FPPPNFPGPPFPPPIFPGPWFPPPPPFRPPPFGPPRFP*
Cyclic dodecapeptide		
Bactenecin	Cow	RLCRIVVIRVCR
Bactenecin	Sheep	RICRIIFLRVCR
β Hairpin		
Protegrin (PG)-1	Pig	RGGRLCYCRRRFCVCVGR*
Protegrin (PG)-4	Pig	RGGRLCYCRGWICFCVGR*
Tryptophan rich		
Indolicidin	Cow	ILPWKWPWWPWRR*
Iritrpticin	Pig	VRRFPWWWPFLRR

In the proline-rich peptide sequences, the proline residues are emboldened to accentuate their motifs. In the other peptide groupings, identical residues are emboldened, and similar residues are underlined. The asterisk (*) signifies carboxy-terminal amidation are separated proteolytically by neutrophil elastase (Scocchi et al. 1992), which also activates cathelicidins in porcine neutrophils (Panyutich et al. 1997; Cole et al. 2001). In contrast, human PMNs activate their cathelicidin, hCAP-18, with another serine protease – protease 3 (Sorensen et al. 2001).

The cytoplasmic storage organelles of human and bovine PMNs differ in morphology and content. In human neutrophils, the primary ('azurophil') granules contain α defensins along with cathepsins, bactericidal/permeability-increasing protein (BPI), lysozyme, and several catalytically active neutral serine proteases (elastase, cathepsin G, and protease 3). The secondary ('specific') granules store hCAP-18, the cathelin-containing precursor of LL-37, along with lactoferrin, additional lysozyme, and B_{12}-binding protein. Bovine PMNs (and those of other ruminants) have an additional class of storage organelles called 'intermediate' granules. (Gennaro et al. 1983; Baggiolini et al. 1985). Intermediate granules serve as the main repositories for cathelicidins, are larger and more numerous than primary or secondary granules, and release their contents in response to phagocytosis or soluble stimuli (Gennaro et al. 1983; Baggiolini et al. 1985).

In an in vitro experimental system wherein hCAP-18 was misdirected into azurophil granules, it underwent premature proteolytic activation and released LL-37 (Bulow et al. 2002). Peptide purification and cloning have revealed at least seven different cathelin-associated antimicrobial peptides in bovine neutrophils: cyclic dodecapeptide, indolicidin, three α-helical peptides (BMAP-27, BMAP-28, and BMAP-37), and two proline-rich molecules (Bac5 and Bac7) (Scocchi et al. 1997). Similar studies in pigs have identified five protegrins, three proline-rich molecules (PR-39, prophenin-1, and prophenin-2), and three α-helical peptides (PMAP-23, PMAP-36, and PMAP-37) (Gennaro and Zanetti 2000; Zanetti et al. 2000).

CATHELICIDINS OF MICE AND MEN

In contrast to numerous cathelicidins in pigs, cattle, and ruminants, the human genome encodes only a single cathelicidin, hCAP-18, the antimicrobial domain of which is the 37-residue, α-helical peptide called LL-37. The gene is expressed constitutively in human neutrophils and the resulting propeptide is stored in its secondary (specific) granules. The murine homologue of hCAP-18 is CRAMP, an acronym for 'cathelin-related antimicrobial peptide (CRAMP)'. Adult mice express CRAMP transcripts in bone marrow, testis, spleen, and stomach. Their CRAMP gene maps to a region of mouse chromosome 9 that is syntenic to the loci of porcine and human cathelicidin genes. NMR spectroscopy of CRAMP in a membrane-mimetic solvent system revealed two amphipathic α helices (Leu4 to Lys10 and Gly16 to Leu33), connected by a flexible region between Gly11 and Gly16. Truncated CRAMP variants that contained its amphipathic carboxy-terminal region (Gly16 to Leu33) retained considerable antibiotic activity.

In human neutrophils, hCAP-18 and lactoferrin are about equally abundant on a molar basis (Sorensen et al. 1997). Other sites of hCAP-18 expression include epididymis, spermatids, various epithelial cells, and some lymphocytes. Expression of hCAP-18 in skin is inducible. The carboxy-terminal domain of murine CRAMP shows considerable homology to LL-37 but is somewhat shorter. Synthetic CRAMP inhibited the growth of a variety of bacterial strains (minimum inhibitory concentrations 0.5–8.0 μmol), and 1.0 μmol CRAMP permeabilized the inner membrane of *E. coli*. Knockout mice that do not express mCRAMP, the murine homolog of LL-37, show undue susceptibility to infection by group A streptococci (Nizet et al. 2001).

In addition to its antimicrobial properties, LL-37 binds bacterial LPS and can induce chemotaxis via the formyl peptide-like receptor-1 (De et al. 2000). A few mammalian α-helical cathelicidin peptides are shorter than LL-37 (e.g. porcine PMAP-23 and bovine BMAP-27), but most are about as long. Whereas the α-helical cathelicidin peptides of cattle and sheep have amidated carboxyl termini, those of rodents and primates do not. Although all the peptides shown in Table 10.1 are cationic, their net positive charges vary from +3 in porcine PMAP-37 to +14 in PMAP-36. Human LL-37 has 11 positively charged lysine and arginines, but its five negatively charged residues reduce its net charge to +6 and contribute to its poor activity against *Staphylococcus aureus* in media with normal or elevated concentrations of NaCl (Zhao et al. 2001a).

CATHELICIDIN GENES

Like other porcine and human cathelicidin genes (Agerberth et al. 1996; Gudmundsson et al. 1996), porcine protegrin and prophenin genes contain four exons and three introns (Zhao et al. 1995a, 1995b). Exon I encodes the signal sequence and the first 37 amino acid residues of the cathelin domain. Exons II and III code for 36 and 24 additional cathelin residues, respectively. Exon IV contains the final few cathelin residues followed by the protegrin sequence. This quadripartite gene structure suggests that expression of structurally diverse antimicrobial peptides on a common, cathelin-containing precursor occurred after mutational translocation of a suitable peptide domain into exon IV. Circumstantial evidence for such events is embedded in the sequences of the PR-39 and prophenin genes (Zhao et al. 1995a).

The upstream region of the PR-39 cathelicidin gene contains several potential recognition sites for NF-IL6 and acute phase response factor (APRF), as well as binding motifs for NF-κB, granulocyte–macrophage colony-stimulating factor (GM-CSF), and NF-1 – factors that regulate gene responsiveness to cytokines and acute phase response factors. Site-directed mutagenesis studies also revealed a negative regulatory element in the 5′-flanking region of the PR-39 gene, suggesting a mechanism for its tissue-specific and age-dependent repression (Wu et al. 2000, 2002).

Bovine or porcine leukocytes each contain at least 10 different cathelicidins (Zanetti et al. 1995) whose structurally diverse C termini contain α-helical, β-sheet, proline-rich, tryptophan-rich, or other molecules (e.g. bactenecin dodecapeptide). In contrast to this polypharmacy, human and murine PMNs each contain a single cathelicidin: hCAP-18 in humans and CRAMP in mice. Neither human nor mice skin cells (keratinocytes) express hCAP-18 or CRAMP constitutively. However, production of both peptides is induced soon after injury (e.g. sterile incision) or infection. As it takes a few hours for epithelial cells to begin substantial cathelicidin production, the rapid infiltration of granulocytes affords protection in the interim (Hoffmann et al. 1996). LL-37 and HBD-2 are abundant in psoriatic skin, but their concentration in atopic skin lesions is considerably lower, perhaps contributing to diminished resistance to *S. aureus* infections in this setting (Ong et al. 2002).

The attributes of LL-37 and other cathelicidins may extend well beyond their core missions of exerting direct antimicrobial activity, and neutralizing the toxicity of LPS. Normal seminal plasma contains levels of hCAP-18 (40–140 μg/ml) that are 70-fold higher than those in blood plasma. Much of this hCAP-18 is on sperm cells, which carry about 6.6 million hCAP-18 molecules each (Andersson et al. 2002). Spermatozoa undoubtedly acquire their hCAP-18 coating in the epididymis, because high level hCAP-18 expression was noted in the body and tail of the epididymis (Malm et al. 2000). As the epididymis of humans (and mice) also expresses β-defensin genes, sperm may start their perilous journey equipped with something of a 'chemical condom' to dissuade any microbial hitchhikers from accompanying them on their journey (von Horsten et al. 2002; Yamaguchi et al. 2002). Alternately, the peptide could participate in later events directly associated with fertilization.

Studies by Oppenheim and associates have delineated a role of LL-37 and defensins as signals that link innate and adaptive immune responses. LL-37 acted via the Gi protein-coupled FPRL-1 (formyl peptide-like receptor-1) (Yang et al. 2001a, b) to induce a chemotactic response in human PMNs, monocytes and lymphocytes. The relatively high concentration of LL-37 needed to induce optimal chemotactic responses in peripheral blood monocytes was 10 μmol/l (about 50 μg/ml) which is likely to occur, if at all, only at sites of inflammation.

LL-37 was detected in freshly isolated lymphocytes and in supernatants of human T and natural killer (NK) cells grown with IL-2 for 5 days in vitro (Agerberth et al. 2000). Reverse transcription-polymerase chain reaction (RT-PCR) demonstrated LL-37 expression in B cells, γ, δ T cells, cloned NK cells, and monocytes, but not in αβ T-cell lines. Transcription and secretion of LL-37 by primary cultures of human lymphocytes responded to IL-6 and interferon-γ. Consequently, LL-37 (and defensins) may also contribute to the antibacterial activity of T cells and NK cells.

Some pathogenic bacteria may undermine host defense by inhibiting local production of antimicrobial peptides, including LL-37, e.g. early in human shigella infections expression of LL-37 and human β-defensin-1 was reduced or eliminated, with shigella plasmid DNA possibly being one of the mediators (Islam et al. 2001). If this were to promote bacterial adherence and invasion, it might enhance virulence.

CONCLUDING REMARKS

Interest in antimicrobial peptides has increased during the past decade, and they are now recognized as fundamental elements of the innate immune system. In addition to having direct effects on microbes, some of these peptides have prominent antiviral properties. In the case of α and θ defensins, our recent (and still largely unpublished) studies have found strong correlations between their antiviral activity and their ability to act as lectins that bind carbohydrate moieties present on viral glycoproteins and their cellular receptors. One wonders if the ability to recognize carbohydrates is also involved in their signaling and co-stimulatory properties. It seems likely that many surprises about the properties of these very old molecules will emerge during the decades to come.

REFERENCES

Agerberth, B., Gunne, H., et al. 1996. PR-39, a proline-rich peptide antibiotic from pig and FALL-39, a tentative human counterpart. *Vet Immunol Immunopathol*, **54**, 127–31.

Agerberth, B., Charo, J., et al. 2000. The human antimicrobial and chemotactic peptides LL-37 and alpha-defensins are expressed by specific lymphocyte and monocyte populations. *Blood*, **96**, 3086–93.

Andersson, E., Sorensen, O.E., et al. 2002. Isolation of human cationic antimicrobial protein-18 from seminal plasma and its association with prostasomes. *Hum Reprod*, **17**, 2529–34.

Arnljots, K., Sorensen, O., et al. 1998. Timing, targeting and sorting of azurophil granule proteins in human myeloid cells. *Leukemia*, **12**, 1789–95.

Ayabe, T., Satchell, D.P., et al. 2000. Secretion of microbicidal alpha-defensins by intestinal Paneth cells in response to bacteria. *Nat Immunol*, **1**, 113–18.

Bach, A.C., Selsted, M.E. and Pardi, A. 1987. Two-dimensional NMR studies of the antimicrobial peptide NP-5. *Biochemistry*, **26**, 4389–97.

Baggiolini, M., Horisberger, U., et al. 1985. Identification of three types of granules in neutrophils of ruminants. Ultrastructure of circulating and maturing cells. *Lab Invest*, **52**, 151–8.

Bastian, A. and Schafer, H. 2001. Human alpha-defensin 1 (HNP-1) inhibits adenoviral infection in vitro. *Regul Pept*, **101**, 157–61.

Bateman, A., MacLeod, R.J., et al. 1996. The isolation and characterization of a novel corticostatin/defensin-like peptide from the kidney. *J Biol Chem*, **271**, 10654–9.

Bellm, L., Lehrer, R.I. and Ganz, T. 2000. Protegrins: new antibiotics of mammalian origin. *Expert Opin Invest Drugs*, **9**, 1731–42.

Boman, H.G. and Hultmark, D. 1987. Cell-free immunity in insects. *Annu Rev Microbiol*, **41**, 103–26.

Broekaert, W.F., Terras, F.R., et al. 1995. Plant defensins: novel antimicrobial peptides as components of the host defense system. *Plant Physiol*, **108**, 1353–8.

Brogden, K.A., Kalfa, V.C., et al. 2001. The ovine cathelicidin SMAP29 kills ovine respiratory pathogens in vitro and in an ovine model of pulmonary infection. *Antimicrob Agents Chemother*, **45**, 331–4.

Bulet, P., Hetru, C., et al. 1999. Antimicrobial peptides in insects; structure and function. *Dev Comp Immunol*, **23**, 329–44.

Bulow, E., Bengtsson, N., et al. 2002. Sorting of neutrophil-specific granule protein human cathelicidin, hCAP-18, when constitutively expressed in myeloid cells. *J Leukoc Biol*, **72**, 147–53.

Chan, Y.R. and Gallo, R.L. 1998. PR-39, a syndecan-inducing antimicrobial peptide, binds and affects p130(Cas). *J Biol Chem*, **273**, 28978–85.

Chertov, O., Michiel, D.F., et al. 1996. Identification of defensin-1, defensin-2 and CAP37/azurocidin as T-cell chemoattractant proteins released from interleukin-8-stimulated neutrophils. *J Biol Chem*, **271**, 2935–40.

Cole, A.M., Shi, J., et al. 2001. Inhibition of neutrophil elastase prevents cathelicidin activation and impairs clearance of bacteria from wounds. *Blood*, **97**, 297–304.

Cole, A.M., Hong, T., et al. 2002. Retrocyclin: a primate peptide that protects cells from infection by T- and M-tropic strains of HIV-1. *Proc Natl Acad Sci USA*, **99**, 1813–18.

Cornet, B., Bonmatin, J.M., et al. 1995. Refined three-dimensional solution structure of insect defensin A. *Structure*, **3**, 435–48.

Cowland, J.B. and Borregaard, N. 1999. The individual regulation of granule protein mRNA levels during neutrophil maturation explains the heterogeneity of neutrophil granules. *J Leukoc Biol*, **66**, 89–995.

Daher, K.A., Selsted, M.E. and Lehrer, R.I. 1986. Direct inactivation of viruses by human granulocyte defensins. *J Virol*, **60**, 1068–74.

Daher, K.A., Lehrer, R.I., et al. 1988. Isolation and characterization of human defensin cDNA clones. *Proc Natl Acad Sci USA*, **85**, 7327–31.

De, Y., Chen, Q., et al. 2000. LL-37, the neutrophil granule- and epithelial cell-derived cathelicidin, utilizes formyl peptide receptor-like 1 (FPRL1) as a receptor to chemoattract human peripheral blood neutrophils, monocytes and T cells. *J Exp Med*, **192**, 1069–74.

Diep, D.B. and Nes, I.F. 2002. Ribosomally synthesized antibacterial peptides in Gram positive bacteria. *Curr Drug Targets*, **3**, 107–22.

Dimarcq, J.L., Bulet, P., et al. 1998. Cysteine-rich antimicrobial peptides in invertebrates. *Biopolymers*, **47**, 465–77.

Duits, L.A., Rademaker, M., et al. 2001. Inhibition of hBD-3, but not hBD-1 and hBD-2, mRNA expression by corticosteroids. *Biochem Biophys Res Commun*, **280**, 522–5.

Eisenhauer, P.B., Harwig, S.S., et al. 1989. Purification and antimicrobial properties of three defensins from rat neutrophils. *Infect Immun*, **57**, 2021–7.

Eisenhauer, P., Harwig, S.S., et al. 1990. Polymorphic expression of defensins in neutrophils from outbred rats. *Infect Immun*, **58**, 3899–902.

Falla, T.J., Karunaratne, D.N. and Hancock, R.E. 1996. Mode of action of the antimicrobial peptide indolicidin. *J Biol Chem*, **271**, 19298–303.

Fant, F., Vranken, W., et al. 1998. Determination of the three-dimensional solution structure of *Raphanus sativus* antifungal protein 1 by 1H NMR. *J Mol Biol*, **279**, 257–70.

Frohlich, O., Po, C. and Young, L.G. 2001. Organization of the human gene encoding the epididymis-specific EP2 protein variants and its relationship to defensin genes. *Biol Reprod*, **64**, 1072–9.

Fromm, J.R., Hileman, R.E., et al. 1995. Differences in the interaction of heparin with arginine and lysine and the importance of these basic amino acids in the binding of heparin to acidic fibroblast growth factor. *Arch Biochem Biophys*, **323**, 279–87.

Frye, M., Bargon, J. and Gropp, R. 2001. Expression of human beta-defensin-1 promotes differentiation of keratinocytes. *J Mol Med*, **79**, 275–82.

Fujii, G., Selsted, M.E. and Eisenberg, D. 1993. Defensins promote fusion and lysis of negatively charged membranes. *Protein Sci*, **2**, 1301–12.

Gallo, R.L., Ono, M., et al. 1994. Syndecans, cell surface heparan sulfate proteoglycans, are induced by a proline-rich antimicrobial peptide from wounds. *Proc Natl Acad Sci USA*, **91**, 11035–9.

Ganz, T. 1987. Extracellular release of antimicrobial defensins by human polymorphonuclear leukocytes. *Infect Immun*, **55**, 568–71.

Ganz, T., Selsted, M.E., et al. 1985. Defensins. Natural peptide antibiotics of human neutrophils. *J Clin Invest*, **76**, 1427–35.

Ganz, T., Rayner, J.R., et al. 1989. The structure of the rabbit macrophage defensin genes and their organ-specific expression. *J Immunol*, **143**, 1358–65.

Garcia-Olmedo, F., Molina, A., et al. 1998. Plant defense peptides. *Biopolymers*, **47**, 479–91.

Gennaro, R. and Zanetti, M. 2000. Structural features and biological activities of the cathelicidin- derived antimicrobial peptides. *Biopolymers*, **55**, 31–49.

Gennaro, R., Dewald, B., et al. 1983. A novel type of cytoplasmic granule in bovine neutrophils. *J Cell Biol*, **96**, 1651–61.

Gera, J.F. and Lichtenstein, A. 1991. Human neutrophil peptide defensins induce single strand DNA breaks in target cells. *Cell Immunol*, **138**, 108–20.

Ghosh, D., Porter, E., et al. 2002. Paneth cell trypsin is the processing enzyme for human defensin-5. *Nat Immunol*, **3**, 583–90.

Groisman, E.A., Chiao, E., et al. 1989. *Salmonella typhimurium* phoP virulence gene is a transcriptional regulator. *Proc Natl Acad Sci USA*, **86**, 7077–81.

Groisman, E.A., Heffron, F. and Solomon, F. 1992. Molecular genetic analysis of the *Escherichia coli* phoP locus. *J Bacteriol*, **174**, 486–91.

Gropp, R., Frye, M., et al. 1999. Epithelial defensins impair adenoviral infection: implication for adenovirus-mediated gene therapy. *Hum Gene Ther*, **10**, 957–64.

Gudmundsson, G.H., Agerberth, B., et al. 1996. The human gene FALL39 and processing of the cathelin precursor to the antibacterial peptide LL-37 in granulocytes. *Eur J Biochem*, **238**, 325–32.

Guina, T., Yi, E.C., et al. 2000. A PhoP-regulated outer membrane protease of *Salmonella enterica* serovar *typhimurium* promotes resistance to alpha-helical antimicrobial peptides. *J Bacteriol*, **182**, 4077–86.

Guo, L., Lim, K.B., et al. 1998. Lipid A acylation and bacterial resistance against vertebrate antimicrobial peptides. *Cell*, **95**, 189–98.

Harder, J., Bartels, J., et al. 1997. A peptide antibiotic from human skin. *Nature*, **387**, 861.

Harder, J., Bartels, J., et al. 2001. Isolation and characterization of human beta-defensin-3, a novel human inducible peptide antibiotic. *J Biol Chem*, **276**, 5707–13.

Harwig, S.S., Park, A.S. and Lehrer, R.I. 1992. Characterization of defensin precursors in mature human neutrophils. *Blood*, **79**, 1532–7.

Harwig, S.S., Swiderek, K.M., et al. 1994. Gallinacins: cysteine-rich antimicrobial peptides of chicken leukocytes. *FEBS Lett*, **342**, 281–5.

Harwig, S.S., Kokryakov, V.N., et al. 1995. Prophenin-1, an exceptionally proline-rich antimicrobial peptide from porcine leukocytes. *FEBS Lett*, **362**, 65–9.

Hileman, R.E., Fromm, J.R., et al. 1998. Glycosaminoglycan-protein interactions: definition of consensus sites in glycosaminoglycan binding proteins. *Bioessays*, **20**, 156–67.

Hoffmann, J.A. and Reichhart, J.M. 2002. Drosophila innate immunity: an evolutionary perspective. *Nat Immunol*, **3**, 121–6.

Hoffmann, J.A., Reichhart, J.M. and Hetru, C. 1996. Innate immunity in higher insects. *Curr Opin Immunol*, **8**, 8–13.

Hoover, D.M., Rajashankar, K.R., et al. 2000. The structure of human beta-defensin-2 shows evidence of higher order oligomerization. *J Biol Chem*, **275**, 32911–18.

Huang, H.J., Ross, C.R. and Blecha, F. 1997. Chemoattractant properties of PR-39, a neutrophil antibacterial peptide. *J Leukoc Biol*, **61**, 624.

Huttner, K.M. and Bevins, C.L. 1999. Antimicrobial peptides as mediators of epithelial host defense. *Pediatr Res*, **45**, 785–94.

Islam, D., Bandholtz, L., et al. 2001. Downregulation of bactericidal peptides in enteric infections: a novel immune escape mechanism with bacterial DNA as a potential regulator. *Nat Med*, **7**, 180–5.

Jones, A.L., Beveridge, T.J. and Woods, D.E. 1996. Intracellular survival of *Burkholderia pseudomallei*. *Infect Immun*, **64**, 782–90.

Kagan, B.L., Selsted, M.E., et al. 1990. Antimicrobial defensin peptides form voltage-dependent ion-permeable channels in planar lipid bilayer membranes. *Proc Natl Acad Sci USA*, **87**, 210–14.

Kalfa, V.C., Jia, H.P., et al. 2001. Congeners of SMAP29 kill ovine pathogens and induce ultrastructural damage in bacterial cells. *Antimicrob Agents Chemother*, **45**, 3256–61.

Kogut, M.H., Tellez, G.I., et al. 1994. Heterophils are decisive components in the early responses of chickens to *Salmonella enteritidis* infections. *Microb Pathog*, **16**, 141–51.

Lawyer, C., Pai, S., et al. 1996. Antimicrobial activity of a 13 amino acid tryptophan-rich peptide derived from a putative porcine precursor protein of a novel family of antibacterial peptides. *FEBS Lett*, **390**, 95–8.

Lehrer, R.I., Selsted, M.E., et al. 1983. Antibacterial activity of microbicidal cationic proteins 1 and 2, natural peptide antibiotics of rabbit lung macrophages. *Infect Immun*, **42**, 10–14.

Lehrer, R.I., Daher, K., et al. 1985. Direct inactivation of viruses by MCP-1 and MCP-2, natural peptide antibiotics from rabbit leukocytes. *J Virol*, **54**, 467–72.

Lehrer, R.I., Ganz, T., et al. 1988. Modulation of the in vitro candidacidal activity of human neutrophil defensins by target cell metabolism and divalent cations. *J Clin Invest*, **81**, 1829–35.

Lehrer, R.I., Barton, A., et al. 1989. Interaction of human defensins with *Escherichia coli*. Mechanism of bactericidal activity. *J Clin Invest*, **84**, 553–61.

Leippe, M. 1999. Antimicrobial and cytolytic polypeptides of amoeboid protozoa-effector molecules of primitive phagocytes. *Dev Comp Immunol*, **23**, 267–79.

Lencer, W.I., Cheung, G., et al. 1997. Induction of epithelial chloride secretion by channel-forming cryptdins 2 and 3. *Proc Natl Acad Sci USA*, **94**, 8585–9.

Leonova, L., Kokryakov, V.N., et al. 2001. Circular minidefensins and posttranslational generation of molecular diversity. *J Leukoc Biol*, **70**, 461–4.

Lichtenstein, A. 1991. Mechanism of mammalian cell lysis mediated by peptide defensins. Evidence for an initial alteration of the plasma membrane. *J Clin Invest*, **88**, 93–100.

Lichtenstein, A., Ganz, T., et al. 1986. In vitro tumor cell cytolysis mediated by peptide defensins of human and rabbit granulocytes. *Blood*, **68**, 1407–10.

Lichtenstein, A.K., Ganz, T., et al. 1988. Mechanism of target cytolysis by peptide defensins. Target cell metabolic activities, possibly involving endocytosis, are crucial for expression of cytotoxicity. *J Immunol*, **140**, 2686–94.

Liu, A.Y., Destoumieux, D., et al. 2002. Human beta-defensin-2 production in keratinocytes is regulated by interleukin-1, bacteria, and the state of differentiation. *J Invest Dermatol*, **118**, 275–81.

Liu, L. and Ganz, T. 1995. The pro region of human neutrophil defensin contains a motif that is essential for normal subcellular sorting. *Blood*, **85**, 1095–103.

Liu, L., Zhao, C., et al. 1997. The human beta-defensin-1 and alpha-defensins are encoded by adjacent genes: two peptide families with differing disulfide topology share a common ancestry. *Genomics*, **43**, 316–20.

Liu, L., Wang, L., et al. 1998. Structure and mapping of the human beta-defensin HBD-2 gene and its expression at sites of inflammation. *Gene*, **222**, 237–44.

Liu, L., Roberts, A.A. and Ganz, T. 2003. By IL-1 signaling, monocyte-derived cells dramatically enhance the epidermal antimicrobial response to lipopolysaccharide. *J Immunol*, **170**, 575–80.

Lohner, K., Latal, A., et al. 1997. Differential scanning microcalorimetry indicates that human defensin, HNP-2, interacts specifically with biomembrane mimetic systems. *Biochemistry*, **36**, 1525–31.

MacLeod, R.J., Hamilton, J.R., et al. 1991. Corticostatic peptides cause nifedipine-sensitive volume reduction in jejunal villus enterocytes. *Proc Natl Acad Sci USA*, **88**, 552–6.

MacMicking, J., Xie, Q.W. and Nathan, C. 1997. Nitric oxide and macrophage function. *Annu Rev Immunol*, **15**, 323–50.

Malm, J., Sorensen, O., et al. 2000. The human cationic antimicrobial protein (hCAP-18) is expressed in the epithelium of human epididymis, is present in seminal plasma at high concentrations, and is attached to spermatozoa. *Infect Immun*, **68**, 4297–302.

Mars, W.M., Patmasiriwat, P., et al. 1995. Inheritance of unequal numbers of the genes encoding the human neutrophil defensins HP-1 and HP-3. *J Biol Chem*, **270**, 30371–6.

Martinez, D.T., Pizarro-Cerda, J., et al. 1995. The outer membranes of *Brucella* spp. are resistant to bactericidal cationic peptides. *Infect Immun*, **63**, 3054–61.

Merlin, D., Yue, G., et al. 2001. Cryptdin-3 induces novel apical conductance(s) in Cl- secretory, including cystic fibrosis, epithelia. *Am J Physiol Cell Physiol*, **280**, C296–302.

Michaelson, D., Rayner, J., et al. 1992. Cationic defensins arise from charge-neutralized propeptides: a mechanism for avoiding leukocyte autocytotoxicity? *J Leukoc Biol*, **51**, 634–9.

Miller, S.I. 1991. PhoP/PhoQ: macrophage-specific modulators of *Salmonella* virulence? *Mol Microbiol*, **5**, 2073–8.

Miller, S.I., Pulkkinen, W.S., et al. 1990. Characterization of defensin resistance phenotypes associated with mutations in the phoP virulence regulon of *Salmonella typhimurium*. *Infect Immun*, **58**, 3706–10.

Nakashima, H., Yamamoto, N., et al. 1993. Defensins inhibit HIV replication in vitro. *AIDS*, **7**, 1129.

Nizet, V., Ohtake, T., et al. 2001. Innate antimicrobial peptide protects the skin from invasive bacterial infection. *Nature*, **414**, 454–7.

O'Connor, E.M. and Shand, R.F. 2002. Halocins and sulfolobicins: the emerging story of archaeal protein and peptide antibiotics. *J Ind Microbiol Biotechnol*, **28**, 23–31.

Olsson, I. 1970. Mucopolysaccharide formation in granulocytes [in Norwegian]. *Nord Med*, **84**, 1567–8.

Ong, P.Y., Ohtake, T., et al. 2002. Endogenous antimicrobial peptides and skin infections in atopic dermatitis. *N Engl J Med*, **347**, 1151–60.

Oren, A., Ganz, T., et al. 2003. In human epidermis, beta-defensin 2 is packaged in lamellar bodies. *Exp Mol Pathol*, **74**, 180–2.

Ouellette, A.J., Greco, R.M., et al. 1989. Developmental regulation of cryptdin, a corticostatin/defensin precursor mRNA in mouse small intestinal crypt epithelium. *J Cell Biol*, **108**, 1687–95.

Pag, U. and Sahl, H.G. 2002. Multiple activities in lantibiotics – models for the design of novel antibiotics? *Curr Pharm Des*, **8**, 815–33.

Panyutich, A. and Ganz, T. 1991. Activated alpha 2-macroglobulin is a principal defensin-binding protein. *Am J Respir Cell Mol Biol*, **5**, 101–6.

Panyutich, A., Shi, J., et al. 1997. Porcine polymorphonuclear leukocytes generate extracellular microbicidal activity by elastase-mediated activation of secreted proprotegrins. *Infect Immun*, **65**, 978–5.

Pardi, A., Hare, D.R., et al. 1988. Solution structures of the rabbit neutrophil defensin NP-5. *J Mol Biol*, **201**, 625–36.

Pardi, A., Zhang, X.L., et al. 1992. NMR studies of defensin antimicrobial peptides. 2. Three-dimensional structures of rabbit NP-2 and human HNP-1. *Biochemistry*, **31**, 11357–64.

Patterson-Delafield, J., Martinez, R.J. and Lehrer, R.I. 1980. Microbicidal cationic proteins in rabbit alveolar macrophages: a potential host defense mechanism. *Infect Immun*, **30**, 180–92.

Patterson-Delafield, J., Szklarek, D., et al. 1981. Microbicidal cationic proteins of rabbit alveolar macrophages: amino acid composition and functional attributes. *Infect Immun*, **31**, 723–31.

Penniall, R. and Spitznagel, J.K. 1975. Chicken neutrophils: oxidative metabolism in phagocytic cells devoid of myeloperoxidase. *Proc Natl Acad Sci USA*, **72**, 5012–15.

Perregaux, D.G., Bhavsar, K., et al. 2002. Antimicrobial peptides initiate IL-1 beta posttranslational processing: a novel role beyond innate immunity. *J Immunol*, **168**, 3024–32.

Peschel, A., Otto, M., et al. 1999. Inactivation of the dlt operon in *Staphylococcus aureus* confers sensitivity to defensins, protegrins, and other antimicrobial peptides. *J Biol Chem*, **274**, 8405–10.

Peschel, A., Jack, R.W., et al. 2001. Staphylococcus aureus resistance to human defensins and evasion of neutrophil killing via the novel virulence factor MprF is based on modification of membrane lipids with l-lysine. *J Exp Med*, **193**, 1067–76.

Qu, X.D., Harwig, S.S., et al. 1996. Susceptibility of *Neisseria gonorrhoeae* to protegrins. *Infect Immun*, **64**, 1240–5.

Rausch, P.G. and Moore, T.G. 1975. Granule enzymes of polymorphonuclear neutrophils: A phylogenetic comparison. *Blood*, **46**, 913–19.

Ryan, L.K., Rhodes, J., et al. 1998. Expression of beta-defensin genes in bovine alveolar macrophages. *Infect Immun*, **66**, 878–81.

Sanchez, J., Hoh, F., et al. 2002a. Structure of the cathelicidin motif of protegrin-3 precursor. Structural insights into the activation mechanism of an antimicrobial protein. *Structure (Camb)*, **10**, 1363.

Sanchez, J.F., Wojcik, F., et al. 2002b. Overexpression and structural study of the cathelicidin motif of the protegrin-3 precursor. *Biochemistry*, **41**, 21–30.

Satoh, Y. 1988. Effect of live and heat-killed bacteria on the secretory activity of Paneth cells in germ-free mice. *Cell Tissue Res*, **251**, 87–93.

Satoh, Y., Ishikawa, K., et al. 1989. Effects of cholecystokinin and carbamylcholine on Paneth cell secretion in mice: a comparison with pancreatic acinar cells. *Anat Rec*, **225**, 124–32.

Sawai, M.V., Jia, H.P., et al. 2001. The NMR structure of human beta-defensin-2 reveals a novel alpha-helical segment. *Biochemistry*, **40**, 3810–16.

Schibli, D.J., Hwang, P.M. and Vogel, H.J. 1999. Structure of the antimicrobial peptide tritrpticin bound to micelles: a distinct membrane-bound peptide fold. *Biochemistry*, **38**, 16749–55.

Schibli, D.J., Hunter, H.N., et al. 2002. The solution structures of the human beta-defensins lead to a better understanding of the potent bactericidal activity of HBD3 against *Staphylococcus aureus*. *J Biol Chem*, **277**, 8279–89.

Schonwetter, B.S., Stolzenberg, E.D. and Zasloff, M.A. 1995. Epithelial antibiotics induced at sites of inflammation. *Science*, **267**, 1645–8.

Schutte, B.C., Mitros, J.P., et al. 2002. Discovery of five conserved beta-defensin gene clusters using a computational search strategy. *Proc Natl Acad Sci USA*, **99**, 2129–33.

Scocchi, M., Skerlavaj, B., et al. 1992. Proteolytic cleavage by neutrophil elastase converts inactive storage proforms to antibacterial bactenecins. *Eur J Biochem*, **209**, 589–95.

Scocchi, M., Wang, S. and Zanetti, M. 1997. Structural organization of the bovine cathelicidin gene family and identification of a novel member. *FEBS Lett*, **417**, 311–15.

Selsted, M.E. and Harwig, S.S. 1989. Determination of the disulfide array in the human defensin HNP-2. A covalently cyclized peptide. *J Biol Chem*, **264**, 4003–7.

Selsted, M.E., Brown, D.M., et al. 1983. Primary structures of MCP-1 and MCP-2, natural peptide antibiotics of rabbit lung macrophages. *J Biol Chem*, **258**, 14485–9.

Selsted, M.E., Szklarek, D. and Lehrer, R.I. 1984. Purification and antibacterial activity of antimicrobial peptides of rabbit granulocytes. *Infect Immun*, **45**, 150–4.

Selsted, M.E., Harwig, S.S., et al. 1985a. Primary structures of three human neutrophil defensins. *J Clin Invest*, **76**, 1436–9.

Selsted, M.E., Szklarek, D., et al. 1985b. Activity of rabbit leukocyte peptides against *Candida albicans*. *Infect Immun*, **49**, 202–6.

Selsted, M.E., Tang, Y.Q., et al. 1993. Purification, primary structures, and antibacterial activities of beta-defensins, a new family of antimicrobial peptides from bovine neutrophils. *J Biol Chem*, **268**, 6641–8.

Sethi, S. and Dikshit, M. 2000. Modulation of polymorphonuclear leukocytes function by nitric oxide. *Thromb Res*, **100**, 223–47.

Shafer, W.M., Qu, X., et al. 1998. Modulation of *Neisseria gonorrhoeae* susceptibility to vertebrate antibacterial peptides due to a member of the resistance/nodulation/division efflux pump family. *Proc Natl Acad Sci USA*, **95**, 1829–33.

Shi, J., Ross, C.R., et al. 1996. PR-39, a proline-rich antibacterial peptide that inhibits phagocyte NADPH oxidase activity by binding to Src homology 3 domains of p47 phox. *Proc Natl Acad Sci USA*, **93**, 6014–18.

Shi, J., Zhang, G., et al. 1999. Porcine epithelial beta-defensin 1 is expressed in the dorsal tongue at antimicrobial concentrations. *Infect Immun*, **67**, 3121–7.

Solomon, S., Hu, J., et al. 1991. Corticostatic peptides. *J Steroid Biochem Mol Biol*, **40**, 391–8.

Sorensen, O., Arnljots, K., et al. 1997. The human antibacterial cathelicidin, hCAP-18, is synthesized in myelocytes and metamyelocytes and localized to specific granules in neutrophils. *Blood*, **90**, 2796–803.

Sorensen, O.E., Follin, P., et al. 2001. Human cathelicidin, hCAP-18, is processed to the antimicrobial peptide LL-37 by extracellular cleavage with proteinase 3. *Blood*, **97**, 3951–9.

Sparkes, R.S., Kronenberg, M., et al. 1989. Assignment of defensin gene(s) to human chromosome 8p23. *Genomics*, **5**, 240–4.

Spicer, S.S., Staley, M.W., et al. 1967. Acid mucosubstance and basic protein in mouse Paneth cells. *J Histochem Cytochem*, **15**, 225–42.

Stabler, J.G., McCormick, T.W., et al. 1994. Avian heterophils and monocytes: phagocytic and bactericidal activities against *Salmonella enteritidis*. *Vet Microbiol*, **38**, 293–305.

Tang, Y.Q. and Selsted, M.E. 1993. Characterization of the disulfide motif in BNBD-12, an antimicrobial beta-defensin peptide from bovine neutrophils. *J Biol Chem*, **268**, 6649–53.

Tang, Y.Q., Yuan, J., et al. 1999. A cyclic antimicrobial peptide produced in primate leukocytes by the ligation of two truncated alpha-defensins. *Science*, **286**, 498–502.

Territo, M.C., Ganz, T., et al. 1989. Monocyte-chemotactic activity of defensins from human neutrophils. *J Clin Invest*, **84**, 2017–20.

Thomma, B.P., Cammue, B.P. and Thevissen, K. 2002. Plant defensins. *Planta*, **216**, 193–202.

Tominaga, T., Fukata, J., et al. 1990. Effects of corticostatin-I on rat adrenal cells in vitro. *J Endocrinol*, **125**, 287–92.

Tominaga, T., Fukata, J., et al. 1992. Distribution and characterization of immunoreactive corticostatin in the hypothalamic–pituitary–adrenal axis. *Endocrinology*, **130**, 1593–8.

Travis, S.M., Anderson, N.N., et al. 2000. Bactericidal activity of mammalian cathelicidin-derived peptides. *Infect Immun*, **68**, 2748–55.

Tzou, P., De Gregorio, E. and Lemaitre, B. 2002. How *Drosophila* combats microbial infection: a model to study innate immunity and host–pathogen interactions. *Curr Opin Microbiol*, **5**, 102–10.

Valore, E.V. and Ganz, T. 1992. Posttranslational processing of defensins in immature human myeloid cells. *Blood*, **79**, 1538–44.

Valore, E.V., Martin, E., et al. 1996. Intramolecular inhibition of human defensin HNP-1 by its propiece. *J Clin Invest*, **97**, 1624–9.

Valore, E.V., Park, C.H., et al. 1998. Human beta-defensin-1: an antimicrobial peptide of urogenital tissues. *J Clin Invest*, **101**, 1633–42.

von Horsten, H.H., Derr, P. and Kirchhoff, C. 2002. Novel antimicrobial peptide of human epididymal duct origin. *Biol Reprod*, **67**, 804–13.

Wang, Y., Griffiths, W.J., et al. 1999. Porcine pulmonary surfactant preparations contain the antibacterial peptide prophenin and a C-terminal 18-residue fragment thereof. *FEBS Lett*, **460**, 257–62.

Wetzel, B.K., Horn, R.G. and Spicer, S.S. 1967. Fine structural studies on the development of heterophil, eosinophil, and basophil granulocytes in rabbits. *Lab Invest*, **16**, 349–82.

Wientjes, F.B. and Segal, A.W. 1995. NADPH oxidase and the respiratory burst. *Semin Cell Biol*, **6**, 357–65.

Wimley, W.C., Selsted, M.E. and White, S.H. 1994. Interactions between human defensins and lipid bilayers: evidence for formation of multimeric pores. *Protein Sci*, **3**, 1362–73.

Wu, H., Zhang, G., et al. 2000. Regulation of cathelicidin gene expression: induction by lipopolysaccharide, interleukin-6, retinoic acid, and *Salmonella enterica* serovar *typhimurium* infection. *Infect Immun*, **68**, 5552–8.

Wu, H., Ross, C.R. and Blecha, F. 2002. Characterization of an upstream open reading frame in the 5′ untranslated region of PR-39, a cathelicidin antimicrobial peptide. *Mol Immunol*, **39**, 9–18.

Yamaguchi, Y., Nagase, T., et al. 2002. Identification of multiple novel epididymis-specific beta-defensin isoforms in humans and mice. *J Immunol*, **169**, 2516–23.

Yang, D., Chertov, O., et al. 1999. Beta-defensins: linking innate and adaptive immunity through dendritic and T cell CCR6. *Science*, **286**, 525–8.

Yang, D., Chen, Q., et al. 2000. Human neutrophil defensins selectively chemoattract naive T and immature dendritic cells. *J Leukoc Biol*, **68**, 9–14.

Yang, D., Chertov, O. and Oppenheim, J.J. 2001a. Participation of mammalian defensins and cathelicidins in anti-microbial immunity: receptors and activities of human defensins and cathelicidin (LL-37). *J Leukoc Biol*, **69**, 691–7.

Yang, D., Chertov, O. and Oppenheim, J.J. 2001b. The role of mammalian antimicrobial peptides and proteins in awakening of innate host defenses and adaptive immunity. *Cell Mol Life Sci*, **58**, 978–89.

Yount, N.Y., Wang, M.S., et al. 1995. Rat neutrophil defensins. Precursor structures and expression during neutrophilic myelopoiesis. *J Immunol*, **155**, 4476–84.

Zanetti, M., Del Sal, G., et al. 1993. The cDNA of the neutrophil antibiotic Bac5 predicts a pro-sequence homologous to a cysteine proteinase inhibitor that is common to other neutrophil antibiotics. *J Biol Chem*, **268**, 522–6.

Zanetti, M., Gennaro, R. and Romeo, D. 1995. Cathelicidins: a novel protein family with a common proregion and a variable C-terminal antimicrobial domain. *FEBS Lett*, **374**, 1–5.

Zanetti, M., Gennaro, R., et al. 2000. Structure and biology of cathelicidins. *Adv Exp Med Biol*, **479**, 203–18.

Zarember, K.A., Katz, S.S., et al. 2002. Host defense functions of proteolytically processed and parent (unprocessed) cathelicidins of rabbit granulocytes. *Infect Immun*, **70**, 569–76.

Zeya, H.I. and Spitznagel, J.K. 1966a. Cationic proteins of polymorphonuclear leukocyte lysosomes. I. Resolution of antibacterial and enzymatic activities. *J Bacteriol*, **91**, 750–4.

Zeya, H.I. and Spitznagel, J.K. 1966b. Cationic proteins of polymorphonuclear leukocyte lysosomes. II. Composition, properties, and mechanism of antibacterial action. *J Bacteriol*, **91**, 755–62.

Zhang, H., Porro, G., et al. 2001. Neutrophil defensins mediate acute inflammatory response and lung dysfunction in dose-related fashion. *Am J Physiol Lung Cell Mol Physiol*, **280**, L947–954.

Zhang, L., Yu, W., et al. 2002. Contribution of human alpha-defensin 1, 2, and 3 to the anti-HIV-1 activity of CD8 antiviral factor. *Science*, **298**, 995–1000.

Zhang, X.L., Selsted, M.E. and Pardi, A. 1992. NMR studies of defensin antimicrobial peptides. 1. Resonance assignment and secondary structure determination of rabbit NP-2 and human HNP-1. *Biochemistry*, **31**, 11348–56.

Zhao, C., Ganz, T. and Lehrer, R.I. 1995a. Structures of genes for two cathelin-associated antimicrobial peptides: prophenin-2 and PR-39. *FEBS Lett*, **376**, 130–4.

Zhao, C., Ganz, T. and Lehrer, R.I. 1995b. The structure of porcine protegrin genes. *FEBS Lett*, **368**, 197–202.

Zhao, C., Nguyen, T., et al. 2001a. RL-37, an alpha-helical antimicrobial peptide of the rhesus monkey. *Antimicrob Agents Chemother*, **45**, 2695–702.

Zhao, C., Nguyen, T., et al. 2001b. Gallinacin-3, an inducible epithelial beta-defensin in the chicken. *Infect Immun*, **69**, 2684–91.

Zhu, Q., Bateman, A., et al. 1989. Isolation and biological activity of corticostatic peptides (anti-ACTH). *Endocr Res*, **15**, 129–49.

Zimmermann, G.R., Legault, P., et al. 1995. Solution structure of bovine neutrophil beta-defensin-12: the peptide fold of the beta-defensins is identical to that of the classical defensins. *Biochemistry*, **34**, 13663–71.

11

Lipid mediators: leukotrienes, prostanoids and other lipids

CHARLES W. PARKER

The lipid mediators are a complex group of biologically active metabolites with diverse effects on cellular metabolism, which particularly target the immune system, airways, and microvasculature. Most of them are produced from arachidonate in response to an immunological or nonimmunological stimulus. They tend to have a short half-life and to act in a paracrine or autocrine fashion. Arachidonate metabolites are typically present as mixtures in areas of immunological inflammation. They vary considerably in their cell(s) of origin, time of appearance, susceptibility to inhibition by pharmacological agents, potency, stability, and biological action, frequently exhibiting antagonistic effects (Parker 1984). None of them is stored in significant quantities and they are primarily products of activated rather than resting cells. They represent an important group of regulatory or modulatory agents whose actions in the control of cellular function are still being unraveled. Although this chapter emphasizes their role in immunological inflammation, gene disruption studies indicate that arachidonate metabolites have functions in virtually every organ, tissue, and cell (Funk 2001).

ARACHIDONATE METABOLITES

Major pathways of arachidonate metabolism

Arachidonate is a C_{20} fatty acid with double bonds at 5–6, 8–9, 11–12, and 14–15 positions (numbering from the carboxyl end). The multiplicity of double bonds helps explain its versatility as a biosynthetic precursor. As discussed below, the two major routes of arachidonate metabolism are the lipoxygenase and cyclooxygenase pathways. Lipoxygenases in mammalian cells act primarily at the 5–6, 12–13, or 15–16 double bonds of arachidonate (termed 5-, 12-, and 15-lipoxygenases, respectively). The five lipoxygenases produce the 5-hydroperoxide eicosatetraenoate (5-HPETE) that is metabolized to the slow-reacting substances (LTC_4, LTD_4, and LTE_4) and LTB_4 (collectively termed 'leukotrienes') (Figure 11.1). Cyclooxygenases oxidize and cyclize arachidonate, producing the endoperoxides PGG_2 and PGH_2 which are metabolized to the D, E, and F prostaglandins (PGD_2, PGE_2, and PGF_2), prostacyclin (PGI_2), and thromboxane A_2 (TxA_2) (Figure 11.2). The term prostanoid is often used to describe the various cyclooxygenase products. As a result of the C_{20} fatty acid structure from which they are derived, the metabolites of arachidonate in the two pathways are collectively termed 'eicosanoids'.

Production of free arachidonate

Lipoxygenases and cyclooxygenases act largely or entirely on nonesterified arachidonate. As almost all of the arachidonate in cells is stored in ester linkage in phospholipids or triglycerides and much of the free arachidonate in the blood is bound to plasma proteins, esterified arachidonate must be released enzymatically at the time of cell activation. Recent evidence indicates

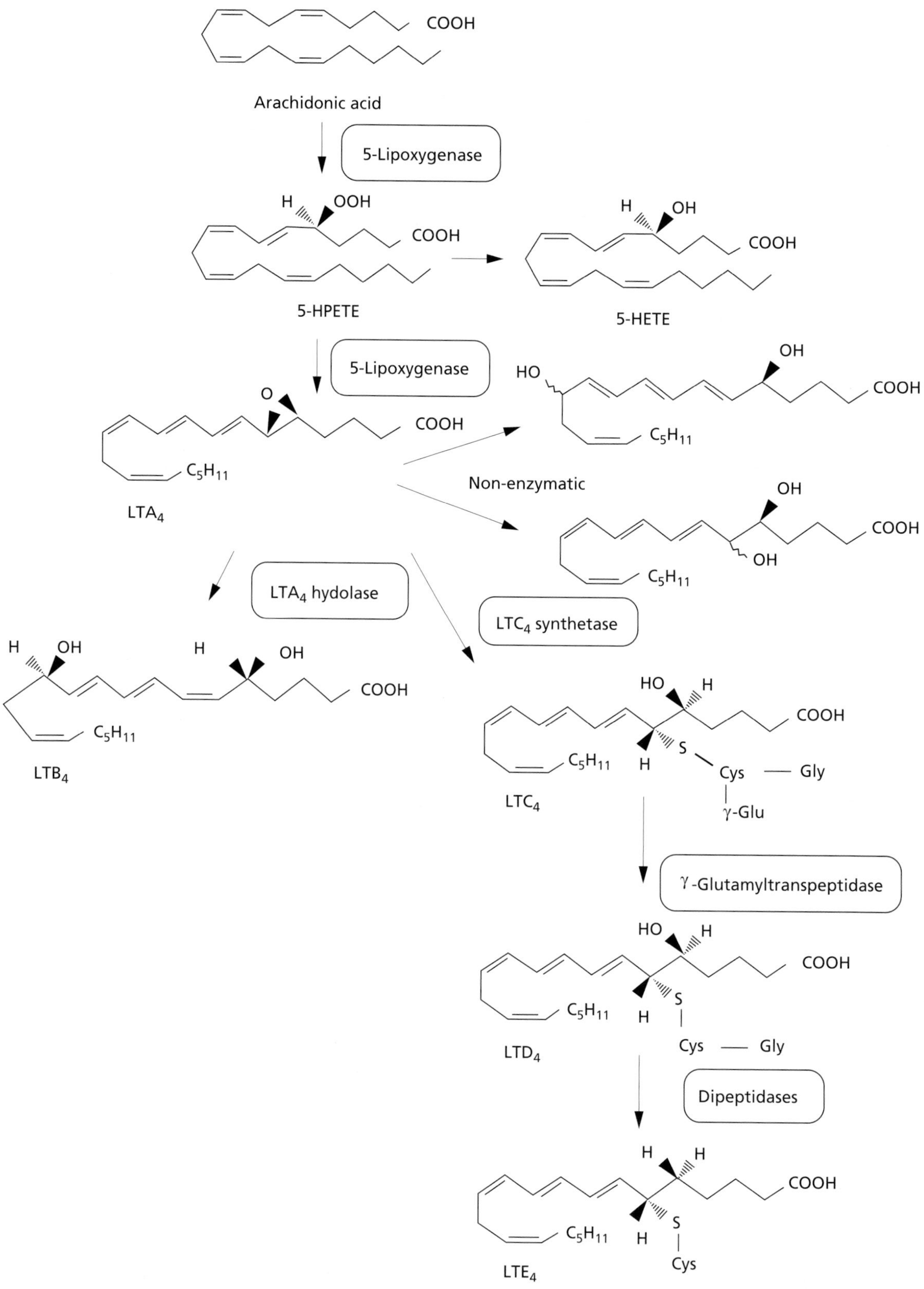

Figure 11.1 *Biosynthesis of leukotrienes. The enzymes involved are shown in boxes. HETE, hydroxyeicosatetraenoic acid; HPETE, hydroperoxide eicosatetraenoate; LT, leukotriene. (Redrawn from Figure 2, p. 5, of Nicosia et al. (2001) with the permission of the publisher Academic Press, Orlando, Florida.)*

that cytosolic phospholipase A_2 is an important enzyme in arachidonate release. Cells lacking this enzyme generally fail to produce eicosanoid metabolites (Funk 2001). Depending on the cell type, cell activation results in

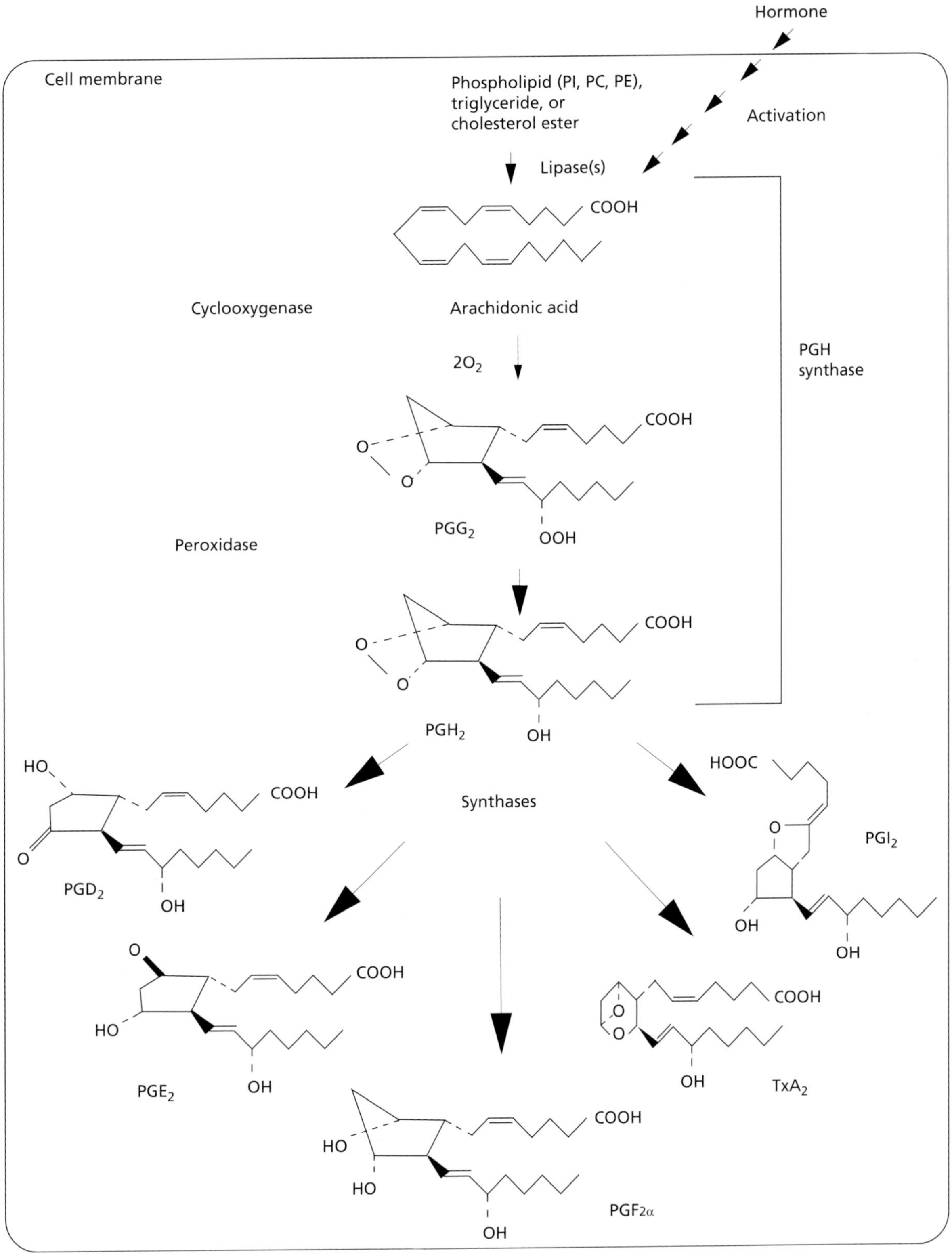

Figure 11.2 *Biosynthesis of prostanoids. The stimulus may be a hormone, antigen (antibody), or cytokine. Pg, prostaglandin; PGI_2, prostacyclin; TxA_2, thromboxane A_2. (Redrawn from Smith and Dewitt (1996), Figure 1, p. 168, with the permission of the publisher Academic Press, Orlando, Florida.)*

localization of this enzyme to the nuclear envelope, Golgi apparatus, or endoplasmic reticulum where it is thought to act locally to release arachidonate to nearby enzymes.

An important mechanism of glucocorticoid action is to inhibit phospholipase A_2 activity, decreasing the availability of free arachidonate, although eicosanoids vary with respect to their susceptibility to steroid inhibition of their biosynthesis (Bisgaard 2000).

Lipoxygenases

Lipoxygenases add molecular oxygen to *cis,cis*-1,4-pentadiene moieties on long chain fatty acids, converting them to hydroperoxides and producing a rearrangement of the double bonds (Galliard 1975). Under special circumstances, fatty acid esters and alcohols are also substrates for these enzymes. The initial enzyme involved in leukotriene biosynthesis is a 5-lipoxygenase (Borgeat and Samuelsson 1979; Jakschik et al. 1977; Parker 1984; Samuelsson et al. 1987). This enzyme is primarily seen in mast cells, macrophages, eosinophils, and polymorphonuclear leukocytes, although basophils, endothelial cells, and epithelial cells also have activity (Parker 1987). It converts arachidonate sequentially to 5-HPETE and the 5,6-epoxide, LTA_4; LTA_4 is in turn converted enzymatically or nonenzymatically to LTC_4 (which has a glutathionyl side chain in thioether linkage at C_6), LTB_4 (a particular 5,12-diHETE diastereoisomer) or other diHETEs (see Figure 11.1). 5-HETE is also formed, probably primarily from 5-HPETE. The relative proportion of products depends on the cell type. Neutrophils contain leukotriene A_4 hydrolase which hydrolyzes LTA_4 to LTB_4, an important product in leukotriene function (Funk 2001). Mast cells contain LTC_4 synthase, which catalyzes the conjugation of LTA_4 to glutathione; neutrophils lack this enzyme and therefore produce little or no LTC_4.

The lipoxygenases that have been carefully studied all contain at least one atom of nonheme iron per enzyme molecule and this is also true of 5-lipoxygenases (Funk 2001). Lipoxygenases are subject to autocatalysis and autoinhibition, probably both caused by peroxides. Lipoxygenase product formation is rapid for the first 5–10 min after cell activation and then stops almost completely, even in the presence of excess exogenous arachidonate. In macrophages pretreated with lipopolysaccharide (LPS), 5-lipoxygenase activity can be downregulated for many hours apparently as a result of induction of nitric oxide synthesis (Coffey et al. 2000). The 5-lipoxygenases that have been characterized are calcium-dependent enzymes with a monomeric molecular weight of about 80 000 (Samuelsson et al. 1987). They have a segment in the N-terminal region capable of binding two calcium ions (Hammarberg et al. 2000). In nonactivated cells, most of the enzyme is in the cytosol in an inactive form, although depending on the cell some of it may be in the nucleoplasm. When the cell is activated and Ca^{2+} enters the cell, cytosolic 5-lipoxygenase presumably binds some of the Ca^{2+} and localizes in the perinuclear membrane where it associates with an activating protein (FLAP) and assumes full activity (Peters-Golden and Brock 2001).

Slow-reacting substances (leukotrienes C, D, and E)

Once LTC_4 is formed it is metabolized by peptidases to LTD_4 (cysteinyl-glycyl leukotriene) and LTE_4 (cysteinyl leukotriene). Collectively LTC_4, LTD_4, and LTE_4 constitute the activity originally described as slow-reacting substance (SRS). SRS was first described in 1938 as an activity obtained from guinea-pig lungs perfused with cobra venom enzymes which produced a characteristic, slowly evolving contraction of isolated guinea-pig ileal smooth muscle (Feldberg and Kellaway 1938). It was later shown to be present in sensitized guinea-pig lungs perfused by antigen. Working with a line of rat basophilic leukemia cells (RBL-1) that contain IgE receptors, our laboratory identified SRS as a mixture of arachidonate metabolites produced through the 5-lipoxygenase pathway (Jakschik et al. 1977; Parker 1982). We later showed that each of the SRS species had a sulfur-containing side chain and identified two of the three side chains as glutathione and cysteine (reviewed in Parker 1982). We also reported that the immunologically and nonimmunologically induced forms of SRS were identical in structure (Watanabe and Parker 1980). Samuelsson and his colleagues placed the sulfur at the 6 position and determined the location of the double bonds (Murphy et al. 1979). Orning et al. (1980) and Morris et al. (1980) definitively identified the cysteinyl-glycyl form of the molecule, for which we had earlier obtained suggestive evidence. Proof of structure and assignment of double bond configuration of LTC_4 were obtained independently by Hammarstrom et al. (1979) and Rokasch et al. (1980) by organic synthesis.

Once LTC_4 is formed, it is rapidly released into the cell medium, where it is normally metabolized to LTD_4 and eventually to LTE_4 by enzymes present in plasma, leukocytes themselves, and tissues (reviewed in Parker 1984). Release into the medium apparently involves the multidrug resistance transporter protein (Qian et al. 2001). The conversion to LTD_4 can involve conventional γ-glutamyl transferases, although recent evidence also implicates a distinct protease with a similar action (Drazen 2000). Once formed, LTD_4 is less rapidly converted to LTE_4 by various dipeptidases. These conversions are associated with substantial changes in biological activity. In chopped lung fragments or isolated leukocytes suspended in medium without serum or plasma proteins, the conversion to LTD_4 is ordinarily well under way within the first 3–5 min and, by 15 min, LTD_4 is the predominant SRS species that is present (Parker 1984). LTE_4 is generally not the most prominent SRS species until after 30 min. The sulfoleukotrienes can also undergo double bond isomerization or oxidation of the sulfur, leading to changes in biological activity; SRS metabolites and SRS itself (particularly LTE_4) are excreted to a significant extent in the urine and bile in humans, and the levels of urinary LTE_4 correlate relatively well with disease activity in patients with asthma, especially if they are aspirin-sensitive (Bisgaard 2000; Nicosia et al. 2001).

The biological activity of SRS that has received most attention is its spasmogenic action on smooth muscle (reviewed in Parker 1983, 1984, 1987). Concentrations of LTD_4 as low as 0.1 pmol/ml produce readily detectable contractile responses on guinea-pig ileal and tracheal smooth muscle strips. On a molar basis, LTD_4 is about 60–100 times more active than histamine on the guinea-pig ileum. LTC_4 and LTE_4 are somewhat less active (by factors of 2 and 10, respectively, in the ileal system) but are still considerably more potent than histamine. In addition to its high potency, SRS produces an exceptionally sustained contractile response normally without tachyphylaxis, raising the possibility of a particularly prolonged action in vivo. Spasmogenic effects are produced on both the central and peripheral airways in humans and animals. LTC_4 and LTD_4 have been reported to constrict and dilate, respectively, cutaneous blood vessels, and decrease systemic blood pressure (Drazen et al. 1980). They also enhance cellular adherence, microvascular edema, mucus hypersecretion, and chemotaxis (especially of eosinophils) (James and Sampson 2001). The cysteinyl leukotrienes also promote granule enzyme release, although they are much less potent than LTB_4 in this regard (Goetzl 1980). Effects of leukotrienes (Öhd et al. 2000) and a 12-HPETE metabolite (Gu et al. 2001) on cell survival have also been described which is of interest with regard to the nuclear localization of active 5-lipoxygenase. The cysteinyl leukotrienes also exert a sustained effect on Purkinje nerve cell activity, which together with other evidence raises the possibility of important effects in the nervous system (Samuelsson et al. 1987).

Two types of receptors for cysteinyl leukotrienes have been identified and characterized: Cys LT1 and Cys LT2 (Drazen 2000; Maekawa et al. 2001). The Cys LT1 receptor is expressed in airway smooth muscle, macrophages, monocytes, eosinophils, and vascular endothelial cells. It has a higher affinity for LTD_4 than the other leukotrienes. The Cys LT2 receptor has an approximately equal affinity for LTD_4 and LTC_4. It is represented in peripheral blood leukocytes including eosinophils as well as in the lung, heart, adrenal medulla, and brain. Both types of receptors are members of the G-protein superfamily. The level of Cys LT1 receptor expression in human monocytes is upregulated by IL-4 and IL-13, suggesting a mechanism by which these cytokines might increase LTD_4 responsiveness and magnify the local response in IgE-mediated allergy (Thivierge et al. 2001).

There has been considerable activity in the pharmaceutical industry to develop drugs that prevent LTC_4 and LTD_4 formation or action. Both 5-lipoxygenase inhibitors and leukotriene LT1 receptor antagonists are now available for treatment of patients with respiratory allergy in Europe and the USA, and have been shown often to help relieve symptoms in chronic and acutely induced asthma (Nicosia et al. 2001). However, not all chronically asthmatic patients respond well and, as standard regimens not using these agents are often effective, more studies are needed for better definition of their precise role in treatment.

Dihydroxyeicosatetraenoic acids

LTB_4 is produced enzymatically from LTA_4 by a specific hydroxylating enzyme, although nonenzymatic hydrolysis may play a minor role (Samuelsson et al. 1987). When LTB_4 is purified from biological samples, several diastereoisomers of LTB_4 can be seen by high-pressure liquid chromatography or thin layer chromatography. These products appear to arise primarily by racemization of LTB_4 during purification. In general, the diastereoisomers are less active in biological systems than LTB_4 (Ford-Hutchinson et al. 1980).

As with cysteinyl leukotrienes, the major cell sources for LTB_4 in vitro are neutrophils, eosinophils, mast cells, monocytes, and basophils (Parker 1987; Nicosia et al. 2001), and the maximal response occurs within the first 5–10 min after cell activation. In neutrophils, much of the LTB_4 produced initially remains associated with the cells, but ultimately the bulk of the LTB_4 appears in the medium either as LTB_4 itself or as one of its metabolites (Stenson and Parker 1979). At 37°C human neutrophils rapidly metabolize LTB_4 to its 20-OH and 20-COOH derivatives, both of which are substantially less active in chemotaxis and granule enzyme release than LTB_4 itself.

LTB_4 stimulates chemokinesis in human neutrophils at concentrations of 1 nmol/ml or even lower (Ford-Hutchinson et al. 1980; Parker 1984), although substantially higher concentrations are required if plasma albumin, which binds LTB_4 is also present. The two major diastereoisomers of LTB_4 are considerably less active in this system. Although neutrophils are especially sensitive to LTB_4, cell movement is also stimulated in eosinophils, lymphocytes, and monocytes, indicating a general effect on leukocyte migration. LTB_4 also stimulates chemotaxis, although higher LTB_4 concentrations are needed (Goetzl 1980). At low nanomoles per milliliter concentrations LTB_4 also enhances lysosomal enzyme release from neutrophils, although as a rule this effect has required the concurrent presence of cytochalasins, casting some doubt on its physiological relevance. LTB_4 has little effect on vascular permeability but can enhance leukocyte adherence and emigration from the vasculature, resulting in part from upregulation of the expression of b_2-integrins (Wallace and Ma 2001).

Although early evidence indicated the presence of specific receptors for LTB_4 on human neutrophils (Kreisle and Parker 1983), it is only recently that the genes involved have been identified. There is a high-affinity receptor termed BLT1 on leukocytes which acts though G-coupled proteins to stimulate chemokinesis, chemotaxis, and granule secretion (Serhan and Prescott 2000). Another LTB receptor, BLT2, has a considerably lower affinity for LTB_4 but is much more widely distributed. Evidence for the importance of LTB_4 and the BLT1 receptor in in vitro models of inflammation has been obtained in genetically manipulated mice that overexpress or fail to express this receptor (Serhan and Prescott 2000). One of the effects of overexpression of the BLT1 receptor was enhanced leukotriene biosynthesis, consistent with other evidence that LTB_4 is primarily a proinflammatory mediator. Specific antagonists for these receptors are under development.

Monohydroxyeicosatetraenoic acids

5-Hydroxyeicosatetraenoic acid (5-HETE) is quantitatively the major 5-lipoxygenase product obtained from leukocytes and mast cells (Parker 1984; Stenson and Parker 1979). It is formed from 5-HPETE and LTA_4 by spontaneous or enzymatic reduction. Peroxidases appear to be the primary enzymes involved in the enzymatic reduction. The mono-HETEs are less potent than SRS and LTB_4 in their known biological activities. Nevertheless, 5-HETE, 5-HPETE, and to a lesser extent the other mono-HETEs have significant chemokinetic and granule enzyme-releasing activities (Goetzl 1980; Stenson and Parker 1980). Although low micromolar concentrations are required to produce these effects, it is possible that the mono-HETEs are primarily active in the cells in which they originate. In neutrophils 5-HETE alone induces the release of specific granule enzymes. In mast cells and basophils, 5-HETE enhances antigen-induced histamine release but is not active by itself. Although the mechanism of 5-HETE action is not known, it and other monohydroxyl C_{20} acids have the very interesting property of being incorporated covalently into phospholipids and triglycerides (Stenson and Parker 1979). Even though the extent of this incorporation appears to be quite limited, localization of 5-HETE containing phospholipids in critical areas of lipid membranes could have important effects on local membrane fluidity and function (Parker 1984).

Other lipoxygenases and their products

The lipoxins are eicosanoids produced primarily in leukocytes by the combined or sequential action of 15- and 5-lipoxygenases (Samuelsson et al. 1987; Levy et al. 2001); 15-lipoxygenase activation is induced as a delayed response in leukocytes during inflammatory responses, caused at least in part by exposure to PGE_2 generated locally during cell activation (Levy et al. 2001). Once 15-HPETE has been produced, it is further metabolized to lipoxins, a group of 5,15-dihydroxy fatty acids with at least one additional hydroxyl group attached to the fatty acid chain; lipoxin formation sometimes involves collaboration between nearby leukocytes containing different lipoxygenases. Similar to PGE_2, lipoxins have both pro- and anti-inflammatory actions. Levy et al. (2001) have emphasized the anti-inflammatory effects of lipoxins proposing that they act primarily in the later stages of inflammation to reduce leukocytic infiltration and function. This may occur in part through an ability of lipoxins to stimulate phagocytosis of apoptotic leukocytes, removing them from the local environment.

Cyclooxygenases

In the cyclooxygenase pathway, oxygen is added enzymatically to arachidonate to form an unstable endoperoxide, PGG_2, with a cyclopentane ring derived from carbons 8–12 and a hydroperoxy group at the 15 position (Moncada et al. 1980; Calder 2001). The hydroperoxy group is then reduced by the same enzyme, producing PGH_2. Cyclooxygenase is frequently abbreviated as COX or PGHS for PGH synthetase. COX activity requires the presence of molecular oxygen and is promoted by a prosthetic heme group bound tightly to the enzyme (Smith and Dewitt 1996). Although COX exists in cells in a proactive state, there appears to be a requirement for at least some peroxide for enzyme activity. As the lipoxygenase system generates hydroperoxy fatty acids, which may in turn be reduced by glutathione peroxidase and other peroxidases, both of these enzymes may indirectly affect COX activity. There are two major classes of COX enzymes: COX-1 and COX-2; COX-1 is primarily a constitutive enzyme broadly represented in organs and tissues (Gianoukakis et al. 2001). It is responsible for basal prostaglandin (PG) synthesis. COX-2 is usually induced by synthesis from scratch of the COX-2 protein by hormones, growth factors, and cytokines. Induction occurs in immunocytes during immunological activation and is the major source of the increase in PGE_2 that accompanies immunological inflammation (Calder 2001). The COX-1 and COX-2 proteins are encoded by two very similar but distinct genes. The crystal structures of the two enzymes are almost identical but a critical amino acid difference leads to a larger substrate-binding pocket in COX-2 (Funk 2001). The two enzymes appear to be primarily localized in the endoplasmic reticulum and nuclear envelope, respectively (Smith and Dewitt 1996; Funk 2001), which may have important functional implications (see below).

PGG_2 and PGH_2 have half-lives in aqueous solution of about 5 min. Depending on the cell or tissue, PGH_2 may be converted to a PG, TxA_2, or PGI_2 and sometimes a mixture of two or more of these products is formed (Kleeberger and Freed 2000). PGG_2 can be metabolized directly to PGD_2. Which of these products is made depends on the presence and level of activity of the appropriate enzyme systems (thromboxane synthetase, prostacyclin synthetase, 11-keto-isomerase, 9-keto-isomerase, and 9-keto-reductase) (reviewed in Parker 1984). In general, nonsteroidal anti-inflammatory agents such as aspirin and indometacin act primarily by blocking the COX, thereby reducing PGG_2 and PGH_2 formation. Therefore, they inhibit the synthesis of all of the eventual COX products. Nevertheless, the PG, TxA_2, and PGI_2 pathways are not necessarily inhibited equally. The degrees of inactivation depend in part on the relative K_ms of the individual enzymes involved in these subsequent metabolic conversions. Aspirin has a unique mechanism of action through acetylation of a critical serine residue on the enzyme. Most COX inhibitors act more or less equally on the COX-1 and COX-2 enzymes. Selective inhibitors of COX-2, rofecoxib (Vioxx) and celecoxib (Celebrex), are now in clinical use and still more selective inhibitors are under development (Funk 2001). The use of the selective COX-2 inhibitors reduces gastrointestinal side effects such as bleeding but the long-term advantages (and disadvantages) of such drugs are still not fully elucidated, particularly in individuals with other chronic diseases. None of the nonsteroidal anti-inflammatory agents can be regarded as completely specific for COX.

Prostaglandin metabolism and actions

The PGs are C_{20} fatty acids with a cyclopentane ring (see Figure 11.2). The E, F, and D PGs vary in the arrangement and type (hydroxy or keto and hydroxy) of substituents on the cyclopentane ring (Moncada et al. 1980). PG formation is associated with the loss of two double bonds, so prostaglandins derived from arachidonate have two remaining double bonds (e.g. PGE_2). PGH_2 is converted to PGD_2 and PGE_2 by a 11-keto-isomerase and 9-keto-isomerase, respectively. Both of these enzymes require glutathione. In addition to PGH_2, PGG_2 may be a substrate for 9-keto-isomerase. To a limited extent these conversions can be nonenzymatic because PGs can be formed by spontaneous breakdown of the endoperoxides. The existence of an isomerase for $PGF_{2\alpha}$ is doubtful. $PGF_{2\alpha}$ may be formed from PGE_2 by 9-keto-reductase or by direct reduction of PGH_2.

The PGs have long been known to affect blood vessel tone and promote smooth muscle contraction or relaxation, and they were originally postulated to be circulating hormones. However, it is now known that most of the PG in the circulation is rapidly metabolized, and it is generally agreed that PGs do not act as hormones affecting distant tissues (Moncada et al. 1980), except perhaps under exceptional circumstances. The major catabolic pathway for PG is by oxidation of the 15-OH group to the corresponding ketone by prostaglandin 15-OH-dehydrogenase (Kleeberger and Freed 2000). The 15-keto metabolite is then reduced to a 13,14-dihydro derivative. Subsequent metabolism is by β and terminal oxidation (Parker 1984). Enzymes that catalyze PG degradation are widely distributed in the body. One of the most active regions is the lung and, for example, more than 90 percent of infused PGE_2 is inactivated during a single passage through the lungs.

Leukocytes show marked differences in their abilities to produce PGs (Parker 1984; Kleeberger and Freed 2000; Funk 2001). Macrophages and monocytes make large amounts of PGE_2, substantial amounts of $PGF_{2\alpha}$, and very little or no PGD_2; neutrophils make moderate amounts of PGE_2 and little or no $PGF_{2\alpha}$ or PGD_2; mast cells make large amounts of PGD_2 and little or no $PGF_{2\alpha}$ or PGE_2. Resting lymphocytes or lymphocytic cell lines have been reported to make PGE_2 and less frequently to make $PGF_{2\alpha}$, but the amounts are quite small relative to monocytes and macrophages, and contamination of unstimulated lymphocyte preparations by monocytes may account for most or all of the PGs that are formed by these cells (Goldyne and Stobo 1979). However, when lymphocytes are stimulated by mitogens or appropriate cytokines, rapid induction of the COX-2 enzyme, with corresponding increases in PGE_2 production, may be seen, although the amounts of PGE_2 formed are not usually large. Originally TNF-α, IL-1, and IFN-γ were found to be stimulatory and IL-4, IL-10, and IL-13 inhibitory to enzyme induction (Berg et al. 2001). There is now evidence that IL-10 can be a potent inducer of COX-2 and PGE_2 production in LPS-stimulated mouse splenocytes. The induction is apparently produced indirectly through increases in cytokines that promote PGE_2 production. Surface stimuli including cytokines and antigens may also promote the production and release of PGs from monocytes and mast cells. As discussed below, the predominant effect of local increases in PGE_2 production may be to down-regulate ongoing immune responses.

One of the problems in interpretation of the data on PG formation has been the variation in results in different laboratories in the quantities or even the spectrum of arachidonate metabolites formed by a given cell type or mixture (Parker 1984). A study in human peripheral blood monocytes done many years ago (Bockman 1981) indicates that some of the discrepancies may involve differences in cellular sources and subsequent handling. The pattern of arachidonate metabolites formed by human peripheral blood monocytes cultured in vitro varied markedly with the duration of the culture following isolation of monocytes by cellular adherence. TxA_2 and PGEs were the major products on the first day of the culture. On the second day, PGEs were the major arachidonate metabolites and TxA_2 production was markedly diminished. Further changes in the spectrum of eicosanoids may be seen because monocytes continue to be maintained in tissue culture (Funk 2001).

Cellular differentiation, selective cell loss, restraints placed on the cells by the nutrient medium provided, and the accumulation of stimulatory and inhibitory cytokines may all affect arachidonate metabolite formation in this situation.

The biological effects of the PGs on immune function are quite diverse. PGE_2 is often the most active of the prostaglandins. In relatively high concentrations PGE_2 induces immature thymocytes and immature B lymphocytes to differentiate and acquire the functional, morphological, and immunological characteristics of mature lymphocytes (reviewed in Parker et al. 1974; Parker 1984), e.g. the addition of exogenous PGE_2 to thymocytes in vitro results in an increase in thymocyte cyclic adenosine monophosphate (cAMP) levels and thymocyte proliferation (Scheid et al. 1975). Other agents raising cAMP in these cells produce a similar response. PGE_2 affects erythropoiesis through direct effects on red cell precursors as well as by releasing erythropoietin from the kidney (Parker 1984). Some leukocyte precursors are not stimulated by PGE_2, e.g. macrophage colony formation is markedly inhibited. PGE_2 may also affect the differentiation of more mature cells, e.g. by the induction of collagenase secretion in apparently mature monocytes.

Once cells have matured, PGE_2 is primarily inhibitory exerting a variety of effects on leukocyte function, limiting inflammation (reviewed in Parker 1984; Calder 2001). PGE_2 has been reported to inhibit: (1) T- and B-cell proliferation; (2) leukocyte chemotaxis, chemokinesis, aggregation, spreading, phagocytosis, and oxidative metabolism; (3) cell-mediated cytotoxicity either by natural killer or cytotoxic T cells; (4) the release of inflammatory mediators from mast cells, basophils, eosinophils, and neutrophils; (5) production of cytokines, particularly IL-1, IL-2, IL-6, TNFα, and IFN-λ (Calder 2001) (although it has been suggested that PGs promote the T-helper (Th)2 cell pathway, in our laboratory PGE_2 and orally effective PGE_1 analogs are rapid and potent inhibitors of murine splenocyte IL-4 production, in vitro, apparently through a direct suppressive effect on IL-4 mRNA levels (Parker et al. 1995); and (6) inhibition of MHC antigen expression. Most of these effects are probably exerted directly on the responding cell preparations but indirect effects involving nearby cytokine producing cells undoubtedly also occur. While some of the inhibitory effects of PGE_2 require relatively high PGE_2 concentrations, others are produced at concentrations likely to be present at inflammatory sites in vivo. In a delicately regulated immune response, even relatively modest inhibitions may be significant, particularly if they are exerted selectively. In pharmacological concentrations in experimental animals, PGE and PGE analogs markedly suppress experimental inflammatory responses such as allograft rejection, immune complex glomerulonephritis, and the Arthus reaction (early work is reviewed in Stenson and Parker 1982). Orally effective PGE_1 analogs are being evaluated for their possible usefulness in a variety of therapeutic situations in humans.

Prostaglandins have proinflammatory as well as anti-inflammatory effects. Exogenously administered PGE_2 induces fever, erythema, increased vascular permeability, and vasodilatation (Moncada et al. 1980). PGE_2 is a very potent vasodilator. The dilatation is exerted throughout much of the microvascular bed. Although exogenously added PGs do not induce pain by themselves, they can markedly potentiate the pain and edema caused by bradykinin and histamine (Parker 1984). PGE_2 is found in increased quantities in inflammatory exudates at concentrations that can produce the classic signs of inflammation. Moreover, PGE_2 appears in experimentally induced inflammatory exudates over a time course consistent with its role as a mediator and PGE_2-binding proteins administered to arthritic joints have been shown to reduce local inflammation. A role for PGE_2 in arthritis seems particularly likely and this is supported by the widespread use of COX inhibitors in therapy in humans. PGs may also play a role in asthma and inflammatory bowel disease (Berg et al. 2001). $PGF_{2\alpha}$, 15-keto- $PGF_{2\alpha}$, and PGD_2 are potent constrictors of bronchial smooth muscle in humans and other animals (O'Byrne 1997). Subthreshold amounts of $PGF_{2\alpha}$ and PGD_2 increase overall airway reactivity. The bronchoconstriction involves both a direct effect on smooth muscle and an indirect effect through cholinergic pathways. PGE_2 and PGI_2 are bronchodilatory: PGE_2 may act in part by inhibiting the release of acetylcholine from airway cholinergic nerves.

By 2001 there were nine known PG receptor subtypes including four binding PGE_2 (EP_1–EP_4), two binding PGD_2 (DP_1 and DP_2), and one each binding $PGF_{2\alpha}$ (FP), PG_2 (IP), and TxA_2 (TP) (Funk 2001). All except DP_2 are members of the G-protein-coupled superfamily with seven transmembrane-spanning domains. Marked interspecies differences have been observed in the cellular distribution and function of some of these receptors (Kleeberger and Freed 2000). Most are located in the plasma membrane but several, including EP_1, are (or can be) in the nuclear envelope (Bhattacharya et al. 1998; Funk 2001). Selective effects involving individual PGE receptors have already been described, and it seems almost certain that the pattern will become more complex as studies continue. PGE_2 exerts most of its physiological effects through changes in intracellular cAMP. In many of the tissues or isolated cell systems in which it has been studied, PGE_2 stimulates adenylyl cyclase and increases intracellular cAMP concentrations. Many of its effects can be mimicked by cAMP agonists and analogs. However, effects through the EP_1 receptor apparently occur via increases in intracellular Ca^{2+} (Funk 2001) and stimulation through the EP_3 receptor is associated with decreases in cAMP. The F-type prostaglandins are generally less effective in raising cAMP than the PGEs and, in a few tissues, stimulate increases in cGMP instead of cAMP; PGI_2, TxA_2, PGH_2, and fatty acid hydroperoxides may also affect cAMP or cGMP levels (Parker 1984).

Changes in the level of expression or location of the prostanoid receptors with time during an immune response in conjunction with evolving patterns of eicosanoid biosynthesis could importantly alter cellular responsiveness. Although PGs are normally thought of as having primarily a paracrine function, the evidence that the COX-2 enzyme is mainly localized in the perinuclear membrane where PG receptors may also be present is of interest for a possible additional autocrine action of PGs in the nucleus, perhaps affecting cellular replication or differentiation (Smith and Dewitt 1996). In this connection, cAMP localization has been demonstrated in the nucleus of human lymphocytes both in adenylyl cyclase studies of isolated nuclei and by cAMP immunofluorescence (Wedner and Parker 1977). Although nuclear cAMP accumulation was not stimulated by PG, only PGE_1 was studied and PG receptors might have been lost during the procedure used for the isolation of nuclei.

Thromboxanes

Thromboxane A_2 is a chemically labile C_{20} fatty acid with a six-membered oxygen-containing ring originally characterized structurally in platelet supernatants by Hamberg and Samuellsson (1974). It is produced from PGH_2 by the enzyme thromboxane synthetase. Thromboxane synthetase also catalyzes the conversion of PGH_2 to 12-hydroxy-5, 8, 10-heptadecatraenoic acid (HHT), a C_{17} hydroxy fatty acid formed by splitting off C9, C10, and C11 of the cyclopentane ring. The two products, TxA_2 and HHT, are formed in comparable amounts; HHT is unique in that it is the only simple hydroxylated eicosanoid that is not a lipoxygenase product. TxA_2 has a half-life in aqueous solution of about 30 s, spontaneously degrading to thromboxane B_2 (TxB_2) by the addition of water. As a result of this lability, it is almost always TxB_2 that is measured when thromboxane metabolism is studied.

Apart from platelets, macrophages and monocytes are the major known biosynthetic sources of TxA_2 (O'Byrne 1997). Mast cells and lymphocytes are poor sources of TxA_2, neutrophils make moderate amounts and platelets can account for about 95 percent of thromboxane detected in serum (Wallace and Ma 2001).

Stable endoperoxides mimicking TxA_2 action, inhibitors of TxA_2 synthetases, and TxA_2 receptor antagonists are now available and have helped to elucidate thromboxane's role (O'Byrne 1997). TxA_2 is a very potent vasoconstrictor, particularly in the rabbit aorta, but is also very effective in constricting tracheal and bronchial smooth muscle and has vasoconstrictor activity throughout the vascular system. Roles in asthma and in early and late bronchial responses to antigen have been suggested, but there appear to be major species differences and the effects of TxA_2 inhibitors in these situations have not been dramatic; TxA_2 has been implicated in late cutaneous responses to antigen in human skin. The best-defined functional action of TxA_2 on circulating cells is its ability to promote platelet aggregation (Hamberg and Samuellsson 1974). It may also have a role in neutrophil adherence. Inhibitors of thromboxane synthesis have been reported to reduce lectin-induced mitogenesis in human T cells in an apparent relationship with their potency as thromboxane inhibitors, raising the possibility that the thromboxanes play a positive role in mitogenesis (Parker 1984), but there has been little recent interest in this possibility. In contrast to PGI_2 and PGE_2, TxA_2 lowers intracellular cAMP concentrations, at least in platelets.

Prostacyclin

Prostacyclin synthetase catalyzes the conversion of PGH_2 to PGI_2, which in turn spontaneously degrades to 6-keto-$PGF_{1\alpha}$ by the addition of water (Moncada et al. 1980). Its half-life in aqueous solution at 37°C and neutral pH is several minutes or less. There is an interesting interaction between the lipoxygenase and cyclooxygenase pathways in that prostacyclin synthetase is inhibited by the hydroperoxy intermediates of the lipoxygenase pathway (Stenson and Parker 1982).

Prostacyclin is formed in vascular endothelium, macrophages, and mast cells (Humes et al. 1977; Kleeberger and Freed 2000). PGI_2 and TxA_2 frequently have adversarial roles and the relative amounts of these two agents may serve as a normal physiological control mechanism. PGI_2 is a potent vasodilator and inhibitor of platelet aggregation and, given intravenously in small quantities, produces systemic hypotension. Levels of the prostacyclin metabolite, 6-keto- $PGF_{1\alpha}$, are elevated in the inflammatory exudates of chronic granulomas (Parker 1984). In addition to its potency as a vasodilator, PGI_2 increases vascular permeability directly and potentiates the increased vascular permeability induced by other inflammatory mediators. PGI_2 is also a potent inducer of pain. Most or all of PGI_2's effects on tissue and cells appear to be mediated through increases in cAMP.

OTHER LIPIDS WITH A KNOWN OR POSSIBLE SIGNALING ROLE

Isoprostanes

Isoprostanes are isomers of conventionally derived PGs, which are produced primarily by a free radical attack on esterified polysaturated fatty acids in cell membranes, especially arachidonate (Pratico et al. 2001). They are generated in situ under conditions of oxidant stress and then released, presumably by phospholipase. The F_2 isoprostanes (isomers of $PGF_{2\alpha}$, designated as F_2-iPs) have been the most frequently studied, but analogous isomers exist for other PGs and LTs. In addition to being markers for lipid peroxidation a number of the isoprostanes have reasonably potent biological activities, e.g. $iPF_{2\alpha}$ III produces bronchoconstriction, vasoconstriction, and platelet aggregation, apparently by stimulation of the TxA_2 receptor, at relatively low concentrations. The role of isoprostanes in inflammatory processes in vivo is still uncertain.

Lipid metabolites resembling eicosanoids

In general, LTs and PGs are produced predominantly from arachidonate. However, long-chain polyunsaturated fatty acids other than arachidonate also have to be considered as sources of biologically active lipids. They are present in cell membranes and may be substrates for enzymes in the various lipoxygenase and COX pathways, depending on their availability for rapid release as free fatty acids, structure (location of the double bonds, number of carbon atoms), and the capabilities of the individual enzymes. The resulting products are as a rule formed in relatively limited quantities. Moreover, they are altered in their double bond structure or number of carbons and tend to be less potent biologically than the usual LTs and PGs (Calder 2001). They may assume increased importance when the fatty acid content of cells has been manipulated in vivo by diet. Animals on diets rich in eicosapentaenoic, docosahexaenoic, oleic, or linoleic acids in general show less active responses in experimental models of inflammation than animals on the usual laboratory diets. Known or suspected mechanisms include decreases in the arachidonate content of cells that reduce its availability as a substrate, competitive inhibition of arachidonate-metabolizing enzymes by nonarachidonate fatty acids and their metabolites, and possible effects through alterations in cellular function, which may include changes in enzyme or receptor expression directly affecting eicosanoid metabolism or action. A considerable literature already exists on the possible usefulness of such diets in treating immunological diseases in humans.

Platelet-activating factor

Platelet-activating factor (PAF) is a family of structurally closely related, chemically stable neutral lipids containing a glyceryl core, a phosphorylcholine head group at the 3 position, one of several long-chain alkyl ethers (especially hexadecyl or octadecyl) at the 1 position, and an esterified acetyl group at the 2 position (Pinckard et al. 1982). 1-Alkyl,2-acyl-phosphatidylcholines, in which the acyl group is oxidatively fragmented, may also have PAF-like activity (Prescott et al. 2000). Studies of the aggregation response of rabbit platelets with analogs of PAF indicate that all three of the groups attached to the glyceryl backbone are important for its aggregating activity (Demopoulos et al. 1979). Replacement of the alkyl group at the 1 position by a carboxylic acid ester of the same chain length results in a 250-fold decrease in activity. The naturally occurring analog of PAF with a 16:0 alkyl group has about five times the activity of 18:0 alkyl-PAF. Replacement of the 2-acetyl group with butyryl reduces activity about 10-fold, whereas lyso-PAF has no activity even at very high concentrations. Removal of the choline or phosphorylcholine group results in a decrease in activity of more than 1000-fold.

Platelet-activating factor is not prestored. There are two known pathways of PAF biosynthesis. One is a pathway from scratch in which the final step is the addition phosphorylcholine to 1-alkyl,2-acetyl-glycerol (Watson and Snapper 1997). Such synthesis can account for most of the low-grade constitutive synthesis of PAF that is seen in some tissues. In the second, generally more important remodeling pathway, preexisting 1-alkyl,2-acyl-phosphatidylcholine is deacylated at the 2 position to form the corresponding lysophosphatidylcholine (or lyso-PAF) which in turn is acetylated by an acetyl-CoA-lyso-PAF-acetyl transferase to form PAF. The remodeling pathway predominates when PAF is generated in response to an acute or chronic cellular stimulus. As with the eicosanoids, cytosolic phospholipase A_2, which preferably acts on *sn*-2-arachidonyl residues in phospholipids, plays a key role (Prescott et al. 2000). Thus eicosanoid and PAF biosynthesis tend to occur together.

Production of PAF in response to cellular stimuli occurs rapidly, with significant activity usually being generated in less than a minute. Originally PAF action was thought to require its release from cells. Although activity does appear in the medium of cells stimulated in vitro and the free PAF is active, the extent of this release varies with the cell type. Vascular endothelial cells retain most of their PAF activity on their surfaces (Prescott et al. 2000). In this position the PAF interacts with PAF receptors on nearby intraluminal leukocytes, resulting in their immobilization and metabolic activation. P-selectin participates importantly in the immobilization process. PAF production tends to fall off rapidly, probably resulting in part from limitations in alkylphospholipid precursor availability, which varies considerably in different tissues. Once formed the PAF is rapidly degraded, much of it within a few minutes. The major mechanism for inactivation both inside and outside the cell is enzymatic deacetylation. Extracellular PAF acetyl hydrolases are present primarily in the lipoprotein fractions of human and animal plasma (Pinckard et al.

1982). At least three isoforms of the enzyme exist intracellularly (Prescott et al. 2000) and all forms of the enzyme are serine proteases inactivated by diisopropylfluorophosphate. As PAF production falls off rapidly with time, PAF is quickly degraded and receptor desensitization tends to occur rapidly, PAF actions typically are brief. However, in ongoing inflammatory responses in vivo newly arrived cells may help continue the response.

Platelet-activating factor is produced in many different cell types and tissues, usually in response to an immunological or nonimmunological stimulus. Immunological stimuli producing PAF include antigen and antibody, cytokines, and other mediators. Immunocytes including monocytes, macrophages, neutrophils, basophils, and eosinophils (Watson and Snapper 1997) are significant sources with small amounts being made by lymphocytes, mast cells, and platelets. Vascular endothelial cells are an important site of PAF production. The best-characterized effects of PAF (and stable PAF-like agonists) are on vascular reactivity and inflammation (Watson and Snapper 1997; Prescott et al. 2000; Wallace and Ma 2001). PAF stimulates: (1) platelet aggregation; (2) leukocyte aggregation, chemotaxis, and secretion; (3) airway and intestinal smooth muscle contraction; and (4) microvascular leakage and spasm. PAF may also induce the production of more effective action by other mediators and cytokines. There is substantial species variation in PAF actions. Aggregation responses of rabbit platelets and neutrophils occur at subnanomolar concentrations of PAF but human platelets are considerably less susceptible. The rapid intravenous infusion of as little as 2.5 μg of PAF in adult rabbits results in the almost immediate induction of marked neutropenia, thrombocytopenia, hypotension, and respiratory obstruction, culminating in respiratory arrest and death within minutes (McManus et al. 1980). At lower, nonfatal doses of PAF, the decreases in circulating platelets and neutrophils are reversible but animals show aggregates of platelets and neutrophils in pulmonary vessels and pulmonary arterial hypertension. Similar changes occur in sensitized rabbits undergoing fatal or nonfatal systemic anaphylaxis. Most of the effects of systemically injected PAF in experimental animals probably do not involve mechanical obstruction as such. In addition to direct effects on vessel walls by PAF, PAF may in part act by stimulating the secretion of TxA_2 and LTs (Pinckard et al. 1982) by platelets and leukocytes. The bronchoconstrictor effects of aerosolized PAF also appear to have complex mechanisms. PAF may have physiologically significant actions on cutaneous vascular reactivity. On a molar basis PAF is 10–1000 times more potent than histamine in producing acute weal-and-flare reactions in human and animal skin. Important actions outside the immune system in the brain and elsewhere are also suspected (Prescott et al. 2000).

The PAF receptor is a G-linked protein that is expressed on the surfaces on a variety of cell types (Prescott et al. 2000) and the receptor has a number of conformational states with various affinities. Most of the available PAF antagonists act by reversibly competing with PAF for the receptor. They include products present in Chinese herbal medicines that have long been used in the treatment of asthma (Watson and Snapper 1997). Despite evidence that PAF may participate in the pathogenesis of asthma, used by themselves, PAF antagonists have not been shown to be consistently helpful in the treatment of asthma.

Despite its potency and diverse actions PAF is produced in association with other mediators and is rapidly metabolized, complicating studies of its role in vivo; however, studies on genetically manipulated animals with increased or absent PAF receptor expression, or impaired PAF degradation, are now available (Prescott et al. 2000). Taken together with pharmacological studies with PAF receptor antagonists and inhibitors of PAF synthesis, they indicate that the PAF system is probably not normally essential for physiological well-being. However, PAF clearly can have substantial modulating roles affecting airway reactivity, anaphylaxis, endotoxemia, and local inflammation. Not enough is known about the role of PAF in local resistance to serious acute and chronic infections. Excess PAF activity is a potential problem and humans with defective PAF catabolism appear to be at increased risk for severe asthma and neonatal necrotizing enterocolitis.

REFERENCES

Berg, D.J., Zhang, J., et al. 2001. IL-10 Is a central regulator of cyclooxygenase-2 expression and prostaglandin production. *J Immunol*, **166**, 2674–80.

Bhattacharya, M., Peri, K.G., et al. 1998. Nuclear localization of prostaglandin E_2 receptors. *Proc Natl Acad Sci USA*, **95**, 15792–7.

Bisgaard, H. 2000. Role of leukotrienes in asthma pathophysiology. *Pediatr Pulmonol*, **30**, 166–76.

Bockman, R.S. 1981. Prostaglandin production by human blood monocytes and mouse peritoneal macrophages: Synthesis dependent on in vitro culture condition. *Prostaglandins*, **21**, 9–30.

Borgeat, P. and Samuelsson, B. 1979. Arachidonic acid metabolism in polymorphonuclear leukocytes: Effects of ionophore A23187. *Proc Natl Acad Sci USA*, **76**, 2148–52.

Calder, P.C. 2001. Polyunsaturated fatty acids, inflammation, and immunity. *Lipids*, **36**, 1007–24.

Coffey, M.J., Phare, S.M. and Peters-Golden, M. 2000. Prolonged exposure to lipopolysaccharide inhibits macrophage 5-lipoxygenase metabolism via induction of nitric oxide synthesis. *J Immunol*, **165**, 3592–8.

Demopoulos, C.A., Pinckard, R.N. and Hanahan, D.J. 1979. Platelet-activating factor. Evidence for 1-O-alkyl-2-acetyl-sn-glyceryl-3-phosphorylcholine as the active component (A new class of lipid chemical mediators). *J Biol Chem*, **254**, 9355–8.

Drazen, J.M. 2000. Leukotrienes. In: Busse, W.W. and Holgate, S.T. (eds), *Asthma and rhinitis*, Vol. 1. . Oxford: Blackwell Science, 1014–25.

Drazen, J.M., Austen, K.F., et al. 1980. Comparative airway and vascular activities of leukotrienes C-1 and D in vivo and in vitro. *Proc Natl Acad Sci USA*, **77**, 4354–8.

Feldberg, W. and Kellaway, C.H. 1938. Liberation of histamine and formation of lysocithin-like substance by cobra venom. *J Physiol*, **94**, 187–226.

Ford-Hutchinson, A.W., Bray, M.A., et al. 1980. Leukotriene B: A potent chemokinetic and aggregating substance released from polymorphonuclear leukocytes. *Nature*, **286**, 264–5.

Funk, C.D. 2001. Prostaglandins and leukotrienes: Advances in eicosanoid biology. *Science*, **294**, 1871–5.

Galliard, T. 1975. Degradation of plant lipids. In: Stumps, P.K. and Conn, E.E. (eds), *Biochemistry of plants*. New York: Academic Press, 335–57.

Gianoukakis, A.G., Cao, J.H., et al. 2001. Prostaglandin endoperoxide H synthase expression in human thyroid epithelial cells. *Am J Physiol Cell Physiol*, **280**, C701–708.

Goetzl, E.J. 1980. Mediators of immune hypersensitivity derived from arachidonic acid. *N Engl J Med*, **303**, 822–5.

Goldyne, M.E. and Stobo, J.D. 1979. Synthesis of prostaglandins by subpopulations of human peripheral blood monocytes. *Prostaglandins*, **18**, 687–95.

Gu, J., Liu, Y., et al. 2001. Evidence that increased 12-lipoxygenase activity induces apoptosis in fibroblasts. *J Cell Physiol*, **186**, 357–65.

Hamberg, M. and Samuellson, B. 1974. Prostaglandin endoperoxides. Novel transformation of arachidonic acid in human platelets. *Proc Natl Acad Sci USA*, **71**, 3400–4.

Hammarberg, T., Provost, P., et al. 2000. The N-terminal domain of 5-lipoxygenase binds calcium and mediates calcium stimulation of enzyme activity. *J Biol Chem*, **275**, 38787–93.

Hammarstrom, S., Murphy, R.C., et al. 1979. Structure of leukotriene C. Identification of the amino acid part. *Biochem Biophys Res Commun*, **91**, 1266–72.

Humes, J.L., Bonney, H.J., et al. 1977. Macrophage synthesis and release of prostaglandins in response to inflammatory stimuli. *Nature*, **269**, 149–51.

Jakschik, B.A., Falkenhein, S. and Parker, C.W. 1977. Precursor role of arachidonic acid in slow-reacting substance from rat basophilic leukemia cells. *Proc Natl Acad Sci USA*, **74**, 4577–81.

James, A.J. and Sampson, A.P. 2001. A tale of two CysLTs. *Clin Exp Allergy*, **31**, 1660–4.

Kleeberger, S.R. and Freed, A.N. 2000. Prostanoids. In: Busse, W.W. and Holgate, S.T. (eds), *Asthma and rhinitis*, Vol. 1. . Oxford: Blackwell Science, 999–1013.

Kreisle, R.A. and Parker, C.W. 1983. Specific binding of leukotriene B_4 to a receptor on human polymorphonuclear leukocytes. *J Exp Med*, **157**, 628–41.

Levy, B.D., Clish, C.B., et al. 2001. Lipid mediator class switching during acute inflammation: signals in resolution. *Nat Immunol*, **2**, 612–19.

McManus, L.H., Hanahan, D.J., et al. 1980. Pathobiology of the intravenous infusion of acetyl glyceryl ether phosphorycholine (AGEPC), a synthetic platelet-activating factor (PAF) in the rabbit. *J Immunol*, **124**, 2919–24.

Maekawa, A., Kanaoka, Y., et al. 2001. Identification in mice of two isoforms of the cysteinyl leukotriene 1 receptor that result from alternative splicing. *Proc Natl Acad Sci USA*, **98**, 2256–61.

Moncada, S., Flower, R.J. and Vane, J.R. 1980. Prostaglandins, prostacyclin and thromboxane A_2. In: Goodman, L.S. and Gilman, A. (eds), *The pharmacological basis of therapeutics*. New York: Macmillan Publishing Co., Inc, 668–81.

Morris, H.R., Taylor, G.W. and Piper, P.J. 1980. Slow-reacting substances (SRSs) from rat basophil leukemia (RBL-1) cells. *Prostaglandins*, **19**, 185–201.

Murphy, R.C., Hammarstrom, S. and Samuelsson, B. 1979. Leukotriene C: A slow-reacting substance from murine mastocytoma cells. *Proc Natl Acad Sci USA*, **76**, 4275–9.

Nicosia, S., Capra, V. and Rovati, G.E. 2001. Leukotrienes as mediators of asthma. *Pulm Pharmacol Therapeut*, **14**, 3–19.

O'Byrne, P.M. 1997. Cyclooxygenase products. In: Barnes, P.J., Grunstein, M.M., Leff, A.R. and Woolcock, A.J. (eds), *Asthma*, Vol. 1. . Lippincott-Raven: Philadelphia, 559–66.

Öhd, J.F., Wikström, K. and Sjölander, A. 2000. Leukotrienes induce cell-survival signaling in intestinal epithelial cells. *Gastroenterology*, **119**, 1007–16.

Orning, L., Hammarstrom, S. and Samuelsson, B. 1980. Leukotriene D: A slow reacting substance from rat basophilic leukemia cells. *Proc Natl Acad Sci USA*, **77**, 2012–17.

Parker, C.W. 1982. The chemical nature of slow-reacting substances. In: Weissman, G. (ed.), *Advances in inflammation research*. New York: Raven Press, 1–24.

Parker, C.W. 1983. Immunopharmacology of slow reacting substances. In: Newball, H.H. (ed.), *Immunopharmacology of the lung*. New York: Marcel Dekker, Inc., 25–53.

Parker, C.W. 1984. Mediators: Release and function. In: Paul, W.E. (ed.), *Fundamental immunology*. New York: Raven Press, 697–747.

Parker, C.W. 1987. 5-Lipoxygenase, leukotrienes, and regulation of inflammatory responses. *Drug Dev Res*, **10**, 277–93.

Parker, C.W., Sullivan, T.J. and Wedner, H.J. 1974. Cyclic AMP and the immune response. In: Robinson, G.A. and Greengard, P. (eds), *Advances in cyclic nucleotide research*, Vol. 4. . New York: Raven Press, 1–79.

Parker, C.W., Huber, M.G. and Godt, S.M. 1995. Modulation of IL-4 production in murine spleen cells by prostaglandins. *Cell Immunol*, **160**, 278–85.

Peters-Golden, M. and Brock, T.G. 2001. Intracellular compartmentalization of leukotriene synthesis: unexpected nuclear secrets. *FEBS Lett*, **487**, 323–6.

Pinckard, R.N., McManus, L.M. and Hanahan, D.J. 1982. Chemistry and biology of acetyl glyceryl ether phosphorylcholine. In: Weissman, G. (ed.), *Advances in inflammation research*, Vol. 4. . New York: Raven Press, 147–80.

Pratico, D., Lawson, J.A., et al. 2001. The isoprostanes in biology and medicine. *Trends Endocrinol Metab*, **12**, 243–7.

Prescott, S.M., Zimmerman, G.A., et al. 2000. Platelet-activating factor and related lipid mediators. *Annu Rev Biochem*, **69**, 419–45.

Qian, Y.-M., Mian, G., et al. 2001. Characterization of binding of leukotriene C_4 by human multidrug resistance protein 1. *J Biol Chem*, **276**, 38636–44.

Rokasch, J., Girard, Y. and Guindon, Y. 1980. The synthesis of a leukotriene with SRS-like activity. *Tetrahedron Lett*, **21**, 1485–8.

Samuelsson, B., Dahlen, S.-E., et al. 1987. Leukotrienes and lipoxins: structures, biosynthesis, and biological effects. *Science*, **237**, 1171–6.

Scheid, M.P., Goldstein, G., et al. 1975. Lymphocyte differentiation from precursor cells in vitro. *Ann NY Acad Sci*, **249**, 531–40.

Serhan, C.N. and Prescott, S.M. 2000. The scent of a phagocyte, advances on leukotriene B receptors. *J Exp Med*, **192**, F5–8.

Smith, W.L. and Dewitt, D.L. 1996. Prostaglandin endoperoxide H synthases-1 and 2. *Adv Immunol*, **62**, 167–215.

Stenson, W.F. and Parker, C.W. 1979. Metabolism of arachidonic acid in ionophore-stimulated neutrophils. *J Clin Invest*, **64**, 1457–65.

Stenson, W. and Parker, C.W. 1980. Monohydroxyeicosatetraenoic acid ($HETE_s$) induce degranulation of human neutrophils. *J Immunol*, **124**, 2100–4.

Stenson, W.F. and Parker, C.W. 1982. Prostaglandins. In: Sirois, P. and Rola-Pleszczynski, M. (eds), *Immunopharmacology*. Amsterdam: Elsevier/North Holland, 75–112.

Thivierge, M., Stankova, J. and Rola-Pleszczynski, M. 2001. IL-13 and IL-4 Up-regulate cysteinyl leukotriene 1 receptor expression in human monocytes and macrophages. *J Immunol*, **167**, 2855–60.

Wallace, J.L. and Ma, L. 2001. Inflammatory mediators in gastrointestinal defense and injury. *Exp Biol Med*, **226**, 1003–15.

Watanabe, S. and Parker, C.W. 1980. Role of arachidonic acid in the biosynthesis of slow-reacting substance of anaphylaxis (SRS-A) from sensitized guinea pig lung fragments. Evidence that SRS-A is very similar or identical structurally to nonimmunologically induced forms of SRS. *J Immunol*, **125**, 946–55.

Watson, P.L. and Snapper, J.R. 1997. Platelet-activating factor and its implications. In: Barnes, P.J., Grunstein, M.M., et al. (eds), *Asthma*. Vol. 1. Philadelphia: Lippincott-Raven, 567–75.

Wedner, J.H. and Parker, C.W. 1977. Adenylate cyclase activity in lymphocyte subcellular fractions. *Biochem J*, **162**, 483–91.

12

The acute phase response

JOHN G. RAYNES

INTRODUCTION

In this chapter the aim is to explain the changes that occur as a local inflammatory response becomes sufficiently strong to start causing systemic changes. The term 'acute phase response' is frequently used to encompass all the changes that occur in different organs when inflammation becomes systemic, indeed some of the most common manifestations of severe illness are components of the acute phase response. Fever, somnolence, and confusion represent some of the behavioral or physiological changes that are easily observed, whereas analysis of the biochemical, immunological, or metabolic alterations has demonstrated an array of changes that take place.

The acute phase response (APR) is a conserved response and it is rare to find individual patients who have an inability to mount components of the response. This is not surprising as the response is vital for homeostatic effects and protection against infection. There is an argument that one of the most powerful selective pressures evolutionarily is infection so that, whether or not the acute phase function response was directly protective or homeostatic, most of the responses seen are likely to counter infection. Over the last few years, the amount of investigation into the APR has been dwarfed by the efforts afforded to the cytokine initiators of the APR. These are the proinflammatory cytokines that generate the APR. These cytokines and other inflammatory mediators, which act at a local level, are also responsible for effects at the systemic level. In this chapter the role of these inducers is reviewed, concentrating on systemic responses rather than purely localized responses. The APR could be considered to include circulating cytokine responses to inflammation because they are also part of the overall systemic inflammatory response. One further aspect of the acute phase response is that many of the changes that occur and are present in an acute episode of inflammation will also be present in a chronic inflammatory disease. Thus, the name acute phase response is not really ideal because it is also a phenomenon of chronic inflammation, and an alternative term is the 'systemic inflammatory response syndrome (SIRS)'. This term is often used to describe severe clinical situations, however, and sepsis is used if the cause is infectious.

One of the most interesting aspects of the APR is the increase in acute phase proteins (APP) synthesized mainly in hepatocytes (Kushner 1982). Although normally considered to be a function of the liver, the definition of APP is not entirely limited to hepatic synthesis, because many APPs are synthesized outside the hepatocyte. Aspects of the APR are found in many different cells and sites in the body.

In this review, the APR to inflammation of any cause is considered although the concentration is on infectious examples where appropriate. It has to be remembered, however, that some of these proteins described are likely to contribute to homeostasis in many noninfectious situations and many may have more than one function. The aim is to cover mechanisms by which responses are stimulated, what is known about the func-

Table 12.1 *Major aspects of the acute phase response*

Metabolic aspects
Loss of muscle and negative nitrogen balance (protein catabolism)
Decreased gluconeogenesis (lactate, etc. no longer converted to glucose)
Osteoporosis (in chronic inflammation)
Increased hepatic lipogenesis
Increased lipolysis in adipose tissue
Increased triglycerides in serum and decreased high-density lipoprotein
Cachexia
Increased requirement for glutamine in fast-dividing immune cells, possibly leading to deficiency of glutamine
Micronutrient changes
Reduced serum zinc, iron, and copper
Reduced plasma retinol
Increased glutathione concentrations
Hemopoietic changes
Reduced red blood cell numbers
Increased neutrophils
Increased platelets
Neuroendocrine changes
Fever
Somnolence
Increased corticotropin-releasing hormone, corticotropin, and cortisol
Increased secretion of arginine vasopressin
Decreased insulin-like growth factor 1
Increased secretion of catecholamines
Hepatic changes
Positive and negative acute phase proteins
Increased metallothionein, heme oxygenase, etc.

tion of these responses, and where responses may malfunction. The major aspects are summarized in Table 12.1.

INDUCTION OF THE ACUTE PHASE RESPONSE

Induction of systemic inflammation

The APR is a nonspecific response in that it can be initiated by many different stimuli although, regardless of stimulus, the magnitude of the response is dependent on the extent of injury. Such injury may be caused by burns, irradiation, surgical or physical trauma of tissue injury or infection. Infection is often a strong inducer of the response, and particularly bacterial infection, because of the range of powerful immune stimulators that bacteria possess. More recently, when more sensitive assays were used to measure markers of inflammation such as C-reactive protein (CRP), associations were observed in a number of diseases that were previously not thought of as inflammatory in nature, such as atherosclerosis (Haverkate et al. 1997; Libby et al. 2002). This may be extended to other diseases in time. At the lower end of the spectrum of stimulus, strenuous exercise such as marathon running (Vider et al. 2001) or some psychiatric illnesses or stress (Maes et al. 1997) may cause a mild APR, at least detectable through the more sensitive indicators of the acute phase.

The initial stimulus for the APR may be physical trauma, through other means of tissue damage, or through adaptive immunological mechanisms including allergen and IgE-mediated mechanisms, immune complex activation of phagocytic cells, or T-cell-mediated recognition. Alternately, infection can be recognized by an increasing range of innate mechanisms such as endotoxin or peptidoglycan activation through Toll-like receptors (TLR) or other pattern recognition molecules. It is now known that such pattern recognition molecules can recognize many different foreign structures including nucleotide, protein, carbohydrate, and lipid structures. Following such stimuli, tissue injury may at first cause changes in vascular permeability through short-lived lipid mediators such as prostaglandins and leukotrienes, which allow fluid to leak from the post-capillary venules into the tissues. This is accompanied by a chemotactic stimulus from a variety of factors that bring inflammatory cells such as neutrophils, and subsequently macrophages, into the inflammatory site. The chemotactic stimulus works in conjunction with expression of adhesion molecules on the endothelium and leukocyte to control this cellular influx. These include the chemokines such as interleukin-8 (IL-8) which attracts neutrophils. The inflammatory cells themselves contain or synthesize a number of proinflammatory activators, many small and short-lived, but in addition some proinflammatory cytokines are generated that have the ability to transmit the inflammatory signal over much larger distances.

Different aspects of the APR take a different length of time to be observed following a defined stimulus. The induction of some of the APPs, for instance, may take between 24 and 72 hours to reach their peak (Figure 12.1b) whereas effects such as fever and malaise may be more rapidly observed. The main reason for such delays is that several rounds of inducible protein synthesis may be required. The proinflammatory cytokines such as tumor necrosis factor-α (TNFα) and interleukin-1 (IL-1α or IL-1β) can be generated within an hour or two of the start of the stimulus. TNFα is usually induced (largely through post-transcriptional regulation) earlier than IL-1β but both then induce a number of other cytokines (Figure 12.1a). If the stimulus for inflammation continues to be present at a sufficient level then the proinflammatory cytokines TNFα and IL-1β (more than IL-1α) are released into the circulation and induce responses at distant sites. In addition to release of such cytokines, early responses involve the release of a range

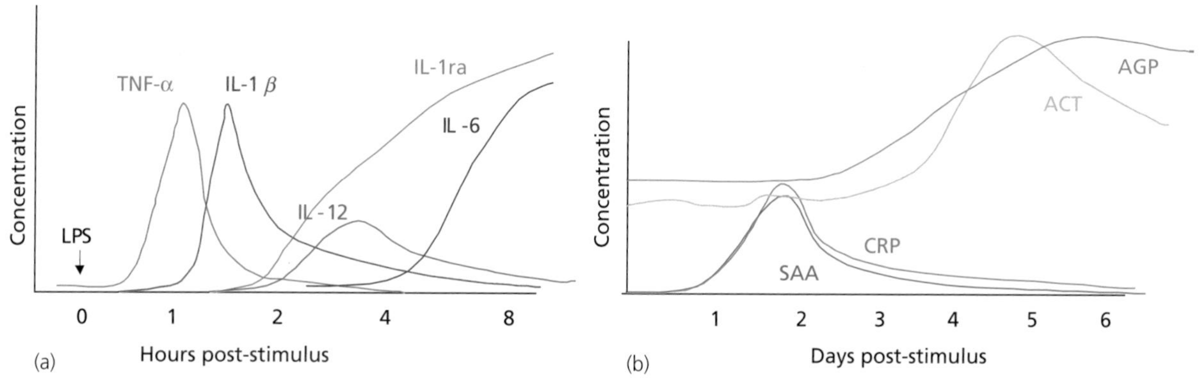

Figure 12.1 *Time course of induction of* **(a)** *cytokines and* **(b)** *acute phase proteins after an acute inflammatory stimulus such as lipopolysaccharide (LPS). ACT, antichymotrypsin; AGP, acid glycoprotein; CRP, C-reactive protein; IL, interleukin; SAA, serum amyloid A; TNF, tumor necrosis factor.*

of different chemokines, each with their own spectrum of cell attraction properties. These chemokines influence the range of cells entering the site of inflammation and thus the course of the inflammatory response. These early cytokines will in turn give rise to other cytokines that they induce at local and distal sites, such as IL-6 which frequently mediate cellular responses (Figure 12.1a). Other cytokines take rather longer to be synthesized and in some cases are no longer proinflammatory and some, such as IL-10 and IL-1 receptor antagonist (IL-1ra), are definitely anti-inflammatory. The overall effect is sometimes referred to as a cytokine 'storm' – a useful phrase because it reflects the battery of new stimuli to which cells are subjected.

Proinflammatory cytokines and the acute phase proteins

As an example of how the APR is generated hepatocyte production of APPs is the main focus because this is comparatively well known. Other aspects are considered later. The induction of the APR in the liver was studied extensively as a model of gene expression. The major cytokine involved in induction of the APR is IL-6. IL-6 was originally also called hepatocyte-stimulating factor (among other names), based on its inducing properties (Gauldie et al. 1987). This cytokine is the most prominent member of a family of cytokines (oncostatin M, leukemia inhibitory factor, ciliary neutrotrophic factor, IL-11, and cardiotropin 1) that can all induce the APR. This family of cytokines binds a family of receptor complexes containing a cytokine-specific receptor component chain, as well as a common component chain called gp130. It is the gp130 that has the major signaling role in the complex, which responds by transmitting a signal when homodimerized (Paonessa et al. 1995). Interestingly, the soluble IL-6R (sIL-6R) acts as an agonist and continues to help induce responses to IL-6 if gp130 is expressed on the cell surface (Mackiewicz et al. 1992). In addition, the sIL-6R–IL-6 complex has a longer half-life, thus stabilizing the activity of IL-6 (Peters et al. 1996). The soluble gp130, on the other hand, inhibits the response (Jostock et al. 2001). The other major inducer of the APR is IL-1. This cytokine family has many members but three are relevant to the induction of APPs. IL-1β is probably the most important inducing form because it is the major serum form of active IL-1. IL-1α is thought to be more important at a local level [illegible] the other form of IL-1 is an antagonist form called inte[illegible] (IL-1ra) which can bind to receptor but does not activate or recruit the accessory chain (Hannum et al. 1990; Greenfeder et al. 1995). IL-1β binds to two receptors: IL-1R1, which is capable of inducing response, and IL-1RII, which is a decoy receptor with no ability to signal (Colotta et al. 1993). Very few receptors need be occupied for a cell to respond to this cytokine but receptor numbers are regulated during the APR. Responses to IL-1 are thus kept under control by a number of systems (Mantovani et al. 2001).

The APPs have been classified as class I or class II based on the cytokines to which they respond (Figure 12.2). The class I APPs are induced by IL-1-type cytokines such as IL-1β or IL-1α (as well as TNFα and TNFβ) and IL-6. The TNF cytokines are included in this definition because they induce some of the same signaling and transcription factors as IL-1. The class II APPs, on the other hand, are induced almost exclusively by IL-6 and other members of that family of cytokines (mainly through IL-6RE which bind the STAT transcription factors). In some cases IL-1 may even reduce responses, for instance although IL-6 induces fibrinogen this is inhibited by IL-1β or TNFα (Rokita et al. 1994). The use of mouse IL-6 knock-out animals has confirmed the important role of IL-6 but this revealed another feature of the APR. Although turpentine-induced inflammation could not induce an APR in these animals, induction with lipopolysaccharide (LPS) led to an almost normal APR. This may be caused by induction of a different range of cytokines that can make up for the lack of IL-6 (Fattori

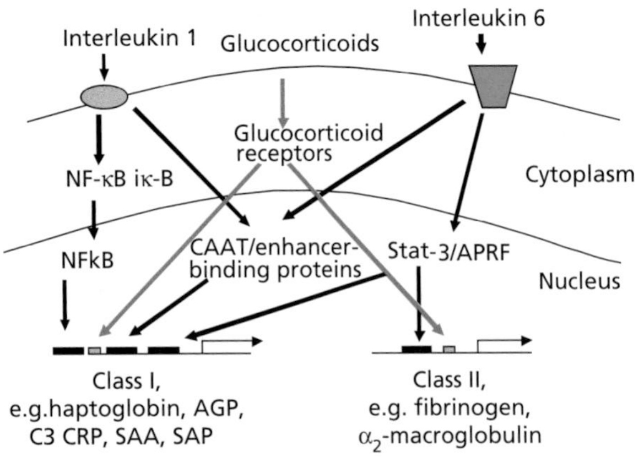

Figure 12.2 *Simplified pathways of induction of acute phase protein genes. AGP, acid glycoprotein; CRP, C-reactive protein; SAA, serum amyloid A; SAP, serum amyloid P.*

et al. 1994; Kopf et al. 1994). The likely candidates are other members of the IL-6 family of cytokines but leukemia inhibitory factor (LIF) and IL-11 are not likely to be involved (Gabay et al. 1996). Interestingly, the same sort of pattern is seen in IL-1β knock-out mice with responses to turpentine being lost but LPS maintained (Zheng et al. 1995). IL-6 production in response to IL-1 is diminished after turpentine injection. Other knock-out mice lacking IL-1-converting enzyme (caspase-1) show no reduction in responses to LPS or local turpentine (Fantuzzi et al. 1997). The loss of the signaling molecule gp130 in mice leads to severe abnormalities in development and immune cells making interpretation difficult. It has been seen, however, that loss of the signaling component STAT3 (downstream of gp130 signaling) leads to complete loss of induction of some class I acute phase genes which have regulatory elements for C/EBP transcription factors. Type II APPs were reduced at 24 hours but earlier responses are maintained (Alonzi et al. 2001). Some APPs (complement C3 and SAA3) have no STAT3 regulatory regions and are not affected by its loss. Adaptor proteins that bind STAT3 such as STAP-2 (BKS) also have significant roles in regulating signaling for APP synthesis (Minoguchi et al. 2003). Synthesis of each APP gene is regulated both transcriptionally and post-transcriptionally. The transcriptional regulation is controlled by the range of nuclear factors that bind to the promoter regions of the protein gene. Some of these are induced by IL-6 such as NF–IL–6 and others such as NF-κB are induced by TNFα or IL-1β (Edbrooke et al. 1989; Akira et al. 1990). Often such factors may act synergistically, e.g. the combinations of IL-6 and IL-1 for synthesis of serum amyloid A (SAA). In addition, some proteins are also strongly regulated post-transcriptionally by stabilization of the mRNA and this occurs for instance for α acid glycoprotein (AGP) (Shiels et al. 1987). The regulation of each protein is, however, complex and unique, e.g. a range of transcription factors has been identified in the induction of SAA genes including NF-κB, C/EBP, AP-2, Sp1 and YY1, and SAF (Uhlar and Whitehead 1999).

Lipopolysaccharide has been reported to activate hepatocytes directly, although it is hard to rule out the possibility that this is an indirect effect through LPS-induced cytokines. Thus, some questions remain that are unresolved with regard to induction of the hepatic response. Can the hepatocyte, if it expresses Toll-like receptor 4 (TLR4), respond to LPS directly? And if not, what role do the nonparenchymal cells of the liver have in directing the hepatocyte response? In particular, what contribution to the IL-6 stimulus to the hepatocyte comes from the Kupffer cell or possibly even the endothelial cell or fibroblast, and what contribution comes from circulating cytokine? Histological studies of mRNA or protein synthesis in liver sections has revealed a pattern of synthesis that involves initial synthesis in periportal regions followed by spread to perilobular, midlobular, and centriolobular regions until, at peak serum CRP, almost all hepatocytes are synthesizing CRP (Kushner and Feldmann 1978) (Figure 12.3). It should also be remembered that control can be exerted at the secretion stage as, for instance, for CRP (Yue et al. 1996). As referred to later, under Protein metabolism, the hepatocyte requires an increased supply of

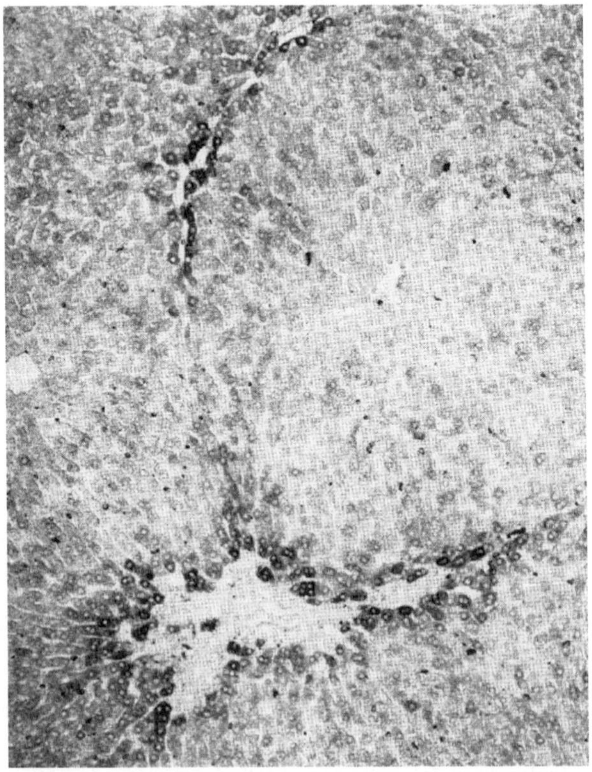

Figure 12.3 *Immunoenzymatic identification of hepatocytes producing C-reactive protein (CRP) 8 h after an inflammatory stimulus. Perilobular and periportal areas show intense cytoplasmic staining. (Reproduced from Kushner and Feldmann 1978, with permission.)*

amino acids for this increased burden of protein synthesis, and thus amino acid uptake by hepatocytes is increased.

Influence of inhibitory or modulating factors on APPs

Although glucocorticoids are generally an anti-inflammatory influence, it is also clear that they enhance synthesis of many APP genes (Baumann et al. 1989). The presence or absence of glucocorticoid response elements controls the extent of response to glucocorticoids which varies between proteins with, for instance, AGP being very strongly dependent on these hormones.

As IL-1 is a major inducing factor, it is not surprising that IL-1Ra would have an inhibitory action because it increases at a later time point in the APR subsequent to IL-1β. IL-1ra can reduce synthesis of APPs (Bevan and Raynes 1991) and, in a mouse model, completely prevented SAA induction, showing that IL-1 is required for SAA synthesis (Grehan et al. 1997). The hepatocyte makes a significant contribution to plasma IL-1ra (Gabay et al. 2001) and would thus be an autocrine regulatory response. The liver makes this IL-1ra in response to IL-6 whereas IL-1ra from other tissue appears to be independent of IL-6 (Gabay et al. 2001).

TNFα has an ability to induce responses in vitro and would clearly do so indirectly in vivo. Transforming growth factor β (TGFβ) and interferon-α and -γ have been demonstrated to have some ability to induce APPs (Ramadori et al. 1988; Mackiewicz et al. 1990). Other factors with an influence are hepatocyte growth factor and retinoic acid (Koj et al. 1995). Insulin has a downregulatory effect on APP synthesis (Campos and Baumann 1992).

It has recently been found that a member of the IL-10 family of cytokines, IL-22, has the ability to induce an APR in hepatocytes. This cytokine, produced mainly by T cells, can interact with IL-22 receptor together with IL-10R2 to induce STAT1 and STAT3 and hence induce a range of proteins such as SAA, haptoglobin, and antichymotrypsin (Dumoutier et al. 2000a, 2000b). As yet the extent of IL-22 contribution to the APR is not known. The effects of IL-22 are also not restricted to the hepatocyte because it has been shown that epithelial cells can also respond and IL-22 may thus have pleiotropic effects. These and the APR induction are antagonized by a soluble receptor which acts as a binding protein or by receptor antagonism (Dumoutier et al. 2001; Wei et al. 2003).

Effects of nutrient deficiency or modulation

Protein synthesis by hepatocytes represents a considerable drain on amino acid precursors and total hepatic protein synthesis during inflammation. It might be expected that it would therefore be absent or greatly reduced in nutritional deficiency. However, this appears not to be the case, because in severe protein malnutrition the APR is often seen in equal or higher levels compared with individuals with normal weight for height, although such studies do not take into account a reduced resistance to infection in such individuals. In fact, when faced with an equivalent stimulus in human studies there is a reduction in response in malnutrition following, for example, immunization protocols (Doherty et al. 1993) or in animal studies (Jennings et al. 1992; Lyoumi et al. 1998). Nevertheless the response is still a strong one and is essentially maintained. The reduction is probably at the level of cytokine production rather than hepatocyte response because serum IL-6 was reduced as well as APPs (Doherty et al. 1994). This provides further evidence for the essential role of the APR and APPs in homeostasis or resistance to infection. It is often assumed that the concentration of the APPs is dependent on the rate of synthesis; however, there is evidence that the rate of clearance may be different in protein malnutrition (Morlese et al. 1998). It is also clear that certain proteins such as fibrinogen may be more severely affected by protein malnutrition than others (Morlese et al. 1998) and that the malnutrition itself, in the absence of other stimuli, may in some cases cause an increase in certain proteins (Lyoumi et al. 1998). The effects of other forms of nutritional deficiency on the APR are less well characterized, although in the reverse direction the APR can certainly alter micronutrient availability (see later, under Micronutrient changes). Low levels of vitamin E may lead to a more pronounced inflammatory response, perhaps because of a reduced ability to control oxidants.

Another factor that can modulate APRs through their effect on cytokine production is the amount of *n*-3 and *n*-6 polyunsaturated fatty acids in the diet. Fish oils that are rich in *n*-3 fatty acids reduce the proinflammatory cytokine production of IL-1 and TNFα in comparison with *n*-6 fatty acids, which increase cytokine responses (Calder and Grimble 2002). The effect of the *n*-3-rich oils is sufficient to improve the status of patients with diseases with inflammatory pathology such as rheumatoid arthritis and psoriasis or asthma and in animal studies with LPS (Calder and Grimble 2002)

Induction of other aspects of the APR

Fever has been shown to be induced by administration of proinflammatory cytokines (called endogenous pyrogens) but appears to need IL-6, which acts downstream of the potent pyrogens IL-1α or IL-1β. When the cytokines reach the central nervous system they generate prostaglandins, particularly PGE_2 in the organum vasculosum of the lamina terminalis, which reset the

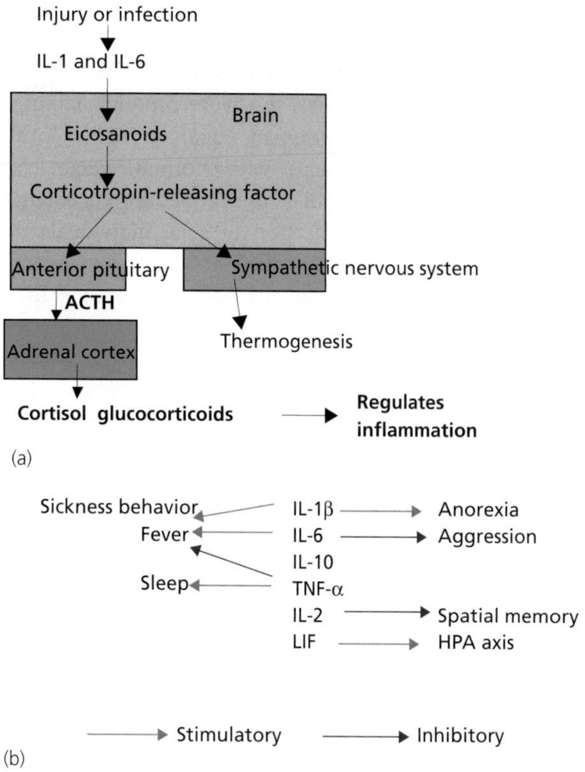

Figure 12.4 *Induction of fever and glucocorticoid downregulation of inflammation through brain responses to proinflammatory cytokines. HPA, hypothalamo–pituitary–adrenal; IL, interleukin; LIF, leukemia inhibitory factor; TNF, tumor necrosis factor.*

temperature set point (Figure 12.4a). Mice lacking the prostaglandin receptor EP_3 are unable to generate a febrile response (Ushikubi et al. 1998). Although other pathways may ultimately also act, they all generate a response in the thermoregulatory center in the anterior hypothalamus. Although the original model suggests that the cytokine originates from the periphery, there are several possible pathways and local cytokine synthesis is likely. It is even possible that endotoxins may act directly in a similar way to that proposed for hepatocyte responses. Responses have been linked to a number of different cytokines using inhibition or addition experiments, but direct effects are difficult to demonstrate. The use of knock-out mice has suggested that IL-6 and IL-1β are involved in the induction of fever (Zheng et al. 1995; Kluger et al. 1998; Netea et al. 2000; Inui 2001) whereas others such as TNFα or IL-10 appear to reduce fever (Leon et al. 1997; Leon 2002). Recently it was shown that vagotomy reduces the extent of fever in response to intra-abdominal IL-1 (Watkins et al. 1995). The sensory input of afferent vagal nerves can thus alter fever responses in the brain and this is dependent on the site and type of stimulation. The interaction between neural and immune inflammation was recently reviewed (Tracy 2002).

Studies using knock-out mice also suggest that anorexia and somnolence are regulated by IL-1β and IL-6 (Figure 12.4b, reviewed in Inui 2001). IL-1 appears to be important for anorexia and TNFα is thought to be needed for sleep responses. Lethargy may be caused by IL-1 because mice lacking type I IL-1 receptor do not show lethargy responses and these responses do not require IL-6 (Leon et al. 1997).

Little information is available on the proinflammatory cytokine regulation of hemopoiesis and they are likely to work through growth factors (see later under Hemopoietic responses). Thrombocytosis is regulated by IL-6 mainly through thrombopoietin (Kaser et al. 2001).

ACUTE PHASE PROTEINS

Acute phase proteins have many different functions and in this review have been organized into functionally related groups, although there is some doubt about the role of many proteins and to which category they should belong. It should be remembered that there is no requirement that a particular protein should only have one function. The choice of whether to include proteins that are made mainly outside the liver or in nonhepatic cells, or when to start considering proteins as part of the acute phase, is a difficult one. In some respects a review of the acute phase should consider TNFα and other cytokines released as early components of this system. However, this review focuses a few hours after the initial stimulus and includes proteins that are increased by at least 25 percent or more during inflammation and that are at least, in part, made in hepatocytes. Also included are proteins that show substantial increases in concentration in human sera and/or increases in several other species, which may be made in other cells that might be used to follow inflammation. It has been shown recently, using oligonucleotide array hybridization, that 7 percent of hepatic genes were responsive to LPS (Yoo and Desiderio 2003), demonstrating the importance of this response in liver function and confirming the impression that many such genes are related to host defense and immunity, metabolism, or coagulation.

Acute phase proteins are produced at a time when the host might be expected to require a downregulatory force on the systemic inflammation that generated the APR. Thus many of the proteins are thought to have an anti-inflammatory function (Tilg et al. 1997). It is interesting that, although similar proteins are found in most species, there is considerable variation between the concentrations of the proteins, and variations between which are strongly or weakly induced, e.g. CRP, haptoglobin, AGP, and α_2-macroglobulin, have very different patterns of expression in humans, mice, rabbits, and rats.

In general APPs are well conserved and many have ancestors in teleosts and elasmobranchs (Bayne and Gerwick 2001). There are some human APP deficiencies

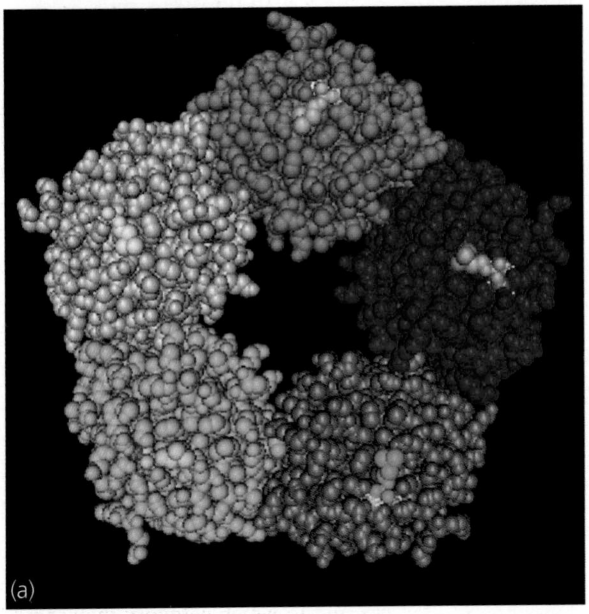

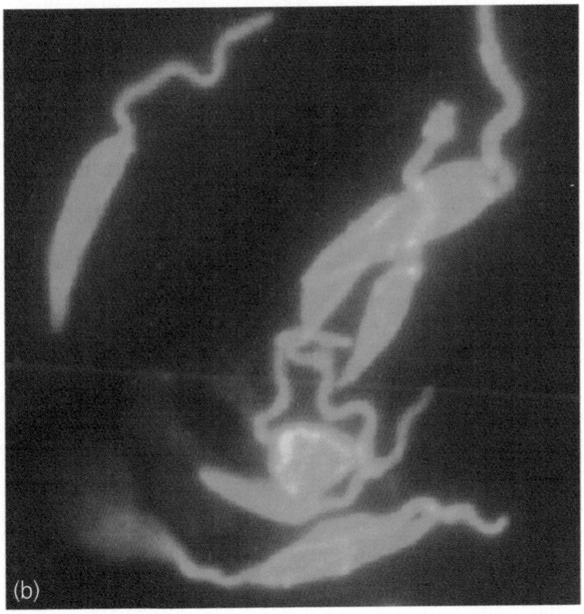

Figure 12.5 (a) *Structure of C-reactive protein (CRP);* **(b)** *binding of CRP to* Leishmania mexicana *demonstrated by immunofluorescence.*

which have provided information about function and knock-out mice have also provided information. APPs will now be considered according to groups with related function.

Innate immune proteins

C-REACTIVE PROTEIN AND OTHER PENTRAXINS

C-reactive protein was originally discovered over 70 years ago and given its name because it interacted with the phosphorylcholine-containing polysaccharide and lipoteichoic acid found on *Streptococcus pneumoniae* (Tillet and Francis 1930). CRP is the best known of the APPs because it is regularly used as a marker of systemic inflammation in clinical settings and can increase from approximately 1 µg/ml to 500 µg/ml in severe inflammation (see later under Clinical use of APPs and inflammation markers). The protein is, however, a member of a family of proteins (pentraxins) that includes homologs of similar size to CRP such as serum amyloid P (SAP) component or homologous domains found as part of larger proteins such as long pentraxins (PTX3). Other species usually show either SAP or CRP to be an APP. In mice, for example, CRP is present at low levels and SAP is a major APP whereas human SAP concentrations change little in inflammation (Pepys and Baltz 1983). CRPs are found in arthropods that lack an acquired immune system and often several copies are found; in the horseshoe crab these have different binding specificities (Iwaki et al. 1999). Human PTX3 demonstrates small increases in concentration during the acute phase (Muller et al. 2001b).

The common feature of these proteins is their structure which is pentameric (see Figure 12.5a). Crystal structures are now available for both CRP and its homolog SAP (Emsley et al. 1994; Shrive et al. 1996). They both possess the ability to bind to phosphorylated ligands such as phosphorylcholine or phosphorylethanolamine in a calcium-dependent manner. However, this is not the only ligand because phosphorylated carbohydrates can also bind (Culley et al. 2000). Such ligands are found on microorganisms including *Leishmania* spp. (see Figure 12.5b) One feature of these interactions is that the avidity of CRP for monomeric ligand is usually low and, only when such ligands are expressed as an array, e.g. on the surface of a microorganism, are high avidities generated. The binding specificity of SAP includes heparin, a 4,6-cyclic acetal of pyruvate, 6-phosphorylated mannose, and 3-sulfated saccharides (Hind et al. 1984; Loveless et al. 1992). CRP, SAP, and PTX3 have all been shown to interact with apoptotic cells (Gershov et al. 2000; Rovere et al. 2000; reviewed in Nauta et al. 2003). The mechanism of binding for CRP may be related to binding to damaged membranes which has been observed in a number of other systems where membrane integrity or composition is altered (Li et al. 1994).

It is clear that CRP can activate complement through the classical pathway but it has been shown that CRP activates the pathway only as far as C5 (Mold et al. 1984). The C1q binding site is found on the opposite face to the phosphorylcholine- or calcium-dependent ligand-binding face. CRP can directly interact with cellular receptors such as FcγRI (Marnell et al. 1995; Bodman-Smith et al. 2002) and perhaps also FcγRII. The result of CRP interaction with a range of microorganisms is increased phagocytosis by cells such as macrophages and neutrophils, either directly or indirectly through complement. These ligands on infectious organisms may allow CRP to be protective against disease as in the case of *Streptococcus pneumoniae* (Yother et al. 1982; Du Clos and Mold 2001), but may not always be so in cases of *Leishmania donovani* when CRP binding to lipophosphoglycan on the parasite increases access to the macrophage as an important part of its life cycle (Culley et al. 1996). There is little or no evidence for opsonization of microorganisms through SAP binding, although recently it has been suggested that SAP can cause phagocytosis of its ligand zymosan through murine Fc receptors (Mold et al. 2001).

The role of slightly higher baseline CRP concentrations as a predictor of heart disease is a fascinating new observation (Haverkate et al. 1997; Libby et al. 2002). It is currently important to discover whether this is a causal observation or merely a marker of some other inflammation-driven cause of atherosclerosis. A potential mechanism may be through low-density lipoprotein (LDL) uptake into monocytes or through activation of endothelial (CRP induces tissue factor) or other cell types at the lesion site.

PTX3 lacks the ability to bind to phosphorylcholine ligand but retains an affinity for carbohydrate and also binds to macrophages and can protect against fungal infection (Garlanda et al. 2002).

COMPLEMENT COMPONENTS

A number of the complement cascade proteins are APPs including the central component C3. The complement cascade acts as an innate immune and acquired immune pathway, being triggered by both antibody and the innate proteins mannose-binding lectin (MBL) and ficolin. The alternative pathway is activated by charged surfaces often presented by microbes. MBL is itself an APP (Ezekovitz et al. 1988). The complement components (see Chapter 9, Complement) that are induced are C1q, C3, C4, C9, factor B, C1 inhibitor, and C4-binding protein. Some of these are required to replenish protein depleted by activation and usage of complement as is observed after, for example, a severe burn injury. APPs such as C4-binding protein are required as controlling proteins.

Mannose-binding lectin is a member of a family of collectins that all bind to carbohydrate on pathogens and direct these pathogens for opsonization through complement after association with a protease called mannose-binding protein-associated serine protease (MASP), which activates C1q (Matsushita and Fujita 1992). This protein is a decamer of units that have globular lectin domains and collagenous tails (Figure 12.6) (Peterson et al. 2001). The binding to a variety of carbohydrate structures such as mannose or *N*-acetylglucosamine on microbes can lead to phagocytosis. Besides activating complement a direct receptor for MBL has been implicated but not defined as yet. A fairly common mutation in one of the alleles leads to large reduction in secreted active protein and such individuals are more at risk of certain infections, particularly at the ages of 2–4 years before an appropriate humoral immunity has been attained (Sumiya et al. 1991). MBL is one of a number of proteins that can lead to improved presentation to T cells (Figure 12.7).

LIPOPOLYSACCHARIDE-BINDING PROTEIN

Lipopolysaccharide-binding protein (LBP) is found constitutively at about 5–10 μg/ml but can increase 10-fold during severe inflammation. LBP has been shown to bind to LPS and transfer it to CD14 and TLR4, and consistent with this LBP can increase the activity of LPS to activate $CD14^+$ cells by more than 100-fold (Schumann et al. 1990). However, LBP also transfers LPS into high-density lipoprotein (HDL) within which environment LPS is almost completely without activating effect (Wurfel et al. 1994). As the LBP interacts mainly with the lipid A portion of the LPS, it is unlikely to bind directly to bacteria and opsonize them. Further information of its role comes from LBP-deficient mice which can clear LPS normally but need LBP for an inflammatory response to LPS. Furthermore, these mice are more susceptible to intraperitoneal salmonella infection (Jack et al. 1997). In the *salmonella* infections, TNFα synthesis was reduced and evidence was presented that LBP contributed towards TNFα activation of polymorphs (Fierer et al. 2002).

SECRETORY PHOSPHOLIPASE A_2

Phospholipase A_2 (PLA_2) is an enzyme that generates fatty acid and a lysophospholipid from phospholipid. The enzyme exists in a cytosolic form and as a secreted version ($sPLA_2$), and there are several different isoforms of each. The products are important for signaling pathways and generation of lipid inflammatory mediators and for this reason have been considered as potential targets for anti-inflammatory drugs. The secreted PLA_2 is an APP (Andreani et al. 2000), of which the most studied form, $sPLA_2$ type IIA, is a potent anti-streptococcal and anti-staphylococcal enzyme (Weinrauch et al. 1998). It is also thought to be coordinated with other prostaglandin synthesis enzymes in order to play a role in inflammation. The effects and potential functions of such enzymes are clearly wide ranging and a range of different receptors is being characterized (reviewed in Lambeau and Lazdunski 1999; Murakami et al. 2000).

Protease inhibitors

There are a number of protease inhibitors present in plasma that have a spectrum of activity and many of

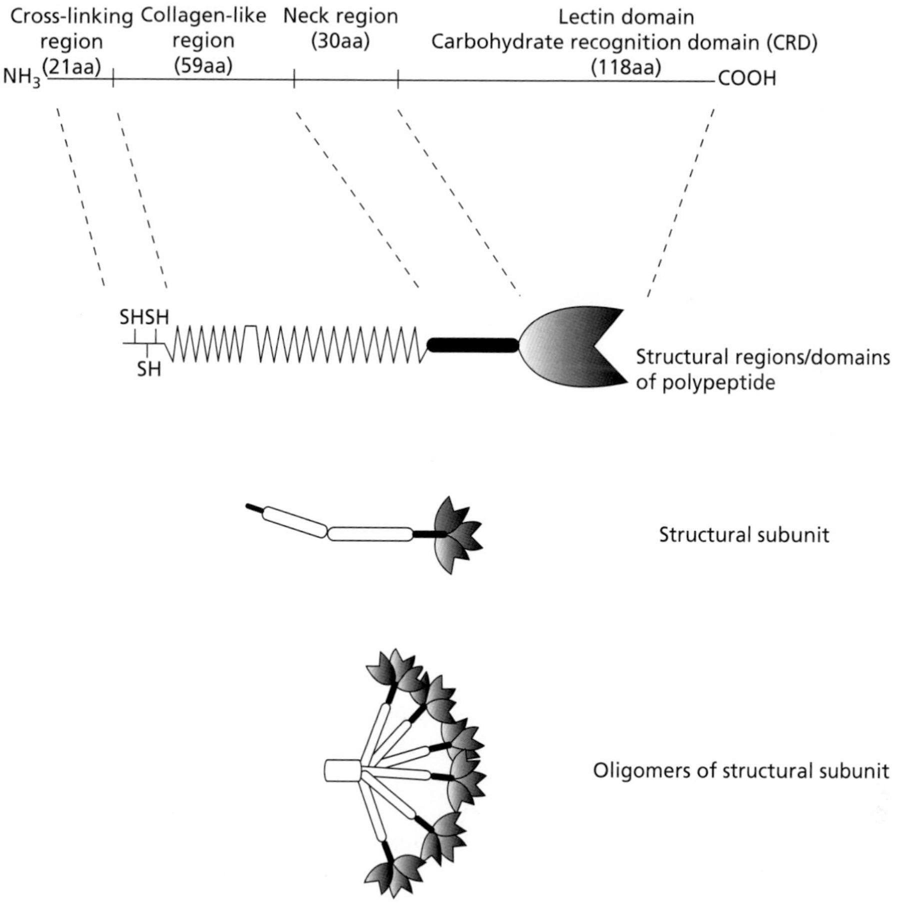

Figure 12.6 *Structure of mannan-binding lectin (MBL) showing structural domains, subunits, and oligomeric organization. (Redrawn from Peterson et al. 2001.)*

which increase in response to inflammation. They generally increase at later time points (2–5 days). Names of the protease inhibitors have often been given on the basis of the protease that allows demonstration of inhibitory activity rather than the actual protease that they

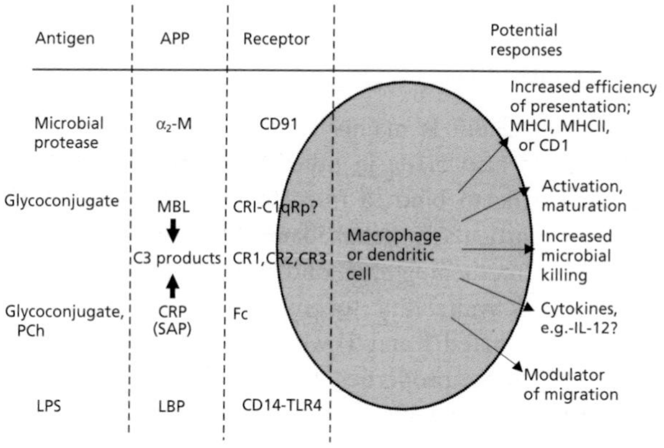

Figure 12.7 *Diagram depicting the different acute phase proteins that deliver particular microbial products to macrophages or dendritic cells. This can have a number of different potential outcomes, all of which have been described for at least one of the uptake pathways.*

inhibit in vivo. Although a major role is to inhibit endogenous proteases and thus control inflammation and tissue clearance before remodeling, it has also been proposed that some functions may relate to control of microbial proteases (Hiemstra 2002). Many of these protease inhibitors are serine protease inhibitors of a family called serpins. Some of these inhibitors have particular functions such as plasminogen activator inhibitor, antithrombin III, and C1q inhibitor which are therefore considered in other sections.

α_1-ANTITRYPSIN OR α_1-PROTEASE INHIBITOR

α_1-Protease inhibitor (α_1-PI) is defined as a serpin because it is structurally related to members of a family of serine protease inhibitors. Already present at approximately 2–3 mg/ml it can increase fourfold. The name α_1-PI is to be preferred to antitrypsin because its actual antiprotease effect is more likely to be on neutrophil elastase and cathepsin G or protease 3. This glycoprotein is synthesized mainly by hepatocytes but also by macrophages and neutrophils. Occasionally we can learn about function from deficiency diseases and this is the case for α_1-PI (Carrell and Lomas 2002). The disease leads to a greatly increased risk of emphysema or liver disease. The emphysema is the result of the lack of control of proteases, and the liver disease also caused by a problem with misfolding and protein aggregates accumulating in the hepatocyte endoplasmic reticulum (Lomas et al. 1992). Thus, a major function of this protein is to prevent degradation of elastase in the lung. Treatment with replacement α_1-PI was able to reduce frequency of lung infection in α_1-PI-deficient patients (Lieberman 2000). After complex formation with protease, a large change in the protease structure is generated (Huntington et al. 2000) and clearance follows by endocytosis through the serpin enzyme complex (SEC) receptor (Perlmutter et al. 1990; Joslin et al. 1992).

α_1-ANTICHYMOTRYPSIN

This protein is increased to a greater extent (up to sixfold) than other slow responding human APPs such as α_1-PI (see Figure 12.1b). Again, the specificity for serine proteases and localization is such that it is more likely to inhibit cathepsin G and mast cell chymases. Interestingly a point mutation in α_1-antichymotrypsin (α_1-ACT) can lead to reduced concentrations in plasma and a deficiency disease similar to that seen with α_1-PI. This is only seen with particular mutations (Faber et al. 1993). As with other serpinopathies (of C1 inhibitor or antithrombin III) many α_1-ACT mutations do not lead to such pathology. This is likely to be because they are produced at 10 percent of the rate and degradative pathways can handle the inappropriately folded protein. Interestingly, the presence of an APR may precipitate pathology when the rate of synthesis is increased, although this is based on a limited number of observations.

α_2-MACROGLOBULIN

This is a very large protein with an interesting mechanism of inhibition. It is so large that it can be visualized by electron microscopy and it acts to trap the protease when the protease cleaves a bond on the internal aspect of one of the faces of the protein. The change in conformation of the α_2-macroglobulin reveals a site for interaction with a receptor called LDL receptor-related protein or CD91 (Moestrup and Gliemann 1989) (see Figure 12.8). CD91 has been identified as a receptor site for heat shock protein (HSP)-mediated binding and endocytosis. The result of this is that α_2-macroglobulin may also be an immune component because it improves adjuvanticity through cross-presentation (Binder et al. 2001) (see Figure 12.7).

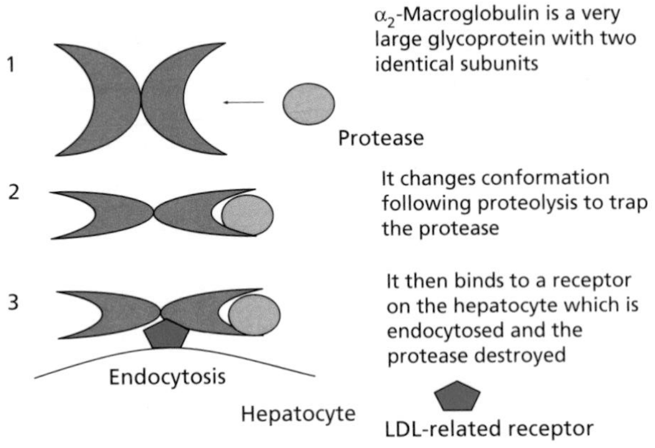

Figure 12.8 *Diagram depicting the mechanism by which α_2-macroglobulin captures proteases and delivers them from endocytosis into macrophages and other cells expressing CD91 or low-density lipoprotein (LDL)-related receptor.*

Transport proteins

FERRITIN

Ferritin is composed of two sorts of protein subunit – H and L – which combine together to form a complex of 24 subunits that form an apoferritin shell which can hold up to 4500 iron atoms. It is present inside the cell and acts mainly as a storage protein rather than a transporter, but smaller amounts are also found in the serum. The serum form is thought to be derived from the L subunit and is normally poor in iron. Hepatocyte cytoplasmic ferritin is also predominantly the L form. Its primary function is to sequester iron and, by reducing availability for microbial growth, this helps control infection. However, ferritin should be considered as a member of a group of proteins that together with transferrin and transferrin receptor work to make available the iron necessary for many of the host of mammalian iron-containing proteins. Ferritin synthesis is induced in a post-transcriptional way by intracellular iron availability. It is also induced by proinflammatory cytokines in a complex way which also involves increased secretion (Torti and Torti 2002), although IL-4 and IL-13 may also regulate ferritin produced in macrophages (Weiss et al. 1997). The function and regulation of iron availability appear to be linked with another APP called hepcidin which is produced by hepatocytes and macrophages (Nemeth et al. 2003)

HAPTOGLOBIN

This glycoprotein is mainly synthesized in hepatocytes but some is also made in other cell types. Its function appears to be to bind to free hemoglobin and prevent damage, particularly renal damage, which would be caused by free hemoglobin, and then to recycle the iron and reduce availability for microbes. There are two alleles (designated 1 and 2) which give rise to polymeric molecules with properties that diverge considerably (Langlois and Delanghe 1996). Allelic associations exist with infections, atherosclerosis, and autoimmune disease. The haptoglobin and hemoglobin complex interacts with a receptor recently identified as CD163 (Kristiansen et al. 2001) which clears the iron mainly to macrophages. However, the haptoglobin-deficient mouse shows no major symptoms until placed under strong hemolytic stress, when it displays renal injury as a result of oxidative damage (Lim et al. 1998). Extrahepatic synthesis in lung macrophages may hint at other functions.

HEMOPEXIN

Hemopexin has the ability to bind heme released from hemoglobin or other heme-containing proteins, thus acting as a second-line defense against hemoglobin damage. As for haptoglobin, this reduces the opportunity for free iron to cause oxidative damage and also reduces the ease with which microorganisms can have access to iron for growth. It has been proposed that, once heme has been bound with high affinity (dissociation constant $K_d < 1$ pmol/l), a site is revealed that allows binding to a hepatocyte receptor; however, it is unclear if this is responsible for the total uptake by hepatocytes (Noyer et al. 1998). Heme would then be catabolized to bilirubin, biliverdin, and iron, with hemopexin and the receptor recirculating. Deletion of the gene for hemopexin generated mice that had normal handling of iron under unchallenged conditions, but the mice were less able to cope with hemolysis (Tolosano et al. 1999). Although haptoglobin- and hemopexin-deficient mice have increased amounts of the other protein (perhaps to compensate) the double knock-out has a similar phenotype to the single knock-outs. The delivery of heme to cells for destruction is part of a system that includes heme oxygenase which acts to reduce oxidative stress from iron inside the cell (see later, under Liver protective responses).

GC GLOBULIN

Group-specific component (Gc globulin), also known as vitamin D-binding protein, is only a very minor acute phase reactant. Its function appears to be twofold: it acts in clearing actin, a protein that has been implicated in the formation of microthrombi (Lee and Galbraith 1992). Increased tissue damage releases large amounts of actin that need to be cleared, and this first function is achieved in conjunction with the muscle cell-derived gelsolin. Initially after trauma, levels are reduced, presumably reflecting functional depletion and subsequently rise following IL-6 effects on hepatocytes. A second function, as its other name suggests, is as a transporter of vitamin D_3 and its major metabolites including the active 1α,25-dihydroxyvitamin D_3 (Daiger et al. 1975). When circulating, only a small percentage of the circulating protein has vitamin D bound; nevertheless it appears to control availability and uptake by cells. Other reports have suggested an immunomodulating function.

Procoagulant/fibrinolytic proteins

In the acute phase, the balance between the different factors that promote or clear clot formation is one that shifts towards the procoagulant. The process of coagulation is linked to inflammation because coagulation increases inflammation and inhibition of this coagulation can reduce the severity of inflammation which involves coagulation. In addition to the proteins mentioned below, factor VIII and von Willebrand factor are APPs induced by IL-6.

FIBRINOGEN

A range of different mutations in humans has led to rare afibrinogenemias where complete lack of fibrinogen is associated with bleeding disorders. Alternately less severe dysfibrinogenemias have different presentations and patterns of pathology. Fibrinogen is composed of two sets of three different sorts of chains – lack of any one of these leads to deficiency (Doolittle 1984). As well as being an important protein for blood clot formation with the platelet plug, it has a role in inflammation, wound healing, cell migration, and cell proliferation. These properties are thought to be related to interactions with integrins on endothelial cells or (CD11b/CD18) on leukocytes.

This protein is required for wound healing and appropriate cell distribution and migration during the wound healing process (Drew et al. 2001), which was studied in knock-out mice. Although mainly synthesized in the liver, extrahepatic synthesis occurs, e.g. in lung epithelial cells.

PLASMINOGEN AND PLASMINOGEN ACTIVATOR

This protein is a zymogen that is cleaved by the plasminogen activators – urokinase (uPA) or tissue type (tPA) – to form plasmin, an enzyme that cleaves fibrin and other extracellular proteins to remove clots. Upregulation of both plasminogen and plasminogen activator and the variety of other coagulation/fibrinolysis proteins does not necessarily favor enhanced thrombosis (Esmon 2000), but may rather represent a replacement of consumed protein.

PROTEIN S

Activated protein C and protein S work together as an anticoagulant and an anti-inflammatory agent. When small microthombi of fibrin and thrombin are deposited in inflammation or infection then thrombin/thrombomodulin activates the protein C (an antithrombotic serine protease). This led to a trial in patients with severe sepsis of an activated protein C that showed a small improvement in mortality from sepsis compared with placebo, a rare finding because many attempts to improve outcome in sepsis have failed (Bernard et al. 2001; see also Chapter 34, Shock/sepsis). Further studies are needed to confirm efficacy.

VITRONECTIN AND PLASMINOGEN ACTIVATOR INHIBITOR TYPE I

Although mostly synthesized in the liver, mRNA for vitronectin is found at lower levels in the brain, heart, and adipose tissues. It is stimulated by IL-6 and protein can increase by two- to threefold (Seiffert et al. 1994). Vitronectin is a multifunctional adhesive glycoprotein that forms a complex with plasminogen activator inhibitor type I (PAI-1), which stabilizes the function of the latter. PAI-1 binds to plasminogen activators such as tPA to generate a stable inactive complex. Vitronectin also helps PAI-1 binding to fibrin. In addition PAI-1 acts as an antiadhesive factor for cell adhesion involving vitronectin and integrins or the urokinase receptor. PAI-1 deficiency in humans is associated with bleeding disorders, indicating a role in stable clot formation.

ANTITHROMBIN III

Antithrombin II is a negative APP, which by its reduction leads to a more procoagulant state. Antithrombin III-deficiency diseases are characterized by thromboembolism (Mackie et al. 1978). It is a serpin that inhibits thrombin and other proteases that cause coagulation.

Regulatory molecules released into the circulation during the APR

IL-1 RECEPTOR ANTAGONIST

The IL-1Ra, as its name implies, prevents IL-1 action by competing for available receptor. Originally found as a cytokine generated by the same cells that make the active form, but temporarily delayed in response, it has more recently been described as an APP under different regulation in hepatocytes (Gabay et al. 2001).

MACROPHAGE MIGRATION INHIBITORY FACTOR

With the similarity of migration inhibitory factor (MIF) to procalcitonin, it appears that MIF acts as an APP in septic or immune inflammation rather than trauma-induced inflammation (Beishuizen et al. 2001). MIF is an interesting protein which appears to have many immune and inflammation-related functions. Its function may relate to reducing glucocorticoid effects on the inflammatory response (Baugh and Bucala 2002). It appears to mediate shock responses in reaction to Gram-positive and -negative bacteria, and mice that lack MIF are resistant to LPS-induced shock (Bozza et al. 1999). The mechanism of action of MIF remains somewhat unclear despite existing in large extracellular amounts, and no cellular membrane receptor has been identified. It is also found intracellularly and an intracellular ligand, Jab1, has been linked to some responses (Kleemann et al. 2000).

SOLUBLE ADHESION MOLECULES

Soluble intercellular adhesion molecule (sICAM) or soluble vascular cell adhesion molecule (svCAM), which are immunoglobulin adhesion molecule family members, and soluble E selectin are all found in increased amounts in plasma after any infectious and inflammatory stimuli that give rise to systemic effects (Kulander et al. 2001; Reinhart et al. 2002). Their function may relate to an ability to inhibit cellular extravasation.

ANGIOTENSINOGEN

Angiotensinogen is largely produced in the liver, although other tissues can make it and it is cleaved by renin to angiotensin II, which is a powerful vasoconstrictor that controls salt and water homeostasis (Morgan et al. 1996). Other studies have suggested that it may also have proinflammatory effects on vascular endothelia (Brasier et al. 2002).

Other APPs of uncertain function

SERUM AMYLOID A

Serum amyloid A (SAA) protein is a major APP in humans but it is unclear what the true function for this protein might be. SAA was first discovered as the serum component precursor of amyloid AA (Rosenthal et al. 1976). Since then several members of the family have been found. Human SAA is a gene family including two acute phase forms, SAA1 and SAA2, as well as a constitutive form SAA4 (Uhlar and Whitehead 1999). During normal conditions the most abundant isoform is SAA4, but during severe inflammation this protein increases only slightly with the major forms becoming SAA2 and particularly SAA1 which can increase 1000-fold up to 500 μg/ml. All forms of the protein are found associated with HDL to which it is reversibly bound (more than 95 percent in complexed form). This association with HDL has led to the idea that SAA function might be linked to that of HDL. When SAA associates with HDL other lipoproteins such as apolipoprotein A1 are displaced (Coetzee et al. 1986). Nevertheless, despite the demonstration that SAA has effects on lipid transport between HDL and various cells and effects on enzyme activities, no clear role has been demonstrated. Changes in lipid metabolism are relatively small and perhaps to be expected from any protein that displaces other proteins and becomes a major protein (up to 50 percent or more) in the total HDL protein in severe inflammation. In vivo cholesterol transport was not altered by SAA1 overexpressed through an adenoviral construct, although the constitutive form did alter lipoprotein profiles (Kindy et al. 2000).

An alternate hypothesis for SAA function is that it is involved in immune function as a chemotactic agent. Evidence for this has been gathered from experiments that show movement of a variety of cells in response to lipid-free SAA (Xu et al. 1995). As further support for this, interaction with a G-protein-coupled receptor FPRL1 has been suggested (Su et al. 1999). Surprisingly HDL inhibits this function and, if this is a major function, it is unclear why hepatocytes would make so much SAA. An interaction with the RAGE receptor has also been suggested for the amyloidogenic form of SAA (Yan et al. 2000).

SAA3 is synthesized extrahepatically in a number of cells such as macrophages and adipose cells (Meek and Benditt 1986). It has recently been demonstrated that adipose cells synthesize SAA3 in response to hyperglycemia (Lin et al. 2001). In addition epithelial tissues were found to express SAA1, SAA2, and SAA4 under normal physiological states (Urieli-Shoval et al. 1998).

α_1-ACID GLYCOPROTEIN

Acid glycoprotein (AGP) (also called orosomucoid) is highly acidic with a p*I* of between 2.8 and 3.8 as a result of approximately 60 percent of its mass being made up of N-linked glycans (Fournier et al. 2000). It is a member of a class of protein called the lipocalins, which also includes α_1-microglobulin and retinol-binding protein. In plasma it is an abundant protein (see Table 12.1), which can increase up to fivefold from 0.3 to 0.6 mg/ml.

A large proportion of the research on this protein is related to its ability to bind and alter the bioavailability of a wide range of drugs. This is because a number of sites are available to interact with drugs of both basic and neutral lipophilic character and even acidic drugs. Some of the more important drugs bound are propranolol, verapamil, and quinine (Israili and Dayton 2001). The fact that AGP increases severalfold during an APR may thus alter the availability of drug and pharmacokinetics in the acute phase as compared with the normal dosage of drug (e.g. quinine). This ability to carry small molecules may be part of AGP's function and certainly AGP can be seen to be associated with steroid hormones such as progesterone. However, several other possible functions exist. The N-linked sugars themselves change during the APR becoming shorter, whereas in pregnancy they are found to be longer, perhaps reflecting the rate of synthesis (Raynes 1982). The glycosyl transferases responsible for full glycosylation of proteins are also induced by cytokines, but their induction takes place over a slow time course (Mackiewicz et al. 1987). This phenomenon is not restricted to AGP. A further change to the carbohydrate that depends on activation status of secreting cells is the presence of a sialyl Lewis X structure on a percentage of AGP glycans, although this too is not restricted to AGP (De Graaf et al. 1993). It is possible that this acts to inhibit selectin-mediated effects at the endothelium. An immunomodulating capacity has been reported; however, this is still contentious and, although AGP is reported to prevent TNFα or LPS septic shock under some circumstances, this is not always observed in different models. Other reported observations include an inhibition of lymphocyte proliferation and a selective alteration in permeability of endothelia.

One alternative possibility that is attractive and for which there is limited evidence is that it may act to bind and inactivate pathogens that would use such N-linked glycans to bind to endothelia or gain entry to cells, e.g. a nonspecific resistance to infections such as that with *Klebsiella pneumoniae* (Hochepied et al. 2000). This may be related to the property of certain pathogen adhesins to bind to N-linked sugars.

CERULOPLASMIN

This protein is named after its blue color as a result of the copper it contains. It requires the copper for function but is not involved in transport of this metal despite the fact that it contains the bulk of plasma copper. Rather it has ferroxidase activity and is involved in the release of iron from stores. This property came to light following the discovery of a neurodegenerative deficiency disease (aceruloplasminemia) (Yoshida et al. 1995; Hellman and Gitlin 2002).

Negative APPs

There is no obvious reason why a protein such as albumin should be reduced in the APR; nevertheless this process is a controlled one in which the synthesis rate is reduced. This active downregulation is through transcriptional and post-transcriptional control (Perlmutter et al. 1986). The most plausible reason for this is that, although there is an overall increase in protein synthesis rate by the hepatocyte during the APR, the required switch towards the upregulated proteins requires extra capacity which can be achieved only by downregulating synthesis of this major serum protein.

Transthyretin was previously called prealbumin and functions to transport retinol-binding protein and thyroxine. Transferrin transports iron but it is reduced in the acute phase, presumably to reduce availability of iron for microorganisms that usually have a greater affinity for the iron it carries. The transferrin receptor is responsible for uptake into those tissues that require the iron.

Liver protective responses

Following inflammatory stimulation the hepatocyte also starts to produce a number of other enzymes and proteins that have host-protective function. Inducible nitric oxide synthase (iNOS) was first identified in hepatocytes and has an ability to protect the hepatocyte against injury in severe sepsis. Raised plasma nitric oxide is observed in a number of inflammatory conditions. Another enzyme produced in hepatocytes, as well as other cells such as endothelial cells, is heme oxygenase which has been demonstrated to have a protective role against stress from oxidative conditions and to reduce inflammation (Willis et al. 1996). This enzyme is responsible for reducing the effects of iron released from heme-containing enzymes (Ferris et al. 1999). Its main role may lie in protecting not only hepatocytes but also endothelial cells from injury.

Metallothionein is an intracellular low-molecular-weight protein that appears to have several functions, including protection against heavy metal and oxidant damage, or metabolism and control of zinc (Coyle et al. 2002). Two isoforms are induced in hepatocytes in response to IL-6, as well as other stimuli such as metals or drugs. An increase in zinc content in hepatocytes is mirrored by a hypozincemia.

Clinical use of APPs and inflammation markers

The most commonly used marker of APR has traditionally been the erythrocyte sedimentation rate (ESR), which is simple to perform but suffers from problems that affect results, such as anemia, and an increase with age. It has been considered that the major factor behind the ESR is the concentration of fibrinogen, which is slower to react than some of the faster APPs. Mainly for these reasons and the increase in sensitivity of assays, CRP is currently the best marker of severity of inflammation. There are, however, exceptions to the rule that CRP reflects inflammation in, for example, systemic lupus erythematosus (SLE) when CRP levels are not increased (Pepys et al. 1982). As a measure of inflammation, SAA may be slightly more sensitive for particular diseases (Malle and de Beer 1996) but is more difficult to measure for a number of technical reasons, including a difficulty in generating good antibodies that are specific for the acute phase form, and do not recognize the constitutive form. Certain cytokines have been reported to have levels that correlate with severity of inflammation but in general they suffer from problems of rapid fluctuation, with the result that even the better ones, such as IL-6, are unlikely to be used in preference to CRP. In the future other markers may be used that provide more information than the current nonspecific ones, e.g. procalcitonin may be useful because it reacts faster than CRP and is induced only by infection and not by other sterile inflammatory stimuli (Chirouze et al. 2002; Reinhart et al. 2002). Alternately, proteins specific for damage to particular organs or cells have been investigated, although to date little improvement on CRP has been found either for any specific inflammatory disease or to be specific to particular cell types or locations. Neonatal tissues also appear capable of an APR and APPs can be used as markers of infection (Dollner et al. 2001).

High-sensitivity CRP assays that measure higher levels within the normal range revealed that higher CRP was a risk factor for coronary heart disease. In addition, statin therapy, which reduces coronary events, also reduces CRP (Ridker et al. 2001). Following this a number of potential markers of vascular inflammation have been examined, e.g. sICAM-1, IL-6, TNFα, and soluble P-selectin, all of which indicate an increased vascular risk in a number of clinical settings (reviewed in Blake and Ridker 2001). The APR is largely unaffected by age although baseline levels of CRP increase slightly with age. CRP has been identified at lesion sites; however, other APPs such a fibrinogen are also associated with atherosclerosis. As CRP is raised in a number of subclinical conditions, the value of such low level CRP determinations may be more than currently appreciated.

The APR may have effects on other markers used to assess, for example, nutritional status. Vitamin A measurement in serum is also somewhat confused by the fact that the carrier transthyretin and retinol-binding protein are negative APPs and thus serum carriage of vitamin A may be reduced as a result. Transferrin receptor and ferritin may be used to measure iron deficiency but transferrin receptor may have the advantage that it is not subject to the confusion caused by potential APP responses of the ferritin.

HEMOPOIETIC RESPONSES

Lymphocytes

The APR includes increases in glucocorticoids and catecholamines, which have considerable effect on the thymus causing a large increase in apoptosis (Haeryfar and Berczi 2001). This may reflect the greater importance of diverting resources to the immediate and innate immune mechanisms rather than promoting long-term adaptive immune responses.

Polymorphonuclear cells

The leukocytosis that occurs in even comparatively mild inflammatory conditions results in an increased release of cells from the bone marrow and a consequent rise in the concentration in the circulation. As the movement from the bone marrow to the circulation under the control of cytokines, such as IL-6, granulocyte–macrophage colony-stimulating factor (GM-CSF), and G-CSF and others, continues and severity of inflammation increases, less mature forms ($CD34^+$) can migrate into the circulation (Liu et al. 1997). The increase in numbers thus outweighs the disappearance of these cells into the site of inflammation or increased apoptosis rates. This response provides rapid supplementation of cells, the function of which is to kill microorganisms. The cytokine control of release of cell type is best seen in asthma or helminth infections. IL-6-deficient mice have normal circulating neutrophil numbers but do not show leukocytosis to *Listeria monocytogenes* and are thus more susceptible to this infection (Dalrymple et al. 1995).

Other cells

Although there are no initial changes in red cell numbers after a prolonged inflammatory response resulting from autoimmune stimuli, chronic infection, or cancer, a reduced number of erythrocytes are seen in circulation which is often called the anemia of chronic disease. This results from a combination of factors such as reduced iron, removal of cells by phagocytosis, reduction in synthesis rate in bone marrow, and reduced erythropoietin, several of which are influenced by proinflammatory cytokines (Bron et al. 2001).

Circulating monocytic cells are increased during the first 24 h and this increase comes from an increased rate of release from the bone marrow, which cannot be caused by the stores of cells because there are limited supplies, but rather result from an increased cell cycle turnover. This is controlled by M-CSF as has been seen in phase I trials of M-CSF (Weiner et al. 1994).

Platelets are also increased during an inflammatory state and thrombocytosis correlates with IL-6. Thombocytosis is controlled by thrombopoietin (TPO), which is removed by platelets themselves. IL-6 does not appear directly to regulate platelet counts but rather induces TPO because IL-6 induction of platelet increases can be prevented by neutralization of TPO (Kaser et al. 2001). TPO may thus be considered an APP (Cerutti et al. 1999).

METABOLIC CHANGES

Lipid metabolism

The lipoprotein changes that occur in different species can vary, so the following references are all to humans except where indicated. One of the major changes is the hypertriglyceridemia, largely because of the increase in very-low-density lipoprotein (VLDL) through reduced clearance or increased production (Feingold et al. 1992). Driven by cytokines such as TNFα, IL-1, and IL-6, the hepatocyte increases synthesis of fatty acid which is esterified and incorporated into VLDL. At high concentrations, LPS from bacterial infection has the ability to inhibit lipoprotein lipase, an enzyme responsible for clearance of triglyceride-rich VLDL (Feingold et al. 1992). There are other changes in the VLDL during inflammation, such as an increased sphingolipid content, which also reduce clearance (Krauss et al. 1990). At the same time there is a decreased hepatic lipase and tissue expression of apolipoprotein E.

HDL and LDL are decreased during an APR whereas VLDL levels are increased. The HDL apolipoproteins apo-AI and apo-AII are both negative APPs and HDL content is decreased and replaced with other proteins such as SAA and apo-J. The role of apo-J is not known. The HDL-cholesterol is thus also reduced. The HDL that circulates is depleted in cholesterol ester but has higher free cholesterol, triglyceride, and sphingolipid (Auerbach and Parks 1989).

During an APR the anti-inflammatory and antioxidative properties of HDL are reduced. The reason for this is not entirely clear but a possible explanation is that it may be related to a decrease in content of certain enzymes such as paraoxanase or PAF acetylhydrolase (Feingold et al. 1998). Equally it may be that HDL takes up a number of inflammatory lipids or oxidized lipids released into the circulation. The cholesterol ester and total cholesterol content of acute phase HDL is lower than normal, although the reason is uncertain and the free cholesterol, triglyceride, and sphingolipid are increased.

Protein metabolism

The most obvious change that occurs dependent on proinflammatory cytokine action is muscle protein degradation, although a decreased rate of both myofibrillar and sarcoplasmic protein synthesis also contributes. There is a negative nitrogen balance that occurs in systemic inflammation which results in body weight loss. The cytokines responsible for this weight loss are thought to be TNFα, IL-1, IL-6, etc. The degradation of muscle protein provides amino acids and the hepatocyte increases amino acid uptake in order to cope with the increased protein synthesis and secretion (reviewed in Fischer et al. 1995). The synthesis of such an array of APPs is thought to give rise to a deficiency in sulfur-containing amino acids which are in particular demand (Grimble and Grimble 1998). Nevertheless, as previously indicated by the fact that the APPs are still synthesized in protein malnutrition states, APP synthesis is largely preserved. Rather the lack of these amino acids tends to affect glutathione synthesis to a greater extent (Grimble and Grimble 1998). Another amino acid of particular importance during inflammation is glutamine, which is essential for immune function in critically ill individuals (Andrews and Griffiths 2002).

Micronutrient changes

There are several levels of interaction between micronutrients and inflammation because the inflammation itself can reduce availability of micronutrients, and in the reverse direction micronutrient deficiency may alter the severity of inflammation and the ability to generate inflammatory mediators. It is perhaps also necessary to say that assessment of micronutrient status is frequently based on blood analysis and this, as has already been shown, is heavily dependent on carrier proteins in the serum. An example of this is vitamin A which is reduced in serum during inflammation because of reduced levels of carrier protein; this must be taken into account when assessing vitamin status. The deficiency of vitamin A does, however, also lead to a more inflammatory response (Wiedermann et al. 1996) – an effect that may be the result of an alteration of cytokines and expansion of myeloid cells (Kuwata et al. 2000).

Other micronutrients affected by inflammation include the levels of zinc, iron, and copper which are all decreased by inflammation. Again many of these reductions may not reflect whole body levels but are likely to reflect available levels for peripheral or immune cells. The decrease is related to the increased production of metallothionein in the liver (Cousins and Leinart 1988). The effect of zinc depletion may have adverse effects on the immune system and may relate to a switch to a more Th2-like phenotypic response to infection (Prasad 2000). Selenium has recently been shown to be important for effective responses, particularly to viral illness (Beck and Levander 2000), and is also reduced during acute inflammation (Maehira et al. 2002); this may also be the reason for reduced glutathione through alteration in selenium availability for selenium-containing antioxidant enzymes such as glutathione peroxidase and thioredoxin reductase. Selenium deficiency appears to reduce the synthesis of a set of hepatocyte-produced proteins in rats (Fischer et al. 2001).

HORMONAL CHANGES

In inflammatory conditions, the major endocrine changes are increased plasma concentration of glucagon, glucocorticoid, and catecholamine. One of the major changes that occurs is stimulation of the hypothalamic, pituitary, and adrenal glands in an ordered manner. This occurs after cytokine stimulation and involves alteration in certain hormones and leads to the induction of the controlling glucocorticoids such as prednisolone or cortisol (see Figure 12.4, p. 198). Loss of mediators such as corticotropin-releasing hormone reduces but does not prevent responses (Jacobson et al. 2000). Cytokines also induce the production of corticotropin-releasing factor (CRF). This has recently been found to be important not just for its ability to generate ACTH in the pituitary and then in turn corticosteroid in the adrenal cortex, but also because it can act on immune cells and has an anti-inflammatory action on a number of immune cells that express one of the receptors for CRF (Casadevall et al. 1999). The changes in such hormones can stimulate the metabolic changes seen in infection or inflammation (Bessey et al. 1984). Although the glucocorticoids increase in the acute phase there is a reduced production of mineralocorticoids and androgens. Triiodothyronine (T3) and thyroxine (T4) are reduced during the acute phase (Woloski and Jamieson 1987). Sex steroids are also changed, with some increased and some decreased.

Immunostimulatory hormones such as prolactin, growth hormone (GH), and insulin-like growth factor 1 (IGF-1) are suppressed. The reduction in the concentrations of GH and IGF-1 or the reduction in the ability of cells to respond may be part of the reason for the protein imbalance that leads to catabolism of muscle and synthesis of APPs.

Arginine vasopressin (AVP) is stimulated by IL-6 and this causes hyponatremia by increasing water reabsorption. AVP is also synthesized within the hypothalamus in response to cytokines and acts in a synergistic way with CRF (Chikanza et al. 2000). Prolactin is synthesized in the pituitary, and both prolactin and AVP have generally proinflammatory effects (Chikanza et al. 2000). CRF also induces α-melanocyte-stimulating hormone (αMSH) in the pituitary, which is an anti-inflammatory hormone acting on several tissues.

Procalcitonin is a 13-kDa precursor of the hormone calcitonin. The gene *calc-1* gives rise to an intracellular protein that can be secreted. Following infection-induced inflammation it becomes elevated about 4 h after endotoxin administration and is back to normal after about 24 h; as previously indicated under Clinical use of APPs and inflammation markers, it may have value in that its induction appears to be specific to infectious inflammation. Under normal conditions, expression is limited to the thyroid but in sepsis all tissues and particularly parenchymal cells produce it (Muller et al. 2001a), although the reason for infection specificity is not clear. Its function is also somewhat unclear, with some reports suggesting that it may have cytokine/chemokine-like properties and others hormonal properties. It appears to reduce survival in models of systemic infection (Nylen et al. 1998).

Leptin is a hormonal protein that is synthesized in the adipocyte which at least in some circumstances appears to behave as an APP. The 16-kDa protein is similar in structure to the IL-6 family (Fantuzzi and Faggioni 2000). The leptin receptor present on target cells also has similarity to IL-6 receptors because it is a gp130-containing complex; despite this leptin has not been shown to have any ability to induce hepatic APP synthesis. The role that led to the gene's discovery in obese mice is one of lipid metabolism control. This relates to the fact that larger fat stores produce more leptin, which then regulate appetite and energy expenditure through specific areas of the brain. Conversely, when leptin is low hunger is stimulated, and this may relate to the fact that hunger is depressed during inflammatory episodes when leptin is stimulated (Faggioni et al. 2001).

However, this is not the only function because the obese leptin-deficient mice have several other defects. It has been demonstrated that immune responses are also inhibited in the absence of leptin such as reduced phagocytosis by macrophages, which leads to a impaired host defense to gram-negative pneumonia (Mancuso et al. 2002).

FEVER AND OTHER BEHAVIORAL CHANGES

The process of fever is thought to be beneficial because overall it is more harmful to the microorganism than the host and may put additional stress on the microorganism inducing, for example, heat shock proteins (Hasday et al. 2000). Some animal models support an increased resistance at higher temperature. An alternate concept is that it favors mammalian membrane function.

It is reasonable to assume that somnolence will reduce energy expenditure to allow redirection of resources to fight infection and for tissue repair. It is possible that similar arguments might also account for anorexia, because a fit host would have sufficient protein resource to survive a sufficient time to control infection.

CONTROL OF SYSTEMIC INFLAMMATION

Current new therapies designed to inhibit inflammation are often intended to have an effect at local level to control damage done to specific organs or structures as, for example, in rheumatoid arthritis. In part this research is driven by the fact that the current most powerful anti-inflammatory drugs are steroids, which have considerable metabolic side effects. It is also clear, however, that these treatments also reduce the inflammation systemically. The range of different approaches to inhibit inflammation has also increased. Recently the use of soluble TNF receptor or humanized monoclonal antibody to TNFα has been shown to be an effective treatment for rheumatoid arthritis, Crohn's disease, and psoriasis (Elliott et al. 1994; Moreland et al. 2001). Currently inhibitors of intracellular signaling pathways such as the MAP kinase pathway are in trial. All of these approaches can reduce the APR including the APPs, leukocyte activation and migration, fever, etc. Not all these approaches will have exactly the same inhibitory effect but, with the reduction in inflammation, there may also come a risk that removal of some of these responses may have deleterious effects. At least at some level all these effects are likely to be beneficial to host function, particularly in terms of response to infection; to remove them may therefore increase risks of infection, although at least for TNFα blockade this appears to be a rare phenomenon.

The statins introduced to reduce cholesterol in atherosclerosis have been found to have an ability not only to reduce LDL cholesterol but also to reduce CRP and other APPs such as fibrinogen and SAA (Staels et al. 1998; Ridker et al. 2001). This control may be exerted through the peroxisome proliferator receptor α (PPARα), which not only alters lipid metabolism but has an anti-inflammatory role. It is possible that such effects are through transcription factors that induce CRP (Kleeman et al. 2003). In any event such treatment may be useful in other diseases that have an inflammatory component such as Alzheimer's disease, diabetes mellitus, or osteoporosis.

DISORDERS OF THE ACUTE PHASE RESPONSE

AA Amyloidosis

Serum amyloid A can, when present in high amounts for sufficient length of time (as, for example, in chronic diseases such as Crohn's disease or rheumatoid arthritis), give rise to deposits of a structurally altered AA amyloid protein that is resistant to degradation. This is thus one of the many forms of the amyloidosis diseases in which stable protein fibrils are deposited in vital organs. Although many of these amyloidoses can resolve they are capable, for example in AA amyloid, of destroying renal function and causing death if the balance remains in favor of deposition. These proteins are linked by the ability to switch conformation towards a β-pleated sheet-rich form that has resistance to degradation. In the case of SAA this is often accompanied by a cleavage of approximately 30 amino acids from the C-terminal end of the protein. Techniques to allow visualization of deposition of amyloid has demonstrated that AA amyloid deposits can regress (Hawkins et al. 1993) and more recently that depletion of the SAP component has the potential to be therapeutically useful (Pepys et al. 2002)

APP deficiences

As previously mentioned, deficiency in some anti-proteases leads to disease (see α_1-Antitrypsin or α_1-protease inhibitor). So far no patient with a deficiency of certain proteins such as CRP has been reported. However, the number of reports of deficiencies of particular APPs is increasing and, together with information from knock-out mice, the role of some of the proteins is in many cases not only confirming previous ideas but also providing some unexpected new observations.

Osteoporosis

Associated with increased proinflammatory cytokine levels, the balance of bone resorption and synthesis moves towards resorption. There is thus a tendency towards osteoporosis. A number of proinflammatory cytokines and some newly discovered members of the TNF family regulate this process (Rodan and Martin 2000).

Systemic inflammation and shock

The ultimate effect of an uncontrolled APR is shock (see Chapter 34, Shock/sepsis). Associated with such severe systemic inflammation, a further complication that may arise is acute respiratory distress syndrome. Sufficiently severe inflammation can also have the effect of apparently reducing immune responses (Lederer et al. 1999; Faunce et al. 2003). Lung function is compromised and so far one of the more promising ways of treating this is the use of neutrophil elastase inhibitors – a number of other potential treatments such as PAF antagonists having failed to have significant effect in clinical trials (Eaton and Martin 2002). There is considerable interest in some proteins that behave as APPs which seem to amplify the systemic inflammation. One such is high mobility group 1 protein (HMGB1) which can activate cells when released from necrotic cells. It is normally a nuclear protein which when released can behave as a cytokine (Andersson et al. 2002; Scaffidi et al. 2002). It is possible that this and other late mediators of inflammation might be more effective targets.

REFERENCES

Akira, S., Isshiki, H., et al. 1990. A nuclear factor for IL-6 expression (NF-IL6) is a member of a C/EBP family. *EMBO J*, **9**, 1897–906.

Alonzi, T., Maritano, D., et al. 2001. Essential role for STAT3 in the control of the acute phase response as revealed by inducible gene activation in the liver. *Mol Cell Biol*, **21**, 1621–32.

Andersson, U., Eriandsson-Harris, H., et al. 2002. HMGB1 as a DNA-binding cytokine. *J Leukocyte Biol*, **72**, 1084–91.

Andreani, M., Olivier, J.L., et al. 2000. Transcriptional regulation of inflammatory secreted phospholipases A(2). *Biochim Biophys Acta*, **31**, 149–58.

Andrews, F.J. and Griffiths, R.D. 2002. Glutamine: essential for immune function in the critically ill. *Br J Nutr*, **87**, S3–8.

Auerbach, B.J. and Parks, J.S. 1989. Lipoprotein abnormalities associated with lipopolysaccharide-induced lecithin: cholesterol acyltransferase and lipase deficiency. *J Biol Chem*, **264**, 10264–70.

Baugh, J.A. and Bucala, R. 2002. Macrophage migration inhibitory factor. *Crit Care Med*, **30**, S27–35.

Baumann, H., Prowse, K.R., et al. 1989. Stimulation of hepatic acute phase response by cytokines and glucocorticoids. *Ann NY Acad Sci*, **557**, 280–95.

Bayne, C.J. and Gerwick, L. 2001. The acute phase response and innate immunity of fish. *Dev Comp Immunol*, **25**, 725–43.

Beck, M.A. and Levander, O.A. 2000. Host nutritional status and its effect on a viral pathogen. *J Infect Dis*, **182**, S93–6.

Beishuizen, A., Thijs, L.G., et al. 2001. Macrophage migration inhibitory factor and hypothalamo-pituitary-adrenal function during critical illness. *J Clin Endocrinol Metab*, **86**, 2811–16.

Bernard, G.R., Vincent, J.L., et al. 2001. Efficacy and safety of recombinant human activated protein, C, for severe sepsis. *N Engl J Med*, **344**, 699–709.

Bessey, P.Q., Watters, J.M., et al. 1984. Combined hormonal infusion stimulates the metabolic response to injury. *Ann Surg*, **200**, 264–81.

Bevan, S. and Raynes, J.G. 1991. IL-1 receptor antagonist regulation of acute phase protein synthesis in human hepatoma cells. *J Immunol*, **147**, 2573–8.

Binder, R.J., Karimeddini, D. and Srivastava, P.K. 2001. Adjuvanticity of α2-macroglobulin, an independent ligand for the heat shock protein receptor CD91. *J Immunol*, **166**, 4968–72.

Blake, G.J. and Ridker, P.M. 2001. Novel clinical markers of vascular wall inflammation. *Circ Res*, **89**, 763–71.

Bodman-Smith, K.B., Melendez, A.J., et al. 2002. C-reactive protein-mediated phagocytosis and phospholipase D signalling through the high-affinity receptor for immunoglobulin G (FcgammaRI). *Immunology*, **107**, 252–60.

Bozza, M., Satoskar, A.R., et al. 1999. Targetted disruption of MIF gene reveals its critical role in sepsis. *J Exp Med*, **189**, 341–6.

Brasier, A.R., Recinos, A. and Eledrisi, M.S. 2002. Vascular inflammation and the renin-angiotensin system. *Arterioscler Thromb Vasc Biol*, **22**, 1257–66.

Bron, D., Meuleman, N. and Mascaux, C. 2001. Biological basis of anemia. *Semin Oncol*, **28**, S1–6.

Calder, P.C. and Grimble, R.F. 2002. Polyunsaturated fatty acids, inflammation and immunity. *Eur J Clin Nutr*, **56**, S14–19.

Campos, S.P. and Baumann, H. 1992. Insulin is a prominent modulator of the cytokine-stimulated expression of acute-phase plasma protein genes. *Mol Cell Biol*, **12**, 1789–97.

Carrell, R.W. and Lomas, D.A. 2002. Alpha1-antitrypsin deficiency – a model for conformational diseases. *N Engl J Med*, **346**, 45–53.

Casadevall, M., Saperas, E., et al. 1999. Mechanisms underlying the anti-inflammatory actions of central corticotropin releasing factor. *Am J Physiol*, **276**, G1016–1026.

Cerutti, A., Custodi, P., et al. 1999. Circulating thrombopoietin in reactive conditions behaves like an acute phase reactant. *Clin Lab Haematol*, **21**, 271–5.

Chikanza, I.C., Petrou, P. and Chrousos, G. 2000. Perturbations of arginine vasopressin secretion during inflammatory stress. Pathophysiologic implications. *Ann NY Acad Sci*, **917**, 825–34.

Chirouze, C., Schuhmacher, H., et al. 2002. Low serum procalcitonin level accurately predicts the absence of bacteraemia in adult patients with acute fever. *Clin Infect Dis*, **35**, 156–61.

Coetzee, G.A., Strachan, A.F., et al. 1986. Serum amyloid A containing human HDL 3. Density, size and apolipoprotein composition. *J Biol Chem*, **261**, 9644–51.

Colotta, F., Re, F., et al. 1993. Interleukin-1 type II receptor: a decoy target for IL-1 that is regulated by IL-4. *Science*, **261**, 472–5.

Cousins, R.J. and Leinart, A.S. 1988. Tissue-specific regulation of zinc metabolism and metallothionein genes by interleukin 1. *FASEB J*, **2**, 2884–90.

Coyle, P., Philcox, J.C., et al. 2002. Metallothionein: the multipurpose protein. *Cell Mol Life Sci*, **59**, 627–47.

Culley, F.J., Harris, R.A., et al. 1996. C-reactive protein binds to a novel ligand on *Leishmania donovani* and increases uptake into human macrophages. *J Immunol*, **156**, 4691–6.

Culley, F.J., Bodman-Smith, K.B., et al. 2000. C-reactive protein binds to phosphorylated carbohydrates. *Glycobiology*, **10**, 59–65.

Daiger, S.P., Schanfield, M.S. and Cavallli-Sforza, L.L. 1975. Group-specific component (Gc) proteins bind vitamin, D, and 25-hydroxyvitamin D. *Proc Natl Acad Sci USA*, **72**, 2076–80.

Dalrymple, S.A., Lucien, L.A., et al. 1995. IL-6 deficient mice are highly susceptible to *L. monocytogenes* infection: correlation with inefficient neutrophilia. *Infect Immunol*, **63**, 2262.

De Graaf, T.W., Van der Stelt, M.E., et al. 1993. Inflammation-induced expression of sialyl Lewis X-containing glycan structures on alpha 1-acid glycoprotein (orosomucoid) in human sera. *J Exp Med*, **177**, 657–66.

Doherty, J.F., Golden, M.H., et al. 1993. Acute-phase protein response is impaired in severely malnourished children. *Clin Sci (Lond)*, **84**, 169–75.

Doherty, J.F., Golden, M.H., et al. 1994. Production of interleukin-6 and tumour necrosis factor-alpha in vitro is reduced in whole blood of severely malnourished children. *Clin Sci*, **86**, 347–51.

Dollner, H., Vatten, L. and Austgulen, R. 2001. Early diagnostic markers for neonatal sepsis: comparing C-reactive protein, interleukin-6, soluble tumour necrosis factor receptors and soluble adhesion molecules. *J Clin Epidemiol*, **54**, 1251–7.

Doolittle, R.F. 1984. Fibrinogen and fibrin. *Annu Rev Biochem*, **53**, 195–229.

Drew, A.F., Liu, H., et al. 2001. Wound-healing defects in mice lacking fibrinogen. *Blood*, **97**, 3691–8.

Du Clos, T.W. and Mold, C. 2001. The role of C-reactive protein in the resolution of bacterial infection. *Curr Opin Infect Dis*, **14**, 289–93.

Dumoutier, L., Van Roost, E., et al. 2000a. Human IL-10-related, T-cell-derived inducible factor; molecular cloning and functional characterization as an hepatocyte stimulating factor. *Proc Natl Acad Sci USA*, **97**, 10144–9.

Dumoutier, L., Louahed, J. and Renauld, J.C. 2000b. Cloning and characterization of IL-10-related, T, cell-derived inducible factor (IL-TIF), a novel cytokine structurally related to IL-10 and inducible by IL-9. *J Immunol*, **164**, 1814–19.

Dumoutier, L., Lejeune, D., et al. 2001. Cloning and characterisation of IL-22 binding protein, a natural antagonist of IL-10 related-T-cell derived inducible factor/IL-22. *J Immunol*, **166**, 7090–5.

Eaton, S. and Martin, G. 2002. Clinical developments for treating ARDS. *Expert Opin Invest Drugs*, **11**, 37–48.

Edbrooke, M.R., Burt, D.W., et al. 1989. Identification of cis-acting sequences responsible for phorbol ester induction of human serum amyloid A gene expression via a nuclear factor kappaB-like transcription factor. *Mol Cell Biol*, **9**, 1908–16.

Elliott, M.J., Maini, R.N., et al. 1994. Randomised double-blind comparison of chimeric monoclonal antibody to tumour necrosis factor alpha (cA2) versus placebo in rheumatoid arthritis. *Lancet*, **344**, 1105–10.

Emsley, J., White, H.E., et al. 1994. Structure of pentameric human serum amyloid P component. *Nature*, **367**, 338–45.

Esmon, C.T. 2000. Does inflammation contribute to thrombotic events? *Haemostasis*, **30**, suppl 2, 34–40.

Ezekovitz, R.A.B., Day, L.E. and Herman, G.A. 1988. A human mannose binding protein is an acute phase phase reactant that shares sequence homology with other vertebrate lectins. *J Exp Med*, **167**, 1034–46.

Faber, J.P., Poller, W., et al. 1993. The molecular basis of α1-antichymotrypsin deficiency in a heterozygote with liver and lung disease. *J Hepatol*, **18**, 313–21.

Faggioni, R., Feingold, K.R. and Grunfeld, C. 2001. Leptin regulation of the immune response and the immunodeficiency of malnutrition. *FASEB J*, **15**, 2565–71.

Fantuzzi, G. and Faggioni, R. 2000. Leptin in the regulation of immunity, inflammation and hematopoiesis. *J Leukocyte Biol*, **68**, 437–46.

Fantuzzi, G., Ku, G., et al. 1997. Response to local inflammation of IL-1 beta-converting enzyme-deficient mice. *J Immunol*, **158**, 1818–24.

Fattori, E., Cappelletti, M., et al. 1994. Defective inflammatory response in IL-6 deficient mice. *J Exp Med*, **180**, 1243–50.

Faunce, D.E., Garnelli, R.L., et al. 2003. A role for CD1d restricted NKT cells in injury associated T cell suppression. *J Leucocyte Biol*, **73**, 747–55.

Feingold, K.R., Staprans, I., et al. 1992. Endotoxin rapidly induces changes in lipid metabolism that produce hypertriglyceridemia: low doses stimulate hepatic triglyceride production while high doses inhibit clearance. *J Lipid Res*, **33**, 1765–76.

Feingold, K.R., Memon, R.A., et al. 1998. Paraoxonase activity in the serum and hepatic mRNA levels decrease during the acute phase response. *Atherosclerosis*, **139**, 307–15.

Ferris, C.D., Jaffrey, S.R., et al. 1999. Haem oxygenase-1 prevents cell death by regulating cellular iron. *Nat Cell Biol*, **1**, 152–7.

Fierer, J., Swancutt, M.A., et al. 2002. The role of lipopolysaccharide binding protein in resistance to *Salmonella* infections in mice. *J Immunol*, **68**, 6396–403.

Fischer, C.P., Bode, B.P., et al. 1995. Hepatic uptake of glutamine and other amino acids during infection and inflammation. *Shock*, **3**, 315–22.

Fischer, A., Paullauf, J., et al. 2001. Effect of selenium and vitamin, A, deficiency on differential gene expression in liver. *Biochem Biophys Res Commun*, **285**, 470–5.

Fournier, T., Medjoubi, N.N. and Porquet, D. 2000. Alpha-1-acid glycoprotein. *Biochim Biophys Acta*, **1482**, 157–71.

Gabay, C., Singwe, M., et al. 1996. Circulating levels of IL-11 and LIF do not significantly participate in the production of acute phase proteins by the liver. *Clin Exp Immunol*, **105**, 260–5.

Gabay, C., Gigley, J., et al. 2001. Production of IL-1 receptor antagonist by hepatocytes is regulated as an acute-phase protein in vivo. *Eur J Immunol*, **31**, 490–9.

Garlanda, C., Hirsch, E., et al. 2002. Non-redundant role of the long pentraxin PTX3 in anti-fungal innate immune response. *Nature*, **420**, 182–6.

Gauldie, J., Richards, C., et al. 1987. Interferon beta 2/B-cell stimulatory factor type 2 shares identity with monocyte-derived hepatocyte-stimulating factor and regulates the major acute phase protein response in liver cells. *Proc Natl Acad Sci USA*, **84**, 7251–5.

Gershov, D., Kim, S., et al. 2000. C-Reactive protein binds to apoptotic cells, protects the cells from assembly of the terminal complement components, and sustains an antiinflammatory innate immune response: implications for systemic autoimmunity. *J Exp Med*, **192**, 1353–64.

Greenfeder, S.A., Nunes, P., et al. 1995. Molecular cloning and characterization of a second subunit of the interleukin 1 receptor complex. *J Biol Chem*, **270**, 13757–65.

Grehan, S., Uhlar, C.M., et al. 1997. Expression of a biologically active recombinant mouse IL-1 receptor antagonist and its use in vivo to modulate aspects of the acute phase response. *J Immunol*, **159**, 369–78.

Grimble, R.F. and Grimble, G.K. 1998. Immunonutrition: role of sulfur amino acids, related amino acids, and polyamines. *Nutrition*, **14**, 605–10.

Haeryfar, S.M. and Berczi, I. 2001. The thymus and the acute phase response. *Cell Mol Biol (Noisy-le-grand)*, **47**, 145–56.

Hannum, C.H., Wilcox, C.J., et al. 1990. Interleukin-1 receptor antagonist activity of a human interleukin-1 inhibitor. *Nature*, **343**, 336–40.

Hasday, J.D., Fairchild, K.D. and Shanholtz, C. 2000. The role of fever in the infected host. *Microbes Infect*, **2**, 1891–904.

Haverkate, F., Thompson, S.G., et al. 1997. Production of C-reactive protein and risk of coronary events in stable and unstable angina. European Concerted Action on Thrombosis and Disabilities Angina Pectoris Study Group. *Lancet*, **349**, 462–6.

Hawkins, P.N., Richardson, S., et al. 1993. Serum amyloid P component scintigraphy and turnover studies for diagnosis and monitoring of AA amyloidosis in juvenile rheumatoid arthritis. *Arthritis Rheum*, **36**, 842–51.

Hellman, N.E. and Gitlin, J.D. 2002. Ceruloplasmin metabolism and function. *Annu Rev Nutr*, **22**, 439–58.

Hiemstra, P.S. 2002. Antimicrobial activity of antiproteinases. *Biochem Soc Trans*, **30**, 116–20.

Hind, C.R., Collins, P.M., et al. 1984. Binding specificity of serum amyloid P component for the pyruvate acetal of galactose. *J Exp Med*, **159**, 1058–69.

Hochepied, T., Van Molle, W., et al. 2000. Involvement of the acute phase protein alpha 1-acid glycoprotein in nonspecific resistance to a lethal gram-negative infection. *J Biol Chem*, **275**, 14903–9.

Huntington, J.A., Read, R.J. and Carrell, R.W. 2000. Structure of a serpin-protease complex shows inhibition by deformation. *Nature*, **407**, 923–6.

Inui, A. 2001. Cytokines and sickness behavior: implications from knockout animal models. *Trends Immunol*, **22**, 469–73.

Israili, Z.H. and Dayton, P.G. 2001. Human alpha-1-glycoprotein and its interactions with drugs. *Drug Metab Rev*, **33**, 161–235.

Iwaki, D., Osaki, T., et al. 1999. Functional and structural diversities of C-reactive protein present in horseshoe crab hemolymph plasma. *Eur J Biochem*, **264**, 314–26.

Jack, R.S., Fan, X., et al. 1997. Lipopolysaccharide-binding protein is required to combat a murine gram-negative bacterial infection. *Nature*, **389**, 742–5.

Jacobson, L., Muglia, L.J., et al. 2000. CRH deficiency impairs but does not block pituitary-adrenal responses to diverse stressors. *Neuroendocrinology*, **71**, 79–87.

Joslin, G., Griffin, G.L., et al. 1992. The serpin-enzyme complex (SEC) receptor mediates the neutrophil chemotactic effect of alpha-1 antitrypsin-elastase complexes and amyloid-beta peptide. *J Clin Invest*, **90**, 1150–4.

Jostock, T., Mullberg, J., et al. 2001. Soluble gp130 is the natural inhibitor of soluble interleukin 6 receptor transsignalling responses. *Eur J Biochem*, **268**, 160–7.

Jennings, G., Bourgeois, C. and Elia, M. 1992. The magnitude of the acute phase protein response is attenuated by protein deficiency in rats. *J Nutr*, **122**, 1325–31.

Kaser, A., Brandacher, G., et al. 2001. Interleukin-6 stimulates thrombopoiesis through thrombopoietin: role in inflammatory thrombocytosis. *Blood*, **98**, 2720–5.

Kindy, M.S., De Beer, M.C., et al. 2000. Expression of mouse acute-phase (SAA1.1) and constitutive (SAA4) serum amyloid A isotypes: influence on lipoprotein profiles. *Arterioscler Thromb Vasc Biol*, **20**, 1543–50.

Kleeman, R., Gervois, P.P., et al. 2003. Fibrates down-regulate IL-1 stimulated C-reactive protein gene expression in hepatocytes by reducing nuclear p50-NFκB-C/EBP-β complex formation. *Blood*, **101**, 545–51.

Kleemann, R., Hausser, A., et al. 2000. Intracellular action of the cytokine MIF to modulate AP-1 activity and the cell cycle through Jab1. *Nature*, **408**, 211–16.

Kluger, M.J., Kozak, W., et al. 1998. The use of knockout mice to understand the role of cytokines in fever. *Clin Exp Pharmacol Physiol*, **25**, 141–4.

Koj, A., Guzdek, A., et al. 1995. Hepatocyte growth factor and retinoic acid exert opposite effects on synthesis of type 1 and type 2 acute phase proteins in rat hepatoma cells. *Int J Biochem Cell Biol*, **27**, 39–46.

Kopf, M., Baumman, H., et al. 1994. Impaired immune and acute phase responses in interleukin-6 deficient mice. *Nature*, **368**, 339–42.

Krauss, R.M., Grunfeld, C., et al. 1990. Tumor necrosis factor acutely increases plasma levels of very low density lipoproteins of normal size and composition. *Endocrinology*, **127**, 1016–21.

Kristiansen, M., Graversen, J.H., et al. 2001. Identification of the haemoglobin scavenger receptor. *Nature*, **409**, 198–201.

Kulander, L., Pauksens, K. and Venge, P. 2001. Soluble adhesion molecules, cytokines and cellular markers in serum in patients with acute infections. *Scand J Infect Dis*, **33**, 290–300.

Kushner, I. 1982. The phenomenon of the acute phase response. *Ann NY Acad Sci*, **389**, 39–48.

Kushner, I. and Feldmann, G. 1978. Control of the acute phase response. Demonstration of C-reactive protein synthesis and secretion by hepatocytes during acute inflammation in the rabbit. *J Exp Med*, **148**, 466–77.

Kuwata, T., Wang, I.M., et al. 2000. Vitamin A deficiency in mice causes a systemic expansion of myeloid cells. *Blood*, **95**, 3349–56.

Lambeau, G. and Lazdunski, M. 1999. Receptors for a growing family of phospholipases A_2. *Trends Pharm Sci*, **20**, 162–70.

Langlois, M.R. and Delanghe, J.R. 1996. Biological and clinical significance of haptoglobin polymorphism in humans. *Clin Chem*, **42**, 1589–600.

Lederer, J.A., Rodrick, M.L. and Mannick, J.A. 1999. The effects of injury on the adaptive immune response. *Shock*, **11**, 153–9.

Lee, W.M. and Galbraith, R.M. 1992. The extracellular actin-scavenger system and actin toxicity. *N Engl J Med*, **326**, 1335–41.

Leon, L.R. 2002. Molecular biology of thermoregulation. invited review of cytokine regulation of fever: studies using gene knockout mice. *J Appl Physiol*, **92**, 2648–55.

Leon, L.R., Kozak, W., et al. 1997. Exacerbated febrile responses to LPS, but not turpentine, in TNF double receptor-knockout mice. *Am J Physiol*, **272**, R563–569.

Li, Y.P., Mold, C. and Du Clos, T.W. 1994. Sublytic complement attack exposes C-reactive protein binding sites on cell membranes. *J Immunol*, **152**, 2995–3005.

Lieberman, J. 2000. Augmentation therapy reduces frequency of lung infections in antitrypsin deficiency: a new hypothesis with supporting data. *Chest*, **118**, 1480–5.

Libby, P., Ridker, P.M. and Maseri, A. 2002. Inflammation and atherosclerosis. *Circulation*, **105**, 1135–43.

Lim, S.K., Kim, H., et al. 1998. Increased susceptibility in Hp knockout mice during acute hemolysis. *Blood*, **92**, 1870–7.

Lin, Y., Rajala, M.W., et al. 2001. Hyperglycemia-induced production of acute phase reactants in adipose tissue. *J Biol Chem*, **276**, 42077–83.

Liu, F., Poursine-Laurent, J., et al. 1997. Interleukin-6 and the granulocyte colony-stimulating factor receptor are major independent regulators of granulopoiesis in vivo but are not required for lineage commitment or terminal differentiation. *Blood*, **90**, 2583–90.

Lomas, D.A., Evans, D.L., et al. 1992. The mechanism of Z alpha 1 antitrypsin in the liver. *Nature*, **357**, 605–7.

Loveless, W., O'Sullivan, G., et al. 1992. Human serum amyloid P is a multispecific adhesive protein whose ligands include 6-phosphorylated mannose and the 3-sulphated saccharides galactose, N-acetylgalactosamine and glucuronic acid. *EMBO J*, **11**, 813–19.

Lyoumi, S., Tamion, F., et al. 1998. Induction and modulation of acute phase response by protein malnutrition in rats; comparative effect of systemic and localised inflammation on IL-6 and acute phase protein synthesis. *J Nutr*, **128**, 166–74.

Mackie, M., Bennett, B., et al. 1978. Familial thrombosis: inherited deficiency of antithrombin III. *BMJ*, **21**, 136–8.

Mackiewicz, A., Ganapathi, M.K., et al. 1987. Monokines regulate glycosylation of acute-phase proteins. *J Exp Med*, **166**, 253–8.

Mackiewicz, A., Ganapathi, M.K., et al. 1990. Transforming growth factor beta 1 regulates production of acute-phase proteins. *Proc Natl Acad Sci USA*, **87**, 1491–5.

Mackiewicz, A., Schooltink, H., et al. 1992. Complex of soluble human IL-6-receptor/IL-6 up-regulates expression of acute-phase proteins. *J Immunol*, **149**, 2021–7.

Maehira, F., Luyo, G.A., et al. 2002. Alterations of serum selenium concentrations in the acute phase of pathological conditions. *Clin Chim Acta*, **316**, 137–46.

Maes, M., Delange, J., et al. 1997. Acute phase proteins in schizophrenia, mania and major depression; modulation by pyschotrophic drugs. *Psychiatry Res*, **66**, 1–11.

Malle, E. and de Beer, F.C. 1996. Human SAA: a prominent acute phase reactant for clinical practice. *Eur J Clin Invest*, **26**, 427–35.

Mancuso, P., Gottschalk, A., et al. 2002. Leptin-deficient mice exhibit impaired host-defense in gram-negative pneumonia. *J Immunol*, **168**, 4018–24.

Mantovani, A., Locati, M., et al. 2001. Decoy receptors: a strategy to regulate inflammatory cytokines and chemokines. *Trends Immunol*, **22**, 328–36.

Marnell, L.L., Mold, C., et al. 1995. C-reactive protein binds to Fc gamma RI in transfected COS cells. *J Immunol*, **155**, 2185–93.

Matsushita, M. and Fujita, T. 1992. Activation of the classical complement pathway by mannose-binding protein in association with a novel C1s-like serine protease. *J Exp Med*, **176**, 1497–502.

Meek, R.L. and Benditt, E.P. 1986. Amyloid A gene family expression in different mouse tissues. *J Exp Med*, **164**, 2006–17.

Minoguchi, M., Minoguchi, S., et al. 2003. STAP-2/BKS an adaptor/docking protein, modulates STAT3 activation in acute phase response through its YXXQ motif. *J Biol Chem*, **278**, 11182–9.

Moestrup, S.K. and Gliemann, J. 1989. Purification of the rat hepatic alpha 2-macroglobulin receptor as an approximately 440 kDa single chain protein. *J Biol Chem*, **264**, 15574–7.

Mold, C., Kingzette, M. and Gewurz, H. 1984. C-reactive protein inhibits pneumococcal activation of the alternative pathway by increasing the interaction between factor H and C3b. *J Immunol*, **133**, 882–5.

Mold, C., Gresham, H.D. and Du Clod, T.W. 2001. Serum amyloid P, component and C-reactive protein mediate phagocytosis through murine FcγRs. *J Immunol*, **166**, 1200–5.

Moreland, L.W., Cohen, S.B., et al. 2001. Long-term safety and efficacy of etanercept in patients with rheumatoid arthritis. *J Rheumatol*, **28**, 1238–44.

Morgan, L., Pipkin, F.B. and Kalsheker, N. 1996. Angiotensinogen: molecular biology, biochemistry and physiology. *Int J Biochem Cell Biol*, **28**, 1211–22.

Morlese, J.F., Forrester, T. and Jahoor, F. 1998. Acute phase protein response to infection in severe malnutrition. *Am J Physiol*, **275**, E112–117, (*Endocrinol Metab*, **38**).

Muller, B., White, J.C.N., et al. 2001a. Ubiquitous expression of the calcitonin 1 gene in multiple tissues in response to sepsis. *J Clin Endocrinol Metab*, **86**, 396–404.

Muller, B., Peri, G., et al. 2001b. Circulating levels of the long pentraxin PTX3 correlate with severity of infection in critically ill patients. *Crit Care Med*, **29**, 1404–7.

Murakami, M., Nakatani, Y., et al. 2000. Cellular components that functionally interact with signaling phospholipase A(2)s. *Biochim Biophys Acta*, **1488**, 159–66.

Nauta, A.J., Daha, M.R., et al. 2003. Recognition and clearance of apoptotic cells: a role for complement and pentraxins. *Trends Immunol*, **24**, 148–54.

Nemeth, E., Valore, E.V., et al. 2003. Hepcidin, a putative mediator of anemia of inflammation, is a type II acute-phase protein. *Blood*, **101**, 2461–3.

Netea, M.G., Kullberg, B.J. and van der Meer, J.W.M. 2000. Circulating cytokines as mediators of fever. *J Infect Dis*, **31**, S178–84.

Noyer, C.M., Immenschuh, S., et al. 1998. Initial heme uptake from albumin by short-term cultured rat hepatocytes is mediated by a transport mechanism differing from that of other organic anions. *Hepatology*, **28**, 150–5.

Nylen, E.S., Whang, K.T., et al. 1998. Mortality is increased by procalcitonin and decreased by an antiserum to procalcitonin in experimental sepsis. *Crit Care Med*, **26**, 1001–6.

Paonessa, G., Graziani, R., et al. 1995. Two distinct and independent sites on IL-6 trigger gp 130 dimer formation and signalling. *EMBO J*, **14**, 1942–51.

Pepys, M.B. and Baltz, M.L. 1983. Acute phase proteins with special reference to C-reactive protein and related proteins (pentaxins) and serum amyloid A protein. *Adv Immunol*, **34**, 141–212.

Pepys, M.B., Lanham, J.G. and de Beer, F.C. 1982. C-reactive protein in SLE. *Clin Rheum Dis*, **8**, 91–103.

Pepys, M.B. and Herbert, J. 2002. Targetted pharmacological depletion of serum amyloid P component for treatment of human amyloidosis. *Nature*, **417**, 231–3.

Perlmutter, D.H., Dinarello, C.A., et al. 1986. Cachectin/tumor necrosis factor regulates hepatic acute-phase gene expression. *J Clin Invest*, **78**, 1349–54.

Perlmutter, D.H., Joslin, G., et al. 1990. Endocytosis and degradation of alpha 1-antitrypsin-protease complexes is mediated by the serpin-enzyme complex (SEC) receptor. *J Biol Chem*, **265**, 16713–16.

Peters, M., Jacobs, S., et al. 1996. The function of the soluble interleukin6 (IL-6) receptor in vivo; sensitisation of human soluble IL-6 receptor transgenic mice towards IL6 and prolongation of the plasma half-life. *J Exp Med*, **183**, 1399–406.

Peterson, S.V., Thiel, S. and Jensenius, J.C. 2001. The mannan binding lectin pathway of complement activation: biology and disease association. *Mol Immunol*, **38**, 133–49.

Prasad, A.S. 2000. Effects of zinc deficiency on Th1 and Th2 cytokine shifts. *J Infect Dis*, **182**, S62–8.

Ramadori, G., Mitsch, A., et al. 1988. Alpha- and gamma-interferon (IFN alpha, IFN gamma) but not interleukin-1 (IL-1) modulate synthesis and secretion of beta 2-microglobulin by hepatocytes. *Eur J Clin Invest*, **18**, 343–51.

Raynes, J. 1982. Variations in the relative proportions of microheterogeneous forms of plasma glycoproteins in pregnancy and disease. *Biomed Pharmacother*, **36**, 77–86.

Reinhart, K., Bayer, O., et al. 2002. Markers of endothelial damage in organ dysfunction and sepsis. *Crit Care Med*, **30**, S302–12.

Ridker, P.M., Rifai, N., et al. 2001. Air Force/Texas Coronary Atherosclerosis Prevention Study Investigators 2001. Measurement of C-reactive protein for the targeting of statin therapy in the primary prevention of acute coronary events. *N Engl J Med*, **344**, 1959–65.

Rodan, G.A. and Martin, T.J. 2000. Therapeutic approaches to bone diseases. *Science*, **289**, 1508–14.

Rokita, H., Loose, L.D., et al. 1994. Synergism of IL-1 and IL-6 induces serum amyloid A production while depressing fibrinogen: a quantitative analysis. *J Rheumatol*, **21**, 400–5.

Rosenthal, C.J., Franklin, E.C., et al. 1976. Isolation and partial characterization of SAA-an amyloid-related protein from human serum. *J Immunol*, **116**, 1415–18.

Rovere, P., Peri, G., et al. 2000. The long pentraxin PTX3 binds to apoptotic cells and regulates their clearance by antigen-presenting dendritic cells. *Blood*, **96**, 4300–6.

Scaffidi, P., Misteli, T. and Bianchi, M.E. 2002. Release of chromatin protein HMGB1 by necrotic cells triggers inflammation. *Nature*, **418**, 191–5.

Schumann, R.R., Leong, S.R., et al. 1990. Structure and function of lipopolysaccharide binding protein. *Science*, **249**, 1429–31.

Seiffert, D., Crain, K., et al. 1994. Vitronectin gene expression in vivo. Evidence for extrahepatic synthesis and acute phase regulation. *J Biol Chem*, **269**, 19836–42.

Shiels, B.R., Northemann, W., et al. 1987. Modified nuclear processing of alpha 1-acid glycoprotein RNA during inflammation. *J Biol Chem*, **262**, 12826–31.

Shrive, A.K., Cheetham, G.M., et al. 1996. Three-dimensional structure of human C-reactive protein. *Nat Struct Biol*, **3**, 346–54.

Su, S.B., Gong, W., et al. 1999. A seven-transmembrane, G protein-coupled receptor, FPRL1, mediates the chemotactic activity of serum amyloid A for human phagocytic cells. *J Exp Med*, **189**, 395–402.

Sumiya, M., Super, M., et al. 1991. Molecular basis of opsonic defect in immunodeficient children. *Lancet*, **337**, 1569–70.

Staels, B., Koenig, W., et al. 1998. Activation of human aortic smooth muscle cells is inhibited by PPAR but no t by PPAR. *Nature*, **393**, 790–3.

Tilg, H., Dinarello, C.A. and Mier, J.W. 1997. IL-6 and APPs: anti-inflammatory and immunosuppressive mediators. *Immunol Today*, **18**, 428–32.

Tillet, W.S. and Francis, T. 1930. Serological reactions in pneumonia with a non-protein somatic fraction of *pneumococcus*. *J Exp Med*, **52**, 561–71.

Tolosano, E., Hirsch, E., et al. 1999. Defective recovery and severe renal damage after acute hemolysis in hemopexin-deficient mice. *Blood*, **94**, 3906–14.

Torti, F.M. and Torti, S.V. 2002. Regulation of ferritin genes and protein. *Blood*, **99**, 3505–16.

Tracy, K.J. 2002. The inflammatory reflex. *Nature*, **420**, 853–9.

Uhlar, C.M. and Whitehead, A.S. 1999. Serum amyloid A the major vertebrate acute phase reactant. *Biochem J*, **265**, 501–23.

Urieli-Shoval, S., Cohen, P., et al. 1998. Widespread expression of serum amyloid A in histologically normal human tissues. Predominant localization to the epithelium. *J Histochem Cytochem*, **46**, 1377–84.

Ushikubi, F., Segi, E., et al. 1998. Impaired febrile response in mice lacking the prostaglandin receptor subtype EP3. *Nature*, **395**, 281–4.

Vider, J., Lehtmaa, J., et al. 2001. Acute immune response in respect to exercise-induced oxidative stress. *Pathophysiology*, **7**, 263–70.

Watkins, L.R., Goehler, L.E., et al. 1995. Blockade of IL-1 induced hyperthermia by subdiaphragmatic vagotomy: evidence for vagal mediation of immune brain communication. *Neurosci Letts*, **183**, 27–31.

Wei, C.C., Ho, T.W., et al. 2003. Cloning and characterisation of mouse IL-22 binding protein. *Genes Immunity*, **4**, 204–11.

Weiner, L.M. and Li, W. 1994. Phase I, trial of recombinant macrophage colony-stimulating factor and recombinant gamma-interferon: toxicity, monocytosis, and clinical effects. *Cancer Res*, **54**, 4084–90.

Weinrauch, Y., Abad, C., et al. 1998. Mobilization of potent plasma bactericidal activity during systemic bacterial challenge; role of group iia phospholipase A_2. *J Clin Invest*, **102**, 633–8.

Weiss, G., Bogdan, C. and Hentze, M.W. 1997. Pathways for the regulation of macrophage iron metabolism by the anti-inflammatory cytokines IL-4 and IL-13. *J Immunol*, **15**, 420–5.

Wiedermann, U., Chen, X.J., et al. 1996. Vitamin A deficiency increases inflammatory responses. *Scand J Immunol*, **44**, 578–84.

Willis, D., Moore, A.R., et al. 1996. Heme oxygenase: a novel target for the modulation of the inflammatory response. *Nat Med*, **2**, 87–90.

Woloski, B.M. and Jamieson, J.C. 1987. Rat corticotropin, insulin and thyroid hormone levels during the acute phase response to inflammation. *Comp Biochem Physiol A*, **86**, 15–19.

Wurfel, M.M., Kunitake, S.T., et al. 1994. Lipopolysaccharide (LPS)-binding protein is carried on lipoproteins and acts as a cofactor in the neutralization of LPS. *J Exp Med*, **180**, 1025–35.

Xu, L., Badolato, R., et al. 1995. A novel biologic function for SAA. Induction of T lymphocyte migration and adhesion. *J Immunol*, **155**, 1184–90.

Yan, S.D., Zhu, H., et al. 2000. Receptor dependent cell stress and amyloid accumulation on systemic amyloidosis. *Nat Med*, **6**, 643–51.

Yoo, J.Y. and Desiderio, S. 2003. Innate and acquired immunity intersect in a global view of the acute phase response. *Proc Natl Acad Sci USA*, **100**, 1157–62.

Yoshida, K., Furihata, K., et al. 1995. A mutation in the ceruloplasmin gene is associated with systemic hemosiderosis in humans. *Nat Genet*, **9**, 267–72.

Yother, J., Volanakis, J.E. and Briles, D.E. 1982. Human C-reactive protein is protective against fatal *Streptococcus pneumoniae* infection in mice. *J Immunol*, **128**, 2374–6.

Yue, C.C., Muller-Greven, J., et al. 1996. Identification of a CR-reactive protein binding site in two hepatic carboxylesterases capable of retaining CRP within the endoplasmic reticulum. *J Biol Chem*, **271**, 22245–50.

Zheng, H., Fletcher, D., et al. 1995. Resistance to fever induction and impaired acute phase protein production in interleukin-1beta deficient mice. *Immunity*, **3**, 9–19.

PART III

SOLUBLE MEDIATORS

13

Chemokines

MARCO BAGGIOLINI AND PIUS LOETSCHER

Chemokine is a short form for chemotactic cytokine. The term was coined at a meeting in Baden near Vienna after the International Immunology Congress of Budapest (Lindley et al. 1993). Only few chemokines were known at that time and receptors for interleukin (IL)-8 had just been cloned and shown to belong to the family of G-protein-coupled receptors (GPCR) (Holmes et al. 1991; Murphy and Tiffany 1991). The importance of the new class of cytokines and their function as chemoattractants was already obvious, but no one in the field had anticipated the enormous and rapid development of research that led to a new understanding of leukocyte traffic (Baggiolini 1998; Loetscher et al. 2000; Sallusto et al. 2000; Gerard and Rollins 2001; Mackay 2001; Moser and Loetscher 2001; Murphy 2001; Thelen 2001). Chemokines are produced by leukocytes and tissue cells either constitutively or after induction, and act locally in a paracrine and possibly autocrine fashion on cells that express the appropriate GPCR. Chemotaxis is their main common effect.

A systematic nomenclature for chemokines was established recently (Zlotnik and Yoshie 2000). It is based on the principle adopted for chemokine receptors, which are defined as CXC, CC, XC, and CX_3C followed by R and a number. Chemokines are defined by the same structure-related acronyms followed by L (for ligand) and their gene number. Chemokine genes were originally designated as *SCY* (for small, secreted cytokines) and numbered chronologically. The systematic nomenclature is particularly useful for chemokines that were discovered in recent years, which have often been given more than one name. For IL-8, the monocyte chemoattractant proteins (MCP), RANTES, the macrophage infectivity potentiators (MIP), and other chemokines of the early days, however, the traditional names are still in current use (Tables 13.1 and 13.2 and Figure 13.1).

CHEMOKINES AND THEIR STRUCTURES

Chemokines are small soluble proteins with four conserved cysteines and molecular weights in the range 7–15 kDa (Baggiolini et al. 1994, 1997). They are synthesized with a leader sequence of 20–25 amino acids, which is cleaved off before release. Two main subfamilies, CXC and CC chemokines, are distinguished according to the position of the first two cysteines, which are adjacent (CC) or separated by one amino acid (CXC). The cysteines form two disulfide bonds linking Cys1 to Cys3 and Cys2 to Cys4, which keep the chemokines in a stable three-dimensional conformation that is required for receptor binding and activation. This structure has been resolved by nuclear magnetic resonance (NMR) in solution and X-ray crystallography. Chemokines have a prominent core made of anti-parallel β strands and the connecting loops, a short, conformationally disordered amino-terminal region (3–10 amino acids) and a carboxy-terminal α helix which usually consists of 20–30 amino acids, but can exceed 50. The NMR structure of stromal cell-derived factor 1 (SDF-1) (CXCL12) is presented as an example in Figure 13.2.

In concentrated solution and on crystallization several chemokines form dimers (Clore et al. 1990; Baldwin

Table 13.1 *Human CXC chemokines and their receptors*

Systematic and original names		Gene locus	Receptor
CXCL1	GRO	4q21.1	CXCR2
CXCL2	GROβ	4q21.1	CXCR2
CXCL3	GROγ	4q21.1	CXCR2
CXCL4	PF4	4q21.1	Unknown
CXCL5	ENA-78	4q21.1	CXCR2
CXCL6	GCP-2	4q21.1	CXCR1, CXCR2
CXCL7	NAP-2	4q21.1	CXCR2
CXCL8	IL-8	4q21.1	CXCR1, CXCR2
CXCL9	Mig	4q21.1	CXCR3
CXCL10	IP10	4q21.1	CXCR3
CXCL11	I-TAC	4q21.1	CXCR3
CXCL12	SDF-1α/β	10q11.21	CXCR4
CXCL13	BCA-1	5q31.1	CXCR5
CXCL14	BRAK	Unknown	Unknown
CXCL16		Unknown	CXCR6

For abbreviations see the text.

et al. 1991). The mode of aggregation is strikingly different for CXC and CC chemokines, as illustrated in Figure 13.3 for IL-8 (CXCL8) and MIP-1α (CCL3). Studies of IL-8 (CXCL8), GROα (CXCL1), and NAP-2 (CXCL7) show that CXC chemokines associate along their first β strands via hydrogen bonds and amino acid side chain interactions (Baggiolini et al. 1997), whereas CC chemokines, e.g. MIP-1β (CCL4) (Lodi et al. 1994) and RANTES (CCL5) (Chung et al. 1995; Skelton et al. 1995) dimerize by interacting with their amino-terminal regions. It is believed that the distribution of hydrophobic areas on the surface, which is different for CXC

Table 13.2 *Human CC chemokines and their receptors*

Systematic and original names		Gene locus	Receptor
CCL1	I-309	17q11.2	CCR8
CCL2	MCP-1	17q11.2	CCR2
CCL3	MIP-1α, LD78	17q12	CCR1, CCR5
CCL3L1	LD78β	17q12	CCR1, CCR5
CCL4	MIP-1β	17q12	CCR5
CCL5	RANTES	17q12	CCR1, CCR3, CCR5
CCL7	MCP-3	17q11.2	CCR1, CCR2, CCR3
CCL8	MCP-2	17q11.2	CCR1, CCR2, CCR3, CCR5
CCL11	Eotaxin-1	17q11.2	CCR3
CCL13	MCP-4	17q11.2	CCR1, CCR2, CCR3
CCL14	HCC-1	17q12	CCR1
CCL15	HCC-2, Lkn-1, MIP-1δ	17q12	CCR1, CCR3
CCL16	HCC-4, LEC	17q12	CCR1
CCL17	TARC	16q13	CCR4
CCL18	PARC, DC-CK1, AMAC1	17q12	Unknown
CCL19	ELC, MIP-3β, exodus-3	9p13.3	CCR7
CCL20	LARC, MIP-3α, exodus-1	2q36.3	CCR6
CCL21	SLC, 6Ckine, exodus-2	9p13.3	CCR7
CCL22	MDC, STCP-1	16q13	CCR4
CCL23	MPIF-1, CKβ8	17q12	CCR1
CCL24	Eotaxin-2, MPIF-2	7q11.23	CCR3
CCL25	TECK	9p13.3	CCR9
CCL26	Eotaxin-3	7q11.23	CCR3
CCL27	CTACK, ILC	9p13.3	CCR10
CCL28	MEC	5p12	CCR3, CCR10

For abbreviations see the text.

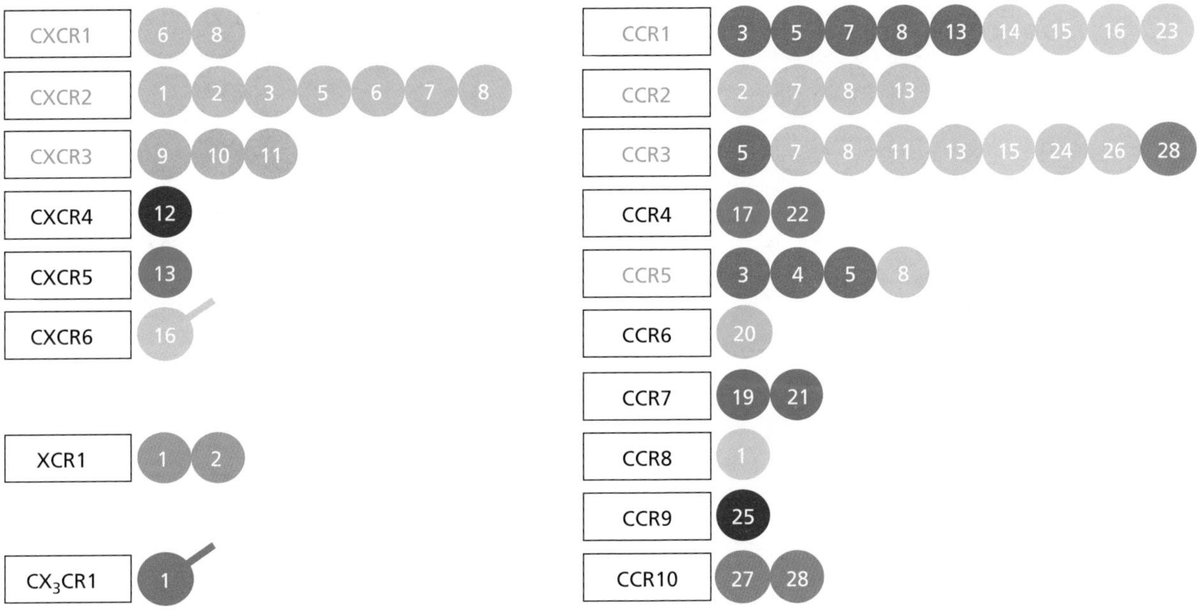

Figure 13.1 *Human chemokines and chemokine receptors: chemokines including the lymphotactins are presented as circles. Circles with a bar represent membrane-anchored chemokines. The numbers within the circles correspond to the chemokine numbers in the systematic nomenclature (see Tables 13.1 and 13.2). The colors of the circles indicate chemokines with structural similarities. Receptors for inflammatory chemokines are presented in red.*

and CC chemokines, determines the mode of dimer formation (Covell et al. 1994; Clore and Gronenborn 1995). The distribution of the inner hydrophobicity clusters, by contrast, is similar for chemokines of both subfamilies, explaining the common mode of folding of monomers.

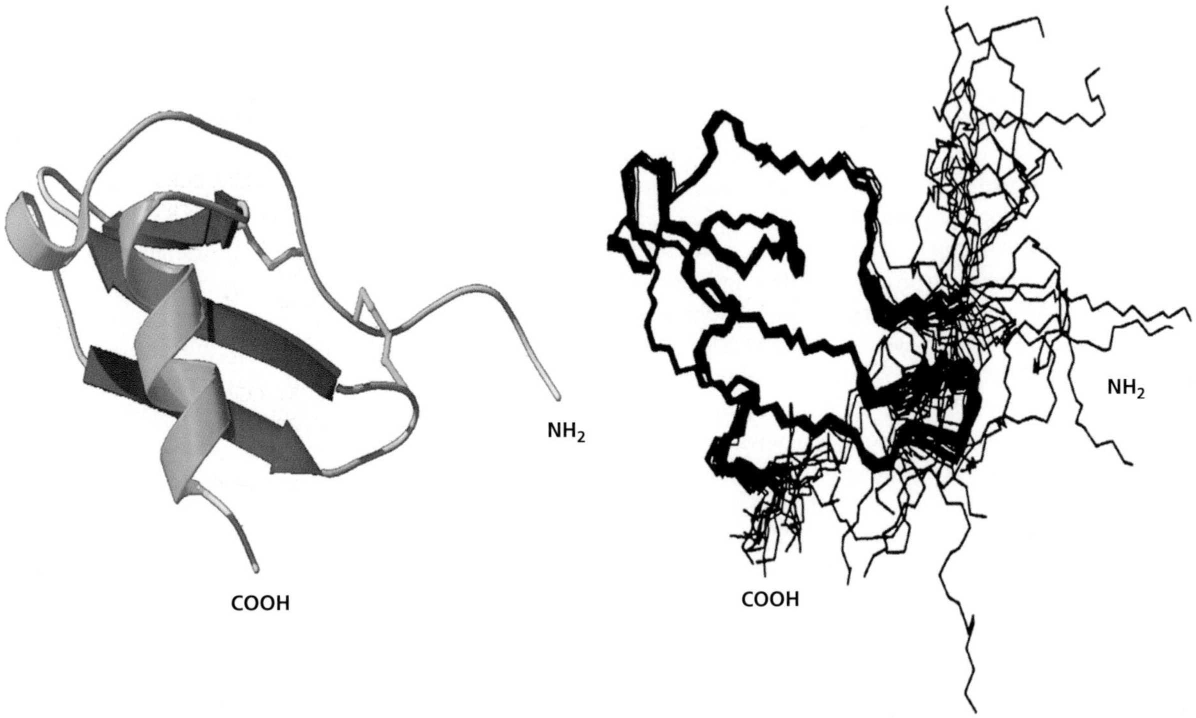

Figure 13.2 *Three-dimensional structure of the CXC chemokine SDF-1 (CXCL12) as obtained by NMR spectroscopy in solution. The model on the left shows the core consisting of anti-parallel β strands and the connecting loops, which is kept together by the disulfide bonds (in yellow), and presents an idealized view of the amino-terminal sequence and the carboxyl-terminal α helix. On the right, 30 single NMR views are projected on to each other. This presentation highlights the rigidity of the core and the structural disorder of the terminal regions. (Reproduced with permission from Crump et al. (1997).)*

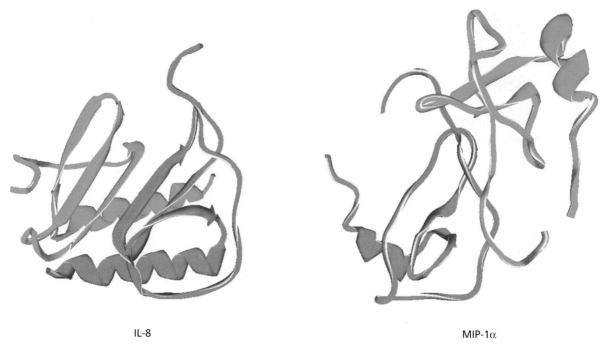

Figure 13.3 *Dimer formation by CXC and CC chemokines as illustrated by IL-8 (CXCL8) and MIP-1α (CCL3). CXC chemokines associate along their first β strands (Gerber et al. 2000), whereas CC chemokines associate by interacting with their amino-terminal regions (Czaplewski et al. 1999). The mode of dimer formation is believed to reflect the different distribution of surface hydrophobicity areas in CXC and CC chemokines. The monomers of both subfamilies, by contrast, fold in the same manner because the distribution of the internal hydrophobicity clusters is similar.*

Aggregation was originally considered an important property and it was suggested that chemokines, like some cytokines, act as dimers (Baggiolini et al. 1997). It was eventually realized, however, that the biological activities of chemokines are observed at nanomolar concentrations, which are too low for stable aggregation to dimers (Burrows et al. 1994; Clark-Lewis et al. 1995). To demonstrate that IL-8 (CXCL8) can function as a monomer, an analogue of the 72 amino acid form was synthesized with *N*-methyl-leucine instead of leucine at position 25 to disturb hydrogen bonding and prevent dimerization. Although the analog remained monomeric, it was as active as wild-type IL-8 (CXCL8) (Rajarathnam et al. 1994). Similar results were obtained with monomeric forms of MIP-1α (CCL3) (Graham et al. 1994) and it was shown that some chemokines, MCP-3 (CCL7) for instance, do not dimerize (Kim et al. 1996). As monomeric chemokines have full biological activity and aggregation occurs at concentrations that are much higher than those required for a chemotactic response, there is little doubt today that the biologically relevant conformation of chemokines is the monomer (Clark-Lewis et al. 1995).

Two variants of the chemokine structure paradigm have been described: lymphotactin (XCL1, XCL2) with two instead of four conserved cysteines (Kennedy et al. 1995) and fractalkine or neurotactin (CX_3CL1), a membrane-bound mucin bearing an amino-terminal chemokine-like domain with three amino acids between the first two cysteines (CX_3C motif) (Bazan et al. 1997; Pan et al. 1997).

RECEPTOR BINDING AND ACTIVATION

The receptor for chemotactic *N*-formyl-methionyl peptides was cloned more than a decade ago (Boulay et al. 1990) and found to have a heptahelical structure and to couple to heterotrimeric GTP-binding proteins. The cloning of the first chemokine receptors, two heptahelical proteins with high affinity for IL-8 (CXCL8), followed soon thereafter (Holmes et al. 1991; Murphy and Tiffany 1991). Meanwhile six human receptors for CXC chemokines and ten for CC chemokines, in addition to the receptors for lymphotactin and fractalkine, have been characterized (Murphy et al. 2000; Murphy 2002). The study of receptor selectivity and expression in different types of leukocytes has provided considerable insight into the mechanism for the specific recruitment of different types of leukocytes and the regulation of leukocyte traffic in health and disease. Blood phagocytes, for instance, express different types and combinations of chemokine receptors. CXCR1 and CXCR2 are found exclusively in neutrophils, the front-line cells for antibacterial defense. Eosinophil and basophil granulocytes as well as monocytes share CCR1, but can be recruited selectively by chemokines acting on CCR3, for eosinophils and basophils, or CCR5 for monocytes (Figure 13.4).

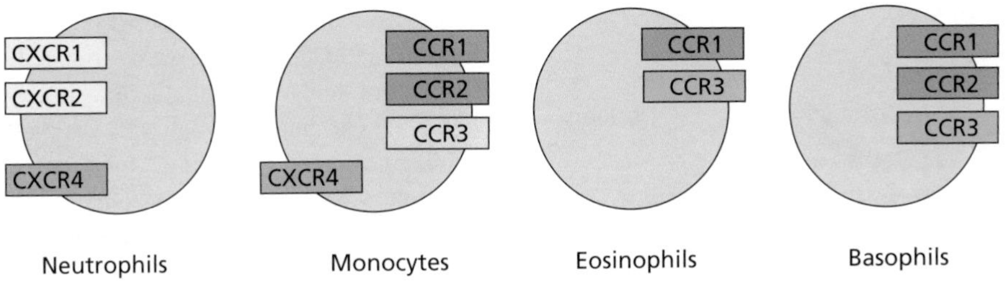

Figure 13.4 *Chemokine receptor expression in human phagocytic leukocytes.*

The search for sequence domains that are involved in receptor recognition and activation began after the characterization of the receptors for IL-8 (CXCL8) and related chemokines. These studies revealed the importance of the amino-terminal region and showed that a sequence of three residues, Glu-Leu-Arg, the so-called ELR motif, immediately preceding the first cysteine, is essential for IL-8 (CXCL8) activity (Clark-Lewis et al. 1991, 1993; Hébert et al. 1991). The ELR motif is conserved in all IL-8 (CXCL8)-related chemokines, the growth-related oncogene (GRO) proteins (CXCL1–3), ENA-78 (CXCL5), granulocyte chemoattractant protein 2 (GCP-2) (CXCL6), and neutrophil-activating protein 2 (NAP-2) (CXCL7), and is necessary for activation of CXCR1 and CXCR2 (Baggiolini et al. 1994, 1997). Neither receptor, however, responds to linear or cyclic oligopeptides enclosing the Glu-Leu-Arg-Cys-X-Cys sequence or to unrelated chemokines such as MCP-1 (CCL2) and interferon-inducible protein 10 (IP10) (CXCL10) that were modified by insertion of an ELR-containing amino-terminal sequence (Clark-Lewis et al. 1993). These observations indicated that other recognition sites are required. Using mutagenesis or chemical synthesis of analogues of the 72-residue form of IL-8 (CXCL8), such sites were identified in the loop region following the second cysteine (residues 10–17) and in the sequence immediately preceding the third cysteine (Clark-Lewis et al. 1994, 1995). Discrete differences between IL-8 (CXCL8) and its analogs, e.g. NAP-2 (CXCL7) and GROα (CXCL1) (Kim et al. 1994), determine the binding selectivity for CXCR1 and CXCR2.

Similar studies performed with several other CC and CXC chemokines confirmed the importance of the amino-terminal region for receptor activation (Loetscher and Clark-Lewis 2001; Fernandez and Lolis 2002). In most cases, however, receptor-triggering motifs could not be unequivocally identified. MCP-1, for instance, requires the entire sequence of 10 amino acids preceding the first cysteine for full activity on CCR2. Potency drops considerably after truncation or elongation of the amino-terminal sequence, but the amino-terminal residue can be replaced by several amino acids without affecting activity (Clark-Lewis et al. 1995). MCP-1, MCP-2, MCP-3, and MCP-4 (CCL2, CCL8, CCL7, and CCL13), which are all potent agonists for CCR2, share the amino-terminal Gln-Pro motif and have other similarities within the first 10 residues. Despite these analogies, the structure–activity relationships are far from clear. In contrast to MCP-1 (CCL2), all three analogs act on additional receptors, CCR3 in particular. On the other hand, MCP-1 (CCL2) itself becomes a high-affinity ligand for CCR3 after deletion of glutamine at the amino terminus, which causes a 50-fold drop in affinity for CCR2 (Weber et al. 1996).

Of particular interest are the structure–activity relations studies on SDF-1 (CXCL12) (Crump et al. 1997; P. Loetscher et al. 1998a), the exclusive ligand for CXCR4, a receptor that is widely expressed in leukocytes and tissue cells and functions as a co-receptor for HIV (Murphy et al. 2000). The first amino-terminal residues of SDF-1 (CXCL12), Lys1-Pro2, are essential for receptor triggering: deletion of Lys1 dramatically decreases activity and the deletion of both amino acids fully inactivates the chemokine. As for IL-8 (CXCL8), some residues in the loop region of SDF-1 (CXCL12) immediately after the second cysteine (residues 12–17, RFFESH motif) are required for receptor binding (Crump et al. 1997). The importance of the amino-terminal domain of SDF-1 is underscored by an astonishing observation: GROα (CXCL1), a selective ligand of CXCR2, and IP10 (CXCL10), a selective ligand of CXCR3, can be converted into agonists for CXCR4 by substituting their amino-terminal domain with the first 17 residues of SDF-1 (CXCL12). Interestingly, CXCR4 triggering was also obtained with an oligopeptide consisting only of the first 17 residues of SDF-1 (P. Loetscher et al. 1998a), which folds in a similar way to the wild-type chemokine (Elisseeva et al. 2000).

All studies of structure–activity relationships indicate the importance of the amino-terminal domain of CXC and CC chemokines for receptor recognition and activation (Clark-Lewis et al. 1995; Loetscher and Clark-Lewis 2001). Two separate or partly overlapping sites of interaction with the receptors can be distinguished, one in the amino-terminal sequence preceding the first cysteine and the other within the exposed, conformationally rigid loop after the second cysteine (N loop). Both sites are small (consisting of few amino acids) and are kept in close proximity by the disulfide bonds (see Figure 13.2). Clark-Lewis and colleagues (Crump et al. 1997) have proposed that the receptor recognizes first the binding site within the loop region, which functions as a *docking*

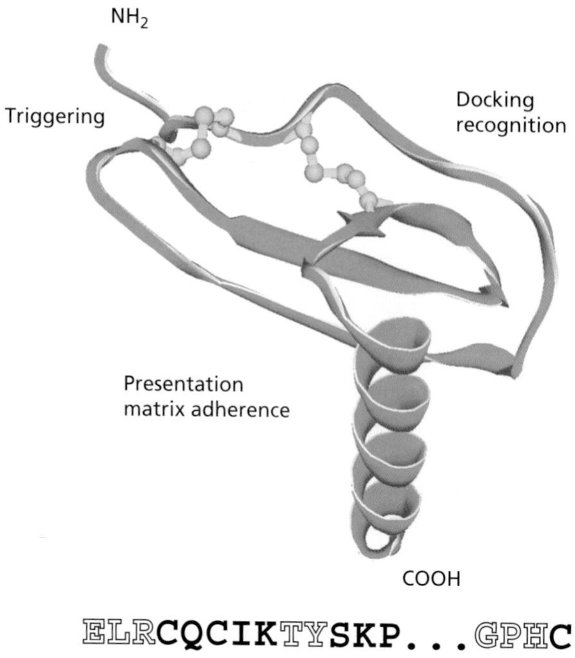

Figure 13.5 *Chemokine-binding domains: chemokines interact with their receptors by means of two discrete, contiguous, or slightly overlapping domains. The receptor is recognized via a binding site within the loop region, which appears to function as* a docking domain. *This interaction restricts the mobility of the chemokine and presumably facilitates the proper orientation of the amino-terminal* triggering domain *which activates the receptor. Chemokines tend to bind to glycosaminoglycans on the surface of cells or in the extracellular matrix via basic residues of the core and the carboxy-terminal region. Bound chemokines retain their full chemotactic activity.*

domain. This interaction restricts the mobility of the chemokine and presumably facilitates the proper orientation of the amino-terminal *triggering domain* that activates the receptor (Figure 13.5).

INTRACELLULAR SIGNALING

Chemokine signaling was first studied in human neutrophils stimulated with IL-8 (CXCL8). It was found that all functional responses were blocked when the cells were pre-treated with *Bordetella pertussis* toxin, indicating that the receptor couples to GTP-binding proteins of the Gi type (Thelen et al. 1988), which eventually turned out to be the rule for all chemokine receptors (Murphy et al. 2000). When a chemokine binds to its receptor, heterotrimeric Gi proteins are activated: GDP, which is bound to the inactive trimeric complex, is exchanged for GTP, and the complex dissociates into its α subunit bound to GTP and the $\beta\gamma$ subunit. The release of the $\beta\gamma$ subunit is essential for the stimulation of chemotaxis (Neptune and Bourne 1997), which involves the activation of the rho GTPases Rac and CDC42, the Wiscott–Aldrich syndrome protein (WASP), and the Arp2/3 complex, and leads to actin polymerization (Cory and Ridley 2002). In addition the $\beta\gamma$ subunit activates two major signal transduction enzymes: a phospholipase C (PLCβ_2 and-β_3) which is specific for phosphatidylinositol, and a phosphatidylinositol-3-hydroxyl kinase (PI3Kγ). The phospholipase cleaves phosphatidylinositol 4,5-bisphosphate, yielding two second messengers: inositol 1,4,5-trisphosphate (IP_3) and diacylglygerol (DAG). IP_3 induces the release of Ca^{2+} from intracellular stores, leading to a characteristic, transient rise of the free calcium concentration, and DAG activates several isoforms of protein kinase C (PKC). The IP_3 kinase generates phosphatidylinositol 3,4,5-trisphosphate and initiates the activation of another kinase, PKB. There is evidence that the $\beta\gamma$ subunit of the Gi protein may activate other signaling kinases, such as the MAP kinase, but the mechanism and the role of this step are still unclear (Thelen 2001). The signaling that is initiated with the exchange of GTP for GDP and the consequent dissociation of the α and $\beta\gamma$ subunits is terminated by the hydrolysis of GTP to GDP and the re-association of the $\beta\gamma$ subunit with the GDP-bound α subunit. Newer findings suggest that the α subunit is more than a binding moiety that regulates the activity of the $\beta\gamma$ subunit, and signals on its own by activating tyrosine kinases (Thelen 2001).

The signal transduction events induced by IL-8 (CXCL8) appear to correspond to those observed after stimulation with the classic chemotactic agonists such as fMet-Leu-Phe (formyl-methionine-leucine-phenylalanine) and C5a (Baggiolini and Kernen 1992). Using Jurkat cells stably transfected with CXCR1 or CXCR2 copy DNA (cDNA), it was shown that both receptors respond equally well to IL-8 (CXCL8), as judged by the activation of p42/p44 MAP kinase (Jones et al. 1995), Ca^{2+} mobilization and chemotaxis (Loetscher et al. 1994a), and that the two IL-8 receptors function independently of each other. By blocking one or the other receptor in neutrophils using monoclonal antibodies it was found that phospholipase D activation and the respiratory burst are mediated by CXCR1 only (Jones et al. 1996). In agreement with these observations, it was reported that phospholipase D is activated by stimulation with IL-8 (CXCL8), but not with GROα (CXCL1) or NAP-2 (CXCL7) (L'Heureux et al. 1995).

In contrast to other chemokines, which induce short-lived responses, SDF-1 (CXCL12) was found to mediate the prolonged activation of protein kinase B and the MAP kinases ERK1/2 via CXCR4 (Tilton et al. 1997). The sustained effect on intracellular signaling reflects the continuous interaction of CXCR4 with its ligand. Such activity may be required for the retention pre-B cells at their sites of maturation within the bone marrow (Ma et al. 1999). Prolonged activation of protein kinase B was shown to protect cells from apoptosis (Marte and Downward 1997). Prolongation of cell survival is an as yet unexplored effect mediated by CXCR4, which is widely expressed in leukocytes and nonhemopoietic cells.

It was recently reported that after stimulation chemokine receptors form homo- or heterodimers (Mellado et al. 2001). Up to now, this mechanism has not received general acceptance and its role in the initiation of chemokine responses has been questioned (Thelen and Baggiolini 2001). The existence of GPCR dimers is documented by studies showing that aggregation may pre-exist or occurs slowly after stimulation (Bouvier 2001; Pierce et al. 2002), suggesting that dimerization is too slow as an initiating event.

ASSESSING CHEMOKINE ACTIVITIES

The most common test for chemokine activity is chemotaxis in a two-well chamber where leukocytes, which are placed in the upper well, migrate through a porous polycarbonate membrane in response to chemokines supplied in the lower well. The cells sense chemokine molecules that diffuse across the membrane and move toward higher concentrations of the attractant. The pores are always smaller than the migrating cells, and their diameter is chosen depending on the properties of the cells, in particular their size and mobility. Migration is assessed by counting the cells that have crossed the membrane and stick to its lower surface or fall into the fluid of the lower well. Coating of the lower membrane surface with collagen is used to increase sticking for the purpose of recovering migrated cells on the lower surface of the filter. The crossing of a polycarbonate membrane is a simple model of diapedesis, the migration of leukocytes through the endothelial layer and the basement membrane of microvessels, which is the first step of the intervention of host-defense cells in infection and inflammation.

The dependence of the chemotaxis response in vitro on chemokine concentration is usually bimodal: the number of migrating cells increases up to an optimum concentration and then falls, because over-stimulation increasingly leads to adherence (Baggiolini et al. 1994). Migration may also be assessed in vivo by monitoring the infiltration of leukocytes into a tissue area or a body cavity where a chemokine is injected. The infiltration can be quantified by image analysis of histology or cytochemistry specimens (Uguccioni et al. 1999), by counting the leukocytes collected in an exudate or by measuring the radioactivity of tissue sites in animals supplied with radioactively labeled leukocytes (Colditz et al. 1989). Furthermore, vital microscopy may be used in microcirculation experiments to observe chemokine-induced rolling and adhesion of leukocytes on the endothelial surface (Stein et al. 2000; Warnock et al. 2000).

The migration across the wall of microvessels and within the tissues along a chemokine concentration gradient is a complex function resulting from the combination of discrete responses. Some of these responses can be measured in real time as in vitro correlates of chemotaxis. Early studies on neutrophils stimulated with IL-8 (CXCL8) have shown that chemokines induce rapid, active changes in cellular shape as a result of the polymerization and depolymerization of actin (Thelen et al. 1988). Other characteristic effects are the upregulation and activation of integrins through which the leukocytes adhere to endothelial cells before emigration (Springer 1994), the release of granule contents, e.g. proteases from neutrophils, monocytes, $CD8^+$ T lymphocytes, and natural killer (NK) cells, histamine from basophils and cytotoxic proteins from eosinophils, the production of bioactive lipids, and the formation of oxygen radicals during the respiratory burst (Baggiolini et al. 1994, 1997). The release responses are observed at higher chemokine concentrations and are enhanced when the leukocytes are exposed to bacterial toxins or inflammatory cytokines. It must be assumed that release occurs once the leukocytes have reached their target, e.g. a site of infection and inflammation, where they stop migrating and perform antimicrobial and other functions in host defense (Baggiolini et al. 1994, 1997).

As already mentioned the second messenger inositol trisphosphate releases Ca^{2+} from intracellular stores, leading to a transient rise of its free concentration in the cytosol, which is one of the earliest cellular responses to chemoattractants (von Tscharner et al. 1986a, 1986b). With appropriate instruments one can measure the rate of the increase of Ca^{2+}-related fluorescence, which reflects the intensity of chemokine effects in real time and is the most reliable method to assess concentration–response relationships. We have used this assay extensively for the analysis of chemokine receptor selectivity and desensitization (Uguccioni et al. 1995, 1996; P. Loetscher et al. 1994b, 1996; Forssmann et al. 1997; Bardi et al. 2001).

CHEMOKINE ACTIONS ON PHAGOCYTES

As shown in Figure 13.4, phagocytes rely on a small repertoire of chemokine receptors, CXCR1 and CXCR2 for neutrophils, CCR1, CCR2, CCR3, and CCR5 for eosinophils, basophils, and monocytes. They are expressed constitutively and are always detectable and functional on the phagocytes that circulate in the blood. The receptors are ready for rapid interventions in response to chemokines induced in endothelial cells and in the tissues under pathological conditions by inflammatory stimuli such as bacterial toxins, inflammatory cytokines, such as IL-1, tumor necrosis factor (TNF), and interferons, hemopoietic growth factors, bioactive lipids, oxygen radicals, etc. (Baggiolini et al. 1994). Even though receptor numbers may change when the cells are activated (Bonecchi et al. 1999, 2000), their repertoire remains characteristic for each type of phagocyte. The system that drives phagocyte recruitment is redundant: most receptors recognize more than one chemokine and several chemokines act on multiple receptors (see

Figure 13.1). CXCR4, the selective receptor for SDF-1 (CXCL12), which is found in neutrophils and monocytes, makes an exception, because its role for these cells is unknown. In addition, phagocytes express several other receptors for nonchemokine ligands, like the complement product C5a, *N*-formyl-methionyl peptides, and several bioactive lipids, which may all contribute to phagocyte recruitment in inflammation (Boulay et al. 1997).

The ligands of CXCR1, CXCR2, CCR1, CCR2, CCR3, and CCR5 are collectively referred to as *inflammatory chemokines* because they are released in pathological conditions and disturbances of tissue homeostasis leading to inflammation. As a rule these chemokines are not detectable in healthy tissues. Numerous publications document the expression of CXC and CC chemokines at sites of inflammation, infection, and immune reactions. The main sources are different types of tissue cells, tissue macrophages, mast cells, but also the phagocytes that enter the inflamed tissues, which amplify in this way inflammatory and host-defense reactions by contributing to further cell recruitment (Baggiolini et al. 1994, 1997).

Inflammatory chemokines act as well on lymphocytes and other effector cells of acquired immunity. $CD4^+$ and $CD8^+$ T cells (Loetscher et al. 2000; Sallusto et al. 2000), NK cells (Maghazachi and Al-Aoukaty 1998), and immature dendritic cells (Sozzani et al. 1999) can express CCR1, CCR2, CCR3, and CCR5, and are thus readily attracted into inflamed tissues. In addition T and NK cells express CXCR3, which is upregulated in lymphocytes together with the other receptors for inflammatory CC chemokines indicated, and respond to a monokine induced by interferon γ (Mig), IP10, and interferon-inducible T-cell α-chemoattractant (I-TAC) (CXCL9, 10, and 11, respectively), which are induced in inflamed tissues by interferon γ (IFN-γ). CXCR3 is the only receptor for inflammatory chemokines that is not found in phagocytes.

CHEMOKINE ACTIONS ON LYMPHOCYTES

Memory and effector functions

In contrast to phagocytes, which leave the bloodstream to enter tissues where they perform host-defense functions and eventually die, but never return to the blood, lymphocytes circulate continuously through lymphoid and nonlymphoid tissues in search of antigens to provide specific protection against pathogens (Mackay 1993; Butcher and Picker 1996). When naïve T cells, in secondary lymphoid tissues, encounter an antigen they are activated, differentiate into effector or memory cells, and proliferate. Unlike their naïve precursors, effector and memory lymphocytes usually migrate into nonlymphoid tissues, which are the prime sites of entry for microorganisms and other foreign antigens. They have, however, the ability to home again into secondary lymphoid tissues for renewed episodes of activation. Recent research has shown that the various re-circulation itineraries are regulated by the expression of chemokine receptors on the lymphocytes and of the appropriate chemokines in the homing areas as well as adhesion molecules (Sallusto et al. 2000; Von Andrian and Mackay 2000; Moser and Loetscher 2001).

Early studies had suggested that T lymphocytes isolated from the blood respond poorly to chemokines. When T cells, however, are kept in culture in the presence of IL-2 the expression of several receptors for inflammatory chemokines, namely CCR1, CCR2, CCR5, and CXCR3, is markedly enhanced and migration in responses to the respective ligands, such as RANTES (CCL5), MCP-1 (CCL2), MIP-1β (CCL4), and IP10 (CXCL10), increases progressively (M. Loetscher et al. 1998; P. Loetscher et al. 1996). IL-4, IL-10, and IL-12 have similar effects but are less potent, whereas other cytokines known to act on T lymphocytes (IL-13, IFN-γ, IL-1β, and TNFα) are inactive. The effect is reversible: Receptor expression and responsiveness are rapidly lost when IL-2 is withdrawn, and are fully restored when it is added again (P. Loetscher et al. 1996). Rapid downregulation of receptors for inflammatory chemokines is also observed when IL-2 is replaced by anti-CD3 alone or in combination with anti-CD28, mimicking activation via the T-cell receptor. These observations created much interest and several laboratories began systematically to study chemokine receptor expression in relation to T-lymphocyte differentiation.

T-lymphocyte-dependent immune responses rely on helper cells of T-helper (Th)1 or Th2 phenotype with different functional properties (Mosmann and Coffman 1989; Abbas et al. 1996), which develop from naïve precursors after antigen recognition and priming. Th1 cells secrete IFN-γ and lymphotoxin and enhance cell-mediated immunity to intracellular pathogens, whereas Th2 cells secrete IL-4 and IL-5, and regulate allergic responses and humoral immunity against parasites. A lymphocyte infiltrate may be of Th1 or Th2 type depending on the pathological conditions, and it was natural to assume that the selective recruitment of cells of either phenotype is driven by the chemokine receptors that they bear and the chemokines expressed in the diseased tissues.

CCR3, a receptor that was originally identified in eosinophils and basophils and that binds several chemokines including the eotaxins (see Figure 13.1), is expressed on a subset of blood T lymphocytes which produce IL-4 and IL-5 and thus qualify as Th2 cells (Sallusto et al. 1997). CCR3 is also expressed at high levels in Th2-type cells, which are obtained by culturing umbilical cord blood lymphocytes activated with phytohemagglutinin in the presence of IL-4 and neutralizing anti-IL-12 antibodies (Sallusto et al. 1997, 1998), and in cloned, allergen-specific T cells with a Th2 phenotype (Gerber et al. 1997). CCR3-positive Th2 cells are recruited together with eosinophils to sites of allergic inflammation, and are likely to support eosinophil survival by secreting IL-4 and IL-5 (Gerber et al. 1997). Without questioning the fact that CCR3 is found in Th2 and not in Th1 cells, it is important to note that the level of CCR3 expression in Th2 lymphocytes was shown in several studies to be moderate and variable, suggesting that CCR3-bearing cells constitute a Th2 subpopulation (Loetscher et al. 2000).

CCR4 and CCR8 are also considered as characteristic for Th2 lymphocytes (D'Ambrosio et al. 1998; Zingoni et al. 1998; Imai et al. 1999). Both receptors are transiently upregulated in Th2 cells after stimulation in culture with anti-CD3 and anti-CD28. In contrast to CCR8, which is present exclusively in activated Th2 cells, CCR4 appears to be expressed constitutively and is also found in Th1 cells on activation with anti-CD3 and anti-CD28 (D'Ambrosio et al. 1998).

CCR5 is expressed preferentially in Th1 cells (Annunziato et al. 1998; Bonecchi et al. 1998; P. Loetscher et al. 1998b; Siveke and Hamann 1998). It is detected in Th1 and Th2 cells obtained from umbilical cord blood by treatments inducing polarization, but is not expressed in cloned Th2 cells (P. Loetscher et al. 1998b; Sallusto et al. 1998). Th1 lymphocytes also express high levels of CXCR3, the receptor for Mig, IP10, and I-TAC (CXCL9, 10, and 11, respectively) (Cole et al. 1998; P. Loetscher et al. 1998b; Qin et al. 1998). We and others have found that CXCR3 is present in both types of helper cells after proliferation induced with IL-2 (Annunziato et al. 1998; P. Loetscher et al. 1998b), whereas preferential expression in Th1 cells has been observed under other conditions (Bonecchi et al. 1998; Sallusto et al. 1998). Cytochemical analysis shows that the abundant Th1 lymphocyte infiltrate in the synovial pannus of rheumatoid arthritis joints is strongly positive for CCR5 and CXCR3, whereas CCR3 is virtually absent (P. Loetscher et al. 1998b; Qin et al. 1998).

A similar chemokine receptor pattern is observed in cytotoxic T cells (Tc): CCR5 is present in Tc1 whereas enhanced levels of transcripts for CCR3, CCR4, and CCR8 are characteristic for Tc2 cells (D'Ambrosio et al. 1998). It was recently reported that CXCR6 is preferentially expressed in blood Th1 and Tc1 cells and that CXCR6-positive $CD4^+$ and $CD8^+$ T cells are enriched in the synovial fluid of rheumatoid arthritis joints (Kim et al. 2001b). Such observations have been confirmed and extended in several studies emphasizing the role of chemokines and their receptors in directing lymphocyte traffic under physiological and pathological conditions (Sallusto et al. 2000; Von Andrian and Mackay 2000; Moser and Loetscher 2001).

A particularly important role in lymphocyte traffic and for the identification of cells with distinct functional properties is ascribed to CCR7. Sallusto et al. (1999) have defined two subsets of human memory T lymphocytes, one comprising cells without immediate effector properties, termed central memory T cells (T_{CM}), which are CCR7 positive, and the other comprising IL-4 and IFN-γ producing, perforin-positive cells, termed effector memory T cells (T_{EM}), which lack CCR7, but bear inflammatory chemokine receptors including CXCR3 and CCR5. The receptor profile underscores the different role played by these cells in a secondary immune response. T_{EM} cells can be recruited rapidly into inflamed tissues for immediate defense, whereas T_{CM} cells, which represent a clonally expanded memory cell pool, enter lymph nodes after a secondary antigen challenge, where they may stimulate dendritic cells to produce IL-12, provide help to antigen-specific B cells, and generate a new wave of effector T cells (Sallusto et al. 1999; Masopust et al. 2001; Reinhardt et al. 2001).

The concept of central and effector memory lymphocytes has recently been questioned in a number of reports. According to the model, CCR7 expression should be lost in memory $CD4^+$ T lymphocytes homing into the skin and the gut, and in fully differentiated, cytokine-producing Th1 and Th2 cells. However, in human blood, most memory $CD4^+$ lymphocytes with skin- or gut-homing markers (CLA^+ and $\alpha4\beta7^+$, respectively) were reported to bear CCR7 (Campbell et al. 2001), and the same was observed for a substantial fraction of IFN-γ- or IL-4-producing effector $CD4^+$ T lymphocytes (Kim et al. 2001c; Debes et al. 2002). It was also reported that CCR7-positive $CD4^+$ and $CD8^+$ memory T lymphocytes, arising in mice after viral infection, produce IFN-γ and exhibit lytic activity, respectively (Unsoeld et al. 2002). As they bear CCR7, such cells retain the capacity to re-circulate through secondary lymphoid tissues. The apparent discrepancy between the original and the subsequent reports should be clarified by further studies.

Much attention has recently been given to CXCR5, the selective receptor for BCA-1 (BLC in the mouse, CXCL13), to identify lymphocytes with distinct homing and effector properties (Mackay 2000; Kim et al. 2001a; Moser et al. 2002). CXCR5 is expressed in mature, circulating B lymphocytes and a subset of memory T cells (Förster et al. 1994; Breitfeld et al. 2000; Schaerli et al. 2000; Kim et al. 2001d). It is present in about 20 percent of the blood $CD4^+CD45RO^+$ T lymphocytes, which also express CCR7 but do not produce effector cytokines, suggesting that they qualify as T_{CM} cells. $CXCR5^+$ and $CCR7^+$ blood lymphocytes are considered as the precursors of the follicular B-helper T (T_{FH}) cells found in the B-cell areas of secondary lymphoid tissues. In the tonsils, most $CD4^+$ memory T cells express CXCR5. They have a B-helper function, which is particularly evident in $CD57^+$ T cells from germinal centers, and markedly enhance antibody production when cocultured with B cells (Breitfeld et al. 2000; Schaerli et al. 2000; Kim et al. 2001d). Naïve blood T lymphocytes rapidly acquire CXCR5 on activation in vitro with antigen-presenting dendritic cells and irreversibly lose expression of this receptor after terminal differentiation to effector cells (Schaerli et al. 2001). Together, these observations show that CXCR5-bearing T lymphocytes constitute a unique subset that is distinct from Th1 and Th2 cells.

Homing into lymphoid tissues

The role of chemokines in lymphocyte homing has already been addressed in the context of immune defense, but it is important to highlight their critical involvement in the formation and the renewal of secondary lymphoid tissues, e.g. lymph nodes and Peyer's patches, through the recruitment of naïve cells, a process that depends on two chemokine receptors, CCR7 and CXCR5, and their ligands (Sallusto et al. 2000; Von Andrian and Mackay 2000; Moser and Loetscher 2001).

The recognition that chemokines direct the homing of lymphocytes into secondary lymphoid tissues goes back to a remarkable experiment by Lipp and colleagues (Förster et al. 1996) who found that deletion of the gene of the then putative chemokine receptor termed 'BLR1' or 'MDR15', which was cloned from Burkitt's lymphoma (Förster et al. 1994) and human monocytes (Barella et al. 1995), resulted in impaired formation of Peyer's patches and inguinal lymph nodes. B cells lacking BLR1 were unable to enter their area of destination. The ligand for BLR1 was soon found to be a chemokine, termed 'BCA-1' or 'BLC' (CXCL13), and the receptor was renamed CXCR5 (Gunn et al. 1998; Legler et al. 1998). BCA-1/BLC (CXCL13) is selectively expressed in the B-cell follicles and deletion of the *BLC* (CXCL13) gene in mice yields the same phenotype as the deletion of the CXCR5 gene (Ansel et al. 2000).

Subsequent studies elucidated the role of CCR7, which binds two chemokines – secondary lymphoid tissue chemokine (SLC) (CCL21) and Epstein–Barr virus-induced receptor ligand chemokine (ELC) (CCL19) – and is expressed in all naïve and part of memory T lymphocytes as well as on B lymphocytes (Loetscher et al. 2000; Sallusto et al. 2000). In response to SLC (CCL21), which is expressed in high-endothelial venules, T lymphocytes enter secondary lymphoid tissues and are then attracted within the parafollicular area by SLC (CCL21) and ELC (CCL19), which are co-expressed there. The receptor and the ligands are essential for the homing and distribution of T lymphocytes as illustrated by deletion of the corresponding genes. Mice lacking CCR7 present morphological abnormalities, reflecting a disturbed homing of T cells into lymph nodes, and are unable to mount adequate antibody and delayed-type hypersensitivity responses (Förster et al. 1999). Similar disturbances are observed in mice with the *plt* (paucity of lymph node T cells) syndrome resulting from defective SLC (CCL21) and ELC (CCL19) expression (Gunn et al. 1999; Stein et al. 2000; Warnock et al. 2000).

Despite the disturbance of T lymphocytes homing, *plt* mice have a nearly normal B-lymphocyte recruitment into secondary lymphoid organs (Nakano et al. 1997). CCR7-deficient B lymphocytes transferred into normal mice, however, accumulate less efficiently in lymph nodes and Peyer's patches (Förster et al. 1999). Using transferred chemokine receptor-deficient and chemokine-desensitized B lymphocytes, it has recently been shown, by intravital microscopy, that B-cell homing into lymph nodes depends on two receptors – CCR7 and CXCR4 – and that, in addition, CXCR5 is important for B-cell homing into Peyer's patches (Okada et al. 2002). As shown by experiments in mice, the positioning of B cells in lymphoid tissues depends on responsiveness to BLC (CXCL13), on the one hand, and ELC and SLC (CCL19, CCL21), on the other, which are expressed in the B- and the T-cell areas, respectively (Reif et al. 2002). Naïve B cells, which bear CXCR5, migrate into the B-cell area in response to BLC (CXCL13). After antigen encounter and activation, however, B cells upregulate CCR7 and are attracted by SLC (CCL21) and ELC (CCL19) to the boundary between the B-and T-cell area (Reif et al. 2002).

In contrast to B2 cells (the conventional B cells), B1 cells home preferentially to the peritoneal and pleural cavities where macrophages and omentum cells constitutively produce BLC. B1 cells are a significant source of serum antibodies and make a major contribution to natural antibody production (low-affinity immunoglobulin M or IgM). In mice lacking BLC (CXCL13), the immigration of B1 cells into the peritoneal and pleural cavities is impaired and the production of natural and antigen-specific antibodies is markedly decreased (Ansel et al. 2002). Additional evidence for the important role of BLC (CXCL13) in homing of B1 cells is provided by the observation that B1 cells accumulate in the kidney and the thymus of aging BWF1 mice as a result of the abnormal expression of BLC (CXCL13) by myeloid dendritic cells (Ishikawa et al. 2001).

Another aspect of homing is the relocation of cells within a lymphoid tissue during maturation and differentiation as observed for thymocytes, which change receptor expression as they move from cortical to intermediate and then medullar sites (Campbell et al. 1999b; Annunziato et al. 2001; Ansel and Cyster 2001). Chemokines that are selectively produced in the different thymic areas are believed to retain the thymocytes as long as they express the proper chemokine receptor. A similar mechanism may operate in lympho- and myelopoiesis. Before being recognized as a chemokine, SDF-1 (CXCL12) was described as a factor with co-stimulatory effects on B-cell precursors (Tashiro et al. 1993; Nagasawa et al. 1994). We found that this chemokine attracts pre- and pro-B cells in contrast to more mature forms, and suggested that it could stimulate lymphopoiesis by attracting maturing cells in the vicinity of growth factor-producing stromal cells (D'Apuzzo et al. 1997; Baggiolini 1998). In agreement with this hypothesis, deletion of CXCR4 in mice resulted in enhanced escape of B-cell precursors into the circulation (Ma et al. 1999).

Homing into nonlymphoid tissues

Chemokines and their receptors are also involved in the regulation of T-cell traffic through nonlymphoid tissues. It has been suggested that memory T cells show a selective tropism for specific peripheral tissues and re-circulate preferentially through the tissues where they have acquired their immunological memory (Mackay 1993). Good examples are the skin-homing and gut-homing memory T cells, which are characterized by the expression of adhesion molecules, the cutaneous lymphocyte-associated antigen (CLA), and the integrin $\alpha_4\beta_7$, which co-determine their homing selectivity. CLA binds to E-selectin expressed on endothelial cells in the skin, whereas $\alpha_4\beta_7$ binds to mucosal addressin-cell adhesion molecule-1 (MadCAM-1) expressed in the endothelia of mucosal tissues. The homing preference of the cells is also reflected by the chemokine receptors that they express, CCR4, CCR9, and CCR10 in particular, and by the production of the corresponding chemokines in the tissues.

CCR4 is present on all CLA-positive and other memory T cells, but absent from $\alpha_4\beta_7$ memory T cells (Campbell et al. 1999a; Andrew et al. 2001). TARC (CCL17), one of CCR4's two selective ligands, is expressed by normal and inflamed endothelium of the skin, but not of the intestine (Campbell et al. 1999a). About a third of CLA^+ T cells also bear CCR10 and thus migrate in response to its two ligands, CTACK (CCL27) and MEC (CCL28) (Morales et al. 1999; Homey et al. 2000, 2002; Pan et al. 2000; Wang et al. 2000). CTACK (CCL27) is a skin-associated chemokine (Morales et al. 1999) that is produced in the basal layers of the epidermis and is upregulated in inflammatory skin diseases (Homey et al. 2002). In two different mouse models of allergen-challenged skin, anti-cutaneous T-cell attracting chemokine (CTACK) antibodies markedly inhibited the recruitment of lymphocytes and tissue swelling (Homey et al. 2002). A role for CCR4 and CCR10 in T-cell recruitment into the inflamed skin is suggested by a recent observation in delayed-type hypersensitivity. The immigration of T lymphocytes was not appreciably affected by antibodies neutralizing the CCR10 ligand CTACK (CCL27), but complete inhibition was observed when transferred CCR4-deficient T cells were used, suggesting that both receptors are involved concomitantly (Reiss et al. 2001).

CCR9 and its ligand thymus-expressed chemokine (TECK) (CCL25) are implicated in the homing of $\alpha_4\beta_7^+$ T cells to the gut (Zabel et al. 1999; Kunkel et al. 2000). CCR9 is expressed in $\alpha_4\beta_7^+$ T cells, and TECK (CCL25) is produced by epithelial cells of the small intestine, in particular in the crypt region, which is closely associated with the vessels involved in lymphocyte recruitment that express MadCAM-1 (Kunkel et al. 2000; Wurbel et al. 2000). TECK (CCL25) is also detected in small intestine endothelial cells (Papadakis et al. 2001). Several investigations have shown that nearly all T cells in the small intestine express CCR9, underscoring the possible importance of CCR9 and TECK (CCL25) for the lymphocyte traffic in the gut (Zabel et al. 1999; Kunkel et al. 2000; Papadakis et al. 2001).

CHEMOKINES IN DISEASE

The analysis of tissues, exudates, and body fluids by immunochemistry, cytofluorimetry, and in situ hybridization highlights the role of chemokines in infectious and inflammatory pathologies. Receptors for inflammatory chemokines are commonly detected in the lesions of chronic inflammatory diseases, such as rheumatoid arthritis, lupus erythematosus, ulcerative colitis, Crohn's disease, multiple sclerosis, chronic bronchitis, sarcoidosis, and arteriosclerosis. The patterns of expression reflect the peculiarities of the underlying pathology: CCR1, CCR2, CCR5, and CXCR3 are highly expressed in chronic lesions with a predominant infiltration of mononuclear phagocytes and Th1 lymphocytes, CCR3 is enhanced in allergic pathologies with participation of eosinophils and Th2 lymphocytes, whereas CXCR1 and CXCR2 dominate in bacterial infections and acute inflammation. Especially in chronic processes the analysis of receptors and their ligands reveals an apparent redundancy of chemokine involvement in pathology. In animal models, deletions of chemokine or receptor genes and selective receptor antagonists have been used to explore the pathophysiological role of single chemokines and receptors. The issue of chemokine hierarchy in host defense and inflammation, which is highly relevant for the design of therapeutic approaches targeting chemokines, is addressed in a recent review (Gerard and Rollins 2001).

Chemokines and viral infections

Although infections by bacteria and fungi elicit inflammatory responses by inducing chemokine production either directly or on mediation by inflammatory cytokines such as IL-1 and TNF, herpes viruses, pox viruses, and retroviruses have evolved means to subvert the chemokine defense system to their own advantage. The genome of these viruses can encode chemokines, chemokine receptors, structurally unrelated chemokine receptor ligands, and chemokine-binding proteins. These gene products may be expressed on the viral surface or by the cells that the viruses infect. The most impressive case of viral interaction with the chemokine system is the mechanism that enables HIV to enter CD4-bearing cells. Gp120, a viral envelope protein with no structural similarity to chemokines, binds first CD4 and then a chemokine receptor, usually CCR5 or CXCR4. This interaction exposes the fusogenic extremity of another surface protein, gp41, initiating the fusion of the viral envelope with the membrane of the target cell, which becomes infected. The interaction process leading to fusion and viral entry has not been clarified beyond the definition of the molecules that are necessary on the surface of the virus and the target cell. Several points of contact are assumed between the interacting moieties and formation of aggregates has been suggested, as recently reviewed (Murphy 2001). Co-receptor recognition, the choice between CCR5 and CXCR4, depends on the structure of the variable region of the V3 loop of gp120. In addition to clarifying the mechanism of HIV entry, the discovery of the second binding site, which remained elusive for long after the recognition that CD4 was important, helped to define R5 and X4 HIV strains, which bind CCR5 and CXCR4, respectively, and strains binding to both co-receptors, termed 'R5X4' (Berger et al. 1999). The relevance of chemokine receptors for the infection with HIV is underscored by the observations that individuals with an inactive form of CCR5 (CCR5Δ32) are resistant.

It was reported that gp120, in addition to docking on to CCR5 or CXCR4, also induces signaling (Davis et al. 1997) and thus may contribute to recruitment of additional target cells and/or influence cellular immune defense. A similar interference is ascribed to another HIV protein, the transcription factor Tat, which is released into tissue fluids and has been reported to attract leukocytes bearing CCR2 or CCR3 and to block CXCR4 (Murphy 2001).

Multiple, more direct interferences with the chemokine system were described for human herpesviruses 6 and 8 (HHV6 and 8), and human *cytomegalovirus* (HCMV) which all encode chemokines and chemokine receptors. The receptors have evolved for broad activities and are either constitutively active, similar to ORF74 encoded by HHV8 and expressed in Kaposi's sarcoma (Arvanitakis et al. 1997), or responsive to multiple human chemokines, such as ORF U51 encoded by HHV6 (Milne et al. 2000) and US28 encoded by HCMV (Gao and Murphy 1994). HCMV encodes two CXC chemokines, vCXC1, which is selective for CXCR2, and vCXC2, which has not been characterized (Penfold et al. 1999). The best known viral chemokines vMIP-I, -II, and-III are encoded by HHV8 and interact, as agonist or antagonists, with several CCRs in addition to CXCR4 (Kledal et al. 1997; Stine et al. 2000).

Studies on inflammatory diseases in animal models

In recognition of the inflammatory nature of arteriosclerosis and the importance of monocytes, which infiltrate the arterial wall and progressively transform into macrophages and foam cells (Ross 1999), research has focused on chemokines attracting monocytes. Although, as in other chronic inflammatory conditions, several chemokines are expressed in arteriosclerotic plaques and the underlying arterial wall tissue, deletion of the genes encoding CCR2 in murine models of the disease results in a marked reduction of fatty streak and plaque formation (Boring et al. 1998; Dawson et al. 1999). Remarkably, the pathological process is also attenuated in animals with a deletion of the MCP-1 gene, indicating that other MCPs cannot compensate for the lack of MCP-1 (CCL2) (Gu et al. 1998; Gosling et al. 1999).

The pathology of experimental allergic encephalomyelitis in mice also appears to depend on chemokines acting on mononuclear cells. Deletion of CCR2, the receptor for MCP-1 (CCL2), MCP-2 (CCL8), MCP-3 (CCL7), and MCP-4 (CCL13), protects the animals against the relapsing central nervous system (CNS) inflammation induced by immunization with myelin components (Fife et al. 2000; Izikson et al. 2000), suggesting that monocytes and T lymphocytes, which respond to CCR2 ligands, are particularly important for disease progression. By contrast the development of the disease was not, or only minimally, affected by deleting the genes for MIP-1α (CCL3), RANTES (CCL5), and other chemokines (Gerard and Rollins 2001). These observations suggest that some chemokines, even if expressed in inflammatory lesions, play only a minor role in pathology or act in subordination to other chemokines. This conclusion is supported by studies showing that the encephalomyelitis was not appreciably affected by deletion of the *CCR1* or the *CCR5* genes, suggesting that neither receptor is important for the recruitment of mononuclear cells (Gerard and Rollins 2001). Unfortunately, the role of CXCR3, a receptor that is exclusively expressed in activated T lymphocytes, and its exclusive ligands, Mig, IP10, and I-TAC (CXCL9, -10, and -11, respectively), has not yet been investigated.

Experimental transplantation is a very useful model because of its close relationship to the clinical situation. The introduction of the graft elicits an almost immediate inflammatory response, which is characterized by the expression of IL-8 (CXCL8), MCP-1 (CCL2), and their analogs. This reaction is not related to the specific process of graft rejection and may be induced by inflammatory mediators produced as a consequence of transplant reperfusion (Hancock et al. 2000a). A reaction against the graft follows after the local induction – in the graft and the host tissue – of chemokines, which attract mononuclear cells via CCR1, CCR2, CCR5, and CXCR3. Deletion of any of these receptors retards graft rejection, but the most pronounced effect is observed after deletion of CXCR3 (Gao et al. 2000; Hancock et al. 2000a, b, 2001), confirming that activated $CD4^+$ and $CD8^+$ T cells, which characteristically express high levels of CXCR3 (M. Loetscher et al. 1996), are essential for the immune reaction leading to rejection. The apparent involvement of CCR1 and CCR2, which are not selective for the effector T-cell population, suggests a role for other players, or simply reflects the concomitant occurrence of an unspecific inflammatory reaction.

An alternate way to assess the role of chemokines in pathology is the use of receptor-blocking agents. In contrast to gene deletion, the intervention with antagonists can be timed at any stage of the pathological process allowing exploration of preventive as well as curative effects. Several models of chronic inflammatory joint diseases, such as the adjuvant-induced arthritis in rats, collagen-induced arthritis in mice, and chronic polyarthritis of the MRL-lpr mouse, are considered as correlates of human rheumatoid arthritis. These models are widely used in the pharmaceutical industry for the assessment of anti-inflammatory drugs, and are of obvious interest for the study of chemokines. Two chemokine receptor antagonists, an amino-terminally truncated MCP-1 (CCL2) (Gong et al. 1997) and Met-RANTES (Met-CCL5) (Plater-Zyberk et al. 1997), were successfully applied in these models to prevent the development of inflammatory lesions and to attenuate the already established disease. These observations confirm the major role of the MCP receptor, CCR2, in the development and maintenance of chronic inflammation, and suggest the involvement of CCR1 and possibly CCR5.

Studies in patients

Despite the frequent, almost obligatory expression of chemokines in diseased tissues, the information about their role in human pathology is rather limited. It follows that the task of chemokine expression studies in human disease is to identify chemokines that are chiefly involved in steering the process of host defense and inflammation for two main reasons: a better understanding of pathogenic mechanisms and the identification of ligands and receptors as targets for therapeutic intervention.

Immunocytochemistry and in situ hybridization of tissue biopsies show that several inflammatory chemokines are usually expressed concomitantly. As chemokines act in the microenvironment of the cells that release them, the study of their potential role in pathology must be based on observations in situ. Discrete evaluation of lesional and nonlesional areas of the same tissue usually discloses important differences and provides a good internal control for the changes occurring in the affected tissues. A random assessment does not take into account the focal nature of inflammation, and measurements of chemokine concentrations in exudates and other body fluids yield only a pale reflection of the disease process. The approach in such investigations may be exemplified by a study of biopsies of inflamed and normal areas of the gut mucosa at different stages of ulcerative colitis (Uguccioni et al. 1999). The local levels of chemokines were quantified by determining the numbers of chemokine-producing cells using image analysis. It was not attempted to quantify the *intensity* of chemokine staining within the cells or in the extracellular space because we found it virtually impossible to obtain reproducible results in standard specimens. Within the lesions, the numbers of cells expressing IL-8 (CXCL8), MCP-1 (CCL2), and MCP-3 (CCL7) were strictly correlated with disease severity, as assessed by clinical criteria, but the frequency of cells producing IL-8 (CXCL8) was about tenfold higher than those producing MCPs. IP10 (CXCL10)-positive cells also increased with pathology, but a significant expression of this chemokine was also observed in nonlesional biopsies, a finding that was not studied further. MIP-1α (CCL3), a chemokine acting via CCR1 and CCR5, was also studied, but no positive cells were detected. These observations indicate that leukocytes bearing CCR2, CXCR1, CXCR2, and CXCR3, i.e. monocytes, activated T cells, and neutrophils, are most likely to be recruited into the lesions, which is confirmed by histology. CCR1 and CCR3, which bind MCP-3 (CCL7), may also be involved in the immigration of mononuclear cells. The redundancy in the expression of inflammatory chemokines is well documented in human disease and animal models. In consideration of the chemokine expression pattern observed in ulcerative colitis, CCR2, the receptor for MCPs, which is expressed in monocytes and all IL-2-activated T cells (Figure 13.6 and see Figure 13.4), appears to be of particular relevance.

The only known chemokine receptor defect in humans results from the expression of an inactive variant of CCR5, CCR5Δ32. The defect is relatively frequent in individuals of Caucasian descent who do not present an increased susceptibility to infectious diseases (see 'Chemokines and viral infections' above). Several studies have shown that carriers of the Δ32 allele are partially resistant to chronic inflammatory diseases. It was found that they have a delayed onset of multiple sclerosis (Barcellos et al. 2000). Even homozygotes, however, can develop the disease, indicating that a functional CCR5 is not essential for the occurrence of this particular pathology (Bennetts et al. 1997). In a comparison of about 700 patients with rheumatoid arthritis, 100 patients with lupus erythematosus, and 800 controls, no difference was found in the frequencies of the normal and defective CCR5 allele, but no patient was homozygous for the defective receptor (Gòmez-Reino et al. 1999). Another study of 163 patients with rheumatoid arthritis revealed no difference in the hetero- and homozygous incidence of the CCR5 defect as compared with the healthy population. Carriers of the Δ32 allele, however, showed a tendency to milder disease (Garred et al. 1998).

Svanborg and her colleagues (Frendeus et al. 2000) have studied the role of IL-8 receptor expression for

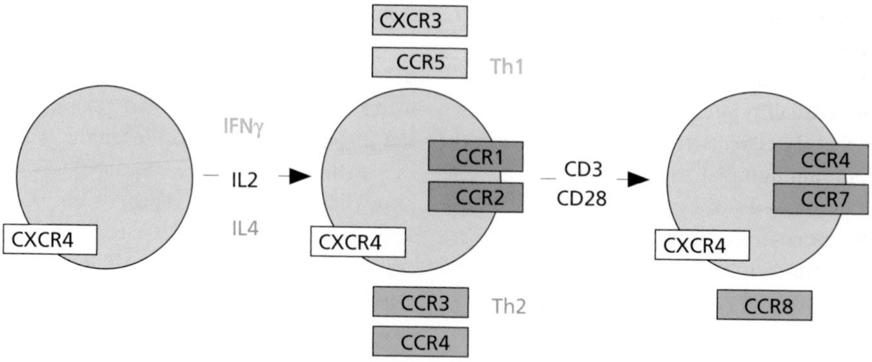

Figure 13.6 Chemokine receptor expression in human T lymphocytes. Blood T lymphocytes usually express low levels of chemokine receptors and respond poorly to chemokines. Receptor expression depends on maturation, activation, and differentiation (see text).

antibacterial defense by comparing the coping of normal and IL-8 receptor-deficient mice with urinary tract infections. The susceptibility of receptor-deficient mice (Godaly et al. 2000; Hang et al. 2000) motivated a study of CXCR1 expression in neutrophils of normal and pyelonephritis-prone children, whose neutrophils were found to have significantly lower CXCR1 levels than those of healthy controls. This observation offers an explanation for the recurrence of pyelonephritis in certain individuals and may lead to the characterization of a genetic polymorphism of CXCR1.

A highly interesting case of chemokine involvement in infection-induced human pathology is documented by a study of chemokine expression in *Helicobacter pylori* gastritis (Mazzucchelli et al. 1999). The comparison of normal and infected mucosa shows that the B-cell-attracting chemokine (BCA-1) (CXCL13) is abundantly and exclusively expressed at the sites of formation of the ectopic follicles, which are characteristic for the disease. The staining for the chemokine coincides with the staining for its receptor, CXCR5, in the immigrated lymphocytes. SLC, by contrast, which is expressed constitutively in the extrafollicular areas of lymphoid tissues together with ELC and is prominent in high-endothelial venules, was not detectable in and around the mucosal follicles, and was restricted to the endothelia of some microvessels. It may have a role in the extravasation of B cells which are then attracted into the ectopic follicles by BCA-1 (CXCL13). Mucosa-associated lymphoid tissue (MALT) lymphomas are a frequent complication of *H. pylori* infection. Interestingly the transformed cells produce high amounts of BCA-1 (CXCL13) and express CXCR5, suggesting that the B-cell-attracting chemokine, in the tumor, may act in an autocrine fashion and influence the proliferation of lymphoma cells. The pathological formation of follicle-like structures was later found to be associated with BCA-1 (CXCL13) expression in Sjögren's syndrome (Amft et al. 2001) and rheumatoid arthritis (Shi et al. 2001) as well.

Luther et al. (2000) have reported the formation of ectopic lymph node-like structures in pancreas islets after expression of BLC, the murine homolog of BCA-1 (CXCL13), in transgenic mice. This study shows that immigrating CXCR5-positive B cells cluster to form follicles. The process of ectopic lymphoid neogenesis, however, goes beyond the accumulation of B cells observed in *H. pylori*-induced gastritis and other human inflammatory diseases. The transgenic animals also express SLC in the parafollicular area leading to the formation of a T-cell zone with high-endothelial venules and lymphotoxin, possibly as a consequence of the exaggerated production of BLC.

CHEMOKINE RECEPTOR ANTAGONISTS

The idea that chemokine antagonists could have therapeutic effects in inflammatory diseases by preventing leukocyte infiltration was proposed soon after the discovery of IL-8 (CXCL8) (Baggiolini et al. 1989). It was then shown that CXCR1 and CXCR2 could be blocked with IL-8 (CXCL8) analogs obtained by truncation or minimal modification of the amino-terminal triggering sequence, and that the same principle could be applied to MCP-1 (CCL2) and RANTES (CCL5) to block the respective CC chemokine receptors (Baggiolini et al. 1994, 1997). The interest in the antagonists grew considerably with the recognition that all chemokines act via heptahelical, Gi-protein-coupled receptors (Murphy et al. 2000) and the discovery that human immunodeficiency viruses bind to chemokine receptors to infect leukocytes and viral entry is prevented by competing chemokines (Berger et al. 1999) and chemokine antagonists (Arenzana-Seisdedos et al. 1996; Simmons et al. 1997). In the same context, chemical substances with known HIV-suppressing activity were tested for chemokine antagonism and it was shown that chemokine receptors could be blocked with small, chemokine-unrelated molecules (De Clercq 2000; Gerlach et al. 2001). These observations boosted the search for nonpeptide chemokine antagonists using high-throughput screening of chemical libraries, with the aim of discovering new drugs for chronic inflammatory diseases.

The hypothesis that antagonists could be effective in the therapy of chronic inflammatory diseases was validated in animal models using amino-terminally modified MCP-1 (CCL2) or RANTES (CCL5). Daily injections of the CCR2 antagonists MCP-1 (9–76), obtained by omission of the first eight amino-terminal residue of synthetic MCP-1 (CCL2), prevented or strongly inhibited the development of the chronic arthritis that arises spontaneously in MRL-lpr mice, and showed considerable anti-inflammatory effects even in animals that had already developed the disease (Gong et al. 1997). Similar preventive and therapeutic effects were observed on repeated injections of Met-RANTES (Met-CCL5) in mice with collagen-induced arthritis (Plater-Zyberk et al. 1997). Met-RANTES also prevented the infiltration of inflammatory cells and significantly reduced vascular injury and tubular damage in renal allografts performed in Lewis RT1 rats (Grone et al. 1999). Met-RANTES is not a true antagonist, because it retains different levels of agonistic activity on the RANTES receptors, CCR1, CCR3, and CCR5 (Proudfoot et al. 1999).

Synthetic, chemokine-unrelated antagonists

The development of chemokine antagonists became a major goal of the pharmaceutical industry. The focus is on receptors that mediate leukocyte infiltration in inflammatory diseases as reflected by the patent applications, which mainly claim activities against CXCR1, CXCR2, CXCR3, CCR1, CCR2, and CCR3. Other, more restricted targets are CXCR4 and CCR5, the two main HIV co-receptors. Several, mostly polycyclic, compounds have been identified in broad screening programs as blockers of single or multiple receptors (Horuk and Ng 2000).

Among the compounds that are ready for studies in patients, the CCR1 antagonist BX471 (Berlex) may soon yield the proof of concept for the use of chemokine antagonists in the therapy of inflammation. It is a potent inhibitor of chemokine activities with K_i values around 1 nmol/l, is apparently selective for CCR1 (Liang et al. 2000), and inactive on adrenergic, muscarinic, dopamine, serotonin, bradykinin, leukotriene B_4 (LTB_4), and neuropeptide receptors. In animal models of disease BX471 was moderately effective in preventing graft rejection in rodents (Horuk et al. 2001b) and was found to act in synergy with the immunosuppressant cyclosporin (Horuk et al. 2001a, 2001b). It also reduced leukocyte infiltration and the development of renal fibrosis after unilateral ureter ligation in mice (Anders et al. 2002). Somewhat related to BX471 is a xanthene derivative, from the Banyu Company, that blocks CCR1 and CCR3. The combination of CCR1 and CCR3 antagonism may be therapeutically desirable for allergic inflammation because both receptors are prominent on eosinophil and basophil leukocytes. Highly selective antagonism for CCR3 was obtained, however, in the same laboratories with benzothiazole derivatives with IC_{50} (concentration of 50 percent inhibition) values for inhibition of binding and function in the low-nanomolar range (Naya et al. 2001; Sabroe et al. 2000). Naphthalene compounds synthesized by Smith Kline Beecham also showed potent blocking effects on CCR3 and only weak interaction with CXCR1, CXCR2, CCR1, CCR7, and the receptors for C5a, C3a, and LTD_4 (White et al. 2000; Dhanak et al. 2001).

Interesting studies were performed with spiropiperidine compounds from Roche (e.g. RS-102895, RS-504393), binding CCR2 but not CCR1, CCR3, or CXCR1 and inhibiting the activity of MCP-1 (CCL2) and its analogs, which are major mediators in chronic inflammatory diseases (Mirzadegan et al. 2000). These compounds were shown to interact with the acidic residue Glu291 at the extracellular end of the seventh transmembrane helix of CCR2, which is important for the high-affinity binding of MCP-1 (CCL2). The compounds, however, were equally or even more potent as blockers for α_1-adrenergic receptors (Mirzadegan et al. 2000), possibly jeopardizing their use as MCP blockers.

In view of their HIV co-receptor function, CCR5 and CXCR4 became prime targets for the development of synthetic antagonists. TAK-799, a compound by Takeda, with high affinity for CCR5 and CCR2 with K_i values of about 1 and 20 nmol/l, respectively, and no effects on CCR1, CCR3, CCR4, and CXCR4 (Baba et al. 1999; Shiraishi et al. 2000) was reported to prevent the binding of the HIV surface protein gp120 by interacting with a cluster of residues at the outer end of the transmembrane helices 1, 2, 3, and 7 of CCR5 (Dragic et al. 2000). CCR5 antagonists without relevant inhibition of CCR2 were synthesized by Ono (Maeda et al. 2001), Schering-Plough (Strizki et al. 2001), and Merck (Finke et al. 2001). Cyclams and bicyclams, on the other hand, are potent antagonists for CXCR4 (De Clercq 2000). Binding-site analysis shows that bicyclams interact with two acidic residues, Asp171 and Asp262, located at the extracellular end of transmembrane domains 4 and 6 of CXCR4, which are both necessary for high-affinity blockade of the ligand-binding pocket (Gerlach et al. 2001).

Missed targets

So far the development of synthetic low-molecular-mass antagonists for CXCR1, CXCR3, and CCR2 has not been as successful. IL-8 (CXCL8), the major ligand for CXCR1, is expressed ubiquitously and most prominently in inflamed tissues, and must be regarded as a primary mediator of neutrophil recruitment in conditions such as infarction and reperfusion, ulcerative colitis, alcoholic hepatitis, early graft rejection, etc., for which CXCR1 antagonists are therapeutically desirable. Antagonists for CXCR3, the receptor for Mig, IP10, and I-TAC

(CXCL9, -10, and -11, respectively) appears equally important, because they would be ideal drugs for preventing the recruitment of activated T lymphocytes in autoimmune diseases and at sites of transplant rejection. Finally the need for selective CCR2 antagonists is underscored by many observations in experimental pathology, including studies on receptor and ligand gene deletions, indicating a primary role for MCP-1 in chronic inflammatory diseases (Gerard and Rollins 2001).

Research and development in this important area of drug discovery have concentrated so far on the search of monoselective compounds. In inflamed tissues, however, one usually observes the concerted expression of several chemokines, suggesting that inhibitors of multiple receptors may be better drugs. Autoimmune inflammation may be treated more efficiently by drugs that block CCR1, CCR2, and CXCR3, rather than with antagonists for a single receptor. Similarly, the combined blockade of CCR1, CCR2, and CCR3 may be the best therapeutic strategy in allergic inflammation. The comparison of the therapeutic efficacy of antagonists for single and multiple receptors in animal models will be useful for directing drug discovery programs.

Natural chemokines as antagonists

Recent observations have shown that some natural chemokines have agonistic as well as antagonistic activities. In a study of chemokines acting on receptors that are differentially expressed in Th1 and Th2 lymphocytes, we found that the agonists for CXCR3, Mig, IP10, and I-TAC (CXCL9,-10, and-11, respectively) are antagonists for CCR3 (Loetscher et al. 2001). They compete for the binding of chemokines to CCR3-bearing cells, and inhibit calcium mobilization and migration induced by CCR3 agonists such as eotaxin-1 (CCL11), eotaxin-2 (CCL24), MCP-2 (CCL8), MCP-3 (CCL7), MCP-4 (CCL13), and RANTES (CCL5). As a result of their dual properties the attractants of Th1 lymphocytes acting via CXCR3 can inhibit the recruitment of Th2 lymphocytes by blocking CCR3, and in this way enhance the polarization of T-cell recruitment. Other natural chemokines with agonistic and antagonistic activities are eotaxin (CCL11), which attracts eosinophils, basophils, and Th2 lymphocytes via CCR3 while blocking CCR2 (Ogilvie et al. 2001), and MCP-3 (CCL7), a potent agonist for CCR1, CCR2, and CCR3 that blocks CCR5 (Blanpain et al. 1999). The inhibition of CCR2-, CCR3-, and CCR5-mediated responses represents a true antagonism as indicated by the fact that binding of the inhibitor does not induce receptor internalization. More work must be done to assess the role of the combination of triggering and inhibiting effects of single chemokines on different receptors, which impresses as a possible mechanism for increasing the selectivity of leukocyte recruitment in disease.

REFERENCES

Abbas, A.K., Murphy, K.M. and Sher, A. 1996. Functional diversity of helper T lymphocytes. *Nature*, **383**, 787–93.

Amft, N., Curnow, S.J., et al. 2001. Ectopic expression of the B cell-attracting chemokine BCA-1 (CXCL13) on endothelial cells and within lymphoid follicles contributes to the establishment of germinal center-like structures in Sjögren's syndrome. *Arthritis Rheum*, **44**, 2633–41.

Anders, H.J., Vielhauer, V., et al. 2002. A chemokine receptor CCR-1 antagonist reduces renal fibrosis after unilateral ureter ligation. *J Clin Invest*, **109**, 251–9.

Andrew, D.P., Ruffing, N., et al. 2001. C-C chemokine receptor 4 expression defines a major subset of circulating nonintestinal memory T cells of both Th1 and Th2 potential. *J Immunol*, **166**, 103–11.

Annunziato, F., Galli, G., et al. 1998. Molecules associated with human Th1 or Th2 cells. *Eur Cytokine Netw*, **9**, 12–16.

Annunziato, F., Romagnani, P., et al. 2001. Chemokines and lymphopoiesis in human thymus. *Trends Immunol*, **22**, 277–81.

Ansel, K.M. and Cyster, J.G. 2001. Chemokines in lymphopoiesis and lymphoid organ development. *Curr Opin Immunol*, **13**, 172–9.

Ansel, K.M., Ngo, V.N., et al. 2000. A chemokine-driven positive feedback loop organizes lymphoid follicles. *Nature*, **406**, 309–14.

Ansel, K.M., Harris, R.B. and Cyster, J.G. 2002. CXCL13 is required for B1 cell homing, natural antibody production, and body cavity immunity. *Immunity*, **16**, 67–76.

Arenzana-Seisdedos, F., Virelizier, J.L., et al. 1996. HIV blocked by chemokine antagonist. *Nature*, **383**, 400.

Arvanitakis, L., Geras-Raaka, E., et al. 1997. Human herpesvirus KSHV encodes a constitutively active G-protein-coupled receptor linked to cell proliferation. *Nature*, **385**, 347–50.

Baba, M., Nishimura, O., et al. 1999. A small-molecule, nonpeptide CCR5 antagonist with highly potent and selective anti-HIV-1 activity. *Proc Natl Acad Sci USA*, **96**, 5698–703.

Baggiolini, M. 1998. Chemokines and leukocyte traffic. *Nature*, **392**, 565–8.

Baggiolini, M. and Kernen, P. 1992. Neutrophil activation: Control of shape change, exocytosis, and respiratory burst. *News Physiol Sci*, **7**, 215–19.

Baggiolini, M., Walz, A. and Kunkel, S.L. 1989. Neutrophil-activating peptide-1/interleukin 8, a novel cytokine that activates neutrophils. *J Clin Invest*, **84**, 1045–9.

Baggiolini, M., Dewald, B. and Moser, B. 1994. Interleukin-8 and related chemotactic cytokines – CXC and CC chemokines. *Adv Immunol*, **55**, 97–179.

Baggiolini, M., Dewald, B. and Moser, B. 1997. Human chemokines: An update. *Annu Rev Immunol*, **15**, 675–705.

Baldwin, E.T., Weber, I.T., et al. 1991. Crystal structure of interleukin 8: Symbiosis of NMR and crystallography. *Proc Natl Acad Sci USA*, **88**, 502–6.

Barcellos, L.F., Schito, A.M., et al. 2000. CC-chemokine receptor 5 polymorphism and age of onset in familial multiple sclerosis. Multiple Sclerosis Genetics Group. *Immunogenetics*, **51**, 281–8.

Bardi, G., Lipp, M., et al. 2001. The T cell chemokine receptor CCR7 is internalized on stimulation with ELC, but not with SLC. *Eur J Immunol*, **31**, 3291–7.

Barella, L., Loetscher, M., et al. 1995. Sequence variation of a novel heptahelical leucocyte receptor through alternative transcript formation. *Biochem J*, **309**, 773–9.

Bazan, J.F., Bacon, K.B., et al. 1997. A new class of membrane-bound chemokine with a CX_3C motif. *Nature*, **385**, 640–4.

Bennetts, B.H., Teutsch, S.M., et al. 1997. The CCR5 deletion mutation fails to protect against multiple sclerosis. *Hum Immunol*, **58**, 52–9.

Berger, E.A., Murphy, P.M. and Farber, J.M. 1999. Chemokine receptors as HIV-1 coreceptors: Roles in viral entry, tropism, and disease. *Annu Rev Immunol*, **17**, 657–700.

Blanpain, C., Migeotte, I., et al. 1999. CCR5 binds multiple CC-chemokines: MCP-3 acts as a natural antagonist. *Blood*, **94**, 1899–905.

Bonecchi, R., Bianchi, G., et al. 1998. Differential expression of chemokine receptors and chemotactic responsiveness of type 1 T helper cells (Th1s) and Th2s. *J Exp Med*, **187**, 129–34.

Bonecchi, R., Polentarutti, N., et al. 1999. Up-regulation of CCR1 and CCR3 and induction of chemotaxis to CC chemokines by IFN-gamma in human neutrophils. *J Immunol*, **162**, 474–9.

Bonecchi, R., Facchetti, F., et al. 2000. Induction of functional IL-8 receptors by IL-4 and IL-13 in human monocytes. *J Immunol*, **164**, 3862–9.

Boring, L., Gosling, J., et al. 1998. Decreased lesion formation in $CCR2^{-/-}$ mice reveals a role for chemokines in the initiation of atherosclerosis. *Nature*, **394**, 894–7.

Boulay, F., Tardif, M., et al. 1990. The human N-formylpeptide receptor. Characterization of two cDNA isolates and evidence for a new subfamily of G-protein-coupled receptors. *Biochemistry*, **29**, 11123–33.

Boulay, F., Naik, N., et al. 1997. Phagocyte chemoattractant receptors. *Ann N Y Acad Sci*, **832**, 69–84.

Bouvier, M. 2001. Oligomerization of G-protein-coupled transmitter receptors. *Nat Rev Neurosci*, **2**, 274–86.

Breitfeld, D., Ohl, L., et al. 2000. Follicular B helper T cells express CXC chemokine receptor 5, localize to B cell follicles, and support immunoglobulin production. *J Exp Med*, **192**, 1545–52.

Burrows, S.D., Doyle, M.L., et al. 1994. Determination of the monomer-dimer equilibrium of interleukin-8 reveals it is a monomer at physiological concentrations. *Biochemistry*, **33**, 12741–5.

Butcher, E.C. and Picker, L.J. 1996. Lymphocyte homing and homeostasis. *Science*, **272**, 60–6.

Campbell, J.J., Haraldsen, G., et al. 1999a. The chemokine receptor CCR4 in vascular recognition by cutaneous but not intestinal memory T cells. *Nature*, **400**, 776–80.

Campbell, J.J., Pan, J.L. and Butcher, E.C. 1999b. Developmental switches in chemokine responses during T cell maturation. *J Immunol*, **163**, 2353.

Campbell, J.J., Murphy, K.E., et al. 2001. CCR7 expression and memory T cell diversity in humans. *J Immunol*, **166**, 877–84.

Chung, C., Cooke, R.M., et al. 1995. The three-dimensional solution structure of RANTES. *Biochemistry*, **34**, 9307–14.

Clark-Lewis, I., Schumacher, C., et al. 1991. Structure-activity relationships of interleukin-8 determined using chemically synthesized analogs. Critical role of NH_2-terminal residues and evidence for uncoupling of neutrophil chemotaxis, exocytosis, and receptor binding activities. *J Biol Chem*, **266**, 23128–34.

Clark-Lewis, I., Dewald, B., et al. 1993. Platelet factor 4 binds to interleukin 8 receptors and activates neutrophils when its N terminus is modified with Glu-Leu-Arg. *Proc Natl Acad Sci USA*, **90**, 3574–7.

Clark-Lewis, I., Dewald, B., et al. 1994. Structural requirements for interleukin-8 function identified by design of analogs and CXC chemokine hybrids. *J Biol Chem*, **269**, 16075–81.

Clark-Lewis, I., Kim, K.-S., et al. 1995. Structure–activity relationships of chemokines. *J Leukocyte Biol*, **57**, 703–11.

Clore, G.M. and Gronenborn, A.M. 1995. Three-dimensional structures of α and β chemokines. *FASEB J*, **9**, 57–62.

Clore, G.M., Appella, E., et al. 1990. Three-dimensional structure of interleukin 8 in solution. *Biochemistry*, **29**, 1689–96.

Colditz, I., Zwahlen, R., et al. 1989. In vivo inflammatory activity of neutrophil-activating factor, a novel chemotactic peptide derived from human monocytes. *Am J Pathol*, **134**, 755–60.

Cole, K.E., Strick, C.A., et al. 1998. Interferon-inducible T cell alpha chemoattractant (I-TAC): A novel non-ELR CXC chemokine with potent activity on activated T cells through selective high affinity binding to CXCR3. *J Exp Med*, **187**, 2009–21.

Cory, G.O. and Ridley, A.J. 2002. Cell motility: Braking WAVEs. *Nature*, **418**, 732–3.

Covell, D.G., Smythers, G.W., et al. 1994. Analysis of hydrophobicity in the α and β chemokine families and its relevance to dimerization. *Protein Sci*, **3**, 2064–72.

Crump, M.P., Gong, J.H., et al. 1997. Solution structure and basis for functional activity of stromal cell-derived factor-1; dissociation of CXCR4 activation from binding and inhibition of HIV-1. *EMBO J*, **16**, 6996–7007.

Czaplewski, L.G., McKeating, J., et al. 1999. Identification of amino acid residues critical for aggregation of human CC chemokines macrophage inflammatory protein (MIP)-1α, MIP-1β and RANTES – characterization of active disaggregated chemokine variants. *J Biol Chem*, **274**, 16077–84.

D'Ambrosio, D., Iellem, A., et al. 1998. Selective up-regulation of chemokine receptors CCR4 and CCR8 upon activation of polarized human type 2 Th cells. *J Immunol*, **161**, 5111–15.

D'Apuzzo, M., Rolink, A., et al. 1997. The chemokine SDF-1, stromal cell-derived factor 1, attracts early stage B cell precursors via the chemokine receptor CXCR4. *Eur J Immunol*, **27**, 1788–93.

Davis, C.B., Dikic, I., et al. 1997. Signal transduction due to HIV-1 envelope interactions with chemokine receptors CXCR4 or CCR5. *J Exp Med*, **186**, 1793–8.

Dawson, T.C., Kuziel, W.A., et al. 1999. Absence of CC chemokine receptor-2 reduces atherosclerosis in apolipoprotein E-deficient mice. *Atherosclerosis*, **143**, 205–11.

De Clercq, E. 2000. Inhibition of HIV infection by bicyclams, highly potent and specific CXCR4 antagonists. *Mol Pharmacol*, **57**, 833–9.

Debes, G.F., Hopken, U.E. and Hamann, A. 2002. In vivo differentiated cytokine-producing CD4(+) T cells express functional CCR7. *J Immunol*, **168**, 5441–7.

Dhanak, D., Christmann, L.T., et al. 2001. Discovery of potent and selective phenylalanine derived CCR3 antagonists. Part 1. *Bioorg Med Chem Lett*, **11**, 1441–4.

Dragic, T., Trkola, A., et al. 2000. A binding pocket for a small molecule inhibitor of HIV-1 entry within the transmembrane helices of CCR5. *Proc Natl Acad Sci USA*, **97**, 5639–44.

Elisseeva, E.L., Slupsky, C.M., et al. 2000. NMR studies of active N-terminal peptides of stromal cell-derived factor-1. Structural basis for receptor binding. *J Biol Chem*, **275**, 26799–2805.

Fernandez, E.J. and Lolis, E. 2002. Structure, function, and inhibition of chemokines. *Annu Rev Pharmacol Toxicol*, **42**, 469–99.

Fife, B.T., Huffnagle, G.B., et al. 2000. CC chemokine receptor 2 is critical for induction of experimental autoimmune encephalomyelitis. *J Exp Med*, **192**, 899–905.

Finke, P.E., Meurer, L.C., et al. 2001. Antagonists of the human CCR5 receptor as anti-HIV-1 agents. Part 2: structure-activity relationships for substituted 2-Aryl-1-[*N*-(methyl)-*N*-(phenylsulfonyl)amino]-4-(piperidin-1-yl)butanes. *Bioorg Med Chem Lett*, **11**, 265–70.

Forssmann, U., Uguccioni, M., et al. 1997. Eotaxin-2, a novel CC chemokine that is selective for the chemokine receptor CCR3, and acts like eotaxin on human eosinophil and basophil leukocytes. *J Exp Med*, **185**, 2171–6.

Förster, R., Emrich, T., et al. 1994. Expression of the G-protein-coupled receptor BLR1 defines mature, recirculating B cells and a subset of T-helper memory cells. *Blood*, **84**, 830–40.

Förster, R., Mattis, A.E., et al. 1996. A putative chemokine receptor, BLR1, directs B cell migration to defined lymphoid organs and specific anatomic compartments of the spleen. *Cell*, **87**, 1037–47.

Förster, R., Schubel, A., et al. 1999. CCR7 coordinates the primary immune response by establishing functional microenvironments in secondary lymphoid organs. *Cell*, **99**, 23–33.

Frendeus, B., Godaly, G., et al. 2000. Interleukin 8 receptor deficiency confers susceptibility to acute experimental pyelonephritis and may have a human counterpart. *J Exp Med*, **192**, 881–90.

Gao, J.-L. and Murphy, P.M. 1994. Human cytomegalovirus open reading frame *US28* encodes a functional β chemokine receptor. *J Biol Chem*, **269**, 28539–42.

Gao, W., Topham, P.S., et al. 2000. Targeting of the chemokine receptor CCR1 suppresses development of acute and chronic cardiac allograft rejection. *J Clin Invest*, **105**, 35–44.

Garred, P., Madsen, H.O., et al. 1998. CC chemokine receptor 5 polymorphism in rheumatoid arthritis. *J Rheumatol*, **25**, 1462–5.

Gerard, C. and Rollins, B.J. 2001. Chemokines and disease. *Nature Immunol*, **2**, 108–15.

Gerber, B.O., Zanni, M.P., et al. 1997. Functional expression of the eotaxin receptor CCR3 in T lymphocytes co-localizing with eosinophils. *Curr Biol*, **7**, 836–43.

Gerber, N., Lowman, H., et al. 2000. Receptor-binding conformation of the 'ELR' motif of IL-8: X-ray structure of the L5C/H33C variant at 2.35 A resolution. *Proteins*, **38**, 361–7.

Gerlach, L.O., Skerlj, R.T., et al. 2001. Molecular interactions of cyclam and bicyclam non-peptide antagonists with the CXCR4 chemokine receptor. *J Biol Chem*, **276**, 14153–60.

Godaly, G., Hang, L., et al. 2000. Transepithelial neutrophil migration is CXCR1 dependent in vitro and is defective in IL-8 receptor knockout mice. *J Immunol*, **165**, 5287–94.

Gong, J.-H., Ratkay, L.G., et al. 1997. An antagonist of monocyte chemoattractant protein 1 (MCP-1) inhibits arthritis in the MRL-*lpr* mouse model. *J Exp Med*, **186**, 131–7.

Gosling, J., Slaymaker, S., et al. 1999. MCP-1 deficiency reduces susceptibility to atherosclerosis in mice that overexpress human apolipoprotein B. *J Clin Invest*, **103**, 773–8.

Gòmez-Reino, J.J., Pablos, J.L., et al. 1999. Association of rheumatoid arthritis with a functional chemokine receptor, CCR5. *Arthritis Rheum*, **42**, 989–92.

Graham, G.J., MacKenzie, J., et al. 1994. Aggregation of the chemokine MIP-1α is a dynamic and reversible phenomenon. Biochemical and biological analyses. *J Biol Chem*, **269**, 4974–8.

Grone, H.J., Weber, C., et al. 1999. Met-RANTES reduces vascular and tubular damage during acute renal transplant rejection: blocking monocyte arrest and recruitment. *FASEB J*, **13**, 1371–83.

Gu, L., Okada, Y., et al. 1998. Absence of monocyte chemoattractant protein-1 reduces atherosclerosis in low density lipoprotein receptor-deficient mice. *Mol Cell*, **2**, 275–81.

Gunn, M.D., Ngo, V.N., et al. 1998. A B-cell-homing chemokine made in lymphoid follicles activates Burkitt's lymphoma receptor-1. *Nature*, **391**, 799–803.

Gunn, M.D., Kyuwa, S., et al. 1999. Mice lacking expression of secondary lymphoid organ chemokine have defects in lymphocyte homing and dendritic cell localization. *J Exp Med*, **189**, 451–60.

Hancock, W.W., Gao, W., et al. 2000a. Chemokines and their receptors in allograft rejection. *Curr Opin Immunol*, **12**, 511–16.

Hancock, W.W., Lu, B., et al. 2000b. Requirement of the chemokine receptor CXCR3 for acute allograft rejection. *J Exp Med*, **192**, 1515–20.

Hancock, W.W., Gao, W., et al. 2001. Donor-derived IP-10 initiates development of acute allograft rejection. *J Exp Med*, **193**, 975–80.

Hang, L., Frendeus, B., et al. 2000. Interleukin-8 receptor knockout mice have subepithelial neutrophil entrapment and renal scarring following acute pyelonephritis. *J Infect Dis*, **182**, 1738–48.

Hébert, C.A., Vitangcol, R.V. and Baker, J.B. 1991. Scanning mutagenesis of interleukin-8 identifies a cluster of residues required for receptor binding. *J Biol Chem*, **266**, 18989–94.

Holmes, W.E., Lee, J., et al. 1991. Structure and functional expression of a human interleukin-8 receptor. *Science*, **253**, 1278–80.

Homey, B., Wang, W., et al. 2000. Cutting edge: the orphan chemokine receptor G protein-coupled receptor-2 (GPR-2, CCR10) binds the skin-associated chemokine CCL27 (CTACK/ALP/ILC). *J Immunol*, **164**, 3465–70.

Homey, B., Alenius, H., et al. 2002. CCL27-CCR10 interactions regulate T cell-mediated skin inflammation. *Nat Med*, **8**, 157–65.

Horuk, R. and Ng, H.P. 2000. Chemokine receptor antagonists. *Med Res Rev*, **20**, 155–68.

Horuk, R., Clayberger, C., et al. 2001a. A non-peptide functional antagonist of the CCR1 chemokine receptor is effective in rat heart transplant rejection. *J Biol Chem*, **276**, 4199–204.

Horuk, R., Shurey, S., et al. 2001b. CCR1-specific non-peptide antagonist: efficacy in a rabbit allograft rejection model. *Immunol Lett*, **76**, 193–201.

Imai, T., Nagira, M., et al. 1999. Selective recruitment of CCR4-bearing T_h2 cells toward antigen-presenting cells by the CC chemokines thymus and activation-regulated chemokine and macrophage-derived chemokine. *Int Immunol*, **11**, 81–8.

Ishikawa, S., Sato, T., et al. 2001. Aberrant high expression of B lymphocyte chemokine (BLC/CXCL13) by C11b+CD11c+ dendritic cells in murine lupus and preferential chemotaxis of B1 cells towards BLC. *J Exp Med*, **193**, 1393–402.

Izikson, L., Klein, R.S., et al. 2000. Resistance to experimental autoimmune encephalomyelitis in mice lacking the CC chemokine receptor (CCR)2. *J Exp Med*, **192**, 1075–80.

Jones, S.A., Moser, B. and Thelen, M. 1995. A comparison of post-receptor signal transduction events in Jurkat cells transfected with either IL-8R1 or IL-8R2: Chemokine mediated activation of p42/p44 MAP-kinase (ERK-2). *FEBS Lett*, **364**, 211–14.

Jones, S.A., Wolf, M., et al. 1996. Different functions for the interleukin 8 receptors (IL-8R) of human neutrophil leukocytes: NADPH oxidase and phospholipase D are activated through IL-8R1 but not IL-8R2. *Proc Natl Acad Sci USA*, **93**, 6682–6.

Kennedy, J., Kelner, G.S., et al. 1995. Molecular cloning and functional characterization of human lymphotactin. *J Immunol*, **155**, 203–9.

Kim, C.H., Campbell, D.J. and Butcher, E.C. 2001a. Nonpolarized memory T cells. *Trends Immunol*, **22**, 527–30.

Kim, C.H., Kunkel, E.J., et al. 2001b. Bonzo/CXCR6 expression defines type 1-polarized T-cell subsets with extralymphoid tissue homing potential. *J Clin Invest*, **107**, 595–601.

Kim, C.H., Rott, L., et al. 2001c. Rules of chemokine receptor association with T cell polarization in vivo. *J Clin Invest*, **108**, 1331–9.

Kim, C.H., Rott, L.S., et al. 2001d. Subspecialization of CXCR5(+) T Cells. B helper activity is focused in a germinal center-localized subset of cxcr5(+) t cells. *J Exp Med*, **193**, 1373–82.

Kim, K.-S., Clark-Lewis, I. and Sykes, B.D. 1994. Solution structure of GRO/melanoma growth stimulatory activity determined by 1H NMR spectroscopy. *J Biol Chem*, **269**, 32909–15.

Kim, K.S., Rajarathnam, K., et al. 1996. Structural characterization of a monomeric chemokine: Monocyte chemoattractant protein-3. *FEBS Lett*, **395**, 277–82.

Kledal, T.N., Rosenkilde, M.M., et al. 1997. A broad-spectrum chemokine antagonist encoded by Kaposi's sarcoma-associated herpesvirus. *Science*, **277**, 1656–9.

Kunkel, E.J., Campbell, J.J., et al. 2000. Lymphocyte CC chemokine receptor 9 and epithelial thymus-expressed chemokine (TECK) expression distinguish the small intestinal immune compartment: Epithelial expression of tissue-specific chemokines as an organizing principle in regional immunity. *J Exp Med*, **192**, 761–8.

L'Heureux, G.P., Bourgoin, S., et al. 1995. Diverging signal transduction pathways activated by interleukin-8 and related chemokines in human neutrophils: Interleukin-8, but not NAP-2 or GROα, stimulates phospholipase D activity. *Blood*, **85**, 522–31.

Legler, D.F., Loetscher, M., et al. 1998. B cell-attracting chemokine 1, a human CXC chemokine expressed in lymphoid tissues, selectively attracts B lymphocytes via BLR1/CXCR5. *J Exp Med*, **187**, 655–60.

Liang, M., Mallari, C., et al. 2000. Identification and characterization of a potent, selective, and orally active antagonist of the CC chemokine receptor-1. *J Biol Chem*, **275**, 19000–8.

Lindley, I.J.D., Westwick, J. and Kunkel, S.L. 1993. Nomenclature announcement – the chemokines. *Immunol Today*, **14**, 24.

Lodi, P.J., Garrett, D.S., et al. 1994. High-resolution solution structure of the β chemokine hMIP-1β by multidimensional NMR. *Science*, **263**, 1762–7.

Loetscher, M., Gerber, B., et al. 1996. Chemokine receptor specific for IP10 and Mig: Structure, function, and expression in activated T-lymphocytes. *J Exp Med*, **184**, 963–9.

Loetscher, M., Loetscher, P., et al. 1998. Lymphocyte-specific chemokine receptor CXCR3: regulation, chemokine binding and gene localization. *Eur J Immunol*, **28**, 3696–705.

Loetscher, P. and Clark-Lewis, I. 2001. Agonistic and antagonistic activities of chemokines. *J Leukoc Biol*, **69**, 881–4.

Loetscher, P., Seitz, M., et al. 1994a. Both interleukin-8 receptors independently mediate chemotaxis. Jurkat cells transfected with IL-8R1 or IL-8R2 migrate in response to IL-8, GROα and NAP-2. *FEBS Lett*, **341**, 187–92.

Loetscher, P., Seitz, M., et al. 1994b. The monocyte chemotactic proteins, MCP-1, MCP-2 and MCP-3, are major attractants for human $CD4^+$ and $CD8^+$ T lymphocytes. *FASEB J*, **8**, 1055–60.

Loetscher, P., Seitz, M., et al. 1996. Interleukin-2 regulates CC chemokine receptor expression and chemotactic responsiveness in T lymphocytes. *J Exp Med*, **184**, 569–77.

Loetscher, P., Gong, J.H., et al. 1998a. N-terminal peptides of stromal cell-derived factor-1 with CXC chemokine receptor 4 agonist and antagonist activities. *J Biol Chem*, **273**, 22279–83.

Loetscher, P., Uguccioni, M., et al. 1998b. CCR5 is characteristic of Th1 lymphocytes. *Nature*, **391**, 344–5.

Loetscher, P., Moser, B. and Baggiolini, M. 2000. Chemokines and their receptors in lymphocyte traffic and HIV infection. *Adv Immunol*, **74**, 127–80.

Loetscher, P., Pellegrino, A., et al. 2001. The ligands of CXC chemokine receptor 3, I-TAC, Mig and IP10, are natural antagonists for CCR3. *J Biol Chem*, **276**, 2986–91.

Luther, S.A., Lopez, T., et al. 2000. BLC expression in pancreatic islets causes B cell recruitment and lymphotoxin-dependent lymphoid neogenesis. *Immunity*, **12**, 471–81.

Ma, Q., Jones, D. and Springer, T.A. 1999. The chemokine receptor CXCR4 is required for the retention of B lineage and granulocytic precursors within the bone marrow microenvironment. *Immunity*, **10**, 463–71.

Mackay, C.R. 1993. Immunological memory. *Adv Immunol*, **53**, 217–65.

Mackay, C.R. 2000. Follicular homing T helper (Th) cells and the Th1/Th2 paradigm. *J Exp Med*, **192**, F31–34.

Mackay, C.R. 2001. Chemokines: immunology's high impact factors. *Nat Immunol*, **2**, 95–101.

Maeda, K., Yoshimura, K., et al. 2001. Novel low molecular weight spirodiketopiperazine derivatives potently inhibit R5 HIV-1 infection through their antagonistic effects on CCR5. *J Biol Chem*, **276**, 35194–200.

Maghazachi, A.A. and Al-Aoukaty, A. 1998. Chemokines activate natural killer cells through heterotrimeric G-proteins: implications for the treatment of AIDS and cancer. *FASEB J*, **12**, 913–24.

Marte, B.M. and Downward, J. 1997. PKB/Akt: connecting phosphoinositide 3-kinase to cell survival and beyond. *Trends Biochem Sci*, **22**, 355–8.

Masopust, D., Vezys, V., et al. 2001. Preferential localization of effector memory cells in nonlymphoid tissue. *Science*, **291**, 2413–17.

Mazzucchelli, L., Blaser, A., et al. 1999. BCA-1 is highly expressed in H*elicobacter pylori*-induced mucosa-associated lymphoid tissue and gastric lymphoma. *J Clin Invest,, R*, **104**, R49–54.

Mellado, M., Rodriguez-Frade, J.M., et al. 2001. Chemokine signaling and functional responses: the role of receptor dimerization and TK pathway activation. *Annu Rev Immunol*, **19**, 397–421.

Milne, R.S., Mattick, C., et al. 2000. RANTES binding and down-regulation by a novel human herpesvirus-6 beta chemokine receptor. *J Immunol*, **164**, 2396–404.

Mirzadegan, T., Diehl, F., et al. 2000. Identification of the binding site for a novel class of CCR2b chemokine receptor antagonists: binding to a common chemokine receptor motif within the helical bundle. *J Biol Chem*, **275**, 25562–71.

Morales, J., Homey, B., et al. 1999. CTACK, a skin-associated chemokine that preferentially attracts skin-homing memory T cells. *Proc Natl Acad Sci USA*, **96**, 14470–5.

Moser, B. and Loetscher, P. 2001. Lymphocyte traffic control by chemokines. *Nat Immunol*, **2**, 123–8.

Moser, B., Schaerli, P. and Loetscher, P. 2002. CXCR5(+) T cells: follicular homing takes center stage in T-helper-cell responses. *Trends Immunol*, **23**, 250–4.

Mosmann, T.R. and Coffman, R.L. 1989. TH1 and TH2 cells: different patterns of lymphokine secretion lead to different functional properties. *Annu Rev Immunol*, **7**, 145–73.

Murphy, P.M. 2001. Viral exploitation and subversion of the immune system through chemokine mimicry. *Nature Immunol*, **2**, 116–22.

Murphy, P.M. 2002. International Union of Pharmacology. XXX. Update on chemokine receptor nomenclature. *Pharmacol Rev*, **54**, 227–9.

Murphy, P.M. and Tiffany, H.L. 1991. Cloning of complementary DNA encoding a functional human interleukin-8 receptor. *Science*, **253**, 1280–3.

Murphy, P.M., Baggiolini, M., et al. 2000. International Union of Pharmacology. XXII. Nomenclature for chemokine receptors. *Pharmacol Rev*, **52**, 145–76.

Nagasawa, T., Kikutani, H. and Kishimoto, T. 1994. Molecular cloning and structure of a pre-B-cell growth-stimulating factor. *Proc Natl Acad Sci USA*, **91**, 2305–9.

Nakano, H., Tamura, T., et al. 1997. Genetic defect in T lymphocyte-specific homing into peripheral lymph nodes. *Eur J Immunol*, **27**, 215–21.

Naya, A., Sagara, Y., et al. 2001. Design, synthesis, and discovery of a novel CCR1 antagonist. *J Med Chem*, **44**, 1429–35.

Neptune, E.R. and Bourne, H.R. 1997. Receptors induce chemotaxis by releasing the βgamma subunit of Gi, not by activating Gq or Gs. *Proc Natl Acad Sci USA*, **94**, 14489–94.

Ogilvie, P., Bardi, G., et al. 2001. Eotaxin is a natural antagonist for CCR2 and an agonist for CCR5. *Blood*, **97**, 1920–4.

Okada, T., Ngo, V.N., et al. 2002. Chemokine requirements for B cell entry to lymph nodes and Peyer's patches. *J Exp Med*, **196**, 65–75.

Pan, J., Kunkel, E.J., et al. 2000. A novel chemokine ligand for CCR10 and CCR3 expressed by epithelial cells in mucosal tissues. *J Immunol*, **165**, 2943–9.

Pan, Y., Lloyd, C., et al. 1997. Neurotactin, a membrane-anchored chemokine upregulated in brain inflammation. *Nature*, **387**, 611–17.

Papadakis, K.A., Prehn, J., et al. 2001. CCR9-positive lymphocytes and thymus-expressed chemokine distinguish small bowel from colonic Crohn's disease. *Gastroenterology*, **121**, 246–54.

Penfold, M.E.T., Dairaghi, D.J., et al. 1999. Cytomegalovirus encodes a potent α chemokine. *Proc Natl Acad Sci USA*, **96**, 9839–44.

Pierce, K.L., Premont, R.T. and Lefkowitz, R.J. 2002. Signalling: Seven-transmembrane receptors. *Nat Rev Mol Cell Biol*, **3**, 639–50.

Plater-Zyberk, C., Hoogewerf, A.J., et al. 1997. Effect of a CC chemokine receptor antagonist on collagen induced arthritis in DBA/1 mice. *Immunol Lett*, **57**, 117–20.

Proudfoot, A.E.I., Buser, R., et al. 1999. Amino-terminally modified RANTES analogues demonstrate differential effects on RANTES receptors. *J Biol Chem*, **274**, 32478–85.

Qin, S., Rottman, J.B., et al. 1998. The chemokine receptors CXCR3 and CCR5 mark subsets of T cells associated with certain inflammatory reactions. *J Clin Invest*, **101**, 746–54.

Rajarathnam, K., Sykes, B.D., et al. 1994. Neutrophil activation by monomeric interleukin-8. *Science*, **264**, 90–2.

Reif, K., Ekland, E.H., et al. 2002. Balanced responsiveness to chemoattractants from adjacent zones determines B-cell position. *Nature*, **416**, 94–9.

Reinhardt, R.L., Khoruts, A., et al. 2001. Visualizing the generation of memory CD4 T cells in the whole body. *Nature*, **410**, 101–5.

Reiss, Y., Proudfoot, A.E., et al. 2001. CC chemokine receptor (CCR)4 and the CCR10 ligand cutaneous T cell-attracting chemokine (CTACK) in lymphocyte trafficking to inflamed skin. *J Exp Med*, **194**, 1541–7.

Ross, R. 1999. Atherosclerosis – an inflammatory disease. *N Engl J Med*, **340**, 115–26.

Sabroe, I., Peck, M.J., et al. 2000. A small molecule antagonist of chemokine receptors CCR1 and CCR3. Potent inhibition of eosinophil function and CCR3-mediated HIV-1 entry. *J Biol Chem*, **275**, 25985–92.

Sallusto, F., Mackay, C.R. and Lanzavecchia, A. 1997. Selective expression of the eotaxin receptor CCR3 by human T helper 2 cells. *Science*, **277**, 2005–7.

Sallusto, F., Lenig, D., et al. 1998. Flexible programs of chemokine receptor expression on human polarized T helper 1 and 2 lymphocytes. *J Exp Med*, **187**, 875–83.

Sallusto, F., Lenig, D., et al. 1999. Two subsets of memory T lymphocytes with distinct homing potentials and effector functions. *Nature*, **401**, 708–12.

Sallusto, F., Mackay, C.R. and Lanzavecchia, A. 2000. The role of chemokine receptors in primary, effector, and memory immune responses [in process citation]. *Annu Rev Immunol*, **18**, 593–620.

Schaerli, P., Willimann, K., et al. 2000. CXC chemokine receptor 5 expression defines follicular homing T cells with B cell helper function [in process citation]. *J Exp Med*, **192**, 1553–62.

Schaerli, P., Loetscher, P. and Moser, B. 2001. Cutting edge: induction of follicular homing precedes effector th cell development. *J Immunol*, **167**, 6082–6.

Shi, K., Hayashida, K., et al. 2001. Lymphoid chemokine B cell-attracting chemokine-1 (CXCL13) is expressed in germinal center of ectopic lymphoid follicles within the synovium of chronic arthritis patients. *J Immunol*, **166**, 650–5.

Shiraishi, M., Aramaki, Y., et al. 2000. Discovery of novel, potent, and selective small-molecule CCR5 antagonists as anti-HIV-1 agents: synthesis and biological evaluation of anilide derivatives with a quaternary ammonium moiety. *J Med Chem*, **43**, 2049–63.

Simmons, G., Clapham, P.R., et al. 1997. Potent inhibition of HIV-1 infectivity in macrophages and lymphocytes by a novel CCR5 antagonist. *Science*, **276**, 276–9.

Siveke, J.T. and Hamann, A. 1998. T helper 1 and T helper 2 cells respond differentially to chemokines. *J Immunol*, **160**, 550–4.

Skelton, N.J., Aspiras, F., et al. 1995. Proton NMR assignments and solution conformation of RANTES, a chemokine of the C-C type. *Biochemistry*, **34**, 5329–42.

Sozzani, S., Allavena, P., et al. 1999. The role of chemokines in the regulation of dendritic cell trafficking. *J Leukoc Biol*, **66**, 1–9.

Springer, T.A. 1994. Traffic signals for lymphocyte recirculation and leukocyte emigration: The multistep paradigm. *Cell*, **76**, 301–14.

Stein, J.V., Rot, A., et al. 2000. The CC chemokine thymus-derived chemotactic agent 4 (TCA-4, secondary lymphoid tissue chemokine, 6Ckine, exodus-2) triggers lymphocyte function-associated antigen 1-mediated arrest of rolling T lymphocytes in peripheral lymph node high endothelial venules. *J Exp Med*, **191**, 61–76.

Stine, J.T., Wood, C., et al. 2000. KSHV-encoded CC chemokine vMIP-III is a CCR4 agonist, stimulates angiogenesis, and selectively chemoattracts TH2 cells. *Blood*, **95**, 1151–7.

Strizki, J.M., Xu, S., et al. 2001. SCH-C (SCH 351125), an orally bioavailable, small molecule antagonist of the chemokine receptor CCR5, is a potent inhibitor of HIV-1 infection in vitro and in vivo. *Proc Natl Acad Sci USA*, **98**, 12718–23.

Tashiro, K., Tada, H., et al. 1993. Signal sequence trap: A cloning strategy for secreted proteins and type I membrane proteins. *Science*, **261**, 600–3.

Thelen, M. 2001. Dancing to the tune of chemokines. *Nat Immunol*, **2**, 129–34.

Thelen, M. and Baggiolini, M. 2001. Is dimerization of chemokine receptors functionally relevant? *Sci STKE*, **PE34**.

Thelen, M., Peveri, P., et al. 1988. Mechanism of neutrophil activation by NAF, a novel monocyte-derived peptide agonist. *FASEB J*, **2**, 2702–6.

Tilton, B., Andjelkovic, M., et al. 1997. G-protein-coupled receptors and Fcgamma-receptors mediate activation of Akt/protein kinase B in human phagocytes. *J Biol Chem*, **272**, 28096–101.

Uguccioni, M., D'Apuzzo, M., et al. 1995. Actions of the chemotactic cytokines MCP-1, MCP-2, MCP-3, RANTES, MIP-1α and MIP-1β on human monocytes. *Eur J Immunol*, **25**, 64–8.

Uguccioni, M., Loetscher, P., et al. 1996. Monocyte chemotactic protein 4 (MCP-4), a novel structural and functional analogue of MCP-3 and eotaxin. *J Exp Med*, **183**, 2379–84.

Uguccioni, M., Gionchetti, P., et al. 1999. Increased expression of IP-10, IL-8, MCP-1 and MCP-3 in ulcerative colitis. *Am J Pathol*, **155**, 331–6.

Unsoeld, H., Krautwald, S., et al. 2002. Cutting edge: CCR7(+) and CCR7(−) memory T cells do not differ in immediate effector cell function. *J Immunol*, **169**, 638–41.

Von Andrian, U.H. and Mackay, C.R. 2000. T-cell function and migration. Two sides of the same coin. *N Engl J Med*, **343**, 1020–34.

von Tscharner, V., Deranleau, D.A. and Baggiolini, M. 1986a. Calcium fluxes and calcium buffering in human neutrophils. *J Biol Chem*, **261**, 10163–8.

von Tscharner, V., Prod'hom, B., et al. 1986b. Ion channels in human neutrophils activated by a rise in free cytosolic calcium concentration. *Nature*, **324**, 369–72.

Wang, W., Soto, H., et al. 2000. Identification of a novel chemokine (CCL28), which binds CCR10 (GPR2). *J Biol Chem*, **275**, 22313–23.

Warnock, R.A., Campbell, J.J., et al. 2000. The role of chemokines in the microenvironmental control of T versus B cell arrest in Peyer's patch high endothelial venules. *J Exp Med*, **191**, 77–88.

Weber, M., Uguccioni, M., et al. 1996. Deletion of the NH2-terminal residue converts monocyte chemotactic protein 1 from an activator of basophil mediator release to an eosinophil chemoattractant. *J Exp Med*, **183**, 681–5.

White, J.R., Lee, J.M., et al. 2000. Identification of potent, selective non-peptide CC chemokine receptor-3 antagonist that inhibits eotaxin-, eotaxin-2-, and monocyte chemotactic protein-4-induced eosinophil migration. *J Biol Chem*, **275**, 36626–31.

Wurbel, M.A., Philippe, J.M., et al. 2000. The chemokine TECK is expressed by thymic and intestinal epithelial cells and attracts double- and single-positive thymocytes expressing the TECK receptor CCR9. *Eur J Immunol*, **30**, 262–71.

Zabel, B.A., Agace, W.W., et al. 1999. Human G protein-coupled receptor GPR-9-G/CC chemokine receptor 9 is selectively expressed on intestinal homing T lymphocytes, mucosal lymphocytes, and thymocytes and is required for thymus-expressed chemokine-mediated chemotaxis. *J Exp Med*, **190**, 1241–55.

Zingoni, A., Soto, H., et al. 1998. The chemokine receptor CCR8 is preferentially expressed in Th2 but not Th1 cells. *J Immunol*, **161**, 547–51.

Zlotnik, A. and Yoshie, O. 2000. Chemokines: a new classification system and their role in immunity. *Immunity*, **12**, 121–7.

14

Type I interferons and receptors

SIDNEY PESTKA

In the 1930s several investigators described the phenomenon of viral interference, whereby the infection of an animal by a virus seemed somehow to protect it against subsequent infection by another virus (Findlay and Mac Callum 1937; Schlesinger 1959; Dianzani 1975). In 1957 Isaacs and Lindenmann (1957; Davies et al. 1982) found an agent of viral interference: a protein, released by cells exposed to a virus, which enabled other cells to resist viral infection. They called it interferon. The great promise of interferon as an antiviral agent was evident from the moment of its discovery, which was supported by an independent report of similar findings by Nagano and Kojima (1958). The promise was enticing because interferon is not directed against any one virus but rather protects cells against a wide range of viruses.

The interferons represent proteins with antiviral activity that are secreted from cells in response to a variety of stimuli (Pestka 1981, 1986; Pestka et al. 1987). There are at least six classes of interferons (IFN): alpha (α), beta (β), gamma (γ), tau (τ), omega (ω), and kappa (κ). The interferons are divided into two groups, designated type I and type II interferons (Pestka et al. 1987). IFN-γ is the only type II interferon whereas the type I interferons consist of five major classes: IFN-α, IFN-β, IFN-ω, IFN-τ, and IFN-κ. There is only one human Hu-IFN-β (Hu-IFN-β), one Hu-IFN-ω, and one Hu-IFN-κ, but a family of multiple IFN-β species exists. It is unlikely that any human IFN-τ exists. IFN-τ was described first as ovine trophoblast protein-1 and is found in ungulates, where it is required for implantation of the ovum (Roberts et al. 1991). Hu-IFN-κ, although it exhibits low specific antiviral activity, is expressed in human keratinocytes (LaFleur et al. 2001).

In general, exposure of human cells to viruses and double-stranded RNAs induces the production of IFN-α and IFN-β species, although IFN-ω and IFN-κ can be produced by appropriate cells. The ratio of IFN-α to IFN-β produced by cells varies with the tissue of origin and the species of the organism. T lymphocytes produce IFN-γ when stimulated with antigens to which they are immune, or when stimulated with mitogens such as staphylococcal enterotoxin A or the combination of phytohemagglutinin and phorbol esters. Most of the interferons in therapeutic use are produced through genetic engineering (Pestka 1981, 1983b, 1986; Pestka et al. 1987). As the first biotherapeutic approved, IFN-α paved the way for the many new biotherapeutics to follow. Nevertheless, we have only touched the surface of understanding the multitude of human interferons.

Many procedures have been described for the partial purification of human and animal interferons (Berg 1982; Pestka 1981, 1983b, 1986; Pestka et al. 1987). Although partial purification of the interferons as bands on a sodium dodecylsulfate–polyacrylamide gel electrophoresis (SDS–PAGE) was reported by a number of groups, it was not until 1978 and thereafter that any interferon was purified to homogeneity in sufficient amounts for its chemical and physical characterization (Rubinstein et al. 1978, 1979a, 1981; Stein et al. 1980; Friesen et al. 1981). The introduction of reverse phase and normal phase high-performance liquid chromatography (HPLC) to the purification of proteins (Rubinstein et al. 1978, 1979a, 1981; Stein et al. 1980; Friesen et al. 1981) led to the first successful purification of these proteins so that sufficient amounts were available without detergent for their chemical, biological, and immunological studies. Various affinity purification techniques, particularly antibody affinity chromatography were utilized to purify human leukocyte (α) and fibroblast (β) interferons (Knight 1976; Berthold et al. 1978; Cabrer et al. 1979; Zoon et al. 1979; Allen and Fantes 1980; Okamura et al. 1980; Berg and Heron 1981; Kawade et al. 1981; Zoon 1981b; Knight and Fahey 1982; Pestka et al. 1987).

PURIFICATION OF HUMAN LEUKOCYTE INTERFERON α

Since their discovery, many attempts have been made to purify the interferons, with little success until 1978. In fact, interferon used in experiments as well as in initial human clinical trials was essentially a crude protein fraction, less than 1 percent of which by weight consisted of interferon. As a result of the use of such crude interferon-containing material, it was not clear what activities of these preparations were caused inherently by the interferon present and what activities were caused by the numerous other contaminating proteins. By definition, the antiviral activity was the result of the interferon. However, these crude preparations exhibited antiprotozoal and antibacterial activities, inhibited cellular growth (antiproliferative activity), and blocked antibody synthesis, and were ascribed many other activities. However, without purified interferon, it was not possible to demonstrate definitively whether or not a particular activity was the result of the interferon protein molecule itself. Accordingly, it was essential to obtain purified interferon to determine what activities were an inherent part of the interferon molecule. As very little was known about the size and structure of the interferons, the isolation of purified interferons established their chemical composition and structure as well as their biological activities.

Production

We began purification of interferon from human leukocytes in 1977. This interferon was produced by incubating human white blood cells with Newcastle disease virus or Sendai virus for 6–24 h (Familletti and Pestka 1981; Familletti et al. 1981a; Hershberg et al. 1981; Waldman et al. 1981). The procedure was a combination of techniques that have previously been reported (Wheelock 1966; Cantell and Tovell 1971). The antiviral activity was found in the cell culture medium after overnight incubation of the leukocytes as illustrated in Figure 14.1. We substituted milk casein for human or bovine serum in the culture medium as had been described (Cantell and Tovell 1971). The use of casein, a single protein, instead of serum, which contains many different and uncharacterized proteins, simplified the initial concentration and purification steps. We used leukocytes from normal donors as well as from patients with chronic myelogenous leukemia. These leukemic cells make large amounts of human leukocyte interferon when induced with Newcastle disease virus or Sendai virus (Hadhazy et al. 1967; Lee et al. 1969; Rubinstein et al. 1979a; Familletti et al. 1981a).

The cytopathic effect inhibition assay for interferon as originally described took 3 days. Other assays for interferon were even longer. A more rapid assay was necessary to proceed with the purification expeditiously. A cytopathic effect inhibition assay that could be done in 12–16 h was developed (Familletti et al., 1981b; S. Rubinstein et al., 1981) and accelerated the purification immensely.

High-performance liquid chromatography for protein purification

As classic techniques for protein purification were not successful in the purification of the human interferons,

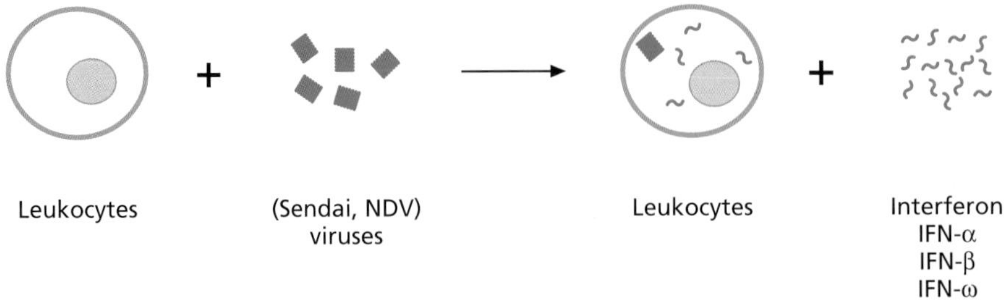

Figure 14.1 *Production of leukocyte interferon with Newcastle disease virus (NDV) and leukocytes. Leukocytes, the white blood cells of peripheral blood, were obtained from normal donors or patients with chronic myelogenous leukemia. The cells were washed, placed in culture medium with Newcastle disease virus (or with Sendai virus), and incubated overnight at 37°C. Interferon is found in the culture medium after incubation. The cells and virus can be removed by centrifugation, leaving the culture medium containing interferon.*

we applied HPLC to the purification process. Udenfriend and co-workers (Udenfriend et al. 1972; Stein et al. 1973; Bohlen et al. 1975) had developed sensitive fluorescent techniques for detection of amino acids and peptides, and had achieved the separation of peptides by reverse-phase HPLC. However, separation of proteins had not yet been accomplished. In the early experiments, there was uniform failure to achieve any purification of proteins with reverse-phase HPLC because the interferon activity was constantly lost. At the time, increasing the ethanol concentration was used to elute proteins and this was tried for interferon and other proteins without success. It was necessary to use a less polar solvent to elute interferon. Although there was initial hesitancy to use *n*-propanol above 20 percent (v/v) and other organic solvents because of the limited solubility of proteins in such solvents, it was found that *n*-propanol gradients effectively eluted interferon and other proteins without noticeable precipitation at the concentrations employed (Rubinstein et al. 1978, 1979b; S. Rubinstein et al. 1981; Rubinstein and Pestka 1981). Furthermore, by changing the pH of the elution buffer, a completely different separation could be achieved during elution of the same reverse-phase column with *n*-propanol. As subsequently demonstrated with fibroblast interferon, (Friesen et al. 1981) a large number of different columns and solvent systems could be used to effect resolution of proteins. By applying normal-phase chromatography with a diol silica column between the two reverse-phase columns, it was possible to use just three sequential HPLC steps to purify human leukocyte interferon to homogeneity. Sufficient amounts were purified in high yield for initial chemical characterization of the protein and for determination of amino acid composition. The amino acid composition of the human leukocyte interferon species γ2 was the first reported for any purified interferon (Rubinstein et al. 1979b).

The initial steps for purification of IFN included selective precipitations and gel filtration (Figure 14.2) followed by HPLC. The HPLC steps were reverse-phase chromatography (Figure 14.3) at pH 7.5 on LiChrosorb RP-8, normal partition chromatography on LiChrosorb Diol (Figure 14.4), and reverse-phase chromatography at pH 4.0 on LiChrosorb RP-8 (Figure 14.5). Gradients of *n*-propanol were used for elution of interferon from these columns (Figures 14.3-14.5). The overall purification was about 80 000-fold and the specific activity of purified interferon was 2–4 × 10^8 units/mg (Rubinstein et al. 1979b). Interferon prepared by this procedure yielded a single band of molecular mass (M_r) 17 500 on PAGE. The antiviral activity was associated with the single protein band (Rubinstein et al. 1978). The specific activity of this peak was 4 × 10^8 units/mg.

Several reports had previously described HPLC of proteins, mainly on ion exchange and size exclusion columns (Chang et al. 1976; Regnier and Noel 1976). However, these systems were either not commercially

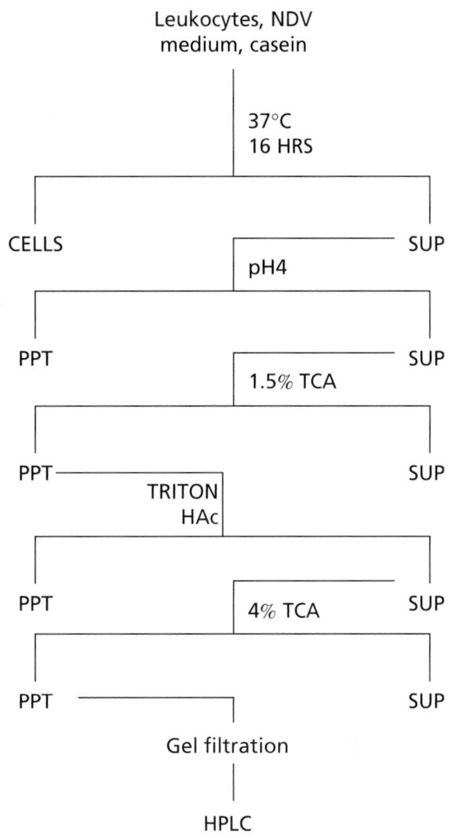

Figure 14.2 *Flow chart of initial steps in purification of leukocyte interferon. Cells and debris were removed by low-speed centrifugation from the medium containing interferon. Casein was used as a serum substitute. By acidification of the medium to pH 4 with hydrochloric acid, the bulk of the casein, which precipitated, was removed from the interferon, which remained in solution. The interferon was concentrated by two steps involving precipitation with trichloroacetic acid. The concentrated solution containing relatively crude interferon was separated into components of different sizes by gel filtration on Sephadex G-100 in the presence of 4 mol/l urea. Details of these procedures have been described (M. Rubinstein et al. 1979b, 1981a; Familletti et al. 1981a; Hershberg et al. 1981; Waldman et al. 1981). HLPC, high-performance liquid chromatography; NDV, Newcastle disease virus; Ppt, precipitate; Sup, supernatant; TCA, trichloroacetic acid.*

available or had a low capacity. With proper choice of eluent and pore size, octyl and octadecyl silica could be used for high-resolution reverse-phase HPLC of both peptides and proteins. Accordingly, with *n*-propanol as eluent, the use of LiChrosorb RP-8 (octyl silica) columns for protein fractionation was a major factor in the success of the purification (Figure 14.5). In addition, LiChrosorb Diol, which is chemically similar to glycophase resins that have been used for exclusion chromatography of proteins, was introduced as a support for normal partition chromatography of proteins (Figure 14.5b). High recoveries of interferon activity were obtained in each chromatographic step, a requirement when small amounts of initial starting material are present. Although the initial experiments were

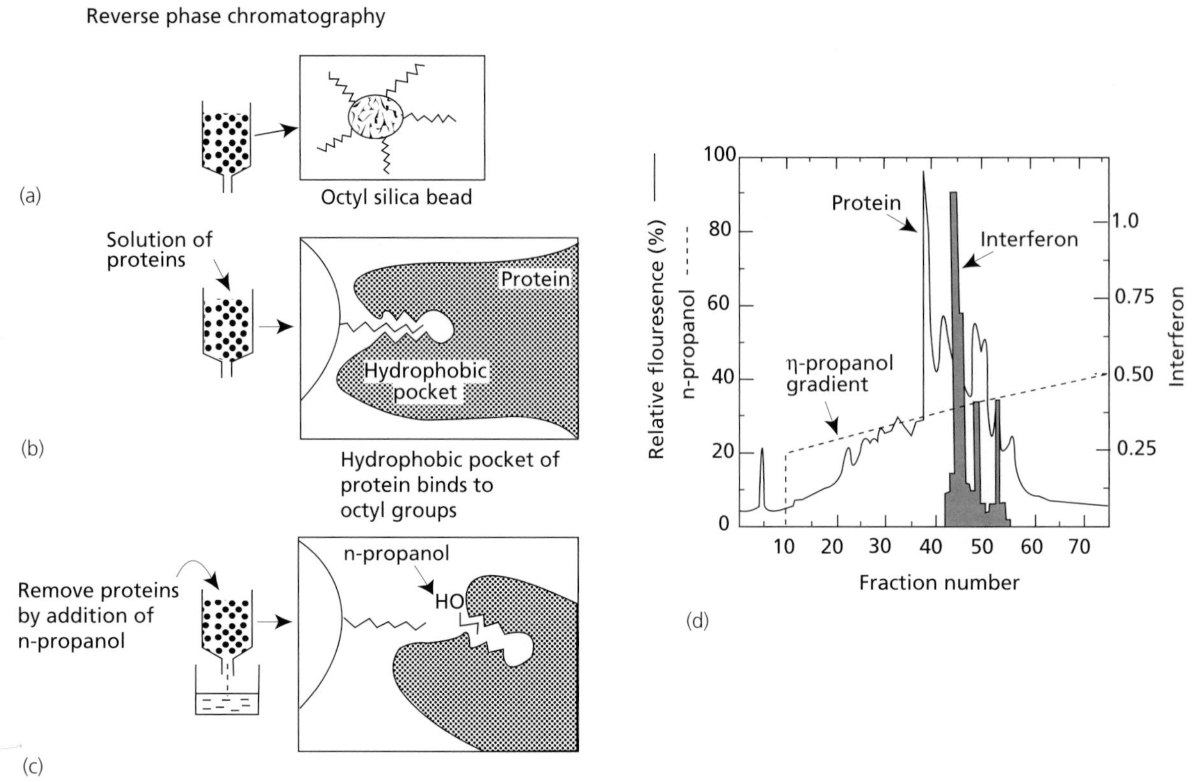

Figure 14.3 *High-performance liquid chromatography of leukocyte interferon on reverse-phase columns. Columns of porous silica to which octyl groups were bound were used to separate leukocyte interferons from other proteins and to resolve the individual leukocyte interferons. The proteins enter the interstices within the silica particles where the hydrophobic areas of the protein bind tightly to the octyl groups. The nonpolar portion of* n-propanol *can interact with interferon, releasing interferon and other proteins from the column. By eluting the proteins with an increasing gradient of* n-propanol*, the proteins are released in order of their increasing hydrophobicity. Those proteins binding most tightly are released only after high concentrations of* n-propanol *or other appropriate organic solvents are used (Pestka 1983b).*

performed with leukocytes from normal donors (Rubinstein et al. 1978, 1979b), it was found that leukocytes from patients with chronic myelogenous leukemia (CML), who were undergoing leukapheresis to lower their peripheral white blood cell counts, were a rich source of interferon that appeared to be essentially identical to the human leukocyte interferon purified from leukocytes from normal donors (Rubinstein et al. 1979a). As with HPLC of interferon from normal leukocytes on the Diol column (Figure 14.5b), three major peaks of activity, labeled α, β, γ^2, were observed with interferon prepared from CML cells. (The natural interferons which were isolated from the mixture present in leukocyte interferon by HPLC (Rubinstein et al. 1978, 1979b, 1981; Pestka 1983b) were then designated α1, α2, β1, β2, β3, γ1, γ2, γ3, γ4, γ5, and δ. Unfortunately, the same Greek letters were later used to designate leukocyte, fibroblast, and immune interferons, respectively, as α, β, γ.) Although the protein profiles were almost identical, the activity profiles showed that the amount of activity under peak γ was lower in preparations from leukemic cells compared with normal leukocytes (Rubinstein et al. 1979a, 1979b). However, even from normal leukocytes, the ratio of peaks α, β, and γ varied from one preparation to another. Human lymphoblastoid interferon produced by suspension cultures of Namalva cells was purified by a combination of immunoaffinity chromatography and other methods by Zoon et al. (1979).

The amino acid composition of human leukocyte interferon purified by HPLC as described above (Rubinstein et al. 1979b) shows similarity with human lymphoblastoid interferon (Zoon et al. 1979) and one of the types of mouse interferon (Cabrer et al. 1979). It should be noted that the terms 'leukocyte' and 'lymphoblastoid' interferons simply designate the source of the interferons. The major component of both these preparations consists of Hu-IFN-α species; a minor component of Hu-IFN-β and Hu-IFN-ω is also present in these preparations. As a result of the fact that multiple interferon classes were present in interferons produced from these cell sources, a new nomenclature was proposed to designate the species of interferon rather than the source of the interferon (Interferon Nomenclature 1980). The designation IFN-α was suggested for the major class of interferons present in leukocyte and lymphoblastoid interferon preparations. Hu-IFN-β was the designation for the major interferon produced by human fibroblasts

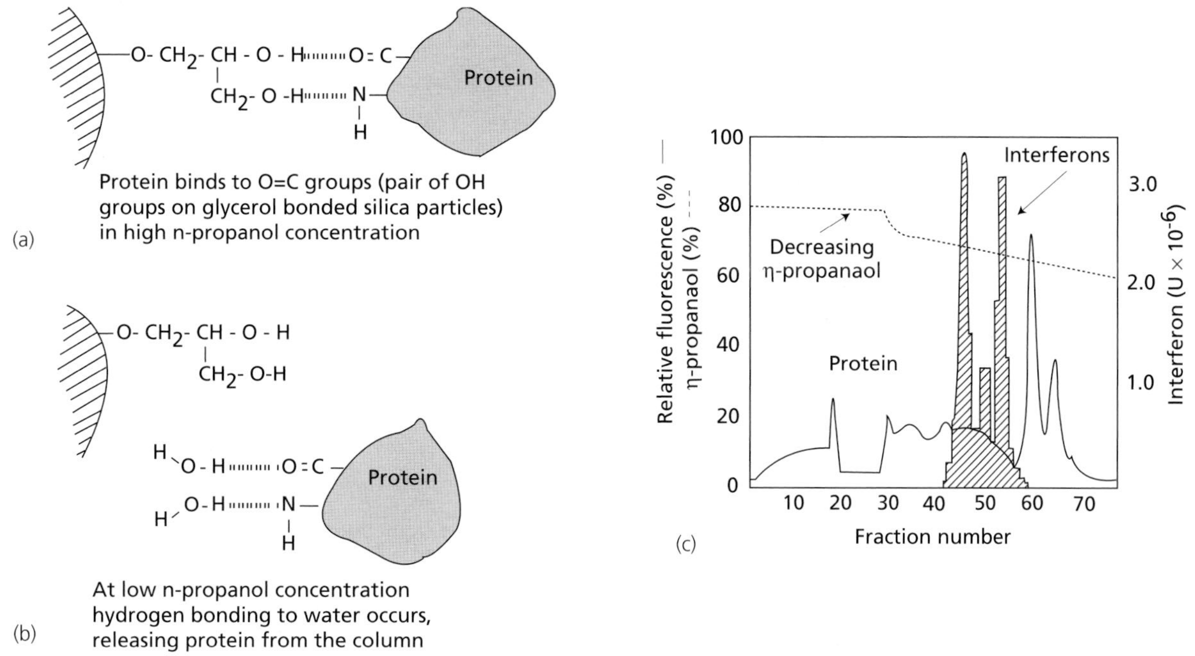

Figure 14.4 *Hydrogen-bonding high-performance liquid chromatography on diol silica. Hydrogen bonding of proteins to columns containing glycerol covalently attached to silica was used to separate interferon species. As hydrogen bonds are relatively weak bonds and are readily made to the water in which the protein is dissolved, in order to force proteins to bind to the diol silica, it was necessary to use very high concentrations of* n-propanol. *Upon reduction of the* n-propanol *concentration, proteins are released from the column in order of their increasing ability to form hydrogen bonds with the diol groups. Those proteins released first form the weakest hydrogen bonds.* **(a)** *Protein binds to diol groups (pair of OH groups on glycerol-bonded silica particles) in high* n-propanol *concentration.* **(b)** *At low* n-propanol *concentration hydrogen bonding to water occurs, releasing protein from the column. Multiple molecular species of human leukocyte interferon (α, β, and γ) are shown in the figure. These designations should not be confused with the subsequent nomenclature of IFN-α, IFN-β, and IFN-γ assigned to leukocyte, fibroblast, and immune interferons, respectively.*

in response to induction with poly(I)·poly(C). Hu-IFN-γ was the designation given for human immune interferon.

Multiple species of leukocyte interferon

During the purification of leukocyte interferon, it became evident that there were multiple species (see Figures 14.4 and 14.5). Ten separate species listed as α1, α2, β1, β2, β3, γ1, γ2, γ3, γ4 and γ5 were purified (Table 14.1). These are all α interferons under the current nomenclature. The designations initially used refer to the peaks obtained on chromatography. It was astonishing at the time, particularly after peptide mapping and sequencing of some of these species, to find a family of proteins that exhibited different activities uncovered (see below).

Human leukocyte interferon is heterogeneous and several bands containing antiviral activity ranging in M_r from 15 000 to 21 000 were observed on SDS–PAGE (Stewart 1974). Heterogeneity of human leukocyte interferon was also observed by isoelectric focusing (Stewart et al. 1977) and several types of chromatographic procedures (Chen et al. 1976; Jankowski et al. 1976; Torma and Paucker 1976; Grob and Chadha 1979; M. Rubinstein et al. 1981). As noted above, our initial work with HPLC revealed three major groups of interferon species that were labeled α, β, and γ according to their order of elution from a LiChrosorb Diol (polar-bonded phase) column (M. Rubinstein et al. 1979b, 1981). These groups were further resolved into several homogeneous components. Although others had reported heterogeneity in crude human leukocyte interferon preparations (Chen et al. 1976; Jankowski et al. 1976; Torma and Paucker 1976; Grob and Chadha 1979), this was not thought to be caused by amino acid sequence heterogeneity. In fact, it had been reported by a number of groups that leukocyte interferon contained carbohydrate and that heterogeneity was the result of differences in the carbohydrate content of the protein (Bose et al. 1976; Bose and Hickman 1977; Bridgen et al. 1977; Stewart et al. 1977). Thus, the well-established heterogeneity of human leukocyte interferon was attributed to differences in the degree of glycosylation. However, five purified species of leukocyte interferon examined contained no detectable carbohydrate: the amino sugar content of each species analyzed (α1, β1, β2, β3, and γ3) was determined to be much less than one residue of either glucosamine or galactosamine per molecule of interferon (M. Rubinstein et al. 1981). Allen and Fantes (1980) also found no carbohydrate on the species of leukocyte interferon that they purified. We therefore concluded that, contrary to the prevailing dogma, human leukocyte interferon is

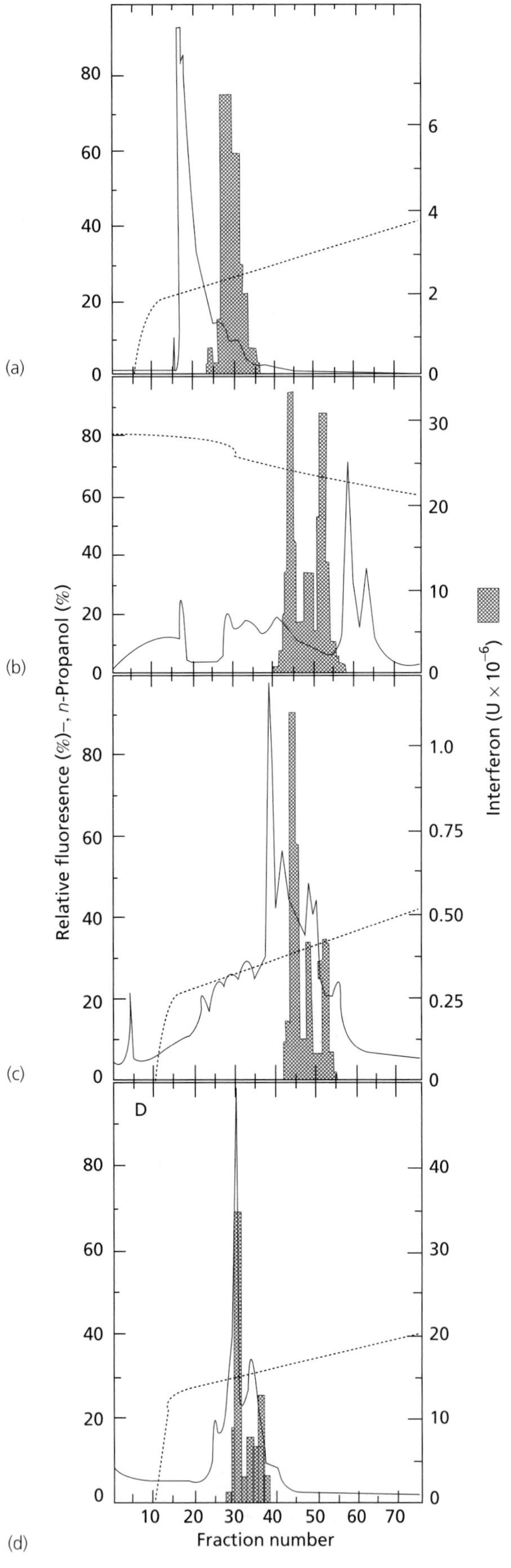

largely devoid of carbohydrate. Furthermore, because peptide mapping and sequencing revealed significant structural differences among the species, we concluded that leukocyte interferon represents a family of homologous proteins. By analogous procedures, additional leukocyte interferon species were isolated from cultured myeloblasts (Hobbs et al. 1981; Hobbs and Pestka 1982). Since our initial purification, other reports (Allen and Fantes 1980; Berg and Heron 1981; Zoon 1981a, b) have also described multiple species of leukocyte interferon.

Amino acid sequences of leukocyte interferons

As only relatively small amounts of each species were isolated in these early experiments, it was difficult to obtain information about their amino acid sequences. Determinations of the amino acid sequences of the amino-terminal end of human IFN-α were reported (Levy et al. 1980; Zoon et al. 1980), and that of IFN-β as well (Knight et al. 1980; Okamura et al. 1980; Stein et al. 1980; Friesen et al. 1981). It was clear that all the amino acid sequences obtained for human fibroblast interferon were identical and that we all had purified and sequenced the same protein. At the time, it was comforting to know that the new microsequencing procedures were dependable. However, it was striking that the amino-terminal sequences of individual species of human leukocyte interferon were different (Levy et al. 1980; Zoon et al. 1980). The differences confirmed that the leukocyte interferons consisted of a family of closely related proteins. We subsequently isolated a human interferon DNA recombinant (Maeda et al. 1980, 1981; Pestka 1983b), the coding sequence of which was virtually identical to the sequence of one of our purified proteins.

Levy et al. (1981) and Shively et al. (1982) reported amino acid sequences of three species of human leukocyte interferon. Additional sequences were reported by Zoon (1981a). Allen and Fantes (1980) reported the sequences of tryptic fragments obtained from a mixture of several leukocyte interferon species. All these sequences were sufficiently different to establish very clearly the concept of a family of closely related proteins. As described above (Maeda et al. 1980; Pestka 1983b), the first clone of human leukocyte interferon isolated in our laboratory was almost identical in

Figure 14.5 *High-performance liquid chromatography of interferon. Chromatography on* **(a)** *LiChrosorb RP-8 at pH 7.5;* **(b)** *LiChrosorb diol at pH 7.5; and* **(c)** *LiChrosorb RP-8 at pH 4.0 of the γ peak of part* **(b)**. **(d)** *Rechromatography on LiChrosorb RP-8 of the major activity peak of* **(c)**. *The conditions were similar to those of step* **(c)**. *Several preparations carried through step* **(c)** *were pooled (1.3 × 10^7 units) and applied to the last column. The gradations on the abscissa correspond to the end of the fractions. The solid lines on the graph represent protein as measured by the fluorescamine method (Rubinstein et al. 1979b; Pestka 1983b).*

Table 14.1 *Human leukocyte interferons first purified*

Species	Molecular mass	Specific activity on bovine MDBK cells (units/mg × 10^{-8})	Specific activity on human AG-1732 cells (units/mg × 10^{-8})
α1	16 500	2.6	2.6
α2	16 200	4	3
β1	16 200	3.4	4.4
β2	16 500	4	2
β3	21 000	4	3
γ1	17 700	2.6	2
γ2	17 700	4	1.5
γ3	17 200	3.5	0.15
γ4	21 000	3.5	4
γ5	16 500	0.9	0.02

Data taken from (M. Rubinstein et al. 1981). The species designations refer to high-performance liquid chromatography peaks not what is now termed IFN-α, IFN-β, and IFN-γ.

sequence to human leukocyte interferon-α2 and interferon-β species, which were, however, 10 amino acids shorter than expected from the DNA sequence. It should be noted that during this time several groups (Iwakura et al. 1978; Kawakita et al. 1978; Maeyer-Guignard et al. 1978; Cabrer et al. 1979; Kawade et al. 1981; Maeyer-Guignard 1981) reported the purification of mouse interferons, and some amino acid sequences were also reported (Taira et al. 1980).

Carbohydrate content

The carbohydrate content of the species of human IFN-α, which were derived from patients with CML and from normal donors, was determined (Labdon et al. 1984). Amino sugar content was measured by HPLC and fluorescamine detection of acid hydrolysates of each sample (Labdon et al. 1984). O-linked glycosylation was also detected by a combination of HPLC, enzymatic analysis, and SDS–PAGE (Adolf et al. 1991). Two species showed significant amounts of glucosamine (Labdon et al. 1984). Most of the purified species of leukocyte interferon from a myeloblast cell line were also tested and two species were found to contain sugar residues. These forms also differed from the CML interferons in that they revealed the presence of greater amounts of galactosamine. The apparent lack of carbohydrate in some of the higher-molecular-mass species of interferon implicated factors other than glycosylation in the molecular-mass differences. The results indicated that some species of IFN-α are glycosylated to various degrees. It was later shown that a natural form of Hu-IFN-α2 was O-glycosylated (Adolf et al. 1991) and that Hu-IFN-ω is glycosylated (Adolf et al. 1990). Considering that the recombinant human IFN-α species produced in *Escherichia coli* do not contain carbohydrate, it was useful to discover that most of the human IFN-α species were devoid of carbohydrate.

PURIFICATION OF HUMAN FIBROBLAST INTERFERON-β

Throughout this chapter, the details focus on Hu-IFN-α because of space limitations. However, sufficient references to the other type I interferons are provided to make the chapter comprehensive.

Native human IFN-β is the major interferon produced by human fibroblasts in response to induction with poly(I)·poly(C) (Havell and Vilcek 1972; Knight 1976; Berthold et al. 1978; Stein et al. 1980; Friesen et al. 1981; Leong and Horoszewicz 1981; Van Damme and Billiau 1981). Figure 14.6 illustrates the production of IFN-β from human fibroblasts. The media from fibroblasts are collected and the native Hu-IFN-β was partially purified by a number of procedures (Knight 1976; Berthold et al. 1978; Cabrer et al. 1979; Stein et al. 1980; Friesen et al. 1981). It was purified to homogeneity with the use of HPLC (Stein et al. 1980; Friesen et al. 1981). Native IFN-β was found to be glycosylated. The partially purified material was used in initial clinical trials, but only after it was produced by recombinant DNA technology did major clinical trials proceed.

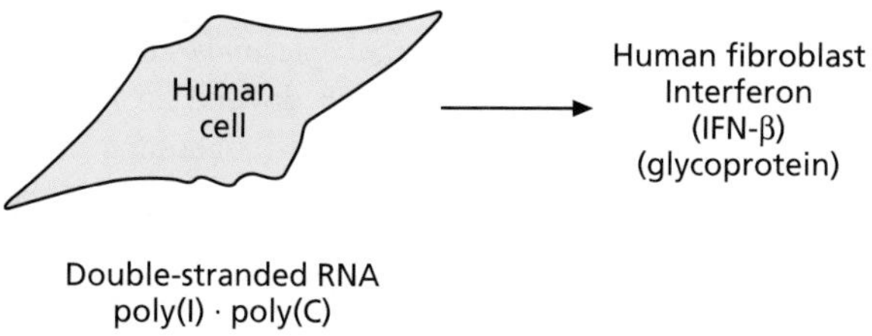

Figure 14.6 *Production of fibroblast interferon (IFN-β). Human fibroblasts were grown in culture and then exposed to the double-stranded RNA, poly(I)·poly(C), and cycloheximide for about 4 h at which time actinomycin D was added. At about 6 h the medium was replaced to remove the poly(I)·poly(C), cycloheximide, and actinomycin D. The culture fluid containing fibroblast interferon was harvested at 24 h.*

The recombinant human IFN-α species

As recombinant DNA technology offered an opportunity to produce large amounts of Hu-IFNs economically, many scientific teams set out to clone them in bacteria. Several groups achieved the isolation of recombinants for several Hu-IFN-α species (Maeda et al. 1980; Nagata et al. 1980) and for IFN-β (Derynck et al. 1980; Goeddel et al. 1980a; Houghton et al. 1980; Maeda et al. 1980; Taniguchi et al. 1980), arriving at their goals by somewhat different but analogous approaches. The cloning and expression of Hu-IFN-αA as an illustration of these procedures are described.

Isolation of Hu-IFN DNA sequences was a formidable task because it meant preparing DNA recombinants from cellular mRNA that was present at a low level. This task had never been accomplished previously from a protein with an unknown structure. In addition, in order to reconstruct DNA recombinants that would express natural IFN, it is useful to know the partial amino acid sequence of the proteins, particularly at the amino- and carboxy-terminal ends. Without this information synthesis of natural Hu-IFN in bacterial cells would not have been possible. Thus, purification of the Hu-IFNs and determination of their structure (M. Rubinstein et al. 1978, 1979b, 1981b; Zoon et al. 1979; Allen and Fantes 1980; Knight et al. 1980; Levy et al. 1981; Hobbs and Pestka 1982; Shively et al. 1982) assisted us in these efforts.

To isolate recombinants containing the human DNA corresponding to IFN-α, we used a number of procedures. First, it was necessary to isolate and measure the IFN mRNA. This was accomplished several years earlier when IFN mRNA was translated in cell-free extracts (Pestka et al. 1975; Thang et al. 1975) and in frog oocytes (Reynolds et al. 1975; Cavalieri and Pestka 1977; Cavalieri et al. 1977a, 1977b). The next step was to prepare sufficient mRNA from cells synthesizing IFN, and this was accomplished with both fibroblasts and leukocytes (Familletti et al. 1981a; McCandliss et al. 1981a). A library of complementary DNA (cDNA) was prepared from a template of partially purified mRNA isolated from human leukocytes synthesizing IFN. The next and hardest part of the procedure was to find in this vast library of recombinant plasmids those that contained DNA encoding IFN. We devised an indirect two-stage procedure to identify clones containing interferon sequences. In the first stage, we screened all the bacterial colonies to find those with cDNA made from the RNA of induced cells; among these there might have been some carrying IFN cDNA. We therefore screened all the recombinants for their ability to bind to mRNA from cells synthesizing IFN (induced cells), but not to mRNA from uninduced cells (those not producing IFN). To do this, individual transformant colonies were screened by colony hybridization for the presence of induced, specific sequences with ^{32P}-labeled IFN mRNA (mRNA from induced cells) as the probe. In the presence of excess mRNA from uninduced cells, recombinants that were representative of mRNA sequences existing only in induced cells should be evident on hybridization. This screening procedure allowed us to discard about 90 percent of the colonies: as their plasmids carried no induced cDNA, these could not encode IFN (Maeda et al. 1980, 1981).

In the second stage, we identified those recombinants containing the IFN DNA sequences among the remaining 10 percent. To do this, we pooled the recombinant plasmids in groups of 10 and examined these for the presence of IFN-specific sequences by an assay that depends on hybridization of IFN mRNA to plasmid DNA (Maeda et al. 1980; McCandliss et al. 1981b). Plasmid DNA from 10 recombinants was isolated and covalently bound to diazobenzyloxymethyl (DBM) paper. The mRNA from induced cells was hybridized to each filter. Unhybridized mRNA was removed by washing. After the specifically hybridized mRNA was eluted, both fractions were translated in *Xenopus laevis* oocytes. Once a positive group had been found (one in which the specifically hybridized mRNA yielded IFN after microinjection into frog oocytes), it was necessary to identify the specific clone or clones containing IFN cDNA. The 10 individual colonies were grown, the plasmid DNAs were prepared, and each individual DNA was examined by mRNA hybridization as above. By these procedures a recombinant, plasmid 104 (p104), containing most of the coding sequence for a Hu-IFN-α was identified (Maeda et al. 1980). The DNA sequence was determined and found to correspond to what was then known of the amino acid sequence of purified Hu-IFN-α (Levy et al. 1980, 1981). The cDNA insert in p104 contained the sequence corresponding to more than 80 percent of the amino acids in IFN-αA, but not for those at its amino-terminal end. It was, therefore, used as a probe for finding a full-length copy of the IFN cDNA sequence which could be used for expression of Hu-IFN-αA in *E. coli*. In addition, p104 DNA was used to isolate DNA sequences corresponding to other IFN-α species directly from a human gene bank.

Examination of the coding regions of the IFN-α genes that were isolated in our laboratory and others have shown that these correspond to a family of homologous proteins, the IFN-α species (Rubinstein et al. 1979b; Pestka 1983b), which are closely related to each other and yet each is unique in its amino acid sequence. Thus, the previously discovered heterogeneity in Hu-IFN-α was shown to be at least in part the result of distinct genes representing each expressed Hu-IFN-α sequence. The cloned Hu-IFN-αA, which was the first one that we isolated, corresponds to the natural Hu-IFN-α species which we purified from the mixture present in IFN-α by HPLC and termed α2 (see above). By similar procedures to those described for 104, p101 was shown to contain the sequence for Hu-IFN-β (Maeda et al. 1980). Thus, the nucleotide sequences coding for Hu-IFN-α and Hu-IFN-β were identified.

The recombinant human IFN-α genes and proteins

A summary of the IFN-α genes and proteins reported is given in Table 14.2. There are in essence 14 human genes that comprise the IFN-α family. Minor variants consisting of one or two amino acid differences account for the multiple alleles (Pestka 1983a, 1983b, 1986; Diaz et al. 1994). Excluding the pseudogene *IFNAP22*, there are 13 genes. One of them, *IFNA10* is also a pseudogene in one allelic form. There are 13 proteins expressed from these genes. The protein produced from gene *IFNA13* is identical to that produced from *IFNA1*. Thus, there are 12 separate IFN-α proteins (and allelic forms) produced from these 14 genes (Table 14.2).

ACTIVITIES OF THE PURIFIED IFN-α SPECIES

After purification of the IFN-α species, we determined their activities (see Table 14.1). It was evident that each interferon species exhibited a distinct profile of antiviral activity (AV) on human AG-1732 and bovine MDBK cells (Evinger et al. 1980a, b, 1981; Pestka et al. 1980a, b; Evinger and Pestka 1981; S. Rubinstein et al. 1981). The overall ratios varied over a range of 200-fold. This presaged the idea that each IFN-α species had a different activity profile. When the profile of activities was expanded to evaluate antiproliferative activity (AP) (Table 14.3) and natural killer (NK) cell stimulatory activity (Table 14.3), it was observed that there was no clear correlation among the activities. Thus, the IFN-α family represents related and homologous proteins each exhibiting a unique activity profile. This is illustrated further below.

After the production and purification of the recombinant IFN-α species, a number of activities were determined. The sequences of various IFN-α species were described (Goeddel et al. 1980b; Goeddel and Pestka 1982, 1989; Henco et al. 1985). As can be seen in Table 14.4, the hybrid IFN-αA and IFN-αD molecules vary markedly in their AV, AP, and NK cell activity (Herberman et al. 1982a; Ortaldo et al. 1982, 1983a, 1983b, 1984; Rehberg et al. 1982). It is possible to change radically the properties of an interferon by making hybrids and generate properties that neither one of the parental molecules exhibits, e.g. the hybrid Hu-IFN-αA/D (*Bgl*) constructed from IFN-αA and IFN-αD exhibits high activity on mouse cells, a property neither of the parental molecules exhibits (Rehberg et al. 1982). As with the natural IFN-α species, the ranges in the activity ratios vary about 100-fold among the hybrid species (Table 14.4). A hybrid between Hu-IFN-αB2 (α8) and Hu-IFN-αD (α1) was constructed (called Hu-IFN-αB/D) and tested in humans with results comparable to the approved recombinant interferons (Gangemi et al. 1989; von Wussow et al. 1991; Hochkeppel et al. 1992; Ritch et al. 1992; Schellekens et al. 1996). Consensus IFN (IFN-con1) is a synthetic, non-naturally

Table 14.2 *Human interferon α genes (14) and proteins (12/13)*

Genes	Proteins
IFNA1	IFN-αD, IFN-α1
IFNA2	IFN-αA (IFN-α2a), IFN-α2 (IFN-α2b), IFN-α2c
IFNA4	IFN-α4a (IFN-α76), IFN-α4b
IFNA5	IFN-αG, IFN-α5, IFNα61
IFNA6	IFN-αK, IFN-α6, IFN-α54
IFNA7	IFN-αJ, IFN-αJ1, IFN-α7
IFNA8	IFN-αB2, IFN-αB, IFN-α8
IFNA10	IFN-αC, IFN-α10, IFN-αL, IFN-α6L
IFNA13	IFN-α13 (sequence identical to IFN-α1)
IFNA14	IFN-αH, IFN-αH1, IFN-α14
IFNA16	IFN-αWA, IFN-α16,IFN-αO
IFNA17	IFN-αI, IFN-α17, IFN-α88
IFNA21	IFN-αF, IFN-α21
IFNAP22	IFN-αE

Table 14.3 *Relative activities of human leukocyte interferons*

Species	AV	AP	NK
α_1	59	22	Low
α_2	68	12	Low
β_1	100	ND	Low
β_2	45	100	High
β_3	68	6	High
γ_1	45	12	High
γ_2	34	47	Low
γ_3	3.4	16	Low
γ_4	91	5	Low
γ_5	0.45	75	Low

AV, relative antiviral activity; AP, relative antiproliferative activity; NK, relative natural killer cell activity; ND, not done. The activities are relative, with the value 100 arbitrarily set for the interferon with the highest activity.

Table 14.4 *Ratio of specific molecular activities*

IFN-α	AV/AP	AV/NK
A	0.38	41
D	0.80	1.3
A/D (*Bgl*)	0.59	95
A/D (*Pvu*)	0.14	3.2
D/A (*Bgl*)	1.7	6.0
D/A (*Pvu*)	0.14	13
A/D/A	0.60	1.8

AV, relative antiviral activity; AP, relative antiproliferative activity; NK, relative natural killer cell activity.

Table 14.5 *Effect of interferons on human natural killer (NK) cell activity*

	IFN-α (units/ml)
αA, α2	2
αB, α8	1
αC, α10	2
αD, α1	7
αF, α21	89
αI, α17	11
αJ, α7	> 10 000
αK, α6	29

The values in the table represent the concentration for 50 percent stimulation of natural killer cell activity. Data from Ortaldo et al. (1984).

occurring IFN-α hybrid designed by assigning each of the most frequently observed amino acids appearing at each position in the Hu-IFN-α subtypes (Klein et al. 1988). For the most part it is almost a hybrid between IFN-αA and IFN-αF with only five differences, several of which were introduced for purposes of cloning. As a result of the large number of amino acid differences between the hybrid IFN-α species and the naturally occurring IFN subtypes, there is the potential for greater immunogenicity than with the natural IFNs in long-term treatment. However, clinical studies with both the IFN-αB/D and IFN-αCon1 molecules suggests that immunogenicity is not a significant problem. Among the normal IFN-α species (Table 14.5), the individual species differ by over 10 000-fold in NK activity alone (Ortaldo et al. 1983a, 1984). IFN-αJ (IFN-α7) exhibits virtually no NK activity (Table 14.5) and can act as an antagonist of NK activity, blocking other IFN-α species from stimulating NK cells (Ortaldo et al. 1984).

FUNCTIONAL UNIT OF IFN-α

As we did not know whether IFN-α functioned as a monomer or a dimer, we used electron bombardment to determine the functional unit (Pestka et al. 1983; Kempner and Pestka 1986). The results are summarized in Figure 14.7. The functional unit of IFN-α was shown to be a monomer, whether the species were produced in *E. coli* or by human leukocytes (Pestka et al. 1983; Kempner and Pestka 1986). The functional unit of IFN-β appears to be a dimer (Pestka et al. 1983; Kempner and Pestka 1986) whereas that of IFN-γ was shown to be a tetramer (Pestka et al. 1983; Kempner and Pestka 1986; Langer et al. 1994). One crystal structure of human IFN-α2b suggested a dimer structure (Radhakrishnan et al. 1996). However, the solution structure is consistent with a monomer (Klaus et al. 1997). These results need to be understood in terms of the receptor–ligand interaction. The structural results suggest that IFN-α and IFN-β interact with the receptor differently,

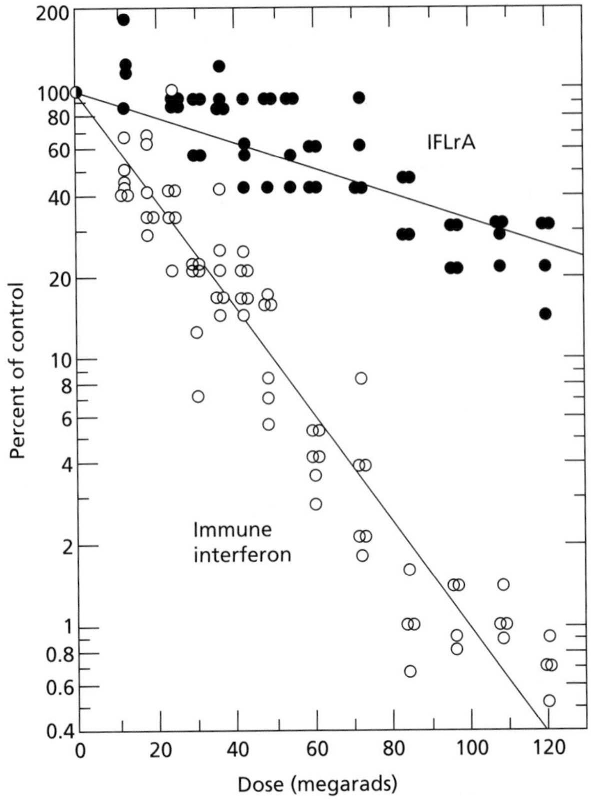

Figure 14.7 *Electron bombardment of recombinant human leukocyte (Hu-IFN-αA) and immune (IFN-γ) interferons. Data from Batcheler et al. (1986) and Fish et al. (1986). The molecular weight estimates for the functional units of the recombinant proteins are as follows: IFN-αA, 20 000; IFN-γ, 73 000. The monomer molecular masses are: IFN-αA, 19 219; IFN-γ, 17 126.*

which will very probably explain some of their functional differences.

General remarks

The IFN-α family consists of 13 expressed alleles producing 12 different proteins that exhibit remarkably different activity profiles. For the most part, the IFN-α species are not glycosylated although some contain carbohydrate. The recombinant proteins produced in *E. coli* have properties essentially equivalent to the proteins produced by human cells. Predominantly, only one recombinant IFN-α protein is used therapeutically (IFN-α2a, IFN-α2b, and IFN-α2c, allelic variants) so that the remaining IFN-α species remain an untapped reservoir of opportunity. Why the body produces so many of these interferons is an unanswered question. As our understanding of the mechanism of their receptor interactions develops, some of these answers should be forthcoming.

Although purification of the interferons to homogeneity remained elusive for about two decades after their discovery, they are now available in purified form. The largest amounts available are the species produced in *E. coli*. For purification, immunoaffinity chromatography has proved to be generally useful both on a laboratory and on a commercial scale. Nevertheless, techniques other than immunoaffinity chromatography have also proved to be successful. The availability of these proteins for laboratory and clinical studies has already catalyzed extensive new developments with them. The interferons are approved therapeutic agents worldwide. As the understanding of these agents becomes more extensive, we will gain new insights into their actions and develop new applications for their use.

RECOMBINANT HUMAN IFN-β

There is only one human IFN-β gene. The IFN-β was cloned by a number of laboratories (Derynck et al. 1980; Goeddel et al. 1980a; Houghton et al. 1980; Taniguchi et al. 1980) and expressed in *E. coli* and in eukaryotic vectors for expression in mammalian cell such as mouse or Chinese hamster ovary (CHO) cells (Canaani and Berg 1982; Zinn et al. 1982; Higashi et al. 1983; Maroteaux et al. 1983). IFN-β is active when expressed with or without carbohydrate. Similar to IFN-α, IFN-β exhibits antiviral and antiproliferative activity. The major use of IFN-β has been in the treatment of multiple sclerosis (Keegan and Noseworthy 2002), but the mechanisms by which it functions to ameliorate this disease are far from understood.

INTERFERON RECEPTORS

As noted above, the interferons are divided into two groups designated type I (IFN-α, IFN-β, IFN-κ, IFN-ω, and IFN-τ) and type II (IFN-γ) (Pestka 1981, 1986, 1997; Pestka et al. 1987; LaFleur et al. 2001). The past and current designations of the interferons are given in Table 14.6. Although leukocyte and fibroblast interferons were the original designations based on the source of the interferons, they usually consisted of multiple components dependent on the method of production. In general, leukocyte interferon obtained from white blood cells predominantly contained IFN-α species, but small quantities of IFN-β and IFN-ω were also present. Human fibroblast interferon consisted of IFN-β when induced by poly(I)·poly(C), but contained both IFN-α and IFN-β when induced by viruses, although IFN-β was predominant.

Similar to most cytokines and growth factors the actions of interferons are mediated by interaction with specific cell-surface receptors and the Jak–Stat signal transduction pathway (Aguet 1980; Lengyel 1982; Pestka et al. 1987; Langer and Pestka 1988; Sen and Lengyel 1992; Darnell et al. 1994; Uzé et al. 1995), although other pathways are increasingly being delineated (Raz et al. 1994; Durbin et al. 2000; Dalod et al. 2002). Competition binding studies demonstrated that type I IFNs share the same receptor complex, whereas type II IFN (IFN-γ) binds to a distinct receptor (Branca and Baglioni 1981; Pestka et al. 1987; Langer and Pestka 1988; Flores et al. 1991; Li and Roberts 1994; Alexenko et al. 1995). Components of both these classes of receptors were cloned. With the cloning of the receptor components, the mechanism of interferon action and the resultant signal transduction events were delineated in remarkable detail. Two transmembrane chains of the type I receptor complex (Uzé et al. 1990; Cleary et al. 1992, 1994; Domanski et al. 1995; Novick et al. 1994; Soh et al. 1994c; Lutfalla et al. 1995; Cook et al. 1996) and two chains of the type II receptor complex (Rashidbaigi et al. 1986; Jung et al. 1987; Aguet et al. 1988; Gray et al. 1989; Hemmi et al. 1989, 1994b; Kumar et al. 1989; Munro and Maniatis 1989; Cofano et al. 1990; Soh et al. 1993, 1994a) were characterized and cloned. As the IFN-γ–receptor complex (type II) has been characterized much better than the type I interferon–receptor complex, the IFN-γ receptor is discussed as a preface to the type I receptor. Understanding of the molecular events from ligand binding to signal transduction has elucidated several new paradigms that provide a basis for understanding the family of multichain cytokine receptors and the specificity of signal transduction. The IFN-γ–receptor complex has thus provided the basic model for other members of the family of class II cytokine receptors including the type I interferon and interleukin (IL) 10 receptor complexes.

Table 14.6 *Classes of interferons*

Original designation	Greek name	Current designation	Type
Leukocyte	Alpha	IFN-α	Type I
Fibroblast	Beta	IFN-β	Type I
Leukocyte (II)	Omega	IFN-ω	Type I
Keratinocyte	Kappa	IFN-κ	Type I
Trophoblast	Tau	IFN-τ	Type I
Immune	Gamma	IFN-γ	Type II

Receptor nomenclature

The designations of the interferon receptor components are given in Tables 14.7 and 14.8. These receptor complexes consist of two or more components. It also appears that the individual components may contribute to one extent or another to ligand binding so that designations such as an α subunit for the ligand-binding component and the β subunit for the signal transduction subunit are not warranted. The subunits are named in the order in which they were cloned and discovered as distinct entities. Alternate designations for the subunits that have been used are also given (Tables 14.7 and 14.8).

Table 14.7 *Designations of human interferon receptor components: type I interferon (α/β/ο/τ) receptor*

Chain or mRNA	Gene	References
Hu-IFN-αR1, Hu-IFN-αR1a	*IFNAR1*	Uzé et al. (1990)
Hu-IFN-αR1s, Hu-IFN-αR1b (splice variant missing exons IV, V)	*IFNAR1*	Cleary et al. (1994); Cook et al. (1996)
Hu-IFN-αR2a (soluble form)	*IFNAR2*	Novick et al. (1994)
Hu-IFN-αR2b (short form)	*IFNAR2*	Novick et al. (1994)
Hu-IFN-αR2c (long form)	*IFNAR2*	Domanski et al. (1995); Lutfalla et al. (1995)
αYAC (F136C5)	*IFNAR1* and *IFNAR2*	Soh et al. (1994c)

Table 14.8 *Designations of human interferon receptor components: type II interferon (IFN-γ) receptor*

Chain	Gene	References
Hu-IFN-γR1 (Hu-IFN-γRα; ligand binding chain of receptor)	*IFNGR1*	Aguet et al. (1988); Kumar et al. (1989); Hemmi et al. (1989); Gray et al. (1989); Munro and Maniatis (1989); Cofano et al. (1990)
Hu-IFN-γR2 (accessory factor-1; AF-1; Hu-IFN-γRβ; second chain of receptor)	*IFNGR2*	Soh et al. (1994a); Hemmi et al. (1994b)

THE TYPE II INTERFERON (IFN-γ) RECEPTOR

Chromosomal localization of the IFN-γ receptor ligand-binding chain and discovery of two chains required for activity

It was shown by study of ligand-binding competition that the IFN-γ receptor was distinct from that of the receptor that bound IFN-α and IFN-β (Branca and Baglioni 1981). Through somatic cell genetic techniques, Rashidbaigi et al. (1986) demonstrated that the gene for the ligand-binding chain of the human IFN-γ receptor was localized to human chromosome 6 (specifically 6q). Nevertheless, although somatic cell hybrids that contain this region of, or the entire, chromosome 6 exhibited excellent binding of IFN-γ, the ligand was unable to initiate any biological activities. This study led Jung et al. (1987, 1988) to the discovery that an additional component located on human chromosome 21 (specifically 21q) was required for function through the IFN-γR1 chain encoded on human chromosome 6. Thus, two species-specific components were involved as part of the functional IFN-γ receptor: the ligand-binding chain of the receptor, IFN-γR1; and the second chain of the receptor, IFN-γR2, we initially designated accessory factor-1 (AF-1) that is required for signal transduction through the receptor. These somatic cell genetic experiments led to the discovery of the location of the ligand-binding chain (IFN-γR1) to chromosome 6 and the location of the second chain, IFN-γR2, to human chromosome 21 and set the stage to isolate and clone these components. The comparable mouse chains were localized to mouse chromosomes 10 and 16, respectively (Mariano et al. 1987, 1996). Tables 14.7 and 14.8 summarize the suggested nomenclature for these chains.

Subsequent to the localization of the ligand-binding chain, both the human (Aguet et al. 1988) and mouse (Gray et al. 1989; Hemmi et al. 1989; Kumar et al. 1989; Munro and Maniatis 1989; Cofano et al. 1990) IFN-γR1 chains were cloned and shown to bind ligand. In addition, these studies confirmed our observations that the ligand-binding component was insufficient for generating a biological response. To generate a biological response, it was necessary to have the ligand-binding chain plus the second chain IFN-γR2 (AF-1). It should be noted that the biological response measured in these assays was induction of class I major histocompatibility complex (MHC) antigen expression. By reconstituting functional activity with the cloned Hu-IFN-γR1 and human chromosome 21, it was definitively demonstrated that the ligand-binding chain was the necessary and sufficient component contributed by human chromosome 6 (Jung et al. 1990). It was thus concluded that the functional receptor consisted of two chains, which are now designated IFN-γR1 and IFN-γR2 (see Table 14.7).

Study of chimeric human and mouse IFN-γR1 chains demonstrated that the ability of mouse and human IFN-γ species to stimulate MHC class I antigen induction in various cells transfected with the chimeric receptors required the homologous extracellular domain of the receptor, e.g. the chimeric receptor HMM (human extracellular, murine transmembrane, and murine intracellular domains, respectively) was able to respond to Hu-IFN-γ only in mouse cells or hamster cells containing human chromosome 21 or 21q (Gibbs et al. 1991; Hemmi et al. 1992; Hibino et al. 1992; Kalina et al. 1993). Modification of the mouse IFN-γR1 chain by site-specific mutation was reported by Lai (1994) to yield an interesting ectodomain mutant chain (His196-Ala) that was able to bind ligand, but was not able to support signal transduction as measured by MHC class I antigen induction, growth inhibition, or activation of Stat1α. This appears to be the first ectodomain mutant that alters signal transduction, but not ligand binding. It should provide some interesting insight into how this His196 of the IFN-γR1 chain is involved in supporting signal transduction. Perhaps, this region of the receptor is required for interaction with the IFN-γR2 chain.

The IFN-γR1 chain

The IFN-γR1 chain serves to bind ligand. The functional architecture of the IFN-γR1 intracellular domain is concentrated in two specific regions. Distal from the membrane, a five-residue sequence ($Y^{457}DKPH^{461}$) is required for all signal transduction (Cook et al. 1992; Farrar et al. 1991, 1992). This sequence is completely conserved in human and mouse receptors. Y^{457} is phosphorylated on ligand binding, and serves as a recruitment site for Stat1α (Greenlund et al. 1994). The function of the other residues in the YDKPH motif are not known, but D^{458} and H^{461} are required (Cook et al. 1992; Farrar et al. 1992). Specific mutations have shown that the carboxy-terminal 29 amino acids have no apparent function (Cook et al. 1992). A membrane-proximal $L^{266}PKS^{269}$ motif is required for receptor activity and Jak-1 binding (Kaplan et al. 1996).

The second receptor chain (IFN-γR2)

The second chain of the IFN-γ receptor was isolated by Soh et al. (1993, 1994a); Cook et al. (1994), and Hemmi et al. (1994b). The cDNA clones encode the necessary species-specific factor and are able to substitute for human chromosome 21 to reconstitute the Hu-IFN-γ receptor-mediated induction of class I HLA antigens. However, the factor encoded by the cDNA does not confer full antiviral protection against encephalomyocarditis virus (EMCV), suggesting that an additional factor encoded on human chromosome 21 may be required for reconstitution of antiviral activity against EMCV (Soh et al. 1993, 1994a; Cook et al. 1994; Lembo et al. 1996). Similar observations were made with the mouse IFN-γR1 and IFN-γR2 chains. Substitution of each of the tyrosine residues of the intracellular domain by phenylalanine did not alter the ability of the mouse IFN-γR2 chain to support signal transduction (Hemmi et al. 1994a). Kotenko et al. (1995) showed that the intracellular domain of the Hu-IFN-γR2 chain lacking the terminal 49 residues was totally inactive in MHC class I antigen induction, Jak1 and Jak2 phosphorylation, Stat1α activation, and tyrosine phosphorylation of the IFN-γR1 chain. Furthermore, cells expressing the Hu-IFN-γR2 chain alone did not crosslink or bind ligand; however, when both Hu-IFN-γR1 and Hu-IFN-γR2 chains were co-expressed in hamster cells, the association constant for binding of ligand increased about threefold and a specific band of a crosslinked Hu-IFN-γ–Hu-IFN-γR2 complex was observed (Kotenko et al. 1995). This indicated that the two chains of the receptor must be in close proximity as suggested by experiments with chimeric receptors noted above. Jak2 was found to associate with the IFN-γR2 intracellular domain (Kotenko et al. 1995). Residues 263–267 and 270–274 of the intracellular domain of IFN-γR2 act as a Jak2-binding site (Bach et al. 1996). The cytoplasmic domains of the IFN-γR2 subunits, similar to the cytoplasmic domains of the IFN-γR1 chains, can be interchanged between species with no loss of biological activity, confirming that the species-specific interaction of the IFN-γR1 and IFN-γR2 chains involves only the extracellular domains of the two proteins (Muthukumaran et al. 1996).

The functional IFN-γ receptor complex

A model for the functional IFN-γ receptor is shown in Figure 14.8. The IFN-γR1 chains bind the ligand whereas the IFN-γR2 chains serve to complete the complex for signal transduction.

Specificity of ligand binding

There are two distinct interactions that underlie species specificity: the binding of ligand to the IFN-γR1 chain, and the interaction of the IFN-γR1 and IFN-γR2, independent of ligand. The interaction of IFN-γ with the IFN-γR1 chain is highly species specific. Human IFN-γ stimulates no activity on rodent cells whatsoever, and rodent IFN-γ exhibits no activity on human cells. This effect is attributed to the interaction of the ligand with the IFN-γR1 chain. The presence of the second chain IFN-γR2 may increase the overall affinity of the ligand to the receptor complex slightly (Lai 1994; Kotenko et al. 1995; Marsters et al. 1995).

Specificity of the interactions of the two chains

Chimeric receptors were constructed between the mouse and human IFN-γR1 chains (Gibbs et al. 1991; Hemmi et al. 1992; Hibino et al. 1992; Kalina et al. 1993). The extracellular, transmembrane and intracellular domains were swapped between the human and mouse IFN-γR1 chains. The chains were introduced into mouse–human and hamster–human somatic cell hybrids that contained human chromosome 21, which expressed the Hu-IFN-γR2 chain. These results established that the extracellular domains of the two chains must be matched from the same species to enable the ligand to initiate signal transduction.

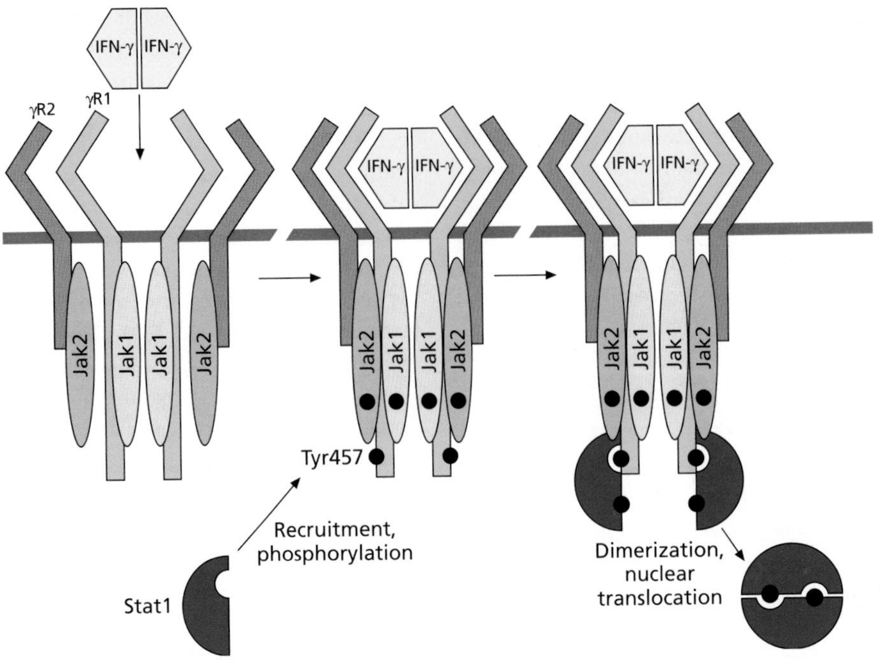

Figure 14.8 *Model of the IFN-γ receptor complex and signal transduction. In the three-dimensional structure it is likely that the extracellular domains of both IFN-γR1 and IFN-γR2 chains contact the ligand, IFN-γ.*

In a complementary series of experiments with hamster–mouse somatic cell hybrid cells, it was shown that mouse IFN-γ could activate the hybrid cells only when the mouse chromosome 16 was present in the hybrids and the IFN-γR1 chain contained the extracellular mouse domain of this chain (Hibino et al. 1992; Mariano et al. 1996).

Specificity of signal transduction

Each cytokine that utilizes the Jak–Stat signal transduction pathway activates a distinct combination of members of the Jak and Stat families. Thus, the Jaks, the Stats, or both could contribute to the specificity of ligand action. With the use of chimeric receptors involving the interferon-γ receptor (IFN-γR) complex as a model system, Kotenko et al. (1996) demonstrated that Jak2 activation is not an absolute requirement for IFN-γ signaling. Other members of the Jak family can functionally substitute for Jak2. IFN-γ can signal through the activation of Jak family members other than Jak2 as measured by Stat1α homodimerization and MHC class I antigen expression (Figure 14.9). This indicates that Jaks are interchangeable in the Jak–Stat signal transduction pathway. The necessity for the activation of one particular kinase during signaling can be overcome by recruiting another kinase to the receptor complex (Figure 14.9). The results suggest that the Jaks do not contribute significantly to the specificity of signal transduction.

The Stats represent proteins containing -SH_2, -SH_3, and DNA-binding domains (for reviews, see Darnell et al. 1994; Fu 1995). The highly selective and specific interaction between Stat -SH_2 domains and the phosphotyrosine-containing Stat recruitment sites on the intracellular domains of the cytokine receptors determines which Stats are to be recruited to a particular receptor complex (Heim et al. 1995; Stahl et al. 1995). Thus, the major specificity of the pathway probably results in large part from the specificity of the Stat recruitment sites on the receptor chains. Other molecules that interact with Jaks and Stats may contribute to the specificity and range of the interaction (Pollack et al. 1995; Collum et al. 2000).

Rationale for the multichain receptor

In the current model, binding of IFN-γ causes oligomerization of the two IFN-γ receptor (IFN-γR) subunits, receptor chain 1 (IFN-γR1, the ligand-binding chain) and the second chain of the receptor (IFN-γR2), and causes activation of two Jak kinases (Jak1 and Jak2) as illustrated in Figure 14.8. In contrast, the erythropoietin receptor (EpoR) requires only one receptor chain and one Jak kinase (Jak2). Chimeras between the EpoR and the IFN-γR1 and IFN-γR2 chains demonstrated that the architecture of the EpoR and the IFN-γR complexes differs significantly (Muthukumaran et al. 1997). Although IFN-γR1 alone cannot initiate signal transduction, both the chimeric EpoR/γR1 (extracellular/intracellular) homodimer and the EpoR/γR1–EpoR/γR2 heterodimer generate responses characteristic of IFN-γ in response to Epo. Thus, the configuration of the extracellular domains influences the architecture of the intracellular domains.

In contrast to the growth hormone (GH) receptor (de Vos et al. 1992) and the EpoR (Watowich et al. 1992)

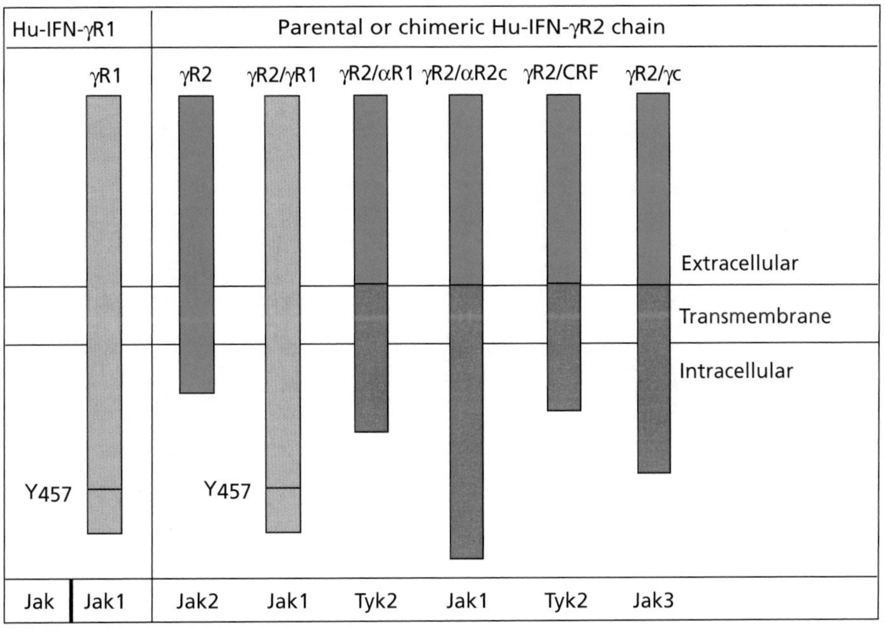

Figure 14.9 *Structure of chimeric receptors. Hu-IFN-γR1 (γR1) and Hu-IFN-γR2 (γR2) are the intact chains of the human IFN-γ receptor complex. All chimeric receptors have the extracellular domain of the human IFN-γR2 and the transmembrane and intracellular domains of different human receptors: γR2/γR1, Hu-IFN-γR1; γR2/αR1, Hu-IFN-αR1 (Uzé et al. 1990); γR2/αR2, Hu-IFN-αR2c (Domanski et al. 1995; Lutfalla et al. 1995); γR2/CRF, CRFB4 (Lutfalla et al. 1993); γR2/γC, IL-2 receptor* γ_C *chain (Takeshita et al. 1992). The short form Hu-IFN-αR2b binds Jak1 (Novick et al. 1994), but does not support signal transduction.*

complexes, when one IFN-γ homodimer binds two IFN-γR1 molecules, the two receptor subunits do not interact with one another and are separated by 2.7 nm (Walter et al. 1995) at their closest point. Therefore, although the IFN-γR1 chain possesses both a Jak1-association site and a Stat1α-recruitment site, alone it is unable to transduce a signal on homodimerization because the two Jak1 kinases are not in physical proximity to permit transphosphorylation (Figure 14.10a). Crystallographic analysis of the IFN-γ–IFN-γR1 complex suggests that each monomer of the IFN-γ homodimer binds one IFN-γR1 and one IFN-γR2 subunit (Walter et al. 1995). Thus the signal-transducing complex of IFN-γ consists of the IFN-γ homodimer bound to two IFN-γR1 and two IFN-γR2 chains (see Figures 14.8 and 14.10b) which recruit Jak1 and Jak2, respectively (Kotenko et al. 1995, 1996; Muthukumaran et al. 1996, 1997) and Jak2 phosphorylates Jak1, after which either kinase phosphorylates Tyr-457 of the IFN-γR1 chain. The phosphorylated segment of each IFN-γR1 chain recruits Stat1α, which is then phosphorylated by Jak1 or Jak2, and released to dimerize and form the active Stat1α. In contrast, with the EpoR/γR1 dimer, two Jak1 kinases are brought sufficiently close together to activate one another (Figure 14.10c). In the case of the EpoR/γR1–EpoR/γR2 dimer, one Jak1 and one Jak2 are in close apposition for Jak2 to phosphorylate Jak1 and initiate efficient downstream signaling events (Figure 14.10d). A major function of receptor dimerization is to bring two receptor-associated kinases together for transactivation and phosphorylation of the receptor chains. The cytoplasmic domain of the IFN-γR2 subunit serves to bring Jak2 kinase into the signal transduction complex (see Figures 14.8 and 14.10b) because the IFN-γR1 chain alone cannot bring Jak1 into sufficient proximity to initiate signal transduction.

For hormones, growth factors, and cytokines, the conversion of the extracellular ligand-binding event to the intracellular signal involves a change in the structure of the receptor. Depending on the ligand, this can take the form of receptor homodimers (Epo, GH), heterodimers (ciliary neurotropic factor (CNTF), leukemia inhibitory factor (LIF)), homotrimers (tumor necrosis factor (TNF)), and more complex assemblies (Stahl and Yancopoulos 1993). The IFN-γR2 subunit is a helper receptor subunit with a Jak2-association site, but no Stat-recruitment site; its intracellular domain can be substituted with the cytoplasmic domain of any receptor subunit that can bring a Jak kinase to the IFN-γ receptor complex to support signal transduction (Kotenko et al. 1996; Muthukumaran et al. 1996).

We propose that the multichain cytokine class II receptors have two major chains exemplified by the IFN-γ receptor complex (see Figure 14.10b). The ligand-binding chain (IFN-γR1) and the accessory chain (AC) (IFN-γR2; helper receptor) serve as a foundation for the functional IFN-γR complex (Kotenko et al. 1995, 1996; Muthukumaran et al. 1996, 1997). The geometry of the IFN-γR1 chain is such that its homodimerization yields a nonfunctional intracellular receptor complex. The accessory chain completes this function (see Figure 14.10b). The question arises of why

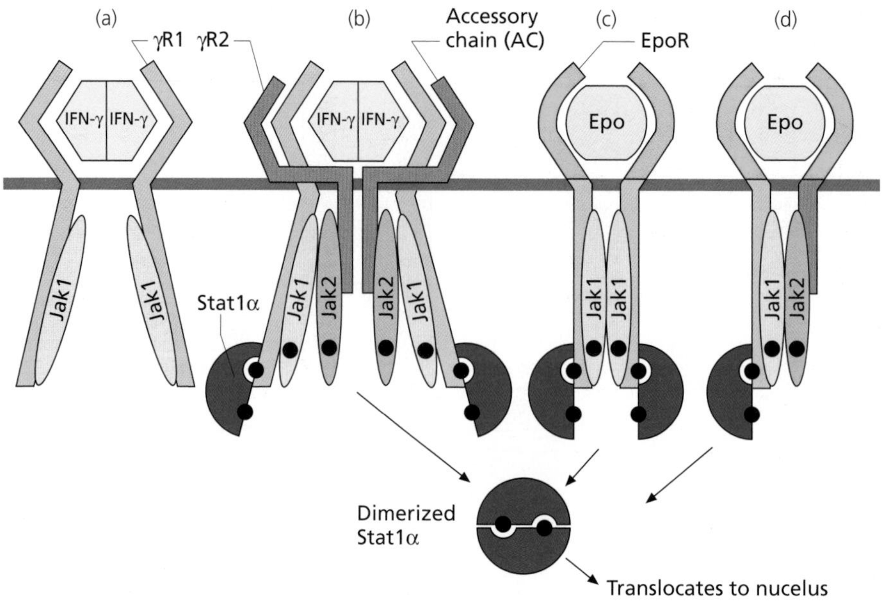

Figure 14.10 *Schematic representation of receptor complexes.* **(a)** *The IFN-γR1 homodimer bound to IFN-γ. The cytoplasmic domains of the two chains are too far apart to permit transactivation of the two Jak1 kinases.* **(b)** *The active heteromeric IFN-γ receptor complex with two IFN-γR1 and two IFN-γR2 subunits per complex. The IFN-γ homodimer binds to two IFN-γR1 chains, followed by its interaction with two IFN-γR2 chains. The associated Jak2 and Jak1 kinases activate one another by transphosphorylation, with subsequent phosphorylation and dimerization of Stat1α.* **(c)** *The EpoR/IFN-γR1 homodimer which, unlike the IFN-γR1 homodimer, permits transactivation of the two Jak1 molecules.* **(d)** *The structure of the heterodimer of EpoR/IFN-γR1 and EpoR/IFN-γR2 which is the putative active receptor complex.*

two separate chains should have evolved when one in the correct configuration would suffice. We postulate that the presence of two distinct chains provides more effective control and fine-tuning of responses to ligand, e.g. the differences in response of T-helper (Th)1 and Th2 cells to IFN-γ results from the lack of expression of the IFN-γR2 chain in the Th1 subset (Adolf et al. 1990, 1991) and allows exquisite fine-tuning of sensitivity to IFN-γ. It is also possible that receptors with multiple chains could recruit additional factors into the complex to generate a wider variety of intracellular signals. This could explain how receptors with multiple subunits could activate a greater number of specific pathways and signals than those with fewer elements in the receptor complex.

THE TYPE I INTERFERON (IFN-α/β/ω) RECEPTOR

Chromosomal localization, antibodies, and cDNA clones

Somatic cell genetic studies with human–rodent hybrid cells containing various combinations of human chromosomes have provided evidence that the presence of human chromosome 21 confers sensitivity of the rodent cells to human type I interferons (Tan et al. 1973; Slate et al. 1978; Epstein et al. 1982; Raziuddin and Gupta 1985). It was also demonstrated that antibodies to human chromosome 21-encoded cell surface components were able to block the action or binding of Hu-IFN-α to cells (Revel et al. 1976; Shulman et al. 1984). Later, Langer et al. (1990) demonstrated that 3x1S irradiation-reduced hamster–human somatic hybrid cells containing about 3 Mb (megabases) of chromosome 21q around 21q22.1 (Jung 1991; Soh et al. 1994c) were able to bind ^{32}P-labeled Hu-IFN-αA and generate a complex of about 150 kDa when crosslinked to the cell surface. During this time, the gene for the Hu-IFN-αR1 receptor chain was mapped to the 3x1S region (21q22.1) (Lutfalla et al. 1990). The paradoxical observation that Chinese hamster ovary 3x1S cells could bind Hu-IFN-αA, whereas the expression of the cloned receptor cDNA (Hu-IFN-αR1) in mouse cells did not confer binding to Hu-IFN-αA, suggested that the 3x1S region of human chromosome 21 contains other subunits of the receptor complex. This assumption was supported by the identification of two separate components after immunoprecipitation of ^{125}I-labeled Hu-IFN-αA–receptor complexes from 3x1S cell extracts with anti-IFN-α receptor antibody (Colamonici et al. 1990, 1992; Colamonici and Domanski 1993). These two subunits differ from the cloned Hu-IFN-αR1. The monoclonal antibodies (MAbs) against one subunit (110 kDa) and the recombinant Hu-IFN-αR1 receptor locked the biological activity of type I interferons whereas MAbs against the second subunit did not (Colamonici et al. 1990, 1992; Benoit et al. 1993; Colamonici and Domanski 1993), suggesting that the type I IFN receptor consists of at least two different subunits. Antibodies to Hu-IFN-αR1 blocked the activity of various type I interferons (Uzé et al. 1991). Thus, it was likely that the Hu-IFN-αR1 molecule was at least one component of the type I IFN receptor.

Mouse cells with functional Hu-IFN type I IFN receptors were first isolated by Jung and Pestka (1986) and Revel et al. (1991). The mouse cells transfected with total human DNA exhibited the properties of a type I interferon receptor (also designated Hu-IFN-αR, Hu-IFN-βR, or Hu-IFN-α/βR) in that they responded to two type I interferons tested: Hu-IFN-α and Hu-IFN-β. Although primary transformants were obtained by these groups, no molecular clone was obtained that provided type I interferon receptor activity. Employing the procedures of Jung and Pestka (1986); Uzé et al. (1990), by switching the selection procedure from Hu-IFN-αA and Hu-IFN-β to Hu-IFN-αB2 (a more species-specific Hu-IFN-α), were able to obtain a molecular clone which they designated the type I IFN receptor. However, as shown by them and other groups, this cDNA clone, when expressed in mouse or hamster cells, did not bind all type I interferons other than Hu-IFN-αB2 and yielded very little response even to Hu-IFN-αB2. However, Hu-IFN-αR1 expressed in xenopus oocytes to minimize the possibility of endogenous receptor components can bind and be covalently crosslinked to Hu-IFN-αA and Hu-IFN-αB, although to a small degree (Lim et al. 1994). None of the other Hu-IFN-α species tested seemed to activate the mouse cells expressing this cDNA clone. During this period, however, a number of groups obtained antibodies, suggesting that the type I receptor consisted of multiple components, a hypothesis consistent with the inability of Jung and Pestka (1986) to obtain stable secondary transformants. A comparison of hamster cells with the 3x1S region of human chromosome 21 and cells transfected with the Hu-IFN-αR1 cDNA showed that other components were involved in the type I interferon receptor. Hamster cells with the 3x1S region of human DNA responded to Hu-IFN-αA and Hu-IFN-β, whereas mouse or hamster cells with the Hu-IFN-αR1 cDNA did not respond to low concentrations of these interferons (Langer et al. 1990; Soh et al. 1994c).

As noted above, cloning of the first human type I IFN receptor chain (IFN-αR1) was reported on the basis of rendering mouse cells sensitive to Hu-IFN-αB2 (Uzé et al. 1990). However, when mouse cells were transfected with the Hu-IFN-αR1 cDNA, they did not exhibit binding and antiviral protection with type I IFN subtypes other than Hu-IFN-αB2. Similarly, human cells transfected with the homologous cloned mouse Mu-IFN-αR1 receptor cDNA showed antiviral protection activity with only Mu-IFN-α11. However, the expression of this Mu-IFN-αR1 cDNA in murine L1210 R101 cells resistant to type I IFNs and lacking mRNA for this Mu-IFN-αR1 receptor component showed antiviral protection in response to all type I Mu-IFNs tested (Uzé et al. 1992). In contrast, it was reported that, when CHO-K1 cells were transfected with the cloned Hu-IFN-αR1 cDNA, no induction of 2′,5′-oligoadenylic acid synthetase activity was observed after treating cells with Hu-IFN-αA and Hu-IFN-αB2 (Revel et al. 1991).

In affinity, crosslinking experiments, ^{125}I-labeled Hu-IFN-α–receptor complexes with an M_r of 80 000 (Hannigan et al. 1986), 210 000 (Colamonici et al. 1992), 260 000 (Vanden Broecke and Pfeffer 1988), or 300 000 (Raziuddin and Gupta 1985) were observed, in addition to the major complex that migrates as a broad band with an M_r of 140 000–150 000. These observations strongly suggested that other subunits, components or accessory proteins, are involved in ligand binding and in signal transduction in response to type I IFNs (Colamonici and Pfeffer 1991; Mariano et al. 1992; Abramovich et al. 1994b) as described for the IFN-γ receptor (Jung et al. 1987; Cook et al. 1992, 1994; Soh et al. 1993, 1994a).

Functional YAC selection and screening

Jung et al. (1987, 1988, 1990; Jung 1991) attempted to obtain the gene and/or cDNA clone for Hu-IFN-γR2 in studies that served as a foundation for isolation of a genomic clone encoding the functional type I IFN receptor complex. However, the use of cDNA expression libraries, cosmid genomic clones, and total human DNA proved inadequate to obtain a molecular clone for Hu-IFN-γR2. We thus turned to the use of yeast artificial chromosomes (YAC) because they contain large inserts of human DNA. YAC cloning techniques allow the cloning of DNA fragments from 100 to 2000 kb. (Burke et al. 1987; Chumakov et al. 1992a). The large insert size not only facilitates physical mapping (Chumakov et al. 1992b), but also makes it possible to express genes that are larger than permitted by conventional cloning procedures and regions of chromosomes containing multiple genes. To use YACs for fusion to mammalian cells and selection, it was necessary to devise and construct plasmids that would insert mammalian markers into the YACs so that the appropriate cells could be selected (Soh et al. 1994b; Emanuel et al. 1995). In addition, we designed vectors that would fragment the YAC clones into more manageable smaller ones (Cook et al. 1993, 1994; Emanuel et al. 1995). By examining a number of YACs containing human DNA inserts from this region, we were able to find one that contained the gene for the Hu-IFN-γR2 chain. Having successfully used this approach to obtain a functional Hu-IFN-γ receptor, we then applied this YAC technology to examine the type I interferon system.

A functional human interferon type I receptor

With the knowledge that the 3x1S region of human chromosome 21 contained the genes for the type I interferon receptor, we screened three YAC clones from this region. Two YACs were initially screened by a primer pair derived from the 524-5P probe (*21S58* locus) near the cloned Hu-IFN-αR1 receptor gene (Lutfalla et al. 1992). Tassone et al. (1990) reported that the two loci (*21S58* and *IFNAR*) were located within 170 kb of each other. It was also reported that the *CRFB4* gene identified by the 524-5P probe was located at less than 35 kb from the Hu-IFN-αR1 gene (Lutfalla et al. 1993). The αYAC containing the gene for the cloned Hu-IFN-αR1 receptor cDNA was selected for expression into hamster cells based on the assumption that all the genes involved in forming a functional type I IFN receptor might be encompassed on this YAC. The objective was to obtain a YAC clone that would support type I human interferon activity when transferred into hamster cells. We found one YAC clone that fit our criteria. It contained the genes for the cloned Hu-IFN-αR1 receptor subunit and other genes in the 3x1S region of chromosome 21. In addition, the introduction of this YAC clone, designated αYAC, into hamster cells rendered the cells much more sensitive to Hu-IFN-αA and Hu-IFN-αB2, and somewhat more sensitive to Hu-IFN-ω and Hu-IFN-β (Soh et al. 1994c). We thus hypothesized that this YAC clone must contain multiple genes required to reconstitute a fully functional type I IFN receptor.

Antiviral protection of hamster cells containing the Hu-IFN-αR1 cDNA or the αYAC

The hamster cells fused to spheroplasts with the αYAC containing the type I interferon receptor complex showed increased sensitivity to Hu-IFN-αA and Hu-IFN-αB2 in antiviral protection against EMCV and vesicular stomatitis virus (VSV) when compared with the parental hamster 16-9 cells or hamster cells transfected with the Hu-IFN-αR1 receptor cDNA (Soh et al. 1994c). The hamster cells containing the αYAC exhibited large increases in sensitivity to Hu-IFN-αA and Hu-IFN-αB2. Furthermore, there was substantial increase in sensitivity to Hu-IFN-β and Hu-IFN-ω. When the sensitivity of the cells to the interferons was evaluated, in all cases hamster cells with the αYAC showed substantial increase in sensitivity to all type I interferons ranging from about threefold to more than 100-fold. There was little or no increased sensitivity of the comparable cells containing the cloned Hu-IFN-αR1 cDNA.

Induction of class I MHC surface antigens

Subclones isolated from transformed hamster 16-9 cells, which express the human HLA-B7 antigen, fused to the αYAC or transfected with the Hu-IFN-αR1 cDNA exhibited HLA-B7 induction as a function of IFN concentration for all of the type I IFNs tested. Hu-IFN-αA, Hu-IFN-αB2, Hu-IFN-β, and Hu-IFN-ω had little or no effect on the parental hamster 16-9 cells or hamster 16-9 cells transfected with the Hu-IFN-αR1 cDNA. However, hamster cells fused to the αYAC showed enhanced levels of HLA-B7 antigens in response to Hu-IFN-αA, Hu-IFN-αB2, Hu-IFN-β, and Hu-IFN-ω. Treatment of hamster cells fused with the αYAC with as little as 1 unit/ml of Hu-IFN-αA, Hu-IFN-αB2, Hu-IFN-ω, or Hu-IFN-β gave a significant HLA-B7 induction whereas parental hamster 16-9 cells or 16-9 cells transfected with the Hu-IFN-αR1 cDNA did not show any significant induction at this level (Soh et al. 1994c).

Cells containing the αYAC can bind ^{32}P-labeled Hu-IFN-αA and ^{32}P-labeled Hu-IFN-αB2

The hamster cells with the αYAC bound ^{32}P-labeled Hu-IFN-αA-P1 and ^{32}P-labeled Hu-IFN-αB2-P quite well. There was a small level of binding of ^{32}P-labeled Hu-IFN-αB2-P to cells containing the Hu-IFN-αR1 cDNA, but no binding of ^{32}P-labeled Hu-IFN-αA-P1 was seen. Furthermore, competition binding studies with ^{32}P-labeled Hu-IFN-αA-P1 as the labeled ligand showed that Hu-IFN-αA, Hu-IFN-αB2, Hu-IFN-β, and Hu-IFN-ω all compete effectively for ^{32}P-labeled Hu-IFN-αA-P1 binding to hamster cells with the αYAC as well as to human Daudi lymphoblastoid cells (Soh et al. 1994c). The specific binding of Hu-IFN-αA and Hu-IFN-αB2 to cells containing the αYAC and the competition by all type I interferon classes together with the activity data indicate that the human DNA insert in this YAC contains the genes encoding the subunits that comprise a functional type I receptor. As the Hu-IFN-αR1 gene is included in this DNA insert, one or more additional genes complementing the cloned Hu-IFN-αR1 receptor encoded on this YAC enable the cells to bind these interferons effectively (Soh et al. 1994c).

Proof that the IFN-αR1 component is part of the type I receptor complex

A large number of experiments were consistent with the concept that the IFN-αR1 chain was one component of the type I receptor complex. IFN-α-resistant K562 cells can bind type I IFNs, but are restored to IFN-α sensitivity by the introduction of Hu-IFN-αR1, without any apparent change in receptor number or affinity, suggesting a role for Hu-IFN-αR1 in cellular signaling (Colamonici et al. 1994a). Evidence for the role of IFN-αR1 in signal transduction includes the enhanced sensitivity to IFNs seen in some transfection studies, sometimes in the absence of enhanced IFN binding (Colamonici et al. 1994a; Constantinescu et al. 1994) and the interaction of IFN-αR1 with the intracellular tyrosine kinase Tyk2, required for IFN-α responses (Velazquez et al. 1992; Barbieri et al. 1994; Colamonici et al. 1994b).

Direct proof of the requirement for the IFN-αR1 chain for type I interferon receptor function was demonstrated by experiments disrupting the IFN-αR1 gene. Homozygous deletions of *IFNAR1* in mice (IFN-$\alpha R^{0/0}$) were reported to cause enhanced susceptibility to several viruses and eliminate antiproliferative activity of IFN-α and IFN-β (Müller et al. 1994; Hwang et al. 1995). Primary embryo fibroblasts from such mice lack type I IFN-stimulated resistance to viruses and inducibility of 2′,5′-oligoadenylic acid synthetase. Using homologous recombination targeted to the αYAC, Cleary et al. (1994) produced a deletion within the human IFN-α receptor (Hu-IFN-αR1) gene which eliminated exon II of the gene. The resultant αYAC was transferred to CHO cells. This deletion effectively eliminated the ability of type I interferons to induce MHC Class I antigens and exhibit antiviral activity, which are properties of the fully functional parental YAC clone (Soh et al. 1994c). By subsequent transfection of the cDNA for Hu-IFN-αR1 into cells containing the αYAC, antiviral activity and ability of Hu-IFN-α to stimulate MHC class I antigens was successfully reconstituted. The Hu-IFN-αR1 subunit thus plays a critical role in the functional human type I IFN receptor complex, the components of which are encoded on this YAC. In addition, as binding of ligands is retained in the cells containing the YAC with the deletion, it was clear that one or more additional subunits encoded on the YAC are responsible for ligand binding and activity.

Proof that the IFN-αR2c chain is required for function of the type I interferon receptor

After our studies describing the αYAC, a second chain, IFN-αR2b, which was suggested as another component of the type I interferon receptor complex, was reported, but it appeared to exhibit no intrinsic activity alone or together with the Hu-IFN-αR1 chain (Novick et al. 1994). The human gene *IFNAR2* encoding this chain is located on the αYAC and also localizes to the 3x1S region of chromosome 21. This Hu-IFN-αR2b chain was reported to bind type I interferons and antibodies to this chain were able to co-immunoprecipitate Jak1 (Novick et al. 1994). However, expression of IFN-αR1 or IFN-αR2b chains, or the combination of both, in hamster cells was not able to reconstitute functional human receptor activity (Mariano et al. 1994; Soh et al. 1994b; Kotenko et al. 1995). In addition, the CHO cells containing the ΔαYAC with the disrupted *IFNAR1* gene retained the ability to bind Hu-IFN-αA and Hu-IFN-αB2 (Cleary et al. 1994). This paradox was partially resolved when U5 cells (Darnell et al. 1994) that do not respond to type I interferons were able to be reconstituted to respond to the interferons by introduction of the αYAC (J. Cook, S. Pestka, I. Kerr, and G. Stark, unpublished data). Unfortunately, no stable transformants were obtained with the αYAC in U5 cells. The data indicated, however, that another component encoded on the αYAC was necessary for response to type I interferons. This component was subsequently cloned (Domanski et al. 1995; Lutfalla et al. 1995) and shown to be a long form of the Hu-IFN-αR2b chain called Hu-IFN-αR2c (see Table 14.7). All three chains (Hu-IFN-αR2a, -αR2b, and -αR2c) are encoded by the same *IFNAR2* gene. The Hu-IFN-αR2c gene contains a large intracellular domain compared with the short domain of the Hu-IFN-αR2c chain. The Hu-IFN-αR2c chain reconstitutes U5 cells for responses to type I interferons. The Hu-IFN-αR2a protein is a soluble form of the receptor consisting of the extracellular domain of the Hu-IFN-αR2b and Hu-IFN-αR2c chains.

Hamster cells containing the αYAC exhibit the properties expected for a functional type I human IFN receptor complex. The YAC provides genes which are necessary and sufficient to encode this functional type I interferon receptor complex as measured by three distinct biological assays and by binding of both ^{32}P-labeled Hu-IFN-αA and ^{32}P-labeled Hu-IFN-αB2 to cells fused to this αYAC.

Diversity of the interaction of type I interferons with the receptor

As noted above CHO cells containing the YAC F136C5 (αYAC) respond to all type I human interferons including IFN-αA, IFN-β, and IFN-ω. The αYAC contains at least two genes encoding IFN-αR chains that are required for response to type I human interferons: Hu-IFN-αR1 and Hu-IFN-αR2c. We previously isolated a splice variant of the Hu-IFN-αR1 chain designated Hu-IFN-αR1s or Hu-IFN-αR1b (Cleary et al. 1992) (see Table 14.7). CHO cells containing the disrupted αYAC, which contains a deletion in the Hu-IFN-αR1 gene, ΔαYAC, were transfected with expression vectors for the Hu-IFN-αR1 and Hu-IFN-αR1s chains. With these cells, two type I interferons were identified that can interact with the splice variant (Hu-IFN-αR1s) and with the Hu-IFN-αR1 chains: Hu-IFN-αA and Hu-IFN-ω. Two other type I interferons – Hu-IFN-αB2 and Hu-IFN-αF – are capable of signaling through the Hu-IFN-αR1 chain only, and cannot utilize the splice variant Hu-IFN-αR1s. Hu-IFN-αR1 and Hu-IFN-αR1s differ in that the latter is missing a single subdomain of the four subdomains of the receptor extracellular domain encoded by exons 4 and 5 of the Hu-IFN-αR1 gene. Therefore, different type I interferons require different subdomains of the Hu-IFN-αR1 receptor chain.

These results with the various forms of the Hu-IFN-α receptor components generally demonstrate differences in interaction of all the type I interferons with the receptor that reflect the differences in the activity profiles of the interferons. Specifically, some type I interferons (e.g. Hu-IFN-B2, Hu-IFN-αF) require the two subdomains absent in the splice variant (Figure 14.11) and some can function without these domains (e.g. Hu-IFN-αA, Hu-IFN-ω) as described by Cook et al. (1996). The results indicate that the various Hu-IFN-α species and other type I interferons interact with the receptor differently, thereby accounting for their differential activities. The conservation of the multitude of type I interferons throughout evolution of the mammals is consistent with unique functional roles for each of the type I interferons.

THE CYTOKINE TYPE 2 RECEPTOR FAMILY

The IFN-αR1, IFN-αR2, CRFB4, IFN-γR1, and IFN-γR2 chains are members of the cytokine type 2 receptor family as described by Bazan (1990a, b) and by Thoreau et al. (1991), who proposed that the interferon receptors as well as other receptors for cytokines and some growth factors are composed of two folding domains that comprise the ligand-binding site, which resides in the crevice between the folds. The primary cytokine–receptor interaction was suggested to involve one face of the ligand whereas another face of the bound cytokine can interact with accessory binding components. A summary of these receptors for the interferon-related receptor components is illustrated in a recent review (Kotenko and Pestka 2000). These homologies relate the interferon receptor components to the fibronectin type III structure, which in turn relates all these structures to the immunoglobulin superfamily.

SIGNAL TRANSDUCTION

All type I IFNs activate Jak1 and Tyk2 tyrosine kinases during signal transduction, leading to formation and activation of ISGF3 (IFN-α-stimulated gene factor 3), DNA-binding complexes consisting of Stat1 and Stat2 transcriptional factors and p48 DNA-binding protein from the IFN regulatory factor (IRF) family of proteins (Fu et al. 1990, 1992; Schindler et al. 1992; Veals et al. 1992; Müller et al. 1993). Two subunits of the type I IFN receptor complex were identified: Hu-IFN-αR1 and Hu-IFN-αR2c and its variants as described above (Novick et al. 1994; Domanski et al. 1995; Lutfalla et al. 1995).

Some Stats are activated by a number of cytokines; others are highly specific. Stat2 has been shown to be activated only in response to type I IFN (Fu et al. 1992). A number of studies were made to define how Stat1 and Stat2 are recruited to the type I IFN receptor complex (Uddin et al. 1995; Domanski and Colamonici 1996; Yan et al. 1996; Li et al. 1997). Although it is clear that both receptors are necessary for signaling of type I IFNs, because disruption of any one of them completely abolishes the ability of cells to respond to type I IFNs (Hwang et al. 1995; Lutfalla et al. 1995), the reports about their role in Stat recruitment were inconclusive. The IFN-αR1 chain as well as both forms of the IFN-αR2 chain, the IFN-αR2c and the IFN-αR2b chain, were reported to associate with Stat proteins (Uddin et al. 1995; Domanski and Colamonici 1996; Krishnan et al. 1996; Yan et al. 1996; Yang et al. 1996).

The difficulty in evaluating the contribution of each chain of the IFN-α receptor complex to signal transduction is the result of the lack of cell lines without the endogenous receptor chains and in the cross-species activity of the type I IFNs. To overcome these limita-

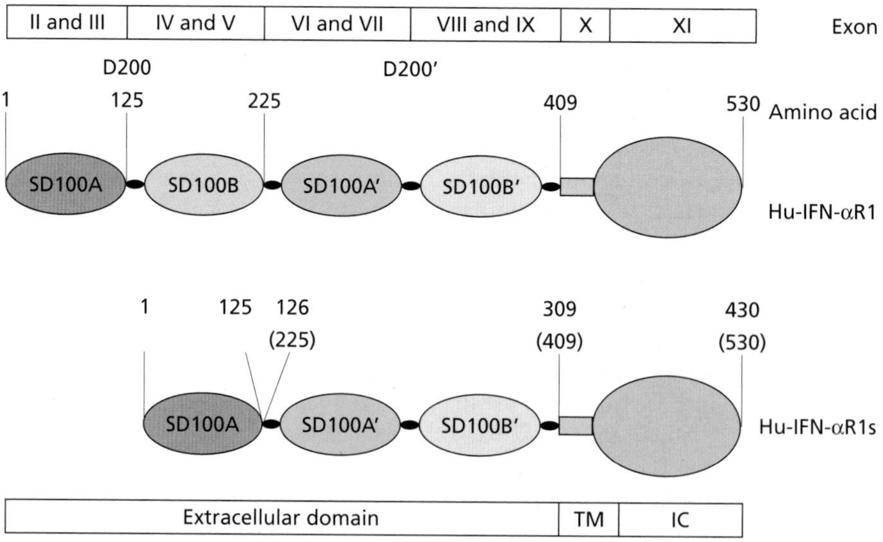

Figure 14.11 *Schematic Illustration of the Hu-IFN-αR1 chain and the splice variant Hu-IFN-αR1s. The domains of the Hu-IFN-αR1 chain are shown. The splice variant chain, Hu-IFN-αR1s, lacks exons 4 and 5.*

tions we used chimeric receptors with the extracellular human IFN-γ receptor chains expressed in hamster cells because Hu-IFN-γ is highly species specific and does not activate the endogenous hamster IFN-γ receptor. This strategy with the use of chimeric receptors (Kotenko et al. 1999) permitted us to show that the IFN-αR2c chain alone is necessary and sufficient for recruitment of Stat1 and Stat2.

Results of other workers have implicated all the receptor subunits of the IFN-α receptor complex (the IFN-αR1, IFN-αR2b, and IFN-αR2c chains) in Stat activation (Uddin et al. 1995; Domanski and Colamonici 1996; Yan et al. 1996; Li et al. 1997). The IFN-αR1 chain was reported to bind Stat2 and Stat3 in a ligand-dependent manner through the phosphorylated Tyr466 and the phosphorylated Tyr527, respectively (Yan et al. 1996; Yang et al. 1996; Li et al. 1997). It was originally demonstrated that the peptide containing phosphorylated Tyr466 (P-Tyr466) can inhibit type I IFN signaling in permeabilized cells and specifically interact with the - SH_2 domain of Stat2, but not of Stat1 (Yan et al. 1996). Later the P-Tyr466 peptide, which was one amino acid longer, was shown to interact with both Stat1 and Stat2 proteins (Li et al. 1997). However, mutation of all four tyrosine residues within the IFN-αR1 intracellular domain to phenylalanine resulted in a functional receptor (Gibbs et al. 1996), demonstrating that phosphorylation of the IFN-αR1 chain is unnecessary for the generation of a biological response. The IFN-αR2c chain was shown to bind both Stat1 and Stat2 in a ligand-independent manner (Domanski and Colamonici 1996; Li et al. 1997). As Stat1 activation by type I IFNs is Stat2 dependent (Improta et al. 1994; Leung et al. 1995), it was proposed that Stat1 is recruited to the complex through Stat2 (Leung et al. 1995; Li et al. 1997). The short form, the IFN-α2b chain, was reported to associate with Stat2 in a ligand-dependent manner (Uddin et al. 1995). However, most experiments were performed in cells where the endogenous type I receptor subunits were present. It is thus likely that endogenous components interacting with the heterologous type I interferon components in the host cells contributed to the results previously reported.

In our experiments with chimeric receptors, we could isolate the contributions of endogenous and exogenous components which was not possible previously (Kotenko et al. 1999). The chimeric receptors with the IFN-γR2 extracellular domain and intracellular αR1 and αR2c intracellular domains were expressed in hamster cells expressing the Hu-IFN-γR1 chain. The γR2/αR1 and γR2/αR2c chimeras rendered 16-9 cells sensitive to Hu-IFN-γ as measured by IFN-γ-induced MHC class I antigen expression and Stat1α activation as did the intact γR2/γR2. The γR2/αR2b was unable to support IFN-γ signaling because the IFN-αR2b intracellular domain does not associate with any kinase as we demonstrated previously (Fu 1995). The IFN-γ-induced activation of Stat1α DNA-binding complexes in hamster cells expressing chimeric receptors correlated with MHC class I antigen induction; however, formation of the IFN-γ-induced ISGF3 DNA-binding complexes was detected only in γR2/αR2c cells (Kotenko et al. 1999). Thus, we demonstrated that the Stat2 protein can be recruited and activated in cells expressing the chimeric receptor complex where the γR2/γR2 chain is substituted by the γR2/αR2c chimeric chain, but not by the γR2/αR1 or the γR2/αR2b chimeric chains, demonstrating that recruitment and activation of Stat2 occur through the intracellular domain of the IFN-αR2c chain. In addition, the γR2/αR2c chimeric chain expressed in these cells was able to support IFN-γ-induced antiviral protection against EMCV.

In the γR2/αR2c cells the presence of the Hu-IFN-γR1 chain, which recruits Stat1α to the receptor complex, did not allow us to answer the question of whether or not the presence of the IFN-αR2c intracellular domain is sufficient only for recruitment, and activation of Stat1α and Stat2 for formation of the ISGF3 DNA-binding complexes and the resultant biological activities. To define the requirements for Stat2 recruitment further, we switched to a hamster cell line expressing the Hu-IFN-γR2 chain which does not recruit any Stats, unlike the IFN-γR1 chain. Thus, the chimeric receptors with the IFN-γR1 extracellular domain expressed in these cells were the only chains that could contribute to Stat recruitment. Therefore, MHC class I antigen induction in these cells could serve as a marker of Stat activation. The cells expressing the γR1/γR1 and γR1/αR2c chimeras demonstrated IFN-γ-induced MHC class I antigen expression, whereas the γR1/γR1 and γR1/αR2b cells did not (Kotenko et al. 1999). Similarly, Stat1α DNA-binding complexes and small amounts of Stat3 DNA-binding complexes were activated in the γR1/γR1 and γR1/αR2c cells, but not in the γR1/γR1 and γR1/αR2b cells (Kotenko et al. 1999). However, ISGF3 DNA-binding complexes were induced only in γR1/αR2c cells (Kotenko et al. 1999). Thus, the presence of the IFN-αR2c intracellular domain as the only Stat-recruiting domain in the chimeric receptor complex is sufficient for Stat1, Stat2, and Stat3 recruitment, ISGF3 DNA-binding complex activation, and induction of MHC class I antigens. Only when the IFN-αR2c intracellular domain was present in the chimeric receptor was IFN-γ able to induce antiviral protection in cells.

We therefore conclude that all Stats activated by type I IFNs, Stat1, Stat2, and Stat3 are activated through the IFN-αR2c intracellular domain (Figure 14.12). The IFN-αR1 intracellular domain does not recruit Stats, but supports type I IFN signal transduction by bringing Tyk2 tyrosine kinase to the receptor complex and modulates type I IFN signaling. Stat recruitment by the type I IFN receptor complex is solely a function of the IFN-αR2c intracellular domain and the IFN-αR2c chain is sufficient and necessary for recruitment of Stat1, Stat2, and Stat3.

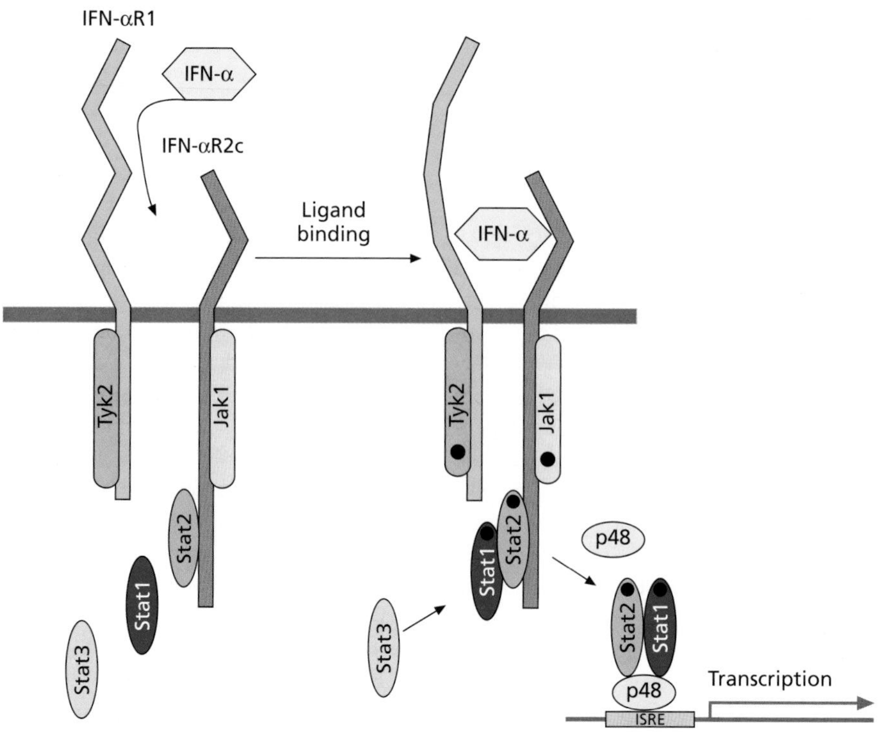

Figure 14.12 *Model of type I interferon (IFN)–receptor complex and signaling. Ligand binding to the subunits of the type I IFN receptor complex, the IFN-αR2c and the IFN-αR1 chains, initiates the cascade of signal transduction events. All Stats involved in IFN-α signaling are activated through the intracellular domain of the IFN-αR2c chain.*

Receptor and signal transduction endnote

Although two major components of the type I interferon receptor have been identified, a number of results suggest that there are other components yet to be delineated (Abramovich et al. 1994a; Cook et al. 1996; Hertzog et al. 1994). The crystal structures of Mu-IFN-β (Mitsui et al. 1993; Senda et al. 1995) and Hu-IFN-α2b (Radhakrishnan et al. 1996) and solution structure (Klaus et al. 1997) provide a foundation to develop an understanding of the interferon–receptor interactions further. The beginning of the elucidation of the type I interferon receptor is just starting with undoubtedly many surprises to come.

THERAPEUTIC USE OF TYPE I INTERFERONS

Interferons have been used in clinical trials for about three decades, but were not approved by regulatory agencies until the 1980s. The recombinant human interferons (IFN-α, IFN-β, and IFN-ω) and bovine IFN-τ have been used in clinical trials since 1981. Hu-IFN-αA (Hu-IFN-α2a) was the first recombinant interferon approved for clinical trial; and both Hu-IFN-αA (Hu-IFN-α2a) and Hu-IFN-α2 (Hu-IFN-α2b) were approved by regulatory agencies in many countries about the same time in the mid-1980s. The first approvals were for hairy cell leukemia and Kaposi's sarcoma. Since that time, they have been found to be useful in a variety of cancers and viral diseases. The Hu-IFN-αs have been approved for the treatment of a broad range of cancers such as CML (Talpaz et al. 1987; Faderl et al. 2000) and metastatic malignant melanoma (Sun and Schuchter 2001; Gray et al. 2002; Kilbridge et al. 2002; Kirkwood 2002; Kirkwood et al. 2002). They have been used in many clinical protocols for the treatment of other cancers with significant effects. In some cancers a small subset of patients seems to respond, but the genotype or phenotype of the responders has not been identified. It would be a major advance if the responders could be identified by genomic or other markers, a goal that many investigators are pursuing. Clinical trials continue in many cancers such as renal cell cancer (Hofmockel et al. 1997; Dutcher et al. 2001; van Herpen and De Mulder 2002) and many others (Cooper 1991; Einhorn and Strander 1993; Portillo Martin et al. 1995; Pfeffer et al. 1998; Ravandi et al. 1999; Borden et al. 2000; Oberg 2000; Eliason 2001; Jonasch and Haluska 2001; Brassard et al. 2002; Nathan and Eisen 2002). A summary of the approved therapeutic indications for interferons is given in Table 14.9. Local regional therapy has been attempted (van Herpen and De Mulder 2000), but effective delivery or sustained-release systems have not yet been developed.

Although interferons were first discovered because of their antiviral activity, they have not yet been used

Table 14.9 *Therapeutic activities of interferons*

Approved therapeutic interventions	
Hairy cell leukemia[a]	Kaposi's sarcoma[a]
Renal cell leukemia[a]	Non-Hodgkin's lymphoma[a]
T-cell lymphoma[a]	Multiple myeloma[a]
Laryngeal papillomatosis[a]	Malignant melanoma[a]
Bladder cell carcinoma[a]	Colon carcinoma[a]
Condyloma scuminatum[a]	Rhinovirus (prevention)[d]
Chronic hepatitis B[a]	Chronic hepatitis C (NANB)[a]
Hemangiomas[a]	Chronic myelogenous leukemia[a]
Malignant carcinoid tumor[a]	Crohn's disease[d]
Chronic granulomatous disease[b]	Diabetic retinopathy[d]
Cervical intraepithelial neoplasia[c]	Multiple sclerosis[c]
Carcinoid tumors[d]	Mycosis fungoides[d]
Ovarian cancer[d]	Polycythemia vera[d]
Skin cancer[d]	Thrombocytosis[d]

a) IFN-α, approval in the USA and/or other countries.
b) IFN-γ, approval in the USA and other countries.
c) IFN-β, approval in the USA and/or other countries.
d) IFN-α, not approved.

generally to treat many viral diseases. However, remarkably, virtually every class of viruses has one or more members that are sensitive to interferon in culture or in animals (Table 14.10). This leaves open the possibility that most viral diseases will be able to be prevented and/or treated with an appropriate interferon.

The interferons have been useful in the treatment of hepatitis. Specifically, the IFN-α species have been used effectively and are approved for the treatment of chronic hepatitis B (Haria and Benfield 1995; Woo and Burnakis 1997; Grob 1998; Marques et al. 1998; Mazzella et al. 1999; Alberti et al. 2002; Perrillo 2002) and hepatitis C (Vithanomsat et al. 1984; Yamamoto et al. 1992; Davis 1994; Iino et al. 1994; Trepo et al. 1994; Weiland 1994; Haria and Benfield 1995; Roffi et al. 1995; Romeo et al. 1995; Saracco and Rizzetto 1995; Zein and Rakela 1995; Jonas 1996; Alberti et al. 1997; Cooksley et al. 1997; Woo and Burnakis 1997; Hanley and Haydon 1998; Barnes et al. 1999; Shiffman 1999; Markland et al. 2000; Pianko and McHutchison 2000; Yasuda et al. 2000; Diamond and Harris 2001; Hu et al. 2001; Lyra and Di Bisceglie 2001; Sagmeister et al. 2001; Wilkinson 2001; Hino et al. 2002; Katze et al. 2002; Anderson and Rahal 2002). Certain strains of hepatitis C virus are more resistant to treatment than others. These can be identified by genotyping the strains (Martell et al. 1992; Okamoto et al. 1992; Hino et al. 1994; Tsubota et al. 1994; Enomoto and Sato 1995a, 1995b; Enomoto et al. 1995, 1996; Gale et al. 1997; Arens 2001). Studies have correlated a region of the hepatitis C viral nonstructural protein 5A (NS5A) with sensitivity and resistance to interferon. Protein NS5A was found to repress interferon-induced protein kinase, PKR, which is one of the mediators of antiviral activity of interferon. Furthermore, it has been possible to begin to correlate single nucleotide polymorphisms in patients with hepatitis C with their ability to respond to interferon (Hijikata et al. 2001). This will probably be improved immensely in the next few years.

Although interferon has been approved for the treatment of few other infectious diseases (e.g. condyloma acuminatum (Rockley and Tyring 1995), genital warts caused by human papilloma virus type 6 and 11, and labial and genital herpes (Ophir et al. 1995; Glezerman et al. 1988)), it has been shown to be effective for the treatment of laryngeal papillomatosis (Deunas et al. 1997; Haglund et al. 1981; Lundquist et al. 1984) and the prevention of common colds produced by rhinoviruses (Scott et al. 1982; Hayden and Gwaltney 1983; Phillpotts et al. 1983, 1984; Hayden et al. 1986; Higgins et al. 1986), although it has not been approved for these and other viral diseases. Very probably the type I interferons would be efficacious in the treatment and prevention of many viral diseases once appropriate delivery systems have been developed. Moreover, it has been suggested that interferon will be used for many infectious diseases in the future because it has potent immunomodulatory activities (Masihi 2000, 2001). That fact that interferon is active in blocking propagation of all classes of viruses (see Table 14.10) is tantalizing and may suggest that it will take some novel initiatives to make better use of the interferons to treat viral diseases, e.g. IFN-α is effective in substantially inhibiting retroviruses in tissue culture (Sen et al. 1984; Sperber et al. 1992), but has little effect in the treatment of diseases caused by retroviruses such as HIV – a paradox that has not been adequately addressed.

IFN-β has been found to be effective in relapsing–remitting multiple sclerosis (Silberberg 1994; Goodin 2001; Calabresi 2002; Keegan and Noseworthy 2002; Wingerchuk and Noseworthy 2002) and is currently approved for treatment. Various preparations of IFN-β are in use and all are effective, although no treatment can eliminate the disease. The mechanism by which interferon works is not clear, but it was suggested that IFN-β inhibits migration of activated T cells into the central nervous system (Leppert et al. 1996).

The detailed biological effector mechanisms that result in the various activities of the interferons are surprisingly not defined in most cases. What has made this exceptionally difficult is that the mechanisms vary from animal species to species and from one cell type to another even in the same species. It is clear that the Jak–Stat pathway is involved in many of the mechanisms, as demonstrated by analysis of mice deficient in various components of this pathway, e.g. Stat1 is required for protection of mice from microbial and viral pathogens (Durbin et al. 1996; Meraz et al. 1996). However, the downstream events required for protection against specific viruses and other pathogens is still not

Table 14.10 *Effect of interferons on viral propagation and in patients*

Virus family	Inhibited by interferons	Major viruses studied with interferon	References
Picornaviridae	Yes	Rhinovirus, cardiovirus (encephalomyocarditis virus)	Scott et al. (1982); Hayden and Gwaltney (1983); Phillpotts et al. (1983, 1984); Hayden et al. (1986); Higgins et al. (1986); Sperber et al. (1993b); Soh et al. (1994c); Yasuda et al. (2000)
Caliciviridae	Yes	Feline calicivirus (FCV)	Fulton and Burge (1985); Mochizuki et al. (1994)
Astroviridae	Not tested		Not tested
Togaviridae	Yes	Sindbis, Semliki forest virus	Imanishi et al. (1981); Weigent et al. (1981); Lloyd et al. (1983); Yasuda et al. (2000)
Flaviviridae	Yes	Hepatitis C virus, Dengue, West Nile, yellow fever	Vithanomsat et al. (1984); Yamamoto et al. (1992); Iino et al. (1994); Trepo et al. (1994); Weiland (1994); Haria and Benfield (1995); Roffi et al. (1995); Romeo et al. (1995); Saracco and Rizzetto (1995); Zein and Rakela (1995); Jonas (1996); Alberti et al. (1997); Cooksley et al. (1997); Woo and Burnakis (1997); Hanley and Haydon (1998); Barnes et al. (1999); Shiffman (1999); Markland et al. (2000); Pianko and McHutchison (2000); Yasuda et al. (2000); Diamond and Harris (2001); Hu et al. (2001); Lyra and Di Bisceglie (2001); Sagmeister et al. (2001); Wilkinson (2001); Anderson and Rahal (2002); Katze et al. (2002); Hino et al. (2002)
Coronaviridae	Yes	Infectious bronchitis virus (IBV; poultry), mouse hepatitis virus	Aurisicchio et al. (2000); Pei et al. (2001)
Arteriviridae	Yes	Porcine reproductive and respiratory syndrome virus (PRRSV)	Albina et al. (1998); Buddaert et al. (1998)
Rhabdoviridae	Yes	Vesicular stomatitis virus	Familletti et al. (1981b); Imanishi et al. (1981); Langford et al. (1981); S. Rubinstein et al. (1981); Arnheiter and Haller (1983); Soh et al. (1994c); Yasuda et al. (2000)
Filoviridae	Yes	Marburg, Ebola	Jahrling et al. (1999); Bray (2001); Kolokol'tsov et al. (2001)
Paramyxoviridae	Yes	Respiratory syncytial virus (human, bovine), Newcastle disease virus	Imanishi et al. (1981); Strube et al. (1985); Marcus and Sekellick (2001)
Orthomyxoviridae	Yes	Influenza viruses	Machida et al. (1980); Imanishi et al. (1981); Sedmak and Grossberg (1981); Isomura et al. (1982); Arnheiter and Haller (1983); Saito et al. (1983); Hayden et al. (1984); Phillpotts et al. (1984); Ransohoff et al. (1985); Sasaki et al. (1985); Strube et al. (1985); Sun et al. (1986); Arnheiter and Haller (1988)
Bunyavididae	Yes	Bunyamwera bunyavirus	Weber and Elliott (2002); Weber et al. (2002)
Arenaviridae	Yes	Lymphocytic choriomeningitis	Andrei and De Clercq (1993); Djavani et al. (2001)
Bornaviridae	Yes	Borna disease virus	von Rheinbaben et al. (1985); Hallensleben and Staeheli (1999); Staeheli et al. (2001)
Reoviridae	Yes	Reovirus, rotavirus	Petersen et al. (1997); Marcus and Sekellick (2001)
Retroviridae	Yes	Human immunodeficiency virus, feline immunodeficiency virus, many others	Sen et al. (1984); Wells et al. (1991); Sperber et al. (1992, 1993a)
Papovaviridae	Yes	SV-40, polyoma virus, papillomavirinae	Gotlieb-Stematsky et al. (1966); Oxman et al. (1967); Mallucci and Taylor-Papadimitriou (1973); Birg and Meyer (1975); Yakobson et al. (1977); Tevethia et al. (1979); Haglund et al. (1981); Brennan and Stark (1983); Lundquist et al. (1984); Strander (1986); Lambropoulos and Koliais (1989); Einhorn et al. (1991); Browder et al. (1992); Melkova and Esteban (1994); Rockley and Tyring (1995); Deunas et al. (1997); Aaltonen et al. (2002)

(*Continued over*)

Table 14.10 *Effect of interferons on viral propagation and in patients (Continued)*

Virus family	Inhibited by interferons	Major viruses studied with interferon	References
Adenoviridae	Yes	Adenovirus	Pusztai and Szabo (1978); Langford et al. (1983); Mistchenko et al. (1987)
Parvoviridae	Yes	Canine parvovirus	Minagawa et al. (1999)
Herpesviridae	Yes	Herpes simplex, Epstein–Barr virus, cytomegalovirus	Falcoff et al. (1968); Langford et al. (1983); Andersson et al. (1985); Batcheler et al. (1986); Domke-Opitz et al. 1986; Babiuk et al. (1987); Fish et al. (1986); Scheck et al. (1986); Leventon-Kriss et al. (1987); Glezerman et al. (1988); Ophir et al. (1995); Ryman et al. 2000; Yasuda et al. (2000); Carr and Noisakran (2002); Cull et al. 2002; Katze et al. (2002)
Poxviridae	Yes	Vaccinia, mouse pox	Rosel and Jungwirth (1983); Rodriguez et al. (1991); Karupiah et al. (1993); Melkova and Esteban (1994); Baron et al. (2002); Katze et al. (2002)
Hepadnaviridae	Yes	Hepatitis B virus	Haria and Benfield (1995); Woo and Burnakis (1997); Grob (1998); Mazzella et al. (1999); Alberti et al. (2002); Perrillo (2002)

defined, and the mechanisms differ from virus to virus. Furthermore, it is becoming increasingly clear that other pathways independent of the Jak–Stat pathway can initiate signal transduction by the type I interferons, e.g. cells from mice lacking Stat1 can still respond to type I interferons: IFN-α and IFN-β can modulate proliferative responses in phagocytes from Stat1-deficient mice (Gil et al. 2001). Understanding of these events is further complicated by the multiplicity of the type I interferons (see Table 14.6) that exhibit different activities (see Tables 14.3-14.5), although they interact with the same receptor. This is an area that needs to be explored in great detail to understand this family of proteins and their mechanisms of action.

The side effects of most biotherapeutics are significant and limit the dose of most cytokines. Interferon is not an exception, with side effects that often require reducing dosage or ceasing treatment (Nathan et al. 2002; Raanani and Ben Bassat 2002). So far the mechanisms by which interferons produce side effects have not been determined. It would be a major advance to have interferon molecules with little or no toxicity.

Patients treated with protein molecules often develop serum antibodies. If the antibodies neutralize the activity of the proteins, they can cause a relapse. This has been shown in many diseases treated with interferons (Nolte et al. 1994; Antonelli et al. 1997; Dianzani and Pestka 1997; Viscomi et al. 1999).

In carrying out clinical trials with interferons, it is useful to follow the activity in patients and in culture by biological assays. A number of these have been developed (Meager 2002), but no single assay or set of assays currently provides a standard assessment of activity in patients. Many molecules have been reported to stimulate production of interferons and other cytokines. One of these, imiquimod, has been approved as a topical agent for the treatment of external and anal genital warts (Dockrell and Kinghorn 2001).

As noted above, interferon is already used extensively for a wide range of diseases. Nevertheless, because the type I interferons have broad activities, it is likely that they will be used to a greater extent in the future, e.g. these interferons activate cytotoxicity of many cells of the immune system such as NK cells, T cells, macrophages, and dendritic cells (Herberman et al. 1981, 1982a, 1982b; Ortaldo et al. 1982, 1983a, 1983b; Li et al. 1990). Interferon has enormous anti-angiogenic activity, perhaps, the highest activity of any known biotherapeutic (White et al. 1989; Appelbaum 1990; White 1990; Kaban et al. 1999; Ozawa et al. 2001). Furthermore, interferons enhance the expression of tumor-associated antigens on the cell surface of cells enormously in culture and in patients (Greiner et al. 1984, 1985, 1987, 1992; Ozzello et al. 1995). This increase in the surface expression of the tumor-associated antigens often turns the heterogeneous population of tumor cells with low levels of the antigens and few cells carrying these surface antigens into a population of cells that are all expressing these surface tumor antigens. The cells are, therefore, recognized more efficiently by the immune system and by cytotoxic cells activated to destroy cells expressing these antigens. Together with the direct antiproliferative activity of interferons on the tumor cells, all these actions make interferon a most promising agent to treat cancers in general. The challenge is to be able to use this enormous potential of the interferons without the debilitating side effects. Appropriate technology to localize the interferons in tumors could overcome the problem of systemic side effects. Overall, it is highly likely that interferon will play a major role in the next generation of novel antitumor and antiviral therapies.

ACKNOWLEDGMENTS

For the work done in my laboratory discussed in this chapter, I thank my many colleagues who have carried out the studies cited. I thank Ellen Feibel for her diligent assistance in the preparation of this manuscript. This author's work was supported in part by US Public Health Services Grants RO1-CA46465 from the National Cancer Institute and RO1 AI36450 and RO1 AI43369 from the National Institute of Allergy and Infectious Diseases.

REFERENCES

Aaltonen, L.M., Rihkanen, H. and Vaheri, A. 2002. Human papillomavirus in larynx. *Laryngoscope*, **112**, 700–7.

Abramovich, C., Chebath, J. and Revel, M. 1994a. The human interferon alpha-receptor protein confers differential responses to human interferon-beta versus interferon-alpha subtypes in mouse and hamster cell transfectants. *Cytokine*, **6**, 414–24.

Abramovich, C., Shulman, L.M., et al. 1994b. Differential tyrosine phosphorylation of the IFNAR chain of the type I interferon receptor and of an associated surface protein in response to IFN-alpha and IFN-beta. *EMBO J*, **13**, 5871–7.

Adolf, G.R., Maurer-Fogy, I., et al. 1990. Purification and characterization of natural human interferon omega 1. Two alternative cleavage sites for the signal peptidase. *J Biol Chem*, **265**, 9290–5.

Adolf, G.R., Kalsner, I., et al. 1991. Natural human interferon-alpha 2 is *O*-glycosylated. *Biochem J*, **276**, Pt 2, 511–18.

Aguet, M. 1980. High-affinity binding of ^{125}I-labeled mouse interferon to a specific cell surface receptor. *Nature*, **284**, 768–70.

Aguet, M., Dembic, Z. and Merlin, G. 1988. Molecular cloning and expression of the human interferon-gamma receptor. *Cell*, **55**, 273–80.

Alberti, A., Chemello, L., et al. 1997. Therapy of hepatitis C: re-treatment with alpha interferon. *Hepatology*, **26**, 3 suppl 1, 137A–42S.

Alberti, A., Brunetto, M.R., et al. 2002. Recent progress and new trends in the treatment of hepatitis B. *J Med Virol*, **67**, 458–62.

Albina, E., Carrat, C. and Charley, B. 1998. Interferon-alpha response to swine arterivirus (PoAV), the porcine reproductive and respiratory syndrome virus. *J Interferon Cytokine Res*, **18**, 485–90.

Alexenko, A.P., Li, J., et al. 1995. Interaction of bovine interferon-τ with the type I interferon receptor on Daudi cells. *J Interferon Cytokine Res*, **15**, suppl 1, S97.

Allen, G. and Fantes, K.H. 1980. A family of structural genes for human lymphoblastoid (leukocyte-type) interferon. *Nature*, **287**, 408–11.

Anderson, J.F. and Rahal, J.J. 2002. Efficacy of interferon alpha-2b and ribavirin against West Nile virus in vitro. *Emerg Infect Dis*, **8**, 107–8.

Andersson, J.P., Andersson, U.G., et al. 1985. Effects of pure interferons on Epstein–Barr virus infection in vitro. *J Virol*, **54**, 615–18.

Andrei, G. and De Clercq, E. 1993. Molecular approaches for the treatment of hemorrhagic fever virus infections. *Antiviral Res*, **22**, 45–75.

Antonelli, G., Simeoni, E., et al. 1997. Interferon antibodies in patients with infectious diseases. Anti-interferon antibodies. *Biotherapy*, **10**, 7–14.

Appelbaum, F.R. 1990. Introduction and overview of interferon alfa in myeloproliferative and hemangiomatous diseases. *Semin Hematol*, **27**, 3 suppl 4, 1–5.

Arens, M. 2001. Clinically relevant sequence-based genotyping of HBV, HCV, CMV and HIV. *J Clin Virol*, **22**, 11–29.

Arnheiter, H. and Haller, O. 1983. Mx gene control of interferon action: different kinetics of the antiviral state against influenza virus and vesicular stomatitis virus. *J Virol*, **47**, 626–30.

Arnheiter, H. and Haller, O. 1988. Antiviral state against influenza virus neutralized by microinjection of antibodies to interferon-induced Mx proteins. *EMBO J*, **7**, 1315–20.

Aurisicchio, L., Delmastro, P., et al. 2000. Liver-specific alpha 2 interferon gene expression results in protection from induced hepatitis. *J Virol*, **74**, 4816–23.

Babiuk, L.A., Lawman, M.J. and Gifford, G.A. 1987. Use of recombinant bovine alpha 1 interferon in reducing respiratory disease induced by bovine herpesvirus type 1. *Antimicrob Agents Chemother*, **31**, 752–7.

Bach, E.A., Tanner, J.W., et al. 1996. Ligand-induced assembly and activation of the gamma interferon receptor in intact cells. *Mol Cell Biol*, **16**, 3214–21.

Barbieri, G., Velazquez, L., et al. 1994. Activation of the protein kinase Tyk2 by Interferon α/β. *Eur J Biochem*, **223**, 427–35.

Barnes, E., Webster, G., et al. 1999. Long-term efficacy of treatment of chronic hepatitis C with alpha interferon or alpha interferon and ribavirin. *J Hepatol*, **31**, suppl 1, 244–9.

Baron, S., Salazar, A., et al. 2002. Smallpox: prevention by IFN and an IFN inducer. *J Interferon Res*, **22**, S86.

Batcheler, L.M., Bonham, D.G., et al. 1986. Topical interferon cream for the treatment of herpes genitalis: a double-blind controlled trial. *Aust NZ J Obstet Gynaecol*, **26**, 239–41.

Bazan, J.F. 1990a. Shared architecture of hormone-binding domains in type I and II interferon receptors. *Cell*, **61**, 753–4.

Bazan, J.F. 1990b. Structural design and molecular evolution of a cytokine receptor superfamily. *Proc Natl Acad Sci USA*, **87**, 6934–8.

Benoit, P., Maguire, D., et al. 1993. A monoclonal antibody to recombinant human IFN-α receptor inhibits biologic activity of several species of human IFN-α,IFN-β and IFN-o: detection of heterogeneity of the cellular type I IFN receptor. *J Immunol*, **150**, 707–16.

Berg, K. 1982. Purification and characterization of murine and human interferons. A review of the literature of the 1970s. *Acta Pathol Microbiol Immunol Scand Suppl*, **279**, 1–136.

Berg, K. and Heron, I. 1981. Antibody affinity chromatography of human leukocyte interferon. *Methods Enzymol*, **78**, Pt A, 487–99.

Berthold, W., Tan, C. and Tan, Y.H. 1978. Purification and in vitro labeling of interferon from a human fibroblastoid cell line. *J Biol Chem*, **253**, 5206–12.

Birg, F. and Meyer, G. 1975. Effect of interferon on induction of S antigen by polyoma virus in BHK 21 cells. *J Gen Virol*, **26**, 201–4.

Bohlen, P., Stein, S., et al. 1975. Automatic monitoring of primary amines in preparative column effluents with fluorescamine. *Anal Biochem*, **67**, 438–45.

Borden, E.C., Lindner, D., et al. 2000. Second-generation interferons for cancer: clinical targets. *Semin Cancer Biol*, **10**, 125–44.

Bose, S. and Hickman, J. 1977. Role of the carbohydrate moiety in determining the survival of interferon in the circulation. *J Biol Chem*, **252**, 8336–7.

Bose, S., Gurari-Rotman, D., et al. 1976. Apparent dispensability of the carbohydrate moiety of human interferon for antiviral activity. *J Biol Chem*, **251**, 1659–62.

Branca, A.A. and Baglioni, C. 1981. Evidence that Type I and II interferons have different receptors. *Nature*, **294**, 768–70.

Brassard, D.L., Grace, M.J. and Bordens, R.W. 2002. Interferon-alpha as an immunotherapeutic protein. *J Leukoc Biol*, **71**, 565–81.

Bray, M. 2001. The role of the type I interferon response in the resistance of mice to filovirus infection. *J Gen Virol*, **82**, Pt 6, 1365–73.

Brennan, M.B. and Stark, G.R. 1983. Interferon pretreatment inhibits simian virus 40 infections by blocking the onset of early transcription. *Cell*, **33**, 811–16.

Bridgen, P.J., Anfinsen, C.B., et al. 1977. Human lymphoblastoid interferon. Large scale production and partial purification. *J Biol Chem*, **252**, 6585–7.

Browder, J.F., Araujo, O.E., et al. 1992. The interferons and their use in condyloma acuminata. *Ann Pharmacother*, **26**, 42–5.

Buddaert, W., Van Reeth, K. and Pensaert, M. 1998. In vivo and in vitro interferon (IFN) studies with the porcine reproductive and respiratory syndrome virus (PRRSV). *Adv Exp Med Biol*, **440**, 461–7.

Burke, G., Carle, G.F. and Olson, M.V. 1987. Cloning of large segments of DNA into yeast by means of artificial chromosome vectors. *Science*, **236**, 806–12.

Cabrer, B., Taira, H., et al. 1979. Structural characteristics of interferons from mouse Ehrlich ascites tumor cells. *J Biol Chem*, **254**, 3681–4.

Calabresi, P.A. 2002. Considerations in the treatment of relapsing–remitting multiple sclerosis. *Neurology*, **58**, 8 suppl 4, S10–22.

Canaani, D. and Berg, P. 1982. Regulated expression of human interferon beta 1 gene after transduction into cultured mouse and rabbit cells. *Proc Natl Acad Sci USA*, **79**, 5166–70.

Cantell, K. and Tovell, D.R. 1971. Substitution of milk for serum in the production of human leukocyte interferon. *Appl Microbiol*, **22**, 625–8.

Carr, D.J. and Noisakran, S. 2002. The antiviral efficacy of the murine alpha-1 interferon transgene against ocular herpes simplex virus type 1 requires the presence of CD4(+), alpha/beta T-cell receptor-positive T lymphocytes with the capacity to produce gamma interferon. *J Virol*, **76**, 9398–406.

Cavalieri, R.L. and Pestka, S. 1977. Synthesis of interferon in heterologous cells, cell-free extracts, and *Xenopus laevis* oocytes. *Tex Rep Biol Med*, **35**, 117–25.

Cavalieri, R.L., Havell, E.A., et al. 1977a. Induction and decay of human fibroblast interferon mRNA. *Proc Natl Acad Sci USA*, **74**, 4415–19.

Cavalieri, R.L., Havell, E.A., et al. 1977b. Synthesis of human interferon by *Xenopus laevis* oocytes: two structural genes for interferons in human cells. *Proc Natl Acad Sci USA*, **74**, 3287–91.

Chang, S., Noel, R. and Regnier, F.E. 1976. High speed ion exchange chromatography of proteins. *Anal Chem*, **48**, 1839–45.

Chen, J.K., Jankowski, W.J., et al. 1976. Nature of the molecular heterogeneity of human leukocyte interferon. *J Virol*, **19**, 425–34.

Chumakov, I., Rigault, P., et al. 1992a. Continuum of overlapping clones spanning the entire human chromosome 21q. *Nature*, **359**, 380–36.

Chumakov, I.M., Le Gall, I., et al. 1992b. Isolation of chromosome 21-specific yeast artificial chromosome from a total human genome library. *Nat Genet*, **1**, 222–5.

Cleary, C.M., Donnelly, R.J. and Pestka, S. 1992. Cloning of an alternatively spliced form of the human interferon alpha receptor. *J Interferon Res*, **12**, S220, (abstract).

Cleary, C.M., Donnelly, R.J., et al. 1994. Knockout and reconstitution of a functional human type I interferon receptor complex. *J Biol Chem*, **269**, 18747–9.

Cofano, F., Moore, S.K., et al. 1990. Affinity purification, peptide analysis and cDNA sequence of the mouse interferon-gamma receptor. *J Biol Chem*, **265**, 4064–71.

Colamonici, O.R. and Domanski, P. 1993. Identification of a novel subunit of the type I interferon receptor localized to human chromosome 21. *J Biol Chem*, **268**, 10895–9.

Colamonici, O.R. and Pfeffer, L.M. 1991. Structure of the human interferon alpha receptor. *Pharmacol Ther*, **52**, 227–33.

Colamonici, O.R., D'Alessandro, F., et al. 1990. Characterization of three monoclonal antibodies that recognize the interferon alpha 2 receptor. *Proc Natl Acad Sci USA*, **87**, 7230–4.

Colamonici, O.R., Pfeffer, L.M., et al. 1992. Multichain structure of the IFN-alpha receptor on hematopoietic cells. *J Immunol*, **148**, 2126–32.

Colamonici, O.R., Porterfield, B., et al. 1994a. Complementation of the interferon alpha response in resistant cells by expression of the cloned subunit of the interferon alpha receptor. A central role of this subunit in interferon alpha signaling. *J Biol Chem*, **269**, 9598–602.

Colamonici, O.R., Uyttendaele, H., et al. 1994b. p135tyk2, an interferon-alpha-activated tyrosine kinase, is physically associated with an interferon-alpha receptor. *J Biol Chem*, **269**, 3518–22.

Collum, R.G., Brutsaert, S., et al. 2000. A Stat3-interacting protein (StIP1) regulates cytokine signal transduction. *Proc Natl Acad Sci USA*, **97**, 10120–5.

Constantinescu, S.N., Croze, E., et al. 1994. Role of interferon alpha/beta receptor chain 1 in the structure and transmembrane signaling of the interferon alpha/beta receptor complex. *Proc Natl Acad Sci USA*, **91**, 9602–6.

Cook, J.R., Jung, V., et al. 1992. Structural analysis of the human interferon gamma receptor: a small segment of the intracellular domain is specifically required for class I major histocompatibility complex antigen induction and antiviral activity. *Proc Natl Acad Sci USA*, **89**, 11317–21.

Cook, J.R., Emanuel, S.L. and Pestka, S. 1993. Yeast artificial chromosome fragmentation vectors that utilize URA3+ selection. *Gene Analysis: Tech Appl*, **10**, 109–12.

Cook, J.R., Emanuel, S.L., et al. 1994. Sublocalization of the human interferon-gamma receptor accessory factor gene and characterization of accessory factor activity by yeast artificial chromosomal fragmentation. *J Biol Chem*, **269**, 7013–18.

Cook, J.R., Cleary, C.M., et al. 1996. Differential responsiveness of a splice variant of the human type I interferon receptor to interferons. *J Biol Chem*, **271**, 13448–53.

Cooksley, W.G., Dudley, F.J. and Watson, K. 1997. Treatment of cirrhotic hepatitis C virus patients with daily doses of interferon-alpha 2a. *J Viral Hepat*, **4**, suppl 2, 75–8.

Cooper, M.R. 1991. A review of the clinical studies of alpha-interferon in the management of multiple myeloma. *Semin Oncol*, **18**, 5 suppl 7, 18–29.

Cull, V.S., Bartlett, E.J. and James, C.M. 2002. Type I interferon gene therapy protects against cytomegalovirus-induced myocarditis. *Immunology*, **106**, 428–37.

Dalod, M., Salazar-Mather, T.P., et al. 2002. Interferon alpha/beta and interleukin 12 responses to viral infections: pathways regulating dendritic cell cytokine expression in vivo. *J Exp Med*, **195**, 517–28.

Darnell, J.E. Jr, Kerr, I.M. and Stark, G.R. 1994. Jak-STAT pathways and transcriptional activation in response to IFNs and other extracellular signaling proteins. *Science*, **264**, 1415–21.

Davies, E.G., Isaacs, D. and Levinsky, R.J. 1982. Defective immune interferon production and natural killer activity associated with poor neutrophil mobility and delayed umbilical cord separation. *Clin Exp Immunol*, **50**, 454–60.

Davis, G.L. 1994. Interferon treatment of chronic hepatitis C. *Am J Med*, **96**, 1A, 41S–6S.

de Vos, A.M., Ultsch, M. and Kossiakoff, A.A. 1992. Human growth hormone and extracellular domain of its receptor: crystal structure of the complex. *Science*, **255**, 306–12.

Derynck, R., Content, J., et al. 1980. Isolation and structure of a human fibroblast interferon gene. *Nature*, **285**, 542–7.

Deunas, L., Alcantud, V., et al. 1997. Use of interferon-alpha in laryngeal papillomatosis: eight years of the Cuban national programme. *J Laryngol Otol*, **111**, 134–40.

Diamond, M.S. and Harris, E. 2001. Interferon inhibits dengue virus infection by preventing translation of viral RNA through a PKR-independent mechanism. *Virology*, **289**, 297–311.

Dianzani, F. 1975. Viral interference and interferon. *Ric Clin Lab*, **5**, 196–213.

Dianzani, F. and Pestka, S. 1997. A review of interferon immunogenicity. *J Interferon Cytokine Res*, **17**, suppl 1, S1– S3.

Diaz, M.O., Pomykala, H.M., et al. 1994. Structure of the human type-I interferon gene cluster determined from a YAC clone contig. *Genomics*, **22**, 540–52.

Djavani, M., Rodas, J., et al. 2001. Role of the promyelocytic leukemia protein PML in the interferon sensitivity of lymphocytic choriomeningitis virus. *J Virol*, **75**, 6204–8.

Dockrell, D.H. and Kinghorn, G.R. 2001. Imiquimod and resiquimod as novel immunomodulators. *J Antimicrob Chemother*, **48**, 751–5.

Domanski, P. and Colamonici, O.R. 1996. The type-I interferon receptor. The long and short of it. *Cytokine Growth Factor Rev*, **7**, 143–51.

Domanski, P., Witte, M., et al. 1995. Cloning and expression of a long form of the β subunit of the interferon α receptor that is required for signaling. *J Biol Chem*, **270**, 21606–11.

Domke-Opitz, I., Straub, P. and Kirchner, H. 1986. Effect of interferon on replication of herpes simplex virus types 1 and 2 in human macrophages. *J Virol*, **60**, 37–42.

Durbin, J.E., Hackenmiller, R., et al. 1996. Targeted disruption of the mouse Stat1 gene results in compromised innate immunity to viral disease. *Cell*, **84**, 443–50.

Durbin, J.E., Fernandez-Sesma, A., et al. 2000. Type I IFN modulates innate and specific antiviral immunity. *J Immunol*, **164**, 4220–8.

Dutcher, J., Atkins, M.B., et al. 2001. Kidney cancer: the Cytokine Working Group experience (1986–2001): part II. Management of IL-2 toxicity and studies with other cytokines. *Med Oncol*, **18**, 209–19.

Einhorn, N., Ling, P., et al. 1991. Treatment of advanced condylomata acuminata with semi-purified and purified human leukocyte interferon. *Acta Oncol*, **30**, 343–5.

Einhorn, S. and Strander, H. 1993. Interferon treatment of human malignancies – a short review. *Med Oncol Tumor Pharmacother*, **10**, 1-2, 25–9.

Eliason, J.F. 2001. Pegylated cytokines: potential application in immunotherapy of cancer. *BioDrugs*, **15**, 705–11.

Emanuel, S.L., Cook, J.R., et al. 1995. New vectors for manipulation and selection of functional yeast artificial chromosomes (YACs) containing human DNA inserts. *Gene*, **155**, 167–74.

Enomoto, N. and Sato, C. 1995a. Clinical relevance of hepatitis C virus quasispecies. *J Viral Hepat*, **2**, 267–72.

Enomoto, N. and Sato, C. 1995b. Hepatitis C virus quasispecies populations during chronic hepatitis C infection. *Trends Microbiol*, **3**, 445–7.

Enomoto, N., Sakuma, I., et al. 1995. Comparison of full-length sequences of interferon-sensitive and resistant hepatitis C virus 1b. Sensitivity to interferon is conferred by amino acid substitutions in the NS5A region. *J Clin Invest*, **96**, 224–30.

Enomoto, N., Sakuma, I., et al. 1996. Mutations in the nonstructural protein 5A gene and response to interferon in patients with chronic hepatitis C virus 1b infection. *N Engl J Med*, **334**, 77–81.

Epstein, C.J., McManus, N.H. and Epstein, L.B. 1982. Direct evidence that the gene product of the human chromosome 21 locus, IFRC, is the interferon-α receptor. *Biochim Biophys Res Commun*, **107**, 1060–6.

Evinger, M. and Pestka, S. 1981. Assay of growth inhibition in lymphoblastoid cell cultures. *Methods Enzymol*, **79**, 362–8.

Evinger, M., Rubinstein, M. and Pestka, S. 1980a. Growth-inhibitory and antiviral activity of purified leukocyte interferon. *Ann NY Acad Sci*, **350**, 399–404.

Evinger, M., Rubinstein, M. and Pestka, S. 1980b. *Interferon: properties and clinical uses*. Dallas, TX: Leland Fikes Foundation Press.

Evinger, M., Rubinstein, M. and Pestka, S. 1981. Antiproliferative and antiviral activities of human leukocyte interferons. *Arch Biochem Biophys*, **210**, 319–29.

Faderl, S., Kantarjian, H.M., et al. 2000. New treatment approaches for chronic myelogenous leukemia. *Semin Oncol*, **27**, 578–86.

Falcoff, R., Falcoff, E., et al. 1968. [Biologic activity of human interferon on the simian species in vitro and in vivo]. *C R Acad Sci Hebd Seances Acad Sci D*, **266**, 297–300.

Familletti, P.C. and Pestka, S. 1981. Cell cultures producing human interferon. *Antimicrob Agents Chemother*, **20**, 1–4.

Familletti, P.C., McCandliss, R. and Pestka, S. 1981a. Production of high levels of human leukocyte interferon from a continuous human myeloblast cell culture. *Antimicrob Agents Chemother*, **20**, 5–9.

Familletti, P.C., Rubinstein, S. and Pestka, S. 1981b. A convenient and rapid cytopathic effect inhibition assay for interferon. *Methods Enzymol*, **78**, 387–94.

Farrar, M.A., Fernandez-Luna, J. and Schreiber, R.D. 1991. Identification of two regions within the cytoplasmic domain of the human interferon-gamma receptor required for function. *J Biol Chem*, **266**, 19626–35.

Farrar, M.A., Campbell, J.D. and Schreiber, R.D. 1992. Identification of a functionally important sequence in the C terminus of the interferon-gamma receptor. *Proc Natl Acad Sci USA*, **89**, 11706–10.

Findlay, G.M. and MacCallum, F.O. 1937. An interference phenomenon in relation to yellow fever and other viruses. *J Pathol Bacteriol*, **44**, 405–24.

Fish, E.N., Banerjee, K., et al. 1986. Antiherpetic effects of a human alpha interferon analog, IFN-alpha Con1, in hamsters. *Antimicrob Agents Chemother*, **30**, 52–6.

Flores, I., Mariano, T.M. and Pestka, S. 1991. Human interferon omega binds to the interferon-α/β receptor. *J Biol Chem*, **266**, 19875–7.

Friesen, H.J., Stein, S., et al. 1981. Purification and molecular characterization of human fibroblast interferon. *Arch Biochem Biophys*, **206**, 432–50.

Fu, X.-Y. 1995. A direct signalling pathway through tyrosine kinases activation of sh2 domain-containing transcriptional factors. *J Leukocyte Biol*, **57**, 529–35.

Fu, X.-Y., Kessler, D.S., et al. 1990. ISGF3, the transcriptional activator induced by interferon-α, consists of multiple interacting polypeptide chains. *Proc Natl Acad Sci USA*, **87**, 8555–9.

Fu, X.Y., Schindler, C., et al. 1992. The proteins of ISGF-3, the interferon α-induced transcriptional activator, define a gene family involved in signal transduction. *Proc Natl Acad Sci USA*, **89**, 7840–3.

Fulton, R.W. and Burge, L.J. 1985. Susceptibility of feline herpesvirus 1 and a feline calicivirus to feline interferon and recombinant human leukocyte interferons. *Antimicrob Agents Chemother*, **28**, 698–9.

Gale, M.J. Jr, Korth, M.J., et al. 1997. Evidence that hepatitis C virus resistance to interferon is mediated through repression of the PKR protein kinase by the nonstructural 5A protein. *Virology*, **230**, 217–27.

Gangemi, J.D., Lazdins, J., et al. 1989. Antiviral activity of a novel recombinant human interferon-alpha B/D hybrid. *J Interferon Res*, **9**, 227–37.

Gibbs, V.C., Williams, S.R., et al. 1991. The extracellular domain of the human interferon gamma receptor interacts with a species-specific signal transducer. *Mol Cell Biol*, **11**, 5860–6.

Gibbs, V.C., Takahashi, M., et al. 1996. A negative regulatory region in the intracellular domain of the human interferon-alpha receptor. *J Biol Chem*, **271**, 28710–16.

Gil, M.P., Bohn, E., et al. 2001. Biologic consequences of Stat1-independent IFN signaling. *Proc Natl Acad Sci USA*, **98**, 6680–5.

Glezerman, M., Lunenfeld, E., et al. 1988. Placebo-controlled trial of topical interferon in labial and genital herpes. *Lancet*, **i**, 150–2.

Goeddel, D.V. and Pestka, S. 1982. Polypeptides, process for their microbial production, intermediates therefore and compositions containing them (patent).

Goeddel, D.V. and Pestka, S. 1989. Microbial production of mature human leukocyte interferon K and L. US Patent 4,801,685 (patent).

Goeddel, D.V., Shepard, H.M., et al. 1980a. Synthesis of human fibroblast interferon by *E. coli*. *Nucleic Acids Res*, **8**, 4057–4.

Goeddel, D.V., Yelverton, E., et al. 1980b. Human leukocyte interferon produced by *E. coli* is biologically active. *Nature*, **287**, 411–16.

Goodin, D.S. 2001. Interferon-beta therapy in multiple sclerosis: evidence for a clinically relevant dose response. *Drugs*, **61**, 1693–703.

Gotlieb-Stematsky, T., Rotem, Z. and Karby, S. 1966. Production and susceptibility to interferon of polyoma virus variants of high and low oncogenic properties. *J Natl Cancer Inst*, **37**, 99–103.

Gray, P.W., Leong, S., et al. 1989. Cloning and expression of the cDNA for the murine interferon gamma receptor. *Proc Natl Acad Sci USA*, **86**, 8497–501.

Gray, R.J., Pockaj, B.A. and Kirkwood, J.M. 2002. An update on adjuvant interferon for melanoma. *Cancer Control*, **9**, 16–21.

Greenlund, A.C., Farrar, M.A., et al. 1994. Ligand-induced IFN gamma receptor tyrosine phosphorylation couples the receptor to its signal transduction system (p91). *EMBO J*, **13**, 1591–600.

Greiner, J.W., Hand, P.H., et al. 1984. Enhanced expression of surface tumor-associated antigens on human breast and colon tumor cells after recombinant human leukocyte α-interferon treatment. *Cancer Res*, **44**, 3208–14.

Greiner, J.W., Schlom, J., et al. 1985. Modulation of tumor associated antigen expression and shedding by recombinant human leukocyte and fibroblast interferons. *Pharmacol Ther*, **31**, 209–36.

Greiner, J.W., Guadagni, F., et al. 1987. Recombinant interferon enhances monoclonal antibody-targeting of carcinoma lesions in vivo. *Science*, **235**, 895–8.

Greiner, J.W., Guadagni, F., et al. 1992. Intraperitoneal administration of interferon-gamma to carcinoma patients enhances expression of tumor-associated glycoprotein-72 and carcinoembryonic antigen on malignant ascites cells. *J Clin Oncol*, **10**, 735–46.

Grob, P.J. 1998. Hepatitis B: virus, pathogenesis and treatment. *Vaccine*, **16**, suppl, S11–16.

Grob, P.M. and Chadha, K.C. 1979. Separation of human leukocyte interferon components by concanavalin A-agarose affinity chromatography and their characterization. *Biochemistry*, **18**, 5782–6.

Hadhazy, C.Y., Gergely, L., et al. 1967. Comparative study on the interferon production by the leukocytes of healthy and leukaemic subjects. *Acta Microbiol Acad Sci Hung*, **14**, 391–7.

Haglund, S., Lundquist, P.G., et al. 1981. Interferon therapy in juvenile laryngeal papillomatosis. *Arch Otolaryngol*, **107**, 327–32.

Hallensleben, W. and Staeheli, P. 1999. Inhibition of Borna disease virus multiplication by interferon: cell line differences in susceptibility. *Arch Virol*, **144**, 1209–16.

Hanley, J.P. and Haydon, G.H. 1998. The biology of interferon-alpha and the clinical significance of anti-interferon antibodies. *Leuk Lymphoma*, **29**, 3-4, 257–68.

Hannigan, G.E., Lau, A.S. and Williams, B.R. 1986. Differential human interferon alpha receptor expression on proliferating and non-proliferating cells. *Eur J Biochem*, **157**, 187–93.

Haria, M. and Benfield, P. 1995. Interferon-alpha-2a. A review of its pharmacological properties and therapeutic use in the management of viral hepatitis. *Drugs*, **50**, 873–96.

Havell, E.A. and Vilcek, J. 1972. Production of high-titered interferon in cultures of human diploid cells. *Antimicrob Agents Chemother*, **2**, 476–84.

Hayden, F.G. and Gwaltney, J.M.J. Jr 1983. Intranasal interferon alpha 2 for prevention of rhinovirus infection and illness. *J Infect Dis*, **148**, 543–50.

Hayden, F.G., Schlepushkin, A.N. and Pushkarskaya, N.L. 1984. Combined interferon-alpha 2, rimantadine hydrochloride, and ribavirin inhibition of influenza virus replication in vitro. *Antimicrob Agents Chemother*, **25**, 53–7.

Hayden, F.G., Albrecht, J.K., et al. 1986. Prevention of natural colds by contact prophylaxis with intranasal alpha 2-interferon. *N Engl J Med*, **314**, 71–5.

Heim, M.H., Kerr, I.M., et al. 1995. Contribution of STAT SH2 groups to specific interferon signaling by the Jak-STAT pathway. *Science*, **267**, 1347–9.

Hemmi, S., Peghini, P., et al. 1989. Cloning of murine interferon gamma receptor cDNAs expression in human cells mediates high-affinity binding but is not sufficient to confer sensitivity to murine interferon gamma. *Proc Natl Acad Sci USA*, **86**, 9901–5.

Hemmi, S., Merlin, G. and Aguet, M. 1992. Functional characterization of a hybrid human-mouse interferon-gamma receptor: evidence for species-specific interaction of the extracellular receptor domain with a putative signal transducer. *Proc Natl Acad Sci USA*, **89**, 2737–41.

Hemmi, S., Bohni, R. and Aguet, M. 1994a. Functional characterization of the cytoplasmic domain of the IFN-γ receptor β chain. *J Interferon Res*, **14**, S94.

Hemmi, S., Bohni, R., et al. 1994b. A novel member of the interferon receptor family complements functionality of the murine interferon gamma receptor in human cells. *Cell*, **76**, 803–10.

Henco, K., Brosius, J., et al. 1985. Structural relationship of human interferon alpha genes and pseudogenes. *J Mol Biol*, **185**, 227–60.

Herberman, R.B., Ortaldo, J.R., et al. 1981. Augmentation of natural and antibody-dependent cell-mediated cytotoxicity by pure human leukocyte interferon. *J Clin Immunol*, **1**, 149–53.

Herberman, R.B., Ortaldo, J.R., et al. 1982a. Effect of human recombinant interferon on cytotoxic activity of natural killer (NK) cells and monocytes. *Cell Immunol*, **67**, 160–7.

Herberman, R.B., Ortaldo, J.R., et al. 1982b. Interferon and natural killer (NK) cells. *Tex Rep Biol Med*, **41**, 590–5.

Hershberg, R.D., Gusciora, E.G., et al. 1981. Induction and production of human interferon with human leukemic cells. *Methods Enzymol*, **78**, 45–8.

Hertzog, P.J., Hwang, S.Y., et al. 1994. A gene on human chromosome 21 located in the region 21q22.2 to 21q22.3 encodes a factor necessary for signal transduction and antiviral response to type I interferons. *J Biol Chem*, **269**, 14088–93.

Hibino, Y., Kumar, C.S., et al. 1992. Chimeric interferon gamma receptors demonstrate that an accessory factor required for activity interacts with the extracellular domain. *J Biol Chem*, **267**, 3741–9.

Higashi, Y., Sokawa, Y., et al. 1983. Structure and expression of a cloned cDNA for mouse interferon-beta. *J Biol Chem*, **258**, 9522–9.

Higgins, P.G., Al Nakib, W., et al. 1986. Interferon-beta ser as prophylaxis against experimental rhinovirus infection in volunteers. *J Interferon Res*, **6**, 153–9.

Hijikata, M., Mishiro, S., et al. 2001. Genetic polymorphism of the MxA gene promoter and interferon responsiveness of hepatitis C patients: revisited by analyzing two SNP sites (-123 and -88) in vivo and in vitro. *Intervirology*, **44**, 379–82.

Hino, K., Sainokami, S., et al. 1994. Genotypes and titers of hepatitis C virus for predicting response to interferon in patients with chronic hepatitis C. *J Med Virol*, **42**, 299–305.

Hino, K., Kitase, A., et al. 2002. Interferon retreatment reduces or delays the incidence of hepatocellular carcinoma in patients with chronic hepatitis C. *J Viral Hepat*, **9**, 370–36.

Hobbs, D.S. and Pestka, S. 1982. Purification and characterization of interferons from a continuous myeloblastic cell line. *J Biol Chem*, **257**, 4071–6.

Hobbs, D.S., Moschera, J., et al. 1981. Purification of human leukocyte interferon produced in a culture of human granulocytes. *Methods Enzymol*, **78**, 472–81.

Hochkeppel, H.K., Gruetter, M., et al. 1992. Human IFN-alpha hybrids. *Drugs of the Future*, **17**, 899–914.

Hofmockel, G., Tack, W. and Frohmuller, H.G. 1997. Cyclic interferon alpha treatment in metastatic renal cell carcinoma: results of a phase II study and review of the literature. *Urol Int*, **58**, 8–12.

Houghton, M., Stewart, A.G., et al. 1980. The amino-terminal sequence of human fibroblast interferon as deduced from reverse transcripts obtained using synthetic oligonucleotide primers. *Nucleic Acids Res*, **8**, 1913–31.

Hu, K.Q., Vierling, J.M. and Redeker, A.G. 2001. Viral, host and interferon-related factors modulating the effect of interferon therapy for hepatitis C virus infection. *J Viral Hepat*, **8**, 1–18.

Hwang, S.Y., Hertzog, P.J., et al. 1995. A null mutation in the gene encoding a type I interferon receptor component eliminates antiproliferative and antiviral responses to interferons alpha and beta and alters macrophage responses. *Proc Natl Acad Sci USA*, **92**, 11284–8.

Iino, S., Hino, K. and Yasuda, K. 1994. Current state of interferon therapy for chronic hepatitis C. *Intervirology*, **37**, 87–100.

Imanishi, J., Hoshino, S., et al. 1981. New simple dye-uptake assay for interferon. *Biken J*, **24**, 103–8.

Improta, T., Schindler, C., et al. 1994. Transcription factor ISGF-3 formation requires phosphorylated Stat91 protein, but Stat113 protein is phosphorylated independently of Stat91 protein. *Proc Natl Acad Sci USA*, **91**, 4776–80.

Interferon nomenclature. 1980. *Nature*, **286**, 110.

Isaacs, A. and Lindenmann, J. 1957. Virus interference: I. The interferon. *Proc R Soc Lond Ser B*, **147**, 258–67.

Isomura, S., Ichikawa, T., et al. 1982. The preventive effect of human interferon-alpha on influenza infection; modification of clinical manifestations of influenza in children in a closed community. *Biken J*, **25**, 131–7.

Iwakura, Y., Yonehara, S. and Kawade, Y. 1978. Purification of mouse L cell interferon. Essentially pure preparations with associated cell growth inhibitory activity. *J Biol Chem*, **253**, 5074–9.

Jahrling, P.B., Geisbert, T.W., et al. 1999. Evaluation of immune globulin and recombinant interferon-alpha2b for treatment of experimental Ebola virus infections. *J Infect Dis*, **179**, suppl 1, S224–34.

Jankowski, W.J., von Muenchhausen, W., et al. 1976. Binding of human interferons to immobilized Cibacron Blue F3GA: The nature of molecular interaction. *Biochemistry*, **15**, 5182–7.

Jonas, M.M. 1996. Hepatitis C virus infection: clinical aspects and treatment with interferon alfa. *Clin Ther*, **18**, suppl B, 110–25.

Jonasch, E. and Haluska, F.G. 2001. Interferon in oncological practice: review of interferon biology, clinical applications, and toxicities. *Oncologist*, **6**, 34–55.

Jung, V. 1991. The human interferon gamma receptor and signal transduction, PhD thesis, Graduate School – New Brunswick, Rutgers, The State University of New Jersey; Graduate School of Biomedical Sciences, Robert Wood Johnson Medical School.

Jung, V. and Pestka, S. 1986. Selection and screening of transformed NIH3T3 cells for enhanced sensitivity to human interferons α and β. *Methods Enzymol*, **11**, 597–611.

Jung, V., Rashidbaigi, A., et al. 1987. Human chromosomes 6 and 21 are required for sensitivity to human interferon gamma. *Proc Natl Acad Sci USA*, **84**, 4151–5.

Jung, V., Jones, C., et al. 1988. Chromosome mapping of biological pathways by fluorescence-activated cell sorting and cell fusion: the human interferon gamma receptor as a model system. *Somat Cell Mol Genet*, **14**, 583–92.

Jung, V., Jones, C., et al. 1990. Expression and reconstitution of a biologically active human interferon gamma receptor in hamster cells. *J Biol Chem*, **265**, 1827–30.

Kaban, L.B., Mulliken, J.B., et al. 1999. Antiangiogenic therapy of a recurrent giant cell tumor of the mandible with interferon alfa-2a. *Pediatrics*, **103**, 6 Pt 1, 1145–9.

Kalina, U., Ozman, L., et al. 1993. The human gamma interferon receptor accessory factor encoded by chromosome 21 transduces the signal for the induction of 2,5-oligoadenylate-synthetase, resistance to virus cytopathic effect, and major histocompatibility complex class I antigens. *J Virol*, **67**, 1702–6.

Kaplan, D.H., Greenlund, A.C., et al. 1996. Identification of an interferon-gamma receptor alpha chain sequence required for JAK-1 binding. *J Biol Chem*, **271**, 9–12.

Karupiah, G., Fredrickson, T.N., et al. 1993. Importance of interferons in recovery from mousepox. *J Virol*, **67**, 4214–26.

Katze, M.G., He, Y. and Gale, M. Jr 2002. Viruses and interferon: a fight for supremacy. *Nat Rev Immunol*, **2**, 675–87.

Kawade, Y., Fujisawa, J., et al. 1981. Purification of L cell interferon. *Methods Enzymol*, **78**, Pt A, 522–35.

Kawakita, M., Cabrer, B., et al. 1978. Purification of interferon from mouse Ehrlich ascites tumor cells. *J Biol Chem*, **253**, 598–602.

Keegan, B.M. and Noseworthy, J.H. 2002. Multiple sclerosis. *Annu Rev Med*, **53**, 285–302.

Kempner, E.S. and Pestka, S. 1986. Radiation inactivation and target size analysis of interferons. *Methods Enzymol*, **119**, 255–60.

Kilbridge, K.L., Cole, B.F., et al. 2002. Quality-of-life-adjusted survival analysis of high-dose adjuvant interferon alpha-2b for high-risk melanoma patients using intergroup clinical trial data. *J Clin Oncol*, **20**, 1311–18.

Kirkwood, J. 2002. Cancer immunotherapy: the interferon-alpha experience. *Semin Oncol*, **29**, 3 suppl 7, 18–26.

Kirkwood, J.M., Ibrahim, J.G., et al. 2002. Interferon alfa-2a for melanoma metastases. *Lancet*, **359**, 978–9.

Klaus, W., Gsell, B., et al. 1997. The three-dimensional high resolution structure of human interferon alpha-2a determined by heteronuclear NMR spectroscopy in solution. *J Mol Biol*, **274**, 661–75.

Klein, M.L., Bartley, T.D., et al. 1988. Structural characterization of recombinant consensus interferon-α. *J Chromatogr*, **454**, 205–15.

Knight, E.J. 1976. Interferon: purification and initial characterization from human diploid cells. *Proc Natl Acad Sci USA*, **73**, 520–3.

Knight, E.J. and Fahey, D. 1982. Human interferon-beta: effects of deglycosylation. *J Interferon Res*, **2**, 421–9.

Knight, E.J., Hunkapiller, M.W., et al. 1980. Human fibroblast interferon: amino acid analysis and amino terminal amino acid sequence. *Science*, **207**, 525–6.

Kolokol'tsov, A.A., Davidovich, I.A., et al. 2001. The use of interferon for emergency prophylaxis of Marburg hemorrhagic fever in monkeys. *Bull Exp Biol Med*, **132**, 686–8.

Kotenko, S.V. and Pestka, S. 2000. Jak-Stat signal transduction pathway through the eyes of cytokine class II receptor complexes. *Oncogene*, **19**, 2557–65.

Kotenko, S.V., Izotova, L.S., et al. 1995. Interaction between the components of the interferon gamma receptor complex. *J Biol Chem*, **270**, 20915–21.

Kotenko, S.V., Izotova, L.S., et al. 1996. Other kinases can substitute for Jak2 in signal transduction by IFN-gamma. *J Biol Chem*, **271**, 17174–82.

Kotenko, S.V., Izotova, L.S., et al. 1999. The intracellular domain of interferon-alpha receptor 2c (IFN-alphaR2c) chain is responsible for Stat activation. *Proc Natl Acad Sci USA*, **96**, 5007–12.

Krishnan, K., Yan, H., et al. 1996. Dimerization of a chimeric CD4-interferon-alpha receptor reconstitutes the signaling events preceding STAT phosphorylation. *Oncogene*, **13**, 125–33.

Kumar, C.S., Muthukumaran, G., et al. 1989. Molecular characterization of the murine interferon gamma receptor cDNA. *J Biol Chem*, **264**, 17939–46.

Labdon, J.E., Gibson, K.D., et al. 1984. Some species of human leukocyte interferon are glycosylated. *Arch Biochem Biophys*, **232**, 422–6.

LaFleur, D.W., Nardelli, B., et al. 2001. Interferon-kappa, a novel type I interferon expressed in human keratinocytes. *J Biol Chem*, **276**, 39765–71.

Lai, D. 1994. The mapping of murine and human interferon gamma receptor, PhD thesis, Graduate School – New Brunswick, Ruttgers, The State University of New Jersey; Graduate School of Biomedical Sciences, Robert Wood Johnson Medical School.

Lambropoulos, A.F. and Koliais, S.I. 1989. Effect of interferon on the accumulation of RNA transcripts of genes coding for cellular and viral proteins. *J Gen Virol*, **70**, Pt 5, 1267–71.

Langer, J.A. and Pestka, S. 1988. Interferon receptors. *Immunol Today*, **9**, 393–400.

Langer, J.A., Rashidbaigi, A., et al. 1990. Sublocalization on chromosome 21 of human interferon-alpha receptor gene and the gene for an interferon-gamma response protein. *Somat Cell Mol Genet*, **16**, 231–40.

Langer, J.A., Rashidbaigi, A., et al. 1994. Radiation inactivation of human gamma-interferon: cellular activation requires two dimers. *Proc Natl Acad Sci USA*, **91**, 5818–22.

Langford, M.P., Weigent, D.A., et al. 1981. Virus plaque-reduction assay for interferon: microplaque and regular macroplaque reduction assays. *Methods Enzymol*, **78**, Pt A, 339–46.

Langford, M.P., Villarreal, A.L. and Stanton, G.J. 1983. Antibody and interferon act synergistically to inhibit enterovirus, adenovirus, and herpes simplex virus infection. *Infect Immun*, **41**, 214–18.

Lee, S.H.S., van Rooyen, C.E. and Ozere, R.L. 1969. Additional studies of interferon production by human leukemic leukocytes in vitro. *Cancer Res*, **29**, 645–52.

Lembo, D., Ricciardi-Castagnoli, P., et al. 1996. Mouse macrophages carrying both subunits of the human interferon-gamma (IFN-gamma) receptor respond to human IFN-gamma but do not acquire full protection against viral cytopathic effect. *J Biol Chem*, **271**, 32659–66.

Lengyel, P. 1982. Biochemistry of interferons and their actions. *Annu Rev Biochem*, **51**, 251–82.

Leong, S.S. and Horoszewicz, J.S. 1981. Production and preparation of human fibroblast interferon for clinical trials. *Methods Enzymol*, **78**, Pt A, 87–101.

Leppert, D., Waubant, E., et al. 1996. Interferon beta-1b inhibits gelatinase secretion and in vitro migration of human T cells: a possible mechanism for treatment efficacy in multiple sclerosis. *Ann Neurol*, **40**, 846–52.

Leung, S., Qureshi, S.A., et al. 1995. Role of STAT2 in the alpha interferon signaling pathway. *Mol Cell Biol*, **15**, 1312–17.

Leventon-Kriss, S., Movshovitz, M., et al. 1987. Sensitivity in vitro of herpes simplex virus isolates to human fibroblast interferon. *Med Microbiol Immunol (Berl)*, **176**, 151–9.

Levy, W.P., Shively, J., et al. 1980. Amino-terminal amino acid sequence of human leukocyte interferon. *Proc Natl Acad Sci USA*, **77**, 5102–4.

Levy, W.P., Rubinstein, M., et al. 1981. Amino acid sequence of a human leukocyte interferon. *Proc Natl Acad Sci USA*, **78**, 6186–90.

Li, B.-L., Zhao, X.-X., et al. 1990. Alpha-interferon structure and natural killer cell stimulatory activity. *Cancer Res*, **50**, 5328–32.

Li, J. and Roberts, R.M. 1994. Interferon-tau and interferon-alpha interact with the same receptors in bovine endometrium. Use of a readily iodinatable form of recombinant interferon-tau for binding studies. *J Biol Chem*, **269**, 13544–50.

Li, X., Leung, S., et al. 1997. Functional subdomains of STAT2 required for preassociation with the alpha interferon receptor and for signaling. *Mol Cell Biol*, **17**, 2048–56.

Lim, J.K., Xiong, J., et al. 1994. Intrinsic ligand binding properties of the human and bovine alpha-interferon receptors. *FEBS Lett*, **350**, 2-3, 281–6.

Lloyd, R.E., Weigent, D.A. and Stanton, G.J. 1983. Microassay for Sindbis virus and interferon activity. *J Clin Microbiol*, **18**, 296–9.

Lundquist, P.G., Haglund, S., et al. 1984. Interferon therapy in juvenile laryngeal papillomatosis. *Otolaryngol Head Neck Surg*, **92**, 386–91.

Lutfalla, G., Roeckel, N., et al. 1990. Assignment of human interferon-α receptor gene to chromosome 21q22.1 by in situ hybridization. *J Interferon Res*, **10**, 515–17.

Lutfalla, G., Gardiner, K., et al. 1992. The structure of the human interferon α/β receptor gene. *J Biol Chem*, **267**, 2802–9.

Lutfalla, G., Gardiner, K. and Uzé, G. 1993. A new member of the cytokine receptor gene family maps on chromosome 21 at less than 35 kb from IFNAR. *Genomics*, **16**, 366–73.

Lutfalla, G., Holland, S.J., et al. 1995. Mutant U5A cells complemented by an interferon-alpha/beta receptor subunit generated by alternative processing of a new member of the cytokine receptor gene cluster. *EMBO J*, **14**, 5100–8.

Lyra, A.C. and Di Bisceglie, A.M. 2001. What is the optimal therapy for chronic hepatitis B? *Minerva Med*, **92**, 431–4.

McCandliss, R., Sloma, A. and Pestka, S. 1981a. Isolation and cell-free translation of human interferon mRNA from fibroblasts and leukocytes. *Methods Enzymol*, **79**, 51–9.

McCandliss, R., Sloma, A. and Pestka, S. 1981b. Use of DNA bound to filters for selection of interferon-specific nucleic acid sequences. *Methods Enzymol*, **79**, 618–22.

Machida, H., Kuninaka, A. and Yoshino, H. 1980. Susceptibility of influenza viruses to interferon and to poly(I). Poly(C) determined by the plaque reduction method. *Microbiol Immunol*, **24**, 725–31.

Maeda, S., McCandliss, R., et al. 1980. Construction and identification of bacterial plasmids containing nucleotide sequence for human leukocyte interferon. *Proc Natl Acad Sci USA*, **77**, 7010–13.

Maeda, S., Gross, M. and Pestka, S. 1981. Screening of colonies by RNA-DNA hybridization with mRNA from induced and uninduced cells. *Methods Enzymol*, **79**, 613–18.

Maeyer-Guignard, J. 1981. Purification of mouse C-243 cell interferon by affinity chromatography and polyacrylamide gel electrophoresis. *Methods Enzymol*, **78**, Pt A, 513–22.

Maeyer-Guignard, J., Tovey, M.G., et al. 1978. Purification of mouse interferon by sequential affinity chromatography on poly(U)- and antibody-agarose columns. *Nature*, **271**, 622–5.

Mallucci, L. and Taylor-Papadimitriou, J. 1973. Inhibition by interferon of polyoma virus-induced cell DNA synthesis in mouse peritoneal macrophages. *J Gen Virol*, **21**, 391–8.

Marcus, P.I. and Sekellick, M.J. 2001. Combined sequential treatment with interferon and dsRNA abrogates virus resistance to interferon action. *J Interferon Cytokine Res*, **21**, 423–9.

Mariano, T.M., Kozak, C.A., et al. 1987. The mouse immune interferon receptor gene is located on chromosome 10. *J Biol Chem*, **262**, 5812–14.

Mariano, T.M., Donnelly, R.J., et al. 1992. Structure and function of the type I interferon receptor. In: Baron, S., et al. (eds), *Interferon: principles and medical applications*. Galveston, TX: University of Texas Medical Branch at Galveston, 129–38.

Mariano, T.M., Soh, J., et al. 1994. Expression of a functional human type i interferon receptor in hamster cells: application of functional YAC screening. *J Interferon Res*, **14**, S92.

Mariano, T.M., Muthukumaran, G., et al. 1996. Genetic mapping of the gene for the mouse interferon-gamma receptor signaling subunit to the distal end of chromosome 16. *Mammalian Genome*, **7**, 321–2.

Markland, W., McQuaid, T.J., et al. 2000. Broad-spectrum antiviral activity of the IMP dehydrogenase inhibitor VX-497: a comparison with ribavirin and demonstration of antiviral additivity with alpha interferon. *Antimicrob Agents Chemother*, **44**, 859–66.

Maroteaux, L., Kahana, C., et al. 1983. Sequences involved in the regulated expression of the human interferon-beta1 gene in recombinant SV40 DNA vectors replicating in monkey cells. *EMBO J*, **2**, 325–32.

Marques, A.R., Lau, D.T., et al. 1998. Combination therapy with famciclovir and interferon-alpha for the treatment of chronic hepatitis B. *J Infect Dis*, **178**, 1483–7.

Marsters, S.A., Pennica, D., et al. 1995. Interferon gamma signals via a high-affinity multisubunit receptor complex that contains two types of polypeptide chain. *Proc Natl Acad Sci USA*, **92**, 5401–5.

Martell, M., Esteban, J.I., et al. 1992. Hepatitis C virus (HCV) circulates as a population of different but closely related genomes: quasispecies nature of HCV genome distribution. *J Virol*, **66**, 3225–9.

Masihi, K.N. 2000. Immunomodulators in infectious diseases: panoply of possibilities. *Int J Immunopharmacol*, **22**, 1083–91.

Masihi, K.N. 2001. Fighting infection using immunomodulatory agents. *Expert Opin Biol Ther*, **1**, 641–53.

Mazzella, G., Saracco, G., et al. 1999. Long-term results with interferon therapy in chronic type B hepatitis: a prospective randomized trial. *Am J Gastroenterol*, **94**, 2246–50.

Meager, A. 2002. Biological assays for interferons. *J Immunol Methods*, **261**, 1-2, 21–36.

Melkova, Z. and Esteban, M. 1994. Interferon-gamma severely inhibits DNA synthesis of vaccinia virus in a macrophage cell line. *Virology*, **198**, 731–5.

Meraz, M.A., White, J.M., et al. 1996. Targeted disruption of the Stat1 gene in mice reveals unexpected physiologic specificity in the JAK-STAT signaling pathway. *Cell*, **84**, 431–42.

Minagawa, T., Ishiwata, K. and Kajimoto, T. 1999. Feline interferon-omega treatment on canine parvovirus infection. *Vet Microbiol*, **69**, 1-2, 51–3.

Mistchenko, A.S., Diez, R.A. and Falcoff, R. 1987. Recombinant human interferon-gamma inhibits adenovirus multiplication without modifying viral penetration. *J Gen Virol*, **68**, Pt 10, 2675–9.

Mitsui, Y., Senda, T., et al. 1993. Structural, functional and evolutionary implications of the three-dimensional crystal structure of murine interferon-l. *Pharmacol Ther*, **58**, 93–132.

Mochizuki, M., Nakatani, H. and Yoshida, M. 1994. Inhibitory effects of recombinant feline interferon on the replication of feline enteropathogenic viruses in vitro. *Vet Microbiol*, **39**, 1-2, 145–52.

Müller, M., Briscoe, J., et al. 1993. The protein tyrosine kinase Jak1 complements defects in interferon-α/l and -l signal transduction. *Nature*, **366**, 129–35.

Müller, U., Steinhoff, U., et al. 1994. Functional role of type I and type II interferons in antiviral defense. *Science*, **264**, 1918–21.

Munro, S. and Maniatis, T. 1989. Expression cloning of the murine interferon gamma receptor, cDNA. *Proc Natl Acad Sci USA*, **86**, 9248–52.

Muthukumaran, G., Donnelly, R.J., et al. 1996. The intracellular domain of the second chain of the interferon-gamma receptor is interchangeable between species. *J Interferon and Cytokine Res*, **16**, 1039–45.

Muthukumaran, G., Kotenko, S., et al. 1997. Chimeric erythropoietin-interferon gamma receptors reveal differences in functional architecture of intracellular domains for signal transduction. *J Biol Chem*, **272**, 4993–9.

Nagano, Y. and Kojima, Y. 1958. Inhibition de l'infection vaccinale par le virus homolog. *C R Seances Soc Biol Filiales*, **152**, 1627–30.

Nagata, S., Taira, H., et al. 1980. Synthesis in *E. coli* of a polypeptide with human leukocyte interferon activity. *Nature*, **284**, 316–20.

Nathan, P.D. and Eisen, T.G. 2002. The biological treatment of renal-cell carcinoma and melanoma. *Lancet Oncol*, **3**, 89–96.

Nathan, P.D., Gore, M.E. and Eisen, T.G. 2002. Unexpected toxicity of combination thalidomide and interferon alpha-2a treatment in metastatic renal cell carcinoma. *J Clin Oncol*, **20**, 1429–30.

Nolte, K.U., Jakschies, D., et al. 1994. Different specificities of SLE-derived and therapy-induced interferon-alpha antibodies. *J Interferon Res*, **14**, 197–9.

Novick, D., Cohen, B. and Rubinstein, M. 1994. The human interferon alpha/beta receptor: characterization and molecular cloning. *Cell*, **77**, 391–400.

Oberg, K. 2000. Interferon in the management of neuroendocrine GEP-tumors: a review. *Digestion*, **62**, suppl 1, 92–7.

Okamoto, H., Sugiyama, Y., et al. 1992. Typing hepatitis C virus by polymerase chain reaction with type-specific primers: application to clinical surveys and tracing infectious sources. *J Gen Virol*, **73**, Pt 3, 673–9.

Okamura, H., Berthold, W., et al. 1980. Human fibroblastoid interferon: immunosorbent column chromatography and N-terminal amino acid sequence. *Biochemistry*, **19**, 3831–5.

Ophir, J., Brenner, S., et al. 1995. Effect of topical interferon-beta on recurrence rates in genital herpes: a double-blind, placebo-controlled, randomized study. *J Interferon Cytokine Res*, **15**, 625–31.

Ortaldo, J.R., Herberman, R.B. and Pestka, S. 1982. Augmentation of human natural killer cells with human leukocyte and human recombinant leukocyte interferon. In: Herberman, R.B. (ed.), *NK cells and other natural effector cells*. New York: Academic Press, 1279–83.

Ortaldo, J.R., Mason, A., et al. 1983a. Effects of recombinant and hybrid recombinant human leukocyte interferons on cytotoxic activity of natural killer cells. *J Biol Chem*, **258**, 15011–15.

Ortaldo, J.R., Mantovani, A., et al. 1983b. Effects of several species of human leukocyte interferon on cytotoxic activity of NK cells and monocytes. *Int J Cancer*, **31**, 285–9.

Ortaldo, J.R., Herberman, R.B., et al. 1984. A species of human α interferon that lacks the ability to boost human natural killer activity. *Proc Natl Acad Sci USA*, **81**, 4926–9.

Oxman, M.N., Baron, S., et al. 1967. The effect of interferon on SV-40 T antigen production in SV-40-transformed cells. *Virology*, **32**, 122.

Ozawa, S., Shinohara, H., et al. 2001. Suppression of angiogenesis and therapy of human colon cancer liver metastasis by systemic administration of interferon-alpha. *Neoplasia*, **3**, 154–64.

Ozzello, L., DeRosa, C.M., et al. 1995. Up-regulation of a tumor-associated antigen (TAG-72) by interferons alpha and gamma in patients with cutaneous breast cancer recurrences. *Intl J Oncol*, **6**, 985–91.

Pei, J., Sekellick, M.J., et al. 2001. Chicken interferon type I inhibits infectious bronchitis virus replication and associated respiratory illness. *J Interferon Cytokine Res*, **21**, 1071–7.

Perrillo, R.P. 2002. How will we use the new antiviral agents for hepatitis B? *Curr Gastroenterol Rep*, **4**, 63–71.

Pestka, S. 1981. Cloning of human interferons. *Methods Enzymol*, **79**, 599–601.

Pestka, S. 1983a. The purification and manufacture of human interferons. *Sci Am*, **249**, 36–43.

Pestka, S. 1983b. The human interferons – from protein purification and sequence to cloning and expression in bacteria: before, between, and beyond. *Arch Biochem Biophys*, **221**, 1–37.

Pestka, S. 1986. Interferon from 1981 to 1986. *Methods Enzymol*, **119**, 3–14.

Pestka, S. 1997. The human interferon alpha species and hybrid proteins. *Semin Oncol*, **24**, suppl 9, S9–4.

Pestka, S., McInnes, J., et al. 1975. Cell-free synthesis of human interferon. *Proc Natl Acad Sci USA*, **72**, 3898–901.

Pestka, S., Evinger, M., et al. 1980a. *Biochemical characterization of lymphokines*. New York: Academic Press.

Pestka, S., Evinger, M., et al. 1980b. *Polypeptide hormones*. New York: Raven Press.

Pestka, S., Kelder, B., et al. 1983. Molecular weight of the functional unit of human leukocyte, fibroblast, and immune interferons. *J Biol Chem*, **258**, 9706–9.

Pestka, S., Langer, J.A., et al. 1987. Interferons and their actions. *Annu Rev Biochem*, **56**, 727–77.

Petersen, C., Bruns, E., et al. 1997. Treatment of extrahepatic biliary atresia with interferon-alpha in a murine infectious model. *Pediatr Res*, **42**, 623–8.

Pfeffer, L.M., Dinarello, C.A., et al. 1998. Biological properties of recombinant alpha-interferons: 40th anniversary of the discovery of interferons. *Cancer Res*, **58**, 2489–99.

Phillpotts, R.J., Scott, G.M., et al. 1983. An effective dosage regimen for prophylaxis against rhinovirus infection by intranasal administration of HuIFN-alpha 2. *Antiviral Res*, **3**, 121–36.

Phillpotts, R.J., Higgins, P.G., et al. 1984. Intranasal lymphoblastoid interferon (Wellferon) prophylaxis against rhinovirus and influenza virus in volunteers. *J Interferon Res*, **4**, 535–41.

Pianko, S. and McHutchison, J.G. 2000. Treatment of hepatitis C with interferon and ribavirin. *J Gastroenterol Hepatol*, **15**, 581–6.

Pollack, B.P., Kotenko, S.V. and Pestka, S. 1995. Use of the yeast two-hybrid system to study interferon signal transduction. *J Interferon Cytokine Res*, **15**, S67, (abstract).

Portillo Martin, J.A., Martin, G.B., et al. 1995. Clinical trial with intravesical alfa-2b interferon for the prevention of T1 transitional carcinoma of the bladder: preliminary results. Review of the bibliography (translation). *Arch Esp Urol*, **48**, 479–88.

Pusztai, R. and Szabo, E. 1978. Sensitivity of formation of adenovirus specific tumour antigen to leukocyte interferon. *Acta Virol*, **22**, 325–8.

Raanani, P. and Ben Bassat, I. 2002. Immune-mediated complications during interferon therapy in hematological patients. *Acta Haematol*, **107**, 133–44.

Radhakrishnan, R., Walter, L.J., et al. 1996. Zinc mediated dimer of human interferon-α2b revealed by X-ray crystallography. *Structure*, **4**, 1453–63.

Ransohoff, R.M., Maroney, P.A., et al. 1985. Effect of human alpha A interferon on influenza virus replication in MDBK cells. *J Virol*, **56**, 1049–52.

Rashidbaigi, A., Langer, J.A., et al. 1986. The gene for the human immune interferon receptor is located on chromosome 6. *Proc Natl Acad Sci USA*, **83**, 384–8.

Ravandi, F., Estrov, Z., et al. 1999. A phase I study of recombinant interferon-beta in patients with advanced malignant disease. *Clin Cancer Res*, **5**, 3990–8.

Raz, R., Durbin, J.E. and Levy, D.E. 1994. Acute phase response factor and additional members of the interferon-stimulated gene factor 3 family integrate diverse signals from cytokines, interferons, and growth factors. *J Biol Chem*, **269**, 24391–5.

Raziuddin, A. and Gupta, S.L. 1985. *The 2-5A system: molecular and clinical aspects of the interferon-regulated pathway*. New York: Alan R. Liss.

Regnier, F.E. and Noel, R. 1976. Glycerolpropylsilane bonded phases in the steric exclusion chromatography of biological macromolecules. *J Chromatogr Sci*, **14**, 316–20.

Rehberg, E., Kelder, B., et al. 1982. Specific molecular activities of recombinant and hybrid leukocyte interferons. *J Biol Chem*, **257**, 11497–502.

Revel, M., Bash, D. and Ruddle, F.H. 1976. Antibodies to a cell-surface component coded by human chromosome 21 inhibit action of interferon. *Nature*, **260**, 139–41.

Revel, M., Cohen, B., et al. 1991. Components of the human type I IFN receptor system. *J Interferon Res*, **11**, suppl, S61.

Reynolds, F.H. Jr, Premkumar, E. and Pitha, P.M. 1975. Interferon activity produced by translation of human interferon messenger RNA in cell-free ribosomal systems and in *Xenopus* oocytes. *Proc Natl Acad Sci USA*, **72**, 4881–5.

Ritch, P.S., Witt, P.L., et al. 1992. Phase I study of IFN alpha BDBB hybrid. *Proc ASCO*, **11**, 252.

Roberts, R.M., Cross, J.C. and Leaman, D.W. 1991. Unique features of the trophoblast interferons. *Pharmacol Ther*, **51**, 329–45.

Rockley, P.F. and Tyring, S.K. 1995. Interferons alpha, beta and gamma therapy of anogenital human papillomavirus infections. *Pharmacol Ther*, **65**, 265–87.

Rodriguez, J.R., Rodriguez, D. and Esteban, M. 1991. Interferon treatment inhibits early events in vaccinia virus gene expression in infected mice. *Virology*, **185**, 929–33.

Roffi, L., Mels, G.C., et al. 1995. Breakthrough during recombinant interferon alfa therapy in patients with chronic hepatitis C virus infection: prevalence, etiology, and management. *Hepatology*, **21**, 645–9.

Romeo, R., Rumi, M. and Colombo, M. 1995. Alpha interferon treatment of chronic hepatitis C. *Biomed Pharmacother*, **49**, 111–15.

Rosel, J. and Jungwirth, C. 1983. Isolation of early viral proteins from poxvirus-infected chick embryo fibroblasts by DNA-cellulose chromatography and inhibition of their synthesis by chicken interferon. *Eur J Biochem*, **132**, 361–7.

Rubinstein, M. and Pestka, S. 1981. Purification and characterization of human leukocyte interferons by high performance liquid chromatography. *Methods Enzymol*, **78**, 464–72.

Rubinstein, M., Rubinstein, S., et al. 1978. Human leukocyte interferon purified to homogeneity. *Science*, **202**, 1289–90.

Rubinstein, M., Rubinstein, S., et al. 1979a. Human leukocyte interferon production and purification to homogeneity by HPLC. In: Gross, E. and Meienhofer, J. (eds), *Peptides: structure and biological function*. Rockford, IL: Pierce Chemical Co, 99–103.

Rubinstein, M., Rubinstein, S., et al. 1979b. Human leukocyte interferon: production, purification to homogeneity, and initial characterization. *Proc Natl Acad Sci USA*, **76**, 640–4.

Rubinstein, M., Levy, W.P., et al. 1981. Human leukocyte interferon: isolation and characterization of several molecular forms. *Arch Biochem Biophys*, **210**, 307–18.

Rubinstein, S., Familletti, P.C. and Pestka, S. 1981. Convenient assay for interferons. *J Virol*, **37**, 755–8.

Ryman, K.D., Klimstra, W.B., et al. 2000. Alpha/beta interferon protects adult mice from fatal Sindbis virus infection and is an important determinant of cell and tissue tropism. *J Virol*, **74**, 3366–78.

Sagmeister, M., Wong, J.B., et al. 2001. A pragmatic and cost-effective strategy of a combination therapy of interferon alpha-2b and ribavirin for the treatment of chronic hepatitis C. *Eur J Gastroenterol Hepatol*, **13**, 483–8.

Saito, N., Suzuki, F. and Ishida, N. 1983. Antiviral effect of interferon on influenza virus infection in mice. *Tohoku J Exp Med*, **139**, 355–63.

Saracco, G. and Rizzetto, M. 1995. The long-term efficacy of interferon alfa in chronic hepatitis C patients: a critical review. *J Gastroenterol Hepatol*, **10**, 668–73.

Sasaki, O., Karaki, T. and Imanishi, J. 1985. Activity of recombinant human alpha interferon against influenza virus infection in mice. *Biken J*, **28**, 3-4, 79–82.

Scheck, A.C., Wigdahl, B., et al. 1986. Prolonged herpes simplex virus latency in vitro after treatment of infected cells with acyclovir and human leukocyte interferon. *Antimicrob Agents Chemother*, **29**, 589–93.

Schellekens, H., Niphuis, H., et al. 1996. The effect of recombinant human interferon alpha B/D compared to interferon alpha 2b on SIV infection in rhesus macaques. *Antiviral Res*, **32**, 1–8.

Schindler, C., Fu, X.Y., et al. 1992. Proteins of transcription factor ISGF-3: one gene encodes the 91- and 84-kDa ISGF-3 proteins that are activated by interferon alpha. *Proc Natl Acad Sci USA*, **89**, 7836–9.

Schlesinger, R.W. 1959. Interference between animal viruses. In: Baret, F.M. and Stanley, W.M. (eds), *The viruses*, 3rd edn. New York City, NY: Academic Press, 157–94.

Scott, G.M., Phillpotts, R.J., et al. 1982. Prevention of rhinovirus colds by human interferon alpha-2 from *Escherichia coli*. *Lancet*, **ii**, 186–8.

Sedmak, J.J. and Grossberg, S.E. 1981. Virus yield-reduction assays for interferon with the influenza virus neuraminidase assay. *Methods Enzymol*, **78**, Pt A, 369–73.

Sen, G.C. and Lengyel, P. 1992. The interferon system. A bird's eye view of its biochemistry. *J Biol Chem*, **267**, 5017–20.

Sen, G.C., Herz, R.E., et al. 1984. Antiviral and protein-inducing activities of recombinant human leukocyte interferons and their hybrids. *J Virol*, **50**, 445–50.

Senda, T., Saitoh, S. and Mitsui, Y. 1995. Refined crystal structure of recombinant murine interferon-l at 2.15l resolution. *J Mol Biol*, **253**, 187–207.

Shiffman, M.L. 1999. Use of high-dose interferon in the treatment of chronic hepatitis C. *Semin Liver Dis*, **19**, suppl 1, 25–33.

Shively, J.E., Del Valle, U., et al. 1982. Microsequence analysis of peptides and proteins. *Anal Biochem*, **126**, 318–26.

Shulman, L.M., Kamarck, M.E., et al. 1984. Antibodies to chromosome 21 coded cell surface components block binding of human alpha interferon but not gamma interferon to human cells. *Virology*, **137**, 422–7.

Silberberg, D.H. 1994. Specific treatment of multiple sclerosis. *Clin Neurosci*, **2**, 3-4, 271–4.

Slate, D.L., Shulman, L., et al. 1978. Presence of human chromosome 21 alone is sufficient for hybrid cell sensitivity to human interferon. *J Virol*, **25**, 319–25.

Soh, J., Donnelly, R.J., et al. 1993. Identification of a yeast artificial chromosome clone encoding an accessory factor for the human interferon gamma receptor: evidence for multiple accessory factors. *Proc Natl Acad Sci USA*, **90**, 8737–41.

Soh, J., Donnelly, R.J., et al. 1994a. Identification and sequence of an accessory factor required for activation of the human interferon gamma receptor. *Cell*, **76**, 793–802.

Soh, J., Mariano, T.M., et al. 1994b. Generation of random internal deletion derivatives of YACs by homologous targeting to Alu sequences. *DNA Cell Biol*, **13**, 301–9.

Soh, J., Mariano, T.M., et al. 1994c. Expression of a functional human type I interferon receptor in hamster cells: application of functional yeast artificial chromosome (YAC) screening. *J Biol Chem*, **269**, 18102–10.

Sperber, S.J., Gocke, D.J., et al. 1992. Anti-HIV-1 activity of recombinant and hybrid species of interferon alpha. *J Interferon Res*, **12**, 363–8.

Sperber, S.J., Gocke, D.J., et al. 1993a. Low-dose oral recombinant interferon-αA in patients with HIV-1 infection: a blinded pilot study. *AIDS*, **7**, 693–7.

Sperber, S.J., Hunger, S.B., et al. 1993b. Anti-rhinoviral activity of recombinant and hybrid species of interferon alpha. *Antiviral Res*, **22**, 121–9.

Staeheli, P., Sentandreu, M., et al. 2001. Alpha/beta interferon promotes transcription and inhibits replication of borna disease virus in persistently infected cells. *J Virol*, **75**, 8216–23.

Stahl, N. and Yancopoulos, G.D. 1993. The alphas, betas, and kinases of cytokine receptor complexes. *Cell*, **74**, 587–90.

Stahl, N., Farruggella, T.J., et al. 1995. Choice of STATs and other substrates specified by modular tyrosine-based motifs in cytokine receptors. *Science*, **267**, 1349–53.

Stein, S., Bohlen, P., et al. 1973. Amino acid analysis with fluorescamine at the picomole level. *Arch Biochem Biophys*, **155**, 202–12.

Stein, S., Kenny, C., et al. 1980. NH2-terminal amino acid sequence of human fibroblast interferon. *Proc Natl Acad Sci USA*, **77**, 5716–19.

Stewart, W.E. 1974. Distinct molecular species of interferons. *Virology*, **61**, 80–6.

Stewart, W.E., Lin, L.S., et al. 1977. Elimination of size and charge heterogeneities of human leukocyte interferons by chemical cleavage. *Proc Natl Acad Sci USA*, **74**, 4200–4.

Strander, H.A. 1986. Interferon in the treatment of human papilloma virus. *Med Clin North Am*, **Suppl**, 19–23.

Strube, M., Bodo, G. and Jungwirth, C. 1985. Sensitivity of ortho- and paramyxovirus replication to human interferon alpha. *Mol Biol Rep*, **10**, 237243.

Sun, C.S., Wilson, S.Z. and Wyde, P.R. 1986. Limited efficacy of aerosolized recombinant alpha interferon against virulent influenza A/HK infection in mice. *Proc Soc Exp Biol Med*, **181**, 298–304.

Sun, W. and Schuchter, L.M. 2001. Metastatic melanoma. *Curr Treat Options Oncol*, **2**, 193–202.

Taira, H., Broeze, R.J., et al. 1980. Mouse interferons: amino terminal amino acid sequences of various species. *Science*, **207**, 528–30.

Takeshita, T., Asao, H., et al. 1992. Cloning of the gamma chain of the human IL-2 receptor. *Science*, **257**, 379–82.

Talpaz, M., Kantarjian, H., et al. 1987. Therapy of chronic myelogenous leukemia. *Cancer*, **59**, 3 suppl, 664–7.

Tan, Y.H., Tischfield, J. and Ruddle, F.H. 1973. The linkage of genes for the human interferon-induced antiviral protein and indophenol oxidase-B traits to chromosome G-21. *J Exp Med*, **137**, 317–30.

Taniguchi, T., Ohno, S., et al. 1980. The nucleotide sequence of human fibroblast interferon cDNA. *Gene*, **10**, 11–15.

Tassone, F., Lutfalla, G., et al. 1990. Macrorestriction mapping of the interferon alpha receptor gene on chromosome 21 and linkage of cystathionine beta synthetase to alpha-crystallin. *Am J Human Genet*, **47**, suppl, A263.

Tevethia, S.S., Greenfield, R.S., et al. 1979. Biology of simian virus 40 (SV40) transplantation antigen (TrAg). IV. Inhibition by human interferon of expression of SV40 TrAg in SV40-infected monkey cells. *Virology*, **95**, 587–92.

Thang, M.N., Thang, D.C., et al. 1975. Biosynthesis of mouse interferon by translation of its messenger RNA in a cell-free system. *Proc Natl Acad Sci USA*, **72**, 3975–7.

Thoreau, E., Petridou, B., et al. 1991. Structural symmetry of the extracellular domain of the cytokine/growth hormone/prolactin receptor family and interferon receptors revealed by hydrophobic cluster analysis. *FEBS Lett*, **282**, 26–31.

Torma, E.T. and Paucker, K. 1976. Purification and characterization of human leukocyte interferon components. *J Biol Chem*, **251**, 4810–16.

Trepo, C., Habersetzer, F., et al. 1994. Interferon therapy for hepatitis C. *Antiviral Res*, **24**, 2-3, 155–63.

Tsubota, A., Chayama, K., et al. 1994. Factors predictive of response to interferon-alpha therapy in hepatitis C virus infection. *Hepatology*, **19**, 1088–94.

Uddin, S., Chamdin, A. and Platanias, L.C. 1995. Interaction of the transcriptional activator Stat-2 with the type I interferon receptor. *J Biol Chem*, **270**, 24627–30.

Udenfriend, S., Stein, S., et al. 1972. Fluorescamine: a reagent for assay of amino acids, peptides, proteins, and primary amines in the picomole range. *Science*, **178**, 871–2.

Uzé, G., Lutfalla, G. and Gresser, I. 1990. Genetic transfer of a functional human interferon alpha receptor into mouse cells: cloning and expression of its cDNA. *Cell*, **60**, 225–34.

Uzé, G., Lutfalla, G., et al. 1991. Murine tumor cells expressing the gene for the human interferon alpha beta receptor elicit antibodies in syngeneic mice to the active form of the receptor. *Eur J Immunol*, **21**, 447–51.

Uzé, G., Lutfalla, G., et al. 1992. Behavior of a cloned murine interferon α/β receptor expressed in homospecific or heterospecific background. *Proc Natl Acad Sci USA*, **89**, 4774–8.

Uzé, G., Lutfalla, G. and Mogensen, K.E. 1995. Alpha and beta interferons and their receptor and their friends and relations. *J Interferon Cytokine Res*, **15**, 3–26.

Van Damme, J. and Billiau, A. 1981. Large-scale production of human fibroblast interferon. *Methods Enzymol*, **78**, Pt A, 101–19.

van Herpen, C.M. and De Mulder, P.H. 2000. Locoregional immunotherapy in cancer patients: review of clinical studies. *Ann Oncol*, **11**, 1229–39.

van Herpen, C.M. and De Mulder, P.H. 2002. Prognostic and predictive factors of immunotherapy in metastatic renal cell carcinoma. *Crit Rev Oncol Hematol*, **41**, 327–34.

Vanden Broecke, C. and Pfeffer, L.M. 1988. Characterization of interferon-alpha binding sites on human cell lines. *J Interferon Res*, **8**, 803–11.

Veals, S.A., Schindler, C., et al. 1992. Subunit of an alpha-interferon-responsive transcription factor is related to interferon regulatory factor and Myb families of DNA-binding proteins. *Mol Cell Biol*, **12**, 3315–24.

Velazquez, L., Fellous, M., et al. 1992. A protein tyrosine kinase in the interferon α/β signalling pathway. *Cell*, **70**, 313–22.

Viscomi, G.C., Antonelli, G., et al. 1999. Antigenic characterization of recombinant, lymphoblastoid, and leukocyte IFN-alpha by monoclonal antibodies. *J Interferon Cytokine Res*, **19**, 319–26.

Vithanomsat, S., Wasi, C., et al. 1984. The effect of interferon on flaviviruses in vitro: a preliminary study. *Southeast Asian J Trop Med Public Health*, **15**, 27–31.

von Rheinbaben, F., Stitz, L. and Rott, R. 1985. Influence of interferon on persistent infection caused by Borna disease virus in vitro. *J Gen Virol*, **66**, Pt 12, 2777–80.

von Wussow, P., Hochkeppel, H.K., et al. 1991. Phase I study of a new recombinant hybrid IFN (alpha1/alpha2). *Proc ASCO*, **32**, 1532, (abstract).

Waldman, A.A., Miller, R.S., et al. 1981. Induction and production of interferon with human leukocytes from normal donors with the use of Newcastle disease virus. *Methods Enzymol*, **78**, 39–44.

Walter, M.R., Windsor, W.T., et al. 1995. Crystal structure of a complex between interferon-gamma and its soluble high-affinity receptor (see comments). *Nature*, **376**, 230–5.

Watowich, S.S., Yoshimura, A., et al. 1992. Homodimerization and constitutive activation of the erythropoietin receptor. *Proc Natl Acad Sci USA*, **89**, 2140–4.

Weber, F. and Elliott, R. 2002. Antigenic drift, antigenic shift and interferon antagonists: how bunyaviruses counteract the immune system. *Virus Res*, **88**, 1-2, 129.

Weber, F., Bridgen, A., et al. 2002. Bunyamwera bunyavirus nonstructural protein NSs counteracts the induction of alpha/beta interferon. *J Virol*, **76**, 7949–55.

Weigent, D.A., Stanton, G.J., et al. 1981. Virus yield-reduction assay for interferon by titration of infectious virus. *Methods Enzymol*, **78**, Pt A, 346–51.

Weiland, O. 1994. Interferon therapy in chronic hepatitis C virus infection. *FEMS Microbiol Rev*, **14**, 279–88.

Wells, D.E., Chatterjee, S., et al. 1991. Inhibition of human immunodeficiency virus type 1-induced cell fusion by recombinant human interferons. *J Virol*, **65**, 6325–630.

Wheelock, E.F. 1966. Virus replication and high-titered interferon production in human leukocyte cultures inoculated with Newcastle disease virus. *J Bacteriol*, **92**, 1415–21.

White, C.W. 1990. Treatment of hemangiomatosis with recombinant interferon alfa. *Semin Hematol*, **27**, 3 suppl 4, 15–22.

White, C.W. and Sondheimer, H.M. 1989. Treatment of pulmonary hemangiomatosis with recombinant interferon alfa-2a. *N Engl J Med*, **320**, 1197–200.

Wilkinson, T. 2001. Hepatitis C virus: prospects for future therapies. *Curr Opin Invest Drugs*, **2**, 1516–22.

Wingerchuk, D.M. and Noseworthy, J.H. 2002. Randomized controlled trials to assess therapies for multiple sclerosis. *Neurology*, **58**, 8 suppl 4, S40–8.

Woo, M.H. and Burnakis, T.G. 1997. Interferon alfa in the treatment of chronic viral hepatitis B and C. *Ann Pharmacother*, **31**, 330–7.

Yakobson, E., Prives, C., et al. 1977. Inhibition of viral protein synthesis in monkey cells treated with interferon late in simian virus 40 lytic cycle. *Cell*, **12**, 73–81.

Yamamoto, H., Hayashi, E., et al. 1992. Interferon therapy for non-A, non-B hepatitis: a pilot study and review of the literature. *Hepatogastroenterology*, **39**, 377–80.

Yan, H., Krishnan, K., et al. 1996. Phosphorylated interferon-alpha receptor 1 subunit (IFNaR1) acts as a docking site for the latent form of the 113 kDa STAT2 protein. *EMBO J*, **15**, 1064–74.

Yang, C.H., Shi, W., et al. 1996. Direct association of STAT3 with the IFNAR-1 chain of the human type I interferon receptor. *J Biol Chem*, **271**, 8057–61.

Yasuda, S., Huffman, J.H., et al. 2000. Spectrum of virus inhibition by consensus interferon YM643. *Antivir Chem Chemother*, **11**, 337–41.

Zein, N.N. and Rakela, J. 1995. Interferon therapy in hepatitis C. *Semin Gastrointest Dis*, **6**, 46–53.

Zinn, K., Mellon, P., et al. 1982. Regulated expression of an extrachromosomal human beta-interferon gene in mouse cells. *Proc Natl Acad Sci USA*, **79**, 4897–901.

Zoon, K.C. 1981a. International meeting. In: De Maeyer, E., Galasso, G. and Schellenkens, H. (eds), *The biology of the interferon system.* Amsterdam: Elsevier/North Holland, 47–55.

Zoon, K.C. 1981b. Purification and characterization of human interferon from lymphoblastoid (Namalva) cultures. *Methods Enzymol*, **78**, Pt A, 457–64.

Zoon, K.C., Smith, M.E., et al. 1979. Purification and partial characterization of human lymphoblast interferon. *Proc Natl Acad Sci USA*, **76**, 5601–5.

Zoon, K.C., Smith, M.E., et al. 1980. Amino terminal sequence of the major component of human lymphoblastoid interferon. *Science*, **207**, 527–8.

15

Cytokines

SERGIO ROMAGNANI

Cytokines are important signaling molecules produced by cells involved in inflammation, immunity, differentiation, cell division, fibrosis repair, and many other functions. Although cytokines share properties in common with hormones that are produced continuously and interact with them, there are also notable distinctions. Hormones are typically produced by specialized cells and released into the bloodstream and so can act at a distance from the source, in an 'endocrine fashion'. In contrast, cytokines usually act at short range, a few cell diameters apart, as in a 'paracrine' or 'autocrine' manner. The major differences between hormones and cytokines are summarized in Figure 15.1.

Today, we are confronted by considerably more than 100 cytokines as structurally identified molecules (Oppenheim and Feldman 2000). A great proportion of these molecules have recently been characterized because of their chemotactic activity and, therefore, they have been named as chemotactic cytokines or chemokines (Zlotnik and Yoshie 2000). These are considered separately (see Chapter 13, Chemokines). Some other cytokines are not discussed here, because either they mainly act as membrane rather than soluble signals or their activity is only minimally involved in the function of the immune system. Usually cytokines are grouped in different families according to structural similarity of ligands and/or receptors. Despite the fact that the same cytokine may exhibit different functions and that the same function may be exerted by different cytokines, we have tried to group cytokines into five different families based on their most impressive or better-known function (Table 15.1). This type of classification is certainly arbitrary and questionable, but it may be of some usefulness from a didactic point of view.

GROWTH FACTORS FOR HEMOPOIETIC PRECURSORS, MYELOID CELLS, AND THROMBOCYTES

Definitive hemopoiesis is a complex cellular process that is regulated, in part, by hemopoietic growth factors (HGF) and the bone marrow microenvironment, which act to promote the survival, proliferation, and differentiation of hemopoietic stem cells (SC) and their progeny. HGFs are produced by accessory or stromal cells (macrophages, fibroblasts, endothelial cells, and adipocytes) in the bone marrow and elsewhere, and interact with specific receptors expressed on hemopoietic cells.

Stem cell factor

The main HGF is stem cell factor (SCF). SCF is also known as steel factor (SF), because it was mapped to the Sl locus, Kit ligand (KL), and mast cell growth factor (MCGF) (Lyman and Jacobsen 1998). SCF is produced in both soluble and membrane-bound forms. These isoforms arise from two differentially spliced complementary DNAs (cDNA). One cDNA encodes a precursor of 273 amino acids that contains a cleavable N-terminal signal peptide of 25 amino acids and gives rise to the transmembrane protein with 248 amino acids. The gene for SCF might be located on the distal end of

← **Gradient** →

Cytokine | **IL-6, M-CSF, EPO** | **Hormone**

Acts locally
Made by many cells, e.g. IL-l, IL-6 almost ubiquitous
Synthesized transiently after cell activation
Usually inactive in serum/plasma

Acts at distance
Made by specialized cells and organs, e.g. pituitary, adrenal
Produced constitutively and continuously
Bioactive in serum/plasma

Common properties: Receptors often homologous (e.g. hemopoietin)
Potent signals

Figure 15.1 *Differences between cytokines and hormones. EPO, erythropoietin; IL, interleukin; M-CSF, macrophage colony-stimulating factor. (Redrawn from Oppenheim and Feldman 2000, with permission.)*

the long arm of human chromosome 12 (Keller and Linnekin 2000).

Analysis of the expression of the gene for SCF in the developing embryo suggests that this gene has multiple functional roles in development, e.g. the gene for SCF is expressed along the migratory pathways for stem cells that give rise to hemopoietic, melanocyte, and germ-cell lineages. Specifically, SCF has been detected in the genital ridge of day 10 embryos, whereas its receptor (SCFR) is expressed in the migrating germ cells. SCF expression in the genital ridge decreases early after the beginning of gestation, but remains high in the developing gonads during sexual differentiation (both in the testes and in the ovary). This pattern of expression suggests that SCF is involved in regulating the migration, proliferation, and differentiation of germ cells (Matsui et al. 1990). Moreover, SCF is expressed in mesenchymal cells located in the limb bud where melanocyte precursors colonize, whereas SCFR is expressed on the migrating cells. The expression of SCF persists during and after stem cell colonization of the limb buds. SCF is also expressed in fetal liver, which is the migratory site for hemopoietic SCs in the developing embryo. As would be predicted, there is a marked reduction in the number of SCFR-positive SCs that migrate to the fetal livers of Sl/Sl embryos (mutants that have deletion of the transmembrane and cytoplasmic domains of SCG). SCF mRNA transcripts have also been detected in other tissues in the developing embryo, including the spinal cord, forebrain, cerebellum, and olfactory bulbs, suggesting that SCF might play a role in the developing CNS. Although there are no gross neurological defects in Sl mutant mice, Sl/Sl mutant mice show a defect in hippocampus-dependent learning (spatial learning). In the adult, SCF is expressed by stromal or accessory cells (endothelial cells, monocytes, and fibroblasts) in the adult, where these cells constitute the hemopoietic microenvironment (Broudy 1997). SCF is also produced by intestinal epithelial cells, Sertoli cells, and follicular cells that surround oocytes in the gonads, thymic stroma, and brain cells, including those that constitute the olfactory bulb, thalamus, cerebellum, and brain. SCF expression has also been detected in human $CD34^+$ cells and keratinocytes in the skin (Ratajczak et al. 1995).

Stem cell factor plays an essential role in the survival, growth, and differentiation of cells responsible for hemo-

Table 15.1 *Classification of cytokines based on their major functional activities*

Growth factors for hemopoietic precursors, myeloid cells and thrombocytes
Stem cell factor (SCF)
Colony-stimulating factors (CSFs): interleukin (IL)-3, granulocyte (G)-CSF, macrophage (M)-CSF, GM-CSF
IL-5
IL-11
Growth and differentiation factors for lymphoid cells
IL-2
IL-4
IL-7
IL-9
IL-15
IL-21
IL-27
Proinflammatory cytokines
IL-1α and IL-1β
IL-6
Tumor necrosis factor (TNF)-α
Lymphotoxins (LT)α and LTβ
Interferon (IFN)-γ
IL-12
IL-16
IL-17 family
IL-18
IL-23
IL-25
Anti-inflammatory and regulatory cytokines
IL-1 receptor antagonist (IL-1Ra)
IL-10
IL-13
Transforming growth factor (TGF)-β
Chemotactic cytokines (chemokines)
(See Chapter 13, Chemokines)

poietic, germ-cell, and melanocyte cell development during both embryonic development and adult life In particular, SCF is essential for the migration and homing of SCs to their appropriate developmental sites; moreover, SCF directly promotes the survival of these stem-cell populations (Keller and Linnekin 2000).

The receptor for SCF, SCFR, is expressed on most hemopoietic progenitors but is not expressed on their differentiated progeny, including mature myeloid and monocytic cells or lymphoid and erythroid cell populations; however, its expression is maintained at high levels on mast cells. In this regard, SCF promotes the survival, proliferation, and differentiation of mast cells in vitro. In addition, SCF, in combination with the interleukin (IL)-3 and IL-4, promotes the proliferation of mast cells and their progenitors. SCF can promote the adhesion of mast cells, hemopoietic progenitor cells, and cell lines to fibronectin or vascular cell adhesion molecule 1 (VCAM-1) expressed on endothelial cells by activating VLA-4 and VLA-5 integrin expression on progenitor cells. A single injection of SCF to normal mice promotes a dose-dependent increase in total number of peripheral blood leukocytes, including neutrophils and immature myeloid cells, but not circulating platelets or red cells (Galli et al. 1994). The in vivo hemopoietic effects of SCF are summarized in Table 15.2.

Although no abnormalities involving the SCF genetic loci have been reported, locally high concentrations of soluble SCF have been found in lesions of human cutaneous mastocytosis. This disease is characterized by accumulations of mast cells, as well as increases in the production of epidermal melanin similar to that observed in transgenic animals which expressed SCF transgenes in keratinocytes. This has led to the hypothesis that locally produced SCF can promote mast cell hyperplasia (Keller and Linnekin 2000).

Table 15.2 *In vivo hemopoietic effects of stem cell factor*

Cell type		Response
LTRC	Expansion	+
	Mobilization	+
Primitive/committed progenitors	Expansion	++
	Mobilization	++
Red blood cells	Reticulocytes	+/NE
	Hematocrit	+/NE
Platelets	Megakaryocytes	+/NE
	Platelets	+/NE
White blood cells	Total number	+
	Granulocytes	+
	Monocytes	+/NE
	Lymphocytes	+/NE
Mast cells	Number	+
	Activation	+
Dendritic cells	Number	NE

+, increase; NE, no effect; +/NE, effect found in some, but not all species investigated.Modified from Lyman and Jacobsen (1998).

Colony-stimulating factors

Hemopoietic activity is also the main activity of the so-called colony-stimulating factors (CSF). CSFs comprise four cytokines, named multi-CSF or IL-3, granulocyte (G)-CSF, CSF-1 or macrophage (M)-CSF, and granulocyte–macrophage (GM)-CSF. The major activity of CSFs is the development of colonies from precursors of the granulocyte and monocyte–macrophage lineage.

INTERLEUKIN 3

IL-3, also known as multi-CSF, is a typical member of the family of four helix-bundle cytokines. The mature human IL-3 is a polypeptide of 133 amino acids and the mature murine IL-3 has 140 amino acids. The human gene for IL-3 is on chromosome 5q21 (Schrader 2000).

IL-3 is synthesized and released by antigen-activated T lymphocytes, as well as by mast cells and eosinophils following antigen crosslinking of cytophilic antibodies bound to Fc receptors present on their surface (Schrader 2000).

IL-3 stimulates the growth, differentiation, and survival of pluripotential hemopoietic SCs and many of their progeny, including multipotential progenitors and progenitors committed to individual cell lineages and mature cells (Bukowski et al. 1996). These include SCs able to originate all lymphohemopoietic cell lineages and multipotential progenitors capable of generating neutrophils, macrophages, megakaryocytes, and erythroid cells. More committed progenitors targeted by IL-3 include those giving rise to in vitro colonies of eosinophils, neutrophils, macrophages, megakaryocytes, mast cells, and erythroid cells. IL-3 also supports the survival of mature mast cells, eosinophils, basophils, and megakaryocytes, and also augments the effector functions of basophils, mast cells, and eosinophils.

The effects of IL-3 depend on where it is released. The local release of IL-3 in mucosal surfaces or in lymph nodes results in the generation of mucosa-type mast cells from undifferentiated, committed, mast-cell progenitors present in these tissues. Systemic release of IL-3 results in increases in the number of hemopoietic progenitor cells and mast cell precursors in the spleen, as well as increases in megakaryocytes, neutrophils, and mast cells.

IL-3 appears to have a role in the response to certain parasites, probably because of its ability to increase the numbers of infection-stimulated mast cells and basophils. Administration of recombinant IL-3 by subcutaneous injection increases the levels of neutrophils and eosinophils, as well platelet counts, lymphocyte numbers and numbers of $CD34^{+}$ cells in the peripheral blood

(Schrader 2000). Side effects induced by IL-3 include headaches, flu-like symptoms, fever, and rashes. In general, clinical application of IL-3 has been poor.

G-CSF

G-CSF is a 25-kDa glycoprotein that regulates production of neutrophilic granulocytes, and activates mature neutrophils. Its gene is located on human chromosome 17q21-q22 (Nagata 2000).

Monocytes, macrophages, endothelial cells, and fibroblasts are induced to express G-CSF by various stimuli (Metcalf and Nicola 1985). Some carcinoma cells and tumor cell lines produce G-CSF constitutively. G-CSF has a unique receptor which mediates colony formation of neutrophilic granulocytes in semi-solid cultures of bone marrow cells.

Unlike other CSFs, such as GM-CSF and IL-3, G-CSF is rather specific to progenitor cells of neutrophilic granulocytes (Nicolas et al. 1983). G-CSF not only stimulates proliferation and differentiation of progenitors, but also prolongs the survival of mature neutrophils and enhances their functional capacity. Mice lacking the G-CSF gene show chronic neutropenia (Figure 15.2), are deficient in granulocyte and macrophage progenitor cells, and show impaired neutrophil mobilization (Lieschke et al. 1994; Basu et al. 2002), whereas administration of G-CSF causes increase in granulocyte numbers (Welte et al. 1987) and long-term exposure to

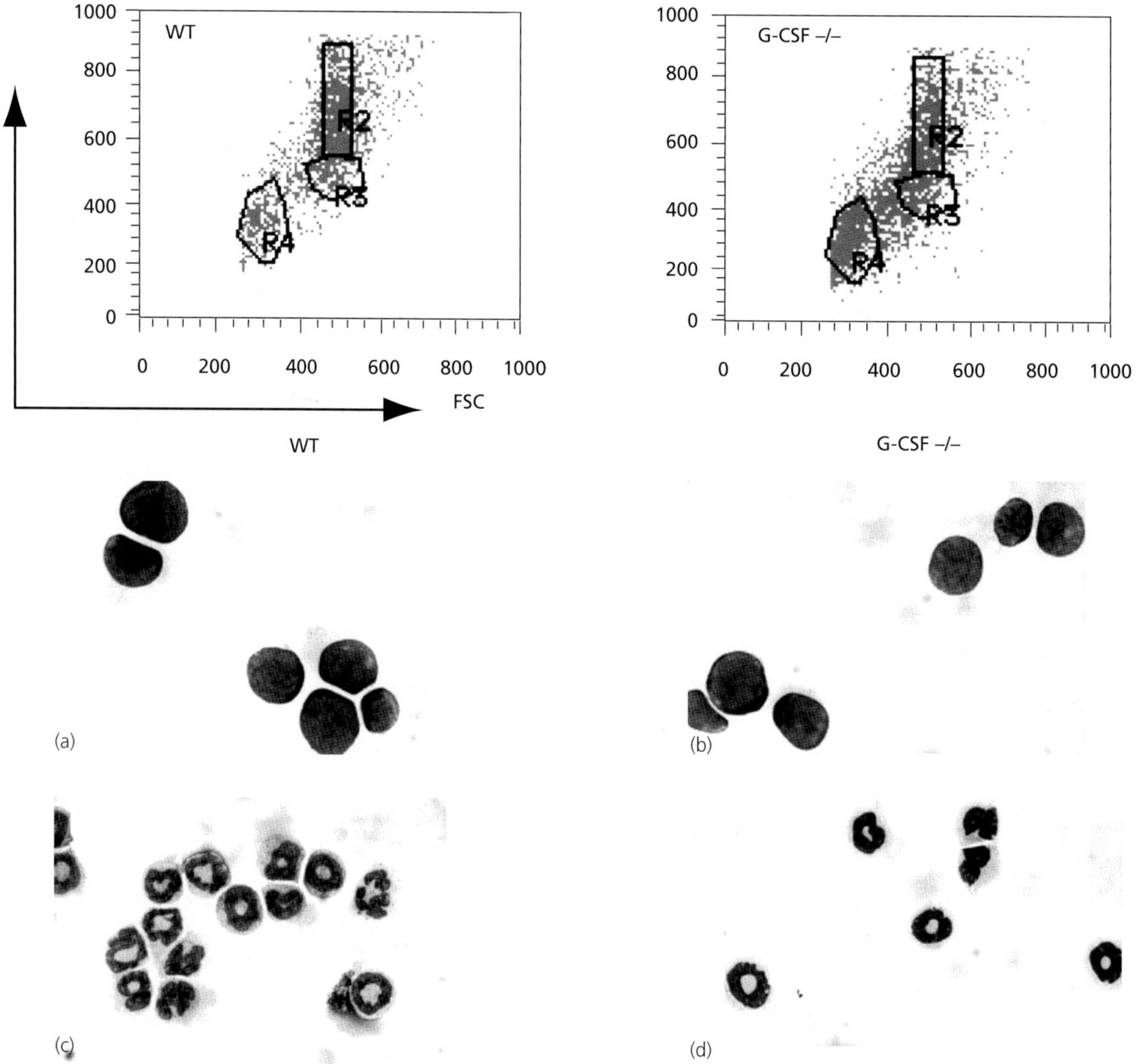

Figure 15.2 *Essential role of G-CSF in neutrophil development. Dot–blot presentation of forward scatter (FSC) versus side scatter (SSC) of bone marrow cells from wild-type (WT) and granulocyte colony-stimulating factor (G-CSF)-deficient (G-CSF$^{-/-}$) mice. R2, granulocytes; R3, blasts; R4, lymphocytes. Cells in regions R2 and R3 were sorted, and cytospin preparations of these cells were stained with May–Grünwald–Giemsa. Panels* **(a)** *and* **(b)** *represent cells in region R3, and panels* **(c)** *and* **(d)** *represent cells in region 2. (Redrawn from Basu et al. 2002, with permission.)*

G-CSF of transgenic mice causes sustained granulocytosis (Chang et al. 1989).

G-CSF is effectively used to stimulate granulopoiesis in neutropenic patients. G-CSF is also being administered to patients with cancer receiving chemotherapy or radiotherapy with or without bone marrow transplantation, to patients receiving immunosuppressive agents after organ transplantation, and to patients with cyclic neutropenia. In these last patients, without altering the cyclic nature of this disease, G-CSF elevates neutrophil levels during the nadir phase and therefore prevents many of the symptoms of the disease (Nagata 2000).

M-CSF

M-CSF, initially known as CSF-1, is a 80- to 100-kDa glycoprotein or 130- to 160-kDa chondroitin sulfate-containing proteoglycan, or it is expressed as a membrane-spanning 68- to 86-kDa glycoprotein on the surface of cells. The human M-CSF gene is approximately 21 kilobases (kb) in length, comprising 10 exons, and is localized to human chromosome 1p13-p21 (Stanley 1994).

M-CSF is expressed in most tissues, including submaxillary gland, lung, spleen, kidney, lymph nodes, brain, liver, testis, and ovary. Several types of normal cells synthesize M-CSF, including fibroblasts, endothelial cells, bone marrow stromal cells, osteoblasts, thymic epithelial cells, keratinocytes, astrocytes, myoblasts, mesothelial cells, liver parenchymal cells, thyrocytes, and adipocytes. M-CSF is also synthesized by ovarian granulosa cells, oviduct epithelium, and in large amounts by uterine epithelial cells during pregnancy (Arceci et al. 1992).

M-CSF is the primary regulator of the survival, proliferation, and differentiation of mononuclear phagocytes, including tissue macrophages and osteoclasts. It has also been shown to stimulate $CD5^+$ B lymphocytes to develop into biphenotypic B/macrophage cells. Cells requiring M-CSF for their development may regulate, via tropic and/or scavenger functions, bone resorption, male fertility, the thickness of the dermis, and neural processing. In the female reproductive system, M-CSF regulates the development of macrophages and the function of nonmononuclear phagocytic cells.

GM-CSF

GM-CSF is a protein of 144 amino acids, containing a leader sequence of 17 amino acids, two intramolecular disulfide bonds, and two potential sites of *N*-glycosylation, as well as sites of *O*-glycosylation. The apparent molecular weight of the mature glycosylated proteins is 13 kDa. The GM-CSF gene maps to chromosome 5q31.1 (Nicolas 2000) and it is very tightly linked to the IL-3 gene. There is also a cluster of cytokine (M-CSF, IL-4, IL-5) and receptor (*c-fms*) genes in the same area.

GM-CSF is a product of activated T lymphocytes, fibroblasts, endothelial cells, macrophages, and stromal cells, but also B lymphocytes, mast cells, eosinophils, blast cells, and osteoblasts. The major stimulant for T-cell production of GM-CSF is engagement of the T-cell receptor (TCR) (TCR) by antigen. In addition, the cytokines IL-1 and IL-2 and infection with the human T-cell lymphotropic virus (HTLV) also increase GM-CSF production by T cells. For B lymphocytes, antigen receptor activation (e.g. by *Staphylococcus aureus*) and bacterial lipopolysaccharide (LPS) or phorbol esters induce GM-CSF synthesis. For mast cells, degranulating agents, such as anti-IgE and calcium ionophores and, for osteoblasts, LPS and parathyroid hormone, are effective. For macrophages, fibroblasts, and endothelial cells, the major inducers of GM-CSF synthesis are LPS, IL-1, and tumor necrosis factor (TNF), as well as phorbol esters (Metcalf and Nicola 1995).

The effects of injected GM-CSF consist of a rapid and profound decrease in white blood cell counts, resulting from sequestration within the lungs followed by a progressive rise in circulating neutrophils, eosinophils, monocytes, and progenitor cells for all lineages (colony-forming cells) (Metcalf and Nicola 1995). These rises are, however, significantly less than those seen with injected G-CSF. GM-CSF has also been used to mobilize hemopoietic SCs into the peripheral blood for subsequent autologous bone marrow transplantation (ABMT). Such SCs induce a more rapid recovery of both neutrophils and platelets than is achieved by ABMT, but G-CSF exhibits a greater mobilizing efficiency than GM-CSF even for this purpose. Some studies have begun to appear in human beings evaluating the use of GM-CSF as an antiviral vaccine adjuvant for immunization against hepatitis B and influenza, with encouraging but preliminary results. Trials have also been initiated in which GM-CSF is administered after surgical resection of melanoma tumors or with passive (antimelanoma or antineuroblastoma antibodies) or active (autologous melanoma cells with BCG) immunization against tumor cells (Nicolas 2000).

Interleukin 5

IL-5 is an important growth and differentiation factor for eosinophil granulocytes. It is a glycoprotein with an M_r of 45 kDa and is unusual among the T-cell-produced cytokines in being a disulfide-linked homodimer (Gretchen et al. 2000). It is the most highly conserved member of a group of evolutionally related cytokines, including IL-3, IL-4, IL-13, and GM-CSF, which are closely linked on human chromosome 5.

T cells are an important source of the cytokine (Sanderson 1992). However, IL-5 mRNA production has also been demonstrated in mast-cell lines and human Epstein–Barr virus (EBV)-transformed B cells. Furthermore, eosinophils themselves have been demonstrated to produce IL-5 (Broide et al. 1992).

IL-5 plays a unique and specific role in the control of eosinophil production and differentiation (eosinophil differentiating factor (EDF)). It is also able to activate basophils, but is probably not the major factor controlling basophil production. The effect on eosinophil production is relatively direct. When IL-5 is expressed, eosinophils are produced, and when IL-5 expression is inhibited by drugs or gene knock-out eosinophil production and survival virtually cease. The role of IL-5 in eosinophilia (Figure 15.3), coupled with a better understanding of the part played by eosinophils in the development of tissue damage in chronic allergy, has made IL-5 a major target for a new generation of antiallergic drugs (Schwenger et al. 2000).

Interleukin 11

IL-11 is an important growth factor for thrombocytes. The mature IL-11 protein is a highly conserved, cationic protein of 178 amino acids. The IL-11 gene consists of five exons and four introns which contain 7 kilobase-pairs (kbp) of genomic DNA. The gene for IL-11 has been localized to the long arm of chromosome 19 at band 19q13.3–q13.4. The IL-11 gene is in close proximity to the gene that codes for the subunit of protein kinase

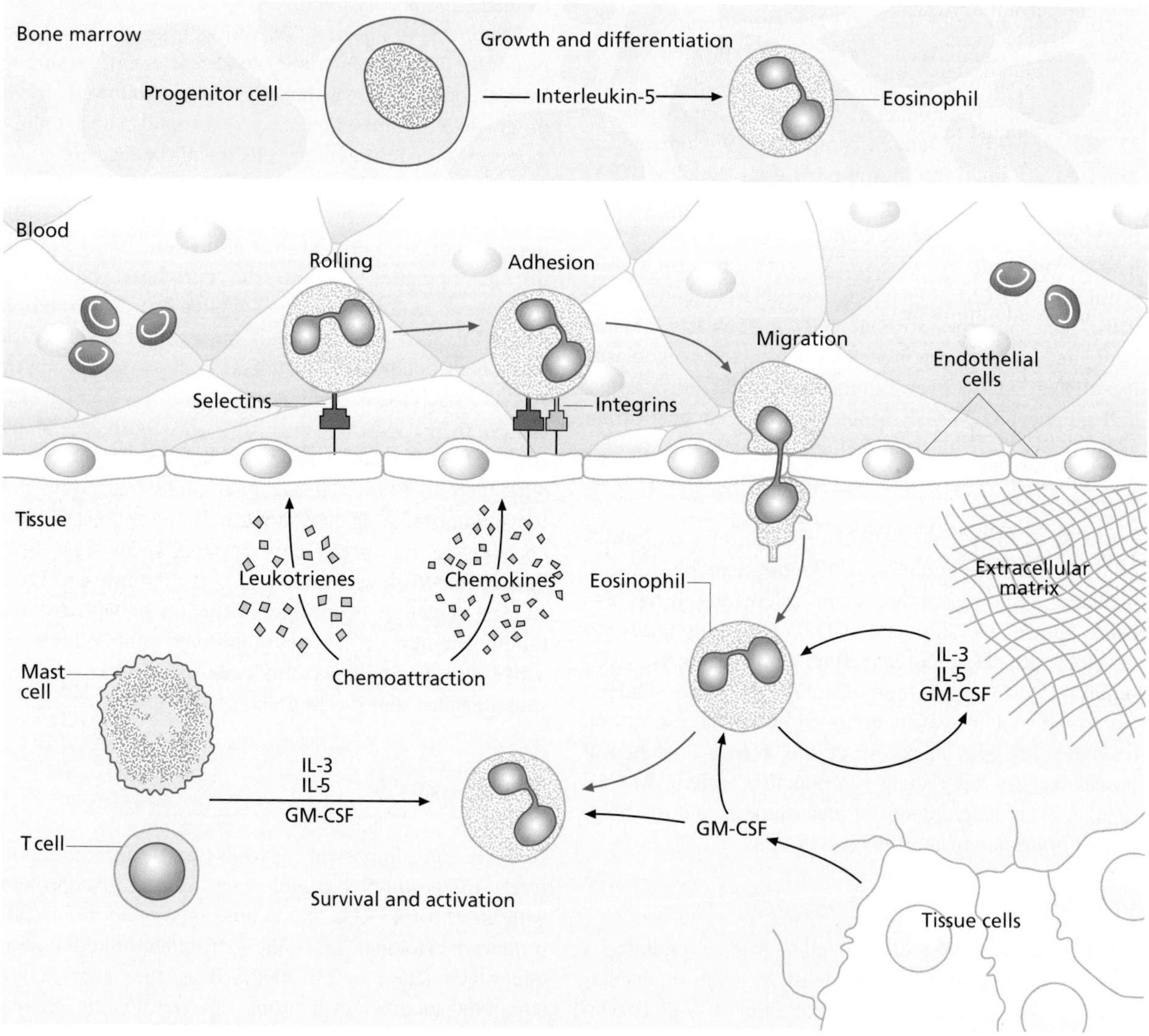

Figure 15.3 *Different activities of interleukin IL-5 on eosinophil granulocytes and in processes involved in eosinophilia. Eosinophilia develops in the bone marrow in response to the stimulation of progenitor cells by IL-5. Mature eosinophils in the blood adhere to endothelial cells through the interaction of selectins and integrins with endothelial receptors for these molecules. On exposure to chemoattractant mediators, eosinophils undergo diapedesis between endothelial cells and migrate into the tissues. The accumulation of eosinophils is regulated by the generation and survival and activation factors (IL-3, IL-5, and granulocyte–macrophage colony-stimulating factor [GM-CSF]) by T cells and mast cells. In response to extracellular matrix components, eosinophils themselves can also generate the cytokines and prolong their survival. (Redrawn from Rothenberg 1998, with permission.)*

C, as well as the genes for several zinc finger proteins (Keith 2000).

Basal and inducible IL-11 mRNA expression can be detected in fibroblasts, epithelial cells, chondrocytes, synoviocytes, keratinocytes, endothelial cells, osteoblasts, and certain tumor cells and cell lines (Table 15.3).

IL-11 has several activities. Human IL-11, in synergy with IL-3, IL-4, IL-6, or SCF, supports murine primitive hemopoietic cell. IL-11 can induce production of the same acute phase proteins (APP) as IL-6. IL-11 also acts on adipocytes and osteoclasts, and reduces proinflammatory mediator production by LPS-activated macrophages. IL-11 plasma levels are significantly elevated in patients with severe thrombocytopenia secondary to myeloablative therapy or in those with immune thrombocytopenia. Platelet counts and endogenous IL-11 levels after myeloablative therapy were inversely related. Therefore, it is suggested that induction of IL-11 expression is a physiological response to thrombocytopenia in humans and that IL-11 plays a role in the regulation of megakaryocytopoiesis and thrombopoiesis during acute thrombocytopenia (Goldman 1995). Although administration of IL-11 as a single agent to normal animals primarily stimulated megakaryocytopoiesis and thrombopoiesis, in myelosuppressed animals IL-11 stimulated multilineage recovery of hemopoietic progenitor cells. Mice receiving subcutaneous human IL-11 before whole-body radiation exposure had increased numbers of surviving crypts. IL-11 produces intestinal mucosal tropic effects in rats with experimental short bowel syndrome. Administration of IL-11 was also shown to enhance survival in a murine model of radiation-induced pulmonary injury (radiation pneumonitis). IL-11 has been recently approved for use in the prevention of the severe thrombocytopenia that occurs after cancer chemotherapy. Studies of cells and tissues from other organ systems indicate that IL-11 is active in protection and restoration of the gastrointestinal mucosa, and has major effects as an immunomodulating agent as well as activity in bone metabolism (Keith 2000).

Table 15.3 *Tissue/cell types expressing interleukin IL-11*

Tissue	Cell type/cell lines
CNS	Hippocampal neurons
	Spinal motor and sympathetic neurons
	Astrocytic glioblastoma
Thymus	Myeloid? (T2)
Lung	Fibroblasts, epithelial cells
Muscle cells	
Bone	Fibroblasts, osteosarcoma cell lines, osteoblasts
Connective tissues	Chondrocytes, synoviocytes
Vein endothelial cells	
Uterus	Trophoblast, endometriotic, and endometrial tissues
Skin	Keratinocytes, melanoma cell lines
Sarcoidosis	Multinucleated giant cells
Testis	Round spermatids

From Du and Williams (1997).

GROWTH AND DIFFERENTIATION FACTORS FOR LYMPHOID CELLS

Interleukin 2

IL-2 was the first interleukin to be identified and characterized at the molecular level. IL-2 is a small (15.5 kDa) globular glycoprotein of 133 amino acids. The IL-2 gene is located in chromosome 4, band q28 (Smith 2000).

For a long time, the only cells known to express the IL-2 gene following antigen or polyclonal stimulation were T cells (Smith 1980). More recently, however, dendritic cells have also been shown to express the IL-2 gene (Granucci et al. 2003). Of note, IL-2 shares a receptor chain (γc) with other cytokines, i.e. IL-4, IL-7, IL-9, IL-15, and IL-21 (Figure 15.4), whereas its α chain (known as TAC) is specific.

One of the major activities of IL-2 is to promote the clonal expansion of both $CD4^+$ T-helper (Th) cells

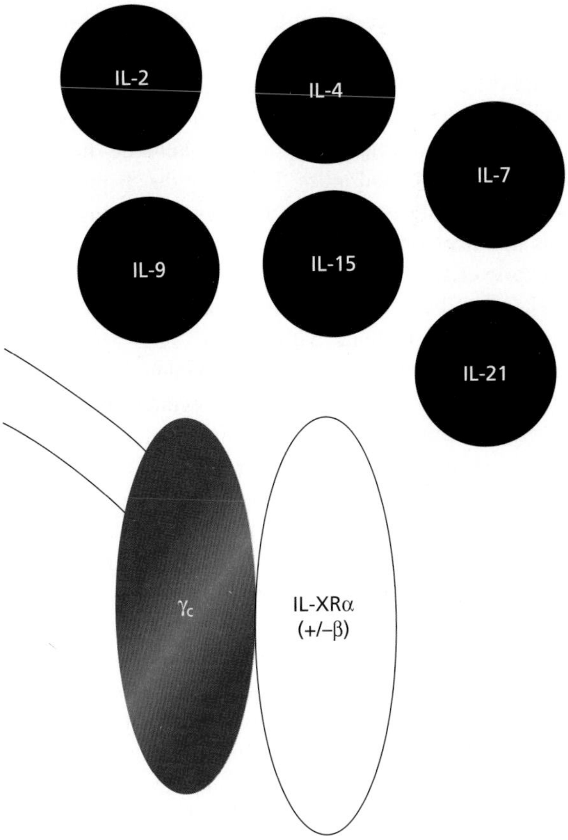

Figure 15.4 *Interleukins IL-2, IL-4, IL-7, IL-9, and IL-15 share the γ chain of their receptor. (Modified from Fry and Mackall 2002.)*

and CD8$^+$ cytotoxic T lymphocytes (CTLs). IL-2 is obligatory for the generation of both type 1 T-helper (Th1) and type 2 (Th2) cells and potentiates the production of the characteristic cytokines released by these differentiated Th cell subsets. IL-2 also synergizes with both interferon-γ (IFN-γ) and IL-12 in augmenting natural killer (NK) cell cytolytic activity. In addition, IL-2 also triggers the feedback downregulation of the expanded, differentiated effector cells. First, IL-2 is produced only transiently after antigen activation and, therefore, its positive effects rapidly disappear. Second, IL-2 withdrawal results in apoptosis, so that many of the antigen-specific effector cells are deleted as soon as there is no longer any antigen-induced IL-2 production. There are also other ways in which IL-2 gives negative signals. One is via the IL-2-promoted expression of CTLA-4, a negative regulator of T-cell receptor signals, which competes with the positive, costimulatory molecule, CD28. Thus, instead of leading to continuous cytokine production, the IL-2-promoted expression of CTLA-4 results in suppression of IL-2 gene expression. Also, IL-2 promotes the expression of Fas ligand (FasL), which activates programmed cell death via Fas, expressed to a greater extent on antigen-activated CD4$^+$ T cells (Smith 2000).

Deletion of the IL-2 gene has no effect on lymphocyte development, so that at birth IL-2 knock-out mice have normal numbers of T cells, B cells, and NK cells in both primary and secondary lymphoid compartments. However, during postnatal development a progressive lymphoid hyperplasia occurs, and cells accumulate in the secondary lymphoid tissues with an activated surface phenotype. Concomitantly, an autoimmune hemolytic anemia ensues, and mice begin to die from anemia within the first few weeks of life. Mice surviving beyond this initial phase subsequently develop colonic enteritis (Schorle et al. 1991)

IL-2 has been the first interleukin to be used therapeutically in patients with cancer. IL-2 was initially administered in these patients at very high doses intravenously. This kind of treatment regimen resulted in severe systemic toxicity ('cytokine syndrome'). IL-2 therapy results in an antitumor response in about 15 percent of individuals suffering from renal cell carcinoma, with about 10 percent of individuals achieving a long-term, complete response (Rosenberg et al. 1987), but the mechanisms responsible for this antitumor response still remain obscure, even after 15 years of IL-2 therapy. More recently, IL-2 has been used in the treatment of individuals infected with HIV (Kovacs et al. 1996). The use of the anti-TAC monoclonal antibody to prevent IL-2 binding to its high-affinity receptor, has recently been shown to be an effective immunosuppressant therapy for the prevention of allograft rejection (Vincenti et al. 1998). Accordingly, all of these approaches underscore the central role of IL-2 in the generation of an effective immune response, and the effectiveness of immunosuppressive therapies that block either IL-2 production or activity.

Interleukin 4

IL-4 is a 20-kDa secreted glycoprotein. The IL-4 gene resides on the long arm of chromosome 5 at position 5q21 within a complex that contains genes for other cytokines. The IL-4 gene is closely linked to the IL-13 gene, which lies immediately downstream of the IL-4 locus. The gene for another Th2 cytokine, IL-5, is also closely linked. The IL-3 and GM-CSF genes are located in this chromosomal region as well. The close proximity of the cytokines IL-4, IL-13, and IL-5 suggests that there may be some type of locus control to allow for coordinate expressions of these cytokines in Th2 cells (Keegan 2000).

IL-4 expression is induced in T cells and highly induced in differentiated Th2 cells and NK1.1$^+$ T cells in response to stimulation via the TCR. IL-4 message is also expressed in mast cells, basophils, and eosinophils in response to stimulation through the cell surface receptor for IgE.

IL-4 can elicit many diverse biological responses. These responses include costimulation of B-cell and T-cell proliferation, the protection of cells from spontaneous and induced apoptosis, and the regulation of chloride ion transport by intestinal epithelial cells. However, the dominant function of IL-4 is its ability to promote the differentiation of naïve CD4$^+$ T cells into the so-called Th2 profile of cytokine production (Figure 15.5). As known, Th2 cells secrete a set of cytokines, including IL-4, IL-5, IL-6, IL-10, and IL-13, that tend to favor a phagocyte-independent immune response while suppressing the phagocyte-dependent immune response controlled by Th1 cells. The second dominant function of IL-4 is its ability to drive immunoglobulin class switching to the IgG1 and IgE isotypes in mice and to the IgG4 and IgE isotypes in humans (Paul 1991). The ability of IL-4 to regulate the Th cell phenotype has direct relevance to the outcome of several diseases. Excessive IL-4 production by Th2 cells has been associated with elevated IgE production and allergy. In addition, a strong tendency towards Th2 cell differentiation can result in a failure to cure certain infections efficiently by intracellular pathogens such as *Leishmania major*, and lead to immunopathology. IL-4 also has a number of effects on monocytes. It increases expression of MHC class II molecules and IL-1Ra, while downregulating production of the proinflammatory cytokines, IL-1, TNF-α, IL-6, and IL-8. IL-4 is a growth and survival factor for mast cells. It enhances VCAM-1 expression on endothelial cells and downregulates IL-8 production. IL-4 induces eotaxin production by lung, and calcium ion secretion by gut, epithelial cells (Keegan 2000).

IL-4 has been used to treat a number of disease models in mice. It has been the most successful at

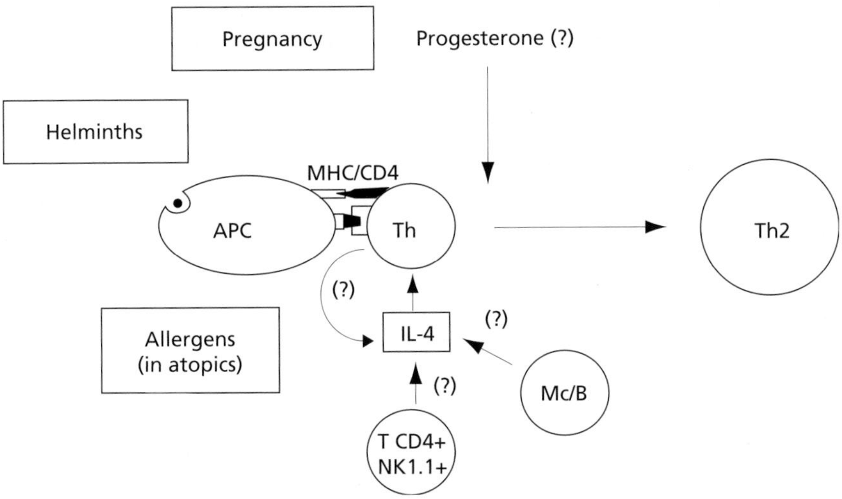

Figure 15.5 *Role of interleukin IL-4 in the differentiation of naïve T-helper (Th) cells into Th2 effectors. IL-4, produced by natural killer NK.1.1$^+$ T cells, mast cells/basophils, but mainly by naïve Th cells themselves, at the beginning of the specific immune response, is required for the differentiation of these last cells into Th2 effectors. APC, antigen-presenting cell. (Redrawn from Romagnani 1998, with permission.)*

ameliorating autoimmune diseases that are caused by activated Th1 cells. IL-4 treatment prevents the development of diabetes in NOD mice, as well the development of experimental autoimmune encephalitis (EAE) or neuritis. Although initially characterized as a growth and survival factor, IL-4 has been shown to suppress the growth of some cancer cells in vivo. This inhibition is seen in the absence of T cells and depends on the infiltration of eosinophil granulocytes and the inhibition of tumor angiogenesis. IL-4 has been used systemically as an aid to cell-based therapy for cancer. Bolus injection of IL-4 results in flu-like symptoms, gastrointestinal upset, asymptomatic liver damage, severe allergy-type symptoms in the nasal mucosa, and vascular leak syndrome. However, IL-4 does not have apparent toxicity if administered locally (Saleh et al. 1999).

Interleukin 7

IL-7 is a single-chain glycoprotein of 25 kDa. The human IL-7 gene is located on chromosome 8, bands q13 (Spits 2000).

The main cell types that express the gene are bone marrow stroma, thymic stroma, intestinal epithelial cells and keratinocytes, mature but not immature dendritic cells, dendritic cells derived from CD34$^+$ cord blood cells cultured with GM-CSF and TNF-α, and platelets (Wiles et al. 1992; Watanabe et al. 1995).

Gene-targeting studies in the mouse have demonstrated that IL-7 is a major factor involved in development of T and B lymphocytes. In humans, IL-7 plays an essential role in the development of T cells (Figure 15.6). IL-7 also has effects on human B-cell precursors, but it does not seem to be essential for human B-cell development. Whether IL-7 is actually a growth factor for immature thymocytes is somewhat controversial, but it is well established that IL-7 acts as a growth/maturation factor for human thymocyte precursors. IL-7 has also been reported directly to augment cytolytic activity in human NK cells, even if less efficiently than IL-2. Several reports have documented effects of IL-7 on both development and function of cells of the myeloid lineages. IL-7 also enhances myeloid colony formation from CD34$^+$ cells in vitro and may play a role in the function of mature monocyte–macrophages by inducing secretion of cytokines and increasing tumoricidal activity (Spits 2000).

The activities of IL-7 on T cells have led to the proposal that IL-7 can be used to overcome immunodeficiencies in certain situations by accelerating T-cell development, expanding the pool of newly developed T cells, and promoting functional maturation of T cells. However, more studies are necessary to evaluate the effects of IL-7 on immune reconstitution.

Interleukin 9

IL-9 protein sequence contains 144 residues with a signal peptide of 18 amino acids. The human IL-9 gene is a single copy gene and was mapped on chromosome 5, in the 5q31q35 region, which contains various growth factor and growth factor receptor genes such as IL-3, IL-4, IL-5, GM-CSF, and CSF-1 receptor (CSF-1R) (Renauld 2000).

So far, IL-9 expression seems to be mainly restricted to activated CD4$^+$CD45RO$^+$ T cells (Houssiau et al. 1995), HTLVI- infected T-cell leukemias (Kelleher et al. 1991), and Hodgkin's cell lines (Merz et al. 1991). Polyclonal T-cell stimulants induce a substantial IL-9 expression by T-cell-enriched lymphocyte populations, and more specifically, by CD4$^+$CD45RO$^+$ T cells. IL-9 expression appears in the late stages of T-cell activation, with a peak at 28 h. IL-2 was identified as a major

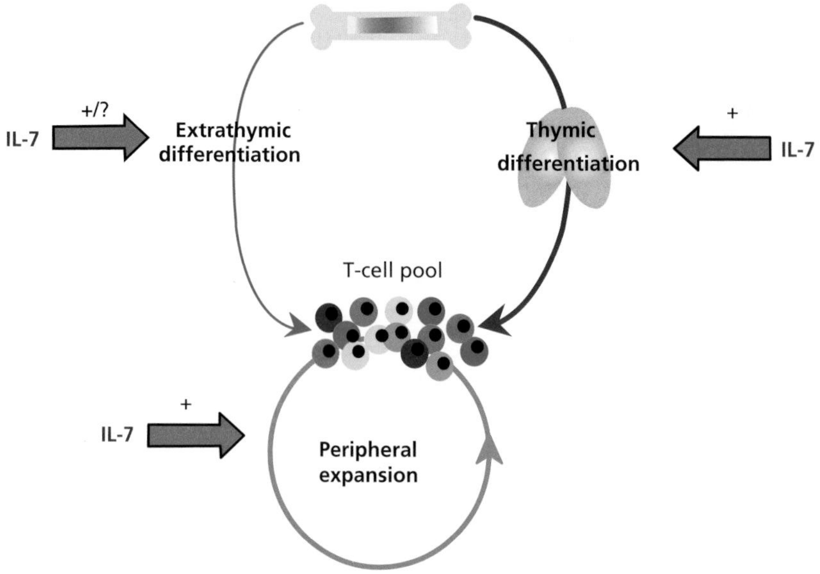

Figure 15.6 *Modulation of T-cell regenerative pathways by the interleukin IL-7. After T-cell depletion, regeneration of the peripheral T-cell pool can occur through multiple mechanisms. Thymic differentiation is the predominant pathway through which new T cells are generated if thymic capacity is sufficient. However, with diminished thymic function related to therapy-related toxicity, or age-related decline, the peripheral expansion of remaining mature T cells can substantially regenerate the T-cell pool. Extrathymic differentiation from bone marrow progenitors is a relatively minor pathway through which new T cells develop. IL-7 can profoundly increase thymic differentiation, peripheral expansion, and potentially extrathymic differentiation pathways to T-cell regeneration. (Redrawn from Fry and Mackall 2002, with permission.)*

mediator of IL-9 expression, because anti-TAC antibodies completely block this process.

Several studies indicate that IL-9 not only is involved in the late growth of T cells, but also induces the proliferation and differentiation of mast cells. Other potential biological targets for IL-9 include B lymphocytes, eosinophils, and hemopoietic progenitors. IL-9 might play an important role in the immune response against intestinal parasites such as helminths, probably by contributing to the development of mucosal mast cell hyperplasia induced by worm infections. Resistance to *Trichuris muris* was found to correlate with the production of IL-5 and IL-9 in mesenteric lymph nodes. The existence of an IL-9-mediated autocrine loop has been suggested for Hodgkin's disease. In addition, both genetic and experimental evidence points to the implication of IL-9 in the pathogenesis of asthma (Figure 15.7). The potential activity of IL-9 in autoimmunity models is illustrated by preliminary data obtained in nonobese diabetic (NOD) mice (Renauld 2000).

Interleukin 15

IL-15 is a 15-kDa glycoprotein whose mature form consists of 114 amino acids. The IL-15 gene was mapped to chromosome 4q31. The classic long (48 amino acids) signal peptide associated with all secreted IL-15 is encoded by a 1.6 kbp cDNA (Waldmann and Tagaya 2000).

There is widespread constitutive expression of IL-15 mRNA in a variety of tissues (Waldmann and Tagaya 2000). IL-15 stimulates the proliferation of activated $CD4^+$ and $CD8^+$ T cells and dendritic epidermal T cells. IL-15 does not have any effect on resting B cells, but it induces proliferation and immunoglobulin synthesis by B cells costimulated with phorbol myristate acetate or an immobilized anti-IgM antibody. However, the most critical function of IL-15 is a pivotal role in the development, survival, and activation of NK cells (Figure 15.8). IL-15 also has unique functions on nonlymphoid cells, including mast cells and muscle, brain, and microglial cells. The action of IL-15 on T cells, B cells, and NK cells can be blocked by selective antibodies to the IL-2/15Rβ chain. IL-15 acting through the IL-2/15Rβ and γc receptors leads to the induction of the expression of IL-2Rα by T lymphocytes.

Failure to produce IL-15 has not been demonstrated in disease states, although presumably it would be associated with the absence of NK cell development. Abnormalities involving increased IL-15 expression have been reported in inflammatory autoimmune diseases. IL-15 may precede tumor necrosis factor-α (TNF-α) in the cytokine cascade and suggest a role for IL-15 in development of rheumatoid arthritis, as well as in other inflammatory diseases, including active ulcerative colitis, Crohn's disease, type C chronic liver disease, sarcoidosis, T-cell-mediated alveolitis, and multiple sclerosis. Furthermore, the observation that IL-15 stimulates mast cell proliferation suggests a potential role for this cytokine in mastocytosis. IL-15 was shown to help correct impaired proliferative responses of $CD4^+$ lymphocytes studied ex vivo from HIV-infected individuals. Thus, as IL-15 is associated with less severe capillary leak syndrome than

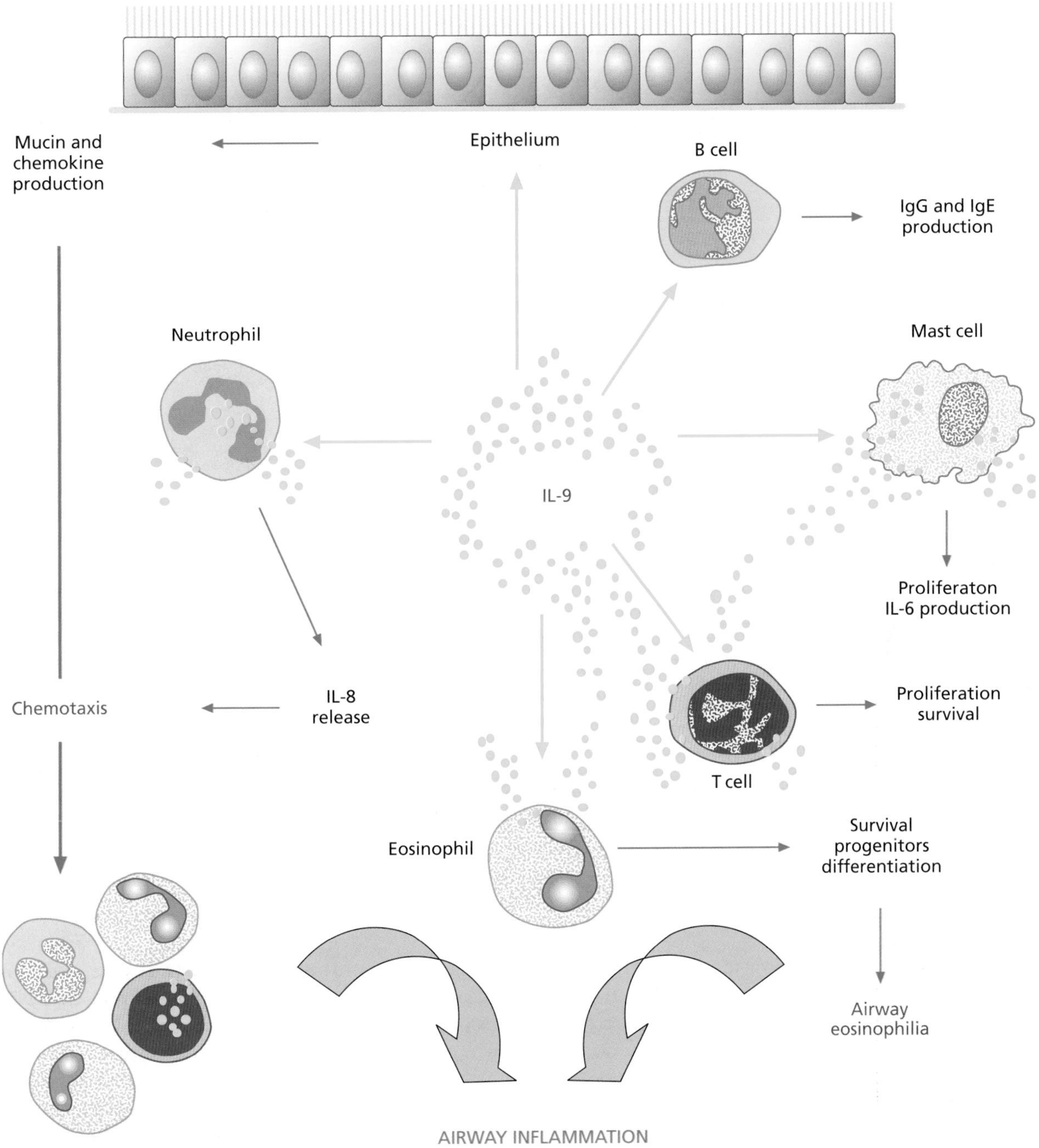

Figure 15.7 *Role of the interleukin IL-9 in pathophysiological manifestations of allergic inflammation and bronchial asthma. IL-9, a T-helper 2 (Th2) cytokine, has a pleiotropic activity on inflammatory and structural cells associated with asthma, such as mast cells, T cells, eosinophils, and epithelial cells. Within the lung, IL-9 is mainly produced by T cells and, to a lesser extent, by granulocytes. The effect of IL-9 leads to various immunological processes, including eosinophil survival, chemokines, and mucus production. These pathways may provide a potential mechanism to explain airway inflammation. (Redrawn from Soussi-Gonoussi et al. 2001, with permission.)*

the IL-2 molecule, it could provide an alternate therapeutic option to IL-2 in the treatment of patients with select tumors or AIDS (Waldmann and Tagaya 2000).

Interleukin 21

IL-21 is a four-helix-bundle cytokine with 131 amino acids that has significant sequence with homology to IL-2, IL-4, and IL-15. The IL-21R has highest homology to the IL-2Rβ chain and the IL-4Rα chain. On ligand binding, IL-21R has been reported to associate with the common γ chain, a property that it shares with receptors for IL-2, IL-4, IL-7, IL-9, and IL-15. The main source for IL-21 seems to be activated T lymphocytes. IL-21 apparently influences the functions of B cells, T cells, and NK cells (Parish-Novak et al. 2000). Moreover,

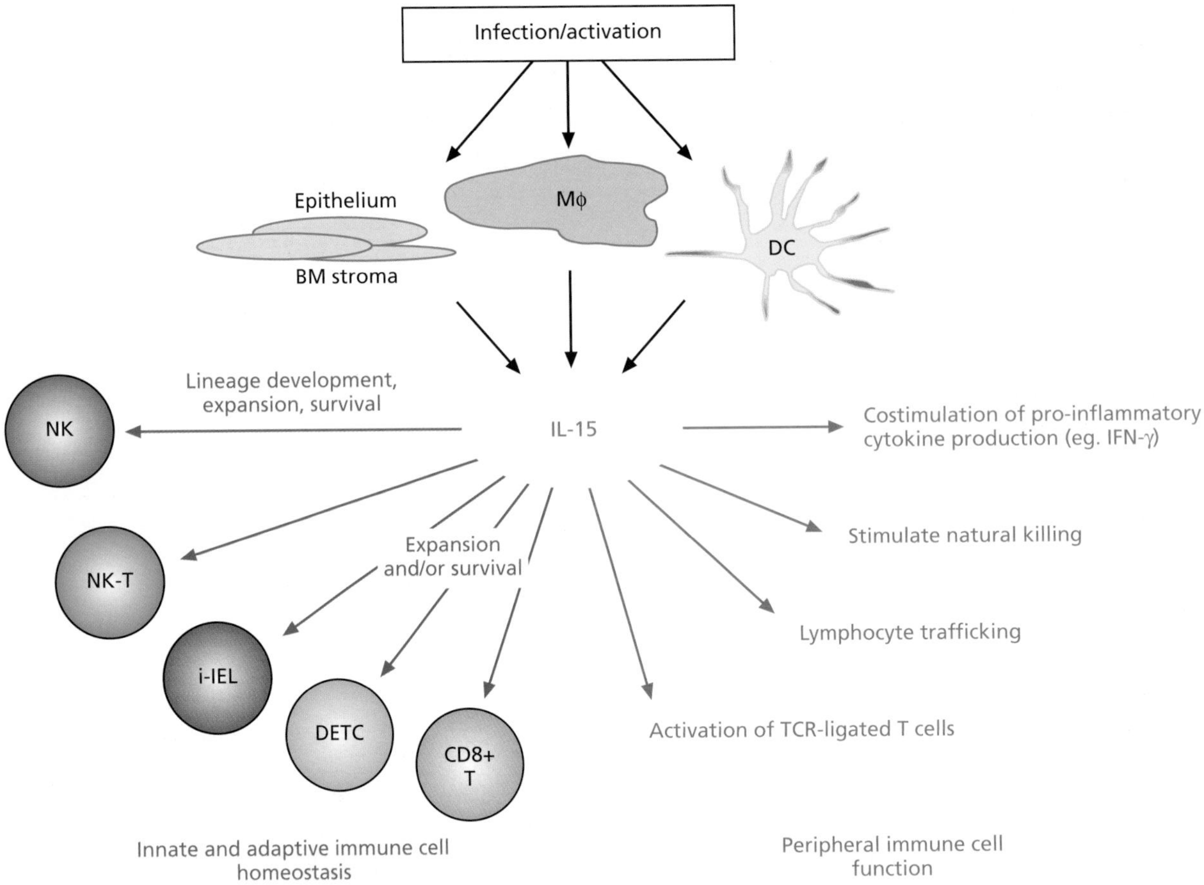

Figure 15.8 *Role of interleukin IL-15 in natural killer (NK) cell development, lymphocytes homeostasis, and peripheral immune functions. Multiple cell types elaborate IL-15, including activated monocytes/macrophages, dendritic cells, and epithelium, as well as constitutive production by bone marrow stromal cells. IL-15 has a critical role in the development of NK lineage, as well as in its survival, expansion, and function. Other innate lymphocyte (NK-T, CD8αα intestinal intraepithelial lymphocytes, TCRγδ DETCs) and memory phenotype CD8$^+$ T cells depend on IL-15 for survival or expansion. DETC, dendritic epidermal T-cells; IFN, interferon; Mϕ, macrophage; TCR, T-cell receptor. (Redrawn from Fehniger and Caligiuri 2001, with permission.)*

IL-21 has recently been shown to exert a proliferative effect on human myeloma cells and to inhibit the apoptosis of the IL-6-dependent human myeloma cell lines with a potency close to that of IL-6 (Brenne et al. 2002).

Interleukin 27

IL-27 is a new heterodimeric cytokine composed of EB13 (an IL-12 p40-related protein) and p28 (a new IL-12 p35-related polypeptide). It represents an early product of activated antigen-presenting cells (APC) and induces the proliferation of naïve, but not memory, CD4$^+$ T cells. It also synergizes with IL-12 for the development of Th1 cells via the receptor TCCR/WSX-1 (Pflanz et al. 2002).

PROINFLAMMATORY CYTOKINES

Interleukin 1

There are two distinct species of IL-1, which have been named as IL-1α and IL-1β, respectively. IL-1α is initially synthesized as a (31-kDa) precursor molecule without a signal peptide, mature IL-1α being a 17.5-kDa molecule. Calpain, a calcium-activated cysteine protease, is responsible for the cleavage of the IL-1α precursor (Dinarello 2000b). IL-1β is initially synthesized as a precursor molecule (31 kDa) without a signal peptide. Mature IL-1β is a 17-kDa molecule. The IL-1β-converting enzyme (ICE) is primarily responsible for cleavage of the precursor intracellularly, but other proteases can also process the IL-1β precursor into an active cytokine (Dinarello 2000a, 2000b).

Blood monocytes and tissue macrophages are the main sources of IL-1α and IL-1β. However, unlike IL-1β, IL-1α is found constitutively expressed also in keratinocytes and other epithelial cells. Virtually all microbes and microbial products induce the production of both IL-1α and IL-1β. The main differences between the two cytokines are summarized in Table 15.4.

IL-1 induces neutrophilia and the production of acute phase proteins (APP), and the injection of modest doses of IL-1 into mice results in fever, anorexia, and the production of circulating IL-6. The most dramatic

Table 15.4 *A comparison of interleukins IL-1α and IL-1β*

IL-1α	IL-1β
Pro-IL-1α is active	Pro-IL-1β is inactive
Active membrane form is IL-1α	Membrane IL-1β not observed
Mature IL-1α does not circulate	Mature IL-1β circulates
Nuclear localization	No nuclear localization
Intracellular role for pro-IL-1α	No intracellular role for pro-IL-1β
Neutralizing autoantibodies	Non-neutralizing autoantibodies
Calpain cleavage of pro-IL-1α	ICE and PR-3 cleavage of pro-IL-1β
No disease link with calpain expression	Disease link with ICE expression
No correlation	Correlation with bone resorption
IL-1α knock-out mice normal	IL-1β knock-out mice resistant to disease
Anti-IL-1α ineffective in CIA	Anti-IL-1β effective in CIA
IL-1α expression in AML absent	IL-1β expression in AML present
No data	ICE inhibition→reduced brain ischemia
No data	ICE inhibition→reduced AML proliferation
No data	ICE antisense→reduced AML proliferation

AML, acute myeloid leukemia; CIA, collagen-induced arthritis; ICE, IL-1β-converting enzyme; PR-3, a compound used for cleavage.
From Dinarello (2000b).

responses to the pharmacological effects of IL-1 are observed in humans. The role of IL-1 in human disease states is best revealed by the response of humans to parenterally administered IL-1. Chills and fever are observed in nearly all patients. The febrile response increases in magnitude with increasing dose, and chills and fever can be abated with indometacin (indomethacin) treatment. IL-1 is also a potent immunoadjuvant for several tumors. IL-1 has been administered to patients during receipt of ABMT. The treatment with IL-1 of ABM or SC transfer resulted in an earlier recovery of thrombocytopenia compared with controls (Dinarello 2000b).

Interleukin 6

Human IL-6 is a protein of 186 amino acids glycosylated at positions 73 and 172. It is synthesized as a precursor protein of 212 amino acids. At least five different molecular forms of IL-6 with molecular masses from 21 to 28 kDa are expressed in monocytes. The IL-6 gene has a length of approximately 5 kb and maps to human chromosome 7p21 between the markers D7S135 and D7S370 (Matsuda and Hirano 2000).

IL-6 is produced by a variety of cell types. The main sources are macrophages, fibroblasts, and endothelial cells, but also T and B cells. The IL-6 receptor consists of two subunits: the α chain (IL-6R), an 80-kDa transmembrane glycoprotein that binds IL-6 with low affinity, and the β chain (gp130), a 130-kDa transmembrane glycoprotein that binds to the IL-6–IL-6R heterodimer to form the high-affinity signal transducing complex (Matsuda and Hirano 2000).

IL-6 induces immunoglobulin production by normal activated or EBV-transformed or leukemic B cells. IL-6 is involved in T-cell activation, growth, and differentiation. IL-6 synergizes with IL-3 to induce the proliferation of murine pluripotent hemopoietic progenitors in vitro. Human megakaryocytes were demonstrated to express IL-6 receptor and produce IL-6, suggesting that IL-6 regulates the terminal maturation of megakaryocytes in an autocrine manner. However, the most important function of IL-6 is to induce the biosynthesis by hepatocytes of APPs, such as fibrinogen, α1-antichymotrypsin, haptoglobulin, serum amyloid A, and C-reactive protein (CRP) (Geiger et al. 1988). As a result of the ability of IL-6 to act as a growth factor for plasmacytoma, myeloma, and hybridoma cells, different inhibitors of IL-6, such as anti-IL-6 monoclonal antibody and mutated IL-6, might be used to treat patients with multiple myeloma, Castleman's disease, and rheumatoid arthritis (Hirano 1998).

TNF-α

TNF-α under denaturing conditions is about 17 kDa. Under native conditions, however, TNF-α is a trimer with an approximate molecular mass of 50 kDa. The TNF-α gene is localized on human chromosome 6 in a region between p23 and q12 (p21.1 and p21.3) (Aggarwal et al. 2000).

Although first isolated from a macrophage-like cell line, it is now clear that TNF is produced by a wide variety of different cell types, including macrophages and monocytes, T, B, and NK cells, astrocytes, fibroblasts, basophils, mast cells, Kupffer cells, smooth muscle cells, and epidermal cells, as well as neoplastic cells from breast tumor, ovarian tumor, prostate tumor, pancreatic cancer, glioblastoma, melanoma, and leukemia. However, monocytes/macrophages are probably the major sources of TNF in most conditions (Aggarwal and Vilcek 1992).

Tumor necrosis factor binds to two different receptors referred to as p60 (also called p55, or type I or CD120a) and p80 (also called p75, or type II or CD120b) based on their molecular weight. These two receptors are homologous in their extracellular domains, but distinct in their intracellular domains. The p60 receptor is expressed on all cell types, whereas the p80 form is expressed chiefly on cells of the hemopoietic and immune system, as well as on endothelial cells. The binding of TNF to its receptor can be displaced by lymphotoxin, suggesting that they have a common receptor.

The true normal physiological role of TNF in vivo is unclear. TNF is an inflammatory cytokine, because of its chemotactic activity on monocytes and neutrophils. Moreover, stimulation with TNF induces phagocytosis, and adherence of these cells to endothelial cells, as well as generation of free radicals of oxygen, superoxide anion, and hydrogen peroxide. Therefore, it is believed that TNF is important for protection against bacterial, fungal, parasitic, and perhaps even viral infections and other stressful stimuli. Besides hemorrhagic necrosis, whether TNF is able to block tumorigenesis and metastasis in vivo is still not fully understood (Lejeune et al. 1998). Administration of TNF to various animals leads to hemorrhage, necrosis, local inflammation, shock, and death. Prolonged exposure to TNF causes anorexia, loss of body weight, dehydration, and loss of body proteins and lipids. This condition, called cachexia, may occur during chronic parasitic, bacterial, and viral infections. The symptoms also appear in cancer patients. The mediator involved in this process was named cachectin, later recognized to be the same as TNF. In severe diseases such as AIDS, the TNF level is significantly increased when the signs and symptoms of cachexia develop. Stimulation of cultured human endothelial cells with TNF induces procoagulant activity. TNF-induced endothelial cell activation leads to the structural reorganization of the endothelium, resulting in vascular leakiness that is partly caused by its capacity to upregulate vascular endothelial growth factor (VEGF). The main activities of TNF-α are summarized in Figure 15.9. TNF is considered as a major mediator of septic shock, because it is overproduced during sepsis and administration of high doses of TNF-inducing LPS causes shock and tissue injury that are identical to sepsis (Aggarwal et al. 2000).

Lymphotoxins

Lymphotoxin (LT) was initially discovered as a secreted cytotoxic/cytostatic factor produced by activated lymphocytes. It was then recognized as a member of a large superfamily (Table 15.5). A distinct cell surface form of LT was defined as a heterotrimer made up of a subunit of LT with a dimer of a 33-kDa protein, designated LTβ, the third member of the family. The soluble LT is known as LTα, which was previously called TNF-β. The cell surface form of LT is formed by two subunits, LTα and LTβ. Two distinct heterotrimers are formed, LTαβ2 (major form) and LTα2β1. LTα is TNF splicing factor (SF)1 and LTβ is TNFSF3. LTα is a secreted glycoprotein of 171 amino acids with a secondary structure of antiparallel sandwich structure which assembles into a relatively compact trimer, a feature common to all members of the TNF superfamily. LTβ is a type II transmembrane glycoprotein (N-terminal cytosolic tail), which lacks a signal cleavage sequence and is retained in the membrane. LTβ is biologically active as a heterotrimer with LTα. The LTαβ ligand remains anchored to the cell membrane and, as such, acts in a localized fashion that requires cell-to-cell contact. By contrast, LTα lacks a retained transmembrane domain and is exclusively secreted as a homotrimer. TNF, LTα, and LTβ form a contiguous cytokine locus that resides on chromosome 6p21.3 (chromosome 17 in mouse) within the major histocompatibility gene complex (MHC). The LTα, LTβ, and TNF genes show similar intron and exon organization (Wallach et al. 1999), which is largely conserved for all members of the TNF superfamily.

The main sources of LTα and LTβ are activated T and B lymphocytes, but LTs are also produced by NK and lymphokine-activated killer (LAK) cells in response to IL-2. LTα binds to the receptors TNFRI and TNFRII with high affinity, and to HVEM with low affinity; LTα2β1 binds to the LTβR, whereas the LTα2β1 complex binds LTβ R weakly (25 nmol/l), but TNFRI and TNFRII with high affinity (Ware et al. 1998).

The in vitro biological responses to LTα and LTβ are very similar. However, based on dose–response curves, LTα is typically less potent compared with TNF in inducing most functions. LTα behaves as a partial agonist of TNF in some assays, such as induction of MHC molecules, intercellular adhesion molecule 1 (ICAM-1), and other types of markers of inflammatory reactions. LTα1β2 displays even weaker potency for induction of proinflammatory markers on various cell types, including endothelial cells. LTs play a role in the initiation of inflammation, which presumably contributes to the protection against microbes. LTα can also induce expression of adhesion molecules and chemokines, whereas LTαβ does not appear to be able to induce adhesion molecules, but can induce chemokines. LTα and LTβ may play normal roles in tumor immunity. LTα induces apoptosis (programmed cell death) in several tumor lines in vitro and LTα1β2 induces killing of a more limited array of tumor cells. This effect is the result of the action of a distinct types of receptor; LTα uses TNFRI, a death domain proapoptotic signaling receptor that directly activates the caspase pathway,

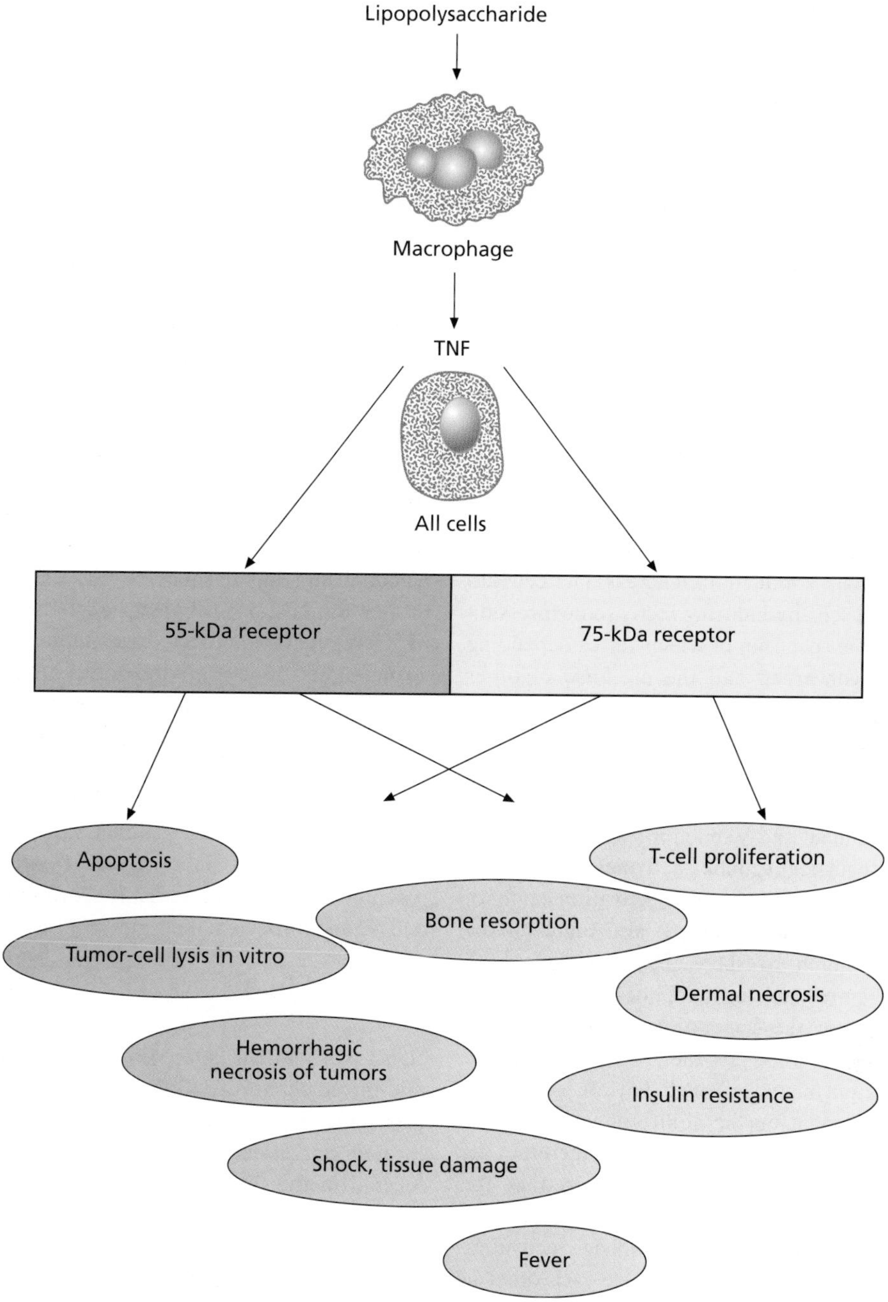

Figure 15.9 *Range of actions of tumor necrosis factor α (TNF-α). In response to inflammatory stimuli, such as lipopolysaccharide (LPS), macrophages produce TNF-α. TNF-α binds to receptors present on virtually all cells throughout the body, causing a variety of reactions. (Redrawn from Bazzoni and Beutler 1996, with permission.)*

whereas LTα1β2 uses the LTβR, a TRAF-binding receptor and a potent activator of apoptotic inhibitory pathways, such as NF-κB transcription factor (Ware et al. 1998). LT gene-deficient mice lack most lymph nodes, do not have Peyer's patches, and have disorganized spleens (Alimzhanov et al. 1997). LTs are elevated in several human diseases, including multiple sclerosis, juvenile rheumatoid arthritis, juvenile spondylarthropathy, and Crohn's disease, suggesting an important role of LTs in these disorders.

Interferon-γ

In its biologically active form, IFN-γ is a 34-kDa homodimer stabilized by noncovalent forces. The IFN-γ gene maps close to the D12S335 and D12S313 microsatellites and shows physical linkage with the *MDM2* oncogene on chromosome band 12q15 (Billiau and Vandenbroeck 2000).

Interferon-γ is a typical lymphokine, being produced almost exclusively by NK cells and certain subpopula-

Table 15.5 *Members of the tumor necrosis factor (TNF) ligand and TNF receptor family*

Ligand	Source of ligand	Receptor	Distribution of receptor
TNF-α	Macrophages	55-kDa	Many cell types
LTα	Macrophages	55-kDa	Many cell types
LTβ	T cells, others	75-kDa	T cells, B cells, others
Fas-L	T cells, others	LTβ receptor	Many cell types
NGF	NA	NGF receptor	Neurons, others
C40L	T cells	NGF receptor	B cells, T cells
CD27L	T cells	CD27	T cells
CD30L	T cells	CD30	T cells, B cells, others
OX-40L	T cells	OX40	T cells
4-1BBL	T cells	4-1BB	T cells

LT, lymphotoxin; NA, not applicable; NGF, nerve growth factor. Reproduced from Bazzoni and Beutler (1996), with permission.

tions of T cells. Both $CD4^+$ and $CD8^+$ lymphocytes can produce IFN-γ, but only Th1 cells produce IFN-γ following appropriate stimulation, whereas Th2 cells do not. IFN-γ acts on cells by inducing increased expression of several genes, the spectrum of which varies depending on the cell type concerned and the presence of other cytokines, some of which (e.g. IFN-γ) synergize with IFN-γ, whereas others (e.g. IL-4) antagonize its activities. Receptors for IFN-γ occur on virtually all cells of the body, so that many organs and systems undergo the action of IFN-γ (Billiau and Vandenbroeck 2000).

Interferon-γ regulates cellular activities responsible for inflammation, in particular the activation state of macrophages and endothelial cells. It also regulates the antigen-specific immune response by affecting both APCs and antigen-recognizing lymphocytes. IFN-γ has an important role in the generation of NO. Another important function of IFN-γ is the induction of MHC class II antigens on many, although not all, cell types, thus enhancing or inducing the ability of these cells to present foreign antigens. IFN-γ can also increase the expression of MHCI antigen. It is recognized as the most important cytokine converting macrophages from a 'resting' to an 'activated' state (macrophage activating factor (MAF)). IFN-γ and IL-4 antagonize each other in a variety of systems, and it has been established that antibody responses in fact depend on the balance between two categories of cytokines, IFN-γ and IL-2 produced by Th1 cells and IL-4, IL-5, IL-6, and IL-10 produced by Th2 cells. In this context, IFN-γ suppresses IgG1 and IgE and stimulates IgG2a antibody formation. Thus IFN-γ is not only important in the initial phase (aspecific inflammatory and antigen presenting) and in the middle phase (expansion and differentiation of antigen-reactive lymphocyte clones), but also in the end phase (sustained or final inflammation) of immune reactions. Defects in the IFN-γ mechanism are associated with severe impairment of resistance to infections caused by viruses and certain bacteria, in particular those normally killed by activated macrophages. Massive production of IFN-γ, occurring as part of so-called acute cytokine release syndromes, is often associated with severe systemic manifestations, such as generalized bleeding and lethal shock. IFN-γ has the potential to protect the host against virus infection, not only because of its regulatory activity on immunocytes, but also by virtue of its direct antiviral effect on most cell types. IFN-γ contributes to protection against tumors, as shown by studies in which the rejection of some immunogenic autologous or isologous tumors was abrogated by administration of neutralizing anti-IFN-γ antibodies. In children suffering from exceptional susceptibility to mycobacterial infections, inherited deficiencies in the IFN-γ receptor system have recently been described (Billiau and Vandenbroeck 2000).

Interleukin-12

IL-12 is a 70-kDa heterodimer composed of two disulfide-linked chains of 35 kDa (p35) and 40 kDa (p40). The genes encoding the two heterologous chains of IL-12 are located on different chromosomes. In humans, p40 is located in the 5q31–q33 region, whereas p35 has been mapped to 3p12–p13.2. Secretion of the biologically active IL-12 heterodimer (p70) is regulated at the level of p40 chain transcription. The p40 gene is highly inducible and expressed only in IL-12-secreting cells, whereas the p35 gene is expressed ubiquitously (Esche et al. 2000).

IL-12 was initially recognized as an inducer of IFN-γ synthesis by resting human peripheral blood mononuclear cells (PBMC) in vitro and as being capable of synergizing with IL-2 to increase cytotoxic lymphocyte responses. IL-12 also represents a growth factor for activated $CD4^+$ T cells, $CD8^+$ T cells, and NK cells, and most importantly it promotes Th1-specific immune responses (Manetti et al. 1994) (Figure 15.10). Thus, IL-12 enhances host defenses against organisms that are controlled by cells mediating the delayed hypersensitivity response of T cells.

Dendritic cells are the most powerful producer of IL-12 when stimulated with CD154 (CD40L) or IL-12. Epidermal Langerhans' cells express IL-12 p40 mRNA,

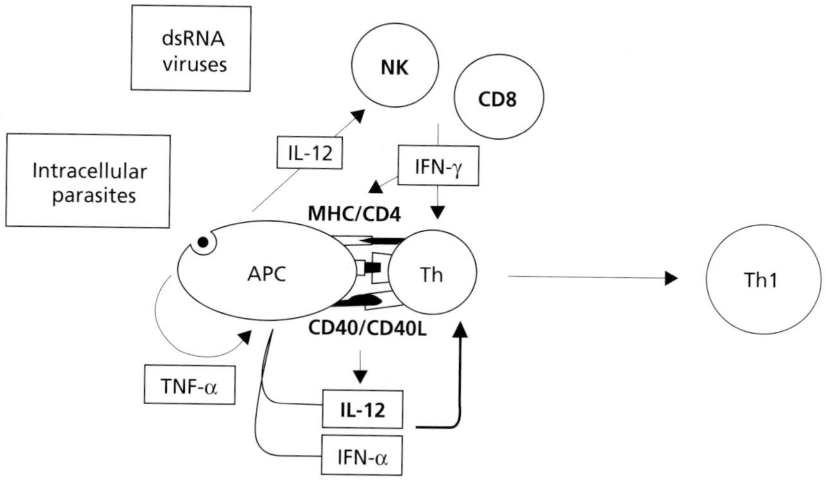

Figure 15.10 *Role of IL-12 in the differentiation of naïve T-helper (Th) cells into Th1 effectors. Intracellular bacteria and some viruses strongly activate dendritic cells and macrophages to produce interferon α (IFN-α) and IL-12, as well as natural killer (NK cells) to produce IFN-γ. Under these microenvironmental conditions and in the absence of IL-4, naïve Th cells responsible for the subsequent specific immune response differentiate into Th1 effectors. (Reproduced from Romagnani 1998, with permission.)*

as well as p40 and functional p70 protein. Stimulated macrophages produce both p40 and p70. Although monomeric p40 is typically secreted in large excess over the p70 heterodimer, only the latter is biologically active. In humans, the homodimer binds with a much lower affinity than the heterodimer and therefore acts as an antagonist only at much higher concentration. IL-12-induced production of large amounts of IFN-γ from resting and activated T and NK cells requires the presence of low levels of both TNF-α and IL-1. IL-12 is also capable of inducing its own inhibitor IL-10, a negative-feedback mechanism that limits ongoing T-cell activation. IL-12 promotes the generation and potentiates the activity of cytotoxic T lymphocytes (CTL) and LAK cells (Trinchieri 1998).

This array of activities suggests clinical potential for IL-12 as an anti-infective and antitumor agent. The lack of IL-12R expression indeed results in a human immunodeficiency characterized by strong reduction in resistance to infections caused by intracellular bacteria. The attempt to administrate IL-12 in patients with cancer has been hampered by adverse events that are mostly IFN-γ dependent and include fever, chills, fatigue, headache, nausea, vomiting, cough, myalgia, dizziness, insomnia, anemia, neutropenia, lymphocytopenia, thrombocytopenia, hyperglycemia, liver function test abnormalities, rhinitis, stomatitis, and colitis. Three deaths have also been reported in renal carcinoma patients receiving IL-12, but prior exposure to IL-12 has been shown to protect against IL-12 toxicity (Leonard et al. 1997).

Interleukin 16

IL-16 is a 55-kDa protein which appears as a single 17-kDa band on sodium dodecylsulfate (SDS) gel electrophoresis, prompting the hypothesis of a monomeric polypeptide autoaggregated into tetramers. The IL-16 gen is located in chromosome 15q26.1 (Center et al. 2000).

IL-16 is synthesized by a variety of cell types although it was first identified as a $CD8^+$ lymphocyte cell product. $CD8^+$ T cells release IL-16 in response to stimulation by mitogens, antigens, or vasoactive amines such as histamine and serotonin (Laberge et al. 1996). For histamine, H_2-type receptors are required based on inhibition of secretion by H_2-, but not H_1-, receptor antagonists. Histamine has no effect on the secretion of IL-16 from $CD4^+$ T cells. Serotonin has similar effects on $CD8^+$ T cells via S2 receptors, but no effect on $CD4^+$ T cells.

IL-16 was initially described as a chemoattractant with specificity for $CD4^+$ T cells. It was later observed that IL-16 is also a potent chemoattractant for all peripheral immune cells expressing CD4, including $CD4^+$ monocytes, eosinophils, and dendritic cells. The role of IL-16 in vivo remains to be elucidated; however, one possibility is that it contributes at least in part to antigen-independent, nonclonal recruitment and priming of $CD4^+$ cells in inflammatory processes, whereas the same cells become unresponsive to specific antigen stimulation. This condition may result in the increase of the number of viable cells recruited to an inflammatory site by reducing the susceptibility of those cells to antigen-induced cell death (AICD). As a result of these activities, IL-16 has to be considered as a proinflammatory cytokine. It may play an important role in the pathogenesis of diseases characterized by $CD4^+$ cellular infiltration, such as bronchial asthma and granulomatous diseases (Center et al. 2000).

Interleukin 17 family

IL-17 is secreted, after cleavage of a signal peptide of 23 amino acids, as a glycoprotein homodimer of

155 amino acids with an M_r ranging from 22 to 15 kDa. IL-17 gene has been mapped to chromosome 2 (2q31).

IL-17 appears to be mostly expressed by activated $CD4^+$ T cells, in particular by $CD4/^+$CD45RO 'memory' T cells. All T-cell activation signals upregulate IL-17 gene transcription. Analysis of T-cell clones suggests that both Th1 and Th2 $CD4^+$ subsets can express IL-17 at comparable levels. The IL-17R is ubiquitously expressed.

IL-17 was found to exert biological effects on cells of hemopoietic origin and stromal cells, to induce the secretion of IL-6 by skin and lung fibroblasts and by normal and rheumatoid synoviocytes. It also stimulates the production of IL-8, PGE_2, G-CSF, and leukemia inhibitory factor (LIF) by rheumatoid synoviocytes, upregulates the expression of ICAM-1 by foreskin fibroblasts, stimulates the production of NO by normal and osteoarthritic human articular chondrocytes, and increases their production of IL-1, IL-6, stromelysin, the inducible NO synthase (iNOS), and cyclooxygenase 2 (COX-2). IL-17 stimulates the production by endothelial and epithelial cells of several chemokines. IL-17 increases the secretion of G-CSF by human synoviocytes and by murine fibroblasts, leading fibroblasts to support the growth and differentiation of $CD34^+$ hemopoietic progenitors into mature neutrophils. IL-17 cooperates with TNF-α, IFN-γ, and IL-1 to induce the secretion of IL-6 by rheumatoid synoviocytes and with IFN-γ to enhance the production of IL-6 and IL-8 and to upregulate the expression of ICAM-1 and HLA-DR by human keratinocytes (Yao et al. 1995a, b). Thus, IL-17 mainly exhibits proinflammatory and hemopoietic activities, which appear to play an upstream role in T-cell-triggered inflammation and hemopoiesis, by stimulating stromal cells to secrete other cytokines and growth factors. The hemopoietic effect of IL-17, and in particular its ability to trigger indirectly an acute neutrophilia, might have therapeutic applications in the context of immunosuppression, i.e. after bone marrow transplantation. On the other side, IL-17 might represent a target for therapeutic inhibition in T-cell-dependent autoimmune diseases, chronic inflammatory conditions of the lung, skin, and intestinal tract, organ graft rejection, and some cancers (Lebecque et al. 2000).

More recently, three IL-17-associated molecules have been described, which have been called IL-17B, IL-17C, and IL-17F. Although also these new members can promote inflammation and hemopoiesis, some of the activities of IL-17B and -C are distinct from those described for IL-17, e.g. IL-17B and -C do not bind to IL-17R and only promote the expression of TNF-α and IL-1β, but not of IL-6, IL-8, and G-CSF. IL-17F-induced substantial increases in the mRNA for inflammatory cytokines and chemokines, including IL-6, IFN-γ, CXCL10, and CXCL9 (Li et al. 2000; Shi et al. 2000; Starnes et al. 2001).

Interleukin 18

IL-18 is a protein consisting of 193 amino acids showing homology with IL-1. IL-18 is processed by a protease-like ICE. Moreover, the receptor for IL-18 was shown to be a member of the IL-1 receptor family. The IL-18 gene is located on chromosome 11q22.2.3, closely linked to the dopamine receptor D2 (DRD2) locus, whereas the IL-18R gene maps to chromosome 2q11, on which human IL-1 family members and IL-1R type I are located (Okamura et al. 1995).

A wide range of cell types, including mononuclear cells, keratinocytes, osteoblastic cells, intestine epithelial cells, dendritic cells, chondrocytes, and neuroblastomas, express IL-18. However, IL-18 is mainly produced by activated macrophages or dendritic cells.

IL-18 was originally discovered as an IFN-γ-inducing factor for $CD4^+$ T cells. IL-18 by itself, as IL-12, induces only small amounts of this cytokine. However, combined stimulation of IL-18 and IL-12 induces remarkably higher production of IFN-γ. The underlying mechanism for this strong synergism is that IL-12 induces the IL-18R on $CD4^+$ T cells. $CD8^+$ T cells are also an important source of IFN-γ, and the same synergistic mechanism with IL-12 seems to be operating on $CD8^+$ T cells, although IL-18 also directly activates the cytotoxicity of $CD8^+$ T cells (Biet et al. 2002). When IL-18 was discovered, it was considered to be another factor that could differentiate naïve Th cells into Th1 effectors, such as IL-12. More recent studies have revealed that IL-18 itself has no ability to drive the differentiation of Th1 cells, but strongly induces them to express their functions and induce synthesis of IFN-γ or Fas ligand. However, surprisingly, it was recently found that IL-18, as IFN-γ, also enhances production of the Th2 cytokine IL-13 in T and NK cells. These findings suggest that IL-18 may be involved in the amplification, as well as the regulation, of Th1 responses through the induction of Th2 cytokine production. As with its actions on T cells, IL-18 alone, as well as IL-12 alone, induces NK cells to produce only a little IFN-γ, but again IL-18 and IL-12 synergize in the induction of IFN-γ by NK cells. The main targets of IL-18 and its mechanisms of action are summarized in Figure 15.11.

Since IL-18 induces IFN-γ production, it is obvious that this cytokine is involved in the defense mechanism against intracellular parasites, such as mycobacteria and *Listeria* spp. Recently, IL-18 was shown to contribute also to host defenses against *Salmonella typhimurium*, *Yersinia enterocolitica*, *Cryptococcus neoformans*, and some viruses, such as Epstein–Barr virus, influenza A virus, Sendai virus, herpes simplex virus, vaccinia, and encephalomyocarditis. Although IL-18 exhibits antitumor activity against several types of cells, the mechanism and mediating factors seem to be different for each type of tumor cell. Tumors transfected with

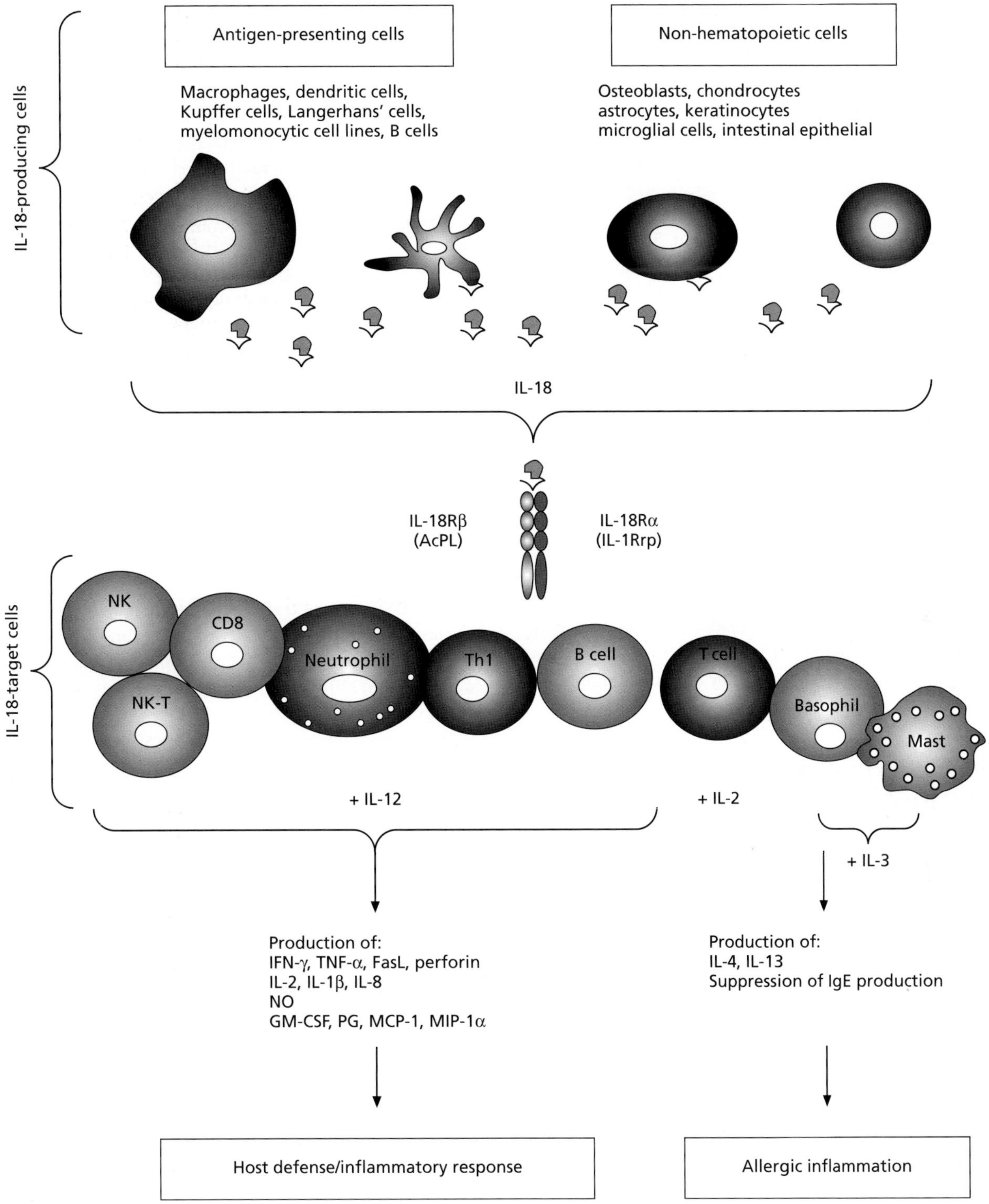

Figure 15.11 *Cellular sources and the targets of interleukin IL-18. Both antigen-presenting cells (APC) and nonhemopoietic cells produce IL-18. Synergy between IL-18 and IL-12 induce T-helper type 1 (Th1) differentiation increases the cytotoxic response of CD8⁺ T cells, natural killer (NK) cells, and NK T cells and their production of interferon γ (IFN-γ), which results in the activation of macrophages. IL-18 has also the potential to induce Th2 cells in a IL-4-independent manner. In response to IL-18 and IL-3, mast cells and basophils produce large amounts of IL-4 and IL-13. Administration of a mixture of IL-12 and IL-18 inhibits IgE production. GM-CSF, granulocyte–macrophage colony-stimulating factor; MCP, monocytic chemotactic protein; MIP, macrophage inflammatory protein; TNF, tumor necrosis factor. (Redrawn from Biet et al. 2002, with permission.)*

IL-18 gene exhibited reduced tumorigenicity and exhibited immunoprotective effects against parental tumor cells in an IFN-γ-dependent manner. IL-18 is also involved in the pathogenesis of chronic inflammatory and autoimmune diseases, such as type 1 diabetes mellitus, experimental autoimmune encephalomyelitis, and chronic active hepatitis (Okamura et al. 2000).

Interleukin 23

The newly discovered cytokine IL-23 shares some in vivo functions with IL-12. This factor, which was termed p19, showed no biological activity itself, but combined with the p40 subunit of IL-12 to form a novel, biologically active compound. IL-23 binds to IL-12Rβ1, but fails to engage IL-12Rβ2 (Oppmann et al. 2000).

IL-23 is secreted by activated dendritic cells, induces the activation of the transcription factor Stat4 in stimulated T cells, a strong proliferation of memory T cells, and IFN-γ production by the same cells (Belladonna et al. 2002).

Interleukin 25

IL-25 is a recently discovered cytokine showing close homology with the other members of IL-17 family. IL-25 gene expression was detected following *Aspergillus* and *Nippostrongylus* infection in the lung and gut.

IL-25 induces responses similar to those mediated by Th2 cells, including IL-4, IL-5, IL-13, and eotaxin production, which is followed by eosinophil infiltrate and airway hyperreactivity (Hurst et al. 2002).

ANTI-INFLAMMATORY AND REGULATORY CYTOKINES

Interleukin receptor antagonist

IL-1R antagonist (IL-1Ra) is a member of the IL-1 family. Three forms of IL-1Ra have been described, two of them being expressed as intracellular proteins (icIL-1RaI and icIL-1RaII) and one being secreted (sIL-1Ra). The three forms of IL-1Ra result from the same gene. The function(s) of the intracellular forms of IL-1Ra are still elusive, whereas sIL-1Ra binds competitively to IL-1RI without inducing signal transduction and thus inhibits IL-1α and IL-1β actions. Mature sIL-1Ra (sIL-1Ra) is a protein of 152 amino acids which is generated by the cleavage of a hydrophobic signal sequence of 25 amino acids from a cytoplasmic precursor of 177 amino acids. The IL-1Ra gene is referred to as IL-1RN and has been mapped in the long arm of chromosome 2 at band q11 (Burger and Dayer 2000).

It is very likely that all cell types able to produce IL-1α and/or IL-1β also express sIL-1Ra or icIL-1Ra or both forms. However, most of the studies have reported the expression of sIL-1Ra in monocyte/macrophages, neutrophils, and fibroblasts and of icIL-1Ra in epithelial cells. In the brain, IL-1Ra is constitutively expressed by cell types other than those expressing IL-1, such as neurons of the paraventricular nucleus and supraoptic nucleus. The sIL-1Ra competitively binds the IL-1RI without inducing signal transduction. It is therefore likely that sIL-1Ra regulates (inhibits) cellular functions affected by IL-1α and/or IL-1β (Figure 15.12). The function(s) of intracellular forms of IL-1Ra are less obvious. One possibility may be that icIL-1Ra counteracts intracellular IL-1α activities and destabilizes and/or degrades mRNAs induced by IL-1α. More recently, it has been shown that resting and cytokine-stimulated human pulmonary epithelial cells release icIL-1RaI in the extracellular space, where it can antagonize cell surface IL-1R. Therefore, icIL-1Ra might be an epithelial store of IL-1Ra liable to immediate release. The role of IL-1Ra in normal physiology of healthy humans remains unclear. The serum levels of sIL-1Ra are elevated in many pathologies (Arend et al. 1998). Therefore, although IL-1Ra was inefficient in sepsis treatment, clinical trials are currently undertaken in inflammatory diseases.

Interleukin 10

IL-10 belongs to the family of long-chain cytokines. The mature IL-10 protein consists of 160 amino acids, Ser1 being the N-terminal residue. The predicted molecular weight of hIL-10 is 18 647 Da and it runs as a single species with an apparent molecular weight of 17 kDa in SDS–polyacrylamide gel electrophoresis (SDS-PAGE). Biologically active IL-10 is a homodimer. IL-10 is located on chromosome 1q. The human IL-10 gene spans 4.7 kb and consists of five exons separated by four introns.

IL-10 is expressed by naïve and memory T cells derived from either peripheral blood or cord blood, from T-cell clones belonging to Th1, Th2, and from T-regulatory 1 (Tr1) subsets, NK cells, and B cells derived from peripheral blood, tonsils, or spleen. A viral homolog of IL-10 has been found in the EBV genome. The EBV-encoded IL-10 (viral IL-10) is located on the BCRF sequence (the gene sequence of the Epstein–Barr virus) and the protein has maintained some, but not all, the biological activities of its cellular counterpart. IL-10 has 90 percent homology at the amino acid level with viral IL-10 (de Waal Malefyt 2000).

IL-10 regulates many aspects of inflammatory and immune responses and acts on both hemopoietic and nonhemopoietic cells. It has dominant suppressive effects on the production of proinflammatory cytokines by monocytes and neutrophils, and downregulates the expression of activating and costimulatory molecules on monocytes and dendritic cells (Fiorentino et al. 1991). This is the reason why it has also been defined as 'macrophage deactivating factor'. IL-10 strongly inhibits the production of cytokines and chemokines by activated monocytes/macrophages. In addition, IL-10 enhances the production of IL-1Ra expression, as well

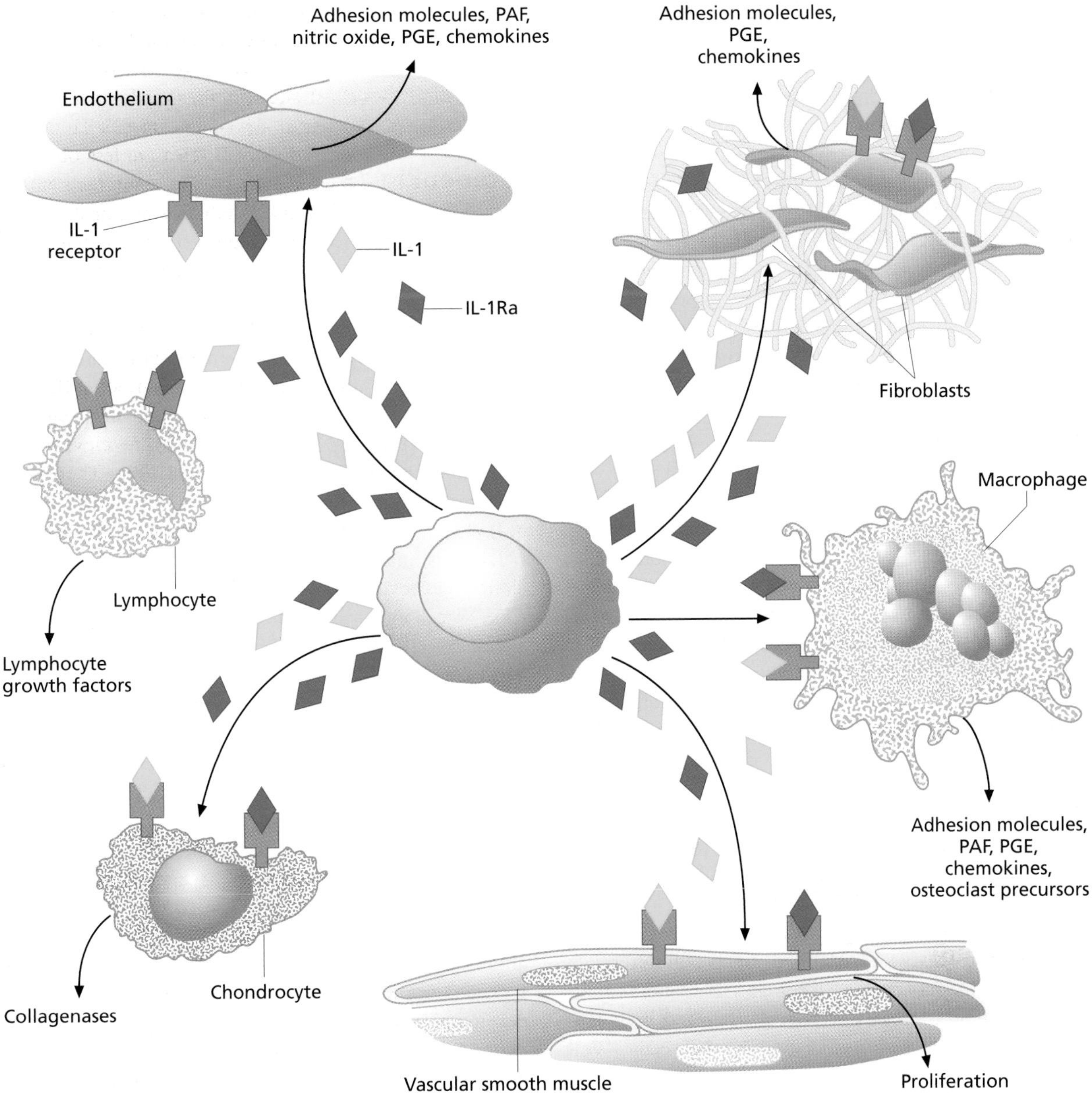

Figure 15.12 *The actions of interleukin 1 (IL-1) and its receptor antagonist (IL-1Ra). IL-1 activates its receptor on cells resulting in various functions. When IL-1R is occupied by the IL-1Ra, IL-1 cannot bind and thus cannot elicit a biological response. This is a natural balance between the proinflammatory activities of IL-1 and the ability of IL-1Ra to keep those activities in check by occupying IL-1Rs. PAF, platelet-activating factor; PGE, prostaglandin E. (Redrawn from Dinarello 2000c, with permission)*

as of soluble p55 and p75 TNFRs, indicating that IL-10 induces a shift from production of proinflammatory to anti-inflammatory mediators. IL-10 also inhibits expression of MHCII antigens, CD54 (ICAM-1), CD80 (B7), and CD86 (B7.2) on monocytes, even following induction of these molecules by IL-4 or IFN. IL-10 inhibits production of PGE_2, another proinflammatory mediator, as well as the ability of monocytes/macrophages to modulate turnover of extracellular matrix, an effect that is mediated by the inhibition of the production of gelatinase and collagenase, and the increase in the production of tissue inhibitor of metalloproteases. IL-10 also inhibits LPS-induced CRP biosynthesis.

Furthermore, IL-10 inhibits production of IL-12 and expression of costimulatory molecules on various types of dendritic cells. IL-10 also inhibits the production of chemokines, proinflammatory cytokines, and mediators of granulocyte survival, thus limiting the duration of inflammatory responses. IL-10 exhibits growth factor activities on B cells and mast cells, and inhibits or enhances the activities of $CD4^+$ and $CD8^+$ T cells depending on their activation conditions. IL-10 enhances the survival of normal human B cells (depending on their activation state), which correlated with increased expression of the antiapoptotic protein Bcl-2 and strongly increases the proliferation of human B-cell precursors and mature activated B cells. Such effects of IL-10 may play a role in pathogenesis of systemic lupus erythematosus (SLE), where positive correlations between serum IL-10 levels and severity of disease, and between the production of IL-10 and autoantibodies by the SLE patient's B cells, have been demonstrated. IL-10 strongly inhibits cytokine production and proliferation of T cells and T-cell clones activated in the presence of APCs. This effect of IL-10 results mostly from its downregulatory effects on APC functions. The effects of IL-10 on individual cell types suggest that it could have potent anti-inflammatory/immunosuppressive activities in vivo in chronic inflammatory disorders, autoimmune disorders, and infectious diseases (de Waal Malefyt 2000).

Interleukin 10-related cytokines

Recently, five novel IL-10-related molecules and their receptors have been identified in blood mononuclear cells. These cytokines have been named IL-19, IL-20, IL-22, IL-24, and IL-26 (Gallagher et al. 2000; Dumoutier et al. 2000, 2001; Blumberg et al. 2001; Caudell et al. 2002; Wolk et al. 2002). Similar to IL-10, they are secreted α-helical proteins, the amino acid sequences of which are up to approximately 30 percent identical to those of IL-10 and comprise a definite position for cysteine. Of note, the encoding genes are located in the humane genome in two clusters, one comprising the genes for IL-10, IL-19, IL-20, and IL-24 on chromosome 1q32, and another comprising the IL-22- and IL-26-encoding genes located on chromosome 12q1 (Dumoutier et al. 2001)

IL-19 and IL-20 were found to be preferentially expressed in monocytes, whereas IL-22 and IL-26 (AK155) expression was exclusively detected in T cells, especially on Th1 polarization, and in NK cells (Wolk et al. 2002). IL-24 (melanoma differentiation-associated gene 7) expression was restricted to monocytes and T cells. Detection of these molecules in lymphocytes was predominantly linked to cellular activation. With regard to T cells, IL-26 was primarily produced by memory cells, and its expression was independent of costimulation.

In contrast to the extensively studied IL-10, the knowledge of the biology of the novel IL-10 homologs is still fragmentary. Preliminary functional data exist for IL-20, IL-22, and IL-24. Overexpression of IL-20 induced neonatal lethality, psoriasis-like skin abnormalities, lack of adipose tissue, and elevated apoptosis of thymic lymphocytes. IL-22 was suggested as playing a role in inflammatory processes through the observation that it induces acute phase reactant production in a hepatoma cell line and in vivo. Overexpression of IL-24 via adenovirus gene transfer induced growth inhibition in various tumor types. No function is known for IL-19 and IL-26 as yet.

However, although immune cells exhibit a differential expression of the IL-10 homologs, in contrast to IL-10 that is produced by and acts on all monocytes, NK cells, B cells, and T cells, these cells do not seem to be the major target population of these molecules.

Interleukin 13

IL-13 is secreted as a monomeric peptide of 10 kDa (McKenzie and Matthews 2000). Of note, the amino acid sequences of IL-13 and IL-4 are approximately 30 percent homologous, a level of similarity that is not evident among any other interleukins. The human IL-13 gene is located on the long arm of human chromosome 5 (5q31), where it is closely linked to the genes encoding IL-4, IL-5, IL-3, and GM-CSF. Indeed, the IL-13 gene maps approximately 12 kb upstream of the IL-4 gene (Figure 15.13) and there is a coordinate regulator of IL-4, IL-13, and IL-5 (Loots et al. 2000).

IL-13 is mainly produced by $CD4^+$ Th2 cells and clones. However, Th1 cell clones, Th0 cell clones, and $CD8^+$ T-cell clones, have also been shown to express IL-13 mRNA. Primary mouse mast cells and mouse and human mast cell lines have also been shown to express IL-13 in response to activation, and primary mouse NK cells and the human NK cell line NK3.3 secrete IL-13 in response to activation. IL-13 gene transcription has also been detected in a number of B-cell malignancies (McKenzie and Heath 1996).

IL-13 has been shown to have anti-inflammatory functions on monocytes and macrophages and to induce B cells to proliferate and isotype switch to the production of IgE. Blockage of IL-13 activity has been shown to inhibit the pathophysiology of asthma. Studies using IL-1 gene-deficient mice have identified impaired Th2 cell development in the absence of IL-13 and indicated an important role for IL-13 in the expulsion of parasitic gastrointestinal helminths. The anti-inflammatory function of IL-13 is manifested in its ability to suppress the expression of cytokines such as IL-1α and IL-1β, TNF-α, IL-8, and IL-12. Significantly, by inhibiting IL-12, it may also act to skew the T-helper populations away from a Th1 phenotype and towards a Th2 phenotype. IL-13 expression correlates strongly with the occurrence of allergic asthma and atopy, and the associated expression of IgE. Recent studies using mouse models of experimental nairway hypersensitivity have demonstrated that IL-13 plays a central role in these responses. On the other side, the anti-inflammatory roles of IL-13 may be important in controlling inflammation, such as that encountered in osteoarthritis. Interestingly, IL-13 has recently been demonstrated to be secreted by, and stimulatory for the growth of, Reed–Sternberg cells. Administration of recombinant IL-13 to IL-13-deficient mice or severe combined immunodeficient (SCID) mice resulted in improved expulsion of *Nippostrongylus brasiliensis* from helminth-infected animals, although the

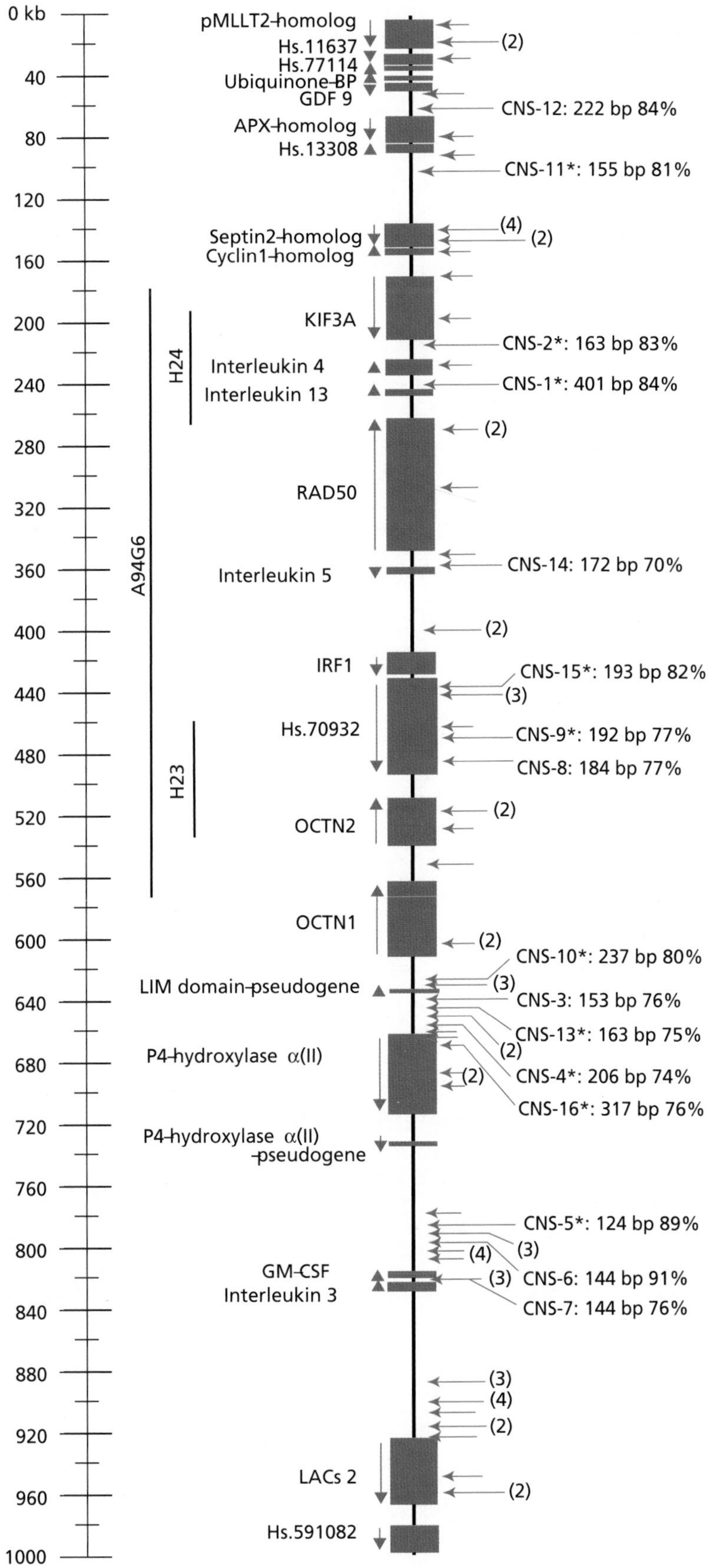

Figure 15.13 *The chromosomal association of interleukin IL-13 with other T-helper type 2 (Th2) cytokines, as shown by the physical map of the 1-Mbp human 5q31 region. (From Loots et al. 2000.)*

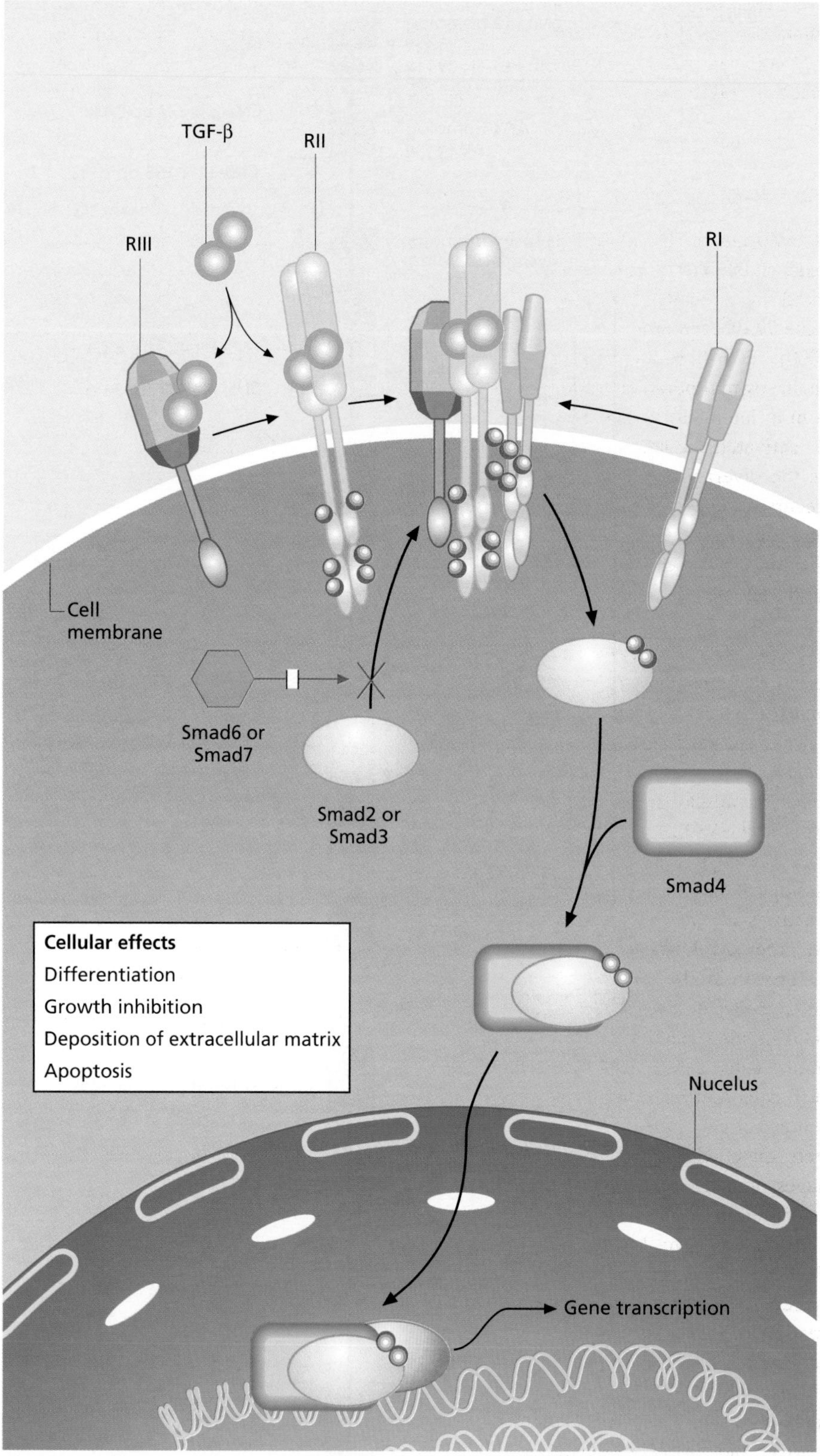

Figure 15.14 *Mechanisms of signal transduction and cellular effects of transforming growth factor β (TGF-β). In the extracellular space TGF-β binds either to the type III TGF-β receptor (RIIi), which presents it to the type II receptor (RII), or directly to RII on the cell membrane. The binding of TGF-β to RII then leads to binding of the type I receptor (RI) to the complex, and the phosphorylation of RI initiates the cascade of transcription factors that regulate the transcription of TGF-β-responsive genes and mediate the effects of TGF-β at the cellular level. (Redrawn from Blobe et al. 2000, with permission.)*

mechanism for this clearance is still unclear. As a result of its anti-inflammatory roles, IL-13 treatment has been used in models of collagen-induced arthritis and uveitis, and LPS-induced endotoxemia (McKenzie and Matthews 2000).

TGF-β

Three different isoforms of TGF-β (TGF-β_1, TGF-β_2, and TGF-β_3) exist as stable 25-kDa homo- or heterodimers crosslinked by a single disulfide bond that is formed by cysteine 77 of each monomeric unit (Flanders and Roberts 2000). TGF-β is secreted in noncovalent association with its own prodomain (latency-associated protein (LAP)) in a 'latent' form that is unable to bind receptors until activated. Whereas in other TGF-β family members the divergent N-terminal region of the unprocessed precursor serves only to facilitate proper folding and secretion of the mature peptides, for the TGF-βs, the LAP protein serves a unique role of conferring latency and effectively masking the receptor-binding domains of the molecule (Gleizes et al. 1997). The three TGF-β species are encoded by unique genes located on different chromosomes. All three genes share a similar intron/exon structure with a total of seven exons spanning greater than 100 kb of genomic DNA.

TGF-β is widely expressed in embryo tissues, whereas the major sources in adults are platelets, bone, and spleen (Thompson et al. 1989).

As almost every cell type can express receptors for TGF-β, its physiological and pathophysiological roles are extensive. The activity of the TGF-βs that distinguishes them from most other cytokines is their ability to limit cell growth. This growth inhibitory action is quite broad, targeting epithelial cells, endothelial cells, and hemopoietic cells. TGF-β also regulates the differentiated function of immune cells, acting as a strong suppressor of activation of T cells and of antibody secretion by B cells. Other major cellular targets for TGF-β action include its effects on chemotaxis (fibroblasts, lymphocytes, macrophages, and neutrophils) and its ability to control cellular differentiation, apoptosis, and extracellular matrix production. The last is the most prominent effect of TGF-β on mesenchymal cells, and is manifested by enhanced expression of extracellular matrix proteins, suppression of expression of matrix-degrading proteases, induction of expression of protease inhibitors, and regulation of expression of integrin receptors. Together, these effects result in increased accumulation of extracellular matrix and in cellular interaction with matrix (Figure 15.14). These many and varied cellular functions of TGF-β underlie its pathophysiological roles in fibrotic diseases, carcinogenesis, wound healing, autoimmune diseases, and parasitic diseases. TGF-β can be either synergistic and antagonistic to the action of other cytokines/growth factors, depending on the cellular context. Thus, TGF-βs play critical roles in normal physiology, most prominently in branching morphogenesis, in the transformation from epithelial to mesenchymal, control of cell growth, chemotaxis, and elaboration of extracellular matrix (Letterio and Roberts 1998).

The widespread expression of TGF-β coupled with its multiple bioactivities leads to its involvement in the pathology of many human diseases, such as fibrotic disorders, acute experimental allergic encephalomyelitis, and collagen-induced arthritis. TGF-β antagonists may be useful not only in these conditions, but mainly in reducing tumor growth, possibly by inhibiting the immunosuppressive effects of TGF-β. Clinical applications for TGF-β are limited by the difficulty to find optimal methods of delivery and ensure its bioavailability (Flanders and Roberts 2000)

REFERENCES

Aggarwal, B.B., Samanta, A. and Feldman, M. 2000. TNF-α. In: Oppenheim, J.J. and Feldman, M. (eds), *Cytokine reference*. London: Academic Press, 413–34.

Aggarwal, B.B. and Vilcek, J. 1992. *Tumor necrosis factor: structure, functions and mechanisms of action*. New York: Marcel Dekker.

Alimzhanov, M.B., Kuprash, D.V. and Kosco-Vilbois, M.H. 1997. Abnormal development of secondary lymphoid tissues in lymphotoxin-deficient mice. *Proc Natl Acad Sci USA*, **94**, 9302–7.

Arceci, R.J., Pampfer, S. and Pollard, J.W. 1992. Role and expression of colony stimulating factor-1 and steel factor receptors and their ligands during pregnancy in the mouse. *Reprod Fertil Dev*, **4**, 619–32.

Arend, W.P., Malyak, M., et al. 1998. Interleukin-1 receptor antagonist: role in biology. *Annu Rev Immunol*, **16**, 27–55.

Basu, S., Hodgson, G., et al. 2002. Evaluation of role of G-CSF in the production, survival, and release of neutrophils from bone marrow into circulation. *Blood*, **100**, 854–61.

Bazzoni, F. and Beutler, B. 1996. The tumor necrosis factor ligand and receptor families. *N Engl J Med*, **334**, 1717–25.

Belladonna, M.L., Renauld, J.-C., et al. 2002. IL-23 and IL-12 have overlapping, but distinct, effects on murine dendritic cells. *J Immunol*, **168**, 5448–54.

Biet, F., Locht, C. and Kremer, L. 2002. Immunoregulatory functions of interleukin 18 and its role in defense against pathogens. *J Mol Med*, **80**, 147–62.

Billiau, A. and Vandenbroeck, K. 2000. IFNγ. In: Oppenheim, J.J. and Feldman, M. (eds), *Cytokine reference*. London: Academic Press, 641–88.

Blobe, G.C., Schiemann, W.P. and Lodish, H.F. 2000. Role of transforming growth factor β in human disease. *N Engl J Med*, **342**, 1350–8.

Blumberg, H., Conklin, D., et al. 2001. Interleukin 20: discovery, receptor identification, and role in epidermal function. *Cell*, **104**, 9–19.

Brenne, A.-T., Baade Ro, T., et al. 2002. Interleukin-21 is a growth factor and survival factor for human myeloma cells. *Blood*, **99**, 3756–62.

Broide, D.H., Paine, M.M. and Firenstein, G.S. 1992. Eosinophils express interleukin-5 and granulocyte macrophage colony-stimulating factor mRNA at sites of allergic inflammation in asthmatics. *J Clin Invest*, **90**, 1414–24.

Broudy, V.C. 1997. Stem cell factor and hemopoiesis. *Blood*, **90**, 1345–64.

Bukowski, R.M., Oleneki, T., et al. 1996. Phase I trial of subcutaneous interleukin-3 in patients with refractory malignancy: haematological, immunological and pharmacodynamic findings. *Clin Cancer Res*, **2**, 347–57.

Burger, D. and Dayer, J.M. 2000. IL-1 Ra. In: Oppenheim, J.J. and Feldman, M. (eds), *Cytokine reference*. London: Academic Press, 319–36.

Caudell, E.G., Mumm, J.B., et al. 2002. The protein product of the tumor suppressor gene, melanoma differentiation-associated gene 7, exhibits immunostimulatory activity and is designated IL-24. *J Immunol*, **168**, 6041–6.

Center, D.M., Kornfeld, H. and Cruikshank, W.W. 2000. IL-16. In: Oppenheim, J.J. and Feldman, M. (eds), *Cytokine reference*. London: Academic Press, 225–40.

Chang, J.M., Metcalf, D., et al. 1989. Long-term exposure to retrovirally expressed granulocyte colony-stimulating factor induces a nonneoplastic granulocytic and progenitor cell hyperplasia without tissue damage in mice. *J Clin Invest*, **84**, 1488–96.

de Waal Malefyt, R. 1685. IL-10. In: Oppenheim, J.J. and Feldman, M. (eds), *Cytokine reference*. London: Academic Press.

Dinarello, C. 2000a. IL-1α. In: Oppenheim, J.J. and Feldman, M. (eds), *Cytokine reference*. London: Academic Press, 308–18.

Dinarello, C. 2000b. IL-1β. In: Oppenheim, J.J. and Feldman, M. (eds), *Cytokine reference*. London: Academic Press, 351–74.

Dinarello, C. 2000c. The role of interleukin-1-receptor antagonist blocking inflammation mediated by interleukin-1. *N Engl J Med*, **343**, 732–4.

Du, X. and Williams, D.A. 1997. Interleukin-11: review of molecular, cell biology and clinical use. *Blood*, **89**, 3893–8.

Dumoutier, L., Louhaed, J. and Renauld, J.C. 2000. Cloning and characterization of IL-10-related T cell-derived inducible factor (IL-TIF), a novel cytokine structurally related to IL-10 and inducible by IL-9. *J Immunol*, **164**, 1814–19.

Dumoutier, L., Lejeune, D., et al. 2001. Cloning and characterization of IL-22 binding protein, a natural antagonist of IL-10-related-derived T cell-derived inducible factor/IL-22. *J Immunol*, **166**, 7090–5.

Esche, C., Sharin, M.R. and Lotze, M.T. 2000. IL-12. In: Oppenheim, J.J. and Feldman, M. (eds), *Cytokine reference*. London: Academic Press, 187–201.

Fehniger, T.A. and Caligiuri, M.A. 2001. Interleukin-15: biology and relevance to human disease. *Blood*, **97**, 14–32.

Fiorentino, D.F., Zlotnik, A., et al. 1991. IL-10 inhibits cytokine production by activated macrophages. *J Immunol*, **147**, 3815–22.

Flanders, C. and Roberts, A.B. 2000. TGF-β. In: Oppenheim, J.J. and Feldman, M. (eds), *Cytokine reference*. London: Academic Press, 719–46.

Fry, T.J. and Mackall, C.L. 2002. Interleukin-7: from bench to clinic. *Blood*, **99**, 3892–904.

Gallagher, G., Dickensheets, H., et al. 2000. Cloning, expression and initial characterization of interleukin 19 (IL-19), a novel homologue of human interleukin-10 (IL-10). *Genes Immunol*, **1**, 442–50.

Galli, S.J., Zsebo, K.M. and Geissler, E.M. 1994. The kit ligand, stem cell factor. *Adv Immunol*, **55**, 1–96.

Geiger, T., Andus, T.J., et al. 1988. Induction of rat acute-phase proteins by interleukin-6 in vivo. *Eur J Immunol*, **18**, 717–23.

Gleizes, P.E., Munger, J.S., et al. 1997. TGF-β latency: biologicalsignificance and mechanisms of activation. *Stem Cells*, **15**, 190–7.

Goldman, S.J. 1995. Preclinical biology of interleukin-11: a multifunctional hematopoietic cytokine with potent thrombopoietic activity. *Stem Cells*, **13**, 462–71.

Granucci, F., Zanoni, I., et al. 2003. Dendritic cell regulation of immune responses: a new role for interleukin 2 at the intersection of innate and adaptive immunata. *Embo J*, **22**, 2546–51.

Gretchen, T.F. et al. 2000. IL-5. In: Oppenheim J.J. and Feldman, M. (eds.), *Cytokine reference*. London: Academic Press, 861–75.

Hirano, T. 1998. Interleukin 6 and its receptor: ten years later. *Int Rev Immunol*, **16**, 249–84.

Houssiau, F., Schandenè, L., et al. 1995. A cascade of cytokines is responsible for IL-9 expression in human T cells: involvement of IL-2. *IL-4 and IL-10. J Immunol*, **154**, 2624–30.

Hurst, S.D., Muchamuel, T., et al. 2002. New IL-17 family members promote Th1 or Th2 responses in the lung: in vivo function of the novel cytokine IL-25. *J Immunol*, **169**, 443–53.

Keegan, A.D. 2000. IL-4. In: Oppenheim, J.J. and Feldman, M. (eds), *Cytokine reference*. London: Academic Press, 128–35.

Keith, J.C. 2000. IL-11. In: Oppenheim, J.J. and Feldman, M. (eds), *Cytokine reference*. London: Academic Press, 565–84.

Kelleher, K., Bean, K., et al. 1991. Human interleukin 9 genomic sequence, chromosomal location, and sequences essential for the expression in human T-cell leukaemia virus (HTLV-1)-transformed human T cells. *Blood*, **77**, 1436–41.

Keller, J.R. and Linnekin, D.M. 2000. Stem cell factor. In: Oppenheim, J.J. and Feldman, M. (eds), *Cytokine reference*. London: Academic Press, 877–97.

Kovacs, J.A., Vogel, S., et al. 1996. Controlled and interleukin-2 infusions in patients infected with the human immunodeficiency virus. *N Engl J Med*, **335**, 1350–6.

Laberge, S., Cruikshank, W.W., et al. 1996. Secretion of IL-16 (lymphocyte chemoattractant factor) from serotonin-stimulated CD8+ T cells in vitro. *J Immunol*, **156**, 310–15.

Lebecque, S., Fossiez, F. and Bates, E. 2000. IL-17. In: Oppenheim, J.J. and Feldman, M. (eds), *Cytokine reference*. London: Academic Press, 241–50.

Lejeune, F.J., Ruegg, C. and Lienard, D. 1998. Clinical applications of TNF-alpha in cancer. *Curr Opin Immunol*, **10**, 573–80.

Leonard, J.P., Shermar, M.L., et al. 1997. Effects of single-dose intrleukin-12 exposure on IL-12-associated toxicity and interferon-gamma production. *Blood*, **90**, 2541–8.

Letterio, J.L. and Roberts, A.B. 1998. Regulation of immune responses by TGFbeta. *Annu Rev Immunol*, **16**, 137–61.

Li, H., Chen, J., et al. 2000. Cloning and characterization of IL-17B and IL-17C, two new members of the IL-17 cytokine family. *Proc Natl Acad Sci USA*, **97**, 773–7.

Lieschke, G.J., Grail, D., et al. 1994. Mice lacking granulocyte colony-stimulating factor have chronic neutropenia, granulocyte and macrophage progenitor cell deficiency, and impaired neutrophil maturation. *Blood*, **84**, 1737–46.

Loots, G.C., Locksley, R.M., et al. 2000. Identification of a coordinate regulator of interleukins, 4, 13, and 5 by cross-species comparisons. *Science*, **288**, 133–40.

Lyman, S.D. and Jacobsen, S.E.W. 1998. c-kit ligand and Ftl3 ligand: stem/progenitor cell factors with overlapping yet distinct activities. *Blood*, **91**, 1101–34.

McKenzie, A.N.J. and Heath, A.W. 1996. Interleukin 13 and related cytokines. In: Whetton, H. and Gordon, J. (eds), *Blood cell biochemistry: hematopoietic cell growth factors and their receptors*. New York: Plenum Press, 41–50.

McKenzie, A.N.J. and Matthews, D.J. 2000. IL-13. In: Oppenheim, J.J. and Feldman, M. (eds), *Cytokine reference*. London: Academic Press, 203–11.

Manetti, R., Parrinchi, P., et al. 1994. Natural killer stimulatory factor (interleukin-12) induces T helper type 1 (Th1)-specific immune responses and inhibits the development of IL-4-producing cells. *J Exp Med*, **177**, 1199–204.

Matsuda, T. and Hirano, T. 2000. IL-6. In: Oppenheim, J.J. and Feldman, M. (eds), *Cytokine reference*. London: Academic Press, 537–63.

Matsui, Y., Zsebo, K.M. and Hogan, B.L. 1990. Embryonic expression of a hematopoietic growth factor encoded by the SI locus and the ligand for SCFR. *Nature*, **347**, 667–9.

Merz, H., Houssiau, F., et al. 1991. IL-9 expression in human malignant lymphomas: unique association with Hodgkin's cells and large anaplastic lymphoma. *Blood*, **78**, 1311–17.

Metcalf, D. and Nicola, N.A. 1985. Synthesis by mouse peritoneal cells of G-CSF, the differentiation inducer for myeloid leukaemia cells: stimulation by endotoxin, M-CSF and multi-CSF. *Leukemia Res*, **1**, 30.

Metcalf, D. and Nicola, N.A. 1995. *The hemopoietic colony-stimulating factors: from biology to clinical application*. Cambridge: Cambridge University Press.

Nagata, S. 2000. G-CSF. In: Oppenheim, J.J. and Feldman, M. (eds), *Cytokine reference.*. London: Academic Press, 936–40.

Nicolas, N.A. 2000. GM–CSF. In: Oppenheim, J.J. and Feldman, M. (eds), *Cytokine reference*. London: Academic Press, 899–910.

Nicolas, N.A., Metcalf, D., et al. 1983. Purification of factor inducing differentiation in murine myelomonocytic leukaemia cells: identification as granulocyte colony stimulating factor. *J Biol Chem*, **258**, 9017–23.

Okamura, H., Tsutsui, H., et al. 1995. Cloning of a new cytokine that induces IFN-gamma production by T cells. *Nature*, **378**, 81.

Okamura, H. and Tsutsui, H. 2000. IL-18. In: Oppenheim, J.J. and Feldman, M. (eds), *Cytokine reference*. London: Academic Press, 337–50.

Oppenheim, J.J. and Feldman, M. (eds) 2000. *Cytokine reference*. London: Academic Press.

Oppmann, B., Lesley, R., et al. 2000. Novel p19 protein engages IL12p40 to form a cytokine, IL-23, with biological activities similar as well as distinct from IL-12. *Immunity*, **13**, 715–25.

Parish-Novak, J., Dilon, S.R., et al. 2000. Interleukin 21 and its receptor are involved in NK cell expansion and regulation of lymphocyte function. *Nature*, **408**, 57–63.

Paul, W.E. 1991. IL-4: a proteolytic immunoregulatory lymphokine. *Blood*, **77**, 1859–70.

Pflanz, S., Timans, J.C., et al. 2002. IL-27, a heterodimeric cytokine composed of EBI3 and p28 protein, induces proliferation of naïve CD4+ T cells. *Immunity*, **16**, 779–90.

Ratajczak, M.Z., Kuczyasaki, W.I., et al. 1995. Expression and physiologic significance of Kit ligand and stem cell tyrosine kinase-I receptor in normal human CD34+, SCFR+ marrow cells. *Blood*, **86**, 2161–7.

Renauld, J.-C. 2000. IL-9. In: Oppenheim, J.J. and Feldman, M. (eds), *Cytokine reference*. London: Academic Press, 156–64.

Romagnani, S. 1998. T-cell subsets (Th1, Th2) and cytokines in autoimmunity. In: Rose, N.R. and Mackay, I.R. (eds), *The autoimmune diseases*. San Diego, CA: Academic Press, 163–91.

Rosenberg, S.A., Lotze, M.T., et al. 1987. A progress report on the treatment of 157 patients with advanced cancer using lymphokine-activated killer cells and interleukin-2. *N Engl J Med*, **316**, 889–97.

Rothenberg, M.E. 1998. Eosinophilia. *N Engl J Med*, **338**, 1592–600.

Saleh, M., Wiegmans, A., et al. 1999. Effect of in situ retroviral interleukin-4 transfer on established intracranial tumors. *J Natl Cancer Inst*, **91**, 438–45.

Sanderson, C.J. 1992. Interleukin-5, eosinophils and disease. *Blood*, **79**, 3101–9.

Schorle, H., Holtschke, T., et al. 1991. Development and function of T cells in mice rendered interleukin-2-deficient by gene targeting. *Nature*, **352**, 621–4.

Schrader, J.W. 2000. IL-3. In: Oppenheim, J.J. and Feldman, M. (eds), *Cytokine reference*. London: Academic Press, 856–9.

Schwenger, G.T.F., Mordvinov, V.A., et al. 2000. IL-5. In: Oppenheim, J.J. and Feldman, M. (eds), *Cytokine reference*. London: Academic Press, 861–74.

Shi, Y., Ulrich, S.J., et al. 2000. A novel cytokine receptor-ligand pair: identification, molecular characterization, and in vivo immunomodulatory activity. *J Biol Chem*, **275**, 19167–76.

Smith, K.A. 1980. T cell growth factor. *Immunol Rev*, **51**, 337–57.

Smith, K.A. 2000. IL-2. In: Oppenheim, J.J. and Feldman, M. (eds), *Cytokine reference*. London: Academic Press, 114–25.

Soussi-Gonoussi, A., Kontolemos, M. and Hamid, Q. 2001. Role of IL-9 in the pathophysiology of allergic diseases. *J Allergy Clin Immunol*, **107**, 575–82.

Spits, H. 2000. IL-7. In: Oppenheim, J.J. and Feldman, M. (eds), *Cytokine reference*. London: Academic Press, 138–53.

Stanley, E.R. 1994. Colony stimulatory factor-1 (macrophage colony stimulating factor). In: Thomson, A.W. (ed.), *The cytokine handbook*. Orlando, FL: Academic Press, 1650–4.

Starnes, T., Robertson, M.J., et al. 2001. IL-17F, a novel cytokine selectively expressed in activated T cells and monocytes, regulates angiogenesis and endothelial cell cytokine production. *J Immunol*, **161**, 4137–40.

Thompson, N.L., Flanders, K.C., et al. 1989. Expression of transforming growth factor-beta 1 in specific cells and tissues of adult and neonatal mice. *J Cell Biol*, **108**, 661–9.

Trinchieri, G. 1998. Interleukin-12: a cytokine at the interface of inflammation and immunity. *Adv Immunol*, **70**, 83–243.

Vincenti, F., Kirkman, R., et al. 1998. Interleukin-2 receptor blockade with Daclizumab Triple Therapy Study Group. *New Engl J Med*, **338**, 161–5.

Waldmann, T.A. and Tagaya, Y. 2000. IL-15. In: Oppenheim, J.J. and Feldman, M. (eds), *Cytokine reference*. London: Academic Press, 214–23.

Wallach, D., Varfolomeev, E.E., et al. 1999. Tumor necrosis factor receptor and Fas signaling mechanisms. *Annu Rev Immunol*, **17**, 331–67.

Ware, C.F., Santee, S. and Glass, A. 1998. Tumor necrosis factor-related ligands and receptors. In: Thompson, A. (ed.), *Cytokine handbook*. San Diego, CA: Academic Press, 549–92.

Watanabe, M., Ueno, Y., et al. 1995. Interleukin 7 is produced by human intestinal epithelial cells and regulates the proliferation of intestinal mucosal lymphocytes. *J Clin Invest*, **95**, 2945–53.

Welte, K., Bonilla, M.A., et al. 1987. Recombinant human granulocyte-colony stimulating factor: In vitro and in vivo effects on myelopoiesis. *Blood Cells*, **13**, 17–30.

Wiles, M.V., Ruiz, P. and Imhof, A.B. 1992. Interleukin-7 expression during mouse thymus development. *Eur J Immunol*, **22**, 1037–42.

Wolk, K., Kunz, S., et al. 2002. Immune cells as sources and targets of the IL-10 family members? *J Immunol*, **168**, 5397–402.

Yao, Z., Pinter, S.L., et al. 1995a. Human IL-17: a novel cytokine derived from T cells. *J Immunol*, **155**, 5483–6.

Yao, Z., Fanslow, W.C., et al. 1995b. Herpesvirus saimiri encodes a new cytokine, IL-17, which binds to a novel cytokine receptor. *Immunity*, **3**, 81–21.

Zlotnik, A. and Yoshie, O. 2000. Chemokines: a new classification system and their role in immunity. *Immunity*, **12**, 121–7.

PART IV

ACQUIRED IMMUNITY

16

Antibodies and B lymphocytes

WILLIAM CUSHLEY AND GILLIAN BORLAND

Antibody molecules are the functional products of the humoral arm of the mammalian immune system. They are glycoprotein molecules found mainly in the γ fraction of serum, and are members of the immunoglobulin (Ig) family of serum proteins. Although Ig molecules exist as five classes, each with distinctive structural and functional properties, all Ig molecules conform to a common unit structural theme, the four-chain model (Figure 16.1), which provides a molecular explanation for their immunological activities. Antibody molecules are synthesized by B lymphocytes.

The humoral response is one arm of the specific, adaptive, immune response, and is characterized by the diversity of individual specific antibodies that it can produce, immunological memory, and production of antibodies of the most appropriate type to combat particular pathogens. The humoral response interacts with the cellular immune response and also interfaces with components of the nonspecific immune system. Thus, the nonspecific immune system, which shows no specificity or immunological memory, possesses potent cytotoxic power in the form of phagocytic cells and the components of the complement cascade. The humoral response has essentially no toxic capacity in its own right, but uses antibody specifically to recruit the cytotoxic power of the nonspecific system and focus it at the pathogen target.

The humoral immune response displays characteristic features. After initial challenge with antigen, levels of antibody of the IgM class rise over some 4–7 days; this is the primary humoral response. If antigenic challenge persists, antibodies of other classes, notably IgG, are produced; this is the secondary response. Second or subsequent challenge with the same antigen elicits a response that is more rapid than the primary response, and generates greater quantities of specific antibody of greater quality (i.e. different class and higher affinity) from those found in the primary response. The capacity to respond to re-challenge by a given antigen is long-lived and resides in memory B cells. The secondary response encompasses antibody responses, the major components of which are of the IgA, IgD, IgE, or IgG classes.

IMMUNOGLOBULIN STRUCTURE

The four-chain model

The four-chain model describes the overall structure of IgG molecules (Porter 1962), and this structural theme is common to all five Ig classes. The general features of the four-chain model are illustrated in Figure 16.1, using human IgG1 as an example. Antibody molecules are composed of two identical heavy chains, disulfide bonded to two identical light chains in such a way that the amino terminus of each heavy and light chain is juxtaposed in three-dimensional terms to generate the

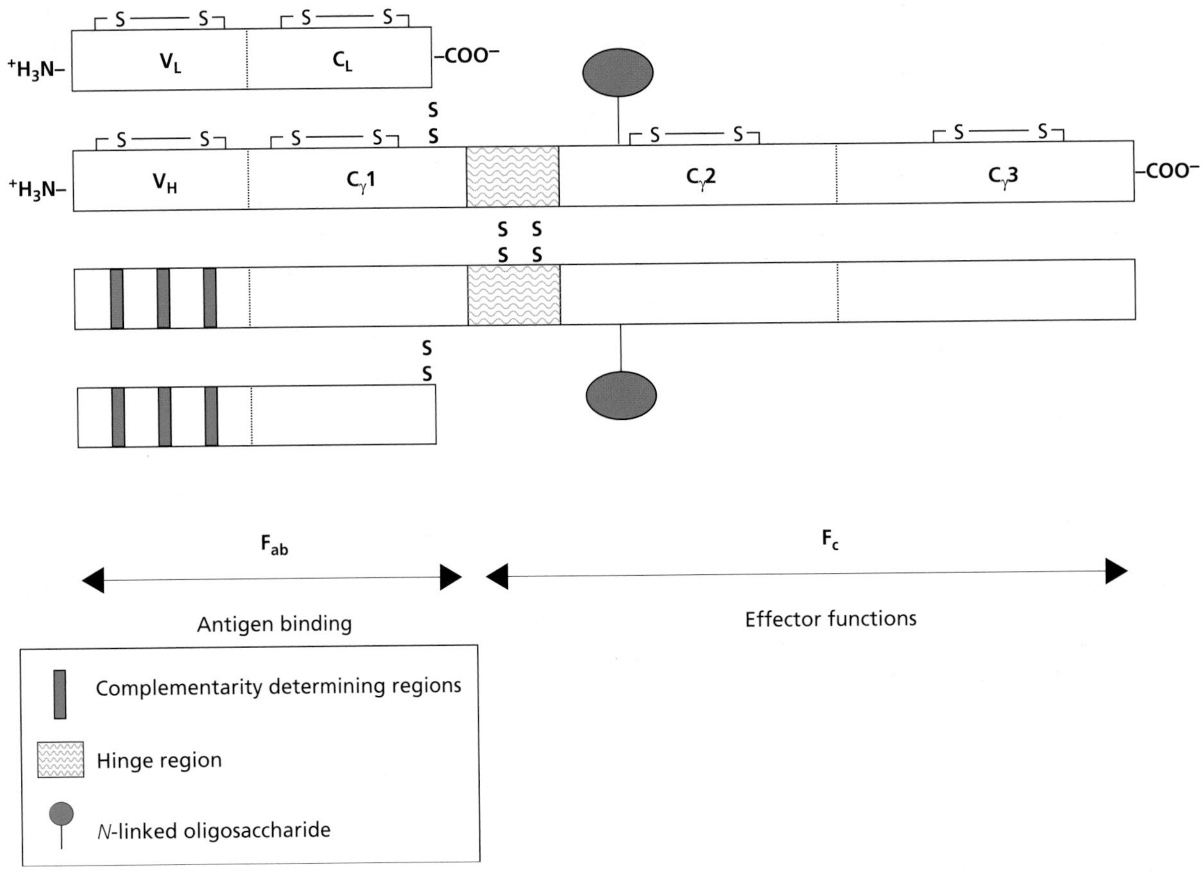

Figure 16.1 The four-chain model: the arrangement of an IgG1 molecule is shown. The hypervariable regions/complementarity determining regions are shown as solid rectangles in the V domains. The hinge region is illustrated as a patterned box and N-linked oligosaccharide by a filled circle. The locations of the Fab and Fc regions are noted.

antibody-combining site. Interchain disulfide bonds link not only the heavy and light chains but also the two heavy chains together. The IgG molecule is bivalent with respect to antigen binding (Edelman and Poulik 1961; Porter 1962).

Controlled proteolysis of IgG molecules has provided insights into structure–function relationships by investigation of the distinct fragments of Ig molecules generated (see Figure 16.1). Papain cleaves the intact IgG molecule to release three fragments of approximately equal molecular weight. Two of these fragments, derived from the amino terminus of the molecule, are identical and, because they retain antigen-binding capacity, are referred to as Fab (fragment antigen binding) fragments. Fab fragments are monovalent with respect to antigen binding and, as such, are unable to form immunoprecipitates in solution or in semi-solid media. The remaining product of papain digestion, the Fc (fragment crystalline) piece, is derived from the C terminus of the intact IgG molecule, and has no antigen-binding capacity. It is, however, of considerable importance in expression of antibody effector functions.

Pepsin digestion of intact IgG yields quite different proteolysis products. A large fragment of about 100 kDa is the main product, the remaining material usually being small peptides. The 100-kDa fragment is derived from the amino terminus of the intact IgG, has antigen-binding capacity, and is bivalent (i.e. possesses two equivalent antigen-combining sites). This is the $F(ab)'_2$ fragment.

Primary structure

Primary protein structure is the linear arrangement of amino acids in the polypeptide chain. Initial sequencing studies of Ig molecules were performed using Bence–Jones proteins, which are monomeric or dimeric light chains derived from the urine of patients with multiple myeloma (Edelman and Gally 1962). Primary sequence analysis of Bence–Jones light chains revealed that they were divisible into two distinct regions of approximately equal size. Thus, from amino acid 1 (the amino-terminal residue) to amino acid 107, the sequence of one Bence–Jones protein was different from that of any other Bence–Jones protein with which it was compared, whereas the sequences from residues 108 to 214 were essentially identical for all Bence–Jones proteins. These observations led to the division of light chains into variable (V) and constant (C) regions on the basis of the variability of amino acid sequence within the protein (Milstein 1966).

A similar structural division can be made for heavy chains. As described for the light chains, the amino-terminal regions of the heavy chains possess considerable variability from one chain to another, but the carboxy-terminal regions are relatively constant. In the case of the heavy chains, however, the variable region extends from residue 1 to residue 113, and the constant region from residue 114 to the carboxyl terminus, which may be some 400 amino acid residues distant in the primary sequence. Furthermore, when the sequences of heavy chain C regions are analyzed, it is clear that there are areas of significant homology of primary sequence along the length of the C region. The sequence can be subdivided into units of homology of approximately 100–110 amino acids. The functional importance of these domains is discussed below in the context of tertiary structure.

The V regions of both heavy (V_H) and light (V_L) chains have numerous amino acid substitutions when individual polypeptide chains are compared. However, plots of variability of amino acid versus position in the primary sequence reveal that the distribution of amino acid substitutions is not random, and that the variability is clustered in small regions of the primary structure. These areas of the V region are the hypervariable regions and they provide a molecular explanation for antibody specificity. Thus, the V_L and V_H regions of an individual antibody molecule are unique and the recognition of antigen by that antibody is similarly distinctive. As the hypervariable regions govern the specificity of the antibody molecule, they are sometimes referred to as complementarity determining regions (CDR).

Both heavy and light chains possess three CDRs. The heavy chain CDRs are located at positions 26–36, 55–65, and 95–105 in the primary sequence, and are referred to as CDR H1–3, respectively. The light chain CDRs (L1–3) are positioned at residues 25–35, 54–67, and 94–108. The above numbering is based on the EU myeloma protein (Edelman et al. 1969). Outwith the hypervariable regions, or CDRs, the primary sequence of the V region is largely conserved between molecules. These conserved regions are crucial in the maintenance of the higher structure of the V_H and V_L regions and are therefore termed ‘framework regions’.

Secondary and tertiary structure

Secondary structure is the relationship between amino acids located some distance apart in the primary structure, the interactions of which give rise to periodic structural motifs in the folded protein molecule (e.g. α helix or β-pleated sheet structures). Ig molecules contain no α-helical structures but are rich in β-pleated sheets. Tertiary structure also describes the spatial relationship of amino acids which are distant in the primary sequence and, for the purposes of this discussion, refers to those cysteine residues in the primary sequence that form intrachain disulfide bridges, giving rise to individual domains within the Ig molecule.

The ‘Ig-like fold’ or domain is a characteristic higher structural motif of Ig structure. The primary structural data indicate that the sequences of Ig chains are divisible into homology units of approximately 110 amino acids in length. Within each of these units lies a single disulfide bridge, enclosing 65–75 residues in the V regions and 52–59 residues in the C-region domains. Clearly, the location of the cysteine residues is critical in domain formation, and this is reflected not only in the conservation of this amino acid at defined positions in the polypeptide chain, but also by the conservation of primary sequences surrounding the cysteine groups participating in intrachain disulfide bond formation.

The domain structure produced by disulfide bond formation is rich in β-sheet structure, with each domain in both the V and the C regions of the Ig molecule containing two β sheets. In each β sheet, the polypeptide structure may be considered as layers of overlapping sequence lying parallel to the long axis of the domain, one layer containing three strands of polypeptide and the other four strands. The polarity of adjacent, individual strands is anti-parallel, and the two layers of β strands are joined by the single disulfide bond. Multiple, hydrophobic, amino acid, side-chain groups protrude into the space between the layers.

Quaternary structure

Quaternary structure reflects the interaction between distinct polypeptide subunits of a multidomain protein. In Ig molecules the interaction between particular domains is well defined and correlates well with biological activity. Thus, V_H and V_L domains interact to yield the correct conformation for generation of the antigen-combining site. C_L and C_H domains also interact. In the C region, like domains interact. Thus, $C\gamma2$ interacts with $C\gamma2$ and $C\gamma3$ with $C\gamma3$. However, the interaction does not always involve direct contact between the faces of the two participating domains. In IgG molecules the $C\gamma2$ domains are separated from each other by the large oligosaccharide unit located in this domain, whereas $C\gamma3$ domains interact via contacts between faces of the two domains.

The forces that stabilize domain–domain interactions are noncovalent in character and involve weak intermolecular physical forces (i.e. hydrophobic interactions, salt bridges, hydrogen bonding). Although the physical forces that mediate domain interaction are identical for V and C domains, the faces of the protein that interact are distinct. Thus, V domains interact via those layers of the domain containing three strands of peptide sequence, whereas the C domains interact via the layers containing four strands of polypeptide.

The detailed higher structure of Ig molecules is discussed in under 'Structural biology of Ig and Ig receptors' below.

Other structural features

The hinge region of IgG molecules is of critical importance to their function; located between the Cγl and Cγ2 domains, it is rich in proline and cysteine residues. The size of the hinge region varies from one IgG subclass to another, being 10–20 residues in length in all subclasses except IgG3 where it is 60 residues long (Figure 16.2). This area of the Ig molecule has considerable segmental flexibility, which is important in the expression of the effector functions of IgG molecules, e.g. the greater the segmental flexibility of a given immunoglobulin isotype, the more likely it is that complement can be effectively fixed (Oi et al. 1984). The positioning of the hinge region is such that it allows the Fab arms of the IgG to adopt a wide range of orientations with respect to each other; this feature also explains the characteristic 'Y' shape of IgG molecules visualized in antigen-binding experiments in the electron microscope (Valentine and Green 1967). The hinge region is the location of the inter-heavy chain disulfide bonds in the IgG molecule, the exact number of which varies between IgG subclasses. Thus, IgG1 and IgG4 have two interchain disulfide bridges, IgG2 has four, and IgG3 15. The region is also exposed to the solvent, with the consequence that proteolytic enzymes may attack it and generate fragments as described earlier in this chapter.

Ig molecules contain varying amounts of carbohydrate. In most instances the glycans are attached to asparagine residues (so-called N-linked oligosaccharides), but carbohydrate is also found linked to the hydroxyl groups of serine or threonine residues (O-linked sugars) in human IgD molecules and in the hinge region of human IgA molecules. In IgG molecules the principal site of glycosylation is asn297, and the N-linked oligosaccharide is usually a complex structure with two branches of linear sugars originating at a single point, although the precise oligosaccharide structure can vary enormously between individual IgG molecules. The presence of certain types of carbohydrate structure has been correlated with particular autoimmune disease states (Parekh et al. 1985), but the role of the N-linked glycans themselves in disease pathogenesis remains unclear. The other Ig isotypes are multiply glycosylated (Winkelhake 1978).

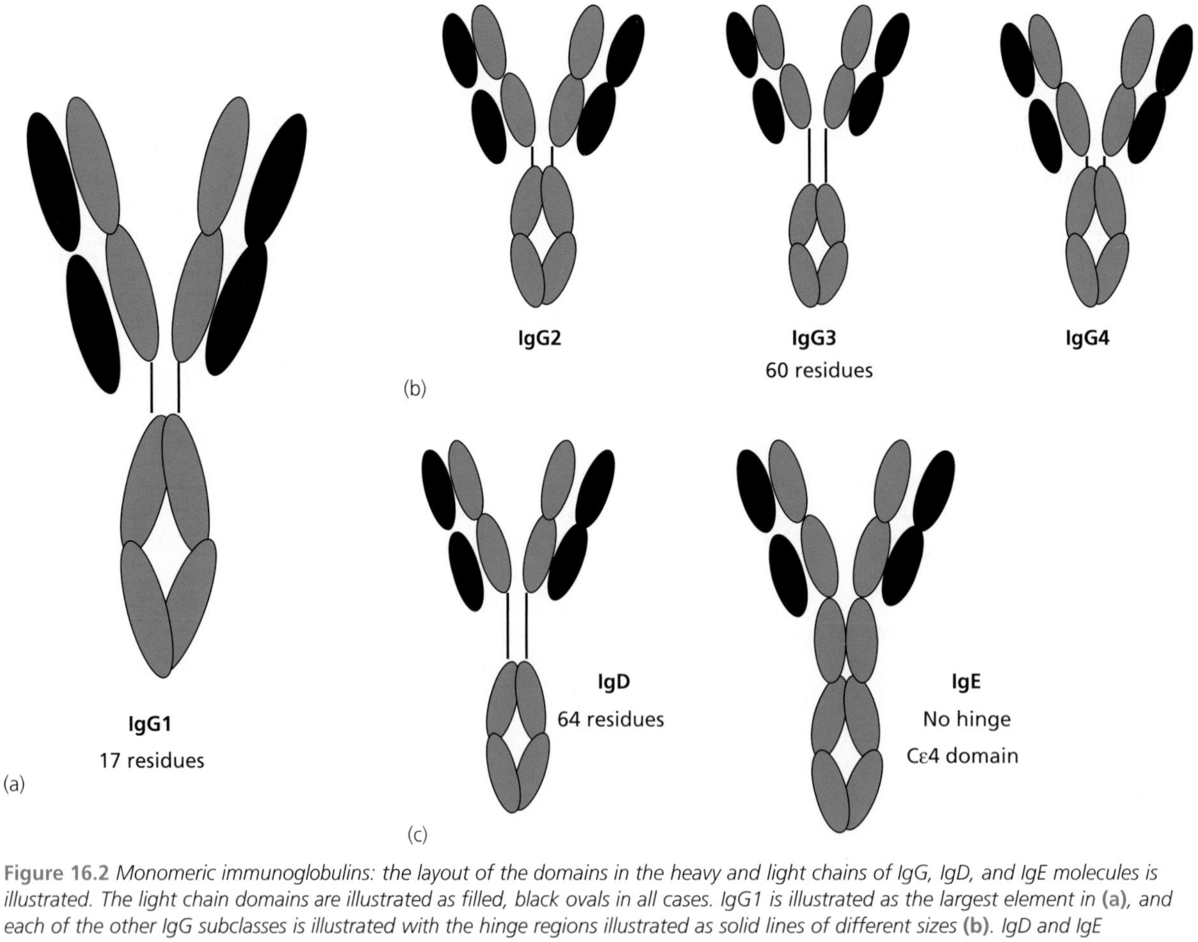

Figure 16.2 Monomeric immunoglobulins: the layout of the domains in the heavy and light chains of IgG, IgD, and IgE molecules is illustrated. The light chain domains are illustrated as filled, black ovals in all cases. IgG1 is illustrated as the largest element in **(a)**, *and each of the other IgG subclasses is illustrated with the hinge regions illustrated as solid lines of different sizes* **(b)**. *IgD and IgE molecules are shown in their 'extended' forms* **(c)**.

IMMUNOGLOBULIN CLASSES

Ig molecules exist as five classes, or isotypes, in humans, each of which has characteristic structural features and particular immunological activities. The serological marker that defines Ig class or subclass is the isotype, and the terms 'isotype' and 'class' (and 'subclass') are used interchangeably. All isotypes have a four-chain unit as their fundamental structural feature, and each class is named for the heavy chain of the molecule. Thus, IgG is named for the γ (gamma) heavy chain, IgM for the μ (mu) chain, and IgA for the α (alpha) chain. The principal molecular properties of the five human Ig classes are detailed in Table 16.1, and are illustrated diagrammatically in Figures 16.2 and 16.3.

IgM

IgM is a pentameric structure comprising five identical four-chain units, i.e. it has 10 identical binding sites. The μ heavy chain has five domains, V_H plus four C regions (Cμl, Cμ2, Cμ3, and Cμ4), and lacks a hinge region. The pentameric structure is stabilized by disulfide bonding between adjacent Cμ3 domains, and by the presence of the J (joining) chain. A single J chain is disulfide bonded close to the C terminus of the IgM pentamer (Chapuis and Koshland 1974). The critical cysteine residue (Cys575) is part of an 18 amino acid carboxy-terminal peptide extension located immediately following the Cμ4 domain, and this residue forms disulfide bonds either with J chain or with cysteines located in an identical position in other μ chains of the pentameric complex (see Figure 16.3).

IgM is the principal component of the primary humoral response. As a result of its large size (970 kDa, 19 S), it is located mainly in the bloodstream. It is decavalent, leading to highly avid binding of antigens (thereby overcoming the potentially low affinity of the antibody–antigen interaction), and is efficient in both opsonization and complement fixation.

IgG

IgG is the main class of Ig in serum. As will be obvious from the detailed discussion of the four-chain model, it exists as a molecule of about 146–160 kDa (7 S) in serum, and is an abundant component of the secondary humoral immune response. This class of Ig is found not only in the bloodstream itself, but also in extravascular spaces. It is transported across the placental membrane and is therefore responsible for passive immunity in the fetus and neonate (see Figure 16.4).

There are four major subclasses of the IgG isotype in humans, each distinguished by minor variations in amino acid sequence in the C region and by the number and location of disulfide bridges (Figure 16.5 and see Figures 16.1 and 16.2). The structural variations have consequences for biological activity. Thus, the IgG1 and IgG3 isotypes are efficient in fixation of complement, whereas IgG2 and IgG4 subclasses are less effective in activating complement. There is a similar hierarchy among IgG subclasses in binding to different types of the Fc receptor (see 'Receptors for immunoglobulin' later).

IgA

IgA is found in two forms in the body: in serum where it occurs as a monomer (160 kDa, 7 S), and on secretory surfaces where it exists as a dimeric molecule (385 kDa, 11 S) (see Figure 16.3). The dimeric form is known as secretory IgA (sIgA) and is found in association with J chain and a secretory component, the latter being involved in transport of the IgA to the secretory surfaces. Secretory component is noncovalently associated with the IgA molecules in the sIgA complex. The α chain has three C domains and, as with μ chains, possesses an 18 amino acid carboxy-terminal sequence allowing disulfide bonding to the J chain. A small hinge region is also present. There are two subclasses of IgA, IgA1, and IgA2, distinguished by their distribution and

Table 16.1 *Molecular properties of immunoglobulins*

	IgM	IgG1	IgG2	IgG3	IgG4	IgA1	IgA2	sIgA	IgD	IgE
Heavy chain	μ	γ_1	γ_2	γ_3	γ_4	α_1	α_2	α_1/α_2	δ	ϵ
Mol. wt (kDa)	65	51	51	60	51	56	52	52 or 56	70	72.5
Assembled form	$(\mu_2L_2)_5$ J[a]	γ_2L_2[b]	γ_2L_2	γ_2L_2	γ_2L_2	α_2L_2	α_2L_2	$(\alpha_2L_2)2$ J SC[c]	δ_2L_2	ϵ_2L_2
Mol. wt. (kDa)	970	146	146	160	146	160	160	385	188	184
Sedimentation co-efficient	19S	7S	7S	7S	7S	7S	7S	11S	7S	8S
Valency for Ag	10	2	2	2	2	2	2	4	2	2
Serum concentration (mg/ml)	1.5	9	3	1	0.5	3	0.5	0.05	0.03	0.00005

a) Mol. wt. of J chain is 15kDa
b) Written as γ_2L_2 for convenience; formal structural formula is $(\gamma_1)_2L_2$
c) Mol. wt of secretory component (SC) is 70 kDa.

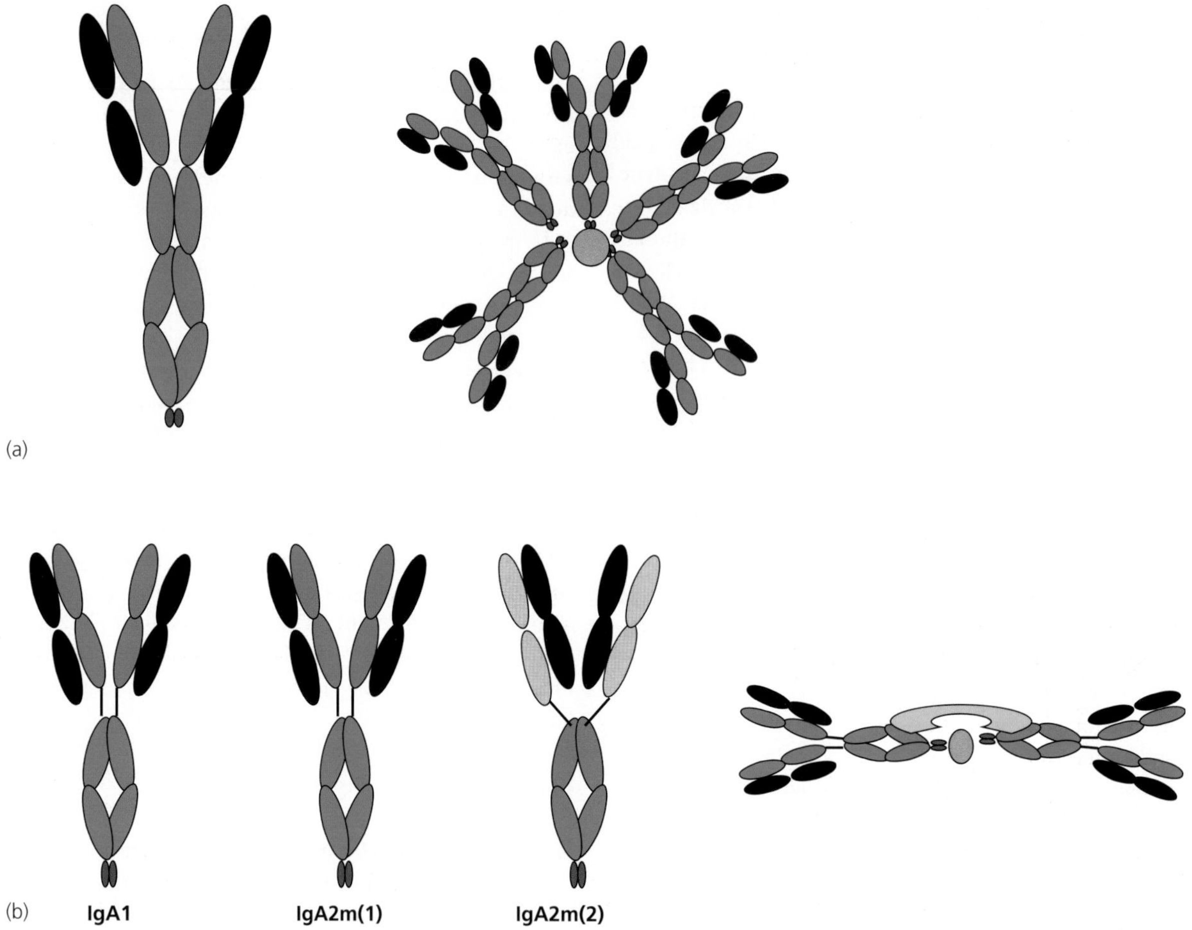

Figure 16.3 *Polymeric immunoglobulins: the monomeric forms of IgM* (a) *and IgA* (b), *based on the four-chain model, are shown. Note the different location of the light chains in the IgA2m(2) molecule (an allele of IgA2). Polymeric forms of both Igs are illustrated, with a pentameric structure for IgM and a dimer for IgA. On polymeric IgM and IgA, J chain is shown as a red circle and on IgA, secretory piece is illustrated as a yellow 'C' shape bridging the two IgA monomers. The μ and α heavy chains each possess a small region of 18–20 residues that facilitates binding of J chain; this is illustrated as a small blue oval on the figures.*

arrangement of disulfide bonds. IgA1 is the predominant form of IgA found in serum (about 85 percent of total), whereas IgA1 and IgA2 isotypes are present in roughly equal proportions in sIgA; both the α1 and α2 heavy chains can interact with J chain and secretory component.

IgA is a component of the secondary humoral response. The principal antigens that elicit an IgA response are microorganisms in the gut (e.g. antigens introduced by foodstuffs) or the airways. IgA cannot cross the placenta, and so has no role in passive immunity in the fetus. However, sIgA can be passed to the neonate during lactation and is therefore of significant protective value because the IgA transferred by the mother will reflect immune responses to pathogens present in the environment throughout the period of breast-feeding.

IgE

IgE (about 184 kDa, 8 S), historically referred to as reaginic antibody, is present in very small amounts in normal individuals, but levels are increased in patients with allergic conditions (e.g. hay fever) or those with parasitic infections. The ε (epsilon) chain has four C domains (see Figures 16.2 and 16.5), and its Fc structure is specialized for interaction with high-affinity receptors for the Fc piece of IgE present on mast cells and basophils. Crosslinking of IgE bound to such Fc receptors leads to degranulation of the cell, with subsequent release of histamine and other pharmacological mediators (Ishizaka et al. 1971; Sutton and Gould 1993; Metzger 1994, 1999), triggering a series of physiological reactions that can result in anaphylaxis. Thus, IgE is a mediator of type I hypersensitivity reactions. IgE may have originally evolved to combat parasitic infestations (e.g. by helminths), and the development of anaphylactic responses was an unfortunate byproduct. IgE does not fix complement via the classic pathway but may activate the alternate pathway. It is found in roughly equal proportions in the bloodstream and extravascular space.

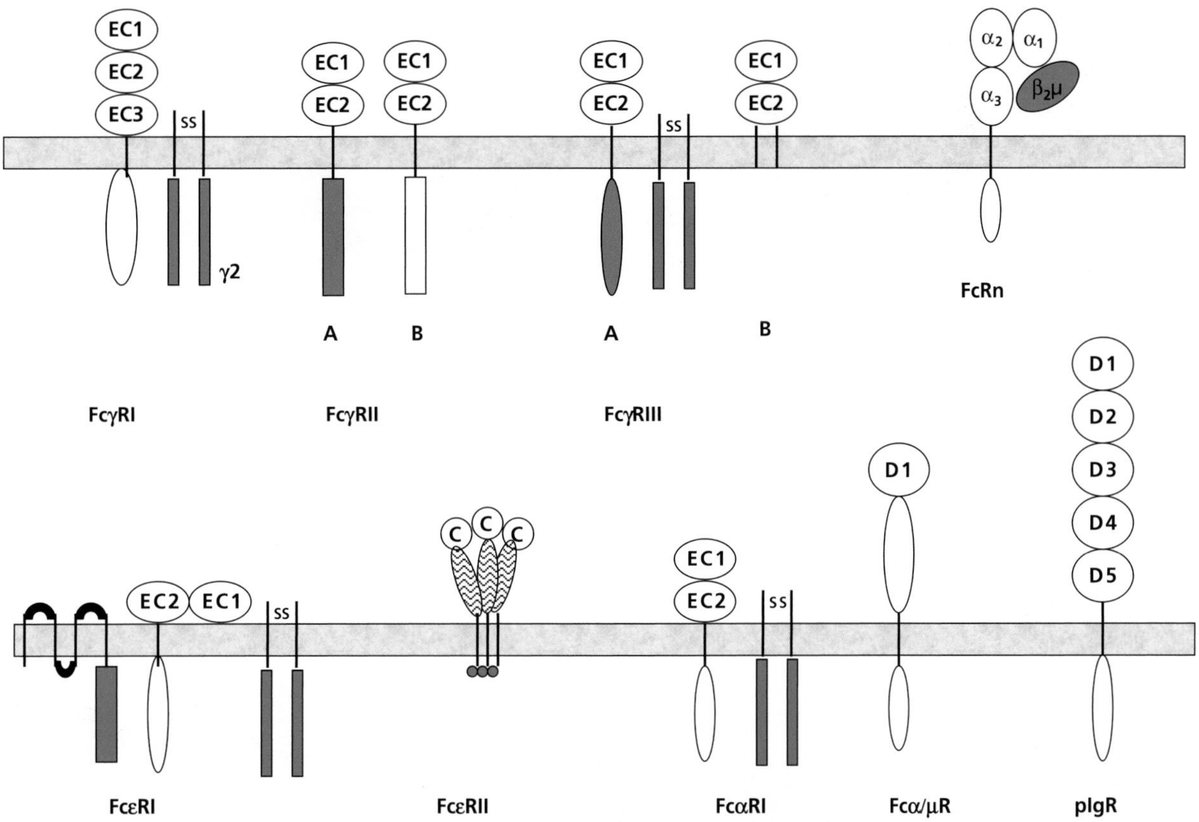

Figure 16.4 *Immunoglobulin receptors: the main classes of Fc receptor for IgG, IgA, IgM and IgE are illustrated. The upper panel shows receptors for IgG, and the lower panel receptors for other Ig isotypes. Each Ig-like extracellular domain (EC, or D in the main text) is shown as a circle, and the domains are numbered from the amino terminus of the receptor molecule. Note that FcγRIIIB is linked to the membrane via a glycophosphatidylinositol (GPI) anchor. ITAM (immunoreceptor tyrosine-based activation motif) and ITIM (immunoreceptor tyrosine-based inhibitory motif) intracellular domains are represented as filled and open rectangles, respectively. Intracellular domains with no or undefined signaling functions are shown as open ovals. FcεRIγ is depicted in a 'lying-down' orientation. For FcεRII, the C-type lectin domain is depicted as 'C' and the oval domain represents the stalk region.*

IgD

IgD is present in very low concentrations in the serum, and its exact functional role is unknown. The human δ heavy chain has three C domains (see Figure 16.2). IgD is most frequently found on the cell membrane of B lymphocytes, where its main function appears to be that of a cell membrane receptor for antigen. Human IgD does have a long hinge region of some 64 residues, and is rich in O-linked oligosaccharide groups; the extent of glycosylation explains its high apparent molecular mass (about 175 kDa). Unusually, the hinge region is encoded by two separate exons in the Cδ gene (White et al. 1985). The mouse, by contrast, has only two constant region domains, Cδ1 and Cδ3 (Preud'-homme et al. 2000). The functions of IgD are not greatly understood, although there are good numbers of IgD^+ plasma cells in nasal and tonsillar tissue. In disease terms, high levels of IgD are found in an autosomal recessive condition, hyper-IgD syndrome, which is linked to a mutation in mevalonate kinase (Drenth et al. 1999), but the links between Ig and isoprenoid synthesis are not clear.

Other immunoglobulin components

Light chains are found in two forms, kappa (κ) and lambda (λ), and any single antibody molecule contains only one type of light chain. The proportion of κ:λ in the human is 2:1, but this ratio varies considerably between species. The κ and λ proteins are products of independent genes located on different chromosomes.

J chain is a glycoprotein of about 15 kDa associated with polymeric Igs (i.e. IgM or IgA, see Figure 16.3), which serves to stabilize the structure of the polymerized immunoglobulins (Chapuis and Koshland 1974). Secretory component is a glycoprotein of about 70 kDa found almost exclusively in sIgA (see Figure 16.3), although association of secretory component with IgM, to yield secretory IgM, has been described in patients with IgA deficiency (Thompson 1970). The association of secretory component with IgM molecules is a reflection of the initial identity of secretory component as a polymeric immunoglobulin receptor (pIgR) on the basolateral surface of epithelial cells. Thus, secretory component, an important component of the sIgA molecule, is not a biosynthetic product of B cells. The immunobiology of

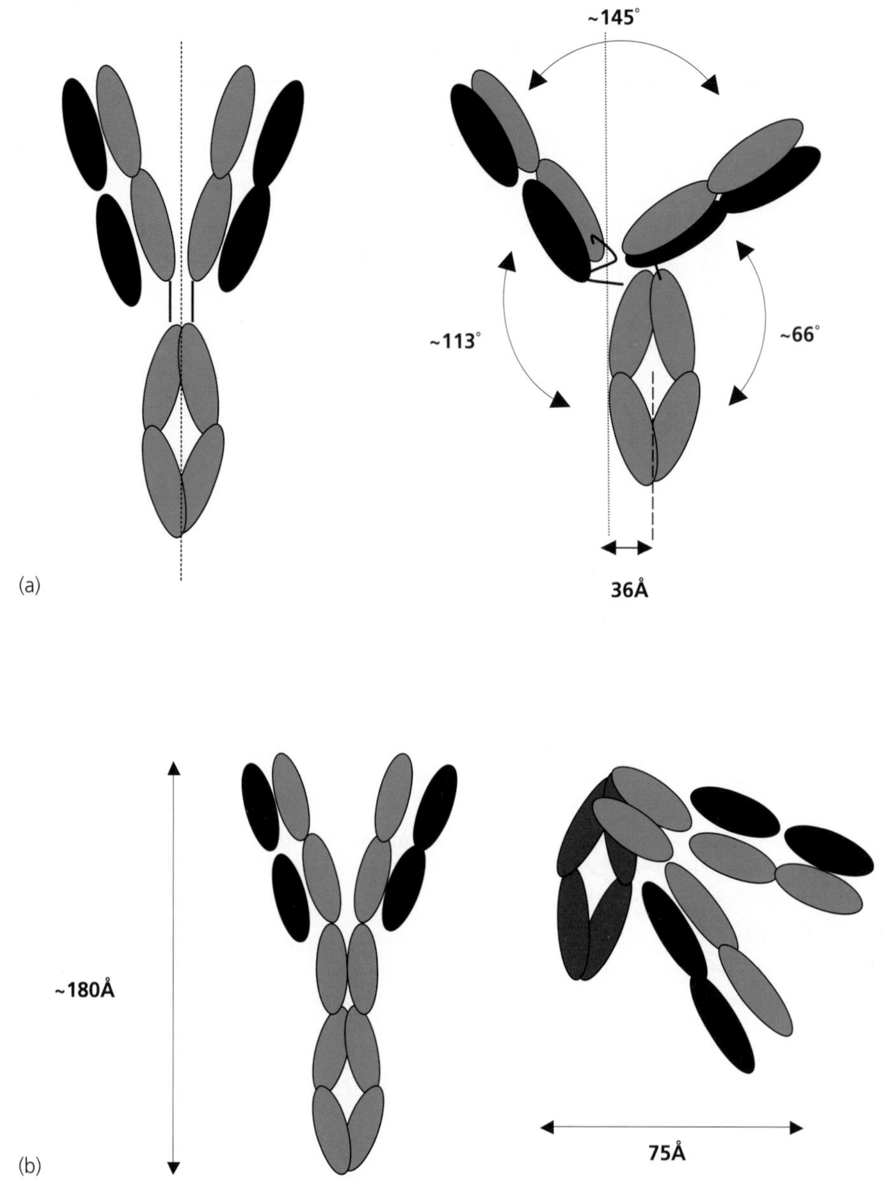

Figure 16.5 *Structures of IgG and IgE re-visited: the disposition of domains on IgG* (a) *based on crystallographic data from the b12 monoclonal antibody (MAb) are sketched and approximate sizes and relative angles of domains illustrated. The broken lines in the IgG cartoons represent the main axis of symmetry through a 'symmetrical' IgG molecule, to illustrate the 3.2 nm offset of the Fc domain in b12. Equivalent cartoons for IgE* (b) *are based on crystallographic analysis of the Cε2/Cε4 Fc region of human IgE. For IgE Cε2–Cε4, the Cε3 and Cε4 domains are shown in blue.*

pIgR is discussed under 'The polymeric immunoglobulin receptor' later).

Immunoglobulin metabolism

Immunoglobulins are being constantly synthesized, secreted into the circulation, and catabolized (Table 16.2). Once secreted into the extracellular environment, each Ig isotype has a characteristic metabolic half-life, with IgG molecules tending to be the longest-lived species, and IgE molecules being most rapidly cleared from the circulation (Table 16.2). The rate of synthesis of IgG molecules in humans is 33 mg/kg per day, i.e. more than 2 g/day for a 70-kg man. IgG molecules are generally relatively long-lived in the circulation, with a half-life of approximately 21 days; IgG3 has a half-life of 7 days. The fractional catabolic rate of IgG molecules, or the percentage turned over per day, is of the order of 17 percent (7 percent for IgG3). During an active immune response, the amount of specific antibody synthesized in terms of micrograms of protein is quite small, and represents only a minor fraction of the total IgG present in the serum. Therefore, initiation of a vigorous humoral immune response does not make a large impact on the total serum concentration of Ig. The catabolism of Ig is regulated by the Fc region and involves both protein and oligosaccharide components (Winkelhake 1978).

Table 16.2 *Metabolism of immunoglobulins*

	IgM	IgG1	IgG2	IgG3	IgG4	IgA1	IgA2	IgD	IgE
Serum concentration (μg/ml)	1500	9000	3000	1000	500	3000	500	30	0.05
Distribution (%)[a]	80	45	45	45	45	42	42	75	50
Synthetic rate (mg/kg per day)	3.3	33	33	33	33	24	24	0.4	0.002
Fractional catabolic rate (%)[b]	8.8	7	7	17	7	25	25	37	71
Half-life (days)	10	21	20	7	20	6	6	3	2

a) Distribution is expressed as the percentage of intravascular immunoglobulin.
b) Fractional catabolic rate is expressed as the percentage of the intravascular pool catabolized per day.

Membrane immunoglobulin

B lymphocytes express a receptor form of antibody, membrane immunoglobulin (mIg), on their cell surfaces. As required by the clonal selection hypothesis, the receptor antibody is identical in essentially all respects to the antibody that will be secreted by the B cell on contact with antigen. The sole difference is the presence of a hydrophobic sequence at the carboxy-terminus of the heavy chain which allows stable insertion into the plasma membrane. The mIg forms part of the B-cell antigen receptor complex (BcR), and is found associated with other proteins at the cell membrane. It should be noted that the mIg molecule is always found as a single four-chain unit; thus, primary B cells synthesizing IgM express a single four-chain mIgM unit at their cell surface although, once activated by antigen, they secrete a polymeric IgM containing five four-chain IgM units. The mIg-associated proteins are transmembrane proteins of 34 kDa (Ig-α) and 37 kDa (Ig-β) which have functions in efficient transport of the mIg molecule to the cell surface and in linking the BcR to the intracellular signaling machinery of the B lymphocyte. The Ig-α and Ig-β proteins form a disulfide-bonded complex with each other, and associate noncovalently with the mIg molecule (Reth 1995). The mechanisms of intracellular signaling triggered by the BcR are extremely complex, and involve recruitment of soluble protein tyrosine kinases, activation of inositol lipid hydrolysis, and calcium mobilization. The biological response of the B cell to binding of antigen to the BcR depends on the state of differentiation of the B cell (see Chapter 17, The B cell antigen receptor).

BIOLOGICAL EFFECTOR FUNCTIONS OF IMMUNOGLOBULINS

Range of effector functions

Antibody molecules by themselves are not directly cytotoxic toward invading pathogens. In most cases, the humoral immune system depends on the recruitment of other cytotoxic systems that can eliminate invading organisms, once specifically directed to the target by antibody. Consequently, antibody molecules participate in a wide variety of effector functions (Table 16.3). These activities are triggered after binding of specific antigen, and can involve a wide range of serum proteins, lymphocytes, and nonspecific inflammatory cells. Thus, the complement cascade is readily activated by immune complexes containing antibodies of particular subclasses. The Fc portion of immunoglobulins can be bound by specific receptors on the plasma membranes of a wide range of cells, and this interaction has consequences for phagocytosis of target organisms, or for direction of antibody-dependent cellular cytotoxicity (ADCC) for the destruction of cellular targets. Studies with fragments of Ig molecules and with monoclonal antibodies (MAb) to specific domains of the IgG molecule have demonstrated convincingly that the expression of

Table 16.3 *Effector functions of immunoglobulins*

	IgM	IgG1	IgG2	IgG3	IgG4	IgA1	IgA2	sIgA	IgD	IgE
Complement fixation	+++	++	+	+++	–	+[a]	–	–	–	–
Placental transfer	–	–	+	–	+	–	–	–	–	–
Binding to Mononuclear cells	–	+	–	+	–	–	–	–	–	–
Polymorphonuclear cells	–	+	–	+	–	–	–	–	–	–
Basophils and mast cells	–	–	–	–	–	–	–	–	–	+++
T and B lymphocytes	+	++	–	++	–	+	+	–	–	+

a) Activation of the alternate pathway.

effector functions is mediated by the Fc portion of the immunoglobulin molecule.

Neutralization

Neutralization is a direct consequence of the binding of antibody to an antigen and is an important means by which antibodies protect the host against disease. Many pathogens mediate their effects by elaborating toxic agents that bind to specific receptors on target tissues to induce a biological response or, in the case of viruses and intracellular bacteria, utilize cell-surface structures to gain entry to cells where replication can occur. In such circumstances, a protective antibody is one that specifically interferes with the interaction of the toxin or pathogen with a cell-surface receptor. In an immune response to a single agent, a large array of antibodies is produced which can bind at distinct sites (called epitopes or determinants) on the foreign protein or pathogen. Taking a toxin as an example, if an antibody binds to the toxin at an epitope that is required by the toxin for interaction with a cell-surface receptor, the antibody sterically hinders this binding of the toxin. The antibody is said to neutralize the biological activity of the toxin because the toxin cannot bind to the receptor and so no pathology or disease develops. The same applies to neutralizing antibodies specific for viruses; if antibody blocks the interaction of a virus with a receptor, the virus cannot enter a cell and consequently no replication occurs and no overt disease develops. A goal of vaccine strategies is therefore to induce the production of neutralizing antibodies in the immunized host. This has been studied at the crystallographic level using the b12 antibody directed against the HIV gp120 protein (Saphire et al. 2001b). The data show clearly that the binding site of the antibody, particularly the CDR3 of the heavy chain, mimics the CD4 natural ligand for gp130 by having a tryptophan residue protruding into space to fill a pocket in gp130 normally occupied by phenylalanine of CD4 (see 'Structure of human IgG1: the b12 anti-HIV-gp120 MAb' later).

Complement fixation

The classic pathway of complement activation is readily triggered by immune complex formation, although not all isotypes are capable of participating in this reaction (see Table 16.3). Thus, IgM is a potent activator of complement but IgA is unable to activate the classic pathway. It should be noted, however, that aggregated IgA, and possibly IgE, molecules may activate the alternate pathway of complement fixation. The capacity to activate the complement cascade depends on the ability to interact with the Clq component and, in the case of IgG molecules, on the segmental flexibility of the molecule.

The point of interaction between IgG and Clq has been mapped to three residues: Glu318, Lys32, and Lys322 in the three-strand face of the Cγ2 domain (Duncan and Winter 1988). The carbohydrate group of IgG, located on Asn297, influences the effectiveness of complement fixation because absence of the oligosaccharide leads to a decrease in activation of the classic pathway, an effect that may be explained by a threefold increase in the dissociation constant for the interaction between IgG and Clq when nonglycosylated IgG molecules are used (Leatherbarrow et al. 1985). The biology of complement is discussed in detail in Chapter 9, Complement.

RECEPTORS FOR IMMUNOGLOBULIN

Antibody molecules express a range of effector functions that are concerned with the elimination of the pathogen or antigen from the host. These functions can range from simple neutralization of function of an invading particle, to bringing about destruction and clearance of a pathogen by either activation of complement or binding to receptors for the Fc regions of individual immunoglobulin isotypes. Fc receptors (FcR) have a range of roles in the immune response, are generally isotype-specific in their binding to Ig, and show a high affinity for binding to the Fc regions of their target Ig (Table 16.4 and see Figure 16.4). Some FcRs show a preference for Ig in immune complexes whereas others can bind monomeric Ig with high affinity, and many FcRs exist, not only as membrane-associated molecules but also as soluble proteins that retain Ig-binding activity and can compete with the cell-surface receptor for Ig binding. Most obviously, perhaps, FcRs can behave as vehicles for mediating uptake of antibody-coated pathogens leading to intracellular destruction of the organisms, although FcRs can also be linked to exocytotic responses that allow cells rapidly to release pharmacological mediators and/or toxic proteins toward a pathogen in a tightly focused manner. Finally, FcRs perform regulatory roles in ongoing immune responses, serving to maintain overall homeostatic control of humoral responses to pathogens.

Receptors for IgG

There are three main subsets of receptors specific for the Fc region of IgG molecules (FcγR), each with distinctive subclass-binding preferences and tissue distributions. Each FcγR type exists in several isoforms, being encoded by separate individual genes located at chromosome 1q and/or by alternate splice variants of those structural genes. All FcγR species belong to the Ig-like domain superfamily and possess two or three extracellular Ig-like domains.

Table 16.4 *Properties of human Fc receptors*

Ig bound	Receptor	CD	Gene	Chromosome	Transcripts	Proteins (kDa)	K_d (l/mol)	Isotype preference	Signaling	Complex
IgM	Fcα/μR			1q32.3		70	3×10^9 (IgM), 3×10^8 (IgA)	IgM > IgA		
IgD	FcδR					70				
IgG	FcγRI	CD64	FcγRIA	1q21	FcγRIa	60–70	10^8–10^9	3 > 1 > 4 >> 2	γ	$\alpha\gamma_2$
			FcγRIB		FcγRIb1	60–70	10^8–10^9			
					FcγRIb2	60–70	10^8–10^9			
			FcγRIC		FcγRIc	60–70	10^8–10^9			
	FcγRII	CD32	FcγRIIA	1q23-4	FcγRIIa1	35–40	10^7	3 > 1 >> 2, 4	ITAM	
					FcγRIIa2	35–40	10^7			
			FcγRIIB		FcγRIIb1	35–40	10^7		ITIM	
					FcγRIIb2	35–40	10^7			
					FcγRIIb3	35–40	10^7			
			FcγRIIC		FcγRIIc	35–40	10^7		ITAM	
	FcγRIII	CD16	FcγRIIIA	1q23-4	FcγRIIIa	25–30	1–3×10^7	1 = 3 >> 2, 4	γ (CD3ζ)	$\alpha\gamma_2$, $\alpha\zeta_2$, $\alpha\zeta\gamma$
			FcγRIIIB		FcγRIIIb	20–25		1 = 3 >> 2, 4		
	FcRn					45 + 12	2–5×10^7			
IgA	FcαR	CD89		19		55–75	10^6		γ	$\alpha\gamma_2$
IgE	FcεRI						10^{10}		γ	$\alpha\beta\gamma_2$
	FcεRII	CD23	FcεRII	19	FcεRIIa	45	10^7			
					FcεRIIb	45	10^7			
IgM, IgA	pIgR					100–105	2×10^9 (IgM), 10^8 (IgA)	IgM > IgA		

ITAM, immunoreceptor tyrosine-based activation motif; ITIM, immunoreceptor tyrosine-based inhibitory motif; pIgR, polymeric Ig receptor.

FcγRI (CD64)

FcγRI (CD64) is the high-affinity IgG receptor, capable of binding monomeric IgG molecules. There are three structural genes encoding FcγRI (CD64), FcγRIA, -B, and -C (Ernst et al. 1992). These genes give rise to primary protein products of 30–40 kDa which are subsequently heavily glycosylated to yield mature glycoproteins of about 60–70 kDa (Ernst et al. 1998). The FcγRIA and -C genes each gives rise to a single transcript and protein product, named FcγRIa and FcγRIc, respectively, whereas the FcγRIB gene directs the synthesis of two RNA and protein products, FcγRIb1 and FcγRIb2 (Ernst et al. 1998). The FcγRIa membrane protein has three extracellular V-like Ig domains (EC1–3), whereas the FcγRIb and FcγRIc proteins possess only two such domains and lack the EC3 domain. FcγRI is the sole member of this family that is capable of binding monomeric IgG molecules, and is regarded as the high-affinity IgG receptor (association constant K_a roughly 10^8–10^9/mol per l) (Allen and Seed 1989; Shopes et al. 1990). FcγRI binds monomeric IgG1, -3, and -4 subclasses, with a preference for IgG3 and IgG1 molecules, but binds IgG2 only very weakly.

FcγRI molecules are type I integral membrane glycoproteins anchored to the cell surface via a single transmembrane helix, and they possess a large intracellular domain (Allen and Seed 1989). However, there are no signaling motifs found in this domain and the FcγRI molecule must associate noncovalently with a disulfide-bonded dimer of the γ chain of the high-affinity IgE receptor, in order to trigger intracellular signaling pathways in FcγRI$^+$ cells (Ernst et al. 1993; Scholl and Geha 1993). The γ chains possess immunoreceptor tyrosine-based activation motifs (ITAM) that recruit the necessary protein tyrosine kinases for initiation of intracellular signaling following receptor cross-linking (see Chapter 17, The B cell antigen receptor). The stoichiometry of the FcγRI receptor complex is $\alpha\gamma_2$. The presence of an ITAM within the FcγRI complex allows this FcγR to function as an 'activating' receptor on monocytes/macrophages, granulocytes, natural killer (NK) cells, platelets, and certain lymphocyte subsets. Interaction of these receptors with IgG activates phagocytosis and uptake of the immune complex (or opsonized target), secretion of inflammatory mediators (cytokines and lipid mediators), and release of other toxic agents required to bring about ADCC. Alterations to patterns of gene expression in activated cells also occur. The principal functions of FcγRI are in uptake of immune complexes, delivery of ADCC to opsonized target, initiation of inflammatory responses, and, in an immunoregulatory context, delivery of antigen in immune complexes into processing pathways for subsequent presentation to T cells.

The binding site on IgG is located in the Cγ2 domain and the lower hinge region of IgG also contributes to FcγRI–IgG interaction. The capacity of IgG to interact with the high-affinity monocyte FcR is a particular property of the Cγ2 domain of the molecule (Woof et al. 1986) and Leu235 in the Cγ2 domain is critical in the interaction (Duncan et al. 1988). As with the IgG–Clq interaction, the carbohydrate groups seem to be necessary for optimal receptor–ligand interaction, because absence of oligosaccharides severely reduces binding of IgG to FcR; the precise molecular role of the oligosaccharides is not well understood. Binding of monomeric IgG to the receptor drives internalization, but the FcγRI-IgG complexes are recycled to the plasma membrane. It is only when FcγRI molecules are cross-linked that the internalized complexes are targeted to intracellular vesicles involved in protein hydrolysis or oxidative killing of organisms (Harrison et al. 1994). The FcγRI–IgG interaction follows a 1:1 stoichiometry.

FcγRII (CD32)

As with the FcγRI family, three independent structural genes at chromosome 1q23-24 encode FcγRII transcripts and proteins (Ernst et al. 1992). The FcγRIIA gene encodes two transcripts (FcγRIIa1 and FcγRIIa2), the FcγRIIB gene three transcripts, whereas the FcγRIIC gene yields only a single transcript (Dijstelbloem et al. 2001). The FcγRII family bind monomeric IgG with relatively low affinity (K_a roughly 10^7/mol per l) and so are unlikely to bind IgG in a monomeric form (Hulett and Hogarth 1994). The mature cell surface receptor glycoproteins have M_r values in the 35 000–41 000 range, with a single transmembrane helix. All isoforms possess two Ig-like extracellular domains and, in striking contrast to FcγRI (and FcγRIII) proteins, the cytoplasmic domains of FcγRII proteins contain ITAM or tyrosine-based inhibitory (ITIM) motifs that allow these receptors to link to intracellular signaling cascades without the need for association with other membrane proteins (Daeron 1995; Van den Herik-Oudijk et al. 1995). The FcγRII proteins display subtle differences in IgG subclass-binding specificity, but there is a general preference for IgG3 and, to a lesser extent, IgG1, with binding of IgG2 and IgG4 being of much lower affinity (Dijstelbloem et al. 2001). As with FcγRI, the binding site on IgG involves the Cγ2 and lower hinge regions of IgG, with residues 234–237 being important for the interaction.

Each FcγRII protein type displays a characteristic pattern of expression. FcγRIIa is expressed at good levels on monocytes and macrophages, and on neutrophils, but is essentially absent from NK cells and lymphoid cells. FcγRIIb proteins are found on monocytes and macrophages, but not on neutrophils, NK cells, or T cells. FcγRIIb is, however, expressed on both B lymphocytes and follicular dendritic cells, where it has key roles in positive and negative regulation of B-cell responses.

FcγRIII (CD16)

The two highly homologous FcγRIII genes are also found at chromosome 1q23-24, and encode mature proteins of quite different character; there are no reports of alternate transcripts from either of the FcγRIIIA or FcγRIIIB genes (Ravetch and Perussia 1989). Both protein products have external regions of about 180 amino acids arranged as two Ig-like domains, have a low to medium affinity for monomeric IgG (K_a roughly 1–3 × 10^7/mol per l) and so are likely to bind IgG only in immune complexes or aggregates (Ghirlando et al. 1995). As with other FcγRs, there is a preference for binding of IgG3 and IgG1 subclasses over the IgG2 and IgG4 isotypes. Receptor–ligand complexes show a 1:1 stoichiometry (Ghirlando et al. 1995), and the target region of IgG for binding of FcγRIII is as described for FcγRI and FcγRII.

The FcγRIIIa protein is a heavily glycosylated transmembrane glycoprotein, containing two extracellular Ig-like domains and a small cytoplasmic domain that lacks ITAM and/or ITIM motifs (Ravetch and Perussia 1989); FcγRIIIa must, therefore, associate with other chains possessing such motifs to gain signaling capability. This is provided either by the γ chain of the high-affinity IgE receptor (Hibbs et al. 1989), as is observed with FcγRI, or by the ζ chain of the CD3–TcR complex (in NK cells – Lanier et al. 1989). FcγRIIIa is expressed on neutrophils and eosinophils and also by NK cells; activated macrophages in the tissues are also FcγRIIIa$^+$, although the receptor is absent from monocytes in the peripheral circulation. FcγRIIIB, by contrast, encodes a smaller protein product, FcγRIIIb, which is associated with the plasma membrane via a glycophosphatidylinositol (GPI) linkage (Ravetch and Perussia 1989), a feature that mandates both a lack of a cytoplasmic domain and ease of release from the membrane via the action of phospholipases. FcγRIIIb is expressed principally by neutrophils, but its expression is also induced in eosinophils by IFNγ.

Neonatal FcRn

A final group of receptors for IgG found on endothelial and epithelial cells in some tissues are the 'neonatal FcR' class (FcRn), so called in recognition of their discovery in intestinal epithelial cells of neonatal rats (Jones and Waldmann 1972). These receptors also possess Ig-like domains, but are strikingly structurally related to MHC class I molecules. The functions of FcRn include transport of IgG from the gut lumen to the bloodstream, transfer of maternal IgG across the placental barrier to the neonatal circulation, and possibly maintenance of overall levels of IgG in the circulation. Uniquely among Fc receptors, the FcRn molecules bind ligand as a homodimeric receptor and show a notable pH dependence for ligand binding.

FcRn

FcRn is a noncovalent heterodimeric complex comprising the FcRn α chain (Simister and Mostov 1989a, b), a type I transmembrane glycoprotein, and the peripheral membrane protein β_2-microglobulin (Simister and Rees 1985). The organization and structural features of FcRn are therefore very similar to those of a class I MHC antigen. The FcRn α chain is 45–50 kDa and has three external domains – α1, α2, and α3 – with the last, most proximal membrane being a classic C-region type Ig domain (Simister and Mostov 1989a, b). The α1 and α2 domains have four β strands and a long α-helical region, highly reminiscent of the peptide-binding grooves of MHC antigens, but the α helices in FcRn are very close together and this precludes formation of a 'groove-like' structure (Raghavan et al. 1993; Burmeister et al. 1994a).

FcRn has an intermediate affinity for monomeric IgG (K_a roughly 2–5 × 10^7/mol per l) (Wallace and Rees 1980; Raghavan et al. 1995) and, unlike other FcγR species, appears to function as a homodimer with a receptor–IgG binding stoichiometry of 2:1. Surface plasmon resonance studies indicate that FcRn monomers have a 100-fold reduced affinity for IgG compared with FcRn dimers (Raghavan et al. 1995). The FcRn dimers are formed via contacts between the α3 and β_2-microglobulin domains and it is believed that dimer formation is dependent on binding of IgG (in a manner similar to that observed in, for example, the growth hormone–growth hormone receptor interaction). Crystallization studies suggest that the FcRn dimer adopts an unusual configuration in its asymmetrical binding of IgG molecules (Burmeister et al. 1994a, 1994b). Thus, receptor contacts with IgG were at the interface of the Cγ2 and Cγ3 domains and were made by only one of the two FcRn molecules in the complex via residues at the edge of the α1/α2 domains and the amino-terminal region of β_2-microglobulin (Burmeister et al. 1994b). The region bound by FcRn is distinct from that bound by other FcγR species and is more akin to that bound by, for example, protein A from the Cowan I strain of *Staphylococcus aureus* (Deisenhofer 1981). The contacts between FcRn and the Cγ2 and Cγ3 interface region involve conserved histidine residues in both partners (His250 and -251 in FcRn and His310 and -433 in IgG) (Burmeister et al. 1994b). The model further suggested that, in order to bind IgG, the dimer of the FcRn molecule would be positioned such that its long axis lay parallel to the plane of the plasma membrane. In this model, the FcRn dimer is 'lying down' in order to capture ligand, and this contrasts with the 'standing up' orientation of class I MHC molecules (and indeed many other FcγR species) where the ligand-binding site projects away from the membrane distal end of the molecule (Burmeister et al. 1994b). Robust evidence that Fc receptors can adopt 'lying down' configurations is provided by the

X-ray crystallographic analysis of the FcεRI–IgE Fc interaction (see 'The interaction of IgE with soluble FcεRIα', below).

FcRn molecules are found in intestinal epithelial cells (Jones and Waldmann 1972), the yolk sac in mice (Ahouse et al. 1993), certain subsets of hepatocytes (at least in rats), and human placenta (Story et al. 1994). FcRn has an intermediate affinity for IgG, but shows a pronounced pH dependence in ligand binding. Binding is optimal and stable at pH 5–6, but is reduced up to 100-fold as pH increases beyond neutrality (Story et al. 1994). This ensures that IgG is bound at the apical (or luminal) surface of intraepithelial lymphocytes (IEL) in the gut where the pH is low, moved across the cell by transcytosis and released by the receptor at the basolateral surface of the cell (blood side) where the pH is neutral. However, there is no pH gradient across the placental barrier and, in this instance, it is proposed that IgG is bound by FcRn in intracellular acidic vesicles which are subsequently targeted to the basolateral face of the cell for release into the fetal circulation (Story et al. 1994). FcγRII is thought to be responsible for the initial binding and uptake of IgG on placental cells and delivery of the IgG to the appropriate intracellular vesicles for interaction with FcRn. The pH sensitivity of FcRn function is explained by the presence of histidine residues in the region of contact between the receptor and IgG. Once IgG is released, the FcRn dimer dissociates and is re-cycled for further rounds of transcytotic delivery of IgG, a situation that contrasts with IgA transport via the polymeric Ig receptor (see 'The polymeric immunoglobulin receptor' below).

IgE receptors

IgE is found at low levels in the blood in normal individuals and, functionally, is responsible for initiating powerful local (and sometimes systemic) acute inflammatory responses (Metzger 1994, 1999; Sutton and Gould 1993). There are two receptors for IgE distinguished by profoundly different structures, cellular functions, tissue distribution, and, importantly, affinities for IgE. The effects of IgE-mediated allergic reactions are almost entirely explained by the biology of the high-affinity IgE receptor, and it is fair to note that the efforts to understand the structure and function of this receptor have driven forward our understanding of receptors for other Ig isotypes.

FcεRI

FcεRI is the high-affinity receptor for IgE, and is a tetrameric complex of three transmembrane glycoprotein chains (Blank et al. 1989): the α chain, responsible for IgE binding, the β chain, and a dimer of the γ chain which is responsible for activation of intracellular signaling via its ITAM motifs. The affinity of FcεRI for IgE is sufficiently high (K_a roughly 10^{10}/mol per l) to dictate that monomeric IgE is bound by the receptor (Beavil et al. 1993); this partly explains the observation that serum IgE levels are low because, in fact, most of the IgE is essentially irreversibly bound to FcεRI$^+$ cells. FcεRI is expressed on mast cells, basophils, and eosinophils, where crosslinking of receptors leads to an exocytotic response, and also on dendritic and monocytic cells where a role in antigen processing and presentation is more likely.

The FcεRI α chain possesses two extracellular Ig-like domains: a transmembrane region and modest cytoplasmic domain of about 25 residues (Kinet et al. 1987). The cytoplasmic domain lacks signaling motifs, but linkage to signaling pathways is provided via the ITAM motifs found in the β and γ chains of the receptor complex (Nadler et al. 2000). The β chain belongs to the tetraspanin family of membrane proteins, passing through the membrane four times, and both the amino and carboxyl termini of the β chain are exposed in the cytoplasm (Kinet et al. 1988). The carboxy-terminal cytoplasmic domain contains an ITAM motif. The γ chain possesses a small extracellular domain, a transmembrane region, and a large cytoplasmic domain that contains ITAM motifs. The dominant FcεRI stoichiometry found on mast cells and basophils is $\alpha\beta\gamma_2$, but other cell types where the IgE receptor may be involved in antigen processing rather than exocytosis (e.g. monocytic cells) show a different FcεRI stoichiometry of $\alpha_{2\gamma}$.

FcεRII (CD23)

FcεRII is the low-affinity receptor for IgE, and is expressed on a range of cells of hemopoietic origin (Delespesse et al. 1992; Bonnefoy et al. 1997). It is a 45-kDa type II transmembrane glycoprotein and is expressed as a noncovalent homotrimeric assembly at the plasma membrane. The affinity for IgE is significantly lower than that of FcεRI (K_a roughly 10^7/mol per l) (Sutton and Gould 1993). FcεRII is encoded by a single gene at chromosome 19p21 (Soilleux et al. 2000) that gives rise to two isoforms – FcεRIIa and FcεRIIb (Yokota et al. 1988) – that differ by six or seven residues at their cytoplasmic amino terminus, and are proposed to be linked to distinct signaling and uptake pathways (Yokota et al. 1992). In human B cells, the two isoforms are subject to distinct patterns of transcriptional regulation (Ewart et al. 2002). FcεRII is unusual among the Fc receptors in that it is not a member of the Ig superfamily, but rather has features that suggest that it is a member of the calcium-dependent family of C-type animal lectins (Delespesse et al. 1992; Bonnefoy et al. 1997). The membrane form of FcεRII/CD23 can be released as several soluble proteins (soluble CD23 or sCD23) and these can act as cytokine-like molecules (Gordon et al. 1989), influencing IgE synthesis and apoptosis in mature B cells (Liu et al. 1991a; Flores-

Romo et al. 1993) and pre-B cells (White et al. 1997), and proinflammatory cytokine synthesis in monocytic cells (Lecoanet-Henchoz et al. 1995; Hermann et al. 1999). The findings of two FcεRII isoforms and cytokine-like activities of sCD23 are apparently unique features of the human FcεRII proteins.

The binding site for FcεRII on IgE is, like that for FcεRI, located in the Cε3 domain of IgE. The precise location of the contact sites for FcεRII is not precisely defined. Soluble CD23 molecules can bind IgE and compete with FcεRI for IgE binding, via simple steric hindrance, thereby providing a degree of antagonism for loading of mast cell FcεRI with IgE. In this context, it is unsurprising that atopic individuals not only have high serum IgE levels, but also have elevated concentrations of sCD23 in their serum (Yanagihara et al. 1990; Wilhelm et al. 1994). FcεRII molecules can bind IgE and on crosslinking can rapidly take up the FcεRII–IgE immune complexes, and FcεRII is required for IgE-dependent antigen processing and presentation. Ligation of FcεRII with IgE–allergen complexes delivers a negative regulatory signal to B cells, downregulating production of IgE (Luo et al. 1991). Mice lacking FcεRII fail to show a negative regulation of IgE antibody responses (Yu et al. 1994). The structural basis for FcεRII function remains to be elucidated.

IgA receptors

IgA is the most abundant Ig class in the body, having a relatively short half-life coupled with a high synthetic rate. IgA functions in several tissue compartments, namely the blood, gut, and airways, and requires receptors both for performance of effector functions and for transport from sites of synthesis to secretory surfaces. IgA therefore interacts with the polymeric Ig receptor (discussed in detail below), an IgM receptor that has specificity for both IgM and IgA (see under IgM receptors), and also with an IgA-specific receptor that assists in the protective functions of IgA. There are also data to suggest that the transferrin receptor can act as a receptor for IgA1 (Moura et al. 2001).

FcαRI (CD89)

FcαRI is an IgA-specific receptor expressed on monocytic cells, neutrophils, and eosinophils (van Egmond et al. 2001). The receptor is a complex comprising the CD89 molecule (the receptor α chain), a transmembrane glycoprotein comprising two Ig-like extracellular domains, a transmembrane helix, and a small cytoplasmic domain (Maliszewski et al. 1990), in noncovalent association with a dimer of the γ chain found in FcεRI, FcγRI, and FcγRIIIa complexes (van Egmond et al. 1999). CD89 is encoded on chromosome 19 (Martin et al. 2002). As in the other receptors, it is the γ chain that is responsible for initiation of signaling in cells following activation of the IgA receptor. The affinity (K_a roughly 10^6/mol per l) is relatively low (Wines et al. 1999), suggesting that IgA will bind to the receptor only in complexes or aggregates rather than in a monomeric form. Both IgA subclasses are bound equally well by FcαRI, a result consistent with the mapping of the binding site, on IgA itself, to the interface between the Cα2 and Cα3 domains (Pleass et al. 1999).

IgA is classically considered to be a 'non'-inflammatory immunoglobulin isotype. However, given the pattern of expression of FcαRI, it is difficult to envisage how FcαRI and FcγRI, both using the γ chain as signal initiator, would generate anti- and proinflammatory responses, respectively, after activation. It is therefore unsurprising that FcαRI$^+$ neutrophils can both phagocytose IgA-coated particles (Weisbart et al. 1988) and generate a subsequent powerful oxidative burst (Keler et al. 2000). FcαRI$^+$ cells can also mediate ADCC-type lysis of tumor cells (Keler et al. 2000), and FcαRI is important in IgA-dependent antigen processing and presentation (Geissmann et al. 2001). The FcαRI complex should therefore be regarded as an 'activatory' FcR in the same way as FcγRI, although FcαRI may act as an overtly proinflammatory receptor in a more limited set of circumstances.

IgM receptors

IgM is the first Ig isotype to be produced in an immune response, and levels of IgM are known to be important in feedback homeostatic regulation of antibody responses. This observation suggests that receptors for IgM are expressed on a range of cell types. There are two main types of IgM receptor, a GPI-linked IgM-binding protein found in activated human B cells and a receptor, Fcα/μR, that binds both IgM and IgA, but is distinct from CD89/FcαRI and, with the exception of a small conserved motif, from pIgR.

Fcα/μR

Fcα/μR is a transmembrane glycoprotein of 535 amino acids, encoded by a gene located at chromosome 1q32.3, with no significant homology to proteins already recorded in public databases, apart from single Ig-like domain in the extracellular region (Shibuya et al. 2000). The protein is heavily glycosylated and has a molecular mass of about 70 kDa. The Ig-like domain of Fcα/μR has a stretch of some 25 residues that shows strong conservation with the polymeric Ig-binding site found in the most membrane distal Ig-like domain of the poly-Ig receptor (pIgR). This site is regarded as a potential binding site on Fcα/μR for IgM and IgA. Overall, however, Fcα/μR has less than 10 percent homology to pIgR.

The Fcα/μR molecule binds IgM with high affinity (K_a roughly 3×10^9/mol per l), and the murine receptor can bind mouse, human and rat IgM molecules with broadly similar affinity. Fcα/μR also binds IgA, but with a lower, intermediate affinity (K_a roughly 3 × 10^8/mol per l). The receptor is capable of mediating endocytic uptake of IgM-coated particles, raising the possibility that this receptor could deliver antigen in IgM immune complexes to the antigen-processing machinery of the cell. It remains unclear whether ligation of Fcα/μR on monocytic cells leads to proinflammatory cytokine synthesis, and whether IgA-coated targets can be internalized by Fcα/μR$^+$ cells (Shibuya et al. 2000). The cytoplasmic domain contains no ITAM/ITIM motifs and it is reasonable to expect that Fcα/μR will associate with other membrane proteins in order to activate intracellular signaling pathways in the cells expressing it. However, there are no data to suggest that Fcα/μR associates with the γ chain found in other FcR complexes. In hemopoietic tissue, the receptor is expressed in B cells, including B-cell precursors, and on macrophages, but is absent from granulocytes, T lymphocytes, and NK cells. In nonlymphoid tissue, Fcα/μR transcripts are detected in liver, kidney, intestinal tissue, testis, and placenta, and also on thymic stroma (Shibuya et al. 2000). The functions of Fcα/μR in these tissues remain to be fully characterized.

IgD receptors

Although the existence of IgD receptors (IgD-R) is well documented, the formal molecular characterization of these binding proteins has proved a difficult problem (Preud'homme et al. 2000). The receptors expressed on human T cells appear to bind both membrane-associated IgD and secreted IgD and, in the case of the latter type, monomeric and polymeric (i.e. complexed or aggregated) forms (Coico et al. 1988b). Thus, monomeric IgD tends to downregulate IgD-R expression, whereas higher oligomers tend to enhance its expression (Coico et al. 1987, 1988a). The molecular mass of the receptor is about 70 kDa in human cells (the murine receptor appears to be different, containing two components), but there are no details of its primary or higher structural features (Tamma and Coico 1992). The receptor species appear to bind to O-linked oligosaccharides of the IgD molecule, a feature that accounts for the ability of IgD-R also to bind IgA1 molecules (Swenson et al. 1998). In the murine system the interaction of IgD-R with Ig requires Ca^{2+}, suggesting a C-type lectin interaction (Swenson et al. 1993). The paucity of molecular details makes difficult the task of defining functions for IgD-R. However, it is likely that the main roles of this receptor are in the antigen presentation process. The observation that monomeric IgD can drive IgD-R downregulation suggests that the receptor protein or complex has at least intermediate affinity for IgD, otherwise monomeric IgD would not bind for a sufficient time to be internalized. If the IgD-R is endocytosed, as seems likely in light of the trafficking of other receptors, crosslinked receptors may be internalized and routed to processing compartments for assembly of peptides into MHC molecules. Other data suggest that IgD-R can interact with glycans on membrane IgD on B cells and so enhance cell–cell contact between T cells and B cells. The molecular basis for all the potential functions of IgD-R requires cloning of receptor complementary DNAs (cDNA).

The polymeric immunoglobulin receptor

The secretory surfaces of the gut and airways are protected by secretory IgA (sIgA) (Johansen et al. 2000) or, in the case of individuals with selective IgA deficiencies, secretory IgM (sIgM) (Thompson 1970). In each case, the newly synthesized Ig must be transported from the site of synthesis across a cellular barrier in order to reach the tissue space where its protective function can be expressed. This transport is achieved via transcytosis and is mediated by the pIgR. In this elegant process, the pIgR collects the polymeric Ig at the basolateral surface of the cell, transports it via the cell cytoplasm to the apical surface, and is then itself cleaved and released from the cell (Mostov et al. 1984; Johansen et al. 2000). The cleaved pIgR molecule remains bound to sIgA (-M) as secretory component (SC) and now offers a degree of protection against proteolysis in the airway or gut microenvironment.

pIgR

Like most other Ig-binding proteins, pIgR is a member of the Ig-domain superfamily. The mature pIgR has a molecular mass of 100–105 kDa, and contains five Ig-like domains in the extracellular region of the receptor (named D1–D5), a transmembrane helix, and a cytoplasmic domain (Mostov et al. 1984). The five extracellular domains are very similar to V-like Ig domains (Mostov et al. 1984), and the cytoplasmic domain contains a targeting motif that ensures targeting of pIgR to the basolateral surface of the cell after biosynthesis (Casanova et al. 1991). There are separate motifs that facilitate rapid endocytosis after binding of pIgR and inhibition of unwanted delivery of the endocytosed complex to lysosomal compartments during transcytosis. The D1 domain is the main site of binding of polymeric Ig, although the remaining extracellular domains also contribute to binding. Pentameric IgM and dimeric IgA bind to pIgR in different ways, and association constants for the interaction of pIgR with each isotype are distinct (K_a roughly 2 × 10^9/mol per l for IgM (Goto and Aki 1984) and roughly 10^8/mol per l for IgA (Kuhn and Kraehenbuhl 1979)). Possession of J chain within the polymeric Ig appears to be a requirement for interaction with pIgR. Polymeric, J-chain-containing IgA molecules bind pIgR via D1 (Coyne et al. 1994), but also appear to require contacts between the α chain and the D2 and D3 domains of pIgR for stable receptor interaction (Norderhaug et al. 1999). A disulfide bond is formed between Cys467 in pIgR and Cys311 in the Cα2 domain of the IgA molecule (Fallgreen-Gebauer et al. 1993), which gives further stability to the complex. In contrast, binding of IgM to the pIgR appears to require only the D1 domain (Roe et al. 1999); there appears to be no need for contacts between the μ chain and D2/D3 domains, nor is a μ chain–pIgR disulfide bond formed (Fallgreen-Gebauer et al. 1993). The site of interaction of IgA α chains with pIgR appears to map to the Cα3 domain, with Cα2 also likely to be involved (Geneste et al. 1986).

Although it is indisputable that J chain is required for interaction of polymeric Igs with pIgR, what is less definitively clear is whether J chain itself makes direct physical contact with pIgR (Johansen et al. 2000). Data from knock-out mice lacking either J chain (Hendrickson et al. 1995) or pIgR (Johansen et al. 1999), in which both strains fail to transport Ig, argue in favor of a direct interaction. The capacity of anti-J-chain antibodies to block the interaction of polymeric IgA and pIgR are also consistent with a direct interaction between pIgR and J chain (Brandtzaeg 1975). However, phage display experiments demonstrating a strong interaction between Cα3 peptides and pIgR argue against a mandatory requirement for J chain for the interaction of polymeric Igs with pIgR (Hexham et al. 1999). The precise role of J chain remains to be defined, but it is possible that it interacts with polymeric Ig to create a conformation that can be bound effectively by pIgR.

STRUCTURAL BIOLOGY OF IMMUNOGLOBULINS AND IMMUNOGLOBULIN RECEPTORS

Elucidation of protein structure via X-ray crystallographic analysis invariably provides great insights into the molecular basis of protein function. The structures provide significant insight into the functions of Ig molecules and their receptors.

Structure of human IgG1: the b12 anti-HIV-gp120 MAb

The b12 human IgG1κ antibody was isolated from a phage-display combinatorial library prepared from bone marrow cells derived from an HIV-positive donor. The antibody recognizes an epitope on the gp120 protein that partially overlaps the site recognized by CD4, and the MAb can neutralize HIV infectivity by many strains both in vitro and in in vivo animal models (Burton et al. 1994).

The b12 IgG1κ molecule is highly asymmetrical in shape and structure (Saphire et al. 2001a,b). The molecule as a whole lies somewhere between a 'T' or 'Y' shape, but the Fc region does not lie centrally beneath the Fab arms. Rather, it is shifted significantly to one side of the central axis of symmetry of a Y-shaped IgG molecule and lies largely under only one of the Fab arms (Figure 16.5). Thus, one Fab arm sits on top of the Fc region and can make physical contact with it (via Cγ2), whereas the second Fab arm makes no contact at all with the Fc domains. In detailed terms (Saphire et al. 2001a, 2001b), the Fab arms lie at an angle of 143–148° relative to each other with a distance between the two apices of the combining sites on the Fab arms of 17.1 nm. The Fc region is offset by 3.2 nm from the central axis of the molecule and is twisted by almost 90° relative to the major axes of the Fab arms. The Fab arms are also rotated relative to each other, such that the light chains appear on opposite sides of the heavy chain in the intact molecule. The V_H–V_L and CH_1–C_L domains in the Fab arms have a unique 'elbow' angle between their individual axes of symmetry.

In the Fc region, the two Cγ3 domains pack closely with essentially complete symmetry, whereas the Cγ2 domains make few protein–protein contacts as a result of the presence of the N-linked oligosaccharides in the space between the domains. The Fc region can show rotational and translation shifts relative to the Fab arms, meaning that different angles exist between this region and the two Fab arms. This has consequences for the disposition of the hinge region where the hinge angle in a single molecule can be quite different. In the case of the b12 IgG1κ molecule, one hinge angle is acute (66°) and the other obtuse (113°) (see Figure 16.5).

The b12 molecule allowed good visualization of the hinge region in an intact human IgG molecule (Saphire et al. 2001a, b). The 17-residue hinge of IgG1 molecules is functionally split into three regions: an upper hinge close to the Cγ1 domain, a core hinge, and a lower hinge immediately proximal to the Cγ2 domain. The upper hinge allows rotation and other movement of the Fab arm, and the lower hinge serves the same function relative to the Fc region; the core hinge is cysteine and proline rich and is therefore involved in interchain disulfide bridging between the γ heavy chains. Surprisingly, however, the crystal structure of IgG1κ reveals that only one of the two possible disulfide bonds in the hinge region actually forms; the Cys226 residues form a disulfide, but the Cys229 residues do not. In general terms, the b12 hinge region appears to have an extended conformation, with the upper and lower hinges being somewhat disordered in the crystal structure and the core hinge having some polyproline helical character.

The combining site structure of the b12 molecule departs from the conventional view of a large flat area available for surface-to-surface contacts between the antibody and the protein antigen. The b12-combining site could be considered as a large 'spike' flanked by two platforms. The spike region is contributed by the long

CD3 of the heavy chain (CDR H3), and one platform of 1.1 nm width is composed of the remaining two heavy chain CDRs and the second platform of 0.7 nm width by the three light chain CDRs. The CDR H3 is longer than normal, a feature common to anti-CD4 neutralizing antibodies and, in the combining site, protrudes 1.5 nm above the plane of the low, light chain 'platform' and is tipped by Trp100 (Saphire et al. 2001b). In complex with the gp120 monomer, 103 nm of gp130 and 104 nm of the b12-combining site are buried, and the intercalating residues on the two proteins are completely complementary. In particular, the Trp100 residue of CDR H3 of the b12 antibody protrudes precisely into the same pocket that would be occupied by a critical residue of CD4 (Phe43) – a feature that helps to explain the capacity of b12 to act as a potent neutralizing antibody.

The availability of the b12 structure allows comparisons to be made with other complete structures (e.g. of murine IgG2a and IgG1 molecules) or partial structures (Saphire et al. 2002). The human structure differs profoundly, but a common feature is the extent of asymmetry in the structures. Thus, although the primary structures of the two 'halves' of the IgG molecules are identical, they have completely different structures. In terms of general layout, murine IgG1 is more Y-shaped, with the angle between the Fab arms being 115°, whereas the murine IgG2a has a more T-like organization with an angle of 172° between the Fab arms. The Fab 'elbow' angles in murine IgG1 appear to be identical, whereas the IgG2a equivalents are slightly different (143° and 159°). Significant differences also exist in the position of the Fc region relative to the Fab arms. Thus, in b12, the Fc region is twisted and offset by 3.2 nm relative to the plane of the Fab arms, whereas murine IgG2a is shifted 2.6 nm and away from both Fab arms such that essentially no contact between the Fc and Fab arms takes place. The Fc 'elbow' angles of the murine IgG1 and IgG2a molecules are in close agreement with the b12 Fc elbow angle, being 177.2° and 176.6°, respectively. The hinges of murine IgG1 (19 residues) and IgG2a (12 residues) are broadly similar to the b12 structures, showing extended conformations with different torsion angles in the two heavy chains. However, in contrast to b12, all three possible interchain disulfide bridges in both murine Ig hinges are formed (Saphire et al. 2002).

Structure of the IgE Fc region

Biophysical studies clearly indicate that the IgE molecule in solution is 'bent' in conformation such that the distance between the tips of the Fab arms and the tail of the Fc region is approximately 7.5 nm (see Figure 16.5), in both free and receptor-bound forms (Zheng et al. 1991, 1992). Recent success in crystallizing the Fc region (Cε2–Cε4) of human IgE provides insight into the structural basis for IgE 'bending' and begins to explain the asymmetry of the interaction of IgE with its high-affinity receptor (Wurzburg et al. 2000; Wan et al. 2002; Wurzburg and Jardetzky 2002).

The IgE Fc region contains three C-type Ig domains and has no hinge region, with the Cε2 domain occupying this position in the IgE molecule. The Cε3 and Cε4 domains can be regarded as broadly similar to the Cγ2 and Cγ3 domains of IgG, with Cε4 domains being essentially symmetrical and making extensive protein–protein contacts, and the Cε3 domains being held apart in space by oligosaccharide groups. In crystals of the Cε3/Cε4 protein (Wurzburg et al. 2000), the Fc region adopts a relatively 'closed' configuration relative to IgG Fc, but this structure 'opens up' somewhat upon interaction with the FcεRI, with the two Cε3 domains moving 1 nm apart (Wurzburg et al. 2000; Garman et al. 2000). The IgE Fc also shows considerably greater flexibility than that described for IgG Fc regions (Wurzburg et al. 2000).

However, it is in the Cε2/Cε4 Fc structure, where a pronounced bend occurs at the region that links the Cε2 domains to Cε3, that the most striking feature of the IgE Fc is found (Wan et al. 2002). The Cε2 domains associate with a high level of symmetry, adopt classic Ig-like folding patterns, but unusually use polar contacts (rather than nonpolar) to stabilize the domain interaction. The linker region between Cε2 and Cε3 is dramatically bent, folding acutely through 62° and back onto the Cε3 and Cε4 domains (Wan et al. 2002) (see Figure 16.5). A consequence of this acute folding back is that the Cε2 domain of one ε chain makes extensive contacts with both the Cε3 and Cε4 domains of the second ε heavy chain, whereas the second Cε2 domain makes rather few contacts with the more carboxy-terminal domains. The contacts made between Cε2 and the Cε3/4 region are therefore highly asymmetrical. The interaction buries a total 39.0 nm^2 of solvent-exposed surface on the Cε2/Cε4 molecule (30.6 nm^2 on Cε3 and 24.1 nm^2 on Cε4, respectively) and a total of six hydrogen bonds and three salt bridges are formed. Experiments with purified Cε2 and Cε3/Cε4 proteins in vitro suggest that the affinity of interaction between these domains is in the micromolar range, a value consistent with the area of surface interaction. A final notable feature of the asymmetry of the IgE Fc region relates to the two disulfide bridges in the Cε2 domains. These disulfides are formed by Cys241 and Cys328 in the ε heavy chain, but, rather than forming 'parallel' bonds, the disulfides 'crossover' in the structure, i.e. in each case, Cys241 interacts with Cys328 to form the disulfide bond (Wan et al. 2002).

The interaction of IgE Fc with soluble FcεRIα

The recent crystallization of a soluble FcεRI α chain–IgE Fc complex reveals the basis for IgE binding to the receptor (Garman et al. 2000). The complex stoichiometry is 1:1, there is no role for carbohydrate groups on either IgE or the receptor in the interaction, and there is little change in the receptor after ligand binding. Contacts are made exclusively between the Cε3 domain and the α chain; although the Cε4 domain provides a dimerization platform for IgE Fc, neither this domain itself nor the Cε3/Cε4 interface region makes physical contact with the receptor. The Cε3 domain binds at two distinct sites on the receptor, the first site being along one edge of the D2 domain, and the second being located at the apex of the interface between the D1 and D2 regions (Garman et al. 2000). These data explain earlier studies which suggested that mutant α chains lacking the D1 domain still bound IgE but with vastly reduced affinity; both sites are needed for high-affinity binding. The binding site along the edge of the D2 domain is centered around tyr131, while site two involves four tryptophan residues located some distance apart in the primary sequence (Trp87, Trp110, Trp113, and Trp156).

IgE adopts an unusual 'bent' conformation in solution, and retains this when bound to FcεRI (Zheng et al. 1991, 1992). The bending of IgE results in the molecule presenting a convex and a concave face, with only the convex face presenting a functional binding site for the FcεRI complex. This explains the observed FcεRI–IgE stoichiometry of 1:1. The data suggest that the FcεRI complex adopts a 'lying-down' conformation on the cell surface such that the Cε2–Cε3 interface region is readily available for interaction with the bent IgE ligand (Garman et al. 2000).

The interaction of IgG Fc with soluble FcγRIII

The molecular basis of the interaction of the Fc region of IgG with an Fc receptor was visualized using a soluble, two-domain form of the FcγRIII molecule (Sondermann et al. 2000). The partners interact with a K_a of roughly 5×10^5/mol per l, which is lower than found with intact proteins. The data obtained are entirely consistent with results from mutagenesis studies identifying particular residues as being critical for the interaction. As with the structural biological analysis of IgG, the analysis of the Fc–FcR interaction again shows a large element of asymmetry in the behavior of the proteins.

In the crystal structure, the FcγRIII molecule uses principally domain 2 to make contact with the Fc molecule, and only two residues from the linker between the first and second receptor domains also participate in making contacts with the Fc piece (Sondermann et al. 2000). The key regions of the Fc piece involved in the receptor interaction are the Cγ2 domain and the lower hinge region; as expected Leu-234 and Leu-235 residues of the Fc piece make contact with receptor elements. The contact between the receptor and the Fc region Cγ2 domains is asymmetrical, with one Cγ2 domain having more surface area buried in the interaction (23.34 nm^2) than the other (18.70 nm^2).

The contact region involves five discrete stretches of three to four amino acids of the receptor domain binding to three regions of the Cγ2 domain: the Leu234–Ser239 region of both lower hinges and an *N*-acetylglucosamine group of the Fc region carbohydrate (Sondermann et al. 2000). The physical interactions are mainly van der Waals' and hydrogen bonds, many of which are contributed by residues 234–239 in the lower hinge. These latter lower hinge regions are one of two main regions of contact in the crystal, the other being Pro329 of one Cγ2 domain which is found in a 'proline sandwich' secured tightly by two tryptophan residues (Trp89 and -110) of the receptor.

The interaction of the Fc piece with the receptor causes large changes in the structures of each participant (Sondermann et al. 2000). In the unliganded receptor, the elbow angle between the two domains is about 70°, but this opens up on interaction with the Fc region to some 80°. The Fc piece also 'opens up' on binding to the receptor, with the tips of the two Cγ2 domains being pushed 0.7 nm further apart than is observed in the free Fc structure. The interaction of the *N*-linked oligosaccharides in the Fc piece is also altered with the terminal mannose residues moving from 0.28 nm to 0.53 nm apart. One consequence of the conformational change and asymmetrical nature of the interaction is that binding of a second FcR molecule to the IgG Fc region is precluded, thereby enforcing a 1:1 stoichiometry of interaction of receptor and IgG.

CELLULAR BASIS OF ANTIBODY PRODUCTION

Theories of antibody production

The primary structural analysis of Ig molecules indicates that the humoral immune system is capable of recognizing a vast array of antigens in a specific manner. Two schools of thought emerged to account for this diversity: instruction of the immune system by each antigen or selection of pre-existing antibody by antigen. Evidence to support the selective theory was provided by studies of denatured and reduced Fab fragments of purified anti-RNAse antibody (Haber 1964). Reactivity to RNAse was always recovered after renaturation in the absence of RNAse, indicating that antigen (RNAse) did not 'instruct' the antibody to recognize it. Thus, the information for antibody specificity must be contained in the primary structure of the immunoglobulin.

The clonal selection theory (Burnet 1959) was developed to provide a framework to explain the synthesis of antibody molecules by B lymphocytes. All B lymphocytes, whether responding to antigen for the first time or daughter memory cells undergoing activation in response to re-challenge, obey the rules of this theory. The principal tenets of this theory are:

- The capacity to respond to a given antigen exists before antigen exposure.
- Each B lymphocyte possesses a single receptor specificity for antigen.
- The binding specificity of the receptor is identical to that of the antibody that the cell will secrete in response to antigen binding.
- Specific antigen is the sole signal for clonal expansion.
- The antibody produced by a cell is subject to allelic exclusion (i.e. only one set of antibody-determining genes is activated).

B lymphocytes are the cellular site of synthesis of antibody molecules. B lymphocytes, like all blood cells in mature mammals, initiate their development in the bone marrow and are derived originally from pluripotent hemopoietic stem cells. Some early B-cell progenitors are found in fetal liver and the yolk sac and, in avian species, B cells develop in the cloacal organ, the bursa of Fabricius. Moreover, in murine models, there are good data demonstrating the development of a self-repopulating B-cell subset (variously called Ly-1$^+$, CD5$^+$, or B-1 B cells) in the peritoneal cavity. In all cases, however, the B-cell development program is a multi-stage process, and regulation of differentiation is achieved by stepwise expression of key genes, accurate rearrangement of Ig genes, cell–cell adhesion and soluble signals from bone marrow stromal elements or other cell types in the periphery, and contact with antigen (Figure 16.6).

Antigen-independent B-cell development

The development of mature B cells from pluripotent hemopoietic stem cells is a complex process during which regulated rearrangement of the germline Ig heavy (*Igh*) and Ig light (*Igl*) genes takes place. B-cell differentiation can be divided into two anatomically and functionally distinct stages. The first phase of development is antigen independent, occurs in the bone marrow, and is concerned with generation of a specific receptor for antigen (i.e. successful somatic recombination of Ig heavy and light chain genes). The second phase of B-

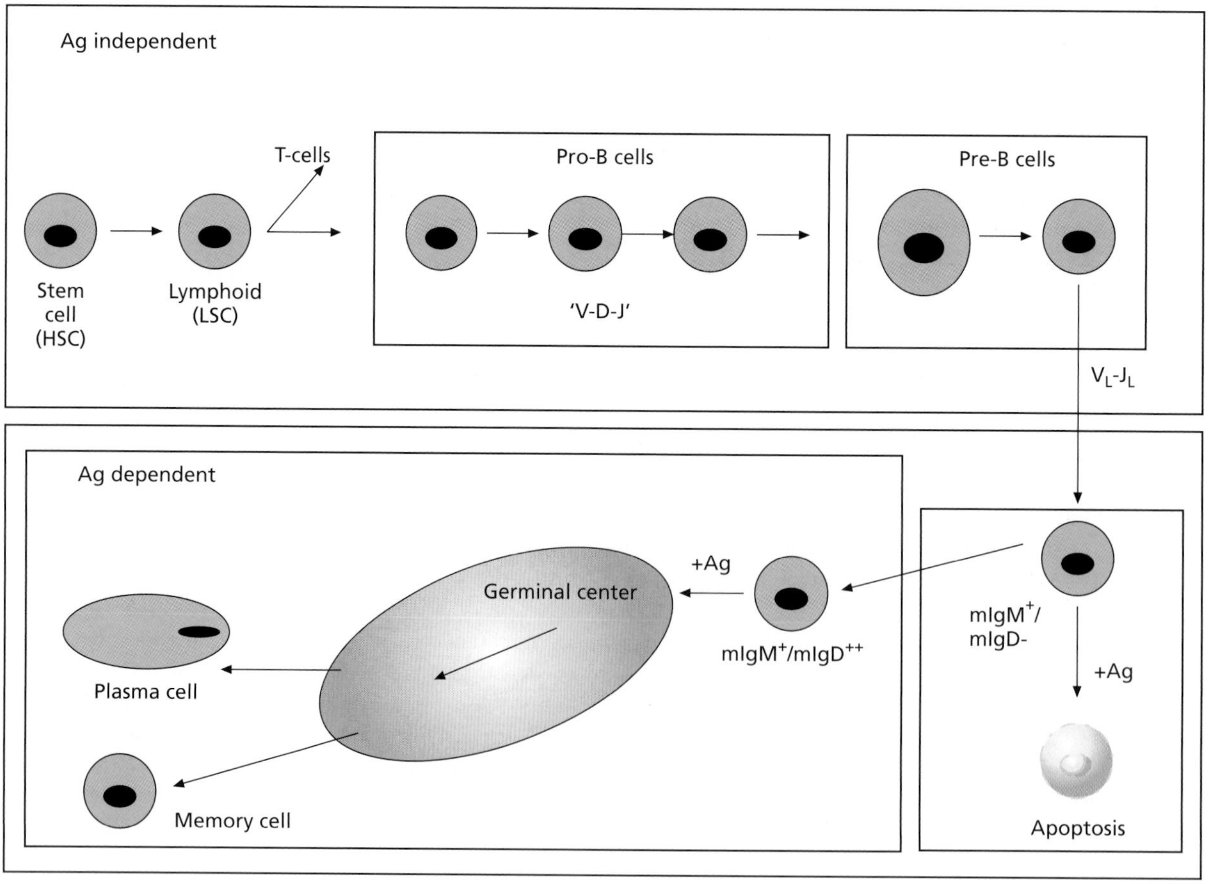

Figure 16.6 *A route map of B-cell differentiation: the main stages of B-cell development are shown. The upper panel illustrates the antigen-independent phase of development, occurring largely in the bone marrow, whereas the lower panel describes antigen-dependent events in the periphery.*

lymphocyte development is antigen dependent and occurs in the peripheral lymphoid system. In this second phase of development, the fate of B cells expressing clonally distributed receptors for antigen (i.e. membrane Ig or 'BcR') is inextricably linked to contact with specific antigen. This contact can result in clonal deletion or anergy, clonal expansion or prevention of apoptosis, and recruitment into the memory B-cell pool, with the outcome being dependent on the stage of differentiation of the B cell upon contact with antigen. A number of checkpoints and selection steps ensure that only cells expressing functional Ig heavy and light chains, which can associate into cell-surface IgM that is not autoreactive, are allowed to progress to the mature B-cell stage.

The first step in progression along the pathway of antigen-independent B-cell development in the bone marrow is differentiation of pluripotent stem cells into $CD34^+$ bipotential lymphoid stem cells (LSC). These LSCs can, depending on the transcription factors activated in this cell, become either a T-cell precursor ($CD2^+$ or $CD7^+$) or a B-cell precursor ($CD19^+$). The earliest stage at which cells committed to the B lineage can be detected is known as the pro-B-cell stage. These cells express some B-cell-specific markers (e.g. CD19), and undergo the process of *Igh* rearrangement (Hardy et al. 1991). Once the *Igh* locus has been successfully rearranged, the resulting μ chain is expressed on the surface as part of the pre-B-cell receptor (pre-BcR, described below), and the cells undergo the burst of rapid proliferation that is characteristic of the early (large) pre-B-cell stage (Kurasuyama et al. 1994). This stage of proliferation means that each productively rearranged IgH chain is duplicated in many daughter cells and has the opportunity to associate with many different IgL chains; the *Igl* locus is rearranged during the next stage of development, that of the small (late) pre-B cell. The cytokine interleukin IL-7, produced by bone marrow stromal cells, is important during these early stages of B-cell development in the mouse, particularly in its ability to stimulate proliferation of the cells (Corcoran et al. 1996). Mice deficient in IL-7, the IL-7 receptor α chain, or the cytokine receptor common γ chain (γc) have severely impaired B-cell development (Peschon et al. 1994; Cao et al. 1995; von Freeden-Jeffry et al. 1995). However, IL-7 appears to be much less important during human B-cell development, and has only a weak proliferative effect on normal human B-cell precursors in vitro (Wolf et al. 1991). One form of the disease severe combined immunodeficiency (SCID) is caused by a lack of the γc chain required for IL-7 signaling, but although they have few T cells or NK cells, patients with this disease have normal peripheral B-cell numbers (Noguchi et al. 1993).

Productive rearrangement of *Igl* leads to the cell surface expression of heavy (μ) and light (κ or λ) chain on the cell surface as intact IgM, at which point the cells enter the immature B-cell stage. This is the stage at which negative selection of autoreactive B cells occurs, resulting in B-cell tolerance. Thus, only non-self-reactive B cells are able to exit the bone marrow and enter the periphery, where they complete their development into mature B cells, which express cell-surface IgM and IgD and can be activated on binding of antigen.

Selection during antigen-independent B-cell development

Selection of B cells occurs throughout their development. One of the most important and best-characterized selection events is for pre-B cells, which are capable of expressing the pre-BcR. Once IgH rearrangement is complete, μ chain is expressed on the cell surface as one component of the pre-BcR; the other components are the surrogate light chains λ_5 and $V_{pre\text{-}B}$, products of B-cell-specific, non-rearranging genes, and the signaling components Igα and Igβ. Only μ chains resulting from in-frame *Igh* recombination and capable of binding κ or λ light chain after *Igl* rearrangement will be able to associate with the rest of the pre-BcR and allow signaling through this receptor. Productive rearrangement and the resulting pre-BcR signaling lead to proliferation of the cells (Kurasuyama et al. 1994); those cells with non-productive rearrangements cannot form the pre-BcR and/or signal through that complex, and so will not progress further through the B-cell developmental pathway. Proliferation induced by pre-BcR signaling appears to be self-limiting, as production of the λ_5 surrogate light chain component ceases once the pre-BcR is expressed on the cell surface. Thus, the expression level of the pre-BcR and the proliferative signals transduced by it reduce as proliferation progresses, until the cells no longer receive the proliferative signal and so exit the cell cycle. No ligand has yet been identified for the pre-BcR, and it has been speculated that no such ligand exists. Thus, it is possible that it is simply the expression of the pre-BcR on the cell surface that causes the complex to signal, rather than binding of an extracellular ligand to the complex.

The importance of signaling through the pre-BcR is demonstrated by the effect of loss of activity of the Bruton's tyrosine kinase (Btk), a defect that results in X-linked agammaglobulinemia (XLA) (Vetrie et al. 1993). Btk is an important component of the pre-BcR (and, indeed, of the mature BcR) signaling pathway and its loss results in a defect in the ability of pro-B cells to progress to the pre-B-cell stage and proliferate (Nomura et al. 2000). Thus, XLA patients have reduced numbers of pre-B cells (and therefore also of mature B cells), with the severity of the reduction in numbers varying depending on the precise Btk mutation inherited by the patient (Hashimoto et al. 1999). Interestingly, loss of Btk function in mice, by either natural mutation or targeted gene disruption, results in a much less severe phenotype than seen in human XLA (Scher 1982;

Kerner et al. 1995). These data suggest a lesser reliance on Btk in early murine B-cell development than in human B-cell development.

Expression of the intact μ chain and the pre-BcR also leads to allelic exclusion at the *Igh* locus; recombinase activating gene products (RAG) 1 and 2 are degraded, and presumably alterations in transcription factor expression at the pro-B- to pre-B-cell transition reduce the accessibility of the *Igh* locus, preventing further recombination (Grawunder et al. 1995). Thus, only a single productively rearranged Igh locus is present in each pre-B cell. The ability of a productively rearranged *Igh* locus to induce allelic exclusion has been convincingly demonstrated using mice transgenic for a particular V_HDJ_H gene combination: the only μ chain expressed is that of the transgene, indicating that its presence and ability to associate in the pre-BcR prevent rearrangement of either of the endogenous IgH alleles (Nussenzweig et al. 1987).

The next stage at which B cell selection takes place is after rearrangement of the *Igl* locus. In a manner similar to that of selection of pre-B cells, which can successfully associate intact μ chain in the pre-BcR, only those cells in which the product of the newly recombined κ or λ light chain gene can associate with existing μ chain to allow expression of IgM on the cell surface in association with Igα and Igβ and form the mature BcR can progress further. The signal resulting in this positive selection is not known, but successfully selected cells go on to become surface-expressing immature B cells, and undergo the next level of selection.

So far, cells have only been selected for the ability to express intact and functional μ and κ/λ chains; there has been no negative selection to remove those cells that express autoreactive receptors. This occurs at the immature cell stage. Interestingly, it seems that not all autoreactive cells are immediately deleted; instead, cells expressing self-reactive surface IgM can enter a process known as 'receptor editing', during which secondary rearrangements at the *Igh* and/or *Igl* loci change the antigen specificity of the BcR expressed (Tiegs et al. 1993). If receptor editing does not succeed, self-reactive immature B cells undergo anergy or apoptosis on encounter with antigen. This contrasts with the ability of mature B cells to become activated on encounter with antigen: mature cells become activated, whereas immature cells die by apoptosis. The differences in signaling mechanisms underlying these radically different responses to antigen at the immature and mature B-cell stages are considered in detail in Chapter 17, The B cell antigen receptor.

Transcriptional control of B-cell development

So far, the mechanisms of B-cell development, but not of the control of the developmental pathway, have been discussed. This takes place through the expression of various transcription factors, which regulate the activation of lineage-appropriate genes, the repression of genes associated with development of other hemopoietic lineages, and through control of the accessibility of the *Igh* and *Igl* loci to the recombination machinery. Several of the most important and best-studied transcription factors are considered here.

PU.1

PU.1 is a member of the Ets family of transcription factors, and is expressed in monocytic, granulocytic, and lymphoid lineages (Klemsz et al. 1990). Ets sites, which can be bound by PU.1 in association with various other proteins, are found in a number of genes important in B-cell development, including *Igh* and *Igl* genes, RAG1, components of the pre-BcR, Btk, and terminal deoxynucleotidyl transferase (TdT) (Kozmik et al. 1992; Omori and Wall 1993; Ha et al. 1994; Fitzsimmons and Hagman 1996; Muller et al. 1996). PU.1-deficient mice lack both B- and T-cell precursors, and die before birth (Scott et al. 1997), but experiments in which $PU.1^{-/-}$ embryonic stem cells or fetal liver cells were transferred to irradiated normal animals suggests that this transcription factor is especially important in the development of a multipotential lymphomyeloid precursor cell (Scott et al. 1997). Although PU.1 is expressed in cells from various hemopoietic lineages in normal animals, it appears to play a role in lineage commitment. Retroviral transfer of PU.1 to $PU.1^{-/-}$ lymphomyeloid progenitor cells from fetal liver rescued development of both B cells and macrophages, but the macrophages expressed significantly higher levels of PU.1 than the B cells (DeKoter and Singh 2000); these experiments also demonstrated that overexpression of PU.1 inhibits B-cell development. Thus, PU.1 operates very early in hemopoietic development, at the level of multipotent precursors and lineage commitment.

IKAROS AND AIOLÖS

Ikaros is mainly expressed in hemopoietic cells, particularly in B-cell precursors, suggesting a role for Ikaros in B-cell development. Ikaros-deficient mice lack fetal B and T cells, but only peripheral B cells are missing from the adult mice (Wang et al. 1996). The block in B-cell development caused by loss of Ikaros is before the pro-B-cell stage (Wang et al. 1996), and Ikaros-binding sites have been identified in the promoters of RAG1, Igα, V_{preB}, λ_5, and TdT genes (Georgopoulos et al. 1997). In the TdT promoter, the Ikaros-binding site overlaps an Ets-binding site, suggesting that Ikaros and Ets transcription factors may compete for binding here (Ernst et al. 1996).

Aiolös is a member of the Ikaros family of proteins but is expressed later in development than Ikaros itself (Morgan et al. 1997). Aiolös is first detected in committed B- and T-cell precursors, and its expression levels increase as the cells mature (Morgan et al. 1997). Aiolös-deficient mice have increased numbers of pro- and pre-B cells, suggesting a defect in differentiation of the cells to the later stages of antigen-independent development (Wang et al. 1998). Such mice also show defects in mature B-cell functions, including isotype switching in the absence of immunization, proliferation in response to very low levels of BcR signaling, and the formation of B-cell lymphomas (Wang et al. 1998). In contrast to Aiolös$^{-/-}$, Ikaros$^{+/+}$ mice, animals that are Aiolös$^{-/-}$ Ikaros$^{+/-}$ have decreased numbers of both pre-B and mature B cells (Cortes et al. 1999), suggesting that these two transcriptional regulatory proteins act together. In fact, the two proteins are expressed in a complex in both developing and mature B-cell populations. Mature B cells in Aiolös$^{-/-}$ Ikaros$^{+/-}$ mice are also more readily activated than those derived from Aiolös$^{-/-}$ Ikaros$^{+/+}$ mice (Cortes et al. 1999), indicating that the two proteins may also act in concert to regulate signaling thresholds for B-cell activation through the BcR.

E2A

Alternate splicing leads to the production of two proteins from the *E2A* gene, known as E12 and E47 (Murre 1994). These basic helix–loop–helix transcription factors are members of the E protein family (also known as class I HLH proteins), the members of which homo- or heterodimerize (to other E proteins or to members of the class II HLH family) to allow binding to the sequence CANNTG, known as an E-box site. This sequence is found in the promoter of a number of B-lineage genes, including Igα and λ_5 (Sigvardsson et al. 1997). E12 and E47 are ubiquitously expressed, but are especially important in B-cell development, where B-cell-specific phosphorylation allows the E47 protein to form a DNA-binding homodimer (Sloane et al. 1996). In other tissues, E proteins such as E12 and E47 usually heterodimerize with class II HLH proteins; thus such homodimerization is tissue specific. E12 and E47 act early in B-cell development, and mice deficient in E2A have B cells that are blocked at the very early pro-B cell stage, before DJ_H rearrangement, and have virtually no mature B cells (Bain et al. 1994). These cells also do not express proteins associated with B-cell commitment and development, such as Igα and RAG1, underlining the important role played in early B-cell development by the E2A proteins (Bain et al. 1994, 1997; Zhuang et al. 1994).

The early and profound block in B-cell development seen in E2A$^{-/-}$ mice means that these mice cannot be used to identify genetic targets of the E12 and E47 transcription factors, or their potential roles in later B-cell development. Thus, alternate strategies, such as transfection of non-B-lineage cell lines with E12 or E47, must be employed. Such studies have shown that, in various cell lines, expression of E47 results in production of germline Ig transcripts, the RAGs and TdT, suggesting an involvement in regulation of Ig rearrangement as well as lineage commitment (Schlissel et al. 1991; Choi et al. 1996; Romanow et al. 2000). Indeed, when E47 and the RAG genes are expressed in a human embryonic kidney carcinoma cell line, both *Igh* DJ and Igκ VJ rearrangements are seen (Romanow et al. 2000). Rather than the transcription factors acting directly in V(D)J recombination, however, it appears that binding of E2A proteins to Ig enhancers increases the accessibility of these loci to the recombination machinery. Transfection of E12 into a macrophage cell line that has rearranged *IgH* and Igκ genes, but which does not express cell surface IgM, results in the induction of a number of B-cell-specific genes, including RAG-1, EBF, λ_5, and *Pax5* (Kee and Murre 1998). It is also notable that there is a gene dosage effect for E2A proteins in B-cell development. Thus E2A$^{+/-}$ mice have 50 percent of the numbers of B cells found in E2A$^{+/+}$ animals (Zhuang et al. 1994). This effect is explained by the Id protein family discussed below.

Another means of investigating the roles of E2A proteins in B-cell development is to transfect members of an E2A-inhibiting family known as Id proteins into E2A-expressing cells. These Id proteins are related to the E proteins, containing the domain that allows them to heterodimerize with E proteins but not the DNA-binding domain (Sun et al. 1991). Thus, expression of Id proteins causes E proteins to be 'trapped' in non-DNA-binding E–Id heterodimers, effectively inhibiting the function of the E proteins. Mice expressing an *Id1* transgene exhibit the same block in B-cell development as E2A-deficient mice, and the severity of the block is dependent on the level of expression of the transgene, i.e. on the amount of E2A proteins that can be sequestered by *Id1* (Sun et al. 1991).

EBF

As mentioned above, transfection of cell lines with E2A proteins has shown that these transcription factors can induce production of early B cell factor (EBF) (Kee and Murre 1998). This is supported by the observation that, although EBF-deficient mice, similar to E2A$^{-/-}$ mice, exhibit an early block in B-cell development (Lin and Grosschedl 1995), the few B-cell precursors that are found express E12 and E47, indicating that E2A expression is not dependent on EBF expression (Lin and Grosschedl 1995). A number of B-cell-specific genes have binding sites for EBF in their promoters, including Igα, Igβ, and λ_5 (Kee and Murre 1998), indicating that expression of these proteins may be directly regulated by EBF. EBF and the E2A transcription factors appear to act together to regulate certain B-cell-specific genes, such as the components of the surrogate light chain, and binding sites for both EBF and E47 are present in the λ_5 promoter (Sigvardsson et al. 1997).

PAX5/BSAP

Expression of the *Pax5* gene, encoding the B-cell stimulatory/activatory protein (BSAP) protein, is regulated by the E2A and EBF transcription factors; EBF binds to a site in the *Pax5* promoter, and activates transcription. The BSAP protein is expressed in all committed B cells from the pro-B stage until activation of mature B cells; plasma cells do not express this transcription factor (Busslinger and Urbanek 1995). Interestingly, BSAP appears to function as both a transcriptional activator and a repressor: it activates genes for B-cell-specific proteins such as CD19 and the surrogate light chains, but represses genes associated with other hemopoietic lineages (Kozmik et al. 1992; Nutt et al. 1998, 1999; Wallin et al. 1998). This dual function is dependent on *Pax5* protein levels in the cell; transcriptional activatory sites have a higher affinity for *Pax5* than repressive sites (Wallin et al. 1998), and so the activation functions of this transcription factor can be carried out when the protein is present at lower levels than is necessary for repression. B-cell development in mice deficient in *Pax5* is blocked at the pro-B-cell stage (Nutt et al. 1997), i.e. slightly later in the differentiation pathway than is seen in the $E2A^{-/-}$ and $EBF^{-/-}$ mice; this is consistent with the regulation of *Pax5* by EBF. The role of *Pax5*/BSAP in B-cell commitment has recently been demonstrated in vitro, using pro-B cells from $Pax5^{-/-}$ mice. Under suitable culture conditions, these cells, which appear to be committed to the B-cell lineage, can differentiate into a variety of other hemopoietic lineages, including macrophages, granulocytes, and T cells (Nutt et al. 1999). Thus, expression of *Pax5* appears to be vital to allow very early B cells to commit irreversibly to the B lineage.

Thus, B-cell commitment and development are controlled by the sequential expression of a number of transcription factors that control the developmental pathway by activating those genes required for B-cell differentiation and repressing lineage-inappropriate genes.

Antigen-dependent B-cell development

Recirculating mature B cells in the periphery die after several weeks or months unless they encounter an antigen containing epitope(s) recognized by the cell's BcR. Numbers of mature B cells are maintained by the continual replacement of 'old' B cells by newly developed cells that have emigrated from the bone marrow.

B cells can be activated in either the presence or absence of help from T cells, depending on the type of antigen encountered. T-independent (TI) antigens can themselves provide the co-stimulatory signals required for B-cell activation, either through binding non-BcR cell-surface receptors that cause B-cell activation, or through extensive crosslinking of the BcR by highly repetitive antigens. TI antigens usually lead to low-affinity IgM responses. Mature B cells that are activated by T-dependent antigen in the presence of co-stimulatory signals undergo further differentiation, which allows the cells to:

- introduce mutations into their IgH and IgL chain genes to increase affinity for the antigen (somatic hypermutation)
- change the isotype of the antibody produced (class or isotype switching)
- become either antibody-secreting plasma cells or memory B cells.

This affinity maturation of B-cell responses occurs in specialized structures within lymph nodes known as germinal centers, and allows the humoral response to become faster and more efficient on future contact with the same antigen.

B-CELL ACTIVATION

Most immune responses require both contact between, and activation of, B and T cells recognizing the same antigen (although not necessarily the same epitope on that antigen). Binding of specific antigen by B cells leads to signaling through the BcR, which activates the B cell. In addition, the antigen–BcR complex is internalized by the B cell; the antigen is processed and then presented on the cell surface in association with MHC class II molecules. In the T-cell area of the lymph node, antigen-presenting B cells interact with antigen-specific $CD4^+$ helper T cells, which have been primed by encounter with the antigen presented on MHC class II by interdigitating dendritic cells in the lymph node. Only B cells that interact with T cells that have been activated by the same antigen will go on to differentiate further.

The interaction of B cells with antigen-specific T cells involves a number of receptor–ligand pairs on the two cell types in addition to the MHC class II–T cell receptor interaction. Various adhesion molecule pairs, such as leukocyte function-associated antigen-1 (LFA-1) and intercellular adhesion molecule 1 (ICAM-1), each of which is expressed on both B and T cells, contribute to stabilizing the interaction. These adhesion molecules can also transduce signals into the cells that contribute to B-cell activation, although the signaling pathway(s) used is not clear.

Perhaps the most important co-stimulatory interaction that takes place during B-cell activation is that of CD40 (on B cells) and its ligand (CD40L or CD154) on activated T cells and follicular dendritic cells (FDC) (Gordon and Pound 2000). Engagement of CD40 by its ligand promotes a variety of functions involved in enhancement of B-cell responses, including proliferation, antibody synthesis, cytokine production, and isotype switching. Once activated, B cells are predisposed to apoptose in the absence of survival signals at various checkpoints during antigen-dependent differentiation;

signaling though the CD40–CD40L interaction is an important survival signal for the cells and inhibits apoptosis of germinal center B cells in vitro. The importance of CD40-mediated signaling is underlined by the effects of a mutation in the gene for CD40L, which results in the immunodeficiency disease X-linked hyper-IgM syndrome (Kroczek et al. 1994). Patients with this disease have impaired antibody responses, mainly caused by an inability of B cells to undergo class switching and affinity maturation, resulting in overproduction of low-affinity IgM antibodies (see 'Mechanisms of somatic recombination' below). Additional signals are received by B cells through interactions between B-cell surface CD80 (B7–1) or CD86 (B7–2) and T-cell CD28 (Jeannin et al. 1997). These interactions are also important in the co-stimulation of T cells by signaling through CD28. CD80 and CD86 are expressed on centrocytes, but not on centroblasts.

Once B cells are activated by encounter with antigen-specific, activated, helper T cells, they can differentiate immediately into antibody-secreting plasma cells. These plasma cells will usually produce only low-affinity antibody, of the IgM isotype, but allow specific antibody to be secreted while other B cells undergo additional differentiation to produce higher-affinity antibodies of different isotypes. Those activated B cells that do not develop into plasma cells at this stage enter the primary follicle in the lymphoid tissue, adjacent to the T-cell area where they have been activated, and initiate the formation of a germinal center (Maclennan 1994). The germinal center consists of a dark zone containing centroblasts (B cells rapidly proliferating and undergoing somatic hypermutation) and a light zone containing centrocytes (B cells undergoing selection for high-affinity BcRs after somatic hypermutation has taken place).

SOMATIC HYPERMUTATION, CLASS SWITCHING, AND SELECTION

The process of somatic hypermutation introduces mutations into the IgH and IgL V(D)J regions; these are usually point mutations, although deletions and duplications are also occasionally found (Goossens et al. 1998). The mechanism by which mutation occurs is not well understood, and although upregulation of the RAG genes is found in germinal center B cells (Han et al. 1996), the type of gene rearrangement seen in earlier stages of B-cell development does not seem to occur. There is some evidence to suggest that mutations are introduced by a form of error-prone, DNA-repair system. Whatever the method used, the process of hypermutation introduces mutations into the V(D)J region at a rate of approximately 1 change per 10^3 basepairs/cell per generation (McKean et al. 1984).

Introduction of mutations does not necessarily lead to increased affinity for the antigen; many mutated BcRs will have reduced affinity or will even become potentially autoreactive. Thus, some form of selection must operate to allow those B cells with increased affinity to survive, and those with reduced affinity or altered antigen specificity to be lost. As mentioned above, germinal center B cells are predisposed to apoptose in the absence of survival signals, and these survival signals are dependent on the ability of the BcR to interact with antigen and of the cell to present antigen to specific T-helper (Th) cells and receive survival signals from them (Liu et al. 1991b). Therefore, after somatic hypermutation has taken place, the centroblasts move from the dark zone of the germinal center to the light zone, where they become centrocytes and can interact with mature FDCs present in this area. These FDCs express a number of cell-surface receptors, including complement receptors and Fc receptors, which allow them to bind large quantities of immune complexes and retain them for long periods of time on the cell surface. Centrocytes compete for access to these immune complexes, resulting in rescue signals (e.g. through the CD40–CD40L interaction (Gordon and Pound 2000)) from the FDCs for only those centrocytes expressing the highest affinity BcRs. Those cells that are selected (i.e. those with high-affinity BcRs) are able to acquire and process the antigen from the FDCs and present it on class II MHC to T cells, receiving a further survival signal from the antigen-specific Th cells at this stage. These two stages of selection ensure that only cells with high-affinity BcRs, which recognize antigen that is also recognized by T cells, are allowed to survive passage through the germinal center; other cells die by apoptosis. This prevents the survival of centrocytes that recognize self-antigen after somatic hypermutation, because, even if the self-antigen is present on FDCs, no T cells specific for that antigen will be present.

As discussed earlier, antibody molecules can carry out different effector functions by utilizing different C regions in the *IgH* gene. Switching is dependent on engagement of B-cell CD40 by its ligand (Kawabe et al. 1994), and the production of different cytokines by Th cells which induce switching to specific Ig isotypes, e.g. activation of B cells in the presence of IL-4 leads to production of IgE (Th2-type response), whereas IFN-γ causes switching to IgG3 and IgG2_2 (Th1-type response). The molecular mechanisms underlying immunoglobulin isotype switching are discussed under 'Class switch recombination' below.

B cells that have undergone somatic hypermutation and class switching can either form high-affinity plasma cells in the lymph nodes or bone marrow, which secrete large amounts of specific, high-affinity antibody of the appropriate isotype for 2–3 weeks before dying, or become long-lived memory B cells. These memory B cells retain the antigen specificity and antibody isotype determined by their differentiation in the germinal center, and remain in the lymph node until they again encounter antigen. At this time, they become activated more quickly than naïve B cells, allowing a faster response to antigen; they also have greater capacity for presenting antigen to T cells, through higher expression of MHC class II and co-stimulatory molecules such as CD80 and CD86.

IMMUNOGLOBULIN GENES AND ANTIBODY DIVERSITY

Antibody diversity

The adaptive immune system must be able to generate a very large number of different antibodies (or BcRs and hence B lymphocytes) in order to recognize all possible antigens that may be encountered by the host. The same is true of T-cell receptors (TcR). However, the size of the genome is finite, and so genetic mechanisms must exist to enable a large number of gene products (Ig chains) to be assembled from a limited number of genes. How is this achieved?

The pioneering experiments of Tonegawa and his colleagues demonstrated that the genetic elements encoding V and C regions of the polypeptide are located some distance from each other in the DNA of non-B cells, but are fused together in antibody-synthesizing B cells (Hozumi and Tonegawa 1976). Indeed, in the case of the genetic material encoding V-region sequences, multiple separate elements were shown to be involved. Thus, for κ chains, there are multiple V genes (250–300) and four functional J 'mini-genes'. V and J genes are separated by a great distance in germline DNA but, in a B cell, one V element is found joined to a single J element, giving a continuous unit of VJ information, i.e. V and J elements undergo somatic recombination. The joining of any V gene to any J gene (or DJ for heavy chains) results in deletion of all intervening DNA. A simple arithmetic calculation reveals that between 1000 and 1200 different VJ units can be formed by somatic recombination at the κ locus. A similar rearrangement of V and J information is observed at the λ locus (Figure 16.7).

At the heavy chain locus, there is an additional mini-gene family located between the V and J genes, called the D (diversity) genes. Two somatic recombination events are therefore required at the heavy chain locus to give a complete and active V gene. These occur in the order of one D and one J element being recombined to give a DJ unit, followed by fusion of this DJ gene to a single V gene to give a continuous *VDJ* gene (Coleclough et al. 1981). Clearly, therefore, the capacity to rearrange members of mini-gene families randomly greatly expands the final number of total genes and proteins available as antibodies or BcRs. Finally, somatic recombination is independent of antigen, and successful recombination on one of the two chromosomes bearing a given Ig gene prevents rearrangement on the other chromosome (allelic exclusion), thus conforming to the rules of the clonal selection theory.

V(D)J recombination: signals and rules

The recombination process is controlled by highly conserved nucleotide sequences flanking the genes to be rearranged. For V genes examination of sequences lying 3′ to the end of the coding elements revealed the presence of a conserved heptameric sequence linked by a spacer to a similarly highly conserved nonameric sequence. These are called recombination signal sequences (RSS). The size of the spacer between the heptanucleotide and nonanucleotide RSSs is always either 12 ± 1 or 23 ± 1 nucleotides, even though the sequence itself is not highly conserved. Indeed, recombination can occur only between mini-genes flanked by RSSs with different-sized spacers, i.e. one partner must have a 12-nucleotide spacer and the other a 23-nucleotide spacer. This is the so-called 12/23 rule. The recombination process is mediated by the RAG products, and is not exact, and shifts in the frame of recombination can increase diversity. In the case of fusion to the D genes, the enzyme terminal deoxyribonucleotidyl transferase can add nucleotides (usually G) to 3′-hydroxyl groups a nontemplate-directed manner; these are referred to as Nucleotide (N) regions. There are also small regions of palindromic repeats found at V(D)J joints and these are referred to as P sequences.

Mechanisms of somatic recombination

The V(D)J recombination process can be divided into four main steps: alteration of chromatin structure to allow access of the recombination machinery; recognition and binding of RSS; cleavage of DNA; and DNA repair and closure of joints. The joints formed are a 'coding joint', which brings together V and J sequences, and a signal joint which forms a closed circle containing the intervening DNA lost as a function of the recombination reaction. Signal joints are always precise, whereas coding joints are variable, a feature that is important in generation of antibody (and TcR) diversity. The proteins participating in V(D)J recombination are drawn from both lymphocyte-specific enzymes required for RSS recognition and cleavage and from ubiquitously expressed proteins involved in DNA repair and chromatin dynamics.

Highly condensed chromatin is likely to impede access of RAG complexes to Ig genes and associated RSS motifs (Roth and Roth 2000). Indeed, in in vitro assays mononucleosomes are able to inhibit the recombination reaction (Kwon et al. 1998; McBlane and Boyes 2000), largely by inhibiting the binding of the RAG complex to the RSS (McBlane and Boyes 2000; Kwon et al. 2000). Studies of histone acetylation have suggested that the

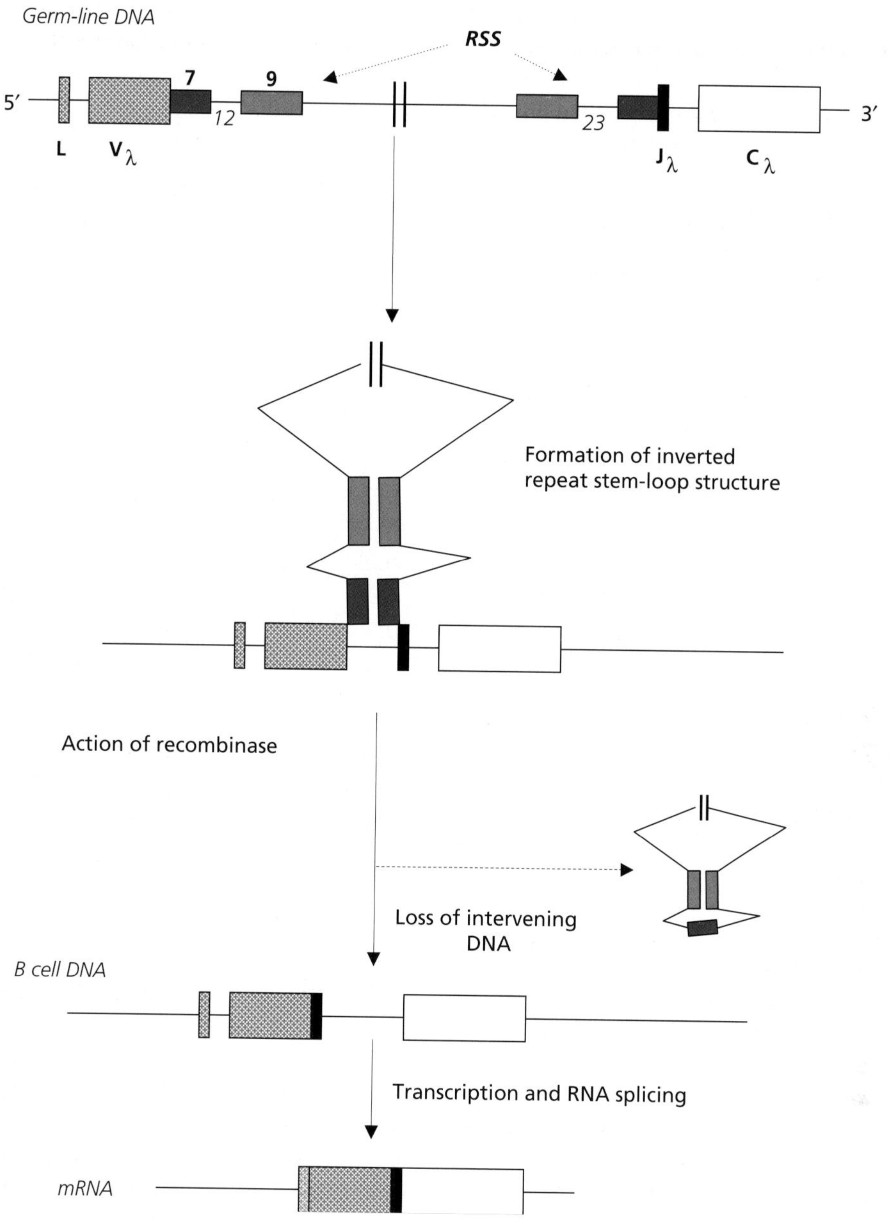

Figure 16.7 *Immunoglobulin λ chain gene rearrangement: the organization of the Igλ locus in germline and B-cell DNA is illustrated. Vλ and its associated leader peptide exon (L) are shown as stippled boxes, Jλ as a solid black box and Cλ as a solid white box. The heptameric and nonameric RSS are shown in blue and red, respectively. Intronic sequences are depicted by the thin line, and exons by boxes.*

level of acetylated histone H3 correlates with the degree of V(D)J recombination observed in vivo, indicating that local chromatin remodeling caused by acetylation favors recombination (McMurry and Krangel 2000). In many models, histone acetylation is greatly increased in those parts of the chromatin where transcription is viable.

Using the λ light gene as the model (see Figure 16.7), a large single-stranded stem-loop structure is formed by pairing of complementary heptanucleotide and nonanucleotide RSSs separated by 12 and 23 spacer sequences. This structure is bound by a tetrameric RAG1–RAG2 protein complex consisting of two molecules of each RAG (Bailin et al. 1999; Sadofsky 2001). RAG1 has demonstrable affinity for the nonanucleotide RSS (Difilippantonio et al. 1996; Mo et al. 1999), but it remains to be demonstrated unequivocally that RAG2 binds DNA (although this seems likely (Mo et al. 1999)). The enzyme complex introduces a single nick in each DNA strand, precisely cleaving the phosphodiester bond between the final base of the coding sequence and the first base of the heptameric RSS (McBlane et al. 1995). The free hydroxyl group at the 3′ of the coding strand now attacks the phosphodiester bond at the same position on the opposite strand, forming a closed hairpin loop at the coding joint. Plainly, hairpins are formed at both the V and the J coding joints, and the remaining products are blunt and 5′-phosphate-bearing ends of the signal joint. The signal joints are precisely closed in a process requiring the RAG proteins, but, more importantly, the normal enzymes of DNA repair (Ku proteins, XRCC4, and DNA ligase IV) (Jeggo 1998).

In order for V-J joining to proceed, the hairpin loops must now be opened. As with signal joints, the RAG and Ku proteins appear to be mandatory for hairpin opening, but the process also requires DNA-dependent protein kinase catalytic subunit (DNA-PKcs) and the Artemis double-stranded DNA repair protein (Schlissel 2002). Artemis itself possesses a Mg^{2+}-dependent exonuclease activity but normally has no endonuclease activity. However, Artemis forms a complex, both in vivo and in vitro, with DNA-PKcs and is a substrate for the kinase activity of DNA-PKcs (Ma et al. 2002). In this complex, phosphorylated Artemis now expresses an endonuclease activity and is capable of opening hairpin loops using water as nucleophile for cleavage of target phosphodiester bonds. Support for the hypothesis that the Artemis–DNA-PKcs complex opens hairpins at V and J coding joints is provided by the rare human condition of radiation-sensitive SCID (RS-SCID). Fibroblasts from RS-SCID patients have a specific defect in V(D)J recombination in that no coding joints are formed, implying an inability to open hairpins; the sole genetic defect in RS-SCID is the Artemis enzyme activity (Moshous et al. 2001).

The action of the Artemis–DNA-PKcs complex opens the hairpin loops, leaving overhanging ends, generally of two to seven nucleotides (Livak and Schatz 1997; Schlissel 1998), bearing 3′-OH groups. These 3′-OH groups are the target for action of other enzymes that can add nucleotides via either template-dependent or nontemplate-directed mechanisms. The enzyme TdT adds bases to free 3′-OH groups in a nontemplate-directed manner, with a preference for guanine; these additional sequences are referred to as N regions. A second group of 'extra' nucleotides (i.e. bases not attributable to the germline V or J sequences) are the P nucleotides. These short stretches of up to four bases are palindromes of sequences at the end of coding joints and are thought to be generated by repair of overhanging ends during hairpin opening. Both N and P nucleotides contribute greatly to junctional diversity and, together with the inherent imprecision of V(D)J joining itself, are an important contribution to maximizing the possible range of antibodies that can be generated from a fixed number of germline mini-genes.

The final stage of VDJ recombination is the closing of the coding joint, and this proceeds by using the ubiquitously expressed enzymes involved in DNA repair and nonhomologous end joining (NHEJ). The key proteins involved are the XRCC4 protein in a complex with DNA ligase IV, as are the members of the Ku autoantigen family (Jeggo 1998). The overhanging ends of the opened hairpins will be repaired, either by exonuclease action to trim the ends or by polymerase action to fill the overhang with complementary nucleotides, before final joining of blunt ends. Any overhanging flaps that remain after trimming or in-filling are removed by flap endonucleases such as the fen endonuclease, or possibly by the RAG enzymes themselves. Ku binds exclusively to ends of DNA molecules in a sequence-independent manner; there are also no structural restrictions on Ku binding and so it can associate with blunt or overhanging ends (Smith and Jackson 1999). Binding of Ku allows other proteins to bind, including DNA-PKcs, and the XRCC4–DNA ligase IV complex and, indeed, Ku promotes the ligase activity of the latter complex (Jones et al. 2001). Recent structural analysis of Ku indicates that it can form a bridge over broken DNA in such a way that not only can it bind the free end of the DNA molecule (Walker et al. 2001; Jones et al. 2001), but it can also allow access of other proteins to the nucleotide strands to be joined and repaired. In V(D)J recombination, Ku is likely to serve to bind the blunt ends of the coding joints and recruit the XRCC4–DNA ligase IV complex to them (Ramsden and Gellert 1998; Nick McElhinny et al. 2000). It is the action of DNA ligase IV that ultimately forms the phosphodiester bond joining the V and J segments to yield a somatically recombined VJ unit.

A number of disease states provide compelling evidence for the involvement in the recombination process of the various proteins discussed above. Thus, there is ample evidence from knock-out mice that absence of *RAG-1* or *RAG-2* genes causes severe immunodeficiency usually manifest as a lack of both B and T cells, and the same is true of human RAG null mutations. However, RAG mutations that result in defective but not inactive proteins give rise to Omenn's syndrome (Villa et al. 1998), an immunodeficiency that is characterized by a lack of B cells and the presence of some T cells (Noordzij et al. 2000). As noted above, Artemis deficiency results in an unusual SCID disease (RS-SCID) and, intriguingly, the original *scid* mice accumulate unopened hairpin coding joints and rarely make coding joints (Roth et al. 1992); the defective gene in *scid* mice encodes DNA-PKcs (Schlissel 2002). Deficiencies in any of the Ku family proteins or in XRCC4 or DNA ligase IV all give rise to striking immunodeficiencies of differing levels of severity, usually coupled with defective DNA-repair and developmental abnormalities in a range of tissues. The data from disease states therefore underscore the importance of both lymphoid-specific and ubiquitous protein factors in V(D)J recombination.

Class switch recombination

Immunological memory in the humoral response is reflected in the production of higher affinity antibodies of non-IgM isotypes (e.g. IgG). The *Igh* locus comprises the V, D, and J gene clusters, plus groups of exons encoding the individual domains of particular heavy chains (Figure 16.8). Increased affinity is a function of somatic hypermutation of V region sequences and selection of antigen-mediated selection of high affinity clones in germinal centers (see 'Antigen-dependent B-cell development' above). Isotype switching at the level of the DNA results from movement of the *VDJ* gene from its original position just 5′ to the Cμ gene to a new position immediately 5′ to, for example, the Cγ gene. All intervening DNA is deleted during this rearrangement process, called switch recombination, but the molecular signals are different from those controlling VDJ and VJ recombination events (Harriman et al. 1993; Kinoshita and Honjo 2001). The exception to this is the simultaneous production of mIgM and mIgD by mature B cells. The synthesis of the δ heavy chain does not involve switch recombination, but is a result of RNA splicing of a long transcript containing *VDJ*, all the Cμ information, and the Cδ gene (Blattner and Tucker 1984).

The 5′-flanking region of each C_H gene cluster contains a 'switch' recombination region (or S region). Unlike V(D)J recombination, there are no tightly defined DNA sequences for the S regions, although these areas do contain many tandemly repeated and palindromic sequences. As class switching always involves changing from synthesis of IgM (and IgD) to a second isotype located 3′ to the Cμ exons, it follows that Sμ is mandatory for pairing with downstream S regions of selected C_H exons. Indeed, deletion of the Sμ region greatly impairs class switching (Luby et al. 2001), and deletion of individual S regions blocks switching to the associated isotype (Gu et al. 1993; Jung et al. 1993; Kinoshita et al. 1998). As indicated in 'Antigen-dependent B-cell development', cytokines direct class switching and, at the molecular level, this is reflected in local alterations in chromatin structure. Thus, IL-4 promotes IgE synthesis and, in B cells undergoing such switching, IL-4 promotes synthesis of a sterile transcript comprising the Iϵ region plus the four Cϵ exons, indicative of a local opening of chromatin structure (Stavnezer-Nordgren and Sirlin 1986; Yancopoulos et al. 1986). Transcription is required for class switching to occur. Similarly, transforming growth factor β stimulation results in transcription of the Iα and Cα domains (Nakamura et al. 1996).

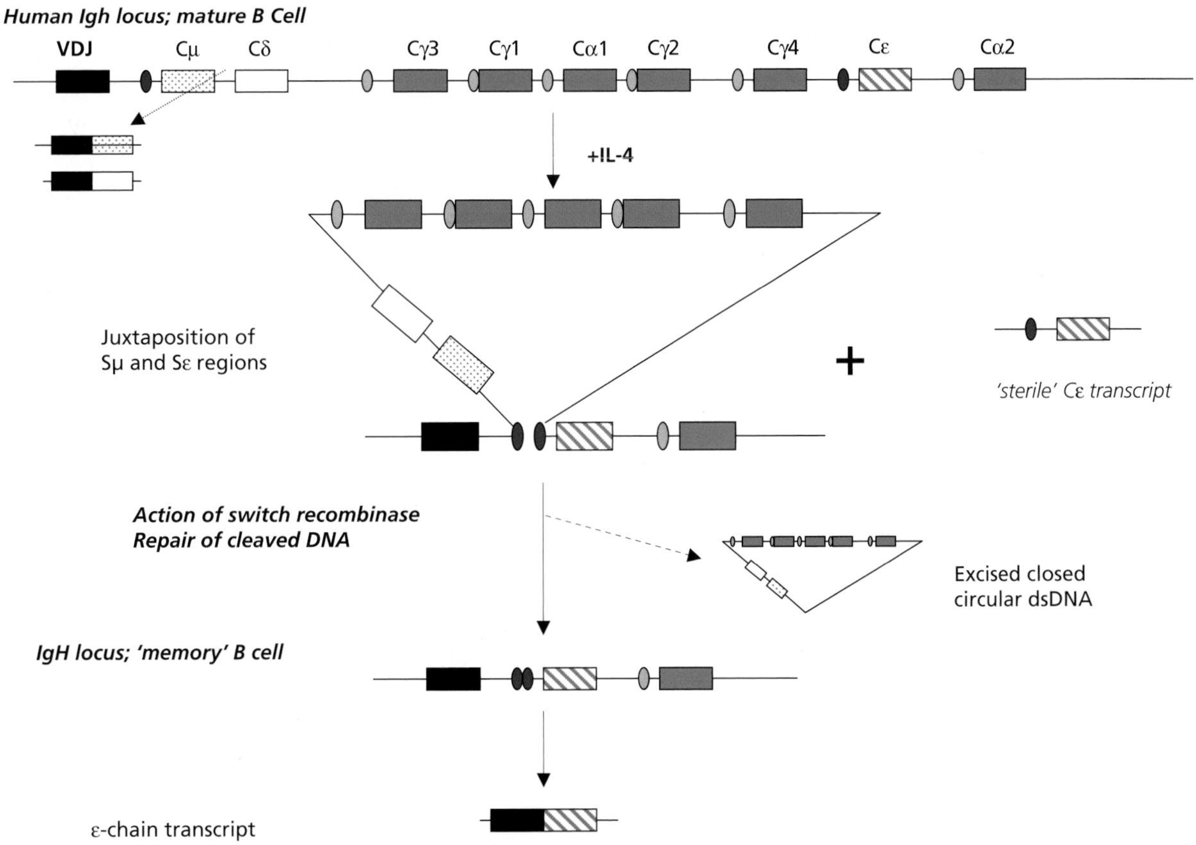

Figure 16.8 *Immunoglobulin isotype switching: the layout of the human* Igh *locus is shown and the S sequences at each C_H gene are illustrated as small red circles except those of Sμ and Sϵ which are blue. The figure depicts switching from IgM(D) synthesis (white and stippled boxes) to IgE production (hatched box) under the influence of interleukin 4 (IL-4) showing movement of the somatically recombined* VDJ *unit from 5′ of Cμ/Cδ to just 5′ of Cϵ, with concomitant loss of intervening DNA. Sterile and productive transcripts from the Ig locus during the isotype switch process are shown.*

Once the target C_H gene has been chosen (e.g. Cϵ), the Sμ and Sϵ regions are brought into close proximity so that the components of the recombination system can act. The putative switch recombinase cleaves the DNA, joins the S regions together (so bringing the *VDJ* unit close to the Cϵ exons), and removes the intervening DNA as a looped-out, closed, circular DNA (see Figure 16.8). The absence of defined 'switch recombination sequences' suggests that the recombinase machinery might recognize higher structural features of the DNA rather than sequence elements (Kinoshita et al. 1998; Tashiro et al. 2001). Current models suggest that the feature recognized is a single-stranded stem-loop structure not dissimilar to that recognized in V(D)J rearrangement. Such structures are favored by the presence of short inverted repeat sequences, such as those found in S regions.

Analysis of the junction regions in switch recombination products indicated the presence of both deletion of DNA sequences and duplication of others at the junctions (Lee et al. 1998; Kinoshita and Honjo 2001). These data indicate that the recombinase machinery introduces staggered cleavages or nicks into the two strands of DNA. Such staggered cleavage products could be acted on by either single-stranded nucleases or error-prone polymerases (e.g. TdT) to repair the ends before closure by the same NHEJ DNA-repair machinery that seals V(D)J joints.

Not only is transcription of the targeted C_H gene required for isotype switching, but *de novo* protein synthesis is also mandatory (Muramatsu et al. 1999), indicating the requirement for transcription and translation of new gene products during the switching process. One such gene is the AID product, whose expression is limited to B cells and, more importantly, to those B cells in germinal centers (Muramatsu et al. 1999). Over-expression of AID enhances class switching in in vitro models, and mice lacking the gene ($AID^{-/-}$) fail to produce IgG, IgA, or IgE, indicating that class switching has been abolished. Moreover, $AID^{-/-}$ animals show essentially no somatic hypermutation in response to immunization, suggesting that AID has a role in both class switching and somatic hypermutation. In humans, the hyper-IgM syndrome (HIM) manifests itself by over-production of IgM and a lack of other Ig isotypes. There are two forms of the disease HIM1: an X-linked condition linked to a failure to produce CD40L (Gordon and Pound 2000), and HIM2, an autosomal recessive condition mapping to 12p13, the location of the AID gene (Revy et al. 1998). $AID^{-/-}$ (Muramatsu et al. 2000) and HIM B cells (Revy et al. 2000) can perform VDJ recombination normally and, on cytokine stimulation, synthesize 'sterile' transcripts, suggesting that AID is required for the latter stages of switch recombination. This is entirely consistent with the cytidine deaminase activity of both murine and human AID (Muramatsu et al. 1999), a function that suggests a potential role for AID in RNA editing.

BcR heavy chains and Ig synthesis

Clonal selection requires the receptor Ig to have the same structure as the antibody that the B cell will later secrete. B cells simultaneously synthesize discrete mRNAs that program the synthesis of the structurally distinct receptor and secretory forms of their heavy chain polypeptide (Singer et al. 1980). This is again accomplished by RNA splicing, in this case by selective use of two small exons located at the 3′ end of the C gene for each heavy chain isotype, which encode hydrophobic sequences allowing stable insertion into the plasma membrane; these are the M (membrane) exons (Alt et al. 1980). Heavy and light chain mRNA molecules are synthesized on distinct membrane-bound polyribosomes and, in common with all secretory and membrane proteins, the nascent chains are guided across the endoplasmic reticulum membrane by a hydrophobic sequence, the signal peptide, which is proteolytically removed during transit across the membrane. Glycosylation of the nascent chain occurs co-translationally and assembly of four-chain units occurs in the lumen of the endoplasmic reticulum; in the case of IgM and IgA molecules, polymerization, and addition of J chains are late events, probably occurring immediately before the final secretory event. Ig synthesis proceeds in different B cells at distinct rates that reflect the state of differentiation of the B cell. Thus, a small resting B cell synthesizes 10^6 Ig molecules per day, mostly for use as receptor Ig, whereas a plasma cell can produce up to 2000 Ig molecules per second, essentially all of which is of the secretory form.

The active Ig gene is transcribed into a primary nuclear RNA (nRNA) transcript that contains not only the coding elements (exons) for V and C regions but also all the noncoding sequences (introns). Introns are found between the recombined VJ or VDJ unit and its appropriate C gene and, in the case of heavy chains only, between the exons that encode the individual domains of the heavy chain polypeptide. Introns are removed by RNA splicing to yield an mRNA molecule where all the V and C information is continuous. This is translated to yield the functional Ig polypeptide.

IMMUNOTECHNOLOGY: GENERATION AND USES OF MONOCLONAL ANTIBODIES

The specificity of antibodies makes them excellent tools for use in diagnostics and therapy. The critical advance that revolutionized the diagnostic and therapeutic application of antibodies was the development of MAbs (Kohler and Milstein 1975, 1976; Kohler et al. 1976). In short, this technology allows the establishment of an immortal cell line that secretes a single antibody of defined specificity. In practical terms, the procedure exploits the enormous specificity present in a sample of normal lymphocytes and the capacity for infinite growth found in B-cell tumors.

In practice, normal lymphocytes from an immunized host are fused to continuously growing tumor cells in vitro to make a hybrid cell. The tumor cells are derived from plasmacytomas, a tumor of myeloma cells, and so have a highly developed secretory apparatus; sublines are generally chosen on the basis of an inability to synthesize their own heavy and light chains. As normal murine B lymphocytes are highly prone to apoptosis in vitro, any that do not fuse to the tumor cells die after a few days in culture. The tumor cells used in the fusion are chosen on the basis of a defect in nucleotide metabolism (a lack of the enzyme hypoxanthine–guanine phosphoribosyl transferase (HGPRT)), which means that addition of nucleotide analogues to the cultures will selectively cause death of the tumor cells. The normal lymphocytes possess HGPRT activity and when fused to a tumor cell contribute both their antibody specificity and their normal nucleotide metabolism to gain the immortal properties of the myeloma. It is this combination that allows only the hybrid cells to survive in the presence of the selecting drug. The hybrids, called 'hybridomas', can be cloned at limiting dilution and screened for the desired MAb specificity. Once a suitable clone is identified, it can be grown in large cultures, and gram quantities of homogeneous antibody produced.

Monoclonal antibodies have found many applications in medicine. Perhaps the most obvious example of an immunodiagnostic product is the pregnancy testing kit available at most pharmacists which employs MAbs to human chorionic gonadotropin (hCG) and yields a definitive result in under 5 min. In this system, MAbs to two distinct epitopes on the hCG molecule are generated, one for 'capture' and the second for detection. The capture MAb is immobilized on a plastic surface and binds any hCG present in a morning urine sample. In contemporary kits, the flow of fluid solubilizes the second MAb, directed against a distinct hCG epitope. This second MAb has an enzyme coupled to it that will convert a colorless substrate also present in the solubilized material into an insoluble product that precipitates around the zone where the first MAb is immobilized. In practice, this is visualized as a colored line. An insoluble precipitate can form only if the second MAb is retained in the 'sensor' area, an event that can occur only if hCG is itself captured by the first MAb. MAbs specific for a range of cell-surface markers are used in the diagnosis of leukemia (e.g. the presence of CD10, or c-ALLA, on cells derived from acute lymphoblastic leukemia patients, or the $CD5^+/CD23^+$ phenotype of B-chronic lymphocytic leukemia cells), and for accurate quantitation of analytes in tissue samples.

The application of MAbs in vivo as a therapeutic agent faces the hurdle of hypersensitivity reactions in the patient. Thus injection of murine Ig into an individual will provoke an anti-murine IgG response that will cause severe immune complex disease on subsequent exposure to the murine MAb (see Chapter 36, Airway hypersensitivity and Chapter 37, Autoimmunity). To overcome this, murine MAbs can be humanized by 'grafting' the CDRs from a useful murine MAb on to the backbone of a human IgG molecule. A similar strategy can be used to take useful sequences from antibody-combining sites selected by phage display methods, to generate a therapeutically useful product (e.g. the b12 IgG1κ molecular discussed earlier). These molecular manipulations go some way to alleviating the potential problems of host hypersensitivity, but this remains a significant factor in management of patients treated with MAbs.

Immunotherapeutics using antibodies envisages infusion of MAbs, either alone or coupled to radionuclides or potent biological toxins, as a means of eliminating tumor cells or alleviating other conditions (see Chapter 18, Monoclonal antibody therapy). Several MAbs have met with notable success in the treatment of neoplastic and other diseases, although it is fair to note that the precise in vivo mechanisms by which they provide clinical benefit remain unclear. In allograft patients, a particular problem is rejection of the grafted tissue by host T cells. Two humanized MAbs, basiliximab and daclizumab, directed against the CD25 molecule (a component of high-affinity IL-2 receptors (Cushley et al. 2002)) have been used to suppress acute rejection in renal allograft patients (Waldmann 2000). The MAbs appear to function by blocking the capacity of IL-2 receptors to send mitogenic signals to host T cells, thereby blocking the early proliferative phase of the T-cell response to the allograft. Neither MAb elicits severe side effects in the patients, and daclizumab is notably effective when used in conjunction with immunosuppressive drugs such as cyclosporin. In the context of neoplasia, rituximab, an anti-CD20-specific reagent is widely used in treatment of non-Hodgkin's lymphoma and other B-cell neoplasias (McLaughlin 2002), with encouraging results. As the MAb appears to act by reducing (neoplastic) B-cell numbers, there are also suggestions that rituximab might be applied to eliminate or reduce the high levels of $CD20^+$ autoreactive B cells in patients with inflammatory autoimmune disease. Finally, in the specific case of rheumatoid arthritis, infliximab, an anti-tumor necrosis factor reagent, is used successfully to ameliorate disease, and finds application in other inflammatory disorders, including Crohn's disease (Graninger and Smolen 2002).

REFERENCES

Ahouse, J.J., Hagerman, C.L., et al. 1993. Mouse MHC class I-like Fc receptor encoded outside the MHC. *J Immunol*, **151**, 6076–88.

Allen, J.M. and Seed, B. 1989. Isolation and expression of functional high-affinity Fc receptor complementary DNAs. *Science*, **243**, 378–81.

Alt, F.W., Bothwell, A.L., et al. 1980. Synthesis of secreted and membrane-bound immunoglobulin mu heavy chains is directed by mRNAs that differ at their 3′ ends. *Cell*, **20**, 293–301.

Bailin, T., Mo, X. and Sadofsky, M.J. 1999. A RAG1 and RAG2 tetramer complex is active in cleavage in V(D)J recombination. *Mol Cell Biol*, **19**, 4664–71.

Bain, G., Maandag, E.C., et al. 1994. E2A proteins are required for proper B cell development and initiation of immunoglobulin gene rearrangements. *Cell*, **79**, 885–92.

Bain, G., Robanus Maandag, E.C., et al. 1997. Both E12 and E47 allow commitment to the B cell lineage. *Immunity*, **6**, 145–54.

Beavil, A.J., Beavil, R.L., et al. 1993. Structural basis of the IgE-Fc epsilon RI interaction. *Biochem Soc Trans*, **21**, 968–72.

Blank, U., Ra, C., et al. 1989. Complete structure and expression in transfected cells of high affinity IgE receptor. *Nature*, **337**, 187–9.

Blattner, F.R. and Tucker, P.W. 1984. The molecular biology of immunoglobulin D. *Nature*, **307**, 417–22.

Bonnefoy, J.-Y., Lecoanet-Henchoz, S., et al. 1997. Structure and functions of CD23. *Int Rev Immunol*, **16**, 113–28.

Brandtzaeg, P. 1975. Blocking effect of J chain and J-chain antibody on the binding of secretory component to human IgA and IgM. *Scand J Immunol*, **4**, 837–42.

Burmeister, W.P., Gastinel, L.N., et al. 1994a. Crystal structure at 2.2-A resolution of the MHC-related neonatal Fc receptor. *Nature*, **372**, 336–43.

Burmeister, W.P., Huber, A.H. and Bjorkman, P.J. 1994b. Crystal structure of the complex of rat neonatal Fc receptor with Fc. *Nature*, **372**, 379–83.

Burnet, F. 1959. *The clonal selection theory of immunity*. New York: Vanderbilt Press.

Burton, D.R., Pyati, J., et al. 1994. Efficient neutralization of primary isolates of HIV-1 by a recombinant human monoclonal antibody. *Science*, **266**, 1024–7.

Busslinger, M. and Urbanek, P. 1995. The role of BSAP (Pax-5) in B cell development. *Curr Opin Genetics Dev*, **5**, 595–601.

Cao, X., Shores, E.W. and Hu-Li, J. 1995. Defective lymphoid development in mice lacking expression of the common cytokine receptor γ chain. *Immunity*, **1995**, 223–8.

Casanova, J.E., Apodaca, G. and Mostov, K.E. 1991. An autonomous signal for basolateral sorting in the cytoplasmic domain of the polymeric immunoglobulin receptor. *Cell*, **66**, 65–75.

Chapuis, R. and Koshland, M. 1974. Mechanisms of IgM polymerisation. *Proc Natl Acad Sci USA*, **71**, 657–61.

Choi, J.K., Shen, C.-P., et al. 1996. E47 activates the Ig-heavy chain and TdT loci in non-B cells. *EMBO Journal*, **15**, 5014–21.

Coico, R.F., Berzofsky, J.A., et al. 1987. Physiology of IgD. VII. Induction of receptors for IgD on cloned T cells by IgD and interleukin 2. *J Immunol*, **138**, 4–6.

Coico, R.F., Finkelman, F., et al. 1988a. Exposure to crosslinked IgD induces receptors for IgD on T cells in vivo and in vitro. *Proc Natl Acad Sci USA*, **85**, 559–63.

Coico, R.F., Siskind, G.W. and Thorbecke, G.J. 1988b. Role of IgD and T delta cells in the regulation of the humoral immune response. *Immunol Rev*, **105**, 45–67.

Coleclough, C., Perry, R.P., et al. 1981. Aberrant rearrangements contribute significantly to the allelic exclusion of immunoglobulin gene expression. *Nature*, **290**, 372–8.

Corcoran, A.E., Smart, F.M., et al. 1996. The interleukin-7 receptor a chain transmits distinct signals for proliferation and differentiation during B lymphopoiesis. *EMBO J*, **15**, 1924–32.

Cortes, M., Wong, E., et al. 1999. Control of lymphocyte development by the Ikaros gene family. *Curr Opin Immunol*, **11**, 167–71.

Coyne, R.S., Siebrecht, M., et al. 1994. Mutational analysis of polymeric immunoglobulin receptor/ligand interactions. Evidence for the involvement of multiple complementarity determining region (CDR)-like loops in receptor domain I. *J Biol Chem*, **269**, 31620–5.

Cushley, W., Curran, J.A., et al. 2002. CD25. In: Creighton, T. (ed.), *Encyclopaedia of molecular medicine*, Vol. 5. London: John Wiley & Sons, 570–4.

Daeron, M. 1995. Intracytoplasmic sequences involved in the biological properties of low-affinity receptors for IgG expressed by murine macrophages. *Braz J Med Biol Res*, **28**, 263–74.

Deisenhofer, J. 1981. Crystallographic refinement and atomic models of a human Fc fragment and its complex with fragment B of protein A from *Staphylococcus aureus* at 2.9- and 2.8-A resolution. *Biochemistry*, **20**, 2361–70.

DeKoter, R.P. and Singh, H. 2000. Regulation of B lymphocyte and macrophage development by graded expression of PU.1. *Science*, **288**, 1439–41.

Delespesse, G., Sarfati, M., et al. 1992. The low affinity receptor for IgE. *Immunol Rev*, **125**, 77–97.

Difilippantonio, M.J., McMahan, C.J., et al. 1996. RAG1 mediates signal sequence recognition and recruitment of RAG2 in V(D)J recombination. *Cell*, **87**, 253–62.

Dijstelbloem, H.M., van de Winkel, J.G. and Kallenberg, C.G. 2001. Inflammation in autoimmunity: receptors for IgG revisited. *Trends Immunol*, **22**, 510–16.

Drenth, J.P., Cuisset, L., et al. 1999. Mutations in the gene encoding mevalonate kinase cause hyper-IgD and periodic fever syndrome. International Hyper-IgD Study Group. *Nat Genet*, **22**, 178–81.

Duncan, A.R. and Winter, G. 1988. The binding site for C1q on IgG. *Nature*, **332**, 738–40.

Duncan, A.R., Woof, J.M., et al. 1988. Localization of the binding site for the human high-affinity Fc receptor on IgG. *Nature*, **332**, 563–4.

Edelman, G. and Gally, J. 1962. The nature of Bence Jones proteins. Chemical similarities to polypeptide chains of myeloma globulins and normal γ-globulins. *J Exp Med*, **116**, 207–27.

Edelman, G. and Poulik, M. 1961. Studies on structural units of the γ-globulins. *J Exp Med*, **113**, 861–84.

Edelman, G.M., Cunningham, B.A., et al. 1969. The covalent structure of an entire gammaG immunoglobulin molecule. *Proc Natl Acad Sci USA*, **63**, 78–85.

Ernst, L.K., van de Winkel, J.G., et al. 1992. Three genes for the human high affinity Fc receptor for IgG (Fc gamma RI) encode four distinct transcription products. *J Biol Chem*, **267**, 15692–700.

Ernst, L.K., Duchemin, A.M. and Anderson, C.L. 1993. Association of the high-affinity receptor for IgG (Fc gamma RI) with the gamma subunit of the IgE receptor. *Proc Natl Acad Sci USA*, **90**, 6023–7.

Ernst, L.K., Duchemin, A.M., et al. 1998. Molecular characterization of six variant Fcgamma receptor class I (CD64) transcripts. *Mol Immunol*, **35**, 943–54.

Ernst, P., Hahm, K., et al. 1996. A potential role for Elf-1 in terminal transferase gene regulation. *Mol Cell Biol*, **16**, 6121–31.

Ewart, M.A., Ozanne, B.W. and Cushley, W. 2002. The CD23a and CD23b proximal promoters display different sensitivities to exogenous stimuli in B lymphocytes. *Genes Immun*, **3**, 158–64.

Fallgreen-Gebauer, E., Gebauer, W., et al. 1993. The covalent linkage of secretory component to IgA. Structure of sIgA. *Biol Chem Hoppe Seyler*, **374**, 1023–8.

Fitzsimmons, D. and Hagman, J. 1996. Regulation of gene expression at early stages of B-cell and T-cell differentiation. *Curr Opin Immunol*, **8**, 166–74.

Flores-Romo, L., Shields, J., et al. 1993. Inhibition of an in vivo antigen specific IgE response by antibodies to CD23. *Science*, **261**, 1038–41.

Garman, S.C., Wurzburg, B.A., et al. 2000. Structure of the Fc fragment of human IgE bound to its high-affinity receptor Fc epsilonRI alpha. *Nature*, **406**, 259–66.

Geissmann, F., Launay, P., et al. 2001. A subset of human dendritic cells expresses IgA Fc receptor (CD89), which mediates internalization and activation upon cross-linking by IgA complexes. *J Immunol*, **166**, 346–52.

Geneste, C., Iscaki, S., et al. 1986. Both Fc alpha domains of human IgA are involved in in vitro interaction between secretory component and dimeric IgA. *Immunol Lett*, **13**, 221–6.

Georgopoulos, K., Winandy, S. and Avitahl, N. 1997. The role of the Ikaros gene in lymphocyte development and homeostasis. *Annu Rev Immunol*, **15**, 155–76.

Ghirlando, R., Keown, M.B., et al. 1995. Stoichiometry and thermodynamics of the interaction between the Fc fragment of human IgG1 and its low-affinity receptor Fc gamma RIII. *Biochemistry*, **34**, 13320–7.

Goossens, T., Klein, U. and Kuppers, R. 1998. Frequent occurrence of deletions and duplications during somatic hypermutation: implications for oncogene translocations and heavy chain disease. *Proc Natl Acad Sci USA*, **95**, 2463–8.

Gordon, J. and Pound, J. 2000. Fortifying B cells with CD154; an engaging tale of many hues. *Immunology*, **100**, 269–80.

Gordon, J., Flores-Romo, L., et al. 1989. CD23: a multi-functional receptor/lymphokine? *Immunol Today*, **10**, 153–6.

Goto, Y. and Aki, K. 1984. Interaction of the fluorescence-labeled secretory component with human polymeric immunoglobulins. *Biochemistry*, **23**, 6736–44.

Graninger, W. and Smolen, J. 2002. Treatment of rheumatoid arthritis by TNF-blocking agents. *Int Arch Allergy Immunol*, **127**, 10–14.

Grawunder, U., Leu, T.M., et al. 1995. Down-regulation of RAG1 and RAG2 gene expression in preB cells after functional immunoglobulin heavy chain rearrangement. *Immunity*, **3**, 601–8.

Gu, H., Zou, Y.R. and Rajewsky, K. 1993. Independent control of immunoglobulin switch recombination at individual switch regions evidenced through Cre-loxP-mediated gene targeting. *Cell*, **73**, 1155–64.

Ha, H.J., Barnoski, B.L., et al. 1994. Structure, chromosomal localization and methylation pattern of human mbn-1 gene. *J Immunol*, **152**, 5749–57.

Haber, E. 1964. Recovery of antigenic specificity after denaturation and complete reduction of disulfides in a papain fragment of antibody. *Proc Natl Acad Sci USA*, **52**, 1099–106.

Han, S., Zheng, B., et al. 1996. Neoteny in lymphocytes: Rag1 and Rag2 expression in germinal centre B cells. *Science*, **274**, 2092–4.

Hardy, R.R., Carmack, C.E., et al. 1991. Resolution and characterization of pro-B and pre-pro-B cell stages in normal mouse bone marrow. *J Exp Med*, **173**, 1213–25.

Harriman, W., Volk, H., et al. 1993. Immunoglobulin class switch recombination. *Annu Rev Immunol*, **11**, 361–84.

Harrison, P.T., Davis, W., et al. 1994. Binding of monomeric immunoglobulin G triggers Fc gamma RI-mediated endocytosis. *J Biol Chem*, **269**, 24396–402.

Hashimoto, S., Miyawaki, T., et al. 1999. Atypical X-linked agammaglobulinaemia diagnosed in three adults. *Intern Med*, **38**, 722–5.

Hendrickson, B.A., Conner, D.A., et al. 1995. Altered hepatic transport of immunoglobulin A in mice lacking the J chain. *J Exp Med*, **182**, 1905–11.

Hermann, P., Armant, M., et al. 1999. The vitronectin receptor and its associated CD47 molecule mediates proinflammatory cytokine synthesis in human monocytes by interaction with soluble CD23. *J Cell Biol*, **144**, 767–75.

Hexham, J.M., White, K.D., et al. 1999. A human immunoglobulin (Ig)A calpha3 domain motif directs polymeric Ig receptor-mediated secretion. *J Exp Med*, **189**, 747–52.

Hibbs, M.L., Selvaraj, P., et al. 1989. Mechanisms for regulating expression of membrane isoforms of Fc gamma RIII (CD16). *Science*, **246**, 1608–11.

Hozumi, N. and Tonegawa, S. 1976. Evidence for somatic rearrangement of immunoglobulin genes coding for variable and constant regions. *Proc Natl Acad Sci USA*, **73**, 3628–32.

Hulett, M.D. and Hogarth, P.M. 1994. Molecular basis of Fc receptor function. *Adv Immunol*, **57**, 1–127.

Ishizaka, T., Tomioka, H. and Ishizaka, K. 1971. Degranulation of human basophil leukocytes by anti-gamma E antibody. *J Immunol*, **106**, 705–10.

Jeannin, P., Delneste, Y., et al. 1997. CD86 (B7-2) on human B cells. *J Biol Chem*, **272**, 15613–19.

Jeggo, P.A. 1998. DNA breakage and repair. *Adv Genet*, **38**, 185–218.

Johansen, F.E., Pekna, M., et al. 1999. Absence of epithelial immunoglobulin A transport, with increased mucosal leakiness, in polymeric immunoglobulin receptor/secretory component-deficient mice. *J Exp Med*, **190**, 915–22.

Johansen, F.E., Braathen, R. and Brandtzaeg, P. 2000. Role of J chain in secretory immunoglobulin formation. *Scand J Immunol*, **52**, 240–8.

Jones, E.A. and Waldmann, T.A. 1972. The mechanism of intestinal uptake and transcellular transport of IgG in the neonatal rat. *J Clin Invest*, **51**, 2916–27.

Jones, J.M., Gellert, M. and Yang, W. 2001. A Ku bridge over broken DNA. *Structure (Camb)*, **9**, 881–4.

Jung, S., Rajewsky, K. and Radbruch, A. 1993. Shutdown of class switch recombination by deletion of a switch region control element. *Science*, **259**, 984–7.

Kawabe, T., Naka, T., et al. 1994. The immune responses in CD40-deficient mice: impaired immunoglobulin class switching and germinal centre formation. *Immunity*, **1**, 67–78.

Kee, B.L. and Murre, C. 1998. Induction of early B cell factor (EBF) and multiple B lineage genes by the basic helix-loop-helix transcription factor. *J Exp Med*, **188**, .

Keler, T., Wallace, P.K., et al. 2000. Differential effect of cytokine treatment on Fc alpha receptor I- and Fc gamma receptor I-mediated tumor cytotoxicity by monocyte-derived macrophages. *J Immunol*, **164**, 5746–52.

Kerner, J.D., Appleby, M.W., et al. 1995. Impaired expansion of mouse B cell progenitors lacking Btk. *Immunity*, **3**, 301–12.

Kinet, J.P., Metzger, H., et al. 1987. A cDNA presumptively coding for the alpha subunit of the receptor with high affinity for immunoglobulin E. *Biochemistry*, **26**, 4605–10.

Kinet, J.P., Blank, U., et al. 1988. Isolation and characterization of cDNAs coding for the beta subunit of the high-affinity receptor for immunoglobulin E. *Proc Natl Acad Sci USA*, **85**, 6483–7.

Kinoshita, K. and Honjo, T. 2001. Linking class-switch recombination with somatic hypermutation. *Nat Rev Mol Cell Biol*, **2**, 493–503.

Kinoshita, K., Tashiro, J., et al. 1998. Target specificity of immunoglobulin class switch recombination is not determined by nucleotide sequences of S regions. *Immunity*, **9**, 849–58.

Klemsz, M., McKercher, S.R., et al. 1990. The macrophage and B cell specific transcription factor PU.1 is related to the ets oncogene. *Cell*, **61**, 113–24.

Kohler, G. and Milstein, C. 1975. Continuous cultures of fused cells secreting antibody of predefined specificity. *Nature*, **256**, 495–7.

Kohler, G. and Milstein, C. 1976. Derivation of specific antibody-producing tissue culture and tumor lines by cell fusion. *Eur J Immunol*, **6**, 511–19.

Kohler, G., Howe, S.C. and Milstein, C. 1976. Fusion between immunoglobulin-secreting and nonsecreting myeloma cell lines. *Eur J Immunol*, **6**, 292–5.

Kozmik, Z., Wang, S., et al. 1992. The promoter of the CD19 gene is a target for the B cell-specific transcription factor BSAP. *Mol Cell Biol*, **12**, 2662–72.

Kroczek, R.A., Graf, D., et al. 1994. Defective expression of CD40 ligand on T cells causes 'X-linked immunodeficiency with hyper-IgM (HIGM1)'. *Immunol Rev*, **138**, 39–59.

Kuhn, L.C. and Kraehenbuhl, J.P. 1979. Interaction of rabbit secretory component with rabbit IgA dimer. *J Biol Chem*, **254**, 11066–71.

Kurasuyama, H., Rolink, A., et al. 1994. The expression of vpre-B/lambda 5 surrogate light chain in early bone marrow precursor B cells and B cell-deficient mutant mice. *Cell*, **77**, 133–43.

Kwon, J., Imbalzano, A.N., et al. 1998. Accessibility of nucleosomal DNA to V(D)J cleavage is modulated by RSS positioning and HMG1. *Mol Cell*, **2**, 829–39.

Kwon, J., Morshead, K.B., et al. 2000. Histone acetylation and hSWI/SNF remodeling act in concert to stimulate V(D)J cleavage of nucleosomal DNA. *Mol Cell*, **6**, 1037–48.

Lanier, L.L., Yu, G. and Phillips, J.H. 1989. Co-association of CD3 zeta with a receptor (CD16) for IgG Fc on human natural killer cells. *Nature*, **342**, 803–5.

Leatherbarrow, R.J., Rademacher, T.W., et al. 1985. Effector functions of a monoclonal aglycosylated mouse IgG2a: binding and activation of complement component C1 and interaction with human monocyte Fc receptor. *Mol Immunol*, **22**, 407–15.

Lecoanet-Henchoz, S., Gauchat, J.-F., et al. 1995. CD23 regulates monocyte activation through a novel interaction with the adhesion molecules CD11b-CD18 and CD11c-CD18. *Immunity*, **2**, 1–20.

Lee, C.G., Kondo, S. and Honjo, T. 1998. Frequent but biased class switch recombination in the S mu flanking regions. *Curr Biol*, **8**, 227–30.

Lin, H. and Grosschedl, R. 1995. Failure of B cell differentiation in mice lacking the transcription factor EBF. *Nature*, **376**, 263–7.

Liu, Y.-J., Cairns, J.A., et al. 1991a. Recombinant 25-kDa CD23 and interleukin-1α promote the survival of germinal centre B cells: evidence for bifurcation in the development of centrocytes rescued from apoptosis. *Eur J Immunol*, **21**, 1107–14.

Liu, Y.-J., Mason, D.Y., et al. 1991b. Germinal centre cells express *bcl-2* protein after activation by signals which prevent their entry into apoptosis. *Eur J Immunol*, **21**, 1905–10.

Livak, F. and Schatz, D.G. 1997. Identification of V(D)J recombination coding end intermediates in normal thymocytes. *J Mol Biol*, **267**, 1–9.

Luby, T.M., Schrader, C.E., et al. 2001. The mu switch region tandem repeats are important, but not required, for antibody class switch recombination. *J Exp Med*, **193**, 159–68.

Luo, H., Hofstetter, H., et al. 1991. Cross-linking of CD23 antigen by its natural ligand (IgE) or by anti-CD23 antibody prevents B lymphocyte proliferation and differentiation. *J Immunol*, **146**, 2122–9.

Ma, Y., Pannicke, U., et al. 2002. Hairpin opening and overhang processing by an Artemis/DNA-dependent protein kinase complex in nonhomologous end joining and V(D)J recombination. *Cell*, **108**, 781–94.

McBlane, F. and Boyes, J. 2000. Stimulation of V(D)J recombination by histone acetylation. *Curr Biol*, **10**, 483–6.

McBlane, J.F., van Gent, D.C., et al. 1995. Cleavage at a V(D)J recombination signal requires only RAG1 and RAG2 proteins and occurs in two steps. *Cell*, **83**, 387–95.

McKean, D., Huppi, K., et al. 1984. Generation of antibody diversity in the immune response of Balb/c mice to influenza virus haemagglutinin. *Proc Natl Acad Sci USA*, **81**, 3180–4.

McLaughlin, P. 2002. Progress and promise in the treatment of indolent lymphomas. *Oncologist*, **7**, 217–25.

Maclennan, I.C. 1994. Germinal centres. *Annu Rev Immunol*, **12**, 117–39.

McMurry, M.T. and Krangel, M.S. 2000. A role for histone acetylation in the developmental regulation of VDJ recombination. *Science*, **287**, 495–8.

Maliszewski, C.R., March, C.J., et al. 1990. Expression cloning of a human Fc receptor for IgA. *J Exp Med*, **172**, 1665–72.

Martin, A.M., Kulski, J.K., et al. 2002. Leukocyte Ig-like receptor complex (LRC) in mice and men. *Trends Immunol*, **23**, 81–8.

Metzger, H. 1994. Immunoglobulin receptors. Handicapping the immune response. *Curr Biol*, **4**, 644–6.

Metzger, H. 1999. It's spring, and thoughts turn to allergies. *Cell*, **97**, 287–90.

Milstein, C. 1966. Variations in amino-acid sequence near the disulphide bridges of Bence Jones proteins. *Nature*, **209**, 370–3.

Mo, X., Bailin, T. and Sadofsky, M.J. 1999. RAG1 and RAG2 cooperate in specific binding to the recombination signal sequence in vitro. *J Biol Chem*, **274**, 7025–31.

Morgan, B., Sun, L., et al. 1997. Aiolos, a lymphoid-restricted transcription factor that interacts with Ikaros to regulate lymphocyte differentiation. *EMBO J*, **16**, 2004–13.

Moshous, D., Callebaut, I., et al. 2001. Artemis, a novel DNA double-strand break repair/V(D)J recombination protein, is mutated in human severe combined immune deficiency. *Cell*, **105**, 177–86.

Mostov, K.E., Friedlander, M. and Blobel, G. 1984. The receptor for transepithelial transport of IgA and IgM contains multiple immunoglobulin-like domains. *Nature*, **308**, 37–43.

Moura, I.C., Centelles, M.N., et al. 2001. Identification of the transferrin receptor as a novel immunoglobulin (Ig)A1 receptor and its enhanced expression on mesangial cells in IgA nephropathy. *J Exp Med*, **194**, 417–25.

Muller, S., Sideras, P., et al. 1996. Cell specific expression of human Bruton's agammaglobulinaemia tyrosine kinase gene (Btk) is regulated by Sp-1 and Spi-1/PU.1 family members. *Oncogene*, **13**, 1955–64.

Muramatsu, M., Sankaranand, V.S., et al. 1999. Specific expression of activation-induced cytidine deaminase (AID), a novel member of the RNA-editing deaminase family in germinal centre B cells. *J Biol Chem*, **271**, 18470–6.

Muramatsu, M., Kinoshita, K., et al. 2000. Class switch recombination and hypermutation require activation-induced cytidine deaminase (AID), a potential RNA-editing enzyme. *Cell*, **102**, 553–63.

Murre, C. 1994. Structure and function of the helix-loop-helix proteins. *Biochim Biophys Acta*, **1218**, 129–35.

Nadler, M.J., Matthews, S.A., et al. 2000. Signal transduction by the high-affinity immunoglobulin E receptor Fc epsilon RI: coupling form to function. *Adv Immunol*, **76**, 325–55.

Nakamura, M., Kondo, S., et al. 1996. High frequency class switching of an IgM+ B lymphoma clone CH12F3 to IgA+ cells. *Int Immunol*, **8**, 193–201.

Nick McElhinny, S.A., Snowden, C.M., et al. 2000. Ku recruits the XRCC4-ligase IV complex to DNA ends. *Mol Cell Biol*, **20**, 2996–3003.

Noguchi, M., Yi, H. and Rosenblatt, H.M. 1993. Interleukin-2 receptor γ chain mutation results in X-linked severe combined immunodeficiency in humans. *Cell*, **73**, 147–57.

Nomura, K., Kanegane, H., et al. 2000. The genetic defect in X-linked agammaglobulinaemia impedes a maturational evolution of pro-B cells into later stages of pre-B cells in B cell differentiation pathway. *Blood*, **96**, 610–17.

Noordzij, J.G., Verkaik, N.S., et al. 2000. N-terminal truncated human RAG1 proteins can direct T-cell receptor but not immunoglobulin gene rearrangements. *Blood*, **96**, 203–9.

Norderhaug, I.N., Johansen, F.E., et al. 1999. Domain deletions in the human polymeric Ig receptor disclose differences between its dimeric IgA and pentameric IgM interaction. *Eur J Immunol*, **29**, 3401–9.

Nussenzweig, M.C., Shaw, A.C., et al. 1987. Allelic exclusion in transgenic mice that express the membrane form of immunoglobulin mu. *Science*, **236**, 816–19.

Nutt, S.L., Urbanek, P., et al. 1997. Essential functions of Pax5 (BSAP) in pro-B cell development: difference between fetal and adult B lymphopoiesis and reduced V-to-DJ recombination. *Immunobiology*, **198**, 227–35.

Nutt, S.L., Morrison, A.M., et al. 1998. Identification of BSAP (Pax-5) target genes in early B cell development by loss- and gain-of-function experiments. *EMBO J*, **17**, 2319–33.

Nutt, S.L., Heavey, B., et al. 1999. Commitment to the B-lymphoid lineage is dependent on the transcription factor Pax5. *Nature*, **401**, 556–62.

Oi, V.T., Vuong, T.M., et al. 1984. Correlation between segmental flexibility and effector function of antibodies. *Nature*, **307**, 136–40.

Omori, S.A. and Wall, R. 1993. Multiple motifs regulate the B-cell-specific promoter of the B29 gene. *Proc Natl Acad Sci USA*, **90**, 11273–7.

Parekh, R.B., Dwek, R.A., et al. 1985. Association of rheumatoid arthritis and primary osteoarthritis with changes in the glycosylation pattern of total serum IgG. *Nature*, **316**, 452–7.

Peschon, J.J., Morrissey, P.J. and Grabstein, K.H. 1994. Early lymphocyte expansion is severely impaired in interleukin-7 receptor-deficient mice. *J Exp Med*, **180**, 1955–60.

Pleass, R.J., Dunlop, J.I., et al. 1999. Identification of residues in the CH2/CH3 domain interface of IgA essential for interaction with the human Fcalpha receptor (FcalphaR) CD89. *J Biol Chem*, **274**, 23508–14.

Porter, R. 1962. Structure of γ-globulins. In: Gelhorn, A. and Hirschberg, E. (eds), *Symposium on basic problems in neoplastic disease*. New York: Columbia University Press, 177.

Preud'homme, J.L., Petit, I., et al. 2000. Structural and functional properties of membrane and secreted IgD. *Mol Immunol*, **37**, 871–87.

Raghavan, M., Gastinel, L.N. and Bjorkman, P.J. 1993. The class I major histocompatibility complex related Fc receptor shows pH-dependent stability differences correlating with immunoglobulin binding and release. *Biochemistry*, **32**, 8654–60.

Raghavan, M., Wang, Y. and Bjorkman, P.J. 1995. Effects of receptor dimerization on the interaction between the class I major histocompatibility complex-related Fc receptor and IgG. *Proc Natl Acad Sci USA*, **92**, 11200–4.

Ramsden, D.A. and Gellert, M. 1998. Ku protein stimulates DNA end joining by mammalian DNA ligases: a direct role for Ku in repair of DNA double-strand breaks. *EMBO J*, **17**, 609–14.

Ravetch, J.V. and Perussia, B. 1989. Alternative membrane forms of Fc gamma RIII(CD16) on human natural killer cells and neutrophils. Cell type-specific expression of two genes that differ in single nucleotide substitutions. *J Exp Med*, **170**, 481–97.

Reth, M. 1995. The B cell antigen receptor complex and co-receptors. *Immunol Today*, **16**, 310–16.

Revy, P., Geissmann, F., et al. 1998. Normal CD40-mediated activation of monocytes and dendritic cells from patients with hyper-IgM syndrome due to a CD40 pathway defect in B cells. *Eur J Immunol*, **28**, 3648–54.

Revy, P., Muto, T., et al. 2000. Activation-induced cytidine deaminase (AID) deficiency causes the autosomal recessive form of the hyper-IgM syndrome (HIGM2). *Cell*, **102**, 565–75.

Roe, M., Norderhaug, I.N., et al. 1999. Fine specificity of ligand-binding domain 1 in the polymeric Ig receptor: importance of the CDR2-containing region for IgM interaction. *J Immunol*, **162**, 6046–52.

Romanow, W.J., Langerak, A.W., et al. 2000. EBF and the V(D)J recombinase act in synergy to generate a diverse immunoglobulin repertoire in non-lymphoid cells. *Mol Cell*, **5**, 343–53.

Roth, D.B. and Roth, S.Y. 2000. Unequal access: regulating V(D)J recombination through chromatin remodeling. *Cell*, **103**, 699–702.

Roth, D.B., Menetski, J.P., et al. 1992. V(D)J recombination: broken DNA molecules with covalently sealed (hairpin) coding ends in scid mouse thymocytes. *Cell*, **70**, 983–91.

Sadofsky, M.J. 2001. The RAG proteins in V(D)J recombination: more than just a nuclease. *Nucleic Acids Res*, **29**, 1399–409.

Saphire, E.O., Parren, P.W., et al. 2001a. Crystallization and preliminary structure determination of an intact human immunoglobulin, b12: an antibody that broadly neutralizes primary isolates of HIV-1. *Acta Crystallogr D Biol Crystallogr*, **57**, 168–71.

Saphire, E.O., Parren, P.W., et al. 2001b. Crystal structure of a neutralizing human IGG against HIV-1: a template for vaccine design. *Science*, **293**, 1155–9.

Saphire, E.O., Stanfield, R.L., et al. 2002. Contrasting IgG structures reveal extreme asymmetry and flexibility. *J Mol Biol*, **319**, 9–18.

Scher, I. 1982. The CBA/N mouse strain: an experimental model illustrating the influence of the X-chromosome on immunity. *Adv Immunol*, **33**, 1–71.

Schlissel, M., Voronova, A. and Baltimore, D. 1991. Helix-loop-helix transcription factor E47 activates germ-line immunoglobulin heavy-chain transcription and rearrangement in a pre-T cell line. *Genes Dev*, **5**, 1367–76.

Schlissel, M.S. 1998. Structure of nonhairpin coding-end DNA breaks in cells undergoing V(D)J recombination. *Mol Cell Biol*, **18**, 2029–37.

Schlissel, M.S. 2002. Does Artemis end the hunt for the hairpin-opening activity in V(D)J recombination? *Cell*, **109**, 1–4.

Scholl, P.R. and Geha, R.S. 1993. Physical association between the high-affinity IgG receptor (Fc gamma RI) and the gamma subunit of the high-affinity IgE receptor (Fc epsilon RI gamma). *Proc Natl Acad Sci USA*, **90**, 8847–50.

Scott, E.W., Fisher, R.C., et al. 1997. PU.1 functions in a cell-autonomous manner to control the differentiation of multipotential lymphoid-myeloid progenitors. *Immunity*, **6**, 437–47.

Shibuya, A., Sakamoto, N., et al. 2000. Fc alpha/mu receptor mediates endocytosis of IgM-coated microbes. *Nat Immunol*, **1**, 441–6.

Shopes, B., Weetall, M., et al. 1990. Recombinant human IgG1-murine IgE chimeric Ig. Construction, expression, and binding to human Fc gamma receptors. *J Immunol*, **145**, 3842–8.

Sigvardsson, M., O'Riordan, M. and Grosschedl, R. 1997. EBF and E47 collaborate to induce expression of the endogenous immunoglobulin surrogate light chain genes. *Immunity*, **7**, 25–36.

Simister, N.E. and Mostov, K.E. 1989a. Cloning and expression of the neonatal rat intestinal Fc receptor, a major histocompatibility complex class I antigen homolog. *Cold Spring Harb Symp Quant Biol*, **54**, 571–80.

Simister, N.E. and Mostov, K.E. 1989b. An Fc receptor structurally related to MHC class I antigens. *Nature*, **337**, 184–7.

Simister, N.E. and Rees, A.R. 1985. Isolation and characterization of an Fc receptor from neonatal rat small intestine. *Eur J Immunol*, **15**, 733–8.

Singer, P.A., Singer, H.H. and Williamson, A.R. 1980. Different species of messenger RNA encode receptor and secretory IgM mu chains differing at their carboxy termini. *Nature*, **285**, 294–300.

Sloane, S.R., Shen, C.P., et al. 1996. Phosphorylation of E47 as a potential determinant of B cell-specific activity. *Mol Cell Biol*, **16**, 6900–8.

Smith, G.C. and Jackson, S.P. 1999. The DNA-dependent protein kinase. *Genes Dev*, **13**, 916–34.

Soilleux, E.J., Barten, R. and Trowsdale, J. 2000. DC-SIGN; a related gene, DC-SIGNR; and CD23 form a cluster on 19p13. *J Immunol*, **165**, 2937–42.

Sondermann, P., Huber, R., et al. 2000. The 3.2-A crystal structure of the human IgG1 Fc fragment-Fc gammaRIII complex. *Nature*, **406**, 267–73.

Stavnezer-Nordgren, J. and Sirlin, S. 1986. Specificity of immunoglobulin heavy chain switch correlates with activity of germline heavy chain genes prior to switching. *EMBO J*, **5**, 95–102.

Story, C.M., Mikulska, J.E. and Simister, N.E. 1994. A major histocompatibility complex class I-like Fc receptor cloned from human placenta: possible role in transfer of immunoglobulin G from mother to fetus. *J Exp Med*, **180**, 2377–81.

Sun, X.-H., Copeland, N.G., et al. 1991. Id proteins, Id1 and Id2, selectively inhibit DNA binding by one class of helix-loop-helix proteins. *Mol Cell Biol*, **11**, 5603–11.

Sutton, B.J. and Gould, H.J. 1993. The human IgE network. *Nature*, **366**, 421–8.

Swenson, C.D., Amin, A.R., et al. 1993. Regulation of IgD-receptor expression on murine T cells. I. Characterization and metabolic requirements of the process leading to their expression. *Cell Immunol*, **152**, 405–21.

Swenson, C.D., Patel, T., et al. 1998. Human T cell IgD receptors react with O-glycans on both human IgD and IgA1. *Eur J Immunol*, **28**, 2366–72.

Tamma, S.M. and Coico, R.F. 1992. IgD-receptor-positive human T lymphocytes. II. Identification and partial characterization of human IgD-binding factor. *J Immunol*, **148**, 2050–7.

Tashiro, J., Kinoshita, K. and Honjo, T. 2001. Palindromic but not G-rich sequences are targets of class switch recombination. *Int Immunol*, **13**, 495–505.

Thompson, R.A. 1970. Secretory piece linked to IgM in individuals deficient in IgA. *Nature*, **226**, 946–8.

Tiegs, S.L., Russell, D.M. and Nemazee, D. 1993. Receptor editing in self-reactive bone marrow B cells. *J Exp Med*, **177**, 1009–20.

Valentine, R.C. and Green, N.M. 1967. Electron microscopy of an antibody-hapten complex. *J Mol Biol*, **27**, 615–17.

Van den Herik-Oudijk, I.E., Ter Bekke, M.W., et al. 1995. Functional differences between two Fc receptor ITAM signaling motifs. *Blood*, **86**, 3302–7.

van Egmond, M., van Vuuren, A.J., et al. 1999. Human immunoglobulin A receptor (FcalphaRI, CD89) function in transgenic mice requires both FcR gamma chain and CR3 (CD11b/CD18). *Blood*, **93**, 4387–94.

van Egmond, M., Damen, C.A., et al. 2001. IgA and the IgA Fc receptor. *Trends Immunol*, **22**, 205–11.

Vetrie, D., Vorechovsky, I., et al. 1993. The gene involved in X-linked agammaglobulinaemia is a member of the src family of protein-tyrosine kinases. *Nature*, **361**, 226–33.

Villa, A., Santagata, S., et al. 1998. Partial V(D)J recombination activity leads to Omenn syndrome. *Cell*, **93**, 885–96.

von Freeden-Jeffry, U., Vieira, P., et al. 1995. Lymphopenia in interleukin (IL)-7 gene-deleted mice identifies IL-7 as a nonredundant cytokine. *J Exp Med*, **181**, 1519–26.

Waldmann, T.A. 2000. T-cell receptors for cytokines: targets for immunotherapy of leukemia/lymphoma. *Ann Oncol*, **11**, 101–6.

Walker, J.R., Corpina, R.A. and Goldberg, J. 2001. Structure of the Ku heterodimer bound to DNA and its implications for double-strand break repair. *Nature*, **412**, 607–14.

Wallace, K.H. and Rees, A.R. 1980. Studies on the immunoglobulin-G Fc-fragment receptor from neonatal rat small intestine. *Biochem J*, **188**, 9–16.

Wallin, J.J., Gackstetter, E.R. and Koshland, M.E. 1998. Dependence of BSAP repressor and activator functions on BSAP concentration. *Science*, **279**, 1961–4.

Wan, T., Beavil, R.L., et al. 2002. The crystal structure of IgE Fc reveals an asymmetrically bent conformation. *Nat Immunol*, **3**, 681–6.

Wang, J.H., Nichogiannopoulou, A., et al. 1996. Selective defects in the development of the fetal and adult lymphoid system in mice with an Ikaros null mutation. *Immunity*, **5**, 537–49.

Wang, J.H., Avitahl, N., et al. 1998. Aiolos regulates B cell activation and maturation to the effector state. *Immunity*, **9**, 543–53.

Weisbart, R.H., Kacena, A., et al. 1988. GM-CSF induces human neutrophil IgA-mediated phagocytosis by an IgA Fc receptor activation mechanism. *Nature*, **332**, 647–8.

White, L.J., Ozanne, B.W., et al. 1997. Inhibition of apoptosis in a human pre-B cell line by CD23 is mediated via a novel receptor. *Blood*, **90**, 234–43.

White, M.B., Shen, A.L., et al. 1985. Human immunoglobulin D: genomic sequence of the delta heavy chain. *Science*, **228**, 733–7.

Wilhelm, D., Klouche, M., et al. 1994. Expression of sCD23 in atopic and non-atopic blood donors: correlation with age, total serum IgE and allergic symptoms. *Allergy*, **49**, 521–5.

Wines, B.D., Hulett, M.D., et al. 1999. Identification of residues in the first domain of human Fc alpha receptor essential for interaction with IgA. *J Immunol*, **162**, 2146–53.

Winkelhake, J.L. 1978. Immunoglobulin structure and effector functions. *Immunochemistry*, **15**, 695–714.

Wolf, M.L., Buckley, J.A., et al. 1991. Development of a bone marrow culture for maintenance and growth of normal human B cell precursors. *J Immunol*, **147**, 3324–30.

Woof, J.M., Partridge, L.J., et al. 1986. Localisation of the monocyte-binding region on human immunoglobulin G. *Mol Immunol*, **23**, 319–30.

Wurzburg, B.A. and Jardetzky, T.S. 2002. Structural insights into the interactions between human IgE and its high affinity receptor FcepsilonRI. *Mol Immunol*, **38**, 1063–72.

Wurzburg, B.A., Garman, S.C. and Jardetzky, T.S. 2000. Structure of the human IgE-Fc C epsilon 3-C epsilon 4 reveals conformational flexibility in the antibody effector domains. *Immunity*, **13**, 375–85.

Yanagihara, Y., Sarfati, M., et al. 1990. Serum levels of IgE binding factor (CD23) in diseases associated with elevated IgE. *Clin Exp Allergy*, **20**, 395–401.

Yancopoulos, G.D., DePinho, R.A., et al. 1986. Secondary genomic rearrangement events in pre-B cells: VHDJH replacement by a LINE-1 sequence and directed class switching. *EMBO J*, **5**, 3259–66.

Yokota, A., Kikutani, H., et al. 1988. Two species of human Fc epsilon receptor II (FcϵRII/CD23): tissue-specific and IL-4 specific regulation of gene expression. *Cell*, **55**, 611–18.

Yokota, A., Yukawa, K., et al. 1992. Two forms of the low affinity receptor for IgE differentially mediate endocytosis and phagocytosis; identification of the critical cytoplasmic domains. *Proc Natl Acad Sci USA*, **89**, 5030–4.

Yu, P., Kosco-Vilbois, M.H., et al. 1994. Negative feedback regulation of IgE synthesis by murine CD23. *Nature*, **369**, 753–6.

Zheng, Y., Shopes, B., et al. 1991. Conformations of IgE bound to its receptor Fc epsilon RI and in solution. *Biochemistry*, **30**, 9125–32.

Zheng, Y., Shopes, B., et al. 1992. Dynamic conformations compared for IgE and IgG1 in solution and bound to receptors. *Biochemistry*, **31**, 7446–56.

Zhuang, Y., Soriano, P. and Weintraub, H. 1994. The helix-loop helix gene E2A is required for B cell formation. *Cell*, **79**, 875–84.

17

The B-cell antigen receptor

ANTHONY L. DEFRANCO

The major function of B lymphocytes is to make antibodies. The control of antibody production is a complex process, but a central element of that control, as initially enunciated by the clonal selection theory, is that contact of antigen by the B-cell antigen receptor (BCR) promotes activation of the B cell, which, if coming in the presence of sufficient additional signals such as those produced by helper T cells, leads to the production of antibodies.

Studies in recent years have revealed that the BCR plays a pervasive role in B-cell biology, driving nearly every step in the development of B-lineage cells into mature B cells, in addition to being a critical element in the triggering of B-cell activation. Also, the BCR plays a key role in promoting B-cell survival at several stages of B-cell life. These functions of the BCR are summarized in Figure 17.1.

STRUCTURE AND SYNTHESIS OF THE BCR

The BCR is a complex between the membrane form of immunoglobulin (mIg) and two signaling chains, called Igα and Igβ (or CD79a and CD79b) (Figure 17.2). Recognition of antigen by the mIg unit of the BCR leads to signaling via the cytoplasmic domains of Igα and Igβ.

The membrane and secreted forms of Ig made by a particular B cell differ only at the carboxy-terminal end of the heavy chain. This is achieved by differential transcriptional termination and RNA-processing events, giving rise to a distinct mRNA for each type of heavy chain. As a result, individual B cells have the same specificity in their antigen receptors and in the antibody that will be secreted after B-cell activation and terminal differentiation to the plasma cell state.

The mRNA encoding the secreted form of the heavy chain is made by usage of the first of two polyadenylation sites. Usage of this site occurs when transcription terminates before the two exons that encode the transmembrane and cytoplasmic exons. This early termination gives rise to an mRNA that encodes the secretory form, whereas usage of the second polyadenylation site permits RNA splicing which cuts out the sequence that is found only in the secretory form and also removes stop codons (Calame 2001). RNA splicing of this longer transcript produces mRNA encoding the membrane form of the heavy chain. The membrane forms of heavy chains contain at their carboxyl terminus a transmembrane domain and a very short cytoplasmic domain, ranging from 3 to 28 amino acids, depending on the isotype of heavy chain (Reth 1992). Whereas naïve B cells make primarily the membrane form of Ig, terminal differentiation of B cells into high rate antibody-secreting cells (plasma cells) leads to synthesis of much more of the secretory form and less of the membrane form, thereby leading to production of secreted antibodies.

Although the short (three amino acids) cytoplasmic domain of mIgM and mIgD is not known to have any function other than positioning the transmembrane domain relative to the membrane, the longer cytoplasmic domains of the switched isotypes could engage signaling components. In transgenic mouse experiments,

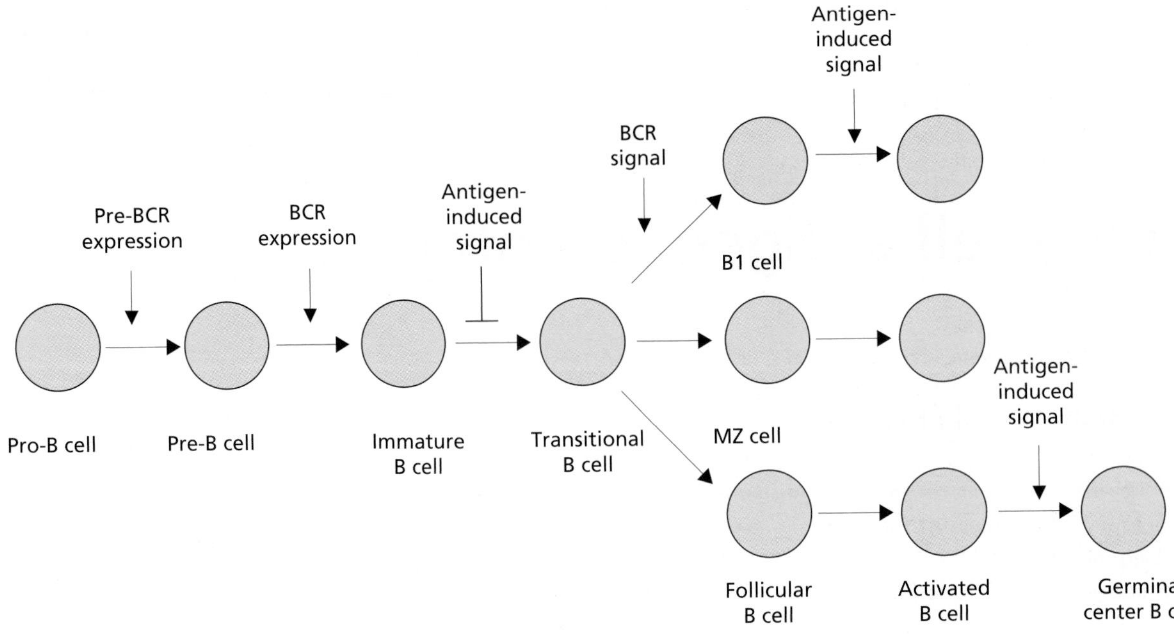

Figure 17.1 *Regulation of B-cell development, survival, tolerance, and activation by the B-cell antigen receptor (BCR). Shown are stages of B-cell development from the pro-B-cell stage (μ chain negative) to the three mature B cell types, B1 cells, marginal zone B cells and follicular B cells. Signals from the pre-BCR or BCR, either generated at a low level as a result of expression ('tonic' signaling) or induced by contact with a self or foreign antigen, regulate the steps shown. Arrows indicate stimulation of the step shown, whereas a perpendicular line indicates inhibition. Low-level BCR signals from weak responsiveness to self-antigens are probably required for maturation of all three B-cell types from transitional B cells, as well as their survival (not shown). Stronger BCR signals ('antigen-induced signal') promote activation of mature B cells, as well as entry of follicular B cells into germinal center reactions and survival of centrocytes.*

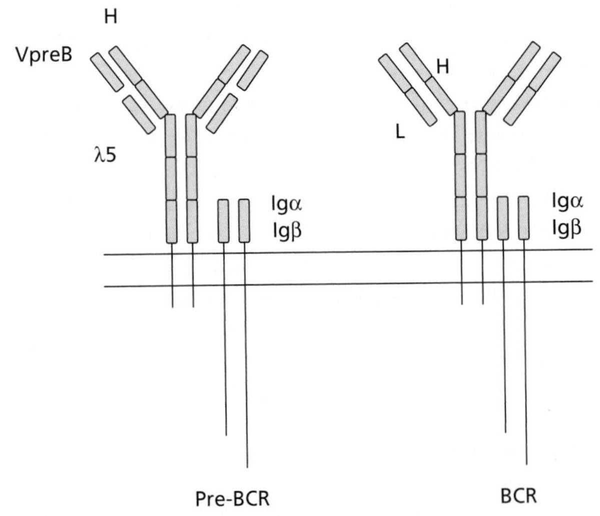

Figure 17.2 *Structure of the pre-BCR and the B-cell antigen receptor (BCR). The pre-BCR consists of a pair of identical μ heavy chains, each of which is bound to the two surrogate light chains, Vpre-B1 and λ5, and to a disulfide-linked heterodimer of Igα and Igβ. The cytoplasmic domains of these latter two molecules have ITAM sequences, which are primarily responsible for mediating signaling. The BCR is a similar structure, with rearranged κ or λ light chains instead of surrogate light chains. In mature B cells, BCRs with μ or δ heavy chains are found and isotype-switched B cells have BCRs with γ, α, or ε heavy chains complexed with light chains and Igα/Igβ.*

anti-lysozyme IgG1 transgenic mice were found to give rise to much larger T-cell-dependent antibody responses than equivalent IgM transgenic mice as a result of a greater proliferative burst and enhanced plasma cell differentiation. These properties could be conferred by the transmembrane domain plus the cytoplasmic tail of the γ1 heavy chain fused to the extracellular domain of the μ heavy chain (Martin and Goodnow 2002). It seems likely that this functional effect depends primarily on the cytoplasmic domains, because gene-targeted mice, in which there has been a deletion of the IgG1 cytoplasmic tail (Kaisho et al. 1997) or the IgE cytoplasmic tail (Achatz et al. 1997), show considerably decreased antibody production of those isotypes. Thus, the longer cytoplasmic tail of the isotype-switched Ig heavy chains promotes B-cell proliferation, survival, and antibody production and may account for the hallmark properties of memory B cells.

The pre-BCR and B-cell development

Pre-B cells have a signaling receptor related to the BCR called the pre-BCR. This receptor is a complex of Igα/Igβ, Ig heavy chain, and two polypeptides that take the place of light chain and hence are called surrogate light chains (see Figure 17.2). These two polypeptides, called λ5 and Vpre-B, each has an Ig domain related to light chain C and V regions, respectively. The pre-BCR plays a critical role during B-cell development by generating a signal to indicate the presence of a properly rearranged heavy chain. When an IgH gene rearrangement occurs that creates an in-frame μ heavy chain gene, this leads to synthesis of Ig heavy chain and formation of the pre-BCR, which then sends a signal inducing further developmental progression toward the B-cell state (see Figure 17.1).

The function of the pre-BCR has been extensively studied by targeted gene mutations in mice (Kurosaki 2002a; Meffre et al. 2000). Ablation of the IgH locus or of the *rag1* or *rag2* genes required for V(D)J recombination causes a complete block in B-cell development in which B220$^+$ (CD45R$^+$) B-cell precursors fail to progress beyond the pro-B-cell stage, characterized as being positive for the S7 epitope of the CD43 molecule. This epitope is created by a specific carbohydrate modification of the CD43 polypeptide backbone (Shiota et al. 1994). Pro-B cells also have the functional property that they will proliferate in contact with suitable stromal cells derived from bone marrow, but will not proliferate in response to interleukin 7 (IL-7) in the absence of contact with stromal cells. Expression of a properly rearranged μ heavy chain and subsequent pre-BCR signaling induces enhanced responsiveness to IL-7 (Reichman-Fried et al. 1993; Fleming and Paige 2001). This developmental transition is also characterized by expression of CD25 (the α chain of the IL-2 receptor), and loss of expression of c-kit, a transmembrane tyrosine kinase receptor for a hemopoietic growth factor. Pre-BCR signaling also retargets the V(D)J recombinase away from the IgH locus and toward the IgL loci (Schlissel and Stanhope-Baker 1997). This is important for insuring that a given B cell expresses only a single Ig heavy chain, a phenomenon referred to as allelic exclusion.

Other mutations that affect pre-BCR assembly or signaling lead to impairment in the developmental transition from pro-B cell to pre-B cell (Figure 17.3). These include mutations of the IgH locus or of λ5, combined deletion of the cytoplasmic domains of Igα and Igβ (Kraus et al. 2001), and mutations in a variety of signaling components (Kurosaki 2002a; Meffre et al. 2000). The last mutations are discussed in greater detail below. Individual deletions of the cytoplasmic domain of Igα or Igβ have partial, but relatively mild, phenotypes, indicating a redundancy in the signaling capabilities of these two BCR-associated proteins.

BCR sequences that mediate intracellular signaling

The BCR complex forms in the endoplasmic reticulum, where mIg and Igα/Igβ subcomplexes are retained by chaperones until assembly occurs. Assembly allows the signaling-competent BCR to traffic to the cell surface. Igα and Igβ each contain an amino-terminal single Ig domain extracellular domain, a transmembrane domain,

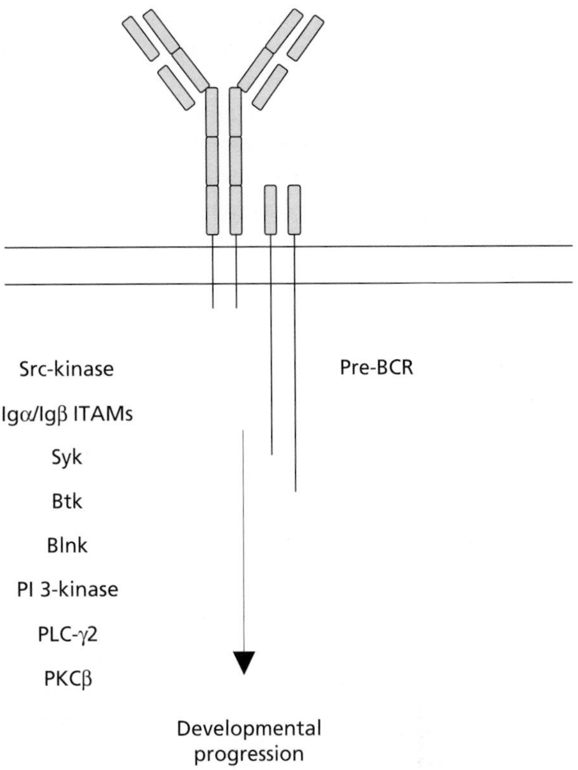

Figure 17.3 *Signaling events required for pre-BCR signaling. Genetic experiments have probed the signaling events required for the pre-BCR to induce developmental progression from the pro-B cell stage to the pre-B cell stage. Signaling components or sequences required for this transition are shown. In addition, μ heavy chain is required as is the λ5 surrogate light chain.*

and a moderate length cytoplasmic domain (about 50 amino acids long) containing immunoreceptor tyrosine-based activation motif (ITAM) sequences. ITAMs are found also in subunits of the T-cell receptor (TCR), the activating Fc receptors, and activating natural killer (NK) and myeloid cell receptors, and are responsible for the signaling functions of these receptors. Signaling is initiated by phosphorylation of the tyrosines in the ITAM motifs, as described in greater detail below. Targeted mutations of mice that mutate ITAM tyrosines of Igα or Igβ lead to defects in B-cell development, presumably as a result of defects in signaling by the pre-BCR and/or the BCR (Kraus et al. 2001; Kurosaki 2002a).

Higher order structure of the BCR

Recent studies have indicated that the BCR exists in the B-cell membrane as a higher oligomer of the basic H_2L_2Igα/β unit (Schamel and Reth 2000; Matsuuchi and Gold 2001; Reth 2001). The number of units within these higher-order structures has not been defined, but unliganded BCR complexes are submicroscopic and thus are probably relatively small oligomers. These oligomers are composed of single isotypes of mIg (e.g. individual oligomers contain all mIgM or all mIgD on a naïve B cell expressing both IgM and IgD).

The functional consequence of the oligomeric structure of the BCR has likewise not been clearly defined, but there are two leading hypotheses. The first is that these oligomers hold the BCR in a conformation that sends a tonic signal which promotes B-cell developmental events and survival of mature B-cell types (see Figure 17.1) (Reth 2001). According to this hypothesis, antigen binding distorts these oligomers and thereby results in a qualitative change in the nature of BCR signaling events. This qualitatively different BCR signal would promote activation of mature B cells or deletion of transitional B cells. The clearest precedent for this model is distortion of IgM pentamers on antigen binding which initiates the complement cascade. However, at this point there is little evidence for two qualitatively distinct modes of BCR signaling.

The alternate hypothesis also holds that, in the absence of antigen, there is a low level of tonic BCR signaling which mediates various developmental transitions and survival of mature B cells. However, this hypothesis postulates that antigen induces clustering of BCRs, which triggers a higher level of the same signaling events. The latter hypothesis has been the more traditional view of how BCR signaling is triggered and in general can explain many of the phenomena regarding the relationship between the oligomeric state of antigens and their ability to induce stronger or weaker immune responses, e.g. antigens able to crosslink the BCR strongly (e.g. capsular polysaccharides of bacteria and capsid proteins of highly ordered virus particles (Mond et al. 1995; Bachmann and Zinkernagel 1996)), can induce antibody responses in the absence of helper T cells, whereas most protein antigens, which have a lesser potential for inducing BCR clustering, require T-cell help to generate an antibody response.

The clustering hypothesis is compatible with the idea that the BCR pre-exists in higher-order oligomers, although clearly it does raise questions about why the oligomers signal at only a low rate, whereas further clustering triggers a much higher amount of signaling. This issue may relate to lipid raft localization, which is triggered by clustering of the BCR with a ligand (see below). Moreover, given the complexity of BCR signaling events (DeFranco 1997; Kurosaki 2002b) and the observations that some signaling events participate in some biological responses to the BCR and not others (Richards et al. 2001), it may be that tonic signaling generates a subset of the signaling reactions induced by antigen-induced clustering, e.g. the signals may have some qualitative differences in addition to quantitative differences.

According to the clustering hypothesis for BCR signaling, what is the purpose of the higher-order oligomeric structure of the BCR before antigen encounter? It is likely that clustering of oligomers instead of monomeric BCR units ($H_2L_2Ig\alpha/\beta$) would amplify the signal at low doses of antigen as clustering would bring together oligomers, each with multiple $Ig\alpha/\beta$ signaling modules (Matsuuchi and Gold 2001). Indeed direct evidence for this possibility has been obtained in experiments using coexpression of two distinguishable forms of Igα, one of which had an external FLAG-epitope tag (Schamel and Reth 2000). Stimulating only the FLAG-tagged BCRs by using an anti-FLAG antibody revealed tyrosine phosphorylation not only of the FLAG-tagged Igα molecules, but also of the untagged Igα molecules. Presumably this is because oligomers contain both types of Igα molecules. Thus, BCRs that are not directly bound by the stimulating antibody are activated to signal.

BCR SIGNALING

Antigen-induced clustering of the BCR leads to rapid tyrosine phosphorylation of the ITAM tyrosines by the Src family tyrosine kinases expressed in B cells, Lyn, Fyn, and Blk. Why this occurs is not clearly established, but it may relate to the microdomains of the plasma membrane referred to as lipid rafts. Lipid rafts are enriched in cholesterol, sphingolipids, and a variety of lipid-modified proteins, all of which associate with one another in a dynamic fashion to form subdomains that vary in size from about 70 nm in diameter to almost 1 μm (Pierce 2002). In unstimulated B cells, these structures are relatively small and dispersed, although they may account for as much as 30 percent of the plasma membrane surface area. Lyn, Fyn and Blk are highly enriched in lipid rafts, whereas before stimulation the BCR is found in the nonraft region of the bilayer. Upon stimulation, the BCR rapidly enters or associates with lipid rafts, and this association apparently does not require phosphorylation of the ITAMs of the BCR (Cheng et al. 2001).

Why antigen-induced multimerization of the BCR induces it to associate with lipid rafts is not known. One hypothesis is that the BCR has a weak affinity for lipid rafts as an oligomer, and multimerization increases that interaction, making it more stable. An argument against this possibility is that the association of antigen-ligated BCRs with lipid rafts occurs in mature B cells but not in immature B cells (Sproul et al. 2000; Chung et al. 2001), suggesting that there is some way of regulating this association. A second hypothesis is that a small subset of BCR molecules are preassociated with lipid rafts and multimerization brings non-lipid draft BCRs together with raft BCRs, with the resulting aggregate now associated with rafts. In this case, a regulated post-translational modification or protein–protein association could be responsible for directing some BCRs to lipid rafts before stimulation.

Activation of protein tyrosine kinases by the BCR

A major consequence of BCR association with lipid rafts is likely to be a closer proximity of the BCR and Src family tyrosine kinases located in the lipid rafts and hence increased tyrosine phosphorylation of the ITAMs. Phosphorylation of both tyrosines of a single ITAM triggers the binding of a second type of intracellular protein tyrosine kinase, Syk (Figure 17.4). This binding is mediated by association of the two SH2 (Src homology 2) domains of Syk with the doubly phosphorylated ITAM sequence. The ITAM sequence is essentially a tandem SH2-binding site, with the amino acids between the two SH2-binding motifs (Y-PxxL/I where Y-P means a phosphorylated tyrosine) extending a sufficient distance to permit the ITAM to bind simultaneously to both SH2 domains of one Syk molecule, as demonstrated by structural studies (Futterer et al. 1998).

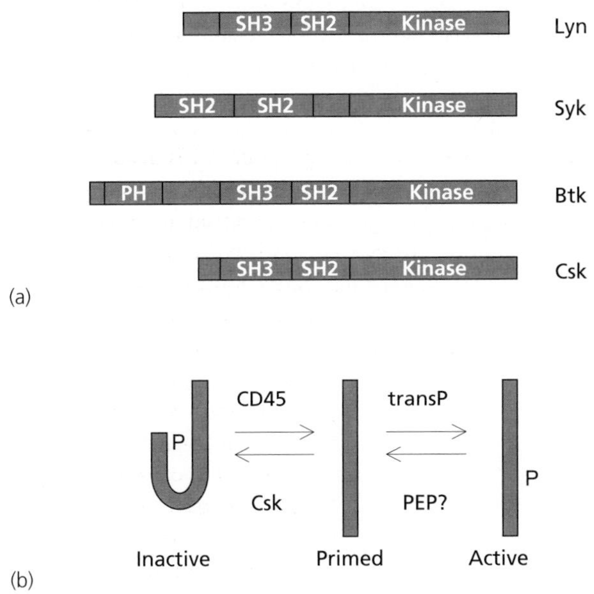

Figure 17.4 *Tyrosine kinases involved in B-cell antigen receptor (BCR) signaling.* **(a)** *Structures of the four major types of intracellular protein tyrosine kinases that participate in or regulate BCR signaling. Lyn, Fyn, and Blk are members of the Src family of tyrosine kinases, which have amino-terminal unique sequences with lipid attachment sites (myristate in all cases and palmitate in the cases of Lyn and Fyn). The unique region is followed by Src homology 3 (SH3) and Src homology 2 (SH2) domains, a kinase domain, and a negative regulatory tyrosine near the carboxyl terminus (not shown). Syk, like ZAP-70 has two SH2 domains, an interdomain region with sites of regulatory tyrosine phosphorylation, and a kinase domain. Btk, a Tec family kinase, has an amino-terminal pleckstrin homology (PH) domain that mediates regulated binding to membranes via* PIP_3*, followed by SH3, SH2, and kinase domains. Csk is responsible for phosphorylating the negative-regulatory site on Src family kinases and has a structure similar to Src, but lacking the amino-terminal fatty acylation sites and the negative regulatory tyrosine.* **(b)** *Regulation of Src family tyrosine kinases by tyrosine phosphorylation. Csk phosphorylation of the carboxy-terminal negative regulatory site of Lyn converts it to an inactive state in which the SH2 domain is bound to the C-terminal tyrosine phosphate and the kinase domain is inactive. CD45 is responsible for removing the carboxy-terminal tyrosine phosphate. Lyn lacking the carboxy-terminal phosphate is in a primed but low activity state. Transphosphorylation of a tyrosine residue in the activation loop of the kinase domain leads to the fully active state. The tyrosine kinase PEP is a leading candidate for removing this activating phosphorylation and it forms a complex with Csk, suggesting coordinate regulation converting active Src family kinases to the inactive state. This inactivation may occur via a feedback inhibition mechanism, because Src family kinases apparently are responsible for phosphorylating Cbp, which recruits Csk to the membrane.*

Once Syk has docked on to the oligomerized BCRs in the lipid rafts, it becomes activated. The binding of an ITAM to the Syk SH2 domains appears to be partly responsible for this activation by allosteric means (Rowley et al. 1995; Shiue et al. 1995). In addition, Syk is activated by tyrosine phosphorylation of a tyrosine in the kinase domain activation loop (Kurosaki et al. 1995). Syk activity appears to increase by at least 10-fold and, of course, Syk activity is also localized by its association with the BCR. Indeed, fluorescence microscopy demonstrates a dramatic movement of Syk from the cytosol to the plasma membrane after BCR crosslinking (Ma et al. 2001), and this association is primarily associated with lipid raft subdomains of the plasma membrane (Gupta and DeFranco 2003). Similarly, a dramatic increase in tyrosine phosphorylation of proteins can also be seen to occur coincident with lipid raft microdomains. Thus, BCR signaling appears to be occurring primarily in or adjacent to lipid rafts.

In addition to the activation of Syk, there is also a rapid increase in the activity of Src family tyrosine kinases on stimulation of the BCR (Saouaf et al. 1994). This increase may result partly from association of Src family tyrosine kinases with ITAM half-sites via their single SH2 domains (Law et al. 1993; Clark et al. 1994). Alternatively, it may relate to decreased inhibition of Src kinase activity by Csk, which phosphorylates the C-terminal negative regulatory tyrosine of Src family kinases (Figure 17.4). Csk localization is regulated and, in T cells, Csk is present initially in lipid rafts bound to a protein called Csk-binding protein (Cbp) (also called PAG). Upon TCR stimulation, Csk is released from Cbp by dephosphorylation of Cbp (Torgersen et al. 2001). Whether or not this occurs in B cells is not yet known. Finally, greater removal of Csk phosphorylations by the transmembrane protein tyrosine phosphatase CD45 could be an important means of regulating activity of Src family tyrosine kinases (Figure 17.4).

Formation of signaling complexes

Once Syk is activated, it phosphorylates the key signaling adapter molecule BLNK (also called SLP-65) (Kelly and Chan 2000; Kurosaki 2002b). BLNK is a cytosolic molecule containing a carboxy-terminal SH2-domain and multiple tyrosines that become phosphorylated and then serve as binding sites for SH2-containing signaling molecules (Fu et al. 1998). How BLNK is localized to signaling receptors is not entirely clear at this point. In TCR signaling, the adapter SLP-76 is closely analogous to BLNK and it is recruited to participate in TCR signaling by binding to a phosphorylated tyrosine in a transmembrane lipid raft-localized protein called linker for activation of T cells (LAT). Genetic evidence demonstrates that both SLP-76 and LAT are required for TCR signaling (Leo and Schraven 2001). Moreover, SLP-76 and LAT, but not either molecule alone, can replace BLNK to permit BCR signaling in DT-40 chicken B cells mutated in BLNK (Wong et al. 2000). These observations suggest that there may be a B-cell-specific equivalent of LAT and a candidate molecule called LAB (linker for activation of B cells) or NTAL (non T-cell activation linker) has been found (Brdicka et al. 2002; Janssen et al. 2003). An alternative possibility is that the BCR itself recruits BLNK to participate in BCR signaling and indeed there is evidence that BLNK's SH2 domain can bind well to a non-ITAM tyrosine (Y204) of Igα when this tyrosine becomes phosphorylated (Engels et al. 2001; Kabak et al. 2002).

The importance of BLNK for BCR signaling has been established by genetic experiments in chickens (Fu et al. 1998) and mice (Pappu et al. 1999; Hayashi et al. 2000; Xu et al. 2000), and by the discovery of rare immunodeficiency patients with agammaglobulinemia who have loss of function mutations of BLNK (Minegishi et al. 1999). Mice lacking BLNK have a strong block in B-cell development at the pro-B cell stage, probably as a result of a defect in pre-BCR signaling. An equivalent defect is seen in mice with genetic ablation of Syk (Cheng et al. 1995; Turner et al. 1995) or of the three main Src family tyrosine kinases expressed in B cells (Lyn, Fyn, and Blk) (Saijo et al. 2003) (see Figure 17.3).

Phosphorylation of BLNK leads to formation of a signaling complex that includes a third type of intracellular protein tyrosine kinase, Btk (see Figure 17.4), and phospholipase Cγ2 (PLCγ2) (Kurosaki 2002b). In this complex, Btk becomes activated, apparently by phosphorylation by Syk, whereupon it phosphorylates PLCγ2, activating its catalytic function. Thus, BLNK both recruits PLCγ2 to the membrane where its substrate phosphatidylinositol 4,5-bisphosphate (PIP_2) is located and promotes its activation (Figure 17.5). These combined actions induce PLCγ2 to hydrolyze PIP_2, yielding diacylglycerol, which activates protein kinase C

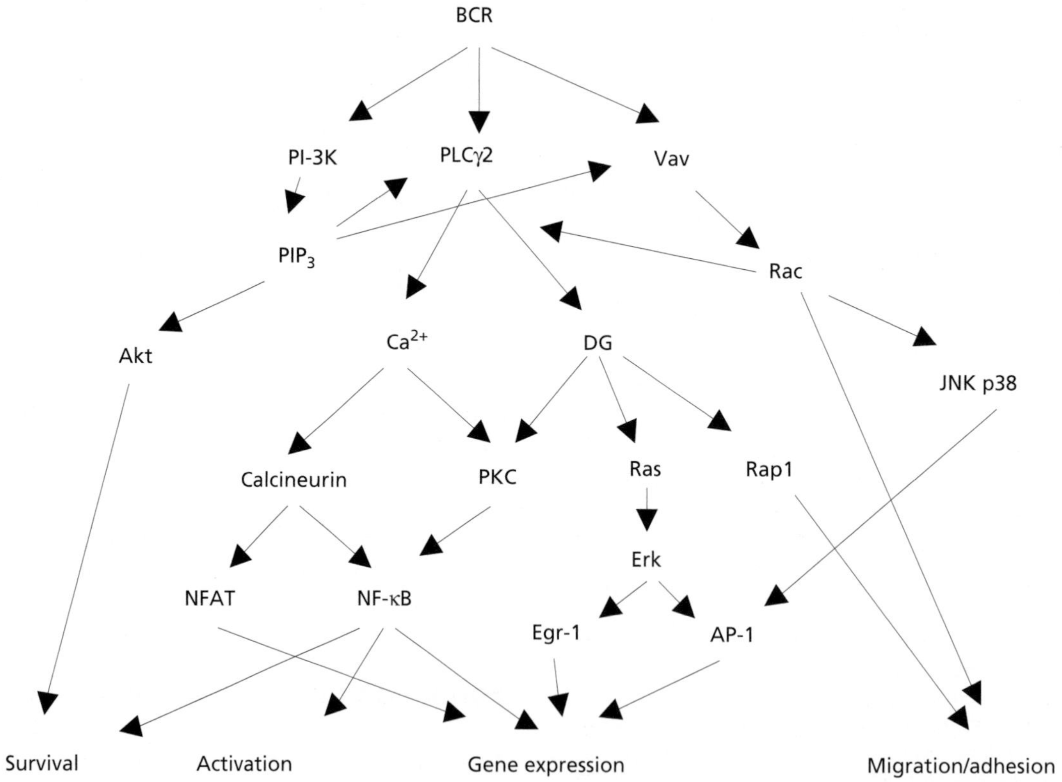

Figure 17.5 *Networks of signaling reactions activated by the B-cell antigen receptor (BCR). Clustering of the BCR causes it to associate with lipid rafts, which contain Lyn, Fyn and Blk. These Src family tyrosine kinases phosphorylate the BCR ITAMs, inducing recruitment of Syk (not shown), with each of its SH2 domains binding to one-half of the phosphorylated ITAM. Activated Syk and/or Src family tyrosine kinases phosphorylate adapter molecules (see text) such as Blnk and BCAP, leading to activation of PI 3-kinase, PLC-γ2 and the guanine nucleotide exchange factor Vav. PIP_3 generated by PI 3-kinase plays an important role in activation of PLC-γ2 and Vav, as well as the protein kinase Akt, which promotes survival. PLC-γ2 hydrolyzes the phospholipid PIP_2, generating calcium and diacylglycerol (DG). These reactions lead to activation of the transcription factors NFAT, NF-κB, and AP-1 and the induced expression of the transcription factor Egr-1. Also activated are the small-molecular-mass GTP-binding proteins Ras, Rac, and Rap1, which regulate gene expression via MAP kinases and also regulate actin networks and integrin adhesiveness, controlling adhesion, and migration.*

(PKC) isoforms, and inositol 1,4,5-trisphosphate (IP_3), which opens channels releasing stored calcium into the cytoplasm. Depletion of intracellular calcium stores results in the opening of plasma membrane Trp1 channels to keep intracellular free calcium levels elevated (Mori et al. 2002).

The recruitment of Btk to the plasma membrane requires not only BLNK but also phosphoinositide 3-kinase (PI 3-kinase) (Kurosaki 2002b). PI 3-kinase phosphorylates PIP_2 to yield phosphatidylinositol 3,4,5-trisphosphate (PIP_3). PIP_3 in turn provides a binding ligand for Btk. Thus, Btk is recruited to participate in BCR signaling by the combined action of BLNK and PI 3-kinase.

Btk and a number of other signaling proteins are attracted to the membrane by PIP_3 via homologous domains, called pleckstrin homology (PH) domains. Among these PH domain- containing signaling proteins are the protein kinase Akt and its upstream activating kinase PDK-1. Akt is thought to be important for promoting B-cell survival.

Mice or humans with mutations in Btk, the PI 3-kinase p85α subunit, or PLCγ2 exhibit impairment in B-cell development that is similar to that seen in the Blnk and Syk deficiencies (Fruman et al. 2000), presumably reflecting the participation of these components in pre-BCR signaling (see Figure 17.3).

Activation of PI 3-kinase

Activation of PI 3-kinase by the BCR is also mediated by adapter proteins. On BCR oligomerization, the transmembrane protein CD19 becomes phosphorylated on tyrosines in its cytoplasmic domain which serve as recruitment sites for PI 3-kinase and another signaling molecule Vav (see below) (Kelly and Chan 2000). CD19 is part of the complement receptor 2 (CR2) complex and acts as a co-receptor for BCR signaling, as discussed below.

A genetic deficiency in CD19 in mice compromises BCR signaling (Engel et al. 1995; Rickert et al. 1995), although less so than mutation of PI 3-kinase or Btk, suggesting that there are other mechanisms for activating PI 3-kinase. Two other adapter proteins have been found to bind PI 3-kinase after BCR stimulation: B-cell adapter for PI 3-kinase (BCAP) (Okada et al. 2000) and Grb-2-associated binding protein 1 (Gab1) (Ingham et al. 2001). PI 3-kinase activation is compromised in BCAP mutants of the chicken DT-40 B-cell line (Okada et al. 2000), but not in splenic B cells from mice lacking BCAP. These mice do exhibit defects in B1 B-cell development, greatly decreased antibody responses to T-independent type II antigens (see below), and somewhat decreased numbers of mature B cells (Yamazaki et al. 2002). Moreover, the BCAP-deficient B cells have poor calcium elevation and poor proliferative responses, although decreased activation of PI 3-kinase was not evident (Yamazaki et al. 2002). These defects are less than those seen in PI 3-kinase p85α subunit or Btk mutant mice. It could be that CD19 and BCAP represent independent routes for BCR-induced activation of PI 3-kinase, or alternately that they act in concert or that BCAP functions for activation of PLC-γ2 independently of PI 3-kinase.

BCR signaling induces phosphorylation of Gab1 along with binding of PI 3-kinase. So far, the effects of removing Gab1 on B-cell function have not been established, but overexpression of Gab1 in the WEHI-231 B-cell line potentiated BCR-induced activation of PI 3-kinase (Ingham et al. 2001). BCR stimulation induces Gab1 translocation from the cytosol to the plasma membrane and this translocation requires the PH domain of Gab1, which binds PIP_3. Therefore it has been proposed that Gab1 is an amplifier of PI 3-kinase activation in BCR signaling. Initial activation of PI 3-kinase via CD19 or BCAP is postulated to result in production of some PIP_3, which would attract Gab1 to the membrane, where it would become tyrosine phosphorylated and recruit additional PI 3-kinase (Ingham et al. 2001).

Signaling events activated by the BCR

As described above, BCR stimulation leads to activation of PI 3-kinase and PIP_2 hydrolysis. BCR stimulation also leads to activation of Vav1, Vav2, and Vav3, which are exchange factors for Rac/Rho family GTPases, activation of Ras, and downstream activation of a variety of transcription factors, including NFAT, NF-κB, AP-1, and Egr-1 (DeFranco 1997; Kurosaki 2002b).

VAV

Vav exists as three isoforms: Vav1, Vav2, and Vav3. Genetic experiments have demonstrated the importance of Vav1 and Vav2 in murine B cells (DeFranco 2001) and Vav3 in DT-40 chicken B cells (Inabe et al. 2002). Vav1 is thought to be activated as a consequence of its recruitment either to the cytoplasmic tail of CD19 or to BLNK, in either case via an SH2-mediated interaction. How Vav2 and Vav3 are activated is less clear. Deficiency of Vav1 in mice leads to loss of B1 B cells, as does loss of CD19, whereas Vav2-deficient mice have decreased T-cell-independent type 2 and T-cell-dependent antibody responses. These findings indicate that Vav1 and Vav2 have distinctive functions (DeFranco 2001). The Vav1/Vav2 double knockout mice have severe defects in B-cell development, maturation in the periphery, and BCR signaling, indicating that many of the functions of Vav1 and Vav2 are overlapping.

The three Vavs all function as activators of Rac family GTPases. Among the downstream consequences of Vav activation are modest activation of the JNK and p38 mitogen-activated protein (MAP) kinases, stimulated actin polymerization, and activation of PIP 5-kinase, which replenishes PIP_2 to permit rapid PIP_2 hydrolysis by PLCγ2. Indeed *vav1*$^{-/-}$*vav2*$^{-/-}$ B cells exhibit very poor calcium responses to BCR stimulation, indicating weak PIP_2 hydrolysis (DeFranco 2001). Vav3 has been reported to activate PI 3-kinase in chicken B cells downstream of activation of Rac1 (Inabe et al. 2002). As Vav has a PH domain that binds to PIP_3 resulting in increased activity for activation of Rac, it may be that Vav activation of PI 3-kinase is part of a positive feedback amplification loop (Kurosaki 2002b).

RAS

Another key signaling reaction activated by the BCR involves the small GTPase Ras. BCR signaling promotes the loading of GTP on to Ras, which converts it to the active configuration (DeFranco 1997; Gold 2002). Activated Ras has a number of different downstream effects, but the best characterized is the activation of the Erk MAP kinases. MAP kinases are involved in activation of a number of transcriptional pathways.

The mechanism by which the BCR activates Ras is not well established. A major mechanism for the activation of Ras by many receptors involves tyrosine phosphorylation of binding sites for the adapter molecule Grb2, either on a receptor or on the adapter molecule Shc. In most cells, Grb2 is pre-bound to Sos, a guanine nucleotide exchange factor for Ras. Recruitment of Sos to the plasma membrane brings it in close proximity to Ras, where it can induce Ras to release GDP and bind GTP. In lymphocytes, however, Grb2 and Sos are not present in a complex before stimulation (Ravichandran et al. 1995; Harmer and DeFranco 1997). BCR stimulation induces a large increase in Shc phosphorylation and there is formation of a Shc/Grb2/Sos complex, which is localized to the plasma membrane (Saxton et al. 1994; Harmer and DeFranco 1997).

Given the important role of Grb2 and Sos in activating Ras in other systems and the strong tyrosine phosphorylation of Shc in response to BCR stimulation, it has been attractive to consider this to be the mechanism by which BCR stimulation leads to Ras activation. However, genetic studies in DT-40 chicken B cells have found that Grb2 and Shc are not necessary for the activation of Ras via the BCR (Nagai et al. 1995). Thus, the importance of Shc for BCR signaling remains unclear. Interestingly, most of the phosphorylated Shc in BCR-stimulated B cells is in a complex with SHIP (Harmer and DeFranco 1999), an SH2-domain containing inositol phosphatase which is active in removing the 5-phosphate from PIP_3, and thereby countering at least some of the actions of PI 3-kinase (see below), so Shc's primary role may reflect feedback inhibitory events rather than Ras pathway activation.

Recently, a second mechanism for activating Ras in some cell types has been established. Diacylglycerol generated from PIP_2 breakdown can recruit a distinct type of guanine nucleotide exchange factor for Ras, called RasGRP (Ebinu et al. 2000). In this activation mode, Ras activation is downstream of PIP_2 hydrolysis. This possible mechanism for BCR activation of Ras is supported by studies in DT-40 cells, which have shown the importance of phospholipase (PLC)γ2 for activation of the Ras pathway (Hashimoto et al. 1998), a result that would not be expected if Shc/Grb2/Sos were responsible for BCR-induced Ras activation.

In addition to Ras, Rac family GTPases are also activated by the BCR, as indicated by Vav activation (Hashimoto et al. 1998). Rac family GTPases regulate actin polymerization and activation of JNK and p38 MAP kinases, as described above.

A third type of small GTPase that is activated by BCR signaling is Rap1 (McLeod et al. 1998). Activated Rap1 increases integrin binding to their ligands and thereby promotes cell adhesion and possibly migration (Gold 2002). Activation of Rap is thought to be a consequence of diacylglycerol elevation resulting from PLC-γ2 activation.

Activation of transcription factors downstream of BCR signaling

A key signaling pathway downstream of the BCR is the activation of the NF-κB transcription factors, which are dimers of two types of subunits: the p50 (p50 or p52) and the p65 type (p65/RelA, c-Rel, or RelB). Mice deficient in the c-Rel and p50 subunits of NF-κB have normal lymphocyte development but are severely defective in B- and T-cell activation (Pohl et al. 2002). Thus, antigen receptor activation of NF-κB is necessary for lymphocyte activation. How antigen receptors activate NF-κB is not well established, but some of the players are known. In T cells, PKCθ is required for TCR activation of NF-κB (Arendt et al. 2002). The analogous function in B cells is performed by PKCβ (Saijo et al. 2002; Su et al. 2002).

Another signaling component that has been found to participate in antigen receptor activation of NF-κB is the adapter molecule Bcl-10. Mice lacking Bcl-10 have a lymphocyte phenotype that is very similar to that of NF-κB knockouts: normal lymphocyte development, but a failure of lymphocyte activation (Ruland et al. 2001). Bcl-10 is an adapter molecule with an amino-terminal domain with considerable homology to caspase recruitment domains (CARD) of other proteins such as Apaf-1. Bcl-10 was initially discovered as being encoded by a gene translocated to the Ig locus in a subset of B-cell lymphomas (Willis et al. 1999), so overexpression of Bcl-10 probably contributes to lymphoma formation. The opposite hypothesis has also been advanced, e.g. that translocation to the Ig locus leads to inactivation of Bcl-10 by somatic mutation (Willis et al. 1999), but translocations are not always accompanied by somatic mutations in Bcl-10, so the model that Bcl-10 overexpression contributes to lymphoma formation, probably via activation of NF-κB, seems most likely.

Bcl-10 is thought to function in a complex with CARD11 (also called CARMA1) or related proteins containing CARD, PDZ, SH3, and guanylate kinase domains (Pomerantz et al. 2002). In addition to CARD11, which is highly expressed in lymphoid tissues, this subgroup of the membrane-associated guanylate kinase (MAGUK) family of molecular scaffolds includes CARD10 (Bimp1), and CARD14 (Bimp2) (Bertin et al. 2000, 2001; Gaide et al. 2001, 2002; McAllister-Lucas et al. 2001; Wang et al. 2001). Other members of this signaling complex are less well defined, but may include a protein with caspase-like, Ig-like, and death domains called mucosa-associated lymphoid tissue 1 (MALT-1) (Akagi et al. 1999; Morgan et al. 1999). The gene for MALT-1, similar to that for Bcl-10, is translocated to the Ig loci in a subset of MALT lymphomas.

As in T cells, elevation of intracellular calcium resulting from BCR engagement leads to activation of NFAT transcription factors (Dolmetsch et al. 1997), although their downstream targets in B cells are not well characterized. One target appears to be the gene encoding CD5 (Berland and Wortis 1998), which is a negative regulator of BCR signaling (see below). Curiously, mice genetically modified to ablate both NFATc1 and NFATc2 have hyperactivated B cells and elevated levels of IgG1 and IgE (Peng et al. 2001). NFATc2 ablation alone resulted in increased B-cell proliferation (Caetano et al. 2002).

Ets transcription factors such as Ets-1 are also likely to be regulated by calcium elevation in B cells (Fisher et al. 1991); in the case of Ets-1, calcium leads to its inactivation. Mice in which the Ets-1 gene has been ablated exhibit elevated numbers of IgM-secreting plasma cells (Bories et al. 1995), indicating that Ets-1 probably plays a role in maintaining B cells in a resting state in the absence of antigenic stimulation. Two other Ets family transcription factors important in B cells are PU.1 and Spi-B (Su et al. 1997), apparently by regulating expression of c-Rel, a NF-κB family member (Hu et al. 2001).

Another transcription factor that plays an important role in mediating the response to BCR signaling is Egr-1, which is an early response gene that is activated via the Ras pathway and serum response element (SRE) sequences in B cells (McMahon and Monroe 1995). Downstream of Egr-1 appear genes encoding two cell adhesion molecules, ICAM-1 and CD44 (Maltzman and Monroe 1996b, 1996a). MEK (or MAP kinase/ERK kinase) inhibitors, which block the Ras/Erk pathway just upstream of Erk, block activation of Egr-1, upregulation of these adhesion molecules, and B-cell proliferation induced by BCR signaling (Richards et al. 2001).

B-cell co-receptors

The concept of co-receptors was initially developed to describe the role of CD4 and CD8 in T-cell activation. Both the TCR and the co-receptors bind to the same ligands, MHC–peptide complexes. Clustering of TCR and co-receptor by binding to the same ligand allows their cytoplasmic domains to cooperate to generate stronger TCR signaling reactions than would occur without the co-receptor. Thus, one can view the role of the co-receptor as providing additional information about the ligand that is being recognized by the TCR. B cells also have co-receptors which provide important additional information about the nature of molecules that bind to the BCR or the type of cell on which the antigen is found.

The CR2 (also called CD21) complex is a positively acting co-receptor for B cells. CR2 forms a complex with CD19 and CD81. If complement fragments are deposited on an antigen, then the antigen is much more effective at inducing an immune response, as a result of the ability of the CR2/CD19/CD81 complex to boost suboptimal BCR signaling, e.g. immunization of mice with a lysozyme fusion protein containing ligands for CR2 allowed it to elicit a strong antibody response at 1000–10 000 × lower concentration of immunizing antigen compared with normal lysozyme (Dempsey et al. 1996). This enhanced B cell activation is thought to result from phosphorylation of the cytoplasmic tail of CD19 on sites that permit recruitment of Vav and PI 3-kinase, two signaling components described above (Fearon and Carroll 2000). CD19 also binds to Lyn and promotes its activation (Fujimoto et al. 2000); it helps maintain the BCR in lipid rafts (Cherukuri et al. 2001b) and enhances loading of antigenic peptides on to class II MHC molecules for antigen presentation to T cells (Cherukuri et al. 2001a).

B cells also express several co-receptors that decrease B-cell activation, analogous to the regulation of NK cell killing by NK cell inhibitory receptors. The best understood example is FcγRIIB. Co-engagement of the BCR and FcγRIIB blocks B-cell activation when a naïve B cell encounters antigen in the form of immune complexes with IgG. This is a circumstance when an immune response has already been made, so FcγRIIB mediates a negative feedback loop, and indeed mice lacking FcγRIIB exhibit enhanced antibody responses, particularly at later times (Takai et al. 1996). The inhibitory function of FcγRIIB is circumvented when a germinal center B cell contacts antigen on the surface of a follicular dendritic cell, probably because these cells have a very high density of FcγRIIB and therefore bind the Fc portions of the IgG in the immune complexes on their surface (Tarlinton and Smith 2000).

The inhibitory effect of co-engagement of FcγRIIB with the BCR is the result of a sequence motif in the cytoplasmic domain of FcγRIIB, called the immunoreceptor tyrosine-based inhibitory motif (ITIM), consisting of I/V/L/SxYxxL/V. When FcγRIIB and the BCR are brought together by an IgG-containing immune complex, kinases associated with the BCR, of which Lyn is the most important (DeFranco et al. 1998), phosphorylate the tyrosine in the FcγRIIB ITIM. This phosphorylation serves as a site to recruit SHIP, a phosphatase that removes the 5-phosphate from PIP_3, and thereby counters the positive action of PI 3-kinase for B-cell activation (Ono et al. 1997; Kurosaki 2002b). SHIP also forms a complex with $p62^{dok}$ and RasGAP, so it appears also directly to downregulate Ras activation. Indeed, mice lacking $p62^{dok}$ fail to suppress Erk activation (Tamir et al. 2000; Yamanashi et al. 2000).

A second established negative co-receptor of B cells is CD22, which is an Ig superfamily member specific for some sialic acid-containing glycoproteins, and thus a member of the family of proteins called Siglecs (Tsubata 1999; Crocker and Varki 2001). Although the role of CD22 in regulating B-cell activation is not well understood, it has been proposed that it inhibits BCR signaling when the B cell recognizes an antigen on the surface of a host cell, rather than on the surface of a microbe that does not express sialic acid (Lanoue et al. 2002).

Other inhibitory receptors on B cells include PIR-B, CD72, and CD5 (expressed by B1 cells and anergic B cells), although their functions remain to be elucidated.

BCR ANTIGEN UPTAKE FUNCTION

The BCR, in addition to its signaling function, also plays a key role in B-cell activation by its function as an uptake receptor, greatly increasing the amount of antigen presented by B cells that can bind the antigen via their BCR versus B cells that cannot. This antigen is routed to the correct intracellular compartment, e.g. the late endosomes, where it is processed to peptides and loaded on to MHC class II molecules. Therefore, the efficient uptake and presentation of antigen allow antigen-specific B cells to present that antigen to helper T cells and thus allow for antigen-specific T cell-dependent antibody responses.

This function of the BCR is heavily dependent on the Igα/Igβ heterodimer and optimally requires the cytoplasmic domains of both these chains. Thus, the cytoplasmic domains of Igα and Igβ seem to provide complementary functions, in addition to the redundant functions of the ITAMs of these two polypeptides (Siemasko and Clark 2001). The mechanisms of these complementary functions for antigen uptake and trafficking to the correct compartment inside the B cell are not known.

FUNCTIONS OF THE BCR IN B-CELL MATURATION AND ACTIVATION

As described above, pre-BCR signaling events are required for B-cell development. In contrast, too much BCR signaling in immature B cells arrests their maturation and blocks exit from the bone marrow. These cells undergo further VJ recombination events at the light chain loci, a process called receptor editing (Nemazee 2000). If antigen specificity is changed by these rearrangements such that the B cell is no longer self-reactive, it can presumably exit the bone marrow and resume maturation. Once in the periphery, transitional B cells must choose between additional tolerance fates (clonal deletion or clonal anergy) and three possible mature cell types: B-1 cells, marginal zone B cells, and follicular recirculating B cells (also called B-2 cells). The BCR is thought to play important roles in all of these cell fate decisions (Meffre et al. 2000; Cariappa and Pillai 2002; Gold 2002; Kurosaki 2002a). How this occurs is poorly understood because it seems unlikely that simple quantitatively different thresholds for each possible fate can explain these different outcomes. In any case, once mature B cells are present, they require a low level of BCR signaling for continued survival (Lam et al. 1997). A higher level of BCR signaling leads to activation of the B cell, as is summarized briefly here.

In mature B cells that encounter antigen, BCR signaling is important for initial activation of the B cell. If the antigen is highly polymeric in nature, such as a repetitive carbohydrate epitope on a bacterial cell surface or a highly repetitive protein determinant on a virion, it will induce very strong signaling reactions and this induces a T-cell-independent mode of B-cell activation. This rapid IgM immune response is produced by marginal zone B cells and B-1 cells, and appears to serve an early defense role in response to infection (Bachmann and Kopf 1999; Martin and Kearney 2001).

Most antigens induce a lower level of BCR signaling, and B-cell activation in this case is dependent on productive interactions with antigen-specific helper T cells. BCR signaling induces follicular B cells to migrate to the outer T-cell zone of the lymph node, Peyer's patch, or splenic white cord. Some of the helper T cells activated by antigen-presenting dendritic cells also migrate to this same region, where they scan B cells for the requisite MHC class II–peptide complexes. If the helper T cell finds a B cell that presents the correct peptide–MHC complex, this leads to a stable interaction lasting many hours. Marginal zone B cells can also participate in T-cell-dependent antibody responses.

Among the signals that the activated helper T cell provides for the antigen-stimulated B cell are CD40L and cytokines such as IL-4 and IL-5. Interestingly, CD40L stimulation, in addition to being a key activation signal, also induces Fas on the B cell and makes it susceptible to Fas-induced apoptosis. BCR signaling protects against Fas-induced death in this circumstance (Rathmell et al. 1995; Rothstein et al. 1995), and this may be one way that anergic B cells are prevented from making T-cell-dependent antibody responses, because anergic B cells signal poorly through their BCR (Cooke et al. 1994).

Another function of CD40L is to induce the B cell to initiate a germinal center reaction, where there is both class switching and somatic hypermutation followed by affinity selection. The affinity selection step is believed to require both BCR signaling function and BCR antigen uptake function. Antigen in the germinal center is held on the surface of follicular dendritic cells and B cells with high-affinity BCRs can interact with this antigen and receive a survival signal. In addition, these B cells extract the antigen from the follicular dendritic cells, take it up and present it to helper T cells, which have also migrated into the germinal center (Batista et al. 2001). These helper T cells provide an essential role in promoting activation of these germinal center B cells. Therefore, the BCR again plays a critical role in the germinal center reaction, the products of which are high-affinity isotype switched antibody produced by long-lived plasma cells and high-affinity memory B cells.

CONCLUSION

The BCR is composed of the membrane-bound form of Ig bound to a heterodimer of Igα and Igβ (CD79a and -b). Membrane Ig has the antigen-binding function of the receptor whereas the cytoplasmic tails of Igα and Igβ mediate the signaling function. Pre-B cells express a related receptor called the pre-BCR, which differs from the BCR in that it has the two surrogate light chains, Vpre-B1 and λ5, in place of the Ig light chains.

The pre-BCR and the BCR function in two ways: by generating tonic signals that induce developmental transitions and/or provide survival signals, and by generating stronger signals on antigen-induced clustering. The latter type of signaling causes developmental arrest of developing B cells in the bone marrow, tolerance-related effects such as deletion and anergy of immature B cells in the periphery, and activation of mature B cells. Little is known about the events important for tonic signaling, with the exception of pre-BCR signaling, which has been genetically studied in detail, as illustrated in Figure 17.3. Antigen (or anti-Ig)-induced signaling is understood in outline and many of the signaling reactions are reasonably well defined. BCR clustering leads to movement of clustered receptors into lipid raft microdomains of the plasma membrane, where signaling molecules such as Src family tyrosine kinases are localized. This leads to phosphorylation of ITAM sequences in the Igα and Igβ cytoplasmic domains, which in turn recruits the Syk tyrosine kinase. Once activated, Syk phosphorylates downstream signaling components that mostly function by assembly into signaling complexes. Signaling events activated include PIP_3 generation, PIP_2 hydrolysis, calcium elevation, activation of small GTPases including Ras, Rac, and Rap1, and eventually activation of transcription factors that lead to alterations in gene expression. Much remains to be learned about how downstream events are mediated, particularly those related to the biological functions of the BCR.

REFERENCES

Achatz, G., Nitschke, L. and Lamers, M.C. 1997. Effect of transmembrane and cytoplasmic domains of IgE on the IgE response. *Science*, **276**, 409–11.

Akagi, T., Motegi, M., et al. 1999. A novel gene, MALT1 at 18q21, is involved in t(11;18) (q21;q21) found in low-grade B-cell lymphoma of mucosa-associated lymphoid tissue. *Oncogene*, **18**, 5785–94.

Arendt, C.W., Albrecht, B., et al. 2002. Protein kinase C-θ: signaling from the center of the T-cell synapse. *Curr Opin Immunol*, **14**, 323–30.

Bachmann, M.F. and Kopf, M. 1999. The role of B cells in acute and chronic infections. *Curr Opin Immunol*, **11**, 332–9.

Bachmann, M.F. and Zinkernagel, R.M. 1996. The influence of virus structure on antibody responses and virus serotype formation. *Immunol Today*, **17**, 553–8.

Batista, F.D., Iber, D. and Neuberger, M.S. 2001. B cells acquire antigen from target cells after synapse formation. *Nature*, **411**, 489–94.

Berland, R. and Wortis, H.H. 1998. An NFAT-dependent enhancer is necessary for anti-IgM-mediated induction of murine CD5 expression in primary splenic B cells. *J Immunol*, **161**, 277–85.

Bertin, J., Guo, Y., et al. 2000. CARD9 is a novel caspase recruitment domain-containing protein that interacts with BCL10/CLAP and activates NF-κB. *J Biol Chem*, **275**, 41082–6.

Bertin, J., Wang, L., et al. 2001. CARD11 and CARD14 are novel caspase recruitment domain (CARD)/membrane-associated guanylate kinase (MAGUK) family members that interact with BCL10 and activate NF-κB. *J Biol Chem*, **276**, 11877–82.

Bories, J.C., Willerford, D.M., et al. 1995. Increased T-cell apoptosis and terminal B-cell differentiation induced by inactivation of the Ets-1 proto-oncogene. *Nature*, **377**, 635–58.

Brdicka, T., Imrich, M., et al. 2002. Non-T cell activation linker (NTAL): a transmembrane adaptor protein involved in immunoreceptor signaling. *J Exp Med*, **196**, 1617–26.

Caetano, M.S., Vieira-De-Abreu, A., et al. 2002. NFATC2 transcription factor regulates cell cycle progression during lymphocyte activation: evidence of its involvement in the control of cyclin gene expression. *FASEB J*, **16**, 1940–2.

Calame, K.L. 2001. Plasma cells: finding new light at the end of B cell development. *Nature Immunol*, **2**, 1103–8.

Cariappa, A. and Pillai, S. 2002. Antigen-dependent B-cell development. *Curr Opin Immunol*, **14**, 241–9.

Cheng, A.M., Rowley, B., et al. 1995. Syk tyrosine kinase required for mouse viability and B-cell development. *Nature*, **378**, 303–6.

Cheng, P.C., Brown, B.K., et al. 2001. Translocation of the B cell antigen receptor into lipid rafts reveals a novel step in signaling. *J Immunol*, **166**, 3693–701.

Cherukuri, A., Cheng, P.C. and Pierce, S.K. 2001a. The role of the CD19/CD21 complex in B cell processing and presentation of complement-tagged antigens. *J Immunol*, **167**, 163–72.

Cherukuri, A., Cheng, P.C., et al. 2001b. The CD19/CD21 complex functions to prolong B cell antigen receptor signaling from lipid rafts. *Immunity*, **14**, 169–79.

Chung, J.B., Baumeister, M.A. and Monroe, J.G. 2001. Cutting edge: differential sequestration of plasma membrane-associated B cell antigen receptor in mature and immature B cells into glycosphingolipid-enriched domains. *J Immunol*, **166**, 736–40.

Clark, M.R., Johnson, S.A. and Cambier, J.C. 1994. Analysis of Ig-α-tyrosine kinase interaction reveals two levels of binding specificity and tyrosine phosphorylated Ig-α stimulation of Fyn activity. *EMBO J*, **13**, 1911–19.

Cooke, M.P., Heath, A.W., et al. 1994. Immunoglobulin signal transduction guides the specificity of B cell–T cell interactions and is blocked in tolerant self-reactive B cells. *J Exp Med*, **179**, 425–38.

Crocker, P.R. and Varki, A. 2001. Siglecs, sialic acids and innate immunity. *Trends Immunol*, **22**, 337–42.

DeFranco, A.L. 1997. The complexity of signaling pathways activated by the BCR. *Curr Opin Immunol*, **9**, 296–308.

DeFranco, A.L. 2001. Vav and the B cell signalosome. *Nature Immunol*, **2**, 482–4.

DeFranco, A.L., Chan, V.W. and Lowell, C.A. 1998. Positive and negative roles of the tyrosine kinase Lyn in B cell function. *Semin Immunol*, **10**, 299–307.

Dempsey, P.W., Allison, M.E.D., et al. 1996. C3d of complement as a molecular adjuvant: Bridging innate and acquired immunity. *Science*, **271**, 348–50.

Dolmetsch, R.E., Lewis, R.S., et al. 1997. Differential activation of transcription factors induced by Ca2+ response amplitude and duration. *Nature*, **386**, 855–8.

Ebinu, J.O., Stang, S.L., et al. 2000. RasGRP links T-cell receptor signaling to Ras. *Blood*, **95**, 3199–203.

Engel, P., Zhou, L.J., et al. 1995. Abnormal B lymphocyte development, activation, and differentiation in mice that lack or overexpress the CD19 signal transduction molecule. *Immunity*, **3**, 39–50.

Engels, N., Wollscheid, B. and Wienands, J. 2001. Association of SLP-65/BLNK with the B cell antigen receptor through a non-ITAM tyrosine of Ig-α. *Eur J Immunol*, **31**, 2126–34.

Fearon, D.T. and Carroll, M.C. 2000. Regulation of B lymphocyte responses to foreign and self-antigens by the CD19/CD21 complex. *Ann Rev Immunol*, **18**, 393–422.

Fisher, C.L., Ghysdael, J. and Cambier, J.C. 1991. Ligation of membrane Ig leads to calcium-mediated phosphorylation of the proto-oncogene product Ets-1. *J Immunol*, **146**, 1743–9.

Fleming, H.E. and Paige, C.J. 2001. Pre-B cell receptor signaling mediates selective response to IL-7 at the pro-B to pre-B cell transition via an ERK/MAP kinase-dependent pathway. *Immunity*, **15**, 521–31.

Fruman, D.A., Satterthwaite, A.B. and Witte, O.N. 2000. Xid-like phenotypes: a B cell signalosome takes shape. *Immunity*, **13**, 1–3.

Fu, C., Turck, C.W., et al. 1998. BLNK: a central linker protein in B cell activation. *Immunity*, **9**, 93–103.

Fujimoto, M., Fujimoto, Y., et al. 2000. CD19 regulates Src family protein tyrosine kinase activation in B lymphocytes through progressive amplification. *Immunity*, **13**, 47–57.

Futterer, K., Wong, J., et al. 1998. Structural basis for Syk tyrosine kinase ubiquity in signal transduction pathways revealed by the crystal structure of its regulatory SH2 domains bound to a dually phosphorylated ITAM peptide. *J Mol Biol*, **281**, 523–37.

Gaide, O., Martinon, F., et al. 2001. Carmal, a CARD-containing binding partner of Bcl10, induces Bcl10 phosphorylation and NF-κB activation. *FEBS Lett*, **496**, 121–7.

Gaide, O., Favier, B., et al. 2002. CARMA1 is a critical lipid raft-associated regulator of TCR-induced NF-κB activation. *Nature Immunol*, **3**, 836–43.

Gold, M.R. 2002. To make antibodies or not: signaling by the B-cell antigen receptor. *Trends Pharmacol Sci*, **23**, 316–24.

Gupta, N. and DeFranco, A.L. 2003. Visualization of lipid raft dynamics and early signaling events during antigen receptor-mediated B cell activation. *Mol Biol Cell*, **14**, 432–44.

Harmer, S.L. and DeFranco, A.L. 1997. Shc contains two Grb2 binding sites needed for efficient formation of complexes with SOS in B lymphocytes. *Mol Cell Biol*, **17**, 4087–95.

Harmer, S.L. and DeFranco, A.L. 1999. The src homology domain 2-containing inositol phosphatase SHIP forms a ternary complex with Shc and Grb2 in antigen receptor-stimulated B lymphocytes. *J Biol Chem*, **274**, 12183–91.

Hashimoto, A., Okada, H., et al. 1998. Involvement of guanosine triphosphatases and phospholipase C-γ2 in extracellular signal-regulated kinase, c-Jun NH2-terminal kinase, and p38 mitogen-activated protein kinase activation by the B cell antigen receptor. *J Exp Med*, **188**, 1287–95.

Hayashi, K., Nittono, R., et al. 2000. The B cell-restricted adaptor BASH is required for normal development and antigen receptor-mediated activation of B cells. *Proc Natl Acad Sci USA*, **97**, 2755–60.

Hu, C.J., Rao, S., et al. 2001. PU.1/Spi-B regulation of c-rel is essential for mature B cell survival. *Immunity*, **15**, 545–55.

Inabe, K., Ishiai, M., et al. 2002. Vav3 modulates B cell receptor responses by regulating phosphoinositide 3-kinase activation. *J Exp Med*, **195**, 189–200.

Ingham, R.J., Santos, L., et al. 2001. The Gab1 docking protein links the B cell antigen receptor to the phosphatidylinositol 3-kinase/Akt signaling pathway and to the SHP2 tyrosine phosphatase. *J Biol Chem*, **276**, 12257–65.

Janssen, E., Zhu, M., et al. 2003. LAB: a new membrane-associated adaptor molecule in B cell activation. *Nat Immunol*, **4**, 117–23.

Kabak, S., Skagg, B.J., et al. 2002. The direct recruitment of BLNK to immunoglobulin α couples the B-cell antigen receptor to distal signaling pathways. *Mol Cell Biol*, **22**, 2524–35.

Kaisho, T., Schwenk, F. and Rajewsky, K. 1997. The roles of γ1 heavy chain membrane expression and cytoplasmic tail in IgG1 responses. *Science*, **276**, 412–15.

Kelly, M.E. and Chan, A.C. 2000. Regulation of B cell function by linker proteins. *Curr Opin Immunol*, **12**, 267–75.

Kraus, M., Pao, L.I., et al. 2001. Interference with immunoglobulin (Ig)α immunoreceptor tyrosine-based activation motif (ITAM) phosphorylation modulates or blocks B cell development, depending on the availability of the Igβ cytoplasmic tail. *J Exp Med*, **194**, 455–69.

Kurosaki, T. 2002a. Regulation of B cell fates by BCR signaling components. *Curr Opin Immunol*, **14**, 341–7.

Kurosaki, T. 2002b. Regulation of B-cell signal transduction by adaptor proteins. *Nature Rev Immunol*, **2**, 354–63.

Kurosaki, T., Johnson, S.A., et al. 1995. Role of the Syk autophosphorylation site and SH2 domains in B cell antigen receptor signaling. *J Exp Med*, **182**, 1815–23.

Lam, K.-P., Kuhn, R. and Rajewsky, K. 1997. In vivo ablation of surface immunoglobulin on mature B cells by inducible gene targeting results in rapid cell death. *Cell*, **90**, 1073–83.

Lanoue, A., Batista, F.D., et al. 2002. Interaction of CD22 with α2, 6-linked sialoglycoconjugates: innate recognition of self to dampen B cell autoreactivity. *Eur J Immunol*, **32**, 348–55.

Law, D.A., Chan, V.W.F., et al. 1993. B-cell antigen receptor motifs have redundant signalling capabilities and bind the tyrosine kinases PTK72, Lyn and Fyn. *Curr Biol*, **3**, 645–57.

Leo, A. and Schraven, B. 2001. Adapters in lymphocyte signaling. *Curr Opin Immunol*, **13**, 307–16.

Ma, H., Yankee, T.M., et al. 2001. Visualization of Syk-antigen receptor interactions using green fluorescent protein: differential roles for Syk and Lyn in the regulation of receptor capping and internalization. *J Immunol*, **2001**, 1507–16.

McAllister-Lucas, L.M., Inohara, N., et al. 2001. Bimp1, a MAGUK family member linking protein kinase C activation to Bcl10-mediated NF-κB induction. *J Biol Chem*, **276**, 30589–97.

McLeod, S.J., Ingham, R.J., et al. 1998. Activation of the Rap1 GTPase by the B cell antigen receptor. *J Biol Chem*, **273**, 29218–23.

McMahon, S.B. and Monroe, J.G. 1995. Activation of the p21ras pathway couples antigen receptor stimulation to induction of the primary response gene egr-1 in B lymphocytes. *J Exp Med*, **181**, 417–22.

Maltzman, J. and Monroe, J.G. 1996a. A role for EGR1 in regulation of stimulus-dependent CD44 transcription in B lymphocytes. *Mol Cell Biol*, **16**, 2283–94.

Maltzman, J. and Monroe, J.G. 1996b. Transcriptional regulation of the Icam-1 gene in antigen receptor and phorbol ester stimulated B lymphocytes: Role for transcription factor EGR1. *J Exp Med*, **183**, 1747–59.

Martin, F. and Kearney, J.F. 2001. B1 cells: similarities and differences with other B cell subsets. *Curr Opin Immunol*, **13**, 195–201.

Martin, S.W. and Goodnow, C.C. 2002. Burst-enhancing role of the IgG membrane tail as a molecular determinant of memory. *Nature Immunol*, **3**, 182–8.

Matsuuchi, L. and Gold, M.R. 2001. New views of BCR structure and organization. *Curr Opin Immunol*, **13**, 270–7.

Meffre, E., Casellas, R. and Nussenzweig, M.C. 2000. Antibody regulation of B cell development. *Nature Immunol*, **1**, 379–85.

Minegishi, Y., Rohrer, J., et al. 1999. An essential role for BLNK in human B cell development. *Science*, **286**, 1954–7.

Mond, J.J., Lees, A. and Snapper, C. 1995. T cell-independent antigens type 2. *Annu Rev Immunol*, **13**, 655–92.

Morgan, J.A., Yin, Y., et al. 1999. Breakpoints of the t(11;18)(q21;q21) in mucosa-associated lymphoid tissue (MALT) lymphoma lie within or near the previously undescribed gene MALT1 in chromosome 18. *Cancer Res*, **59**, 6205–13.

Mori, Y., Wakamori, M., et al. 2002. Transient receptor potential 1 regulates capacitative Ca^{2+} entry and Ca^{2+} release from endoplasmic reticulum in B lymphocytes. *J Exp Med*, **195**, 673–81.

Nagai, K., Takata, M., et al. 1995. Tyrosine phosphorylation of Shc is mediated through Lyn and Syk in B cell receptor signaling. *J Biol Chem*, **270**, 6824–9.

Nemazee, D. 2000. Receptor selection in B and T lymphocytes. *Ann Rev Immunol*, **18**, 19–51.

Okada, T., Maeda, A., et al. 2000. BCAP: the tyrosine kinase substrate that connects B cell receptor to phosphoinositide 3-kinase activation. *Immunity*, **13**, 817–27.

Ono, M., Okada, H., et al. 1997. Deletion of SHIP or SHP-1 reveals two distinct pathways for inhibitory signaling. *Cell*, **90**, 293–301.

Pappu, R., Cheng, A.M., et al. 1999. Requirement for B cell linker protein (BLNK) in B cell development. *Science*, **286**, 1949–54.

Peng, S.L., Gerth, A.J., et al. 2001. NFATc1 and NFATc2 together control T and B cell activation and differentiation. *Immunity*, **14**, 13–20.

Pierce, S.K. 2002. Lipid rafts and B-cell activation. *Nature Rev Immunol*, **2**, 96–105.

Pohl, T., Gugasyan, R., et al. 2002. The combined absence of NF-κB1 and c-Rel reveals that overlapping roles for these transcription factors in the B cell lineage are restricted to the activation and function of mature cells. *Proc Natl Acad Sci USA*, **99**, 4514–19.

Pomerantz, J.L., Denny, E.M. and Baltimore, D. 2002. CARD11 mediates factor-specific activation of NF-κB1 by the T cell receptor complex. *EMBO J*, **21**, 5184–94.

Rathmell, J.C., Cooke, M.P., et al. 1995. CD95 (Fas)-dependent elimination of self-reactive B cells upon interaction with CD4+ T cells. *Nature*, **376**, 181–4.

Ravichandran, K.S., Lorenz, U., et al. 1995. Interaction of Shc with Grb2 regulates association of Grb2 with mSOS. *Mol Cell Biol*, **15**, 593–600.

Reichman-Fried, M., Bosma, M.J. and Hardy, R.R. 1993. B-lineage cells in μ-transgenic scid mice proliferate in response to IL-7 but fail to show evidence of immunoglobulin light chain gene rearrangement. *Int Immunol*, **5**, 303–10.

Reth, M. 1992. Antigen receptors on B lymphocytes. *Ann Rev Immunol*, **10**, 97–121.

Reth, M. 2001. Oligomeric antigen receptors: a new view on signaling for the selection of lymphocytes. *Trends Immunol*, **22**, 356–60.

Richards, J.D., Dave, S.H., et al. 2001. Inhibition of the MEK/ERK signaling pathway blocks a subset of B cell responses to antigen. *J Immunol*, **166**, 3855–64.

Rickert, R.C., Rajewsky, K. and Roes, J. 1995. Impairment of T-cell-dependent B-cell responses and B-1 cell development in CD19-deficient mice. *Nature*, **376**, 352–5.

Rothstein, T.L., Wang, J.K., et al. 1995. Protection against Fas-dependent Th1-mediated apoptosis by antigen receptor engagement in B cells. *Nature*, **374**, 163–5.

Rowley, R.B., Burkhardt, A.L., et al. 1995. Syk protein-tyrosine kinase is regulated by tyrosine-phosphorylated Igα/Igβ immunoreceptor tyrosine activation motif binding and autophosphorylation. *J Biol Chem*, **270**, 11590–4.

Ruland, J., Duncan, G.S., et al. 2001. Bcl10 is a positive regulator of antigen receptor-induced activation of NF-κB1 and neural tube closure. *Cell*, **104**, 33–42.

Saijo, K., Mecklenbrauker, I., et al. 2002. Protein kinase C β controls nuclear factor κB activation in B cells through selective regulation of the IκB kinase α. *J Exp Med*, **195**, 1647–52.

Saijo, K., Schmedt, C., et al. 2003. Essential role of Src-family protein tyrosine kinases in NF-κB activation during B cell development. *Nat Immunol*, **4**, 274–9.

Saouaf, S.J., Mahajan, S., et al. 1994. Temporal differences in the activation of the three classes of non-transmembrane protein tyrosine kinases following B-cell antigen receptor surface engagement. *Proc Natl Acad Sci USA*, **91**, 9524–8.

Saxton, T.M., van Oostveen, I., et al. 1994. B cell antigen receptor cross-linking induces phosphorylation of the p21*ras* oncoprotein activators SHC and mSOS1 as well as assembly of complexes containing SHC, GRB-2, mSOS1 and a 145-kDa tyrosine-phosphorylated protein. *J Immunol*, **153**, 623–36.

Schamel, W.W. and Reth, M. 2000. Monomeric and oligomeric complexes of the B cell antigen receptor. *Immunity*, **13**, 5–14.

Schlissel, M.S. and Stanhope-Baker, P. 1997. Accessibility and the developmental regulation of V(D)J recombination. *Semin Immunol*, **9**, 161–70.

Shiota, J., Nishimura, H., et al. 1994. A unique murine CD43 epitope Lp-3: distinct distribution from another CD43 epitope S7. *Cell Immunol*, **155**, 402–13.

Shiue, L., Zoller, M.J. and Brugge, J.S. 1995. Syk is activated by phosphotyrosine-containing peptides representing the tyrosine-based activation motifs of the high affinity receptor for IgE. *J Biol Chem*, **270**, 10498–502.

Siemasko, K. and Clark, M.R. 2001. The control and facilitation of MHC class II antigen processing by the BCR. *Curr Opin Immunol*, **13**, 32–6.

Sproul, T.W., Malapati, S., et al. 2000. Cutting edge: B cell antigen receptor signaling occurs outside lipid rafts in immature B cells. *J Immunol*, **165**, 6020–3.

Su, G.H., Chen, H.M., et al. 1997. Defective B cell receptor-mediated responses in mice lacking the Ets protein, Spi-B. *EMBO J*, **16**, 7118–29.

Su, T.T., Guo, B., et al. 2002. PKC-β controls I κB kinase lipid raft recruitment and activation in response to BCR signaling. *Nat Immunol*, **3**, 780–6.

Takai, T., Ono, M., et al. 1996. Augmented humoral and anaphylactic responses in FcγRII-deficient mice. *Nature*, **379**, 346–9.

Tamir, I., Stolpa, J.C., et al. 2000. The RasGAP-binding protein $p62^{dok}$ is a mediator of inhibitory FcγRIIB signals in B cells. *Immunity*, **12**, 347–58.

Tarlinton, D.M. and Smith, K.G. 2000. Dissecting affinity maturation: a model explaining selection of antibody-forming cells and memory B cells in the germinal centre. *Immunol Today*, **21**, 436–41.

Torgersen, K.M., Vang, T., et al. 2001. Release from tonic inhibition of T cell activation through transient displacement of C-terminal Src kinase (Csk) from lipid rafts. *J Biol Chem*, **276**, 29313–18.

Tsubata, T. 1999. Co-receptors on B lymphocytes. *Curr Opin Immunol*, **11**, 249–55.

Turner, M., Mee, P.J., et al. 1995. Perinatal lethality and a block in the development of B cells in mice lacking the tyrosine kinase p72syk. *Nature*, **378**, 298–302.

Wang, L., Guo, Y., et al. 2001. Card10 is a novel caspase recruitment domain/membrane-associated guanylate kinase family member that interacts with BCL10 and activates NF-κB. *J Biol Chem*, **276**, 21405–9.

Willis, T.G., Jadayel, D.M., et al. 1999. Bcl10 is involved in t(1;14)(p22;q32) of MALT B cell lymphoma and mutated in multiple tumor types. *Cell*, **96**, 35–45.

Wong, J., Ishiai, M., et al. 2000. Functional complementation of BLNK by SLP-76 and LAT linker proteins. *J Biol Chem*, **275**, 33116–22.

Xu, S., Tan, J.E., et al. 2000. B cell development and activation defects resulting in xid-like immunodeficiency in BLNK/SLP-65-deficient mice. *Int Immunol*, **12**, 397–404.

Yamanashi, Y., Tamura, T., et al. 2000. Role of the rasGAP-associated docking protein p62dok in negative regulation of B cell receptor-mediated signaling. *Genes Dev*, **14**, 11–16.

Yamazaki, T., Takeda, K., et al. 2002. Essential immunoregulatory role for BCAP in B cell development and function. *J Exp Med*, **195**, 535–45.

18

Monoclonal antibody therapy

ANDREW J.T. GEORGE

INTRODUCTION

The possibility of using antibodies in the treatment of diseases was first recognized in the 1890s when it was shown that antibodies to bacterial exotoxins were responsible for immunity to tetanus and diphtheria, and that antisera to cholera vibrios could transfer immunity to naive animals (Silverstein 1988). At the start of the twentieth century, until the advent of microbial chemotherapy, antibodies played a major role in the treatment of a wide range of infectious diseases. More recently polyclonal antibodies are routinely used for tetanus, rabies, hepatitis B, and other infectious diseases (Oral and Akdis 2000), as well as for the prevention of immunization of the mother in cases of rhesus incompatibility (Moise 2002).

Therapy in most cases has been with polyclonal antibodies, produced either by immunization of animals with the appropriate antigen or by purification of human immunoglobulin (Ig). A new opportunity was offered by the invention in 1975 of the hybridoma approach to isolating monoclonal antibodies of a desired specificity (see Chapter 16, Antibodies and B lymphocytes) (Kohler and Milstein 1975). It is worth noting (see below) that monoclonal antibodies are not inherently better than polyclonal antibodies; indeed for many applications polyclonal antibodies are more potent. The big advantage of monoclonal antibodies is that it is possible to produce essentially unlimited amounts of antibody with a predetermined specificity.

Polyclonal antibodies versus monoclonal antibodies

It is often assumed that monoclonal antibodies are to be preferred to polyclonal antibodies for most clinical applications. However, although there are very good practical reasons to opt for monoclonal antibodies, there can be advantages to using polyclonal antibodies. Hybridoma technology is one of the possible ways of generating monoclonal antibodies; there are others, such as phage display, which are discussed below. Indeed tumors of antibody-producing cells produce monoclonal antibodies, although normally of unknown specificity. Monoclonal antibodies, as implied by their name, are derived from a single clone of B cells. As such they react with a single epitope on the target. Polyclonal antibodies, on the other hand, react with a range of epitopes. This has the advantage that it is harder for the target (e.g. an infectious pathogen or neoplastic cell) to mutate in order to escape from attack by a polyclonal antibody, because it would need to alter many epitopes. It also makes polyclonal antibodies more robust at reacting with different strains of infectious agent. The ability of polyclonal antibodies to bind to multiple epitopes makes it easier for them to precipitate out molecules from solution, because they can form a lattice with the target molecules. In general the target can also get coated with more antibody molecules (including those of different isotypes) when a polyclonal antibody is used, making recruitment of effector mechanisms more efficient.

The main advantage of monoclonal antibodies produced by hybridoma technology is that it is possible to make large quantities of the antibody. Polyclonal antibodies are derived by bleeding immunized animals and purifying the antibodies obtained from the sera. The amount of antibody that can be obtained from one animal is limited, and once it has been used up the process has to be repeated – resulting in considerable batch-to-batch variability. This also militates against a thorough characterization of the antibody, because much of it would be used in the characterization process. In the case of a monoclonal antibody it is worth investing considerable time and effort into characterizing the antibody specificity because it is possible to generate as much antibody as is required. In addition, monoclonal antibodies are valuable when an antibody against a single antigen that is difficult to isolate in a pure enough form to immunize an animal is required. Finally, the use of monoclonal antibodies that can be produced in defined cell lines in vitro obviates many of the safety considerations inherent in using antibodies isolated from animals (including humans) that may carry infectious organisms.

When monoclonal antibodies were first described there was considerable optimism that they would form the next generation of therapeutic agent, acting as 'magic bullets' that could be used to seek out and destroy target cells. This was fuelled by early data from lymphoma, in which the first patient treated with an anti-idiotypic antibody specific for his tumor cells went into long-term complete remission (Miller et al. 1982). However, after a period in which there was considerable investment in antibody-based therapies with little return, disillusionment spread and there was a belief that those antibodies would play little role in the clinic. In recent years the picture has changed (Glennie and Johnson 2000; Carter 2001). There has been a considerable increase in the number of antibody molecules licensed by the US Food and Drug Administration (FDA) (Table 18.1) and the antibody field is now one of the fastest growing areas of the pharmaceutical industry.

One of the problems with our thinking about the use of antibodies is probably with the term 'magic bullet', which has been overused in many papers, grant applications, and business proposals over the years. It is a somewhat unfortunate term, even if originally coined by the father of antibody therapy, Paul Ehrlich, to describe the targeting of toxic substances with antibodies. The term 'magic bullets' suggests a guided missile, and that if such an antibody was injected into a patient it would somehow sense where its target is and home to, and kill, it. In fact, administration of antibodies to a patient results in their distribution throughout the body, and if they happen to bump into their target they will bind to it (for a while). It could be argued that this inappropriate term has befuddled our way of thinking about antibody therapy.

In this chapter, some of the reasons why it has taken 25 years for antibodies to make an impact are discussed, and some of the more futuristic applications of these molecules considered.

HOW ANTIBODIES KILL TARGETS

One of the important questions in antibody therapy is how antibodies work in therapeutic settings. In general this can be divided into three categories: those that rely on the natural functions recruited by antibodies, those that use the ability of antibodies to bind to soluble or cell surface receptors, and those that harness artificial effectors.

Recruitment of natural effectors

COMPLEMENT

The Fc region of antibody molecules is capable of recruiting the complement cascade, as described in much more detail in Chapter 9, Complement and reviewed in Walport (2001a, b). This has several consequences, including the release of soluble mediators such as C5a, which act as proinflammatory anaphylatoxins, and the coating of the target with molecules such as C3b, which serve as opsonins, aiding recognition and phagocytosis by macrophages and other phagocytes. In addition, the deposition of the membrane attack complex (the final step of which involves polymerization of C9) can lead to osmotic lysis of the target cell.

In addition to promoting inflammation and destruction of the target cells, complement has a number of other important functions. Complement deposition can reduce the size of immune complexes that form between antibodies and antigens (Miller and Nussenzweig 1975). In addition complement is involved in the processing and clearance of immune complexes, e.g. in patients with C2 deficiency no splenic uptake of immune complexes is observed (Davies et al. 1993). More recently complement has been implicated in the clearance of apoptotic bodies (Taylor et al. 2000). Finally, complement deposition is also important in the generation of antibody responses after immunization (Pepys 1974), in part because of the presence of complement receptors on the surface of follicular dendritic cells and also because the binding of C3d by CD21 (complexed to CD19) on B cells is important in B-cell activation (Fearon and Carroll 2000).

Thus, complement activation is important not only because of its potential direct role in the destruction of the target pathogen, but also because it is involved in the clearance of the resulting debris from the body and the immunization of the individual against the pathogen.

Fc RECEPTOR-MEDIATED KILLING

A wide range of cells expresses receptors for the Fc region of the antibody molecule (FcR), and interaction of the Fc with the FcR has a range of effects (Ravetch and Bolland 2001). These can include the promotion of phagocytosis (e.g. by macrophages and other phagocytes; see Chapter 3, Phagocytes part 1: Macrophages), the induction of antibody-directed cellular cytotoxicity (ADDC) (by natural killer (NK) cells; see Chapter 6, Natural killer cells), the release of inflammatory mediators (e.g. following interaction through the FcεR of mast

Table 18.1 *Antibodies approved for clinical use*[a]

Trade name **(Proper name)**	**Indications for use**	**Specificity**	**Nature**	**Manufacturer**	**Date approved**
Avastin (Bevacizumab)	Metastatic colorectal cancer	VEGF (vascular endothelial growth factor)	Humanized	Genentech	2004
Bexxar Tositumab and I^{131} Tositumab	$CD20^{+}$ NHL	CD20	^{131}I labeled / unlabeled murine	Corixa	2003
Campath (Alemtuzumab)	B-CLL	CD52	Humanized	ILEX	2001
CEA-scan (Arcitumomab)	Imaging colorectal carcinoma	CEA	^{99m}Tc labeled Fab′ murine	Immunomedics	1996
Erbitux (Cetuximab)	Colorectal cancer	Epidermal growth factor receptor	Chimeric	ImClone	2004
Herceptin (Trastuzumab)	Breast cancer	HER–2/*erb* B2	Humanized	Genentech	1998
Humira (Adalimumab)	Rheumatoid arthritis	TNF	Human (phage derived)	Abbott Laboratories	2002
Leukoscan (Sulesomab)	Imaging inflammation/ infection in osteomyelitis	NCA 90 (granulocyte marker)	^{99m}Tc labeled Fab murine	Immunomedics	1997 EU
Myoscint (Imciromab pentetate)	Cardiac imaging	Cardiac myosin	^{111}In labeled Fab murine	Centocor	1996
Oncoscint (Satumomab pendetide)	Imaging colorectal/ovarian carcinomas	TAG-72	^{111}In labeled murine	Cytogen	1992
Orthoclone (muromonab-CD3)	Renal allograft rejection	CD3	Murine	Ortho	1986
Panorex (Edrecolomab)	Rectal/colon cancer	17-1A	Murine	Johnson & Johnson	1995 (Germany)
Prostascint (Capromab pendetide)	Imaging prostatic cancer	Prostate-specific membrane antigen	^{111}In labeled murine IgG	Cytogen Corp	1996

(*Continued over*)

Table 18.1 *Antibodies approved for clinical use[a] (Continued)*

Trade name (Proper name)	Indications for use	Specificity	Nature	Manufacturer	Date approved
Raptiva (Efalizumab)	Psoriasis	CD11a	Humanized	Genentech	2003
Remicade (Infliximab)	Rheumatoid arthritis and Crohn's disease	TNF	Chimeric	Centocor	1999
ReoPro (Abciximab)	Cardiac intervention, unstable angina	Glycoprotein IIb/IIIa (GPIIb/IIIa) receptor of human platelets	Fab fragment of chimeric antibody	Centocor	1997
Rituxan/Mabthera (Rituximab)	Non-Hodgkins lymphoma	CD20	Chimeric	Genentech/Hoffman La-Roche	1997
Simulect (Baxsiliximab)	Renal transplantation	CD25	Chimeric	Novartis	1998
Synagis (Palivizumab)	Respiratory syncytial viral infection (RSV)	F protein of RSV	Humanized	MedImmune (USA)Abbot (EU)	1998
Verluma (Nofetumomab)	Imaging small cell lung cancer	40 kDa carcinoma associated antigen	^{99m}Tc labeled Fab fragment of murine antibody	Dr Karl Thomae GmbH	1996
Xolair (Omalizumab)	Asthma	IgE	Humanized	Genentech	2003
Zenapax (Daclizumab)	Renal allograft rejection	CD25	Humanized	Hoffman La Roche	1997
Zevalin (Ibritumomab Tiuxetan)	Non Hodgkins lymphoma	CD20	^{111}In and ^{90}Y labeled murine antibody	IDEC	2002

a) The table lists the majority of current approved drugs (withdrawn drugs not given) as of 2004. The date of first approval is shown, there may have been subsequent approvals for other indications. Approval date is shown for the USA unless otherwise indicated. Data from web and personal communications.

cells and basophils; see Chapter 5, Basophils and eosinophils), and clearance from the circulation by cells of the reticuloendothelial system (see Chapter 3, Phagocytes part 1: Macrophages). In some cases these functions will be enhanced by complement activation. In addition the interaction of the Fc region with FcRs is important in controlling humoral immunity (Ravetch and Bolland 2001).

GENERAL CONSIDERATIONS FOR THE RECRUITMENT OF NATURAL EFFECTORS

One of the features of the use of monoclonal antibodies is that a single Ig isotype is employed. This is either of rodent origin or, after antibody engineering, may be a human isotype. It is clearly important to select an appropriate isotype for the recruitment of the appropriate effector functions. This assumes that the important effector function is known and often this can be difficult to determine, e.g. in the case of neoplastic disease there is still little consensus as to whether recruitment of complement or ADCC is important in treatment. The ability of different rodent or human Fc regions to recruit human effectors has been well described; however, the situation is not simple. There are polymorphisms in FcR that influence their ability to bind to particular subclasses of antibody; e.g. the FcγRII (CD32) receptor is polymorphic in the human population, with one form (H131) binding to IgG2 and the other (R131) not (Warmerdam et al. 1990). The allotype of the antibody can also be important in its ability to bind to FcR (Greenwood and Greenwood 1993). Other factors can also determine the ability of an antibody to recruit an effector function, such as the distance from the epitope to the cell surface, as well as the orientation and density of the epitope (Bindon et al. 1988). It is therefore important to determine for each individual antibody what effector functions it can recruit.

Blocking or activation by antibodies

Until recently the main focus has been on the use of antibodies as killing agents, using natural or artificial effector mechanisms. More recently we have come to an appreciation that they can act to modulate cellular responses, either by blocking the interaction of soluble molecules, such as cytokines, with their receptors, or by binding to molecules on the cell surface that then signal to the cell.

BLOCKING BY ANTIBODIES

Antibodies are widely used in experimental settings to block the action of cytokines or other soluble molecules. This can be done using either antibodies against the soluble molecule or a blocking antibody against the receptor.

In the clinic, the most advanced version of this application for cytokines is the administration of antibodies to tumor necrosis factor-α (TNF-α) in the treatment of rheumatoid arthritis and other inflammatory disorders (Taylor 2000). The first such trial involved a chimeric anti-TNF-α antibody (cA2, infliximab) (Elliott et al. 1993), which was followed by a number of trials (some in combination with drug therapy (Elliott et al. 1994a, b; Maini et al. 1999; reviewed in Feldmann and Maini 2001). The overall picture is that most patients (50–60 percent) respond rapidly to treatment with infliximab, with an improvement in both symptoms and clinical signs of disease. However, when treatment is stopped patients eventually relapse, necessitating prolonged or repeated therapy. A range of anti-TNF-α agents has been produced, including humanized antibodies (CDP571), phage-derived antibodies (D2E7), and fusion proteins between the Fc region of the antibody with the p75 (etanercept) or p55 (lenercept) TNF receptors (reviewed in Feldmann and Maini 2001). TNF-α blockade has also been shown to have benefit in other inflammatory diseases, including Crohn's disease (Targan et al. 1997) and Jarisch–Herxheimer reactions (Fekade et al. 1996). Similar strategies have also been used in septic shock, although with less success (McCloskey et al. 1994), whereas treatment of multiple sclerosis with TNF-α-blocking agents appears to be deleterious (Lenercept Multiple Sclerosis Study Group and the University of British Columbia MS/MRI Analysis Group 1999).

Antibodies have also been used against other cytokines, such as interleukin-2 (IL-2). The alternative approach is to target the receptor for the cytokine, such as the CD25 receptor for IL-2, which has been used to downregulate immune responses in graft rejection. An antibody against endotoxin (HA-1A, Centoxin) was developed for use in septic shock, but was withdrawn when phase III trials demonstrated an increased mortality in patients treated with the antibody (McCloskey et al. 1994). Antibodies are also routinely used to reverse drug toxicities (such as ouabain).

As well as the modulation of cytokines, antibodies can block the access of toxins (such as diphtheria and tetanus) to receptors on cells. Similar blocking can prevent molecules on the surface of viruses from engaging receptors on the surface of cells. However, in many cases the viruses 'hide' the interaction site on their protein either in a buried location or by masking it with another protein. One of the advantages of some of the antibody engineering approaches outlined below is that it may be possible to make artificial antibodies that can bind to these buried interaction sites.

Antibodies can also block interactions between cell surface receptors. Anti-CD3 was the first antibody licensed for clinical use, and is used to block T-cell responses during graft rejection. In experimental settings, nondepleting antibodies against CD4 will block

T-cell responses by interfering in the signaling events leading to T-cell activation, whereas antibodies to adhesion molecules on either endothelial cells or leukocytes will block the recruitment of inflammatory cells.

SIGNALING BY ANTIBODIES

Antibodies are also able to signal cells by cross-linking surface receptors. The importance of this in therapy was realized in patients treated with anti-idiotypic antibody for lymphoma. It was shown in a retrospective study that cells from patients who responded to treatment with antibody showed evidence of signaling (tyrosine phosphorylation) after binding of anti-idiotypic antibody to tumor cells, whereas those that showed little or no clinical benefit did not show such signaling (Vuist et al. 1994). It is also likely that the actions of rituximab (anti-CD20) in lymphoma and trastuzumab (anti-Her2/neu) in solid tumors are in large part the result of their ability to signal to the neoplastic cells (Johnson and Glennie 2001; Yarden and Sliwkowski 2001). This can lead to synergy with other forms of therapy, such as chemotherapy, because the signaling can sensitize the tumor cells to the drug (Demidem et al. 1997).

In addition to direct signaling on the target cell, it is also possible to see an effect resulting from signaling to a nontarget cell, e.g. in an animal model of lymphoma it was shown that anti-CD40 antibodies were highly effective in tumor treatment, but only in situations when the animals had a high tumor burden (French et al. 1999; Tutt et al. 2002). Dissection of the mechanisms involved demonstrated that this was because the anti-CD40 antibody was interacting with CD40 on dendritic cells, rather than the tumor cells. The dendritic cells were activated by this interaction, and then presented tumor antigens to T cells – efficiently immunizing the mice against the lymphoma. Similar strategies could be considered in other settings where immunization is needed.

It should be noted that the signaling function can be reduced by the generation of $F(ab')_2$ molecules which lack the Fc region. The reason for this is that the Fc region can help in the signaling effect by interaction with FcR^+ cells that cross-link the antibody, so increasing its potency (Lane et al. 1991).

Artificial effector functions

The concept of antibodies as delivery agents has proved highly attractive. Thus antibodies have been conjugated to a wide range of toxic agents or other molecules in order to target the molecule to where it is needed. Some of the most common of these are discussed below. The main drawbacks with this approach are that antibody targeting, although capable of high specificity, is relatively poor at delivering large numbers of antibody molecules to the target site. In clinical trials in neoplastic disease, typically 0.01 percent of the injected dose localizes per gram of tissue (Esteban et al. 1987). This is one of those times when the concept of the antibody as a magic bullet is perhaps misleading because it suggests that a large proportion of the antibody molecules administered will reach the target site. Thus, the molecule being targeted needs to be capable of being effective in low amounts. The other side of this equation is that most of the antibody never reaches the target site. Thus, if the antibody is conjugated to a toxic molecule there is the possibility of nonspecific damage to healthy tissues.

TOXINS AND DRUGS

Toxins are one of the most obvious types of molecule to target with antibodies (Figure 18.1). There is a vast range of such toxins, derived from plants (e.g. ricin, saporin, gelonin), from bacteria (e.g. diphtheria and pseudomonas exotoxins), and from fungi (e.g. α-sarcin) (Thrush et al. 1996; Kreitman 1999). These molecules typically enzymatically inactivate protein synthesis, and so are highly potent, with one molecule of the toxin being capable of killing a cell. These toxins have been conjugated to antibodies, to form immunotoxins, using either chemical or genetic means.

The major problem faced with the use of immunotoxins is that it is not sufficient simply to deliver the toxin to the surface of the cell; it must enter the cytosol to be effective. Natural toxins have a range of mechanisms by which they do this, e.g. ricin, which is probably the most commonly used plant-derived toxin, is made of two chains joined by a disulfide bond (Olsnes and Kozlov 2001). The A chain is the enzymatically active chain. The B chain binds to the cell surface and facilitates entry of the A chain into the cytosol. If immunotoxins are made that consist of an intact A and B chain, they are effective, but also show considerable nontargeted toxicity because the B chain binds to all cells. However, if the B chain is removed, the toxin no longer binds to irrelevant cells, but the immunotoxin is relatively poor at entering the target cells. Several strategies have been used to block or modify the cell-binding chain, while leaving the internalization functions of the B chain intact (Thrush et al. 1996). Similar approaches have also been used with the bacterially derived toxins, although the binding, internalization, and enzymatic regions are normally found on the same polypeptide chain.

The importance of cytosolic entry also means that some antigens are better for immunotoxin delivery than others. These antigens generally internalize after binding of antibodies into endosomes. After acidification of the endosomes, toxins can escape into the cytosol. However, this remains an inefficient process, e.g. in in vitro experiments carried out using bispecific antibodies to target a toxin, saporin to lymphoma cells, it was shown that

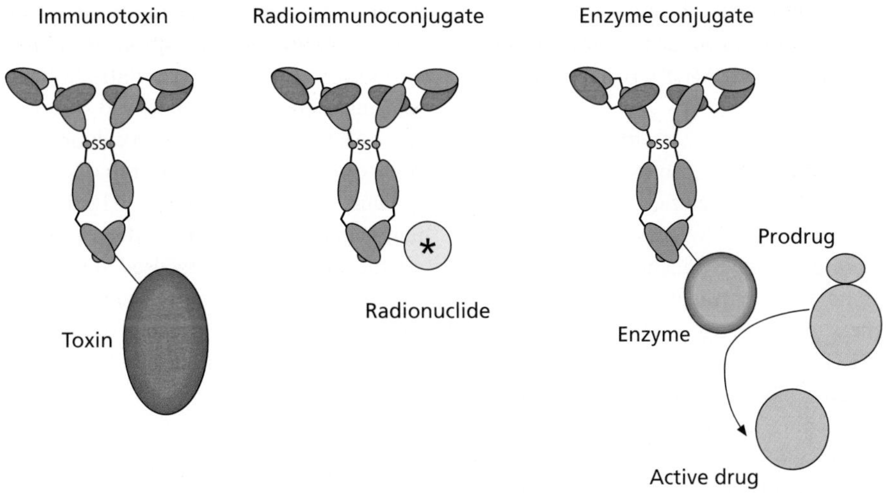

Figure 18.1 *Immunoconjugates: in the text three basic types of immunoconjugate are described. The first is the immunotoxin, in which the antibody is conjugated to a toxin molecule. This can lead to selective delivery of the toxin to the target cell. The second are radioimmunoconjugates, in which a radioisotope (suitable for therapy or imaging) is used. Although the targeting of the conjugate to the target is specific, the effect of the radiation will spread from that site, depending on the pathlength. Finally antibody–enzyme conjugates can be used to convert harmless prodrugs into active drugs at the target site. This leads to amplification of the targeting effect, with many copies of the drug created by each enzyme.*

constructs directed against CD22 were highly effective at killing, whereas those against CD19, CD37, and surface Ig less so. For 50 percent killing of the tumor cells it was necessary to target around 1 000 toxin molecules per cell using CD22. With the other targets, far more toxin was needed – more than 90 000 molecules in the case of CD37 (Bonardi et al. 1993). Therefore, claims about the potency of the toxins used in immunotoxins need to be treated with caution; they are incredibly toxic but only once they are in the cytosol of the cell.

The second problem about many of these toxins is that they are very immunogenic (see below for why immunogenicity is a problem). Indeed in laboratories making ricin, hypersensitivity reactions to the toxin are more problematic than the toxicity. This limits the number of times an immunotoxin can be administered. For this reason there is increasing interest in mammalian DNase and RNase molecules which have low immunogenicity (Newton and Rybak 2001). These work by degrading all the DNA or RNA in the cell, and again are highly potent if they can enter the cell.

A final problem with immunotoxins is that many of them have side effects, e.g. a limiting feature of treatment with ricin A chain is vascular leak syndrome, caused by interactions of the toxin with endothelial cells (Schindler et al. 2001). Elegant mutational analysis has allowed identification of the regions involved in this, and it may prove possible to mutate out this feature of the molecules.

In a similar manner to toxins, a number of research groups have targeted drugs using antibodies. However, a drawback of this approach is that normally a relatively large number of drug molecules is needed to see an effect. In some cases it may be possible to target enough of the drug to improve the therapeutic window of efficacy.

RADIOIMMUNOCONJUGATES

Conjugation of radionuclides to antibodies can be used for two purposes: therapy and imaging (see Figure 18.1). In the case of therapy a radionuclide with a short pathlength (e.g. β emitters) is used so that the damage is limited to the targeted area. For imaging, radionuclides with long pathlengths are used (γ emitters), which can be detected by an appropriate camera.

One feature of radioimmunoconjugates is that, even if the antibody is targeted specifically to a cell bearing the appropriate antigen, the killing mechanism spreads from that targeted cell. This can lead to unwanted toxicity to normal tissues. However, it can be an advantage because the radiation may kill cells that need to be killed, but are not targeted by the antibody. This might include the blood vessels feeding a tumor or tumor cells that the antibody cannot reach.

Imaging with antibodies may prove useful in a number of settings. It may localize where disease activity is, monitor its response to therapy, or even assess the nature of the disease, using specific antibodies. In most cases the antibodies used are directed against tumor cells. One exciting alternative is to image E-selectin expression on endothelial cells. E-selectin is an adhesion molecule that is expressed only on activated endothelium, seen at sites of inflammation. Not only is it a highly specific marker of inflammation, but, being expressed on the luminal surface of endothelium, it is highly accessible to antibodies in the vasculature. Antibodies to E-selectin have been used to image rheumatoid arthritis and inflammatory bowel disease, as well as to locate occult infection in patients with acquired immunodeficiency syndrome (AIDS) (Chapman et al. 1996).

Most imaging is done with γ-emitting antibodies, which can be detected with a gamma camera, using standard nuclear medicine facilities such as single photon emission computed tomography (SPECT). However, there are alternatives, including the delivery of positron emitters for positron emission tomography (PET) and magnetic contrast agents for magnetic resonance imaging (MRI) (Weissleder and Mahmood 2001). Antibodies have even been conjugated onto bubbles, with a view of developing targetable contrast agents for ultrasonography (Villanueva et al. 1998). Each imaging modality has particular advantages, giving complementary information for clinical diagnosis. The ability to use antibodies to localize the expression of molecules on cells has enormous potential not only for clinical diagnosis but also for the careful monitoring of novel therapies.

ENZYME CONJUGATES

One of the most promising, although also complex, forms of immunotherapy relies on targeting an enzyme within a tumor, often termed 'ADEPT'. Once the enzyme–antibody conjugate has been allowed to localize to the target site, an inactive prodrug is given that is converted by the enzyme into its active form (see Figure 18.1). There are several such enzyme–prodrug combinations that have been developed (Niculescu-Duvaz et al. 1999; Syrigos and Epenetos 1999). In many cases the prodrug is a modified version of a standard drug already in use.

There are several advantages to this approach. The first is that both agents administered to the patient (antibody–enzyme conjugate and prodrug) are essentially nontoxic, and only become toxic when combined. If a drug is chosen that has a short half-life, the toxicity is limited to close to the site of activation. The second is that targeting a single enzyme molecule can facilitate the production of thousands of drug molecules; there is therefore an inbuilt amplification step. In addition in most cases (in neoplastic disease) the drug is more cytopathic to tumor cells than normal cells, so reducing the toxicity to normal tissue around the activation site. At the very least, this approach should improve the therapeutic window of drugs.

The drawback to this approach is the complexity. Not only are there two agents that need to be optimized, but also the timing of the administration of the antibody–enzyme conjugate and the prodrug needs to be optimized. The prodrug cannot be administered while there is free antibody–enzyme in circulation, otherwise drug activation will not be localized to the tumor. To avoid waiting a long time for unbound conjugate to clear, most groups are devising methods to clear the antibody–enzyme from the circulation. Administering a second antibody (e.g. anti-enzyme, anti-idiotypic, or anti-mouse) that binds to the conjugate and causes clearance can do this. Alternatively, the glycosylation status of the antibody can be used to ensure rapid hepatic clearance.

Thus, although attractive, ADEPT has still to make a major impact in the clinic. It is perhaps surprising that all the attention has focused on neoplastic disease for this approach to therapy. It might be thought that this would be useful for focusing the action of anti-parasitic or anti-inflammatory drugs to sites where they are needed.

BISPECIFIC ANTIBODIES

Natural antibodies are monospecific, i.e. they have a single form of the antigen-binding site. Bispecific antibodies are an artificial form of the antibody that has two distinct antigen-binding sites (Figure 18.2).

There are three ways to prepare bispecific antibodies: chemical, hybrid hybridoma, and recombinant. Chemical methods (reviewed in Segal et al. 1992) range from relatively crude crosslinking with molecules, such as *N*-succinimidyl-3-(2-pyridyldithio) propionate (SPDP), which yield a heterogeneous product, to highly precise production of clinical grade material, e.g. by conjugation through the hinge-region cysteines of Fab′ molecules (Glennie et al. 1987). Hybrid hydridoma technology relies on the fusion of two monoclonal antibody-producing hybridomas (Milstein and Cuello 1983). The advantage over the chemical approach is that the result is a cell line that secretes the bispecific antibody on a permanent basis. However, because of random assortment of the two heavy and two light chain domains, a large number of antibody species is produced – only one of which is bispecific. It is necessary to find ways of purifying the desired molecule from the others. The final way to generate bispecific antibodies is by recombinant DNA technology (George and Huston 1997); a number of constructs have been made, mostly based on the basic scFv unit (as discussed below). The final choice as to which method is used will depend on the amount of material needed, the grade it has to be made to, and also whether it is important that the molecule is monovalent or polyvalent to the antigens (i.e. the number of antigen-binding sites present).

Bispecific antibodies can be specific for soluble molecules (Figure 18.2). In this way they are essentially acting as immunoconjugates, and toxins, drugs, and radionuclides have also been targeted in this way (French et al. 1995). It is not necessary to make a conjugate between the antibody and the other effector molecule, which can damage the effector. It would theoretically be possible to administer the bispecific antibody and the effector molecule separately, which, if the effector has a short half-life, should reduce toxicity.

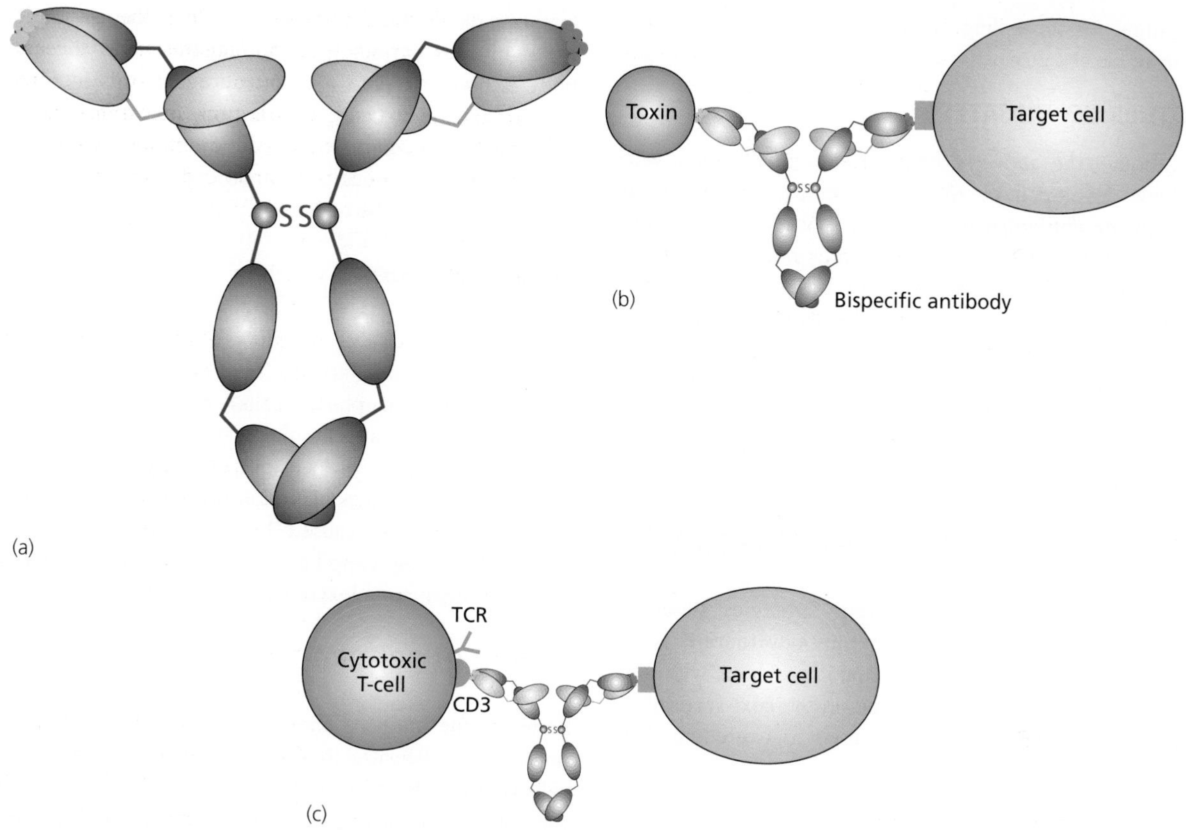

Figure 18.2 *Bispecific antibodies have two distinct antigen-binding sites, as illustrated here* **(a)** *using different colours for the CDR regions. They can be used to target soluble molecules or effector cells to the target site as shown for* **(b)** *targeting toxins and* **(c)** *cellular cytotoxicity.*

However, the pharmacokinetics of antibody delivery would mean that this is an inefficient process. This process is also highly dependent on the affinity and kinetics of the bispecific antibody to both the target cell and the therapeutic molecule (George et al. 1995a).

In addition to targeting effector molecules, bispecific antibodies can also be used to target immunogens to antigen-presenting cells, to boost immune responses (Snider and Segal 1989), e.g. bispecific antibodies specific for hen egg lysozyme and major histocompatibility (MHC) class II molecules on antigen-presenting cells (as well as some other molecules) have been shown to be effective in vivo at immunizing animals (Snider et al. 1990).

The above applications for bispecific antibodies are essentially similar to those for immunoconjugates. However, one way in which bispecific antibodies can be used is to target cells (Karpovsky et al. 1984; Perez et al. 1985) (Figure 18.2). In this case the bispecific antibody has to be specific for a molecule on the effector and the target cells. The effector cell could include T cells, neutrophils, NK cells, or any other cell capable of mediating an appropriate response. The bispecific antibody serves not only to bring the two cells together, but also to trigger the effector cell. For that reason the antibody must interact with a 'trigger molecule' on the effector cell, such as CD3 on T cells or FcγRIII (CD16) on NK cells.

The main application of this approach is to kill neoplastic or virally infected cells. The advantage of this strategy is that the effector cells are appropriate for the targets (e.g. the main function of CD8 cells is to kill virally infected cells). They are therefore efficient at the task.

Bispecific antibodies can also be used to activate cells, e.g. combinations of bispecific antibodies can be used that engage not only the trigger molecule on the effector cells, but a co-stimulatory molecule to activate the cell (such as CD28) (Grosse-Hovest et al. 1999). It is even possible to generate trispecific antibodies that engage two molecules on the effector cell, a triggering molecule and an activating molecule (Tutt et al. 1991).

There have been a number of clinical trials using bispecific antibodies (Segal et al. 1999; van Spriel et al. 2000). Some of these have shown promising results; however, progress is slow. The reasons for this are likely to lie in the complex nature of the therapy being attempted; it is necessary to ensure that the antibody and the effector cells both reach the target tissue and that the effector cells are adequately activated. However, the ability to target effector cells that are optimal for the killing of the target cell remains highly attractive.

OTHER CONJUGATES

Although the above strategies represent the main ones being developed or used for therapy, the ability to conjugate antibodies using chemical or molecular techniques can be applied to an enormous range of partners, e.g. antibodies linked to magnetic beads can be used to purge bone marrow of malignant cells (Gee et al. 1992). Antibodies have also been used to target cytokines such as IL-2 to stimulate immune cells at specific sites (Boleti et al. 1995). In addition antibodies can also be used to target gene therapy vectors, both viral (Harari et al. 1999) and nonviral (Tan et al. 2003), to specific cells.

PROBLEMS WITH ANTIBODY THERAPY

Given the plethora of different strategies described above, it has to be asked why antibody therapy is not more successful. Some of the major problems with antibody therapy are given here and, in the next section, the genetic strategies that can be used to overcome these are considered.

Immunogenicity

Nearly all monoclonal antibodies produced by hybridoma technology are of mouse or rat origin. This means that when they are introduced into patients they are immunogenic. They therefore elicit an immune response, which can be seen as a human anti-mouse (or rat) antibody (HAMA) response. The production of HAMA has two consequences. First, the antibodies bind to the therapeutic antibody, making it ineffective by blocking it and removing it from circulation. Second, the formation of immune complexes with the antibody can lead to serum sickness (type III hypersensitivity). Similar responses against the effector molecule in immunoconjugates (such as toxin molecules) can have a similar effect. The result of this is that it is frequently impossible to give repeated administrations of antibodies to patients.

Pharmacokinetics

Antibodies are large molecules compared with most drugs (around 150 kDa). This means that they are relatively poor at penetrating solid tissue, especially in cases where the tissue has a high interstitial pressure (such as tumors). This limits their ability to get to where they are needed. In addition the large size of antibodies (as well as their interaction with the Brambell receptor FcRn – Junghans 1997) means that they have a long half-life ($t_{1/2}$). The $t_{1/2}$ of a human IgG1 antibody in a patient is around 21 days. Although most murine antibodies have a shorter half-life in patients, this means that large amounts of unbound antibody remain in the circulation for significant periods after administration. If the antibody is conjugated to a cytotoxic agent, this increases the nonspecific toxicity. In addition, for other applications, such as imaging, the unbound antibody provides a background that needs to clear in order for the specific bound antibody to be detected.

Loss of antigen

If the target loses the antigen recognized by the antibody, it can escape attack. This can occur (for both pathogens and neoplastic cells) by mutation of the antigen. In some parasites there are well-described strategies for switching surface antigens to enable them to escape antibody attack. In addition, the loss of antigen can be temporary, caused by modulation of surface antigen (patching, capping, and internalization or shedding of antigen complexed with antibody).

Nature of antigen

Some of the antigens chosen for antibody therapy are not effective because they are not expressed on all the cells (perhaps because of differential expression through the cell cycle). In addition, as discussed above for the immunotoxins (see section on Toxins and drugs), some antigens are better at delivering effector molecules to the cell than others. Expression of the same (or cross-reactive) epitopes on other cells can also cause problems, e.g. ricin A chain containing-immunotoxin was infused into five patients with breast cancer, most of whom developed marked fluid overload and debilitating sensorimotor neuropathies. This was probably the result of an unexpected recognition by the antibody of a molecule on Schwann cells, which resulted in demyelination of the patients' neurons (Gould et al. 1989).

GENETIC ENGINEERING

Many of the problems outlined above have been tackled using the tools of antibody genetic engineering. There are three aspects of antibody production that genetic engineering has influenced: the selection of novel antibodies, the design and construction of 'improved' antibody molecules, and the inexpensive production of antibodies using mammalian, eukarytotic, and prokaryotic cells (outside the scope of this chapter, but reviewed in Verma et al. 1998).

Production of new antibodies

Hybridoma technology has proved a powerful tool for generating monoclonal antibodies. However, it has some severe limitations. The first of these is that it is limited to the production of mouse, rat, or hamster antibodies. Although some groups have been able to use hybridoma technology to make antibodies from other species (including humans), for a variety of technical reasons (difficulty of immunizing, problems with fusion partners) this has never been routine.

The second problem relates to the way in which hybridoma technology is used to screen for antibodies. This relies on screening individual wells containing hybridomas to see whether they contain an antibody of the desired specificity. This process is inherently inefficient, and so it is difficult to obtain antibodies that are rare. To give a practical illustration of this, if we want to isolate a hybridoma that is present at a frequency of 1/10 000 one would need to screen in the order of 100 96-well plates in order to find it, and that is assuming that every well contains one hybridoma.

This has led to a number of approaches for generating novel antibodies, such as phage display (McCafferty et al. 1990; Clackson et al. 1991) and ribosome display (Hanes and Pluckthun 1997; He and Taussig 1997). Of these, phage display is the most commonly used. In addition, transgenic mouse technology has allowed the production of human antibodies using conventional hybridoma technology (Bruggemann et al. 1991).

PHAGE DISPLAY

Filamentous bacteriophages (such as M13) are single-stranded DNA viruses that infect bacteria such as *E. coli*. They are long phages, typically 1 μm, and around 6–7 nm in diameter. The single-stranded DNA is covered with coat proteins, in particular the major coat protein pVIII, which is present at around 2 700 copies per phage, and a number of minor coat proteins of which the most important for our purposes is pIII, which is present at around three to five copies at one end of the phage.

To carry out phage display it is necessary to make recombinant antibody fragments (see section on Antibody fragments) fused to one of the coat proteins of the phage (for a review of this technology, see Winter et al. 1994; George and Epenetos 1996). Several fragments have been fused to a number of coat proteins, but, for simplicity, scFv fragments fused to pIII are considered here. This is probably the most commonly used format, although many groups use Fab fragments.

In the basic protocol (Figure 18.3), B cells are used as a source of mRNA. This is reverse transcribed to cDNA and polymerase chain reaction (PCR) used to isolate the gene fragments encoding the heavy and light chain variable domains. These are cloned into the phage as scFv (or Fab) fragments fused to the gene encoding pIII. When these phages are expressed in bacteria they are generated as phage particles that express antibody fragments on their surface (McCafferty et al. 1990). The result of this is a library of phages expressing a large number of antibody molecules. It is now possible to take this library and incubate it with immobilized antigen (e.g. coated onto plastic). Phages expressing the antibody of interest will bind to the antigen; the rest will be washed away. Repeating this panning procedure allows the isolation of phages bearing the appropriate antibody (and also containing the gene encoding for that antibody) (Clackson et al. 1991).

Looking at the steps in the process in some more detail, the source of variable region gene can be B cells from any species from which it is possible to amplify the genes – including humans. In addition, the animal can be either immunized or 'naïve' to the antigen in question. In many cases the source of the genes is synthetic, using artificial sequences. Indeed some groups have moved beyond the antibody, and are making antigen-binding molecules based on different scaffolds, such as fibronectin-derived domains (Koide et al. 1998). This opens up the possibility of making antigen binders with a different number of complementarity-determining regions (CDR) regions, or with different sized CDR regions (long protuberant CDR may be useful to bind to buried epitopes on viruses as discussed earlier).

The size of the library is a very important factor in the process. Typical libraries will have 10^7–10^9 different antibody molecules. It is also possible to use genetic tricks to make libraries that have close to 10^{11} different antibody molecules (Griffiths et al. 1994). To put that in context, the number of different B cells in a mouse is probably around 10^8. Given that a mouse is capable of making an antibody against just about any foreign antigen, this means that it is highly likely that a library will contain an antibody of the desired specificity. The other advantage of large libraries is that the antibodies isolated are of higher affinity than those isolated from smaller libraries (Griffiths et al. 1994).

The affinity selection can take place in a number of ways. In general, purified antigen is coated on to plastic plates. Alternatively, selection can be done in solution, using biotinylated antigen followed by the addition of streptavidin-coated beads to pull the antigen–phage complex out of solution. However, selection can be done on the surface of cells (Palmer et al. 1997), on crude extracts, tissue sections (Owens et al. 2000), and even in vivo, after injection of the library into an animal (Johns et al. 2000). This latter approach allows the isolation of antibodies reactive with tissue-specific markers on endothelium. Selection can also involve negative selection steps, to remove unwanted specificities, or sequential selection on different antigens (e.g. different strains of human immunodeficiency virus (HIV) to deliberately select for antibodies capable of cross-reacting with both antigens or the use of blocking antibodies to direct the antibodies away from a particular epitope (Ditzel et al. 1995).

Once the antibody has been selected it can be modified to give it appropriate effector functions (see 'Effector functions'). However, in many cases, especially

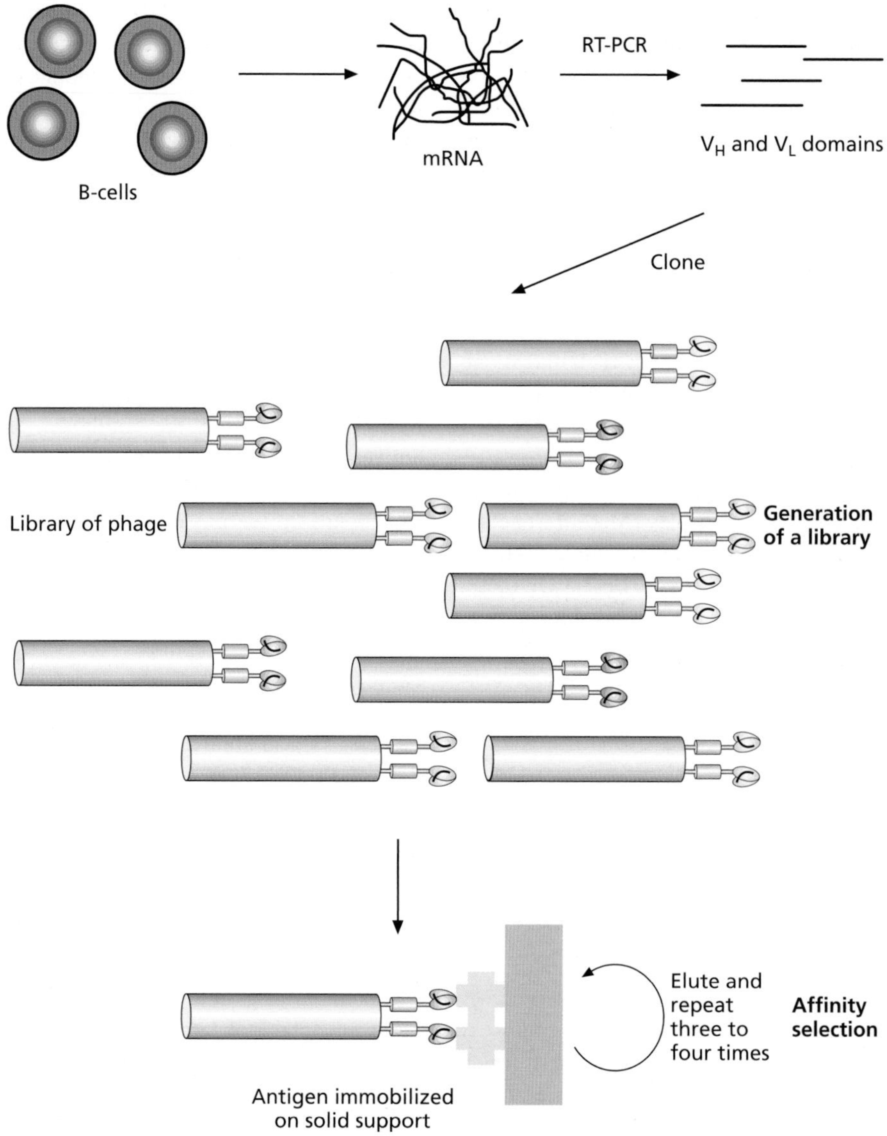

Figure 18.3 *In phage display technology V region genes are isolated from B cells (or artificially made) and are constructed to form a library of antibody fragments (illustrated here as scFv), displayed on the surface of filamentous phage as a fusion with a coat protein (in this case pIII). The library consists of a large number of phages, each with different antibodies on their surface, and carrying in the genome of the phage particle, the gene encoding that antibody. As a result, if affinity selection techniques are used, it is possible to isolate phage-expressing antibodies that bind to the antigen in question. This allows isolation of the gene for that antibody. The selection process has to be repeated a number of times, resulting in the isolation of an antibody specific for the antigen. RT-PCR, reverse transcriptase polymerase chain reaction.*

from small libraries, the affinity of the antibody is too low for practical use. It is possible to improve the affinity by random mutation of the antibody (using error-prone PCR or passing the phage through a mutator strain of bacteria), followed by further selection on antigen (Marks et al. 1992b). In addition, shuffling the heavy and light chains with novel heavy and light chains, and repeating the selection, can also improve affinity (Marks et al. 1992a). This process can be highly effective; in one case the affinity of anti-HIV antibodies was improved using a variety of mutational approaches from the already high affinity of 6.3 nmol/l to 15 pmol/l (Yang et al. 1995).

The process described above is highly reminiscent of the natural life history of B cells and antibody production. In the bone marrow a large library of naïve B cells is produced with different antibodies on their surface. Antigens are used to affinity select those B cells with the appropriate specificity. These are then randomly mutated and subject to further selection to affinity mature the response. The shuffling of heavy and light chains is even similar to the process of receptor editing, which may play a role in the improvement of antibody affinity (George and Gray 1999).

What are the advantages of phage display? The ability to use human or even artificial antibodies is important.

The process is also better at the isolation of rare antibodies. As antibodies are selected using an affinity technique, so long as the selection system is robust, it is possible to isolate very rare antibodies quickly. In addition, the library has never undergone negative selection or tolerance in vivo. It is therefore possible to isolate antibodies against antigens to which the animals are tolerant (Griffiths et al. 1993). In some cases this has made it possible to produce antibodies that recognize the same antigen in a variety of species (Palmer et al. 1999).

TRANSGENIC ANIMALS

One method for producing human antibodies using hybridoma technology has been to make animals in which their native Ig loci have been replaced using knockout and transgenic approaches with the human counterparts (Lonberg et al. 1994; Bruggemann and Neuberger 1996; Mendez et al. 1997; Nicholson et al. 1999; Tomizuka et al. 2000). These animals, when immunized, produce human antibodies. The antibodies undergo somatic mutation and, if the genes for the appropriate heavy chain isotype are present, can class switch. It is therefore simple to use such immunized animals to generate human monoclonal antibodies using conventional hybridoma technology.

If such transgenic approaches could be applied to larger animals, such as pigs, sheep, or cattle, it might be possible to use them as a source of therapeutic polyclonal human antibodies. It would be conceivable to immunize such animals with virus or toxoids, and to harvest the antibody from them. This should have the advantage of reducing the risks of using material derived from humans, as well as allowing the production of large quantities of defined material.

Immunogenicity

Among the first constructs to be made were those aimed at tackling the immunogenicity of rodent (mostly murine) antibody molecules. The most commonly used methods for doing this are chimerization and humanization, although other procedures such as veneering have been described. There are additional strategies for reducing the immunogenicity, including the production of nonbinding antibody molecules and removal of T-cell epitopes (termed 'deimmunization').

CHIMERIZATION

The structure of the antibody molecule is made up of domains, which essentially fold as independent units. It is therefore relatively easy to swap domains from one antibody to another. Chimeric antibodies are created by replacing all the rodent constant region domains with those of humans, resulting in a molecule where 8 of 12 of the domains are human (Figure 18.4) (Boulianne et al. 1984; Morrison et al. 1984). These antibodies have considerably reduced immunogenicity in patients when compared with their murine counterpart. In addition, the antibodies have human Fc regions (which can be chosen at will), and so will in general be better at interacting with human effector mechanisms than murine Fc regions.

HUMANIZATION

Although the majority of a chimeric antibody is human in sequence, the variable domains remain rodent in origin. However, most of the variable domains serve no antigen-binding function, but act as a platform for the six CDRs (or hypervariable loops) to form the antigen-binding site. This has led to the process of humanization, in which just the hypervariable loops from the rodent antibody are transferred onto human variable domains (Jones et al. 1986; Reichmann et al. 1988). The result is an antibody that is essentially totally human.

The process of humanization relies first on the identification of human variable domains that are similar in structure to the original rodent variable domains. The CDRs can then be transferred using standard recombinant approaches. When this is done, it is often found that the antibodies have a lower affinity than the parental antibody. Judicious mutation of some of the framework residues that interact with the CDRs will normally restore the affinity. Although this process was originally somewhat hit and miss, there is now a considerable body of experience that ensures that humanization is a robust and relatively routine procedure (Emery and Harris 1995).

Although humanization might seem optimal, it is important to note that the resulting antibodies are still immunogenic (Clark 2000). This is because the antigen-binding site is immunogenic and capable of eliciting an anti-idiotypic response. This is not unique, of course, to humanized antibodies; natural human antibodies are equally capable of inducing anti-idiotypic antibodies. There is no evidence that the CDRs of humanized antibodies are any more (or less) immunogenic than the CDRs of human antibodies. It is also important to realize that, although there might be theoretical advantages of humanization over chimerization, there is little evidence that the humanized antibodies are better than chimeric antibodies (Clark 2000). The immunogenicity of the six CDR loops is probably considerably greater than that of the relatively few framework residues that differ between rodent and human.

VENEERING AND DEIMMUNIZATION

Veneering antibodies relies on the realization that, if the surface of a murine antibody variable domain is compared with its human equivalent (and ignoring the

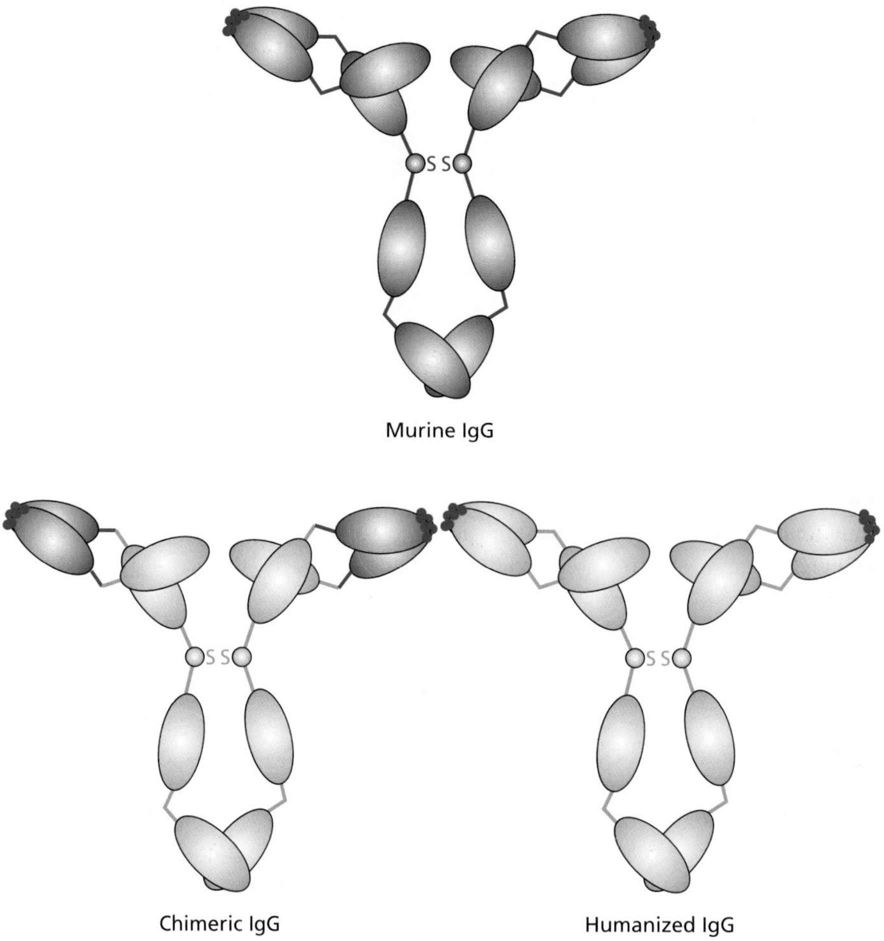

Figure 18.4 *Reducing immunogenicity: most monoclonal antibodies are totally rodent in origin (shown as blue). However, it is possible to replace parts of the molecule with human sequences (red). In the simplest form chimeric antibodies contain the rodent variable domains and human constant domains. In humanized antibodies all the domains are human in sequence, but the complementarity-determining regions (CDR), shown as circles, are replaced by those from the parental antibody.*

CDR regions), relatively few residues are different (Padlan 1991). Given that HAMA will recognize the surface of these domains, mutation of these few residues from the mouse to the human sequence should abolish the ability of HAMA to bind to the antibodies (Roguska et al. 1994). This approach has been termed 'veneering', because it is similar to the practice in furniture making of covering cheap wood with a veneer of expensive wood. The mouse variable domain is covered with a veneer of human amino acids.

The complementary approach to this has been termed 'deimmunization', in which it has been reasoned that to generate a HAMA response it is necessary for the relevant B cells to obtain T-cell help. As the T-helper cells will see peptide bound in the groove of MHC II molecules, and as this binding is dependent on motifs of amino acids, it should be possible to mutate out these MHC-binding motifs, making an antibody that it invisible to T cells.

Both of these approaches are elegant. However, given the success of humanization and chimerization, it is likely that they will not have a major impact except, possibly, as a way to overcome restrictive patents on the other strategies. It is possible that deimmunization may be effective in preventing anti-idiotypic responses (which require T-cell help), in which case there would be a clear advantage for this approach. However, this has yet to be shown.

TOLERANCE INDUCTION

All of the approaches outlined above are designed to make the antibody invisible to the immune system. An alternative would be to tolerize the patient to the antibody being given. One approach to this is based on the observation that the administration of soluble antibodies to patients (or animals) is normally tolerogenic. However, administration of antibodies that bind to cell surfaces is immunogenic. It is possible to produce antibodies that have mutations in their CDR loops and so no longer bind to their antigen. Intravenous injection of these antibodies (at least in animal models) tolerizes the animal to the antibody, allowing subsequent administration of the complete antigen-binding antibody with no induction of HAMA (Gilliland et al. 1999).

Antibody fragments

As noted above the large size of antibody molecules ensures that they have a long half-life and are relatively poor at penetrating solid tissue. For many circumstances this is an advantage, e.g. if the object is to maintain high levels of a blocking antibody for prolonged periods. However, in many cases it would be preferable to have antibodies that are cleared rapidly. The main approach to doing this has been to make recombinant antibody fragments, which are smaller than the native molecule.

It is fairly easy to make the range of antibody fragments (Fab, Fab′, F(ab′)$_2$ – Figure 18.5) that are available using conventional enzymatic digestion of antibodies. It is also possible to make novel molecules, normally based on the Fv fragment of an antibody that consists of the two variable domains of an antibody. This is the smallest antibody fragment that retains an intact antigen-binding site (25 kDa, as compared with 150 kDa for IgG). It is possible to make Fv fragments by enzymatic digestion of some antibodies (Inbar et al. 1972); however, the molecules are normally unstable because the two domains are free to dissociate (in an Fab fragment the heavy and light chains are held together by a disulfide bonds as well as noncovalent interactions that are predominantly between the two constant domains). There has been interest, therefore, in strategies to make artificial Fv-based molecules.

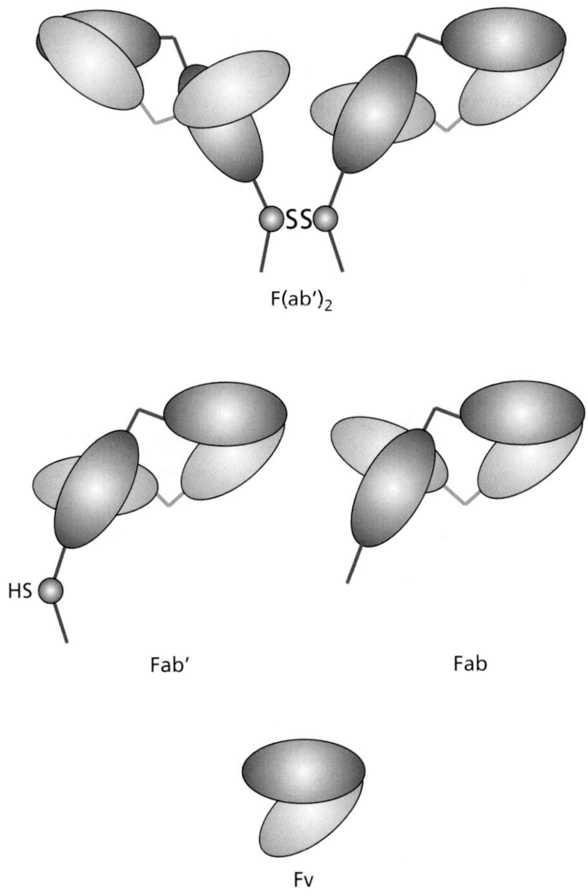

Figure 18.5 Antibody fragments: the whole immunoglobulin IgG molecule can be enzymatically digested to produce F(ab′)$_2$, Fab′, Fab, and Fv fragments of the molecule, which contain intact antigen-binding sites but are smaller than the parental molecule. These are also accessible using recombinant approaches. However, the Fv in particular is unstable, because there are no disulfide bonds and only weak noncovalent interactions to prevent the two chains from dissociating.

Fv-BASED CONSTRUCTS

The aim of all Fv-based constructs is to stabilize the interactions between the two variable domains without destroying the antibody-binding site. The first type of molecule in which this was achieved was the single chain Fv (scFv or sFv, commonly referred to as a single chain antibody). In this molecule a peptide linker is used to join the C terminus of one domain with the N terminus of the other (Bird et al. 1988; Huston et al. 1988) (Figure 18.6). The (linear) distance that needs to be spanned is around 3–4 nm (Huston et al. 1996a), and to do this the linker is typically around 15 amino acids; it has been designed or selected to be highly flexible (the archetypal sequence being (Gly$_4$Ser)$_3$, with the glycines providing maximal flexibility – Huston et al. 1988). However, many other linker sequences have been designed or selected by phage display (Turner et al. 1997). The format of the scFv can be V_H–linker–V_L, or V_L–linker–V_H, whereas some scFvs perform better in one orientation than the other; in most cases the choice is unimportant.

The scFv has the advantage of being a robust building block for the generation of targeting molecules, in large part because of its simplicity; it is a single polypeptide chain encoded by a single gene construct. The pharmacokinetics of the scFv are as might be expected from its small

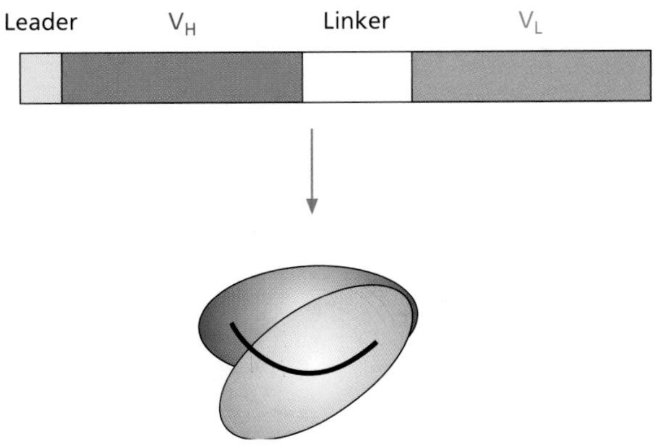

Figure 18.6 The single chain Fv (scFv) consists of the V_H and V_L domains of the antibody, stabilized by a peptide spacer between the N terminus of one domain and the C terminus of the other. The molecule is encoded by a single gene, which translates into a single polypeptide chain.

Table 18.2 *Half-lives of antibody fragments*

	$t_{1/2\alpha}$ (min)	$t_{1/2\beta}$ (h)
IgG	39	113
$F(ab')_2$	26	12
Fab′	9.2	88 min
scFv	3.7	90 min

The data taken from Milenic et al. (1991) shows the half-life of different versions of the CC49 antibody. These are given as two phases, the α phase (roughly corresponding to equilibration into the extravascular volume) and the β phase (clearance from the body). The scFv and Fab′ fragments show much more rapid equilibration and clearance.

size, with a very short clearance rate (Table 18.2) (Milenic et al. 1991) and good penetration of solid tissue. A phage-derived scFv with specificity for carcinoembryonic antigen has been used to image patients with neoplastic disease, with a half-life of around 5 h (Begent et al. 1996). In this case the antibody was better at imaging tumors than conventional antibodies. Similarly, a scFv specific for the C5 component of complement has a half-life of 7–14 h in patients (Fitch et al. 1999).

Other Fv-based molecules have been produced. The main alternative is the disulfide-stabilized Fv (dsFv) (Figure 18.7). In this molecule single mutations have been made that have changed an amino acid residue on the interface between the two variable domains into cysteine (Glockshuber et al. 1990). The molecules are then free to pair and make a disulfide bond that stabilizes the interaction between the two domains. Clinical trials have been described in which dsFvs fused to toxins have been administered to patients with hematological malignancies (Kreitman et al. 2001).

SMALLER FRAGMENTS

Although the Fv is the smallest fragment of a human antibody that retains an intact antigen-binding site, attempts have been made to decrease the size of recombinant antibodies still further. Although an intact antigen-binding site has six CDRs that can contribute to the interaction with antigen, in many cases not all are needed. Thus, some antibodies show preferential usage of the heavy chain CDRs. This has led to the production of single domain antibodies (dAb), in which just one variable domain (normally the V_H) is produced (Ward et al. 1989). In some cases, dAbs show binding to antigen. However, there are two drawbacks to this approach. The first is that there is likely to be a loss of affinity as half the CDRs are removed. This might be overcome by techniques such as phage display. The major problem is that the dAb contains a surface that is normally hidden by interaction with the other variable domain, and this surface contains hydrophobic amino acids that normally contribute to stabilization of the interaction between the domains. However, in a dAb they can cause the fragment to become highly ‘sticky’ and also prone to aggregate.

One solution to this has come from the realization that members of the cammelid family (camels and llamas) have antibodies that consist of just the heavy chain (Hamers-Casterman et al. 1993). This feature is

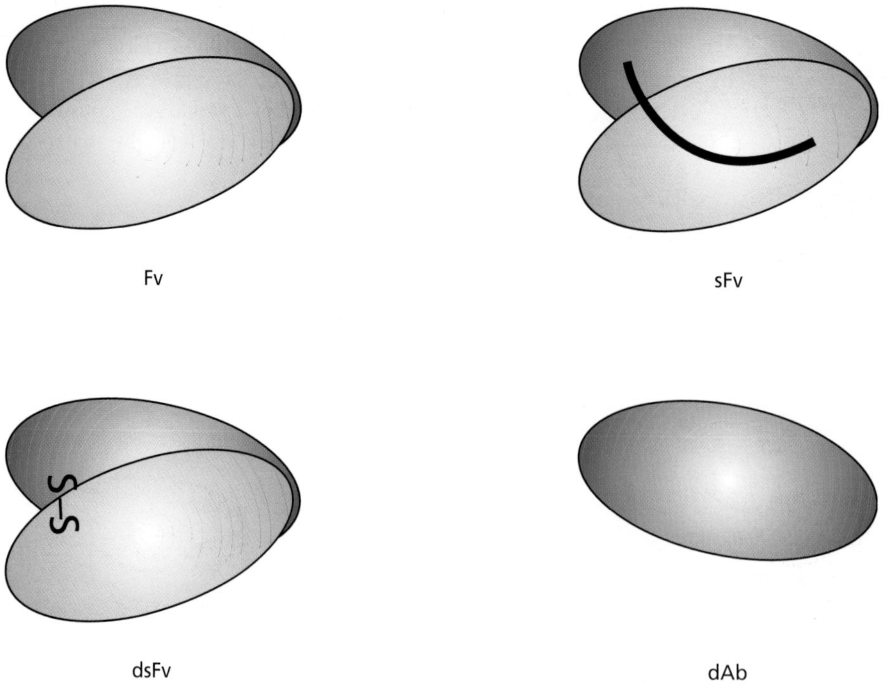

Figure 18.7 *Other Fv-based molecules: in addition to the scFv other molecules have been made with the aim of exploiting the antigen-binding site of the Fv. These include the disulfide-stabilized Fv (dsFv) in which a disulfide bond in the interface of the two domains prevents the V_H and V_L from dissociating. In addition the single domain antibody (dAb) contains just one domain (normally the V_H).*

also seen in other species such as sharks (Pilstrom 2002). The equivalent surface of the heavy chain variable domain is adapted to working in the absence of a partner V_L, and so is not 'sticky'. It is therefore possible to make dAbs from such species, as well as to consider mutating the human V_H domain to make it more 'camel like' (Davies and Riechmann 1994),

The ultimate in small recognition units is a single CDR. Several groups have devised peptide sequences based on the CDR of an antibody that retains a degree of antigen binding (Zhang et al. 1996; Laune et al. 1997; Park et al. 2000). In most cases these peptides are cyclic, thus somewhat constraining their conformation. In most cases the affinity of the peptides for their antigen is relatively low. However, they are inexpensive to make and can be administered in large quantities to compensate for this. Although it is unlikely that they will replace antibody-like molecules for most targeting purposes, the use of antibody technologies to identify and isolate CDRs that can be used for specialized applications (such as blocking viral entry) is an interesting route to drug development.

Effector functions

The small antibody fragments described above have the ability to target their antigen, but carry no effector function (other than blocking). In addition, most of the fragments described above are monovalent and so are not capable of cross-linking their antigen (and also suffer from a loss of avidity). It is therefore necessary to modify them, normally by fusing them to alternative molecules. In the following section, several examples normally based on the scFv molecule (as that is the most commonly used) are given. However, most of the approaches can also be applied to other fragments (Fab, dsFv, dAb, etc.).

FUSION PROTEINS

The simplest way to endow an antibody fragment with function is to fuse it to the molecule with the desired function (Figure 18.8) (Neuberger et al. 1984). The scFv is very tolerant of fusions to both the N terminus and C terminus (or indeed both), retaining its affinity for antigen, although this is not always true of the fusion partner.

The partner protein can be just about any protein, including toxins (Chaudhary et al. 1989), enzymes, and cytokines (Boleti et al. 1995), as described earlier for conventional conjugates. They can also be viral coat proteins (e.g. pIII in filamentous phage, see section on Phage display). In some cases it is also possible to use peptides with a function, e.g. a short peptide has been designed that chelates the radioisotope ^{99m}Tc (George et al. 1995b). The scFv incorporating this peptide can, in a single, rapid, one-tube process, bind to and chelate the radioisotope. The interaction is highly stable and allows the site-specific labeling of recombinant scFv (or other proteins), making them highly suitable for imaging applications (George et al. 1995b; Huston et al. 1996b).

RECOMBINANT BISPECIFIC ANTIBODIES

Conventional methods of making bispecific antibodies have been described above, but recombinant antibody fragments also offer very convenient building blocks for making these molecules (George and Huston 1997). A variety of fragments has been described, some of which are shown in Figure 18.9.

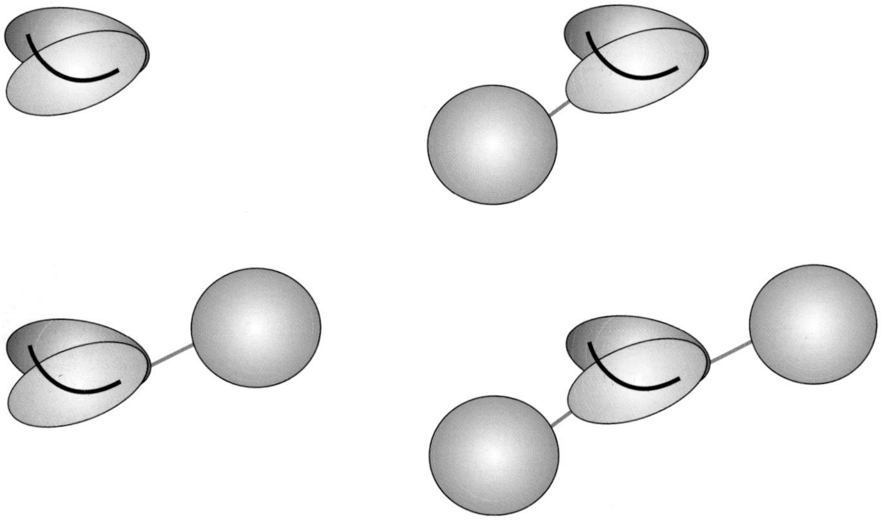

Figure 18.8 *Fusions with scFv: functional properties can be given to the scFv antibody by fusing the molecule with another protein or peptide (shown in green). This fusion can be N- or C-terminal to the scFv (or even at both ends). In general the scFv is tolerant to such additions, although the function of the effector protein may depend on the orientation.*

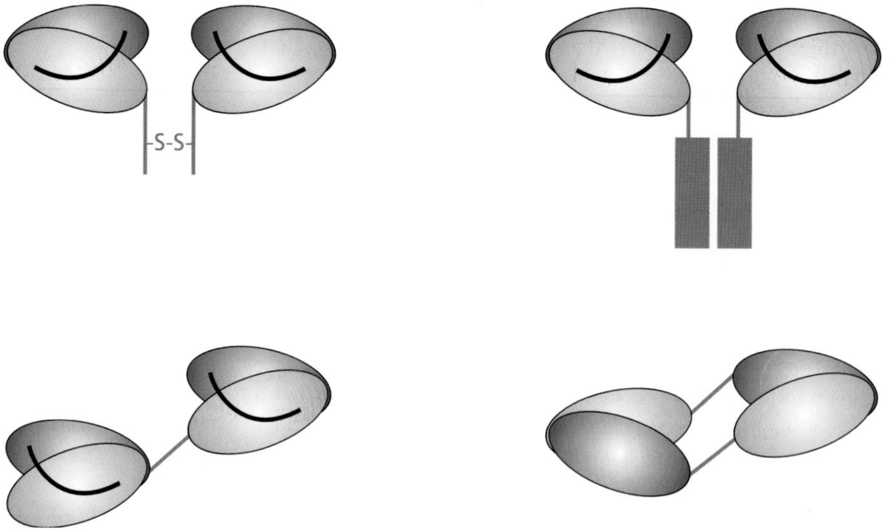

Figure 18.9 *Recombinant bispecific constructs: there are several ways in which the scFv (or equivalent) antibody fragments can be used to generate bispecific antibodies. These include using disulfide bonds to join two fragments together, fusion to domains (such as leucine zippers) that cause heterodimerization, use of a peptide linker to join two scFvs, or the formation of diabodies in which two polypeptide chains associate in a head-to-tail conformation.*

The simplest approach is to add a cysteine residue to the scFv to allow dimerization (or chemical conjugation) (McCartney et al. 1995). It is possible to fuse the scFv with domains in order to encourage heterodimerization, as opposed to homodimerization. These are often based on leucine zipper motifs, such as jun and fos, which naturally heterodimerize. Fusion of scFv or other antibody fragments with such zippers results in the formation of bispecific antibodies (Kostelny et al. 1992; de-Kruif and Logtenberg 1996).

The second approach is simply to fuse two scFv together, to form a single chain bispecific antibody, which is expressed on a single polypeptide chain. Although this is an elegant approach, in many cases the yields of such molecules are low (Andrew et al. 1991; Huston et al. 1991; Kurucz et al. 1995).

The final approach that is described is the formation of diabodies (Holliger et al. 1993; Whitlow et al. 1994). The scFv molecule is designed with a long enough linker so that the V_H and V_L domains interact with each other. However, if the linker is shortened this is not possible, and in such cases the domains interact with their partner domains on other molecules, forming two chain diabodies. With the appropriate choice of molecule, it is possible to generate bispecific diabodies. Indeed, this approach can be taken further to create trivalent triabodies (Hudson and Kortt 1999).

All of the strategies described above for generating bispecific antibodies can also be used to make bivalent scFv. This might have advantages in terms of the affinity of the interaction with cell surfaces (Adams et al. 1998), and also allow cross-linking of the target molecules and therefore signaling.

MODIFICATION OF TARGET CELLS

The above approaches all rely on administering the recombinant antibody as a protein. However, it is also possible genetically to modify cells so that they express the antibody of interest in a manner that modulates their phenotype or function. One example of this is to express scFv fragments as fusion proteins with molecules involved in signaling (such as the ζ chain of the T-cell receptor (TCR)–CD3 complex) (Eshhar et al. 1993; Eshhar 1997). If such a scFv-ζ fusion is expressed in a T cell, the T cell can become activated upon encounter with the antibody (so-called T bodies). This approach has been applied to other cell types, and may form a useful therapy for neoplastic disease as well as against virally infected cells.

The scFv can also be expressed in an intracellular localization, where they can bind to their antigens. They are directed to the appropriate site by fusion with signal peptides (e.g. KDEL which retains or retrieves the molecule to the endoplasmic reticulum). This can result in 'knocking out' expression of a particular protein or blocking the function of that molecule (Figure 18.10) (Richardson et al. 1995). However, in the context of infectious disease it can also be used to block viral infection (often termed 'intracellular immunization'). This has been considerably developed in the context of plant infections, but has also been applied to human settings, e.g. in the case of HIV, intracellular antibodies have been generated to a wide range of the viral proteins. Expression of these proteins can prevent functional virions being assembled and so block infection (Mhashilkar et al. 1995; Marasco et al. 1999; Poznansky et al. 1999). This opens the possibility of gene therapy in

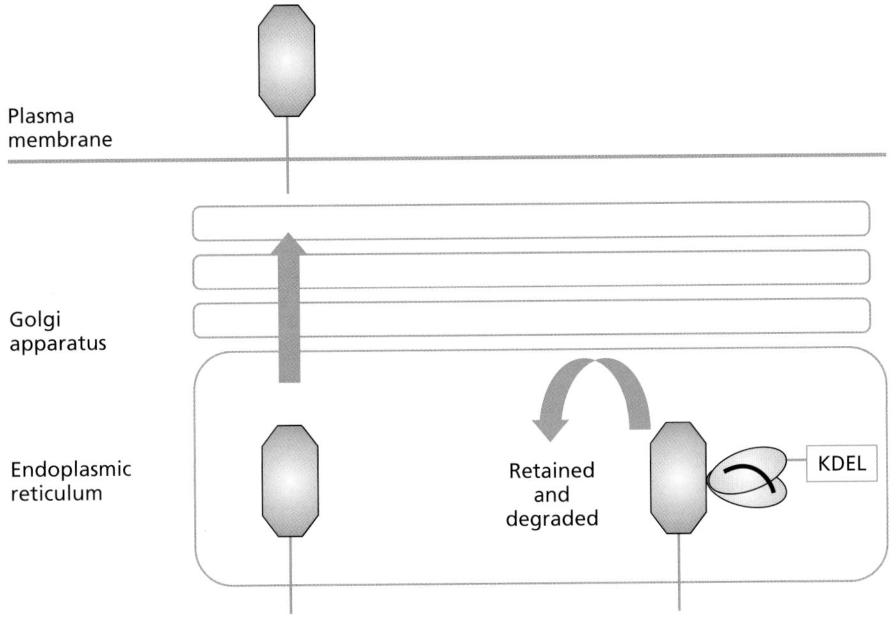

Figure 18.10 *Intracellular antibodies: normally (shown on left) molecules destined for secretion from a cell or expression on the cell membrane are synthesized in the endoplasmic reticulum. They then pass through the Golgi apparatus to the cell surface. On the right is shown the intervention possible using an intracellular antibody. An antibody (scFv in this example) is expressed in the cell fused to the KDEL sequence. This causes the scFv to be retained in or retrieved to the endoplasmic reticulum. There they bind their target antigen, preventing them from moving to the Golgi and to the cell surface – eventually targeting them for degradation.*

which bone marrow cells are made resistant to infection by expression of intracellular antibodies.

CONCLUSION

A quarter of a century after the description of a generally applicable method for making monoclonal antibodies, they are only now beginning to take their place in the clinic. Why did this process take so long? Many of the reasons were scientific, and the problems and solutions have been discussed above. In addition, there are many commercial obstacles that scientists and clinicians are often rather naïve about, which slow down the development of antibodies (for a fascinating account of the development of one antibody, CAMPATH-1, see Hale and Waldmann 2000). It should perhaps be remembered that it does take time to develop new classes of therapeutic agent. Even penicillin, which is often seen as a remarkable wonder drug that achieved widespread and rapid acceptance, took some time to be developed. Alexander Fleming first noted the death of bacteria on the Petri dish in 1928. It was first tested in patients in 1941 and was in routine clinical use by 1945. This represented a period of scientific advance (including the isolation of the active molecule) as well as industrial development (to produce the product in large enough amounts), which was accelerated by the wartime demands. One of the problems with the cycles of hype and cynicism that surround new forms of therapy is that it can disrupt the steady and sustained effort that is needed to achieve success.

What does the future hold? The current antibodies that have achieved licensing by the FDA are mostly relatively conventional (albeit humanized or chimerized). In the pipeline are the products of phage display and more radical antibody engineering. These are likely to start to make an impact over the next decade, although it is difficult to tell how great this will be. Although the tools of molecular biology do offer really exciting possibilities, it should be remembered that technology developed in the nineteenth century (polyclonal antibodies) is still the most commonly used for the production of clinical reagents. We must adopt the new technologies where appropriate, while not being dazzled by their novelty into applying them in an inappropriate manner.

REFERENCES

Adams, G.P., Schier, R., et al. 1998. Increased affinity leads to improved selective tumor delivery of single-chain Fv antibodies. *Cancer Res*, **58**, 485–90.

Andrew, S.M., Perez, P., et al. 1991. Production of a single chain bispecific antibody by recombinant DNA technology. In: Romet-Lemonne, J.-P., Fanger, N.W. and Segal, D.M. (eds), *Bispecific antibodies and targeted cellular cytotoxicity*. Les Ulis, France: Fondation Nationale de Transfusion Sanguine, 197–9.

Begent, R.H., Verhaar, J., et al. 1996. Clinical evidence of efficient tumor targeting based on single-chain Fv antibody selected from a combinatorial library. *Nat Med*, **2**, 979–84.

Bindon, C.I., Hale, G. and Waldmann, H. 1988. Importance of antigen specificity for complement-mediated lysis by monoclonal antibodies. *Eur J Immunol*, **18**, 1507–14.

Bird, R.E., Hardman, K.D., et al. 1988. Single-chain antigen-binding proteins. *Science*, **242**, 423–6.

Boleti, E., Deonarain, M., et al. 1995. Construction, expression and characterization of a single-chain anti-tumor antibody-IL-2 fusion protein. *Ann Oncol*, **6**, 945–7.
Bonardi, M.A., French, R.R., et al. 1993. Delivery of saporin to human B-cell lymphoma using bispecific antibody: targeting via CD22 but not CD19, CD37, or immunoglobulin results in efficient killing. *Cancer Res*, **53**, 3015–21.
Boulianne, G.L., Hozumi, N. and Shulman, M.J. 1984. Production of functional chimaeric mouse/human antibody. *Nature*, **312**, 643–6.
Bruggemann, M. and Neuberger, M.S. 1996. Strategies for expressing human antibody repertoires in transgenic mice. *Immunol Today*, **17**, 391–7.
Bruggemann, M., Spicer, C., et al. 1991. Human antibody production in transgenic mice: expression from 100 kb of the human IgH locus. *Eur J Immunol*, **21**, 1323–6.
Carter, P. 2001. Improving the efficacy of antibody-based cancer therapies. *Nat Rev Cancer*, **1**, 118–29.
Chapman, P.T., Jamar, F., et al. 1996. Use of a radiolabeled monoclonal antibody against E-selectin for imaging of endothelial activation in rheumatoid arthritis. *Arthritis Rheum*, **39**, 1371–5.
Chaudhary, V.K., Queen, C., et al. 1989. A recombinant immunotoxin consisting of two antibody variable domains fused to *Pseudomonas* exotoxin. *Nature*, **339**, 394–7.
Clackson, T., Hoogenboom, R., et al. 1991. Making antibody fragments using phage display libraries. *Nature*, **352**, 624–8.
Clark, M. 2000. Antibody humanization: a case of the 'Emperor's new clothes'? *Immunol Today*, **21**, 397–402.
Davies, J. and Riechmann, L. 1994. 'Camelising' human antibody fragments: NMR studies on VH domains. *FEBS Lett*, **339**, 285–90.
Davies, K.A., Erlandsson, K., et al. 1993. Splenic uptake of immune complexes in man is complement-dependent. *J Immunol*, **151**, 3866–73.
de-Kruif, J. and Logtenberg, T. 1996. Leucine zipper dimerized bivalent and bispecific scFv antibodies from a semi-synthetic antibody phage display library. *J Biol Chem*, **271**, 7630–4.
Demidem, A., Lam, T., et al. 1997. Chimeric anti-CD20 (IDEC-C2B8) monoclonal antibody sensitizes a B cell lymphoma cell line to cell killing by cytotoxic drugs. *Cancer Biother Radiopharm*, **12**, 177–86.
Ditzel, H.J., Binley, J.M., et al. 1995. Neutralizing recombinant human antibodies to a conformational V2- and CD4-binding site-sensitive epitope of HIV-1 gp120 isolated by using an epitope-masking procedure. *J Immunol*, **154**, 893–906.
Elliott, M.J., Maini, R.N., et al. 1993. Treatment of rheumatoid arthritis with chimeric monoclonal antibodies to tumor necrosis factor alpha. *Arthritis Rheum*, **36**, 1681-9, 0.
Elliott, M.J., Maini, R.N., et al. 1994a. Randomised double-blind comparison of chimeric monoclonal antibody to tumor necrosis factor alpha (cA2) versus placebo in rheumatoid arthritis. *Lancet*, **344**, 1105–10.
Elliott, M.J., Maini, R.N., et al. 1994b. Repeated therapy with monoclonal antibody to tumor necrosis factor alpha (cA2) in patients with rheumatoid arthritis. *Lancet*, **344**, 1125–7.
Emery, S.C. and Harris, W.J. 1995. Strategies for humanizing antibodies. In: Borrebaeck, C.A.K. (ed.), *Antibody engineering*. Oxford: Oxford University Press, 159–83.
Eshhar, Z. 1997. Tumor-specific T-bodies: towards clinical application. *Cancer Immunol Immunother*, **45**, 131–6.
Eshhar, Z., Waks, T., et al. 1993. Specific activation and targeting of cytotoxic lymphocytes through chimeric single chains consisting of antibody-binding domains and the γ or z subunits of the immunoglobulin and T-cell receptors. *Proc Natl Acad Sci USA*, **90**, 720–4.
Esteban, J.M., Colcher, D., et al. 1987. Quantitative and qualitative aspects of radiolocalization in colon cancer patients of intravenously administered MAb B72.3. *Int J Cancer*, **39**, 50–9.
Fearon, D.T. and Carroll, M.C. 2000. Regulation of B lymphocyte responses to foreign and self-antigens by the CD19/CD21 complex. *Annu Rev Immunol*, **18**, 393–422.
Fekade, D., Knox, K., et al. 1996. Prevention of Jarisch-Herxheimer reactions by treatment with antibodies against tumor necrosis factor alpha. *N Engl J Med*, **335**, 311–15.
Feldmann, M. and Maini, R.N. 2001. Anti-TNF alpha therapy of rheumatoid arthritis: what have we learned? *Annu Rev Immunol*, **19**, 163–96.
Fitch, J.C., Rollins, S., et al. 1999. Pharmacology and biological efficacy of a recombinant, humanized, single-chain antibody C5 complement inhibitor in patients undergoing coronary artery bypass graft surgery with cardiopulmonary bypass. *Circulation*, **100**, 2499–506.
French, R.R., Chan, H.T., et al. 1999. CD40 antibody evokes a cytotoxic T-cell response that eradicates lymphoma and bypasses T-cell help. *Nat Med*, **5**, 548–53.
French, R.R., Hamblin, T.J., et al. 1995. Treatment of B-cell lymphomas with combination of bispecific antibodies and saporin. *Lancet*, **346**, 223–4.
Gee, A., Moss, T., et al. 1992. Large-scale immunomagnetic separation system for the removal of tumor cells from bone marrow. *Prog Clin Biol Res*, **377**, 181–7.
George, A.J.T. and Epenetos, A.A. 1996. Advances in antibody engineering. *Expert Opinion on Therapeutic Patents*, **6**, 441–56.
George, A.J.T. and Gray, D. 1999. Receptor editing during affinity maturation. *Immunol Today*, **20**, 196.
George, A.J.T. and Huston, J.S. 1997. Bispecific antibody engineering. In: Zanetti, M. and Capra, J.D. (eds), *The antibodies*. Luxembourg: Harwood Academic Publishers, 99–141.
George, A.J.T., French, R.R. and Glennie, M.J. 1995a. Measurement of kinetic binding constants of a panel of anti-saporin antibodies using a resonant mirror biosensor. *J Immunol Methods*, **183**, 51–63.
George, A.J.T., Jamar, F., et al. 1995b. Radiometal labeling of recombinant proteins by a genetically engineered minimal chelation site: technetium-99m coordination by single-chain Fv antibody fusion proteins through a C-terminal cysteinyl peptide. *Proc Natl Acad Sci USA*, **92**, 8358–63.
Gilliland, L.K., Walsh, L.A., et al. 1999. Elimination of the immunogenicity of therapeutic antibodies. *J Immunol*, **162**, 3663–71.
Glennie, M.J. and Johnson, P.W. 2000. Clinical trials of antibody therapy. *Immunol Today*, **21**, 403–10.
Glennie, M.J., McBride, H.M., et al. 1987. Preparation and performance of bispecific $F(ab' \gamma)_2$ antibody containing thioether-linked Fab′ γ fragments. *J Immunol*, **139**, 2367–75.
Glockshuber, R., Malia, M., et al. 1990. A comparison of strategies to stabilize immunoglobulin Fv-fragments. *Biochemistry*, **29**, 1362–7.
Gould, B.J., Borowitz, M.J., et al. 1989. Phase I study of an anti-breast cancer immunotoxin by continuous infusion: report of a targeted toxic effect not predicted by animal studies. *J Natl Cancer Inst*, **81**, 775–81.
Greenwood, J. and Greenwood, C.M. 1993. Effector functions of matched sets of recombinant human IgG subclass antibodies. In: Greenwod, C.M. (ed.), *Protein engineering of antibody molecules for prophylactic and therapeutic applications in man*. Nottingham: Academic Titles, 85–100.
Griffiths, A.D., Malmqvist, M., et al. 1993. Human anti-self antibodies with high specificity from phage display libraries. *EMBO J*, **12**, 725–34.
Griffiths, A.D., Williams, S.C., et al. 1994. Isolation of high affinity human antibodies directly from large synthetic repertoires. *EMBO J*, **13**, 3245–60.
Grosse-Hovest, L., Brandl, M., et al. 1999. Tumor-growth inhibition with bispecific antibody fragments in a syngeneic mouse melanoma model: the role of targeted T-cell co-stimulation via CD28. *Int J Cancer*, **80**, 138–44.
Hale, G. and Waldmann, H. 2000. From laboratory to clinic. The story of CAMPATH-1. In: George, A.J.T. and Urch, C.E. (eds), *Diagnostic and therapeutic antibodies*. Totowa, NJ: Humana Press, 243–66.
Hamers-Casterman, C., Atarhouch, T., et al. 1993. Naturally occurring antibodies devoid of light chains. *Nature*, **363**, 446–8.
Hanes, J. and Pluckthun, A. 1997. In vitro selection and evolution of functional proteins by using ribosome display. *Proc Natl Acad Sci USA*, **94**, 4937–42.

Harari, O.A., Wickham, T.J., et al. 1999. Targeting an adenoviral gene vector to cytokine-activated vascular endothelium via E-selectin. *Gene Ther*, **6**, 801–7.

He, M. and Taussig, M.J. 1997. Antibody-ribosome-mRNA (ARM) complexes as efficient selection particles for in vitro display and evolution of antibody combining sites. *Nucleic Acids Res*, **25**, 5132–4.

Holliger, P., Prospero, T. and Winter, G. 1993. 'Diabodies': small bivalent and bispecific antibody fragments. *Proc Natl Acad Sci USA*, **90**, 6444–8.

Hudson, P.J. and Kortt, A.A. 1999. High avidity scFv multimers; diabodies and triabodies. *J Immunol Methods*, **231**, 177–89.

Huston, J.S., Levinson, D., et al. 1988. Protein engineering of antibody binding sites: recovery of specific activity in an anti-digoxin single-chain Fv analogue produced in *Escherichia coli*. *Proc Natl Acad Sci USA*, **85**, 5879–83.

Huston, J.S., Mudgett-Hunter, M., et al. 1991. Protein engineering of single-chain Fv analogs and fusion proteins. *Methods Enzymol*, **203**, 46–88.

Huston, J.S., George, A.J.T., et al. 1996a. Single-chain Fv radioimmunotargeting. *Q J Nucl Med*, **40**, 320–33.

Huston, J.S., Margolies, M.N. and Haber, E. 1996b. Antibody binding sites. *Adv Protein Chem*, **49**, 329–450.

Inbar, D., Hochman, J. and Givol, D. 1972. Localization of antibody-combining sites within the variable portions of heavy and light chains. *Proc Natl Acad Sci USA*, **69**, 2659–62.

Johns, M., George, A.J.T. and Ritter, M.A. 2000. In vivo selection of sFv from phage display libraries. *J Immunol Methods*, **239**, 137–51.

Johnson, P.W. and Glennie, M.J. 2001. Rituximab: mechanisms and applications. *Br J Cancer*, **85**, 1619–23.

Jones, P.T., Dear, P.H., et al. 1986. Replacing the complementarity-determining regions in a human antibody with those from a mouse. *Nature*, **321**, 522–5.

Junghans, R.P. 1997. Finally! The Brambell receptor (FcRB). Mediator of transmission of immunity and protection from catabolism for IgG. *Immunol Res*, **16**, 29–57.

Karpovsky, B., Titus, J.A., et al. 1984. Production of target-specific effector cells using hetero-cross-linked aggregates containing anti-target cell and anti-Fc gamma receptor antibodies. *J Exp Med*, **160**, 1686–701.

Kohler, G. and Milstein, C. 1975. Continuous cultures of fused cells secreting antibody of predefined specificity. *Nature*, **256**, 495–7.

Koide, A., Bailey, C.W., et al. 1998. The fibronectin type III domain as a scaffold for novel binding proteins. *J Mol Biol*, **28**, 1141–51.

Kostelny, S.A., Cole, M.S. and Tso, J.Y. 1992. Formation of a bispecific antibody by the use of leucine zippers. *J Immunol*, **148**, 1547–53.

Kreitman, R.J. 1999. Immunotoxins in cancer therapy. *Curr Opin Immunol*, **11**, 570–8.

Kreitman, R.J., Wilson, W.H., et al. 2001. Efficacy of the anti-CD22 recombinant immunotoxin BL22 in chemotherapy-resistant hairy-cell leukemia. *N Engl J Med*, **345**, 241–7.

Kurucz, I., Titus, J.A., et al. 1995. Retargeting of CTL by an efficiently refolded bispecific single-chain Fv dimer produced in bacteria. *J Immunol*, **154**, 4576–82.

Lane, A.C., Foroozan, S., et al. 1991. Enhanced modulation of antibodies coating guinea pig leukemic cells in vitro and in vivo. The role of Fc gamma R expressing cells. *J Immunol*, **146**, 2461–8.

Laune, D., Molina, F., et al. 1997. Systematic exploration of the antigen binding activity of synthetic peptides isolated from the variable regions of immunoglobulins. *J Biol Chem*, **272**, 30937–44.

Lenercept Multiple Sclerosis Study Group and the University of British Columbia MS/MRI Analysis Group, 1999. TNF neutralization in MS: results of a randomized, placebo-controlled multicenter study. The Lenercept Multiple Sclerosis Study Group and The University of British Columbia MS/MRI Analysis Group. *Neurology*, **53**, 457–65.

Lonberg, N., Taylor, L.D., et al. 1994. Antigen-specific human antibodies from mice comprising four distinct genetic modifications. *Nature*, **368**, 856–9.

McCafferty, J., Griffiths, A.D., et al. 1990. Phage antibodies: filamentous phage displaying antibody variable domains. *Nature*, **348**, 552–4.

McCartney, J.E., Tai, M.S., et al. 1995. Engineering disulfide-linked single chain Fv dimers [$(sFv')_2$] with improved solution and targeting properties: anti-digoxin $(sFv')_2$ and anti-c-erbB-2 741F8 $(sFv')_2$ made by protein folding and bonded through C-terminal cysteinyl peptides. *Protein Eng*, **8**, 301-14, 26–10.

McCloskey, R.V., Straube, R.C., et al. 1994. Treatment of septic shock with human monoclonal antibody HA-1A. A randomized, double-blind, placebo-controlled trial. CHESS Trial Study Group. *Ann Intern Med*, **121**, 1–5.

Maini, R., St Clair, E.W., et al. 1999. Infliximab (chimeric anti-tumor necrosis factor alpha monoclonal antibody) versus placebo in rheumatoid arthritis patients receiving concomitant methotrexate: a randomised phase III trial. ATTRACT Study Group. *Lancet*, **354**, 1932–9.

Marasco, W.A., LaVecchio, J. and Winkler, A. 1999. Human anti-HIV-1 tat sFv intrabodies for gene therapy of advanced HIV-1-infection and AIDS. *J Immunol Methods*, **231**, 223–38.

Marks, J.D., Griffiths, A.D., et al. 1992a. By-passing immunization: building high affinity human antibodies by chain shuffling. *Bio/technology*, **10**, 779–83.

Marks, J.D., Hoogenboom, H.R., et al. 1992b. Molecular evolution of proteins on filamentous phage. Mimicking the strategy of the immune system. *J Biol Chem*, **267**, 16007–10.

Mendez, M.J., Green, L.L., et al. 1997. Functional transplant of megabase human immunoglobulin loci recapitulates human antibody response in mice. *Nat Genet*, **15**, 146–56.

Mhashilkar, A.M., Bagley, J., et al. 1995. Inhibition of HIV-1 Tat-mediated LTR transactivation and HIV-1 infection by anti-Tat single chain intrabodies. *EMBO J*, **14**, 1542–51.

Milenic, D.E., Yokota, T., et al. 1991. Construction, binding properties, metabolism, and tumor targeting of a single-chain Fv derived from the pancarcinoma monoclonal antibody CC49. *Cancer Res*, **51**, 6363–71.

Miller, G.W. and Nussenzweig, V. 1975. A new complement function: solubilization of antigen-antibody aggregates. *Proc Natl Acad Sci USA*, **72**, 418–22.

Miller, R.A., Maloney, D.G., et al. 1982. Treatment of B-cell lymphoma with monoclonal anti-idiotype antibody. *N Engl J Med*, **306**, 517–22.

Milstein, C. and Cuello, A.C. 1983. Hybrid hybridomas and their use in immunohistochemistry. *Nature*, **305**, 537–40.

Moise, K.J. Jr. 2002. Management of rhesus alloimmunization in pregnancy. *Obstet Gynecol*, **100**, 600–11.

Morrison, S.L., Johnson, M.J., et al. 1984. Chimeric human antibody molecules: mouse antigen-binding domains with human constant region domains. *Proc Natl Acad Sci USA*, **81**, 6851–5.

Neuberger, M.S., Williams, G.T. and Fox, R.O. 1984. Recombinant antibodies possessing novel effector functions. *Nature*, **312**, 604–8.

Newton, D.L. and Rybak, S.M. 2001. Preparation and preclinical characterization of RNase-based immunofusion proteins. *Methods Mol Biol*, **160**, 387–406.

Nicholson, I.C., Zou, X., et al. 1999. Antibody repertoires of four- and five-feature translocus mice carrying human immunoglobulin heavy chain and κ and λ light chain yeast artificial chromosomes. *J Immunol*, **163**, 6898–906.

Niculescu-Duvaz, I., Friedlos, F., et al. 1999. Prodrugs for antibody- and gene-directed enzyme prodrug therapies (ADEPT and GDEPT). *Anticancer Drug Dev*, **14**, 517–38.

Olsnes, S. and Kozlov, J.V. 2001. Ricin. *Toxicon*, **39**, 1723–8.

Oral, H.B. and Akdis, C.A. 2000. Antibody-based therapies in infectious diseases. In: George, A.J.T. and Urch, C.E. (eds), *Diagnostic and therapeutic antibodies*. Totowa, NJ: Humana Press, 157–78.

Owens, G.P., Williamson, R.A., et al. 2000. Cloning the antibody response in humans with chronic inflammatory disease: immunopanning of subacute sclerosing panencephalitis (SSPE) brain sections with antibody phage libraries prepared from SSPE brain enriches for antibody recognizing measles virus antigens in situ. *J Virol*, **74**, 1533–7.

Padlan, E.A. 1991. A possible procedure for reducing the immunogenicity of antibody variable domains while preserving their ligand-binding properties. *Mol Immunol*, **28**, 489–98.

Palmer, D.B., George, A.J.T. and Ritter, M.A. 1997. Selection of antibodies to cell surface determinants on mouse thymic epithelial cells using a phage display library. *Immunology*, **91**, 473–8.

Palmer, D.B., Crompton, T., et al. 1999. Intrathymic function of the human cortical epithelial cell surface antigen gp200-MR6: single chain antibodies to evolutionarily conserved determinants disrupt mouse thymus development. *Immunology*, **96**, 236–45.

Park, B.W., Zhang, H.T., et al. 2000. Rationally designed anti-HER2/neu peptide mimetic disables P185HER2/neu tyrosine kinases in vitro and in vivo. *Nat Biotechnol*, **18**, 194–8.

Pepys, M.B. 1974. Role of complement in induction of antibody production in vivo. Effect of cobra factor and other C3-reactive agents on thymus-dependent and thymus-independent antibody responses. *J Exp Med*, **140**, 126–45.

Perez, P., Hoffman, W., et al. 1985. Specific targeting of cytotoxic T cells by anti-T3 linked to anti-target cell antibody. *Nature*, **316**, 354–6.

Pilstrom, L. 2002. The mysterious immunoglobulin light chain. *Dev Comp Immunol*, **26**, 207–15.

Poznansky, M.C., La Vecchio, J., et al. 1999. Inhibition of human immunodeficiency virus replication and growth advantage of CD4+ T cells and monocytes derived from CD34+ cells transduced with an intracellular antibody directed against human immunodeficiency virus type 1 Tat. *Hum Gene Ther*, **10**, 2505–14.

Ravetch, J.V. and Bolland, S. 2001. IgG Fc receptors. *Annu Rev Immunol*, **19**, 275–90.

Reichmann, L., Clark, M., et al. 1988. Reshaping human antibodies for therapy. *Nature*, **322**, 323–7.

Richardson, J.H., Sodroski, J.G., et al. 1995. Phenotypic knockout of the high-affinity human interleukin 2 receptor by intracellular single-chain antibodies against the alpha subunit of the receptor. *Proc Natl Acad Sci USA*, **92**, 3137–41.

Roguska, M.A., Pedersen, J.T., et al. 1994. Humanization of murine monoclonal antibodies through variable domain resurfacing. *Proc Natl Acad Sci USA*, **91**, 969–73.

Schindler, J., Sausville, E., et al. 2001. The toxicity of deglycosylated ricin A chain-containing immunotoxins in patients with non-Hodgkin's lymphoma is exacerbated by prior radiotherapy: a retrospective analysis of patients in five clinical trials. *Clin Cancer Res*, **7**, 255–8.

Segal, D.M., Urch, C.E., et al. 1992. Bispecific antibodies in cancer treatment. In: DeVita, V.T.J., Hellman, S. and Rosenberg, S.A. (eds), *Biologic therapy of cancer updates*. Philadelphia: Lippincott, 1–12.

Segal, D.M., Weiner, G.J. and Weiner, L.M. 1999. Bispecific antibodies in cancer therapy. *Curr Opin Immunol*, **11**, 558–62.

Silverstein, A.M. 1988. *A history of immunology*. San Diego, CA: Academic Press.

Snider, D.P. and Segal, D.M. 1989. Efficiency of antigen presentation after antigen targeting to surface IgD, IgM, MHC, FcγRII and B220 molecules on murine splenic B cells. *J Immunol*, **143**, 59–65.

Snider, D.P., Kaubisch, A. and Segal, D.M. 1990. Enhanced antigen immunogenicity induced by bispecific antibodies. *J Exp Med*, **171**, 1957–63.

Syrigos, K.N. and Epenetos, A.A. 1999. Antibody directed enzyme prodrug therapy (ADEPT): a review of the experimental and clinical considerations. *Anticancer Res*, **19**, 605–13.

Tan, P.H., Manunta, M., et al. 2003. Antibody targeted gene transfer to endothelium. *J Gene Med*, **5**, 311–23.

Targan, S.R., Hanauer, S.B., et al. 1997. A short-term study of chimeric monoclonal antibody cA2 to tumor necrosis factor alpha for Crohn's disease. Crohn's Disease cA2 Study Group. *N Engl J Med*, **337**, 1029–35.

Taylor, P.C. 2000. Antibodies for inflammatory disease. In: George, A.J.T. and Urch, C.E. (eds), *Diagnostic and therapeutic antibodies*. Totowa, NJ: Humana Press, 115–39.

Taylor, P.R., Carugati, A., et al. 2000. A hierarchical role for classical pathway complement proteins in the clearance of apoptotic cells in vivo. *J Exp Med*, **192**, 359–66.

Thrush, G.R., Lark, L.R., et al. 1996. Immunotoxins: an update. *Annu Rev Immunol*, **14**, 49–71.

Tomizuka, K., Shinohara, T., et al. 2000. Double trans-chromosomic mice: maintenance of two individual human chromosome fragments containing Ig heavy and kappa loci and expression of fully human antibodies. *Proc Natl Acad Sci USA*, **97**, 722–7.

Turner, D.J., Ritter, M.A. and George, A.J.T. 1997. Importance of the linker in expression of single-chain Fv antibody fragments: optimisation of peptide sequence using phage display technology. *J Immunol Methods*, **205**, 43–54.

Tutt, A., Stevenson, G.T. and Glennie, M.J. 1991. Trispecific $F(ab')_3$ derivatives that use cooperative signaling via the TCR/CD3 complex and CD2 to activate and redirect resting cytotoxic T cells. *J Immunol*, **147**, 60–9.

Tutt, A.L., O'Brien, L., et al. 2002. T cell immunity to lymphoma following treatment with anti-CD40 monoclonal antibody. *J Immunol*, **168**, 2720–8.

van Spriel, A.B., van Ojik, H.H. and van De Winkel, J.G. 2000. Immunotherapeutic perspective for bispecific antibodies. *Immunol Today*, **21**, 391–7.

Verma, R., Boleti, E. and George, A.J.T. 1998. Antibody engineering: comparison of bacterial, yeast, insect and mammalian expression systems. *J Immunol Methods*, **216**, 165–81.

Villanueva, F.S., Janowski, R.J., et al. 1998. Microbubbles targeted to intercellular adhesion molecule-1 bind to activated coronary artery endothelial cells. *Circulation*, **98**, 1–5.

Vuist, W.M., Levy, R. and Maloney, D.G. 1994. Lymphoma regression induced by monoclonal anti-idiotypic antibodies correlates with their ability to induce Ig signal transduction and is not prevented by tumor expression of high levels of bcl-2 protein. *Blood*, **83**, 899–906.

Walport, M.J. 2001a. Complement. First of two parts. *N Engl J Med*, **344**, 1058–66.

Walport, M.J. 2001b. Complement. Second of two parts. *N Engl J Med*, **344**, 1140–4.

Ward, E.S., Güssow, D., et al. 1989. Binding activity of a repertoire of single immunoglobulin variable domains secreted from *Escherichia coli*. *Nature*, **341**, 544–6.

Warmerdam, P.A., van der Winkel, J.G., et al. 1990. Molecular basis for a polymorphism of human Fc gamma receptor II (CD32). *J Exp Med*, **172**, 19–25.

Weissleder, R. and Mahmood, U. 2001. Molecular imaging. *Radiology*, **219**, 316–33.

Whitlow, M., Filpula, D., et al. 1994. Multivalent Fvs: characterization of single-chain Fv oligomers and preparation of a bispecific Fv. *Protein Eng*, **7**, 1017–26.

Winter, G., Griffiths, A.D., et al. 1994. Making antibodies by phage display technology. *Annu Rev Immunol*, **12**, 433–55.

Yang, W.P., Green, K., et al. 1995. CDR walking mutagenesis for the affinity maturation of a potent human anti-HIV-1 antibody into the picomolar range. *J Mol Biol*, **254**, 392–403.

Yarden, Y. and Sliwkowski, M.X. 2001. Untangling the ErbB signaling network. *Nat Rev Mol Cell Biol*, **2**, 127–37.

Zhang, X., Piatier-Tonneau, D., et al. 1996. Synthetic CD4 exocyclic peptides antagonize CD4 holoreceptor binding and T cell activation. *Nat Biotechnol*, **14**, 472–5.

19

Processing and presentation of antigen by the class II histocompatibility system

EMIL R. UNANUE

INTRODUCTION

Antigen presentation involves the interaction between the T cell and an antigen-presenting cell (APC) responsible for the uptake and intracellular handling of the protein. All T cells recognize antigen molecules that are presented in the context of histocompatibility molecules. The molecules encoded in the major histocompatibility gene complex (MHC) bind peptides derived from the fragmentation of the protein antigen and present these to T cells. It is the peptide–MHC complex, which constitutes the antigenic determinant, that the T cell recognizes. It follows that all proteins need to be processed by an APC in order for peptides to be generated. Without antigen presentation there is no recognition of the protein by the lymphocyte system (for a historical summary, see Unanue 2002). The two major stable sets of T cells, the CD4 and the CD8 T cells, each recognize peptides that are bound to different sets of MHC molecules. The set of MHC class I (MHCI) molecules present peptides to the CD8 T cells, whereas the MHCII molecules present peptides to the CD4 T cells. The MHCI molecules, examined in (see Chapter 21, MHC class I antigen processing system), mainly sample the cytosol of the APCs, whereas in contrast the MHCII molecules preferentially sample the vesicular system. In this way, the MHC molecules contain peptides from proteins that have entered the two major cellular compartments of the APCs. Thus, viruses, intracellular bacteria, or parasites that enter the cytosol are recognized primarily by the CD8 T cells which recognize the peptide antigen–MHCI complex (Rock and Goldberg 1999; Yewdell and Bennink 1999). In contrast, soluble proteins or proteins derived from phagocytosed organisms are presented to CD4 T cells that recognize the peptide–MHCII complex. There are other MHC molecules expressed in lower amounts which can present certain unique molecules, e.g. the MHCI-like molecule H-2M3, binds to small hydrophobic peptides that contain formlymethionine at its amino terminus (Lindahl et al. 1997). The CD1 molecules bind to glycolipids, including those derived from *Mycobacterium tuberculosis* (Porcelli et al. 1992). T cells directed to these MHC complexes may have a role in antimicrobial immunity. This chapter, based on a previous review (Unanue 2001), considers antigen processing and presentation by the MHCII molecules.

It is important, in the context of microbial immunity, to understand how the immune system has evolved to deal with either protein or polysaccharide antigens. The former involve the T cells, as indicated above, by recognition of products of antigen processing, as well as B cells, which can recognize the proteins before catabolism. The end result of a productive encounter with protein antigens is both the production of antibody and the development of a T-cell response – cellular immunity. The T-cell response is long-lived and heightens on repeated immunization, a fundamental feature of prophylactic immunization – the recall response associated with immunization. With the T-cell response

Table 19.1 *Responses to carbohydrates and protein antigens*

	Pure polysaccharide	Protein
B-cell recognition	Yes	Yes
T-cell recognition	No	Yes
Binding to MHC molecules	No	Yes
Activation of CD4 T cells	No	Yes
T-cell memory	No	Yes
Delayed sensitivity response	No	Yes
Antibody affinity changes	No	Yes

there follows the capacity to activate macrophages and to form the immune granulomas. An important clinical demonstration of the T-cell response is the 'delayed sensitivity' skin reaction that takes place on injection of a minute amount of the antigen into the skin of the immunized individual. This small indurated lesion indicates that the patient has encountered the microbe, and has activated T cells. With regard to the B-cell response, it is characterized by high-affinity antibodies of the various subclasses, which is an indication of affinity-driven maturation by T-cell 'help'.

In contrast, pure carbohydates do not stimulate T cells and only induce a B-cell response that is limited in the range of its response. Immunological memory is poor. There is no delayed sensitivity response. The antibody response shows poor affinity maturation and is mostly represented by IgM antibodies.

This difference in T-cell responses between proteins and pure polysaccharides is explained because carbohydrates do not interact with MHC molecules (Harding et al. 1991; Ishioka et al. 1992). Without an MHC molecule to serve as a carrier of the foreign entity, T cells will not recognize it. Knowing this difference, vaccines against bacterial polysaccharides are now produced by conjugating the carbohydrate to an immunogenic 'carrier' protein, in order also to elicit a T-cell response (Schneerson et al. 1980; Insel and Anderson 1986). Table 19.1 compares both responses.

THE INNATE SYSTEM OF DEFENSE, APCS, AND SYMBIOSIS WITH T CELLS

The APC cellular system is essential for antigen presentation. Three main cells are involved in presentation; two are derived from the monocyte lineage: the dendritic cells (DC) and the macrophages. They belong to the 'innate' cellular system that operates independently of the lymphocyte lineage (Janeway and Medzhitov 2002). These cells sample and handle moieties from the extracellular milieu, and are therefore essential APCs. The second APCs are the B cells which are involved in the interaction with CD4 T cells during antibody formation.

There is an intimate, truly symbiotic relationship between the innate cellular system and the lymphocyte (Unanue 1981, 1997). The innate system is represented by cells of monocyte lineage: the granulocytes and the natural killer (NK) cells. Only those cells derived from the monocytes are APCs. The cells of the innate system sample the environment, constituting the earliest system of defense that reacts to the presence of diverse pathogens. The innate system is phylogenetically older and represented by the amebocytes and phagocytes of invertebrates (Hoffmann et al. 1999). This is the cellular system first described by Metchnikoff in his classic studies of the phagocytes as an essential defense cellular system (Metchnikoff 1968). In vertebrates, the innate system can effectively handle a number of pathogens but it is incapable of resolving the infections entirely, and importantly will show the property of neither specificity in recognition nor immunological memory.

The phagocytes recognize many bacteria and microorganisms through 'pattern recognition' in which the polysaccharides, lipoproteins, and other moieties are seen as a whole (see Chapter 7, Pattern recognition). Phagocytes contain a number of cell surface molecules that allow them to handle a wide range of pathogens (see below). Phagocytes, and in general the cells of the innate system, obey chemical signals from a variety of secreted polypeptides – the family of cytokines and chemokines produced by the lymphocytes (Buchmeier and Schreiber 1985; reviewed in Luster 2002). As a result, the innate system heightens its capacity to deal with, and eliminates, a number of pathogens once the lymphocyte enters the scene. The lymphocyte system, on the other hand, can effectively eliminate pathogens, have exquisite specificity of recognition, and importantly shows memory – the basis of prophylactic immunization. The operation is, however, truly symbiotic, inasmuch as the lymphocyte is blind to antigens unless the antigen molecules are presented by the phagocytes (referring to DCs and macrophages), by way of their MHC molecules, during antigen presentation. During handling of the antigen molecules, the phagocytes also release a number of cytokines, which help in the early recruitment and activation of the lymphocytes (Hsieh et al. 1993) (Figure 19.1). As the phagocyte system needs to be 'activated' through a number of cytokines elaborated by the lymphocytes, the loop of cell-to-cell interaction is evident, each cell critically depending on the other. The communication between the two interacting cellular systems is by way of antigen presentation via MHCII molecules as well as by cytokines. It is antigen presentation that imparts specificity to the system because the recognition of the presenting antigens recruits the specific clones of T cells. A comparison of the two recognition systems is shown in Table 19.2.

A highly informative experimental model of infection that brings out the symbiotic relationship between the innate and adaptive system is that of *Listeria mono-*

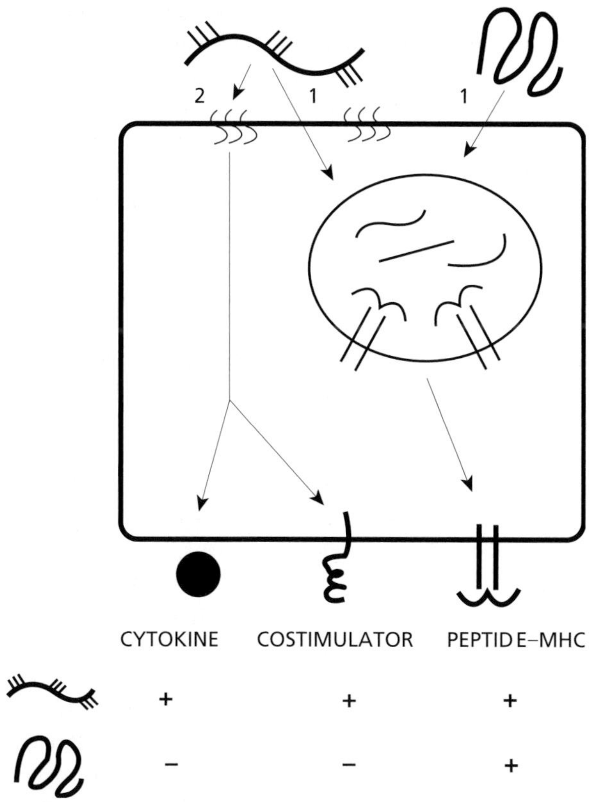

Figure 19.1 *Graphic representation of the results of two kinds of interactions of an antigen-presenting cell (APC). A bacterium (left side, top) will generate peptides after it is internalized (pathway indicated as 1), but will also activate (pathway 2) Toll-like receptors (TLRs). Pathway 1 will yield peptide–MHC complex to T-cell recognition. Pathway 2 will result in secretion of soluble cytokines and the presence of membrane costimulatory molecules. All three components are required for optimal T-cell activation. A protein (right, top) will give rise to peptide–MHC complex after it is processed, but will not induce cytokine or costimulation and will not productively activate T cells.*

cytogenes infection in the inbred mouse (Mackanness 1962; reviewed in Unanue 1997). *Listeria* species is an intracellular pathogen that is taken up by macrophages where it escapes from the phagocytic vacuole to multiply in the cytoplasm. *Listeria* infection proceeds through various stages: first there is an early neutrophil component that partially contains the growth particularly in the liver; this is followed by a phase in which the macrophages curb *Listeria* replication while also releasing inflammatory cytokines such as the interleukins IL-1, IL-12, and IL-18 and tumor necrosis factor (TNF). These cytokines then lead to an activation of various cells including NK cells as well as CD4 and CD8 T cells. The last are activated by presentation of *Listeria* antigens and then participate in the complete elimination of the bacteria. Mice that only have an innate system, as happens in mice with the severe combined immunodeficiency (SCID) mutation, which lack lymphocytes, will not result in sterilizing immunity although the growth of *Listeria* monocytogen is partially contained. SCID mice will become carriers of the infection but will eliminate *Listeria* sp. completely if reconstituted with T cells. Both CD4 and CD8 kill *Listeria* monocytogen found in phagocytes or epithelial or mesenchymal cells.

With regard to APCs, four conditions are required for them to be effective in antigen presentation. First, the cells must have the capacity to take up proteins, which they do by various molecular systems. Second, the APCs must have the internal cellular machinery to enable them to process proteins. All cells have a lysosomal system that allows them to handle endocytosed proteins. Thus, as far as their capacity to present is concerned, it will depend to a major extent whether the MHC molecules are expressed. Indeed, many cell lines that do not express MHCII molecules will do so if transfected with the genes encoding MHC genes. Lastly, for effective antigen presentation APCs must also express other molecules that allow for stimulation of the T cell.

Dendritic cells derive from the blood monocyte and inhabit many tissues, where they are highly effective in antigen presentation (Inaba et al. 1983; Banchereau and Steinman 1998; Lanzavecchia and Sallusto 2001; Guermonprez et al. 2002). DCs circulate in small numbers in blood and are rapidly mobilized to sites of infection. Monocytes also differentiate to DCs as they cross into the tissues. In the lymphoid organs, DCs constitute a network of interdigitating cells located mainly in the deep cortex of the lymph nodes, or the periarteriolar sheath of the spleen. DCs express receptors for some chemokines such as CCR7 which regulates their migration into lymphoid organs (Tang and Cyster 1999). DCs are found in the skin, as Langerhans' cells, situated between the keratinocytes: on interaction with antigens that contact the skin, they migrate into the draining node and there recruit specific T cells. DCs are also found in the thymus where they play a vital role in the process of presentation of autologous proteins. DCs are divided into two subsets called myeloid and lymphoid,

Table 19.2 *Comparison of innate and adaptive immunity*

	Innate	Adaptive: B cell	Adaptive: T cell
Antigen recognition	Nonclonal	Clonal	Clonal
Antigen receptors	Many	Single	Single
MHC involvement for recognition	No	No	Yes
Memory	No	Yes	Yes

A clonal system refers to B and T cells, each of which express only one set of antigen receptors having unique specificity. The adaptive system is therefore a selection by antigen of those B and T cells with receptors of high affinity. The cells of the innate system can identify more than one foreign antigen.

distinguished by the presence of the C8 α protein, in the latter.

Dendritic cells are highly effective in interacting with T cells (Lanzavecchia and Sallusto 2001). Their expression of both class I and II MHC molecules is high and constitutive. DCs also express adhesion and costimulatory molecules. DCs show long cytoplasmic extensions which favor the intimate physical contact with T cells. DCs can be generated from bone marrow cells in the presence of the cytokine granulocyte–macrophage colony-stimulating factor (GM-CSF) (Inaba et al. 1992; Sallusto and Lanzavecchia 1994). These in vitro cells can present antigens and have been used in transplantation studies to immunize, particularly in cancer immunotherapy (Nestle et al. 2001).

Dendritic cells evolve through various stages of maturation (Thery and Amigorena 2001; Guermonprez et al. 2002). The immature DCs express low levels of adhesion and costimulatory molecules, although their processing of antigens is not impaired. On interaction with a variety of stimuli, DCs increase their expression of the adhesion and costimulatory molecules and become more effective in antigen presentation. Among the stimuli are cytokines such as TNF-α or IL-1, both gram-positive and -negative bacteria, and their products, such as endotoxins, double-stranded RNA, and interaction with the CD40 ligand (Inaba et al. 1993; Cella et al. 1996, 1999; Randolph et al. 1998).

Macrophages were the first cells to be identified as APCs (Unanue 2002). Derived from monocytes by way of interaction with the cytokine CSF-1 (or M-CSF), macrophages inhabit many tissues, particularly around blood vessels where they sample the extracellular fluid (see Chapter 3, Phagocytes part 1: macrophages). Macrophages have an important effector function in their uptake and handling of microbes. Their microbicidal activity is readily enhanced by contact with cytokines particularly with interferon-γ and TNF. Macrophages secrete a large number of important cytokines that are involved in the early stages of an immune response. Macrophages differentiate in tissues influenced by the local environment of the tissue. They express low levels of MHC molecules and their antigen-presenting function can be limited unless activated by interferon, which markedly increases their expression.

B cells express constitutively both class I and II molecules and have an important antigen-presenting role in the interaction with CD4 T cells (Chesnut et al. 1982; MacPherson et al. 1999). This interaction leads to antibody formation in a two-step process: first, B cells bind the antigen by way of their specific membrane-bound antibody (Lanzavecchia 1990), after which the protein is processed, leading to the expression and presentation of the peptide–MHC complex; second the cloned T cell then recognizes the complex leading to their reciprocal activation. The final result is a reciprocal activation of both cells: the T lymphocyte will continue its activation while the B cell proliferates and differentiates, evolving into an antibody-forming cell. The end product is the release of antibody molecules that are identical in their specificity to the original antibody on the B-cell surface. These antibodies can be directed to conformational determinants of the protein. Thus, the result is the release of antibodies to conformational determinants of the protein and T cells that recognize linear sequences of the same. Immature B cells have limited antigen-presenting capacity, which increases as the B cell is activated.

ANTIGEN PRESENTATION IN THYMUS AND PERIPHERAL LYMPHOID ORGANS

Antigen presentation takes place during the response to foreign molecules that enter the tissues, including the lymphoid tissues. The encounter of the phagocytes with antigen results in the selection of T cell, with complementary receptors to the peptide–MHC complex displayed on the APC surface. The exact events involve several steps where cytokines and chemokines are released, resulting in increases in vascular permeability and cell migration to the foci of antigen–APC interaction. The end result is the recruitment of the antigen-specific T-cell clones, leading to their proliferation and the release of cytokines. Clonal enlargement results in an increase in specific lymphocytes and a more effective process for elimination of the foreign antigen. The cytokines released by T cells markedly influence the cellular environment, fostering growth and differentiation as well as activation of phagocytes. From this process, the phagocytes change their behavior to a cell more active in cytocidal activity and capable of eliminating a range of microorganisms.

T cells also encounter peptide–MHC during their normal process of maturation in the thymus gland. The nature of this encounter is very different from that described above, in that the peptides that form the complex do not derive from foreign molecules (which normally do not enter the thymus gland), but from the processing of self-proteins. It is this encounter that influences the fate of the early T cells during its normal process of differentiation. The thymus contains in its cortex a network of epithelial cells that express MHCII molecules (in contrast to most epithelial cells which do not). It also contains DCs particularly in the area between cortex and medulla, and in the medullary area itself. As the thymocyte matures, it expresses by random rearrangements of its receptor genes, antigen receptors (T-cell receptor (TCR)) that may or may not have specific complementarity to the autologous peptide–MHC complexes. This normally engages amino acid residues from the peptide, and also segments of the MHC molecules itself, around the area that binds the peptide. Thus, it is a receptor with a dual specificity (Garcia et al. 1996; Garboczi et al. 1996; Reinherz et al. 1999).

Three developments take place during the differentiation of the T cell, depending on the nature of the TCR and the MHC molecules with which it can interact (reviewed in von Boehmer 1990; Robey and Fowlkes 1994; Jameson et al. 1995; Borowski et al. 2002). A T cell with a TCR that does not match or complement the autologous peptide–MHC dies by 'neglect'. A T cell that encounters a perfect match will also die, a process called 'negative selection' (Kappler et al. 1987; Kisielow et al. 1988a, 1988b). Through this negative selection event, a number of autoreactive T cells are eliminated and therefore autoimmunity is prevented. In both these processes the T cell dies by apoptosis. Finally, a T cell with a receptor that matches the MHC, but matches the peptide poorly, matures, leaves the thymus, enters the recirculating pool of blood T cells, and seeds the lymphoid organs (Kisielow et al. 1988b). This process of 'positive selection' results in the survival and selection of T cells with TCRs that interact with self-MHC molecules, and particularly with peptides other than the autologous ones presented in the thymus, i.e. peptides from foreign proteins.

This process of T-cell maturation, in which T cells are selected to recognize a peptide and its own MHC molecule, explains the important phenomenon known as 'MHC restriction', which is characteristic of antigen presentation (Rosenthal and Shevach 1973; Zinkernagel and Doherty 1974). The mature T cells only recognize peptides derived from proteins presented by an APC that displays its own MHC molecules. In an outbred population, where the MHC shows marked allelic polymorphism, a T cell with specificity for a protein processed by its own APCs will not recognize the protein presented by an APC of a different individual. The fundamental reason is that the T cell is constrained as a result of the nature of the thymic selection process in recognizing its own MHC proteins. The phenomenon of MHC restriction was discovered for both CD4 and CD8 T cells when antigen-specific cells from one inbred strain of experimental animals were combined in culture with APCs of strains with different MHC alleles. (The experiments that discovered restriction in the MHCII molecule are shown in Table 19.3.) The same results were obtained when studying T- and B-cell interactions (Katz and Unanue 1973). Apart from the fact that this phenomenon was instrumental in pointing to the basic rules of APC–T-cell interaction, it also has practical applications. The clinical relevance is to the use of antigen-specific T cells for immunotherapy of patients with infectious diseases. For example, specific T-cell clones that can be generated ex vivo will not be useful unless they are transplanted in individuals who share the same MHC alleles.

MHCII MOLECULES

Every species contains an MHC gene complex that encodes for a number of class I and class II molecules. In humans, the complex is the HLA gene complex encoded in chromosome 6. The HLA gene complex includes genes that encode for the α and β chains of MHCII molecules, for the heavy chain of several MHCI molecules and genes for several complement proteins. The MHCII molecules contain two transmembrane chains, termed α and β, that assemble to create the peptide-binding site. The MHC of the mouse is H-2, discovered first by transplantation biologists who identified it as a system of cell-surface antigens with multiple alleles, responsible for tissue rejection.

The major function of class I and II molecules is to bind peptides, creating the complex that forms the substrate for T-cell recognition (Babbitt et al. 1985). One important feature of the MHC gene complex is its large degree of allelic polymorphism. The allelic differences are accounted for by several amino acids located in the region of the molecules that bind to peptides. The evolutionary pressure for diversification of the MHC and its selection is probably accounted for by microbial and parasitic infections (reviewed in Klein et al. 1993; Dawkins et al. 1999; Parham 1999). The argument goes

Table 19.3 *Rosenthal–Shevach experiment showing major histocompatibility complex (MHC) restriction for the presentation of purified protein derivative (PPD)*

Macrophages		T lymphocytes (cpm × 10^{-3})		
Strain	PPD	Strain 2	Strain 13	Strain (2 × 13) F1
2	–	0.9	5.7	1.6
2	+	26.4	8.6	7.0
13	–	4.6	1.7	1.8
13	+	3.1	19.9	7.8
(2 × 13) F1	–	1.9	4.3	1.7
(2 × 13) F1	+	12.4	11.8	12.6

The two inbred strains of guinea pigs, named 2 and 13, differ at their class II MHC gene locus. The guinea pigs were immunized with dried tubercle bacillus in water in oil emulsion. Their T cells were isolated and cultured with macrophages from normal guinea pigs, in the absence or presence of PPD of *Mycobacterium tuberculosis*. Strain 2 lymphocytes responded only to PPD presented by macrophages of strain 2, and the same applied to lymphocytes from strain 13. Note the mild mixed lymphocytic reaction when lymphocytes from 2 or 13 are incubated with macrophages of strains 13 or 2, respectively. Modified from Rosenthal and Shevach (1973).

that the more polymorphism there is in the species, the more the diversity of peptides is selected from microbes, and the better protected is the species to face infectious agents. Examples are known of HLA alleles favoring protection against malaria and leprosy (Piazza et al. 1973; Hill et al. 1991). Conversely, situations in nature that have reduced MHC polymorphism translate into enhanced susceptibility to infection (O'Brien and Yuhki 1999). This occurs in some examples of cheetahs, tigers, and Florida panthers (O'Brien and Yuhki 1999).

MHC molecules are peptide-binding molecules that select peptides from intracellular digestion of the protein (Babbitt et al. 1985; Bjorkman et al. 1987b; Unanue 2002). Both MHC molecules contain a single binding site that accommodates peptides of varying lengths. The MHCI molecule is made up of a single transmembrane glycopolypeptide – a heavy chain of about 44 kDa that folds in its amino terminus to create the binding site. It also contains a small polypeptide called β_2-microglobulin that gives structure to the heavy chain. The MHCII molecules contain two extracellular transmembrane chains, α and β, of about 20–30 kDa, which together create the binding site. The binding site of both class I and II molecules is similar with a platform of β-pleated sheets and two helical walls, between which is located the peptide (Bjorkman et al. 1987a, 1987b; Stern et al. 1994; Madden 1995).

Each MHC molecule binds one peptide, usually in the range of a nanomolar or micromolar affinity constant. The interaction of MHC molecules with peptides has been studied in binding interactions using purified molecules and peptides (Babbitt et al. 1985, 1986; Buus et al. 1987a, 1987b). By creating single or multiple changes in the composition of the peptides, the specificity of the interactions and the contributions of a given residue to binding strength can be determined. Peptides usually bind with a slow on-rate but, once bound, the dissociation rate from the complex is slow. It translates into peptides in the live APCs being maintained for a relatively long period of time.

The structural studies of MHC molecules containing peptides are important for understanding the nature of the binding (Brown et al. 1993; Stern et al. 1994; Fremont et al. 1998a, 1998b; Scott et al. 1998; Latek and Unanue 1999). In the MHC molecules, the various residues responsible for the allelic differences are situated in sites combining class I and II MHC molecules. These various residues constitute allele-specific binding sites or 'pockets' which accommodate different amino acids from the peptide. For each MHC allelic form, there are usually four to five sites: P1, P4, P6, P7, and P9. These accommodate the various side chains of the peptide, which is stretched through the combining site. For many alleles one or two of these pocket sites are mainly responsible for both binding the peptide and its specificity. The binding results from two main interactions, that of the peptide amino acid side chains with the pockets and that of the peptide backbone with conserved residues of the MHC binding sites, through which a large network of hydrogen bonds is created (Chicz et al. 1992; Hammer et al. 1992; Hunt et al. 1992; Sinigaglia and Hammer 1995; Suri et al. 2002).

What are the features of peptides presented by the class II molecules that CD4 T cells recognize? Peptides presented by class II MHC molecules are usually longer than 10 amino acids whereas those presented by class I are eight to nine residues in length. The peptides contain a 'core' of nine amino acids and flanking residues of varying lengths (reviewed in Latek and Unanue 1999). In the peptide core sequence, some amino acid side chains interact with the allele-specific pockets, mentioned above. The flank residues are important in contributing to binding strength and to the stability of the MHC–peptide complex. Class II peptides vary in the length of their flanks; in fact many peptides are selected as families made of the core with flanks of varying length. Two to three amino acid side chains of the peptide are solvent exposed and potentially capable of binding to the TCR.

It is important to note that the MHC molecules bind to self and foreign peptides equally well (Babbitt et al. 1986). This is evident from the description of thymic maturation, which involves interaction with self-peptides. It follows that, because self-proteins are always normally being processed, there is always the potential to develop autoimmunity. Indeed, a series of autoimmune diseases are known to develop in which autoreactive T cells recognize self-peptides bound to MHC molecules.

The process of protein processing and presentation between class I and II molecules differs in important respects. Suffice it to state here that class I molecules have evolved to recognize peptides resulting from cytosolic catabolism, which are then taken into the endoplasmic reticulum where the complex is assembled (Townsend et al. 1986). Class II molecules, as indicated before, mainly recognize peptides derived from the intravesicular processing and are loaded in acid lysosomal-like compartments. The nature of the peptides recognized by both systems differs.

Peptides bind with different degrees of affinity, depending on their constellation of amino acid side chains and the nature of the particular class II molecule. Some do not bind at all and to these the immune system will not mount an immune response (Levine et al. 1963; McDevitt and Sela 1965; reviewed in Benacerraf 1981; McDevitt 2002). It is the fact that some MHC alleles bind peptides poorly whereas others bind strongly that led to the discovery of the role of the MHC gene complex in the immune response. The MHC had been previously examined only in the context of nonphysiological reactions, those of tissue transplantation. When studying responses to small polypeptides of limited heterogeneity, it soon became apparent that some inbred strains of mice responded strongly whereas others made poor responses

(McDevitt 2002). Such a trait was found to be autosomal dominant and mapped to H-2, and in particular to a new region, later found to encode for the murine class II molecules (McDevitt and Chinitz 1969). These studies were seminal in calling attention to the importance of H-2 in regulating immune responses to proteins.

The nature of the peptides bound to MHC molecules during processing can now be studied by electrospray tandem mass spectrometry (Chicz et al. 1992; Hunt et al. 1992) (Figure 19.2). MHC molecules are isolated from APCs and denatured to release the peptides, which are then analyzed and sequenced. One can identify peptide families with as many as 40 members, and some represented in very large amounts (Latek and Unanue 1999). This approach has now been used to identify the precise peptides selected during the processing of viruses and bacteria. Examination of peptides selected by different MHC alleles indicates the preference for each allele to select peptides based on particular sequence motifs. These motifs are based on the presence of amino acids in which side chains enter into interaction with the specific binding loci. For any given protein, some peptide segments are selected during processing and bound to the MHC molecules whereas others are not recognized or recognized very weakly, and rapidly dissociate.

The peptides bound to MHCII molecules derive from extracellular proteins, as expected. Most peptides derive from the processing of membrane proteins, e.g. transferrin receptor or invariant chain, or even from the α and β chain of the class II molecule itself. Peptides also derive from proteins of the cytosol. These probably enter the vesicles by autophagy.

As the peptides bind to class II molecules, a number of the side chains of their component amino acids become solvent exposed and can potentially contact the TCR (Allen et al. 1987). In class II-bound peptides, these solvent-exposed residues are consistently placed at the P1, P2, P3, P5, and P8 positions (the MHC anchors placed at P1, P4, P6, P7, and P9). The TCR interacts with some of the residues of the solvent-exposed residues. Their interactions tend to be of low affinity. Structural studies indicate that both the peptide and the MHC are contacted by the two chains of the TCR (Garboczi et al. 1996; Garcia et al. 1996; Reinherz et al. 1999; Hennecke and Wiley 2001; Rudolph and Wilson 2002). The TCR adopts a canonical conformation in which its long contact axis is diagonal or orthogonal to the peptide–MHC. Part of the TCR contacts the helices of the MHC, particularly the complementary determinant regions (CDR) 1 and 2, which are germline encoded. (The CDRs are the regions of the TCR responsible for their binding specificity.) On the other hand, the CDR3 segment, where extensive variations exist, contacts the middle regions of the peptide. The structural studies have therefore validated the concepts derived from the findings of MHC restriction that the TCR has double specificity, one for the MHC, another for the peptide. One interpretation is that the contacts of CDR1 and CDR2 are responsible for positive selection, whereas it is CDR3 interaction that offers the peptide specificity.

STAGES IN ANTIGEN PRESENTATION

There are several stages in presentation. The antigen molecules need to be taken into vacuoles where they are processed, resulting in the generation and display of the

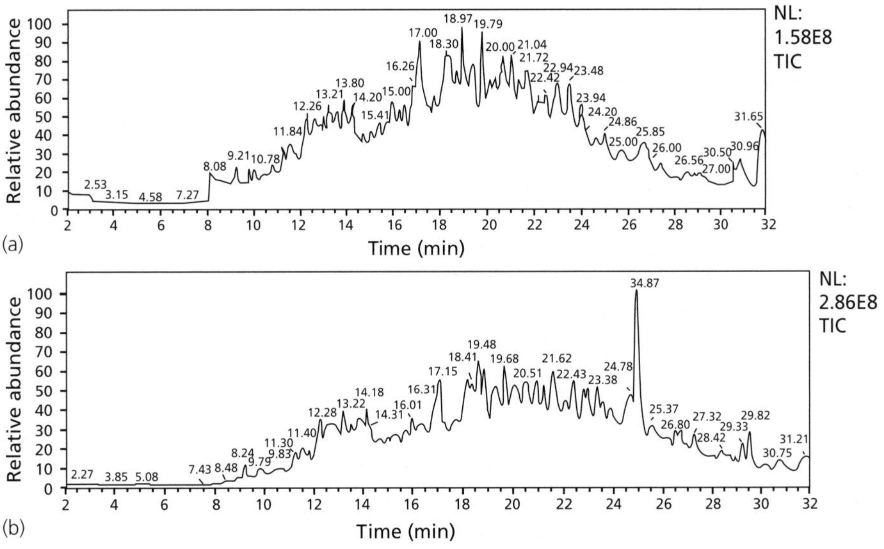

Figure 19.2 *Biochemical analysis of peptides extracted from the class II MHC molecule I-A^k. The two panels represent the separation of peptides by reverse phase chromatography. The top panel indicates the many peptides are bound to class II molecules. In the lower panel, the antigen-presenting cells (APC) were given lysozyme. Note the large peak at 25 min: it is the dominant peptide processed from lysozyme. (Redrawn from Gugasyan et al. 2000, with permission.)*

peptide–MHC complex. Following the display, there is the encounter with the T cells that have receptors specific for the complex. Recognition by the T cell is followed by activation depending on a number of important variables.

Antigen-presenting cells can present peptides from free proteins, or from proteins that form part of the structure of microbes or unicellular organisms. APCs can also interact directly with peptides found in extracellular fluids, and can also present proteins from cells or cell material that has been phagocytosed. (The term 'crosspresentation' or 'crosspriming' has been used to describe T-cell activation by a cell that lacks MHC molecules, but can be taken up when dead by an APC, which then presents its antigens.)

Protein antigen can enter the APC by fluid phase endocytosis or by ligand receptor internalization (reviewed in Unanue 2001). Under both conditions, the internalized protein eventually encounters the MHCII molecules, although the amount of uptake is favored in the case of receptor-mediated uptake. Uptake of viruses, bacteria, or other pathogens can be mediated by a variety of receptors such as the Fc and the complement receptors; or other surface receptors such as the scavenging receptor or those that recognize various polysaccharides. Together with bacteria, an important component of the recognition is the Toll-like receptor (TLR) (Medzhitov et al. 1997; Takeuchi et al. 1999; reviewed in Krutzik et al. 2001; Janeway and Medzhitov 2002). TLRs are involved in signaling during the interaction of the bacterium or its products with the surface of the phagocytes. Each TLR has a preference for the microbial ligands.

For B cells, the receptor for the protein antigen can be the specific membrane-bound immunoglobulin (Lanzavecchia 1990). Uptake by specific B cells can increase the efficiency of presentation by about a 1000-fold over uptake by fluid phase endocytosis. It is the uptake of antigen by specific immunoglobulin of B cells, and the subsequent presentation of its peptides to T cells, that form the basis of B cell–T cell interaction that leads to antibody formation.

The processing of proteins and the loading of MHC molecules with peptides are fast events (Table 19.4). Usually by an hour or less after uptake, complexes of peptide and MHCII molecules can be found on the cell surface (Ziegler and Unanue 1981; Cresswell 1994; Watts 1997, 2001). The proteins are usually processed in deep vesicular compartments of the APC, which are rich in lysosomal proteases as well as having a reducing activity. A number of lysosomal proteases are involved in the proteolytic processing (reviewed in Villadangos et al. 1999; Watts 2001). Alkalinization of the acid proteases of the APC results in inhibition of antigen processing (Table 19.4). The protein antigens have to be denatured and/or partially fragmented before interaction with MHC molecules. A scenario is that the protein, or a large polypeptide derived from it, is unfolded, after which the MHC binds to a preferred segment. The peptide segment is then protected from catabolism (Donermeyer and Allen 1989). Enzymes with amino- and carboxy-peptidase activity proceed to trim the segment of the polypeptide that extends beyond the combining site (Nelson et al. 1997). The reduction and partial fragmentation of the protein give it sufficient conformational flexibility to allow for binding to class II molecules. Although peptides and partially denatured proteins can be bound by class II molecules, most globular proteins in their native state do not bind. As indicated in Table 19.4, peptides can bind to class II molecules and these do not require any further handling. In fact, peptides can bind to surface MHCII molecules directly.

Proteins that are denatured meet the nascent MHCII molecules, recently arrived from the endoplasmic reticulum (ER) via Golgi vesicles (reviewed in Pieters 2000; Unanue 2002). The lysosomal vesicle that receives the antigen also receives the nascent MHCII molecules. MHCII molecules are transported from ER–Golgi to the loading vesicle together with another polypeptide called

Table 19.4 *Experiments indicating the processing of protein antigens for class II major histocompatibility complex (MHC) presentation*

	Antigen-presenting cell display				
Protein	**Peptide**	**Time (min)**	**Treatment**	**Fixation**	**Peptide–MHC**
1 +	–	0	–	–	No presentation
2 +	–	60	–	–	++++
3 +	–	60	Chloroquine	–	+/–
4 +	–	60	–	Fix at time 0	No presentation
5 +	–	60	–	Fix at 60 min	+++
6 –	+	0	–	–	+++
7 –	+	0	Chloroquine	–	+++
8 –	+	0	–	Fix at time 0	++

A protein antigen requires a period of time (indicated as 60 min) before presentation takes place to T cells. Inhibition of intracellular proteolysis by alkalinization of the vesicular pH by chloroquine inhibits presentation (no. 3). Cells that processed the protein and displayed it in their surface MHC molecules can be fixed and still present to T cells (no. 4). Peptides do not need processing (nos 6–8).

the invariant chain (so called because it does not show the allelic polymorphism of the class II molecules). The invariant chain is about 33 kDa, but shows some heterogeneity, with post-translational changes and various different splicing forms (Cresswell 1996). Three invariant chain forms a complex with three α–β dimers of MHCII. The function of the invariant chain is to direct the MHC molecule to the loading vesicle (Lotteau et al. 1990). It also folds over the peptide-binding site, and in this way blocks the binding to it of peptides found in the ER (Roche and Cresswell 1990). Once the proteins arrive at the loading vesicle, the invariant chain is degraded by acid proteases, particularly involving cathepsin S (Riese et al. 1996), liberating the peptide-binding site of the class II molecules, which can then receive peptides from its surrounding (Villadangos et al. 1997).

Peptide loading is markedly favored by a second MHC-like molecule named HLA-DM (Cho et al. 1991; Kelly et al. 1991). DM interacts with class II but does not bind peptides (it is also made of two chains, but has a combining site that is closed) (Fremont et al. 1996; Mosyak et al. 1998). The function of DM is a catalytic one, favoring the rapid dissociation of weak peptides and fostering the binding and stability of strong binding ones. In this way, DM serves to edit peptide selection, favoring the binding of peptides with strong affinities (Morris et al. 1994; Sloan et al. 1995).

Finally, it should be noted that microbes affect intracellular processing, attempting to divert the presentation to T cells. One mechanism is to inhibit fusion of the phagocytic vacuole with lysosomes avoiding processing. This inhibition occurs most notably with *Mycobacterium tuberculosis* (Armstrong and Hart 1975; Ferrari et al. 1999). A number of viruses affect primarily the processing by way of MHCI presentation.

APC INTERACTIONS WITH T CELLS

T cells contact the APC bearing the peptide–MHC complex and establish firm contact that lasts for several hours. During the time of contact, molecular events take place in the T cell that lead to their activation. This contact is in the immunological synapse. At the synapse, there is an early and rapid rearrangement of the TCR, and its accompanying components, with their coalescence into a tight compact area (Shaw and Dustin 1997; Grakoui et al. 1999; Shaw and Allen 2001; Krummel and Davis 2002). Likewise, the peptide–MHC complex of the APC also reorganizes into a single large aggregate. In the synapse, the TCR moves towards the center of it whereas molecules that favor adhesion, such as the intercellular adhesion molecule (ICAM), move towards the periphery of the complex. This segregation of the membrane molecules allows for effective contact of each of the complementing pairs of molecules of the T cell and the APC. The relatively small TCR and the peptide–MHC spans about 12 nm, whereas very large molecules such as CD43, CD44, and CD45 move toward the periphery of the synapse and, by doing this, do not hinder the interaction. The synapse forms part of the events that favor the transcriptional activation of the TCR (Lee et al. 2002). The thinking behind this is that the TCR may contact the complexes several times in a cycle of binding/dissociation. Eventually, the TCRs are internalized and lost (Lanzavecchia et al. 1999).

The amounts of peptide–MHC complex that stimulate a T cell have been determined in some systems (Latek and Unanue 1999). They vary depending on the state of activation of the T cell. In unstimulated T cells the amounts are about 200–300 complexes per APC. This number is reduced greatly, to about 10 or even less, in already activated or 'memory' T cells. Note should be made of the high sensitivity of the immature thymocyte to MHC–peptide complexes. The estimates are that only two or three are needed for negative selection and killing of an immature thymocyte. Thus, central thymic recognition is highly susceptible to low numbers of complexes, as expected for a system that needs to eliminate self-reactive T cells.

The presentation of a peptide–MHC complex by an APC, and its engagement by a specific TCR, result in the activation of the T cell only under suitable conditions of cellular activation brought about by an inflammatory response. These conditions are those that lead to a change in the APC, in turn leading it to express a number of auxiliary molecules that foster the subsequent activation of the T cell. In situations where the number of peptide–MHC complexes is limiting and the APC is in a 'resting' state, the T cell will not respond or even undergoes a process of negative response called anergy (see Figure 19.1, p. 377).

The current thinking follows the 'two-signal hypothesis' (Bretscher and Cohn 1970): TCR engagement by itself is not sufficient to drive the T cell into proliferation and differentiation, and the additional participation of auxiliary molecules plays a role in what is a highly complex series of cellular events. Note that, in cell cultures, engagement of the TCR, say with an antibody, will not suffice to drive the T cell to proliferate unless a second antibody is added to one of the costimulator molecules (in this example to CD28). Engagement of the TCR without costimulation may result in anergy (Jenkins and Schwartz 1987).

Three sets of molecules foster the activation of a T cell on interaction with an APC: the membrane 'costimulator' molecules, which drive the T cell to enter the DNA cycle, activate some cytokine genes, and maintain their viability; adhesion molecules which serve to maintain the physical interaction of the two cells; and the cytokines which are released by the activated APCs and modulate the activation and differentiation of the T cell.

A number of cell surface molecules have been identified and are known to play an important role as costimulators (Linsley et al. 1990; Gross et al. 1990; Turka et al.

1990; Gimmi et al. 1991; Linsley and Ledbetter 1993; Sperling and Bluestone 1996). The CD28 molecule, a homodimer with a single immunoglobulin-like domain, is expressed on the T cell in small amounts, but increases during the activation process (Sharpe and Freeman 2002). The complementary ligand of CD28 is made up of two molecules on the APC, termed B7-1 (CD80) and B7-2 (CD86). Both are expressed in small amounts, but markedly increase their expression if the APCs are activated. Engagement of CD28 fosters T cell–APC adhesion, and increases the transcription of a number of cytokine genes, by activating a number of intracellular transcription systems including the Lck and itk molecules and the Jun and NF-κB pathways. Engagement of CD28 also increases the survival of the T cell through the expression of antiapoptotic molecules (such as BCl-xL). The end-result is a stronger response of the T cell in terms of both its growth survival and its production of cytokines such as IL-2. Mice with created mutations of the CD28 or B7 molecules respond poorly to antigen molecules.

Expression of the B7 family is fostered by activation of the APCs, by cytokines, particularly by TNF, and importantly by interaction with microbes and their products through the TLR molecules that activate the NF-κB pathways of transcription. B7-1 and B7-2 are also induced as a result of interactions involving another critical pair of surface molecules, the CD40 molecule expressed on B cells, DCs, and monocytes (Grewal and Flavell 1998). CD40 has structural homology to the TNF receptor family. Its complementary molecule is a member of the TNF family, the CD40-ligand molecule expressed on T cells in small amounts. Engagement of CD40 on DCs leads to a heightened expression of B7-1 and B7-2. Engagement of CD40 on the B cells is a critical step, because it results in their proliferation and differentiation to antibody-secreting cells. (The importance of the CD40–CD40-ligand molecules can best be found in children with mutations in the gene for the CD40-ligand, called 'hyper-IgM syndrome': its T cells are poor in providing helper activity, which clinically translates into problems in antibody formation against infections with a number of microbes.)

Other surface molecules are involved in fostering the APC interaction with T cells. In humans, the CD2 molecules on T cells also play a critical role akin to CD28. Also participating in the interaction are molecules that foster the adherence of the various cells. Among the adhesion molecules, the intercellular adhesion molecule 1 (ICAM) molecule in APCs is particularly important, fostering the contact with the α_2-β_1-integrins of T cells.

Soluble molecules also influence the outcome of the T cell–APC interaction. Cytokines produced by the APC influence the program of gene expression on T cells in important ways (Hsieh et al. 1993). Among the cytokines that are released on interaction of APCs with microbes, particularly bacterial products, are TNF, IL-1, IL-12, and IL-18. The last two influence the expression of interferon-γ by the CD4 T cell, a program of differentiation called 'Th1' (which contrasts with situations in which the cytokine Il-4 drives the expression of IL-4) (reviewed in Farrar et al. 2002; Murphy and Reiner 2002).

Finally, it is critical to stop the APC–T-cell interaction and regulate the extent of activation of the T cell. The interaction ends, of course, as the stimulus, the antigen molecules, becomes progressively more limiting and finally disappears. Also controlling the interaction are negative regulatory molecules. The molecule CTLA-4 is expressed briefly in the activated T cell. Its engagement by the B-7 molecules on APCs dampens T-cell activation. (Mouse strains with an absence of functional CTLA-4 show marked hyperproliferation of lymphocytes (Thompson and Allison 1997).) Cytokines also dampen the activity of APCs, and this most prominently includes IL-10 and transforming growth factor β.

REFERENCES

Allen, P.M., Matsueda, G.R., et al. 1987. Identification of the T-cell and Ia contact residues of a T-cell antigenic epitope. *Nature*, **327**, 713–15.

Armstrong, J.A. and Hart, P.D. 1975. Phagosome-lysosome interactions in cultured macrophages infected with virulent tubercle bacilli. Reversal of the usual non-fusion pattern and observation in bacterial survival. *J Exp Med*, **142**, 1–16.

Babbitt, B.P., Allen, P.M., et al. 1985. Binding of immunogenic peptides to Ia histocompatibility molecules. *Nature*, **317**, 359–61.

Babbitt, B.P., Matsueda, G., et al. 1986. Antigenic competition at the level of peptide – Ia binding. *Proc Natl Acad Sci USA*, **83**, 4509–13.

Bancherau, J. and Steinman, R.M. 1998. Dendritic cells and the control of immunity. *Nature*, **392**, 245.

Benacerraf, B. 1981. Role of MHC gene products in immune regulation. *Science*, **212**, 1229–38.

Bjorkman, P.J., Saper, M.A., et al. 1987a. Structure of the human class I histocompatibility antigen, HLA-A2. *Nature*, **329**, 506–12.

Bjorkman, P.J., Saper, B., et al. 1987b. The foreign antigen binding site and T cell recognition regions of class I histocompatibility regions. *Nature*, **329**, 512–15.

Borowski, C., Martin, C., et al. 2002. On the brink of becoming a T cell. *Curr Opin Immunol*, **14**, 200–6.

Bretscher, P. and Cohn, M. 1970. A theory of self–non-self discrimination. *Science*, **169**, 1042–9.

Brown, J.H., Jardetzky, T.S., et al. 1993. Three-dimensional structure of the human class II histocompatibility antigen HLA-DR1 [see comments]. *Nature*, **364**, 33–9.

Buchmeier, N.A. and Schreiber, R.D. 1985. Requirement of endogenous interferon-gamma production for resolution of *Listeria monocytogenes* infection. *Proc Natl Acad Sci USA*, **82**, 7404–8.

Buus, S., Sette, A., et al. 1987a. The relation between major histocompatibility complex (MHC) restriction and the capacity of Ia to bind immunogenic peptides. *Science*, **235**, 1353–8.

Buus, S., Sette, A. and Grey, H.M. 1987b. The interaction between protein-derived immunogenic peptides and Ia. *Immunol Rev*, **98**, 115–41.

Cella, M., Schneidegger, D., et al. 1996. Ligation of CD40 on dendritic cells triggers production of high levels of interleukin-12 and enhances T cell stimulatory capacity: T-T help via APC activation. *J Exp Med*, **184**, 747–52.

Cella, M., Salio, M., et al. 1999. Maturation, activation, and protection of dendritic cells induced by double-stranded RNA. *J Exp Med*, **189**, 821–9.

Chesnut, R.W., Colon, S.M. and Grey, H.M. 1982. Requirements for the processing of antigens by antigen-presenting B cells. I. Functional comparison of B cell tumors and macrophages. *J Immunol*, **129**, 2382–8.

Chicz, R.M., Urban, R.G., et al. 1992. Predominant naturally processed peptides bound to HLA-DR1 are derived from MHC-related molecules and are heterogeneous in size. *Nature*, **358**, 764–8.

Cho, S.G., Attaya, M. and Monaco, J.J. 1991. New class II-like genes in the murine MHC. *Nature*, **353**, 573–6.

Cresswell, P. 1994. Assembly, transport, and function of MHC class II molecules. *Annu Rev Immunol*, **12**, 259–93.

Cresswell, P. 1996. Invariant chain structure and MHC class II function. *Cell*, **84**, 505–7.

Dawkins, R., Leelayuwat, C., et al. 1999. Genomics of the major histocompatibility complex: haplotypes, duplication, retroviruses and disease. *Immunol Rev*, **167**, 275–304.

Donermeyer, D.L. and Allen, P.M. 1989. Binding to Ia protects an immunogenic peptide from proteolytic degradation. *J Immunol*, **142**, 1063–8.

Farrar, J.D., Asnagli, H. and Murphy, K.M. 2002. T helper subset development: roles of instruction, selection, and transcription. *J Clin Invest*, **109**, 431–5.

Ferrari, G., Naito, M., et al. 1999. A coat protein on phagosomes involved in the intracellular survival of Mycobacteria. *Cell*, **97**, 435–47.

Fremont, D.H., Hendrickson, W.A., et al. 1996. Structures of an MHC class II molecule with covalently bound single peptides. *Science*, **272**, 1001–4.

Fremont, D.H., Crawford, F., et al. 1998a. Crystal structure of mouse H2-M. *Immunity*, **9**, 385–93.

Fremont, D.H., Monnaie, D., et al. 1998b. Crystal structure of I-A^k in complex with a dominant epitope of lysozyme. *Immunity*, **8**, 305–17.

Garboczi, D.N., Ghosh, P., et al. 1996. Structure of the complex between human T-cell receptor, viral peptide and HLA-A2 [comment]. *Nature*, **384**, 134–41.

Garcia, K.C., Degano, M., et al. 1996. An αβ T cell receptor structure at 2.5 A and its orientation in the TCR-MHC complex. *Science*, **274**, 209–19.

Gimmi, C.D., Freeman, G.J., et al. 1991. B cell surface antigen B7 provides a costimulatory signal that induces T cells to proliferate and secrete interleukin 2. *Proc Natl Acad Sci USA*, **88**, 6575–90.

Grakoui, A., Bromley, S.K. and Sumen, C. 1999. The immunological synapse: a molecular machine controlling T cell activation. *Science*, **285**, 221–7.

Grewal, I.S. and Flavell, R.A. 1998. CD40 and CD154 in cell-mediated immunity. *Annu Rev Immunol*, **16**, 111–35.

Gross, J.A., St. John, T. and Allison, J.P. 1990. The murine homologue of the T lymphocyte antigen CD28. Molecular cloning and cell surface expression. *J Immunol*, **144**, 3201–10.

Guermonprez, P., Valladeu, J., et al. 2002. Antigen presentation and T cell stimulation by dendritic cells. *Annu Rev Immunol*, **20**, 621–68.

Gugasyan, R., Velazquez, C., et al. 2000. Independent selection by I-A^k molecules of two epitopes found in tandem in an extended polypeptide. *J Immunol*, **165**, 3206–13.

Hammer, J., Takacs, B. and Sinigaglia, F. 1992. Identification of a motif for HLA-DR1 binding peptides using M13 display libraries. *J Exp Med*, **176**, 1007–13.

Harding, C.V., Roof, R.W., et al. 1991. Effects of pH and polysaccharides on peptide binding to class II major histocompatibility complex molecules. *Proc Natl Acad Sci USA*, **88**, 2740–4.

Hennecke, J. and Wiley, D.C. 2001. T cell receptor-MHC interaction up close. *Cell*, **104**, 1–4.

Hill, A.V.S., Allsopp, C.E.M., et al. 1991. Common West African HLA antigens are associated with protection from severe malaria. *Nature*, **352**, 595–600.

Hoffmann, J.A., Kafatos, F.C., et al. 1999. Phylogenetic perspectives in innate immunity. *Science*, **284**, 1313–18.

Hsieh, C.S., Macatonia, S.E., et al. 1993. Development of Th1 CD4+ T cells through IL-12 produced by *Listeria*-induced macrophages. *Science*, **260**, 547–9.

Hunt, D.F., Michel, H., et al. 1992. Peptides presented to the immune system by the murine class II major histocompatibility complex molecule I-A^d. *Science*, **256**, 1817–20.

Inaba, K., Steinman, R.M., et al. 1983. Dendritic cells are critical accessory cells for thymus-dependent antibody responses in mouse and in man. *Proc Natl Acad Sci USA*, **80**, 6041–5.

Inaba, K., Inaba, M., et al. 1992. Generations of large numbers of dendritic cells from mouse bone marrow cultures supplemented with granulocyte/macrophage colony-stimulating factor. *J Exp Med*, **176**, 1693–705.

Inaba, K., Inaba, M., et al. 1993. Dendritic cell progenitors phagocytose particulates, including bacillus Calmette-Guérin organisms, and sensitize mice to mycobacterial antigens in vivo. *J Exp Med*, **178**, 479–88.

Insel, R.A. and Anderson, P. 1986. Oligosaccharide-protein conjugate vaccines induce and prime for oligoclonal IgG antibody responses to the *H influenzae b* capsular polysaccharide in human infants. *J Exp Med*, **163**, 262–9.

Ishioka, G.Y., Lamont, A.G., et al. 1992. MHC interaction and T cell recognition of carbohydrates and glycopeptides. *J Immunol*, **148**, 2446–53.

Jameson, S.C., Hogquist, K.A. and Bevan, M.J. 1995. Positive selection of thymocytes. *Annu Rev Immunol*, **13**, 93–126.

Janeway, C.A. and Medzhitov, R. 2002. Innate immune recognition. *Annu Rev Immunol*, **20**, 197–216.

Jenkins, M.K. and Schwartz, R.H. 1987. Antigen presentation by chemically modified splenocytes induces antigen-specific T cell unresponsiveness in vitro and in vivo. *J Exp Med*, **165**, 302–19.

Kappler, J.W., Wade, T., et al. 1987. A T cell receptor Vβ segment that imparts reactivity to a class II major histocompatibility complex product. *Cell*, **49**, 263–71.

Katz, D.H. and Unanue, E.R. 1973. Critical role of determinant presentation in the induction of specific responses in immunocompetent lymphocytes. *J Exp Med*, **137**, 967–90.

Kelly, A.P., Monaco, J.J., et al. 1991. A new human HLA class II-related locus DM. *Nature*, **353**, 571–3.

Kisielow, P., Blüthmann, H., et al. 1988a. Tolerance in T cell receptor transgenic mice involves deletion of non-mature $CD4^+8^-$ thymocytes. *Nature*, **333**, 742–7.

Kisielow, P., Teh, H.S., et al. 1988b. Positive selection of antigen-specific T cells in thymus by restricting MHC molecules. *Nature*, **335**, 730–4.

Klein, J., Satta, Y., et al. 1993. The molecular descent of the Major Histocompatibilty Complex. *Annu Rev Immunol*, **11**, 269–96.

Krummel, M.F. and Davis, M.M. 2002. Dynamics of the immunological synapse: finding, establishing and solidifying a connection. *Curr Opin Immunol*, **14**, 66–74.

Krutzik, S.R., Sieling, P.A. and Modlin, R.L. 2001. The role of Toll-link receptors in host defense against microbial infection. *Curr Opin Immunol*, **13**, 104–8.

Lanzavecchia, A. 1990. Receptor-mediated antigen uptake and its effect on antigen presentation to class II-restricted T lymphocytes. *Annu Rev Immunol*, **8**, 773–93.

Lanzavecchia, A. and Sallusto, F. 2001. The instructive role of dendritic cells on T cell responses: lineages, plasticity and kinetics. *Curr Opin Immunol*, **13**, 291–8.

Lanzavecchia, A., Lezzi, G. and Viola, A. 1999. From TCR engagement to T cell activation: a kinetic view of T cell behavior. *Cell*, **96**, 1–4.

Latek, R.R. and Unanue, E.R. 1999. Mechanisms of consequences of peptide selection by the I-A^k class II molecule. *Immunol Rev*, **172**, 209–28.

Lee, K.H., Holdorf, A.D., et al. 2002. T cell receptor signalling precedes immunological synapse formation. *Science*, **295**, 1539–42.

Levine, B.B., Ojeda, A. and Benacerraf, B. 1963. Studies on artificial antigens. III. The genetic control of the immune response to hapten-poly L-lysine conjugates in guinea pigs. *J Exp Med*, **118**, 953–61.

Lindahl, K.F., Byers, D.E., et al. 1997. H2-M3, a full service class 1b histocompatibility antigen. *Annu Rev Immunol*, **15**, 851–79.

Linsley, P.S. and Ledbetter, J.A. 1993. The role of the CD28 receptor during T cell responses to antigen. *Annu Rev Immunol*, **11**, 191–212.

Linsley, P.S., Clark, E.A. and Ledbetter, J.A. 1990. T cell antigen CD28 mediates adhesion with B cells by interacting with activation antigen B7/BB1. *Proc Natl Acad Sci USA*, **87**, 5031–5.

Lotteau, V., Teyton, L., et al. 1990. Intracellular transport of class II MHC molecules directed by invariant chain. *Nature*, **348**, 600–5.

Luster, A.D. 2002. The role of chemokines in linking innate and adaptive immunity. *Curr Opin Immunol*, **14**, 129–35.

McDevitt, H.O. 2002. The discovery of linkage between the MHC and genetic control of the immune response. *Immunol Rev*, **18**, 69–77.

McDevitt, H.O. and Chinitz, A. 1969. Genetic control of the antibody response: relationship between immune response and histocompatibility (H-2) type. *Science*, **163**, 1207–8.

McDevitt, H.O. and Sela, M. 1965. Genetic control of the antibody response. I. Demonstration of determinant-specific differences in response to synthetic polypeptide antigens in two strains of inbred mice. *J Exp Med*, **122**, 517–31.

Mackanness, G.B. 1962. Cellular resistance to infection. *J Exp Med*, **116**, 381–90.

MacPherson, G., Kushnir, N. and Wykes, M. 1999. Dendritic cells, B cells and the regulation of antibody synthesis. *Immun Rev*, **172**, 325–34.

Madden, D.R. 1995. The three dimensional structure of peptide-MHC complex. *Annu Rev Immunol*, **13**, 587–622.

Medzhitov, R., Preston-Hurlburt, P. and Janeway, C.A. Jr. 1997. A human homologue of the Drosophila Toll protein signals activation of adaptive immunity. *Nature*, **388**, 394–7.

Metchnikoff, E. 1968. *Lectures on the comparative pathology of inflammation*. New York: Dover Publications.

Morris, P., Shaman, J., et al. 1994. An essential role for HLA-DM in antigen presentation by class II major histocompatibility molecules. *Nature*, **368**, 551–4.

Mosyak, L., Zaller, D.M. and Wiley, D.C. 1998. The structure of HLA-DM, the peptide exchange catalyst that loads antigen onto class II MHC molecules during antigen presentation. *Immunity*, **9**, 377–83.

Murphy, K.M. and Reiner, S.L. 2002. Decision-making in the immune system: The lineage decisions of helper T cells. *Nat Rev Immunol*, **2**, 933–44.

Nelson, C.A., Vidavsky, I., et al. 1997. Amino-terminal trimming of peptides for presentation on major histocompatibility complex class II molecules. *Proc Natl Acad Sci USA*,, **94**, 628–33.

Nestle, F.O., Banchereau, J. and Hart, D. 2001. Dendritic cells: on the move from bench to bedside. *Nature Med*, **7**, 761–5.

O'Brien, S.J. and Yuhki, N. 1999. Comparative genome organization of the major histocompatibility complex: lessons from Felidae. *Immunol Rev*, **167**, 133–44.

Parham, P. 1999. Virtual reality in the MHC. *Immunol Rev*, **167**, 5–16.

Piazza, A., Belevedere, M.C., et al. 1973. HL-A variation in four Sardinian villages under differential selective pressure by malaria. In: Dausset, J. and Colombani, J. (eds), *Histocompatibility testing*. Copenhagen: Munksgaard, 73.

Pieters, J. 2000. MHC class II-restricted antigen processing and presentation. *Adv Immunol*, **75**, 159–208.

Porcelli, S., Morita, C.T. and Brenner, M.B. 1992. CD1b restricts the response of human CD-T lymphocytes to a microbial antigen. *Nature*, **360**, 593-7, 4–8.

Randolph, G.J., Beaulieu, S., et al. 1998. Differentiation of monocytes into dendritic cells in a model of transendothelial trafficking. *Science*, **282**, 480–3.

Reinherz, E., Tan, K., et al. 1999. The crystal structure of a T cell receptor in complex with peptide and MHC class II. *Science*, **286**, 1913–20.

Riese, R.J., Wolf, P., et al. 1996. Essential role for cathepsin S in MHC class II-associated invariant chain processing and peptide loading. *Immunity*, **4**, 357–66.

Robey, E. and Fowlkes, B.J. 1994. Selective events in T cell development. *Annu Rev Immunol*, **12**, 521–3.

Roche, P.A. and Cresswell, P. 1990. Invariant chain association with HLA-DR molecules inhibits immunogenic peptide binding. *Nature*, **345**, 615–18.

Rock, K.L. and Goldberg, A.L. 1999. Degradation of cell proteins and the generation of MHC class-I presented peptides. *Annu Rev Immunol*, **17**, 739–79.

Rosenthal, A.S. and Shevach, E.M. 1973. Function of macrophages in antigen recognition by guinea pig T lymphocytes. I. Requirement for histocompatible macrophages and lymphocytes. *J Exp Med*, **138**, 1194–212.

Rudolph, M.G. and Wilson, I.A. 2002. The specificity of TCR/pMHC interaction. *Curr Opin Immunol*, **14**, 52–65.

Sallusto, F. and Lanzavecchia, A. 1994. Efficient presentation of soluble antigen by cultured human dendritic cells is maintained by granulocyte/macrophage colony-stimulating factor plus interleukin 4 and downregulated by tumor necrosis factor alpha. *J Exp Med*, **179**, 1109–18.

Schneerson, R., Barrera, O., et al. 1980. Preparation, characterization and immunogenicity of *H influenzae b* polysaccharide-protein conjugates. *J Exp Med*, **152**, 361–7.

Scott, C.A., Peterson, P.A., et al. 1998. Crystal structures of two I-Ad-peptide complexes reveal that high affinity can be achieved without large anchor residues [published erratum appears in *Immunity*, 1998; **8**, 531]. *Immunity*, **8**, 319–29.

Sharpe, A.H. and Freeman, G.J. 2002. The B7-CD28 superfamily. *Nature Rev Immunol*, **2**, 116–26.

Shaw, A.S. and Dustin, M.L. 1997. Making the T cell receptor go the distance: a topological view of T cell activation. *Immunity*, **6**, 361–9.

Shaw, A.S. and Allen, P.M. 2001. Kissing cousins: immunological and neurological synapses. *Nat Immunol*, **2**, 575–6.

Sinigaglia, F. and Hammer, J. 1995. Motifs and supermotifs for MHC class II binding peptides. *J Exp Med*, **181**, 449–51.

Sloan, V.S., Cameron, P., et al. 1995. Mediation by HLA-DM of dissociation of peptides from HLA-DR. *Nature*, **375**, 802–6.

Sperling, A.I. and Bluestone, J.A. 1996. The complexities of T cell co-stimulation: CD28 and beyond. *Immunol Rev*, **153**, 155–82.

Stern, L., Brown, G., et al. 1994. Crystal structure of the human class II MHC protein HLA-DR1 complexed with an antigenic peptide from influenza virus. *Nature*, **368**, 215–21.

Suri, A., Vidavsky, I., et al. 2002. In antigen presenting cells, the autologous peptides selected by the diabetogenic I-A^{g7} molecules are unique and determined by the amino acid changes in the P9 pocket. *J Immunol*, **168**, 1235–43.

Takeuchi, O., Hoshino, K., et al. 1999. Differential roles of TLR2 and TLR4 in recognition of Gram-negative and Gram-positive bacterial cell wall components. *Immunity*, **11**, 443–51.

Tang, H.L. and Cyster, J.G. 1999. Chemokine up-regulation and activated T cell attraction by maturing dendritic cells. *Science*, **284**, 819–22.

Thery, C. and Amigorena, S. 2001. The cell biology of antigen presentation in dendritic cells. *Curr Opin Immunol*, **13**, 45–51.

Thompson, C.B. and Allison, J.P. 1997. The emerging role of CTLA-4 as an immune attenuator. *Immunity*, **7**, 445–50.

Townsend, A.R.M., Rothbard, J., et al. 1986. The epitopes of influenza nucleoprotein recognized by cytotoxic T lymphocytes can be defined with short synthetic peptides. *Cell*, **44**, 959–68.

Turka, L.A., Ledbetter, J.A., et al. 1990. CD28 is an inducible T cell surface antigen that transduces a proliferative signal in CD3+ mature thymocytes. *J Immunol*, **144**, 1646–53.

Unanue, E.R. 1981. The regulatory role of macrophages in antigenic stimulation. II. Symbiotic relationship between lymphocytes and macrophages. *Adv Immunol*, **31**, 1–48.

Unanue, E.R. 1997. Studies in listeriosis show the strong symbiosis between the innate cellular system and the T cell response. *Immunol Rev*, **158**, 11–25.

Unanue, E.R. 2001. Antigen processing and presentation. In: Austen, K.F., Atkinson, J.P. and Cantor, H. (eds), *Samter's immunological diseases*. Philadelphia, PA: Lippincott, Williams & Wilkins, 53–64.

Unanue, E.R. 2002. Perspective on antigen processing and presentation. *Immunol Rev*, **185**, 86–102.

Villadangos, J.A., Riese, R.J., et al. 1997. Degradation of mouse invariant chain: roles of cathepsins S and D and the influence of major histocompatibility complex polymorphism. *J Exp Med*, **186**, 549–60.

Villadangos, J.A., Bryant, R.A., et al. 1999. Proteases involved in MHC class II antigen presentation. *Immunol Rev*, **172**, 109–20.

von Boehmer, H. 1990. Developmental biology of T cells in T-cell receptor transgenic mice. *Annu Rev Immunol*, **8**, 531–56.

Watts, C. 1997. Capture and processing of exogenous antigens for presentation on MHC molecules. *Annu Rev Immunol*, **15**, 821–50.

Watts, C. 2001. Antigen processing in the endocytic compartment. *Curr Opin Immunol*, **13**, 26–31.

Yewdell, J.W. and Bennink, J.R. 1999. Immunodominance in Major Histocompatibility Complex Class-I restricted T lymphocyte responses. *Annu Rev Immunol*, **17**, 51–88.

Ziegler, K. and Unanue, E.R. 1981. Identification of a macrophage antigen-processing event required for I-region-restricted antigen presentation to lymphocytes. *J Immunol*, **127**, 1869–77.

Zinkernagel, R.M. and Doherty, P.C. 1974. Immunological surveillance against altered self components by sensitised T lymphocytes in lymphocytic choriomeningitis. *Nature*, **251**, 574–8.

20

CD4⁺ T lymphocytes

ALLAN M. MOWAT AND PAUL GARSIDE

INTRODUCTION

CD4⁺ T cells are the conductors of the immunological orchestra, being not only responsible for many important effector functions, but also necessary for the activation of many other aspects of the immune response, including B lymphocytes, CD8⁺ T lymphocytes, macrophages, and other inflammatory cells (Figure 20.1) (Boes and Ploegh 2004). Thus, there are few immune responses that do not involve CD4⁺ T cells at some stage, a role that is underlined by the life-threatening susceptibility to infection seen in patients with a deficiency of this population in, for example, human immunodeficiency virus (HIV) infection.

NATURE AND ROLE OF CD4⁺ T LYMPHOCYTES

CD4⁺ T cells account for 60–70 percent of the T lymphocytes found in the bloodstream and in most organized lymphoid organs, including the spleen and lymph nodes, as well as the lymphoid tissues associated with the mucosal surfaces such as the Peyer's patches, appendix, and tonsils. Mature CD4⁺ T cells are characterized by the expression of CD3, an αβ T-cell receptor (TCR) and the CD4 molecule, a four-domain monomeric member of the immunoglobulin (Ig) superfamily that binds major histocompatibility complex class II (MHC II). CD4 is also the primary receptor for HIV entry, binding the gp120 surface protein. Most resting CD4⁺ T cells also express other pan-T-cell markers such as CD2, CD5, and CD28, many of which are important during the process of activation (see below). Unlike immature T cells in the thymus, mature CD4⁺ T cells cannot express the CD8 molecule.

By virtue of the presence of CD4, the vast majority of this population recognizes peptide antigen when presented by MHC II molecules on the surface of an accessory cell, although there is an unusual subset of 'natural' CD4⁺ T cells that accounts for less than 5 percent of the population and which recognizes nonclassic major histocompatibility complex (MHC) molecules such as CD1 (see below). Only a few cell types can be involved in the activation of CD4⁺ T cells by foreign antigen – dendritic cells (DC), B lymphocytes, and activated macrophages. During inflammation,

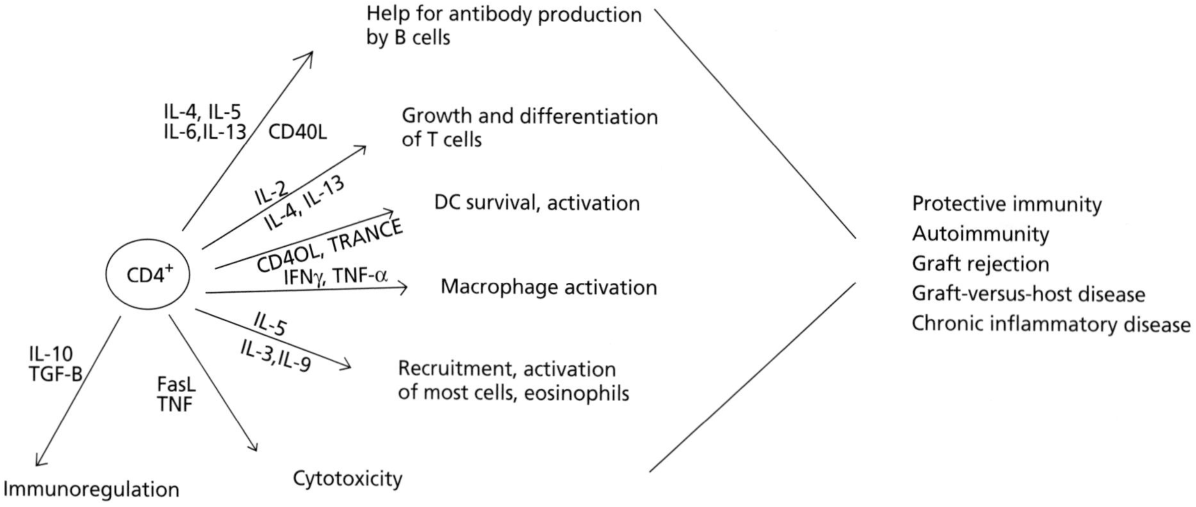

Figure 20.1 *Functions and roles of CD4+ T lymphocytes in protective immunity and immunopathology. DC, dendritic cell; IFN, interferon; IL, interleukin; TGF, transforming growth factor; TNF, tumor necrosis factor.*

other cell types can be induced to express MHC II, but the role of these cells in presenting antigen to CD4+ T cells in vivo is unclear.

As discussed elsewhere in this volume, antigens that are presented on MHC II molecules are derived from proteolytic processing mechanisms that generate 12–24 amino acid peptides within the endocytic pathway of the antigen-presenting cell (APC). As a result, CD4+ T cells are geared to recognize antigens that are taken up into APCs by phagocytosis, endocytosis, or pinocytosis. Thus, CD4+ T cells are important in protective immunity against extracellular pathogens such as pyogenic bacteria, large parasites, and other free-living organisms. In addition, intracellular pathogens such as *Mycobacterium*, *Salmonella*, and *Leishmania* spp., which survive in and colonize endosomes or phagosomes, can be recognized by CD4+ T cells (Boes and Ploegh 2004). Indeed, it is this group of infections that causes the biggest problem in CD4 deficiency states. Nevertheless, it is important to note that CD4+ T cells also play a prominent and often essential role in responses to other types of intracellular pathogens, which do not invade endosomes and characteristically stimulate MHC I-restricted T-cell responses (e.g. viruses). This may be secondary to the uptake of infected and/or damaged cells by phagocytic cells such as DCs or macrophages, or to the recycling of surface-expressed viral proteins via the endocytic pathway.

CD4+ T cells also play critical roles in most immune responses of pathological importance, including organ-specific autoimmune disease, chronic inflammatory disease, and other hypersensitivity disorders. In addition, alone or together with other lymphocytes, CD4+ T cells are important in the rejection of allogeneic transplants and in graft-versus-host disease after bone marrow transplantation (Figure 20.1).

LIFE HISTORY OF CD4+ T LYMPHOCYTES

Similar to all peripheral αβ T cells, CD4+ T cells differentiate from common lymphoid progenitor cells in the thymus, mostly during fetal and early postnatal life (Figure 20.2). The thymic processes of negative and positive selection ensure that the only CD4+ T cells that survive and are exported to the periphery have a TCR that can recognize foreign antigens when presented by self MHC II antigens, but cannot recognize self-tissue antigens (reviewed in Goldrath and Bevan 1999; Starr et al. 2003; Mathis and Benoist 2004). Positive selection occurs because maturing T cells are programmed to die by apoptosis unless they receive a signal from their TCR after it has interacted with self-peptides presented by self-MHC molecules, probably on the network of epithelial cells present in the thymic cortex. In turn, if the TCR has a very high affinity for self-MHC and peptide presented by thymic DCs, the cell will undergo negative selection ('deletion'), again by the induction of apoptosis. The exact timing of these events and their precise anatomical location are still somewhat controversial, but both selection processes occur soon after the T cell has acquired a CD3–TCR complex and when it still expresses both CD4 and CD8 markers ('double positives'). Thereafter, one of these markers is lost permanently as a result of silencing of the appropriate promoter; T cells with a TCR that recognizes peptides on MHC II molecules lose CD8 and retain the CD4 molecule; conversely, T cells with a TCR that recognizes peptides on MHC I molecules lose CD4 and retain CD8 (Figure 20.2). After commitment to the CD4 lineage, the single positive T cells enter the thymic medulla, where they spend a further period of 5–6 days, before emigrating to the thymus-dependent

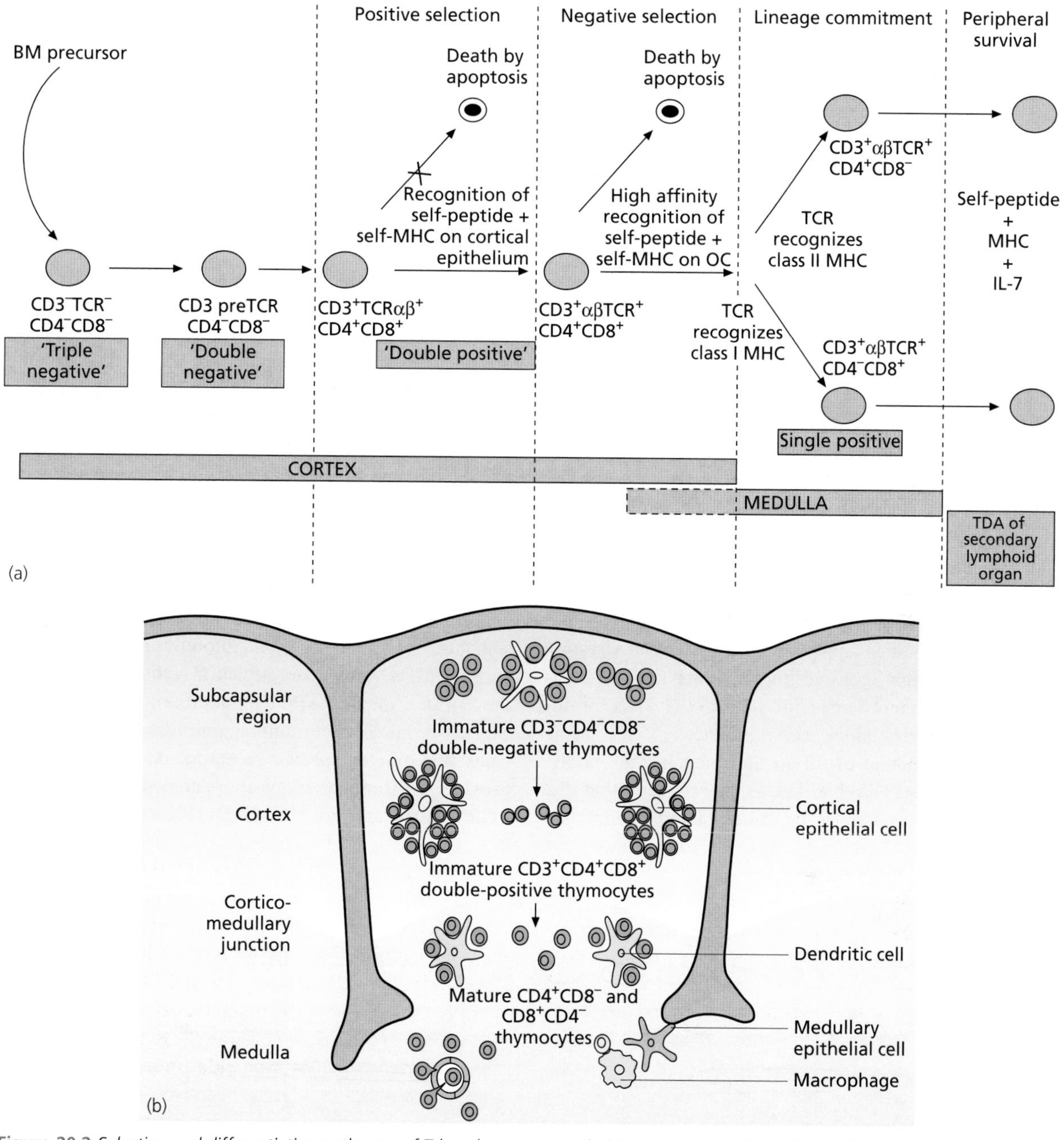

Figure 20.2 *Selection and differentiation pathways of T lymphocytes. Lymphoid precursor cells derived from the bone marrow enter the thymic cortex during fetal life and are induced to begin expansion and differentiation under the influence of soluble mediators and cell-surface molecules expressed by cortical epithelial cells and mesenchymal cells. At this time, the cells do not express a T-cell receptor (TCR), CD3, or CD4 and CD8 ('triple negative'), but they then rapidly acquire a pre-TCR composed of a TCR β chain and the pre-Tα chain, together with low levels of CD3 ('double negative'). Successful expression of this pre-TCR induces expression of both CD4 and CD8, and the mature αβ TCR replaces the pre-TCR. These 'double-positive' cells are now subjected to positive and negative selection, in which only those T cells expressing a TCR capable of recognizing self-peptides + self-MHC on cortical epithelium (positive selection), but which cannot recognize self-peptides + self-MHC strongly on dendritic cells (negative selection), are allowed to survive. This small fraction of cells (2–3 percent of total output) is then restricted to recognizing peptides from foreign antigens that are in complex with self-MHC molecules, but cannot recognize self-antigens with sufficient strength to cause autoimmunity. These selection processes probably occur mainly in the thymic cortex* **(b)**, *although the medulla may also play a role. After selection, T cells with a TCR that recognizes MHC I down-regulate the CD4 molecule and retain CD8 expression, whereas T cells with a TCR that recognizes MHC II down-regulate the CD8 molecule and retain CD4 expression. The resulting single positive T cells now remain in the medulla for a short period of further maturation, before exiting the thymus to recirculate from blood to the thymus-dependent areas (TDA) of secondary lymphoid organs. There they are maintained alive by continual low-level stimulation of their TCR ('tickling') by self-peptide + self-MHC on antigen-presenting cells in the tissues and by the cytokine interleukin 7 (IL-7). The insets show the histological appearance of the normal thymus, illustrating the cortex (C) and medulla (M), and a schematic representation of the local differentiation events. (From Janeway et al. 2001.)*

areas (TDA) of secondary lymphoid organs via the bloodstream.

At this time, the CD4+ T cells are referred to as 'naive', because they have not yet encountered antigen; naive T cells are in a resting state and can survive in this way for many years without stimulation by foreign antigen, or without constant output from the thymus. It was previously believed that outside stimuli were not required for this long-term persistence and that it was an inherent property of naive T cells. However, it is now clear that such T cells require continual stimulation via their TCRs to survive in the periphery (Goldrath and Bevan 1999). This does not involve foreign antigen, but seems to require recognition of the same self-peptide–MHC II complex that was responsible for positively selecting the T cell in the thymus. It is believed that DCs in secondary lymphoid organs are responsible for presenting these complexes and other factors, including cytokines such as interleukin (IL) 7 may also be involved (Figure 20.2) (Marrack and Kappler 2004; Stockinger et al. 2004). As a result of this 'tickling' by self-antigen under physiological conditions, the T cell does not usually undergo clonal expansion or become fully activated; instead it receives survival signals that allow it to persist in the peripheral tissues in a resting state. Interestingly, however, if the same CD4+ T cells are in an immunocompromised host, they can proliferate extensively under the influence of the same signals in an attempt to fill up the space in the 'empty' immune system. This has led to the concept that the normal immune system is tightly regulated to maintain a pre-set number of T cells and that this is determined by competition for a finite amount of MHC–peptide ligands and other survival signals. The phenomenon of 'homeostatic proliferation' is also important in understanding how the immune system may compensate for insults such as irradiation, chemotherapy, or HIV infection especially in adults, where the thymus is almost inactive.

ACTIVATION OF CD4+ T LYMPHOCYTES

Inappropriate CD4+ T cell activation can have serious consequences for the body because of the effects that these cells can have on surrounding tissues via the production of cytokines and activation of nonspecific effector cells. For these reasons, the activation of naive CD4+ T cells is subject to a number of stringent controls, including restrictions in the type and location of cells that can present antigen with MHC II, as well as a requirement for a sequence of highly defined signals to occur before full stimulation of the T cell is achieved (Boes and Ploegh 2004). For a complex antigen to be recognized by CD4+ T cells, it must be internalized by an appropriate APC, degraded into peptides in an endosomal compartment, and loaded on to newly synthesized class II MHC molecules, which are then expressed on the surface of the APC. In addition, the APC must express a number of nonpolymorphic accessory molecules that trigger specific receptors on the T cell and provide 'co-stimulation' of the signal obtained via the TCR (Sharpe and Freeman 2002) (Figure 20.3).

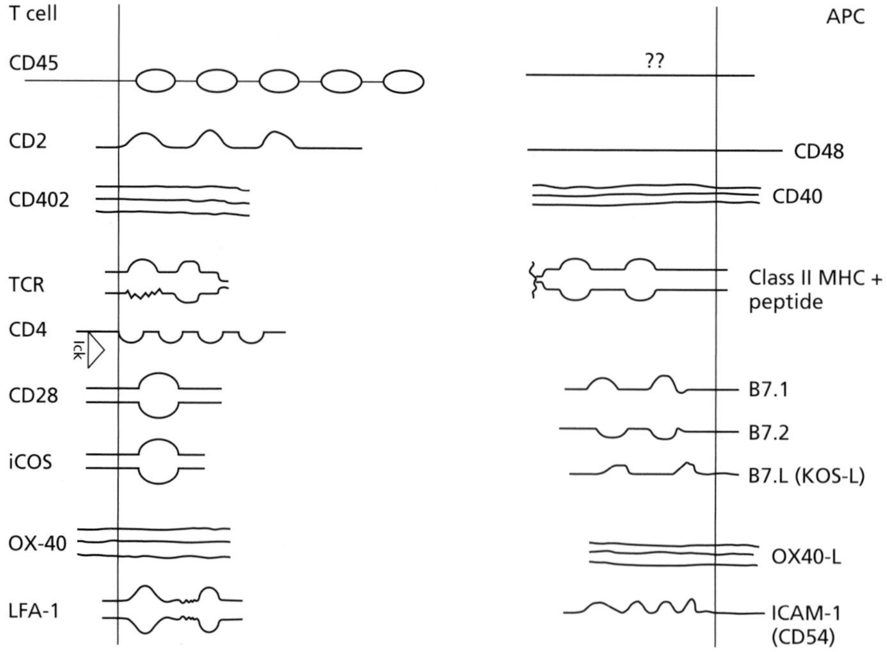

Figure 20.3 Co-stimulatory molecules involved in T cell–antigen-presenting cell (APC) interactions and in the formation of the immunological synapse. ICAM, intercellular adhesion molecule; iCOS, inducible co-stimulatory molecule; MHC, major histocompatibility complex; TCR, T-cell receptor. See text for details.

DENDRITIC CELLS AND PRIMING OF CD4⁺ T LYMPHOCYTES

In most immune responses, priming of CD4⁺ T cells occurs in the thymus-dependent areas (TDA) of secondary lymphoid tissues and the APCs are DCs. DCs are a specialized group of MHC II expressing leukocytes, which can be found in most tissues of the body, but they are most prominent in secondary lymphoid organs. There may be a number of different DC subsets and their exact functions may vary with their anatomical location, but their overall properties make them ideal candidates for initiating and directing CD4⁺ T-cell responses. They have several distinct, but related, roles (Banchereau et al. 2000; Guermonprez et al. 2002; Steinman et al. 2003). First, they are extremely effective at taking up and processing complex antigens for MHC II-restricted presentation. In addition, they are unique among APCs in their ability to patrol the tissues and solid organs of the body, before carrying antigen to the TDA of lymphoid organs where they meet naive T cells (Itano et al. 2003; Boes and Ploegh 2004). DCs are also capable of expressing a wide range of co-stimulatory molecules and can secrete soluble mediators that help in the activation and differentiation of T cells. Finally, and perhaps most importantly, all these DC functions are exquisitely sensitive to modulation by environmental signals derived from pathogens and damaged tissues, allowing DCs to act as the critical cell in linking innate and adaptive immunity. Essentially, they recognize threats to the body ('danger') and translate them into inflammatory signals that, together with specific antigen, the immune system can respond to in an appropriate manner (Banchereau et al. 2000).

The life history and functions of DCs have been elucidated in recent years, using a combination of in vivo and in vitro approaches (Figure 20.4). The tissue-resident DC is typified by the Langerhans' cell (LC) found in the epidermis of the skin, but analogous cells can be found in other epithelial surfaces and in solid organs. These cells are relatively immature, quiescent cells that are derived from a common myeloid precursor circulating in blood, the role of which is to continually sample the local environment. This reflects an extremely high and constitutive ability to take up exogenous materials by a variety of different mechanisms, including endocytosis, phagocytosis, and macrophagocytosis. However, at this stage, LCs and equivalent DCs are not effective APCs. Although they express MHC II, most of this is retained intracellularly within vesicular compartments and the small amount that reaches the cell surface is recycled rapidly. DCs remain in this quiescent state until exposed to products of pathogens or other inflammatory stimuli (Table 20.1). These include bacterial cell wall components such as flagellin, lipopolysaccharide (LPS), and other glycolipids, as well as bacterial DNA, viral nucleic acids, heat shock proteins, and a variety of cytokines released by infected or damaged cells, including IL-1, IL-6, and tumor necrosis factor (TNF) α. By binding to appropriate Toll-like receptors (TLR) (Barton and Medzhitov 2002) or cytokine receptors, these so-called 'danger signals' alert the DCs to the presence of potential harm and stimulate a number of coordinated, activation-related events in the DCs (Banchereau et al. 2000). Endosomal pH levels fall and acidic endosomal protease activity is increased, leading to increased availability of antigenic peptides as a result of enhanced processing of ingested antigen. Stable peptide–MHC II complexes are then exported to the cell surface and remain there for considerable periods of time (48 h or more). In parallel, the endocytic activities of the DCs fall dramatically, meaning that the cell focuses its MHC II processing and presentation activities on the antigen(s) that have provoked the threat of danger. At the same time as these changes in intracellular function, the DCs become motile and alter their expression of chemokine receptors, so that they leave the tissue via afferent lymphatic vessels and migrate to the draining lymph node. The most important chemokine receptor involved in these processes is CCR7, which binds the chemokines CCL (ELC) and CCL (SLC), which are produced in the TDA of lymphoid organs, and are responsible for recruiting

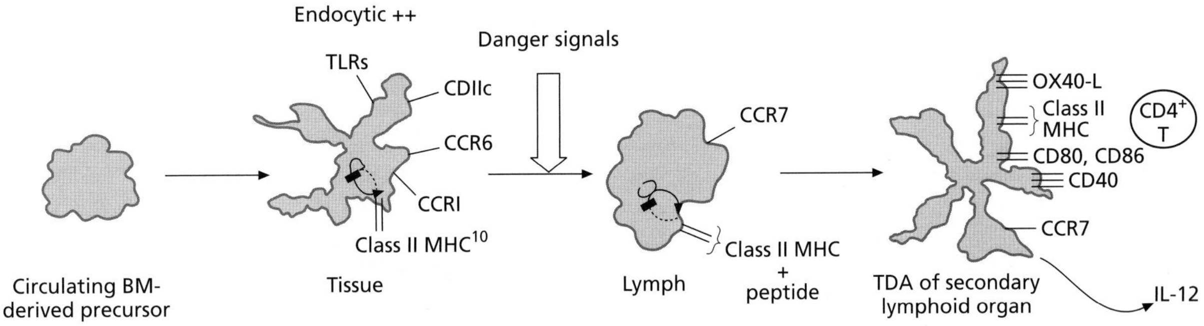

Figure 20.4 *Life history of dendritic cells (DCs). DCs derived from circulating bone marrow-derived precursors (myeloid or lymphoid) enter tissues in a relatively immature state; stimulation by pathogen-derived factors or inflammatory mediators then induces them to mature and emigrate from the tissue to the thymus-dependent area (TDA) of draining lymphoid organs via the afferent lymphatics. BM, bone marrow; IL, interleukin; MHC, major histocompatibility complex; TLR, Toll-like receptor. See text for details.*

Table 20.1 *Danger signals for dendritic cells*[a]

	Receptor
Pathogen associated molecule	
Bacterial lipopeptide	TLR-1
Bacterial lipopolysaccharide	TLR-2, TLR-4, CD14
Double-stranded RNA	TLR-3
Flagellin	TLR-5
Peptidoglycan	TLR-6
Bacterial DNA	TLR-9
Endogenous molecule	
Heat shock proteins	CD91
TNF-α	Type 1 TNF receptor (p55)
IL-1	IL-1 receptor
Histamine	H_1 histamine receptor

IL, interleukin; TNF, tumor necrosis factor.
a) These may be pathogen-associated molecular patterns (PAMPS) that normally interact with members of the Toll-like receptor (TLR) family, or endogenous mediators released during tissue.

both DCs and naive $CD4^+$ T cells to this site (Randolph 2001). Quiescent DCs in tissues do not express CCR7, but have receptors for chemokines produced by tissue cells such as keratinocytes and intestinal epithelial cells (CCR6), as well as for chemokines produced during inflammation (CCR1, CCR2, CCR5). After activation, the expression of these receptors is inhibited, partly because activated DCs produce inflammatory chemokines that induce downregulation of their own receptors; in parallel, CCR7 expression is induced. As a result, the activated DC loses its ability to localize in tissues or inflamed sites and acquires the ability to migrate specifically to the TDA of lymph nodes (Figure 20.4).

The other important effect of DC activation is to induce the expression of the co-stimulatory molecules required for full activation of T lymphocytes, including CD80 (B7.1), CD86 (B7.2), and CD40. In addition, they become capable of producing immunomodulatory cytokines such as IL-12 (Figure 20.4). Together with all the other changes discussed above, the result is that DCs arriving in the TDA of lymphoid organs are now fully competent to activate and polarize effector T-cell responses. In return, the DCs receive signals from the T cell that promote DC survival and activate them further, much of which is mediated by CD40 ligand, which is in turn upregulated on the activated T cell (Banchereau et al. 2000).

DCs are not a homogeneous population and a number of different subsets have been described on the basis of origin, tissue distribution, differentiation status, and function (Banchereau et al. 2000; Guermonprez et al. 2002). In many species, it appears that DCs may develop from either myeloid or lymphoid precursors and in humans these are referred to as 'monocyte-derived' and 'plasmacytoid' DCs. The exact relationship between the subsets is not yet clear, but their potential importance is that different populations of DCs may have distinct effects on $CD4^+$ T cells, selectively stimulating T-helper (Th) 1 or Th2 responses, or even T-cell tolerance. In addition, they may localize preferentially in different tissues.

OTHER TYPES OF ANTIGEN-PRESENTING CELL

It is now considered that DCs are the principal, if not the only, APCs capable of priming $CD4^+$ T cells in vivo. However, other MHC II-expressing cells can act as APCs under some circumstances, especially in the later stages of primary immune responses or in secondary responses. Although macrophages normally degrade materials to the amino acid level, macrophages activated by microbial stimuli and/or interferon (IFN)-γ express high levels of MHC II and co-stimulatory molecules. Such macrophages may be able to sustain ongoing $CD4^+$ T-cell responses, or even initiate them. B lymphocytes possess many of the features of APCs, including the constitutive expression of MHC II, the ability to process proteins in the endocytic pathway, and the expression of co-stimulatory molecules. In practice, the resting B lymphocytes found in normal lymphoid tissues cannot prime naive $CD4^+$ T cells, but, as the response matures, direct presentation of antigen by activated B cells in germinal centers is essential for previously primed $CD4^+$ T cells to help the differentiation of antibody-producing B lymphocytes. This presentation reflects the very high efficiency of antigen-specific B cells in internalizing and processing their cognate antigen via surface Ig. As the frequency of antigen-specific B cells is increased after primary immunization, these cells may also contribute to the initiation of secondary immune responses by presentation to $CD4^+$ T cells.

Many tissue cells can express MHC II during inflammation, probably under the influence of IFNγ. This is exemplified by epithelial cells in the intestine, stomach, kidney, and thyroid during chronic inflammation, as well as by the β cells of the pancreatic islets in type 1 diabetes and by vascular endothelial cells in many different organs. The role of these cells in T-cell-mediated immune responses is controversial, because they usually do not express co-stimulatory molecules. Nevertheless, previously activated $CD4^+$ T cells do not require as much co-stimulation as naive T cells and therefore MHC II-expressing tissue cells may sustain ongoing inflammation or protective immunity. Alternately, some workers believe that presentation of antigen by such APCs represents an attempt to downregulate the immune response by inactivating $CD4^+$ T cells (see below) (Schwartz 2003).

SUPERANTIGENS

A specialized group of proteins can activate $CD4^+$ T cells in an MHC II-restricted fashion, without the need for processing or co-stimulation. These are the 'superantigens', which act by forming a direct connection between nonpolymorphic regions on the MHC II molecule and certain families of TCR (Sundberg et al. 2002). Both $CD4^+$ and $CD8^+$ T cells can be activated in this way, but most superantigens act predominantly on $CD4^+$ T cells. Most are also microbial products and they are capable of activating up to 25 percent of all T cells because of their ability to bind to framework regions on the TCR distant from the MHC–peptide-binding site. Although their recognition by T cells does not require proteolytic processing, superantigens must be presented with appropriate MHC molecules on the surface of APCs, in the same way as conventional peptide antigens. Superantigens have proved extremely useful experimental tools for dissecting T-cell functions and tolerance, as the responding families of T cells can be readily identified using appropriate specific antibodies. In addition, they may contribute to the pathogenesis of the infections caused by the various organisms by virtue of their ability to activate large numbers of T cells, stimulating the production of large amounts of proinflammatory cytokines. The best example is TSST-A, which causes the toxic shock syndrome associated with vaginal infection by *Staphylococcus aureus* after chronic tampon retention, and the others may have analogous effects.

ACCESSORY MOLECULES AND $CD4^+$ T-CELL ACTIVATION

As we have noted, several nonpolymorphic molecules on $CD4^+$ T cells are essential for effective activation by appropriate peptide–MHC complexes (see Figure 20.3). This partly reflects the fact that the TCR itself does not undergo major conformational change after binding to antigen and also has very short cytoplasmic regions, meaning that it is incapable of initiating intracellular signaling on its own. In addition, each TCR–MHC–peptide interaction is of relatively low affinity and may be extremely transient. Thus, additional molecules are required both to stabilize the binding of the T cell to an APC carrying specific antigen and to assist the biochemical signaling pathways.

The CD3 complex that is physically linked to the TCR on all T cells is critical to T-cell signaling, but does not contribute to the interaction with the APC and its functions are considered in Chapter 24, T cell receptors. CD4 itself is the most important of the other molecules involved in these functions. It is a single chain molecule of 55 kDa, comprising four Ig superfamily domains, the outermost of which binds to nonpolymorphic residues on the α_2 domain of the MHC II molecule, distant from the peptide-binding groove. It is likely that each CD4 molecule may bind two separate MHC II molecules, each of which may bind a specific TCR, thus leading to the formation of 'pseudo-dimers'.

The binding of CD4 has two major effects on the T cell. First, it stabilizes the binding between the T cell and the APC, effectively increasing the affinity of the TCR for MHC–peptide and reducing the off-rate of this interaction. The second critical function of CD4 is to initiate tyrosine kinase-mediated signaling via the TCR. CD4 associates with the lck tyrosine kinase in the cell membrane and, after binding to the same MHC II as that bound by the TCR, CD4 brings lck into contact with the CD3–TCR complex, allowing lck to phosphorylate and activate the CD3ζ chain. This is the first and critical step in TCR-mediated signaling (see Chapter 24, T cell receptors) and an analogous function is served by CD8 binding to MHC I on $CD8^+$ T cells.

Many of the remaining nonpolymorphic co-stimulatory molecules belong to the CD28 or TNF/TNF receptor families (Sharpe and Freeman 2002; Croft 2003). CD28 is present on all mature $CD4^+$ T cells and is a homodimeric molecule; each of the chains of this molecule is a 44-kDa Ig superfamily molecule comprising a proximal Ig C-like domain and a distal Ig V-like domain. It binds to two related ligands present on professional APCs: B7.1 (CD80) and B7.2 (CD86). They are homologous to each other and to CD28. The B7 molecules appear to dimerize on the APCs, each unit binding a separate CD28 molecule, creating a zipper-like binding lattice that provides a highly stable and effective cell–cell interaction.

Co-ligation of CD28 after TCR–peptide–MHC binding is essential for most aspects of $CD4^+$ T-cell activation, including clonal expansion, effector T-cell differentiation, germinal center formation, and memory cell generation. The exact mechanisms of action of CD28 are still unclear, but it is a potent signaling molecule that can activate a number of intracellular pathways in the T cell, some of which are unique to CD28, including the activation of phosphatidylinositol-3-kinase. Together, these effects amplify and sustain signaling via the TCR pathway, leading to increased IL-2 production, prolongation in the lifespan of IL-2 mRNA, and improved $CD4^+$ T-cell survival, probably involving upregulation of anti-apoptotic molecules such as bcl_{XL} and of the telomerase enzyme that assists telomere repair in dividing cells. In the absence of these CD28-mediated effects, productive T-cell activation does not occur and $CD4^+$ T cells are effectively blinded to the antigen.

A molecule related to CD28, which plays somewhat similar roles at a different stage of the immune response, is the inducible co-stimulatory molecule (iCOS). It is highly homologous to CD28, but is expressed only after CD28-mediated activation of $CD4^+$ T cells and binds to a B7-related ligand (B7RP1) on B lymphocytes. The primary function of iCOS appears to be in promoting the differentiation of effector T cells after initial clonal expansion has occurred and it co-stimulates the production of cytokines such as IFNγ, IL-4, IL-5 and IL-10, but not IL-2. It is also important in determining the outcome of T-cell–B-cell cooperation and in germinal center formation.

CD40 ligand (CD40L) is the most critical of the TNF-related molecules involved in $CD4^+$ T-cell activation. A homotrimeric molecule expressed on activated $CD4^+$ T cells, it binds CD40 on DCs and B cells, and is required for T-cell help of B-cell differentiation (see below), as well as for the production of IL-12 and differentiation of IFNγ-producing Th1 cells in most immune responses. Its expression on $CD4^+$ T cells requires activation via TCR and CD28, and ligation of CD40 on DCs or macrophages stimulates the expression of B7 molecules and the production of IL-12. Thus, CD40L plays an essential role in positive feedback stimulation of $CD4^+$ T cells and APCs, as well as in delivery of effector T-cell function. Mice lacking CD40L have a severe deficiency in IL-12 production and Th1-mediated defenses against intracellular pathogens.

Other related molecules involved in the co-stimulation of $CD4^+$ T cells include OX40, 4-1BBL, and TRANCE, which bind the DC molecules OX40L, 4-BB, and RANK respectively. The specific functions of these molecules are still under investigation, but they may overlap or synergize with those of the CD40L–CD40 interaction. In addition, ligation of RANK by TRANCE appears to play a unique role as a survival signal for DCs after interaction with antigen-specific T cells.

A number of adhesion molecules act as accessory factors during $CD4^+$ T cell–APC interactions, particularly in the initial, antigen-independent stage before specific TCR–peptide–MHC binding. These include intercellular adhesion molecule (ICAM)-3, and its interaction with its ligand DC-SIGN may be the first event in the binding of T cells to DCs. Leukocyte function antigen 1 (LFA-1) and its ligand ICAM-1 (CD54) are expressed on both T cells and APCs, and they play an essential role in forming the highly organized binding complex (the 'immunological synapse') that is responsible for focusing the TCR on relevant MHC II–peptide complexes (see Chapter 19, Processing and presentation of antigen by the Class II histocompatibility system). Other accessory molecules include CD2, which is expressed on all T cells and binds to ICAM-3 and CD48 on APCs. As well as acting as adhesion molecules, ligation of all these receptors can also enhance signaling within the T cell.

TOLERANCE AND IMMUNITY AS ALTERNATIVE OUTCOMES OF CD4+ T-CELL ENCOUNTER WITH ANTIGEN

Productive activation of $CD4^+$ T cells is not the only possible consequence of presentation of MHC II–peptide complexes and, under some circumstances, the T cell may be inactivated, leading to the phenomenon of specific immunological tolerance. In this situation, the T cell not only fails to make an effective primary response to antigen, but is also unresponsive to subsequent restimulation with the same antigen, even if it is presented under conditions that would normally induce a strong immune response. Tolerance is critical for preventing immune responses to tissue antigens by self-reactive $CD4^+$ T cells that have escaped deletion in the thymus. It is also useful for preventing inappropriate responses to harmless foreign antigens, particularly when such responses could lead to tissue damage. Antigens of this kind include the fetus, food proteins, aerosol antigens, and commensal bacteria.

There are many theories and mechanisms to explain the induction of tolerance rather than productive immunity in $CD4^+$ T cells (Table 20.2). As all the antigens (self and foreign) that induce tolerance share the property of not stimulating inflammation and so not inducing the activation of APCs, it seems that tolerance develops when the antigen is presented by APCs that lack appropriate co-stimulatory molecules. Under these conditions, the $CD4^+$ T cell is partly activated after recognizing its specific peptide–MHC II complex on the APC, but does not receive the additional accessory stimuli necessary for full IL-2 production (Schwartz 2003). As a result, the T cell undergoes cell cycle arrest, probably mediated in part by accumulation of inhibitory factors within the cytoplasm, and it fails to make sufficient cell divisions to ensure an adequate primary response. In addition, the aberrant signaling in the T cell renders it unable to respond to subsequent stimulation via the TCR, permanently preventing effector cell differentiation. Despite these defects, these so-called 'anergic' T cells may also retain some functional capabilities, including the production of cytokines such as IL-10 and transforming growth factor (TGF) β, allowing them to inhibit the functions of other T cells and APCs. Such 'regulatory T cells' (T_{reg}) appear to play an important role in maintaining many forms of tolerance in vivo, because they can prevent the activation of naive, fully responsive $CD4^+$ T cells when antigen is next encountered (Maloy and Powrie 2001). A number of such T_{reg} cells have been described, of which the most studied recently is the $CD4^+CD25^+$ subset, which appears to be a naturally occurring regulatory cell derived from the thymus and which controls immune responses to self-antigens in peripheral tissues by as yet ill-defined mechanisms (Sakaguchi 2004). Others include the Tr1 cell, which differentiates in response to foreign antigen under the influence of environmental IL-10 and acts by producing IL-10 itself (Roncarolo et al. 2001).

Current evidence suggests that the APCs responsible for inducing tolerance in $CD4^+$ T cells may not be completely lacking in accessory molecules and that the process requires an alternate set of co-stimulatory events (Greenwald et al. 2002). Of these, the best understood is that involving CTLA-4, a homolog of CD28 that is expressed mainly on activated $CD4^+$ T cells, but which also can be involved in the earliest phase of T-cell interaction with APCs. Similar to CD28,

Table 20.2 *Potential mechanisms of tolerance*

Mechanisms	
Clonal deletion	Self-antigens in thymus
	Very high doses of peripheral antigens?
	Apoptosis after ligation of TCR
Clonal anergy	Self-antigens in thymus
	Self-antigens in periphery
	Harmless foreign antigens in periphery (foods, commensals, etc.)
	TCR ligation in absence of co-stimulation (or with dominant negative co-stimulation by, for example, CTLA-4) → partial activation, failure to transcribe IL-2 gene, defective clonal expansion, and no proliferation/IL-2 production on challenge
Regulatory T cells	T cells actively inhibit priming/functions of other, naive T cells
	Self-antigens in thymus – $CD4^+CD25^+$ T cells
	Self + foreign antigens in periphery
	$CD4^+CD25^+$ T cells generated by aberrant selection in thymus
	Regulatory T cells induced in periphery by resting APCs or APCs conditioned by, for example, IL-10
	$CD4^+CD25^+$ T cells act by cytokines, cell-cell contact
	Peripheral T_{reg} act by producing IL-10/TGF-β (Tr1, Th3)
Clonal ignorance	Antigen sequestered from T cell and not recognized by TCR
	Self-antigens such as lens protein, testis
	Specific T cells still present and potentially reactive

See text for details.
APC, antigen-presenting cell; IL, interleukin; TCR, T-cell receptor; TGF, transforming growth factor.

CTLA-4 binds CD80 and CD86 and was originally thought to have identical co-stimulatory functions. However, the observation that CTLA-4 knock-out mice developed fatal a lymphoproliferative disease led to the recognition that the principal role of CTLA-4 is to downregulate $CD4^+$ T-cell responses. The exact mechanisms responsible for this effect are not yet known, but it is clear that ligation of CTLA-4 transmits an inhibitory signal to the T cell and that this dominates over other, potentially stimulatory, signals. This can occur late in T-cell responses, when it is important to prevent over-activation of the immune response; this is probably the explanation for the high expression of CTLA-4 on activated T cells, when CD28 is also decreasing. In addition, CTLA-4 has higher affinity for CD80 and CD86 than CD28, meaning that CTLA-4 binding will predominate when the co-stimulatory molecules are expressed at low levels on APCs. As discussed, this is most likely to occur when APCs have not been activated adequately and it has been shown that the induction of tolerance in $CD4^+$ T cells requires early ligation of CTLA-4. Thus, CTLA-4 and CD28 play overlapping, but opposing, roles in the response of $CD4^+$ T cells to antigen, allowing the T cell to discriminate between dangerous antigen presented in the context of inflammation and self or harmless foreign antigens to which tolerance is necessary.

An additional co-stimulatory molecule on T cells that appears to play a preferential role in the induction of tolerance in $CD4^+$ T cells is PD-1, which is a CD28/CTLA-4 homolog that binds PDL-1 and PDL-2 on APCs. Its functions are not yet fully understood, but seem to involve activation of intracellular phosphatases that inactivate the tyrosine kinase signaling pathways of TCR-mediated activation.

DIFFERENTIATION AND FUNCTIONS OF TH1 AND TH2 CELLS

As noted above, $CD4^+$ Th cells are central to the normal immune response and are essential for protective immunity against a wide range of potentially pathogenic organisms. However, $CD4^+$ T cells can be further subdivided depending on the pattern of cytokines they produce and the type of immune response they support. The cardinal marker of Th1 T cells is the secretion of IFNγ. This cytokine is essential for the cell-mediated immune responses generally required for protection against intracellular pathogens such as *Leishmania* spp. and mycobacteria. In contrast, Th2 cells were defined by their production of IL-4 and a role in helping humoral immunity and responses against extracellular pathogens such as helminths (Abbas et al. 1996). Th1 and Th2 responses tend to be reciprocally regulated and their importance has been highlighted in a number of disease models where susceptibility or resistance to a particular pathogen is dependent on the ability to mount the appropriate Th1 versus Th2 response. Dysregulation of these responses may also be involved in a number of inflammatory disorders.

A number of models have been proposed to explain the process by which a naive precursor $CD4^+$ T cell can become either a Th1 or a Th2 cell (Murphy and Reiner 2002; O'Garra and Robinson 2004). Distinct precursors may exist and must become either Th1 or Th2. Alternately, cells could switch between the Th1 and Th2 phenotype, but can express only one particular phenotype at a time. However, it appears from studies in a number of TCR transgenic systems, where cells of the same specificity can mount a Th1 or a Th2 response, depending on the priming conditions, that the most likely explanation is that a common precursor exists which can differentiate into either Th1 or Th2 (Figure 20.5).

A large body of work has shown that cytokines are centrally important in causing naive $CD4^+$ T cells to differentiate into IL-4- or IFNγ-producing cells. Cytokines may exert their polarizing influence by acting directly on T cells or via APCs, and may have one or all of the following effects: promote differentiation of precursor Th cell towards a particular phenotype, cause preferential proliferation of a particular phenotype (i.e. expansion not differentiation), or inhibit either of the above for a particular subset, thereby leading to dominance of the other.

The heterodimeric cytokine IL-12 is a potent inducer of IFNγ production by both natural killer (NK) cells and T cells, and is the principal Th1-inducing cytokine. Many adjuvants and microbial products stimulate IL-12 production from macrophages and DCs and it interacts directly with naive Th cells. Indeed, functional receptors for IL-12 are present on recently activated, uncommitted cells and Th1 cells but are lost from differentiated Th2 cells. IL-18 is an IL-1-related cytokine that assists the IL-12-induced differentiation of Th1 cells, although it may also enhance Th2 responses under some conditions. Other cytokines that may be involved in Th1 cell development are IL-23 and IL-27, both of which are partly related to IL-12. IFNγ also plays a role in the development of Th1 and Th2, partly because it inhibits the clonal expansion of IL-4-producing Th2 cells and

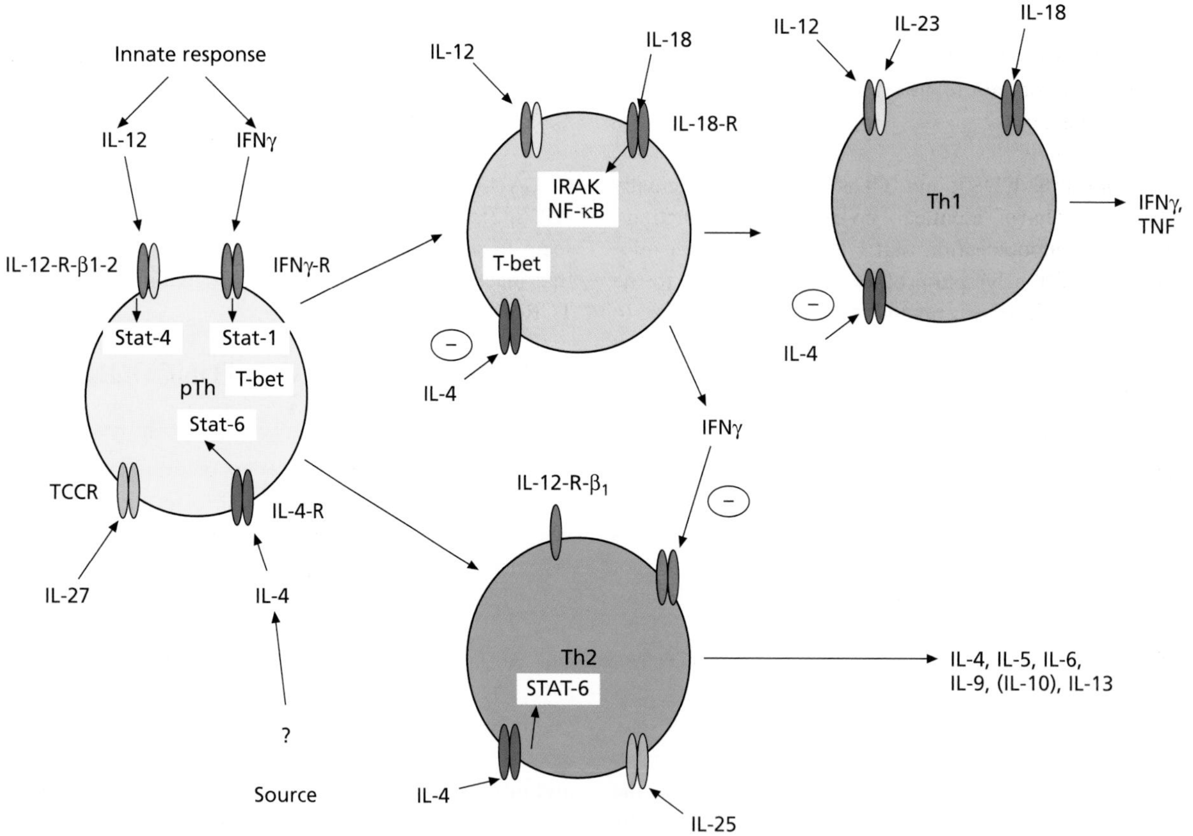

Figure 20.5 *Naive $CD4^+$ T cells can differentiate into either T-helper 1 (Th1) or 2 (Th2) cells after recognition of antigen, depending on signals derived from the local microenvironment. Interleukin IL-12 released by macrophages and dendritic cells (DCs) in response to, for example, intracellular pathogens binds to the IL-12-R-β1/-2 receptor, triggering signaling through Stat-4 and the consequent production of interferon-γ (IFNγ) and activation of the T-bet transcription factor. This leads to increased expression of the IL-18-R, allowing IL-18 released from a wide variety of cell types (including potential APCs) to enhance the production of IFNγ and further differentiation to the Th1 lineage via activation of NF-κB. Th1 cells maintain expression of the IL-12-R-β1/-2 chains, allowing continued positive feedback via IL-12 and the synergistic effects of IL-23 derived from cells such as macrophages and DCs. Th2 differentiation is dependent on IL-4, but its source early in the response is unknown. IL-4 acts by activating transcription factors such as Stat-6 and GATA-3. Developing Th2 cells lose expression of the IL-12-R-β-2 chain making them unresponsive to IL-12/IL-23, but maintain expression of the IFNγ-R, which accounts for the inhibitory effect of IFNγ on Th2 cell differentiation.*

also because it enhances IL-12 production by APCs and maintains the expression of functional IL-12 receptors on CD4+ T cells.

IL-4-producing Th2 cells emerge if IL-4 is present during priming, particularly if this is accompanied by the suppression of the appearance of IFNγ-producing cells. IL-4 appears to act directly on T cells and, once established, the IL-4-producing phenotype appears to be very stable. Another Th2 product, IL-10, diminishes IL-2 and IFNγ production by primed T cells, but, in contrast to IL-4, it appears that IL-10 acts via the APCs by suppressing production of the Th1-polarizing cytokine IL-12. Overall, it appears that IL-10 may contribute to the differentiation towards Th2 but it is not essential; this is supported by the fact that IL-10 knockout mice are capable of mounting Th2 responses.

WHAT ARE THE SOURCES OF THE CYTOKINES THAT POLARIZE TH1 AND TH2 RESPONSES IN VIVO?

Dendritic cells and to some extent macrophages are the sources of the IL-12 essential for the development of Th1 cells. However the in vivo source of IL-4 to promote differentiation into Th2 is more contentious. Naive T cells do not make appreciable amounts of IL-4 and differentiated Th2 cells would make a contribution only in an already primed animal. However, NK1.1+ T cells, which recognize antigens presented in association with the nonpolymorphic β_2-microglobulin-associated molecule, CD1, can produce considerable amounts of IL-4 very rapidly on activation (Chen et al. 1997). However, the role of these cells remains controversial because Th2 responses can still be induced in the absence of these cells. Alternately, cells of the mast cell/basophil lineage may be the source of IL-4, possibly after triggering of the FcεRI or FcγRII/III receptors. Although this would require pre-existing IgE or IgG1 antibodies, mast cells and basophils can be activated nonspecifically by agents such as helminth products.

OTHER FACTORS IN CONTROL OF CD4+ T-CELL DIFFERENTIATION

A number of factors have been implicated in the polarization of naive CD4+ T cells into Th1 or Th2 cells, including the nature of the APC, the dose of antigen, and the co-stimulatory molecules involved (O'Garra and Robinson 2004).

Initial ideas suggested that DCs were responsible for polarizing Th1-cell responses, whereas presentation of antigen by B lymphocytes induced Th2-cell responses preferentially. However, it now appears that all APCs can initiate either form of T-cell response, although different populations of APCs may influence the subsequent maintenance of the distinct forms of response. This may reflect differential production of and/or response to polarizing cytokines, or via the expression of different co-stimulatory molecules (see below). Recently it has been proposed that the distinct lineages of DCs (lymphoid vs myeloid: DC1 vs DC2) may promote the selective differentiation of Th1 and Th2 respectively.

However, again it seems that this is an oversimplification and that all DC subsets may promote either Th1 or Th2 responses under appropriate circumstances. Recent studies indicate that DCs exposed to the cytokine thymic stromal lymphopoietin, produced by tissue cells from atopic individuals, induce Th2 differentiation, suggesting that this may be a corollary for IL-12 and Th1 differentiation in allergic disease (Soumelis et al. 2002). Indeed by altering the affinity of the peptide interaction with the class II molecule or the TCR it has been found that an overall lower affinity favors Th2 priming, whereas Th1 responses dominate if there is high affinity. These findings can be summarized as follows:

Co-stimulation

It has already been suggested that APCs may play a role in the differentiation of Th subsets and that they may do this via their expression of co-stimulatory molecules. Most work in this area has concentrated on the interaction of the well-known co-stimulatory molecules CD28 and CTLA-4 with their ligands B7-1 (CD80) and B7-2 (CD86). However, a variety of blocking or 'knock-out' studies in a wide range of experimental models in vitro and in vivo have yielded conflicting results (O'Garra and Robinson 2004). The confusion is probably related to the fact that, as noted above, the initial interaction of CD28 (or CTLA-4) with its B7 ligands is required for T-cell priming but it may then have differential effects in the expansion and persistence of Th1 and Th2 responses. The role of CTLA-4 in Th1/-2 polarization is also complicated by the negative regulatory effects of this molecule.

It has become apparent recently that a third signal may also be required to elicit co-stimulation for T cells and this may be mediated by iCOS, which is a homolog of CD28, and does not bind either B7-1 or B7-2 but rather interacts with B7-related protein 1 (B7RP-1). This ICOS is not present on naive T cells but is induced on all activated T cells. The signaling of iCOS appears to be involved the generation and maintenance of both Th1 and Th2 responses, but may be of heightened importance in the latter because iCOS expression is sustained on Th2 cells after chronic stimulation.

Thus, the overall affinity of the interaction resulting from the net effects of ligand density, affinity with APCs and TCR, and co-stimulation may be important in determining the type of response initiated but must be viewed in the context of the cytokine environment induced in vivo. It now seems likely that the convergence point for all of these influences is the signal transduction across the cell membrane and this is discussed in greater detail in Chapter 24, T cell receptors.

Genetic background

A final, and relatively poorly defined, influence on Th polarization is that of non-MHC genes. Different inbred strains of mice have long been known to express distinct resistant or susceptible phenotypes to a variety of infections (e.g. *Leishmania major*, *Trichuris muris*) even when they are of the same MHC genotype, implying that genetic influences other than the MHC may be important. Studies using TCR transgenic animals backcrossed onto congenic strains that have the same MHC II antigens but different background genes have demonstrated that these genes influence naive T-cell polarization. The effect in this system appeared to be at the level of the T cell because mixing APCs and T cells from the different strains always led to the production of the cytokine profile associated with the T cell rather than the APC. Thus, it appears that T cells on a BALB/c background default to a Th2 phenotype as a result of greater initial IL-4 production and a decrease in IL-12 responsiveness resulting from the loss of IL-12-Rβ_2 expression. In contrast, animals on the congenic B10.D2 background do not display early IL-4 production and maintain IL-12-Rβ_2 expression and IL-12 responsiveness to develop a default Th1 phenotype.

PHENOTYPIC MARKERS OF TH1 AND TH2 CELLS

One of the major hindrances to progress in the study of Th1 and Th2 polarization has been the lack of reliable phenotypic markers of the two subsets. However, recent studies have identified several candidate molecules (Sallusto et al. 1998). The ligands for P- and E-selectin are preferentially expressed on Th1 cells and facilitate differential migration of these cells into inflammatory sites such as inflamed joints or sensitized skin (Austrup et al. 1997). The migration of Th2 cells, eosinophils, and basophils into tissues undergoing allergic reactions appears to be mediated by the eotaxin (a chemokine) receptor, CCR3, which is expressed on all of these cells but not Th1 cells (Sallusto et al. 1998). Another chemokine receptor, CCR5, may be restricted to Th1 cells whereas the IL-1-R homolog, ST2L, may occur only on differentiated Th2 cells.

B-CELL HELPER FUNCTION OF CD4$^+$ T CELLS – THE GERMINAL CENTER REACTION

The antibody response is an essential component of the immunological armory. In many cases the development of antibody-producing plasma cells from B cells is highly dependent on help from T cells, as evidenced by the lack of B-cell responses in congenitally athymic animals that lack T cells. For an antibody response to occur, rare antigen-specific T and B cells must encounter the antigen that they both recognize and each other. This is achieved in germinal centers in the secondary lymphoid organs (MacLennan 1994).

As discussed above, following exposure to antigen it is transported to the secondary lymphoid tissues, either in blood/lymph or by specialized antigen-transporting cells (e.g. Langerhans' cells in skin). The activated, laden APC has now upregulated receptors (e.g. CCR7) for chemokines (e.g. CCL19, CCL21), which are produced by the stromal cells and other APCs in the thymus-dependent T cell area of the lymph node (paracortex), and is thus attracted to this area. Recirculating naive T cells also express CCR7 and therefore also localize in the paracortex, optimizing the chance of them encountering their cognate antigen (Sallusto et al. 2000). The naive T cell can now 'see' antigenic peptide presented to it in the context of MHC II by the antigen-laden APC. This results in upregulation of co-stimulatory molecules such as CD40L, the production of cytokines, and further migration. Naive B cells also recirculate but they express a chemokine receptor (CXCR5) that is specific for a chemokine (CXCL13). CXCL13 is preferentially produced by the network of follicular DCs that forms the basic structure underlying the B-cell areas of the lymph nodes or primary follicles. Within the specialized B-cell follicle, the naive B cell has also acquired antigen via its surface immunoglobulin (sIg) by this stage, which leads to its activation. It is important to note that although there are very few B cells of any particular antigen specificity they have an enhanced capacity to acquire specific antigen because of their surface receptor. The activated B cells now upregulate their expression of CCR7 and are drawn towards the T-cell area of the lymph node. Antigen-specific T and B cells now meet at the border between the paracortex (Garside et al. 1998) and the follicle, as a result of what has been termed 'a balanced responsiveness' to chemokines produced in each area. Thus, sampling and transport of foreign molecules from all over the body to secondary lymphoid 'depots' that are under constant surveillance by recirculating, naive lymphocytes has maximized the opportunity for these cells to encounter their specific antigen. Furthermore, coordinated expression of chemokines and their receptors has brought activated antigen-specific T and B cells into close proximity within the lymph node (Cyster 2003).

A range of membrane-associated and soluble molecules is now employed to help T and B lymphocytes 'talk' to each other in a variety of ways. Most of these 'conversations' take place within and around the developing germinal center (Cyster 2003). Germinal centers are the specialized anatomical microenvironment where activated B cells proliferate and attempt to increase the affinity of their antibody for the eliciting antigen in the process known as affinity maturation (MacLennan 1994).

Germinal centers are derived from the primary follicles, which, as noted above, are the sites to which naive recirculating B cells migrate as they pass through the lymphoid tissue. Primary follicles contain resting B cells clustered around a network of processes extending from follicular dendritic cells (FDC) (Cyster 2003). FDCs are important in attracting B cells to follicles, but also play an important role in affinity maturation by holding intact antigen and/or antigen–antibody complexes on their surfaces for long periods of time.

To make an antibody response a B cell needs to hypermutate, survive, proliferate (clonally expand), differentiate, and secrete antibody. T cells help B cells to do all of these things. B cells that have acquired antigen via their specific receptor (sIg) are now further activated by presenting peptides from that antigen on their surface and undergoing a cognate interaction with Th cells specific for the same antigen. The necessity for this cognate interaction is demonstrated by the facts that the correct antigen and restriction element (MHC II) are required to elicit T-cell help for B cells. This is important to prevent nonspecific bystander activation of B cells, which could lead to autoantibody production. These activated B cells within the primary lymphoid follicle now start dividing to form germinal centers, and these tightly packed, proliferating B lymphocytes, which no longer express sIg, are referred to as centroblasts, and form the dark zone of the germinal center (MacLennan 1994).

For affinity maturation to occur, variability is randomly generated in the B-cell receptors and those with the highest affinity are selected. Random point mutations are targeted to the V-region genes of the rapidly dividing centroblasts in the process of somatic hypermutation. Newly configured mutant receptors are now expressed as sIg on the progeny of the centroblasts, which are known as centrocytes. Centrocytes subsequently migrate towards the FDC network in the light zone of the germinal center where they can encounter Th cells that have also migrated there. Centrocytes die by apoptosis within a short time of expressing their new sIg unless it is bound by antigen; then they are contacted by an activated Th cell expressing the survival signal CD40 ligand (CD40L). The random process of somatic hypermutation also means that the sIg expressed on the centrocytes derived from a particular progenitor may bind and take up antigen more or less efficiently than that expressed on its precursor. Centrocytes with mutations that result in a loss of the ability to bind antigen die by apoptosis. However, if the mutant sIg binds antigen well, the centrocyte is induced to express the *bcl-xl* gene, the product of which inhibits apoptotic cell death, and the cell is rescued. It is in this competitive environment that centrocytes with the highest affinity receptors bind and take up antigen and move to the outer edge of the light zone, where activated Th cells expressing CD40L are concentrated, whereas those with low-affinity receptors lose out and die by apoptosis (Rathmell et al. 1996). If the centrocyte and Th cell are specific for epitopes from the same antigen, they undergo a cognate interaction during which they exchange signals that promote their further proliferation and differentiation. The B cells become either memory cells or antibody-secreting plasma cells and may have also undergone isotype switching in response to cytokines secreted by Th cells. The involvement of T cells in the selective process in the germinal center prevents survival of centrocytes that have acquired specificity for self-antigens.

REFERENCES

Abbas, A.K., Murphy, K.M. and Sher, A. 1996. A functional diversity of helper T lymphocytes. *Nature*, **383**, 787–93.

Austrup, F., Vestweber, D., et al. 1997. P- and E-selectin mediate recruitment of T-helper-1 but not T-helper-2 cells into inflamed tissues. *Nature*, **385**, 81–3.

Banchereau, J., Briere, F., et al. 2000. Immunobiology of dendritic cells. *Annu Rev Immunol*, **18**, 767–811.

Barton, G.M. and Medzhitov, R. 2002. Control of adaptive immune responses by Toll-like receptors. *Curr Opin Immunol*, **14**, 380–3.

Boes, M. and Ploegh, H.L. 2004. Translating cell biology in vitro to immunity in vivo. *Nature*, **430**, 264–71.

Chen, Y.H., Chiu, N.M., et al. 1997. Impaired NK1+ T cell development and early IL-4 production in CD1-deficient mice. *Immunity*, **6**, 459–67.

Croft, M. 2003. Co-stimulatory members of the TNFR family: keys to effective T-cell immunity? *Nat Rev Immunol*, **3**, 609–20.

Cyster, J.G. 2003. Lymphoid organ development and cell migration. *Immunol Rev*, **195**, 5–14.

Garside, P., Ingulli, E., et al. 1998. Visualization of specific B and T lymphocyte interactions in the lymph node. *Science*, **281**, 96–9.

Goldrath, A.W. and Bevan, M.J. 1999. Selecting and maintaining a diverse T-cell repertoire. *Nature*, **402**, 255–63.

Greenwald, R.J., Latchma, Y.E. and Sharpe, A.H. 2002. Negative co-receptors on lymphocytes. *Curr Opin Immunol*, **14**, 391–6.

Guermonprez, P., Valladeau, J., et al. 2002. Antigen presentation and T cell stimulation by dendritic cells. *Annu Rev Immunol*, **20**, 621–67.

Itano, A.A., McSorley, S.J., et al. 2003. Distinct dendritic cell populations sequentially present antigen to CD4 T cells and stimulate different aspects of cell-mediated immunity. *Immunity*, **19**, 47–57.

Janeway, C.A., Travers, P., et al. 2001. *Immunobiology: The immune system in health and disease*, 5th edn. New York: Garland Publishing.

MacLennan, I.C.M. 1994. Germinal centres. *Annu Rev Immunol*, **12**, 117–39.

Maloy, K.J. and Powrie, F. 2001. Regulatory T cells in the control of immune pathology. *Nat Immunol*, **2**, 816–22.

Marrack, P. and Kappler, J. 2004. Control of T cell viability. *Annu Rev Immunol*, **22**, 765–87.

Mathis, D. and Benoist, C. 2004. Back to central tolerance. *Immunity*, **20**, 509–16.

Murphy, K.M. and Reiner, S.L. 2002. The lineage decisions of helper T cells. *Nat Rev Immunol*, **2**, 933–44.

O'Garra, A. and Robinson, D. 2004. Development and function of T helper 1 cells. *Adv Immunol*, **83**, 133–62.

Randolph, G.J. 2001. Dendritic cell migration to lymph nodes: cytokines, chemokines, and lipid mediators. *Semin Immunol*, **13**, 267–74.

Rathmell, J.C., Townsend, S.E., et al. 1996. Expansion or elimination of B cells in vivo: Dual roles for CD40- and Fas (CD95)-ligands modulated by the B cell Ag receptor. *Cell*, **87**, 319–29.

Roncarolo, M.G., Bacchetta, R., et al. 2001. Type 1 T regulatory cells. *Immunol Rev*, **182**, 68–79.

Sakaguchi, S. 2004. Naturally arising CD4+ regulatory T cells for immunologic self-tolerance and negative control of immune responses. *Annu Rev Immunol*, **22**, 531–62.

Sallusto, F., Lanzavecchia, A. and MacKay, C.R. 1998. Chemokines and chemokine receptors in T-cell priming and Th1/Th2-mediated responses. *Immunol Today*, **19**, 568–74.

Sallusto, F., MacKay, C.R. and Lanzavecchia, A. 2000. The role of chemokine receptors in primary, effector and memory immune responses. *Annu Rev Immunol*, **18**, 593–620.

Schwartz, R.H. 2003. T cell anergy. *Annu Rev Immunol*, **21**, 305–34.

Sharpe, A.H. and Freeman, G.J. 2002. The B7-CD28 superfamily. *Nat Rev Immunol*, **2**, 116–26.

Soumelis, V., Reche, P.A., et al. 2002. Human epithelial cells trigger dendritic cell mediated allergic inflammation by producing TSLP. *Nat Immunol*, **3**, 673–80.

Starr, T.K., Jameson, S.C. and Hogquist, K.A. 2003. Positive and negative selection of T cells. *Annu Rev Immunol*, **21**, 139–76.

Steinman, R.M., Hawiger, D. and Nussenzweig, M.C. 2003. Tolerogenic dendritic cells. *Annu Rev Immunol*, **21**, 685–711.

Stockinger, B., Barthlott, T. and Kassiotis, G. 2004. The concept of space and competition in immune regulation. *Immunology*, **111**, 241–7.

Sundberg, E.J., Li, Y. and Mariuzza, R.A. 2002. So many ways of getting in the way: diversity in the molecular architecture of superantigen-dependent T-cell signaling complexes. *Curr Opin Immunol*, **14**, 36–44.

21

MHC class I antigen processing system

JONATHAN W. YEWDELL

EVOLUTIONARY CONTEXT: OVERVIEW OF THE ADAPTIVE CELLULAR IMMUNE SYSTEM

Many infectious agents are obligate intracellular parasites. All viruses meet this description, as do many pathogenic prokaryotes and unicellular eukaryotes. Cellular organisms can also be opportunistic intracellular interlopers, particularly if it enables them to escape the clutches of the humoral immune system. Cells are not wholly defenseless against intracellular microorganisms, although the capacity of such innate immune mechanisms is relatively limited.

An important part of the innate response of infected cells is the manufacture and release of cytokines (most commonly α- and β interferons). In many circumstances, this provides the initial warning of the invasion to the organism. At this juncture two strategies are conceivable: the immune system could indiscriminately target the general vicinity of the infected cell and implement an anti-pathogen program akin to carpet bombing. As immune effector mechanisms can have deleterious effects on cells (the ultimate being death, of course) this would come with a high cost in collateral damage. Alternately, the immune system can selectively target infected cells for individual attention. This is a sufficiently attractive possibility for vertebrate organisms to make an enormous evolutionary investment to achieve it.

The essential problem faced by the immune system is the efficient identification of infected cells in a spatially complex organ. Any reasonable solution entails endowing immune cells with the ability to detect the presence of intracellular pathogens without disrupting the integrity of cells harboring the agent. This was achieved by the evolution of a molecule that carries small bits of information encoded by the pathogen to the surface of the infected cell for perusal by immune cells bristling with receptors which co-evolved the capacity to decode the information. The information-carrying molecule is known as a major histocompatibility complex (MHC) class I molecule. The information takes the form of pathogen-encoded oligopeptides (usually 8–11 residues in length). These are generated by the antigen-processing machinery, which, like class I molecules, is constitutively expressed by virtually all cells in a vertebrate organism. Decoding is performed by a receptor (the αβ T-cell receptor (TCR) expressed by cells (the $CD8^+$ T cell) charged with the task of finding and modifying cells expressing nonself peptides.

This is an impressive achievement, but the system has a potential flaw: pathogens can evolve to mimic self-peptides and avoid detection. To discourage this, an additional level of complexity was added. The value added by this modification is best illustrated by its high cost. Alleles of MHC class I genes evolved that present distinct sets of peptides. Such alleles are present in the population of most vertebrate species at sufficient frequencies to make it likely that any two individuals present substantially different sets of peptides on their class I molecules. This is the inexpensive part.

As every American parent with college-age children painfully knows, life's real expense comes in education. Since the immune system in any individual cannot anticipate which class I molecules it must recognize, its TCRs cannot be hard-wired into the genome. Rather, evolution invented thymic selection to select, among T-cell clones expressing different TCRs, for those that are capable of recognizing self class I molecules with the proper affinity.

The thymus is more akin to a mortuary than a kindergarten, because the vast majority of T cells entering cannot meet the exacting standard of expressing a TCR that binds to class I molecules with the intermediate affinity required to enable self–nonself discrimination. Given that humans can generate up to 10^9 T cells per day (at birth, the peak of thymic activity), which represents 2–5 percent of immature thymocytes entering the thymus, the daily carnage amounts to perhaps 2×10^{10} cells (50 g or so) (Haynes et al. 2000)! Waste is a theme that we return to when discussing the generation of antigenic peptides.

$CD8^+$ T cells are but half of a dynamic duo, their partners being $CD4^+$ T cells. The siblings are charged with largely distinct tasks. $CD8^+$ T cells serve as a principal immune effector mechanism for fighting viruses and other intracellular parasites. $CD4^+$ T cells are preoccupied with regulating the activities of other immune cells, including their $CD8^+$ T-cell siblings. $CD4^+$ T cells also recognize oligopeptides (occasionally the same peptides as $CD8^+$ T cells), but presented by MHC class II molecules (dead ringers for class I molecules structurally, but very different in primary sequence). $CD8^+$ and $CD4^+$ T cells acquire their TCRs from a single gene pool. The discrimination of class I versus class II molecules results from the expression of the CD8 versus CD4 co-receptors. The interaction of CD8 and CD4 with class I and class II molecules, respectively, is required for positive thymic selection, and also enhances the interaction of mature $CD4^+$ and $CD8^+$ T cells with antigen-presenting cells (APC).

Humans possess about 10^{11} mature T cells, representing approximately 10^8 clones with distinct TCRs (making an average clone size of 1000) (Arstila et al. 1999; Img et al. 2000). Each T cell expresses approximately 10^5 TCRs. T cells can be triggered by APCs expressing about 10–100 class I molecules containing an appropriate peptide. This is truly an amazing feat because, first, the T cell must sort through the roughly 10^5 class I molecules on the APC surface that contain inappropriate peptides, and, second, the affinity of the TCR for its cognate peptide–class I complex is such that contact is maintained only for the order of a few seconds to minutes.

It is important to distinguish two types of $CD8^+$ T-cell activation. 'Afferent' refers to the activation of resting naïve or memory $CD8^+$ T cells. 'Efferent' refers to the activation of $CD8^+$ T-cell effector function by target cells. In both cases activation requires ligation of the TCR by an appropriate MHC–peptide complex. Afferent activation requires additional 'co-stimulatory' signals that are transmitted by molecules normally expressed only by professional APCs (pAPC). The most important co-stimulatory interaction is that of CD28 on the $CD8^+$ T cells with CD80 or CD86 on the pAPC. The pAPCs are bone marrow-derived cells that normally activate $CD8^+$ T cells in lymphoid organs, typically a local draining node or the spleen. These include macrophages, B cells, and dendritic cells (DC). Unlike other cell types, pAPCs constitutively express MHC class II molecules, which enables them to present antigens to $CD4^+$ T cells, and to serve as a bridge between $CD4^+$ and $CD8^+$ T cells.

DCs are believed to play a particularly important role in generating $CD8^+$ T-cell responses. Large numbers are present in tissues, where they can form an interdigitating network. Such networks have been shown to exist in the skin (where the DCs are known as Langerhans' cells) and the respiratory tract. At the early stages of inflammation DCs 'mature', altering their phenotype and physiology as they migrate via lymphatics to local draining lymph nodes, where they activate T cells. Importantly, pAPCs are able to present both 'endogenous' viral antigens, i.e. peptides synthesized by the cell as a result of viral infection, as well as 'exogenous antigens', peptides, or polypeptides acquired from other virus-infected cells. This latter pathway is known as 'crosspriming', and it appears to be the principal pathway used to induce $CD8^+$ T cells when viruses are unable to initiate infection in pAPCs, or when viruses express gene products that interfere with antigen presentation by infected pAPCs.

A critical feature of $CD8^+$ T-cell responses to viruses (and probably other pathogens) is that only a tiny fraction (ranging from a few to perhaps 50 or so) of the thousands to hundreds of thousands of different peptides (depending on the complexity of the virus) generated by infected cells induce measurable $CD8^+$ T-cell responses. This phenomenon, known as immunodominance, is caused by a number of factors (Yewdell and Bennink 1999). The most important is that that only about 0.5 percent of peptides of the correct length bind to any given class I molecule allele with sufficient affinity ($K_D > 5\ (10^{-7})$ to produce enough complexes to trigger $CD8^+$ T-cell activation. Second, the TCR repertoire can distinguish as foreign only about 50 percent of viral peptides that bind to class I molecules at or above this threshold affinity. Third, the antigen-processing machinery is limiting for production of 80 percent of the determinants that bind to class I molecules, mostly as a result of difficulties in proteolytic generation of determinants. Fourth, strong $CD8^+$ T-cell responses to a given determinant suppress responses to other determinants (this is known as immunodomination). Finally, to maximize replication, many viruses shut down the synthesis of host proteins, including class I molecules. If the supply of class I molecules is limiting, determinants from viral proteins expressed late in the infectious cycle will have no means of presentation to $CD8^+$ T cells (this applies only to cases in which $CD8^+$ T-cell activation requires presentation of endogenous antigens by pAPCs).

ANTIGEN PROCESSING: STEP BY STEP

The tripartite complex

CLASS I STRUCTURE

Class I molecules recognized by TCRs have three noncovalently bound chains. In order of size they consist of an oligopeptide of 8–12 residues, an invariant small soluble subunit (termed 'β_2-microglobulin'), and a membrane-bound integral membrane glycoprotein (termed 'α chain') encoded by highly variable genes. α chains consist of a short carboxy-terminal short domain, a typical transmembrane hydrophobic region, a relatively large extracellular domain, and an amino-terminal signal peptide that is cleaved upon import of class I molecules into the endoplasmic reticulum (ER). The three-dimensional structures of the extracellular domains of numerous class I allomorphs have been determined at high resolution by X-ray crystallography (the intracellular and transmembrane domains are excluded to enable crystal formation) (Madden 1995) (Figure 21.1). The stalk of the molecule is formed by the domain most proximal to the membrane, which is composed of residues encoded by the third of the seven exons that encode the α chain (and therefore termed the 'α3 domain'). The α3 domain makes important contacts with β_2-microglobulin and is the region that interacts with CD8. Residues from the first two exons (α1 and α2) combine to form the region most distal from the membrane, which is at its tip and contains the peptide-binding groove. The groove consists of two anti-parallel α helices which border a floor consisting of 7-β sheets. This region of the molecule contains most of the polymorphic residues, which are concentrated in areas of the groove that contact peptides.

α Chains are encoded by the MHC, termed human leukocyte antigen (HLA) in humans (Figure 21.2) and H-2 in mice, located, respectively on chromosomes 6 and 17. Three loci in the HLA encode class I genes, termed HLA-A, -B, and -C, whereas H-2 has two or three such loci (depending on the strain), termed H-2K, -D, or -L. At each α chain locus there are thousands of alleles present at appreciable frequencies in the entire

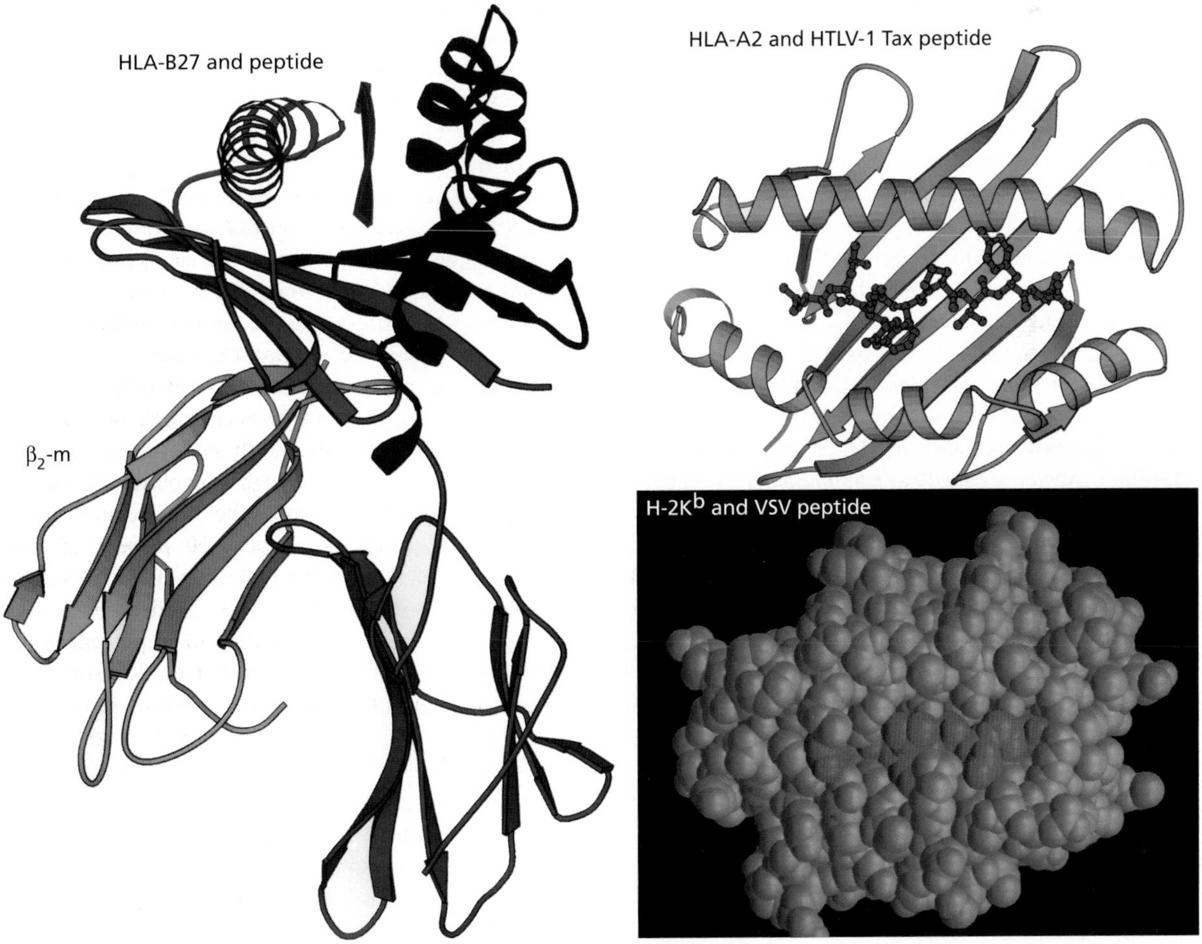

Figure 21.1 *Three-dimensional structure of MHC class I and class II molecules: structure of α-carbon backbone of HLA-B27 molecule (left) bearing an antigenic peptide (short red ribbon) in the groove, as determined by X-ray crystallography of water-soluble molecules released from the cell surface by protease digestion. Molecule is oriented with top toward the T-cell receptor (TCR). On the right are ribbon (top) and space-filling (bottom) models of peptides snug in the grooves of the class I molecules as they would be seen by the TCR.*

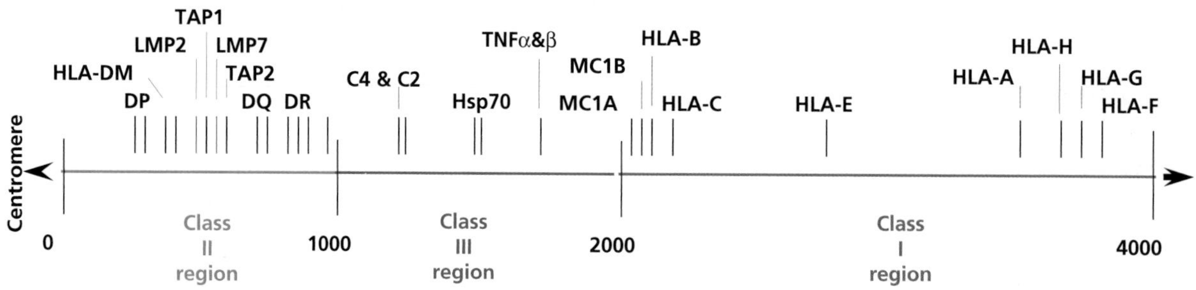

Figure 21.2 *Genetic map of HLA complex.*

human population. Individual ethnic groups often possess certain alleles that are present at higher frequencies than in the overall population. As the functions of HLA-A, -B, and -C molecules are similar, it is useful to lump together all the alleles produced by the three loci under the term 'allomorph'. HLA allomorphs are designated by a logical series of numbers (mercifully) that distinguish allelic alterations in nonsynonymous and synonymous alteration in coding regions and alterations in noncoding regions (see Table 21.1), whereas H-2 allomorphs are identified by a bewildering array of capital letters and superscripts, a nomenclature worthy of Torquemada.

The α chains under discussion are components of 'classical' class I molecules, also known as class Ia molecules (referred to throughout this chapter simply as class I molecules). In addition, there are a number of other homologous genes encoding α chains that generate 'nonclassic' or class Ib molecules. In general, class Ib genes are much less polymorphic than class Ia genes (although there are exceptions). The HLA encodes five such molecules: HLA-E, -F, and -G, which bind β_2-microglobulin, and MHC class I chain-related (MIC) gene products MICA and MICB, which do not (MIC is also of interest because its genes are highly polymorphic). All these genes have immunological functions that for are the most part independent of recognition by T cells with αβ TCRs. In addition, genes outside the MHC encode class Ib molecules: these include genes with immunological functions (such as *CD1*) and those apparently without direct immune function (such as *HFE*, which functions in iron metabolism). Mice have more than 40 genes encoding class Ib α chains; current understanding of the functions of these molecules ranges from fragmentary to nil.

CLASS I PEPTIDE LIGANDS

Binding rules

Peptides recovered from class I molecules are a highly heterogeneous mixture. Given a cell with 10^5 class I molecules of a given allomorph, there will be perhaps 10 000 distinct peptides presented. The dominant anchor residues of peptides bound by numerous HLA class I allomorphs have been determined by Edman sequencing of peptide pools recovered from purified molecules (Engelhard 1994; Rammensee et al. 1995) (the exact sequence of peptides of sufficient abundance can be determined directly by mass spectroscopy). In recent years, mass spectroscopy has been increasingly used to identify peptide ligands, as a result of the rapid technical advances in mass spectroscopy and greater access to advanced mass spectrometers. To date, however, only a few antigenic peptides from viruses have been identified in this manner.

The binding of peptides to class I molecules displays two important features. First, main chain atoms at the carboxyl and amino termini of the peptide make energetically important bonds with invariant residues at the ends of the groove (Bouvier and Wiley 1994). Peptides of fewer than eight residues cannot simultaneously contact both ends of the groove. Elongation of peptides also prevents these interactions because only a limited amount of kinking is allowed. Consequently, class I peptides exhibit little size heterogeneity, with about 90 percent of the peptides recovered from class I molecules falling within the range 8–11 residues in length, depending on the class I allomorph and the ability of peptides to bend in the groove. Second, the residues that demonstrate the most polymorphism among allomorphs form two to three deep pockets in the bottom of the groove which accommodate a highly restricted set of amino acids from bound peptides. As a result, each class I allomorph demonstrates a distinct preference for peptides that possess the complementary 'dominant anchor' residues, one of which is usually located at the carboxyl terminus (Table 21.1).

If antiviral $CD8^+$ T cells are known to be specific for a given viral protein presented by an allomorph with defined anchor residues, predictive algorithms (based largely on dominant anchor residues) can be used to identify a reasonably small number of candidate peptides from the protein (depending on the size of the viral protein, there are usually two to five such peptides) (Rammensee et al. 1997). These peptides can then be synthesized and used to determine the precise peptide recognized by virus-specific $CD8^+$ T cells. This method is used routinely, and is able to identify about 50 percent

Table 21.1 *Human MHC class I-binding peptide motifs*

HLA molecule	Position									
	1	2	3	4	5	6	7	8	9	10
HLA-A1			D, E						Y	
HLA-A*0201		L							L	
HLA-A*0205									L	
HLA-A3		L, V, M							K, Y, F	
HLA-A*1101									K	K
HLA-A24		Y							I, L, F	
HLA-A*3101,2									R	
HLA-A68.1		V, T							R, K	
HLA-B7		P							L, F	
HLA-B8			K		K, R				L	
HLA-B*2702		R							F, Y, I, L, W	
HLA-B*2705		R							L, F	
HLA-B*3501		P							Y, F, M, L, I	Y
HLA-B*3701		D						F, M, L	I, L	
HLA-B*3801									F, L	
HLA-B*39011		R, H							L	
HLA-B*3902		K, Q							L	
HLA-B40		E							L	
HLA-B*4402,3		E							F, Y	
HLA-B*5101,2,3		A, P, G							F, I, V	
HLA-B*5201								I, V	I, V	
HLA-B53		P								
HLA-B*5801		A, S, T							F, W	
HLA-B60 (B*40012)		E							L	
HLA-B61 (B*4006)		E							V	
HLA-B62 (B*1501)		Q, L							F, Y	
HLA-B*7801		P, A, G								
HLA-Cw*0301									L	
HLA-Cw*0401		Y, P, F							L, F	
HLA-Cw*0602									L	
HLA-Cw*0702									Y	

Human MHC molecules are termed 'human leukocyte antigens' (HLA). There are three loci encoding class I molecules, HLA-A, B, and C. Originally HLA molecules were typed serologically; such antigenically defined gene products are identified by one or two digits. More recently, HLA gene products are identified indirectly by genotyping. This provides much greater precision and revealed that previously identified alleles comprised a number of closely related genes. HLA genes (as opposed to gene products) are designated by an asterisk, and are numbered with up to seven digits. Closely related alleles share the first two digits and are discriminated by the last two digits (the remaining three digits are used to designate synonymous alterations in coding regions, or changes in noncoding regions), e.g. there are 30 known genes closely related to the canonical HLA-A2; these are numbered A0201 to A0230. HLA-C genes are given a gratuitous 'w' to avoid confusion with complement components. The anchor residues favor binding to various human class I allomorphs as determined by pooled sequencing of peptides eluted from purified class I molecules. The presence of anchor residues at consecutive positions at residues at consecutive positions at the carboxyl terminus reflects heterogeneity in peptide length, and not consecutive anchor positions.

of the determinants recognized by antiviral $CD8^+$ T cells. If this method fails, overlapping peptides covering the entire protein can be screened for activity. Empirically it has been found that peptides of 13 residues overlapping by 9–10 residues work well.

Exogenous peptide presentation: practical issues

All cells expressing class I molecules possess cell-surface class I molecules capable of binding peptides present in the extracellular fluids. Free peptides are probably rarely present in sufficient concentrations in vivo during a virus infection to sensitize bystander cells. Although the physiological significance of such peptide-receptive (PR) cell surface class I molecules is uncertain, PR class I molecules enable the use of synthetic peptides to sensitize cells to activate $CD8^+$ T cells for in vitro assays (lysis, intracellular cytokine staining, ELISPOT), and to stimulate secondary in vitro responses (an oft-used method to generate $CD8^+$ T cells specific for a known peptide, and an alternate method for determining which peptides are recognized by $CD8^+$ T cells). The expression of cell surface PR molecules can be enhanced by culturing cells at 25–28°C in media supplemented with 2–5 μg/ml human β_2-microglobulin.

Immunogenic peptides typically bind to class I molecules with a K_D of $<10^{-7}$ mol/l. Using optimized systems, most antiviral effector $CD8^+$ T cells require only 10–1000 peptide–class I complexes for activation. Translated into practical terms, incubating cells with sub-nanomolar (often picomolar) concentrations of peptide is sufficient for activation of effector $CD8^+$ T cells. This enables screening of peptides with 13 residues, based on the generation of fragments by serum proteases in culture media (Kozlowski et al. 1992), or low-affinity binding of extended suboptimal peptides. It also means that for screening purposes highly purified peptides need not be used (though, if impure peptides are used to generate $CD8^+$ T cells, they may induce $CD8^+$ T cells that are specific for contaminants (Chen et al. 1996)). Note that great care has to be taken when working with synthetic peptides corresponding to naturally processed peptides, which when present in a 1 mmol/l stock solution often represent a billionfold excess. Care must also be taken when weighing out the peptides, which are notoriously susceptible to floating away on errant air currents, where the tiniest speck can contaminate fluids. If possible, the balance should not be located in rooms used to perform assays or culture target cells. Incubation of cells with a vast excess of peptide can lead to spurious recognition by $CD8^+$ T cells specific for other determinants. Consequently, it is important to establish that $CD8^+$ T cells recognize cells sensitized with a concentration of peptide that results in the generation of a physiological number of peptide–class I complexes; usually this means incubating cells with sub-nanomolar peptide concentrations. Ultimately, definitive evidence that $CD8^+$ T cells recognize a given determinant in a protein requires the demonstration that mutating the corresponding residues in a protein modifies antigenicity. Lamentably, this rigorous approach is rarely applied.

Determinants that fail to be identified using synthetic peptides may possess post-translational modifications required for binding to class I molecules and/or recognition by the cognate TCR. These include phosphorylation, glycosylation, or deglycosylation of N-linked oligosaccharides, which converts asparagine residues that serve as the branch point for N-linked oligosaccharides into aspartic acid (Skipper et al. 1996; Andersen et al. 1999; Zarling et al. 2000). Cysteine-containing peptides (about 15 percent of all antigenic peptides) present special challenges as a result of the highly reactive nature of the free sulfhydryl group. $CD8^+$ T cells may recognize cysteine-crosslinked peptide dimers, cysteinylated peptides, or other undefined post-translational modifications (Meadows et al. 1997; Chen et al. 1999). Another potential reason for failing to locate a determinant in a protein is that the peptide is encoded by an alternate reading frame (Mayrand and Green 1998).

Although the basis for the antigenicity of synthetic peptides is nearly always their binding to cell-surface PR molecules, unless the cells are incubated with peptides at low temperature, peptides will traffic to endosomal compartments as a result of constitutive endocytosis and also to the ER (Day et al. 1997), where they can associate with resident PR molecules.

CLASS I ASSEMBLY AND SURFACE EXPRESSION

As with most integral membrane proteins, α chains are co-translationally inserted into the ER via the translocon. HLA α chains acquire a single N-linked oligosaccharide during translocation, whereas H-2 α chains are either di- or triglycyosylated. Newly synthesized α chains initially bind to calnexin, an abundant general purpose ER molecular chaperone which, like other chaperones, is thought to facilitate proper folding by preventing inappropriate interactions between hydrophobic domains (Williams and Watts 1995) (Figure 21.3). Within 5–10 min, α chains associate with β_2-microglobulin, and are transferred from calnexin to a complex of calreticulin, ERp56 (two more general purpose chaperones), and tapasin, a chaperone dedicated to class I molecules (Pamer and Cresswell 1998). ERp56 catalyzes the proper disulfide bond formation in α chains (Hughes and Cresswell 1998), whereas tapasin mediates the binding of the assembly complex to transporter associated with antigen processing (TAP). $\alpha\beta_2$-microglobulin heterodimers remain in the ER tethered to TAP until their release is triggered by peptide binding (Ortmann et al. 1994; Suh et al. 1994). Class I departure from the ER appears to be subject to further quality control inspection at ER exit sites (Spiliotis et al. 2001). Depending on the class I allomorph and the supply of peptides (and probably other undefined factors), class I export from the ER can take between 10 min and several hours. Transport to the cell surface via the Golgi complex occurs over a period of 10–20 min. The degree of association of class I molecules with tapasin (and therefore TAP) varies considerably among allomorphs (Peh et al. 1998). Why this should be remains an interesting mystery. Although tapasin is not absolutely required for peptide binding, it facilitates the loading of high-affinity peptides through an undefined mechanism (Garbi et al. 2000; Grandea et al. 2000).

'High-affinity' peptide binding refers to a K_D of $<10^{-7}$ mol/l. Peptide ligands that bind with this affinity will not dissociate from class I heterodimers for hours, and those with higher affinities will on average probably remain bound to class I until the molecule is shed from the cell surface or destroyed after internalization into lysosomes, which occurs with a half-time of the order of tens of hours. It is likely, however, that a substantial portion of peptides binds class I molecules less stably. Once peptides dissociate from cell surface class I molecules, class I molecules are unstable and unfold with a time of about 10 min. Just before unfolding β_2-microglobulin dissociates from heavy chains, which denature rapidly in its absence. This process is reversible, which is why β_2-microglobulin promotes the formation of PR molecules. β_2-Microglobulin is naturally present in human and mouse serum and plasma (and fetal bovine serum) at concentrations that create such PR class I molecules. Increasing the β_2-microglobulin concentration enhances the formation of PR molecules, as discussed above. Human β_2-microglobulin is preferred for this purpose because of its commercial availability and because it binds more tightly to both human and mouse α chains than mouse β_2-microglobulin, and it is thus more efficient at creating PR class I molecules.

Generating peptide ligands from biosynthesized proteins

SOURCE OF ANTIGENIC PEPTIDES

The process by which peptides are derived from proteins and delivered to class I molecules (or, for that matter, MHC class II molecules) is termed 'antigen processing' (Yewdell and Bennink 1992; Germain and Margulies 1993; Heemels and Ploegh 1995; Pamer and Cresswell 1998; Yewdell et al. 1999a). The classic class I antigen-processing pathway begins in the cytosol (see Figure 21.3). Proteins can reach the cytosol by virtue of being either synthesized by ribosomes (endogenous antigens) or physically introduced into the cytosol from extracellular fluids (exogenous antigens).

Antigenic peptides can be derived from any type of viral or cellular protein, including those located in the cytosol, nucleus, mitochondria, and various membranes. Even secreted proteins can be highly antigenic. How are peptides generated from these disparate protein sources? A possible clue comes from the kinetics of presentation of newly synthesized viral proteins to $CD8^+$ T cells, which can occur within an hour of adding a virus to cells. Given the time needed for viral penetration and transcription (using DNA or negative strand RNA viruses) and transport of class I–peptide complexes from the ER to the cell surface, this leaves only about 30 min for the virus to begin to synthesize its proteins. If viral proteins were simply entering the steady-state pool of proteins present in a cell, and had to compete with cellular proteins for access to class I molecules, it is difficult to understand how presentation could occur so rapidly.

One potential solution would be that peptides are derived from viral proteins that are much less stable than the cellular proteins with which they compete for access to MHC class I molecules. But, in fact, antigenic peptides are usually derived from viral proteins that are extremely stable when measured by standard means. Another solution, originally proposed by Van Pel and Boon (1989), is that antigenic peptides are derived from short-lived, misbegotten out-of-frame polypeptides that result from errors in transcription or translation. This probably occurs (Mayrand and Green 1998), but it does not account for the vast majority of peptide ligands that are translated in the correct reading frame (Rammensee et al. 1997).

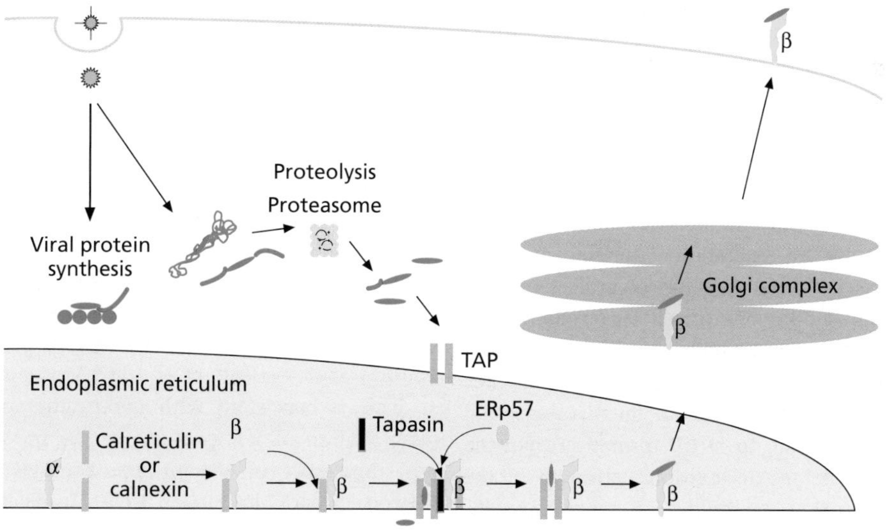

Figure 21.3 *Class I antigen-processing pathway: at the top left of the figure, a virion is shown entering the cell via endocytosis, and beneath it a viral capsid (blue burr with white border) is shown entering the cytosol (with enveloped viruses this is a consequence of fusion of viral and endosomal membranes; with nonenveloped viruses, the virus directly breaches the cellular membrane). In most situations, the major source of antigenic peptides (green oval) is protein synthesis (major arrow emanating from capsid), but peptides can be derived from capsid proteins if sufficient quantities are delivered to the cytosol. Many, and perhaps most, peptides are probably derived from defective forms of newly synthesized proteins (Schubert et al. 2000). Proteasomes are the major producer of peptide in the cytosol, but other proteases may also contribute. In particular, aminopeptidases can trim proteasome products. Cytosolic peptides of 8–17 amino acids are transported into the endoplasmic reticulum (ER) by TAP (transporter associated with antigen processing), where trimming by aminopeptidases can also occur. Peptides bind to newly synthesized class I $\alpha\beta_2$-microglobulin heterodimers, which are released from TAP and transported via the Golgi complex to the cell surface for immune perusal.*

An alternate solution is that protein biosynthesis, like all biological processes, is imperfect. A certain percentage of ribosomal products must be defective in some way and not reach their stable conformation. It has been known for years that introducing alterations in proteins, which increases their degradation in cells, increases their presentation to $CD8^+$ T cells (Tevethia et al. 1983; Townsend et al. 1986, 1988), with the implication that imperfect forms of proteins generated from wild-type genes would be a preferred source of antigenic peptides. Many different types of errors can be envisaged in mRNA generation (misincorporation of nucleotides, missplicing), or in the process of protein synthesis itself that results in the misincorporation of amino acids, premature termination, or deletion of residues. In addition, many proteins are members of multi-subunit complexes, and there must be imbalances in synthesis that result in an excess of certain subunits which are unstable in the absence of their normal partners. Additional mistakes must be made in protein targeting, such that proteins are delivered to the wrong organelle, where they misfold and are targeted for destruction. The folding of nascent proteins in the crowded environment of the cytosol is more difficult than folding in a homogeneous solution in vitro, and there are ample opportunities for the process to go awry, particularly for large multi-domain proteins.

The products of these errors can be grouped together as a source of antigenic peptides, because they will all presumably be degraded by proteasomes and other cellular proteases contributing to quality control. Such substrates have been termed defective ribosomal products (DRiP) (Yewdell et al. 1996). The beauty of DRiPs for the immune system is that they enable MHC class I molecules to monitor protein synthesis rates in cells and not protein concentrations. In this way, viral infections could be detected as soon as possible, particularly as many viruses rapidly monopolize the protein synthesis machinery to produce their own gene products. This would explain the rapid detection of virus-infected cells by $CD8^+$ T cells and also the generation of antigenic peptides from a huge variety of viral proteins, regardless of their apparent metabolic stability or intracellular targeting.

Note that DRiPs are not exclusively limited to viral proteins, but rather they are an inevitable consequence of synthesizing *any* protein. Indeed, the average viral protein may be less prone to DRiP formation than the average cellular protein. An additional strength of the DRiP hypothesis is that it provides an explanation for why class I peptide ligands are not biased toward originating from metabolically unstable proteins. There is experimental evidence to support the idea that DRiPs provide a significant source of peptide ligands to MHC class I molecules. First, 30 percent or more of the total pool of newly synthesized cellular proteins appear to be degraded within a few minutes of their synthesis, as inferred by the increased recovery of radiolabeled proteins from cells treated with proteasome inhibitors. An increased fraction of newly synthesized proteins recovered from proteasome inhibitor-treated cells were polyubiquitylated, as predicted (the ubiquitin–proteasome system is discussed below) (Schubert et al. 2000). Second, blocking protein synthesis reduces the supply of peptide ligands for TAP or class I molecules (Reits et al. 2000; Schubert et al. 2000). Third, using cells expressing a gene under the control of a repressible promoter, the rate of peptide generation from the gene is proportional to the amount of mRNA, not the level of the source protein (Khan et al. 2001). Fourth, presentation of viral peptides is tightly linked to the rate of translation of the source gene product and not the steady state level of stable protein (Princiotta et al. 2003).

This is not to say that DRiPs are the only source of antigenic peptides; clearly they are not. For all we know, on average, peptides might be more efficiently produced from long-lived proteins. Indeed, it is to be expected that the DRiP rate will vary tremendously between different proteins. For proteins with low DRiP rates, the bulk of peptides will probably be derived from the classic turnover of proteins, and vice versa for proteins with high DRiP rates.

What about secreted proteins?

Many viral proteins are targeted to the ER for secretion or insertion into membranes used for viral maturation. Depending on the cell type, a high percentage of cellular proteins can be similarly targeted. Despite their targeting, antigenic peptides can be derived from these proteins with similar efficiency as nuclear or cytosolic proteins. How are such proteins processed?

As discussed below, the secretory pathway has a limited capacity for generating peptides from full-length proteins. Consequently, in a high percentage of cases, processing of ER-targeted proteins occurs in the cytosol (this represents a subset of DRiPs). There are two general mechanisms for delivering such proteins to the cytosol: either they are diverted to the cytosol on their way to the ER or they are returned to the cytosol after visiting the ER. Although only a few studies have examined this question, it appears that the latter route is the more traveled (Bacik et al. 1997; Mosse et al. 1998).

This is consistent with the recent appreciation that degradation of ER proteins occurs in the cytosol after the re-export of the protein through the translocon (Brodsky and McCracken 1999). Ironically, even class I molecules are degraded through this mechanism (Hughes et al. 1997), a process greatly accelerated by the action of some viral proteins (Wiertz et al. 1996).

THE UBIQUITIN–PROTEASOME PATHWAY

The axe

Proteasomes are the principal mechanism used by eukaryotic cells to degrade proteins. In so doing, they provide a major source of class I peptide ligands or their precursors (Rock and Goldberg 1999). Proteasomes are ancient structures, present in all eukaryotes and in many prokaryotic species as well (Voges et al. 1999). They are abundant in eukaryotic cells, e.g. HeLa cells contain approximately 500 000. They are present in both the nucleus and the cytosol, where many bind to the ER: where they may be involved in process of retro-translocation of misfolded ER proteins to the cytosol.

Proteasomes are remarkable machines, capable of degrading a wide variety of protein substrates; indeed, few proteins (if any) are known to be resistant to the action of proteasomes. The cleavage reactions occur in a barrel-like structure known as the 20-S proteasome, and regulatory subunits that attach to each end of the 20-S proteasome. The 20-S proteasomes contain 14 distinct subunits arrayed in a four-ring structure of the type, $\alpha_7\beta_7\beta_7\alpha_7$. Three of the β subunits in each inner ring are known to be catalytically active, with their active sites facing a central chamber in which proteins are degraded.

Given their ability to degrade virtually anything, 20-S proteasomes are potentially extremely dangerous to cells, and safeguards prevent such proteolytic rampages. The catalytic subunits are synthesized with presequences that must be cleaved during the assembly process to activate proteolytic activity. The barrels are closed at both ends, and they must bind to a 19-S regulatory particle for protein substrates to gain access to the central chamber. The 20-S subunits bind to one 19-S subunit on each end to form the 26-S proteasome – the active form of proteasomes in cells. Why proteasomes exhibit dyad symmetry is unclear. The generation of a proteolytic chamber from symmetrical components is a parsimonious solution which is used by organisms to generate other barrel-like assemblies used for protein degradation or folding. The binding of two 19-S subunits may simply follow from the symmetry of 20-S proteasomes and not add much to proteasome function. Alternately, if the 19-S subunit processing of the protein is the rate-limiting step in protein degradation, having two 19-S submits may optimize the use of the 20-S subunit.

Unlike most proteases, the 26-S proteasome degrades substrates in an energy-dependent manner that utilizes adenosine triphosphate (ATP). ATP is exclusively consumed by the 19-S subunit, which recognizes potential substrates bearing polyubiquitin chains, unfolds the substrates, and feeds them, spaghetti like, into the barrel of the 20-S proteasome via the narrow portal that is opened as part of the process (Glickman et al. 1999). At some point before this event, the polyubiquitin chains are removed from the substrate and the ubiquitin is returned to the pool of ubiquitin monomers for reuse.

Proteasomes come in multiple forms. Indeed, the initial evidence implicating proteasomes in antigen processing was the discovery of the MHC-encoded proteasome subunits and that their expression (and that of a third subunit) is enhanced by exposure of cells to interferon γ (IFN)-γ or tumor necrosis factor (TNF)-α, the predominant cytokines released by activated $CD8^+$ T cells (Monaco and Nandi 1995) (these cytokines upregulate transcription of genes encoding each of the components of the class I processing pathway, which share common promoter elements). When induced, these subunits replace constitutively expressed subunits to create 20-S 'immunoproteasomes', which appear to be better at producing peptides favored by MHC class I molecules (Tanaka and Kasahara 1998). Such immunoproteasomes can be created only from scratch, because subunit exchange in mature proteasomes is not known to occur. As proteasomes are extremely long lived (half-life of about 10 days), cells exposed to cytokines will possess a mixture of standard proteasomes and immunoproteasomes for a very long time. Although some defined determinants are produced more efficiently by immunoproteasomes, other determinants are produced less efficiently.

Cytokine-exposed cells also produce 11-S regulators, which can take the place of 19-S regulators on 20-S proteasomes. Expression of 11-S regulators has been shown to favor antigen presentation through undefined mechanisms (Rechsteiner et al. 2000). It has been proposed that 11-S and 19-S regulators bind to a single 20-S subunit to form hybrid proteasomes, with the 11-S regulator serving to attach proteasomes to TAP and thereby increase the efficiency of peptide delivery.

The handle

Ubiquitin is a 76-residue protein that is remarkably well conserved among eukaryotes – yeast ubiquitin differs from human ubiquitin by only three conservative substitutions. It is extremely abundant in cells (about 10^8 copies per HeLa cell (Haas and Bright 1985)), and its many known cellular functions that revolve around covalent conjugation to the ϵ-NH_2 groups of lysine residues (or the amino terminus of proteins) via its carboxyl terminus (Hershko and Ciechanover 1998). Ubiquitin itself is ubiquitylated and, when polyubiquitin 'trees' containing four or more ubiquitins are present on proteins, they bind to 19-S regulators that deliver the protein to proteasomes for destruction, whereas the ubiquitin is recycled (Thrower et al. 2000). Given its dire consequences, polyubiquitylation of proteins would be expected to be a highly regulated and complicated affair and, indeed, numerous gene products are devoted to ubiquitin conjugation. For obscure reasons, cells are not content to add a single ubiquitin tree to proteins destined for destruction. Rather, polyubiquitylation is highly heterogeneous, and trees of different sizes are added to multiple substrate sites in what appears to be an irregular manner, such that polyubiquitylated proteins usually migrate as a ladder (or smear) in sodium dodecylsulfate–polyacrylamide gel electrophoresis (SDS-PAGE). Moreover, the process is not irreversible, and enzymes capable of removing ubiquitin from proteins (ubiquitin hydrolases) are highly active in cells (Wilkinson 2000). Polyubiquitylation is not an absolute prerequisite for protein degradation by proteasomes. There are only a few specific examples of such ubiquitin-independent targeting at present, but this could well prove to be a major source of proteasome substrates (Verma and Deshaies 2000; Benaroudj et al. 2001).

Role of proteasomes in generating antigenic peptides

The contributions of proteasomes to antigen processing, and indeed mammalian cell physiology, have been defined largely through the use of membrane-permeant, low-molecular-weight inhibitors of the proteolytic activities of 26-S proteasomes (Bogyo et al. 1997; Goldberg and Rock 2002). These include natural products of microorganisms and synthetic oligopeptide-based compounds. The former usually exhibit far more specificity for the proteasome than the latter. There are two major problems in using proteasome inhibitors to study cellular processes. First, proteasome inhibitors, like other inhibitors, cannot be absolutely specific for a single target, and they must interact with other cellular targets. It is possible to control for nonproteasome-related effects in that proteasome inhibitors with distinct chemical structures give similar results. Second, proteasomes play a key role in many cellular processes, and blocking them rapidly induces a number of serious secondary effects. These effects include depletion of the pool of free ubiquitin available for protein conjugation, induction of molecular chaperones, inhibition of protein synthesis, and interference with the cell cycle and signaling. That some of these effects are likely to be caused by an accumulation of ubiquitylated substrates awaiting destruction does not simplify matters. These effects can be minimized (although not necessarily made insignificant) by minimizing the time for which cells are exposed to proteasome inhibitors.

Proteasome inhibitors have been used to demonstrate that proteasomes are the principal cytosolic protease used by cells for generating MHC class I peptide ligands (Rock et al. 1994; Rock and Goldberg 1999). Peptide generation is maintained, however, in the presence of proteasome inhibitors, but at a lower rate. This varies in a class I allomorph-specific manner. There are many examples of antigenic peptides whose generation is unimpeded or even enhanced by proteasome inhibitors. In the latter case it has been documented for several examples that proteasomes can function to destroy determinants. These findings have two interpretations that are not mutually exclusive. First, alternate cellular endoproteases may participate in antigen processing. Second, it may not be possible completely to block proteasome function with the inhibitors currently in use. This may be the result of either resistant activities in individual proteasomes or the existence of a subset of proteasomes immune to the effects of the inhibitors, resulting perhaps from inaccessibility.

In vitro studies with isolated 20-S proteasomes have shown that proteasomes can generate the precise peptides presented by MHC class I molecules. This process is not very efficient, however, and extended versions, particularly peptides with amino-terminal extensions, are more likely to be produced. The 20-S proteasomes from yeast generate a similar set of peptides to mammalian proteasomes, deflating the hopes of immunologists that proteasomes (at least standard proteasomes) evolved for the purpose of generating antigenic peptides. Given its numerous subunits, it might be expected that proteasomal cleavage be governed by complex rules. Proteasomes do not disappoint in this regard. Proteasome activity for individual peptide bonds is influenced by amino acids on both sides of the cleavage site, as wells as flanking residues, with the greatest influence mediated by those within five residues of the cleavage sites. Work is progressing on developing predictive algorithms for the peptides that are liberated by proteasomes (Altuvia and Margalit 2000; Kuttler et al. 2000).

ROLE OF NONPROTEASOMAL CYTOSOLIC PROTEASES IN ANTIGEN PROCESSING

Trimming enzymes

Proteasomes need not generate the precise peptides presented by class I molecules. A considerable body of evidence indicates that peptides can be trimmed by aminopeptidases in the cytosol (York et al. 1999) and ER (Yewdell et al. 1999a), whereas carboxypeptidase trimming seems to be highly unusual. A candidate cytosolic aminopeptidase is leucyl aminopeptidase, because its expression is enhanced by IFN-γ and TNF (Beninga et al. 1998). Other aminopeptidases (bleomycin hydrolase and puromycin-sensitive aminopeptidases) are known to be capable of trimming amino-terminal extensions from defined antigenic peptides (Stoltze et al. 2000). The ER contains two aminopeptidases (ERAP1 and ERAP2) that are largely, if not exclusively, dedicated to trimming antigenic peptides (Serwold et al. 2002; York et al. 2002).

One of the most striking features of antigen processing is that the recovery of antigenic peptides from cells is dependent on expression of a class I molecule that binds the peptide with more than the threshold affinity. Two mechanisms potentially contribute to this phenomenon (Falk et al. 1990):

1. class I molecules are required for the generation of antigenic peptides by serving as a template for the action of trimming exopeptidases
2. peptides are rapidly destroyed unless they are protected by class I molecules.

It appears that the second possibility plays a major role in the phenomenon. Class I molecules are still required for the recovery of antigenic peptides when the antigenic peptides are synthesized as cytosolic minigene products corresponding to the exact peptide. Moreover, peptides are rapidly degraded by cytosolic extracts and rapidly exported from the ER unless they bind to class I molecules. Peptides can be destroyed by the very aminopeptidases involved in trimming, and also by endopeptidases active on oligopeptides. One such endopeptidase known to be capable of degrading antigenic peptides and their precursors is thimet oligopeptidase (Silva et al. 1999). Peptide destruction is probably a major contributor to the low efficiency of antigen processing discussed above.

Proteasome understudy?

As mentioned above, the generation of many class I peptide ligands is insensitive to proteasome inhibitors. Two groups reported that it is even possible to adapt cells to resist the cytotoxic effects of proteasome inhibitors (Glas et al. 1998; Geier et al. 1999). In both studies the adapted cells demonstrated enhanced expression of tripeptidyl peptidase (TPPII), which was proposed as a substitute for the functions of the proteasome. This was unexpected because proteasomes are essential for the viability of yeast. Subsequently it was shown that cells adapted to proteasome inhibitors retain proteasome activity and that such activity contributes to antigen processing and protein degradation and is required for viability (Princiotta et al. 2001). School is still out on the possible contributions of TPPII to antigen processing and overall protein degradation, though a recent report suggests that a majority of proteasome products must be further degraded by TPPII to be eligible for binding to class I molecules (Reits et al. 2004).

SHEPHERDING PEPTIDES TO THE PROMISED LAND: TAP

Endoplasmic reticulum trimming by aminopeptidases is possible because extended peptides have access to the ER. Peptides are transported from the cytosol to the ER by TAP, which is a member of a large family of prokaryotic and eukaryotic proteins (the ABC, or ATP-binding cassette, family) that function in the transmembrane transport of a wide variety of substrates (Elliott 1997). TAP is formed by the association of two homologous subunits termed TAP1 and TAP2 which rapidly assemble in the ER. Each subunit possesses multiple (9–10), short, membrane-spanning domains attached to a globular carboxy-terminal, cytosolic, nucleotide-binding domain.

As with other family members, TAP-mediated peptide transport is driven by hydrolysis of ATP or other trinucleotides. TAP preferentially transports the types of peptides favored by class I molecules, particularly in its requirements that peptides be at least eight residues in length. The upper limit of peptide length is messier, but the efficiency drops off considerably when peptides are longer than 16 residues or so, although even those with 40 residues may be transported at low efficiency (Koopmann et al. 1996).

TAP does not transport all peptides with equal efficiencies. Alterations at all positions can influence TAP-mediated transport. The greatest preferences are demonstrated for carboxy-terminal residues; indeed TAP from different species demonstrates a marked preference for the types of carboxyl termini preferred by their respective class I molecules (in humans, hydrophobic or positively charged residues) (Momburg et al. 1994; Schumacher et al. 1994). Thus, longer peptides transported into the ER by TAP are more likely to possess amino-terminal extensions than carboxy-terminal ones. Next in importance are the first three residues from the amino terminus. Similar preferences exist for peptides of different lengths. This suggests a model in which efficient TAP recognition of peptides entails interaction with the peptide's three amino-terminal residues and carboxy-terminal residue, and the presence of no less than 4, and no more than 12, internal spacer residues. Interestingly, despite the fact that proline at position 2 is a dominant anchor residue for numerous human class I allomorphs, this greatly disfavors TAP-mediated transport of many peptides. This suggests that, for these peptides, trimming of amino-terminal extensions in the ER is particularly important.

TAP polymorphism in rats greatly influences the peptides delivered to class I molecules (Howard 1995). Although human TAP genes display limited polymorphism, the known alleles do not appear to differ greatly in their specificities (Obst et al. 1995). Thus, it does not appear that TAP polymorphism plays a major role in influencing the response of individuals to viral proteins. A splice variant of human TAP2 has been described that possesses an altered carboxyl terminus (Yan et al. 1999). This looks to modify the specificity of TAP, but its effects in vivo await further characterization.

TAP-INDEPENDENT PROCESSING OF ENDOGENOUS ANTIGENS

As mentioned above, class I molecules are bound to TAP (via tapasin) until released by peptide binding. It is thought that this facilitates their association with peptides transported by the same complex, thereby greatly increasing the effective peptide concentration. TAP is not, however, essential for peptide loading on to class I molecules. Peptides targeted to the ER are able to associate efficiently with class I molecules in cells lacking TAP (Anderson et al. 1991). Indeed, in studies using recombinant vaccinia virus expressing various forms of a peptide antigen, peptides targeted to the ER have been found to be more immunogenic in mice than cytosolic peptides biosynthesized in similar amounts, or the full-length gene viral proteins products that are the natural source of the peptides (Restifo et al. 1995). It has also been found that cytosolic antigens can be presented to a limited extent in a TAP-independent manner by an unknown mechanism. Although these exceptions are interesting and possibly of practical importance (using ER-targeted peptides for immunization), it should be emphasized that TAP plays a critical role in the presentation of most viral determinants. TAP is also crucial for T-cell development, because TAP-deficient individuals demonstrate greatly decreased levels of T cells (de la Salle et al. 1994; Gadola et al. 2000). Curiously, such individuals are relatively healthy, having mainly recurrent localized bacterial infections.

CONTRIBUTION OF SECRETORY PROTEASES TO ANTIGEN PROCESSING

Many proteins targeted to the ER immediately lose their amino-terminal signal sequences, presumably as a result of the action of signal peptidase. Further proteolysis of these peptides enables their binding to class I molecules, particularly if class I allomorphs favor binding of hydrophobic peptides. HLA-A2 is the prototype for these allomorphs, and many of the peptides that it presents are derived from signal sequences. Signal sequence presentation is central to the function of some class Ib molecules, which present leader peptides from class I molecules to natural killer (NK) cells.

The presentation of such leader peptides can be either TAP independent or TAP dependent. In the latter case, presentation can be either proteasome dependent or independent. Thus, signal peptides can be produced strictly by secretory proteases or a combination of secretory and cytosolic proteases.

From a functional standpoint, using ERAP the ER is able to trim amino-terminal extensions of TAP-transported peptides efficiently, while still having a very limited capacity for removing carboxy-terminal residues. Peptides transported into the ER independently of TAP appear to be handled in a similar manner.

The secretory pathway displays a limited capacity for generating determinants from very large substrates, presumably as a result of endopeptidases acting in concert with aminopeptidases. Such endopeptidases are not necessarily limited to the ER: furin, an endopeptidase activated only in the trans-Golgi complex, is involved in the generation of several defined peptides, which are presumably generated and loaded in the trans-Golgi complex (Gil-Torregrosa et al. 2000).

Generating peptide ligands from exogenous proteins

As mentioned at the start, the activation of naïve $CD8^+$ T cells requires pAPCs that express the proper co-stimulatory molecules (at least according to dogma). Obviously, such cells will present peptides from endogenous antigens synthesized during a viral infection. But, what if the virus cannot (or will not) infect the appropriate APC? And what about nonviral pathogens that do not hijack host ribosomes for their own nefarious ends? Can naïve $CD8^+$ T cells respond under these conditions?

The answer to this question is yes. This pathway was initially discovered by Bevan, who reported that $CD8^+$ T cells can be induced against antigens introduced into mice by adoptive transfer of MHC-mismatched cells, terming the phenomenon 'crosspriming' (Bevan 1976). Underlying this are a number of potential mechanisms that also serve as the basis for the immunogenicity of protein-based vaccines that elicit $CD8^+$ T-cell responses. The true nature of the crosspriming pathway in vivo remains to be determined, although it is likely that it reflects the operation of many (or all) of the mechanisms defined below.

TWO PATHS TO RIGHTEOUSNESS

The processing of exogenous antigens can be divided into two distinct pathways. First, antigens can access the cytosol where they are treated in a manner similar to endogenous antigens. Three basic routes into the cytosol are possible.

The first is traversing cell membranes as a result of properties associated with the substance, e.g. viruses or liposomes can fuse with cell membranes, delivering their contents to the cytosol. Other viruses directly penetrate cellular membranes. In the case of abundant viral core proteins, a sufficient quantity may enter the cytosol to produce enough MHC–class I complexes to trigger $CD8^+$ T cells (Yewdell et al. 1988; Riddell et al. 1991). Bacteria that reside in endosomal compartments secrete proteins that translocate endosomal members to gain access to the cytosol where they can alter cellular function (Pamer et al. 1991). Some proteins have sequences that enable them to cross the plasma membrane (Chikh et al. 2001). These sequences can enable even large proteins to cross membranes.

The second route entails entry from endosomes that leak by accident or by design. Highly active phagocytic cells create macropinosomes which enable substrate access to the cytosol (Norbury et al. 1995). DCs possess an apparently unique endocytic compartment that delivers substances of about 40 kDa to the cytosol (Rodriguez et al. 1999).

The third route is retrograde transport from endosomes to the Golgi complex and then to the ER, where they follow the route traversed by endoplasmic reticulum-associated degradation (ERAD) substrates back to the cytosol. Many toxins are thought to enter cells via this route (Lord and Roberts 1998).

Peptides can also be generated from exogenous antigens outside the APC or in endosomal compartments of

APCs and loaded on to cell surface or endosomal PR class I molecules. This pathway resembles the classic class II antigen-processing pathway. The pAPCs are particularly adept at such nonclassic class I antigen processing.

GENERATION AND TRAFFICKING OF PR CLASS I MOLECULES

Within 60 min of their departure from the ER, a substantial fraction of class I molecules lacks peptide ligands. These molecules may never have been loaded, may have been loaded with a lower affinity ligand, or may have suboptimally bound a peptide that normally binds with higher affinity. This is the source of PR class I molecules, the properties of which are described above. Interference with peptide supply by blocking proteasomes or inactivating TAP actually *decreases* the number of PR class I molecules (Day et al. 1995), presumably because less poorly loaded class I molecules leave the ER. The percentage of such poorly loaded molecules can be very high, representing even 95 percent of class I molecules exported from the ER (Su and Miller 2001).

Such PR molecules are present throughout the secretory pathway. As discussed above, exogenous β_2-microglobulin and/or low temperatures stabilize PR molecules. PR molecules stabilized in this manner also participate in the presentation of exogenous antigens processed in endosomal compartments (Song and Harding 1996; Schirmbeck et al. 1997). This latter statement alludes to the trafficking of class I molecules to endosomes. Class I molecules derived from the cell surface have been found in endosomal compartments that contain class II molecules in a number of cell types, including DCs (Geuze et al. 1985; Chiu et al. 1999; Gromme et al. 1999; Castellino et al. 2000; Kleijmeer et al. 2001; MacAry et al. 2001). A number of class I allomorphs have been reported to bind peptides at the acidic pH characteristic of endosomes (Stryhn et al. 1996), and the generation of peptide class I complexes in endosomes has been visualized (Castellino et al. 2000).

It is uncertain how class I molecules are targeted to endosomal compartments. Several class I allomorphs have been reported to associate with the invariant chain (Cerundolo et al. 1992), and the invariant chain has been reported to direct HLA-B27 to endosomal compartments (Sugita and Brenner 1995). The trafficking of class I molecules from endosomes to the plasma membrane of DCs is upregulated upon DC maturation (MacAry et al. 2001). The mechanism underlying this and nearly every aspect of the intracellular trafficking of class I molecules to and from endosomes remains to be characterized.

Class I molecules are also present in exosomes: small vesicles generated in the lumen of large endosomes by a pinching-off process with the topological consequence of orienting luminal domains of integral membrane proteins (similar to class I molecules) on the outer surface of the exosome. After the fusion of multivesicular endosomes with the plasma membrane, exosomes are released by cells. Originally described in reticulocytes, exosomes are also known to be produced by B cells and DCs. Exosomes are rich in MHC class II and co-stimulatory molecules, and are able to able to stimulate $CD4^+$ (Raposo et al. 1996) and $CD8^+$ T cells (Zitvogel et al. 1998). The physiological significance of exosomes in immune responses remains to be established.

ANTIGEN PROCESSING IN ENDOSOMAL COMPARTMENTS

The possibility of endosomal processing of MHC class I antigens was first shown using antigen coupled to beads (Rock et al. 1990), and has now been extended to a large number of antigens, including bacteria, viruses, virus-like particles, and aggregated proteins (reviewed in Yewdell et al. 1999b). Although 'peptide regurgitation' (i.e. cell-surface PR class I binding of peptides generated in endosomal compartments) (Pfeifer et al. 1993) has been shown to occur under some conditions, it is likely that peptides generated in endosomes bind to endosomal class I molecules. Although every cell type is probably capable of endosomal processing, it occurs more efficiently in pAPCs. The extent to which this is caused by the increased endocytosis versus enhanced trafficking of class I molecules to and from endosomes versus enhanced peptide generation versus facilitated loading remains to be established. Indeed, precious little is known about endosomal processing of class I peptides, and the nature of the proteases and mechanism of peptide loading are completely undefined.

WHAT DO MOLECULAR CHAPERONES DO?

In searching for factors that are able to prime the immune system to reject transplanted tumors, Srivastava and colleagues discovered that the molecular chaperone gp96 purified from tumor cells is able to induce protective immunity against tumor challenge (Li et al. 2002). These findings have been extended to show that several different molecular chaperones are able to induce $CD8^+$ T-cell responses to defined antigens when the chaperones are purified from cells expressing the antigen or loaded with antigenic peptides (Li et al. 2002). Notably, the responses induced by molecular chaperones are quite weak in comparison to virus infections, and even to other exogenous antigen preparations. The jury is still out on the physiological role of molecular chaperones in the crosspriming phenomenon (Wallin et al. 2002), though recent evidence disfavors their participation in crosspriming (Norbury et al. 2004; Wolkers et al. 2004).

REFERENCES

Altuvia, Y. and Margalit, H. 2000. Sequence signals for generation of antigenic peptides by the proteasome: implications for proteasomal cleavage mechanism. *J Mol Biol*, **295**, 879–90.

Andersen, M.H., Bonfill, J.E., et al. 1999. Phosphorylated peptides can be transported by TAP molecules, presented by class I MHC molecules, and recognized by phosphopeptide-specific CTL. *J Immunol*, **163**, 3812–18.

Anderson, K., Cresswell, P., et al. 1991. Endogenously synthesized peptide with an endoplasmic reticulum signal sequence sensitizes antigen processing mutant cells to class I-restricted cell-mediated lysis. *J Exp Med*, **174**, 489–92.

Arstila, T.P., Casrouge, A., et al. 1999. A direct estimate of the human T cell receptor diversity. *Science*, **286**, 958–61.

Bacik, I., Snyder, H.L., et al. 1997. Introduction of a glycosylation site into a secreted protein provides evidence for an alternative antigen processing pathway: transport of precursors of major histocompatibility complex class I-restricted peptides from the endoplasmic reticulum to the cytosol. *J Exp Med*, **186**, 479–87.

Benaroudj, N., Tarcsa, E., et al. 2001. The unfolding of substrates and ubiquitin-independent protein degradation by proteasomes. *Biochimie*, **83**, 3-4, 311–18.

Beninga, J., Rock, K.L. and Goldberg, A.L. 1998. Interferon-gamma can stimulate post-proteasomal trimming of the N terminus of an antigenic peptide by inducing leucine aminopeptidase. *J Biol Chem*, **273**, 18734–42.

Bevan, M.J. 1976. Cross-priming for a secondary cytotoxic response to minor H antigens with H-2 congenic cells which do not cross-react in the cytotoxic assay. *J Exp Med*, **143**, 1283.

Bogyo, M., Gaczynska, M. and Ploegh, H.L. 1997. Proteasome inhibitors and antigen presentation. *Biopolymers*, **43**, 269–80.

Bouvier, M. and Wiley, D.C. 1994. Importance of peptide amino and carboxyl termini to the stability of MHC class I molecules. *Science*, **265**, 398–402.

Brodsky, J.L. and McCracken, A.A. 1999. ER protein quality control and proteasome-mediated protein degradation. *Semin Cell Dev Biol*, **10**, 507–13.

Castellino, F., Boucher, P.E., et al. 2000. Receptor-mediated uptake of antigen/heat shock protein complexes results in major histocompatibility complex class I antigen presentation via two distinct processing pathways. *J Exp Med*, **191**, 1957–64.

Cerundolo, V., Elliot, T., et al. 1992. Association of the human invariant chain with H-2 D^b class I molecules. *Eur J Immunol*, **22**, 2243–8.

Chen, W., Ede, N.J., et al. 1996. CTL recognition of an altered peptide associated with asparagine bond rearrangement. Implications for immunity and vaccine design. *J Immunol*, **157**, 1000–5.

Chen, W., Yewdell, J.W., et al. 1999. Modification of cysteine residues in vitro and in vivo affects the immunogenicity and antigenicity of major histocompatibility complex class I-restricted viral determinants. *J Exp Med*, **189**, 1757–64.

Chikh, G.G., Kong, S., et al. 2001. Efficient delivery of *Antennapedia* homeodomain fused to CTL epitope with liposomes into dendritic cells results in the activation of CD8+ T cells. *J Immunol*, **167**, 6462–70.

Chiu, I., Davis, D.M. and Strominger, J.L. 1999. Trafficking of spontaneously endocytosed MHC proteins. *Proc Natl Acad Sci USA*, **96**, 13944–9.

Day, P.M., Esquivel, F., et al. 1995. Effect of TAP on the generation and intracellular trafficking of peptide-receptive major histocompatibility complex class I molecules. *Immunity*, **2**, 137–47.

Day, P.M., Yewdell, J.W., et al. 1997. Direct delivery of exogenous MHC class I molecule-binding oligopeptides to the endoplasmic reticulum of viable cells. *Proc Natl Acad Sci USA*, **94**, 8064–9.

de la Salle, H., Hanau, D., et al. 1994. Homozygous human TAP peptide transporter mutation in HLA class I deficiency. *Science*, **265**, 237–41.

Elliott, T. 1997. Transporter associated with antigen processing. *Adv Immunol*, **65**, 47–109.

Engelhard, V.H. 1994. Structure of peptides associated with MHC class I molecules. *Curr Opin Immunol*, **6**, 13–23.

Falk, K., Rötzschke, O. and Rammensee, H.-G. 1990. Cellular peptide composition governed by major histocompatibility complex class I molecules. *Nature*, **348**, 248–51.

Gadola, S.D., Moins-Teisserenc, H.T., et al. 2000. TAP deficiency syndrome. *Clin Exp Immunol*, **121**, 173–8.

Garbi, N., Tan, P., et al. 2000. Impaired immune responses and altered peptide repertoire in tapasin-deficient mice. *Nat Immunol*, **1**, 234–8.

Geier, E., Pfeifer, G., et al. 1999. A giant protease with potential to substitute for some functions of the proteasome. *Science*, **283**, 978–81.

Germain, R.N. and Margulies, D.H. 1993. The biochemistry and cell biology of antigen processing and presentation. *Annu Rev Immunol*, **11**, 403–50.

Geuze, H.J., Slot, J.W., et al. 1985. Possible pathways for lysosomal enzyme delivery. *J Cell Biol*, **101**, 2253–62.

Gil-Torregrosa, B.C., Castano, A.R., et al. 2000. Generation of MHC class I peptide antigens by protein processing in the secretory route by furin. *Traffic*, **1**, 641–51.

Glas, R., Bogyo, M., et al. 1998. A proteolytic system that compensates for loss of proteasome function. *Nature*, **392**, 618–22.

Glickman, M.H., Rubin, D.M., et al. 1999. Functional analysis of the proteasome regulatory particle. *Mol Biol Rep*, **26**, 1-2, 21–8.

Goldberg, A.L. and Rock, K. 2002. Not just research tools – proteasome inhibitors offer therapeutic promise. *Nat Med*, **8**, 338–40.

Grandea III, A.G., Golovina, T.N., et al. 2000. Impaired assembly yet normal trafficking of MHC class I molecules in Tapasin mutant mice. *Immunity*, **13**, 213–22.

Gromme, M., Uytdehaag, F.G., et al. 1999. Recycling MHC class I molecules and endosomal peptide loading. *Proc Natl Acad Sci USA*, **96**, 10326–31.

Haas, A.L. and Bright, P.M. 1985. The immunochemical detection and quantitation of intracellular ubiquitin-protein conjugates. *J Biol Chem*, **260**, 12464–73.

Haynes, B.F., Markert, M.L., et al. 2000. The role of the thymus in immune reconstitution in aging, bone marrow transplantation and HIV-1 infection. *Annu Rev Immunol*, **18**, 529–60.

Heemels, M.-T. and Ploegh, H. 1995. Generation, translocation, and presentation of MHC class-I restricted peptides. *Annu Rev Biochem*, **64**, 463–91.

Hershko, A. and Ciechanover, A. 1998. The ubiquitin system. *Annu Rev Biochem*, **67**, 425–79.

Howard, J.C. 1995. Supply and transport of peptides presented by class I MHC molecules. *Curr Opin Immunol*, **7**, 69–76.

Hughes, E.A. and Cresswell, P. 1998. The thiol oxidoreductase ERp57 is a component of the MHC class I peptide-loading complex. *Curr Biol*, **8**, 709–12.

Hughes, E.A., Hammond, C. and Cresswell, P. 1997. Misfolded major histocompatibility complex class I heavy chains are translocated into the cytoplasm and degraded by the proteasome. *Proc Natl Acad Sci USA*, **94**, 1896–901.

Img, S.R.C., de Borghans, J.B., et al. 2000. Diversity of human T cell receptors. *Science*, **288**, 1135a.

Khan, S., de Giuli, R., et al. 2001. Cutting edge: neosynthesis is required for the presentation of a T cell epitope from a long-lived viral protein. *J Immunol*, **167**, 4801–4.

Kleijmeer, M.J., Escola, J.M., et al. 2001. Antigen loading of MHC class I molecules in the endocytic tract. *Traffic*, **2**, 124–37.

Koopmann, J.-O., Post, M., et al. 1996. Translocation of long peptides by transporters associated with antigen processing (TAP). *Eur J Biochem*, **26**, 1720–8.

Kozlowski, S., Corr, M., et al. 1992. Serum angiotensin-1 converting enzyme activity processes a human immunodeficiency virus 1 gp160 peptide for presentation by major histocompatibility complex class I molecules. *J Exp Med*, **175**, 1417–22.

Kuttler, C., Nussbaum, A.K., et al. 2000. An algorithm for the prediction of proteasomal cleavages. *J Mol Biol*, **298**, 417–29.

Li, Z., Menoret, A. and Srivastava, P. 2002. Roles of heat-shock proteins in antigen presentation and cross-presentation. *Curr Opin Immunol*, **14**, 45–51.

Lord, J.M. and Roberts, L.M. 1998. Toxin entry: retrograde transport through the secretory pathway. *J Cell Biol*, **140**, 733–6.

MacAry, P.A., Lindsay, M., et al. 2001. Mobilization of MHC class I molecules from late endosomes to the cell surface following activation of CD34-derived human Langerhans cells. *Proc Natl Acad Sci USA*, **98**, 3982–7.

Madden, D.R. 1995. The three-dimensional structure of peptide-MHC complexes. *Annu Rev Immunol*, **13**, 587–622.

Mayrand, S.M. and Green, W.R. 1998. Non-traditionally derived CTL epitopes: exceptions that prove the rules? *Immunol Today*, **19**, 551–6.

Meadows, L., Wang, W., et al. 1997. The HLA-A*0201-restricted H-Y antigen contains a posttranslationally modified cysteine that significantly affects T cell recognition. *Immunity*, **6**, 273–81.

Momburg, F., Roelse, J., et al. 1994. Selectivity of MHC-encoded peptide transporter from human, mouse and rat. *Nature*, **367**, 648–51.

Monaco, J.J. and Nandi, D. 1995. The genetics of proteasomes and antigen processing. *Annu Rev Genet*, **29**, 729–54.

Mosse, C.A., Meadows, L., et al. 1998. The class I antigen-processing pathway for the membrane protein tyrosinase involves translation in the endoplasmic reticulum and processing in the cytosol. *J Exp Med*, **187**, 37–48.

Norbury, C.C., Hewlett, L.J., et al. 1995. Class I MHC presentation of exogenous soluble antigen via macropinocytosis in bone marrow macrophages. *Immunity*, **3**, 783–91.

Norbury, C.C., Basta, S., et al. 2004. CD8+ T cell cross-priming via transfer of proteasome substrates. *Science*, **304**, 1318–21.

Obst, R., Armandola, E.A., et al. 1995. TAP polymorphism does not influence transport of peptide variants in mice and humans. *Eur J Immunol*, **25**, 2170–6.

Ortmann, B., Androlewicz, M.J. and Cresswell, P. 1994. MHC class I/β_2-microglobulin complexes associate with TAP transporters before peptide binding. *Nature*, **368**, 864–7.

Pamer, E. and Cresswell, P. 1998. Mechanisms of MHC class I-restricted antigen processing. *Annu Rev Immunol*, **16**, 323–58.

Pamer, E.G., Harty, J.T. and Bevan, M.J. 1991. Precise prediction of a dominant class I MHC-restricted epitope of *Listeria monocytogenes*. *Nature*, **353**, 852–5.

Peh, C.A., Burrows, S.R., et al. 1998. HLA-B27-restricted antigen presentation in the absence of tapasin reveals polymorphism in mechanisms of HLA class I peptide loading. *Immunity*, **8**, 531–42.

Pfeifer, J.D., Wick, M.J., et al. 1993. Phagocytic processing of bacterial antigens for class I MHC presentation to T cells. *Nature*, **361**, 359–62.

Princiotta, M.F., Schubert, U., et al. 2001. Cells adapted to the proteasome inhibitor 4-hydroxy-5-iodo-3-nitrophenylacetyl-Leu-Leu-leucinal-vinyl sulfone require enzymatically active proteasomes for continued survival. *Proc Natl Acad Sci USA*, **98**, 513–18.

Princiotta, M.F., Finzi, D., et al. 2003. Quantitating protein synthesis, degradation, and endogenous antigen processing. *Immunity*, **18**, 343–54.

Rammensee, H.-G., Friede, T. and Stevanovic, S. 1995. MHC ligands and peptide motifs: first listing. *Immunogenetics*, **41**, 178–228.

Rammensee, H.-G., Bachmann, J. and Stevanovic, S. 1997. *MHC ligands and peptide motifs*. Austin, TX: Landes Bioscience.

Raposo, G., Nijman, H.W., et al. 1996. B lymphocytes secrete antigen-presenting vesicles. *J Exp Med*, **183**, 1161–72.

Rechsteiner, M., Realini, C. and Ustrell, V. 2000. The proteasome activator 11 S REG (PA28) and class I antigen presentation. *Biochem J*, **345**, Pt 1, 1–15.

Reits, E.A., Vos, J.C., et al. 2000. The major substrates for TAP in vivo are derived from newly synthesized proteins. *Nature*, **404**, 774–8.

Reits, E., Neijssen, J., et al. 2004. A major role for TPPII in trimming proteasomal degradation products for MHC class I antigen presentation. *Immunity*, **20**, 495–506.

Restifo, N.P., Bacík, I., et al. 1995. Antigen processing in vivo and the elicitation of primary CTL responses. *J Immunol*, **154**, 4414–22.

Riddell, S.R., Rabin, M., et al. 1991. Class I MHC-restricted cytotoxic T lymphocyte recognition of cells infected with human cytomegalovirus does not require endogenous viral gene expression. *J Immunol*, **146**, 2795–804.

Rock, K.L. and Goldberg, A.L. 1999. Degradation of cell proteins and the generation of MHC class I-presented peptides. *Annu Rev Immunol*, **17**, 739–.

Rock, K.L., Gamble, S. and Rothstein, L. 1990. Presentation of exogenous antigen with class I major histocompatibility complex molecules. *Science*, **249**, 918–21.

Rock, K.L., Gramm, C., et al. 1994. Inhibitors of the proteasome block the degradation of most cell proteins and the generation of peptides presented on MHC class I molecules. *Cell*, **78**, 761–71.

Rodriguez, A., Regnault, A., et al. 1999. Selective transport of internalized antigens to the cytosol for MHC class I presentation in dendritic cells. *Nat Cell Biol*, **1**, 362–8.

Schirmbeck, R., Thoma, S. and Reimann, J. 1997. Processing of exogenous hepatitis B surface antigen particles for L^d-restricted epitope presentation depends on exogenous β2-microglobulin. *Eur J Immunol*, **27**, 3471–84.

Schubert, U., Anton, L.C., et al. 2000. Rapid degradation of a large fraction of newly synthesized proteins by proteasomes. *Nature*, **404**, 770–4.

Schumacher, T.N.M., Kantesaria, D.V., et al. 1994. Peptide length and sequence specificity of the mouse TAP1/TAP2 translocator. *J Exp Med*, **179**, 533–40.

Serwold, T., Gonzalez, F., et al. 2002. ERAAP customizes peptides for MHC class I molecules in the endoplasmic reticulum. *Nature*, **419**, 480–3.

Silva, C.L., Portaro, F.C., et al. 1999. Thimet oligopeptidase (EC 3.4.24.15), a novel protein on the route of MHC class I antigen presentation. *Biochem Biophys Res Commun*, **255**, 591–5.

Skipper, J.C.A., Hendrickson, R.C., et al. 1996. An HLA-A2-restricted tyrosinase antigen on melanoma cells results from posttranslational modification and suggests a novel pathway for processing of membrane proteins. *J Exp Med*, **183**, 527–34.

Song, R. and Harding, C.V. 1996. Roles of proteosomes, transporter for antigen presentation (TAP), and β2-microglobulin in the processing of bacterial or particulate antigens via an alternate class I MHC processing pathway. *J Immunol*, **156**, 4182–90.

Spiliotis, E.T., Manley, H., et al. 2001. Selective export of MHC class I molecules from the ER after their dissociation from TAP. *Immunity*, **14**, 205.

Stoltze, L., Schirle, M., et al. 2000. Two new proteases in the MHC class I processing pathway. *Nat Immunol*, **1**, 413–18.

Stryhn, A., Pedersen, L.O., et al. 1996. pH dependence of MHC class I-restricted peptide presentation. *J Immunol*, **156**, 4191–7.

Su, R.C. and Miller, R.G. 2001. Stability of surface H-2K(b), H-2D(b), and peptide-receptive H-2K(b) on splenocytes. *J Immunol*, **167**, 4869–77.

Sugita, M. and Brenner, M.B. 1995. Association of the invariant chain with major histocompatibility complex class I molecules directs trafficking to endocytic compartments. *J Biol Chem*, **270**, 1443–8.

Suh, W.-K., Cohen-Doyle, M.F., et al. 1994. Interaction of MHC class I molecules with the transporter associated with antigen processing. *Science*, **264**, 1322–6.

Tanaka, K. and Kasahara, M. 1998. The MHC class I ligand-generating system: roles of immunoproteasomes and the interferon-gamma-inducible proteasome activator PA28. *Immunol Rev*, **163**, 161–76.

Tevethia, S., Tevethia, M., et al. 1983. Biology of simian virus 40 (SV40) transplantation antigen (TrAg). IX. Analysis of TrAg in mouse cells synthesizing truncated SV40 large T antigen. *Virology*, **128**, 319–30.

Thrower, J.S., Hoffman, L., et al. 2000. Recognition of the polyubiquitin proteolytic signal. *EMBO J*, **19**, 94–102.

Townsend, A.R.M., Bastin, J., et al. 1986. Cytotoxic T lymphocytes recognize influenza hemagglutinin that lacks a signal sequence. *Nature*, **324**, 575–7.

Townsend, A., Bastin, J., et al. 1988. Defective presentation to class I-restricted cytotoxic T lymphocytes in vaccinia-infected cells is overcome by enhanced degradation of antigen. *J Exp Med*, **168**, 1211–24.

Van Pel, A. and Boon, T. 1989. T cell-recognized antigenic peptides derived from the cellular genome are not protein degradation products but can be generated directly by transcription and translation of short subgenic regions. A hypothesis. *Immunogenetics*, **29**, 75–9.

Verma, R. and Deshaies, R.J. 2000. A proteasome howdunit: the case of the missing signal. *Cell*, **101**, 341–4.

Voges, D., Zwickl, P. and Baumeister, W. 1999. The 26S proteasome: a molecular machine designed for controlled proteolysis. *Annu Rev Biochem*, **68**, 1015–68.

Wallin, R.P., Lundqvist, A., et al. 2002. Heat-shock proteins as activators of the innate immune system. *Trends Immunol*, **23**, 130–5.

Wiertz, E.J.H., Jones, T.R., et al. 1996. The human cytomegalovirus US11 gene product dislocates MHC class I heavy chains from the endoplasmic reticulum of the cytosol. *Cell*, **84**, 769–79.

Wilkinson, K.D. 2000. Ubiquitination and deubiquitination: targeting of proteins for degradation by the proteasome (in process citation). *Semin Cell Dev Biol*, **11**, 141–8.

Williams, D.B. and Watts, T.H. 1995. Molecular chaperones in antigen presentation. *Current Opinion in Immunol*, **7**, 77–85.

Wolkers, M.C., Brouwenstijn, N., et al. 2004. Antigen bias in T cell cross-priming. *Science*, **304**, 1314–17.

Yan, G., Shi, L. and Faustman, D. 1999. Novel splicing of the human MHC-encoded peptide transporter confers unique properties. *J Immunol*, **162**, 852–9.

Yewdell, J.W. and Bennink, J.R. 1992. Cell biology of antigen processing and presentation to MHC class I molecule-restricted T lymphocytes. *Adv Immunol*, **52**, 1–123.

Yewdell, J.W. and Bennink, J.R. 1999. Immunodominance in major histocompatibility complex class I-restricted T lymphocyte responses. *Annu Rev Immunol*, **17**, 51–88.

Yewdell, J.W., Bennink, J.R. and Hosaka, Y. 1988. Cells process exogenous proteins for recognition by cytotoxic T lymphocytes. *Science*, **239**, 637–40.

Yewdell, J.W., Antón, L.C. and Bennink, J.R. 1996. Defective ribosomal products (DRiPs). A major source of antigenic peptides for MHC class I molecules? *J Immunol*, **157**, 1823–6.

Yewdell, J., Anton, L.C., et al. 1999a. Generating MHC class I ligands from viral gene products. *Immunol Rev*, **172**, 97–108.

Yewdell, J.W., Norbury, C.C. and Bennink, J.R. 1999b. Mechanisms of exogenous antigen presentation by MHC class I molecules in vitro and in vivo: implications for generating CD8+ T cell responses to infectious agents, tumors, transplants, and vaccines. *Adv Immunol*, **73**, 1–77.

York, I.A., Goldberg, A.L., et al. 1999. Proteolysis and class I major histocompatibility complex antigen presentation. *Immunol Rev*, **172**, 49–66.

York, I.A., Chang, S.C., et al. 2002. The ER aminopeptidase ERAP1 enhances or limits antigen presentation by trimming epitopes to 8–9 residues. *Nat Immunol*, **3**, 1177–84.

Zarling, A.L., Ficarro, S.B., et al. 2000. Phosphorylated peptides are naturally processed and presented by major histocompatibility complex class I molecules in vivo. *J Exp Med*, **192**, 12, 1755–62.

Zitvogel, L., Regnault, A., et al. 1998. Eradication of established murine tumors using a novel cell-free vaccine: dendritic cell-derived exosomes. *Nat Med*, **4**, 594–600.

22

The role of CD8 T cells in the control of infectious disease and malignancies

SHIOU-CHIH HSU (STEPHEN)

INTRODUCTION

CD8 T cells are a subset of T lymphocytes that are responsible for cellular immune responses. CD8 T cells recognize specific peptide epitopes presented by class I major histocompatibility complexes (MHC) on the surface of pathogen-infected or malignant cells using T-cell receptors (TCR) and CD8 molecules. TCRs consist of α and β chains, which associate with CD3 molecules. TCRs associating with CD3 bind to peptide and the polymorphic region of MHC, whereas CD8 binds to the nonpolymorphic region. After recognition of peptide–MHCI complexes and binding to several adhesion molecules on pathogen-infected and malignant cells, CD8 T cells are able to protect against pathogens and malignancies by secreting soluble mediators and inducing cytotoxicity. In this chapter, the role of CD8 T cells in the control of infectious diseases and malignancies, the induction of CD8 T-cell responses, and the protective mechanisms mediated by CD8 T cells are discussed.

CD8 T LYMPHOCYTES IN THE CONTROL OF INFECTIOUS DISEASES

CD8 T-cell immunity to viruses

Unlike extracellular pathogens, viruses are obligate intracellular pathogens, the multiplication of which occurs inside infected cells; once released from infected cells, mature virions will infect other normal cells. Although virus-specific antibodies can clear extracellular virus particles by neutralization or other mechanisms, antibodies may not be able to effectively eliminate intracellular virus, particularly as some viruses can be transmitted by fusion between infected and normal cells (Spickett et al. 1989; Rausch et al. 1992; Kahn et al. 1999). When virus infection occurs, viral antigens are processed into short peptides, which are presented by MHCI molecules (Townsend and Bodmer 1989), CD8 T cells are able to recognize these peptide epitopes presented by MHCI molecules. The level of CD8 T-cell responses also increases earlier than that of other adaptive immune responses. The level of CD8 cytotoxic T-lymphocyte (CTL) activity can be measured by in vitro cytotoxicity assays or cytokine analysis. After recognition of peptide–MHC complexes presented by virus-infected cells, CD8 CTLs are capable of inhibiting intracellular virus proliferation by cytotoxicity or the activity of secreted cytokines (Guidotti and Chisari 2001). Virus-specific CD8 CTL responses induced by different vaccine constructs have been demonstrated to protect against several virus infections in animal models (Schulz et al. 1991; Ciernik et al. 1996; Hsu et al. 1998, 1999; Leifert et al. 2001; Li et al. 2001a; Nass et al. 2001; Gierynska et al. 2002). Whether or not the level of CTL activity or the frequency of CD8 CTLs is important in conferring protection needs further investigation in situations where protective immune responses have been induced after immunization.

Different viruses also have a variety of ways to escape CD8 T-cell responses (Phillips et al. 1991; Goulder et al. 1997; McMichael and Phillips 1997; McMichael and Rowland-Jones 2001), which could result in persistence of virus infection or reinfection within the population. Viruses with a potentially high mutation rate, such as human immunodeficiency virus (HIV), simian immunodeficiency virus (SIV), hepatitis C virus (HCV), and influenza virus with antigenic variations within the epitopes, are able to avoid CTL recognition. These observations demonstrate the protective role of CD8 CTLs (Price et al. 2000; Erickson et al. 2001; McMichael and Rowland-Jones 2001). Herpesviruses can interfere with the MHCI processing and presentation pathway (Yamashita et al. 1993; Hill et al. 1995) and respiratory syncytial virus infection can suppress CD8 T-cell memory responses (Chang and Braciale 2002). HIV, adenovirus, and cytomegalovirus (CMV) can down-regulate MHCI molecule expression on the cell surface (Yamashita et al. 1993; Pereira et al. 1995; Mahr and Gooding 1999; Reusch et al. 1999; McMichael and Rowland-Jones 2001). However, little is known about the dynamics of immune responses after infection with mutant viruses. Specificity, cytokine expression and frequency of CD8 T-cell responses to wild-type viruses may be different from those to mutant viruses during infection. The results of studies of the differences in CD8 T-cell responses after infection with wild-type virus and mutant virus could help in the design of promising and effective vaccine constructs and new immunization strategies.

CD8 T-cell immunity to bacteria

Most pathogenic bacteria can survive and proliferate outside cells. However, when intracellular bacteria, such as mycobacteria and *Listeria* spp., cause infection, CD8 T cells could play an important protective role (Gellin and Broome 1989; Harty et al. 1992; Clemens and Horwitz 1996; Sturgill-Koszycki et al. 1996). Mycobacteria are acid-fast intracellular pathogens and, after infection, they can survive in certain endosomal compartments (Sturgill-Koszycki et al. 1996). Mycobacterial antigens are processed in these compartments into peptide fragments that are presented by MHCI molecules to CD8 T cells. Both αβ- and γδ T cells have been shown to play a protective role against mycobacterial infections (Ladel et al. 1995; D'Souza et al. 1997). CD8 CTLs can mediate protective immunity against mycobacteria by granule-mediated cytolysis or by the release of cytokines, such as interferon-γ (IFN-γ) (Harty et al. 1992; Ehrt et al. 2001). IFN-γ and interleukin-12 (IL-12) are also involved in granulomatosis and the generation of protective cellular immune responses (Cooper et al. 1997). Protective CD8 CTL responses against mycobacteria can be induced by a variety of vaccine preparations, including recombinant viral vaccines and DNA vaccines (Lowrie et al. 1997; Zhu et al. 1997).

Listeria monocytogenes is a gram-positive intracellular bacterium that causes listeriosis (Gellin and Broome 1989). Infection with live *L. monocytogenes* induces antigen-specific CD8 T-cell responses, with peak responses 7–9 days and 5 days after reinfection (Busch et al. 1998). Antigen-specific CD8 T-cell responses induced by live *L. monocytogenes* provides protective immunity against subsequent infection. On the other hand, immunization with heat-inactivated *L. monocytogenes* could not provide effective protection against subsequent infections, although the size of the antigen-specific CD8 T-cell population was increased to the same extent as that in immune animals (Von Koenig et al. 1982; Lauvau et al. 2001). However, in situations where CD8 T-cell responses did confer protective immunity against intracellular bacteria after infection or immunization, the soluble mediators secreted by CD8 T cells participating in protection still remain unknown.

CD8 T-cell immunity to parasites

Most pathogenic parasites have complicated life cycles with different developmental stages (Markell and Voge 1981). After infection with intracellular parasites, parasitic antigens are processed and presented as MHCI–peptide complexes in infected cells, which are recognized by CD8 T cells at certain stages in some cases. Thus, CD8 T cells are able to protect against malaria infection at the liver stages (Hoffman et al. 1989; Romero et al. 1989; Charest et al. 2000). Antigen-specific CD8 T-cell responses protect against *Toxoplasma gondii* parasites after immunization (Khan et al. 1994; Nielsen et al. 1991, 1999). In CD8-deficient or CD8-depleted animals, the growth of leishmania parasites cannot be controlled, which indicates the protective role of CD8 T cells in this infection (Belkaid et al. 2002). The protective ability of CD8 T cells against a variety of parasitic infections has also been demonstrated by the adoptive transfer of parasite-specific CD8 T cells from immune animals (Nielsen et al. 1991). As a result of their complicated life cycles, many parasitic antigens from parasites are expressed in different stages and, as an added complication, malaria parasites can also infect red blood cells, which are cells that do not express MHCI–peptide complexes (Urban et al. 1999). The question of whether there are malaria antigens expressed in red blood cells capable of regulating CD8 T-cell responses has yet to be answered.

Parasites have also developed different ways of escaping immune responses (Borst 1991; Hall and Joiner 1991; Barral-Netto et al. 1992), including antigenic variation, modulation of cytokine expression, avoidance of killing by oxygen metabolites or hydrolase, and alteration of the function of antigen-presenting cells (APC). Whether certain parasites have also developed the same strategies as used by viruses to escape CD8 T-cell responses remains to be investigated.

CD8 T LYMPHOCYTES IN THE CONTROL OF MALIGNANCIES

CD8 T-cell immunity to tumors

Historically, several lines of evidence have shown the existence of tumor-specific immunity. Clinical evidence has also shown that tumors sometimes regressed in cancer patients after bacterial infection and the growth of tumors is suppressed after transplantation into an MHC-incompatible host in experimental models. The immune surveillance hypothesis was proposed to explain the role of immune responses in the control of tumors (Boon et al. 1994). Although immune responses are able to control tumors, they always eventually escape immune attack in the absence of the use of further and better treatment (Marincola et al. 2000). In contrast to MHCII molecules, which are mainly expressed on specialized APCs, most cells express MHCI molecules, including tumor cells. With their ability to recognize specific peptide–MHC complexes, CD8 CTLs are considered to be important effectors of cellular immunity against tumor cells. To induce specific CD8 CTL responses against tumor cells, the identification of tumor antigens is important and this also has importance for the development of immunotherapeutic approaches. Several tumor antigens have been identified that have the ability to induce protective tumor-specific CD8 CTL responses, e.g. the melanoma antigens, MAGE, BAGE, and GAGE, are expressed in melanoma cells but not in normal cells (Boon et al. 1994). Many of the melanoma-associated antigens are derived from normal nonmutated melanocyte differentiation antigens, including MART-1, gp-100, and tyrosine-related protein-2 (Zeh et al. 1999).

The lack of appropriate tumor antigens has impeded the development of effective immunotherapeutic approaches to other tumors. To induce protective CD8 T-cell immunity to other tumors, tumor-associated antigens that are overexpressed selfantigens in other tumors, such as mdm and WT-1, have been used in attempts to generate protective tumor immunity (Sadovinikova and Stauss 1996; Gao et al. 2000; Ohminami et al. 2000; Oka et al. 2000). As these overexpressed tumor antigens are expressed in normal cells at lower levels, there is a possibility that deleterious autoimmune responses could be induced when effective tumor-specific T-cell responses are generated against them. Furthermore, the induction of tolerance could also impair the maintenance of T-cell responses against tumors using these overexpressed self-proteins as tumor antigens.

Tumor immunotherapy by CD8 T cells

Tumor immunotherapy can provide an alternative method to traditional therapeutic approaches. Several immunotherapeutic approaches have been developed to generate humoral or cellular immunity to tumors, including the induction of protective cellular immune responses by immunization with tumor antigens and the generation of tumor-specific CTL lines or clones with APCs expressing tumor antigens (Matis et al. 1986). Different tumor antigen preparations have been developed for immunization purposes (Oka et al. 2000). Tumor antigens formulated in different adjuvants, expressed in viral vectors or nucleic acids, and expressed in specialized APCs have been used to induce tumor-specific CD8 CTL responses (Ciernik et al. 1996). CD8 CTL peptide epitopes identified from tumor antigens have been used to generate CD8 CTL lines or clones for tumor immunotherapy (Sadovinikova and Stauss 1996; Zeh et al. 1999). CD8 CTL epitopes have also been used for the construction of vaccines to generate protective CD8 CTL responses. Several vaccine preparations and immunization approaches, including the induction of CD4 T-cell responses and the inclusion of cytokines, chemokines, and costimulatory molecules in the vaccine design, have been used to improve the effectiveness of tumor-specific CD8 CTL responses. In animal models, the induction of tumor-specific CD8 CTL responses by immunization and the transfer of tumor-specific CTL lines or clones have had some success in the control of tumor growth, although the control of growth was not complete. Variations in the effectiveness of immunotherapy to different tumors using CD8 T cells have also been described. Similar to pathogens in some aspects, tumors are also able to avoid immune responses by modulating the expression of MHC molecules, cell surface molecules, and cytokines (Marincola et al. 2000; Buggins et al. 2001; Ibrahim et al. 2001). The investigation of the mechanisms used by specific cells to evade immune responses could lead to the design of better therapeutic strategies. However, the mechanisms used by CD8 CTL to control tumor cells are also not clear other than their cytolytic activity and cytokine expression.

THE PROTECTIVE MECHANISMS INVOLVING CD8 T LYMPHOCYTES

Soluble mediators secreted by CD8 T cells

CD8 T cells protect against infection by intracellular pathogens via cytolytic and noncytolytic mechanisms (Barth et al. 1991; Tuttle et al. 1993; Yang and Walker 1997; Guidotti and Chisari 2001; Binder and Griffin 2001; Russell and Ley 2002). The noncytolytic mechanisms are mediated by cytokines, chemokines, and other

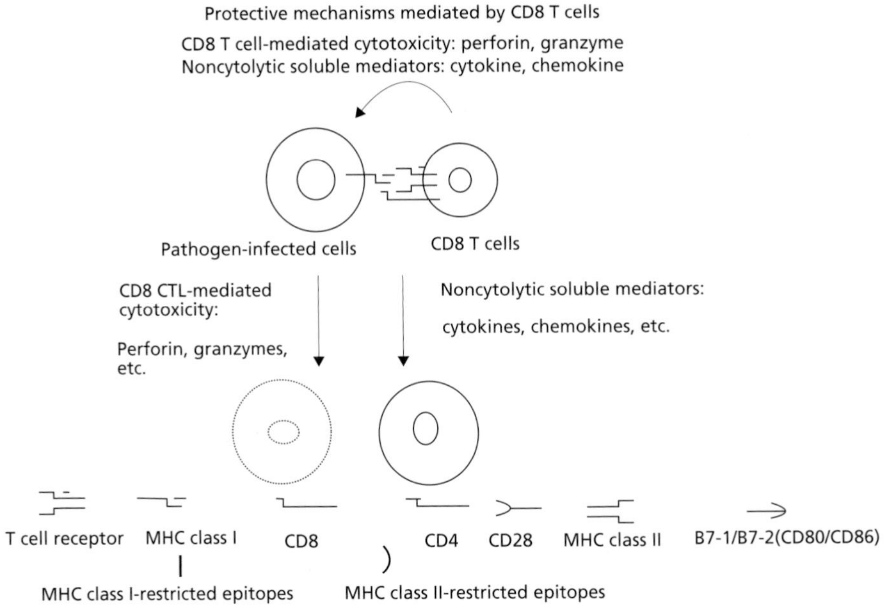

Figure 22.1 *CD8 T cells can protect against pathogens by secreted noncytolytic soluble mediators or granule-mediated cytolysis. Noncytolytic soluble mediators include cytokines or chemokines that inhibit proliferation or infection of intracellular pathogens. Granules containing perforins, granzymes, etc. induce cytolysis of pathogen-infected cells. CTL, cytotoxic T lymphocyte.*

soluble mediators secreted from CD8 T cells (Figure 22.1). The involvement of these noncytolytic mechanisms in protection against pathogens was observed in experiments by using particular cytokine gene-deficient animals or depletion of particular cytokines by a specific antibody in animal models (Klavinskis et al. 1989; Tishon et al. 1995; Hsu et al. 1998). Using these approaches, it has been shown that certain cytokine-deficient CD8 T cells are less efficient in the control of infection with some pathogens than with others (Harty et al. 1992; Tishon et al. 1995). CD8 T cells secrete several antiviral cytokines after infection or peptide epitope stimulation (Klavinskis et al. 1989; Hsu et al. 1998; Patterson et al. 2002). IFN-γ and tumor necrosis factor α (TNF-α) secreted by CD8 T cells are able to reduce virus infection by intracellular or extracellular mechanisms, to recruit and activate macrophages, T cells, or natural killer (NK) cells to perform their effector function. IFN can directly inhibit virus replication by activating the oligoadenylate synthetases, Mx proteins, double-stranded-RNA-activated protein kinase, and the double-stranded-RNA-specific adenosine deaminase systems (Silverman 1994; Patterson et al. 1995; Haller et al. 1998; Terenzi et al. 1999). Oligoadenylate synthetases suppress viral replication by induction of several cellular RNases that degrade viral transcripts. Double-stranded-RNA-activated protein kinase and adenosine deaminase inhibit viral protein synthesis. IFN-γ and TNF-α are also able to regulate antigen processing and presentation, enhance the expression of MHC molecules on the cell surface, and recruit macrophages, NK cells, and T cells into virus infection sites to perform their antipathogen effector function.

During pathogen infection, CD8 T cells are capable of making and secreting many cytokines, chemokines, and other soluble mediators with as yet unknown functions (Toso et al. 1995; Wagner et al. 1998). Anti-HIV-specific CD8 T cells can produce unidentified noncytolytic factors that suppress HIV viral replication in vitro after antigen recognition (Toso et al. 1995). Intracellular bacteria and parasites are also inhibited by several cytokines secreted from CD8 T cells. The detailed intracellular events that inhibit intracellular bacteria or parasites are less clear than those that inhibit intracellular viruses. Although the intracellular mechanisms that inhibit viral replication have been well studied, there are still intracellular events that are not very clear other than the suppression of viral RNA or protein synthesis. The induction of the expression by intracellular molecules, which play an important role in the inhibition of intracellular bacteria and parasites, has been suggested by several authors (Seguin et al. 1994; Scheller et al. 1997). Further investigation of the intracellular events that protect against infection of intracellular bacteria, parasites, or viruses by cytokines could lead to the design of effective therapeutic approaches. Whether there are unidentified soluble molecules produced by CD8 T cells that protect against different virus infections represents a new area to be explored.

CD8 T-cell-mediated cytotoxicity

CD8 CTLs can mediate cytolysis of pathogen-infected or malignant cells by granule exocytosis of perforin, granzymes, and other molecules (Russell and Ley 2002). CD8 CTLs are also able to lyse the pathogen-infected or malignant cells by the Fas/Fas ligand pathway (Figure 22.1). After T-cell activation, granules including perforin, granzyme, and other components are synthesized and reside in the cytoplasm. In the recognition of pathogen-infected cells, granules are fused with cell membranes at the contact sites of the tight junction between CD8 T cells and target cells. Once granules are released from CD8 T cells, perforin polymerizes to insert into the cell membrane and induces membrane damage in the presence of calcium (Tschopp et al. 1989; Muller and Tschopp 1994). Although the function of perforin is similar to that of complement in inducing membrane damage, perforin alone is not sufficient to induce apoptosis of the target cells. Perforin alone was thought to be capable of causing apoptosis of the target cells; however, several authors have suggested that the pore created by perforin is too small to allow large molecules, granzymes, and other components to pass into the target cells to induce apoptosis (Podack et al. 1985; Browne et al. 1999). This debate does not change the fact that the function of perforin is to induce membrane damage. However, the role of perforin in cytotoxicity mechanisms induced by granule exocytosis remains to be defined.

Granzymes are serine proteases in the cytotoxic granules: granzyme A is the tryptase that prefers to cleave protein substrates in the position of arginine or lysine residues (Odake et al. 1991). Granzyme B is similar to the capases that prefer to cleave protein substrates in the position after aspartic acid residues (Odake et al. 1991). The function of granzyme A and other granzymes in cytotoxic granules has not been defined. Granzyme B cleaves procapase-3 and other procaspases in vitro (Sarin et al. 1998; Yang et al. 1998; Sutton et al. 2000), which could also be required for activation of caspase-3 to cleave other substrates in the target cells. After granule exocytosis by CD8 CTL, the cascade effect of substrate digestion by granzymes could result in apoptosis of target cells. Granzyme B induces nuclear DNA fragmentation in cells that are functionally caspase deficient, which suggests that this enzyme can directly activate apoptotic nucleases (Sutton et al. 2000). One of the apoptotic nucleases was identified as caspase-activated DNase (Enari et al. 1998). Granzyme B can enter the nucleus without the involvement of perforin or the alteration of the nuclear pore (Jans et al. 1996). In one of the pathways of granzyme-induced apoptosis, the involvement of mitochondria has been suggested because Bcl-2 can block death induced by perforin and granzymes (Russell and Ley 2002).

Granzyme A is less efficient at inducing apoptosis than granzyme B and the cellular pathways used by granzyme A to induce apoptosis are different from those by granzyme B. Granzyme A neither activates caspases nor induces cleavage of granzyme B substrates, caspase-3, DNA-dependent protein kinase (DNA-PK), or Poly-ADP-ribose-polymerase (PARP). Granzyme A does not result in oligonucleosomal DNA degradation, but only induces single DNA breaks, indicating that granzyme A activates different nucleases from those activated by granzyme B (Shi et al. 1992). The mechanisms used by CD8 CTLs to avoid cell death after granule exocytosis have been studied for many years and CD8 CTLs contain an inhibitor of granzyme, B, known as protease inhibitor 9 (PI-9) (Sun et al. 2001). When murine homologues of this inhibitor, SPI-6 and PI-9 are overexpressed in target cells, they protect these cells from death (Medema et al. 2001). The detailed mechanisms of the intracellular cascade events resulting in the induction of apoptosis of target cells are still unclear. Several viruses can encode inhibitors of granzyme B to inhibit both Fas- and granzyme-mediated lysis, including the poxvirus-encoded cytokine response modifier A (CrmA) and the granzyme B inhibitor which interacts with granzyme B and several capases to inhibit CTL-mediated lysis (Tewari et al. 1995). A study of the mechanisms used by viruses or tumor cells to evade CTL-mediated lysis by granzymes may well provide information that could help in the design of better immunization and therapeutic approaches.

THE DEVELOPMENT OF VACCINES FOR THE INDUCTION OF CD8 T-CELL RESPONSES

Inactivated vaccines

For many years, inactivated vaccines have been prepared from whole virions treated with chemicals, such as formalin, that reduce their infectivity and maintain their ability to stimulate protective immunity (Eller 1969; Fulginiti et al. 1969; Kapikian et al. 1969; Kim et al. 1969). Inactivated pathogens are the only vaccines available to stimulate protective antibody responses for many diseases. Although inactivated vaccines were thought to maintain the immunogenicity to stimulate immune responses with minor damage to the structure of viral proteins, formalin-inactivated vaccines are ineffective at generating protective, conformation-dependent, antibody responses and cellular immune responses mediated by CD8 CTLs (Chargelegue et al. 1998; Hsu et al. 1999). There are also other disadvantages of inactivated vaccines: virulent pathogens could still be infectious if the quality of vaccine preparation is not well controlled; and the contamination of vaccine preparations with materials derived from tissue culture could result in hypersensitivity reactions (Eller 1969; Chanock et al. 1992; Wertz and Sullender 1992). Indeed, the use of formalin-inactivated respiratory syncytial virus vaccines induced exacerbated disease during a subsequent epidemic (Fulginiti et al. 1969) and the pathological effects induced by formalin-inactivated respiratory syncytial virus vaccine have been extensively studied

(Openshaw et al. 2001). A detailed analysis of the factors that result in pathological consequences following the use of formalin-inactivated vaccines is important for the development of new vaccines and immunization strategies to generate protective immunity without exacerbated diseases.

Attenuated vaccines

Attenuated vaccines are mutant live pathogens that have similar antigenicity to wild-type pathogens and induce no pathogenic effects (Wegmann et al. 1986). Mutant live pathogens are selected by attenuating strains of wild-type pathogens in serial cell culture or by genetic manipulation (Beck et al. 1986; Wertz and Sullender 1992; Khattar et al. 2001; Bukreyev et al. 1999, 2001; Stittelaar et al. 2002). Many of the currently available vaccines to prevent infectious diseases are live attenuated vaccines (Table 22.1) that are considered to induce protective humoral and cellular immune responses similar to those induced by the wild-type virus but without pathogenic consequences. In contrast to inactivated vaccines, live attenuated vaccines are able to induce pathogen-specific CD8 CTL responses. There is very little information about the differences in cellular immune responses mediated by CD8 CTL responses generated by attenuated vaccines and wild-type pathogens, and a comparison of these differences will facilitate the development of better vaccines and immunization approaches to avoid any pathogenic consequences of immunization.

Genetic manipulation approaches can be used to insert foreign genes with immunoregulatory functions, such as cytokines, into the pathogen genome, to delete the genes related to pathogenic effects, to introduce mutations into the genome of pathogens to enhance protective immunity, and to avoid exacerbated pathogenesis (Bukreyev et al. 1999, 2001; Khattar et al. 2001). Although the attenuated vaccines currently in use have given encouraging results in conferring protective immune responses against many infectious diseases, there is an urgent need to develop alternative vaccines to prevent infection with mutant pathogens. There is a possibility that attenuated vaccines may revert to the virulent strain or could be contaminated with virulent pathogens after serial cultivation in tissue culture or in the infected population. Investigations into the long-term pathogenic effects of immunization with attenuated vaccines will be important for the design of improved vaccines.

Subunit vaccines

Subunit vaccines mainly comprise protein or carbohydrates expressed by pathogens that are recognized by antibodies, T lymphocytes, or other immune cells (Zuckerman 1986; Jones et al. 1996; Lingappa et al. 2001). Many viral proteins expressed on the surface of virions have been selected as subunit vaccines for the induction of protective antibody responses (Zuckerman 1986; Schirmbeck et al. 1994; Li et al. 1998; Bembridge et al. 2000). Surface and internal virus proteins are capable of generating protective T-cell responses (Schirmbeck et al. 1994; Li et al. 1998; Bembridge et al. 2000). Although capsular carbohydrate antigens are used as subunit vaccines to generate immune responses (Jones et al. 1996; Lingappa et al. 2001), they are not effective at generating antibody responses without the inclusion of a protein carrier or appropriate adjuvant formulations. Designing appropriate immunization strategies and vaccine constructs to generate anticarbohydrate immune responses is important for the development of vaccines against pathogenic bacteria with capsular carbohydrate antigens. T-cell recognition of carbohydrates has also been suggested by several authors (Carbone and Gleeson 1997; Galli-Stampino et al. 1997; Deck et al. 1999; Haurum et al. 1999), and that MHCI molecules present glycopeptides to CD8 T cells. Immunization with MHC-restricted binding glycopeptides generates

Table 22.1 *Vaccines in use to prevent infectious diseases*

Prevention of infectious diseases	Vaccines in use	Route of immunization	CD8 CTL induction
Poliomyelitis	Live attenuated	Oral	Yes (++++)
MMR			
Measles	Live attenuated	Parenteral	Yes (++++)
Mumps	Live attenuated	Parenteral	Yes (++++)
Rubella	Live attenuated	Parenteral	Yes (++++)
Hepatitis B	Subunit vaccines	Intramuscular	(−)?
Purified HBsAg from healthy carrier			
HBsAg from recombinant DNA in yeast			
Haemophilus influenzae b	Subunit vaccines		(−)?
Capsular carbohydrate conjugate vaccine			
Meningococcal C	Subunit vaccines		(−)?
Capsular carbohydrate conjugate vaccine			

(++++), vaccines are efficient at induction of CD8 CTL responses. (−)?, considered to be inefficient at inducing CD8 CTL responses. The ability of the vaccines (hepatitis B subunit vaccines) to induce CD8 CTL responses is not conclusive in the literature. HBsAg, hepatitis B surface antigen.

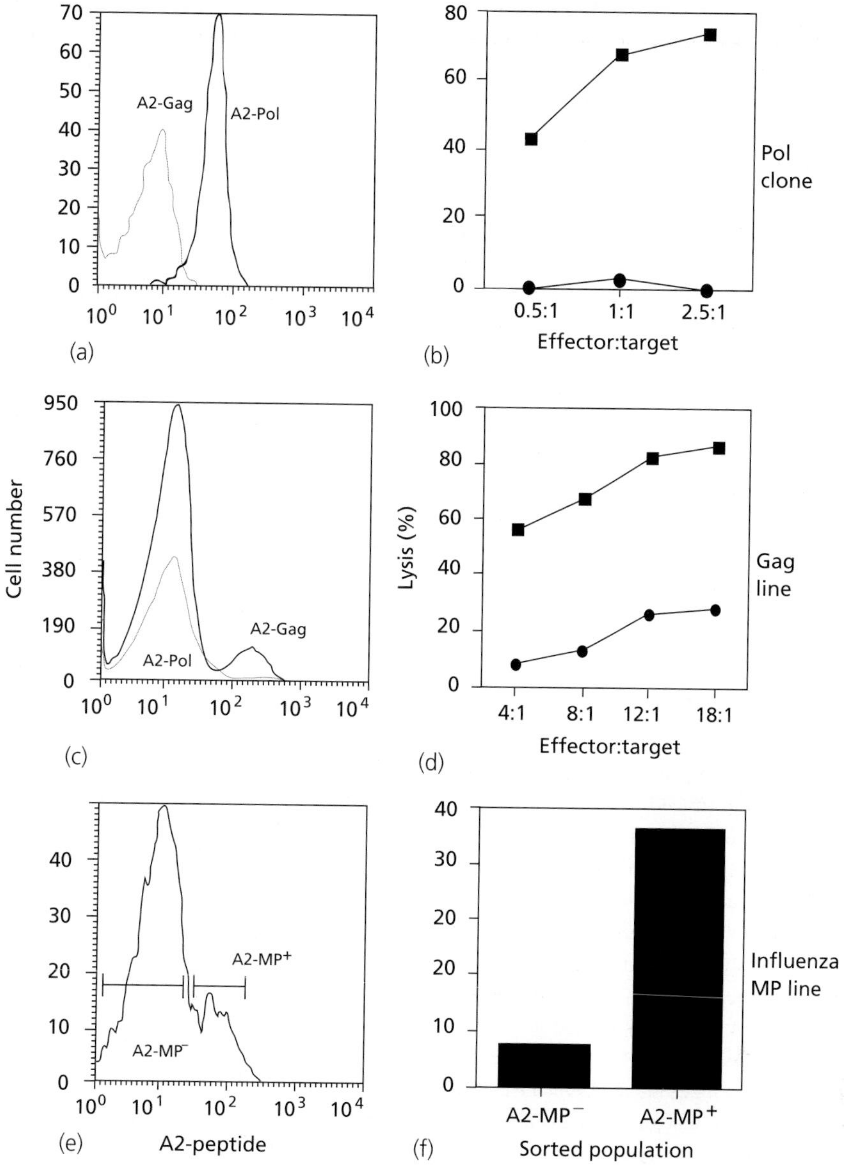

Figure 22.2 *Staining by MHC–peptide tetramers correlates with peptide-dependent cytotoxicity. Flow cytometric analysis (18) of CD8+ T cells (17, 20, 30) from* **(a)** *clone 20 stained with A2-Pol (solid line) and A2-Gag (dotted line) tetramers,* **(c)** *HIV-Gag-specific cytoxic T lymphocyte (CTL) line 868 stained with A2-Gag (solid line) and A2-Pol (dotted line) tetramers, and* **(e)** *an HLA-A2-restricted influenza matrix peptide CTL line (PG-001), stained with A2-MP tetramers and sorted into A2-MP+ and A2-MP− populations, as indicated. Cytotoxicity assays with* **(b)** *clone 20 showed specific killing of autologous* Epstein–Barr virus-*transformed B cells pulsed with Pol peptide (closed squares), but not target cells without added peptide (closed circles).* **(d)** *The 868 Gag-specific CTL line killed cells pulsed with the Gag peptide (closed squares) but not target cells without added peptide (closed circles).* **(f)** *The sorted populations from* **(e)** *were assayed for killing of MP-pulsed target cells at an effector:target ratio of 1:1. The same ratio, in cells not treated with peptide, with no killing of target cells was seen. (From Altman et al. 1996 with permission.)*

glycopeptide-specific, MHC-restricted, CD8 CTLs (Speir et al. 1999); however, the function of glycopeptide-specific CD8 T cells in the control of infection with pathogens expressing carbohydrates is not completely understood.

Advances in molecular biology have facilitated the development of subunit vaccines in which the proteins of pathogens are purified as protein subunit vaccines, expressed with other proteins as fusion protein subunit vaccines, or inserted into a variety of vectors as recombinant subunit vaccines (Gherardi et al. 1999; Berzofsky et al. 2001). However, immunization with purified soluble proteins from pathogens is not effective at inducing CD8 T-cell responses in the absence of appropriate adjuvant formulation (Schirmbeck et al. 1994; Speidel et al. 1997; Sheikh et al. 1999). The use of some subunit proteins has resulted in the induction of exacerbated disease after infection.

Priming with G protein derived from respiratory syncytial virus resulted in eosinophilia during subsequent infection (Openshaw et al. 1992). Although different genetic, physical, or chemical modifications of purified proteins have been used to improve humoral and cellular immune responses after immunization, these approaches have tended to enhance one arm of immune responses while inhibiting the other (Speidel et al. 1997). Whether antigen processing and presentation of fusion protein vaccines are similar to those of protein antigens expressed on pathogens is not clear. The conformation of epitopes of fusion proteins may also be different from that of protein antigens expressed on pathogens. Pathogen proteins are inserted and expressed in different vectors, including viral, bacterial, and plasmid DNA vectors, as recombinant subunit vaccines. Recombinant subunit vaccines using live viral or bacterial vectors have the disadvantage that the boosting is ineffective because immune responses could be directed to the vectors rather than to the expressed pathogen proteins (Fuller et al. 2002; Harrington et al. 2002). Mutant pathogens with antigenic variations could also escape from the immune responses generated by recombinant vaccines expressing proteins from wild-type pathogens.

Epitope-based vaccines

Epitopes are small fragments of antigens that are recognized by specific antibodies produced from B lymphocytes (B-cell epitopes) or presented by MHC to TCRs of T lymphocytes (T-cell epitopes). Most epitopes are peptides derived from proteins of pathogens or specific antigens. CD8 T-cell peptide epitopes consist of 8–12 amino acids that bind to MHCI molecules (Townsend et al. 1989). Epitope-based vaccines consist of T- or B-cell epitopes that are made as synthetic peptides or synthetic oligonucleotides expressed by plasmid DNA or a variety of recombinant vectors (Chargelegue et al. 1998; Hsu et al. 1998, 1999; Berzofsky et al. 2001; Wee et al. 2002). Synthetic peptides, epitope-based DNA, or recombinant vectors expressing T-cell epitopes have all been shown to be capable of inducing protective CD8 CTL responses.

Synthetic peptides alone are often not able to induce effective immune responses without modification by the inclusion of additional sequences or the use of specific adjuvant formulations. Several sequence modifications and different adjuvants have been applied to the enhancement of induction of CD8 CTL responses (Gao et al. 1991; Hsu et al. 1995; Franke et al. 1997). Thus, the addition of T-helper epitopes, fusion peptide, lipophilic molecules, and signal peptides to CD8 CTL epitopes has resulted in enhanced specific CD8 CTL responses (Shirai et al. 1994; Hsu et al. 1995; Hiranuma et al. 1999). One of the advantages of the use of epitope-based vaccines is to allow T-cell epitopes to bind to MHC molecules bypassing some of the steps in protein antigen processing and presentation pathways. The flexibility of the design of epitope-based vaccines also allows peptide epitopes to be delivered to particular intracellular organelles to activate specific protective immune responses. Epitope-based immunization strategies could also be used to explore several unclear areas in immunology at the intercellular level, such as the extent of the TCR repertoire, the importance of the affinity–avidity of T-cell recognition, and the role of CD4–CD8 and CD8–APC interactions. The information from these areas can aid the design of a new generation of epitope-based vaccines and immunization strategies.

THE INDUCTION OF CD8 T-CELL RESPONSES

The role of CD4 T cells

In contrast to CD8 T cells, CD4 T cells recognize peptide epitopes bound to MHCII molecules presented by specialized APCs, such as dendritic cells or macrophages (Allen et al. 1985). CD4 T cells are able to improve CD8 T-cell immunity against pathogens and malignant cells after infection or immunization (Berzofsky et al. 2001); however, the mechanisms used by CD4 T cells to increase CD8 T-cell activity are not clear. CD4 T cells could simply expand the frequency of CD8 T cells or alter the function of CD8 T cells and vice versa. Indeed, CD8 T-cell responses can be expanded or suppressed via the action of cytokines or other soluble mediators from different types of CD4 T cells (Aung and Graham 2000; Aung et al. 1999; Sato et al. 2001). Specialized APCs express MHCI and MHCII molecules that are capable of presenting peptide epitopes to CD4 and CD8 T cells (Figure 22.3). CD8 T-cell responses could also be augmented by the microenviroments of cell–cell contacts between CD8 T cells, CD4 T cells, and specialized APCs. Induction of protective CD8 T-cell immunity by specialized APCs in the absence of CD4 T-cell responses has also been described (Sato et al. 2001; Wang et al. 2001; Diehl et al. 2002). Different vaccine preparations have been used to induce specific CD8 T-cell responses and, in many cases, vaccines including components for the induction of CD4 T-cell responses have resulted in enhanced specific CD8 CTL responses. It should be noted that CD8 CTL responses could also be induced in the absence of CD4 T-cell responses (Figure 22.3). The induction of CD8 T-cell responses with peptides bound with higher affinity to MHCI molecules depends less on the presence of exogenous CD4 T-cell peptide epitopes than CD8 epitopes bound with lower affinity to MHCI molecules. Whether or not other factors contribute to the induction of effective CD8 T-cell immunity by specialized APCs without CD4 T cells needs further investigation.

The role of antigen-presenting cells

CD8 T cells can recognize APCs expressing MHCI–peptide molecules on the cell surface. Several APCs,

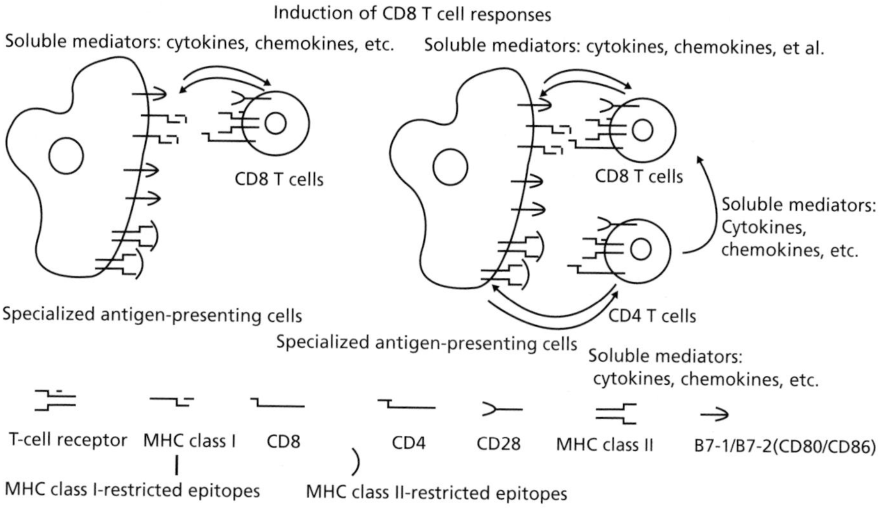

Figure 22.3 *Specialized antigen-presenting cells (APC) present MHCI- and MHCII-restricted epitopes to CD8 and CD4 T cells. CD8 T-cell responses are induced by cell-to-cell contact of CD4, CD8, and specialized APCs upon costimulatory signals or be soluble mediators, CD8 T-cell responses are also capable of being induced in the absence of CD4 T cells.*

such as fibroblasts, epithelial cells, endothelial cells, and different specific cells, are recognized and lysed by CD8 CTLs in vitro using CTL assays (Bennink et al. 1982; Gooding and O'Connell 1983; Townsend et al. 1986; Li et al. 2001b). MHCI-restricted antigen processing and presentation by specialized APCs, such as dendritic cells or macrophages, is required to induce and activate CD8 T-cell responses, as indicated in many publications. In these studies, several different ways to prepare and purify dendritic cells were used to induce protective CD8 T-cell responses (Steinman 1991; Galibert et al. 2001; Manz et al. 2001). There is limited information available to determine whether variations in methods for generation and purification of dendritic cells could alter their immunological function.

Specialized APCs, which some pathogens can directly infect, are capable of presenting MHC–peptide complexes to CD8 T cells through the endogenous MHCI processing and presentation pathway (Bennink et al. 1982; Townsend et al. 1986, 1989; Moore et al. 1988; Pamer and Cresswell 1998; Rock and Goldberg 1999). For other pathogens and particulate antigens, specialized APCs could present MHCI–peptide complexes to CD8 T cells via exogenous pathways that normally present MHCII–peptide complexes to CD4 T cells (Yewdell et al. 1988; Schirmbeck et al. 1995; Rock and Goldberg 1999; Pamer and Creswell 1998; Rock and Goldberg 1999; Stober et al. 2002). In classic MHCI endogenous antigen processing pathways, cytoplasmic antigens are processed into peptides by ubiquitin- and proteosome-mediated proteolysis (Rock et al. 1994; Rock and Goldberg 1999). Processed peptides are transported into the endoplasmic reticulum by TAP-dependent or TAP-independent pathways. After peptide epitopes are selected and bound to MHCI molecules, MHCI–peptide molecules are transported to the Golgi body and then to the cell surface. In the alternate exogenous MHCI pathway, exogenous antigens are endocytosed by specialized APCs into endosomal compartments. Protein antigens are processed by endosomal proteases into peptide fragments and processed peptides are transported into the cytoplasm to enter the endoplasmic reticulum or into other organelle compartments to associate with MHCI molecules. The detailed intracellular pathways of MHCI molecules are not totally clear, and whether the peptide repertoires produced by classic endogenous pathways are different from those produced by alternate exogenous pathways is not known. Specialized APCs stimulate effective specific CD8 CTL responses against pathogens or tumors, when pulsed with peptides and particulate protein antigens or by transfection with recombinant vectors in vivo or in vitro (Porgador and Gilboa 1995; Schirmbeck et al. 1995; Luft et al. 2002; Stober et al. 2002). Specialized APCs are able to express MHCI, MHCII, costimulatory, and other surface molecules. A knowledge of the differences in expression of surface molecules and cytokines between specialized APCs and other APCs is required in order to regulate the immunostimulatory function of specialized APCs for immunotherapy and the generation of protective immunity.

The role of cytokines

Several cytokines are involved in the induction of CD8 T-cell responses after pathogen infection or immunization. Many cytokines have already been included in the design of vaccines and adjuvant formulations to enhance the induction of CD8 CTL responses (Ahlers et al. 2001; Sato et al. 2001; Staats et al. 2001; Cho et al. 2002; Luft et al. 2002; Padovan et al. 2002). Some cytokines, such as interleukin 2 (IL-2), directly stimulate CD8 T-cell proliferation and activation. Granulocyte–monocyte colony-stimulating factor (GM-CSF) and IL-12 are able to upregulate the expression of receptors or surface molecules on CD8 T cells, to induce T-helper cell responses or to induce the cascade effects of cytokine expression from other cells (Gerrard et al. 1987; Ahlers et al. 2001; Berzofsky et al. 2001). IL-12 is able to enhance the induction of CD8 CTL responses and the production of IFN-γ Gately et al. 1994) and GM-CSF increases the number of infiltrating APCs and enhances the expression of IFN-γ and IL-12 receptors (Ahlers et al. 2001; Bukreyev et al. 2001). In addition, cytokines can also act synergistically on the induction of CD8 T cell responses (Mehrotra et al. 1995; Ahlers et al. 2001; Berzofsky et al. 2001). Type 1 IFNs are required for bone marrow- or resident monocyte-derived dendritic cells to stimulate CD8 CTL responses (Palmer et al. 2000; Luft et al. 2002; Montoya et al. 2002; Padovan et al. 2002). Both type 1 and type 2 IFNs regulate MHCI-restricted antigen processing and presentation (Atta et al. 1995; Keskinen et al. 1997). IL-4 has been found to suppress or enhance CD8 CTL activity in different experimental conditions (Bembridge et al. 1998; Aung et al. 1999; Aung and Graham 2000). Finally, cytokines are also involved in pathogenesis of diseases after pathogen infection (Peebles et al. 2000; Openshaw 2002).

Whether cytokines enhance the induction of CD8 CTL responses through the regulation of antigen processing and presentation is an important area to be explored. In several publications, a significant effect on immune responses was observed in the situation of IFN-γ deficiency, which is consistent with the observation that IFN-γ has an effect on the antigen processing and presentation pathway (Hsu et al. 1998; Guidotti and Chisari 2001; Nakajima et al. 2001), and induces the expression of subunits of proteasomes that are responsible for proteolysis in the MHCI-processing pathway (York and Rock 1996; Pamer and Cresswell 1998; Rock and Goldberg 1999). Type 1 IFNs increase the expression of MHCI and MHCII molecules and activate the effector function of T cells, NK cells, and macrophages (Guidotti and Chisari 2001). Whether the mechanisms by which type 1 IFN regulate MHCI expression are similar to those mediated by IFN-γ is not clear.

The role of co-stimulatory and surface molecules

T-cell activation requires the signal derived from the recognition of specific MHC–peptide complexes by TCRs and also additional costimulatory signals provided by accessory molecules on T cells and specialized APCs. CD28 is a well-known costimulatory molecule expressed on naïve or primed T cells, which bind to B7-1 (CD80) or B7-2 (CD86) on APCs (Schwartz 1992; Azuma et al. 1993; Freeman et al. 1993; Lenschow et al. 1996; Alegre et al. 2001). After recognition of specific MHC–peptides and costimulatory molecules, T cells proliferate and produce IL-2. In the absence of costimulatory signals, the engagement of TCRs and MHC–peptide complexes could result in anergic T cells. Costimulatory signals also promote T-cell survival by inducing the expression of antiapoptotic Bcl-2 (Boise et al. 1993). The mechanisms by which costimulatory signals provided by CD28–B7 ligation facilitate T-cell proliferation and differentiation are still not clear. The signals from CD28–B7 ligation may increase the TCR signaling pathway or stimulate different pathways from TCR signaling (Vola and Lanzavecchia 1996). Costimulatory signals were found to reduce the number of TCRs required for stimulation of cytokine production and proliferation at the cellular level. There are other positive signals provided by activating receptors including NKG2D to facilitate CD8 T-cell responses and tumor immunity (Diefenbach et al. 2001). Besides positive costimulatory signals, inhibitory receptors including CTLA-4 were also found to inhibit T-cell activation by suppressing IL-2 and IL-2 receptor expression (Alegre et al. 2001).

The movement of T or B lymphocytes into lymphoid organs is mediated by adhesion molecules on lymphocytes interacting with receptors on the high endothelial venules (HEV). Many experiments prove that T or B cells prefer localization to specific tissues. Lymphocytes isolated from gut-associated lymphoid tissue tend to localize to Peyer's patches after being reinfused, whereas splenocytes prefer migrating to the spleen. Immune responses in nonlymphoid tissues induce the movement of lymphocytes into nonlymphoid tissues. Cytokines induce the expression of adhesion molecules on endothelium which mediate the migration of lymphocytes into the inflammation tissues (Issekutz 1992). Different cytokines induce expression of different adhesion molecules that control different stages of lymphocyte migration (Issekutz 1990). ICAM-1 (CD54) and ICAM-2 (CD102) expressed on endothelial cells are receptors for LFA-1 on leukocytes (Bevilacqua 1993). The expression of adhesion molecules can improve the interaction of T cells with endothelium and target cells. Several publications have indicated that the lack of expression of some adhesion molecules resulted in diminished immune responses.

THE MAJOR HISTOCOMPATIBILITY COMPLEXES AND TCRS

The binding affinity of peptides to MHC

MHCI molecules consist of a heavy chain and β^2-microglobulin. β^2-Microglobulin associates noncovalently with the extracellular region of the heavy chain to form the peptide-binding region. After peptide binding, stable peptide–MHCI complexes are presented on the cell surface. In TAP-deficient RMA-S cells, MHCI complexes are not stable at 37°C without optimal peptide binding (Townsend et al. 1989; Cerundolo et al. 1990). MHCI molecules are detectable at 26°C with specific antibody in RMA-S cells, which are used to screen H-2 K^b-binding peptides. To measure the binding affinity of peptides to MHC, MHCI heavy chains are purified to associate with β^2-microglobulin and labeled peptides (Quesnel et al. 1996). The alternative approaches are to label heavy chain or β^2-microglobulin for the measurement of peptide-binding affinity. The binding affinity of peptides to MHC and the stability of MHC–peptide complexes have been shown to affect the number of MHC–peptide complexes expressed on the cell surface. The binding affinity to MHC also affects the immunogenicity of peptide epitopes for the induction of CD8 CTL responses (Sette et al. 1994; van der Burg et al. 1996). The actual amino acid residues that are important for the binding of peptide epitopes to MHC with appropriate affinity need further investigation. The minimal number of specific MHC–peptide complexes required for activation of CD8 CTL-mediated cytolysis has been suggested to be from one to a few hundred (Christinck et al. 1991; Kageyama et al. 1995; Sykulev et al. 1996). Several factors affect the antigenicity and immunogenicity of peptide epitopes, including the density and number of specific MHC–peptide complexes; however, the number and density of these complexes required for the induction of CD8 CTL responses and CD8 CTL-mediated lysis of target cells are not clear.

The binding affinity and avidity of MHC–peptide complexes to TCRs

Soluble MHC–peptide complexes can be produced with purified MHC heavy chain, β^2-microglobulin, and peptides, and the binding affinity between TCRs and MHC–peptide complexes has been measured with purified MHC–peptide complexes and TCRs. The binding affinity between TCRs and MHC–peptide complexes is lower than that between antibody and antigen (Matsui et al. 1991). The detection of the number of specific CD8 T cells is difficult using specific monomeric MHC–peptide complexes resulting from low binding affinity. Although the number and density of MHC–peptide complexes required for the activation of CD8 CTL-mediated lysis of target cells are not clear, T-cell recognition of specific MHC–peptide complexes could involve multiple binding of TCRs (Altman et al. 1996; Reich et al. 1997; Rubio-Godoy et al. 2001; Demotte et al. 2002; Dutoit et al. 2002; Knabel et al. 2002; Valmori et al. 2002; Wu et al. 2002). Multimeric MHC–peptide complexes have been developed to measure the frequency of specific CD8 T cells (Altman et al. 1996; Rubio-Godoy et al. 2001; Dutoit et al. 2002; Knabel et al. 2002; Valmori et al. 2002) (see Figure 22.2, p. 425). However, appropriate methodology to measure the avidity of T-cell recognition of specific MHC–peptide complexes on the surface of target cells by TCRs is still not available. In several studies, high-avidity CD8 CTL lines or clones that recognize the target cells pulsed with lower concentration of specific peptides have been suggested to provide better protection in vivo (Alexander-Miller et al. 1996; Herbert et al. 1999; Derby et al. 2001). Many hypotheses have also been proposed to explain the avidity of the recognition of MHC–peptide complexes by CD8 CTL, including the binding affinity of TCR to MHC–peptide complexes, maturation of the functional avidity of T-cell recognition and the number of TCRs required for recognition (Vola and Lanzavecchia 1996; Reich et al. 1997; Holler et al. 2001; Slifka and Whitton 2001). The mechanisms by which avidity plays a role in the recognition of MHC–peptide complexes by CD8 T cells and the mediation of cytolysis and cytokine production remain to be defined.

REFERENCES

Ahlers, J.D., Belyakov, I.M., et al. 2001. Mechanisms of cytokine synergy essential for vaccine protection against viral challenge. *Int Immunol*, **13**, 897–908.

Alegre, M.L., Frauwirth, K.A. and Thompson, C.B. 2001. T-cell regulation by CD28 and CTLA-4. *Nat Rev Immunol*, **1**, 220–8.

Alexander-Miller, M.A., Leggatt, G.R. and Berzofsky, J.A. 1996. Selective expansion of high- or low-avidity cytotoxic T lymphocytes and efficacy for adoptive immunotherapy. *Proc Natl Acad Sci USA*, **93**, 4102–7.

Allen, P.M., Mckean, D.J., et al. 1985. Direct evidence that a class II molecule and a simple globular protein generate multiple determinants. *J Exp Med*, **162**, 1264–74.

Altman, J.D., Moss, P.A., et al. 1996. Phenotypic analysis of antigen-specific T lymphocytes. *Science*, **274**, 94–6.

Atta, M.S., Irving, W.L., et al. 1995. Enhanced expression of MHC class I molecules on cultured human thyroid follicular cells infected with reovirus through induction of type 1 interferons. *Clin Exp Immunol*, **101**, 121–6.

Aung, S. and Graham, B.S. 2000. IL-4 diminishes perforin-mediated and increases Fas ligand-mediated cytotoxicity In vivo. *J Immunol*, **164**, 3487–93.

Aung, S., Tang, Y.W. and Graham, B.S. 1999. Interleukin-4 diminishes CD8(+) respiratory syncytial virus-specific cytotoxic T-lymphocyte activity in vivo. *J Virol*, **73**, 8944–9.

Azuma, M., Ito, D., et al. 1993. B70 antigen is a second ligand for CTLA-4 and CD28. *Nature*, **366**, 76–9.

Barral-Netto, M., Barral, A., et al. 1992. Transforming growth factor-beta in leishmanial infection: a parasite escape mechanism. *Science*, **257**, 545–8.

Barth, R.J. Jr, Mule, J.J., et al. 1991. Interferon gamma and tumor necrosis factor have a role in tumor regressions mediated by murine CD8+ tumor-infiltrating lymphocytes. *J Exp Med*, **173**, 647–58.

Beck, M., Smerdel, S., et al. 1986. Immune response to Edmonston-Zagreb measles virus strain in monovalent and combined MMR vaccine. *Dev Biol Stand*, **65**, 95–100.

Belkaid, Y., Von Stebut, E., et al. 2002. CD8+ T cells are required for primary immunity in C57BL/6 mice following low-dose, intradermal challenge with *Leishmania major*. *J Immunol*, **168**, 3992–4000.

Bembridge, G.P., Lopez, J.A., et al. 1998. Recombinant vaccinia virus coexpressing the F protein of respiratory syncytial virus (RSV) and interleukin-4 (IL-4) does not inhibit the development of RSV-specific memory cytotoxic T lymphocytes, whereas priming is diminished in the presence of high levels of IL-2 or gamma interferon. *J Virol*, **72**, 4080–7.

Bembridge, G.P., Rodriguez, N., et al. 2000. DNA encoding the attachment (G) or fusion (F) protein of respiratory syncytial virus induces protection in the absence of pulmonary inflammation. *J Gen Virol*, **81**, 2519–23.

Bennink, J.R., Yewdell, J.W. and Gerhard, W. 1982. A viral polymerase involved in recognition of influenza virus-infected cells by a cytotoxic T-cell clone. *Nature*, **296**, 75–6.

Berzofsky, J.A., Ahlers, J.D. and Belyakov, I.M. 2001. Strategies for designing and optimizing new generation vaccines. *Nature Immunol Rev*, **1**, 209–19.

Bevilacqua, M.P. 1993. Endothelial-leukocyte adhesion molecules. *Annu Rev Immunol*, **11**, 767.

Binder, G.K. and Griffin, D.E. 2001. Interferon-gamma-mediated site-specific clearance of alphavirus from CNS neurons. *Science*, **293**, 303–6.

Boise, L.H., Gonzalez-Garcia, M., et al. 1993. Bcl-x, a Bcl-2-related gene that functions as a dominant regulator of apoptotic cell death. *Cell*, **74**, 597–608.

Boon, T., Cerottini, J.C., et al. 1994. Tumor antigens recognized by T lymphocytes. *Annu Rev Immunol*, **12**, 337–65.

Borst, P. 1991. Molecular genetics of antigenic variation. *Immunol Today*, **12**, A29–33.

Browne, K.A., Blink, E., et al. 1999. Cytosolic delivery of granzyme B by bacterial toxins: evidence that endosomal disruption, in addition to transmembrane pore formation, is an important function of perforin. *Mol Cell Biol*, **19**, 8604–15.

Buggins, A.G., Milojkovic, D., et al. 2001. Microenvironment produced by acute myeloid leukemia cells prevents T cell activation and proliferation by inhibition of NF-kappaB, c-Myc, and pRb pathways. *J Immunol*, **167**, 6021–30.

Bukreyev, A., Whitehead, S.S., et al. 1999. Interferon gamma expressed by a recombinant respiratory syncytial virus attenuates virus replication in mice without compromising immunogenicity. *Proc Natl Acad Sci USA*, **96**, 2367–72.

Bukreyev, A., Belyakov, I.M., et al. 2001. Granulocyte–macrophage colony-stimulating factor expressed by recombinant respiratory syncytial virus attenuates viral replication and increases the level of pulmonary antigen-presenting cells. *J Virol*, **75**, 12128–40.

Busch, D.H., Pilip, I.M., et al. 1998. Coordinate regulation of complex T cell populations responding to bacterial infection. *Immunity*, **8**, 353–62.

Carbone, F.R. and Gleeson, P.A. 1997. Carbohydrates and antigen recognition by T cells. *Glycobiology*, **7**, 725–30.

Cerundolo, V., Alexander, J., et al. 1990. Presentation of viral antigen controlled by a gene in the major histocompatibility complex. *Nature*, **345**, 449–52.

Chang, J. and Braciale, T.J. 2002. Respiratory syncytial virus infection suppresses lung CD8+ T-cell effector activity and peripheral CD8+ T-cell memory in the respiratory tract. *Nat Med*, **8**, 54–60.

Chanock, R.M., Parrott, R.H., et al. 1992. Serious respiratory tract disease caused by respiratory syncytial virus: prospects for improved therapy and effective immunization. *Pediatrics*, **90**, 1 Pt 2, 137–43.

Charest, H., Sedegah, M., et al. 2000. Recombinant attenuated *Toxoplasma gondii* expressing the *Plasmodium yoelii* circumsporozoite protein provides highly effective priming for CD8+ T cell-dependent protective immunity against malaria. *J Immunol*, **165**, 2084–92.

Chargelegue, D., Obeid, O.E., et al. 1998. A peptide mimic of a protective epitope of respiratory syncytial virus selected from a combinatorial library induces virus-neutralizing antibodies and reduces viral load in vivo. *J Virol*, **72**, 2040–6.

Cho, H.J., Hayashi, T., et al. 2002. IFN-alpha beta promote priming of antigen-specific CD8+ and CD4+ T lymphocytes by immunostimulatory DNA-based vaccines. *J Immunol*, **168**, 4907–13.

Christinck, E.R., Luscher, M.A., et al. 1991. Peptide binding to class I MHC on living cells and quantitation of complexes required for CTL lysis. *Nature*, **352**, 67–70.

Ciernik, I.F., Berzofsky, J.A. and Carbone, D.P. 1996. Induction of cytotoxic T lymphocytes and antitumor immunity with DNA vaccines expressing single T cell epitopes. *J Immunol*, **156**, 2369–75.

Clemens, D.L. and Horwitz, M.A. 1996. The *Mycobacterium tuberculosis* phagosome interacts with early endosomes and is accessible to exogenously administered transferrin. *J Exp Med*, **184**, 1349–55.

Cooper, A.M., Magram, J., et al. 1997. Interleukin 12 (IL-12) is crucial to the development of protective immunity in mice intravenously infected with *Mycobacterium tuberculosis*. *J Exp Med*, **186**, 39–45.

D'Souza, C.D., Cooper, A.M., et al. 1997. An anti-inflammatory role for gamma delta T lymphocytes in acquired immunity to *Mycobacterium tuberculosis*. *J Immunol*, **158**, 1217–21.

Deck, M.B., Sjolin, P., et al. 1999. MHC-restricted, glycopeptide-specific T cells show specificity for both carbohydrate and peptide residues. *J Immunol*, **162**, 4740–4.

Demotte, N., Colau, D., et al. 2002. A reversible functional defect of CD8+ T lymphocytes involving loss of tetramer labeling. *Eur J Immunol*, **32**, 1688–97.

Derby, M.A., Alexander-Miller, M.A., et al. 2001. High-avidity CTL exploit two complementary mechanisms to provide better protection against viral infection than low-avidity CTL. *J Immunol*, **166**, 1690–7.

Diefenbach, A., Jensen, E.R., et al. 2001. Rae1 and H60 ligands of the NKG2D receptor stimulate tumour immunity. *Nature*, **413**, 165–71.

Diehl, L., Van Mierlo, G.J., et al. 2002. In vivo triggering through BB enables Th-independent priming of CTL in the presence of an intact CD28 costimulatory pathway. *J Immunol*, **168**, 3755-62, 4–1.

Dutoit, V., Rubio-Godoy, V., et al. 2002. Functional avidity of tumor antigen-specific CTL recognition directly correlates with the stability of MHC/peptide multimer binding to TCR. *J Immunol*, **168**, 1167–71.

Ehrt, S., Schnappinger, D., et al. 2001. Reprogramming of the macrophage transcriptome in response to interferon-gamma and *Mycobacterium tuberculosis*: signaling roles of nitric oxide synthase-2 and phagocyte oxidase. *J Exp Med*, **194**, 1123–40.

Eller, J.J. 1969. Inactivated myxovirus vaccines, atypical illness, and delayed hypersensitivity. *J Pediatr*, **74**, 664–6.

Enari, M., Sakahira, H., et al. 1998. A caspase-activated DNase that degrades DNA during apoptosis and its inhibitor ICAD. *Nature*, **391**, 43–50.

Erickson, A.L., Kimura, Y., et al. 2001. The outcome of hepatitis C virus infection is predicted by escape mutations in epitopes targeted by cytotoxic T lymphocytes. *Immunity*, **15**, 883–95.

Franke, E.D., Corradin, G. and Hoffman, S.L. 1997. Induction of protective CTL responses against the *Plasmodium yoelii* circumsporozoite protein by immunization with peptides. *J Immunol*, **159**, 3424–33.

Freeman, G.J., Gribben, J.G., et al. 1993. Cloning of B7-2: a CTLA-4 counter-receptor that costimulates human T cell proliferation. *Science*, **262**, 909–11.

Fulginiti, V.A., Eller, J.J., et al. 1969. Respiratory virus immunization. I. A field trial of two inactivated respiratory virus vaccines; an aqueous trivalent parainfluenza virus vaccine and an alum-precipitated respiratory syncytial virus vaccine. *Am J Epidemiol*, **89**, 435–48.

Fuller, D.H., Rajakumar, P.A., et al. 2002. Induction of mucosal protection against primary, heterologous simian immunodeficiency virus by a DNA vaccine. *J Virol*, **76**, 3309-17.

Galibert, L., Maliszewski, C.R. and Vandenabeele, S. 2001. Plasmacytoid monocytes/T cells: a dendritic cell lineage? *Semin Immunol*, **13**, 283–9.

Galli-Stampino, L., Meinjohanns, E., et al. 1997. T-cell recognition of tumor-associated carbohydrates: the nature of the glycan moiety plays a decisive role in determining glycopeptide immunogenicity. *Cancer Res*, **57**, 3214–22.

Gao, X.M., Zheng, B., et al. 1991. Priming of influenza virus-specific cytotoxic T lymphocytes in vivo by short synthetic peptides. *J Immunol*, **147**, 3268–73.

Gao, L., Bellantuona, I., et al. 2000. Selective elimination of leukemic CD34(+) progenitor cells by cytotoxic T lymphocytes specific for WT1. *Blood*, **95**, 2198–203.

Gately, M.K., Warrier, R.R., et al. 1994. Administration of recombinant IL-12 to normal mice enhances cytolytic lymphocyte activity and induces production of IFN-gamma in vivo. *Int Immunol*, **6**, 157–67.

Gellin, B.G. and Broome, C.V. 1989. Listeriosis. *JAMA*, **261**, 1313–20.

Gerrard, T.L., Siegel, J.P., et al. 1987. Differential effects of interferon-alpha and interferon-gamma on interleukin 1 secretion by monocytes. *J Immunol*, **138**, 2535–40.

Gherardi, M.M., Ramirez, J.C., et al. 1999. IL-12 delivery from recombinant vaccinia virus attenuates the vector and enhances the cellular immune response against HIV-1 Env in a dose-dependent manner. *J Immunol*, **162**, 6724–33.

Gierynska, M., Kumaraguru, U., et al. 2002. Induction of CD8 T-cell-specific systemic and mucosal immunity against herpes simplex virus with CpG-peptide complexes. *J Virol*, **76**, 6568–76.

Gooding, L.R. and O'Connell, K.A. 1983. Recognition by cytotoxic T lymphocytes of cells expressing fragments of the SV40 tumor antigen. *J Immunol*, **131**, 2580–6.

Goulder, P.J., Phillips, R.E., et al. 1997. Late escape from an immunodominant cytotoxic T-lymphocyte response associated with progression to AIDS. *Nat Med*, **3**, 212–17.

Guidotti, L.G. and Chisari, F.V. 2001. Noncytolytic control of viral infections by the innate and adaptive immune response. *Annu Rev Immunol*, **19**, 65–91.

Hall, B.F. and Joiner, K.A. 1991. Strategies of obligate intracellular parasites for evading host defences. *Immunol Today*, **12**, A22–27.

Haller, O., Frese, M. and Kochs, G. 1998. Mx proteins: mediators of innate resistance to RNA viruses. *Rev Sci Technol*, **17**, 220–30.

Harrington, L.E., Most Rv, R., et al. 2002. Recombinant vaccinia virus-induced T-cell immunity: quantitation of the response to the virus vector and the foreign epitope. *J Virol*, **76**, 3329–37.

Harty, J.T., Schreiber, R.D. and Bevan, M.J. 1992. CD8 T cells can protect against an intracellular bacterium in an interferon gamma-independent fashion. *Proc Natl Acad Sci USA*, **89**, 11612–16.

Haurum, J.S., Hoier, I.B., et al. 1999. Presentation of cytosolic glycosylated peptides by human class I major histocompatibility complex molecules in vivo. *J Exp Med*, **190**, 145–50.

Herbert, J., Zeh III, H.J., et al. 1999. High avidity CTLs for two self-antigens demonstrate superior in vitro and in vivo antitumor efficacy. *J Immunol*, **162**, 989–94.

Hill, A., Jugovic, P., et al. 1995. Herpes simplex virus turns off the TAP to evade host immunity. *Nature*, **375**, 411–15.

Hiranuma, K., Tamaki, S., et al. 1999. Helper T cell determinant peptide contributes to induction of cellular immune responses by peptide vaccines against hepatitis C virus. *J Gen Virol*, **80**, 187–93.

Hoffman, S.L., Isenbarger, D., et al. 1989. Sporozoite vaccine induces genetically restricted T cell elimination of malaria from hepatocytes. *Science*, **244**, 1078–81.

Holler, P.D., Lim, A.R., et al. 2001. CD8(-) T cell transfectants that express a high affinity T cell receptor exhibit enhanced peptide-dependent activation. *J Exp Med*, **194**, 1043–52.

Hsu, S.C., Shaw, D.M. and Steward, M.W. 1995. The induction of respiratory syncytial virus-specific cytotoxic T-cell responses following immunization with a synthetic peptide containing a fusion peptide linked to a cytotoxic T lymphocyte epitope. *Immunology*, **85**, 347–50.

Hsu, S.C., Obeid, O.E., et al. 1998. Protective cytotoxic T lymphocyte responses against paramyxoviruses induced by epitope-based DNA vaccines: involvement of IFN-gamma. *Int Immunol*, **10**, 1441–7.

Hsu, S.C., Chargelegue, D., et al. 1999. Synergistic effect of immunization with a peptide cocktail inducing antibody, helper and cytotoxic T-cell responses on protection against respiratory syncytial virus. *J Gen Virol*, **80**, 1401–5.

Ibrahim, E.C. and Guerra, N. 2001. Tumor-specific up-regulation of the nonclassical class I HLA-G antigen expression in renal carcinoma. *Cancer Res*, **61**, 6838–45.

Issekutz, T.B. 1990. Effects of six different cytokines on lymphocyte adhesion to microvascular endothelium and in vivo lymphocyte migration in rat. *J immunol*, **144**, 2140.

Issekutz, T.B. 1992. Lymphocyte homing to sites of inflammation. *Curr Opin Immunol*, **4**, 287.

Jans, D.A., Jans, P., et al. 1996. Nuclear transport of granzyme B (Fragmentin-2). *J Biol Chem*, **271**, 30781–9.

Jones, C., Crane, D.T., et al. 1996. Physicochemical studies of the structure and stability of polysaccharide-protein conjugate vaccines. *Dev Biol Stand*, **87**, 143–51.

Kageyama, S., Tsomides, T.J., et al. 1995. Variations in the number of peptide-MHC class I complexes required to activate cytotoxic T cell responses. *J Immunol*, **154**, 567–76.

Kahn, J.S., Schnell, M.J., et al. 1999. Recombinant vesicular stomatitis virus expressing respiratory syncytial virus (RSV) glycoproteins: RSV fusion protein can mediate infection and cell fusion. *Virology*, **254**, 81–91.

Kapikian, A.Z., Mitchell, R.H., et al. 1969. An epidemiologic study of altered clinical reactivity to respiratory syncytial (RS) virus infection in children previously vaccinated with an inactivated RS virus vaccine. *Am J Epidemiol*, **89**, 405–21.

Keskinen, P., Ronni, T., et al. 1997. Regulation of HLA class I and II expression by interferons and influenza A virus in human peripheral blood mononuclear cells. *Immunology*, **91**, 421–9.

Khan, I.A., Ely, K.H. and Kasper, L.H. 1994. Antigen-specific CD8+ T cell clone protects against acute Toxoplasma gondii infection in mice. *J Immunol*, **154**, 1856–60.

Khattar, S.K., Yunus, A.S., et al. 2001. Deletion and substitution analysis defines regions and residues within the phosphoprotein of bovine respiratory syncytial virus that affect transcription, RNA replication, and interaction with the nucleoprotein. *Virology*, **285**, 253–69.

Kim, H.W., Canchola, J.G., et al. 1969. Respiratory syncytial virus disease in infants despite prior administration of antigenic inactivated vaccine. *Am J Epidemiol*, **89**, 422–34.

Klavinskis, L.S., Geckeler, R. and Oldstone, M.B.A. 1989. Cytotoxic T lymphocyte control of acute lymphocytic choriomeningitis virus infection: interferon gamma, but not tumor necrosis factor alpha, displays antiviral activity in vivo. *J Gen Virol*, **70**, 3317–25.

Knabel, M., Franz, T.J., et al. 2002. Reversible MHC multimer staining for functional isolation of T-cell populations and effective adoptive transfer. *Nat Med*, **8**, 631–7.

Ladel, C.H., Blum, C., et al. 1995. Protective role of gamma/delta T cells and alpha/beta T cells in tuberculosis. *Eur J Immunol*, **25**, 2877–81.

Lauvau, G., Vijh, S., et al. 2001. Priming of memory but not effector CD8 T cells by a killed bacterial vaccine. *Science*, **294**, 1735–9.

Leifert, J.A., Lindencrona, J.A., et al. 2001. Enhancing T cell activation and antiviral protection by introducing the HIV-1 protein transduction domain into a DNA vaccine. *Hum Gene Ther*, **12**, 1881–92.

Lenschow, D.J., Walunas, T.L. and Bluestone, J.A. 1996. CD28/B7 system of T cell costimulation. *Annu Rev Immunol*, **14**, 233–58.

Li, H., Haviv, Y.S., et al. 2001a. Human immunodeficiency virus type 1-mediated syncytium formation is compatible with adenovirus replication and facilitates efficient dispersion of viral gene products and de novo-synthesized virus particles. *Hum Gene Ther*, **12**, 2155–65.

Li, M., Davey, G.M., et al. 2001b. Cell-associated ovalbumin is cross-presented much more efficiently than soluble ovalbumin in vivo. *J Immunol*, **166**, 6099–103.

Li, X., Sambhara, S., et al. 1998. Protection against respiratory syncytial virus infection by DNA immunization. *J Exp Med*, **18**, 681–8.

Lingappa, J.R., Rosenstein, N., et al. 2001. Surveillance for meningococcal disease and strategies for use of conjugate meningococcal vaccines in the United States. *Vaccine*, **19**, 4566–75.

Lowrie, D.B., Silva, C.L., et al. 1997. Protection against tuberculosis by a plasmid DNA vaccine. *Vaccine*, **15**, 834–8.

Luft, T., Luetjens, P., et al. 2002. IFN-alpha enhances CD40 ligand-mediated activation of immature monocyte-derived dendritic cells. *Int Immunol*, **14**, 367–80.

McMichael, A.J. and Phillips, R.E. 1997. Escape of human immunodeficiency virus from immune control. *Annu Rev Immunol*, **15**, 271–96.

McMichael, A.J. and Rowland-Jones, S.L. 2001. Cellular immune responses to HIV. *Nature*, **410**, 980–7.

Mahr, J.A. and Gooding, L.R. 1999. Immune evasion by adenoviruses. *Immunol Rev*, **168**, 121–30.

Manz, M.G., Traver, D., et al. 2001. Dendritic cell development from common myeloid progenitors. *Ann NY Acad Sci*, **938**, 167–73.

Marincola, F.M., Jaffee, E.M., et al. 2000. Escape of human solid tumors from T-cell recognition: molecular mechanisms and functional significance. *Adv Immunol*, **74**, 181–273.

Markell, E.K. and Voge, M. 1981. *Medical parasitology*. Philadelphia: Saunders.

Matis, L.A., Shu, S., et al. 1986. Adoptive immunotherapy of a syngeneic murine leukemia with a tumor-specific cytotoxic T cell clone and recombinant human interleukin 2: correlation with clonal IL 2 receptor expression. *J Immunol*, **136**, 3496–501.

Matsui, K., Boniface, J.J., et al. 1991. Low affinity interaction of peptide-MHC complexes with T cell receptors. *Science*, **254**, 1788–91.

Medema, J.P., De Jong, J., et al. 2001. Blockade of the granzyme B/perforin pathway through overexpression of the serine protease inhibitor PI-9/SPI-6 constitutes a mechanism for immune escape by tumors. *Proc Natl Acad Sci USA*, **98**, 11515–20.

Mehrotra, P.T., Grant, A.J. and Siegel, J.P. 1995. Synergistic effects of IL-7 and IL-12 on human T cell activation. *J Immunol*, **154**, 5093–102.

Montoya, M., Schiavoni, G., et al. 2002. Type I interferons produced by dendritic cells promote their phenotypic and functional activation. *Blood*, **99**, 3263–71.

Moore, M.W., Carbone, F.R. and Bevan, M.J. 1988. Introduction of soluble protein into class 1 pathway of antigen processing and presentation. *Cell*, **54**, 777–85.

Muller, C. and Tschopp, J. 1994. Resistance of CTL to perforin-mediated lysis. *J Immunol*, **153**, 2470–8.

Nakajima, C., Uekusa, Y., et al. 2001. A role of interferon-gamma (IFN-gamma) in tumor immunity: T cells with the capacity to reject tumor cells are generated but fail to migrate to tumor sites in IFN-gamma-deficient mice. *Cancer Res*, **61**, 3399–405.

Nass, P.H., Elkins, K.L. and Weir, J.P. 2001. Protective immunity against herpes simplex virus generated by DNA vaccination compared to natural infection. *Vaccine*, **19**, 1538–46.

Nielsen, H.V., Lauemoller, S.L., et al. 1991. Human and murine cytotoxic T lymphocyte serine proteases: subsite mapping with peptide thioester substrates and inhibition of enzyme activity and cytolysis by isocoumarins. *Biochemistry*, **30**, 2217–27.

Nielsen, H.V., Lauemoller, S.L., et al. 1999. Complete protection against lethal *Toxoplasma gondii* infection in mice immunized with a plasmid encoding the SAG1 gene. *Infect Immun*, **67**, 6358–63.

Odake, S. and Kam, C.M. 1991. Human and murine cytotoxic T-lymphocyte serine proteases: subsite mapping with peptide thioester substrates and inhibition of enzyme activity and cytolysis by isocoumarins. *Biochemistry*, **30**, 2217–27.

Ohminami, H., Yasukawa, M. and Fujita, S. 2000. HLA class I-restricted lysis of leukemia cells by a CD8(+) cytotoxic T-lymphocyte clone specific for WT1 peptide. *Blood*, **95**, 286–93.

Oka, Y., Udaka, K., et al. 2000. Cancer immunotherapy targeting Wilms' tumor gene WT1 product. *J Immunol*, **164**, 1873–80.

Openshaw, P.J. 2002. Potential therapeutic implications of new insights into respiratory syncytial virus disease. *Respir Res*, **3**, suppl 1, S15–20.

Openshaw, P.J., Clarke, S.L. and Record, F.M. 1992. Pulmonary eosinophilic responses to respiratory syncytial virus infection in mice sensitized to the major surface glycoprotein G. *Int Immunol*, **4**, 493–500.

Openshaw, P.J., Culley, F.J. and Olszewska, W. 2001. Immunopathogenesis of vaccine-enhanced RSV disease. *Vaccine*, **20**, suppl 1, S27–31.

Padovan, E., Spagnoli, G.C., et al. 2002. IFN-alpha2a induces IP-10/CXCL10 and MIG/CXCL9 production in monocyte-derived dendritic cells and enhances their capacity to attract and stimulate CD8+ effector T cells. *J Leukoc Biol*, **71**, 669–76.

Palmer, K.J., Harries, M., et al. 2000. Interferon-alpha (IFN-alpha) stimulates anti-melanoma cytotoxic T lymphocyte (CTL) generation in mixed lymphocyte tumour cultures (MLTC). *Clin Exp Immunol*, **119**, 412–18.

Pamer, E. and Cresswell, P. 1998. Mechanisms of MHC class 1-restricted antigen processing. *Annu Rev Immunol*, **16**, 323–58.

Patterson, C.E., Lawrence, D.M., et al. 2002. Immune-mediated protection from measles virus-induced central nervous system disease is noncytolytic and gamma interferon dependent. *J Virol*, **76**, 4497–506.

Patterson, J.B., Thomis, D.C., et al. 1995. Mechanism of interferon action: double-strand RNA-specific adenosine deaminase from human cells is inducible by alpha and gamma interferons. *Virology*, **210**, 508–11.

Peebles, R.S. jr, Sheller, J.R., et al. 2000. Respiratory syncytial virus (RSV)-induced airway hyperresponsiveness in allergically sensitized mice is inhibited by live RSV and exacerbated by formalin-inactivated RSV. *J Infect Dis*, **182**, 671–7.

Pereira, D.S., Rosenthal, K.L. and Graham, F.L. 1995. Identification of adenovirus E1A regions which affect MHC class I expression and susceptibility to cytotoxic T lymphocytes. *Virology*, **211**, 268–77.

Phillips, R.E., Rowland-Jones, S., et al. 1991. Human immunodeficiency virus genetic variation that can escape cytotoxic T cell recognition. *Nature*, **354**, 453–9.

Podack, E.R., Young, J.D. and Cohn, Z.A. 1985. Isolation and biochemical and functional characterization of perforin from cytolytic T cell granules. *Proc Natl Acad Sci USA*, **82**, 8629–33.

Porgador, A. and Gilboa, E. 1995. Bone marrow-generated dendritic cells pulsed with a class I-restricted peptide are potent inducers of cytotoxic T lymphocytes. *J Exp Med*, **182**, 255–60.

Price, G.E., Ou, R., et al. 2000. Viral escape by selection of cytotoxic T cell-resistant variants in influenza A virus pneumonia. *J Exp Med*, **191**, 1853–67.

Quesnel, A., Hsu, S.C., et al. 1996. Efficient binding to the MHC class I K(d) molecule of synthetic peptides in which the anchoring position 2 does not fit the consensus motif. *FEBS Lett*, **387**, 42–6.

Rausch, D.M., Lifson, J.D., et al. 1992. CD4(81-92)-based peptide derivatives. Structural requirements for blockade of HIV infection, blockade of HIV-induced syncytium formation, and virostatic activity in vitro. *Biochem Pharmacol*, **43**, 1785–96.

Reich, Z., Boniface, J.J., et al. 1997. Ligand-specific oligomerization of T-cell receptor molecules. *Nature*, **387**, 617–20.

Reusch, U., Muranyi, W., et al. 1999. A cytomegalovirus glycoprotein reroutes MHC Class 1 complexes to lysosome for degradation. *EMBO J*, **18**, 1081–91.

Rock, K.L. and Goldberg, A.L. 1999. Degradation of cell proteins and generation of MHC class 1-presented peptides. *Annu Rev Immunol*, **17**, 739–79.

Rock, K.L., Gramm, C., et al. 1994. Inhibitors of the proteasome block the degradation of most cell proteins and the generation of peptides presented by MHC class 1 molecules. *Cell*, **78**, 761–71.

Romero, P., Maryanski, J.L., et al. 1989. Cloned cytotoxic T cells recognize an epitope in the circumsporozoite protein and protect against malaria. *Nature*, **341**, 323–6.

Rubio-Godoy, V., Dutoit, V., et al. 2001. Discrepancy between ELISPOT IFN-gamma secretion and binding of A2/peptide multimers to TCR reveals interclonal dissociation of CTL effector function from TCR-peptide/MHC complexes half-life. *Proc Natl Acad Sci USA*, **98**, 10302–7.

Russell, J.H. and Ley, T.J. 2002. Lymphocyte-mediated cytotoxicity. *Annu Rev Immunol*, **20**, 323–70.

Sadovnikova, E. and Stauss, H.J. 1996. Peptide-specific cytotoxic T lymphocytes restricted by nonself major histocompatibility complex class I molecules: reagents for tumor immunotherapy. *Proc Natl Acad Sci USA*, **93**, 13114–18.

Sarin, A., Haddad, E. and Henkart, P.A. 1998. Caspase dependence of target cell damage induced by cytotoxic lymphocytes. *J Immunol*, **161**, 2810–16.

Sato, M., Chamoto, K., et al. 2001. Th1 cytokine-conditioned bone marrow-derived dendritic cells can bypass the requirement for Th functions during the generation of CD8+ CTL. *J Immunol*, **167**, 3687–91.

Scheller, L.F., Green, S.J. and Azad, A.F. 1997. Inhibition of nitric oxide interrupts the accumulation of CD8+ T cells surrounding *Plasmodium berghei*-infected hepatocytes. *Infect Immun*, **65**, 3882–8.

Schirmbeck, R., Melberk, K., et al. 1994. Selective stimulation of murine cytotoxic T cell and antibody responses by particulate or monomeric hepatitis B virus surface (S) antigen. *Eur J Immunol*, **24**, 1088–96.

Schirmbeck, R., Bohm, W., et al. 1995. Processing of exogenous heat-aggregated (denatured) and particulate (native) hepatitis B surface antigen for class I-restricted epitope presentation. *J Immunol*, **155**, 4676–84.

Schulz, M., Zinkernagel, R.M. and Hengartner, H. 1991. Peptide-induced antiviral protection by cytotoxic T cells. *Proc Natl Acad Sci USA*, **88**, 991–3.

Schwartz, R.H. 1992. Costimulation of T lymphocytes: the role of CD28, CTLA-4 and B7/BB1 in interleukin-2 production and immunotherapy. *Cell*, **71**, 1065–8.

Seguin, M.C., Klotz, F.W., et al. 1994. Induction of nitric oxide synthase protects against malaria in mice exposed to irradiated *Plasmodium berghei* infected mosquitoes: involvement of interferon gamma and CD8+ T cells. *J Exp Med*, **180**, 353–8.

Sette, A., Vitiello, A., et al. 1994. The relationship between class I binding affinity and immunogenicity of potential cytotoxic T cell epitopes. *J Immunol*, **153**, 5586–92.

Sheikh, N.A., Rajananthanan, P., et al. 1999. Generation of antigen specific CD8+ cytotoxic T cells following immunization with soluble protein formulated with novel glycoside adjuvants. *Vaccine*, **17**, 2974–82.

Shi, L., Kam, C.M., et al. 1992. Purification of three cytotoxic lymphocyte granule serine proteases that induce apoptosis through distinct substrate and target cell interactions. *J Exp Med*, **176**, 1521–9.

Shirai, M., Pendleton, C.D., et al. 1994. Helper-cytotoxic T lymphocyte (CTL) determinant linkage required for priming of anti-HIV CD8+ CTL in vivo with peptide vaccine constructs. *J Immunol*, **152**, 549–56.

Silverman, R.H. 1994. Fascination with 2-5 A-dependent RNase: a unique enzyme that functions in interferon action. *J Interferon Res*, **14**, 101–4.

Slifka, M.K. and Whitton, J.L. 2001. Functional avidity maturation of CD8(+) T cells without selection of higher affinity TCR. *Nat Immunol*, **2**, 711–17.

Speidel, K., Osen, W., et al. 1997. Priming of cytotoxic T lymphocyte by five heat-aggregated antigens in vivo: conditions, efficiency, and relation to antibody responses. *Eur J Immunol*, **27**, 2391–9.

Speir, J.A., Abdel-Motal, U.M., et al. 1999. Crystal structure of an MHC class I presented glycopeptide that generates carbohydrate-specific CTL. *Immunity*, **10**, 51–61.

Spickett, G., Beattie, R.E., et al. 1989. Quantitation of HIV-1 activity in tissue culture supernatants: effects of culture condition on syncytial assays and virus production. *J Virol Methods*, **24**, 67–76.

Staats, H.F., Bradney, C.P., et al. 2001. Cytokine requirements for induction of systemic and mucosal CTL after nasal immunization. *J Immunol*, **167**, 5386–94.

Steiman, R.M. 1991. The dendritic cell system and its role in immunogenicity. *Annu Rev Immunol*, **9**, 271–96.

Stittelaar, K.J., de Swart, R.L., et al. 2002. Enteric administration of a live attenuated measles vaccine does not induce protective immunity in a macaque model. *Vaccine*, **20**, 2906–12.

Stober, D., Trobonjaca, Z., et al. 2002. Dendritic cells pulsed with exogenous hepatitis B surface antigen particles efficiently present epitopes to MHC class I-restricted cytotoxic T cells. *Eur J Immunol*, **32**, 1099–108.

Sturgill-Koszycki, S., Schaible, U.E. and Russell, D.G. 1996. *Mycobacterium*-containing phagosomes are accessible to early endosomes and reflect a transitional state in normal phagosome biogenesis. *EMBO J*, **15**, 6960–8.

Sun, J., Whisstock, J.C., et al. 2001. Importance of the P4(residue in human granzyme B inhibitors and substrates revealed by scanning mutagenesis of the proteinase inhibitor 9 reactive center loop. *J Biol Chem*, **276**, 15177–84.

Sutton, V.R., Davis, J.E., et al. 2000. Initiation of apoptosis by granzyme B requires direct cleavage of Bid, but not direct granzyme B-mediated caspase activation. *J Exp Med*, **192**, 1403–13.

Sykulev, Y., Joo, M., et al. 1996. Evidence that a single peptide-MHC complex on a target cell can elicit a cytolytic T cell response. *Immunity*, **4**, 565–71.

Terenzi, F., de Veer, M.J., et al. 1999. The antiviral enzymes PKR and Rnase L suppress gene expression from viral and non-viral based vectors. *Nucleic Acid Res*, **27**, 4369–75.

Tewari, M., Telford, W.G., et al. 1995. CrmA, a poxvirus-encoded serpin, inhibits cytotoxic T-lymphocyte-mediated apoptosis. *J Biol Chem*, **270**, 22705–8.

Tishon, A., Lewiski, H., et al. 1995. An essential role for type 1 interferon-gamma in terminating persistent viral infection. *Virology*, **212**, 244–50.

Toso, J.F., Chen, C.H., et al. 1995. Oligoclonal CD8 lymphocytes from persons with asymptomatic human immunodeficiency virus (HIV) type 1 infection inhibit HIV-1 replication. *J Infect Dis*, **172**, 964–73.

Townsend, A. and Bodmer, H. 1989. Antigen recognition by class I-restricted lymphocytes. *Annu Rev Immunol*, **7**, 601.

Townsend, A.R., Bastin, J., et al. 1986. Cytotoxic T lymphocytes recognize influenza haemagglutinin that lack a signal sequence. *Nature*, **324**, 575–7.

Townsend, A., Ohlen, C., et al. 1989. A mutant cell in which association of class I heavy and light chains is induced by viral peptides. *Cold Spring Harb Symp Quant Biol*, **54**, 299–308.

Tschopp, J., Schafer, S., et al. 1989. Phosphorylcholine acts as a Ca^{2+} dependent receptor molecule for lymphocyte perforin. *Nature*, **337**, 272–4.

Tuttle, T.M., McCrady, C.W., et al. 1993. gamma-Interferon plays a key role in T-cell-induced tumor regression. *Cancer Res*, **53**, 833–9.

Urban, B.C., Ferguson, D.J., et al. 1999. Plasmodium falciparum-infected erythrocytes modulate the maturation of dendritic cells. *Nature*, **400**, 73–7.

Valmori, D., Dutoit, V., et al. 2002. Vaccination with a Melan-A peptide selects an oligoclonal T cell population with increased functional avidity and tumor reactivity. *J Immunol*, **168**, 4231–40.

van der Burg, S.H., Visseren, M.J., et al. 1996. Immunogenicity of peptides bound to MHC class I molecules depends on the MHC-peptide complex stability. *J Immunol*, **156**, 3308–14.

Vola, A. and Lanzavecchia, A. 1996. T cell activation determined by T cell receptor number and tunable thresholds. *Science*, **273**, 104–6.

Von Koenig, C.H., Finger, H. and Hof, H. 1982. Failure of killed *Listeria monocytogenes* vaccine to produce protective immunity. *Nature*, **297**, 233–4.

Wagner, L., Yang, O.O., et al. 1998. Beta-chemokines are released from HIV-1-specific cytolytic T-cell granules complexed to proteoglycans. *Nature*, **391**, 908–11.

Wang, B., Norbury, C.C., et al. 2001. Multiple paths for activation of naive CD8+ T cells: CD4-independent help. *J Immunol*, **167**, 1283–9.

Wee, E.G., Patel, S., et al. 2002. A DNA/MVA-based candidate human immunodeficiency virus vaccine for Kenya induces multi-specific T cell responses in rhesus macaques. *J Gen Virol*, **83**, 75–80.

Wegmann, A., Gluck, R., et al. 1986. Comparative study and evaluation of further attenuated, live measles vaccines alone and in combination with mumps and rubella vaccines. *Dev Biol Stand*, **65**, 69–74.

Wertz, G.W. and Sullender, M.W. 1992. Approaches to immunization against respiratory syncytial virus. In: Eltis, R.W. (ed.), *Vaccines: new approaches to immunological problems*. Boston, MA: Butterworth-Heinemann, 151–76.

Wu, L.C., Tuot, D.S., et al. 2002. Two-step binding mechanism for T-cell receptor recognition of peptide MHC. *Nature*, **418**, 552–6.

Yamashita, Y., Shimokata, K., et al. 1993. Down-regulation of the surface expression of class I MHC antigens by human cytomegalovirus. *Virology*, **193**, 727–36.

Yang, O.O. and Walker, B.D. 1997. CD8+ cells in human immunodeficiency virus type I pathogenesis: cytolytic and noncytolytic inhibition of viral replication. *Adv Immunol*, **66**, 273–311.

Yang, X., Stennicke, H.R., et al. 1998. Granzyme B mimics apical caspases. *J Biol Chem*, **273**, 278–83.

Yewdell, J.W., Bennink, J.R. and Hosaka, Y. 1988. Cells process exogenous proteins for recognition by cytotoxic T lymphocytes. *Science*, **239**, 637–40.

York, I.A. and Rock, K.L. 1996. Antigen processing and presentation by the class 1 major histocompatibility complexes. *Annu Rev Immunol*, **14**, 369–96.

Zeh III, H.J., Perry-Lalley, D., et al. 1999. High avidity CTLs for two self-antigens demonstrate superior in vitro and in vivo antitumor efficacy. *J Immunol*, **162**, 989–94.

Zhu, X., Venkataprasad, N., et al. 1997. Vaccination with recombinant vaccinia viruses protects mice against *Mycobacterium tuberculosis* infection. *Immunology*, **92**, 6–9.

Zuckerman, A.J. 1986. Novel hepatitis B vaccines. *J Infect*, **13**, suppl A, 61–71.

23

Unconventional T cells

ADRIAN HAYDAY AND CARRIE STEELE

DEFINING UNCONVENTIONAL T CELLS

It is now evident that both B lymphocytes and T lymphocytes need to be subdivided into distinct classes. For B cells, these classes comprise B1 cells commonly enriched in the peritoneum, and circulating B2 cells. As the distinct features of B1 cells have only become apparent in the past 25 years, as their functions remain enigmatic, and as B2 cells fully satisfy conventional assays for B-lymphocyte activity, B2 cells are most commonly regarded as 'conventional B cells', with B1 cells being viewed as 'unconventional'. This view of B1 cells as peripheral to core B-cell function is encouraged by their apparently varied representation in different species, and their presence in humans is still uncertain. Likewise, it is now common to view T cells as comprising 'conventional', circulating $\alpha\beta$ T cells, defined by expression of the heterodimeric $\alpha\beta$ T-cell receptor (TCR), and 'unconventional T cells' which, like B1 cells, are of enigmatic function and highly varied in their representation in different species. Nevertheless, any view of immunology that discounts unconventional T cells from playing critical roles in host defense is ill-judged, ignoring their evolutionary conservation over at least 400 million years, and the emerging evidence that they have potent immunoprotective and immunoregulatory roles that are germane to infectious disease, tumor surveillance, and autoimmunity.

The contrast of unconventional T cells with conventional T cells inevitably requires clear operational criteria for conventional T-cell activity. These are: (1) recognition of peptide antigens presented by highly polymorphic major histocompatibility complex (MHC) proteins; (2) negative selection during development by high-affinity engagement of self-antigens; (3) antigen priming in the secondary lymphoid tissues (lymph nodes and spleen) by 'professional' antigen-presenting cells (APC); and (4) commitment of a subset of the primed T-cell repertoire to the long-term memory pool that composes cellular immunity. Collectively, unconventional T cells appear to fail most (perhaps all) of these four criteria. Thus, (1) they are not restricted by conventional, highly polymorphic MHC; (2) it is not certain that they are negatively selected by engagement of autoantigens during development, but rather may be positively selected; (3) their patterns of systemic circulation are commonly (perhaps invariably) distinct, with greater constitutive association with tissues rather than with lymph nodes, spleen, and bone marrow; and (4) the evidence that they contribute to long-term memory is equivocal, with the greater mass of data implying that their primary contribution is to the early phases of immune responses, preceding the activation of conventional T cells.

By these operational criteria, the activities of unconventional T cells would seem complementary to those of conventional T cells. Such complementarity could provide a powerful argument for the cells' evolutionary conservation. At the same time it is unwise to view unconventional and conventional T cells as operating entirely independently in their contributions to immune responses. Growing evidence indicates that unconventional T cells have a potent capacity to regulate conventional T-cell responses, and are thus important factors to consider in the understanding and treatment of immunopathologies such as inflammation, allergy, and antigen-specific autoimmunity.

SUBTYPES OF UNCONVENTIONAL T CELLS: $\gamma\delta$ T CELLS

Perhaps the most galvanizing development in the recognition of T-cell heterogeneity was the discovery in 1984 of a TCR gene cDNA (complementary DNA), TCR γ, that encoded neither the TCR α chain nor the TCR β chain (Saito et al. 1984). Within 3 years, the existence of TCR$\gamma\delta^+$ cells was firmly established. Antigen recognition by TCR$\gamma\delta$ is critically different from that of conventional $\alpha\beta$ T cells. In particular, mice that are deficient in polymorphic MHC class I and/or II molecules show substantial defects in circulating $\alpha\beta$ T cells, whereas the $\gamma\delta$ cell compartment is largely unaffected (Correa et al. 1992; Bigby et al. 1993). The fact that before 1984 no one had predicted the existence of $\gamma\delta$ cells strongly suggested that conventional assays for T-cell activity – primarily the development of antigen-specific immunity – were fully satisfied by $\alpha\beta$ T cells. In turn, this suggested from the outset that $\gamma\delta$ cells use their unconventional TCR specificities to contribute to immune responses in unconventional ways: much work over the past 15 years has supported this idea. To consider $\gamma\delta$ cells more clearly, one must recognize that the $\gamma\delta$ cell compartment itself is made up of several distinct subcompartments.

TCR$\gamma\delta^+$ dendritic epidermal T cells

Murine dendritic epidermal T cells (DETC) are arguably the prototypical nonconventional T cell, and their study introduces many features of nonconventional T cells more broadly. DETCs are an example of intraepithelial lymphocytes (IEL): rather than circulating, they are constitutively associated with a single tissue, which, in the case of DETCs, is the epidermis. Unlike conventional T cells, which are round cells dominated by their nucleus, DETCs appear in situ as dendritic cells that collectively form an anastomosing network in contact with the majority of basal keratinocytes. Several experiments over the past decade have demonstrated that DETCs can directly engage heat-shocked or malignantly transformed keratinocytes, provoking cytokine release and/or target cell killing (Havran et al. 1991). Thus, DETCs as well as other IELs have been considered to contribute to a 'first line of defense' (Janeway et al. 1988). There is, by contrast, little evidence that DETCs interact with professional APCs, such as Langerhans' cells which prime the conventional T-cell response.

DETC progenitors are the first to colonize the murine fetal thymus (Havran and Allison 1988) and, consistent with their failure to engage conventional class I or class II MHC, they complete development without the acquisition of CD4 and CD8 expression which is a signatory feature of conventional $\alpha\beta$ T-cell development. Seemingly, they leave the thymus after positive selection, but until their TCR ligand is characterized the details of this event will remain opaque. The basis for homing to and residence within the skin has also not been elucidated, but it is likely that different molecules contribute to the two processes. Once the perinatal wave of skin colonization by DETCs has occurred, the thymus loses its capacity to regenerate DETCs (Ikuta et al. 1990). Possibly, stem cells from which DETCs can be replenished exist in some compartment of the skin (e.g. the dermis), but if this is the case, those progenitors, like DETC themselves, are vulnerable to surface ultraviolet irradiation, because such treatment causes long-term DETC ablation (Aberer et al. 1986).

Similar to other thymocytes, developing DETC progenitors utilize recombinase-activating gene (RAG)-mediated somatic DNA recombination to generate a TCR. By the quasi-random and imprecise joining of any one of a large number of variable (V) gene segments with any one of a large number of diversity (D) gene segments, which is in turn joined to any one of a large number of junctional (J) gene segments, RAG-mediated recombination can generate immensely diverse receptor repertoires characteristic of the T- and B-cell compartments (Tonegawa 1983). In curious contrast, DETCs express a monomorphic Vγ5/Vδ1 TCR (Asarnow et al. 1988).

Although its ligand is currently not elucidated, the simplicity of the DETC TCR is consistent with the hypothesis that DETCs recognize a generic self-antigen, induced on infected or transformed epithelial cells by a wide range of cellular insult (Janeway et al. 1988). The basis for this hypothesis is that IELs resident within epithelia will not have the opportunity to sample millions of different antigens presented by APCs in the lymph nodes of infected mice, but must therefore rely on activation by a self-antigen that is expressed selectively on infected or transformed epithelial cells.

The TCR is not the only lymphocyte surface molecule that may be engaged in this fashion. Activated DETCs, along with other cytolytic T cells and natural killer (NK) cells, express an activating receptor, NKG2D, that engages any one of a number of nonconventional MHC class IB gene products, e.g. Rae-1 (mouse and human), H60 (mouse), ULBP (human), and MICA/MICB (human) (Bauer et al. 1999; Cerwenka et al. 2000; Diefenbach et al. 2000; Cosman et al. 2001). These molecules resemble conventional MHC class I proteins in general structural features, but most probably do not present antigenic peptides (Li et al. 1999, 2002). As peptide binding stabilizes conventional class I and II MHC proteins, the stable display of peptide–MHC complexes by an APC signifies its 'immunological visibility' to conventional T cells. By contrast, the immunological visibility of cells expressing peptide-independent MHC-related molecules to NKG2D$^+$ lymphocytes is regulated at least in part by strictly inducible gene expression.

Thus, Rae-1 is expressed primarily in the embryo (Zou et al. 1996), and at negligible levels in normal adult tissue (Cerwenka et al. 2000; Diefenbach et al. 2000), but its expression increases in vivo in skin epithelial cells exposed to transforming chemicals (Girardi et al. 2001). Likewise, the expression of MICA/B is upregulated on heat-shocked or transformed epithelial cells of the human gut (Groh et al. 1996, 1999) where there is an additional population of resident TCR$\gamma\delta^+$ cells (see below). Currently, the cell signaling pathways that tightly regulate the expression of 'stress-inducible' class IB MHC are unknown.

DETCs can also express receptors, notably Ly49E (Van Beneden et al. 2002), that are associated with NK cells, and not commonly expressed by conventional T cells. The engagement of such receptors limits T-cell activation, implying that the immunological visibility of skin epithelial cells also relies on overcoming the engagement of inhibitory receptors, either by reducing or altering the expression of their ligands, or by quantitatively overwhelming the cell via activating receptor engagement.

There has to date been little effective testing of the roles of DETCs in the protection of mouse skin against infection. Nevertheless, the physiological relevance of DETC engagement of transformed keratinocytes was strongly implied by the finding that TCR$\gamma\delta$-deficient mice are substantially more susceptible to multiple, diverse protocols for the induction of squamous cell carcinoma (Girardi et al. 2001). Indeed, the mice are more reproducibly susceptible than are TCR $\alpha\beta$–deficient mice. These studies potentially provide a model for the protective activities of TCR$\gamma\delta^+$ IELs against the development of solid tumors in humans (see below).

Once activated, DETCs, as with many other nonconventional T cells, display a clear potential for cytolytic and T-helper (Th)1-type effector responses that can account for their local protective activities. In addition, DETCs and other IELs express well-characterized chemokines, such as RANTES and lymphotactin (Boismenu et al. 1996), as well as enigmatic molecules such as thymosin β4 (Shires et al. 2001), which have potent anti-inflammatory activities in certain assays. Perhaps consistent with this, DETCs and other IELs have immunoregulatory activity and, on certain genetic backgrounds, DETC deficiency leads to striking pathological inflammatory infiltrates of the skin which are provoked by $\alpha\beta$ T-cell responses to environmental antigens (Girardi et al. 2002). Indeed, on particular genetic backgrounds, the pathognomonic outward appearance of TCR$\gamma\delta^{-/-}$ mice is visible to the naked eye. Although the TCR is apparently involved in immunoregulation by DETCs, the relevant ligand is again unelucidated. Indeed, immunoregulation might occur following direct interaction of DETCs with activated infiltrating lymphoid cells, or as an indirect by-product of TCR-mediated DETC engagement of activated epithelial cells.

Importantly, the phenotypic analysis of TCR$\gamma\delta^{-/-}$ mice informs us that DETCs provide a multifaceted protection of epithelial integrity, ranging from the eradication of dysregulated epithelial cells to the inhibition of tissue disruption by systemic lymphoid cells. A further contribution of DETC activity to the maintenance of epithelial integrity is evident in the reported expression by DETCs of fibroblast growth factors that promote keratinocyte growth (Boismenu and Havran 1994; Jameson et al. 2002). Although this may appear paradoxical given the capacity of DETCs to kill epithelial cells, the data are collectively interpreted to suggest that, after target cell eradication, DETCs subsequently contribute to wound healing.

Clearly, the initial view of DETCs as cells that use a monomorphic TCR to target dysregulated epithelial cells as part of a pseudo-innate immune response is insufficient to accommodate the complexity of DETC functions. Conceivably, despite their expression of a single TCR, DETCs may comprise functionally distinct subsets, capable of cytolysis, immunoregulation, and epithelial cell growth promotion, respectively. This hypothesis is being tested at present.

Although DETCs capably illustrate the impressive functional potential of 'local', tissue-associated T cells, the general relevance of the lessons learned has been questioned, given that DETCs are not obviously conserved in humans. Indeed, some have wondered whether 'DETC functions' are an idiosyncrasy of relatively short-lived mammals, such as rodents, which have large litter sizes, placing less emphasis on the long-term survival of the individual (sometimes cited as the key provision of antigen-specific memory in the conventional adaptive immune system). This is clearly not the case, because DETCs are conserved in cattle, large mammals with long lifespans that are more similar to humans than to mice. Therefore, the probability exists that 'local immune functions' exist in human skin, but are provided by other cell types. Thus, it has been reported that a unique TCR $\gamma\delta^+$ subset resides in the dermis of healthy human skin (Holtmeier et al. 2001), and there are increases in cutaneous $\gamma\delta$ cells in scleroderma, an inflammatory pathology characterized in part by fibrotic wound healing, and possibly promoted by human $\gamma\delta$ cells. Given the potential of DETCs to be activated via the NKG2D receptor, it is also possible that local immune function in human skin is provided by NK cells or myeloid cells that can likewise use the NKG2D pathway to respond to epithelial cell dysregulation and/or activated inflammatory infiltrates. In sum, the study of DETCs emphasizes the need for better understanding of local immune function in cutaneous immune responses in humans.

A second important contribution of DETCs to the study of human immunology is the potential to improve our understanding of other epithelia that also harbor TCR$\gamma\delta^+$ IELs, both in mice and in humans.

TCR$\gamma\delta^+$ IELs in other tissues in mice and humans

In mice, the functional and molecular relatedness of IELs that characterize different epithelia – the skin, reproductive tissue, tongue, intestine, and (reportedly) lung – has yet to be firmly established. Unlike the case of DETCs, direct equivalents of such cells are evident in certain human tissues, e.g. the human small intestine. Given the very large surface area of the human gut (>200 m^2), it is likely that IELs will account numerically for a major fraction of human T cells.

Similar to DETCs, the TCRs of IELs in different tissues show limited diversity. Murine vaginal and tongue-associated IELs express a single predominant Vγ chain (Vγ6) (Lafaille et al. 1989) distinct from that in skin (Vγ5) (Asarnow et al. 1988) and the gut (Vγ7) (Bonneville et al. 1988; Goodman and Lefrancois 1988; Kyes et al. 1989; Takagaki et al. 1989). In the human gut, IELs express Vγ1 (Deusch et al. 1991), by contrast to Vγ2 expressed by most systemic $\gamma\delta$ cells. The intestinal IELs of mice and humans show some junctional diversity and some variation in Vδ usage, but the biological significance of this vis-à-vis antigen recognition is unresolved.

In the mouse, the IELs that populate the different tissues develop in sequential 'waves' in the fetal and neonatal thymus, with those in the skin preceding those in the reproductive tissue, which precede those in the gut (Havran and Allison 1988). Thus, it has been proposed that the association of particular TCRs (especially Vγ genes) with particular tissues reflects the sequential activation of gene segment usage. Whether or not this is true, the same association has quite naturally provoked the concept that each TCR recognizes a tissue-specific 'stress antigen' that would serve as a generic beacon of epithelial distress. The likelihood that each class of $\gamma\delta$ TCR recognizes a clearly distinct entity is high because, by contrast to the usual situation in conventional T cells and B cells, individual Vγ genes share little homology and are very distinct from each other in the complementarity determining regions (CDR) CDR1 and CDR2 which would be predicted to form part of the antigen-binding surfaces (Arden et al. 1995b).

As was the case with DETC, there is scant evidence for a critical immunoprotective role of TCR$\gamma\delta^+$ IELs against pathogens that either enter or reside within epithelia. Indeed, whereas $\alpha\beta$ T-cell-deficient mice showed high susceptibility toward a natural parasitic infection of the intestinal epithelium, the immunoprotective role of $\gamma\delta$ cells was only exposed in mice that also lacked $\alpha\beta$ T cells (Smith and Hayday 2000). Such data have encouraged some scientists to regard TCR$\gamma\delta^+$ cells as inferior to $\alpha\beta$ T cells in their value to the host. However, when infected with a natural parasite of the intestinal epithelium, $\gamma\delta$-cell-deficient mice are not without phenotype: rather, they primarily show a defect in immunoregulation, manifest in aggressive $\alpha\beta$ T-cell-dependent immunopathology (Roberts et al. 1996).

Also paralleling the findings with DETCs, human Vγ1/Vδ1$^+$ IELs isolated from surgical specimens of bowel cancer would kill the cancer cells after engagement of the NKG2D ligand, MICA (Groh et al. 1998). Vγ2/Vδ2$^+$ cells would not do this, provoking the concept that MICA engages TCR$\gamma\delta$ as well as NKG2D (Groh et al. 1998; Wu et al. 2002). A precedent for such ligand promiscuity might be found in the binding of conventional MHC class I simultaneously to TCR$\alpha\beta$ and to CD8, or in the binding of human HLA-C or murine Qa-1 to TCR$\alpha\beta$ and to NK receptors (see below). Indeed, cytolysis by Vδ1$^+$ IELs could be inhibited with anti-MICA and anti-TCR$\gamma\delta$ monoclonal antibodies. To clarify the capacity of the Vγ1/Vδ1 TCRs to bind MICA, a T-cell line that does not express NKG2D was transfected with TCR chains from MICA-responsive $\gamma\delta$ clones or MICA-unresponsive clones (Wu et al. 2002). Cells expressing TCRs derived from responsive clones bound MICA tetramers, whereas those transfected with TCRs derived from unresponsive clones did not. Clearly, if these data are correctly interpreted, it should be possible to demonstrate direct binding of MICA to a soluble Vγ1/Vδ1 TCR by surface plasmon resonance.

The same experimental approach might usefully support the evidence that human T-cell clones expressing collectively Vγ1 paired with Vδ1.4 or Vδ2 bind to CD1c (Spada et al. 2000). CD1 proteins constitute a further subset of nonpolymorphic class IB MHC molecules. There are two groups of CD1 proteins: group 1 includes CD1a, Cd1b, and Cd1c, which collectively are found in humans but not in mice; group 2 includes CD1d which is conserved (Gumperz and Brenner 2001). All CD1 proteins have deep hydrophobic grooves that permit them to present lipid molecules to reactive TCRs (see below).

In sum, TCR$\gamma\delta^+$ IELs in the gut display both protective and immunoregulatory functions. The molecular potential for such actions was readily revealed by the comprehensive cataloguing of genes expressed by murine gut TCR$\gamma\delta^+$ IELs. These analyses undertaken by microchip array and by serial analysis of gene expression (SAGE) have shown that more than 2 percent of IEL mRNA is devoted to the expression of the cytolytic effector molecules, granzymes A and B, and the immunoregulatory chemokine, RANTES (Shires et al. 2001).

Systemic $\gamma\delta$ cells

$\gamma\delta$ cells can be found in the peripheral blood, spleen, and lymph nodes, but again their representation varies greatly from very rare (humans and mice) to more than 50 percent of systemic CD3$^+$ cells (calves). Nevertheless, the low numbers of systemic $\gamma\delta$ cells in humans can increase substantially, particularly during bacterial infections, to more than 40 percent of $CD3^+$ (PBL). Systemic $\gamma\delta$ cells, similar to $TCR\gamma\delta^+$ IELs, use limited Vγ and Vδ pairings, but, as these pairings are dissimilar from those used by $TCR\gamma\delta^+$ IELs, systemic $\gamma\delta$ cells and $TCR\gamma\delta^+$ IELs may recognize distinct classes of antigen. Moreover, in contrast to $TCR\gamma\delta^+$ IELs, systemic $\gamma\delta$ cells often display substantial junctional diversity in their TCRs. Indeed, the junctional diversity of TCR$\gamma\delta$ may be more diverse than either TCR$\alpha\beta$ or Ig.

Additional evidence that systemic $\gamma\delta$ cells may not be limited to the recognition of MHC-like structures is provided by an indepth analysis of TCR structure. The CDR1 and CDR2 regions of γ and δ chains are longer than those of TCRα and -β (Arden et al. 1995a; Clark et al. 1995), and although the CDR3 regions of TCRα and -β chains are limited to 6–12 nucleotides (interpreted as the constraint imposed by binding to the relatively 'flat' peptide/MHC surface), the CDR3 of TCRδ, similar to that of IgH, is extremely varied, (6–22 nucleotides), suggesting no constraining topology of $\gamma\delta$ ligands (Rock et al. 1994). Nevertheless, how such diversity translates into antigen specificity is not yet clear.

The crystal structure of an isolated human Vδ3 chain showed that CDR1 and CDR3 assumed a conformation similar to TCR$\alpha\beta$, whereas CDR2 assumed a conformation more like IgH (Li et al. 1998). More recently, a structure of a complete human Vγ2Vδ2 TCR confirmed that CDR2 of Vδ2 more closely resembled IgH than TCR$\alpha\beta$, although the significance of this with respect to antigen binding is also unclear (Allison et al. 2001).

Consistent with their failure to recognize antigen restricted by polymorphic MHC class I or II, systemic $\gamma\delta$ cells in mice and humans usually express neither CD4 nor CD8, and derive directly from $CD4^-CD8^-$ ('double-negative') thymocytes. In humans, the bulk of systemic $\gamma\delta$ cells arise from fetal thymic progenitors.

In the mouse, about 0.5 percent of systemic $\gamma\delta$ cells bind to the nonconventional, peptide-independent β_2-microglobulin-associated MHC class 1B molecule, T10/T22 (Crowley et al. 2000). To date, this is the only $\gamma\delta$ TCR reactivity for which a direct biochemical interaction has been shown. Using a murine $\gamma\delta$ T-cell hybridoma, a reactivity to MHC class II has also been reported, although recognition does not focus on the peptide-containing $\alpha1\alpha2$ helical groove that is seen by TCR$\alpha\beta$ (Chien et al. 1996). Systemic murine $\gamma\delta$ cells have also been proposed to recognize the nonclassic class I molecule, Qa-1 (Vidovic et al. 1989), although this was in the context of presenting a nominal, nonphysiological antigen comprising a mixture of polymers of glutamic acid, aspartic acid, and tyrosine.

In humans but not mice, a highly unconventional TCR specificity has been reported in the capacity of peripheral blood, $V\gamma2V\delta2^+$ cells to be stimulated by low-molecular-mass, nonpeptidic chemicals such as isopentenyl pyrophosphate (Tanaka et al. 1995) and, at much higher concentrations, alkylamines (Bukowski et al. 1999) (Figure 23.1). These chemicals can be isolated from extracts of bacteria, parasites, and algae, but at least some are absent from vertebrates. Although direct chemical binding to the TCR has not been shown, the possibility exists that these chemicals are relatives of 'true' high-affinity antigens which, when clearly identified, will permit direct binding to be shown. In this vein, human $V\gamma2V\delta2^+$ cells are strikingly responsive to a mutant strain of *Escherichia coli* defective in the *lytB* gene, an essential enzyme in the 2-C-methylerythritol-4-phosphate (MEP) pathway of isoprenoid biosynthesis (Altincicek et al. 2001). The hyperresponsiveness presumably reflects reactivity toward an accumulated, biologically active intermediate that has been identified as a pyrophosphated molecule of 262 Da (Eberl et al. 2002).

Such specificities may enable systemic $V\gamma2V\delta2^+$ cells to recognize microbial products directly, but, if this is the case, it remains uncertain how the low-molecular-mass, hapten-like antigens can activate the T cell, conventionally achieved via TCR crosslinking of at least a TCR dimer. Likewise, how would an activated T cell focus in on a target, now thought to require synapse formation with an engaged cell? Possibly the low-molecular-mass antigens are presented by a novel antigen presentation system. Consistent with this hypothesis, the recognition by human $\gamma\delta$ cells of another class of low-molecular-mass chemicals, the aminobisphosphonates, requires a myeloid-presenting cell (Miyagawa et al. 2001).

As well as being produced by microbes, some low-molecular-mass chemicals that stimulate systemic $\gamma\delta$ cells may be products of increased metabolism, e.g. intermediates in protein farnesylation in actively growing cells. Moreover, alkylamines can be generated by catabolism of the amino acid theamine, which exists in tea. The biological relevance of these aspects is not elucidated, although it has been proposed that peripheral blood $\gamma\delta$ cells might be primed by dietary components to respond rapidly to microbes and/or transformed cells. Reactivity of peripheral blood $\gamma\delta$ cells to tumors was reported over a decade ago in the recognition of Daudi B-cell lymphomas by $V\gamma2V\delta2^+$ cells (Fisch et al. 1990). However, in this case the recognition was proposed to be of surface-bound heat shock proteins (HSP).

Murine $\gamma\delta$ cells derived from the thymus have also been reported to recognize HSPs (O'Brien et al. 1989), although there is again no biochemical evidence for this as yet. Moreover, it has become increasingly clear that surface-bound HSPs can be engaged by a variety of non-TCR receptors on lymphoid and/or myeloid cells (Srivastava 2002). Thus, the mechanism and significance of HSP recognition by $\gamma\delta$ cells remains uncertain. As systemic $\gamma\delta$ cells are much more abundant in bovine

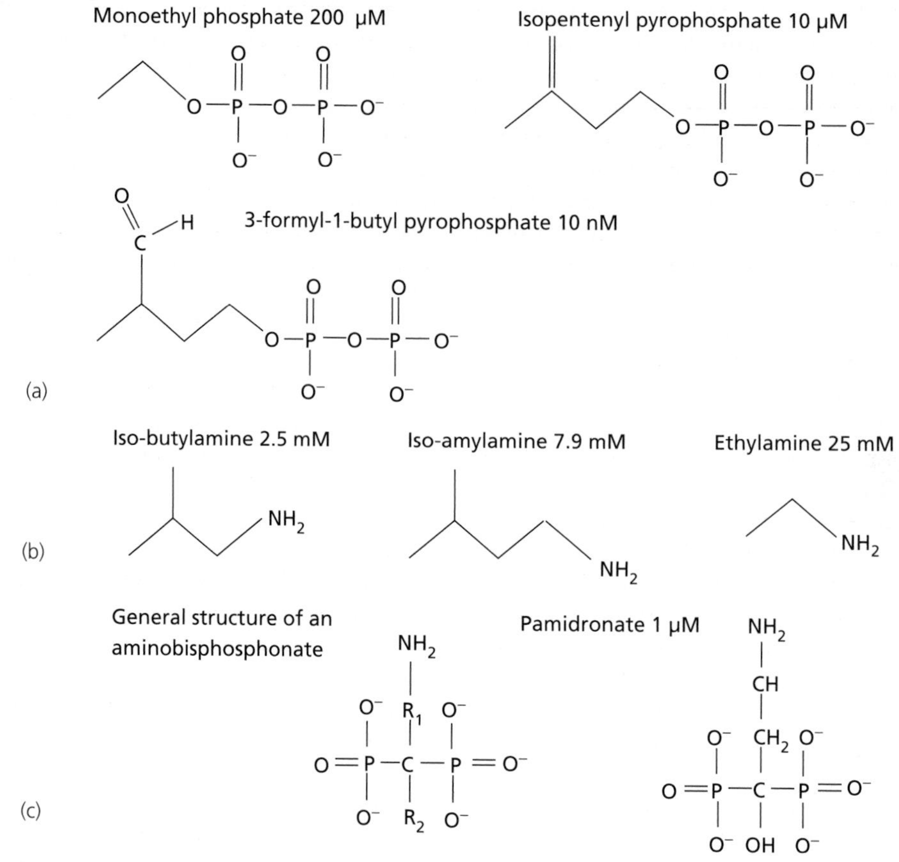

Figure 23.1 *Low-molecular-mass antigens for γδ cells. Structures of* **(a)** *phosphate antigens,* **(b)** *alkylamines, and* **(c)** *aminobisphosphonates. Active concentrations are indicated.*

species, particularly during the first year of life, it would be interesting to determine those cells' reactivities. Although such studies are ongoing, emerging data suggest that those cells too are unconventional, not restricted to conventional MHC.

The biological functions of systemic γδ cells have again been assigned as cytolytic and/or immunoregulatory. In certain strains of mice infected with Coxsackie virus B3, a Th1-mediated myocardial inflammation develops that is dependent on γδ cells. Rather than being directly causative of the inflammation, the role of γδ cells is to eradicate, by fas-mediated cytolysis, virus-responsive Th2 cells (Huber et al. 1999). A broader involvement of unconventional cytolytic T cells in immune regulation is apparent from the identification of regulatory $CD8^+$ αβ T cells, described in a later section.

The activation of human $TCR\gamma\delta^+$ PBLs by low-molecular-mass microbial antigens has been linked to the dramatic expansions that the cells may show in cases of bacterial infection. Human γδ cells reactive to low-molecular-mass mycobacterial antigens express cytolytic chemicals such as granulysin, and may target mycobacteria-infected macrophages. Although a critical contribution of systemic γδ cells to protection against mycobacteria has not been clearly validated, and although no mouse γδ cells have been identified that respond to low-molecular-mass chemicals, γδ-deficient mice inoculated with mycobacteria via aerosols showed altered, disseminated granulomas, consistent with the cells' role in regulating activities of other cells of the immune system (D'Souza et al. 1997). Thus, there are good grounds for viewing γδ cells as an important component of the host response to mycobacteria in mice and humans.

In the rare instances that critical contributions of γδ cells to host protection have been documented in the mouse, they primarily expose a role for γδ cells early in infection, before the priming and expansion of conventional MHC-restricted T cells in the lymph nodes. Thus, it can be considered that such nonconventional T cells collaborate with NK cells in limiting the spread of infection, before the development of antigen-specific immunity. In support of this, there has as yet been no identification of a cloned murine γδ cell line that will transfer antigen-specific immunity upon adoptive transfer to a naïve recipient. Recently, the presence of immunoprotective, mycobacteria-reactive $TCR\gamma\delta^+$ memory cells was reported in primates (Shen et al. 2002), but until we have an improved molecular definition of memory cells (that will probably emerge from contemporary genomic and proteomic studies), the contribution of γδ cells to a memory pool remains uncertain.

Moreover, one possibility relating to γδ cells and other nonconventional T cells is that they are positively selected on autoantigens in the thymus, rather than the negative selection imposed on conventional T cells that are autoreactive. Were this to be the case, the cells could emerge from the thymus in a primed state, capable of very rapid responses to antigen in the periphery. Such a situation has recently been described for unconventional *Listeria*-reactive αβ T cells (see below). Clearly, rapid responses cannot depend on extensive clonal expression of an effector cell (because there would not be time to achieve this). Consistent with this, γδ cell responses to putative antigens, such as low-molecular-mass chemicals or HSPs, seem to occur at the population rather than at the clonal level. Such behavior is consistent with the hypothesis (discussed above) that the fundamental contribution to antigen recognition may be conferred by the CDR1 and CDR2 regions of the Vγ and Vδ gene segments used by the responding populations.

SUBTYPES OF UNCONVENTIONAL T CELLS: αβ T CELLS

TCRαβ$^+$ IELs

The murine intestinal IEL compartment is composed numerically of three main subsets: TCRγδ$^+$ IELs, and two subsets of αβT cells expressing the CD8αα homodimer and the CD8αβ heterodimer, respectively. The CD8αβ heterodimer is the form of CD8 expressed by conventional, systemic, MHC class-I-restricted αβ T cells. Consistent with this, TCRαβ$^+$ CD8αβ$^+$ IELs share many properties with conventional T cells. By contrast, CD8αα expression on systemic T cells is rare and, by several criteria, TCRαβ$^+$CD8αα$^+$ IELs are non-conventional T cells, with much in common with TCRγδ$^+$ IELs. Again, their representation in different species varies, with these IELs being rarer than TCRγδ$^+$ IELs in the adult human gut.

TCRαβ$^+$CD8αα IELs are not restricted by conventional class I or II MHC. Although there are as yet no biochemical data on TCRαβ$^+$CD8αα specificity, the cells, like TCRγδ$^+$ IELs, may recognize nonclassic MHC proteins, transcriptionally upregulated as part of a response to 'stress'. Indeed, their development is strongly regulated by Qa-2 (Das et al. 2000), an MHC class 1B molecule, which similar to MICA and Rae-1 does not require peptide loading by transport associated with antigen processing (TAP) but, unlike MICA and Rae-1, is paired with β_2-microglobulin.

To date, no examples of pathogen-specific, TCRαβ$^+$CD8αα$^+$ IELs have been described. Like TCRγδ$^+$ IELs, some TCRαβ$^+$CD8αα$^+$ IELs may mature in situ, in extrathymic cryptopatches that were recently identified in the murine small intestine (Kanamori et al. 1996). However, under normal circumstances, most probably develop in the thymus. The cells' gene expression profile, sampled as a population, is almost identical to that of TCRγδ$^+$ IELs, with strong potential for cytolysis, and the production of Th1 cytokines and chemokines. In addition, both sets of nonconventional T cells express poorly characterized molecules (e.g. interleukin (IL) 16 and Toll-like receptor (TLR) 8) that may contribute substantially to the delivery and regulation of their effector function (Shires et al. 2001). Not surprisingly, analyses of animal physiology have shown that TCRαβ$^+$CD8αα$^+$ IELs (similar to TCRγδ$^+$ IELs of the gut and of the skin) downregulate tissue inflammation provoked by conventional αβ T cells (Poussier et al. 2002). Both nonconventional TCR αβ$^+$ IELs, and TCR γδ$^+$ IELs may be regulated in part by inhibitory NK cell receptors, such as Ly49E which are expressed on a subset of each cell type.

Unconventional systemic αβ T cells: CD1d-reactive cells

The prototypic αβ T cell exhibiting limited TCR diversity is the NKT cell that expresses the NK1.1 marker (CD161) and that in mice and humans recognizes the conserved group 2 CD1 antigen, CD1d. Most NKT cells express an invariant TCRα chain (Vα14/Jα281 in mouse; Vα21/JαQ in humans), paired with a limited repertoire of TCRβ chains (MacDonald 2002). The development of multivalent CD1d reagents has identified CD1d reactivity in a broader set of cells than those expressing only the signatory TCR and NK1.1. Moreover, not all NK1.1$^+$ cells react to CD1d. Thus, the value of the term 'NKT' is operationally useful, but should not be over-interpreted.

Following the identification of murine NKT cells, autoreactive against CD1d (Bendelac et al. 1995), it was observed that the cells' responses were enhanced by the glycosylated sphingolipid α-galactosylceramide (α-GalCer), a model antigen derived from a marine sponge (Kawano et al. 1997) (Figure 23.2). Other α-linked glycolipids activate NKT cells, whereas β-linked glycolipids, which more closely resemble mammalian lipids, do not. α-linked glycolipids are not normally found in mammalian cells, but may be found in particular fetal tissue, in the kidney or intestine, or in transformed cells (Gumperz and Brenner 2001). Physiological antigens presented by CD1d are only now being identified (Zhou et al. 2004), although at least some are thought likely to be self-encoded because NKT cells are present at essentially normal levels in germ-free mice. The prospect that more than one self-antigen may be recognized is suggested by the fact that a panel of NKT clones showed quite different responses to cells transfected with CD1d,

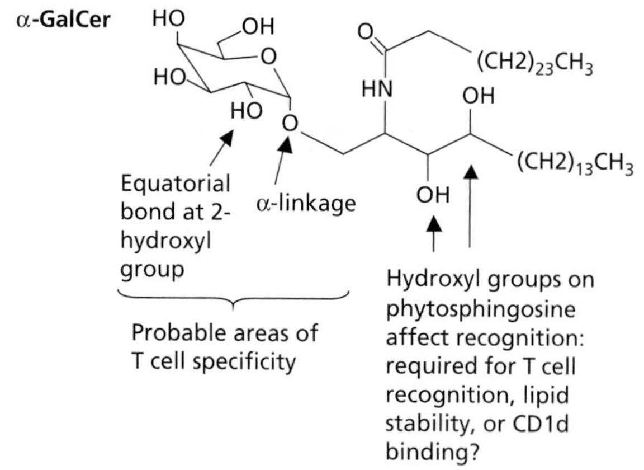

Figure 23.2 *Murine NKT cells are reactive to α-galactosylceramide (α-GalCer) presented by CD1d. NKT cells show fine specificity for the α anomer of galactose, and for an equatorial hydroxyl group at carbon 2. Removal of the hydroxyl groups at positions 2 and 3 of the phytosphingosine also prevented recognition, but this could be the result of decreased lipid stability or CD1d presentation.*

probably reflecting a spectrum of reactivities to different CD1d–lipid complexes displayed by the different transfectants.

CD1d-reactive cells have been assigned a plethora of functions, with a capacity to secrete large amounts of cytokines, including IL-4, IL-10, and interferon γ (IFN-γ) implicating the cell in immunoregulation (Gumperz and Brenner 2001). The NKT cytokine spectrum also implies that some nonconventional T cells are not constrained by the Th1/Th2 paradigm. Altered development of autoimmune disease has been reported in NKT-deficient animals such as CD1d$^{-/-}$ mice, on the appropriate genetic backgrounds. After infection with *Borrelia burgdorferi* (the etiological agent of Lyme disease), CD1d$^{-/-}$ mice displayed an altered (rather than a diminished) immune response (Kumar et al. 2000). Collectively, these data have strongly suggested that NKT cells respond rapidly to perturbation (e.g. infected or transformed cells), by coordinating the actions of other cells of the immune system. Thus, as with γδ cells, these unconventional T cells may make use of limited TCR diversity to recognize generic beacons of host dysregulation and activate immune responses, in a manner not dissimilar from the actions of dendritic cells or macrophages. Interestingly, large numbers of NKT cells are found in the liver, which is the organ responsible for releasing acute phase response mediators.

This notwithstanding, the biology of NKT cells may differ from that commonly attributed to γδ cells in that NKT cells emerge relatively late in thymic ontogeny, compared with the fetal and perinatal emergence of TCRγδ$^+$ IELs. Given this, the raison d'être of NKT cells may be to regulate conventional αβ T cells, rather than to contribute intrinsic immunoprotective capacities, as has been proposed for TCRγδ$^+$ cells. Perhaps consistent with this, the positive selection of NKT cells in the thymus is critically influenced by CD4$^+$CD8$^+$ 'double-positive' thymocytes, which are signatory progenitors of conventional αβ T cells (Bendelac 1995).

CD1a, -b, -c reactive αβ T cells

Numerous T cells have been identified that are specific for various glycolipid antigens presented by CD1a, CD1b, or CD1c. The cells express diverse TCRs, and have high specificity for the surface-exposed carbohydrate heads of glycolipid antigens that are anchored by their acyl chains deep within the hydrophobic core of the antigen-presenting pocket (Figure 23.3). CD1b will present mycobacterial cell wall-derived glycolipids, but CD1 molecules may also present endogenous ligands. In sum, the biological distinction between self and nonself that is a core parameter of conventional αβ T-cell activity remains enigmatic for the bulk of CD1-reactive T cells, as it does for γδ cells.

Like γδ cells, unconventional CD1-reactive T cells are primarily Th1/cytolytic CD4$^-$CD8$^-$ (double-negative (DN)) cells, but are not exclusively so. Hence, their true representation, based exclusively on the analysis of the DN T-cell population, may have been underestimated, particularly in infections. As CD1a, -b, and -c genes are absent from the mouse genome, a role for CD1-reactive cells in infection has been inferred from human studies showing that cells reactive to CD1-presented mycobacterial isoprenoid lipid antigens are readily detectable in people with recent *Mycobacteria tuberculosis* infections. Of note, efficacious immune responses to mycobacteria have been associated with group 1 CD1 antigen expression by dendritic cells (DC).

Unlike expression of MHC class II recognized by conventional T cells, CD1 is highly expressed on immature DCs, before their activation and migration from the periphery to the lymph nodes. The potential therefore exists to activate CD1-reactive T cells directly in peripheral tissues, further supporting the view that unconventional T cells complement conventional T-cell activities by contributing locally to an early phase of the immune response. Interestingly, the different forms of CD1 appear to associate with lipid antigens in different intracellular compartments (Jayawardena-Wolf and Bendelac 2001; Winau et al. 2004), suggesting that a spectrum of antigen-processing events may stimulate different subsets of CD1-reactive cells to respond to either endogenously synthesized antigen (in transformed or infected cells) or exogenously acquired antigen (after phagocytosis).

In sum, CD1-reactive cells compose a potent and versatile response repertoire, and it therefore seems all the more surprising that this system is not conserved in mice. Arguably, the relatively higher abundance of γδ$^+$ cells in mice may partially substitute for the function of

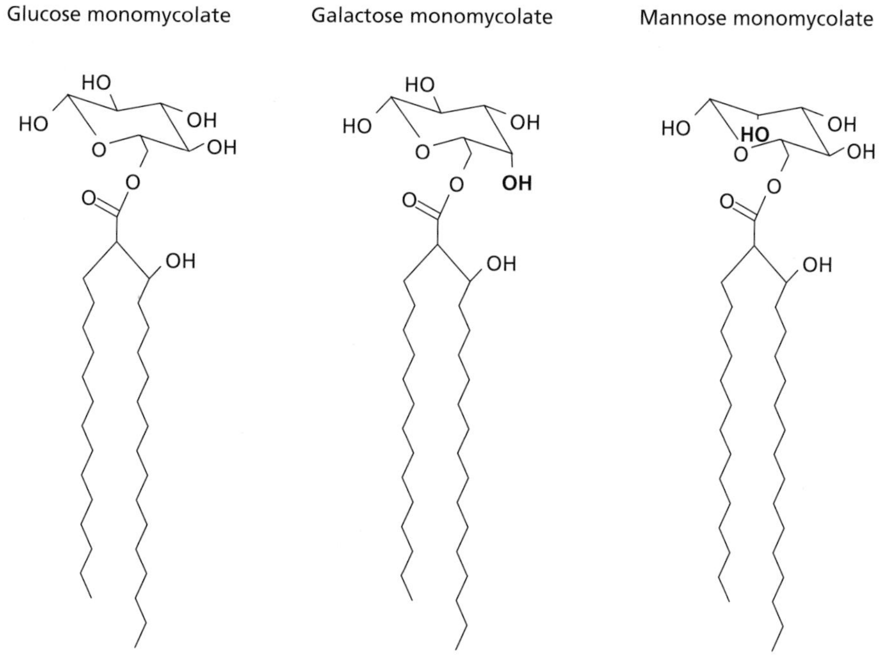

Figure 23.3 αβ T cells exhibit fine specificity for glycolipid antigens presented by CD1b. Some αβ T cells recognize derivatives of mycolic acid, but not mycolic acid derivatized with galactose or mannose, which are stereoisomers of glucose and differ from glucose in the orientation of a single hydroxyl group.

CD1-reactive cells, and CD1 reactivity of $\gamma\delta^+$ cells has been reported, ironically in humans (see above). Nevertheless, the reason that the specific constitutions of unconventional T-cell repertoires seem so variable across species remains poorly understood.

MR1-reactive αβ T cells

Another population of unconventional αβ T cells has been described in the lamina propria of the intestine in mice, humans, and cattle. These T cells express an invariant Vα7Jα33 TCR in humans (the homologous Vα19Jα33 in mice and cattle) (Tilloy et al. 1999). It was noted that this population was present in MHC class I and CD1 double-deficient mice, MHC class II-deficient mice, and TAP-deficient mice, but was missing in $\beta_2m^{-/-}$ mice. Therefore, candidate nonclassic MHC class I molecules were tested as potential ligands. As a result, this invariant T-cell population was found to be dependent on the presence of the nonclassic MHC class I molecule MR1 (Treiner et al. 2003). MR1 mRNA was previously reported to be expressed ubiquitously (Yamaguchi et al. 1997), although no antibody was available to confirm the distribution of the MR1 protein. It has since been found that, despite widespread mRNA expression, the MR1 protein is expressed only on the surface of activated B cells in the lamina propria. These B cells expressing MR1 activate the invariant Vα7Vα19 T cells to secrete transforming growth factor-β (TGF-β), which causes the B cells to class switch to IgA, the appropriate isotype for mucosal surfaces (Lantz, unpublished) (Figure 23.4). These recent findings concerning MR1-reactive αβ T cells parallel the findings from γδ cell biology in emphasizing the association of unconventional T cells with tissues and tissue-specific processes.

Qa-1 reactive/HLA-E reactive CD8αβ⁺ αβ T cells

Other αβ T-cell populations are restricted by MHC class IB molecules of the H-2Q region, the counterpart of which in the human is the HLA-E molecule. After infection of mice with *Salmonella typhimurium*, large numbers of H-2Qa-1 reactive cells were described, whereas HLA-E-reactive T cells have been described in humans infected with *Mycobacterium tuberculosis*. Commonly, such unconventional MHC class Ib-reactive $CD8\alpha\beta^+$ αβ T cells appear to be constitutively activated, before infection, and may thus be primed to contribute to primary protection at early times after infection (see next section). However, an additional role has been proposed for MHC class Ib-reactive $CD8\alpha\beta^+$ αβ T cells, following the identification in the mouse of cells that respond to a Vβ8-derived peptide presented by Qa-1 on seemingly conventional $V\beta8^+$ $CD4^+$ $TCR\alpha\beta^+$ T-helper cells (Jiang and Chess 2000) (Figure 23.5). This $CD8\alpha\beta^+$ αβ T-cell response, which can likewise be elicited by irrelevant cells co-transfected with the Qa-1 and TCR Vβ8 chain genes, results in the cytolysis of the $CD4^+$ T cell, thus downregulating the associated immune effector response.

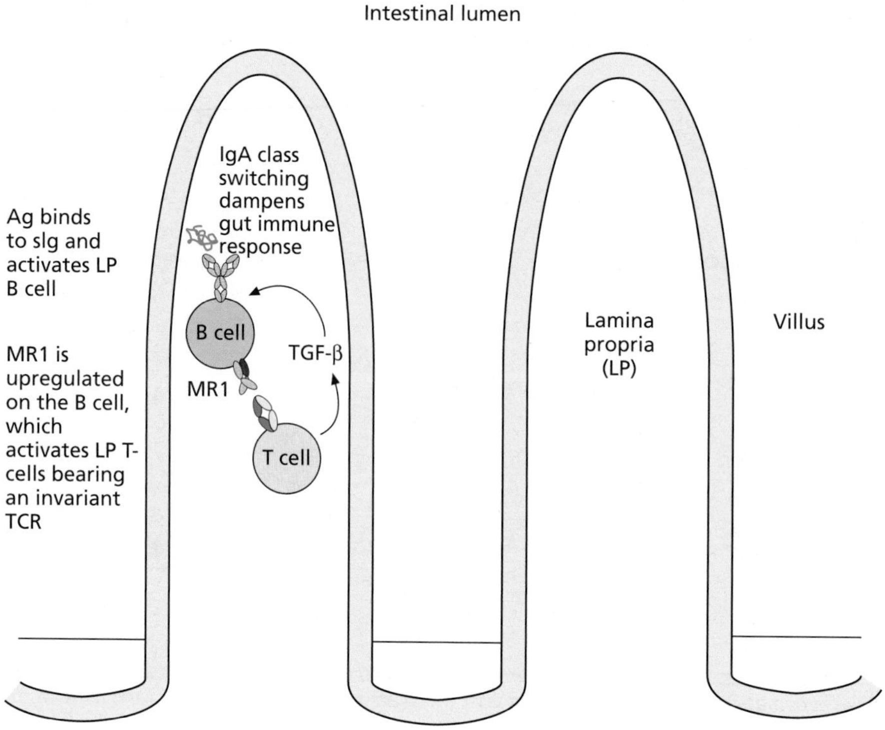

Figure 23.4 *MR1 is a ligand for a conserved population of lamina propria T cells. Expression of MR1 is upregulated on B cells on antigen binding to surface immunoglobulin. MR1 is recognized by T cells expressing an invariant Vα7Jα33 in humans (the homologous Vα19Jα33 in mice and cattle). On MR1 recognition, these T cells produce transforming growth factor β (TGFβ), which induces class switching to IgA, the appropriate isotype for the intestine; as well as preventing hyperactivation of the gut immune system. Ag, antigen; sIg, surface immunoglobulin.*

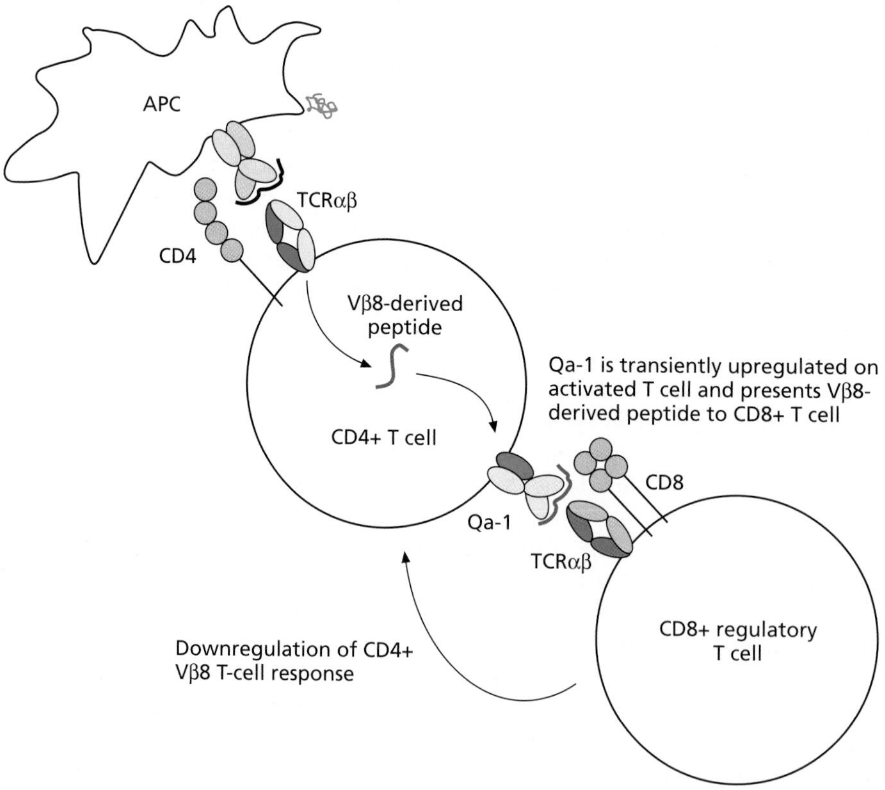

Figure 23.5 *Recognition by regulatory CD8$^+$ T cells of T-cell receptor (TCR)-derived peptides presented on Qa-1. Activated CD4$^+$ T cells transiently upregulate the nonclassic MHC class I molecule Qa-1, which presents peptides derived from the TCR Vβ8 chain. Qa-1 peptide complexes are recognized by CD8$^+$ regulatory T cells which downregulate the CD4 T-cell response. APC, antigen-presenting cell.*

Evidence that $CD8^+$ cytolytic T cells downregulate immune responses to self and to foreign antigens has been presented in many experimental systems for many years, e.g. mice induced to develop experimental allergic encephalomyelitis (in many regards, an animal model for multiple sclerosis (MS)) by immunization with myelin basic protein peptides conventionally show marked periods of disease remission, reminiscent of those that characterize MS and other autoimmune diseases in humans. These are eradicated by either antibody-mediated, or genetic depletion of, $CD8^+$ T cells, leading to unrelenting disease progression (Jiang et al. 1992; Koh et al. 1992). The prospect that such $CD8^+$ T-cell-mediated regulation might target $CD4^+$ T cells in an antigen receptor-specific fashion was emphasized by the finding that the immune response to hen egg lysozyme is reduced in strains of mice that, paradoxically, have more TCR Vβ genes. This immune deficiency is rescued by depletion of $CD8^+$ T cells, indicating that the regulatory cells are targeting $CD4^+$ T cells that express particular TCR Vβ genes (Jiang and Chess 2000).

One would assume, from first principles, that the cytolysis of $CD4^+$ $TCR\alpha\beta^+$ T-helper cells must be carefully regulated. In this light, Qa-1 has some interesting properties. First, it is only expressed on $CD4^+$ T cells after activation and, second, its expression is transient, thereby limiting the potential for regulation to a short window. Third, Qa-1 presenting leader peptides of conventional MHC class I molecules (Qdm) in addition engages an NKG2A/CD94 NK inhibitory receptor that is commonly expressed on activated $CD8^+$ T cells (Aldrich et al. 1994). The same is true for HLA-E, in humans. Thus, one might envision that, when a $CD4^+$ T cell expresses an excess of Qa-1.Qdm over Qa-1.TCR, the regulatory $CD8^+$ T cell is inhibited, whereas, when Qa-1.TCR is in excess, it is activated to target the $CD4^+$ T cell. Interestingly, immune regulation by $CD8^+$ T cells seems primarily to target $CD4^+$ Th1 cells rather than $CD4^+$ Th2 cells. The opposite has been claimed for the *fas*-mediated downregulation of autoreactive Th2 cells by systemic γδ cells (see above).

Unconventional peptide-reactive αβ T cells

Contemporary genomics analyses have revealed an increasing number of unconventional, MHC class 1B genes that are candidate ligands for further unconventional T-cell reactivities. One such reactivity is the αβ T-cell response to bacterial *N*-formylated peptides (Nfp), presented by H2-M3. As the initiator methionine groups in eukaryotic proteins are very rarely *N*-formylated, the recognition of Nfp might be regarded as a form of pathogen-associated molecular pattern recognition.

H2-M3 Nfp-reactive cells have been described in mice infected with *Mycobacterium tuberculosis* and *Listeria monocytogenes* and they may form a part of the T-cell response to a broad spectrum of bacteria. In *Listeria*-infected mice, multivalent cell-staining reagents comprising H2-M3 Nfp tetramers detected reactive αβ T cells early in the response, before the clonal expansion of conventional, MHC-peptide reactive αβ T cells. Consistent with this, the cells constitutively display markers of activation (e.g. $CD44^{hi}$). Two additional aspects of the tetramer-reactive cells are reminiscent of other unconventional T cells: (1) they have cytolytic and Th1 effector potential; and (2) they contribute substantially to primary responses, but, after secondary infection, their contribution is eclipsed by the effector responses of conventional $CD8\alpha\beta^+$ αβ T cells (Kerksiek et al. 1999). Also complying with the hypothesis that unconventional T cells differ from conventional T cells in their selection during development, it was recently shown that the progenitors of H2-M3 Nfp-reactive cells will positively select on autologous MHC class Ib antigens expressed in the thymus by hemopoietic cells, and that, contingent upon this, the cells immediately acquire an activated phenotype before thymic emigration (Urdahl et al. 2002).

Unconventional 'β-only' T cells

When a mutation was experimentally introduced into the mouse TCRα chain, by gene-by-gene knockout technology, a small population of peripheral, $CD4^+$ $TCR\beta^+$ cells was found in the resultant mice (Mombaerts et al. 1992). The potential for TCR β chain expression in the absence of TCRα exists via the formation of either TCRβ/β homodimers, or a complex of TCRβ with an alternately spliced product of the pre-Tα chain which can ordinarily pair with TCRβ during thymocyte development (Barber et al. 1998). As for other nonconventional T cells, these 'β-only' cells have potent Th1 activity and are in part responsible for pathogen-responsive bowel inflammations that develop in $TCR\alpha^{-/-}$ mice but not in $TCR\beta^{-/-}$ mice, which would lack $TCR\beta^{+\alpha-}$ cells.

Naturally, β-only cells have generally been regarded as an idiosyncrasy of $TCR\alpha^{-/-}$ mice, but their existence in normal animals should not be discounted. In thymocyte development, TCRβ-gene rearrangement precedes TCRα-gene rearrangement and the formal possibility therefore exists for cells that do not productively rearrange either TCRα-chain allele to mature as β-only cells. Although such cells would be thought unlikely to receive essential signals for positive selection on MHC, the fact that such cells are present in the periphery of $TCR\alpha^{-/-}$ mice clearly indicates the potential for some 'β-only cells' to mature. Given their functional potency, particularly their capacity to respond to microbial antigens, their existence in humans needs to be more thoroughly tested.

Regulatory CD4$^+$ CD25$^+$ $\alpha\beta$ T cells: putative unconventional T cells

The diversity of unconventional T cells that has been considered in this chapter provokes the concept that unconventional T cells are not particularly rare, and that there may be other sets of T cells that are currently poorly understood, which may ultimately be assigned as unconventional. In this regard, much attention has recently been paid to a set of immunosuppressive T cells that can be found in mice and humans within the CD4$^+$CD25^{hi} subset. Although these markers alone are insufficient to identify a pure population of regulatory T cells (e.g. they also identify activated effector cells), they identify a subset of cells in the thymus that seemingly acquires an activated phenotype immediately on maturation. Perinatal thymectomy in certain strains of mice (e.g. Balb/c) selectively ablates such cells, provoking spontaneous, multiorgan, autoimmune disease. There remains much to learn about these regulatory cells, and there is a high likelihood that they are heterogeneous in phenotype. Nevertheless, evidence is gathering that at least some of them may comply with the operating definitions of unconventional T cells proposed at the beginning of this chapter. Specifically: their antigen specificity may be primarily selfreactive, not necessarily restricted to conventional MHC; their development, as stated, seems to be distinct from that of conventional $\alpha\beta$ T cells; their recirculation patterns are ill-defined but evidence suggests that they may function primarily within tissues; and their potential to contribute to antigen-specific memory is also as yet unclear. The potential that such cells, with proven capacity to regulate immune responses in vivo would be assigned to the unconventional T-cell compartment further highlights the prudence of paying greater attention to the representation of unconventional T-cell subsets in health and disease.

REFERENCES

Aberer, W., Romani, N., et al. 1986. Effects of physicochemical agents on murine epidermal Langerhans cells and Thy-1-positive dendritic epidermal cells. *J Immunol*, **136**, 1210–16.

Aldrich, C.J., DeCloux, A., et al. 1994. Identification of a Tap-dependent leader peptide recognized by alloreactive T cells specific for a class Ib antigen. *Cell*, **79**, 649–58.

Allison, T.J., Winter, C.C., et al. 2001. Structure of a human gamma delta T-cell antigen receptor. *Nature*, **411**, 820–4.

Altincicek, B., Moll, J., et al. 2001. Cutting edge: human gamma delta T cells are activated by intermediates of the 2-C-methyl-D-erythritol 4-phosphate pathway of isoprenoid biosynthesis. *J Immunol*, **166**, 3655–8.

Arden, B., Clark, S.P., et al. 1995a. Human T-cell receptor variable gene segment families. *Immunogenetics*, **42**, 455–500.

Arden, B., Clark, S.P., et al. 1995b. Mouse T-cell receptor variable gene segment families. *Immunogenetics*, **42**, 501–30.

Asarnow, D.M., Kuziel, W.A., et al. 1988. Limited diversity of gamma delta antigen receptor genes of Thy-1+ dendritic epidermal cells. *Cell*, **55**, 837–47.

Barber, D.F., Passoni, L., et al. 1998. The expression in vivo of a second isoform of pT alpha: implications for the mechanism of pT alpha action. *J Immunol*, **161**, 11–16.

Bauer, S., Groh, V., et al. 1999. Activation of NK cells and T cells by NKG2D, a receptor for stress-inducible MICA. *Science*, **285**, 727–9.

Bendelac, A. 1995. Positive selection of mouse NK1.1(+) T cells by CD1-expressing cortical thymocytes. *J Exp Med*, **182**, 2901–6.

Bendelac, A., Lantz, O., et al. 1995. CD1 recognition by mouse NK1+ T lymphocytes. *Science*, **268**, 863–5.

Bigby, M., Markowitz, J.S., et al. 1993. Most gamma delta T cells develop normally in the absence of MHC class II molecules. *J Immunol*, **151**, 4465–75.

Boismenu, R. and Havran, W.L. 1994. Modulation of epithelial cell growth by intraepithelial gamma delta T cells. *Science*, **266**, 1253–5.

Boismenu, R., Feng, L., et al. 1996. Chemokine expression by intraepithelial gamma delta T cells. Implications for the recruitment of inflammatory cells to damaged epithelia. *J Immunol*, **157**, 985–92.

Bonneville, M., Janeway, C.A. Jr, et al. 1988. Intestinal intraepithelial lymphocytes are a distinct set of gamma delta T cells. *Nature*, **336**, 479–81.

Bukowski, J.F., Morita, C.T. and Brenner, M.B. 1999. Human gamma delta T cells recognize alkylamines derived from microbes, edible plants, and tea: implications for innate immunity. *Immunity*, **11**, 57–65.

Cerwenka, A., Bakker, A.B., et al. 2000. Retinoic acid early inducible genes define a ligand family for the activating NKG2D receptor in mice. *Immunity*, **12**, 721–7.

Chien, Y.H., Jores, R. and Crowley, M.P. 1996. Recognition by gamma/delta T cells. *Annu Rev Immunol*, **14**, 511–32.

Clark, S.P., Arden, B., et al. 1995. Comparison of human and mouse T-cell receptor variable gene segment subfamilies. *Immunogenetics*, **42**, 531–40.

Correa, I., Bix, M., et al. 1992. Most gamma delta T cells develop normally in beta 2-microglobulin-deficient mice. *Proc Natl Acad Sci USA*, **89**, 653–7.

Cosman, D., Mullberg, J., et al. 2001. ULBPs, novel MHC class I-related molecules, bind to CMV glycoprotein UL16 and stimulate NK cytotoxicity through the NKG2D receptor. *Immunity*, **14**, 123–33.

Crowley, M.P., Fahrer, A.M., et al. 2000. A population of murine gamma delta T cells that recognize an inducible MHC class Ib molecule. *Science*, **287**, 314–16.

Das, G., Gould, D.S., et al. 2000. Qa-2-dependent selection of CD8alpha/alpha T cell receptor alpha/beta(+) cells in murine intestinal intraepithelial lymphocytes. *J Exp Med*, **192**, 1521–8.

Deusch, K., Luling, F., et al. 1991. A major fraction of human intraepithelial lymphocytes simultaneously expresses the gamma/delta T cell receptor, the CD8 accessory molecule and preferentially uses the V delta 1 gene segment. *Eur J Immunol*, **21**, 1053–9.

Diefenbach, A., Jamieson, A.M., et al. 2000. Ligands for the murine NKG2D receptor: expression by tumor cells and activation of NK cells and macrophages. *Nat Immunol*, **1**, 119–26.

D'Souza, C.D., Copper, A.M., et al. 1997. An anti-inflammatory role $\gamma\alpha$ T cells in acquired immunity to *Mycobacterium tuberculosis*. *J Immunol*, **158**, 1217–21.

Eberl, M., Altincicek, B., et al. 2002. Accumulation of a potent gamma delta T-cell stimulator after deletion of the lytB gene in *Escherichia coli*. *Immunology*, **106**, 200–11.

Fisch, P., Malkovsky, M., et al. 1990. Recognition by human V gamma 9/V delta 2 T cells of a GroEL homolog on Daudi Burkitt's lymphoma cells. *Science*, **250**, 1269–73.

Girardi, M., Oppenheim, D.E., et al. 2001. Regulation of cutaneous malignancy by gamma delta T cells. *Science*, **294**, 605–9.

Girardi, M., Lewis, J., et al. 2002. Resident skin-specific gamma delta T cells provide local, nonredundant regulation of cutaneous inflammation. *J Exp Med*, **195**, 855–67.

Goodman, T. and Lefrancois, L. 1988. Expression of the gamma-delta T-cell receptor on intestinal CD8+ intraepithelial lymphocytes. *Nature*, **333**, 855–8.

Groh, V., Bahram, S., et al. 1996. Cell stress-regulated human major histocompatibility complex class I gene expressed in gastrointestinal epithelium. *Proc Natl Acad Sci USA*, **93**, 12445–50.

Groh, V., Steinle, A., et al. 1998. Recognition of stress-induced MHC molecules by intestinal epithelial gammadelta T cells. *Science*, **279**, 1737–40.

Groh, V., Rhinehart, R., et al. 1999. Broad tumor-associated expression and recognition by tumor-derived gamma delta T cells of MICA and MICB. *Proc Natl Acad Sci USA*, **96**, 6879–84.

Gumperz, J.E. and Brenner, M.B. 2001. CD1-specific T cells in microbial immunity. *Curr Opin Immunol*, **13**, 471–8.

Havran, W.L. and Allison, J.P. 1988. Developmentally ordered appearance of thymocytes expressing different T-cell antigen receptors. *Nature*, **335**, 443–5.

Havran, W.L., Chien, Y.H. and Allison, J.P. 1991. Recognition of self antigens by skin-derived T cells with invariant gamma delta antigen receptors. *Science*, **252**, 1430–2.

Holtmeier, W., Pfander, M., et al. 2001. The TCR-delta repertoire in normal human skin is restricted and distinct from the TCR-delta repertoire in the peripheral blood. *J Invest Dermatol*, **116**, 275–80.

Huber, S.A., Budd, R.C., et al. 1999. Apoptosis in coxsackie virus B3-induced myocarditis and dilated cardiomyopathy. *Ann N Y Acad Sci*, **887**, 181–90.

Ikuta, K., Kina, T., et al. 1990. A developmental switch in thymic lymphocyte maturation potential occurs at the level of hematopoietic stem cells. *Cell*, **62**, 863–74.

Jameson, J., Ugarte, K., et al. 2002. A role for skin gamma delta T cells in wound repair. *Science*, **296**, 747–9.

Janeway, C.A. Jr, Jones, B. and Hayday, A. 1988. Specificity and function of T cells bearing gamma delta receptors. *Immunol Today*, **9**, 73–6.

Jayawardena-Wolf, J. and Bendelac, A. 2001. CD1 and lipid antigens: intracellular pathways for antigen presentation. *Curr Opin Immunol*, **13**, 109–13.

Jiang, H. and Chess, L. 2000. The specific regulation of immune responses by CD8+ T cells restricted by the MHC class Ib molecule, Qa-1. *Annu Rev Immunol*, **18**, 185–216.

Jiang, H., Zhang, S.I. and Pernis, B. 1992. Role of CD8+ T cells in murine experimental allergic encephalomyelitis. *Science*, **256**, 1213–15.

Kanamori, Y., Ishimaru, K., et al. 1996. Identification of novel lymphoid tissues in murine intestinal mucosa where clusters of c-kit(+), IL-7R(+), Thy1(+) lympho-hemopoietic progenitors develop. *J Exp Med*, **184**, 1449–59.

Kawano, T., Cui, J., et al. 1997. CD1d-restricted and TCR-mediated activation of valpha14 NKT cells by glycosylceramides. *Science*, **278**, 1626–9.

Kerksiek, K.M., Busch, D.H., et al. 1999. H2-M3-restricted T cells in bacterial infection: rapid primary but diminished memory responses. *J Exp Med*, **190**, 195–204.

Koh, D.R., Fung-Leung, W.P., et al. 1992. Less mortality but more relapses in experimental allergic encephalomyelitis in CD8-/- mice. *Science*, **256**, 1210–13.

Kumar, H., Belperron, A., et al. 2000. Cutting edge: CD1d deficiency impairs murine host defense against the spirochete, Borrelia burgdorferi. *J Immunol*, **165**, 4797–801.

Kyes, S., Carew, E., et al. 1989. Diversity in T-cell receptor gamma gene usage in the intestinal. *Proc Natl Acad Sci USA*, **86**, 5527–31.

Lafaille, J.J., DeCloux, A., et al. 1989. Junctional sequences of T cell receptor gamma delta genes: implications for gamma delta T cell lineages and for a novel intermediate of V-(D)-J joining. *Cell*, **59**, 859–70.

Li, H., Lebedeva, M.I., et al. 1998. Structure of the Vdelta domain of a human gamma delta T-cell antigen receptor. *Nature*, **391**, 502–506.

Li, P., Willie, S.T., et al. 1999. Crystal structure of the MHC class I homolog MIC-A, a gamma delta T cell ligand. *Immunity*, **10**, 577–84.

Li, P., McDermott, G. and Strong, R.K. 2002. Crystal structures of RAE-1beta and its complex with the activating immunoreceptor NKG2D. *Immunity*, **16**, 77–86.

MacDonald, H.R. 2002. Development and selection of NKT cells. *Curr Opin Immunol*, **14**, 250–4.

Miyagawa, F., Tanaka, Y., et al. 2001. Essential requirement of antigen presentation by monocyte lineage cells for the activation of primary human gamma delta T cells by aminobisphosphonate antigen. *J Immunol*, **166**, 5508–14.

Mombaerts, P., Clarke, A.R., et al. 1992. Mutations in T-cell antigen receptor genes alpha and beta block thymocyte development at different stages. *Nature*, **360**, 225–31.

O'Brien, R.L., Happ, M.P., et al. 1989. Stimulation of a major subset of lymphocytes expressing T cell receptor gamma delta by an antigen derived from *Mycobacterium tuberculosis*. *Cell*, **57**, 667–74.

Poussier, P., Ning, T., et al. 2002. A unique subset of self-specific intraintestinal T cells maintains gut integrity. *J Exp Med*, **195**, 1491–7.

Roberts, S.J., Smith, A.L., et al. 1996. T-cell alpha beta+ and gamma delta+ deficient mice display abnormal but distinct phenotypes toward a natural, widespread infection of the intestinal epithelium. *Proc Natl Acad Sci USA*, **93**, 11774–9.

Rock, E.P., Sibbald, P.R., et al. 1994. CDR3 length in antigen-specific immune receptors. *J Exp Med*, **179**, 323–8.

Saito, H., Kranz, D.M., et al. 1984. A third rearranged and expressed gene in a clone of cytotoxic T lymphocytes. *Nature*, **312**, 36–40.

Shen, Y., Zhou, D., et al. 2002. Adaptive immune response of Vgamma2 Vdelta2+ T cells during mycobacterial infections. *Science*, **295**, 2255–8.

Shires, J., Theodoridis, E. and Hayday, A.C. 2001. Biological insights into TCRgammadelta+ and TCRalphabeta+ intraepithelial lymphocytes provided by serial analysis of gene expression (SAGE). *Immunity*, **15**, 419–34.

Smith, A. and Hayday, A. 2000. An alpha beta T-cell independent immunoprotective response toward gut coccidia is supported by gamma delta cells. *Immunology*, **101**, 325–32.

Spada, F.M., Grant, E.P., et al. 2000. Self-recognition of CD1 by gamma/delta T cells: implications for innate immunity. *J Exp Med*, **191**, 937–48.

Srivastava, P. 2002. Interaction of heat shock proteins with peptides and antigen presenting cells: chaperoning of the innate and adaptive immune responses. *Annu Rev Immunol*, **20**, 395–425.

Takagaki, Y., DeCloux, A., et al. 1989. Diversity of gamma delta T-cell receptors on murine intestinal intra-epithelial lymphocytes. *Nature*, **339**, 712–14.

Tanaka, Y., Morita, C.T., et al. 1995. Natural and synthetic non-peptide antigens recognized by human gamma delta T cells. *Nature*, **375**, 155–8.

Tilloy, F., Treiner, E., et al. 1999. An invariant T cell receptor alpha chain defines a novel TAP-independent major histocompatibility complex class Ib-restricted alpha/beta T cell subpopulation in mammals. *J Exp Med*, **189**, 1907–21.

Tonegawa, S. 1983. Somatic generation of antibody diversity. *Nature*, **302**, 575–81.

Treiner, E., Duban, L., et al. 2003. Selection of evolutionarily conserved mucosal-associated invariant T cells by MR1. *Nature*, **422**, 164–9.

Urdahl, K.B., Sun, J.C. and Bevan, M.J. 2002. Positive selection of MHC class Ib-restricted CD8(+) T cells on hematopoietic cells. *Nat Immunol*, **3**, 772–9.

Van Beneden, K., De Creus, A., et al. 2002. Expression of inhibitory receptors Ly49E and CD94/NKG2 on fetal thymic and adult epidermal TCR V gamma 3 lymphocytes. *J Immunol*, **168**, 3295–302.

Vidovic, D., Roglic, M., et al. 1989. Qa-1 restricted recognition of foreign antigen by a gamma delta T-cell hybridoma. *Nature*, **340**, 646–50.

Winau, F., Schwierzeck, V., et al. 2004. Saposin C is required for lipid presentation by human CD1b. *Nat Immunol*, **5**, 169–74.

Wu, J., Groh, V. and Spies, T. 2002. T cell antigen receptor engagement and specificity in the recognition of stress-inducible MHC class I-related chains by human epithelial gamma delta T cells. *J Immunol*, **169**, 1236–40.

Yamaguchi, H., Hirai, M., et al. 1997. A highly conserved major histocompatibility complex class I-related gene in mammals. *Biochem Biophys Res Commun*, **238**, 697–702.

Zhou, D., Cantu 3rd, C., et al. 2004. Editing of CD1d-bound lipid antigens by endosomal lipid transfer proteins. *Science*, **303**, 523–7.

Zou, Z., Nomura, M., et al. 1996. Isolation and characterization of retinoic acid-inducible cDNA clones in F9 cells: a novel cDNA family encodes cell surface proteins sharing partial homology with MHC class I molecules. *J Biochem (Tokyo)*, **119**, 319–28.

24

T-cell receptors

MARC BONNEVILLE

Even long after the characterization of immunoglobulins and B-cell receptors, the molecular basis of antigen recognition by T cells has remained a major enigma for immunologists. Both the exquisite antigen specificity of T cells and their ability to mount memory responses suggested that, as with B cells, T cells recognized antigens through structurally diverse and clonally distributed receptors, then referred to as T-cell receptors (TCR). However, the unsuccessful attempts to identify idiotypic determinants shared by antibodies and TCRs and the fundamental difference between B-cell and T-cell antigen recognition processes, unveiled by the work of Zinkernagel and Doherty, fostered intensive debates in the 1970s about the TCR nature and structure. Addressing this issue turned out to be particularly challenging but was finally settled in the 1980s with the molecular characterization of the TCR genes. During the last decade, biophysical studies of TCR–pMHC (peptide major histocompatibility complex) interactions and structural analyses of trimolecular TCR–peptide–MHC complexes have brought insights into the fine mechanism of TCR recognition and T-cell activation, which are now viewed as dynamic processes relying on TCR conformational fits and complex interplays between immune receptors and signaling molecules within specialized supramolecular arrangements.

ISOLATION OF T-CELL RECEPTORS: AN HISTORICAL OVERVIEW

In several early 1970s studies, Zinkernagel and Doherty demonstrated that T-cell recognition of virally infected cells requires both viral antigens and expression of self-major histocompatibility complex (MHC) molecules by infected cells (Zinkernagel and Doherty 1974). By analyzing the responses of hybridomas obtained by fusion of T cells with distinct antigen and MHC specificities, Kappler and Marrack's group then showed, in agreement with the so-called 'altered self-model', that this 'self-MHC restriction' involves a single receptor that is able to recognize self-MHC molecules modified by or complexed to the antigen (Kappler et al. 1981). The first hints at the TCR structure were obtained by Allison and colleagues, who generated antisera specific to surface receptors expressed by restricted sets of T-cell clones and demonstrated the heterodimeric nature of these 'clonotypic' receptors (McIntyre and Allison 1983). Several groups showed later on that these heterodimeric receptors, called TCRαβ, were tightly associated on the cell surface with a multimeric transduction complex called CD3 (for a review, see Clevers et al. 1988). Identification of the first TCR gene was achieved in 1984 by the groups of Davis and Mak (Hedrick et al. 1984; Yanagi et al. 1984). The elegant strategy designed by Davis and colleagues to isolate candidate TCR genes relied on two main assumptions: first that the putative TCR genes should be specifically transcribed in T cells and, second, that as with immunoglobulin (Ig) genes, TCR genes should undergo somatic rearrangement. Thus they prepared complementary DNA (cDNA) from a T-cell clone and enriched for T-cell-specific genes by removing the cDNA species that hybridized to B-cell messenger RNA (mRNA). The remaining cDNAs were then used as probes to detect, by Southern blot analysis, genes with patterns that are specifically modified in mature T cells. Following this approach, this group isolated a cDNA showing significant sequence homology with Ig genes, which turned out to encode the TCRβ chain. While looking for the missing α-chain gene (which was isolated a few months later), Tonegawa and colleagues fortuitously identified, in the same year, another gene specifically rearranged in T cells called γ (Saito et al. 1984). Discovery of this 'orphan' gene suggested the existence of new class of TCR, which was totally unexpected from previous immunological studies, and the existence of which remained elusive during the following 2 years. Postulating that, as with the αβ TCR, the γ gene product should form a TCR associated with the CD3 complex, Brenner and colleagues used CD3-specific monoclonal antibodies to immunoprecipitate a new heterodimeric receptor expressed on a distinct set of T cells (Brenner et al. 1986). The TCR gene coding for the missing δ chain was finally identified in 1987 by Davis's group (Chien et al. 1987).

GENOMIC ORGANIZATION AND SOURCE OF TCR DIVERSITY

As for Ig genes, functional TCR genes are generated through somatic recombination of gene segments that are originally separated on the chromosome. This rearrangement process, which is tightly controlled in a lineage- and stage-specific manner, allows the production of myriads of distinct receptors. Similar to antibodies, TCR diversity originates both from the combinatorial usage of VDJ gene segments picked out from a repertoire of distinct elements and from extensive sequence modifications of the rearranged VDJ genes which are mediated by the recombination machinery.

Organization of TCR loci

There are four TCR gene loci in the germline DNA, each comprising arrays of distinct V, J, and in some cases D elements. V elements can be grouped into families, which correspond by convention to sets of V genes with nucleotide sequences that exhibit more than 75 percent homology. V-gene segments have two exons, D and J segments a single exon, and C-gene segments three to five exons. A schematic representation of the organization of TCR loci is represented in Figure 24.1. Detailed description of the VDJ sequences and nomenclatures can be obtained from the ImmunoGenetics database (www.imgt.cnusc.fr:8104).

THE TCRβ LOCUS

The TCRβ locus is located on chromosome 6 in the mouse and 7 in humans. It encompasses a region of grossly 600 kb in humans. All Vβ genes are clustered in the same chromosomal region except *BV30*, which is located downstream of the Cβ2 element and in opposite transcriptional orientation. In humans, there are 67 Vβ elements (of which 41–47 are functional) clustered into 32 Vβ families (Rowen et al. 1996). The 3′ part of the TCRβ locus corresponds to a duplication of an ancestral region comprising one Dβ segment, six functional Jβ segments, and a Cβ gene. The two Cβ genes differ by four amino

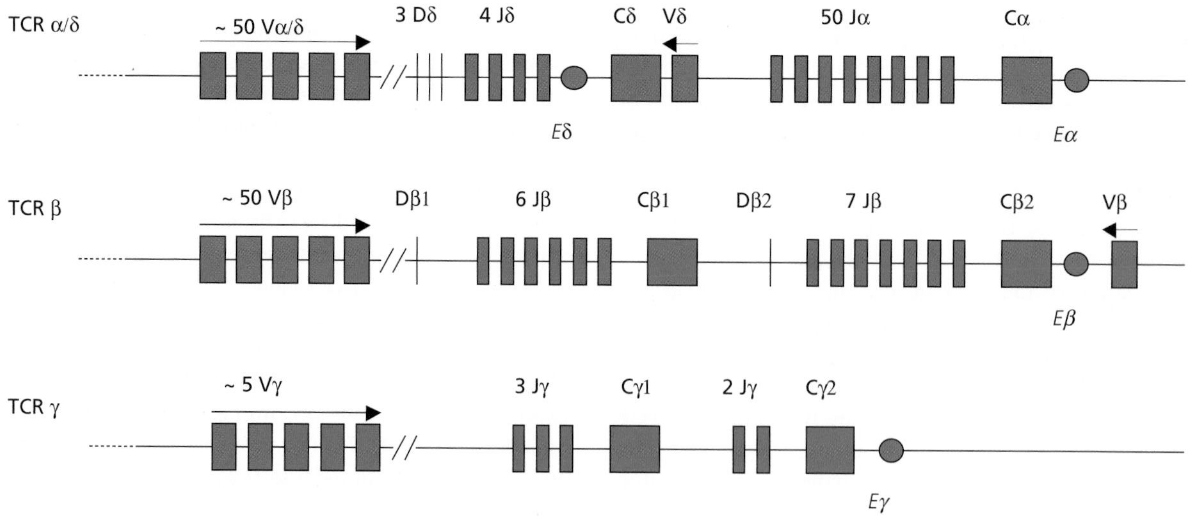

Figure 24.1 *Genomic organization of human T-cell receptor (TCR) gene loci. See the text for details. The numbers mentioned in the figure take into account functional V- and J-gene segments only. V-gene transcriptional orientation is indicated by arrows. Circles correspond to enhancer elements.*

acids only, and appear functionally equivalent. In this regard, unlike Ig genes, rearranged TCR genes do not undergo isotype switching (which consists of replacing the constant region of a rearranged Ig gene by another constant region, generally endowed with distinct functional properties). A β enhancer, which plays a key role in the control of TCRβ locus transcription and rearrangement (see 'Control of TCR gene assembly' below), is located between the Cβ2 element and the downstream BV30 element (Gottschalk and Leiden 1990).

THE TCRα/δ LOCUS

The TCRαδ locus is located on chromosome 14 in rodents and humans, and encompasses a chromosomal region of roughly 1 Mb. It comprises 45–47 functional Vα segments grouped into 41 families in humans. There are 50 functional Jα elements and a single Cα gene. The TCRδ locus is located within the α locus, between the Vα and Jα segments. This peculiar location has important implications because any VJα rearrangement leads to deletion of the δ locus. Together with transcriptional regulation processes detailed below, this mechanism prevents co-expression of α and δ chains and ensures mutual expression of αβ and γδ TCR in a given T cell. The human δ locus comprises three Dδ segments (two in rodents), four Jδ segments (two in rodents), and one Cδ segment. The Vδ and Vα elements are interspersed, which theoretically permits their rearrangement to either DJδ or Jα elements. Although this happens to be the case for some V segments (Miossec et al. 1990), the sets of Vα/δ elements used to form αβ and γδ TCR are generally distinct and only eight Vα/δ elements are used to a significant extent by γδ cells. Among these, one Vδ segment (DV3) is located between the Cδ and Jα elements, in an opposite transcriptional orientation. The rules governing usage of V-gene segments by either the α or δ chain are still unclear but presumably complex. It is likely that both cell-selection processes and locus accessibility constraints contribute to the biased expression of particular Vδ regions by most γδ T cells (see below). Several regulatory sequences controlling TCRα/δ locus transcription and rearrangement have been identified: a TCRα enhancer located downstream to the Cα gene (Ho et al. 1989), the T-early α (TEA) element (which controls rearrangements involving the most upstream Jα segments) between the Cδ and Jα elements (de Chasseval and De Villartay 1993; Wilson et al. 1996), a TCRα silencer (called BEAD-1 for blocking element α–δ 1) immediately upstream from TEA (Zhong and Krangel 1997) and a TCRδ enhancer upstream from the Cδ gene (Redondo et al. 1990).

THE TCRγ LOCUS

Located on chromosome 13 in the mouse and 7 in humans, the γ locus is spread over 160 kb in humans and 200 kb in the mouse. Its genomic organization significantly differs between these two species. In the mouse, there are four clusters presumably resulting from duplication events, which each comprise a single J and C segment together with one to four Vγ segments. A γ enhancer is found downstream to Cγ1 and Cγ3 and upstream from Cγ2 (Vernooij et al. 1993). The human γ locus comprises 11–14 Vγ segments (of which four to six are functional) grouped into four families, and two downstream clusters of J- and C-gene segments (Lefranc and Rabbitts 1989). A γ enhancer and two silencers are found downstream to Cγ2 (Lefranc and Alexandre 1995).

TCR rearrangements

Each TCR chain is encoded by multiple VDJ gene segments which are originally separated on the chromosome. During T-cell development these elements are joined to form a single exon coding for the variable domain of each recognition subunit. The V domain of TCRα and γ chains, like Ig light chains, is encoded by V and J elements, whereas the V domain of TCRβ and δ chains, like Ig heavy chains, is encoded by V, D, and J elements. V(D)J recombination is initiated by recognition and cleavage of double-stranded DNA at conserved sites, named recombination signal sequences (RSS), that immediately flank the V, D, and J elements (Tonegawa 1983). The RSSs are highly conserved in TCR and Ig genes, and each consist of a palindromic 7-base-pair (bp) sequence (consensus 5′-CACAGTG) and an A/T-rich 9-bp sequence (consensus 5′-ACAAAAACC), separated by a poorly conserved spacer, the length of which is either 12 ∓ 1 or 23 ∓ 1 bp (Figure 24.2a). As for Ig genes, recombination between two TCR-gene segments follows the 12/23 rule, i.e. recombination occurs only between an RSS with a 12-bp spacer and one with a 23-bp spacer (Early et al. 1980) (Figure 24.2b). The enzymatic machinery mediating TCR and Ig gene rearrangements involves both lymphoid cell-specific recombinases called RAG1 and RAG2 (Schatz et al. 1989; Oettinger et al. 1990), and ubiquitous enzymes of the DNA-repair machinery (for recent reviews, see Grawunder et al. 1998; Fugmann et al. 2000). The recombination process is outlined below and depicted in Figure 24.3.

V(D)J assembly is initiated by the recognition of the 12-bp and 23-bp RSSs by the RAG proteins, which bring the RSS into close juxtaposition (synapsis) (step no. 1). This step involves two ubiquitous enzymes promoting DNA bending (called high mobility group (HMG)-1 and -2 proteins), which stabilize interactions between RAG proteins and RSSs and ensure the 12/23 rule (Van Gent et al. 1997). RAG proteins then introduce a precise nick on one DNA strand between the RSSs and its flanking element, rapidly followed by cleavage of the other strand (step no. 2). At the end of this first phase, the

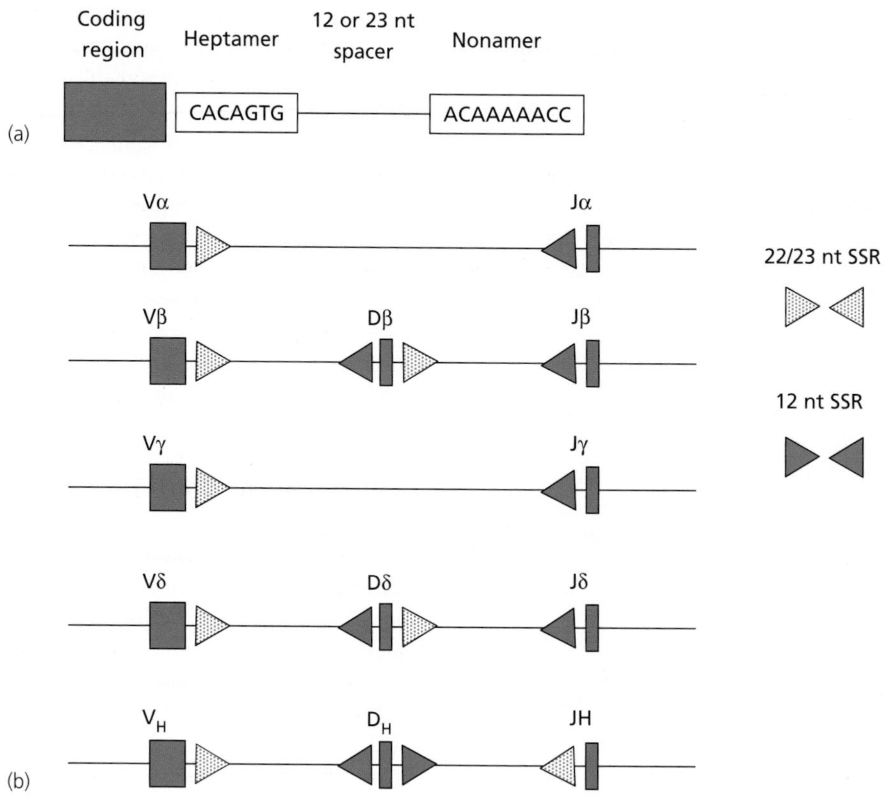

Figure 24.2 *Structure of recombination signal sequences and distribution within the T-cell receptor (TCR) and immunoglobulin (Ig) gene loci. See the text for details.*

recombinases catalyze by a transesterification mechanism both the generation of two open signal strands and the formation of a hairpin between the two open coding strands (McBlane et al. 1995).

The second phase of the recombination reaction is more complex and involves both the recombinases and a larger set of enzymes involved in the repair of DNA double-stranded breaks. The signal ends are joined

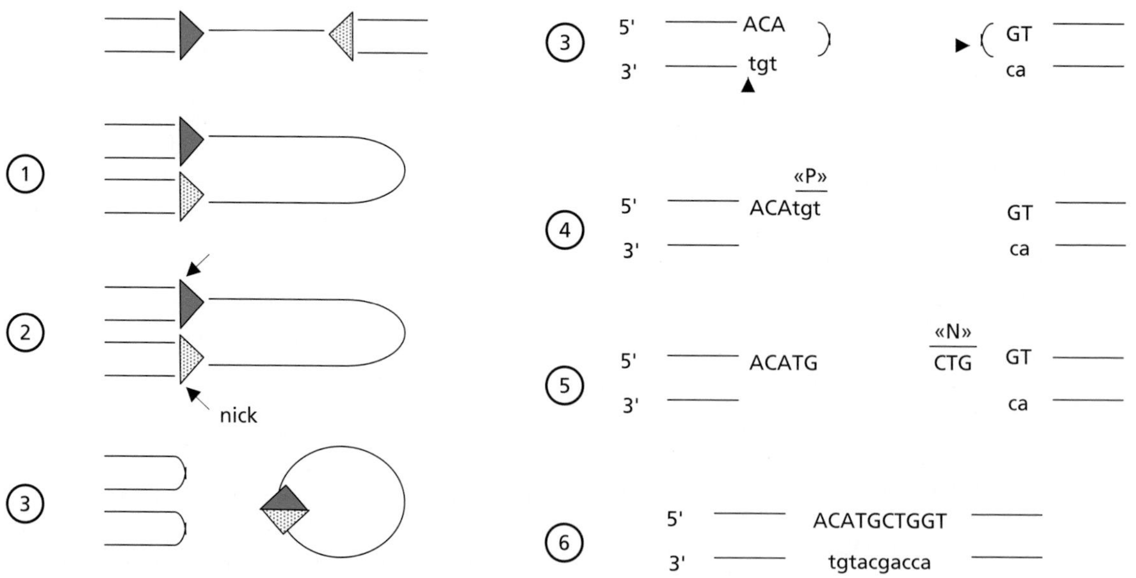

Figure 24.3 *The V(D)J gene recombination reaction. See the text for details. Dark and light triangles correspond to 12 bp and 23 bp recombination signal sequence (RSS). Step 1: synapsis. Step 2: nicking of the RSS. Step 3 (bottom left): generation of hairpins at the coding ends, formation of signal joints in excised circular DNA. Step 3 (up right): hairpin nicking resulting in nibbling of coding ends or addition of 'P' nucleotides (step 4). Step 5: addition of 'N' nucleotides. Step 6: filling and ligation of the coding joints.*

head to head, leading to formation of a 'signal joint' (step no. 3). This process is catalyzed by the RAG proteins and the ubiquitous HMG and Ku DNA-repair proteins (Agrawal and Schatz 1997). On the other side of the recombination complex, the hairpin formed between the two coding ends is opened through introduction of a nick, possibly catalyzed by the recombinases themselves (Shockett and Schatz 1999) (step no. 3). This nicking process is quite imprecise because it occurs at the tip of the hairpin, the coding strand, or the noncoding strand. This generates, respectively, full-length coding ends, deletions on the coding end, or addition of so-called palindromic (or 'P') nucleotides derived from the noncoding strand (Lafaille et al. 1989; Lieber 1991) (step no. 4). In mice deficient for the catalytic subunit of DNA–protein kinase (DNA-PKcs) or for Ku proteins, there is an almost complete abrogation of T- and B-cell production, accompanied by accumulation of uncleaved hairpin coding ends in developing lymphocytes (Lieber et al. 1988; Zhu et al. 1996). This indicates that DNA-PKcs and Ku proteins are both required for RAG-mediated hairpin opening, and probably act by stabilizing interactions between the RAG protein and the coding end-complex. After hairpin opening, the coding ends may undergo an exonucleolytic processing controlled in part by the DNA-PK, which results in significant nibbling of the rearranged VDJ elements. Variable numbers of so-called 'N' nucleotides may be added in a template-independent fashion at the coding ends (step no. 5). This reaction is catalyzed by a lymphoid cell-specific polymerase called terminal deoxynucleotidyl transferase (TdT) (Komori et al. 1993), which acts in conjunction with DNA-PKcs and Ku proteins (Bogue et al. 1997). As for B cells, TdT expression is repressed during embryonic life, resulting in lack of 'N' additions within the rearranged TCR genes produced at that stage. The physiological significance of the regulated expression of TdT during development is still unclear. As suggested by analysis of fetal γδ T-cell development in in vitro thymic organ cultures, TdT repression may favor generation of particular fetal T-cell subsets with conserved TCR and possibly mandatory functions (Ikuta et al. 1990). Alternately lack of TdT activity may prevent development of particular lymphoid subsets which might be deleterious during fetal life.

In the last step of the recombination reaction, the sense and antisense strands of the processed coding ends tend to align along short homologous regions of two to three nucleotides (homology-guided recombination) (Feeney 1992). As discussed earlier, the homology-guided recombination process favors the production of TCR with particular junctional sequences, which may represent a significant fraction of the fetal TCR repertoire (Itohara et al. 1993). The double-stranded DNA junctions are reconstituted through the combined action of yet undefined polymerases and nucleases (step no. 6). Final ligation of the coding strands is performed by the ligase IV/XRCC4 complex, presumably recruited by the Ku proteins (Nick McElhinny et al. 2000).

Modalities of TCR recombination

As for Ig genes, the intervening DNA sequence separating the rearranged TCR gene segments has two possible outcomes (Figure 24.4). When the rearrangement involves

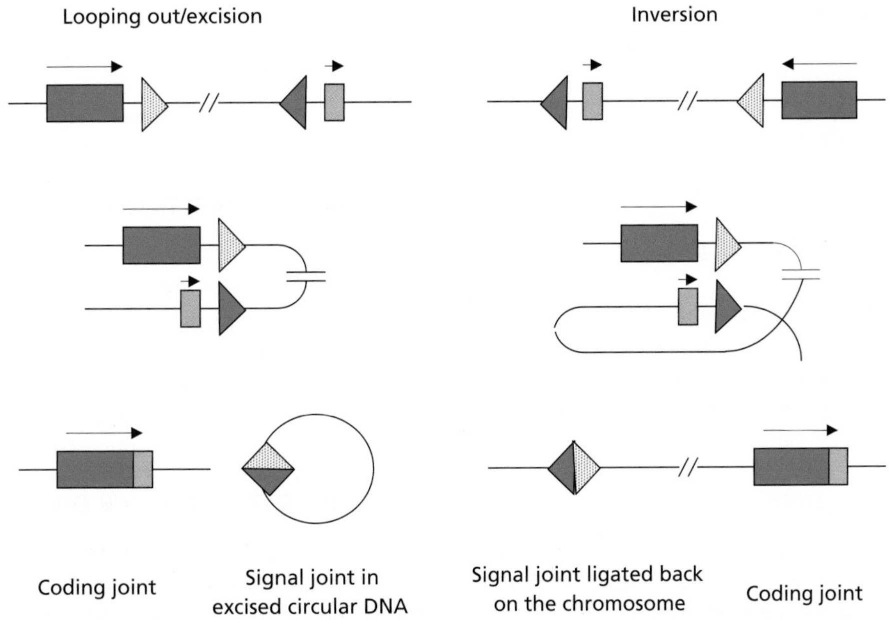

Figure 24.4 *Recombination modalities. See the text for details. Rectangles: coding regions. Triangles: recombination signal sequences (RSSs). Arrows: transcriptional orientation.*

elements in the same transcriptional orientation, which is the classic situation, the intervening DNA stretch between the rearranged gene segments is removed in the form of circular excision products, generated on head-to-head ligation of the RSS (looping out/excision model) (Okazaki et al. 1997). These circular DNAs are specifically found within developing lymphocytes and, thus, can be used as markers to follow T-cell regeneration, e.g. in HIV patients and bone marrow recipients. When the rearrangement involves gene segments in opposite transcriptional orientation (as is the case for the most downstream V elements in the TCRβ and TCRδ loci), the intervening DNA is ligated back and translocated on the chromosome through a chromosomal inversion mechanism (Malissen et al. 1986).

Although recombination events classically involve gene segments belonging to the same locus, they sometimes occur between distinct TCR loci, TCR and Ig loci, or TCR or Ig loci and other genomic elements. These interlocus recombinations or 'trans-rearrangements' are mediated through recognition of classic RSS and/or related or cryptic RSS motifs that are present throughout the genome. The peculiar configuration of the TCRα/δ locus naturally favors rearrangements of a given Vα/δ element to either DJδ or Jα segments (Miossec et al. 1990). Rearrangements between human TCRβ and TCRγ loci, which are both located on chromosome 7 but in distinct regions and in opposite orientations, may occur at high frequencies in T cells from healthy donors and patients with ataxia telangiectasia (Lipkowitz et al. 1990). These trans-rearrangements lead to expression of functional Vγ(Dβ)JβCβ chains that pair with classic TCRα chains, and thus significantly contribute to TCR repertoire diversification (Davodeau et al. 1994; Retière et al. 1999). Finally some lymphoid tumors may originate from illegitimate recombinations between an RSS within a TCR or Ig locus and a cryptic signal sequence close to an oncogene, e.g. Burkitt's lymphomas result from rearrangements between the protooncogene *c-myc* and RSS flanking Jα segments, leading to constitutive expression of *c-myc* expression under the control of the α enhancer (Bernard et al. 1988).

Sources of TCR diversity

Although the number of germline V(D)J elements is much lower in TCRs than in Ig loci, several mechanisms operate during TCR gene assembly to yield a high degree of diversity within the junctional regions of the rearranged VJ or VDJ genes.

COMBINATORIAL DIVERSITY

TCR combinatorial diversity is determined by the number of random V(D)J combinations yielding an αβ or γδ TCR. Although lower than Ig, the combinatorial diversity of αβ TCR appears to be much higher than that of γδ TCR. The random assembly of TCR VJα and VDJβ genes can generate, grossly, 2500 (i.e. 50×50) and 1200 (i.e. $50 \times 2 \times 12$) possible combinations respectively. Considering a random association of α and β chains, this yields up to 3×10^6 distinct TCRs. By contrast, the total number of VJγ/VDJδ combinations is around 3000 only (i.e. $(6 \times 5) \times (10 \times 3 \times 4)$) in humans. An additional source of combinatorial diversity is provided by the peculiar arrangement of the 12- and 23-bp RSSs in TCR genes which permits, unlike Ig genes, joining of several D-gene segments in tandem (see Figure 24.2b). Such joining events, yielding VDDJ or even VDDDJ junctions, are frequently seen within rearranged TCRδ genes and drastically broaden the junctional length distribution of the δ chains (Chien et al. 1996).

JUNCTIONAL DIVERSITY

VDJ assembly is associated with important modifications of the coding ends of the rearranged segments (see Figure 24.3). First, the imprecise cleavage of hairpin coding ends may lead to either 'P' nucleotide additions or nibbling of V(D)J sequences. Second, further VDJ nibbling may occur at a later stage of the recombination reaction by exonucleolytic processing. Third, addition of variable numbers of 'N' nucleotides by TdT may further increase junctional sequence diversity. All these mechanisms operate in both TCR and Ig gene rearrangements. However, although 'N' additions occur in rearranged Ig heavy chain genes only, they are observed in all rearranged TCR genes. Reading frame changes resulting from nucleotide addition and trimming may generate nonproductive rearrangements but, in the case of VDJ rearrangements, they may also generate new junctional sequences encoded by alternate reading frames. In this regard, unlike D_H segments, both the Dβ and Dδ segments can be read in all three reading frames. Altogether nucleotide addition and nibbling at the V(D)J joints generate an enormous diversity in these regions. Considering that up to six nucleotides can be added at each junction, the number of distinct junctional sequences that can be produced in the order of 10^7 to 10^{11}.

SOMATIC HYPERMUTATION

In B cells, additional diversity is generated in the rearranged V(D)J genes by somatic hypermutation (see Chapter 16, Antibodies and B Lymphocytes). By contrast, TCR genes do not undergo somatic hypermutation. This probably ensures that the T-cell repertoire is not modified after its thymic selection and avoids generation of cells with unwanted self-reactivity.

FACTORS RESTRICTING TCR DIVERSITY

The combined effects of combinatorial and junctional diversification processes theoretically permit the production of up to 10^{16} distinct TCRs in a given individual. However, this number is probably largely overestimated for several reasons. Assembly of V(D)J segments is not random because, in general, not all gene segments are equally accessible to the recombination machinery at a given time point. In particular the most downstream V and upstream J elements tend to be rearranged first during ontogeny (Thompson et al. 1990), probably reflecting progressive 'opening' of the TCR locus under the control of proximal *cis*-acting elements. This is also illustrated by the programmed rearrangement of different sets of VDJ gene segments at particular T-cell developmental stages (Goldman et al. 1993; Itohara et al. 1993), which favors generation of distinct waves of γδ TCR with restricted combinations of VJγ and VDJδ elements. Finally, both the repression of TdT activity during fetal life and homology-guided recombination further restrict the diversity of the fetal repertoire, which is sometimes dominated by few 'canonical' TCR sequences (Itohara et al. 1993).

CONTROL OF TCR GENE ASSEMBLY

Assembly of TCR and Ig V(D)J segments is regulated in a tissue-, lineage-, and stage-specific fashion. The restricted expression of RAG proteins in lymphoid cells at a particular stage of their development confers both the tissue- and stage-specificity of the recombination process. In addition, the restricted activation of Ig and TCR gene rearrangements in respectively T and B cells is controlled by *cis*- and *trans*-acting elements that regulate the 'accessibility' of TCR and Ig gene loci to the recombinases (Sleckman et al. 1996).

Regulation of TCR gene assembly during T-cell development

T-cell development is a highly complex and ordered epigenetic process that allows efficient generation and highly restricted TCR expression in the appropriate cell lineage, as well as selection of TCR with 'useful' (i.e. self-MHC-restricted) and 'harmless' (i.e. nonself-reactive) specificities. Importantly a tight control of the accessibility of the various TCR loci to the recombination machinery, which is transiently activated during the pre-T-cell stage, leads to a highly ordered activation of TCR rearrangements in the developing T cell (Figure 24.5) and early commitment of precursor cells to either the αβ or the γδ lineage (Figure 24.6).

INITIATION OF TCR REARRANGEMENTS AND PRE-TCR FORMATION

Intrathymic T-cell maturation can be subdivided into discrete developmental stages characterized by a particular TCR rearrangement status and phenotypic profile (Shortman and Wu 1996). In the mouse the earliest precursors, which are CD4/CD8 double negative (DN), are further split into four subsets based on CD44 and CD25 expression. RAG protein expression is initiated in $CD44^+CD25^-$ (DN I) precursors (Wilson et al. 1994). VJγ, partial VDδ or DJδ and few complete VDJδ rearrangements are first detected at the $CD44^+CD25^+$ (DN II) stage (Livak et al. 1999). Most VJγ, VDJδ, and partial DJβ rearrangements take place during transition to the $CD44^-CD25^+$ (DN III) stage (Tourigny et al. 1997). Complete VDJβ rearrangements are initiated in $CD44^+CD25^+$ cells and are completed in $CD44^-CD25^-$ (DN IV) cells, where productive VDJβ rearrangements are primarily found. VJα rearrangements are first detected in $CD44^-CD25^-$ cells but mainly take place at the following $CD4^+CD8^+$ stage.

A similarly ordered rearrangement of TCRδ, γ, β, and α genes has been more recently documented in human thymocytes (Blom et al. 1999). The TCRβ chains, which are produced at a stage when the α locus is still in germline configuration, pair with a surrogate α chain called

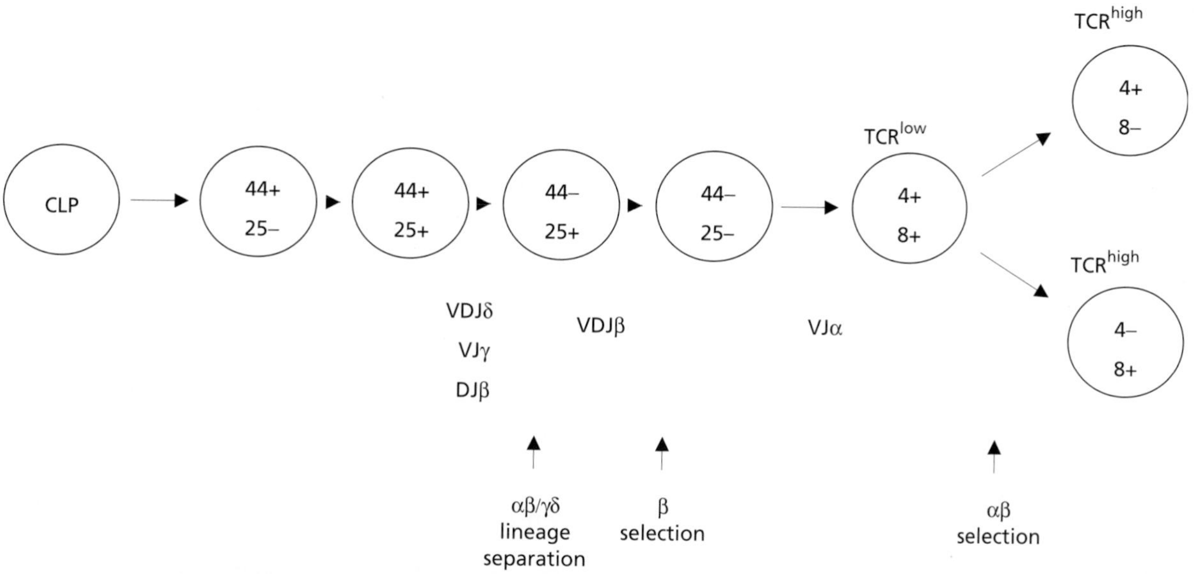

Figure 24.5 *Intrathymic development of murine T cells. See the text for details. CLP, common lymphoid progenitor.*

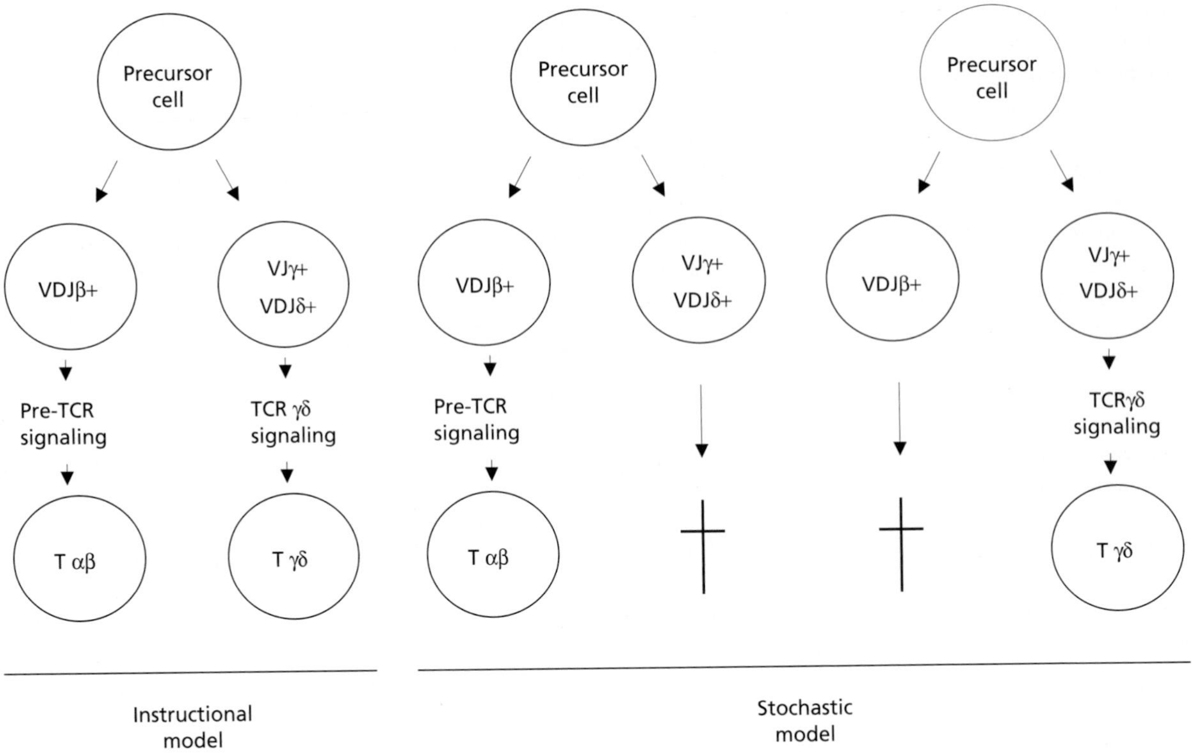

Figure 24.6 *Models of αβ/γδ lineage separation. See the text for details.*

pTα to form a 'pre-TCR' (Saint Ruf et al. 1994). The pTα is encoded by a non-rearranging gene, the expression of which is transiently switched on during T-cell development. It comprises a single Ig-like ectodomain, a transmembrane region with a positively charged amino acid, and a short intracytoplasmic region. Similar to the TCR, the pre-TCR is associated with a complex of CD3 subunits that mediates signal transduction (see 'TCR structure' below). Signaling through the CD3/pre-TCR complex induces transient but massive thymocyte proliferation, paralleled by rapid loss of CD25 and acquisition of CD4, CD8, CD2, CD5, and CD69 markers (Levelt et al. 1995). The mere expression of pre-TCR/CD3 complexes (i.e. without engagement by a putative thymic ligand) is probably sufficient to induce the transition from the DN to the $CD4^+CD8^+$ stage (Irving et al. 1998). Signaling through the pre-TCR (also called 'β selection') represents a key developmental checkpoint, which permits selective expansion and subsequent maturation of T-cell precursors that have generated a functional TCRβ chain. Consistent with a such a critical role played by the pre-TCR, T-cell development is arrested at the $CD44^-CD25^+$ stage in mice deficient for the RAG, β, pTα, CD3γ, or CD3ε proteins (for a recent review, see Sebzda et al. 1999).

EXPRESSION AND INTRATHYMIC SELECTION OF αβ TCR

During the proliferation phase induced by pre-TCR signaling, recombinase activity is drastically reduced as a result of phosphorylation and accelerated degradation of the RAG2 protein (Lin and Desiderio 1994). Re-expression of RAG proteins at this stage seems to be controlled by specific *cis*-acting elements located upstream of the RAG2 promoter (Yu et al. 1999). RAG expression and 'opening' of the α loci allow VJα rearrangements and expression of αβ TCR, which then undergo intrathymic selection. According to the widely accepted affinity/avidity model, the outcome of the $CD4^+CD8^+$ thymocyte will depend on the strength of the avidity signal delivered by its TCR, which integrates both the affinity of the TCR for self-pMHC complexes and the number or density of TCR/pMHC interactions. Below a given avidity threshold, the thymocyte dies by neglect. Above it, the thymocyte is positively selected, i.e. it receives a maturation signal that triggers RAG protein shut-off, TCR upregulation, and modulation of either CD4 or CD8 co-receptors. Finally thymocytes showing very high avidity for self-pMHC are negatively selected, i.e. they receive an apoptotic or inactivating signal leading to their deletion or anergization. Altogether these thymic selection processes, while avoiding production of self-reactive T cells, allow generation of a functional T-cell repertoire with significant affinity for self-MHC (Sebzda et al. 1999).

TCR ALLELIC EXCLUSION

As a result of their diploid nature, T-cell precursors can produce up to four distinct αβ TCRs. T-cell clones generally express a single β chain, which indicates that, similar to Ig genes, the TCRβ locus exhibits allelic exclusion (for a review, see Malissen et al. 1992). Endogenous VDJβ, but not DJβ, gene rearrangements are inhibited in mice expressing a functional TCRβ transgene, suggesting a tight exclusion mechanism whereby generation of a productive VDJβ rearrangement blocks subsequent V to DJβ rearrangement on the other allele (Uematsu et al. 1988). The increased frequency of precursors carrying two complete VDJβ rearrangements in pTα-deficient mice suggests a key implication of the pre-TCR in the negative feedback loop leading to allelic exclusion (Aifantis et al. 1997). Therefore TCRβ exclusion can be explained by the fact that, in the presence of pTα, any functional β chain, irrespective of its specificity, forms a pre-TCR that systematically generates an allelic exclusion signal. Its precise mechanism is still unclear but probably relies on both a transient reduction of the recombinase activity during the proliferation phase that follows pre-TCR signaling and concomitant inhibition of β locus accessibility to recombinases (Sleckman et al. 1996). Unlike β chains, expression of two distinct α chains is quite frequent within mature T-cell clones, indicating a less stringent rearrangement control in the α loci (Padovan et al. 1993). Accordingly, T cells from mice expressing a functional TCRα transgene frequently express endogenous α genes (Borgulya et al. 1992). TCRα allelic inclusion is explained by the fact that the TCRα rearrangement arrest signal, which leads to recombinase shut off in the developing thymocyte, is only generated after TCR engagement by a positively selecting ligand (Turka et al. 1991). Therefore in a T cell that expresses two distinct αβ TCRs, only one is likely to be functional, i.e. restricted by self-MHC molecules.

αβ/γδ LINEAGE SEPARATION

Targeted inactivation of pTα or β genes in the mouse abrogates development of αβ T cells and drastically inhibits production of double-positive thymocytes. By contrast it has no effect on the generation of γδ T cells, which indicates that γδ T-cell development does not require a pre-TCR (Fehling et al. 1995). Accordingly, unlike β and α genes, activation of γ and δ gene rearrangements occurs concomitantly during development, suggesting that γδ T cells do not undergo a 'preselection' process. αβ and γδ T cells derive from a common progenitor and probably diverge during the transition from the DN III to the DN IV stage (Mertsching et al. 1997). Analyses of the TCR rearrangement status of developing and mature T cells suggest several models of αβ/γδ lineage separation (see Figure 24.6). According to the 'stochastic' model, precursor cells are precommitted to one or the other lineage before TCR rearrangement and expression. This assumption is supported by studies documenting transcriptional silencing of pTα or α genes in γδ T-cell precursors (Capone et al. 1993; Mertsching et al. 1997) or silencing of some γ genes in αβ T cells (Ishida et al. 1990).

'Instructive' models postulate that the fate of a given precursor is determined by the expressed TCR, i.e. generation of productive γ and δ rearrangements and subsequent expression of γδ TCR engage the precursor toward the γδ lineage, whereas generation of a productive β rearrangement and pre-TCR expression engage the precursor toward the αβ lineage. Among these last models, the 'separate lineage' model proposes that αβ T cells primarily develop from precursor cells that have failed to produce a functional γδ TCR, assuming that VJγ and VDJδ rearrangements precede VDJβ rearrangements during ontogeny (Dudley et al. 1995). According to the 'competitive' model, which seems better supported by recent studies (Livak et al. 1995; Aifantis et al. 1998), VJγ, VDJδ, and VDJβ gene rearrangements take place concomitantly in the same precursor cell, the fate of which is determined by the TCR or pre-TCR that is first produced. Actually, none of these models provides fully satisfactory explanations for all the experimental data obtained so far. It seems likely that the modalities of αβ/γδ lineage separation differ from one subset to another and are possibly determined by a mix of stochastic and instructive events, as is the case for the differentiation of $CD4^+CD8^+$ thymocytes into either $CD4^+CD8^-$ or $CD4^-CD8^+$ cells (see Chapter 20, $CD4^+$ T lymphocytes and Chapter 22, The role of CD8 T cells in the control of infectious disease and malignancies).

Factors controlling TCR accessibility to recombinases

Expression of transfected RAG proteins in nonlymphoid cells leads to rearrangement of plasmid-like recombination substrates, but not to endogenous TCR or Ig genes (Schatz et al. 1992). Thus, unlike developing lymphocytes, the antigen-receptor genes of nonlymphoid cells are not accessible to the recombination machinery. The fact the Ig and TCR gene rearrangements are restricted respectively to B and T cells suggests differential control of the accessibility of these antigen receptor loci in the corresponding lymphoid precursors (Sleckman et al. 1996). The mechanisms controlling TCR locus accessibility are not completely understood. VDJ recombination closely correlates with changes in chromatin structure, changes in gene methylation status, and transcriptional activation of TCR (or Ig) gene loci (Sleckman et al. 1996). Active transcription of germline V segments coincides with their rearrangement, as clearly illustrated by analysis of the TCRγ locus, where production of germline Vγ transcripts tightly correlates with the ordered rearrangement of these segments during development (Goldman et al. 1993). Along this line analyses of transgenic recombination substrates suggest a key role played by *cis*-acting transcriptional enhancer elements in regulating, in a tissue-, lineage- and stage-specific fashion, recombination of a given TCR or Ig gene locus, e.g. rearrangements of endogenous α genes occur at a later developmental stage than for endogenous β genes. Accordingly β transgenes carrying an α enhancer rearrange later than the same transgenes with a β enhancer, suggesting a direct role of enhancer elements in dictating the stage specificity of VDJ recombination (Capone et al. 1993). However, recombination and rearrangement are not always strictly correlated. In particular, deletion of the β enhancer inhibits both TCRβ transcription and rearrangements. However, RAG-mediated cleavage of VDJβ elements still occurs but ligation of the coding end is prevented. This suggests that the β enhancer regulates the late stages of the recombination reaction but to a lesser extent the locus accessibility to recombinases (Hempel et al. 1998).

Transcriptional regulation is mediated in part by interactions between *trans*-acting DNA-binding proteins with specific motifs in *cis*-acting promoter and enhancer elements. This process turns out to be particularly complex and involves the combinatorial action of several ubiquitous transcriptional factors (Ernst and Smale 1995). As a result of this complexity, it has not been possible yet to identify specific combinations of transcriptional factors able to regulate, in a lineage- or stage-specific fashion, TCR or Ig gene rearrangements, e.g. mutations in the binding sites for *c-myb* and CBF/PEBP2 transcription factors within the δ enhancer abrogate recombination of a TCRδ minilocus. However, replacement of the δ enhancer by a DNA fragment carrying both *c-myb* and CBF/PEBP2 sites does not restore recombination, indicating the need for additional factors for proper regulation of δ rearrangements (Lauzurica et al. 1997).

Besides transcriptional activation, occurrence of VDJ rearrangements is tightly associated with remodeling of chromatin structure, possibly under the direct control of TCR enhancers. In particular histone hyperacetylation and associated chromatin decondensation strongly correlate with activation and/or completion of VDJ rearrangements (McMurry and Krangel 2000). Gene methylation, which is associated with transcriptional silencing, also prevents TCR rearrangements (Hsieh and Lieber 1992). TCR locus demethylation, which is concomitant to VDJ recombination, seems again directly regulated by the enhancers (Kirillov et al. 1996).

Finally *cis*-acting elements blocking TCR accessibility have been identified in the TCRα and γ loci (Ishida et al. 1990). These 'silencers' may selectively repress, in either a stochastic or instructive manner recombination of a given locus in precursor cells committed to the reciprocal cell lineage (see 'Regulation of TCR gene assembly during T-cell development' above).

TCR STRUCTURE

Overall structure of the T-cell recognition complex

TCR CHAINS

αβ and γδ TCRs are expressed in a mutually exclusive fashion on T cells. In adult thymus, blood, spleen, and lymph nodes, the vast majority of T cells express αβ TCRs in rodents and primates. By contrast γδ T cells are greatly enriched in epithelial sites where they sometimes make up all $CD3^+$ T cells (see Chapter 23, Unconventional T cells). The apparent molecular mass (M_r) of α and β chains, which are both glycosylated, is around 42–48 kDs (Clevers et al. 1988). The M_r of γ and δ chains ranges from 30 to 60 kDa and from 40 to 60 kDa, respectively. The isoelectric point of γ and β chains is basic and that of α and δ chains acidic. Each TCR chain possesses a short cytoplasmic tail, a hydrophobic transmembrane region and a large extracellular portion comprising two Ig-like domains, a variable and a constant domain which are respectively distal and proximal to the membrane (Figure 24.7).

As with Ig, the variable domain is encoded by two to three gene segments that form a single exon after somatic rearrangement (Figure 24.8). The amino-terminal part of the variable domain is encoded by the V-gene segment whereas its carboxy-terminal part is encoded by either a single J segment (for α and γ) or D and J segments (for β and δ chains). The length of the V region is around 75–95 amino acids, the J region 15 amino acids, and the D region 5 amino acids. The constant domain is encoded by a C gene comprising three to four exons. The first exon codes for the globular domain stabilized by an intrachain disulfide bond, which is slightly longer (125–135 amino acids for β) or shorter (85 amino acids for α) than the Ig domain (around 110 amino acids). The second exon codes for a 'connecting' region of six amino acids, which frequently comprises a cysteine involved in the covalent binding of the two TCR chains. This cysteine is absent in the duplicated or triplicated exon II of the human Cγ2 gene, but the corresponding γ chain can still form functional TCR by pairing noncovalently with the TCRδ chain (Lefranc and Rabbitts 1989). The transmembrane region of each TCR subunit (21–22 amino acids long) is encoded by a third exon. Although strongly hydrophobic, this region comprises one or two positively charged residues that establish electrostatic interactions with acidic residues located in the transmembrane region of several subunits of the CD3 signal transduction complex. Mutation of these residues abrogates CD3/TCR assembly (Hall et al. 1991). The short TCR chain intracytoplasmic region (4–12 amino acids) is

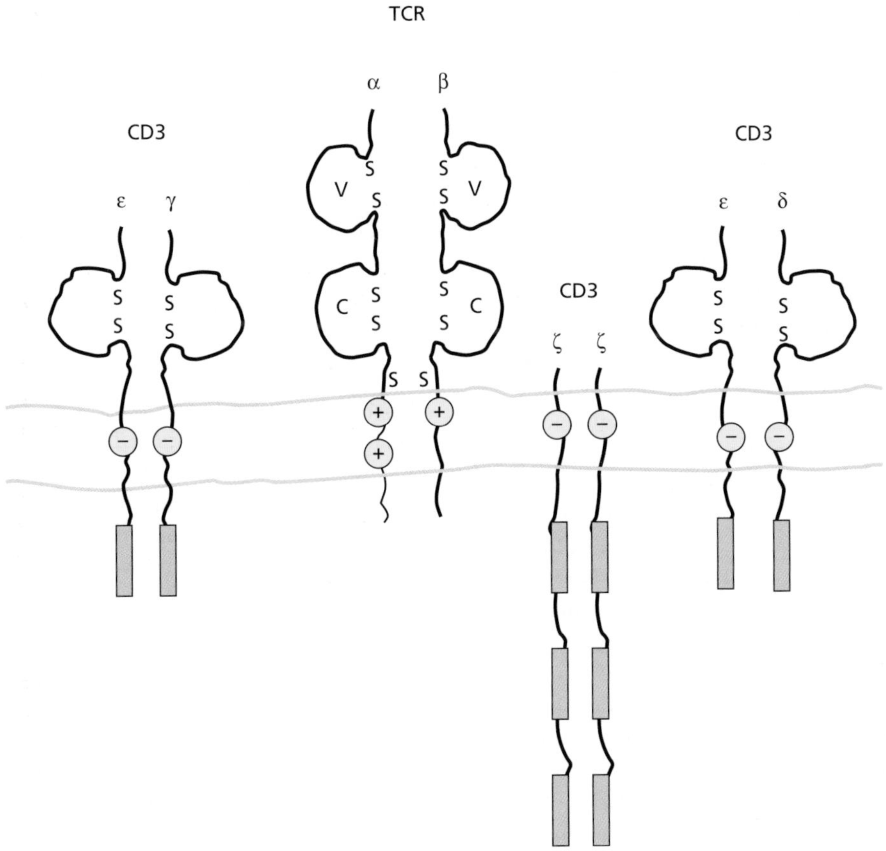

Figure 24.7 *Overall structure of the T-cell receptor (TCR)/CD3 complex. See the text for details. – and + symbols correspond to acidic and basic residues located within the transmembrane region of TCR and CD3 chains. ITAMs located on the intracellular portion of CD3 subunits are symbolized by rectangles. S-S, disulfide bridges.*

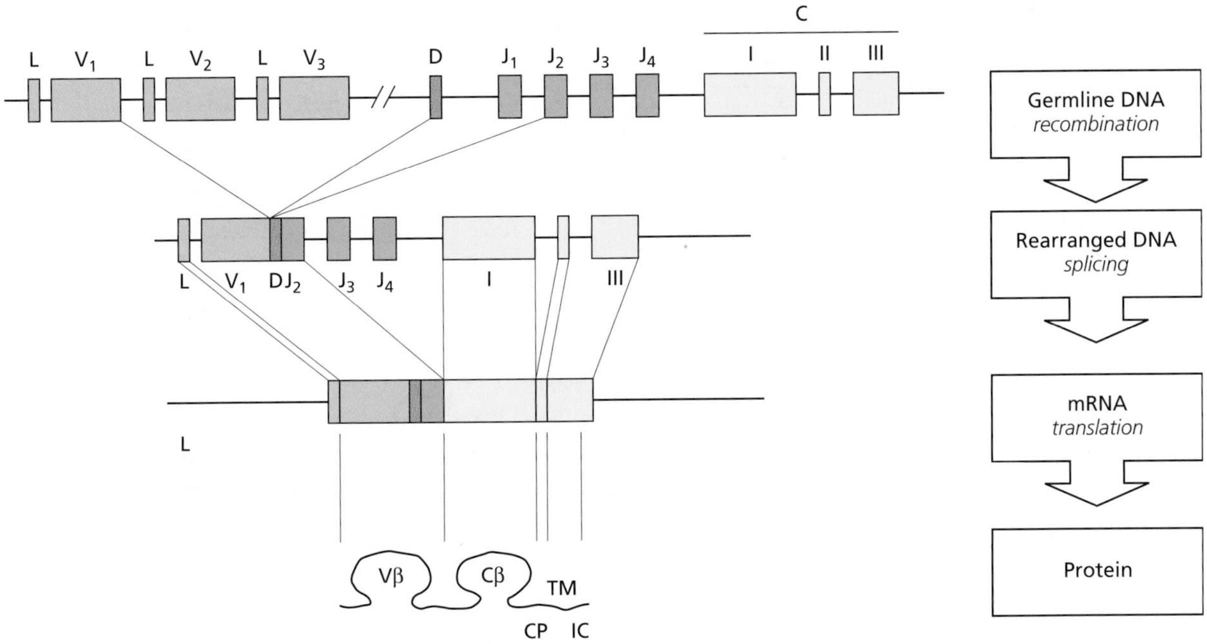

Figure 24.8 *Biosynthesis of a T-cell receptor (TCR)β chain. See the text for details. I, II, III, exons of the Cb gene; CP, connecting peptide; IC, intracytoplasmic region; TM, transmembrane region.*

encoded by either exon III (for Cβ genes) or a fourth exon (for Cα genes) (Figure 24.8).

THE CD3 TRANSDUCTION COMPLEX

None of the TCR subunits possesses a cytoplasmic tail long enough to permit signal transduction after antigen recognition. This function is mediated by a multimeric complex called CD3, which is closely associated with the αβ and γδ TCR and required for TCR surface expression (Sussman et al. 1988; Hall et al. 1991) (see Figure 24.7). In this way, the TCR complex appears very similar to the BCR complex, which consists of an antigen recognition unit (the membrane-bound immunoglobulin) associated with a transduction complex composed of Igα and Igβ subunits (see Chapter 16, Antibodies and B lymphocytes). Five distinct CD3 subunits, called γ, δ, ε, ζ, and ν, have been biochemically identified within the CD3 complex (Borst et al. 1983). In most instances, the CD3 complex is composed of four distinct subunits (γ, δ, ε, and ζ) that are organized in three dimeric transduction modules: γε, δε, and ζζ (Alarcon et al. 1991). CD3γ, -δ, and -ε are encoded by highly homologous genes located within a 50-kb region on chromosome 11 in human and 9 in the mouse (Letourneur et al. 1989). The CD3ζ gene is located on chromosome 1 and can undergo an alternate splicing in the mouse, which leads to generation of either a CD3ζ or a CD3ν protein (Jin et al. 1990). Although the CD3 γ, δ, and ε chains possess a single Ig-like ectodomain of 80 amino acids, the CD3-ζ and ν chains have a very short (nine amino acids) extracellular region. All CD3 subunits contain a negatively charged acidic residue (Asp) in their transmembrane region, which ensures proper assembly of the CD3/TCR complex (see above). The intracytoplasmic tail of all CD3 subunits contain one (for CD3γ, -δ, or -ε) to three (for CD3ζ) consensus motifs called immuno-tyrosine-based activation motif (ITAM) (Reth 1989). These motifs, also found in a variety of other immune receptors (such as Igα/β and some Fc receptors), play a key role in signal transduction by interacting, once phosphorylated, with specific tyrosine kinases required for the initiation of the signaling cascade (like ZAP-70 in T cells) (see also Chapter 17, The B cell antigen receptor). The composition and stoichiometry of CD3 complexes may differ from one T cell to another. In the mouse, about 5–10 percent of $CD3^+$ lymphocytes express ζν heterodimers instead of ζζ homodimers (Baniyash et al. 1988). Although ν is not found on human T cells, some $CD3^+$ T cells in both species may utilize the FcεRIγ subunit instead of the ζ chain (Koyasu et al. 1992). The qualitative/quantitative differences of the signals initiated by CD3 complexes containing ζζ, ζν, or FcεRIγ dimers are still unclear. Finally the composition of CD3 complexes associated with αβ and γδ TCR show differences: unlike αβ TCR complexes, γδ TCR complexes lack CD3δ and rapidly recruit FcεRIγ on T-cell activation (Hayes and Love 2002).

THE CD4 AND CD8 CO-RECEPTORS

Interactions between the αβ TCR and pMHC complexes are classically strengthened by the CD4 or CD8 co-receptors, which bind to the conserved part of MHC class II and class I molecules respectively. As detailed in Chapters 20, CD4+ T lymphocytes and 22, The role of CD8 T cells in the control of infectious disease and malignancies, these co-receptors also play a key role in the initiation of signal transduction by recruiting $p56^{lck}$, which then mediates early phosphorylation of ITAM on the CD3 subunits. As the CD4 and CD8 co-receptors modulate the avidity of TCR/pMHC interactions, they play a critical function during the intrathymic selection of the TCR repertoire and the terminal maturation of CD4/CD8 double-positive thymocytes into CD4 or CD8 single-positive T cells (Ellmeier et al. 1999).

TCR crystallographic analyses

αβ TCRS

Although Ig can interact with high affinity with a wide variety of native antigen, αβ TCRs must recognize subtle differences between MHC molecules loaded with distinct peptidic antigen. This task is facilitated by the concentration of the TCR structural diversity at the center of the TCR/pMHC interface. As with Ig, diversity of rearranged TCR genes is not evenly distributed within the variable region but is instead clustered in so-called hypervariable (HV) regions. There are two HV regions within the V gene segment (HV1, HV2) and a third one corresponding to the V(D)J junction. These three regions code, respectively, for the complementarity determining regions (CDR)-1, -2 and -3 that form the antigen-binding site (see below). A fourth hypervariable region (HV) 4 has been identified in the V region, which forms an additional loop involved in superantigen binding (see 'Structural basis of T-cell antigen recognition' below and see Chapter 29, Superantigens). Consistent with earlier predictions, the overall TCR structure is very similar to that of an Ig Fab fragment (Figure 24.9) (for a recent review, see Garcia et al. 1999).

The C and V domains of both TCR chains adopt a classic 'Ig fold' composed of a sandwich of two β sheets with five inner and four outer β strands for the V domains, and four inner and three outer strands for the carboxyl domains (see also Chapter 16, Antibodies and B lymphocytes, and Chapter 17, The B cell antigen receptor). As for Ig, the CDR loops protrude on top of the V domains to form the antigen-binding site. TCRs also show several distinctive structural features, listed below. The Cβ domain carries a large protruding loop

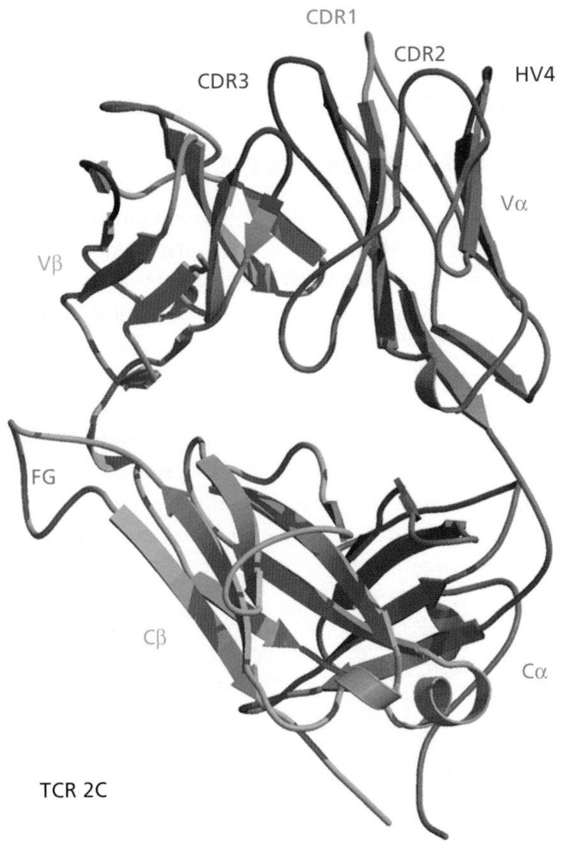

Figure 24.9 *Three-dimensional structure of an αβ T-cell receptor (TCR). See the text for details. Structure of a murine TCR. (Kindly provided by J.B. Reiser and D. Housset, Grenoble, France.)*

between the F and G strands, the significance of which remains unclear. It may facilitate interactions with either some CD3 subunits (Ghendler et al. 1996) or co-receptors. The elbow angle between Vβ and Cβ is fairly constant (between 140° and 150°) contrasting with the much higher flexibility of Ig, with elbow angles ranging from 120° to 225°. Furthermore, the Cα domain shows some structural differences with canonical Ig folds and in particular lacks a C′ and C″ strand. This unusual feature is anticipated from the primary Cα sequence because only 50 amino acids separate the two cysteines, forming the intradomain disulfide bridge in the Cα domain, compared with around 65 amino acids for the Cβ or Ig constant domains. The antigen-binding site of αβ TCR is made of six hypervariable (CDR) loops, three from each Vα and Vβ domain. CDR1 and CDR2 are located in the periphery whereas the two CDR3 are located centrally. While the CDR1 and CDR2 from the Vα and Vβ domains seem to adopt a limited set of canonical conformations, the CDR3α and CDR3β show substantially different conformations and undergo extensive conformational changes upon pMHC bin ing (see below). In this regard, the lack of canonical CDR3 structures is fully consistent with the extensive sequence diversity of the VJα and VDJβ joints (see 'Genomic organization and source of TCR diversity' above).

γδ TCRS

The sole γδ TCR structure resolved so far (Allison et al. 2001) has a highly distinctive overall shape, when compared with αβ TCR or Fab fragments. This unusual shape is produced by a small elbow angle and a small VγCγ interdomain angle, which are both the smallest ever seen within Fabs and TCR structures. Both the Cδ and Cγ domains adopt a canonical Ig fold but the Cγ domain, which is more homologous to Cβ than Cα, does not have the long FG loop found in the Cβ domain. The antigen-binding surface of the γδ TCR appears much rougher than that of αβ TCR. This peculiar feature seems to result mainly from the unusual positioning of the CDR2δ (also seen in crystals of another Vδ domain (Li et al. 1998)), and to large protrusions formed by the CDR3γ and CDR3δ loops. Together with parts of the CDR1 and CDR2 loops, the CDR3 loops form a deep cleft that may constitute the antigen-binding site. Consistent with an Ig-like mode of antigen recognition by γδ TCRs (Chien et al. 1996; see Chapter 23, Unconventional T cells), the jagged antigen-binding surface of the γδ TCR resembles that of an antibody specific to small proteins. However, general predictions about the topology of γδ TCR/antigen interactions, based on analysis of a single unbound γδ TCR, should be taken with caution, particularly in light of the dramatic conformational modifications occurring on the CDR3 loops of several αβ TCR on binding to their pMHC complexes (Reiser et al. 2002).

STRUCTURAL BASIS OF T-CELL ANTIGEN RECOGNITION

Crystallographic analysis of antibody TCR bound to pMHC complexes

As the vast majority of amino acid variations lie in the V(D)J junctional regions, which are equivalent to the centrally located CDR3 within the Ig antigen-binding site, it has been proposed that the CDR3β loops from the Vα and Vβ domains line up above the antigenic peptide, whereas the less diverse CDR1 and CDR2 interact with the MHC molecule (Davis and Bjorkman 1988). As suggested by TCR and MHC mutagenesis studies (Jorgensen et al. 1992; Sant'Angelo et al. 1996) and more recently confirmed by crystallographic analyses of several TCR/pMHC structures (Garcia et al. 1999), some but not all of these assumptions proved to be correct.

Determination of the crystal structure of TCR/pMHC complexes has represented a particularly challenging task, not only because of the difficulties in producing and purifying large quantities of TCR and pMHC and generating stable trimolecular complexes, but also because of the crystallographic problems associated with analysis of such large macromolecular complexes. This explains why only a handful of high-resolution TCR/

pMHC complex structures have been reported so far. Despite this, several general principles for recognition of pMHC by TCR can already be drawn from the few structures determined to date (Figure 24.10).

OVERALL TOPOLOGY

The TCR adopts a diagonal orientation over the pMHC complex in all the TCR/pMHC class I and class II structures resolved so far (Garcia et al. 1996, 1999) (Figure 24.10a, b). This particular topology probably maximizes the cooptation between the MHC and TCR surfaces, because it allows the relatively flat TCR binding surface to lie between the two opposite high points of the MHC α helices (Garboczi et al. 1996). In all instances, the Vα domain is located over the amino-terminal half of the peptide and the Vβ domain over the carboxy-terminal half. Here again this orientation is likely to be conserved, in order to ensure proper positioning of the CD4 and CD8 co-receptors within the TCR/pMHC complex.

CDR FOOTPRINTS ON THE PMHC

Both CDR3 loops lie centrally and establish contacts almost exclusively with the antigenic peptide (Figure 24.10a, b). The CDR1α and β interact with both MHC and peptide residues whereas the CDR2 contacts almost exclusively the MHC α helices. Early crystallographic studies suggested a dominant contribution of the Vα (over the Vβ) CDRs to TCR/pMHC interaction, and frequent involvement of conserved residues at the tip of CDR1α and CDR2α loops in TCR/MHC contacts at conserved MHC areas, thus supporting a key role for

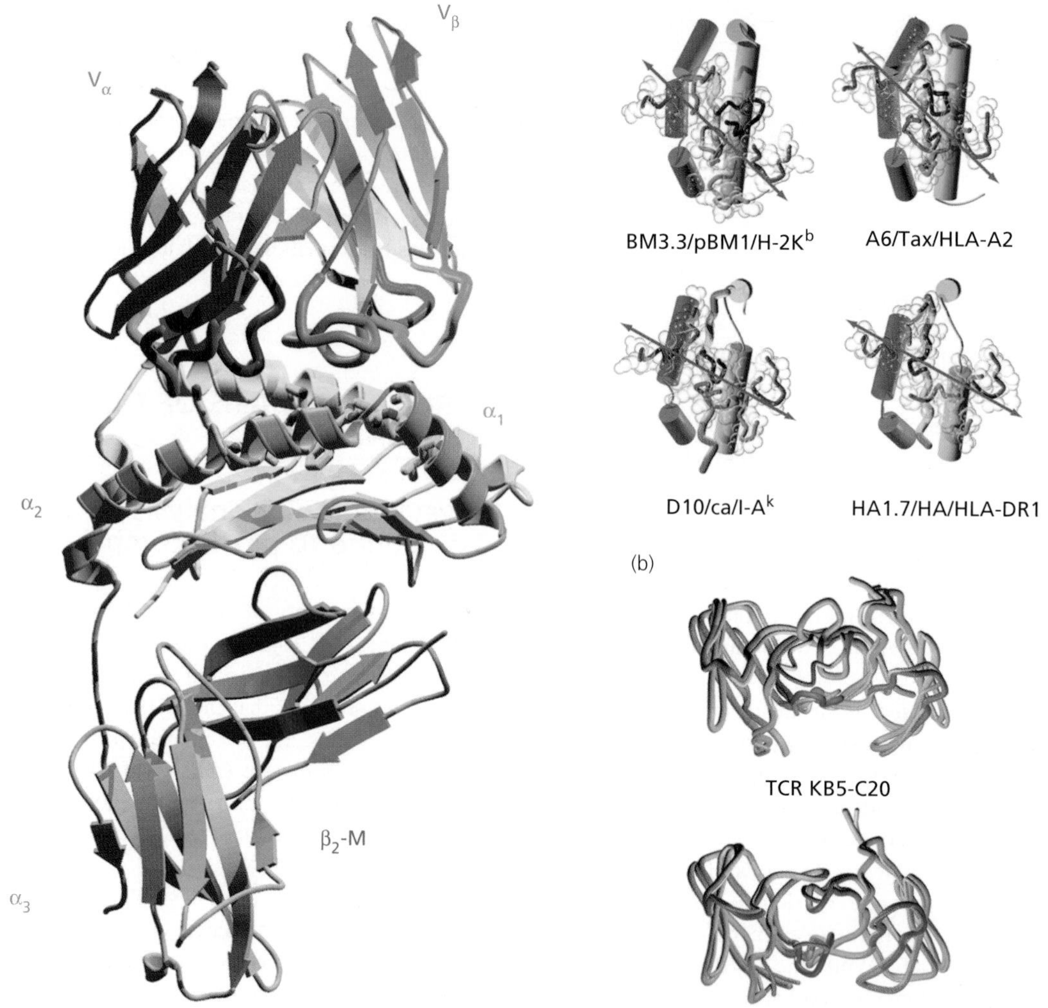

Figure 24.10 *Structure and overall topology of the T-cell receptor (TCR)/pMHC complex. See the text for details.* **(a)** *Overall structure of a TCR/pMHC complex (CDR1 in green, CDR2 in red, CDR3 in blue, peptide in yellow).* **(b)** *Diagonal orientation of TCR over pMHC. Upper left: murine TCR/pMHC class I, upper right: human TCR/pMHC class I, lower left: murine TCR/pMHC class II, lower right: human TCR/pMHC class II (for CDRs and peptide, same color code as in* **(a)***).* **(c)** *Comparison of the CDR conformation of TCR either unbound (gray) or bound to pMHC (same color code as in* **(a)** *and* **(b)***). Note the significant conformational modifications of the CDR3. (Kindly provided by J.B. Reiser and D. Housset, Grenoble, France.)*

the Vα domain in driving the TCR orientation over the pMHC complex (Garcia et al. 1998). This hypothesis has been more recently challenged by the balanced contribution of Vα and Vβ domains to pMHC interaction observed in additional structures, and the significant tilting of the TCR over the 'MHC saddle' from one complex to another (Reiser et al. 2000, 2002). Importantly these studies have failed to identify a truly conserved TCR footprint on the MHC shared by all TCR/pMHC class I complexes. Thus, there is so far no straightforward structural explanation for the inherent MHC reactivity of the TCR documented by biological studies (Zerrahn et al. 1997).

MHC VS PEPTIDE INTERFACE

Clearly the dominance of TCR contacts with the MHC helices should provide enough binding energy between the TCR and MHC heavy chain to allow proper TCR docking on the complex and subsequent scanning of its peptide content (see below). Furthermore comparison of bound versus unbound TCR indicates large conformational changes occurring mainly on the CDR3 loops, which may compensate for the relatively poor shape complementarity between the peptide and the TCR loops (Garcia et al. 1998; Reiser et al. 2002) (Figure 24.10c). Hence, this suggests an important plasticity of the T-cell recognition process, and provides a likely molecular explanation for the ability of a given T cell to recognize, in a degenerate fashion, large sets of peptides during its intrathymic positive selection or its peripheral activation.

ALLOREACTIVITY

A large fraction of T cells (up to several percent) cross-reacts to allogeneic MHC molecules. The molecular basis of this phenomenon, called alloreactivity, has been deciphered during the last decade and turns out to cover distinct types of interactions. In most cases, recognition of allogeneic cells appears mildly affected by the peptidic content of the recognized MHC molecules, suggesting highly degenerate low-affinity interactions between TCR and a large fraction of allogeneic pMHC complexes. Some alloreactive TCRs may also recognize, with much higher affinity and in a more peptide-dependent fashion, allogeneic MHC alleles related to self-MHC (Obst et al. 2000). Comparison of TCR bound to a positively selecting pMHC complex or an allogeneic pMHC suggests that some interactions with MHC in the former case can be 'mimicked' by interactions occurring with the peptide in the latter case (Garcia et al. 1998; Reiser et al. 2000). As a result of the heterogeneity of alloreactive responses documented by biological studies (see above), other molecular explanations (such as weak cooptation between the TCR and pMHC surfaces associated with increased peptide degeneracy) seem highly likely although they need confirmation through resolution of additional structures.

Structure of αβ TCR/superantigen complexes

Antigens are not always recognized in a form of MHC-bound peptide because some of them may directly bind to the TCR and MHC class II molecules in a native form. This particular class of TCR ligands, which is produced by a variety of microbial and viral pathogens, are called superantigens (SAg) because they can activate a substantial fraction of naive T cells. As briefly mentioned below and detailed in Chapter 29, Superantigens, the TCR-binding modes of antigen and SAg are drastically different because MHC class II-bound SAgs can engage all TCRs sharing a particular Vβ (or Vγ) region, irrespective of their Vα (or Vδ) regions and their VDJβ (or VJγ) junctional sequences. This explains why a given SAg can activate up to several percent of the total T-cell repertoire in naïve individuals. Crystallographic analysis of TCR/SAg and SAg/MHC class II complexes has clearly confirmed the peculiar topology of these interactions (Li et al. 1999). Although different SAgs bind to class II MHC in very different ways, their mode of interaction with the TCR appears quite conserved: in most instances, SAgs establish contacts with the HV4 as well as the CDR1 and CDR2 loops of the Vβ chain. This is in stark contrast with TCR/pMHC complexes, for which pMHC contacts involve residues located on all six CDRs but not HV4 (see above). Importantly the orientation of the TCR over the MHC molecule within the TCR/SAg/MHC complex is very different from that in TCR/pMHC complexes, and does not permit proper interaction with the bound peptide, which is consistent with previous observations demonstrating TCR/SAg/MHC interactions irrespective of the bound peptide (Li et al. 1999).

A DYNAMIC VIEW OF THE T-CELL ANTIGEN RECOGNITION PROCESS

Analysis of TCR/pMHC interactions

AGONISM VS ANTAGONISM

TCR engagement by pMHC complexes does not always lead to full T-cell activation. In particular alteration of the antigenic peptide sequence may affect T-cell functions in very different ways. Although some peptide mutants referred to as full agonists retain the ability to activate all T-cell effector functions, others referred to as weak or partial agonists may induce decreased T-cell responses or some but not all effector functions (Evavold and Allen 1991). In extreme cases, T-cell response to agonist peptides may be inhibited after exposure to some altered peptide ligands referred to as antagonists (for a review, see Sloan-Lancaster and Allen 1996). The physiological relevance of these nonproductive or suboptimal TCR/pMHC interactions is still unclear. They may affect T-cell responses against infections and/or may contribute to the selection of the T-cell repertoire as well as peripheral T-cell homeostasis. From a mechanistic point of view, antagonist peptides do not seem to compete with agonist peptides for binding to MHC molecules. Instead antagonists may engage either sterile or abortive TCR interactions (Sloan-Lancaster et al. 1994; Madrenas et al. 1995), thus decreasing the number of productive TCR/agonist interactions and/or triggering an inhibitory signal that dominates the activating signal induced by the agonist. Some biophysical studies, detailed below, have brought important insights into this phenomenon although we do not have yet a clear picture of what precisely is going on.

αβ TCR/PMHC-BINDING STUDIES

Analyses of TCR/pMHC interactions have lagged far behind those of antigen–antibody interactions because of two major technical obstacles. First, the membrane-bound nature of the TCR and MHC molecules, and the relative instability of TCR heterodimers when expressed under soluble forms, have greatly hampered their large-scale production and purification. A second problem lies in the affinity of pMHC/TCR interactions, which have turned out to be in the lower micromolar range, and measurable only using recently available surface plasmon resonance technologies. Indeed the affinity of TCR/pMHC interactions (K_d values in the order of 10^{-4}–10^{-7}) is on average lower than that of antibody–antigen interactions (K_d values of 10^{-6}–10^{-10}). Although the on-rates of TCR/pMHC interactions are quite heterogeneous (from 10^3 to 2.10^5 mol/l per s), their off-rates are very fast and remain in a relatively narrow range (from 0.2 to 0.005/s at 25°C). These fast off-rates have led to the proposal that T-cell activation by a small number of pMHC complexes would be made possible by the transient engagement of many different TCRs within a short time lag (Valitutti et al. 1995). However, the correlation between the strength of the T-cell response and the off-rates of TCR/pMHC interactions is still being debated. In their 'serial TCR engagement' model, Lanzavecchia and colleagues propose that lower TCR/pMHC off-rates should lead to reduced T-cell activation as a result of decreased numbers of serially engaged TCR within a given time frame (Viola and Lanzavecchia 1996). However, this hypothesis is difficult to reconcile with the inverse correlation observed by other groups between TCR/pMHC dissociation rates and T-cell responsiveness (for a recent review, see Davis et al. 1998). Indeed the TCR-binding affinity for strong pMHC agonists appears to be generally much higher than for antagonists. Furthermore, binding of TCRs to weak agonists and antagonists may show very similar affinities but different dissociation rates, which can be up to 10-fold higher in the latter than in the former case (Matsui et al. 1994; Lyons et al. 1996). Molecular explanations for this phenomenon are still pending but recent studies suggest that antagonist peptides prevent efficient TCR clustering and subsequent maturation of the immunological synapse (see above).

Although crystallographic studies allow identification of all the residues involved in a given interaction, many of these interactions can be neutral (i.e. mutation of the corresponding residues may have no impact on the binding affinity). Systematic mutagenesis analyses performed on either the TCR or the pMHC complex have allowed mapping of energetic 'hotspots' involving only a small fraction of interacting residues identified by X-ray analyses (Baker et al. 2001). Interestingly, the nature of TCR/MHC and TCR/peptide interactions may fundamentally differ, as suggested by another recent mutagenesis study (Wu et al. 2002). Mutations introduced within the antigenic peptide have a dramatic effect on the stability of the TCR/pMHC complex. This decreased affinity, when measurable, seems mainly accounted for by a marked increase of the dissociation constant, with only a minor effect on the association constant. By contrast, mutations on the MHC molecule have significantly less impact on the stability of pMHC/TCR interaction and, in most instances, this effect results from a decrease of the association constant. These results suggest a two-step mechanism for T-cell antigenic recognition. In a first step, interactions between TCR residues on the CDR1 and CDR2 loops and MHC residues would permit docking of the TCR on the MHC molecule, and scanning of its peptide content. In a second step pMHC/TCR binding would be stabilized on forming a complex via an induced conformational fit of the CDR3 loops, already documented in several crystallographic studies (Garcia et al. 1998; Reiser et al. 2002). This two-step process is also consistent with the entropic changes of TCR/pMHC interactions reported in several thermodynamic analyses (Willcox et al. 1999; Boniface et al. 1999).

γδ TCR/ANTIGEN-BINDING STUDIES

Unlike αβ T cells, γδ T cells do not generally recognize peptide antigens bound to classic MHC class I and class II molecules. As detailed in Chapter 25, Lymphocyte mediated cytotoxicity, γδ TCRs seem to interact with native antigen in an Ig-like fashion. This assumption is consistent with the extensive structural heterogeneity of the TCRγδ ligands identified so far, which include native MHC or MHC-like proteins, viral glycoproteins, Ig, heat shock protein (HSP), and small phosphorylated esters commonly produced by microorganisms (Chien et al. 1996). The sole biophysical binding study performed to date with a $\gamma\delta$ TCR directed against an 'empty' MHC class I-like molecule has revealed several unusual features. The affinity of this interaction appears much higher than that of $\alpha\beta$ TCR/pMHC interactions, resulting mainly from a very low dissociation rate (Crowley et al. 2000). As, in this particular case, the MHC class I-like molecules recognized by the $\gamma\delta$ TCR are expressed at high densities on target cells, $\gamma\delta$ T-cell activation is probably induced after stable engagement of a large number of TCRs by their ligands. These high avidity/high affinity interactions might be common within nonconventional T cells, as suggested by another recent binding study performed with an $\alpha\beta$ TCR specific for CD1d/glycolipid complexes (Sidobre et al. 2002).

The immunological synapse

Although the half-lives of TCR interactions are of the order of seconds, the duration of signaling required for T-cell activation is of the order of hours, thus suggesting specific mechanisms permitting sustained TCR interactions with their specific pMHC complex. This is achieved through the formation of supramolecular activation clusters (SMAC), which consist in a highly organized clustering of TCR, co-receptors, co-stimulatory, and adhesion receptors as well as signaling molecules within lipid rafts enriched for glycolipids and glycosphingolipids (Monks et al. 1998; Grakoui et al. 1999) (Figure 24.11). These SMACs of immunological receptors, which form within minutes after contact between the T cell and the antigen-presenting cell (APC), are classically referred to as the immunological synapse. Although a detailed description of the formation and function of the immunological synapse is clearly beyond the scope of the present chapter, several general features of the immunological synapse are outlined here.

T-cell activation and immunological synapse formation can be grossly split into four distinct temporal stages corresponding to: (1) the initial T-cell polarization events taking place shortly after APC encounter; (2) the segregation of adhesion molecules within early supramolecular clusters leading to enhanced T-cell adhesion to APC; (3) early TCR-signaling leading to formation of the immature immunological synapse; and finally (4) immunological synapse maturation associated with sustained TCR signaling (Bromley et al. 2001).

T-CELL POLARIZATION

Initial adhesion of the T cell to the APC is accompanied by rapid membrane reorganization and T-cell polarization, presumably in response to chemokines (Sanchez-Madrid and del Pozo 1999). Subsequent signaling through heterotrimeric G protein then triggers actin polymerization and integrin activation. The engaged integrins can in turn promote the formation of membrane protrusions tipped by TCR-enriched membranes, which are probably involved in the initial scanning of pMHC complexes and set the initial stages of immunological synapse formation (Dustin and Cooper 2000).

T-CELL ADHESION TO APCS

Effective adhesion between the T cell and the APC requires rapid segregation of adhesion and recognition receptors within these early supramolecular arrangements. Although surface molecules with large extracellular domains (such as CD43 and CD45) are excluded, smaller adhesion receptors such as CD2 and LFA1 are clustered in the center of the structure and form tight interactions with their counterreceptors (CD58 and intercellular adhesion molecule 1 (ICAM-1), respectively) (Sperling et al. 1998; Grakoui et al. 1999; Leupin et al. 2000).

IMMUNOLOGICAL SYNAPSE FORMATION AND MATURATION

In its initial stage, the immunological synapse is made up of an adhesion molecule cluster surrounded by a ring of engaged TCRs. Along immunological synapse maturation, the structure is inverted: the engaged TCR/pMHC complexes progressively move toward the center of the SMAC (cSMAC) whereas the adhesion molecules move to its periphery (pSMAC) (Grakoui et al. 1999). Although it seems clear that the earliest TCR signaling events induce the cytoskeletal changes required for immunological synapse maturation, the parameters (quantitative or qualitative) controlling sustained signaling within the mature immunological synapse are still poorly defined. Stable formation of the immunological synapse seems to be associated with the recruitment of specific kinases required for full T-cell activation (such as protein kinase C) (Monks et al. 1998). Furthermore CD28, which segregates within the cSMAC in the mature immunological synapse, probably plays an important role in the potentiation of TCR signaling because its co-engagement with the TCR has been shown to sustain TCR-induced tyrosine phosphorylations (Viola et al. 1999). As already mentioned, nonproductive TCR/pMHC interactions (e.g. with high off-rates as observed with some antagonist peptides) may dramatically reduce the density of TCR/pMHC complexes within the mature immunological synapse and thus affect sustained signaling.

CONCLUDING REMARKS

Recent studies are shedding light on several common principles that underlie T-cell antigen recognition and its translation into particular biological outcomes. Recognition of pMHC by TCRs turns out to be a complex multistep process, which involves induction of conformational changes of TCRs on binding and rapid recruitment of adhesion and co-stimulatory receptors within highly

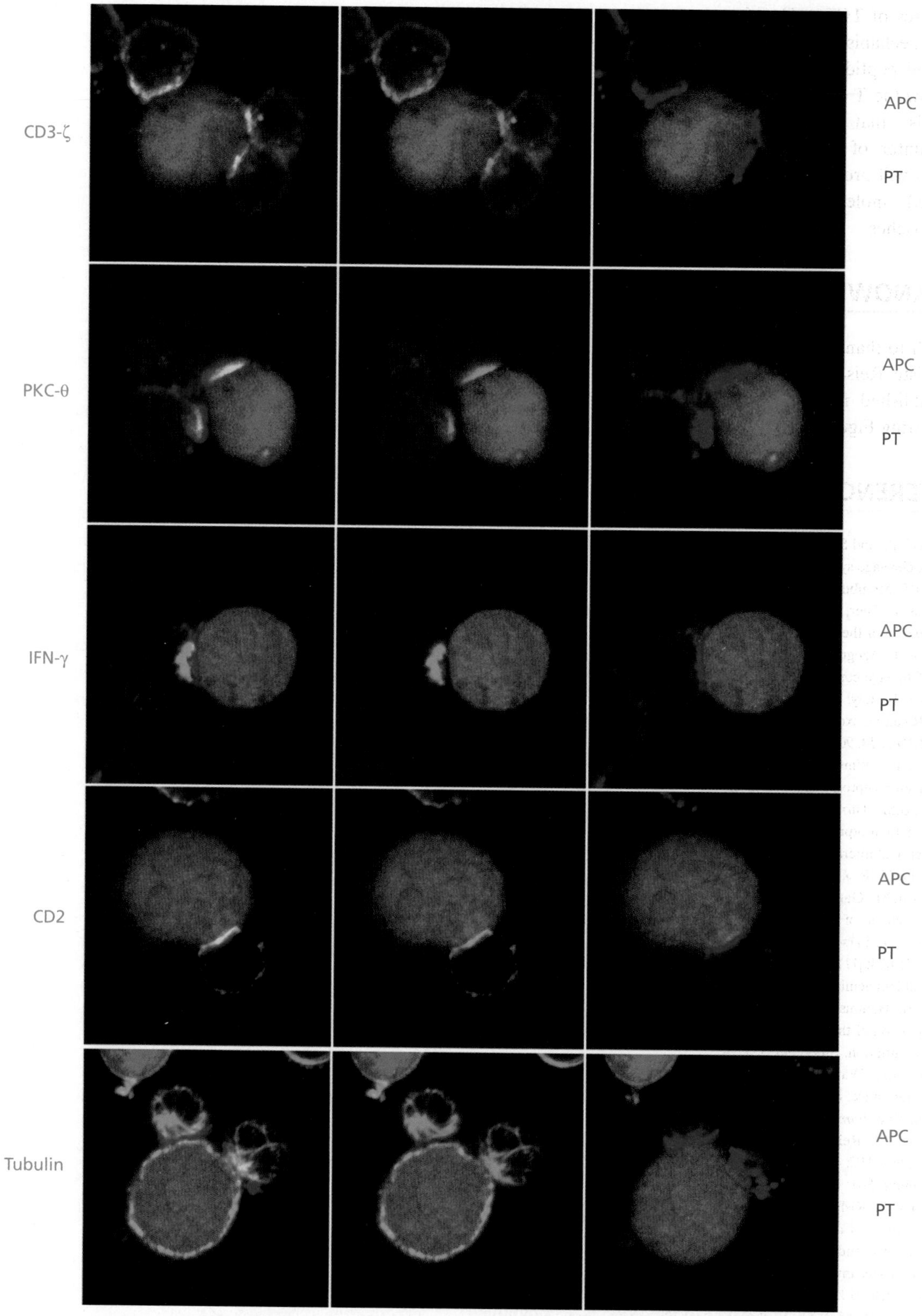

Figure 24.11 *Clustering of surface receptors and signaling molecules within the immunological synapse. See the text for details. APC, antigen-presenting cell (in red). PT, phosphotyrosine (in blue). Note the co-clustering (light blue) of several surface receptors (CD3-ζ, CD2) and phosphorylated tyrosine kinases (protein kinase CΘ) at the contact point between the T cell and the APC, and the polarized secretion of interferon IFN-γ. (Kindly provided by S. Mueller and S. Valitutti, Toulouse, France.)*

organized membrane receptor clusters. Naturally, there are still several challenging issues that should be addressed by future work. Structural explanations for the inherent MHC reactivity of TCR are still lacking and will certainly need resolution of additional TCR/pMHC structures. Biophysical and thermodynamic analyses of TCR/pMHC interactions should help clarify the mechanisms underlying the biological effects of altered peptide ligands. Finally a precise understanding of how the T cell integrates the activating and inhibitory signals that are concomitantly generated during encounter of APCs will be another major challenge, which will probably require the combined use of sophisticated molecular, biochemical, and morphological approaches.

ACKNOWLEDGMENTS

I wish to thank Sabina Mueller, Salvatore Valitutti, Jean Baptiste Reiser, and Dominique Housset for providing unpublished material and for their invaluable help in preparing Figures 19.9-19.11.

REFERENCES

Agrawal, A. and Schatz, D.G. 1997. RAG1 and RAG2 form a stable post-cleavage synaptic complex with DNA containing signal ends in V(D)J recombination. *Cell*, **89**, 43–53.

Aifantis, I., Buer, J., et al. 1997. Essential role of the pre-TCR in allelic exclusion of the TCRβ locus. *Immunity*, **7**, 601–7.

Aifantis, I., Azogui, O., et al. 1998. On the role of the pre-TCR in αβ vs γδ T lineage commitment. *Immunity*, **9**, 649–55.

Alarcon, B., Ley, S.C., et al. 1991. The CD3γ and CD3δ subunits of the TCR can be expressed within distinct functional TCR/CD3 complexes. *EMBO J*, **10**, 903–12.

Allison, T.J., Winter, C.C., et al. 2001. Structure of a human γδ T cell antigen receptor. *Nature*, **411**, 820–4.

Baker, B.M., Turner, R.V., et al. 2001. Identification of a crucial energetic footprint on the α1 helix of human HLA-A2 that provides functional interactions for recognition by Tax peptide/HLA-A2-specific TCR. *J Exp Med*, **193**, 551–62.

Baniyash, M., Garcia-Morales, P., et al. 1988. Disulfide linkage of the ζ and ν chains of the TCR. *J Biol Chem*, **263**, 9874–8.

Bernard, O., Larsen, C.J., et al. 1988. Molecular mechanisms of a t(8;14)(q24;q11) translocation juxtaposing c-myc and TCRα genes in a T cell leukaemia. *Oncogene*, **2**, 195–200.

Blom, B., Hemmskerk, M.H., et al. 1999. TCR gene rearrangements and expression of the pre-TCR complex during human T cell differentiation. *Blood*, **93**, 3033–43.

Bogue, M.A., Wang, C., et al. 1997. V(D)J recombination in Ku86-deficient mice: distinct effects on coding, signal and hybrid joint formation. *Immunity*, **7**, 37–47.

Boniface, I.J., Reich, Z., et al. 1999. Thermodynamics of TCR binding to peptide-MHC: evidence for a general mechanism of molecular scanning. *Proc Natl Acad Sci USA*, **96**, 11446–51.

Borgulya, P., Kishi, H., et al. 1992. Exclusion and inclusion of α and β TCR alleles. *Cell*, **69**, 529–37.

Borst, J., Alexander, S., et al. 1983. The T3 complex on human T lymphocytes involves four structurally distinct glycoproteins. *J Biol Chem*, **258**, 5135–41.

Brenner, M.B., McLean, J., et al. 1986. Identification of a putative second TCR. *Nature*, **322**, 145–8.

Bromley, S.K., Burack, W.R., et al. 2001. The immunological synapse. *Annu Rev Immunol*, **19**, 375–96.

Capone, M., Watrin, F., et al. 1993. TCRα and TCRβ gene enhancers confer tissue- and stage-specificity on V(D)J recombination events. *EMBO J*, **12**, 4335–446.

Clevers, H., Alarcon, B., et al. 1988. The TCR/CD3 complex: a dynamic protein ensemble. *Annu Rev Immunol*, **6**, 629–62.

Chien, Y.H., Iwashima, M., et al. 1987. A new TCR gene located within the α locus and expressed early in T cell differentiation. *Nature*, **327**, 677–82.

Chien, Y.H., Jores, R. and Crowley, M.P. 1996. Recognition by γδ T cells. *Annu Rev Immunol*, **14**, 511–32.

Crowley, M.P., Fahrer, A.M., et al. 2000. A population of murine γδ T cells that recognize an inducible MHC class Ib molecule. *Science*, **287**, 314–16.

de Chasseval, R. and de Villartay, J.P. 1993. Functional characterization of the promoter for the human germline TCR early α (TEA) transcript. *Eur J Immunol*, **23**, 1294–8.

Davis, M.M. and Bjorkman, P.J. 1988. T cell antigen receptor genes and T cell recognition. *Nature*, **334**, 395–402.

Davis, M.M., Boniface, J.J., et al. 1998. Ligand recognition by alpha/beta T cell receptors. *Annu Rev Immunol*, **16**, 523–44.

Davodeau, F., Peyrat, M.A., et al. 1994. Surface expression of functional TCR chains formed by interlocus recombination on human T lymphocytes. *J Exp Med*, **180**, 1685–91.

Dudley, E.C., Girardi, M., et al. 1995. αβ and γδ T cells can share a late common precursor. *Curr Biol*, **5**, 659–69.

Dustin, M.L. and Cooper, J.A. 2000. The actin cytoskeleton and the immunological synapse: molecular hardware for T cell signaling. *Nat Immunol*, **1**, 23–9.

Early, P., Huang, H., et al. 1980. An immunoglobulin heavy chain variable region gene is generated from 3 segments of DNA, V_H, D and J_H. *Cell*, **19**, 981–92.

Ellmeier, W., Sawada, S. and Littman, D. 1999. The regulation of CD4 and CD8 coreceptor gene expression during T cell development. *Annu Rev Immunol*, **17**, 523–54.

Ernst, P. and Smale, S.T. 1995. Combinatorial regulation of transcription. *Immunity*, **2**, 311–19.

Evavold, B.D. and Allen, P.M. 1991. Separation of IL4 production from Th cell proliferation by an altered TCR ligand. *Science*, **252**, 1308–10.

Feeney, A.J. 1992. Predominance of V_HDJ_H junctions occurring at sites of short sequence homology results in limited junctional diversity in neonatal antibodies. *J Immunol*, **149**, 222–9.

Fehling, H.J., Krotkova, A., et al. 1995. Crucial role of the pre-TCRα gene in development of αβ but not γδ T cells. *Nature*, **375**, 795–8.

Fugmann, S.D., Lee, A.I., et al. 2000. The RAG proteins and V(D)J recombination: complexes, ends and transposition. *Annu Rev Immunol*, **18**, 495–527.

Garboczi, D.N., Ghosh, P., et al. 1996. Structure of the complex between human TCR, viral peptide and HLA-A2. *Nature*, **384**, 134–41.

Garcia, K.C., Degano, M., et al. 1996. An αβ TCR structure at 2.5 A and its orientation in the TCR-MHC complex. *Science*, **274**, 209–19.

Garcia, K.C., Degano, M., et al. 1998. Structural basis of plasticity in TCR recognition of a self-peptide MHC antigen. *Science*, **279**, 1166–72.

Garcia, K.C., Teyton, L. and Wilson, I.A. 1999. Structural basis of T cell recognition. *Annu Rev Immunol*, **17**, 369–97.

Ghendler, Y., Smolyar, A., et al. 1996. One of the CD3ε subunits within a TCR complex lies in close proximity to the Cβ FG loop. *J Exp Med*, **187**, 1529–36.

Goldman, J.P., Spencer, D.M. and Raulet, D.H. 1993. Ordered rearrangement of variable region genes of the TCR γ locus correlates with transcription of the unrearranged genes. *J Exp Med*, **177**, 729–39.

Gottschalk, L.R. and Leiden, J.M. 1990. Identification and functional characterization of the human TCRβ gene transcriptional enhancer. *Mol Cell Biol*, **10**, 5486–95.

Grakoui, A., Bromley, S.K., et al. 1999. The immunological synapse: a molecular machine controlling T cell activation. *Science*, **285**, 221–7.

Grawunder, U., West, R.B. and Lieber, M.R. 1998. Antigen receptor gene rearrangement. *Curr Opin Immunol*, **10**, 172–80.

Hall, C., Berkhout, B., et al. 1991. Requirements for cell surface expression of the human TCR/CD3 complex in non T cells. *Int Immunol*, **3**, 359–68.

Hayes, S.M. and Love, P.E. 2002. Distinct structure and signaling potential of the γδ TCR complex. *Immunity*, **16**, 827–38.

Hedrick, S.M., Cohen, D.I., et al. 1984. Isolation of cDNA clones encoding T cell-specific membrane-associated proteins. *Nature*, **308**, 149–53.

Hempel, W.M., Stanhope-Baker, P., et al. 1998. Enhancer control of V(D)J recombination at the TCR β locus: differential effects on DNA cleavage and joining. *Genes Dev*, **12**, 2305–17.

Ho, I.C., Yang, L.H., et al. 1989. A T-cell specific transcriptional enhancer element 3' of Cα in the human TCRα locus. *Proc Natl Acad Sci USA*, **86**, 6714–18.

Hsieh, C.L. and Lieber, M.R. 1992. CpG methylated minichromosomes become inaccessible for V(D)J recombination after undergoing replication. *EMBO J*, **11**, 315–25.

Ikuta, K., Kina, T., et al. 1990. A developmental switch in thymic lymphocyte maturation potential occurs at the level of hematopoietic cells. *Cell*, **62**, 863–74.

Irving, B.A., Alt, F.W. and Killeen, N. 1998. Thymocyte development in the absence of pre-T cell receptor extracellular immunoglobulin domains. *Science*, **280**, 905–8.

Ishida, I., Verbeek, S., et al. 1990. TCRγδ and γ transgenic mice suggest a role of a γ gene silencer in the generation of αβ T cells. *Proc Natl Acad Sci USA*, **87**, 3067–71.

Itohara, S., Mombaerts, P., et al. 1993. TCR δ gene mutant mice: independent generation of αβ T cells and programmed rearrangements of γδ TCR genes. *Cell*, **72**, 337–48.

Jin, Y.J., Clayton, L.K., et al. 1990. Molecular cloning of the CD3ν subunit identifies a CD3ζ-related product in thymus-derived cells. *Proc Natl Acad Sci USA*, **87**, 3319–23.

Jorgensen, J.L., Esser, U., et al. 1992. Mapping TCR peptide contacts by variant peptide immunization of single chain transgenics. *Nature*, **355**, 224–30.

Kappler, J.W., Skidmore, B., et al. 1981. Antigen-inducible, H-2 restricted, interleukin-2-producing hybridomas: lack of independent antigen and H-2 recognition. *J Exp Med*, **153**, 1198–214.

Kirillov, A., Kistler, B., et al. 1996. A role for nuclear NFkB in B cell specific demethylation of the Igk locus. *Nat Genet*, **13**, 435–41.

Komori, T., Okada, A., et al. 1993. Lack of N regions in antigen receptor variable region genes of TdT-deficient lymphocytes. *Science*, **261**, 1171–5.

Koyasu, S., D'adamio, L., et al. 1992. TCR complexes containing FcεRIγ homodimers in lieu of CD3ζ and CD3ν components. *J Exp Med*, **175**, 203–9.

Lafaille, J.J., Decloux, A., et al. 1989. Junctional sequences of TCRγ genes: implications for γδ T cell lineages and for a novel intermediate of V(D)J joining. *Cell*, **59**, 859–70.

Lauzurica, P., Zhong, X.P., et al. 1997. Regulation of TCRδ gene rearrangement by CBF/PEBP2. *J Exp Med*, **185**, 1193–201.

Lefranc, M.P. and Alexandre, D. 1995. γd lineage-specific transcription of human TCRγ genes by a combination of a non-lineage-specific enhancer and silencers. *Eur J Immunol*, **25**, 617–22.

Lefranc, M.P. and Rabbitts, T.H. 1989. The human TCRγ genes. *Trends Biochem Sci*, **14**, 214–18.

Letourneur, F., Mattei, M.G. and Malissen, B. 1989. The mouse CD3γ, δ and ϵ genes reside within 50 kilobases on chromosome 9, whereas CD3ζ maps to chromosome 1. *Immunogenetics*, **29**, 265–8.

Leupin, O., Zaru, R., et al. 2000. Exclusion of CD45 from the T-cell receptor signaling area in antigen-stimulated T lymphocytes. *Curr Biol*, **10**, 277–80.

Levelt, C.N., Wang, B., et al. 1995. Regulation of TCRβ locus allelic exclusion and initiation of TCRα locus rearrangement in immature thymocytes by signalling through the CD3 complex. *Eur J Immunol*, **25**, 1257–61.

Li, H., Lebedeva, M.I., et al. 1998. Structure of the Vδ domain of a human γδ TCR. *Nature*, **391**, 502–6.

Li, H., Llera, A., et al. 1999. The structural basis of T cell activation by superantigens. *Annu Rev Immunol*, **17**, 435–66.

Lieber, M.R. 1991. Site-specific recombination in the immune system. *FASEB J*, **5**, 2934–44.

Lieber, M.R., Hesse, J.E., et al. 1988. The defect in murine severe combined immunodeficiency: joining of signal sequences but not coding segments in V(D)J recombination. *Cell*, **55**, 7–16.

Lin, W.C. and Desiderio, S. 1994. Cell cycle regulation of V(D)J recombination-activating protein RAG-2. *Proc Natl Acad Sci USA*, **91**, 2733–7.

Lipkowitz, S., Stern, M.H. and Kirsch, I.R. 1990. Hybrid TCR genes formed by interlocus recombination in normal and ataxia-telangiectasia lymphocytes. *J Exp Med*, **172**, 409–18.

Livak, F., Petrie, H.T., et al. 1995. In frame TCRδ gene rearrangements play a critical role in the αβ/γδ T cell lineage decision. *Immunity*, **2**, 617–27.

Livak, F., Tourigny, M., et al. 1999. Characterization of TCR gene rearrangements during adult murine T cell development. *J Immunol*, **162**, 2575–80.

Lyons, D.S., Liebermann, S.A., et al. 1996. TCR binding to antagonist peptide/MHC complexes exhibits lower affinities and faster dissociation rates than to agonist ligands. *Immunity*, **5**, 53–61.

McBlane, J.F., Van Gent, D.C., et al. 1995. Cleavage at a V(D)J recombination signal requires only RAG1 and RAG2 proteins and occurs in two steps. *Cell*, **83**, 387–95.

McIntyre, B.W. and Allison, J.P. 1983. The mouse TCR: structural heterogeneity of molecules of normal T cells defined by xenoantiserum. *Cell*, **34**, 739–46.

McMurry, M.T. and Krangel, M.S. 2000. A role for histone acetylation in the developmental regulation of VDJ recombination. *Science*, **287**, 495–8.

Madrenas, J., Wange, R.L., et al. 1995. ζ phosphorylation without ZAP70 activation induced by TCR antagonists or partial agonists. *Science*, **267**, 515–18.

Malissen, M., McCoy, C., et al. 1986. Direct evidence for chromosomal inversion during TCRβ gene rearrangements. *Nature*, **319**, 28–33.

Malissen, M., Trucy, J., et al. 1992. Regulation of TCRα and β gene allelic exclusion during T cell development. *Immunol Today*, **13**, 315–22.

Matsui, K., Boniface, J.J., et al. 1994. Kinetics of TCR binding to peptide-MHC complexes: correlation of the dissociation rate with T cell responsiveness. *Proc Natl Acad Sci USA*, **91**, 862–6.

Mertsching, E., Wilson, A., et al. 1997. TCRα gene rearrangement and transcription in adult thymic γδ cells. *Eur J Immunol*, **27**, 389–96.

Miossec, C., Faure, F., et al. 1990. The Vδ1 gene segment is expressed with either Cα or Cδ. *J Exp Med*, **171**, 1171–88.

Monks, C.R., Freiberg, B.A., et al. 1998. Three-dimensional segregation of supramolecular activation clusters in T cells. *Nature*, **395**, 82–96.

Nick McElhinny, S.A., Snowden, C.M., et al. 2000. Ku recruits the XRCC4-ligase IV complex to DNA ends. *Mol Cell Biol*, **20**, 2996–3003.

Obst, R., Netuschil, N., et al. 2000. The role of peptides in T cell alloreactivity is determined by self-major histocompatibility complex molecules. *J Exp Med*, **191**, 805–12.

Oettinger, M.A., Schatz, D.G., et al. 1990. RAG-1 and RAG-2, adjacent genes that synergistically activate V(D)J recombination. *Science*, **248**, 1517–23.

Okazaki, K., Davis, D.D. and Sakano, H. 1997. TCRβ gene sequences in the circular DNA of thymocyte nuclei: direct evidence for intramolecular DNA deletion in VDJ joining. *Cell*, **49**, 477–85.

Padovan, E., Casorati, G., et al. 1993. Expression of two TCRα chains: dual receptor T cells. *Science*, **262**, 422–4.

Redondo, J.M., Hata, S., et al. 1990. A T cell specific transcriptional enhancer within the human TCRδ locus. *Science*, **247**, 1225–9.

Reiser, J.B., Darnault, C., et al. 2000. Crystal structure of a TCR bound to an allogeneic MHC molecule. *Nat Immunol*, **1**, 291–7.

Reiser, J.B., Grégoire, C., et al. 2002. A TCR CDR3β loop undergoes conformational changes of unprecedented magnitude upon binding to a peptide/MHC class I complex. *Immunity*, **16**, 345–54.

Reth, M. 1989. Antigen receptor tail clue. *Nature*, **338**, 383–4.

Retière, C., Halary, F., et al. 1999. The mechanism of chromosome 7 inversion in human lymphocytes expressing chimeric γβ TCR. *J Immunol*, **162**, 903–10.

Rowen, L., Koop, B.F. and Hood, L. 1996. The complete 685-kilobase DNA sequence of the human β TCR locus. *Science*, **272**, 1755–62.

Saint-Ruf, C., Ungewiss, K., et al. 1994. Analysis and expression of a cloned pre-T cell receptor gene. *Science*, **266**, 1208–12.

Saito, H., Kranz, D.M., et al. 1984. Complete primary structure of a heterodimeric TCR deduced from cDNA sequence. *Nature*, **309**, 757–62.

Sanchez-Madrid, F. and del Pozo, M.A. 1999. Leukocyte polarization in cell migration and immune interactions. *EMBO J*, **18**, 501–11.

Sant'Angelo, D.B., Waterbury, G., et al. 1996. The specificity and orientation of a TCR to its peptide-MHC class II ligands. *Immunity*, **4**, 367–76.

Schatz, D.G., Oettinger, M.A. and Baltimore, D. 1989. The V(D)J recombination activating gene RAG-1. *Cell*, **59**, 1035–48.

Schatz, D.G., Oettinger, M.A. and Schlissel, M.S. 1992. V(D)J recombination: molecular biology and regulation. *Annu Rev Immunol*, **10**, 359–83.

Sebzda, E., Mariathasan, S., et al. 1999. Selection of the T cell repertoire. *Annu Rev Immunol*, **17**, 829–74.

Shockett, P.E. and Schatz, D.G. 1999. DNA hairpin opening mediated by the RAG1 and RAG2 proteins. *Mol Cell Biol*, **19**, 4159–466.

Shortman, K. and Wu, L. 1996. Early T lymphocyte progenitors. *Annu Rev Immunol*, **14**, 29–47.

Sidobre, S., Naidenko, O.V., et al. 2002. The Vα14 NKT cell TCR exhibits high-affinity binding to a glycolipid/CD1d complex. *J Immunol*, **169**, 1340–8.

Sleckman, B.P., Gorman, J.R. and Alt, F.W. 1996. Accessibility control of antigen-receptor variable region gene assembly: role of *cis*-acting elements. *Annu Rev Immunol*, **14**, 459–81.

Sloan-Lancaster, J. and Allen, P.M. 1996. Altered peptide ligand-induced partial T cell activation: molecular mechanism and role in T cell biology. *Annu Rev Immunol*, **14**, 1–27.

Sloan-Lancaster, J., Shaw, A.S., et al. 1994. Partial T cell signaling: altered phospho-ζ and lack of ZAP70 recruitment in APL-induced T cell anergy. *Cell*, **79**, 913–22.

Sperling, A.I., Sedy, J.R., et al. 1998. TCR signaling induces selective exclusion of CD43 from the T cell-antigen-presenting cell contact site. *J Immunol*, **161**, 6459–62.

Sussman, J.J., Bonifacino, J.S., et al. 1988. Failure to synthesize the T cell CD3ζ chain: structure and function of a partial TCR complex. *Cell*, **52**, 85–95.

Thompson, S.D., Pelkonen, J. and Hurwitz, J.L. 1990. First TCRα gene rearrangements during T cell ontogeny skew to the 5' region of the Jα locus. *J Immunol*, **145**, 2347–52.

Tonegawa, S. 1983. Somatic generation of antibody diversity. *Nature*, **302**, 575–81.

Tourigny, M.R., Mazel, S., et al. 1997. TCRβ gene recombination: dissociation from cell cycle regulation and developmental progression during T cell ontogeny. *J Exp Med*, **185**, 1549–56.

Turka, L.A., Schatz, D.G., et al. 1991. Thymocyte expression of RAG-1 and RAG-2: termination by TCR cross-linking. *Science*, **253**, 778–81.

Uematsu, Y., Ryser, S., et al. 1988. In transgenic mice the introduced functional TCRβ gene prevents expression of endogenous β genes. *Cell*, **52**, 831–41.

Valitutti, S., Muller, S., et al. 1995. Serial triggering of many TCRs by a few MHC-peptide complexes. *Nature*, **375**, 148–51.

Van Gent, D.C., Hiom, K., et al. 1997. Stimulation of V(D)J cleavage by high mobility group proteins. *EMBO J*, **16**, 2665–70.

Vernooij, B.T., Lenstra, J.A., et al. 1993. Organization of the murine TCRγ locus. *Genomics*, **17**, 566–74.

Viola, A. and Lanzavecchia, A. 1996. T cell activation determined by TCR number and tunable thresholds. *Science*, **273**, 104–6.

Viola, A., Schroeder, S., et al. 1999. T lymphocyte costimulation mediated by reorganization of membrane microdomains. *Science*, **283**, 680–2.

Willcox, B.E., Gao, G.F., et al. 1999. TCR binding to peptide MHC stabilizes a flexible recognition interface. *Immunity*, **10**, 357–65.

Wilson, A., Held, W. and MacDonald, H.R. 1994. Two waves of recombinase gene expression in developing thymocytes. *J Exp Med*, **179**, 1355–60.

Wilson, A., de Villartay, J.P. and MacDonald, H.R. 1996. TCRα gene rearrangement and T early α (TEA) expression in immature αβ lineage thymocytes. *Immunity*, **4**, 37–45.

Wu, L.C., Tuot, D.S., et al. 2002. Two-step binding mechanism for TCR recognition of peptide-MHC. *Nature*, **418**, 552–6.

Yanagi, Y., Yoshikai, Y., et al. 1984. A human T cell-specific cDNA clone encodes a protein having extensive homology to immunoglobulin chains. *Nature*, **308**, 145–9.

Yu, W., Misulovin, Z., et al. 1999. Coordinate regulation of RAG1 and RAG2 by cell type-specific DNA elements 5′ of RAG2. *Science*, **285**, 1080–4.

Zerrahn, J., Held, W. and Raulet, D.H. 1997. The MHC reactivity of the T cell repertoire prior to positive and negative selection. *Cell*, **88**, 627–36.

Zhong, X.P. and Krangel, M.S. 1997. An enhancer-blocking element between α and δ gene segments within the human TCR α/δ locus. *Proc Natl Acad Sci USA*, **94**, 5219–24.

Zhu, C., Bogue, M.A., et al. 1996. Ku86-deficient mice exhibit severe combined immunodeficiency and defective processing of V(D)J recombination intermediates. *Cell*, **86**, 379–89.

Zinkernagel, R.M. and Doherty, P.C. 1974. Restriction of in vitro T cell mediated cytotoxicitiy in lymphocytic choriomeningitis within a syngeneic or semiallogeneic system. *Nature*, **248**, 701–2.

25

Lymphocyte-mediated cytotoxicity

ECKHARD R. PODACK

Cytotoxic lymphocytes and their killing machinery, the cytolytic granule, are a critical component of the immune response. They are required for the removal of intracellular pathogens and for immune surveillance against tumors. This function necessitates the use of a fail-safe system, embodied by perforin and granzymes that act cooperatively in the clearance of even non-cooperative cells, such as virus-infected and transformed tumor cells. Although cytotoxicity and perforin have a well-understood functional role in the effector pathway of cyototoxic lymphocyte (CTL) and natural killer (NK) cells, it is only now being appreciated that perforin also has important functions in the induction of the adaptive CTL response. Finally, perforin and the granule exocytosis pathway of cytotoxicity are also critical for maintaining homeostasis of the CD8 T-cell compartment and downregulation of CTL memory responses. Cytotoxicity and perforin thus play a complex role in induction of CTL, in their effector function, and in the homeostasis of the CTL response. We are only beginning to understand the implications of these observations. Controlling and manipulating cytotoxicity are the holy grail of tumor immunology and antiviral therapy; there is every hope that further understanding of cytotoxicity will bring this goal within our grasp.

CYTOTOXIC LYMPHOCYTES

Two types of lymphocytes exist with regard to cytotoxicity: constitutively cytotoxic cells and inducibly cytotoxic lymphocytes. NK, NK-T, and γ,δ-T cells have constitutive cytotoxic activity and are able to kill targets without the need for induction. In contrast, naïve CD4 and CD8 T cells require activation and clonal expansion, accompanied by differentiation into CTLs. This process is driven by antigen stimulation with the help of several co-stimulatory molecules, and is accompanied by the acquisition of cytoplasmic granules containing the molecules responsible for target cell lysis, principally perforin and granzymes. Memory CTLs are similar to naïve T cells with regard to cytotoxic activity, except that their reacquisition of cytotoxicity is much more rapid than that of naïve cells.

The ability to kill a given target cell is determined by the specificity of cell surface receptors, whereas the killing process itself is unspecific. Once a killer cell has recognized a cell as a target, the killing machinery (the cytolytic granules) is engaged and kills the target indiscriminately and independently of target cooperation. The decision to kill is made by recognition rather than by downstream events. This decision tree is quite unlike the decision of a target to commit apoptosis, which depends on apoptotic receptor engagement *and* downstream signaling events. Apoptotic receptor engagement can indeed result in cell proliferation via NFκB activation. Targets recognized by CTLs or NK cells are not asked for compliance in dying; they are killed by multiple lytic, apoptotic, and nonapoptotic pathways without recourse to protection.

Recognition of targets by CTLs is achieved by the T-cell receptor binding to major histocompatibility complex (MHC) peptide complexes, triggering tight binding to the target, and killing by granule exocytosis. NK cells, NK-T cells, and γ,δ-T cells recognize a variety of surface molecules, not all of which have been defined. Killing by NK cells is, however, primarily determined by the engagement, or lack thereof, of dominant NK cell inhibitory receptors binding to the MHC class I molecules. If the target expresses normal levels of MHC the dominant killer cell inhibitory receptors will prevent activation of the cytolytic program by dephosporylation of intracellular substrates, even when positively signaling receptors are engaged. CTLs thus kill by MHC recognition whereas NK cells kill only in the absence of MHC molecules. This complementarity of recognition by CTLs and NK cells is an important mechanism to prevent the evasion of virally infected cells from the immune response.

Viruses must express viral genes and proteins during replication and some of the viral peptides will be presented by MHC and detected by CTLs. Virus-mediated downregulation of MHC molecules effectively prevents detection by T cells; however, absence of MHC allows NK cell killing. Viruses are therefore challenged to evolve mechanisms by which both NK cell and CTL evasion is achieved. Two mechanisms are known: cytomegalovirus (CMV) downregulates MHC expression of infected cells, thereby avoiding T-cell detection; in order to avoid killing by NK cells, CMV encodes a viral class I MHC molecule that is expressed on the infected cell and recognized by the inhibitory receptors of the NK cell, thereby inhibiting the killing activity. HIV nef downregulates HLA-A and -B molecules but not HLA-C molecules. As T-cell responses are primarily restricted by HLA-A and -B, CTLs will not be able to recognize HIV-infected cells; as HLA-C engages a large pool of NK cells through the inhibitory receptors, HIV-infected cells are also protected from NK cell attack.

It is evident from these examples that the primary function of cytotoxic lymphocytes is to clear our body of virus-infected cells and other intracellular parasites; this biological task is under continued evolutionary pressure by evolving pathogens. As the genesis of tumors is accompanied by multiple mutations and generation of neoantigens, oncogenic transformation may also be considered as parasitization of cells. As we shall see this process is under surveillance by cytotoxic cells protecting us from carcinogens and spontaneous tumor formation. Autoimmunity is the result of dysregulated immune responses and is frequently accompanied by infiltration of tissues with cytotoxic cells. Cytotoxic cells are generated after allogeneic bone marrow transplantation and contribute to graft-versus-host disease. In allogeneic organ transplantation invasion of cytotoxic cells is one of the hallmarks of organ rejection.

CTLS AND NK CELL MORPHOLOGY AND FUNCTION

Cytotoxicity is a specialized secretory process and CTLs and NK cells are secretory cells (Dennert and Podack 1983; Podack and Dennert 1983; Henkart et al. 1984; Podack and Konigsberg 1984; Henkart 1985; Podack 1985, 1989; Podack and Kupfer 1991; Podack et al. 1991; Kagi et al. 1994, 1996; Berke 1995; Liu et al. 1995; Podack, 1995a, b; Griffiths 1997; Zhang et al. 2001; Blott and Griffiths 2002; Djeu et al. 2002. Secretion of stored granules, also known as granule exocytosis, is the hallmark of the cytolytic process. Secretory cells come in three flavors (Figure 25.1):

1. Constitutively secreting cells: constitutive secretion describes a secretory process occurring continuously without external trigger. Antibody secretion by B cells is the classic example. Membrane-bound vesicles containing the cargo bud of the trans-Golgi network fuse with the plasma membrane, releasing their cargo or inserting membrane proteins into the plasma membrane.
2. Regulated secretion of storage granules is dependent on triggers and Ca^{2+} signals for release of intracellularly stored products. Secretory vesicles budding of the trans-Golgi network fuse with the secretory granule, where the cargo materials are concentrated with the aid of proteoglycans. This type of secretion is typical for endocrine and exocrine glands. In these cells lysosomes and granules are clearly distinct and distinguishable organelles receiving input from the Golgi apparatus by separate vesicular pathways.
3. Regulated secretion of secretory lysosomes (granulosomes) is the process used by cytolytic lymphocytes. Although all cells have lysosomes, only specialized cells have secretory lysosomes. Secretion is triggered by external stimuli and Ca^{2+} signals. Secretory lysosomes are specialized organelles receiving input from the Golgi body through the mannose-6-phosphate receptor pathway used by lysosomes and from the plasma membrane through endocytic vesicles and endosomes. Only lymphocytes, granulocytes, mast cells, platelets, melanocytes, and some renal epithelial cells are equipped with secretory lysosomes (Dennert and Podack 1983; Griffiths 1997; Pham and Ley 1997; Simon et al. 1997).

CTLs and NK cells are indistinguishable by electron microscopic morphology (Figure 25.2) (Henkart et al.

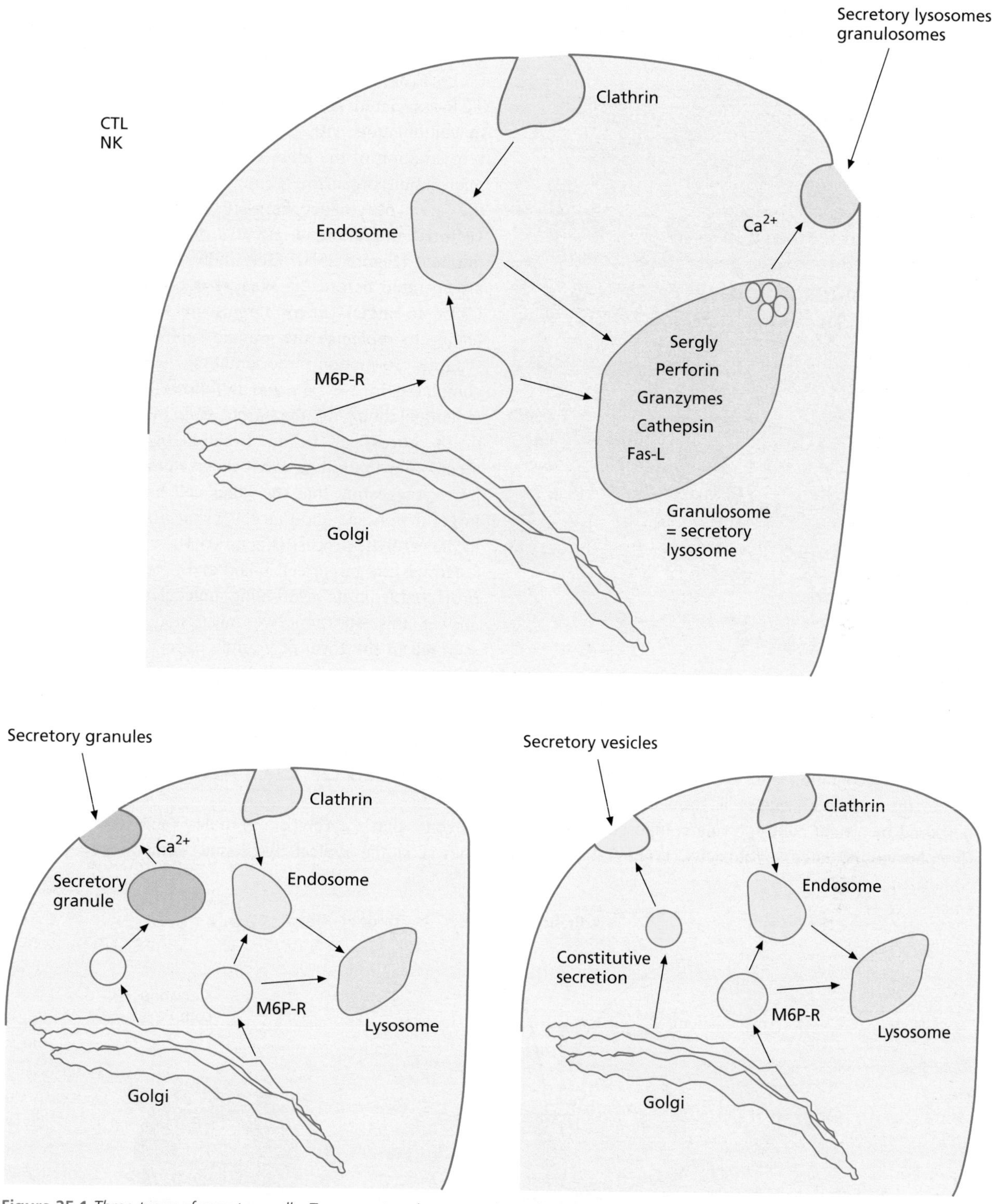

Figure 25.1 *Three types of secretory cells. Top: secretory lysosomes (granulosomes), this type of regulated secretion is used by cytotoxic lymphocytes (CTLs) and natural killer (NK) cells. Lower left: regulated secretion of storage granules, used by exocrine and endocrine glands. Lower right: constitutive secretion used, for example, by antibody-secreting B cells.*

1984; Podack 1995b; Uellner et al. 1997). The cells are characterized by a reniform or lobed nucleus, a well-developed active endoplasmic reticulum, a pronounced Golgi apparatus, and large granules (secretory lysosomes, granulosomes). The granulosomes are characterized by a dense core and areas containing vesicular, apparently membrane material. The significance of the vesicular material is not known; however, it may indicate storage of membrane-bound mediators such as the Fas ligand (Fas-L).

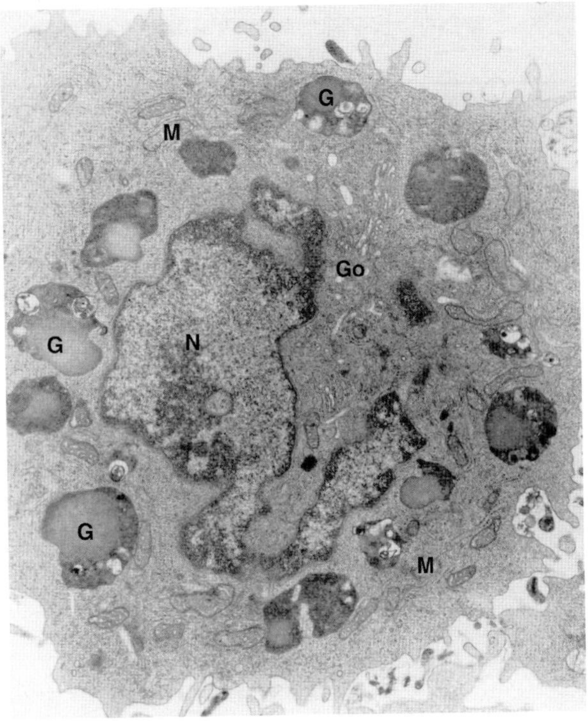

Figure 25.2 *Morphology of cytotoxic lymphocyte. G, granulosome; Go, Golgi body; M, mitochondria; N, nucleus.*

KILLING

On target recognition and T-cell receptor (TCR) triggering the cytolytic synapse is formed. The synapse is bordered by a tight adhesion ring composed of integrins (lymphocyte-mediated cytotoxicity 1 (LFA-1)) on the CTL side and of corresponding ligands (intercellular adhesion molecule 1 (ICAM)) on the target. The integrins are anchored via talin to the cytoskeleton of the CTLs. From inside the adhesion ring signals emanate via TCR-associated kinases and activate Erk-kinase, which in combination with Ca^{2+} fluxes results in a complex reorientation of the killer cells. The Golgi body and the microtubule-organizing center (MTOC) are brought to the area of contact between killer and target, and vectorial migration of granules toward the synapse is initiated (Figure 25.3). Only individual or few granules are secreted before the synapse is broken, allowing the CTLs to attack many targets in succession without having to replenish the granule supply. The process of synapse formation, reorientation, and secretion is completed in 2–3 min and is followed immediately by violent blebbing of the target cell, indicating that the death process has begun. Isolation of membrane fragments after the killing event shows numerous membrane pores, suggesting that the killer cell has perforated the target membrane and that this event is a critical element in the cytolytic process (Figure 25.4).

How is the target cell killed and how is the killer cell protected from its own killing molecules? Before we can answer this question, we must study what is being secreted in the form of granule exocytosis to cause this violent and rapid demise of the target cell.

COMPOSITION OF CYTOLYTIC GRANULES OF CTLS AND NK CELLS

Given that cytolytic granules are granulosomes they contain typical lysosomal components such as

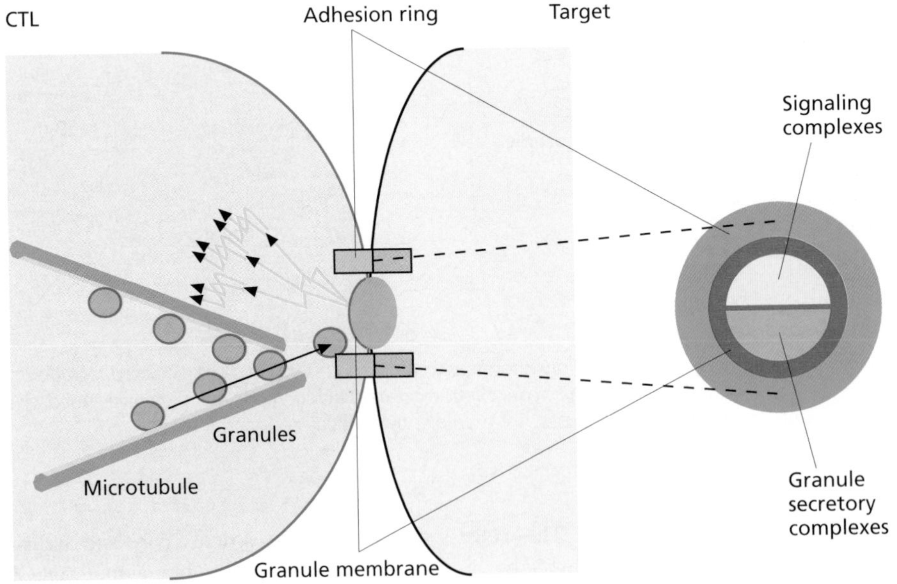

Figure 25.3 *Cytolytic synapse: the adhesion ring is depicted in side view (left) and en face (right panel). Inside the adhesion ring the localization of granule components and signaling components is shown. The granule membrane, lining the synapse on the cytotoxic lymphocyte (CTL) side, is shown in red.*

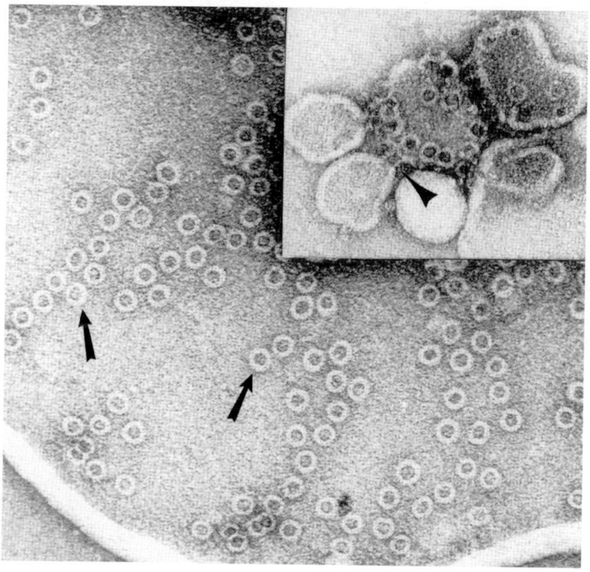

Figure 25.4 *Poly-perforin complexes on target membranes visualized by negative staining electron microscopy. Arrow: complex seen in top view; arrow head on inset: complex seen in side view (profile view).*

cathepsins, glucosaminidase, hexosaminidase, and other acid hydrolases. In addition granulosomes contain specific components not found in lysosomes that are designed for the killing process. The CTL and NK cell-specific components are perforin, the granzymes, Fas-L, granulysin, and serglycine as packing material.

Serglycine

Serglycine is a proteoglycan with a 14-kDa peptide core, which is heavily glycosylated with highly negatively charged chondroitin sulfate and heparan sulfate side chains, in a 250-kDa complex. Serglycine, similar to other granule proteoglycans, packed into dense highly concentrated packages allows condensation of granule contents, mainly granzymes and perforin. This effect is achieved through the formation of salt bridges between the negative charges of the proteoglycan, with positive charges on granzymes and perforin eliminating water molecules and reducing the colloid osmotic pressure. Granule contents are, then, large heteromultimeric complexes composed of the proteoglycan core with complexed perforin and granzymes, which are secreted en bloc.

Perforin

Perforin is a pore-forming protein sharing homology with complement components C6, C7, C8α, C8β, and C9 (Podack and Tschopp 1982; Henkart et al. 1984; Young et al. 1986; Podack and Kupfer 1991; Henkart 1997; Ponting 1999; Rukavina and Podack 2000; Smyth and Trapani 2001). The region of homology has been named the membrane attack complex/perforin (MACPF) domain; modeling studies suggest that this domain forms two amphipathic helices which are involved in transmembrane insertion and channel formation. Genome sequencing of several organisms has revealed additional MACPF-containing proteins and that the MACPF domain has been conserved from prokaryotes through plants and *Drosophila* spp. to the vertebrate system (Figure 25.5). Interestingly, the only prokaryotes containing proteins with MACPF domains to date are *Chlamydia pneumoniae* and *C. trachomatis*, both highly pathogenic organisms with intracellular localization.

Perforin is a 70-kDa protein synthesized as a hydrophilic, glycosylated monomer and it is directed from the trans-Golgi to the granulosome using as yet undefined targeting signals. Perforin on its C-terminus contains a C2 domain that is 100 amino acids long, which is characteristic for phospholipid-binding proteins (Jiang et al. 2001). On secretion and exposure to Ca^{2+} perforin binds to phospholipid head groups, triggering its ability to form multimers and insert itself into the hydrocarbon core of the membrane (Figure 25.6). Polymerization and membrane insertion have to go hand in hand, because, once polymerized, poly-perforin is unable spontaneously to insert into phospholipid bilayers. Perforin shares with the complement proteins above the remarkable biochemical ability to undergo a dramatic hydrophilic-to-amphiphilic transition which allows it to form transmembrane pores. The fully assembled pore is made up of about 20 perforin protomers, forming a tubular (cylindrical) complex that harbors a 16 nm-wide aqueous core. The poly-perforin cylinder is about 16 nm tall and inserted 4–6 nm deep in the membrane.

Perforin pores may be formed with as few as two or as many as 20 perforin molecules. Membrane pores allow the equilibration of ionic gradients, including Ca^{2+}, across the plasma membrane and result in the loss of membrane potential. Larger pores allow the efflux even of macromolecular cellular constituents. Membrane pores must be repaired, or else the cell would die via disruption of the normal cellular homeostasis. Membrane repair is achieved by endocytosis of the membrane patch containing the pore. The signal for the repair process comes from the Ca^{2+} influx across the pore. Endocytosis has two consequences: first, it is accompanied by pinocytosis of the liquid adjacent to the pore which will now be filling the endosome. As this liquid originates from the exocytosed granulosome and contains granzymes and other products, these components are now internalized in the target cell. Second, the pore formed by perforin persists in the endosome, interfering with acidification and normal endosome traffic, and may be responsible for endosomolysis which releases the endosome contents into the cytoplasm of the target cell where they initiate apoptotic and nonapoptotic cell death (Masson et al. 1986).

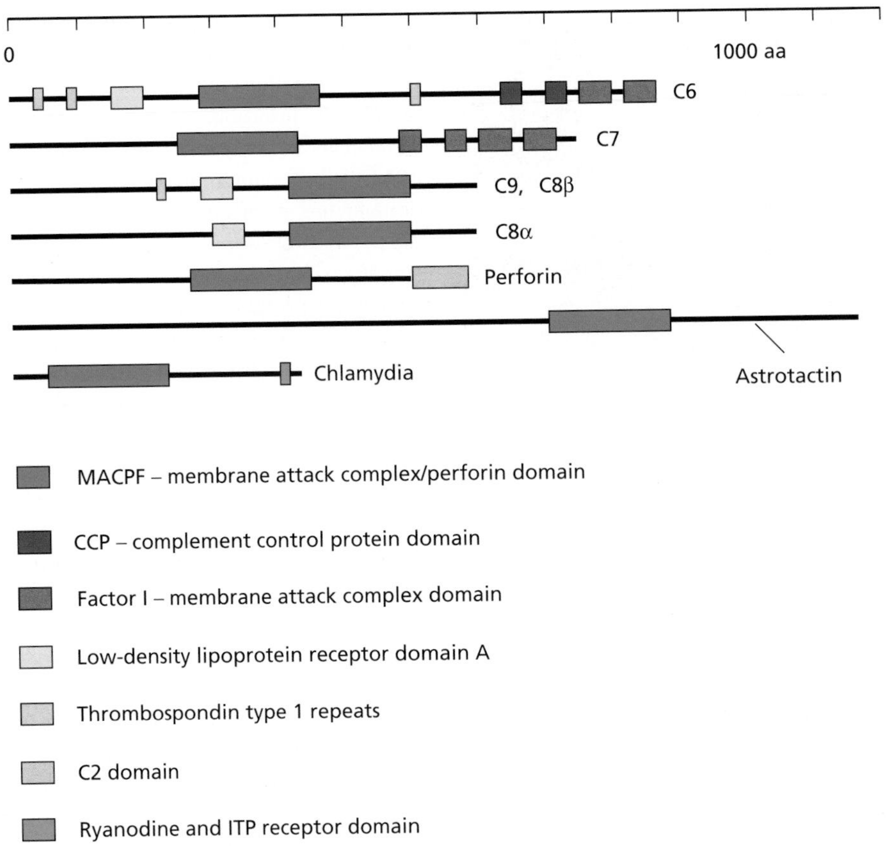

Figure 25.5 *Proteins sharing the membrane attack complex/perforin (MACPF) domain.*

Granzymes

Granzymes make up quantitatively the largest mass of the granule contents (Masson et al. 1986; Masson and Tschopp 1987; Shiver et al. 1992; Berke 1995; Beresford et al. 1997; Henkart 1997; Shiver et al. 1992; Darmon et al. 1996; Froelich et al. 1996; Atkinson et al. 1998; Kataoka et al. 1998; Metkar et al. 2002; Wallich et al. 2001; Zhang et al. 2001). Granzymes are serine esterases with narrow substrate specificities. They are transported to granulosomes by the mannose-6-phosphate receptor pathway typical for other lysosomal components including cathepsins, glycosylases, and other lysosomal enzymes. After exocytosis, granzymes gain entry into the target cell cytoplasm via perforin-dependent endocytosis and endosomolysis. In the target cytoplasm are the specific substrates for the granzymes. Granzymes always act in concert, depending on the collection of granzymes contained in the cytolytic granule. Humans have five granzymes, described below.

Granzyme B is a serine esterase with specificity of cleavage next to acidic (aspartate) residues (Masson et al. 1986; Masson and Tschopp 1987). Within the target cell it cleaves caspases and Bid (BH3 domain binding B-cell lymphoma [bcl]-2-like proapoptotic protein) and CAD (caspase-dominated DNAase) and sets off the apoptotic cascade including the mitochondrial pathway and the direct pathway of ICAD/CAD activation resulting in internucleasomal DNA cleavage and the generation of typical DNA ladders. The downstream activation of apoptotic mediators by granzyme B avoids some of the upstream regulators of apoptosis but is subject to blockade by bcl-2 and crmA. Granzyme B can bind to mannose-6-phosphate receptors expressed by certain cells and enter the cell by receptor-mediated endocytosis. However, in order for granzyme B to exit the endosome into the cytoplasm, perforin-mediated endosomolysis is essential.

Granzymes A and K (Masson et al. 1986; Masson and Tschopp 1987; Nakajima et al. 1995; Mullbacher et al. 1996; Beresford et al. 1997; Wilharm et al. 1999; Davis et al. 2001; Fan et al. 2002) are esterases with specificity for basic residues (arginine, lysine). They enter the target cell in a perforin-dependent process together with granzyme B and other granule components. Granzyme A mediates target apoptosis, including membrane blebbing and disruption of the nucleus. However, caspases are not activated and DNA laddering is not observed. Instead single-stranded DNA breaks are responsible for DNA breakdown. Granzyme A interacts with the nucleosome assembly complex that is involved in altering chromatin structure, to make it accessible for transcription and for single-stranded DNA excision-repair enzymes. It appears that the last activity is altered

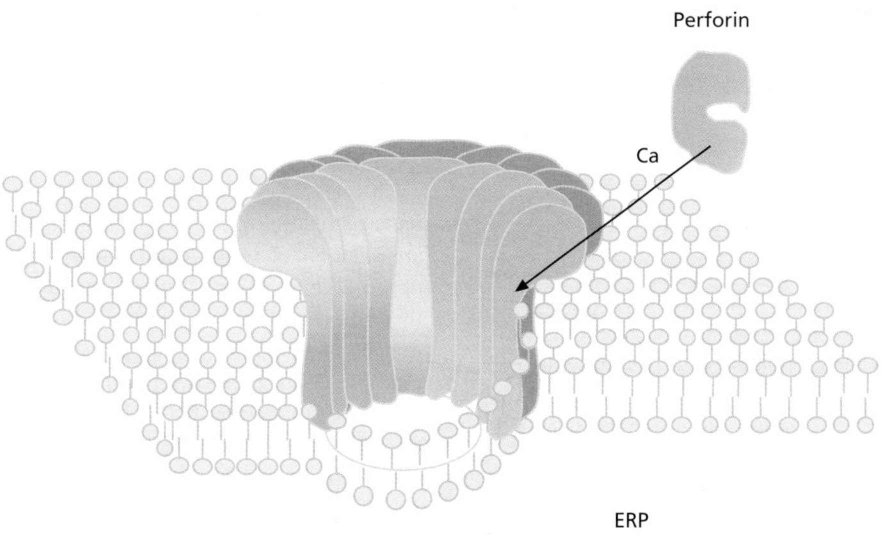

Figure 25.6 *Schematic view of perforin binding to phospholipid via Ca^{2+} and inserting itself as polymeric complex into the lipid bilayer.*

by granzyme A and results in single-stranded DNA breaks. Although granzyme K has similar enzymatic specificity to granzyme A, it is not known what its intracellular substrates are.

Granzymes H and M have chymotryptic specificity, with granzyme M also cleaving next to methionines. Granzyme H is expressed primarily by CTLs whereas granzyme M is exclusively expressed by NK cells. Granzyme H has been reported not to mediate cell death or apoptosis on internalization by target cells. Its function, similar to that of granzyme M, remains to be defined.

Mice, in addition to granzymes A, B, K, and M, express granzymes C, D, E, F, and G, but not granzyme H. This greater polymorphism suggests that mice have to combat a larger array of intracellular pathogens than humans.

Granulysin

Granulysin is found only in human granules. It is distantly related to saponins and has antibacterial activity for mycobacteria. It acts via membrane association and disordering of the lipid bilayer through ionic interaction. On delivery into cells it has specificity for mitochondria and triggers apoptosis and disrupts electron transport.

Fas ligand

Fas-L mediates apoptosis on Fas engagement by activation of caspase 8, and is the classic apoptotic mediator (Takahashi et al. 1994; Nagata and Suda 1995; Nagata 1996; Kataoka et al. 1998; Nagata 1998; Bossi and Griffiths 1999; Barry and Bleackley 2002). Apoptosis is a carefully regulated process subject to multiple regulatory checkpoints. Fas-L has two different localizations for expression. In granulosome-containing CTLs Fas-L is routed from the Golgi to the granule. The targeting information is contained in the proline-rich intracellular domain of Fas-L. In other cells Fas-L is found on the cell membrane. This distinct distribution explains why Fas-L killing of targets by CTLs is MHC restricted because it is exocytosed similar to or together with granule exocytosis only on appropriate signaling by the TCR. In other cells the surface expression of Fas-L allows triggering of apoptosis in Fas-carrying cells without additional triggering. The presence of Fas-L in cytolytic granules links this apoptotic mechanism directly to granule exocytosis.

KILLER CELL SELF-PROTECTION

How is the CTL or NK cell protected from perforin and the highly toxic molecules secreted during the cytotoxic event? First, the microanatomy of the cytolytic synapse confines the action of perforin and directs it toward the target membrane. The adhesion ring around the synapse is so dense that lateral diffusion will be restricted. Therefore, only the granule membrane lines the synapse on the CTL side. It is likely that the granule membrane is impervious to perforin action, and this hypothesis has recently been attributed to cathepsin B which is found coating the granule membrane and not allowing perforin to insert (Balaji et al. 2002). Second, the half-life of perforin after exposure to Ca^{2+} is very short and measured in seconds, because Ca^{2+} induces polymerization and polymerized perforin is not membrane active. Polymerization and membrane insertion have to proceed in a concerted action. Finally, CTLs and other hemopoietic cells express many serpins. Serpins are serine protease inhibitors first described and analyzed in serum as trypsin and thrombin inhibitors. They form 1:1 covalent complexes with the protease that are resistant to dissociation by denaturing agents. Serpins are highly specific substrates for the respective serine protease. On cleavage of a loop in the serpin, a dramatic and rapid conformational change takes place in the serpin molecule, which distorts the active site of the protease to such an extent that the cleavage dissociation reaction cannot take place and the protease remains trapped in the complex. PI-9 is a human intracellular serpin, expressed by killer cells, dendritic cells, and other hemopoietic cells, that inhibits granzyme B with high specificity (Hirst et al. 2001). Surprisingly, although caspases and granzyme B have similar substrate specificities, PI-9 is a much better inhibitor for granzyme B than for caspases. In the mouse at least six additional serpins have been identified, and it is likely that there may be a specific serpin for each of the granzymes described above.

TARGET CELL DEATH

CTL- and NK cell-mediated killing unleashes several cell death pathways simultaneously via the granule exocytosis mechanism (Figure 25.7). The mechanism by which perforin mediates entry of other granule components into the target cytoplasm may be compared with a very sophisticated injection mechanism entailing plasma membrane pore formation and endosomolysis. Receptor-mediated endocytosis of granule contents is also possible but perforin is still required to liberate the granule contents and allow their exit into the cytoplasm where they mediate destruction. The following events, each potentially leading to death, occur contemporaneously upon granule exocytosis:

- Perforin pore formation alone, if extensive enough, can kill cells. More commonly, however, perforin is the catalyst for uptake of granule components and their release into the target cytoplasm.
- Granzyme A mediates cell death by single-stranded DNA breaks, and interference with DNA repair and nucleosome assembly.
- Granzyme B results in caspase and Bid cleavage, setting off two apoptotic cascades that result in CAD activation and DNA laddering.
- Granzymes H, K, and M (NK) are likely to contribute to cell death although their mode of action is as yet unknown.
- Granulysin sets off mitochondrial death and disruption of energy generation by associating with the outer mitochondrial membrane.
- Not studied yet are the effects of typical lysosomal constituents, including acid hydrolases which presumably gain entry into the target cell and may well have lethal effects.
- Finally, in concert with perforin and the pathways depending on it, Fas-L is exocytosed and gains surface expression to engage the Fas receptor in order to trigger conventional apoptosis; the Fas ligand pathway, in contrast to the molecular pathways described above, is not dependent on the availability of perforin.

This listing, presumably still incomplete, shows the barrage of biological weapons brought to bear on the annihilation of target cells. Target cells are recognized because they are parasitized by viruses or oncogenes that strive to evade death and to make the target noncompliant to normal apoptotic signals. By employing multiple death pathways it will be very difficult for the virus, or other parasite, to block all pathways simultaneously, and noncompliance can be overcome by the killer cell.

ROLE OF PERFORIN IN THE INDUCTION OF CTL ACTIVATION

CTLs and NK cells are effector cells mediating effector responses in the efferent arm of immunity by killing target cells via perforin and producing cytokines, principally IFN-γ (Beresford et al. 1997; Bossi and Griffiths 1999; Smyth et al. 2000; Haddad et al. 2001; Hirst et al. 2001). Both cytotoxicity and IFN-γ production are essential for tumor rejection and viral clearance. However, perhaps surprisingly, cytotoxic activity mediated by NK cells is also required in the afferent arm of immunity for induction of CTL responses. Two mechanisms have been defined: (1) CD70-expressing tumor cells are killed by NK cells via CD27 engagement. Killing by NK and IFN-γ production is absolutely required for the induction of a CTL response and establishment of tumor-specific memory (Smyth et al. 2001; Kelly et al. 2002). (2) Heat shock proteins are released on trauma or necrosis and chaperone peptides including potential antigens. Dendritic cells and macrophages have receptors for heat shock proteins, thereby endocytosing the molecules along with bound peptides. The peptides are channeled into the class I MHC antigen-presenting pathway and are available for CTL recognition. However, T-cell activation requires the presence of NK cells and the action of perforin and IFN-γ. In the absence of perforin-containing NK cells, a CTL response does not ensue; NK and dendritic cells undergo reciprocal activation which is needed to permit T-cell activation and clonal expansion.

PERFORIN FUNCTION IN HOMEOSTASIS

During and after an immune response T cells need to expand and contract rapidly, respectively. Clonal contraction is part of the homeostatic regulation required to maintain a balanced T-cell repertoire. Fas and Fas-L, other tumor necrosis factor (TNF) receptors, and cytokines participate in homeostatic regulation of T

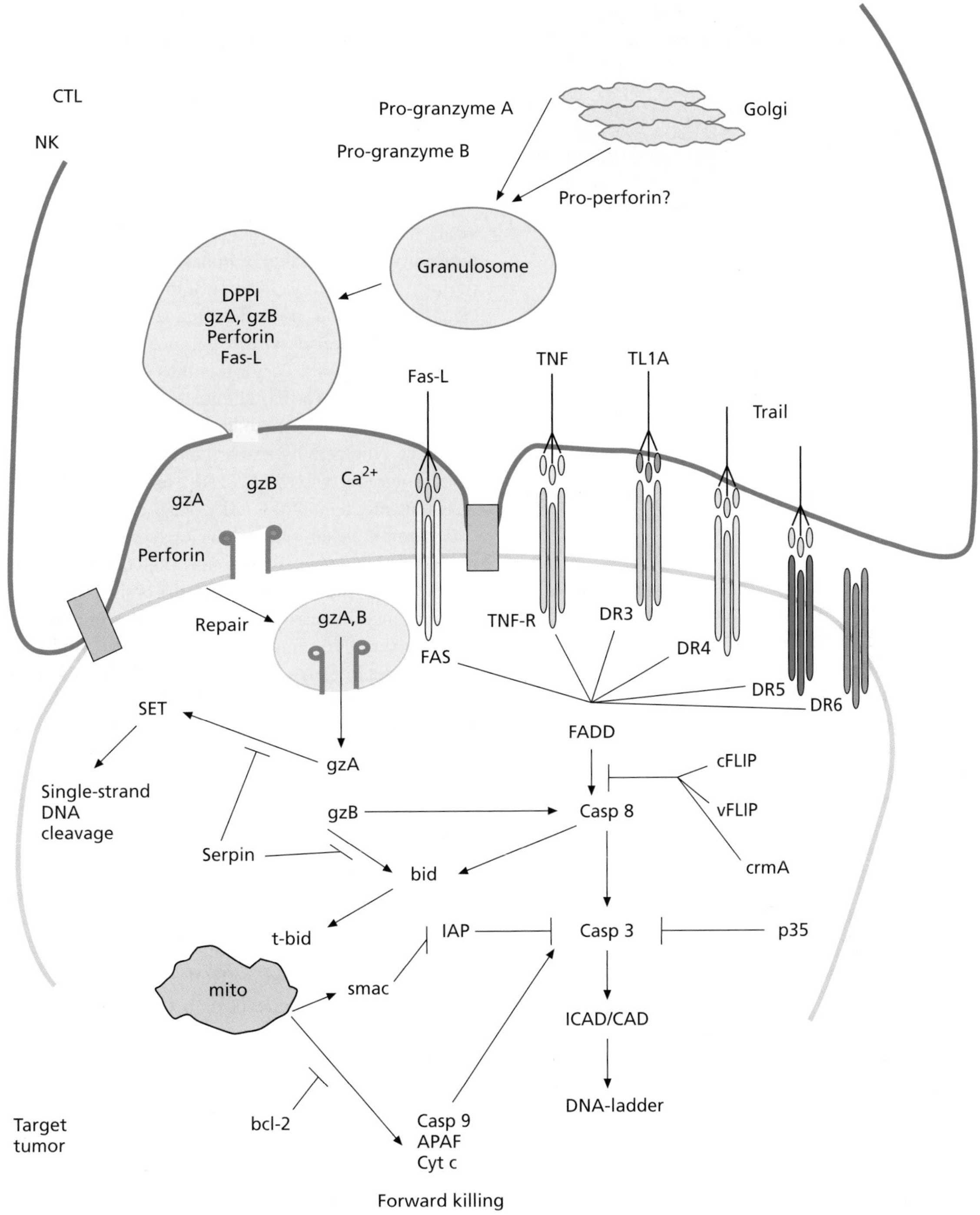

Figure 25.7 *Granule-mediated target killing: events in the target cell. See text for abbreviations.*

and B cells. Cytotoxicity mediated by perforin and associated with granules is required for homeostasis of CD8 CTLs and monocytes/macrophages. This function of perforin is seen only after viral challenge or in combination with other genetic defects. In murine models, the combined deficiency of perforin with Fas-L or Fas is much more severe than that of Fas-L or Fas deficiency alone (Spielman et al. 1998). Perforin/Fas-L deficiency results in early death and organ infiltration with CD8 cells and macrophages, indicating a critical role for perforin in their homeostasis (Figure 25.8). Similarly, perforin deficiency in humans causes childhood death by lymphoproliferation of CD8 cells and macrophage-type cells called histiocytes (see below) (Stepp et al. 1999; Fadeel et al. 2001). Homeostatic dysregulation in perforin deficiency is noted only after repeated antigenic (viral) challenge, suggesting dysregulation of the memory CTL pool.

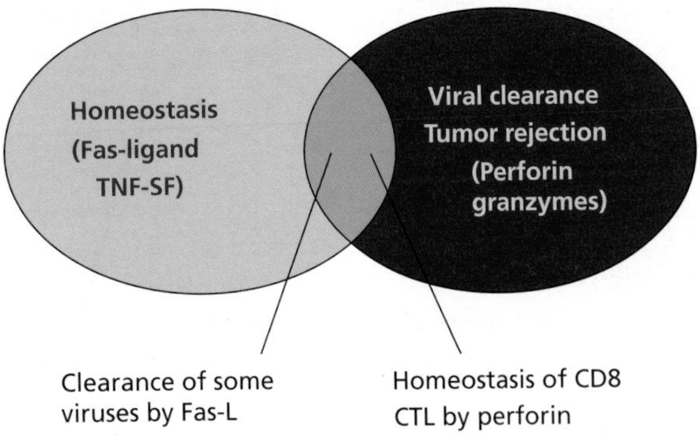

Figure 25.8 *Diagram of separate functions of perforin and Fas ligand (Fas-L) in immune defense and homeostatic regulation. Overlapping function in clearance of some viruses by Fas-L, and homeostatic regulation of CD8 cytotoxic lymphocytes (CTLs) by perforin.*

HOMEOSTATIC FUNCTION OF FAS AND FAS-L

Fas-L can induce apoptosis in Fas-expressing cells. Fas or Fas-L deficiency in mice results in lymphoproliferation and grossly enlarged lymph nodes by 6–12 months of age (Nagata and Suda 1995). Lymphoproliferation can be associated with autoimmunity in certain genetic backgrounds. The largest group of expanded T cells is found in the CD4/CD8$^-$, B220$^+$ population. Cells of the monocyte/macrophage lineage are only moderately expanded. Fas and Fas-L are important for antigen-induced cell death during secondary stimulation of T cells, and are believed to facilitate and maintain peripheral tolerance of T cells for self-antigens. CD4 cells are more susceptible to Fas-L-mediated deletion than CD8 cells, and Fas/Fas-L may be more important for CD4 T-cell homeostasis than for CD8 T cells. In humans, mutations in Fas or Fas-L give rise to autoimmune syndromes. The dysregulated removal of activated T cells results in the maintenance of selfreactive cells causing autoimmunity. It is not clear at the current time which cell types need to express Fas-L to maintain homeostasis; candidates are T cells or antigen-presenting cells.

GENETIC DEFECTS OF CYTOTOXICITY

Perforin deficiency in mice

Perforin is constitutively expressed in NK cells, NK-T cells, and γδ-T cells, all of which comprise a segment of the innate immune system. Although NK-T and γδ-T cells have TCRs, the TCR chains are relatively invariant and do not recognize MHC peptide complexes, although they recognize relatively invariant MHC class Ib molecules in association with lipids or carbohydrates. In αβ-T cells perforin is induced on T-cell activation and clonal expansion. The site with the highest level of perforin expression under physiological conditions is the decidua in the pregnant uterus. The decidua is enriched with decidual NK cells which express very high levels of perforin and may contribute to protection against infection. Perforin deficiency in mice that are kept free of pathogens has no obvious phenotype and does not disrupt the process of a normal pregnancy. However, on viral challenge perforin-deficient mice exhibit increased morbidity and mortality, emphasizing the importance of perforin in protection from viral infection. Perforin-deficient cells exhibit normal clonal expansion and tissue infiltration; however, viral clearance is impaired in the absence of perforin. Perforin is thus critical for the cytolytic process in vivo that eliminates the viruses. Perforin-deficient CTLs and NK cells in vitro have greatly diminished cytolytic activity and are only able to induce apoptosis in targets via Fas-L, TNF, or TNF-related apoptosis-inducing ligand (TRAIL) (Kagi et al. 1996).

Perforin-deficient mice develop spontaneous tumors with high incidence, lymphomas, and adenocarcinomas of the lung, indicating that perforin is important for immune surveillance against spontaneous tumors (Smyth et al. 2000; Smyth and Trapani 2001). Perforin-deficient mice are unable to reject challenge with immunogenic tumors when compared with wild-type mice. Controlled treatment with carcinogens demonstrates a higher frequency and earlier incidence of tumors in perforin-deficient mice in comparison to wild-type mice (van den Broek and Hengartner 2000; van den Broek et al. 1996). It is evident from these observations that perforin is an important mediator of tumor immunity.

Perforin is frequently found expressed at sites of autoimmune reactivity. Accordingly perforin deficiency can ameliorate certain autoimmune states, e.g. perforin-deficient non-obese diabetic (NOD) mice have a much lower and later incidence of diabetes than perforin-sufficient NOD.

Allogeneic bone marrow transplantation is complicated by the development of graft-versus-host disease arising from grafted T cells activated by the recipient's alloantigens. By transplanting perforin-deficient T cells the onset of graft-versus-host disease is dramatically delayed but then sets in with full force and lethality, suggesting that perforin contributes to the initiation of the immune response (Baker et al. 1996, 1997; Jiang et al. 2001). In allogeneic organ transplantation, perforin-expressing cells are found during transplant rejection. However, perforin deficiency does not noticeably affect organ rejection, indicating multiple redundant pathways (Atkinson et al. 1998; Kataoka et al. 1998; Ponting 1999).

Perforin-deficient mice have an impaired ability to downregulate CTLs on chronic infection and repeated in vivo stimulation, indicating a participation of perforin in CD8 CTL homeostasis (Edwards et al. 1999; Harty et al. 2000). This is more apparent when perforin deficiency is combined with Fas or Fas-L deficiency. Perforin/Fas-L double-deficient mice die at about 10 weeks of age of an autoimmune syndrome characterized by organ infiltration with macrophages and expansion of CD8 and CD4 cells, with an inversion of the normal CD4:CD8 ratio (Spielman et al. 1998). The mechanism by which perforin contributes to CTL downregulation is not clear, but two hypotheses have been discussed:

FRATRICIDE

On CTL killing of target cells, the CTLs can pick up target antigens, process the antigens, present them via MHC-I, and thereby become a target itself for other CTLs. In the presence of perforin CTLs would kill each other and thereby downregulate their activity.

KILLING OF ANTIGEN-PRESENTING CELLS

CTL activation and clonal expansion is mediated by antigen-presenting cells. On acquisition of cytotoxicity CTLs are perfectly able to kill antigen-presenting cells, thereby removing the initial signal for their own generation. In the absence of perforin the elimination of antigen-presenting cells is impaired, thereby providing chronic stimulation of CTLs and disruption of CTL homeostasis.

PERFORIN DEFICIENCY AND DEFECTS IN CYTOTOXICITY IN HUMANS

The syndrome of familial hemophagocytic lymphohistiocytosis (FHL) is a lethal inheritable disease associated with dysfunctional cytotoxicity of NK cells and CTLs (Stepp et al. 1999). The disease is characterized by early childhood onset, frequently after viral infections, and accompanied by lymphocytic proliferation and infiltration of tissues with histiocytes. The last cell type represents a late-stage monocyte/macrophage-derived cell characteristic for this syndrome. Recently, several etiological causes of the syndrome have been identified and can be subgrouped into several categories.

About 30 percent of the cases of FHL are caused by perforin deficiency. The remaining cases come from several disorders associated with dysfunctional secretory lysosomes, including granulosomes. Secretory lysosomes are found in lymphocytes and NK cells, granulocytes, mast cells, platelets, and melanocytes. Dysfunction of the secretory or trafficking pathway of secretory lysosomes may therefore affect other cellular systems, in addition to the cytolytic machinery.

The Chédiak–Higashi syndrome is an autosomal recessive disorder causing hypopigmentation of the skin, eyes, and hair, prolonged bleeding times, recurrent infections, abnormal NK cell function, and peripheral neuropathy. Morbidity results from patients succumbing to frequent bacterial infections or to lymphoproliferation. The *CHS1/LYST* gene encoding a cytosolic protein of 430 kDa is dysfunctional. The exact function of this gene is not known except that it participates in the biogenesis/secretion of secretory lysosomes. A similar defect is found in Beige mice. NK cells and polymorphonuclear granulocytes (Figure 25.9) have grotesquely enlarged granules which, however, cannot be secreted and hence NK cell activity is diminished. The inability of granule secretion is associated with the inability to use perforin for killing and in this regard appears as functional perforin deficiency with the same consequence of hemophagocytic lymphohistiocytosis resulting in death.

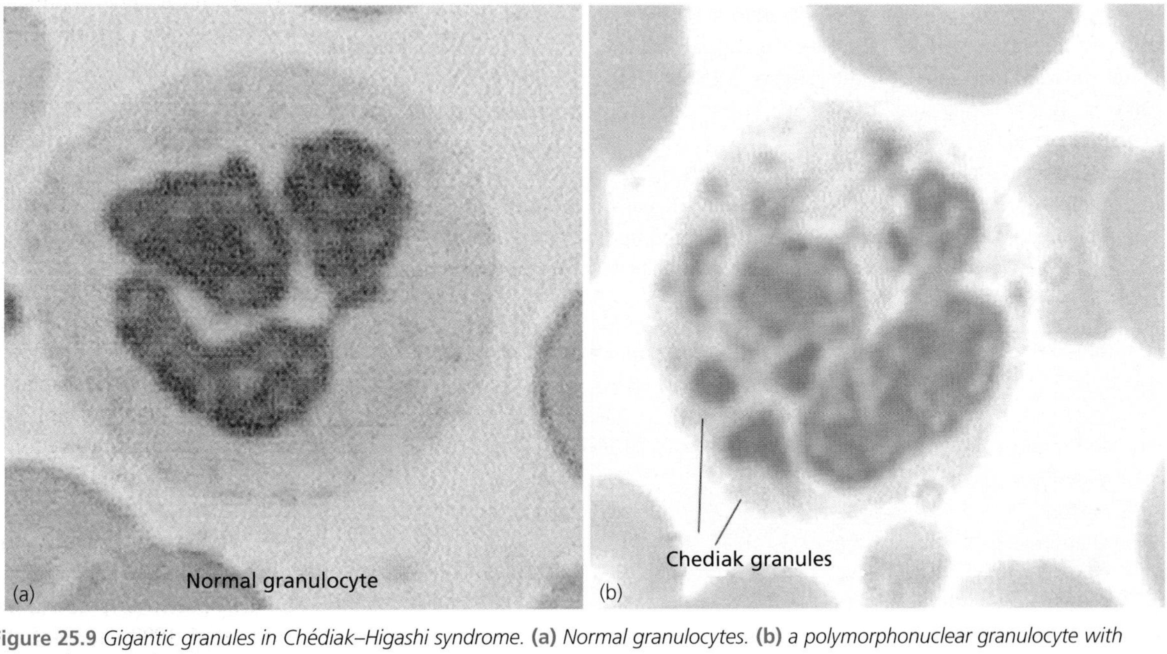

Figure 25.9 *Gigantic granules in Chédiak–Higashi syndrome.* **(a)** *Normal granulocytes.* **(b)** *a polymorphonuclear granulocyte with enlarged granules is shown.*

Griscelli's disease is an autosomal recessive disorder associated with hypopigmentation and occurrence of acute phases of uncontrolled lymphocyte and macrophage activation, ultimately causing death. Several genetic variations of the disease exist. One form of the disease is caused by mutations in Rab27a, a protein involved in vesicle traffic and required for granule exocytosis in lymphocytes and for melanocyte function. Evidence in Ashen mice suggests that Rab27b can substitute for Rab27a, but that Rab27b is not expressed in lymphocytes and melanocytes. CTL granules appear normal in Griscelli's syndrome; they migrate to the cytotoxic synapse; exocytosis does not take place, however, as a result of the absence of Rab27a (Haddad et al. 2001; Stinchcombe et al. 2001).

Patients with Hermansky–Pudlak disease have primarily bleeding abnormalities and ocular albinism. The syndrome includes mutations of at least three different gene products affecting vesicular traffic. One of the mutations in the Rab geranylgeranyl transferase α subunit reduces Rab prenylation and is responsible for defects in platelet granule synthesis. Cytolytic CTL granules fail to polarize properly, although their exocytosis appears normal. The murine model for this disease is found in gunmetal mice.

GRANZYME DEFICIENCIES

Granzyme deficiencies have been created in mice by gene targeting but so far have not been described in human populations. Granzyme A and granzyme B deletions have been described in the literature (Pham and Ley 1997; Simon et al. 1997). However, as granzyme B is on the same chromosome with, and upstream of, granzymes C, D, E, and F, the insertion of a neocassette also inactivated downstream granzyme expression. Re-examination of the granzyme B targeting using the Cre/lox system showed that most of the effects attributed to granzyme B knockout may have been caused by the concurrent extinction of granzyme C.

Granzyme A-deficient mice have no overt phenotype and no defect in the cytotoxic activity of T and NK cells. Similarly, granzyme B-deficient mice appear normal and their cytotoxic activity in vitro is not diminished. However, when DNA release is measured by using granzyme A- or B-deficient CTLs a reduction and delay in DNA release is observed, indicating impaired DNA degradation.

As mentioned above, it is likely that granzymes have evolved to defeat viral escape mechanisms. Therefore it might be expected that granzyme deficiencies may be associated with increased susceptibility to certain viral infections and mortality. Indeed, by titrating the viral dose and measuring disease and mortality, an important function for granzymes in antiviral defense can be demonstrated. Ectromelia is the mouse pox virus which is highly virulent in mice. Wild-type mice are susceptible to infection, but lethality requires an infective dose of more than a million viral units. Perforin-deficient mice are highly susceptible and succumb to disease from as little as one viral unit. Granzyme A- and B-deficient mice exhibit susceptibility between these two extremes (Mullbacher et al. 1996, 1999). Interestingly, the ability to clear virus infection and to reject tumors does not correlate (Table 25.1). Although granzymes clearly are important for viral protection they seem to be dispensable for tumor rejection. RMAS is an MHC-negative tumor that requires NK cells for rejection whereas the K1735 melanoma is rejected by CTLs. In both cases and in immune surveillance against methylcholanthrene-induced carcinomas, perforin is required but granzymes A and B are not.

DPP1 DEFICIENCY (CATHEPSIN C)

Dipeptidyl peptidase is required for the cleavage of the pro-dipeptide of all granzymes. In the absence of this cleavage granzymes remain inactive as zymogens. CTLs with deficiency of the dipeptidyl peptidase have the hallmarks of combined granzyme A/B deficiency. However, dipeptidyl peptidase is also important for activation of proteases in mast cells, granulocytes, and other cells. In humans dipeptidyl peptidase deficiency, the Papillon–Lefevre syndrome, or keratosis palmoplantaris with periodontopathia is an autosomal recessive disorder. Patients suffer early loss of teeth, apparently from chronic infection of the periodontium.

Table 25.1 *Role of perforin and granzymes in viral clearance and tumor rejection*

Deficiency	Lethal viral dose (mouse pox virus)	Rejection of RMAS tumor	Rejection of K1735 melanoma	Immune surveillance, carcinogenesis
Wild type	$>10^6$	Yes	Yes	Normal
Perforin	1	No	No	Impaired
Granzyme A	10^5	Yes	Yes	Normal
Granzyme B[a]	10^4	Yes	Yes	Normal
Granzyme A + B[a]	1	Yes	Yes	Normal

a) Granzyme B deficiency includes cluster deficiency.

Cytotoxicity and antiviral defense

Viruses are intracellular parasites infecting the victim's own cells. Antibodies and pattern recognition receptors used for recognition and defense against extracellular parasites, primarily bacteria and bacilli, are not much use against intracellular parasites, which can be removed only by the destruction of the infected cells. This is achieved in two ways: by suicide (apoptosis) of the infected cell and, in the case of failure of suicide, by the cytotoxic lymphocyte (Mullbacher et al. 1996; Edwards et al. 1999; Harty et al. 2000; Wallich et al. 2001).

A primary defense system against viral spread is the interferon system. Double-stranded RNA or DNA of the viruses is recognized by DNA- or RNA-dependent protein kinase which turns on INF-α and -β with the resultant interferon secretion signaling via interferon receptors to the infected and neighboring cells. The signals result in shutdown of protein synthesis and transcription of antiviral genes that block viral replication and viral clearance, or in apoptosis of the infected cell. Many virus infections are contained at this stage. Other viruses have evolved to overcome the initial antiviral response and block apoptosis of the infected cell. The interferon secretion, however, also activates NK cells which are attracted and activated and begin killing infected cells that fail to undergo apoptosis. It is apparent that successful killing must overcome the anti-apoptotic activities of the virus that have allowed it to begin to replicate. How does the NK cell recognize the infected cell? First, some viruses downregulate MHC molecules to avoid T-cell detection; this is the signal for NK cells to start killing such cells. Second, infected cells frequently express new gene products (stress genes, e.g. Rae-1β) that are recognized by positively signaling receptors on the NK cell (NKG2D) and initiate cytotoxicity. NK cell killing and antigen release, together with IFN-γ production, bring dendritic cells to the site of action. Dendritic cells further activate NK cells and recruit the CTL response. The fact that the virus has survived in the infected cell up to this point is testimony to its ability to block apoptotic pathways. The virus now needs to focus on evading detection by NK and T cells and/or to block the cytotoxic assault. Herpes viruses have very large genomes devoted largely to the purpose of evading immune recognition and to thwarting the cytotoxic response. Indeed many herpes viruses are never totally eliminated and persist as latent infections that can flare up at any time that the CTL response is suppressed by medical immune suppression or other natural causes. Pox viruses focus on blocking cytotoxicity; they express powerful inhibitors for caspases (crmA) and granzymes (serpin homologues). However, the evolution of several granzymes in the arsenal of the cytotoxic response seems to be the response to this family of viruses allowing survival of the host, even though with great difficulty.

It is self-evident that only those species able to resist and overcome viral attack were able to survive and reproduce, and likewise that viruses had to continue to evolve new strategies to prevent obliteration. This struggle continues today, best exemplified in the HIV epidemic and the trend of new viruses emerging.

CYTOTOXICITY AND ANTI-TUMOR DEFENSE

Perforin is a critical part of immune surveillance against spontaneous tumors and protection against carcinogens. In addition perforin is required for the rejection of tumors by NK cells and CTLs whereas granzymes appear dispensable. One might conclude that it is easier to kill tumor cells than virus-infected cells. So, then, why are tumors not eliminated by the immune system? The answer is that the tumor has developed elaborate pathways to evade or suppress the immune system. Tumors do not secrete interferons that would alert the NK response; indeed the lack of an interferon response makes many tumors susceptible to viruses that are easily suppressed by normal cells. The lack of arousal of an NK response seriously hampers the harnessing of dendritic cells and a CTL response. The lack of signals emanating from the tumor also prevents CTLs from homing in on the tumor. The tumor, unlike viral infection, is not perceived by the immune system as dangerous. Again, unlike viral infection and replication, tumor progression and stepwise mutation are slow. Tumors express many negative regulators of the immune response. CTL responses to viruses entail a rapid burst of clonal expansion followed by an equally rapid clonal contraction, leaving behind a few memory cells that can respond again and faster in a second viral attack. The clonal contraction, mediated for CD8 CTL cells by perforin and for CD4 cells by Fas-L, is absolutely necessary to avoid autoimmunity and lymphoproliferation. Tumors express genes that can interfere with clonal expansion and/or cause premature clonal contraction and downregulate cytotoxic activity, thereby allowing their continued survival. The challenge for tumor immunologists is the ability not only to develop vaccines that generate activated NK cells and specific CTLs, but also to find ways to direct these cells to the tumor site.

REFERENCES

Atkinson, E.A., Barry, M., et al. 1998. Cytotoxic T lymphocyte-assisted suicide. Caspase 3 activation is primarily the result of the direct action of granzyme B. *J Biol Chem*, **273**, 21261–6.

Baker, M.B., Altman, N.H., et al. 1996. The role of cell-mediated cytotoxicity in acute GVHD after MHC-matched allogeneic bone marrow transplantation in mice. *J Exp Med*, **183**, 2645–56.

Baker, M.B., Riley, R.L., et al. 1997. Graft-versus-host-disease-associated lymphoid hypoplasia and B cell dysfunction is dependent upon donor T cell-mediated Fas-ligand function, but not perforin function. *Proc Natl Acad Sci USA*, **94**, 1366–71.

Balaji, K.N., Schaschke, N., et al. 2002. Surface cathepsin B protects cytotoxic lymphocytes from self-destruction after degranulation. *J Exp Med*, **196**, 493–503.

Barry, M. and Bleackley, R.C. 2002. Cytotoxic T lymphocytes: all roads lead to death. *Nat Rev Immunol*, **2**, 401–9.

Beresford, P.J., Kam, C.M., et al. 1997. Recombinant human granzyme A binds to two putative HLA-associated proteins and cleaves one of them. *Proc Natl Acad Sci USA*, **94**, 9285–90.

Berke, G. 1995. PELs and the perforin and granzyme independent mechanism of CTL-mediated lysis. *Immunol Rev*, **146**, 21–31.

Blott, E.J. and Griffiths, G.M. 2002. Secretory lysosomes. *Nat Rev Mol Cell Biol*, **3**, 122–31.

Bossi, G. and Griffiths, G.M. 1999. Degranulation plays an essential part in regulating cell surface expression of Fas ligand in T cells and natural killer cells. *Nat Med*, **5**, 90–6.

Darmon, A.J., Ley, T.J., et al. 1996. Cleavage of CPP32 by granzyme B represents a critical role for granzyme B in the induction of target cell DNA fragmentation. *J Biol Chem*, **271**, 21709–12.

Davis, J.E., Smyth, M.J. and Trapani, J.A. 2001. Granzyme A and B-deficient killer lymphocytes are defective in eliciting DNA fragmentation but retain potent in vivo anti-tumor capacity. *Eur J Immunol*, **31**, 39–47.

Dennert, G. and Podack, E.R. 1983. Cytolysis by H-2-specific T killer cells. Assembly of tubular complexes on target membranes. *J Exp Med*, **157**, 1483–95.

Djeu, J.Y., Jiang, K. and Wei, S. 2002. A view to a kill: signals triggering cytotoxicity. *Clin Cancer Res*, **8**, 636–40.

Edwards, K.M., Davis, J.E., et al. 1999. Anti-viral strategies of cytotoxic T lymphocytes are manifested through a variety of granule-bound pathways of apoptosis induction. *Immunol Cell Biol*, **77**, 76–89.

Fadeel, B., Orrenius, S. and Henter, J.I. 2001. Familial hemophagocytic lymphohistiocytosis: too little cell death can seriously damage your health. *Leuk Lymphoma*, **42**, 13–20.

Fan, Z., Beresford, P.J., et al. 2002. HMG2 interacts with the nucleosome assembly protein SET and is a target of the cytotoxic T-lymphocyte protease granzyme A. *Mol Cell Biol*, **22**, 2810–20.

Froelich, C.J., Orth, K., et al. 1996. New paradigm for lymphocyte granule-mediated cytotoxicity. Target cells bind and internalize granzyme B, but an endosomolytic agent is necessary for cytosolic delivery and subsequent apoptosis. *J Biol Chem*, **271**, 29073–9.

Griffiths, G.M. 1997. Protein sorting and secretion during CTL killing. *Semin Immunol*, **9**, 10–159.

Haddad, E.K., Wu, X., et al. 2001. Defective granule exocytosis in Rab27a-deficient lymphocytes from Ashen mice. *J Cell Biol*, **152**, 835–42.

Harty, J.T., Tvinnereim, A.R. and White, D.W. 2000. CD8+ T cell effector mechanisms in resistance to infection. *Annu Rev Immunol*, **18**, 275–308.

Henkart, P.A. 1985. Mechanism of lymphocyte-mediated cytotoxicity. *Annu Rev Immunol*, **3**, 31–58.

Henkart, P.A. 1997. CTL effector functions. *Semin Immunol*, **9**, 85–6.

Henkart, P.A., Millard, P.J., et al. 1984. Cytolytic activity of purified cytoplasmic granules from cytotoxic rat large granular lymphocyte tumors. *J Exp Med*, **160**, 75–93.

Hirst, C.E., Buzza, M.S., et al. 2001. Perforin-independent expression of granzyme B and proteinase inhibitor 9 in human testis and placenta suggests a role for granzyme B-mediated proteolysis in reproduction. *Mol Hum Reprod*, **7**, 1133–42.

Jiang, Z., Podack, E. and Levy, R.B. 2001. Major histocompatibility complex-mismatched allogeneic bone marrow transplantation using perforin and/or Fas ligand double-defective CD4(+) donor T cells: involvement of cytotoxic function by donor lymphocytes prior to graft-versus-host disease pathogenesis. *Blood*, **98**, 390–7.

Kagi, D., Ledermann, B., et al. 1994. Cytotoxicity mediated by T cells and natural killer cells is greatly impaired in perforin-deficient mice. *Nature*, **369**, 31–7.

Kagi, D., Ledermann, B., et al. 1996. Molecular mechanisms of lymphocyte-mediated cytotoxicity and their role in immunological protection and pathogenesis in vivo. *Annu Rev Immunol*, **14**, 207–32.

Kataoka, T., Schroter, M., et al. 1998. FLIP prevents apoptosis induced by death receptors but not by perforin/granzyme B, chemotherapeutic drugs, and gamma irradiation. *J Immunol*, **161**, 3936–42.

Kelly, J.M., Darcy, P.K., et al. 2002. Induction of tumor-specific T cell memory by NK cell-mediated tumor rejection. *Nat Immunol*, **3**, 83–90.

Liu, C.C., Persechini, P.M. and Young, J.D. 1995. Perforin and lymphocyte-mediated cytolysis. *Immunol Rev*, **146**, 145–75.

Masson, D. and Tschopp, J. 1987. A family of serine esterases in lytic granules of cytolytic T lymphocytes. *Cell*, **49**, 679–85.

Masson, D., Zamai, M. and Tschopp, J. 1986. Identification of granzyme A isolated from cytotoxic T-lymphocyte-granules as one of the proteases encoded by CTL-specific genes. *FEBS Lett*, **208**, 84–8.

Metkar, S.S., Wang, B., et al. 2002. Cytotoxic cell granule-mediated apoptosis: perforin delivers granzyme B-serglycin complexes into target cells without plasma membrane pore formation. *Immunity*, **16**, 417–28.

Mullbacher, A., Ebnet, K., et al. 1996. Granzyme A is critical for recovery of mice from infection with the natural cytopathic viral pathogen, ectromelia. *Proc Natl Acad Sci USA*, **93**, 5783–7.

Mullbacher, A., Hla, R.T., et al. 1999. Perforin is essential for control of ectromelia virus but not related poxviruses in mice. *J Virol*, **73**, 1665–7.

Nagata, S. 1996. Apoptosis mediated by the Fas system. *Prog Mol Subcell Biol*, **16**, 87–103.

Nagata, S. 1998. Human autoimmune lymphoproliferative syndrome, a defect in the apoptosis-inducing Fas receptor: a lesson from the mouse model. *J Hum Genet*, **43**, 2–8.

Nagata, S. and Suda, T. 1995. Fas and Fas ligand: lpr and gld mutations. *Immunol Today*, **16**, 39–43.

Nakajima, H., Park, H.L. and Henkart, P.A. 1995. Synergistic roles of granzymes A and B in mediating target cell death by rat basophilic leukemia mast cell tumors also expressing cytolysin/perforin. *J Exp Med*, **181**, 1037–46.

Pham, C.T. and Ley, T.J. 1997. The role of granzyme B cluster proteases in cell-mediated cytotoxicity. *Semin Immunol*, **9**, 127–33.

Podack, E.R. 1985. The molecular mechanism of lymphocyte-mediated tumor lysis. *Immunol Today*, **6**, 21–7.

Podack, E.R. 1989. Killer lymphocytes and how they kill. *Curr Opin Cell Biol*, **1**, 929–33.

Podack, E.R. 1995a. Functional significance of two cytolytic pathways of cytotoxic T lymphocytes. *J Leukoc Biol*, **57**, 548–52.

Podack, E.R. 1995b. Execution and suicide: cytotoxic lymphocytes enforce Draconian laws through separate molecular pathways. *Curr Opin Immunol*, **7**, 11–16.

Podack, E.R. 1999. How to induce involuntary suicide: the need for dipeptidyl peptidase 1. *Proc Natl Acad Sci USA*, **96**, 8312–14.

Podack, E.R. and Dennert, G. 1983. Assembly of two types of tubules with putative cytolytic function by cloned natural killer cells. *Nature*, **302**, 442–5.

Podack, E.R. and Konigsberg, P.J. 1984. Cytolytic T cell granules. Isolation, structural, biochemical, and functional characterization. *J Exp Med*, **160**, 695–710.

Podack, E.R. and Kupfer, A. 1991. T-cell effector functions: mechanisms for delivery of cytotoxicity and help. *Annu Rev Cell Biol*, **7**, 479–504.

Podack, E.R. and Tschopp, J. 1982. Circular polymerization of the ninth component of complement. Ring closure of the tubular complex confers resistance to detergent dissociation and to proteolytic degradation. *J Biol Chem*, **257**, 15204–12.

Podack, E.R., Hengartner, H. and Lichtenheld, M.G. 1991. A central role of perforin in cytolysis? *Annu Rev Immunol*, **9**, 129–57.

Ponting, C.P. 1999. Chlamydial homologues of the MACPF (MAC/perforin) domain. *Curr Biol*, **9**, R911–13.

Rukavina, D. and Podack, E.R. 2000. Abundant perforin expression at the maternal-fetal interface: guarding the semiallogeneic transplant? *Immunol Today*, **21**, 160–3.

Russell, J.H. and Ley, T.J. 2002. Lymphocyte-mediated cytotoxicity. *Annu Rev Immunol*, **20**, 323–70.

Shiver, J.W., Su, L. and Henkart, P.A. 1992. Cytotoxicity with target DNA breakdown by rat basophilic leukemia cells expressing both cytolysin and granzyme A. *Cell*, **71**, 315–22.

Simon, M.M., Hausmann, M., et al. 1997. In vitro- and ex vivo-derived cytolytic leukocytes from granzyme A x B double knockout mice are defective in granule-mediated apoptosis but not lysis of target cells. *J Exp Med*, **186**, 1781–6.

Smyth, M.J. and Trapani, J.A. 2001. Lymphocyte-mediated immunosurveillance of epithelial cancers? *Trends Immunol*, **22**, 409–11.

Smyth, M.J., Thia, K.Y., et al. 2000. Perforin-mediated cytotoxicity is critical for surveillance of spontaneous lymphoma. *J Exp Med*, **192**, 755–60.

Smyth, M.J., Kelly, J.M., et al. 2001. Unlocking the secrets of cytotoxic granule proteins. *J Leukoc Biol*, **70**, 18–29.

Spielman, J.R., Lee, K., et al. 1998. Perforin/Fas ligand double deficiency is associated with macrophage expansion and severe pancreatitis. *J Immunol*, **161**, 7063–70.

Stepp, S.E., Dufourcq-Lagelouse, R., et al. 1999. Perforin gene defects in familial hemophagocytic lymphohistiocytosis. *Science*, **256**, 1957–9.

Stinchcombe, J.C., Barral, D.C., et al. 2001. Rab27a is required for regulated secretion in cytotoxic T lymphocytes. *J Cell Biol*, **152**, 825–34.

Takahashi, T., Tanaka, M., et al. 1994. Generalized lymphoproliferative disease in mice, caused by a point mutation in the Fas ligand. *Cell*, **76**, 969–76.

Uellner, R., Zvelebil, M.J., et al. 1997. Perforin is activated by a proteolytic cleavage during biosynthesis which reveals a phospholipid-binding C2 domain. *EMBO J*, **16**, 7287–96.

van den Broek, M.E., Kagi, D., et al. 1996. Decreased tumor surveillance in perforin-deficient mice. *J Exp Med*, **184**, 1781–90.

van den Broek, M.F. and Hengartner, H. 2000. The role of perforin in infections and tumour surveillance. *Exp Physiol*, **85**, 681–5.

Wallich, R., Simon, M.M. and Mullbacher, A. 2001. Virulence of mousepox virus is independent of serpin-mediated control of cellular cytotoxicity. *Viral Immunol*, **14**, 71–81.

Wilharm, E., Tschopp, J. and Jenne, D.E. 1999. Biological activities of granzyme K are conserved in the mouse and account for residual Z-Lys-SBzl activity in granzyme A-deficient mice. *FEBS Lett*, **459**, 139–42.

Wolters, P.J., Pham, C.T., et al. 2001. Dipeptidyl peptidase 1 is essential for activation of mast cell chymases, but not tryptases, in mice. *J Biol Chem*, **276**, 18551–6.

Young, J.D., Cohn, Z.A. and Podack, E.R. 1986. The ninth component of complement and the pore-forming protein (perforin 1) from cytotoxic T cells: structural, immunological, and functional similarities. *Science*, **233**, 184–90.

Zhang, D., Pasternack, M.S., et al. 2001. Induction of rapid histone degradation by the cytotoxic T lymphocyte protease Granzyme A. *J Biol Chem*, **276**, 3683–90.

26

Immunological memory

SHANE CROTTY AND RAFI AHMED

The primary function of the immune system is to defend against microbial pathogens. It accomplishes this task at two levels: first, by generating a specific immune response against the invading pathogen and controlling the infection; and second, by remembering this first encounter and mounting an accelerated immune response upon re-exposure to the same pathogen. This rapid recall response can either completely prevent disease or greatly lessen the severity of clinical symptoms. The first documentation of 'immune memory' dates back to the time of the Greek historian Thucydides, who recorded that the 'same man was never attacked twice' while describing the plague of Athens in 430BC (Finley 1951). It is remarkable that we knew nothing about the immune system or about microbes when Thucydides made his astute observations on immune memory; it would be more than 2000 years before we gained an appreciation of the immune system and learnt that microbes cause infectious diseases. However, it is now well established that memory and specificity constitute the two defining features of adaptive immune responses.

The focus of this chapter is on the principles of immune memory. This chapter is divided into four parts: (1) a historical perspective of vaccination; (2) an overview of protective immunity to microbes; (3) a discussion of the current models of memory T- and B-cell differentiation; and (4) an overview of the mechanisms involved in maintaining immunological memory.

HISTORY OF VACCINATION

Immunological memory is the basis for vaccination; the discipline of vaccinology originated from the observation that previous exposure to a disease conferred resistance to a subsequent episode. Thus, the principle of vaccinology was that, if somehow the first episode of a disease could be attenuated, one would be protected against the more severe form of the disease. The earliest recorded attempts to put this into practice were made in China and India around AD 1500 when pustular material from smallpox patients was inoculated into healthy people (Fenner et al. 1988). This process, called 'variolation', caused smallpox but, for reasons that are not fully understood, the disease was usually milder. More importantly, 'variolated' individuals were protected against naturally acquired smallpox. However, this approach did not gain popularity and was eventually discontinued because the degree of morbidity and mortality associated with variolation was simply too variable and too high to be acceptable.

The major breakthrough came with the classic experiments of Jenner in 1796. Jenner had noticed that milkmaids who were commonly infected with cowpox were spared the ravages of smallpox. Jenner reasoned that inoculation of cowpox pustular material might prevent smallpox. In many ways, vaccinology was born in 1796 when Jenner inoculated young James Phipps with cowpox virus and subsequently prevented smallpox, thereby showing that exposure to a related but less pathogenic virus could confer protection against a more virulent virus. However, despite this remarkable achievement, the field of vaccinology stood still for the next 50–75 years. This lack of progress was primarily the result of the fact that it was still not proven that microbes caused smallpox, or any disease. Thus, there was no clear scientific basis for developing additional vaccines.

Things changed dramatically in the second half of the nineteenth century as a result of the pioneering work of Pasteur, Koch, Ross, von Behring, Ehrlich, and others. These scientific giants not only proved that microbes cause infectious diseases, thus laying the foundations of immunology and microbiology, but their work also resulted in the development of successful vaccines against rabies, typhoid, cholera, plague, and diphtheria (Plotkin and Orenstein 1999). It is only fitting that the first Nobel Prize in Medicine and Physiology, given in 1901, was awarded to von Behring for his work on diphtheria. Several additional vaccines were developed during the first half of the twentieth century, including the highly effective yellow fever virus vaccine by Theiler, for which he was awarded the Nobel Prize in 1951.

Until 1950 all viral vaccines were prepared in either mammalian or avian whole tissues. In that year Enders and colleagues showed that viruses can be grown in vitro in cell culture, which opened enormous scientific possibilities and facilitated the development of many of our currently used vaccines (Table 26.1), including vaccines against polio virus, measles, mumps, and rubella. This technology continues to be the most common method of manufacturing viral vaccines to this day.

Major advances have occurred during the past 25 years in our ability to 'cut and paste' genes, yet only two currently licensed vaccines are made using recombinant DNA technology – the hepatitis B vaccine and the Lyme disease vaccine. However, it is expected that almost all future vaccines will rely on recombinant DNA technology to some extent. A multitude of expression vectors (bacterial, viral, 'naked' DNA) have been developed and considerable effort has gone into optimizing their in vivo expression and methods/routes of immunization (Table 26.2; see Part VII: Vaccines). It is likely that these will become the main technologies for our future vaccines. Indeed, several recombinant vaccines are currently in human clinical trials. It remains to be seen which of these vectors will prove to be the most effective. The crucial properties will be the ability to target antigen-presenting cells (APC), the level and duration of gene expression in vivo, the ease of constructing the vector, and issues such as cost and safety of the vectors.

Table 26.1 *General approaches for vaccines*

Type of vaccine	Comments	Examples	
		Viral	Bacterial
Live attenuated organism	The organism is attenuated such that it does not produce clinical disease but still retains sufficient immunogenicity and replicative capacity to induce protective immunity	Polio (Sabin, OPV), measles, mumps, rubella, yellow fever, varicella (chickenpox)	Bacilius Calmette–Guérin (BCG)
Killed organism	The vaccine consists of the whole organism, which has been chemically inactivated to prevent replication, but the immunogenic structure of the organism is preserved	Polio (Salk, IPV), influenza, Japanese encephalitis, rabies, hepatitis A	Pertussis (whole), cholera
Antigenically related organism	This is the strategy used by the original vaccine	Cowpox or vaccinia, for smallpox	None
Subunit vaccines	The vaccine consists of subcomponents of the organism. These subcomponents are usually either surface proteins of a virus, or proteins and/or polysaccharides of bacteria	Hepatitis B	*Haemophilus influenza*b, pneumococci, meningococci, typhoid, pertussis (acellular), Lyme disease
Antitoxins	The vaccine consists of inactivated toxin (toxoid) that is no longer toxic but still retains its immunogenic structure	None	Tetanus, diphtheria, anthrax
Vectored vaccines	These vaccines are currently in development. These strategies use known immunogenic and safe viruses or bacteria as engineered vectors to express immunogenic proteins from pathogens of interest (see Table 26.2)	None licensed, but several in phase I and II clinical trials	
Nuclei acid (DNA) vaccines	These vaccines are currently in development. The vaccine consists of plasmid DNA capable of expressing the antigen of interest when introduced into cells	None licensed, but several in phase I clinical trials	

Table 26.2 *Recombinant delivery systems for future vaccines*[a]

Delivery systems
Plasmid 'naked' DNA
Bacterial vectors
Listeria spp.
Mycobacterium spp.
Salmonella spp.
Shigella spp.
Viral vectors
Adenoviruses
Alphaviruses
Lentiviruses
Picornaviruses
Poxviruses
Retroviruses

a) This is a partial list of the many bacterial and viral vectors currently being tested.

PROTECTIVE IMMUNITY

There has been great interest in determining the relative importance of humoral versus cellular responses in protective immunity. This has resulted in much debate and considerable experimentation to assess the role of T- and B-cell responses in protection from reinfection. When examining this issue, one must remember that antibodies and T cells have evolved to perform entirely different functions. The business of antibodies is to deal with the microbe itself (i.e. free virus particles, bacteria, and parasites) and that of T cells is to deal with infected cells. As T cells can only recognize microbial antigens in association with host MHC molecules, the free virus particles or bacteria are invisible to them. Thus, antibody provides our only specific defense against free microbial organisms, and therefore the importance of pre-existing antibody in protective immunity against infectious diseases cannot be overemphasized. In fact, antibody is likely to be the sole mechanism of protective immunity against bacteria and parasites that have an exclusively extracellular lifestyle. However, the equation begins to change for viruses and for those bacteria and parasites that can survive or replicate intracellularly. Although antibody again provides the first line of defense against such infections, frequently the inoculum is not entirely neutralized by the pre-existing antibody. This is where the T cells come into play, because their main function is surveillance of infected cells. T cells are divided into two subsets, $CD4^+$ and $CD8^+$ T cells, and both of these subsets play a role in protective immunity. They do this by either killing the infected cell and/or by releasing cytokines that stop or slow growth of the microbe. In addition to these effector functions carried out by both $CD4^+$ and $CD8^+$ T cells, $CD4^+$ T cells also play an important role in providing help for antibody production and help for generating $CD8^+$ T-cell responses.

Thus, based on these basic principles, protective immunity to extracellular pathogens depends primarily upon B cells and $CD4^+$ T cells (as helpers), whereas a concerted effort by B cells, $CD4^+$ T cells (as both helpers and effectors), and $CD8^+$ T cells is required to control intracellular pathogens. Although this generalization is reasonably accurate, there are several examples where microbial infections have been controlled exclusively by antibody (i.e. passive antibody transfer) or by $CD8^+$ T cells (i.e. after immunization by a vaccine containing only the $CD8^+$ T-cell epitopes) (Ahmed and Biron 1999). These experiments clearly show that there are situations where either humoral or cellular immunity can be sufficient for protection. The correct conclusion from such experiments is that, in the given situation, just the $CD8^+$ T-cell response or the antibody response was adequate for protection. However, it is crucial to realize that it is misleading to conclude from this type of experiment that the missing response does not play a role in protective immunity. The danger of reaching such a conclusion is that potentially useful immune responses may get excluded from the design of a vaccine.

Similarly, when designing a vaccine it is prudent to look beyond the type of immunity generated during the natural infection, e.g. antibody plays a minimal role in controlling an acute primary lymphocytic choriomeningitis virus (LCMV) infection in mice, or in conferring protection from re-infection ($CD8^+$ T cells are the major players in both instances) (Buchmeier and Zajac 1999). Yet, passive transfer of neutralizing antibody can confer a reasonable degree of protection (Buchmeier and Zajac 1999). A similar situation exists for *Listeria monocytogenes*. *Listeria* species has long been considered to be an infection controlled exclusively by T cells, but a recent study has shown that antibody is also effective in eliminating it (Edelson et al. 1999). These findings have obvious implications for vaccine design, e.g. although very little neutralizing antibody is generated during the course of HIV infection, immunization with the right form of HIV envelope protein may induce neutralizing antibody that would be useful in conferring protective immunity (Mascola et al. 2000; Burton 2002). Thus, the right strategy for a HIV vaccine would be to stimulate both the humoral and cellular arms of the immune system.

What is the basis of protective immunity? Is it protection from infection or from disease? In the strictest sense, protection from infection would mean that there was sufficient pre-existing antibody to neutralize/opsonize all of the pathogen in the inoculum and there was no further amplification of the microbe. This is frequently referred to as sterilizing immunity. Does this ever happen? The precise answer is not known, but it is likely that it does happen regularly when the inoculum size of a pathogen is very low. However, when challenged with a substantial inoculum of pathogen, it is more likely that a substantial fraction of the virus/

bacteria gets neutralized and the remaining fraction that is able to initiate infection is quickly controlled by the rapid anamnestic response of memory T cells and/or memory B cells (Ahmed and Gray 1996; McChesney et al. 1997). Overall, this is a pretty good scenario. First, the infection is rapidly controlled and there is no disease; second, the virus is fully eliminated by the memory response; and third, this low-grade, transient, subclinical infection serves as a natural 'booster' to the immune system.

MEMORY T- AND B-CELL DIFFERENTIATION

Before considering models of memory B- and T-cell differentiation it is important to appreciate a fundamental difference between cellular and humoral immunity. Microbial infections usually induce both T- and B-cell long-term memory. However, the nature of T- and B-cell memory is different (Figure 26.1 and Table 26.3). B-cell memory is usually manifested by continuous antibody production, even after resolution of the disease. Prolonged antibody production, lasting for several years after infection or immunization, has been observed in humans as well as in experimental systems (Scheibel et al. 1966; Simonsen et al. 1984; Kjeldsen et al. 1985; Cohen et al. 1994; Slifka et al. 1995; Bottiger et al. 1998; Crotty et al. 2003; Hammarlund et al. 2003). In contrast, the effector phase of the T-cell response is short-lived (a few weeks), and 'memory' in the T-cell compartment results from the presence of quiescent memory T cells, which are found at higher frequencies than naïve cells and can respond faster and develop into effector cells (i.e. cytoxic T lymphocyte (CTL) or cytokine producers) more efficiently than can naïve T cells (Kedl and Mescher 1998; Bachmann et al. 1999a; Cho et al. 1999; Zimmermann et al. 1999; Barber et al. 2003). This dichotomy in effector function in the humoral and cellular memory pools is a feature of most immune responses to immunizations or acute infections, and it makes teleological sense. Sustained secretion or overproduction of cytokines can have deleterious effects, and the presence of fully active killer memory T cells could result in severe immunopathological damage if some of these CTLs were crossreactive with selfantigens. Thus, maintenance of T-cell immunity by sustaining the effector phase would carry a high price tag. As memory T cells can rapidly develop into effectors and quickly gain access to sites of infection, it is not essential in most instances to maintain effector T cells to provide protection.

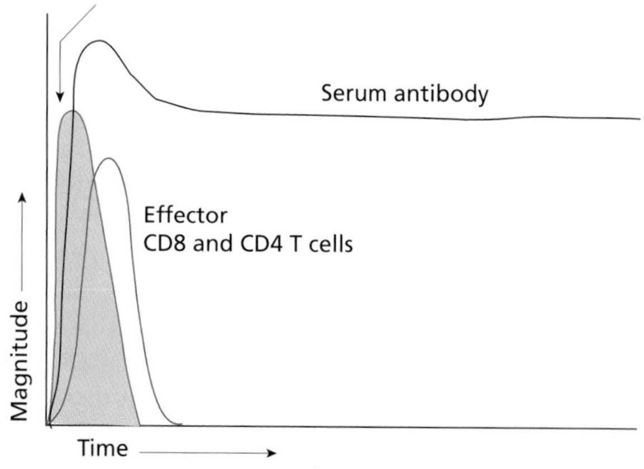

Figure 26.1 *The nature of effector T- and B-cell responses is different. Most microbial infections induce prolonged serum antibody responses that can persist for months or years after resolution of the infection. In contrast, effector T-cell responses (i.e. active killer cells and cytokine producers) are short-lived and are seen only during the acute phase of infection.*

Table 26.3 *Distinction between effector B and T cells*

Effector B cells	Plasma cells are end-stage-differentiated cells that constitutively produce antibody in the absence of antigen.[a] A proportion of plasma cells can live for extended periods in the bone marrow. These long-lived plasma cells are an important source of antibody in the serum and can also contribute to antibody in the mucosa. This pre-existing antibody forms the first line of defense against infection and is a key aspect of protective immunity against microbial infections
Effector T cells	Effector T cells secrete cytokines and can kill infected cells. In contrast to plasma cells, T cells maintain effector functions only in the presence of antigen. In the absence of antigen, effector T cells either die or differentiate into memory T cells. This also contrasts with plasma cells that are fully differentiated end-stage cells. Plasma cells do not give rise to memory B cells

a) Antigen is needed for differentiation of naïve or memory B cells into antibody-secreting plasma cells but is not required for maintaining antibody production by fully differentiated plasma cells.

B-cell memory

The two critical cell types involved in B-cell memory are memory B cells and plasma cells. The major differences in naïve B cells, memory B cells, and plasma cells are summarized in Tables 26.4 and 26.5 and the lineage interrelationships of these three cell types are shown in Figure 26.2. In this simple model, after the initial activation of naïve B cells (by antigen and T-cell help), activated B cells undergo clonal expansion. This initial proliferation is observable as histologically defined regions of B-cell clusters, known as extrafollicular foci, within the T-cell-rich areas of secondary lymphoid organs. During this initial phase of activation, B cells can class switch from IgM to IgG or other isotypes if stimulated strongly. In addition, it is generally thought that there is no or minimal somatic mutation/affinity maturation of the B-cell receptor at this stage of the B-cell response (Jacob and Kelsoe 1992; MacLennan

Table 26.4 *Differences between naïve and memory B cells, in humans*

Naïve B cells	Memory B cells
No somatic mutation or affinity maturation of B-cell receptor	Somatic mutation and affinity maturation of B-cell receptor
Not isotype switched; mostly IgM^+ IgD^+	~40% isotype switched; ~60% IgD^-: 40% IgM^+ IgD^+ 40% IgG^+ or IgA^+, IgD^- 20% IgM^+ IgD-
$CD27^-$	$CD27^+$
	More efficient antigen-induced proliferation? (Martin and Goodnow 2002)

1994); however, this has been challenged by a recent study in an autoimmune mouse model (William et al. 2002). Importantly, most of the antibody-secreting plasma cells generated from B cells in extrafollicular foci are thought to be short-lived, with a half-life of 3–7 days (McHeyzer-Williams 1997; Ho et al. 1986).

An important aspect of the model described in Figure 26.2 is affinity maturation of memory B cells and the generation of long-lived plasma cells. After the initial phase of B-cell proliferation and differentiation in extrafollicular foci, some B cells migrate back to the follicle (the B-cell regions of secondary lymphoid organs), and there is a second phase of clonal expansion of activated B cells within the specialized microenvironment of a germinal center (GC) (Jacob and Kelsoe 1992; MacLennan 1994; Tsiagbe and Thorbecke 1998). It is normally within the GCs that affinity maturation occurs, and B cells selected within the GC mature into memory B cells or plasma cells (Berek et al. 1985; Jacob et al. 1991). Additional class switching occurs in the GC. GCs contain antigen-specific CD4 T cells, and follicular dendritic cells (FDC) that retain depots of antigen for stimulation and selection of high-affinity B cells. Germinal center B cells proliferate rapidly (of the order of 6–7 h per division – Liu et al. 1991) and undergo positive selection by B-cell receptor binding to antigen attached to FDCs, as well as by B-cell interactions with antigen-specific CD4 T cells (Kosco et al. 1988; MacLennan 1994). A great deal of B-cell apoptosis occurs in GCs, as many of the B cells that undergo somatic hypermutation end up with nonantigen-specific or nonfunctional B-cell receptors (MacLennan 1994; McHeyzer-Williams et al. 2001; Ho et al. 1986).

There is evidence to suggest that plasma cells derived from high-affinity, isotype switched B cells tend to be longer-lived and reside in the bone marrow (Manz et al. 1997, 1998; Slifka et al. 1998). Teleologically, the basic model of a B-cell response generating short-lived plasma cells first and long-lived plasma cells and memory B cells later is appealing because, in an infection, it is valuable to get antipathogen antibodies produced as rapidly as possible (which is done by those antigen-specific B cells that differentiate into plasma cells early in extrafollicular foci). But it is also important to evolve high-

Table 26.5 *Differences between memory B cells and plasma cells*

	Memory B cell	Plasma cell
Location	Reside primarily in the secondary lymphoid organs	Reside primarily in the bone marrow
Function	Important for replenishing the pool of plasma cells and memory B cells. Do not actively secrete antibody, but respond to antigen by rapidly dividing and giving rise to more memory B cells and also differentiating into plasma cells	Terminally differentiated cells that constitutively produce antibody. Not stimulated by antigen (low to no surface B cell receptor). Do not divide
Markers[a]		
Surface Ig	++++	+/–
B220 (mouse only)	++++	+/–
CD19	++++	+/–
CD20 (human only)	++++	+/–
MHC class II	++++	+/–
CD138 (syndecan-1)	–	++++
Blimp-1	–	++++

a) List of markers commonly used to distinguish between memory B cells and plasma cells in mice and humans (not a comprehensive listing). All of the markers listed here except for Blimp-1 are expressed at the cell surface and can be used to separate plasma cells from memory B cells.

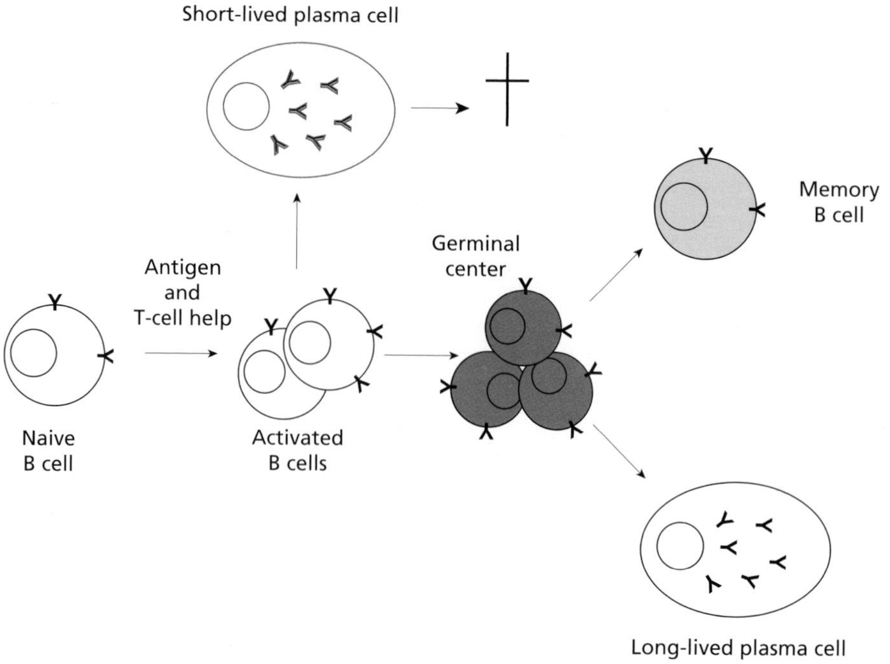

Figure 26.2 *Model of memory B-cell differentiation. After antigenic stimulation, naïve B cells undergo clonal expansion and form clusters of activated B cells known as extrafollicular foci. These activated B cells can either differentiate into short-lived plasma cells or migrate back into the follicle and initiate a germinal center reaction. After proliferation and affinity maturation, germinal center B cells produce both long-lived plasma cells, which in turn produce high-affinity antibodies, and memory B cells which have high-affinity B-cell receptors.*

affinity antibodies that are much more efficient at controlling and eliminating the pathogen (which is done by the antigen-specific B cells that initiate GCs).

The kinetics and anatomical location of antibody production after an acute viral infection in mice are shown in Figure 26.3. The IgM response is transient but the serum IgG response is long-lived and can persist for several years. Antibody is initially produced by short-lived plasma cells present in the secondary lymphoid organs. The plasma cell response in these tissues peaks during the first 2 weeks and then declines within 2–4 weeks after infection (Slifka et al. 1995). As splenic plasma cell populations decline, antigen-specific plasma cells begin to migrate to and/or accumulate in the bone marrow compartment. After the GC reaction subsides, the bone marrow becomes the predominant site of antibody production, with 80–90 percent of the host's plasma cells located in this compartment (Slifka et al. 1995, 1998).

Upon reinfection, antibody responses occur rapidly in the spleen and lymph nodes, because most of the memory B cells reside in these organs. After secondary infection, the memory B cells in spleen and lymph nodes proliferate and/or differentiate into plasma cells, resulting in a transient increase in the number of antibody-secreting cells (ASC) in the spleen. However, once the secondary infection has cleared, this response subsides and, once again, the bone marrow becomes the predominant site of antibody production. It is worth noting the anatomical segregation between plasma cells and memory B cells. One way of looking at this is to consider the spleen and lymph nodes as 'factories' where

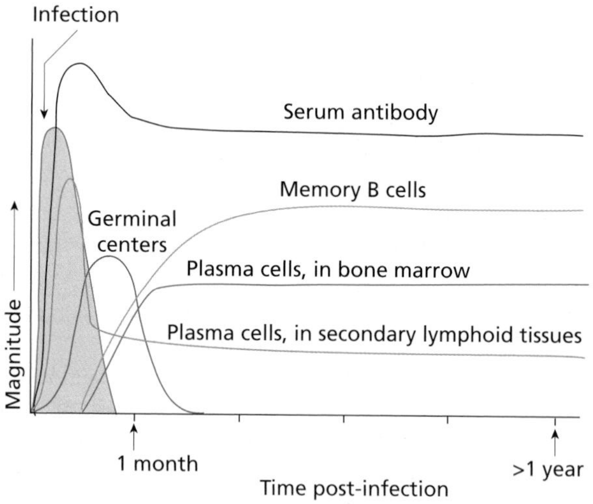

Figure 26.3 *Kinetics and anatomical site of B-cell responses after infection. Initial antibody production is by short-lived plasma cells in the spleen and lymph nodes. Germinal centers form and are maintained for approximately 2–6 weeks after antigen clearance. Long-lived plasma cells and memory B cells are produced from the germinal centers. Most of the long-lived plasma cells migrate to and reside in the bone marrow, though some stay in secondary lymphoid organs. Long-lived plasma cells in the bone marrow are generally responsible for most of the maintenance of serum antibody levels. Most of the memory B cells reside in secondary lymphoid organs long term, although some migrate to and reside in the bone marrow.*

B-cell differentiation into plasma cells occurs, and the bone marrow as the storehouse where the products (i.e. plasma cells) are kept. It makes sense that memory B cells should reside in the vicinity of the factories so that they can be quickly mobilized into action as the need arises, and that the plasma cells are shipped out to the bone marrow to make room in the factory. Plasma cells residing in the bone marrow go on with their business of making antibody, which ends up in the blood and can protect against reinfection. Note that some plasma cells are expected to reside in mucosal tissues and produce IgG and IgA which is secreted to protect the mucosal surfaces, and it should also be pointed out that serum antibody (IgG) can enter the mucosa by transudation and it is therefore possible that plasma cells residing in the bone marrow also contribute to the antibody present at mucosal sites.

The factors that are critical for generation of B-cell memory and plasma cells can be divided into three groups: (1) genes essential for FDC development, (2) B-cell intrinsic factors, and (3) CD4 T-cell intrinsic factors. TNFR1, LTα, and LTβ are essential for FDC development. CD40, CD19, and AID are examples of critical B-cell intrinsic factors (see Tsiagbe and Thorbecke 1998, for a more extensive list). CD28, B7-1/2, ICOS, and CD40L are examples of CD4 T-cell intrinsic factors required for the generation of GCs and development of B-cell memory (McAdam et al. 2001; Tafuri et al. 2001; Borriello et al. 1997; Xu et al. 1994). Interestingly, the intracellular signaling protein SAP (SLAM-associated protein; also known as SH2D1A), which is defective in individuals with the genetic disease X-linked lymphoproliferative (XLP), is essential in CD4 T cells for the generation of GCs and B-cell memory, but not for most other CD4 T-cell functions (Crotty et al. 2003b).

A separate set of genes has been identified that is specifically required for plasma cell differentiation, and XBP-1 and Blimp-1 are two critical B-cell transcription factors controlling the plasma cell differentiation program (Shaffer et al. 2001, 2002; Zhan et al. 2002). Within GCs, multiple factors play a role in determining the ratio of memory B cell versus plasma cell production, including Bcl-6, interleukin 10 (IL-10), OX40, and others (Tsiagbe and Thorbecke 1998).

In summary, immunological memory in the B-cell compartment consists of memory B cells and plasma cells – two distinct cell types with different anatomical locations and very different functions (Table 26.5). Memory B cells are located primarily in the secondary lymphoid organs and are present at much higher frequencies than naïve B cells of the same specificity. In addition to this quantitative advantage over naïve B cells, memory B cells are also qualitatively different and produce antibody of much higher affinity. However, memory B cells do not actively secrete antibody (i.e. they are not effector cells). Their major function is to make rapid recall responses to infection by quickly dividing and differentiating into plasma cells, as well as initiating new GCs. The rapid rise in antibody concentration upon reinfection is the result of memory B-cell differentiation into new antibody-secreting plasma cells. In contrast to memory B cells, plasma cells cannot be stimulated by antigen either to divide or to increase their rate of antibody production. These plasma cells are terminally differentiated cells that constitutively produce and secrete antibody. Plasma cells are extraordinarily efficient in their ability to make antibody; it has been estimated that plasma cells can secrete >1000 antibody molecules per second (Helmreich et al. 1961; Hibi and Dosch 1986). As pre-existing antibody provides the first line of defense against infection by microbial pathogens, the importance of plasma cells in protective immunity cannot be overstated. In fact, it could be argued that plasma cells may be the single most important cell type in protective immunity to infections.

T-cell memory

T-cell memory does not have a plasma cell equivalent, i.e. an effector cell that can continue its effector function in the absence of antigenic stimulation. In contrast to plasma cells, effector T cells elaborate their effector functions (i.e. cytokine secretion and killing of infected cells by release of secretory granules containing perforin/granzymes) only in the presence of antigen (see Figure 26.1 and Table 26.3). These cells exhibit an on–off lifestyle with antigen regulating this switch (Badovinac et al. 2000; Slifka and Whitton 2000). If effector T-cell responses are only transient, then what is the cellular basis of long-term T-cell immunity? It is well established that T-cell memory, as assessed by accelerated recall responses in vivo, is long-lived and is seen after most microbial infections (Ahmed and Gray 1996; Zinkernagel et al. 1996; Dutton et al. 1998; Freitas and Rocha 2000). These rapid recall responses to reinfection are the result of both quantitative and qualitative changes in the pathogen-specific T cells. On primary infection there is substantial expansion of the pool of both CD8 and CD4 T cells specific to the pathogen (Figure 26.4). Several studies have shown that the size of the memory T-cell pool is determined by the burst size during the expansion phase (Figure 26.5) (Hou et al. 1994; Busch et al. 1998; Murali-Krishna et al. 1998; Butz et al. 1998). In the case of some acute viral infections, the increase in the number of antigen-specific T cells can be as great as 1000- to 5000-fold (Murali-Krishna et al. 1998; Ahmed and Biron 1999). This numerical advantage alone can make an enormous difference to the recall response, but recent studies have shown that memory T cells are also qualitatively distinct from naïve T cells and can respond with much quicker cytokine secretion and killing on re-exposure to antigen (Zimmerman et al. 1996; Kedl and Mescher 1998; Bach-

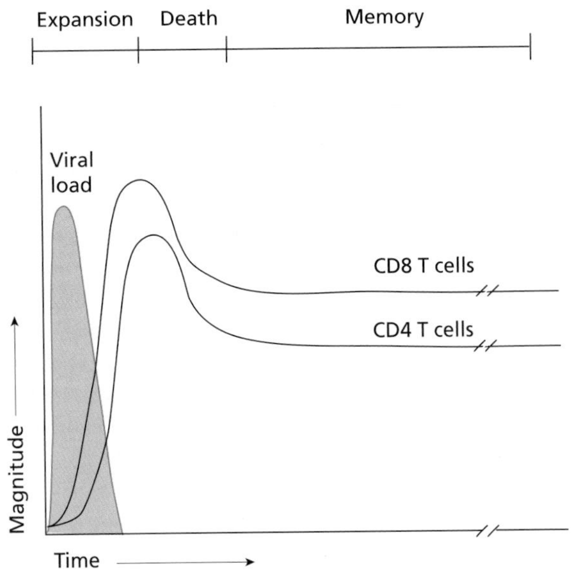

Figure 26.4 Antiviral CD8 and CD4 T-cell responses. The three phases of the immune response are indicated at the top. The increase in cell number during the 'expansion' phase is the result of clones of T cells undergoing cell division. Soon after the virus is cleared, there is a 'death' phase characterized by decreasing numbers of virus-specific T cells caused by apoptosis. Following the death phase, the number of virus-specific T cells stabilizes and can be maintained for extended periods. This is the 'memory' phase. The CD4 T-cell response is similar to the CD8 T-cell response except that the magnitude of the CD4 response is usually lower and slightly delayed, and the death phase can be more protracted than the CD8 response.

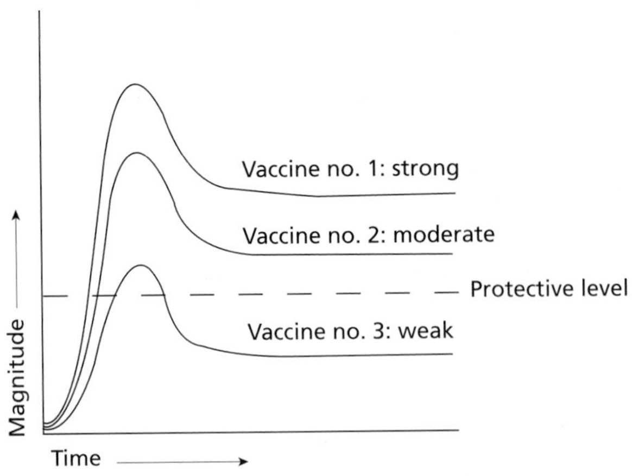

Figure 26.5 The size of the memory T-cell pool is determined by the clonal burst size during the expansion phase. In this figure, the lines represent the T-cell responses induced by three different vaccines. Vaccine number 1 induces the largest expansion of T cells and hence generates the largest pool of memory T cells, vaccine no. 2 is next, and vaccine no. 3 is the weakest. The asterisk denotes the minimum number of antigen-specific T cells required for protective immunity. In this scenario, vaccines nos 1 and 2 will confer long-term immunity whereas protective immunity induced by vaccine no. 3 will be of short duration. The main reason for the failure of vaccine no. 3 is a smaller burst size during the expansion phase. Note that the maintenance of the memory T-cell pool is similar for all three vaccines.

mann et al. 1999a, 1999b; Cho et al. 1999; Barber et al. 2003).

In fact, this faster responsiveness is clearly the defining functional characteristic of memory T cells (Table 26.6). Another important property of memory T cells is their ability to extravasate into nonlymphoid tissues; several recent studies have shown that a subset of memory T cells (termed 'effector' memory) are present in many peripheral tissues and also at mucosal sites (Sallusto et al. 1999; Masopust et al. 2001; Reinhardt et al. 2001). Thus, it is the combination of increased numbers of antigen-specific T cells, their faster responsiveness, and their better location (i.e. near sites of microbial entry) that underpins T-cell memory, and explains how memory T cells confer long-term protective immunity (Lau et al. 1994; Ahmed and Gray 1996; Zinkernagel et al. 1996; Dutton et al. 1998; Freitas and Rocha 2000).

It is well established that memory B cells and plasma cells differentiate along separate arms of a bifurcated pathway, and some of the conditions and signals that direct naïve B cells into the memory versus effector pathways are being defined (McHeyzer-Williams and Ahmed 1999; Calame 2001; Fearon et al. 2001). Our understanding of the memory T-cell differentiation pathway is less clear, but over the past few years there has been substantial progress in defining the lineage interrelationships of naive, effector, and memory T cells (Champagne et al. 2001; Lanzavecchia and Sallusto 2001; Kaech et al. 2003). Also, several markers have been identified that distinguish these three cell types (Table 26.7) (Ahmed and Gray 1996; Zinkernagel et al. 1996; Dutton et al. 1998; Freitas and Rocha 2000;

Table 26.6 Defining characteristics of memory B and T cells

Memory B cells

The hallmark of memory B cells is affinity maturation of the B-cell receptor. This means that the antibody produced by these cells (after their differentiation into antibody secreting cells) is of higher affinity. Thus, the fundamental difference between naïve and memory B cells is that the memory B cells can make a better 'product'. It is also likely that memory B cells respond to antigen stimulation more efficiently than naïve B cells

Memory T cells

The hallmark of memory T cells is faster responsiveness on re-encountering the antigen. In some instances the response is so rapid (i.e. cytokine production in less than 4 h) that memory T cells give the illusion of being effector cells. The effector molecules (cytokines, perforin, granzymes, etc.) of naïve and memory T cells are identical. Thus, the fundamental difference between memory and naïve T cells is that the memory T cells are a much more efficient 'factory' than naïve cells, although the product is the same. Also, unlike naïve T cells, which are located mostly in lymphoid tissues, a subset of memory T cells ($CD62^{lo}$ $CCR7^{-}$) is present in nonlymphoid tissues and at mucosal sites and can immediately confront the invading pathogen

Harrington et al. 2000). Possible models of memory T-cell differentiation are shown in Figure 26.6. It is unlikely that the 'divergent pathway' (model 1 – Figure 26.6a) represents a major pathway of memory T-cell differentiation because recent experimental evidence favors the linear differentiation model (model 2 – Figure 26.6b). Studies using transgenic T cells, or genetic techniques to mark antigen-specific T cells, have shown that memory T cells are derived from effector cells (Jacob and Baltimore 1999; Opferman et al. 1999). However, this simple linear differentiation model does not directly account for the fact that most effector cells undergo apoptosis and only a fraction (about 10 percent) of these cells survive to become memory cells. A second approach, using experiments involving adoptive transfer of effector T cells into naïve mice, showed that memory T cells probably arise directly from this population (Opferman et al. 1999; Hu et al. 2001; Kaech et al. 2003).

The 'decreasing potential hypothesis' (model 3 – Figure 26.6c) incorporates a mechanism for discriminating between effectors that preferentially die and those that preferentially survive and differentiate into memory cells (Kaech et al. 2002). According to this model the balance between effector cells and memory cells is governed by the duration and level of antigenic stimulation. Cells become more and more terminally differentiated with prolonged antigenic stimulation and this is accompanied by an increasing susceptibility to apoptosis and a decreasing potential for memory cell development. This model also explains the phenomenon of clonal deletion/exhaustion that occurs during chronic viral infections with a high antigen load (Moskophidis et al. 1993; Zajac et al. 1998; Ahmed and Biron 1999). Finally, the last memory differentiation model we would like to discuss incorporates the development of 'central' and 'effector' memory T cells (Figure 26.7) (Sallusto et al. 1999). In this model, a shorter duration of antigenic stimulation favors the development of 'central' memory cells whereas longer duration favors 'effector' memory cells. 'Effector' memory cells ($CCR7^-$, $CD62L^{lo}$) are characterized by rapid acquisition of effector function and are found predominantly in nonlymphoid tissues, whereas 'central' memory cells ($CCR7^+$, $CD62L^{hi}$) are located within lymphoid tissues and presumably respond slower than 'effector' memory cells. However, it should be noted that even the 'central' memory cells respond much faster than naïve T cells. There are some interesting parallels between the 'decreasing potential' model and the model incorporating the development of 'central' and 'effector' memory T-cell subsets. In both models, the duration of antigenic stimulus regulates differentiation and a more prolonged antigenic stimulus favors cells with a more effector phenotype (i.e. terminally differentiated cell) (Kaech et al. 2002).

MAINTENANCE OF IMMUNOLOGICAL MEMORY

How is immunological memory maintained? This question has fascinated immunologists, microbiologists, and infectious disease specialists for many years, and there has been great interest in understanding the mechanisms that maintain long-term protective immunity. This infor-

Table 26.7 *Markers that distinguish naïve, effector, and memory T cells*[a]

	Naive	Effector	Memory
Group A			
CD44	Low	High	High
CD11a (LFA-1)	Low	High	High
Ly-6C	Low	High	High
CD122 (IL-2Rβ)	Low	High	High
Group B			
CD25 (IL-2Rα)	Low	High	Low
CD43 (high M_r form)	Low	High	Low
CD80 (B7-1)	Low	High	Low
CD38	Low	High	Low
MHC class II	Low	High	Low
Group C			
CD62L (L-selectin)	High	Low	High/Low
CCR7	High	Low	High/Low
CD45RA	High	Low	High/Low
CD45RO	Low	High	Low/High

a) Not a comprehensive list but illustrates the three patterns of changes seen as naïve T cells go through the naïve→effector→memory transition. Some surface markers (group A) are expressed at low levels in naïve cells, then upregulated upon antigen activation (effector cells) and maintained at high levels in memory T cells. Other markers as shown in group B are only transiently upregulated in effector cells and can be useful in discriminating between memory and effector T cells. Finally, a third group of markers (group C) show a much more gradual change during the effector-to-memory transition and have turned out to be very useful in identifying different subsets of memory T cells, i.e. lymphoid versus nonlymphoid. This group of markers may also be useful in identifying the various stages of memory T-cell differentiation.

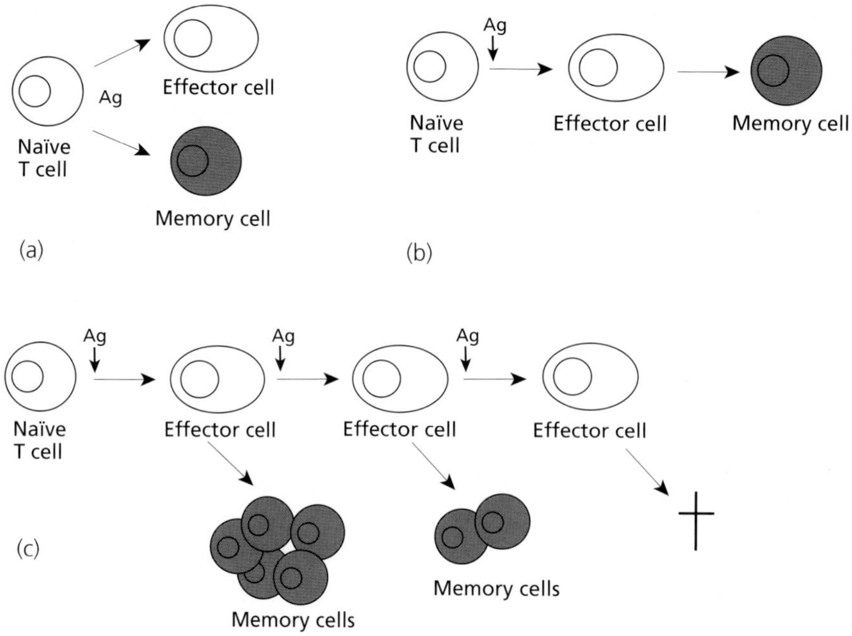

Figure 26.6 *Models of memory T-cell differentiation.* **(a)** *Model 1 represents the B-cell/germinal center paradigm of dichotomy in memory and effector pathways.* **(b)** *Model 2 is the more traditional view of memory T-cell differentiation representing a linear differentiation pathway.* **(c)** *Model 3 is a variation of model 2 and takes into account the finding that only 5–10 percent of the effector cells survive to become memory T cells. In this model, progress toward terminal differentiation (driven by antigen – Ag) is accompanied by increased susceptibility to apoptosis and a decreased potential for memory cell development. In all of these models the effector cell represents a transient population whereas the memory cells survive for long periods. On re-exposure to antigen, the memory T cells can develop into effector cells and also generate more memory cells.*

mation is important for a fundamental understanding of both immunological memory and vaccine development.

The mechanisms involved in sustaining immunological memory are listed in Table 26.8. These can be divided into two categories: antigen dependent and antigen independent. One of the most effective means of maintaining immunity is periodic re-exposure to the pathogen. Such reinfections are usually asymptomatic or produce only mild clinical symptoms and serve as a natural 'booster' to the immune system. The importance of this mechanism is documented by epidemiological studies which show that protective immunity is maintained for longer periods in individuals living in areas endemic for a given disease. Having said this, it is equally, if not more, important to point out that there are several striking examples of long-term protective immunity in the absence of re-exposure to the pathogen. Three such examples are given in Table 26.9. These observations were crucial in shaping our ideas about immunological memory because they showed that the immune system could remember an encounter that occurred many years before and that there are mechanisms for sustaining this long-term memory (Panum 1847; Paul et al. 1951; Sawyer 1931).

Among the 'not reinfection' mechanisms of maintaining immunity, two are antigen dependent: microbial

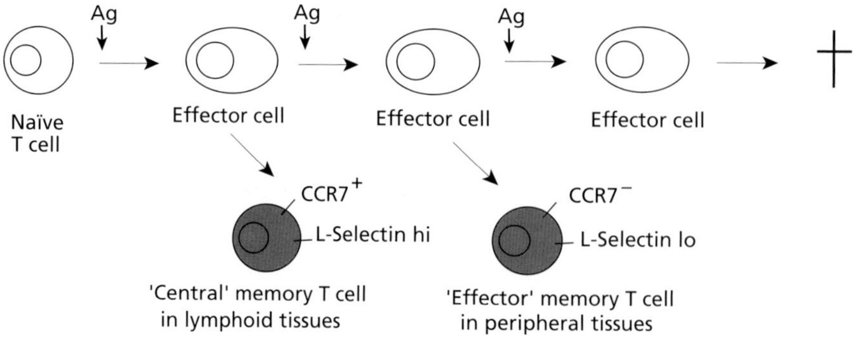

Figure 26.7 *Model of memory T-cell differentiation incorporating the development of 'central' and 'effector' memory T cells. In this model a short duration of antigenic stimulation favors the development of 'central' memory cells whereas longer duration favors differentiation to 'effector' memory T cells. Ag, antigen.*

Table 26.8 *Maintenance of immunological memory*

Antigen-dependent
1. Re-exposure to pathogen can serve as a periodic natural booster to the immune system
2. Low grade chronic/latent infection. Many pathogens can persist at low levels and provide a continuous/intermittent stimulus to memory T and B cells
3. Antigen–antibody complexes on follicular dendritic cells can persist for extended periods and provide a reservoir of antigen that possibly stimulates memory B cells and CD4 T cells
Antigen-independent
1. Long-lived plasma cells can constitutively produce antibody, sustaining serum antibody levels in the absence of antigen
2. Memory B and T cells can persist and maintain their numbers in an antigen-free environment. Memory T cells can undergo homeostatic proliferation to replenish their pool; this homeostatic proliferation does not require stimulation with antigen
3. Memory CD8 and CD4 T cells can retain their rapid responsiveness in the absence of antigen and are able to confer protective immunity

There are antigen-dependent and antigen-independent mechanisms of maintaining long-term immunity to infection.

persistence and antigen depots. A number of microbes can persist at low levels in healthy individuals and this chronicity can provide either a continuous or an intermittent antigenic stimulus to the immune system. This can be an effective mechanism of maintaining a higher frequency of antigen-specific T and B cells but requires a careful balance between pathogen levels and immune responses. This critical balance is necessary to avoid excessive immunopathology and also to avoid overstimulation of the antigen-specific T cells to such an extent that these cells get deleted or functionally exhausted (Moskophidis et al. 1993; Zajac et al. 1998). Pathogens that cause latent infection with periodic reactivation, such as the herpesviruses (Epstein–Barr virus (EBV), herpes simplex virus (HSV), varicella-zoster virus (VZV)) exhibit a lifestyle that is perhaps most conducive to providing an antigenic stimulus for maintaining long-term immunity.

The second antigen-dependent mechanism, antigen depots, relies on the ability of FDCs to trap antigen–antibody complexes on their cell surface and retain them for extended periods of time (Mandel et al. 1980; MacLennan 1994; Bachmann et al. 1996; Zinkernagel et al. 1996; Dutton et al. 1998; Ahmed and Biron 1999; Freitas and Rocha 2000). FDCs express Fc receptors on their cell surface and antigen–antibody complexes can bind to these Fc receptors. It appears that FDCs do not internalize these antigen–antibody complexes but instead display them on their cell surface for long periods, thus promoting maintenance of GCs and continued affinity maturation of B cells. It is generally agreed that antigen is required to maintain GC reactions, to sustain the rapid B-cell proliferation, provide a substrate for positive selection, and prevent apoptosis (MacLennan 1994). Some studies have suggested that antigen can persist on FDCs for more than a year (Mandel et al. 1980). Data from the only study directly tracking antigen in GCs after a viral infection suggest that GCs are sustained by antigen on FDCs for about 30 days after clearance of the virus, after which there is a greater than 90 percent drop in the number of GCs and a greater than 90 percent drop in the amount of viral antigen bound by the FDCs (Bachmann et al. 1996).

It is unlikely that viral particles or protein antigens in vivo can survive the wear and tear of antibody binding for long before being broken into pieces or destroyed. It has been postulated that this trapped antigen directly stimulates the specific B cells and can also be acquired by the B cells, processed and then presented via MHC class II molecules to CD4 T cells (Mandel et al. 1980; MacLennan 1994). Thus, it appears that FDC-trapped antigen can be used for stimulating both memory B cells and CD4 T cells. Many interesting questions about FDCs remain unanswered. What is their half-life? Do these cells divide? What prevents the antigen–antibody complexes from being degraded and/or internalized by the FDCs? What is the half-life of antigen presented by an FDC? It will be important to study FDCs in more detail for better understanding of their role in maintaining B- and T-cell memory.

During the past decade major advances have been made in identifying antigen-independent mechanisms of maintaining immunological memory (Ahmed and Gray 1996; Dutton et al. 1998; Freitas and Rocha 2000; Marrack et al. 2000; Lanzavecchia and Sallusto 2001; Sprent and Surh 2001). These studies were greatly facilitated by the development of new and sensitive techni-

Table 26.9 *Long-term immunity in the absence of re-exposure to the pathogen*

Infection	Duration of immunity (years)	Reference
Measles on the Faroe Islands	65	Panum (1847)
Yellow fever virus in Norfolk, VA, USA	75	Sawyer (1931)
Polio in remote Eskimo villages	40	Paul et al. (1951)
Inactivated poliovirus immunization in Sweden	30+	Bottiger et al. (1998)
Immune memory after smallpox vaccination	30–70+	Crotty et al. (2003a), Hammerlund (2003)

ques for assessing T- and B-cell functions at the single cell level and, even more importantly, by the ability physically to identify antigen-specific T cells using MHC class I and class II tetramers (Altman et al. 1996; Crawford et al. 1998; Murali-Krishna et al. 1998; Butz and Bevan 1998). Also, the use of transgenic T and B cells in mouse model systems has allowed us to monitor the immune response in vivo as naïve cells get activated and differentiate into effector and memory cells (Kearney et al. 1994; Zimmermann et al. 1999). Using a combination of these approaches to analyze a variety of immune responses in mice (using both infectious and noninfectious model systems), it is now clear that both memory CD4 and CD8 T cells, as well as memory B cells, can persist in the absence of antigen (Hou et al. 1994; Lau et al. 1994; Mullbacher 1994; Ahmed and Gray 1996; Tanchot et al. 1997; Dutton et al. 1998; Markiewicz et al. 1998; Murali-Krishna et al. 1999; Swain et al. 1999; Freitas and Rocha 2000; Marrack et al. 2000; Maruyama et al. 2000; Lanzavecchia and Sallusto 2001; Sprent and Surh 2001). It has also been shown that memory T cells can undergo homeostatic proliferation to replenish their numbers and that this proliferative renewal does not require stimulation with antigen (Tanchot et al. 1997; Murali-Krishna et al. 1999; Swain et al. 1999; Sprent and Surh 2001; Kassiotis et al. 2002). Taken together, these experimental studies done in mice have unequivocally shown that memory B and T cells can persist for extended periods (2 years or more) in the absence of antigen.

What about the situation in humans? Here the results are less definitive, but there are data showing long-term memory under conditions where antigen persistence is unlikely, e.g. it has been shown that vaccinia virus-specific memory CD8 T cells can be detected in individuals immunized more than 30 years earlier (Demkowicz et al. 1996; Crotty et al. 2003a; Hammarlund et al. 2003). It is unlikely that this long-term CTL memory is the result of antigenic stimulation, because vaccinia virus does not cause a chronic or latent infection in humans and there is no possibility of re-exposure to vaccinia virus, because vaccination against smallpox virus was discontinued in 1977. There are also studies documenting persistence of memory CD4 T cells to tetanus toxoid many years after immunization (Helms et al. 2000). There is also data showing that memory B cells persist for greater than 50 years after smallpox vaccination (Crotty et al. 2003a). Nevertheless, there is clearly a need for more detailed analysis of memory responses in humans. It would also be worthwhile to pursue such studies in nonhuman primates.

What factors control antigen-independent maintenance of memory B and T cells? The answer to this question is unclear for memory B cells, but this issue of homeostatic maintenance of memory has received a great deal of interest in the study of memory T cells, and it is now clear that cytokines (such as IL-15 and IL-7) play a major role in controlling homeostatic proliferation (Sprent and Surh 2001; Becker et al. 2002; Goldrath et al. 2002; Kaech et al. 2002; Kieper et al. 2002; Tan et al. 2002).

It is clear that there are antigen-independent mechanisms for maintaining memory B and T cells, but what about antibody production? The traditional view has been that plasma cells are short-lived cells (half-life estimates ranging from 3 days to at most 2–3 weeks), and that continuous antigenic stimulation of memory B cells is essential to replenish the pool of rapidly dying plasma cells and thereby maintain antibody production. This view has been challenged by recent studies showing that plasma cells can live for extended periods and that some plasma cells can survive for the life of the mouse (Manz et al. 1997, 1998; Slifka et al. 1998; Helms et al. 2000). This finding may provide an explanation for the remarkable longevity of antibody responses seen in humans after certain acute infections and immunizations (Ahmed and Gray 1996; Slifka and Ahmed 1998). Many acute viral infections induce serum antibody responses that persist for decades (Plotkin and Orenstein 1999), but what is even more striking is that some nonreplicating antigens can also induce long-term humoral immunity. Perhaps the most impressive demonstration of this phenomenon is the large study of poliovirus immunity done in Sweden (Bottiger et al. 1998). The Swedish population is almost ideal for such a study, for several reasons: (1) poliomyelitis has been eliminated in Sweden since 1962; (2) only inactivated poliovirus vaccine (IPV) (the Salk vaccine) has ever been used in the Swedish population; (3) the vaccine is provided by a single, standardized supplier; (4) the final booster immunization is given at the young age of 5 years; (5) the enterovirus infection burden in Sweden is extremely low, and there are relatively few opportunities for introduction of poliovirus from foreign sources; and (6) Sweden has excellent healthcare records and public health surveillance. Given these factors, it is striking to see that, when the Swedish population was surveyed for poliovirus immunity in 1991, substantial antipoliovirus antibody titers were detected in all age groups (Bottiger et al. 1998). Interestingly, there was virtually no difference in serum antibody titers among the different age groups (all at >10 years after immunization), indicating that antipoliovirus antibody titers are stably maintained in the absence of additional immunizations or exposure to live virus (Bottiger et al. 1998). In addition, it is well described that people immunized with diphtheria or tetanus toxoid can have circulating antibody for more than 25, or even 50, years (Scheibel et al. 1966; Simonsen et al. 1984; Kjeldsen et al. 1985; Cohen et al. 1994; Bottiger et al. 1998).

CONCLUSION

Not all infections and vaccines induce long-term antibody responses and there are several instances where antibody responses decay rapidly (Plotkin and Orenstein

1999). The underlying reasons for this are not well understood. Are there only certain conditions and/or antigen formulations that can result in the generation of long-lived plasma cells? One possibility is that T-cell help is necessary and that only high-affinity B cells can differentiate into long-lived plasma cells, whereas low-affinity B cells give rise to short-lived plasma cells. What are the factors that regulate plasma cell survival? Is residence in the bone marrow essential for plasma cell survival? These issues about plasma cells need to be addressed to gain a better understanding of long-term humoral immunity.

In conclusion, in this chapter we have attempted to give an overview of the principles of immunological memory to infection. This remains one of the most exciting areas of immunology and infectious diseases and there are many challenges ahead. Although considerable progress has been made in the past few years, and some of our questions have been answered, many more remain, e.g. what is the molecular definition of a memory T cell? Are there memory specific genes? How are these cells 'wired', making them so different from naïve cells (Bachmann et al. 1999b)? What controls the homeostasis of memory T and B cells? How many memory cells can we accommodate as we age and encounter multiple infections (Selin et al. 1999)? What signals regulate the differentiation program of memory cells (Kaech and Ahmed 2001; Lanzavecchia and Sallusto 2001; van Stipdonk et al. 2001; Wong and Pamer 2001)? Answers to these and many other questions are needed to define the cellular and molecular basis of immunological memory.

REFERENCES

Ahmed, R. and Biron, C.A. 1999. Immunity to viruses. In: Paul, W.E. (ed.), *Fundamental immunology, 4th edn*. Philadelphia, PA: Lippincott-Raven,, 1295–335.

Ahmed, R. and Gray, D. 1996. Immunological memory and protective immunity: understanding their relation. *Science*, **272**, 54–60.

Altman, J.D., Moss, P.A., et al. 1996. Phenotypic analysis of antigen-specific T lymphocytes. *Science*, **274**, 94–6.

Bachmann, M.F., Odermatt, B., et al. 1996. Induction of long-lived germinal centers associated with persisting antigen after viral infection. *J Exp Med*, **183**, 2259–69.

Bachmann, M.F., Barner, M., et al. 1999a. Distinct kinetics of cytokine production and cytolysis in effector and memory T cells after viral infection. *Eur J Immunol*, **29**, 291–9.

Bachmann, M.F., Gallimore, A., et al. 1999b. Developmental regulation of Lck targeting to the CD8 coreceptor controls signaling in naive and memory T cells. *J Exp Med*, **189**, 1521–30.

Badovinac, V.P., Corbin, G.A. and Harty, J.T. 2000. Cutting edge: OFF cycling of TNF production by antigen-specific CD8+ T cells is antigen independent. *J Immunol*, **165**, 5387–91.

Barber, D.L., Wherry, E.J. and Ahmed, R. 2003. Cutting edge: rapid in vivo killing by memory CD8 T cells. *J Immunol*, **171**, 27–31.

Becker, T.C., Wherry, E.J., et al. 2002. Interleukin 15 is required for proliferative renewal of virus-specific memory CD8 T cells. *J Exp Med*, **195**, 1541–8.

Berek, C., Griffiths, G.M. and Milstein, C. 1985. Molecular events during maturation of the immune response to oxazolone. *Nature*, **316**, 412–18.

Borriello, F., Sethna, M.P., et al. 1997. B7-1 and B7-2 have overlapping, critical roles in immunoglobulin class switching and germinal center formation. *Immunity*, **6**, 303–13.

Bottiger, M., Gustavsson, O. and Svensson, A. 1998. Immunity to tetanus, diphtheria and poliomyelitis in the adult population of Sweden in 1991. *Int J Epidemiol*, **27**, 916–25.

Buchmeier, M.J. and Zajac, A.J. 1999. Lymphocytic choriomeningitis virus. In: Ahmed, R. and Chen, I.S.Y. (eds), *Persistent viral infections*. Chichester: John Wiley & Son, 575–605.

Burton, D.R. 2002. Antibodies, viruses and vaccines. *Nat Rev Immunol*, **2**, 706–13.

Busch, D.H., Pilip, I.M., et al. 1998. Coordinate regulation of complex T cell populations responding to bacterial infection. *Immunity*, **8**, 353–62.

Butz, E.A. and Bevan, M.J. 1998. Massive expansion of antigen-specific CD8+ T cells during an acute virus infection. *Immunity*, **8**, 167–75.

Calame, K.L. 2001. Plasma cells: finding new light at the end of B cell development. *Nat Immunol*, **2**, 1103–8.

Champagne, P., Ogg, G.S., et al. 2001. Skewed maturation of memory HIV-specific CD8 T lymphocytes. *Nature*, **410**, 106–11.

Cho, B.K., Wang, C., et al. 1999. Functional differences between memory and naive CD8 T cells. *Proc Natl Acad Sci USA*, **96**, 2976–81.

Cohen, D., Green, M.S., et al. 1994. Long-term persistence of anti-diphtheria toxin antibodies among adults in Israel. Implications for vaccine policy. *Eur J Epidemiol*, **10**, 267–70.

Crawford, F., Kozono, H., et al. 1998. Detection of antigen-specific T cells with multivalent soluble class II MHC covalent peptide complexes. *Immunity*, **8**, 675–82.

Crotty, S., Felgner, P., et al. 2003a. Cutting edge: long term B cell memory in humans after smallpox vaccination. *J Immunol*, **171**, 4969–73.

Crotty, S., Kersh, E.N., et al. 2003b. SAP is required for generating long-term humoral immunity. *Nature*, **421**, 282–7.

Demkowicz, W.E. Jr, Littaua, R.A., et al. 1996. Human cytotoxic T-cell memory: long-lived responses to vaccinia virus. *J Virol*, **70**, 2627–31.

Dutton, R.W., Bradley, L.M. and Swain, S.L. 1998. T cell memory. *Annu Rev Immunol*, **16**, 201–23.

Edelson, B.T., Cossart, P. and Unanue, E.R. 1999. Cutting edge: paradigm revisited: antibody provides resistance to *Listeria* infection. *J Immunol*, **163**, 4087–90.

Fearon, D.T., Manders, P. and Wagner, S.D. 2001. Arrested differentiation, the self-renewing memory lymphocyte, and vaccination. *Science*, **293**, 248–50.

Fenner, F., Henderson, D.A., et al. 1988. *Smallpox and its eradication*. Geneva: World Health Organization, 1460.

Finley, J.H. 1951. *The complete writings of Thucydides: The Peloponnesian War*. New York: Modern Library.

Freitas, A.A. and Rocha, B. 2000. Population biology of lymphocytes: the flight for survival. *Annu Rev Immunol*, **18**, 83–111.

Goldrath, A.W., Sivakumar, P.V., et al. 2002. Cytokine requirements for acute and basal homeostatic proliferation of naive and memory CD8+ T cells. *J Exp Med*, **195**, 1515–22.

Hammarlund, E., Lewis, M.W., et al. 2003. Duration of antiviral immunity after smallpox vaccination. *Nat Med*, **9**, 1131–7.

Harrington, L.E., Galvan, M., et al. 2000. Differentiating between memory and effector CD8 T cells by altered expression of cell surface O-glycans. *J Exp Med*, **191**, 1241–6.

Helmreich, E., Kern, M. and Eisen, H.N. 1961. The secretion of antibody by isolated lymph node cells. *J Biochem*, **236**, 464–73.

Helms, T., Boehm, B.O., et al. 2000. Direct visualization of cytokine-producing recall antigen-specific CD4 memory T cells in healthy individuals and HIV patients. *J Immunol*, **164**, 3723–32.

Hibi, T. and Dosch, H.M. 1986. Limiting dilution analysis of the B cell compartment in human bone marrow. *Eur J Immunol*, **16**, 139–45.

Ho, F., Lortan, J.E., et al. 1986. Distinct short-lived and long-lived antibody-producing cell populations. *Eur J Immunol*, **16**, 1296–301.

Hou, S., Hyland, L., et al. 1994. Virus-specific CD8+ T-cell memory determined by clonal burst size. *Nature*, **369**, 652–4.

Hu, H., Huston, G., et al. 2001. CD4(+) T cell effectors can become memory cells with high efficiency and without further division. *Nat Immunol*, **2**, 705–10.

Jacob, J. and Baltimore, D. 1999. Modelling T-cell memory by genetic marking of memory T cells in vivo. *Nature*, **399**, 593–7.

Jacob, J. and Kelsoe, G. 1992. In situ studies of the primary immune response to (4-hydroxy-3-nitrophenyl)acetyl. II. A common clonal origin for periarteriolar lymphoid sheath-associated foci and germinal centers. *J Exp Med*, **176**, 679–87.

Jacob, J., Kelsoe, G., et al. 1991. Intraclonal generation of antibody mutants in germinal centres. *Nature*, **354**, 389–92.

Kaech, S.M. and Ahmed, R. 2001. Memory CD8+ T cell differentiation: initial antigen encounter triggers a developmental program in naive cells. *Nat Immunol*, **2**, 415–22.

Kaech, S.M., Wherry, E.J. and Ahmed, R. 2002. Effector and memory T-cell differentiation: implications for vaccine development. *Nat Rev Immunol*, **2**, 251–62.

Kaech, S.M., Hemby, S., et al. 2003. Molecular and functional profiling of memory CD8 T cell differentiation. *Cell*, **111**, 837–51.

Kassiotis, G., Garcia, S., et al. 2002. Impairment of immunological memory in the absence of MHC despite survival of memory T cells. *Nat Immunol*, **3**, 244–50.

Kearney, E.R., Pape, K.A., et al. 1994. Visualization of peptide-specific T cell immunity and peripheral tolerance induction in vivo. *Immunity*, **1**, 327–39.

Kedl, R.M. and Mescher, M.F. 1998. Qualitative differences between naive and memory T cells make a major contribution to the more rapid and efficient memory CD8+ T cell response. *J Immunol*, **161**, 674–83.

Kieper, W.C., Tan, J.T., et al. 2002. Overexpression of interleukin (IL)-7 leads to IL-15-independent generation of memory phenotype CD8+ T cells. *J Exp Med*, **195**, 1533–9.

Kjeldsen, K., Simonsen, O. and Heron, I. 1985. Immunity against diphtheria 25–30 years after primary vaccination in childhood. *Lancet*, **i**, 900–2.

Kosco, M.H., Monfalcone, A.P., et al. 1988. Germinal center B cells present antigen obtained in vivo to T cells in vitro and stimulate mixed lymphocyte reactions. *Adv Exp Med Biol*, **237**, 883–8.

Lanzavecchia, A. and Sallusto, F. 2001. Antigen decoding by T lymphocytes: from synapses to fate determination. *Nat Immunol*, **2**, 487–92.

Lau, L.L., Jamieson, B.D., et al. 1994. Cytotoxic T-cell memory without antigen. *Nature*, **369**, 648–52.

Liu, Y.J., Zhang, J., et al. 1991. Sites of specific B cell activation in primary and secondary responses to T cell-dependent and T cell-independent antigens. *Eur J Immunol*, **21**, 2951–62.

MacLennan, I.C. 1994. Germinal centers. *Annu Rev Immunol*, **12**, 117–39.

Mandel, T.E., Phipps, R.P., et al. 1980. The follicular dendritic cell: long term antigen retention during immunity. *Immunol Rev*, **53**, 29–59.

Manz, R.A., Thiel, A. and Radbruch, A. 1997. Lifetime of plasma cells in the bone marrow. *Nature*, **388**, 133–4.

Manz, R.A., Lohning, M., et al. 1998. Survival of long-lived plasma cells is independent of antigen. *Int Immunol*, **10**, 1703–11.

Markiewicz, M.A., Girao, C., et al. 1998. Long-term T cell memory requires the surface expression of self-peptide/major histocompatibility complex molecules. *Proc Natl Acad Sci USA*, **95**, 3065–70.

Marrack, P., Bender, J., et al. 2000. Homeostasis of alpha beta TCR+ T cells. *Nat Immunol*, **1**, 107–11.

Martin, S.W. and Goodnow, C.C. 2002. Burst-enhancing role of the IgG membrane tail as a molecular determinant of memory. *Nat Immunol*, **3**, 182–8.

Maruyama, M., Lam, K.P. and Rajewsky, K. 2000. Memory B-cell persistence is independent of persisting immunizing antigen. *Nature*, **407**, 636–42.

Mascola, J.R., Stiegler, G., et al. 2000. Protection of macaques against vaginal transmission of a pathogenic HIV-1/SIV chimeric virus by passive infusion of neutralizing antibodies. *Nat Med*, **6**, 207–10.

Masopust, D., Vezys, V., et al. 2001. Preferential localization of effector memory cells in nonlymphoid tissue. *Science*, **291**, 2413–17.

McAdam, A.J., Greenwald, R.J., et al. 2001. ICOS is critical for CD40-mediated antibody class switching. *Nature*, **409**, 102–5.

McChesney, M.B., Miller, C.J., et al. 1997. Experimental measles. I. Pathogenesis in the normal and the immunized host. *Virology*, **233**, 74–84.

McHeyzer-Williams, M.G. 1997. Immune response decisions at the single cell level. *Semin Immunol*, **9**, 219–27.

McHeyzer-Williams, M.G. and Ahmed, R. 1999. B cell memory and the long-lived plasma cell. *Curr Opin Immunol*, **11**, 172–9.

McHeyzer-Williams, L.J., Driver, D.J. and McHeyzer-Williams, M.G. 2001. Germinal center reaction. *Curr Opin Hematol*, **8**, 52–9.

Moskophidis, D., Lechner, F., et al. 1993. Virus persistence in acutely infected immunocompetent mice by exhaustion of antiviral cytotoxic effector T cells. *Nature*, **362**, 758–61.

Mullbacher, A. 1994. The long-term maintenance of cytotoxic T cell memory does not require persistence of antigen. *J Exp Med*, **179**, 317–21.

Murali-Krishna, K., Altman, J.D., et al. 1998. Counting antigen-specific CD8 T cells: a reevaluation of bystander activation during viral infection. *Immunity*, **8**, 177–87.

Murali-Krishna, K., Lau, L.L., et al. 1999. Persistence of memory CD8 T cells in MHC class I-deficient mice. *Science*, **286**, 1377–81.

Opferman, J.T., Ober, B.T. and Ashton-Rickardt, P.G. 1999. Linear differentiation of cytotoxic effectors into memory T lymphocytes. *Science*, **283**, 1745–8.

Panum, P.L. 1847. Beobachtungen uber das Maserncontagium. *Virchows Arch*, **1**, 492–503.

Paul, J.R., Riordan, J.T. and Melnick, J.L. 1951. Antibodies to three different antigenic types of poliomyelitis virus in sera from North Alaskan Eskimos. *Am J Hyg*, **54**, 275–85.

Plotkin, S.A. and Orenstein, W.A. 1999. *Vaccines*, 3rd edn. Philadelphia, PA: W.B. Saunders Co..

Reinhardt, R.L., Khoruts, A., et al. 2001. Visualizing the generation of memory CD4 T cells in the whole body. *Nature*, **410**, 101–5.

Sallusto, F., Lenig, D., et al. 1999. Two subsets of memory T lymphocytes with distinct homing potentials and effector functions. *Nature*, **401**, 708–12.

Sawyer, W.A. 1931. Persistence of yellow fever immunity. *J Prev Med*, **5**, 413–28.

Scheibel, I., Bentzon, M.W., et al. 1966. Duration of immunity to diphtheria and tetanus after active immunization. *Acta Pathol Microbiol Scand*, **67**, 380–92.

Selin, L.K., Lin, M.Y., et al. 1999. Attrition of T cell memory: selective loss of LCMV epitope-specific memory CD8 T cells following infections with heterologous viruses. *Immunity*, **11**, 733–42.

Shaffer, A.L., Rosenwald, A., et al. 2001. Signatures of the immune response. *Immunity*, **15**, 375–85.

Shaffer, A.L., Lin, K.I., et al. 2002. Blimp-1 orchestrates plasma cell differentiation by extinguishing the mature B cell gene expression program. *Immunity*, **17**, 51–62.

Simonsen, O., Kjeldsen, K. and Heron, I. 1984. Immunity against tetanus and effect of revaccination 25–30 years after primary vaccination. *Lancet*, **ii**, 1240–2.

Slifka, M.K. and Ahmed, R. 1998. Long-lived plasma cells: a mechanism for maintaining persistent antibody production. *Curr Opin Immunol*, **10**, 252–8.

Slifka, M.K. and Whitton, J.L. 2000. Activated and memory CD8+ T cells can be distinguished by their cytokine profiles and phenotypic markers. *J Immunol*, **164**, 208–16.

Slifka, M.K., Matloubian, M. and Ahmed, R. 1995. Bone marrow is a major site of long-term antibody production after acute viral infection. *J Virol*, **69**, 1895–902.

Slifka, M.K., Antia, R., et al. 1998. Humoral immunity due to long-lived plasma cells. *Immunity*, **8**, 363–72.

Sprent, J. and Surh, C.D. 2001. Generation and maintenance of memory T cells. *Curr Opin Immunol*, **13**, 248–54.

Swain, S.L., Hu, H. and Huston, G. 1999. Class II-independent generation of CD4 memory T cells from effectors. *Science*, **286**, 1381–3.

Tafuri, A., Shahinian, A., et al. 2001. ICOS is essential for effective T-helper-cell responses. *Nature*, **409**, 105–9.

Tan, J.T., Ernst, B., et al. 2002. Interleukin (IL)-15 and IL-7 jointly regulate homeostatic proliferation of memory phenotype CD8+ cells but are not required for memory phenotype CD4+ cells. *J Exp Med*, **195**, 1523–32.

Tanchot, C., Lemonnier, F.A., et al. 1997. Differential requirements for survival and proliferation of CD8 naive or memory T cells. *Science*, **276**, 2057–62.

Tsiagbe, V.K. and Thorbecke, G.J. 1998. Overview of germinal center function and structure in normal and genetically engineered mice. In: Thorbecke, G.J. and Tsiagbe, V.K. (eds), *The biology of germinal centers in lymphoid tissue*. Berlin: Springer-Verlag, 1–103.

van Stipdonk, M.J., Lemmens, E.E. and Schoenberger, S.P. 2001. Naive CTLs require a single brief period of antigenic stimulation for clonal expansion and differentiation. *Nat Immunol*, **2**, 423–9.

William, J., Euler, C., Christensen, S. and Shlomchik, M.J. 2002. Evolution of autoantibody responses via somatic hypermutation outside of germinal centers. *Science*, **297**, 2066–70.

Wong, P. and Pamer, E.G. 2001. Cutting edge: antigen-independent cd8 T cell proliferation. *J Immunol*, **166**, 5864–8.

Xu, J., Foy, T.M., et al. 1994. Mice deficient for the CD40 ligand. *Immunity*, **1**, 423–31.

Zajac, A.J., Blattman, J.N., et al. 1998. Viral immune evasion due to persistence of activated T cells without effector function. *J Exp Med*, **188**, 2205–13.

Zhan, F., Tian, E., et al. 2002. Gene expression profiling of human plasma cell differentiation and classification of multiple myeloma based on similarities to distinct stages of late stage B-cell development. *Blood*, **101**, 128–40.

Zimmerman, C., Brduscha-Riem, K., et al. 1996. Visualization, characterization, and turnover of CD8+ memory T cells in virus-infected hosts. *J Exp Med*, **183**, 1367–75.

Zimmermann, C., Prevost-Blondel, A., et al. 1999. Kinetics of the response of naive and memory CD8 T cells to antigen: similarities and differences. *Eur J Immunol*, **29**, 284–90.

Zinkernagel, R.M., Bachmann, M.F., et al. 1996. On immunological memory. *Annu Rev Immunol*, **14**, 333–67.

27

Lymphocyte homing

MICHEL AURRAND-LIONS AND BEAT A. IMHOF

THE CONCEPT OF RECIRCULATION: LYMPHOCYTES VERSUS LEUKOCYTES

The immune system protects the body from invading microorganisms and parasites and surveys the tissues for expression of aberrant selfantigens. The principal players in this defense system are the leukocytes, and they are well equipped to cope with virtually any pathogen. However, most pathogens have the advantage of an extremely high proliferation rate, and prevention of systemic infections and damage requires appropriate rapid responses from innate and adaptive immune systems. Although all the cells of the innate immune system are able to mount fast responses against various antigens, the response of the adaptive, specific branch is greatly hampered by the low number of cells specific for a given antigen. To counterbalance this disadvantage, cells of the adaptive immune system, i.e. lymphocytes, follow distinct migration and recirculation routes in order to maximize a possible encounter with their cognate antigens and to be strategically positioned at sites of antigen entry.

Cells of the innate immune system are the first effector cells that arrive at the site of infection or tissue damage. As they constitute a uniform antigen nonspecific pool, they can be rapidly recruited in large numbers and, having exerted their function, they are deleted. The recirculation of lymphoid cells contrasts markedly to the unidirectional migration of cells of the innate immune system from blood into tissue. Lymphocytes have a complex migration pattern that is strongly dependent on their state of activation and memory. They have the ability to recirculate, i.e. to re-enter the systemic blood circulation from tissues and migrate to a distant site in the body (Figure 27.1). The reason for this recirculation behavior is presumably the relatively low number of antigen-specific lymphocytes that can be generated for each of the millions of antigens. Positive and negative selections of antigen receptors produce a vast number of specificities, but necessarily only a very small number of cells for any given specificity. Therefore, the migration of lymphocytes is highly organized to ensure an efficient exposure of lymphocytes to their cognate antigens in secondary lymphoid organs. Moreover, clones with relevant specificities, i.e. receptors that recognize antigenic epitopes of foreign organisms, are not lost after their engagement, but are preserved as memory cells for more rapid and stronger responses on reinfection with the same organism. This generation of memory within the specific immune system is the rationale for immunization and it can persist and protect an organism for the rest of its life. Thus, the constitutive recirculation of lymphocytes through secondary lymphoid tissues is distinct from the leukocyte recruitment occurring at sites of inflammation where vascularized tissues respond to damages.

MIGRATION OF LYMPHOCYTES

The initial experiments to study the origin of cells in the lymph (hence the name lymphocytes) were conducted

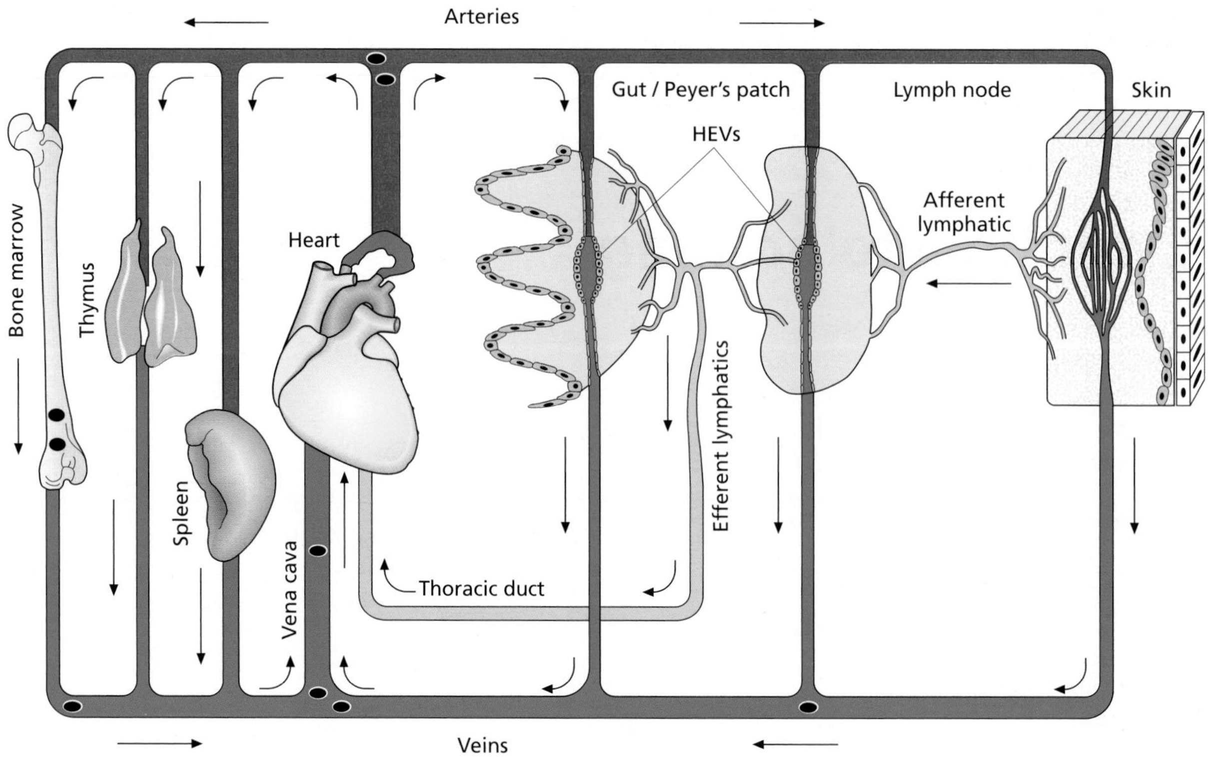

Figure 27.1 *Routes of lymphocyte migration and recirculation. The diagram depicts blood and lymphatic connections between primary and secondary lymphoid organs. The naïve lymphoid cells are located in the thymus (T cells) or bone marrow (B cells) and reach the secondary lymphoid organs as indicated. Lymphoid cells circulating through the blood system enter in organs through postcapillaries venules (skin) or high endothelial venules (HEVs) in Peyer's patches and lymph nodes. The second system used by lymphocytes is the lymphatic system (in black), which drains immune cells from peripheral tissues through lymph nodes and mucosa-associated tissues (MALT) back to the blood via the thoracic duct.*

by James Gowans and colleagues (Gowans 1957; Gowans and Knight 1964). They were the first to show that cells in the lymphatics are blood-borne cells that have the ability to circulate between blood and lymph in order to seek out their cognate antigen, constituting the so-called immune surveillance (Pabst and Binns 1989; Salmi and Jalkanen 1997). Westermann and Pabst have estimated that, in humans, about 5×10^{11} lymphocytes leave the blood each day to enter various organs and then return to the blood (Westermann and Pabst 1990, 1996). In lymphoid organs, lymphocyte extravasation occurs in the postcapillary venules (Gowans and Knight 1964) at specialized postcapillary vascular sites called high endothelial venules (HEV) (Anderson and Anderson 1976; Anderson et al. 1976). These represent the major constitutive extravasation route in vivo (Lasky 1992), and most recirculating lymphocytes selectively bind to the endothelium of HEVs, while ignoring normal vascular endothelium (Mackay et al. 1990). In humans, HEVs are found in all secondary lymphoid organs except the spleen. Endothelial cells of HEVs have a cuboidal appearance that differs considerably from the flat morphology of other endothelial cells (Girard and Springer 1995). In addition to this characteristic morphology, endothelial cells of HEVs differ from others by the specific expression of several genes increasing their adhesive properties for lymphocytes (Girard et al. 1999). Consequently, leukocytes are more likely to collide with, adhere to, and migrate across endothelial cells of HEVs than any other nonstimulated resting endothelial cells (Bjerknes et al. 1986; Johnson-Leger et al. 2000). This constitutive specialization of HEVs to sustain leukocyte recirculation contrasts sharply with the situation at inflamed sites, where the damaged tissue triggers new adhesive properties in the adjacent endothelium in order to induce directional migration of lymphocytes toward the site where the immune effector function takes place (Muller 2002).

STRUCTURE AND ORGANIZATION OF LYMPHOID TISSUES

Lymphoid structures are divided into primary and secondary lymphoid organs. The primary lymphoid organs are the thymus and the bone marrow in mammals, which constitute the respective sites of differentiation for T and B cells. Their function is to sustain the lymphoid differentiation toward the stage of acquisition of immunocompetence, e.g. expression of functional antigen-specific receptors on the surface of lymphoid cells. Such cells are named naïve. Precursor lymphoid cells, also termed 'stem cells', are located in the bone marrow and differentiate in B cells or T-precursor cells, before leaving this organ and seeding secondary lymphoid organs in the case of B cells or thymus in the case of T-precursor cells. Although the migration of T-precursor cells to the thymus is essential for T-cell differentiation, studies of the molecular mechanisms of homing have been hampered by the minute number of precursor T cells leaving the bone marrow and seeding the thymus. Once naïve cells have completed their differentiation in primary lymphoid organs, they specifically migrate to secondary lymphoid organs.

The secondary lymphoid organs encompass the spleen, peripheral and mesenteric lymph nodes, mucosa-associated lymphoid tissue (MALT) including tonsils, and gut-associated lymphoid tissue (GALT) such as Peyer's patches and the appendix. Functionally, the lymphoid organs can be classified into three distinct groups: MALT traps antigens that enter the body through various mucous membrane surfaces, peripheral lymph nodes (PLN) collect antigen from the intercellular tissue fluids, whereas the spleen filters blood-borne antigens (see Figure 27.1). Although important morphological differences exist among the different secondary lymphoid organs, they all have the common function of concentrating B, T and antigen-presenting cells at unique sites in order to mount efficient immune responses. This is reflected by the presence of discrete structures named lymphoid follicles that can be distinguished histologically in all secondary lymphoid organs. They are especially abundant in mucosal surfaces and consist of aggregates of various lymphoid cells surrounded by a network of draining lymphatic capillaries. These structures are surrounded by a fibrous capsule and contain distinct regions of B- and T-cell activity. Lymph nodes are the most complex secondary lymphoid organs, organized in distinct microenvironments for antigen presentation and lymphocyte recirculation. Afferent lymphatic vessels collect the lymph, antigen-presenting cells (dendritic cells), and lymphocytes from tissue and drain them to peripheral lymph nodes or to intestinal/mesenteric lymph nodes. At the same time, blood-borne lymphocytes enter these lymph nodes via specialized postcapillary venules, the HEVs, in order to encounter the resident cells as well as the cells entering via the afferent lymph. The lymph nodes thus constitute a point where the pathways for antigens and specific effector cells converge. Efferent lymphatic vessels drain the nodes and carry lymph and lymphocytes via the thoracic duct back to the systemic blood circulation into the subclavian vein.

The spleen is adapted to respond to systemic infections by filtering the blood and trapping blood-borne antigens. In contrast to all the other secondary lymphoid organs, the spleen is not connected to the lymphatics and therefore does not directly communicate with the tissues. Furthermore, the spleen lacks HEVs: circulating cells and antigens have unhampered access to this organ through arterioles that terminate open-ended in the sinuses of the marginal zone and through the lack of HEVs. As a result of the high blood flow, the spleen has by far the highest lymphocyte throughput of all lymphoid organs and thus is the organ that lymphocytes pass most frequently.

MOLECULAR MECHANISMS OF LYMPHOCYTE MIGRATION

The multistep paradigm

In the early 1990s, Eugene Butcher and Tim Springer (Butcher 1991; Springer 1994) proposed a multistep paradigm for leukocyte recruitment governed by a different class of adhesion molecules. Although specific molecular interactions have been demonstrated for subsets of leukocytes, and resting and inflammatory situations, leukocyte recruitment always occurs in four different steps, namely: tethering and rolling, triggering, firm adhesion, and transmigration (Butcher 1992). The four different steps involve different classes of adhesion molecules with specific properties. Although additional adhesion molecules have been involved in the initial step, leukocyte rolling is mainly mediated by weak interaction of selectins with their carbohydrate ligands on opposing cells. The rolling is a reversible step but is a prerequisite to the following triggering step by chemokines, leading to leukocyte integrin activation and firm adhesion. This is followed by the final transmigration step, also called diapedesis, which consists of ameboid movement of leukocytes between tightly apposed endothelial cells. This final step involves an active remodeling of interendothelial junctions and has recently received new insights with the discovery of proteins specifically involved in transmigration (Vestweber 2002). Although the models for constitutive and inflammatory lymphocyte recruitment are similar, different adhesion molecules are specifically expressed at sites of constitutive lymphocyte recirculation (HEV) or at sites of inflammatory-induced lymphocyte recruitment (Dailey 1998; von Andrian and Mackay 2000). The specific migration route taken by lymphocytes is controlled by the combined vascular expression of L-selectin ligands, E- and P-selectins, chemokines, integrin ligands, and inter-endothelial junctional molecules. Mirroring this endothelial diversification, lymphocyte subpopulations express themselves as specific sets of selectin, selectin ligands, chemokine receptors, integrins, and integrin ligands.

Tethering/rolling

The initial rolling step of lymphocytes along the vessel wall is known to depend mainly on weak interactions between selectins and their ligands. Three selectins, named respectively L-, E-, and P- selectins for leukocytic, endothelial, and platelet selectins, have been identified (Vestweber and Blanks 1999). They all interact with carbohydrate structures and are involved in the regulation of both naive and effector/memory lymphocyte migration. As a result of their anchorage to the actin cytoskeleton, they initiate the adhesion cascade by slowing down the leukocyte along the vascular bed (Dwir et al. 2001) in order to allow the triggering and firm adhesion to occur. In addition, the engagement of selectins leads to signal transduction inside the rolling cells, which may participate in integrin activation (Sikorski et al. 1996; Simon et al. 2000). In contrast to the specific involvement of selectins in lymphocyte rolling, the integrin $\alpha_4\beta_7$ can contribute either to lymphocyte rolling or to firm adhesion (Holzmann et al. 1989; Berlin et al. 1993).

Tethering/rolling of naive lymphocytes

L-selectin is constitutively expressed on virtually all naïve lymphocytes, a portion of memory T cells, neutrophils, eosinophils, and monocytes (Lewinsohn et al. 1987), and is responsible for trafficking of naïve lymphocytes through lymph nodes (Berg et al. 1989). More precisely, L-selectin is implicated in the rolling of naïve lymphocytes along HEVs as demonstrated by real-time intravital video microscopy studies in animals treated with antibody against L-selectin (von Andrian 1996). This C-type lectin interacts with sialyl-Lewis^x structures (sLe^x) found on peripheral lymph node addressins (PNAd) expressed on HEVs such as GlyCAM-1, CD34, podocalyxin, Sgp200, and MAdCAM-1. The optimal binding of L-selectin to its ligands requires sialylation, fucosylation, and carbohydrate sulfation of these ligands by enzymes expressed in HEVs, as demonstrated by the reduced lymphocyte homing to lymph nodes observed in animals deficient for α(1,3)-fucosyltransferase (FucTVII) or *N*-acetyl glycosamine-6-sulfotransferase (HEC-GlcNAc6ST) (Maly et al. 1996; Hemmerich et al. 2001). It is therefore important to consider that optimal L-selectin activity requires expression of PNAd core proteins and post-translational modifying enzymes. Although interaction of L-selectin with its ligands accounts for most lymphocyte entry in lymph nodes, the homing to the mucosal associated tissue in the gut (gut-associated lymphoid tissue or GALT), especially to the Peyer's patches, is only moderately affected in animals deficient for L-selectin, fucosyl, or sulfotransferases (Arbones et al. 1994; Maly et al. 1996; Hemmerich et al. 2001). This is the result of the binding of $\alpha_4\beta_7$ integrin to MAdCAM-1 and to the expression of MAdCAM-1 by HEVs of Peyer's patches (Berlin et al. 1993). Indeed, mesenteric lymph nodes present the features of Peyer's patches and peripheral lymph nodes because they express only MAdCAM-1 on some HEVs, whereas others express MadCAM and L-selectin (Streeter et al. 1988a, 1988b; Berg et al. 1993). However, one could keep in mind that integrin $\alpha_4\beta_7$ represents one of the rare exceptions in which an integrin is used by lymphocytes for rolling.

The significance of integrin $\alpha_4\beta_7$ in lymphocyte homing is best shown in mice that are deficient in the integrin β_7 subunit. The GALT in these mice is severely impaired as a result of the failure of lymphocytes to migrate into the lamina propria, Peyer's patches, and the intraepithelial lymphocyte (IEL) compartment (Wagner et al. 1996). This lymphocyte's homing deficiency is not caused by a defect on HEVs, because naïve β_7-deficient lymphocytes transferred into normal mice normally home to peripheral and mesenteric lymph nodes via L-selectin, but fail to migrate to mucosal effector sites of the gut, i.e. Peyer's patches, lamina propria, and the IEL compartment (Lefrancois et al. 1999).

Tethering/rolling of antigen-primed lymphocytes

Once a naïve lymphocyte encounters its cognate antigen in lymphoid organs, it activates and undergoes dramatic changes in the expression of surface adhesion molecules as it differentiates into an effector or memory lymphocyte (Jung et al. 1988; Picker et al. 1990b; Williams and Butcher 1997). Although subtle differences in expression of adhesion molecules can be found between different effector/memory cell subpopulations (Sallusto et al. 1999; Campbell et al. 2001), the loss of L-selectin expression and the upregulation of ligands for E- and P-selectin by antigen-experienced cells prevent their entry into lymphoid organs (Rigby and Dailey 2000; Hafezi-Moghadam et al. 2001). Notably, this dogma has been recently revised with the identification of memory cell subpopulations that express high levels of L-selectin, migrate toward lymphoid organs, and are called central memory cells (Sallusto et al. 1999; Campbell et al. 2001). Upon leukocyte activation, the downregulation of L-selectin involves transcriptional regulation and protein shedding by surface metalloproteases (Kishimoto et al. 1989; Preece et al. 1996). According to these changes, tethering and rolling of lymphocytes in inflammatory conditions mainly involve P- and E-selectins induced on vascular endothelium by inflammatory stimuli. P-selectin was originally identified in α granules of platelets and later found to be expressed in Weibel–Palade bodies of endothelial cells (Hsu-Lin et al. 1984; McEver et al. 1989). On appropriate stimulation with inflammatory factors such as histamine or thrombin, degranulation of these compartments leads to the rapid expression of P-selectin on the vascular cell surface (Hattori et al. 1989) making it available for interacting with the ligand P-selectin glycoprotein ligand-1 (PSGL-1) or CD24 (the old name was heat stable antigen or HSA) expressed on the surface of effector lymphocyte subpopulations (Aigner et al. 1995; Borges et al. 1997). Although P-selectin is expressed within minutes of stimulation on the cell surface, E-selectin expression on endothelial cells is transcriptionally regulated by inflammatory cytokines such as tumor necrosis factor α (TNF-α), interleukin 1 (IL-1), or lipopolysaccharide (LPS), leading to expression within 4–24 h (Bevilacqua et al. 1987). Once expressed on the cell surface, E-selectin interacts with ligands expressed on leukocytes, namely E-selectin ligand-1 (ESL-1), PSGL-1, or L-selectin (Vestweber and Blanks 1999). Therefore one important aspect of lymphocyte migration toward the site of inflammation is the expression of E- and P-selectin ligands, among which PSGL-1 is the best characterized. Similar to the binding of L-selectin to the sugar moiety of PNAds, the binding of E-selectins to PSGL-1 requires carbohydrate modifications whereas P-selectin binding requires additional tyrosine sulfations (Pouyani and Seed 1995).

The physiological importance of post-translational modifications of PSGL-1 on lymphocytes is best demonstrated by the functional characterization of an inducible carbohydrate epitope expressed on PSGL-1 and named cutaneous lymphocyte-associated antigen (CLA) (Picker et al. 1990a; Berg et al. 1991). Expression of CLA on T-memory lymphocytes has been found to correlate with the ability of these cells to home to inflamed skin. CLA is a carbohydrate epitope attached to PSGL-1 by fucosyltransferase VII (Fuhlbrigge et al. 1997). The CLA-epitope mediates cell binding to E-selectin expressed on endothelial cells in inflamed skin (Picker et al. 1991) and thereby the recruitment of memory T cells. Differential regulation of CLA seems to occur during the activation of naïve T lymphocytes in peripheral lymph nodes (Borowitz et al. 1993; Picker et al. 1993). Following these initial findings, several studies have shown that the expression of L-selectin and E- and P-selectin ligands, in combination with chemokine receptor expression, can be used to subdivide the different effector and memory lymphocytes subsets upon antigenic challenge (Tietz et al. 1998; Sallusto et al. 1999; Campbell et al. 2001).

This contrasts with integrin β_7 expression which appears sufficient to sustain the migration of lymphocytes to the GALT upon antigenic activation (Rott et al. 1997, 2000; Williams and Butcher 1997; Rose et al. 1998). The unique migration pattern of $\alpha_4\beta_7$-expressing cells is confirmed by the fact that orally administrated antigens result in a higher incidence of antigen-specific cells expressing $\alpha_4\beta_7$ compared with systemic antigen exposure which generates antigen-specific cells within the L-selectin expressing compartment (Lakew et al. 1995; Kantele et al. 1997).

Although this is beyond the scope of this chapter, the reader should be aware that additional adhesion molecules have been implicated in the initial rolling step of lymphocytes (Table 27.1). This has been demonstrated by using blocking reagents for L-selectin function and the discovery of alternate molecular pathways using CD44, VAP-1, or α_4 integrins (Stoolman 1989; Picker et al. 1989; Alon et al. 1995; Salmi et al. 1997). Although $\alpha_4\beta_1$, CD44, and VAP-1 are all involved in adhesion of lymphocytes on inflammatory endothelium (Elices et al. 1990; Salmi et al. 1993; Maiti et al. 1998), their relative contributions to constitutive versus antigen-primed lymphocyte rolling remain to be formally established in vivo.

FIRM ADHESION: INTEGRINS GUIDE TO THE 'NO RETURN POINT'

In contrast to the rolling step supported by several classes of adhesion molecules, the subsequent lymphocyte arrest is almost exclusively mediated by activated integrin receptors (see Table 27.1). They constitute the most versatile adhesion molecules because their adhesive properties are regulated with the state of cell activation and because of the nature of activation signals to which leukocytes are exposed (Alon and Feigelson 2002). Integrins are formed of an α and a β subunit, and activation signals change their shape leading to increased affinity of integrins for their ligands (Shimaoka et al. 2002). This is known as a mechanism of inside-out signaling. At the same time, ligand engagement by integrins leads to signal transduction inside the cells in a process called outside-in signaling. Integrin activation occurs within fractions of seconds on chemokine triggering or ligand engagement, implying that most of the circulating lymphocytes express integrins in a nonactivated, resting state. Therefore, leukocyte integrins are exclusively triggered if the rolling step has occurred and if chemokines and endothelial ligands are locally expressed at the site of lymphocyte extravasation.

Among the different heterodimers, $\alpha_L\beta_2$ (LFA-1, CD11a/CD18), $\alpha_4\beta_1$ (VLA-4), and $\alpha_4\beta_7$ (LPAM-1) integrins are the key molecules that mediate firm adhesion of rolling lymphocytes by engagement with their counter-receptors, which include members of the immunoglobulin superfamily (IgSf) (Staunton et al. 1988). The latter can be tentatively classified into two groups: IgSf molecules that are constitutively expressed by endothelial cells at specific sites, such as MAdCAM-1 or intercellular adhesion molecule 2 (ICAM-2) (Staunton et al. 1989; Briskin et al. 1993), and those that are induced by inflammatory stimuli on endothelial cells such as vascular cell adhesion molecule 1 (VCAM-1) or intercellular adhesion molecule 1 (ICAM-1) (Marlin and Springer 1987; Elices et al. 1990). However, it has become clear that this classification is not absolute because constitutive expression of ICAM-1 and VCAM-1 on HEVs has been reported (Tamatani et al. 1991; Sasaki et al. 1996; Faveeuw et al. 2000). ICAM-1, ICAM-2, and intercellular adhesion molecule 3 (ICAM-3) are counterreceptors for $\alpha_L\beta_2$ integrin whereas VCAM-1 binds weakly to $\alpha_4\beta_7$ and is the main ligand

Table 27.1 *Cell adhesion molecules involved in lymphocyte homing*

Cell adhesion molecule	Expression	Ligand	Adhesion step	Implicated in
Integrins				
LFA-1 ($\alpha_L\beta_2$, CD11a/CD18)	Most leukocytes	ICAM-1, -2, -3	Tight adhesion	General role in extravasation
$\alpha_4\beta_1$ (VLA-4)	Lymphocytes	VCAM-1, fibronectin	Tethering and tight adhesion	Leukocyte homing to inflamed tissue
$\alpha_4\beta_7$	Lymphocytes	MadCAM-1, fibronectin, VCAM-1	Tethering and tight adhesion	Lymphocyte homing to MALT
Selectins				
L-Selectin (MEL-14, CD62L)	Most nonactivated leukocytes	sLe^x on GlyCAM, CD34 and MadCAM-1	Tethering	Lymphocyte homing to LNs, leukocyte homing to inflamed tissue
P-Selectin (CD62)	Activated platelets, inflammatory endothelium	PSGL-1	Tethering	Leukocyte recruitment by inflamed tissue
E-Selectin (CD62E)	Inflammatory endothelium	CLA, PSGL-1, ESL-1	Tethering	Leukocyte recruitment by inflamed tissue
Ig superfamily				
ICAM-1	Inflammatory endothelium, activated lymphocytes	LFA-1, $\alpha_M\beta_2$	Tight adhesion	Leukocyte recruitment by inflamed tissue
ICAM-2	Endothelium and resting lymphocytes	LFA-1	Tight adhesion	General role in leukocyte extravasation
VCAM-1	Inflammatory endothelium	$\alpha_4\beta_1$, $\alpha_4\beta_1$	Tight adhesion	Leukocyte recruitment by inflamed tissue
MAdCAM-1	Mucosal endothelium	L-selectin, $\alpha_4\beta_7$	Tethering and tight adhesion	Lymphocyte recruitment to mucosal tissue
PECAM	Endothelium, leukocytes, platelets	PECAM, $\alpha_V\beta_3$	Diapedesis	Monocyte recruitment to inflamed tissues
JAM-1	Endothelium, epithelium, leukocytes, platelets	JAM-1, LFA-1	Tight adhesion and diapedesis	General role in leukocyte extravasation
JAM-2 (also called JAM3)	Endothelium, activated lymphocytes, platelets	JAM-2, VE-JAM, Mac-1	Adhesion and diapedesis	General role in leukocyte extravasation
Carbohydrate ligands of selectins				
GlyCAM (glycosylation dependent CAM)	High endothelial venules	L-Selectin	Tethering	Recruitment of naïve lymphocytes to lymph nodes
CD34	Endothelium	L-Selectin	Tethering	Recruitment of naïve lymphocytes to lymph nodes and inflamed tissue
CLA (cutaneous lymphocyte antigen, carbohydrate structure on PSGL-1)	Activated lymphocytes	E-Selectin	Tethering	Homing of lymphocytes to inflamed skin
MAdCAM-1 (mucosal addressin CAM)	Mucosal endothelium	L-Selectin	Tethering	Recruitment of lymphocytes to MALT
PSGL-1 (P-selectin glycoligand-1)	Myeloid, lymphoid and dendritic lineages	P-Selectin, E-selectin	Tethering	Homing to inflamed tissue
Others				
CD43	All leukocytes except mature B cells	Sialoadhesin-1	Negative regulation of tethering	Leukocyte migration and activation
CD44	Broad distribution	Hyaluronan	Tethering	Function in cell migration to inflamed areas
VAP-1	High endothelial venules, inflammatory endothelium	Amine oxidase activity on primary amino groups	Tethering	Recruitment of naïve lymphocytes to lymph nodes and inflamed tissue

Subdivisions are presented according to the molecular nature of the different protein, and their classification in different protein families. Although different classes of adhesion molecules mediate tethering, firm adhesion and diapedesis of lymphocytes involve exclusively integrins and their counterreceptors. See text for abbreviations.

(with fibronectin) for $\alpha_4\beta_1$ integrin. Therefore, $\alpha_4\beta_1$ is predominantly involved in the migration of lymphocytes to sites of effector functions, whereas $\alpha_L\beta_2$ plays a dual role in constitutive and inflammatory induced migration.

Firm adhesion of naïve lymphocytes

The importance of $\alpha_L\beta_2$ (LFA-1) integrin in homeostatic homing of lymphocytes has been demonstrated in α_L-deficient mice that show reduced numbers of lymphocytes in PLNs (Berlin-Rufenach et al. 1999). LFA-1-mediated adhesion is clearly a downstream event of rolling mediated by L-selectin and does not occur with nonrolling cells (Warnock et al. 1998). Interestingly, residual homing to lymph nodes in LFA-1-deficient mice appears to depend on lymphocyte α_4 integrins ($\alpha_4\beta_1$ and $\alpha_4\beta_7$) and VCAM-1 expressed by HEVs. However, the expression of VCAM-1 on HEVs under noninflammatory conditions is still controversial (Hahne et al. 1993; May et al. 1993; Berlin et al. 1995; Henninger et al. 1997). Real-time video microscopy studies have shown that the sticking fraction of lymphocytes on HEVs of peripheral lymph nodes (which do not express MAdCAM-1 and cannot undergo $\alpha_4\beta_7$-mediated adhesion) is not affected by blocking antibodies against α_4 integrin (Warnock et al. 1998).

In contrast to $\alpha_4\beta_1$, the dual role of $\alpha_4\beta_7$ integrin in rolling and firm adhesion of naïve lymphocytes on MAdCAM-1 is clearly established (Berlin et al. 1995). This was demonstrated using preactivated naïve lymphocytes which require only $\alpha_4\beta_7$ for arrest on the HEVs of Peyer's patches (Bargatze et al. 1995). Therefore, the specific engagement $\alpha_L\beta_2$ or $\alpha_4\beta_7$ with its respective ligand depends mainly on activation signals received by transmigrating cells (Campbell et al. 1998), as illustrated by numerous studies showing that the signals required for integrin clustering and stable adhesion differ between integrin α_4 and integrin β_2 (Constantin et al. 2000; Ding et al. 2001; Shamri et al. 2002).

Firm adhesion of antigen-primed lymphocytes

Once lymphocytes are activated in secondary lymphoid organs, they change their expression pattern of chemokine receptors and adhesion molecules, as demonstrated by phenotypic analysis of surface antigenic markers. Although the original names 'Very late Antigens, VLA' are no longer relevant for most integrins, $\alpha_4\beta_1$ (VLA-4) expression increases after long-term T-cell activation (Hemler 1990). In contrast, $\alpha_L\beta_2$ (lymphocyte function antigen-1 (LFA-1)) was initially identified as a T-cell costimulatory molecule involved in T-cell effector function (Kaufmann et al. 1982), before being shown to participate in lymphocyte adhesion to ICAM-1 and ICAM-2 on endothelial cells (Dustin and Springer 1988; van Kooyk and Figdor 2000). Therefore, in addition to selectin, the migration of lymphocytes at sites of inflammation is regulated by integrin engagement with their ligands ICAM-1 and VCAM-1. The latter are expressed within hours on endothelial cells stimulated by inflammatory chemokines, but their expression peaks within days (Haraldsen et al. 1996). The importance of ICAM-1 and VCAM-1 in lymphocyte migration at inflammatory sites has been formally demonstrated using antibodies and small molecules that inhibit the ligand-binding activities of the integrins $\alpha_L\beta_2$ and $\alpha_4\beta_1$, thus dampening inflammatory reactions (Isobe et al. 1992; Kakimoto et al. 1992; Yednock et al. 1992; Issekutz 1993). The central role of LFA-1 engagement with its counter-receptor ICAM-1 in inflammatory reactions is further demonstrated by the decrease in allogeneic response and delayed-type hypersensitivity in mice with a genetically engineered ICAM-1 expression deficiency (Sligh et al. 1993; Xu et al. 1994). The same transgenic approach has also been used to inactivate the different integrin chains (β_2, α_L, α_4, and β_1) and VCAM-1, confirming to some extent the role of these molecules in lymphocyte migration and inflammatory reactions (Arroyo et al. 1996; 1999; Coxon et al. 1996; Huleatt and Lefrancois 1996; Berlin-Rufenach et al. 1999; Potocnik et al. 2000). However, in the cases of α_4 and VCAM-1 deficiencies, unexpected defects in placental and heart development have also been reported (Kwee et al. 1995; Yang et al. 1995), suggesting a pleiotropic role of integrins in cell migration, differentiation, and organogenesis.

CHEMOKINES SHOW THE WAY

Although selectins and integrins are key mediators of cell arrest along the vasculature, they are not sufficient in determining the specificity of lymphocyte migration. The ability of a circulating leukocyte to employ integrins for tight adhesion is determined by the expression of chemokine receptors that, on ligand binding, signal to and thereby activate the available integrins (Table 27.2). Interestingly, chemokines and their receptors show a much higher degree of tissue specificity than the adhesion molecules. As a result of the slow, selectin-mediated rolling (see above), the lymphocyte's chemokine receptors interact with chemokines presented by the glycocalyx of the endothelium. This mechanism collects the tissue-specific information by triggering $G_{\alpha i}$-protein-linked signaling events which activate the leukocyte integrins. Activated integrins then mediate tight adhesion of the lymphocyte to vascular endothelium of tissue specific lymphoid organs, and this is followed by migration into the tissue (Pachynski et al. 1998). The secretion of chemokines by inflammatory tissue may bypass tissue homeostatic lymphocyte homing. This can occur anywhere in the body and it efficiently redirects the migration of lymphocytes. Furthermore, the ability of lymphocytes to respond to

Table 27.2 *Chemokine receptors and their ligands*

Receptor	Ligands (old name)	Expression profile lymphocytes	Functional role for lymphocytes	Condition of function
CXCR3	CXCL9 (MIG)	Activated Th1 cells < Th2, B cells	Recruitment of lymphocytes to Th1-type inflammation	Inflammation
	CXCL10 (IP-10)	NK cells		
	CXCL11 (I-TAC)			
CXCR4	CXCL12 (SDF-1)	Progenitor cells, resting T and B cells	Emigration of B cells from bone marrow, stem cell, and thymocyte homing	Constitutive
CXCR5	CXCL13 (BCA-1, BLC)	B cells, memory T cells	Lymphocyte migration to B-cell follicles	Constitutive
CXCR6	CXCL16	Memory T cells	Migration of Th1 cells to inflammatory tissue	Inflammation
CCR1	CCL3 (MIP-1α)	Memory T cells	Migration of T cells to inflammatory tissue	Inflammation
	CCL5 (RANTES)			
	CCL7 (MCP-3, MARC)			
	CCL14 (HCC-1, CKβ1)			
	CCL15 (MIP-5, HCC-2, Lkn-1)			
	CCL16 (HCC-4, LEC, Mtn-1, LCC-1)			
	CCL23 (MPIF-1, ckβ8-1, ckβ-8)			
CCR3	CCL5 (RANTES)	Activated Th2 > Th1 cells	Migration of T cells to Th2-type inflammation	Inflammation
	CCL7 (MCP-3, MARC)			
	CCL8 (MCP-2)			
	CCL13 (MCP-4)			
	CCL15 (HCC-2, Lkn-1, MIP-5)			
	CCL24 (MPIF-2, eotaxin-2)			
	CCL26 (MIP-4α, eotaxin-3)			
CCR4	CCL17 (TARC)	Activate Th2 > Th1 cells	Migration of T cells to Th2-type inflammation	Inflammation
	CCL22 (MDC, STCP1, abcd-1)			
CCR5	CCL3 (MIP-1α)	Progenitors, activated Th1 cells	Migration to Th2-type inflammation	Inflammation
	CCL4 (MIP-1β)			
	CCL5 (RANTES)			
CCR6	CCL20 (LARC, MIP-3αEXODUS)	Memory T cells	Migration to inflammatory skin and other tissue	Inflammation
CCR7	CCL19 (ELC, MIP-3β, β11)	Resting and activated T cells, B cells	Migration to secondary lymphoid organs	Constitutive
	CCL21 (6Ckine, SLC, ckβ9)			
CCR8	CCL1 (I-309)	Th2 cells	Migration to Th2-type inflammation	Inflammation
	CCL4 (MIP-1β)			
CCR9	CCL25 (TECK, ckβ15)	$\alpha_4\beta_7^+$ T cells, thymocytes, IgA-secreting B cells	Homing to the gut, thymocyte selection	Constitutive
CCR10	CCL27 (CTACK, ILC, ESkine)	CLA$^+$ T cells	Homing to skin	Constitutive
XCR1	XCL1 (lymphotactin, ATAC)	Recent activated T cells, B cells		Inflammation
	XCL2			
CX3CR1	CX3CL1 (fractalkine, neurotactin)	Activated T cells	Migration to inflammatory tissue	Inflammation

Chemokine receptors are proteins that contain a seven-transmembrane ('serpentine') spanning domain, which can associate with trimeric G-proteins of the Gαi family. Upon chemokine binding, these receptors trigger a $G_{\alpha i}$-mediated signaling cascade that can lead to the activation of leukocyte integrins (Zlotnik and Yoshie 2000). See text for abbreviations.

chemokines depends on the expression of the appropriate chemokine receptor (Table 27.2).

Homeostatic homing of lymphocytes

MIGRATION OF NAÏVE LYMPHOCYTES TO SECONDARY LYMPHOID TISSUE

On the search for antigens, thymus-emigrating naïve T cells have to enter secondary lymphoid organs. They enter through postcapillary venules made of high cuboidal cells, the HEVs. The HEVs themselves and nonlymphoid cells in T-cell-rich areas of lymph nodes, spleen, and Peyer's patches produce the chemokine CCL21/SLC (Gunn et al. 1998b). It triggers rapid activation of integrins LFA-1 and $\alpha_4\beta_7$ and arrests rolling lymphocytes by signaling through the CCL21/SLC receptor CCR7. T lymphocytes deficient in CCR7 show very poor homing to lymph nodes and Peyer's patches (Nakano et al. 1997; Campbell et al. 1998; Gunn et al. 1998b, 1999) and plt mice, which lack CCL21/SLC, show impaired lymphocyte homing (Gunn et al. 1999). After entering the lymphoid organ T cells they have to be correctly positioned. The chemokine receptor CCR7 is also involved in this positioning mechanism but here it uses both ligands, CCL21/SLC and CCL19/ELC (Cyster 1999). Endothelial and stromal cells in T-cell zones produce CCL21/SLC, and dendritic cells and macrophages in T-cell areas make CCL19/ELC. Some of the CCL19/ELC, however, is transcytosed across to HEVs and has also a small effect on T-cell entry into the organ (Baekkevold et al. 2001).

The chemokine responsible for entrance of naïve B cells into lymphoid organs is not known. It is certainly different from CCL21/SLC because absence of CCR7 and/or CCL21/SLC does not dramatically change B-cell homing (Forster et al. 1996; Gunn et al. 1999). Inside the organ, however, B cells use CXCL13/BLC and its receptor CXCR5 to migrate into lymphoid follicles (Forster et al. 1994, 1996; Ansel et al. 2000). Stromal cells and follicular dendritic cells produce CXCL13/BLC in B-cell-rich lymphoid follicles (Gunn et al. 1998a). On B-cell activation the expression of the CXCL13/BLC receptor, CXCR5, is downregulated, probably allowing emigration – release of activated or memory B cells from follicular zones and lymphoid organs.

Polarization and tissue-specific imprinting of lymphocytes in secondary lymphoid organs

NAÏVE LYMPHOCYTES

Naïve lymphocytes enter the different secondary lymphoid organs such as spleen, lymph nodes, Peyer's patches, or tonsils more or less randomly via the chemokine CCL21/SLC and its receptor CCR7. Encounter of antigens leads to activated/memory lymphocytes and to reprogramming of homing properties corresponding to the lymphoid organ microenvironment (Campbell and Butcher 2002; Kunkel and Butcher 2002). It is therefore conceivable that leukocyte subset-specific expression of chemokine receptors may help selectively to recruit only certain subsets of cells to peripheral or lymphoid tissues, e.g. T-cell activation in mucosal lymph nodes induces loss of CCR7 and the expression of CCR9, a receptor for the chemokine CCL25/TECK. This chemokine is abundantly produced by the small intestine and partly by the thymus, and leads to homing of activated or memory T cells to the gut. Alternately, T-cell activation in skin-draining lymph nodes leads to expression of CLA (a skin-specific selectin-binding molecule – see above) and the chemokine receptors CCR4 and CCR10 (Campbell et al. 1999; Kunkel and Butcher 2002). These receptors bind the chemokines CCL17/TARC and CCL27/CTACK respectively. Both chemokines are constitutively produced by cutaneous epithelial cells and induce skin homing of lymphocytes expressing CCR4 and CCR10.

ANTIGEN-ACTIVATED LYMPHOCYTES

Activated/memory T cells were first thought to be mostly CCR7, i.e. unable to re-enter lymphoid organs. This was revised by the finding that $CCR7^+$ and $CCR7^-$ cells existed in these populations and led to the concept that central and effector memory T cells exist (Sallusto and Lanzavecchia 2000). In addition to the tissue-specific chemokine receptors, central memory cells retain their expression of CCR7 and L-selectin and can home back to lymphoid organs to participate in activation of naïve B and T cells. However, this concept has recently been challenged by the finding that cytokine-producing effector cells express CCR7 and migrate back to lymphoid organs (Kim et al. 2001; Debes et al. 2002; Unsoeld et al. 2002). Nevertheless, a large proportion of effector memory or long-term-activated cells lack CCR7 and L-selectin, and migrate to peripheral organs. Both populations may migrate to sites of inflammatory reactions. The $CD4^+$ T cells are of either central or effector subtype whereas $CD8^+$ T cells are mostly of effector type.

T-HELPER 1 VERSUS T-HELPER 2 LYMPHOCYTES

In addition to tissue-specific imprinting activated/memory, CD4 T cells in lymphoid organs polarize their function into T-helper 1 (Th1) and T-helper 2 (Th2) cells (Kim et al. 2001). The Th1 cells secrete cytokines such as lymphotoxin and IFN-γ to promote mainly antiviral cellular immune responses. Th2 cells release IL-4, IL-5, IL-6 and IL-13 to stimulate humoral immunity and allergic reactions, and to augment innate immune reactions. The expression pattern of chemokine receptors not only distinguishes the major lymphocyte subsets from one another, but might also be in fact the key for differential migration characteristics of Th1 versus Th2 cells (Sallusto et al. 1998). Analysis of chemokine receptors on in vitro cultured lymphocytes has attributed expression of CXCR3 and CCR5 to Th1 and of CCR3 and CCR4 to Th2 (Sallusto et al. 1999). However, analysis of primary human T-helper cells revealed a chemokine expression pattern that was slightly more complex (Kim et al. 2001). It showed that the only chemokine receptors that defined helper cell populations were CXCR3 on Th1 cells, and nonexclusive but prevalent expression of CCR4 on Th2 cells. Different subgroups of Th1 cells showed various expression levels of CCR2, CCR5, and CXCR6. With the exception of CCR4 none of the chemokine receptors was exclusive for Th2 cells, including CCR3 for which data are controversial (Imai et al. 1999; Romagnani et al. 1999). The receptors CXCR5, CCR7, and CCR6 were negatively regulated in respect to T-cell polarization, i.e. these receptors are expressed by T cells with reduced polarity such as Th0 cells. Recent data also showed that there are more $CCR7^+$ than $CCR7^-$ T-helper cells in the blood, and the authors concluded that CCR7 expression may be sufficient to enter lymphoid tissue but its presence did not prevent homing of polarized cells into peripheral, nonlymphoid tissue (Kim et al. 2001).

B LYMPHOCYTES

B lymphocytes show less subtle polarization than T cells. However, when B-cell precursors mature into antibody-secreting plasma cells they home to the splenic red pulp, lymph node medullary cords, and bone marrow, where they become resident. Upon differentiation plasma cells express the CXCL12/SDF receptor CXCR4 and they downregulate the CXCL13/BLC and CCL19/ELC receptors, CXCR5 and CCR7, respectively (Wehrli et al. 2001; Hauser et al. 2002; Kunkel and Butcher 2002). Thus, responsiveness to CXCL12/SDF-1 allows B plasma cells to home to secondary lymphoid organs and the bone marrow. Natural antibody-producing B1 cells, however, maintain CXCL13/BLC receptors and use them for migration to the peritoneal cavity and the omentum (Ansel et al. 2002).

Migration of antigen-primed lymphocytes to inflammatory tissue

Inflammatory reactions locally induce the production of inflammatory chemokines by endothelial cells, epithelial cells, dendritic cells, resident macrophages, or other cells. Thereby, the type of inflammatory response is important and selects for the type of chemokines to be produced, e.g. acute Th1 reactions start by bacterial or viral infections that induce the secretion of IFN-γ, TNF-α, IL-1, or IL-12. These inflammatory cytokines stimulate the production of the CXCR3-binding chemokines CXCL10/IP-10, CXCL9/MIG, and CXCL11/I-TAC, and they attract mainly CXCR3-expressing Th1 cells. In contrast, allergic Th2 inflammatory reactions are induced by the cytokine IL-4 which leads to the production of the CCR4-binding chemokines CCL22/MDC or CCL17/TARC, attracting CCR4-expressing Th2 cells. However, subgroups of Th1 and Th2 cells express additional chemokine receptors that are less exclusive (see above). This has the consequence that lymphocytes recruited by inflammatory reactions show mixed populations with prevalent tissue-specific Th1 or Th2, skin- or gut-seeking cells.

DIAPEDESIS

Following rolling, triggering and firm adhesion is a final irreversible step of transmigration, also called diapedesis. The pathway used by transmigrating cells to cross the vascular barrier is still a matter of debate because there is evidence for both transcellular and paracellular migration of leukocytes (Muller 2001; Indrasingh et al. 2002). Therefore, the molecular mechanisms involved in this final step are still poorly understood even if recent findings suggest that molecules concentrated at interendothelial junctions regulate leukocyte transmigration, thus favoring the hypothesis that lymphocyte transmigration occurs at interendothelial contacts (Dejana et al. 2001; Aurrand-Lions et al. 2002; Luscinskas et al. 2002; Vestweber 2002). So far, interendothelial adhesion molecules playing a role in the control of leukocyte transmigration can be classified as follows:

- Proteins concentrated in intercellular contacts and interacting with counterreceptors on transmigrating cells such as PECAM-1/CD31, CD99 and JAMs (Muller et al. 1993; Martin-Padura et al. 1998; Cunningham et al. 2002; Schenkel et al. 2002).
- Structural molecules specifically incorporated in endothelial adherens or tight junctions which are involved in endothelial barrier function, such as VE-cadherin, occludin, or claudins (Allport et al. 2000; Burns et al. 2000; Kucharzik et al. 2001).

In contrast to claudin and JAM family members, which are not equally expressed by all endothelial cells (Morita et al. 1999; Palmeri et al. 2000; Aurrand-Lions et al. 2001; Liang et al. 2002), CD99 and VE-cadherin may play a role in both constitutive and inflammatory lymphocyte recirculation because they are expressed by the entire vascular tree. Therefore, one current hypothesis is that there is heterogeneity in the molecular composition of interendothelial junctions which are more or less permissive to lymphocyte transendothelial migration. Furthermore, the combination of intercellular adhesion molecules found in interendothelial contacts varies with endothelial activation such as inflammation. Indeed, it has been described that inflammatory activation induces interendothelial junctional remodeling and

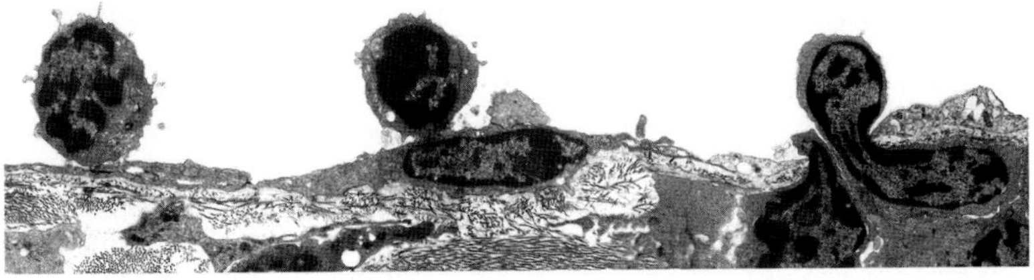

	Rolling	Triggering	Adhesion
LN	L-Selectin/PNAd	CCR7/CCL21	LFA-1/ICAM-2
GALT	L-Selectin/MAdCAM-1 Integrin $\alpha_4\beta_7$/MAdCAM-1	CCR7/CCL21 CCR9/CCL25	LFA-1/ICAM-2 Integrin $\alpha_4\beta_7$/MAdCAM-1
Skin	CLA/E-selectin	CCR4/CCL17 CCR10/CCL27	LFA-1/ICAM-2
Inflammation	PSGL-1/P-, E-selectin	CXCR3/CXCL9,10,11 CCR4/CCL17, 22	LFA-1/ICAM-1, -2 $\alpha_4\beta_1$/ VCAM-1

Figure 27.2 *The multistep paradigm. In the first step, cell adhesion molecules on leukocytes interact loosely with their ligands on the endothelial surface, leading to rolling and slowing down of the leukocyte in the bloodstream. This allows chemokines presented by the endothelial glycocalyx to bind to leukocyte chemokine receptors, thereby triggering the activation of leukocyte integrins. Such activated integrins bind to their respective ligands on the endothelial cells, arrest the leukocyte, and eventually mediate diapedesis. In this sequential process, each step depends on the preceding step, starting with the tethering that induces leukocyte rolling. Therefore, only the expression of a distinct combination of chemokine receptors and cell adhesion molecules allows a leukocyte to adhere to and transmigrate the endothelium at a given site. Inversely, the endothelium can selectively recruit a certain leukocyte subset by expressing the appropriate combination of cell adhesion molecules and chemokines. The boxes below the flow scheme indicate the cell adhesion molecules and chemokine receptors and their ligands (leukocyte/endothelium) implicated in each step of this adhesion cascade in different tissues. LN, lymph nodes; GALT, gut-associated lymphoid tissue; infl., skin and general inflammatory situations.*

redistribution of VE-cadherin, PECAM-1, and JAM away from interendothelial contacts (Romer et al. 1995; Rival et al. 1996; Ozaki et al. 1999; Wong et al. 1999; Shaw et al. 2001). This contributes to the specific regulation of lymphocyte emigration. Such a concept has been reinforced by the findings that JAM is a ligand for the lymphocyte integrin $\alpha_L\beta_2$ (LFA-1), and that its subcellular redistribution to the apical surface of endothelial cells influences its function in lymphocyte transendothelial migration (Ostermann et al. 2002). In contrast to the adhesive interaction of JAM with LFA-1, PECAM-1 homophilic interaction regulates integrin activation in endothelial cells or transmigrating leukocytes (Tanaka et al. 1992; Piali et al. 1993; Zhao and Newman 2001), suggesting that interactions between endothelial and transmigrating cells may have a dual role in adhesion and cellular signaling. Dissecting the specific and sequential contribution of adhesion molecules to this complex signaling network will certainly improve our understanding of the specificity of lymphocyte recirculation.

CONCLUSION

The scope of this chapter was to outline the concept and mechanisms of lymphocyte homing and recirculation and to discuss the underlying molecular functions of cell adhesion molecules, chemokines, and chemokine receptors. As suggested by the pioneering studies on lymphocyte recirculation, the integrated function of the immune system requires highly efficient and specific adhesive mechanisms. These properties are illustrated by the multistep paradigm where a lymphocyte can proceed to the next step only if the previous one occurred successfully. The repertoire of molecular specificity is given by the panel of adhesion molecules that support rolling and firm adhesion, but is also greatly enhanced by the complex network of chemokines/chemokine receptors (Figure 27.2), which constitute the fine-tuning of the specific migration. Finally, the last transmigration step starts to be analyzed with molecular tools, but its contribution to specificity, irreversibility, and control of lymphocyte recirculation is still poorly understood.

REFERENCES

Aigner, S., Ruppert, M., et al. 1995. Heat stable antigen (mouse CD24) supports myeloid cell binding to endothelial and platelet P-selectin. *Int Immunol*, **7**, 1557–65.

Allport, J.R., Muller, W.A. and Luscinskas, F.W. 2000. Monocytes induce reversible focal changes in vascular endothelial cadherin complex during transendothelial migration under flow. *J Cell Biol*, **148**, 203–16.

Alon, R. and Feigelson, S. 2002. From rolling to arrest on blood vessels: leukocyte tap dancing on endothelial integrin ligands and chemokines at sub-second contacts. *Semin Immunol*, **14**, 93–104.

Alon, R., Kassner, P.D., et al. 1995. The integrin VLA-4 supports tethering and rolling in flow on VCAM-1. *J Cell Biol*, **128**, 1243–53.

Anderson, A.O. and Anderson, N.D. 1976. Lymphocyte emigration from high endothelial venules in rat lymph nodes. *Immunology*, **31**, 731–48.

Anderson, N.D., Anderson, A.O. and Wyllie, R.G. 1976. Specialized structure and metabolic activities of high endothelial venules in rat lymphatic tissues. *Immunology*, **31**, 455–73.

Ansel, K.M., Ngo, V.N., et al. 2000. A chemokine-driven positive feedback loop organizes lymphoid follicles. *Nature*, **406**, 309–14.

Ansel, K.M., Harris, R.B. and Cyster, J.G. 2002. CXCL13 is required for B1 cell homing, natural antibody production, and body cavity immunity. *Immunity*, **16**, 67–76.

Arbones, M.L., Ord, D.C., et al. 1994. Lymphocyte homing and leukocyte rolling and migration are impaired in L- selectin-deficient mice. *Immunity*, **1**, 247–60.

Arroyo, A.G., Yang, J.T., et al. 1996. Differential requirements for alpha4 integrins during fetal and adult hematopoiesis. *Cell*, **85**, 997–1008.

Arroyo, A.G., Yang, J.T., et al. 1999. Alpha4 integrins regulate the proliferation/differentiation balance of multilineage hematopoietic progenitors in vivo. *Immunity*, **11**, 555–66.

Aurrand-Lions, M., Johnson-Leger, C., et al. 2001. Heterogeneity of endothelial junctions is reflected by differential expression and specific subcellular localization of the three JAM family members. *Blood*, **98**, 3699–707.

Aurrand-Lions, M., Johnson-Leger, C. and Imhof, B.A. 2002. The last molecular fortress in leukocyte trans-endothelial migration. *Nat Immunol*, **3**, 116–18.

Baekkevold, E.S., Yamanaka, T., et al. 2001. The CCR7 ligand elc (CCL19) is transcytosed in high endothelial venules and mediates T cell recruitment. *J Exp Med*, **193**, 1105–12.

Bargatze, R.F., Jutila, M.A. and Butcher, E.C. 1995. Distinct roles of L-selectin and integrins alpha 4 beta 7 and LFA-1 in lymphocyte homing to Peyer's patch-HEV in situ: the multistep model confirmed and refined. *Immunity*, **3**, 99–108.

Berg, E.L., Goldstein, L.A., et al. 1989. Homing receptors and vascular addressins: cell adhesion molecules that direct lymphocyte traffic. *Immunol Rev*, **108**, 5–18.

Berg, E.L., Yoshino, T., et al. 1991. The cutaneous lymphocyte antigen is a skin lymphocyte homing receptor for the vascular lectin endothelial cell-leukocyte adhesion molecule 1. *J Exp Med*, **174**, 1461–6.

Berg, E.L., McEvoy, L.M., et al. 1993. L-selectin-mediated lymphocyte rolling on MAdCAM-1. *Nature*, **366**, 695–8.

Berlin, C., Berg, E.L., et al. 1993. Alpha 4 beta 7 integrin mediates lymphocyte binding to the mucosal vascular addressin MAdCAM-1. *Cell*, **74**, 185.

Berlin, C., Bargatze, R.F., et al. 1995. Alpha 4 integrins mediate lymphocyte attachment and rolling under physiologic flow. *Cell*, **80**, 413–22.

Berlin-Rufenach, C., Otto, F., et al. 1999. Lymphocyte migration in lymphocyte function-associated antigen (LFA)-1-deficient mice. *J Exp Med*, **189**, 1467–78.

Bevilacqua, M.P., Pober, J.S., et al. 1987. Identification of an inducible endothelial-leukocyte adhesion molecule. *Proc Natl Acad Sci USA*, **84**, 9238–42.

Bjerknes, M., Cheng, H. and Ottaway, C.A. 1986. Dynamics of lymphocyte-endothelial interactions in vivo. *Science*, **231**, 402–5.

Borges, E., Tietz, W., et al. 1997. P-selectin glycoprotein ligand-1 (PSGL-1) on T helper 1 but not on T helper 2 cells binds to P-selectin and supports migration into inflamed skin. *J Exp Med*, **185**, 573–8.

Borowitz, M.J., Weidner, A., et al. 1993. Abnormalities of circulating T-cell subpopulations in patients with cutaneous T-cell lymphoma: cutaneous lymphocyte-associated antigen expression on T cells correlates with extent of disease. *Leukemia*, **7**, 859–63.

Briskin, M.J., McEvoy, L.M. and Butcher, E.C. 1993. MAdCAM-1 has homology to immunoglobulin and mucin-like adhesion receptors and to IgA1. *Nature*, **363**, 461–4.

Burns, A.R., Bowden, R.A., et al. 2000. Analysis of tight junctions during neutrophil transendothelial migration. *J Cell Sci*, **113**, 45–57.

Butcher, E.C. 1991. Leukocyte-endothelial cell recognition: three (or more) steps to specificity and diversity. *Cell*, **67**, 1033–6.

Butcher, E.C. 1992. Leukocyte-endothelial cell adhesion as an active, multi-step process: a combinatorial mechanism for specificity and diversity in leukocyte targeting. *Adv Exp Med Biol*, **323**, 181–94.

Campbell, D.J. and Butcher, E.C. 2002. Rapid acquisition of tissue-specific homing phenotypes by CD4(+) T cells activated in cutaneous or mucosal lymphoid tissues. *J Exp Med*, **195**, 135–41.

Campbell, D.J., Kim, C.H. and Butcher, E.C. 2001. Separable effector T cell populations specialized for B cell help or tissue inflammation. *Nat Immunol*, **2**, 876–81.

Campbell, J.J., Hedrick, J., et al. 1998. Chemokines and the arrest of lymphocytes rolling under flow conditions. *Science*, **279**, 381–4.

Campbell, J.J., Haraldsen, G., et al. 1999. The chemokine receptor CCR4 in vascular recognition by cutaneous but not intestinal memory T cells. *Nature*, **400**, 776–80.

Constantin, G., Majeed, M., et al. 2000. Chemokines trigger immediate beta2 integrin affinity and mobility changes: differential regulation and roles in lymphocyte arrest under flow. *Immunity*, **13**, 759–69.

Coxon, A., Rieu, P., et al. 1996. A novel role for the beta 2 integrin CD11b/CD18 in neutrophil apoptosis: a homeostatic mechanism in inflammation. *Immunity*, **5**, 653–66.

Cunningham, S.A., Rodriguez, J.M., et al. 2002. JAM2 Interacts with alpha 4beta 1. Facilitation by JAM3. *J Biol Chem*, **277**, 27589–92.

Cyster, J.G. 1999. Chemokines and cell migration in secondary lymphoid organs. *Science*, **286**, 2098–102.

Dailey, M.O. 1998. Expression of T lymphocyte adhesion molecules: regulation during antigen-induced T cell activation and differentiation. *Crit Rev Immunol*, **18**, 153–84.

Debes, G.F., Hopken, U.E. and Hamann, A. 2002. In vivo differentiated cytokine-producing CD4(+) T cells express functional CCR7. *J Immunol*, **168**, 5441–7.

Dejana, E., Spagnuolo, R. and Bazzoni, G. 2001. Interendothelial junctions and their role in the control of angiogenesis, vascular permeability and leukocyte transmigration. *Thromb Haemost*, **86**, 308–15.

Ding, Z., Xiong, K. and Issekutz, T.B. 2001. Chemokines stimulate human T lymphocyte transendothelial migration to utilize VLA-4 in addition to LFA-1. *J Leukoc Biol*, **69**, 458–66.

Dustin, M.L. and Springer, T.A. 1988. Lymphocyte function-associated antigen-1 (LFA-1) interaction with intercellular adhesion molecule-1 (ICAM-1) is one of at least three mechanisms for lymphocyte adhesion to cultured endothelial cells. *J Cell Biol*, **107**, 321–31.

Dwir, O., Kansas, G.S. and Alon, R. 2001. Cytoplasmic anchorage of L-selectin controls leukocyte capture and rolling by increasing the mechanical stability of the selectin tether. *J Cell Biol*, **155**, 145–56.

Elices, M.J., Osborn, L., et al. 1990. VCAM-1 on activated endothelium interacts with the leukocyte integrin VLA-4 at a site distinct from the VLA-4/fibronectin binding site. *Cell*, **60**, 577–84.

Faveeuw, C., Di Mauro, M.E., et al. 2000. Roles of alpha(4) integrins/VCAM-1 and LFA-1/ICAM-1 in the binding and transendothelial migration of T lymphocytes and T lymphoblasts across high endothelial venules. *Int Immunol*, **12**, 241–51.

Forster, R., Emrich, T., et al. 1994. Expression of the G-protein-coupled receptor BLR1 defines mature, recirculating B cells and a subset of T-helper memory cells. *Blood*, **84**, 830–40.

Forster, R., Mattis, A.E., et al. 1996. A putative chemokine receptor, BLR1, directs B cell migration to defined lymphoid organs and specific anatomic compartments of the spleen. *Cell*, **87**, 1037–47.

Fuhlbrigge, R.C., Kieffer, J.D., et al. 1997. Cutaneous lymphocyte antigen is a specialized form of PSGL-1 expressed on skin-homing T cells. *Nature*, **389**, 978–81.

Girard, J.P. and Springer, T.A. 1995. High endothelial venules (HEVs): specialized endothelium for lymphocyte migration. *Immunol Today*, **16**, 449–57.

Girard, J.P., Baekkevold, E.S., et al. 1999. Heterogeneity of endothelial cells: the specialized phenotype of human high endothelial venules characterized by suppression subtractive hybridization. *Am J Pathol*, **155**, 2043–55.

Gowans, J.L. 1957. The effect of the continuous re-infusion of lymph and lymphocytes on the output of lymphocytes from the thoracic duct of unanesthetized rats. *Br J Exp Pathol*, **38**, 67–78.

Gowans, J.L. and Knight, E.J. 1964. The route of recirculation of lymphocytes in the rat. *Proc R Soc London Biol*, **159**, 257–82.

Gunn, M.D., Ngo, V.N., et al. 1998a. A B-cell-homing chemokine made in lymphoid follicles activates Burkitt's lymphoma receptor-1. *Nature*, **391**, 799–803.

Gunn, M.D., Tangemann, K., et al. 1998b. A chemokine expressed in lymphoid high endothelial venules promotes the adhesion and chemotaxis of naive T lymphocytes. *Proc Natl Acad Sci USA*, **95**, 258–63.

Gunn, M.D., Kyuwa, S., et al. 1999. Mice lacking expression of secondary lymphoid organ chemokine have defects in lymphocyte homing and dendritic cell localization [see comments]. *J Exp Med*, **189**, 451–60.

Hafezi-Moghadam, A., Thomas, K.L., et al. 2001. L-selectin shedding regulates leukocyte recruitment. *J Exp Med*, **193**, 863–72.

Hahne, M., Lenter, M., et al. 1993. VCAM-1 is not involved in LPAM-1 (alpha 4 beta p/alpha 4 beta 7) mediated binding of lymphoma cells to high endothelial venules of mucosa-associated lymph nodes. *Eur J Cell Biol*, **61**, 290–8.

Haraldsen, G., Kvale, D., et al. 1996. Cytokine-regulated expression of E-selectin, intercellular adhesion molecule-1 (ICAM-1), and vascular cell adhesion molecule-1 (VCAM-1) in human microvascular endothelial cells. *J Immunol*, **156**, 2558–65.

Hattori, R., Hamilton, K.K., et al. 1989. Stimulated secretion of endothelial von Willebrand factor is accompanied by rapid redistribution to the cell surface of the intracellular granule membrane protein GMP-140. *J Biol Chem*, **264**, 7768–71.

Hauser, A.E., Debes, G.F., et al. 2002. Chemotactic responsiveness toward ligands for CXCR3 and CXCR4 is regulated on plasma blasts during the time course of a memory immune response. *J Immunol*, **169**, 1277–82.

Hemler, M.E. 1990. VLA proteins in the integrin family: structures, functions, and their role on leukocytes. *Annu Rev Immunol*, **8**, 365–400.

Hemmerich, S., Bistrup, A., et al. 2001. Sulfation of L-selectin ligands by an HEV-restricted sulfotransferase regulates lymphocyte homing to lymph nodes. *Immunity*, **15**, 237–47.

Henninger, D.D., Panes, J., et al. 1997. Cytokine-induced VCAM-1 and ICAM-1 expression in different organs of the mouse. *J Immunol*, **158**, 1825–32.

Holzmann, B., McIntyre, B.W. and Weissman, I.L. 1989. Identification of a murine Peyer's patch-specific lymphocyte homing receptor as an integrin molecule with an alpha chain homologous to human VLA-4 alpha. *Cell*, **56**, 37–46.

Hsu-Lin, S., Berman, C.L., et al. 1984. A platelet membrane protein expressed during platelet activation and secretion. Studies using a monoclonal antibody specific for thrombin-activated platelets. *J Biol Chem*, **259**, 9121–6.

Huleatt, J.W. and Lefrancois, L. 1996. Beta2 integrins and ICAM-1 are involved in establishment of the intestinal mucosal T cell compartment. *Immunity*, **5**, 263–73.

Imai, T., Nagira, M., et al. 1999. Selective recruitment of CCR4-bearing Th2 cells toward antigen-presenting cells by the CC chemokines thymus and activation-regulated chemokine and macrophage-derived chemokine. *Int Immunol*, **11**, 81–8.

Indrasingh, I., Chandi, G. and Vettivel, S. 2002. Route of lymphocyte migration through the high endothelial venule (HEV) in human palatine tonsil. *Ann Anat*, **184**, 77–84.

Isobe, M., Yagita, H., et al. 1992. Specific acceptance of cardiac allograft after treatment with antibodies to ICAM-1 and LFA-1. *Science*, **255**, 1125–7.

Issekutz, T.B. 1993. Dual inhibition of VLA-4 and LFA-1 maximally inhibits cutaneous delayed- type hypersensitivity-induced inflammation. *Am J Pathol*, **143**, 1286–93.

Johnson-Leger, C., Aurrand-Lions, M. and Imhof, B.A. 2000. The parting of the endothelium: miracle, or simply a junctional affair? *J Cell Sci*, **113**, Pt6, 921–33.

Jung, T.M., Gallatin, W.M., et al. 1988. Down-regulation of homing receptors after T cell activation. *J Immunol*, **141**, 4110–17.

Kakimoto, K., Nakamura, T., et al. 1992. The effect of anti-adhesion molecule antibody on the development of collagen-induced arthritis. *Cell Immunol*, **142**, 326–37.

Kantele, A., Kantele, J.M., et al. 1997. Homing potentials of circulating lymphocytes in humans depend on the site of activation: oral, but not parenteral, typhoid vaccination induces circulating antibody-secreting cells that all bear homing receptors directing them to the gut. *J Immunol*, **158**, 574–9.

Kaufmann, Y., Golstein, P., et al. 1982. LFA-1 but not Lyt-2 is associated with killing activity of cytotoxic T lymphocyte hybridomas. *Nature*, **300**, 357–60.

Kim, C.H., Rott, L., et al. 2001. Rules of chemokine receptor association with T cell polarization in vivo. *J Clin Invest*, **108**, 1331–9.

Kishimoto, T.K., Jutila, M.A., et al. 1989. Neutrophil Mac-1 and MEL-14 adhesion proteins inversely regulated by chemotactic factors. *Science*, **245**, 1238–41.

Kucharzik, T., Walsh, S.V., et al. 2001. Neutrophil transmigration in inflammatory bowel disease is associated with differential expression of epithelial intercellular junction proteins. *Am J Pathol*, **159**, 2001–9.

Kunkel, E.J. and Butcher, E.C. 2002. Chemokines and the tissue-specific migration of lymphocytes. *Immunity*, **16**, 1–4.

Kwee, L., Baldwin, H.S., et al. 1995. Defective development of the embryonic and extraembryonic circulatory systems in vascular cell adhesion molecule (VCAM-1) deficient mice. *Development*, **121**, 489–503.

Lakew, M., Nordstrom, I., et al. 1995. Phenotypic characterization of circulating antibody-secreting cells after mucosal and systemic immunizations in humans. *Adv Exp Med Biol*, **3**, 1451–3.

Lasky, L.A. 1992. Selectins: interpreters of cell-specific carbohydrate information during inflammation. *Science*, **258**, 964–9.

Lefrancois, L., Parker, C.M., et al. 1999. The role of beta7 integrins in CD8 T cell trafficking during an antiviral immune response. *J Exp Med*, **189**, 1631–8.

Lewinsohn, D.M., Bargatze, R.F. and Butcher, E.C. 1987. Leukocyte-endothelial cell recognition: evidence of a common molecular mechanism shared by neutrophils, lymphocytes, and other leukocytes. *J Immunol*, **138**, 4313–21.

Liang, T.W., Chiu, H.H., et al. 2002. Vascular endothelial-junctional adhesion molecule (VE-JAM)/JAM 2 interacts with T, NK, and dendritic cells through JAM 3. *J Immunol*, **168**, 1618–26.

Luscinskas, F.W., Ma, S., et al. 2002. Leukocyte transendothelial migration: A junctional affair. *Semin Immunol*, **14**, 105–13.

McEver, R.P., Beckstead, J.H., et al. 1989. GMP-140, a platelet alpha-granule membrane protein, is also synthesized by vascular endothelial cells and is localized in Weibel-Palade bodies. *J Clin Invest*, **84**, 92–9.

Mackay, C.R., Marston, W.L. and Dudler, L. 1990. Naive and memory T cells show distinct pathways of lymphocyte recirculation. *J Exp Med*, **171**, 801–17.

Maiti, A., Maki, G. and Johnson, P. 1998. TNF-alpha induction of CD44-mediated leukocyte adhesion by sulfation. *Science*, **282**, 941–3.

Maly, P., Thall, A., et al. 1996. The alpha(1,3)fucosyltransferase Fuc-TVII controls leukocyte trafficking through an essential role in L-, E- and P-selectin ligand biosynthesis. *Cell*, **86**, 643–53.

Marlin, S.D. and Springer, T.A. 1987. Purified intercellular adhesion molecule-1 (ICAM-1) is a ligand for lymphocyte function-associated antigen 1 (LFA-1). *Cell*, **51**, 813–19.

Martin-Padura, I., Lostaglio, S., et al. 1998. Junctional adhesion molecule, a novel member of the immunoglobulin superfamily that distributes at intercellular junctions and modulates monocyte transmigration. *J Cell Biol*, **142**, 117–27.

May, M.J., Entwistle, G., et al. 1993. VCAM-1 is a CS1 peptide-inhibitable adhesion molecule expressed by lymph node high endothelium. *J Cell Sci*, **106**, 109–19.

Morita, K., Sasaki, H., et al. 1999. Endothelial claudin: claudin-5/TMVCF constitutes tight junction strands in endothelial cells. *J Cell Biol*, **147**, 185–94.

Muller, W.A. 2001. Migration of leukocytes across endothelial junctions: some concepts and controversies. *Microcirculation*, **8**, 181–93.

Muller, W.A. 2002. Leukocyte-endothelial cell interactions in the inflammatory response. *Lab Invest*, **82**, 521–33.

Muller, W.A., Weigl, S.A., et al. 1993. PECAM-1 is required for transendothelial migration of leukocytes. *J Exp Med*, **178**, 449–60.

Nakano, H., Tamura, T., et al. 1997. Genetic defect in T lymphocyte-specific homing into peripheral lymph nodes. *Eur J Immunol*, **27**, 215–21.

Ostermann, G., Weber, K.S., et al. 2002. JAM-1 is a ligand of the beta2 integrin LFA-1 involved in transendothelial migration of leukocytes. *Nat Immunol*, **14**, 14.

Ozaki, H., Ishii, K., et al. 1999. Cutting edge: combined treatment of TNF-alpha and IFN-gamma causes redistribution of junctional adhesion molecule in human endothelial cells. *J Immunol*, **163**, 553–7.

Pabst, R. and Binns, R.M. 1989. Heterogeneity of lymphocyte homing physiology: several mechanisms operate in the control of migration to lymphoid and non-lymphoid organs in vivo. *Immunol Rev*, **108**, 83–109.

Pachynski, R.K., Wu, S.W., et al. 1998. Secondary lymphoid-tissue chemokine (SLC) stimulates integrin alpha 4 beta 7-mediated adhesion of lymphocytes to mucosal addressin cell adhesion molecule-1 (MAdCAM-1) under flow. *J Immunol*, **161**, 952–6.

Palmeri, D., van Zante, A., et al. 2000. Vascular endothelial junction-associated molecule, a novel member of the immunoglobulin superfamily, is localized to intercellular boundaries of endothelial cells. *J Biol Chem*, **275**, 19139–45.

Piali, L., Albelda, S.M., et al. 1993. Murine platelet endothelial cell adhesion molecule (PECAM-1)/CD31 modulates beta 2 integrins on lymphokine-activated killer cells. *Eur J Immunol*, **23**, 2464–71.

Picker, L.J., Nakache, M. and Butcher, E.C. 1989. Monoclonal antibodies to human lymphocyte homing receptors define a novel class of adhesion molecules on diverse cell types. *J Cell Biol*, **109**, 927–37.

Picker, L.J., Michie, S.A., et al. 1990a. A unique phenotype of skin-associated lymphocytes in humans. Preferential expression of the HECA-452 epitope by benign and malignant T cells at cutaneous sites. *Am J Pathol*, **136**, 1053–68.

Picker, L.J., Terstappen, L.W., et al. 1990b. Differential expression of homing-associated adhesion molecules by T cell subsets in man. *J Immunol*, **145**, 3247–55.

Picker, L.J., Kishimoto, T.K., et al. 1991. ELAM-1 is an adhesion molecule for skin-homing T cells. *Nature*, **349**, 796–9.

Picker, L.J., Treer, J.R., et al. 1993. Control of lymphocyte recirculation in man. II. Differential regulation of the cutaneous lymphocyte-associated antigen, a tissue-selective homing receptor for skin-homing T cells. *J Immunol*, **150**, 1122–36.

Potocnik, A.J., Brakebusch, C. and Fassler, R. 2000. Fetal and adult hematopoietic stem cells require beta1 integrin function for colonizing fetal liver, spleen, and bone marrow. *Immunity*, **12**, 653–63.

Pouyani, T. and Seed, B. 1995. PSGL-1 recognition of P-selectin is controlled by a tyrosine sulfation consensus at the PSGL-1 amino terminus. *Cell*, **83**, 333–43.

Preece, G., Murphy, G. and Ager, A. 1996. Metalloproteinase-mediated regulation of L-selectin levels on leucocytes. *J Biol Chem*, **271**, 11634–40.

Rigby, S. and Dailey, M.O. 2000. Traffic of L-selectin-negative T cells to sites of inflammation. *Eur J Immunol*, **30**, 98–107.

Rival, Y., Del Maschio, A., et al. 1996. Inhibition of platelet endothelial cell adhesion molecule-1 synthesis and leukocyte transmigration in endothelial cells by the combined action of TNF-alpha and IFN-gamma. *J Immunol*, **157**, 1233–41.

Romagnani, P., De Paulis, A., et al. 1999. Tryptase-chymase double-positive human mast cells express the eotaxin receptor CCR3 and are attracted by CCR3-binding chemokines. *Am J Pathol*, **155**, 1195–204.

Romer, L.H., McLean, N.V., et al. 1995. IFN-gamma and TNF-alpha induce redistribution of PECAM-1 (CD31) on human endothelial cells. *J Immunol*, **154**, 6582–92.

Rose, J.R., Williams, M.B., et al. 1998. Expression of the mucosal homing receptor alpha4beta7 correlates with the ability of CD8+ memory T cells to clear rotavirus infection. *J Virol*, **72**, 726–30.

Rott, L.S., Rose, J.R., et al. 1997. Expression of mucosal homing receptor alpha4beta7 by circulating CD4+ cells with memory for intestinal rotavirus. *J Clin Invest*, **100**, 1204–8.

Rott, L.S., Briskin, M.J. and Butcher, E.C. 2000. Expression of alpha4beta7 and E-selectin ligand by circulating memory B cells: implications for targeted trafficking to mucosal and systemic sites. *J Leukoc Biol*, **68**, 807–14.

Sallusto, F. and Lanzavecchia, A. 2000. Understanding dendritic cell and T-lymphocyte traffic through the analysis of chemokine receptor expression. *Immunol Rev*, **177**, 134–40.

Sallusto, F., Lanzavecchia, A. and Mackay, C.R. 1998. Chemokines and chemokine receptors in T-cell priming and Th1/Th2- mediated responses. *Immunol Today*, **19**, 568–74.

Sallusto, F., Lenig, D., et al. 1999. Two subsets of memory T lymphocytes with distinct homing potentials and effector functions [In Process Citation]. *Nature*, **401**, 708–12.

Salmi, M. and Jalkanen, S. 1997. How do lymphocytes know where to go: current concepts and enigmas of lymphocyte homing. *Adv Immunol*, **64**, 139–218.

Salmi, M., Kalimo, K. and Jalkanen, S. 1993. Induction and function of vascular adhesion protein-1 at sites of inflammation. *J Exp Med*, **178**, 2255–60.

Salmi, M., Tohka, S., et al. 1997. Vascular adhesion protein 1 (VAP-1) mediates lymphocyte subtype- specific, selectin-independent recognition of vascular endothelium in human lymph nodes. *J Exp Med*, **186**, 589–600.

Sasaki, K., Okouchi, Y., et al. 1996. Ultrastructural localization of the intercellular adhesion molecule (ICAM-1) on the cell surface of high endothelial venules in lymph nodes. *Anat Rec*, **244**, 105–11.

Schenkel, A.R., Mamdouh, Z., et al. 2002. CD99 plays a major role in the migration of monocytes through endothelial junctions. *Nat Immunol*, **3**, 143–50.

Shamri, R., Grabovsky, V., et al. 2002. Chemokine-stimulation of lymphocyte a4 integrin avidity but not of LFA- 1 avidity to endothelial ligands under shear flow requires cholesterol membrane rafts. *J Biol Chem*, **5**, 5.

Shaw, S.K., Perkins, B.N., et al. 2001. Reduced expression of junctional adhesion molecule and platelet/endothelial cell adhesion molecule-1 (CD31) at human vascular endothelial junctions by cytokines tumor necrosis factor-alpha plus interferon-gamma does not reduce leukocyte transmigration under flow. *Am J Pathol*, **159**, 2281–91.

Shimaoka, M., Takagi, J. and Springer, T.A. 2002. Conformational regulation of integrin structure and function. *Annu Rev Biophys Biomol Struct*, **31**, 485–516.

Sikorski, M.A., Staunton, D.E. and Mier, J.W. 1996. L-selectin crosslinking induces integrin-dependent adhesion: evidence for a signaling pathway involving PTK but not PKC. *Cell Adhes Commun*, **4**, 355–67.

Simon, S.I., Hu, Y., et al. 2000. Neutrophil tethering on E-selectin activates beta 2 integrin binding to ICAM-1 through a mitogen-activated protein kinase signal transduction pathway. *J Immunol*, **164**, 4348–58.

Sligh, J.E. Jr., Ballantyne, C.M., et al. 1993. Inflammatory and immune responses are impaired in mice deficient in intercellular adhesion molecule 1. *Proc Natl Acad Sci USA*, **90**, 8529–33.

Springer, T.A. 1994. Traffic signals for lymphocyte recirculation and leukocyte emigration: the multistep paradigm. *Cell*, **76**, 301–14.

Staunton, D.E., Marlin, S.D., et al. 1988. Primary structure of ICAM-1 demonstrates interaction between members of the immunoglobulin and integrin supergene families. *Cell*, **52**, 925–33.

Staunton, D.E., Dustin, M.L. and Springer, T.A. 1989. Functional cloning of ICAM-2, a cell adhesion ligand for LFA-1 homologous to ICAM-1. *Nature*, **339**, 61–4.

Stoolman, L.M. 1989. Adhesion molecules controlling lymphocyte migration. *Cell*, **56**, 907–10.

Streeter, P.R., Berg, E.L., et al. 1988a. A tissue-specific endothelial cell molecule involved in lymphocyte homing. *Nature*, **331**, 41–6.

Streeter, P.R., Rouse, B.T. and Butcher, E.C. 1988b. Immunohistologic and functional characterization of a vascular addressin involved in lymphocyte homing into peripheral lymph nodes. *J Cell Biol*, **107**, 1853–62.

Tamatani, T., Kotani, M., et al. 1991. Molecular mechanisms underlying lymphocyte recirculation. II. Differential regulation of LFA-1 in the interaction between lymphocytes and high endothelial cells. *Eur J Immunol*, **21**, 855–8.

Tanaka, Y., Albelda, S.M., et al. 1992. CD31 expressed on distinctive T cell subsets is a preferential amplifier of beta 1 integrin-mediated adhesion. *J Exp Med*, **176**, 245–53.

Tietz, W., Allemand, Y., et al. 1998. CD4+ T cells migrate into inflamed skin only if they express ligands for E- and P-selectin. *J Immunol*, **161**, 963–70.

Unsoeld, H., Krautwald, S., et al. 2002. Cutting edge: CCR7+ and CCR7- memory T cells do not differ in immediate effector cell function. *J Immunol*, **169**, 638–41.

van Kooyk, Y. and Figdor, C.G. 2000. Avidity regulation of integrins: the driving force in leukocyte adhesion. *Curr Opin Cell Biol*, **12**, 542–7.

Vestweber, D. 2002. Regulation of endothelial cell contacts during leukocyte extravasation. *Curr Op Cell Biol*, **14**, 587–93.

Vestweber, D. and Blanks, J.E. 1999. Mechanisms that regulate the function of the selectins and their ligands. *Physiol Rev*, **79**, 181–213.

von Andrian, U.H. 1996. Intravital microscopy of the peripheral lymph node microcirculation in mice. *Microcirculation*, **3**, 287–300.

von Andrian, U.H. and Mackay, C.R. 2000. T-cell function and migration. Two sides of the same coin. *N Engl J Med*, **343**, 1020–34.

Wagner, N., Lohler, J., et al. 1996. Critical role for beta7 integrins in formation of the gut-associated lymphoid tissue. *Nature*, **382**, 366–70.

Warnock, R.A., Askari, S., et al. 1998. Molecular mechanisms of lymphocyte homing to peripheral lymph nodes. *J Exp Med*, **187**, 205–16.

Wehrli, N., Legler, D.F., et al. 2001. Changing responsiveness to chemokines allows medullary plasmablasts to leave lymph nodes. *Eur J Immunol*, **31**, 609–16.

Westermann, J. and Pabst, R. 1990. Lymphocyte subsets in the blood: a diagnostic window on the lymphoid system? [see comments]. *Immunol Today*, **11**, 406–10.

Westermann, J. and Pabst, R. 1996. How organ-specific is the migration of 'naive' and 'memory' T cells? [see comments]. *Immunol Today*, **17**, 278–82.

Williams, M.B. and Butcher, E.C. 1997. Homing of naive and memory T lymphocyte subsets to Peyer's patches, lymph nodes, and spleen. *J Immunol*, **159**, 1746–52.

Wong, R.K., Baldwin, A.L. and Heimark, R.L. 1999. Cadherin-5 redistribution at sites of TNF-alpha and IFN-gamma-induced permeability in mesenteric venules. *Am J Physiol*, **276**, H736–48.

Xu, H., Gonzalo, J.A., et al. 1994. Leukocytosis and resistance to septic shock in intercellular adhesion molecule 1-deficient mice. *J Exp Med*, **180**, 95–109.

Yang, J.T., Rayburn, H. and Hynes, R.O. 1995. Cell adhesion events mediated by alpha 4 integrins are essential in placental and cardiac development. *Development*, **121**, 549–60.

Yednock, T.A., Cannon, C., et al. 1992. Prevention of experimental autoimmune encephalomyelitis by antibodies against alpha 4 beta 1 integrin. *Nature*, **356**, 63–6.

Zhao, T. and Newman, P.J. 2001. Integrin activation by regulated dimerization and oligomerization of platelet endothelial cell adhesion molecule (PECAM)-1 from within the cell. *J Cell Biol*, **152**, 65–73.

Zlotnik, A. and Yoshie, O. 2000. Chemokines: a new classification system and their role in immunity. *Immunity*, **12**, 121–7.

28

The mucosal immune response

KOHTARO FUJIHASHI, PROSPER N. BOYAKA AND JERRY R. MCGHEE

INTRODUCTION

That a highly integrated and finely regulated mucosal immune system exists alongside and separate from the peripheral immune system might at first seem redundant and puzzling. Why should such a separate and sophisticated system be necessary when the peripheral immune system already seems to ensure immunity for the host? The mucosal areas exceed over 400 m^2, which is 200 times larger than the skin surface, and this large area is consistently exposed to environmental antigens, allergens, and pathogenic microorganisms (McGhee et al. 1999). Thus, the mucosal immune system provides the first line of defense for the host. It is not, therefore, difficult to imagine that effective mucosal immune responses represents a central pathway to combat infectious diseases, including bioagents of mass destruction, e.g. category A microorganisms/exotoxins. There can be no doubt about the sophistication and elegance of the mucosal immune system. It presents a well-tuned, two-part defense, one more structured and localized and another more diffuse. In the first, foreign antigens are encountered and selectively taken up into highly structured sites for the initiation of both mucosal and systemic immune responses. In the second, diffuse collections of effector cells such as B and T lymphocytes, differentiated plasma cells, macrophages (MΦ), and dendritic cells (DC), as well as eosinophils, basophils, and especially mast cells, come into play. Together, the two produce either mucosal and serum antibody responses and T-cell-mediated immunity (CMI), on one hand, or systemic anergy, commonly termed 'oral' or 'nasal tolerance', on the other. Such a separate and sophisticated immune system may well have evolved as a major defense mechanism against mucosally encountered infectious agents as well as to attenuate mucosal inflammation through tolerance induction. This chapter focuses on the cellular and molecular aspects of the mucosal immune response, including the innate and acquired responses as well as cross-talk between them.

THE INNATE MUCOSAL DEFENSE SYSTEM

Innate defenses comprise a network of cells and molecules that encounter foreign antigens before the acquired immune response. Innate mucosal immunity includes the physical barrier provided by epithelial cells and cilia movement, mucus production, secreted molecules with antibacterial activity, and the cytolytic activity of natural killer (NK) cells. In concert, these innate mechanisms provide a first line of defense against exogenous antigens, allergens, and invading pathogens. These mechanisms also set the stage for the development of antigen-specific immune responses to antigens/pathogens that can be eliminated at the level of the epithelium itself.

Antimicrobial peptide defensins

A growing number of antimicrobial molecules, generally termed 'defensins', are produced by cells of the mucosal epithelium which contribute to the natural protection of mucosal surfaces. Defensins exhibit antimicrobial effects similar to antibiotics. These molecules are β-sheet peptides that generally contain between 30 and 40 amino acid residues and can be divided into α- and β-defensins (Figure 28.1). The α-defensins are smaller, because of two contiguous cysteine residues, whereas β-defensins have cysteines separated by six amino acids; as a result of disulfide bonding the defensins are complexly folded microcyclic molecules. Paneth cells in the crypt regions of the small intestine possess secretory granules that are rich in α-defensins, often termed 'cryptidins', and additional antimicrobial peptides are secreted into the lumen of the crypts. It should be noted that the crypt regions are normally sterile; however, infection, e.g. by gram-negative pathogens, may result in cryptidin production to combat the pathogen. Two α-defensins, the human intestinal defensins (HD) HD-5 and HD-6, were identified in Paneth cells and the human reproductive tract (Ouellette 1997; Porter et al. 1997) (Figure 28.1). α-defensins are also secreted by tracheal epithelial cells and they are homologous to peptides that function as mediators of nonoxidative microbial cell killing in human neutrophils (human neutrophil peptides (HNP)) (Ouellette 1997; Porter et al. 1997). The β-defensins, and in particular human β-defensin (HBD)-1, are expressed in the oral mucosa, trachea, and bronchi, as well as mammary and salivary gland epithelial cells in humans (Zhao et al. 1996; Singh et al. 1998; Mathews et al. 1999) (Figure 28.1).

Defensins contribute to the protection of mucosal surfaces through their direct antimicrobial activity. It has been shown that two to four defensin molecules interact to form multimers that insert into the cell membrane of the target bacteria, where they induce membrane disruption. The resultant channel formation allows leakage of essential bacterial components and leads to death. The fact that adenovirus infection is impaired in cells expressing HBD-1 or HD-5 suggests that the microbicidal activity of mucosal defensins also applies to viruses (Gropp et al. 1999). There is abundant evidence that defensin expression is upregulated during infection, e.g. although bronchoalveolar lavage (BAL) fluids from normal patients express only HBD-1, those of patients

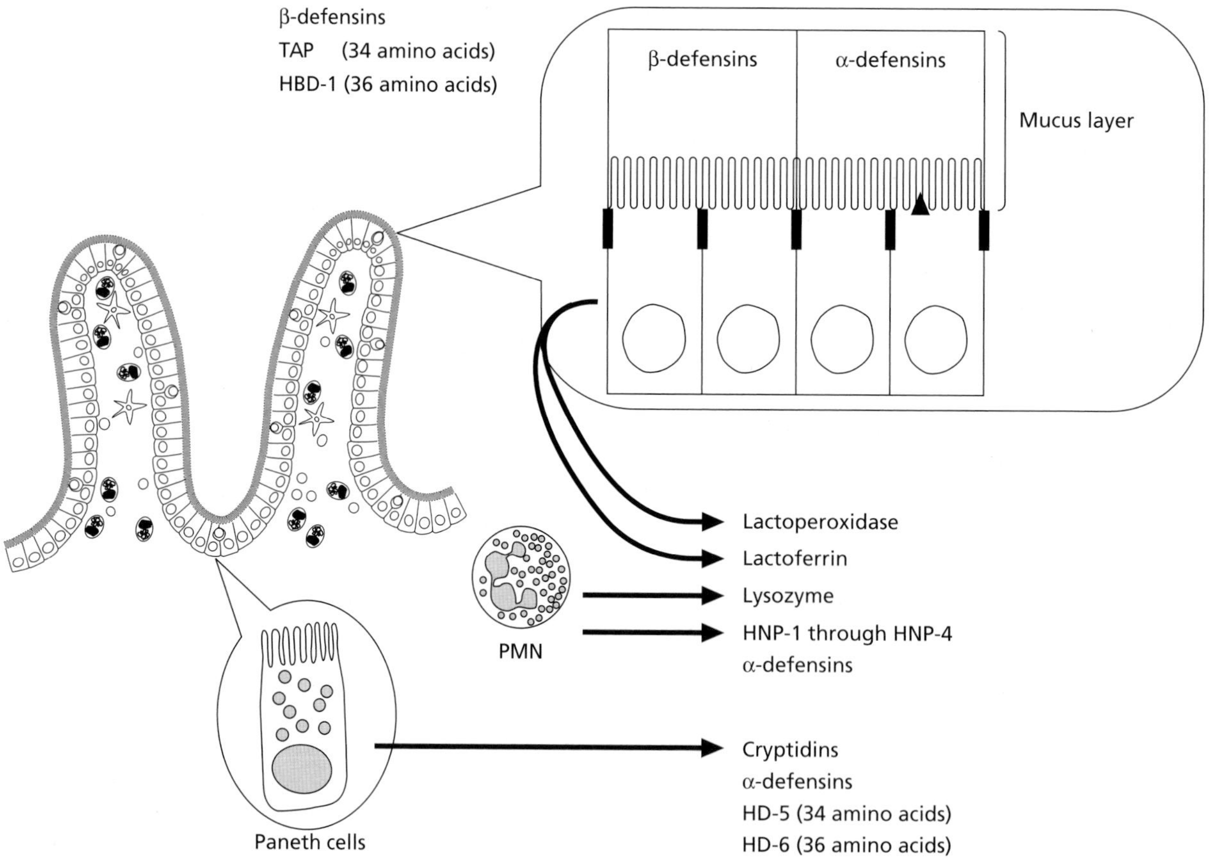

Figure 28.1 *Innate mucosal host defense factors: a thick coat of mucus prevents penetration of macromolecules and potential pathogens. The crypt regions contain Paneth cells, which produce cryptins (α-defensins). The β-defensins are products of epithelial cells and form a defensin network. Other innate factors such as lysozyme, lactoperoxidase, lactoferrin, and secretory leukocyte protease inhibitor (SLIP) also serve in antimicrobial defense. HBD, human β defensin; HD, human defensin; HNP, human neutrophil peptide.*

with cystic fibrosis (CF) or inflammatory lung diseases express both HBD-1 and HBD-2 (Singh et al. 1998). This expression of both HBD-1 versus HBD-2 in CF patients suggests a protective role for HBD-2 in inflammation. On the other hand, normal expression of HBD-1 may protect in the absence of inflammation. Mechanisms that control activation of defensins are poorly understood. Inflammatory cytokines, such as interleukin (IL)-1, tumor necrosis factor α (TNF-α), and lipopolysaccharide (LPS) have been shown to play a role in the induction of some defensins (Singh et al. 1998; Mathews et al. 1999). Metalloprotease matrilysin was recently reported to co-localize with α-defensins in murine Paneth cells (Wilson et al. 1999). Matrilysin was found to cleave the pro-segment from cryptidin precursors (Wilson et al. 1999), suggesting that this molecule regulates the antimicrobial activity of intestinal defensins. Recent studies showed that trypsin plays an important role as a prodefensin convertase in human Paneth cells in the regulation of innate immunity in the small intestine (Ghosh et al. 2002).

Lactoferrin, lysozyme, lactoperoxidase, and antimicrobial innate defense molecules

Other potent antimicrobial innate defense molecules are produced by epithelial cells and serve in natural host defense. These molecules include lactoferrin, lysozyme, the peroxidases, secretory phospholipase A_2, and cathelin-associated peptides. Some of these molecules are secreted by intestinal Paneth cells; all are produced by polymorphonuclear leukocytes (PMN), suggesting that both cell types play important roles in innate defense of mucosal surfaces. Lactoferrin is a member of the transferrin family and shares structural homologies with transferrin and ovotransferrin. This molecule is found in exocrine secretions including milk and saliva, and in lymphocytes of many species where it mediates a number of biological effects including antimicrobial properties. Epithelial cells do not produce lactoferrin; however, they express the lactoferrin receptor. Gastric pepsin hydrolysis of either human or bovine lactoferrin generates a 25-residue peptide called lactoferricin with potent antimicrobial activity (Bellamy et al. 1992). However, not all the 25 residues of lactoferricin are required for antimicrobial activity because an 11-residue peptide containing 5 of the 8 basic residues in bovine lactoferricin displays antimicrobial properties similar to those of the 25-residue peptide (Kang et al. 1996).

Lysozyme is a highly cationic, low-molecular-weight protein that enzymatically cleaves the bonds between *N*-acetylglucosamine and *N*-acetylmuramic acid which stabilizes bacterial peptidoglycans. High concentrations of lysozyme (1 209–1 325 μg/ml) are found in tears. Other secretions that contain lysozyme include saliva, human colostrum, serum, and urine (Pruitt et al. 1990). Human milk is particularly enriched in lysozyme with concentrations ranging from 20 to 245 μg/ml depending on the lactation period (Goldman et al. 1982). These concentrations are about 3000-fold higher than those found in cows' milk. Gram-positive bacteria are most susceptible to the antimicrobial activity of lysozyme, whereas gram-negative bacteria are generally resistant to this effect largely as a result of the protective effects of the outer membrane of LPS that masks the underlying peptidoglycan layer.

Peroxidase activity measured in many mucosal secretions is derived from an enzyme, human lactoperoxidase (hLPO), synthesized in the exocrine glands and secreted into mucosal surfaces. The PMNs also contribute to the peroxidase activity through secretion of myeloperoxidase (MPO) and eosinophil peroxidase (EPO). In this regard, human milk contains at least two peroxidases, the MPO from milk leukocytes and the hLPO produced by mammary gland ductal cells; both display similar properties to the human salivary peroxidases (hSPO) (Pruitt et al. 1991). Peroxidases protect by catalyzing the peroxidation of halides (Cl^-, Br^-, and I^-) and thiocyanate (SCN^-) ions to generate reactive products with potent antimicrobial properties. In the absence of halides and SCN^-, peroxidases can behave as catalases. These two properties of peroxidases prevent the accumulation of toxic products of oxygen reduction.

Secretory leukocyte protease inhibitor (SLPI), a 12-kDa nonglycosylated serine antiprotease, is a potent elastase, trypsin, and chymotrypsin inhibitor found in fluids lining mucosal surfaces, including the respiratory tract, salivary glands, and nasal and cervical mucosa (Mooren et al. 1983; Thompson and Ohlsson 1986; Franken et al. 1989; Hubbard and Crystal 1991; Westin et al. 1994). Thus, it has been shown that SLPI is produced by mucosal epithelial cells as well as goblet cells (Fryksmark et al. 1982; Maruyama et al. 1994; Asano et al. 1995). SLPI has been extensively studied for the protection it gives to the large airway epithelium of the human lung against neutrophil elastase. Thus, it has been suggested that SLPI would be a potential therapeutic tool in inflammatory lung diseases such as CF and pulmonary emphysema (Stolk et al. 1995). Further, SLPI-directed therapeutic genes showed potential roles for directing toxicity to carcinoma tissues (Garver et al. 1994).

Recently, human saliva itself showed an inhibitory effect for adherent primary monocytes infected with HIV-1Ba-L, and it has been shown that this anti-HIV activity was caused by SLPI (McNeely et al. 1995). In this regard, SLPI proved to be a potent inhibitor of translation in vitro. The mechanism of translation inhibition was deduced from in vitro experiments showing that SLPI bound to mRNA and interfered with the interaction of RNA-metabolizing enzymes, such as RNase (Miller et al. 1989). Furthermore, it has been suggested that several inflammatory mediators such as TNF-α and phorbol myristate acetate (PMA) enhanced SLPI mRNA levels (Maruyama et al. 1994); however, the precise regulatory mechanism for the production of SLPI, such as the contribution of immune regulatory T cells and their derived cytokines, still remains unclear.

THE MUCOSAL EPITHELIUM BRIDGES INNATE WITH ACQUIRED MUCOSAL IMMUNITY

A major hallmark of the mucosal immune system is the presence of a mucosal intranet consisting of epithelial cells, αβT-cell receptor positive (TCR^+) T-helper 1 (Th1), T-helper 2 (Th2) cells, $\gamma\delta TCR^+$ T cells and IgA-committed B cells for the induction and regulation of antigen (Ag)-specific secretory IgA (S-IgA) antibodies (Ab) in external secretions. The epithelium that covers mucosal surfaces largely consists of columnar epithelial cells because it is the major point of contact between localized environmental Ags in the gastrointestinal (GI) tract lumen and the underlying mucosal immune system. Epithelial cells not only provide a physical barrier but also produce and express a variety of glycoproteins, peptides, cytokines, and receptors that are important components of mucosal immunity. In addition, this epithelial layer contains a large number of $CD3^+$ T cells commonly termed intraepithelial lymphocytes (IEL). Both intestinal epithelial cells (IEC) and IELs are considered key players in the mucosal intranet and their contact leads to inter- and intracellular molecular communication. Thus, lymphoepithelial interactions contribute both to the maintenance of mucosal immunity and to homeostasis against infection.

Epithelial cells as a physical barrier

Mucosal surfaces are covered by a layer of epithelial cells that prevent the entry of exogenous antigens into the host. The physical protection of the largest mucosal surface, the GI tract, involves a monolayer of tightly joined absorptive epithelial cells termed 'enterocytes' which constitute a highly specialized selective barrier that allows the absorption of nutrients while preventing the entry of pathogens (Fujihashi and Ernst 1999). The intestinal epithelium also contains goblet cells, Paneth cells, and tuft cells, as well as undifferentiated crypt epithelial cells and IELs which contribute to the homeostasis of the epithelium and also serve physical barrier functions. The barrier effect of IECs is facilitated by the mucus blanket covering these cells and prevents the penetration of microorganisms and diffusion of molecules toward the intestinal surface. Mucus consists of glycoproteins of various molecular sizes (Roussel et al. 1988) secreted by goblet cells. These molecules resemble glycoprotein and glycolipid receptors that occur on enterocyte membranes and thus they tend to interfere with the attachment of microorganisms. In the human GI tract, the mucus blanket is approximately 100 μm in thickness. In the stomach and colon, however, this mucus blanket may range from 50 to 450 or 110 to 160 μm, respectively (Kerss et al. 1982; Sandzen et al. 1988). The continuous renewal of the epithelial cell layer also contributes to the barrier effect because damaged or infected enterocytes are replaced by crypt epithelial cells which differentiate into enterocytes as they migrate toward the desquamation zone at the villus tip. This process results in the complete renewal of the absorptive enterocyte layer every 2–3 days.

The epithelia of the other mucosal surfaces, including the oral cavity, pharynx, tonsils, urethra, and vagina, are covered by multilayered squamous epithelial cells. These epithelia lack tight junctions but provide a permeability barrier by secretion of a coating of glycolipoprotein into the intercellular space of the lower stratified layers (Farbman et al. 1988). A mucus blanket of approximately 2 μm covers the respiratory epithelium. Additional barrier effects are provided by the renewal of exposed epithelial cell layers by cells from subjacent layers. The final barrier provided by epithelial cells involves their transport of polymeric IgA (pIgA) via the pIg receptor (pIgR) with intracellular neutralization of viral particles (see below).

Cytokine and chemokine responses to mucosal pathogens

It has now been established that freshly isolated human colonic epithelial cells expressed mRNA for IL-6 and IL-8 (Jung et al. 1995). Further, epithelial cell lines have been useful for investigating the mechanisms that lead to proinflammatory cytokine and chemokine responses following a mucosal infection with pathogenic bacteria or viruses (Figure 28.2). In response to stimuli such as an *Escherichia coli* infection, epithelial cell lines of both intestinal (HT-29 and Caco-2) and urinary tract origin (A-498 and J82) produce IL-6 (Hedges et al. 1992; Agace et al. 1993). Further, fimbriae from *E. coli* also induce IL-6 production in these cell lines, suggesting that adhesive properties of the bacteria play an important role in the induction of this inflammatory cytokine (Figure 28.2). In addition, it has been shown that mucosal epithelial cell lines produce IL-8 after stimulation with *E. coli*, *Salmonella* spp., or *Listeria monocytogenes* (Agace et al. 1993; Eckmann et al. 1993a) (Figure 28.2). Others have shown that the adhesion of *S. typhimurium* to T84 human colonic epithelial cell lines induces the production of IL-8 (McCormick et al. 1993) and is associated with an increased transepithelial migration of neutrophils, although this process appears not to be regulated by IL-8 (McCormick et al. 1993). In addition, it has been reported that the mouse small intestinal

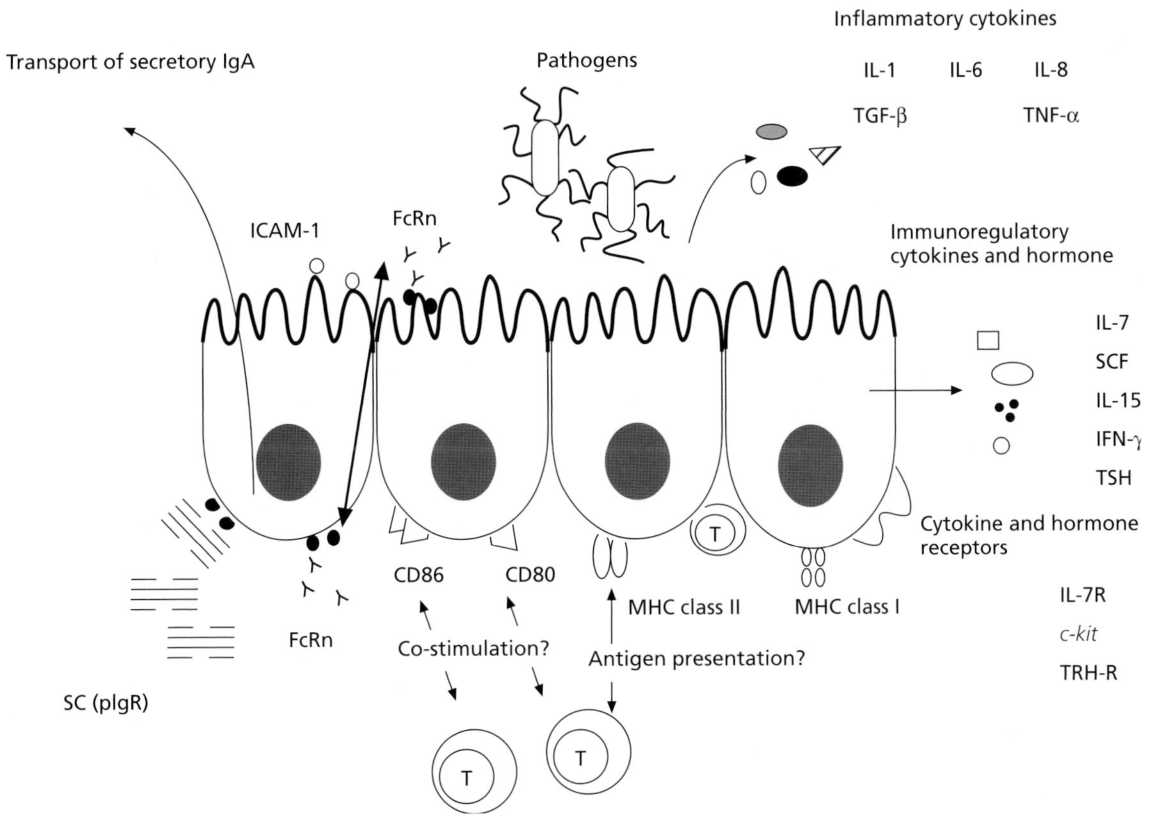

Figure 28.2 *Molecular interactions at the epithelial surface: the mucosal epithelial cells are essential for bridging innate and acquired immunity. The epithelial cells play important roles in both innate and acquired immunity. Cytokines and chemokines are induced by pathogens. Toll-like receptors (TLRs), which play key roles for pathogen-associated virulence factors are expressed by mucosal epithelial cells. The epithelial cells express accessory molecules (major histocompatibility complex [MHC] class I, II, CD80, CD86, CD1, and TL) and serve for antigen-presenting cell (APC) functions. Finally, antigen-specific secretory antibody (S-IgA) as well as IgG transport functions of the epithelial cells indicate essential roles in acquired immunity. ICAM, intercellular adhesion molecule; IFN, interferon; SC, secretory component; SCF, stem cell factor; TGF, transforming growth factor; TNF, tumor necrosis factor; TRH, thyroid-releasing hormone; TSH, thyroid-stimulating hormone.*

cell line, MODE-K, produces stem cell factor (SCF) when infected with *S. typhimurium* (Klimpel et al. 1996) (Figure 28.2). Furthermore, invasive strains of bacteria, such as *S. dublin*, *Shigella dysenteriae*, *Yersinia enterocolitica*, *L. monocytogenes*, and enteroinvasive *E. coli*, induce colonic epithelial cell lines (T84, HT29, and Caco-2) to produce a characteristic array of proinflammatory cytokines, including IL-8, monocyte chemotactic protein-1 (MCP-1), granulocyte–macrophage colony-stimulating factor (GM-CSF), and TNF-α shortly after infection/stimulation (Jung et al. 1995) (Figure 28.2). A similar cytokine array was produced after infection with *Chlamydia*, but chemokine production was delayed and was dependent on infection of cultured cells (Rasmussen et al. 1997). *Helicobacter pylori* infection of gastric epithelium cell lines (Kato III, AGS, or MKN28), but not nongastric epithelial cell lines, induced IL-8 mRNA and protein synthesis (Crowe et al. 1995; Sharma et al. 1995). Immunohistochemical staining of human colon has demonstrated that IECs can express IL-6 and isolated IECs stimulated with LPS have been shown to contain mRNA for both IL-1 and IL-6 (Mayer et al. 1990). It was also shown that cholera toxin (CT)-induced inflammatory cytokines, such as IL-1 and IL-6, in the rat IEC line, IEC-17 (Bromander et al. 1993). Further, increased levels of SCF were also produced by the MODE-K cell line when stimulated with CT (Klimpel et al. 1995). Finally, respiratory syncytial virus (RSV) induced selective production of the chemokine RANTES in upper airway epithelial cells (Saito et al. 1997). Taken together, these studies suggest that epithelial cells are major players in both the inflammatory process and immunity, where they produce anti-inflammatory cytokine pathways.

The secretion of these factors is likely to be mediated initially in large part by interactions between components of microbes and pattern recognition receptors on the cell surface of the epithelium, which stimulate intracellular signals to initiate transcription of genes associated with the inflammatory cascade (Fearon and Locksley 1996). Recently, Toll-like receptors (TLR) have been shown to be key molecules for pathogen-associated virulence factors (e.g. LPS, peptidoglycan, and lipoprotein) and are considered to be major players in innate immunity (Medzhitov et al. 1997; Gerard 1998). In this regard, it has been shown that TLRs are expressed by mucosal epithelial cells in the oral cavity, and the GI and respiratory tracts (Cario et al. 2000; Akira 2001; Asai et al. 2001; Wang et al. 2002) (Figure 28.2), e.g. individual bacterial components bind to specific TLRs, such as peptidoglycan (TLR-2 and TLR-4), lipoteichoic acid (TLR-2), or LPS (TLR-4) (Hoshino et al. 1999; Qureshi et al. 1999; Shimazu et al. 1999; Yoshimura et al. 1999). In addition, other TLRs bind to lipoteichoic acids from gram-positive bacteria (TLR-3), bacterial flagellin (TLR-5), and microbial CpG motifs of DNA (TLR-9) (Akira 2001). In the case of TLR-4, LPS recognition is coupled to CD14 binding wherein LPS bound to CD14 interacts with a TLR-4/MD-2 protein heterodimer (Asai et al. 2001). As breast milk contains soluble CD14 for the innate recognition of bacteria, it is possible that $CD14^-$ epithelial cells recognize LPS through soluble CD14 from milk (Labéta et al. 2000). The TLRs initiate an intracellular signaling cascade and induce activation of NF-κB, which regulates the epithelial cell cycle and subsequent production of soluble mediators (Aradhya and Nelson 2001).

Epithelial cell accessory molecules and antigen-presenting cell functions

In addition to the production of cytokines, IEC lines express adhesion molecules known to be required for antigen-presenting cell (APC) interactions with lymphocytes (see Figure 28.2). Both intercellular adhesion molecule-1 (ICAM-1) and lymphocyte function-associated antigen (LFA)-3 were constitutively expressed at low levels by human intestinal epithelial cell lines and expression of ICAM-1 was enhanced by exposure to the inflammatory cytokines interferon γ (IFN-γ), TNF-α, IL-1β, and IL-6 (Kvale et al. 1992). It was also shown that ICAM-1 expression on the apical side of epithelial cells was upregulated after infection with invasive pathogenic bacteria (Huang et al. 1996). Furthermore, gastric epithelial cell lines, as well as freshly isolated gastric epithelial cells, expressed both B7-1 (CD80) and B7-2 (CD86) (Ye et al. 1997) (see Figure 28.2). Thus, B7-2 expression was increased after crosslinking major histocompatibility complex (MHC) class II on IFN-γ-treated epithelial cells and in cells pretreated with IFN-γ and infected with *H. pylori*. These observations provide support for the finding that rat IECs present processed antigen to antigen-specific $CD4^+$ T cells (Brandeis et al. 1994). Taken together, the findings that epithelial cells express the adhesion molecules ICAM-1 and LFA-3 as well as B7-1 and B7-2, and present antigen to sensitized $CD4^+$ T cells, suggests that IECs probably play an important role in the maintenance of mucosal immune responses in mucosal effector sites and especially in the IEL compartment. It is also likely that IECs exhibit APC functions responsible for some forms of T-cell anergy in mucosal tolerance.

It has been shown that both intestinal and respiratory epithelial cells present antigen in both classic and nonclassic fashions to mucosal T cells (see Figure 28.2). Immunohistochemical analysis revealed that normal human IECs from the small intestine expressed HLA-DR, but less HLA-DP, and this MHC II expression was increased in inflammatory bowel disease (Mayer et al. 1991). Further, direct evidence for APC function was provided with studies of freshly isolated rat IECs and transfected epithelial cell lines, which presented a soluble allopeptide to primed T cells in an MHC II-restricted manner (Brandeis et al. 1994). Although uptake of antigen occurred at both apical (normal) and basal (inflammation) sides of IECs, peptide presentation to T cells through MHC II was seen only at the basolateral surface (Hershberg et al. 1998). Finally, nonclassic MHC I-restricted IEC presentation has been described. Thus, IECs express CD1d constitutively, which in turn is regulated by IFN-γ that also enhances classic MHC I and II molecule expression (Blumberg et al. 1991; Sydora et al. 1996a). The murine CD1 (mCD1) homolog of human CD1d may also bind to peptide antigen (Sydora et al. 1996b). Further, it was shown that mCD1 can bind to $CD8^+$ IELs, i.e. γδ and αβ TCR^+ T cells which express CD8αα homodimers (Sydora et al. 1996b; Gapin et al. 1999). Low numbers of CD1d-restricted NK T cells have been defined in the epithelium using CD1d tetramers (Matsuda et al. 2000). Other nonclassic MHC I molecules expressed by IECs have been directly linked to novel forms of co-stimulation (Leishman et al. 2001; Roberts et al. 2001). The expression of the thymus leukemia (TL) antigen by mouse IEC has been linked to ligation of CD8αα expressed on a subset of IELs, which then delivers a growth-promoting signal to the epithelium (Leishman et al. 2001).

Polymeric IgA and IgM, and monomeric IgG epithelial cell transport

A major function of epithelial cells in mucosal immune responses is the active transcellular transport of pIgA produced in mucosal and glandular tissues to the mucosal surface (see Figure 28.2). The molecule responsible for transport of pIgA into mucosal secretions is the pIgR (Mostov et al. 1980, 1984; Krajci et al. 1992). A major hallmark of the mucosal immune response is the presence of Ag-specific S-IgA Abs in external secretions. As discussed above, S-IgA Abs in humans occur as S-IgA1 and S-IgA2 subclasses, with a preponderance of the former in the upper respiratory tract (URT) and upper GI tract (GIT), and the latter in the lower ileum and large intestine (Mestecky and McGhee 1987; Brandtzaeg 1994). Plasma cells in lamina propria and acinar regions of exocrine glands produce pIgA associated with the 15.6-kDa peptide J chain (Brandtzaeg 1974; Mestecky and McGhee 1987). Initially, it was thought that J chain was involved in polymerization of intracellular monomeric IgA (mIgA) or IgM (mIgM) (Brandtzaeg and Prydz 1984); however, recent studies indicate that aberrant polymers of IgM occur in the absence of J chain (Niles et al. 1995). Further, J chain knock-out mice exhibit IgA in external secretions; however, only mIgA is transported in this mouse (Hendrickson et al. 1995, 1996). Taken together, this suggests that J chain is required in the formation of pIgA and the correct pentameric form of IgM that enables the molecule to bind to pIgR on the basolateral side of the epithelium (Brandtzaeg 1974; Brandtzaeg and Prydz 1984; Hendrickson et al. 1995, 1996; Niles et al. 1995).

As indicated above, epithelial cells in glands and in basolateral crypts of the GIT and URT produce the full-length 100-kDa pIgR which associates with the nonserosal surface of epithelial cells (Mostov 1994). The binding of pIgA/pIgM is followed by endocytosis and transcytosis across the epithelial cell (Eckmann et al. 1993a). During transcytosis, disulfide bonds form between pIgR and pIgA and secretion of S-IgA follows cleavage of a 20-kDa component of pIgR and exocytosis – the entire process requiring less than an hour (Mestecky and McGhee 1987; Mostov 1994) (see Figure 28.1). The disulfide-bonded portion of the pIgR remains attached to the Ab molecule, termed secretory component (SC), stabilizes S-IgA and S-IgM, and renders the molecule more resistant to proteolytic digestion (Mestecky and McGhee 1987; Mostov 1994). This transport process is highly efficient and a normal adult produces 2.8–3.0 g S-IgA/day in the GIT alone.

A number of studies have provided evidence that IEC lines produce cytokines and express cytokine receptors and adhesion molecules that may affect the induction of mucosal immune responses. When human IECs were examined for their ability to produce cytokines, both cell lines and freshly isolated human IECs were shown to produce IL-8 (Eckmann et al. 1993a, b; Schüerer-Maly et al. 1994), and the former also expressed mRNA for IL-1α, IL-1β, IL-10, and TNF-α, but not for IL-2, IL-4, IL-5, IL-6, or IFN-γ (Eckmann et al. 1993a, b). It has now been shown that IFN-γ and TNF-α induced HT-29 cells to increase membrane-associated pIgR (Sollid et al. 1987; Kvale et al. 1988). Further, IL-4 enhanced the expression of surface pIgR, and this cytokine acted in synergy with IFN-γ to induce high levels of pIgR on HT-29 cells (Phillips et al. 1990). Taken together, these results suggest that IECs have the ability to produce cytokines that could play a role in the induction and maintenance of mucosal immune responses and inflammation.

The epithelium also expresses the neonatal Fc receptor for IgG (FcRn). It has been shown that FcRn is responsible for the passive acquisition of IgG neonatally in rodents (Israel et al. 1997; Zhu et al. 2001). Thus, it was predicted that FcRn expression was strictly limited to neonatal life. However, recent evidence indicates that this molecule is also expressed by adult human epithelium and by Mϕs in the intestinal lamina propria. When expressed postnatally in adult humans, FcRn may serve in a capacity to provide for the continuous presence of IgG Abs to prevent microbial infections. The FcRn binds monomeric IgG in a pH-dependent process (pH 6 on, pH 7.4 off) because of histidine residues in the Fc region of IgG. In contrast to the transport associated with pIgR, the pathway associated with FcRn goes from basal to apical as well as from apical to basal (Dickinson et al. 1999) (see Figure 28.2). In addition, the FcRn is not associated with proteolytic cleavage and is thus available for several rounds of transport. It is predicted, therefore, that the FcRn is a major player in the steady-state distribution of IgG on both sides of the epithelial barrier. Most feel that paracellular transport of this macromolecule does not occur because of the molecular exclusion of the tight junctions.

AN IEL–IEC INTRANET

Origin and function of intestinal IELs

The mucosal epithelium, an important interface between the host and its environment, contains a large number of CD3$^+$ T cells which are commonly termed IELs (Ernst et al. 1985; LeFrançois 1991; McGhee et al. 1994) (Figure 28.3). As the name IEL indicates, these lymphocytes reside on the basolateral surface of epithelial cells covering the GI, nasal, and reproductive tracts. It has been estimated that one IEL can be found for every four to six epithelial cells (Ferguson and Parrott 1972; Crowe and Marsh 1994). Thus, tremendous numbers of CD3$^+$ T cells are situated in the mucosal epithelium where they are continuously exposed to mucosally encountered antigens. Although human IELs share several unique features with mouse IELs, the phenotype of cell surface antigens is different, e.g. the most striking characteristic of mouse IELs is the presence of high numbers of $\gamma\delta$ T cells (Ernst et al. 1985; McGhee et al. 1994); however, most human IELs express oligoclonal $\alpha\beta$TCRs (Ebert 1994; Halstensen and Brandtzaeg 1994) (Figure 28.3). Despite the numerous studies that have focused on a better understanding of the ontogeny of murine IELs, only limited information is currently available about the origin and development of human IELs. Morphological studies have suggested that human IELs originate from cells in the lamina propria. Thus, it has been shown that they possess trailing cytoplasmic pseudopods in the direction of lamina propria (Orlic and Lev 1977). Further, the epithelial basement membrane around the site of IEL migration has specific pores

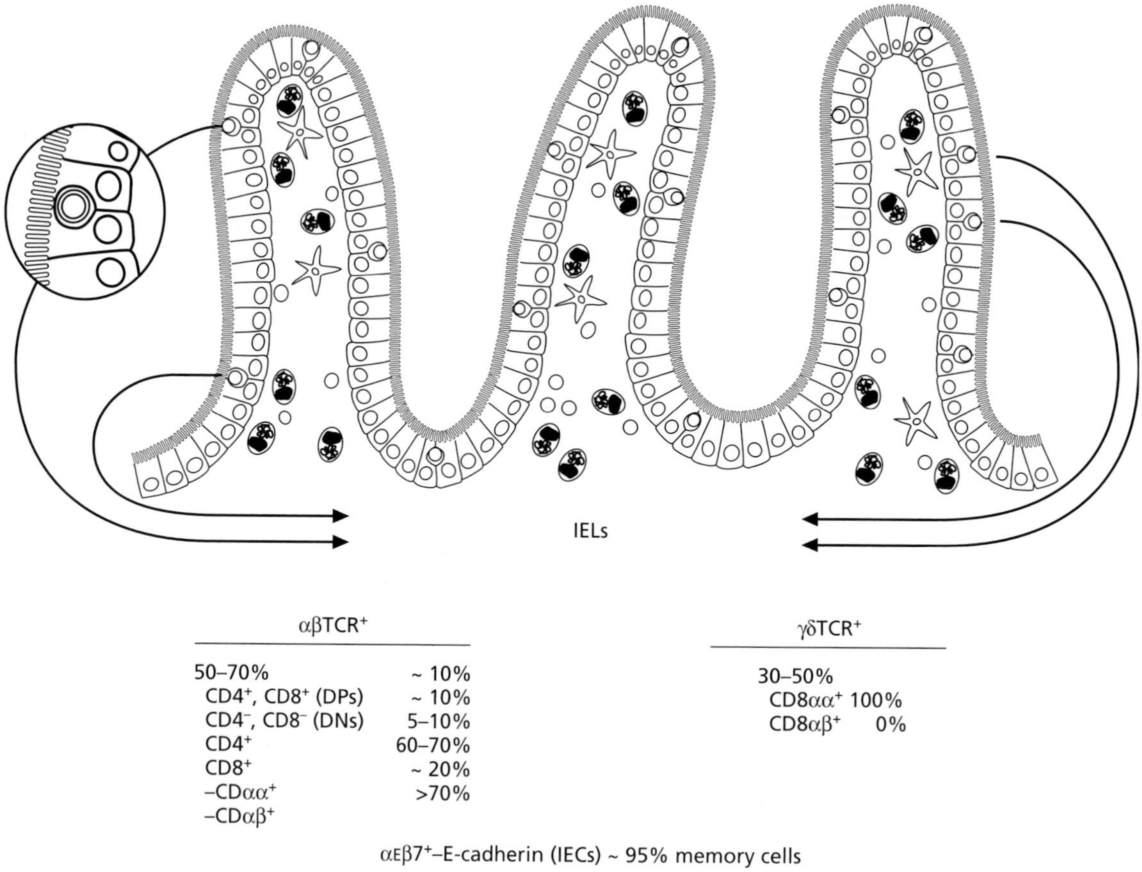

Figure 28.3 *Intraepithelial lymphocytes (IELs). Unique effector T-cell subsets are present in the epithelium. In this regard, the origin and immunological functions of IELs are distinct from other mature T cells. IECs, intestinal epithelial cells; TCR, T-cell receptor.*

(Toner and Ferguson 1971). These findings suggest that human IELs not only migrate from the lamina propria, but also have the potential to migrate back to this region. These observations further suggest that potential extrathymic development of human IELs may occur. Indeed, human IELs express CD7 (Fcμ receptor) which is also expressed on $CD3^-$ pre-T cells in the thymus (Malizia et al. 1985). These $CD7^+$ IELs contain small but significant numbers of $CD3^-$ IELs. In the case of γδ T cells in human IELs, Vδ2 expression also supports the possibility of extrathymic development. It has been shown that this T-cell population is rare in the gut although most fetal γδ IELs express the Vδ2 segment (Spencer and MacDonald 1994). In contrast, other reports showed that human IELs contain an equal frequency of Vδ1 and Vδ2. Despite the lack of a clear answer for the origin of human IELs, recent reports strongly suggest that patches that occur in the crypt region, termed 'cryptopatches', in the intestinal lamina propria of mice do not express lineage markers, including CD3, B220, Mac-1, Gr-1, and TER119, or *c-kit*$^+$ cells that allow differentiation into either αβ or γδ IELs (Kanamori et al. 1996; Saito et al. 1998).

IELs may be assumed to be a primary source of effector T cells in the natural environment of the mucosal epithelium. Such effector cells form a first line of defense against translocation of the mucosal microflora and invading microbial pathogens. The $CD8^+$/IEL T-cell subset is associated with cytotoxic activity (Ernst et al. 1985; LeFrançois 1991; McGhee et al. 1994), e.g. human $CD8^+$ IELs possess cytotoxic activity and kill a tumor epithelial cell line by mechanisms that are totally different from NK-type activity (Ebert 1994; Spencer and MacDonald 1994). It is important to note that cytotoxic activity in human $CD8^+$ IELs is restricted to epithelial cells. These findings clearly suggest that human $CD8^+$ IELs play an immune surveillance role in order to identify and remove defective or infected IECs. Cytotoxic activity in IELs has also been studied in detail in the mouse system. Thus, CTL activity for both αβ and γδ IELs was shown by use of a re-directed cytotoxic cell assay in hybridoma cell lines producing monoclonal antibodies (mAb) specific for $CD3^+$, $αβTCR^+$, or $γδTCR^+$ cells as targets (LeFrançois and Goodman 1989; Guy-Grand et al. 1991). Furthermore, it has been shown that MHC I-restricted virus-specific cytoxic T lymphocytes (CTL) can be induced in the intestinal epithelium of mice (London et al. 1987; Offit and Dudzik 1989).

Certain subsets of IEL T cells have been shown to contribute to regional host defense against intestinal infections with bacterial pathogens (Yamamoto et al. 1993; Emoto et al. 1996; Roberts et al. 1996). During

Listeria monocytogenes infection, IFN-γ production and target cell lysis by $CD8^+$ αβ T cells were essential for complete (sterile) clearance of this pathogen (Kaufmann 1993). It was also shown that both $CD4^+$ αβ and γδ T cells contribute to optimal protection after systemic challenge with *L. monocytogenes* (Kaufmann 1993). Studies in TCR-deficient mice suggest an important role for γδ T cells in immune responses to both intracellular bacteria and parasites (Mombaerts et al. 1993; Tsuji et al. 1994; Ladel et al. 1995). The γδ T cells were required for control of mycobacterial infection (Mombaerts et al. 1993) and also contributed to immunity after *Plasmodium yoelii* immunization, because γδ T-cell-defective ($TCR\delta^{-/-}$) mice failed to respond to these intracellular pathogens and succumbed to infection (Tsuji et al. 1994). The γδ T cells also play an accessory role in the late stages of protective immune responses to *Mycobacterium bovis* Bacillus Calmette–Guérin (BCG) (Ladel et al. 1995). Taken together, these findings show that intraepithelial T cells can serve as effector cells to protect from mucosal parasitic, bacterial, and viral infections.

The vast majority of γδ T cells occur in the epithelium of the small intestine of normal mice and as such could provide a key role in the maintenance of mucosal immunohomeostasis, in addition to regulation of immune responses to intracellular bacteria and parasites. Our previous studies suggested that γδ IEL T cells are important for the maintenance of mucosal IgA Ab responses in the presence of systemic unresponsiveness (or oral tolerance) induced by oral immunization (Fujihashi et al. 1992). Indeed, it was shown that γδ T cells serve an important regulatory role for mucosal IgA responses, because $TCR\delta^{-/-}$ mice possess normal numbers of functional αβ T cells, but display markedly decreased IgA Ab responses after oral immunization (Fujihashi et al. 1996b). Furthermore, recent studies have suggested that γδ T cells play distinct roles in the induction of both low- and high-dose oral tolerance (Ke et al. 1997; Fujihashi et al. 1999). Thus, γδ T cells play a significant immunoregulatory role in IL-10-mediated, low-dose oral tolerance induction, but are not essential participants in the induction of systemic tolerance to orally introduced Ags given in larger doses (Fujihashi et al. 1999).

IEL and IEC crosstalk at the intestinal mucosal barrier

It is logical to consider that epithelial cells and IEL T cells in mucosal tissues cross-regulate each other in order to provide a cellular and molecular network to induce and maintain appropriate immunological homeostasis. Thus, as discussed above, IECs and $CD8^+$ IEL T cells elicit increased levels of MHC I and CTL activity, respectively, after infection by pathogenic viruses. It has been shown that IEL T cells are also capable of producing an array of cytokines including transforming growth factor β (TGF-β) and IFN-γ which in turn induce high levels of MHC expression on IECs (Taguchi et al. 1990b; Barrett et al. 1992; Fujihashi et al. 1993a, b). Further, IEL T-cell-derived cytokines, including IFN-γ, IL-4, and TNF-α, have been shown to influence IEC functions such as the production of the pIgR (Kvale et al. 1988; Phillips et al. 1990). Intraepithelial γδ but not αβ T cells have been shown to moderate the growth and differentiation of IECs by the production of keratinocyte growth factor (Boismenu and Havran 1994) (Figure 28.4). Studies in $TCR\delta^{-/-}$ mice have emphasized the important role played by IEL γδ T cells in IEC growth. In $TCR\delta^{-/-}$ mice, the turnover of IECs in intestinal villi and the levels of MHC II expression were both lower than in mice of the same genetic background (Komano et al. 1995). These findings suggest that intraepithelial γδ T cells provide cytokines essential for the growth and proper functioning of IECs.

Regulation is bi-directional, because epithelial cells can also influence γδ T-cell development and function. It was recently demonstrated that cytokine signaling between IL-7 and its receptor (IL-7R) contributes to development and activation of IEL γδ T cells. It was shown that both human and murine IECs contain specific mRNA for IL-7 (Watanabe et al. 1995; Fujihashi et al. 1996a) (Figure 28.4). Flow cytometry analysis of IL-7R expression revealed that a subset of γδ T cells exhibit high mRNA levels (Fujihashi et al. 1996a) (Figure 28.4). Thus, co-cultivation of intestinal γδ T cells and recombinant IL-7 results in the activation of T cells for proliferative responses (Fujihashi et al. 1996a). Stimulatory signals provided by IL-7, and by the IL-7R pathway (between epithelial cells and γδ T cells), also induce IL-2R expression on γδ T cells. In addition, IL-2 provides a synergistic activation signal for further activation of γδ T cells. Mice that lack the common cytokine receptor γ chain (γc), which is a part of both IL-2R and IL-7R (Noguchi et al. 1993), manifest complete loss of γδ T cells (Cao et al. 1995; He and Malek 1996; Maki et al. 1996). Furthermore, although studies have also provided evidence for a lack of γδ T cells in IL-7 and IL-7R gene-deleted ($IL\text{-}7^{-/-}$ and $IL\text{-}7R^{-/-}$) mice (Cao et al. 1995; He and Malek 1996; Maki et al. 1996; Moore et al. 1996), direct comparison of $IL\text{-}7^{-/-}$ and $IL\text{-}7R^{-/-}$ mice provides a unique opportunity to demonstrate the importance of this pathway for intestinal γδ T-cell development. Intestinal γδ T cells were reduced when the IL-7 gene was deleted and completely disappeared in the absence of IL-7R (Fujihashi et al. 1997). These findings support the idea that epithelial cell-derived IL-7 is an essential cytokine for the development and activation of neighboring $IL\text{-}7R^+$ γδ T cells.

In addition to the IL-7-corresponding receptor cascade, a study with WBB6/F1-*W/W*^{v} (*c-kit*) and WCB6/F1-*Sl/Sl*^{d} (SCF) mutant mice has suggested that

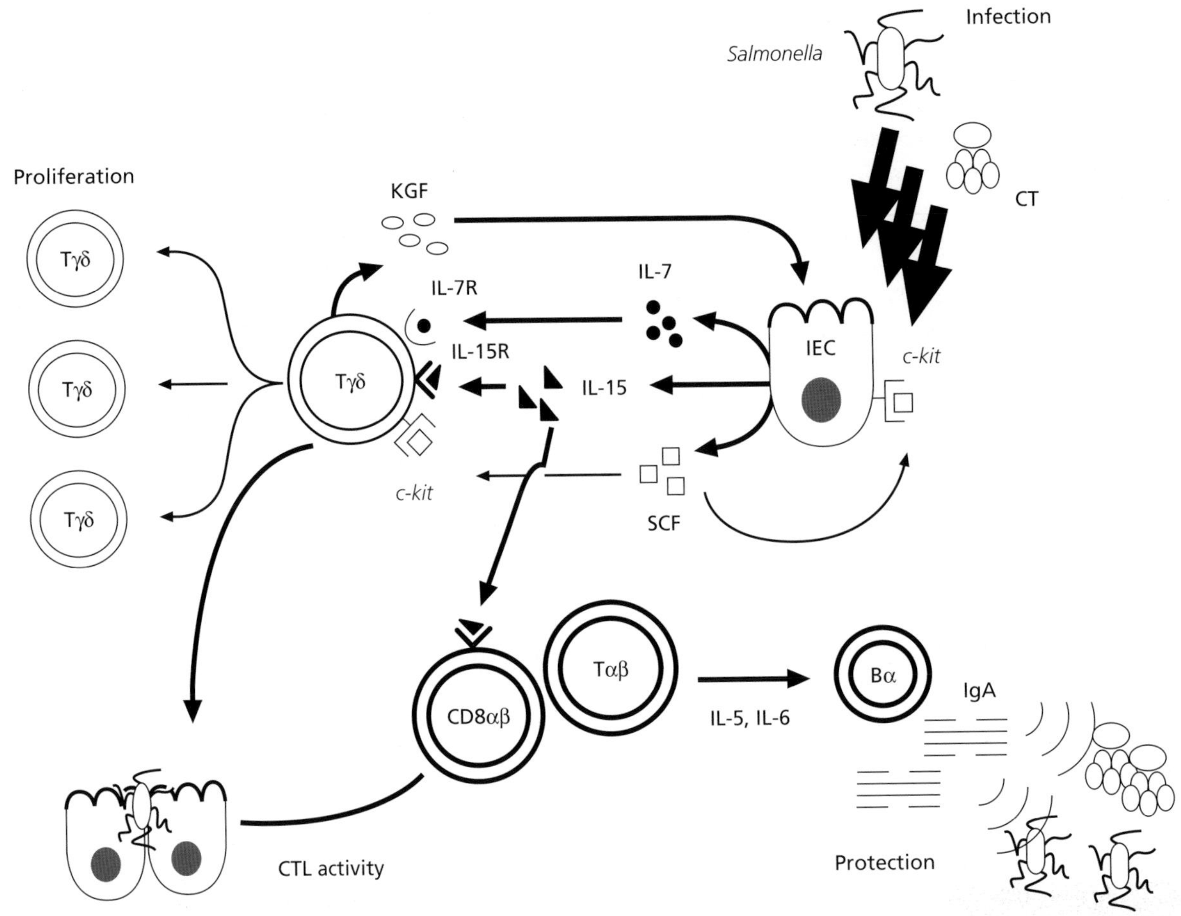

Figure 28.4 *The molecular intranet: a cytokine and growth factor intranet between epithelial cells and intraepithelial lymphocytes (IELs). Bi-directional regulation occurs between epithelial cells and γδ T cells for development and function. Intraepithelial γδ T cells have been shown to moderate the growth and differentiation of epithelial cells by the production of keratinocyte growth factor (KGF). Further, epithelial cells provide essential cytokines, interleukin IL-7, stem cell factor (SCF), IL-15 for γδ T cells, and thyroid-stimulating hormone (TSH) and IL-15 for CD8 αβ T cells. CTLs, cytotoxic T lymphocytes; IECs, intraepithelial cells.*

SCF and *c-kit* interactions also play important roles in the development and maintenance of IELs γδ T cells (Puddington et al. 1994) (Figure 28.4). Further, this study demonstrates that neighboring epithelial cells were able to produce SCF (Puddington et al. 1994) (Figure 28.4). Thus, although normal levels of γδ T cells were detected in IELs of both SCF and *c-kit* mutant mice at 4–8 weeks of age, decreased numbers of this T-cell subset were noted at 16 weeks of age (Puddington et al. 1994). These observations indicate that cross-talk between γδ IELs and IECs is essential for homeostasis of the mucosal immune system in the GIT. As SCF and *c-kit* are the products of IECs and IELs, respectively, this cytokine-signaling pathway from epithelial cells to intestinal γδ T cells is essential for the growth of mucosal γδ T cells.

The SCF and *c-kit* network has also been shown to be important for intestinal fluid secretion induced by *Vibrio cholerae* (Klimpel et al. 1995). Using a ligated intestinal loop model, it was shown that both *Sl/Sld* and *W/Wv* mice produced significantly less intestinal fluid in response to CT challenge than did control mice. The interaction of SCF with its receptor was further shown to be important in salmonella infections (Klimpel et al. 1996). Both human and murine IEC lines show enhanced SCF synthesis and expression of mRNA after exposure to *Salmonella* spp. (Klimpel et al. 1996). Thus, pretreatment of these cell lines with SCF increased their resistance to salmonella invasion (Klimpel et al. 1996). Further, when *c-kit* mutant and control mice were challenged with oral *S. typhimurium*, *W/Wv* mice were more susceptible to infection than were controls (Klimpel et al. 1996). These results show that interactions between SCF and *c-kit* play an essential role as a first line of defense at the mucosal epithelium. In the case of salmonella infection, it has been shown that IL-15 preferentially induces T-cell growth in peritoneal γδ T cells (Nishimura et al. 1996). These studies suggest that IL-15 is a potential growth factor for intestinal IEL γδ T cells. Indeed, other studies showed that IL-15 promoted the growth of IEL γδ T cells (Inagaki-Ohara et al. 1997). Further, it has been shown that gene deletion of the

IL-15 and IL-15R pathway resulted in reduced numbers of IEL γδ T cells in the intestinal epithelium (Lodolce et al. 1998; Kennedy et al. 2000).

Although IEC and IEL γδ T-cell interactions have thus far been the focus of this discussion, the role of IEL αβ T cells should not be ignored. This T-cell subset has the capacity to respond to IL-7 and SCF produced by IECs. In addition to participating in these cytokine signal pathways, IEL αβ T cells and IECs form a unique local hormone network (Wang et al. 1997). Thus, neuroendocrine hormones play an important role in the development of IEL $CD8\alpha\beta^+$, αβ T cells (Wang and Klein 1994, 1995). Mouse IECs express thyrotropin-releasing hormone (TRH) receptor and produce thyroid-stimulating hormone (TSH) upon TRH signal transduction, whereas IELs express TSH receptor (TSH-R)-specific mRNA (Wang et al. 1997). The phenotypic analysis of IELs in *hyt/hyt* mice, which have congenital point mutation in the TSH-R gene, revealed significant reductions in CD8αβ and αβ T-cell subsets but not the CD8αα fraction (Wang et al. 1997). In addition, recent studies showed significant development of $CD8\alpha\beta^+$, $NK1.1^+$ T cells in the IELs and subsequent induction of small intestinal inflammation by intestinal epithelium-specific IL-15 transgenic mice (Ohta et al. 2002). These results suggest the existence of additional important lymphoepithelial interactions, especially those involving intraepithelial $CD8\alpha\beta^+$, αβ T cells, and their important role in mucosal homeostasis and immunity. Taken together, epithelial cells and intraepithelial T cells are major players in the formation of a mucosal intranet and can reciprocally regulate each other via select cytokines and corresponding receptor interactions in order to provide and maintain an effective host defense system in the mucosal environment.

INDUCTIVE AND EFFECTOR LYMPHOEPITHELIAL SITES OF THE MUCOSAL IMMUNE SYSTEM

Organization of the mucosal immune system

The mammalian host has evolved organized secondary lymphoid tissues in the URT and GIT regions which facilitate antigen uptake, processing and presentation for induction of mucosal immune responses. Collectively, these tissues are termed 'mucosal inductive sites' (Figure 28.5). Although the gut-associated

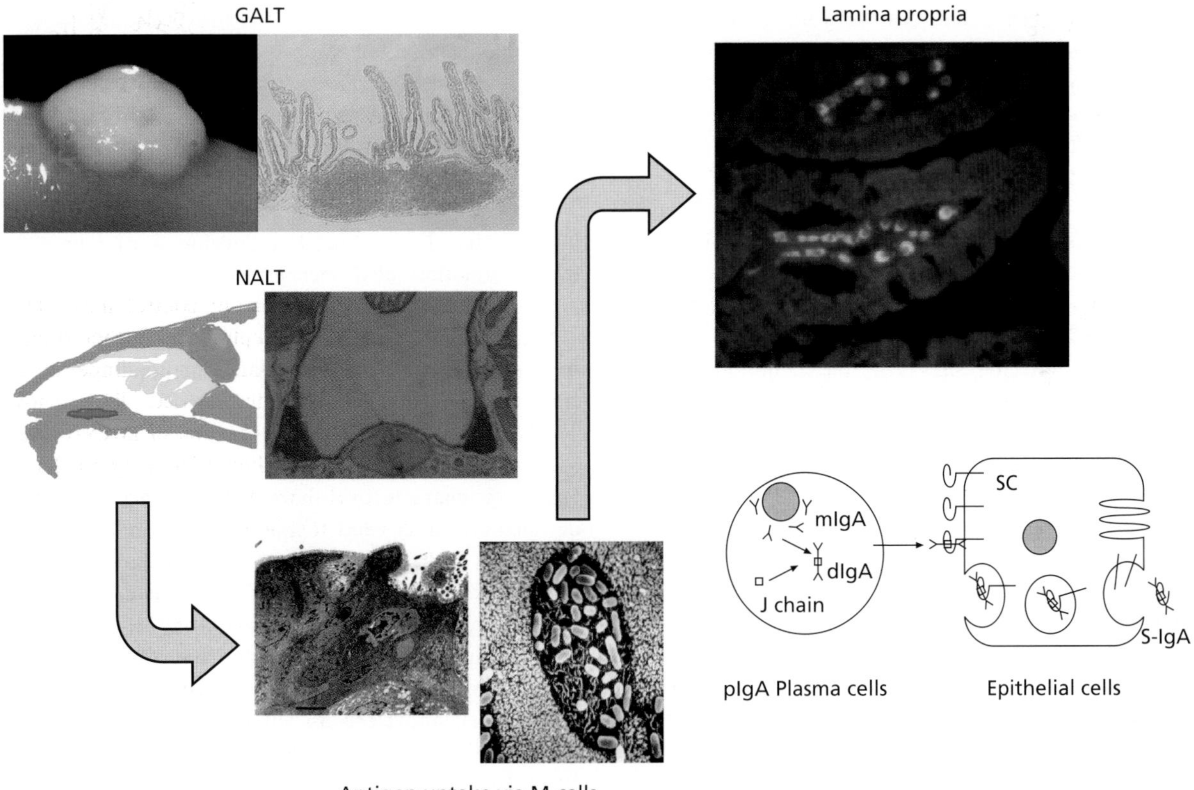

Figure 28.5 *The common mucosal immune system (CMIS): the mammalian host has evolved organized secondary lymphoid tissues, termed inductive sites in the upper respiratory and gastrointestinal tract regions which facilitate antigen uptake, processing, and presentation for induction of mucosal immune responses. Subsequently, antigen-activated and memory B- and T-cell populations emigrate from the inductive environment via lymphatic drainage, circulate through the bloodstream, and home to mucosal effector sites. SC, secretory component; S-IgA, antigen-specific secretory IgA antibody.*

lymphoepithelial tissues (GALT), e.g. Peyer's patches, the appendix, and smaller lymphoid aggregates called solitary lymph nodes (SLN), appear to be major inductive sites in all of the most common experimental mammalian systems, the degree of bronchus-associated lymphoepithelial tissue (BALT) developed at airway branches for defense against intranasal/inhaled antigens differs considerably among species (Pabst 1992; Kolopp-Sarda et al. 1994). Instead, the major inductive tissues for nasal/inhaled antigens in humans, primates, mice, and rats appear to be the palatine tonsils and adenoids (nasopharyngeal tonsils), which together form a physical barrier of lymphoid tissues termed 'Waldeyer's ring', now more frequently referred to as a nasopharyngeal-associated lymphoepithelial tissue (NALT) (Bernstein 1992; Kuper et al. 1992). To summarize, NALT and GALT in humans, mice, and primates and NALT, BALT, and GALT in other experimental mammalian systems comprise a mucosa-associated lymphoepithelial tissue (MALT) network (Bienenstock et al. 1978; Mestecky and McGhee 1987), the integration of which is only partly understood.

There are two major features that distinguish MALT from the other systemic lymphoid tissues. First, the epithelium that separates the tissue from the lumen contains a specialized cell type now called a microfold or M cell which is closely associated with lymphoid cells. Together this epithelial cell network is termed the follicle-associated epithelium (FAE). Second, MALT contains organized regions that include a subepithelial area (dome), B-cell zones with germinal centers containing IgA-committed B cells (surface IgA^+ ($sIgA^+$) B cells) and adjacent T-cell regions with APCs and high endothelial venules (HEV). Naive, recirculating B and T lymphocytes enter MALT through HEVs. Antigen-activated and memory B- and T-cell populations then emigrate from the inductive environment via lymphatic drainage, circulate through the bloodstream, and home to mucosal effector sites (via the common mucosal immune system (CMIS)) (Figure 28.5). These effector sites include more diffuse tissues where antigen-specific T and B lymphocytes ultimately reside and perform their respective functions (i.e. CMI, CTL, and regulatory functions or antibody synthesis) to protect mucosal surfaces.

Mucosal inductive sites

Mucosal inductive sites of the GIT include Peyer's patches, the appendix and SLNs, which collectively comprise the GALT (Bienenstock et al. 1978; Mestecky and McGhee 1987), while the tonsils and adenoids, or NALT, probably serve as the mucosal inductive sites for the URT, the nasal/oral cavity, and the genitourinary tract (Bernstein 1992; Kuper et al. 1992). The most extensively studied mucosal inductive tissues are the Peyer's patches of the murine GI tract, although, in recent years, several groups have also characterized NALT, albeit to a lesser extent than GALT, and salient characteristics of both are presented.

GUT-ASSOCIATED LYMPHOEPITHELIAL TISSUE

The initial steps involved in murine Peyer's patch development have been studied in some detail in mice. A cluster of $VCAM\text{-}1^+$/$ICAM\text{-}1^+$ cells occurs in the upper small intestine beginning at embryonic day –15 to –16 followed by the presence of cells expressing the IL-7 receptor ($IL\text{-}7R\alpha^+$) at day –17.5 (Adachi et al. 1997, 1998; Yoshida et al. 1999) which appear to be the anlage of the patch. Mice defective in IL-7Rα gene expression fail to form mature GALT (Yoshida et al. 1999). It now appears that IL-7–IL-7R triggering results in upregulation of $LT\alpha_1\beta_2$ membrane expression by lymphoid cells, including those in developing Peyer's patches (Rennert et al. 1996; Alimzhanov et al. 1997; Koni et al. 1997; Futterer et al. 1998). Further, mice that lack LT-α_1, LT-β_2 or that have been treated in utero with a fusion protein of LT-β receptor Ig (LT-β-R-Ig) fail to develop Peyer's patches or systemic lymph nodes (De Togni et al. 1994; Rennert et al. 1996; Alimzhanov et al. 1997; Koni et al. 1997; Futterer et al. 1998). In addition, lymphoplasia (*aly/aly*) mice, with a mutation in the NF-κB-inducing kinase (Shinkura et al. 1999), which appears to act downstream of LT-$\alpha_1\beta_2$-LT-βR signaling, also fail to develop Peyer's patches (Shinkura et al. 1999). There is recent evidence that a lymphoid progenitor cell from fetal liver expresses $\alpha 4\beta 7$ and migrates to the Peyer's patch anlage where they ultimately develop into T cells, NK cells, DCs, and lymphotoxin (LT)-lineage cells (Yoshida et al. 2001). In humans, the Peyer's patches develop during prenatal life, a situation also seen in sheep, pigs, dogs, and horses (Griebel and Hein 1996).

Murine Peyer's patches contain a dome, underlying follicles (B-cell zones with germinal centers) (Figure 28.6a), and parafollicular regions enriched with T cells (Figure 28.6b). Originally, the specialized epithelial cell covering MALT was termed a 'FAE cell' because it characterized the organized lymphoid tissues in the GI tract and exhibited pinocytotic activity (Bockman and Cooper 1973). However, the M cell was later named for its unique topical morphology (microfold/membranous) (Owen and Jones 1974) and others now commonly describe the epithelium covering MALT as an FAE type because of characteristic M cells, lack of goblet cells, and close association with lymphoid cells (Wolf and Bye 1984; Farstad et al. 1994; Gebert et al. 1996; Neutra et al. 1996). The surface of the dome region is covered by the specialized FAE, 10–20 percent of which is made up of M cells that exhibit thin extensions around lymphoid cells (Bockman and Cooper 1973; Owen and Jones 1974; Wolf and Bye 1984; Farstad et al. 1994; Gebert et al. 1996; Neutra et al. 1996). These

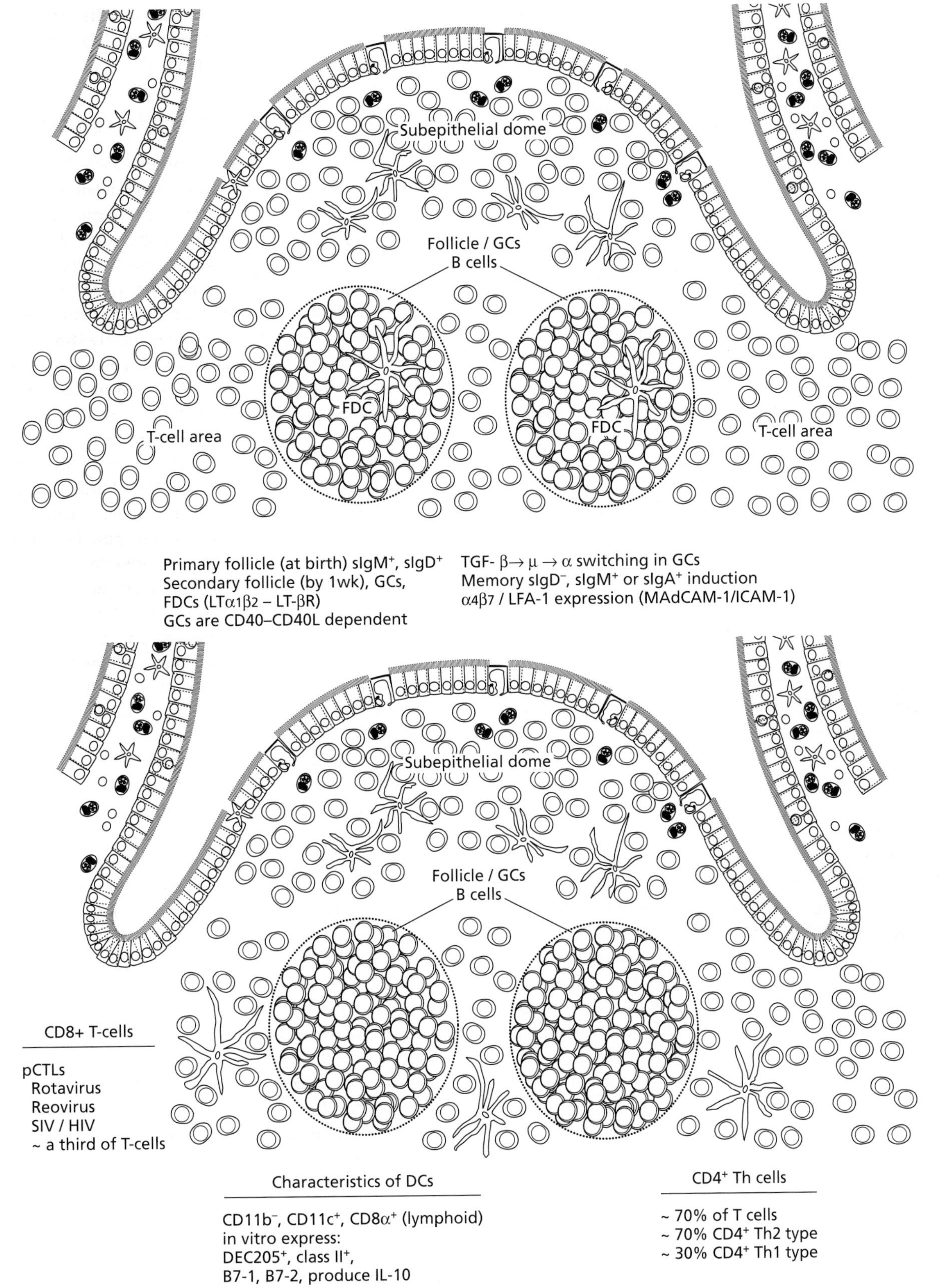

Figure 28.6 *Mucosal inductive sites: the immunological features of typical gut-associated lymphoreticular tissue (GALT), i.e. Peyer's patches.* **(a)** *B-cell zones are located beneath the dome area of the Peyer's patches and contain germinal centers (GCs) where significant B-cell division is seen.* **(b)** *All major mature T-cell subsets are found in the parafollicular area. Over 97 percent of T cells express the $\alpha\beta$ T-cell receptor. FDC, follicular dendritic cell; ICAM, intercellular adhesion molecule; LFA, lymphocyte function-associated antigen; MIP, macrophage inflammatory protein; SIV, simian immunodeficiency virus; Th, T-helper cell; TGF, transforming growth factor.*

extensions, which almost surround B and T lymphocytes and occasional macrophages (MΦ), form an apparent pocket (Farstad et al. 1994; Gebert et al. 1996; Neutra et al. 1996). The M cells, which have short microvilli, small cytoplasmic vesicles, and few lysosomes, are adept at uptake and transport of luminal antigens, including proteins and particulates such as viruses, bacteria, small parasites, and microspheres (Wolf and Bye 1984; Ermak et al. 1995; Gebert et al. 1996; Neutra et al. 1996). Investigators in this field disagree on whether M cells are able to process and present antigen. Some believe that antigen uptake by M cells and transcellular passage result in delivery of intact antigen into the underlying lymphoid tissue (Wolf and Bye 1984; Gebert et al. 1996). Others, however, contend that findings such as M-cell expression of MHC II molecules and acidic endosomal–lysosomal compartments suggest that M cells may also be involved in antigen processing and presentation (Allan et al. 1993). It is possible that the nature of endocytosed antigen influences M-cell activation and their potential to express MHC II molecules. In an important and elegant in vitro study, human Caco-2 cells, which are more immature enterocytes, differentiated into M-like cells when treated with mouse Peyer's patch T and B cells or with a human B-cell line (Raji) (Kerneis et al. 1997). Mice that lack B cells (termed μMT) were also shown to exhibit fewer M cells and less well-developed FAE and Peyer's patches than normal mice (Golovkina et al. 1999). These findings suggest that lymphocytes and especially B cells possess signaling molecules that induce M-cell differentiation.

In addition to serving as a means of transport for luminal antigens, the M cells also provide an entry way for pathogens. Invasive strains of *S. typhimurium* initiate murine infection by invading the M cells of the Peyer's patches (Jones et al. 1994). Although M cells are able to transport luminal antigen, noninvasive strains of *S. typhimurium* cannot penetrate M cells and thus are avirulent. Reoviruses also initiate infection of the mouse through the M cell (Wolf et al. 1981), an ability that has been associated with the reovirus sigma protein (Nibert et al. 1991). As discussed in more detail below, NALT also has a lymphoepithelium with M cells, and the tubercle bacillus *M. tuberculosis* uses this cell type for entry into the host with subsequent uptake in draining lymph nodes (Teitelbaum et al. 1999). Identification of bacterial and viral virulence factors associated with invasion or infection of M cells may provide tools to construct more efficient attenuated bacterial or viral vectors (see below) or to target mucosal vaccines to the inductive environment of MALT. Further, it is possible that M cells are also involved in the induction of mucosally-induced tolerance (e.g. oral tolerance). If antigen deposition via MALT is essential for induction of systemic unresponsiveness, it is likely that optimization of antigen delivery vehicles (including live vectors) that target M cells may improve immunization schema for development of mucosally induced tolerance.

The underlying dome region of the Peyer's patch consists of sparse plasma cells, as well as B and T lymphocytes (Gebert et al. 1996; Adachi et al. 1997), and this suggests that immediate antigen presentation may occur in the dome area after antigen uptake. It is also possible that T- and B-cell interactions in the dome area provide necessary protection for the Peyer's patch. The presence of MΦs (Sminia and van der Ende 1991) including the tingible body type suggests that significant apoptosis occurs, but is not yet proven. An immunohistological study has called into question whether dome MΦs are indeed a major cell type (Kelsall and Strober 1996). This important study has described a major APC population in the dome with characteristics of DCs (Kelsall and Strober 1996) (Figure 28.7). Interestingly, the dome DCs were N418$^+$ (anti-CD11c) and could be differentiated from more classic DCs present in the interfollicular area (T-cell zone), demonstrating that at least two DC subsets occur in key antigen-sampling areas of the Peyer's patch (Kelsall and Strober 1996). This study also suggested that fewer numbers of B220$^+$ B cells occur in the dome area of mouse GALT. Studies of the lymphocyte populations associated with human M-cell pockets, the area where luminal antigen may first be recognized by T and B lymphocytes, have also provided evidence for a characteristic T-cell distribution, e.g. M-cell pockets in human GALT contain approximately equal numbers of CD3$^+$ T and CD19$^+$/CD20$^+$ B lymphocytes with fewer CD68$^+$ macrophages (Farstad et al. 1994). Of the T cells in this location, approximately 75 percent exhibited a T-helper cell phenotype.

Distinct follicles (B-cell zones) are located beneath the dome area of the Peyer's patches and contain germinal centers where significant B-cell division is seen (Figure 28.6a). These germinal centers, which contain most of the sIgA$^+$ B cells (Butcher et al. 1982; Lebman et al. 1987; George and Cebra 1991; Weinstein and Cebra 1991; Weinstein et al. 1991), are considered to be sites where frequent B-cell switches to IgA and affinity maturation occur. However, unlike immune lymph nodes and the spleen in the systemic compartment, plasma cell development does not occur. All major T-cell subsets are found in the T-cell-dependent areas adjacent to follicles. The parafollicular T cells are mature and more than 97 percent of these T cells use the αβ heterodimer form of the TCR (Figure 28.6b). Approximately two-thirds of Peyer's patch αβ TCR$^+$ T cells are CD4$^+$, CD8$^-$ and exhibit properties of Th cells, including support for IgA responses (Kiyono et al. 1982a). Approximately one-third of the αβ T cells in GALT are CD4$^-$, CD8$^+$; this T-cell subset contains precursors of CTLs (London et al. 1987, 1990), whereas other CD8$^+$ T-cell subsets appear to contribute to mucosally-induced tolerance (see below).

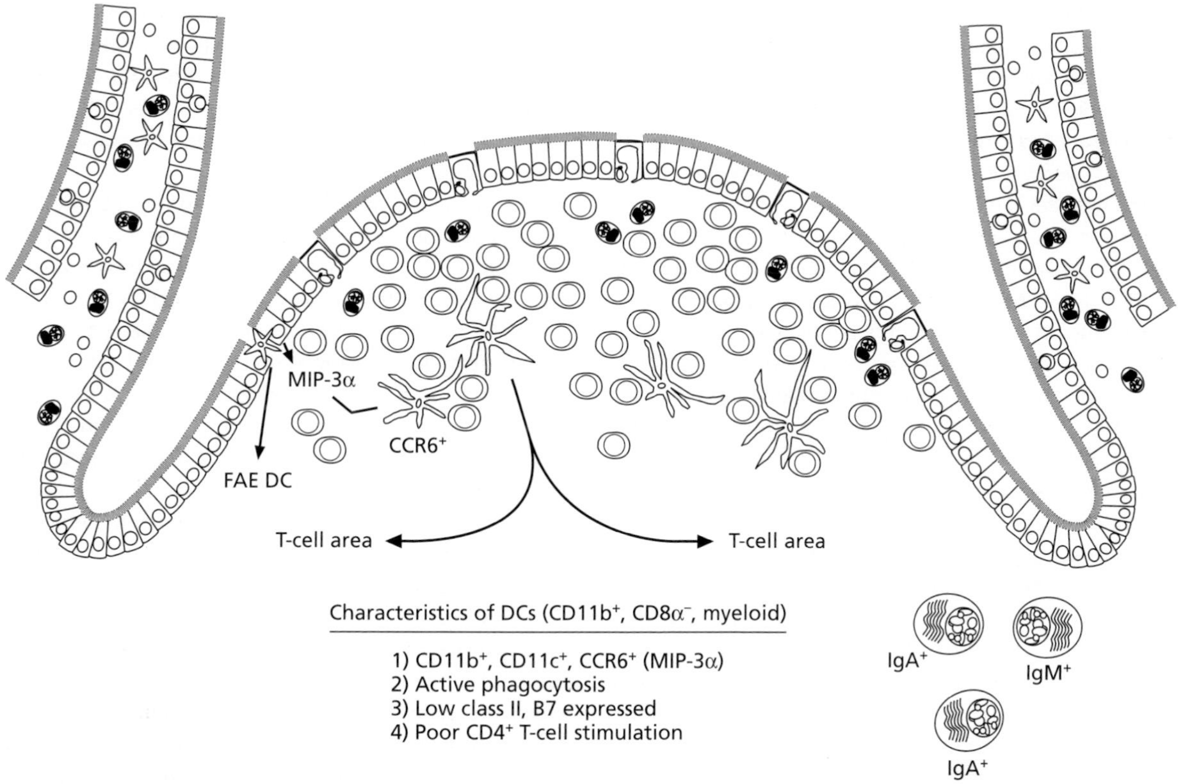

Figure 28.7 *Gut-associated lymphoreticular tissue (GALT) compartments: the subepithelial dome region of the Peyer's patch consists of sparse plasma cells, as well as B and T lymphocytes. A major antigen-presenting cell (APC) population in the subepithelial dome with characteristics of dendritic cells (DCs) plays a role in immediate antigen presentation in the dome area after antigen uptake. FAE, follicle-associated epithelium.*

NASAL-ASSOCIATED LYMPHOEPITHELIAL TISSUE

Although the mouse has been the major model used to study Peyer's patches, the human tonsils are the most accessible secondary lymphoid tissue for study of NALT and, as such, a great deal is known about the component cells (see Figure 28.5). Although the palatine and nasopharyngeal tonsils (adenoids) are largely covered by a squamous epithelium and are often not appreciated as mucosal tissues, the palatine tonsils usually contain 10–20 crypts that increase their surface area. The deeper regions of these crypts contain M cells, which may take up encountered antigens (Owen and Nemanic 1978; Allan et al. 1993). The tonsils contain all major classes of APCs including DCs and Langerhans' cells, MΦs, class II^+ B cells and antigen-retaining, follicular DCs in B-cell germinal centers (see Figure 28.2). Tonsillar APCs are capable of inducing T-cell proliferative and cytokine responses following in vitro restimulation with appropriate vaccines such as tetanus and diphtheria toxoid and purified protein derivative (PPD) of *M. tuberculosis*.

Approximately half of tonsillar cells are B lymphocytes and mainly occur in follicle-containing germinal centers. Most human tonsillar B cells are actually surface IgG-positive ($sIgG^+$); however, significant numbers of $sIgM^+$ and $sIgA^+$ B cells are also present. Further, in situ staining of B-cell blasts/plasma cells indicate a predominance of IgG blasts in germinal centers and of plasma cells in the parafollicular area. The overall ratio of Ig^+ cells was 65:30 for IgG versus IgA (Brandtzaeg et al. 1978; Boyaka et al. 2000). The human palatine tonsil also contains a distinct subepithelial B-cell population which differs from both germinal center and follicular mantle B cells (Dono et al. 1996a, b). This subset may represent the homolog of the extrafollicular B cells of the splenic marginal zone (Dono et al. 1996a, b). It is not accurate to suggest that the tonsils are only a mucosal IgA-inductive site, because of the presence of B cells committed to other isotypes, especially for IgG subclasses. Approximately 40 percent of tonsillar cells are T cells and more than 98 percent express the αβ TCR. Further, somewhat higher CD4:CD8 ratios are found in tonsils (3:1) when compared with peripheral blood or murine Peyer's patches. In summary, the tonsils clearly exhibit not only features of mucosal inductive sites, but also characteristics of effector sites with high numbers of plasma cells. The role of the tonsils in host mucosal immunity after intranasal immunization is not yet established.

To understand the precise contribution of NALT to the induction of IgA responses to inhaled antigens, studies in both mice and rats have established a NALT-like structure (Kuper et al. 1992; Asanuma et al. 1995;

Wu et al. 1996). The NALT consists of bilateral strips of nonencapsulated lymphoid tissue underlying the epithelium on the ventral aspect of the posterior nasal tract and exhibits a bell-like shape in cross-sections (Kilian and Russell 1994; Wu et al. 1997; Hiroi et al. 1998). Although dense aggregates of lymphocytes have been observed in the NALT of normal mice, germinal centers are absent, but could be induced by nasal application of antigen (Hiroi et al. 1998). Thus, uncommitted B cells ($sIgM^+$) have been found in high proportions (80–85 percent), whereas low numbers of $sIgA^+$ and $sIgG^+$ B cells (3–4 percent and 0–1 percent, respectively) have been noted in mononuclear cells isolated from NALT (Wu et al. 1996; Hiroi et al. 1998). In contrast to GALT where a high frequency (10–15 percent) of $sIgA^+$ B cells occur, NALT was found to contain fewer IgA-committed B cells. Despite this, nasal immunization induces much higher numbers of IgA^+ than IgG^+ NALT B cells in the memory compartment, showing the propensity of NALT for mucosal S-IgA Ab responses (McGhee et al. 1989). Characterization of isolated NALT mononuclear cells revealed that approximately 30–40 percent of these cells are $CD3^+$ T cells with a CD4/CD8 ratio of about 3.0 (Wu et al. 1996, 1997; Hiroi et al. 1998). The majority of NALT $CD3^+$ T cells co-express CD45RB, suggestive of naïve, resting T cells (Wu et al. 1996, 1997; Hiroi et al. 1998). As transcriptional single cell analysis revealed the expression of mRNA for both Th1 and Th2 cytokines, the majority of $CD4^+$ T cells are considered to be Thp or Th0 types (Hiroi et al. 1998). Further, stimulation via the TCR–CD3 complex resulted in differentiation of both Th1- and Th2-type cells. These results support the notion that NALT exhibits characteristics of mucosal inductive sites.

Mucosal effector tissues

After initial exposure to antigen in MALT, mucosal lymphocytes leave the inductive site and home to mucosal effector tissues. This pathway, which results in immunity at several mucous membrane sites, is referred to as the common mucosal immune system (CMIS) (see Figure 28.5). Effector sites for mucosal immune responses include the lymphoid cells in the lamina propria (LP) regions of the GI, URT, and reproductive tracts as well as secretory glandular tissues such as mammary, salivary, and lacrimal glands (Adachi et al. 1997). In addition, most evidence suggests that the lymphocytes that reside in the epithelium (i.e. IELs) also serve as effector cells; however, it has been difficult to define IEL functions precisely (see Figure 28.3). Antigen-specific mucosal effector cells include IgA-producing plasma cells as well as B and T lymphocytes. IgA is the primary Ig involved in protecting mucosal surfaces and is locally produced in effector tissues (Adachi et al. 1997). Again, the presence of antigen-specific S-IgA Abs at mucosal surfaces other than the inductive site where antigen uptake initially occurred is definitive evidence of the CMIS. Thus, it would suggest that immunization of either NALT or GALT could induce mucosal immune responses in all mucosal effector tissues.

Effector mechanisms employed to protect mucosal surfaces include CTLs, as well as effector $CD4^+$ Th cells for CMI (Th1) and for S-IgA Ab (Th2) responses (McGhee et al. 1989; Kilian and Russell 1994). Indeed, both CTL and S-IgA Ab responses have been associated with protection against infection at mucosal surfaces and both may be important for resistance to, or more importantly prevention of, mucosal infection with viruses including HIV (Staats et al. 1994). Although little information about protective $CD4^+$ Th1-CMI responses is available, mucosal CMI responses appear to be important in tolerance and in control of infections by intracellular pathogens.

It must be remembered, however, that effector sites, which must serve as a barrier against numerous environmental foreign antigens and mucosal pathogens with which the inductive sites need not contend, will offer mechanisms of protection significantly different from those seen in the inductive sites. The high concentration of IgA plasma cells (estimated at $>10^{10}$ IgA plasma cells per meter of human small intestine (Brandtzaeg and Farstad 1999)) has traditionally been viewed as the most distinctive trait of the immunity offered at these effector sites (Figure 28.8). As discussed below, the murine GI lamina propria has an almost equal distribution of peritoneal B1 B-cell-derived IgA plasma cells. Further, the lamina propria of the gut also contains more than 50 percent IgA plasma cells that are B2 GALT B-cell derived (see below). However, as important, if not more so, are the large numbers of B and T lymphocytes (e.g. lamina propria lymphocytes (LPL)), more than 60 percent of which are T cells (James et al. 1986; Abreu-Martin and Targan 1996). The importance of these cell types is discussed in detail below.

When presented with an environmental antigen, epithelial cells endocytose it and in some cases themselves express MHC II molecules, processing antigens with subsequent association of immunogenic peptides with MHC II (Mayer and Shlien 1987). It has also been shown that Langerhans-like cells occur on the luminal side of the intestine at epithelial junctions between epithelial cells which could also provide accessory functions (Huang et al. 2000). When confronted with microorganisms and even with soluble proteins that can transverse the tight junctions between epithelial cells, the APCs at the effector sites may process them and so induce B- and T-cell responses. Some have suggested that MHC II^+ $sIgA^+$ B cells may bind antigen through endocytic pathways, process, and present peptides to $CD4^+$ Th cells. Macrophages in LP regions could also function in this manner for more complex antigens.

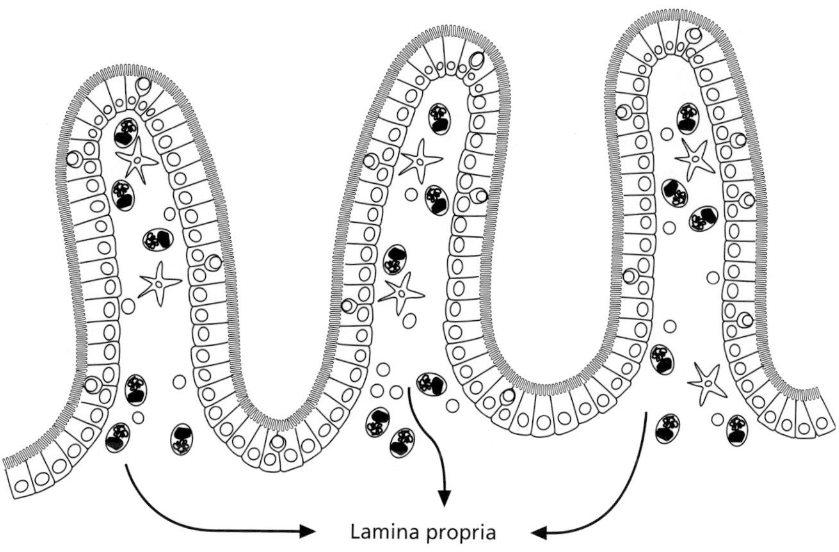

B lineage	
CD5⁺	~ 50%
CD5⁻	~ 50%
Memory	~ 90%
Naive	<5%
Plasma cells	20%
IgA⁺	79–90%
IgM⁺	11–18%
IgG⁺	3–5%

T lineage	
$\alpha\beta$TCR⁺	95–75%
$\gamma\delta$TCR⁺	3–5%
CD4⁺ Th:	60–70%
Th1	~ 40%
Th2	~ 60%
CD8⁺ CTL	30–40%
Memory	~ 95%
Naive	~ 5%
Activated, CD25⁺ blasts	20%

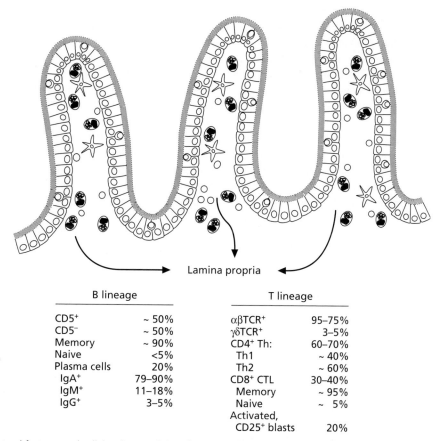

Figure 28.8 *Structural features and cellular characteristics of mucosal effector sites. The lamina propria is equally populated by B1 and B2 cells, both of which differentiate into IgA⁺ plasma cells. Note that memory B and T lymphocytes occur in this compartment.*

Freshly isolated mouse intestinal LP CD4⁺ T cells contain high numbers of IL-5-secreting Th2-type cells in addition to IFN-γ-secreting Th1-type cells, suggesting that the effector regions of the mucosal immune system are somewhat biased toward a Th2 phenotype (Taguchi et al. 1990a, b). Further, recent findings obtained by a single cell reverse transcriptase polymerase chain reaction (RT-PCR) analysis of CD4⁺ T cells from murine nasal passages revealed a high frequency of CD4⁺ T cells expressing Th2 cytokine-specific mRNA (Hiroi et al. 1998). In summary, mucosal effector tissues contain all the necessary cellular components including epithelial cells, Th1/Th2 type CD4⁺ T cells, CTLs, and IgA-producing cells for a multilayer barrier against the numerous environmental foreign antigens and mucosal pathogens.

MUCOSAL T CELLS AND CYTOKINES

T cells and cytokines that influence IgA switching

It is known that cytokines exert profound influences on B-cell switching from sIgM, sIgD expression to downstream isotypes including IgG subclasses, IgE, and IgA. Clear evidence was presented that clones of T cells from murine GALT, when mixed with noncommitted sIgM⁺ B cells, induced isotype switching to B cells expressing sIgA (Kawanishi et al. 1983a, b) (see Figure 28.6a). More recent studies have revealed that T-cell–B-cell interactions support B-cell switches and have postulated a major role for the CD40 receptor on germinal center B cells with CD40L on activated T cells (Fuleihan et al. 1993; Banchereau et al. 1994; MacLennan 1994). In terms of cytokines involved in IgA switching, the most definitive studies to date suggest that transforming growth factor-β1 (TGF-β1) is the major cytokine (Coffman et al. 1989; Sonoda et al. 1989) (see Figure 28.6a). The first studies showed that addition of TGF-β1 to LPS-triggered mouse splenic B-cell cultures resulted in switching to IgA, and IgA synthesis was markedly enhanced by IL-2 (Lebman et al. 1990a) and IL-5 (Sonoda et al. 1989). The effect of TGF-β1 was on sIgM⁺, sIgA⁻ B cells and was not the result of selective induction of terminal B-cell differentiation. It was shown that TGF-β1 induced sterile Cα germline transcripts (Coffman et al. 1989; Lebman et al. 1990b), an event that clearly precedes actual switching to IgA. Importantly, TGF-$\beta^{-/-}$ mice exhibit low levels of IgA⁺ plasma cells in effector sites and of S-IgA in external secretions, providing evidence that TGF-β1 is also important for $\mu \rightarrow \alpha$ switching in vivo (van Ginkel et al. 1999).

Although many presume that isotype switching to IgA (i.e. $\mu \rightarrow \alpha$) occurs in mucosal inductive sites such as GALT, and that terminal differentiation into plasma cells producing IgA is a major event in effector sites, only indirect evidence is at hand to support these assumptions. In this regard, most studies of $\mu \rightarrow \alpha$ switching have been performed with nonmucosal lymphoid cells, e.g. splenic B cells, whereas in vitro studies of B-cell differentiation to IgA synthesis normally employ Peyer's patch B cells (a mucosal inductive site) to support the idea that this also occurs in effector mucosal sites, such as LP and exocrine glands. Moreover, cytokine knock-out mice have been employed to determine the relevance of particular cytokines for mucosal immunity, an approach discussed below. That this dogma of $\mu \rightarrow \alpha$ switching occurs only in mucosal inductive sites is challenged by several recent findings. The activation-induced cytokine deaminaseAID) gene, initially discovered in germinal center B cells (Muramatsu etal. 1999) has been cloned from B-lymphoma cells stimulated with CD40L, IL-4, and TGF-β1 which were undergoing $\mu \rightarrow \alpha$ switches (Muramatsu etal. 2000). Over-expression of AID in μ^+ B-lymphoma cells resulted in spontaneous class switching from IgM to IgA in the complete absence of TGF-β1 or other cytokines (Muramatsu etal. 2000). Mice defective in the AID gene ($AID^{-/-}$) and humans with AID deficiency exhibit a hyper-IgM syndrome with no evidence of downstream switching (Muramatsu et al. 2000; Revy et al. 2000). However, recent studies revealed that $AID^{-/-}$ mice have a subset of $B220^+$ surface IgA^+ B cells in lamina propria (an effector site), and the presence of circles of 'looped out' DNA suggest that $\mu \rightarrow \alpha$ switching had just occurred in this site (Fagarasan et al. 2001). Most recent reports have shown the presence of isolated lymphocyte follicles (ILF) in the LP that contain $sIgA^+$ B cells (Hamada et al. 2002). Thus, it is still possible that these ILFs are the sites of IgA switching. Along these lines, it was also recently revealed that B-cell-deficient, μMT mice also exhibit LP IgA^+ plasma cells, suggesting that switches to IgA can occur even during pre-B-cell development (Macpherson et al. 2001). These intriguing studies have used mouse models where class switching in germinal centers is absent. Thus, $\mu \rightarrow \alpha$ B-cell switches may occur throughout the mucosal immune system and in the complete absence of germinal centers.

T cells and their derived cyokines for IgA synthesis

$CD4^+$ T cells and cytokines are essential for the generation of IgA-producing cells, e.g. depletion of $CD4^+$ T-cell subsets in vivo with mAbs or by knockout of the CD4 co-receptor gene markedly affects mucosal immune responses (Mega et al. 1991; Hörnquist et al. 1995). Loss of $CD4^+$ T cells is associated with diminished levels of IgA^+ plasma cells (Mega et al. 1991) and with deficient Th-cell-regulated IgA responses (Hörnquist et al. 1995). For B-cell terminal differentiation, IL-5 and especially IL-6, possibly in combination with other cytokines, appear essential for the continued presence of plasma cells undergoing high-rate secretion of IgA antibodies (Beagley et al. 1988, 1989; Harriman et al. 1988) (see Figure 28.6a).

Earlier studies revealed that addition of culture supernatants from DC–T-cell clusters, T-cell clones, or T-cell hybridomas to cultures of Peyer's patch or splenic B cells resulted in enhanced secretion of IgA (Spalding et al. 1984; Kiyono et al. 1985). One cytokine responsible for this activity was subsequently shown to be IL-5 (Coffman et al. 1987; Murray et al. 1987; Beagley et al. 1988; Harriman et al. 1988; Lebman and Coffman 1988; Lebman et al. 1990a). Removal of $sIgA^+$ B cells from Peyer's patch (PP) B-cell cultures abrogated IgA synthesis, demonstrating that this cytokine affected post-switched, IgA-committed B cells (Murray et al. 1987). No in vitro stimulus was required for Peyer's patch B cells and IL-4 did not further enhance the effect of IL-5 (Lebman and Coffman 1988). Taken together, these results suggest that IL-5 induces $sIgA^+$ B cells that are in cell cycle (blasts) to differentiate into IgA-producing plasma cells (Figure 28.9). Interestingly, another B-cell population, the peritoneal cavity B-1 cells, has been shown to contain precursors of lamina propria IgA^+ plasma cells (Kroese et al. 1989). Human IL-5 is thought to act mainly as an eosinophil differentiation factor and thus may have little effect on B-cell isotype switching and differentiation. It has been reported, however, that human B cells, when stimulated with the bacterium *Moraxella (Branhamella) catarrhalis*, could be induced by IL-5 to secrete IgA, and also possibly to undergo isotype switching to IgA (Benson et al. 1990). This effect could not be demonstrated using other more conventional B-cell mitogens, a finding that demonstrates the importance of the primary in vitro activation signal for B-cell switching.

The cytokine IL-6, when added to Peyer's patch B cells in the absence of any in vitro stimulus, causes a marked increase in IgA secretion with little effect on either IgM or IgG synthesis (Beagley et al. 1989) (Figure 28.9). In these studies, IL-6 induced two- to threefold more IgA than IL-5 (Beagley et al. 1989). The removal of $sIgA^+$ B cells abolished the effect of IL-6, demonstrating that, similar to IL-5, this cytokine also acted on post-switched B cells. Of relevance was the finding that human appendix $sIgA^+$ B cells express IL-6 receptors, whereas other B-cell subsets present do not. Further, appendix B cells were induced by IL-6 to secrete both IgA1 and IgA2 in the absence of any in

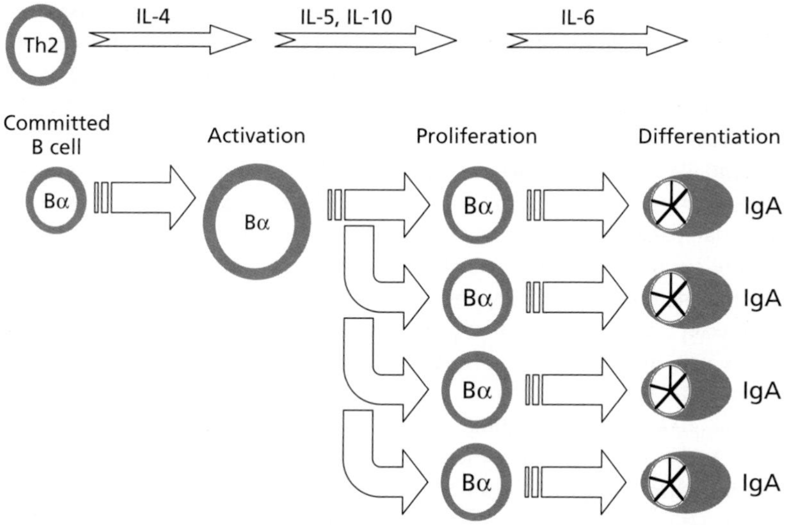

Figure 28.9 *Cytokine cascades in mucosal IgA immunity. T-helper 2 (Th2)-type cyokines clearly support the induction of IgA antibody responses. Interleukin-4 (IL-4) activates post-switched IgA-committed B cells and IL-5 induces sIgA$^+$ B cells which are in cell cycle (blasts) to differentiate into IgA-producing cells. IL-6 induces a marked increase in IgA secretion (two- to three-fold more IgA secretion than IL-5) when added to Peyer's patch B cells in the absence of any in vitro stimulus.*

vitro activation (Fujihashi et al. 1991) (Figure 28.9). This effect was also shown in IgA-committed B cells, again demonstrating the importance of IL-6 for inducing the terminal differentiation of sIgA$^+$ B cells into IgA-producing plasma cells. An additional Th2 cell cytokine, IL-10, has also been shown to play an important role in the induction of IgA synthesis in humans (DeFrance et al. 1992; Nonoyama et al. 1993; Briere et al. 1994). Taken together, these findings demonstrate that Th2 cell cytokines, such as IL-5, IL-6, and IL-10, all play major roles in the induction of IgA plasma cell responses.

INDUCTION OF MUCOSAL IMMUNITY AND VACCINES

Immune responses expressed in mucosal tissues are typified by S-IgA Abs (McGhee et al. 1999). This S-IgA constitutes the predominant Ig class in human external secretions, and is the best-known entity providing specific immune protection for mucosal tissues (Figure 28.10). The resistance of S-IgA Abs to endogenous proteases makes Abs of this isotype uniquely well suited to protect mucosal surfaces. Specific S-IgA

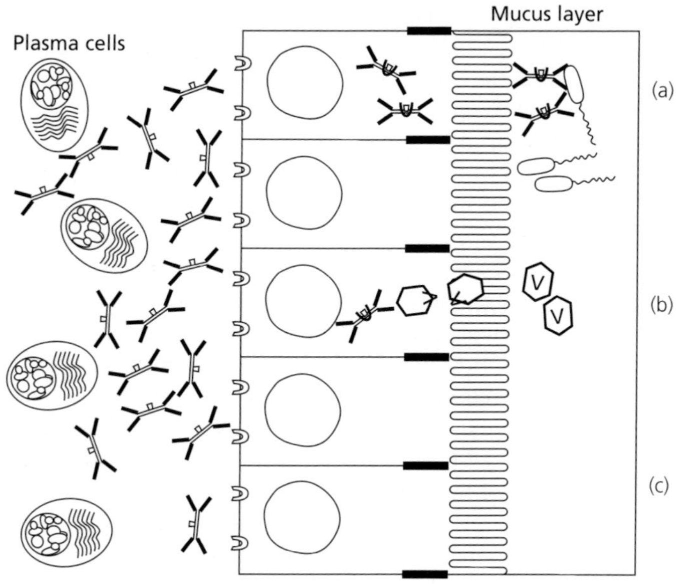

Figure 28.10 *The multiple functions of IgA: immunobiological function of antigen-specific secretory IgA antibody (S-IgA) for mucosal immunity. S-IgA constitutes the predominant immunoglobulin class in human external secretions and is the best-known entity providing specific immune protection for mucosal tissues.* **(a)** *Inhibition of adherence:* S. mutans, Vibrio cholerae, Shigella *spp.*, Escherichia coli, Giardia *spp.*, Haemophilus influenzae, *others;* **(b)** *Intracellular neutralization of:* rotavirus, Sendai virus, reovirus; **(c)** *removal of pIgA immune complexes.*

Abs provide classic 'immune exclusion' of noxious antigens. In addition, S-IgA prevents adherence of bacterial pathogens to epithelial cells and may also neutralize viral particles. Mucosal S-IgA Abs can serve as antitoxins to neutralize bacterial exotoxins, including enterotoxins and other potentially harmful molecules. In addition, S-IgA Abs may interfere with the utilization of growth factors for bacterial pathogens in the mucosal environment. Furthermore, it now appears that pIgA Abs, in the process of transport through the epithelial cell via the polymeric Ig receptor (pIgR), can also function to neutralize viruses and may also transport Ag–IgA complexes into external secretions (Ostov and Kaetzel 1999; Zhang et al. 2000). Taken together, it is essential to induce S-IgA Ab responses in order to provide effective mucosal immunity to environmental antigens, allergens, and infectious pathogens.

Mucosal APCs

Antigen presentation in mucosal tissues reflects the complexity of immune responses that occur in these sites. Indeed, the site of mucosal antigen uptake (i.e. M cells or epithelial cells) and the nature of antigen presentation that takes place will determine the outcome of the immune response. It is now well accepted that large macromolecules are taken up by M cells in the GI tract. It is controversial as to whether M cells express MHC II molecules and present antigen to immune effector cells (Hirata et al. 1986; Bjerke et al. 1993). However, as mentioned earlier, the presence of all three major APC types (i.e. memory B cells, MΦs, and DCs) in the dome epithelium of Peyer's patches make it likely that antigen uptake occurs immediately after release from M cells. Immunohistology of murine Peyer's patches have shown that $N418^+$, $2A1^+$, NLDC-145^-, $M342^-$ DCs form a dense layer of cells in the subepithelial dome (SED), just beneath the follicle epithelium where $CD3^+$ and $CD4^+$, but not $CD8^+$, T cells occur (Kelsall and Strober 1996) (see Figure 28.7). Another subset of DCs, $N418^+$, $2A1^+$, NLDC-145^+, and $M342^+$ DCs, was identified in the interfollicular T-cell regions where $CD3^+$, $CD4^+$, and $CD8^+$ T cells reside (Kelsall and Strober 1996). In contrast with DCs in the dome region, which express the phenotype of immature DCs (i.e. high endocytic activity and low levels of MHC and B7 molecule expression), those in the T-cell areas are mature, interdigitating DCs with low endocytic activity and high levels of MHC I and II as well as B7 molecules (Kelsall and Strober 1996). The presence of these separate populations of DCs suggest that antigen is taken up by M cells and is first endocytosed in the dome region by DCs which may migrate to T-cell areas to become mature DCs.

It has recently been shown that Peyer's patch DCs preferentially promote Th2-type cells (Iwasaki and Kelsall 1999), suggesting that these cells also influence the nature of immune responses initiated in the gut. Few MΦs occur in the SED; however, both B cells and MΦs were found in the interfollicular T regions of Peyer's patches and lamina propria of intestinal villi. In addition, memory B and T cells occur in the pockets formed by M cells, and may be initial sites of immune responses (Yamanaka et al. 2001). DCs are also found in the NALT where they seem to play the same role as in the GALT. In fact, DCs are found in human tonsils (Bernstein 1999). It has been shown that DCs are recruited into the respiratory epithelium during acute immune responses induced by bacterial, viral, and protein antigens (McWilliam et al. 1996). In this regard, although freshly isolated rat respiratory DCs preferentially supported $CD4^+$ Th2-type responses, induction of Th1-type cytokine-mediated immune responses was also seen after stimulation with antigens (Stumbles et al. 1998). Studies of this nature suggest a further compartmentalization/specialization for antigen presentation by classic mucosal APCs; however, much is still unknown about the transport of antigen from M cells to DCs, MΦs, and memory B cells.

Mucosal immunization

It is generally agreed that mucosal adjuvants or delivery systems are essential in order to induce mucosal immune responses. In this regard, two bacterial enterotoxins (i.e. CT and LT from *E. coli*) are now established as very effective mucosal adjuvants for the induction of both mucosal and systemic immunity to co-administered protein antigens. To circumvent toxicity linked to these enterotoxins, mutant CT (mCT) and mutant LT (mLT) molecules devoid of their toxic activity were generated by site-directed mutagenesis. This approach involves the introduction of single amino acid substitutions in the active site (i.e. the site responsible for the ADP-ribosylation activity) of the A subunit of CT or LT or in the protease-sensitive loop of LT. Further, attenuated pathogenic bacteria such as recombinant (r) *Salmonella* were also used as a mucosal delivery system for the induction of S-IgA Ab responses to delivered antigen.

It is now realized that the nature of the delivery system as well as the route of immunization influences the nature of Th cell subsets induced and markedly affect the outcome of systemic and mucosal immunity, e.g. use of native CT or nontoxic mutants of CT with vaccines given orally tends to induce $CD4^+$ Th2-type cells with characteristic serum IgG1, IgG2b, IgE, and IgA as well as mucosal S-IgA Ab responses (Xu-Amano et al. 1993; Marinaro et al. 1995) (Figure 28.11). On the other hand, oral immunization with recombinant bacteria, e.g. r*Salmonella*-expressing proteins, tends to induce not only $CD4^+$ Th1-type cells and CMI responses but characteristic $CD4^+$ Th cells as well. These $CD4^+$ Th cells produce cytokines such as IFN-γ and IL-10 which appear to support mucosal S-IgA Ab responses

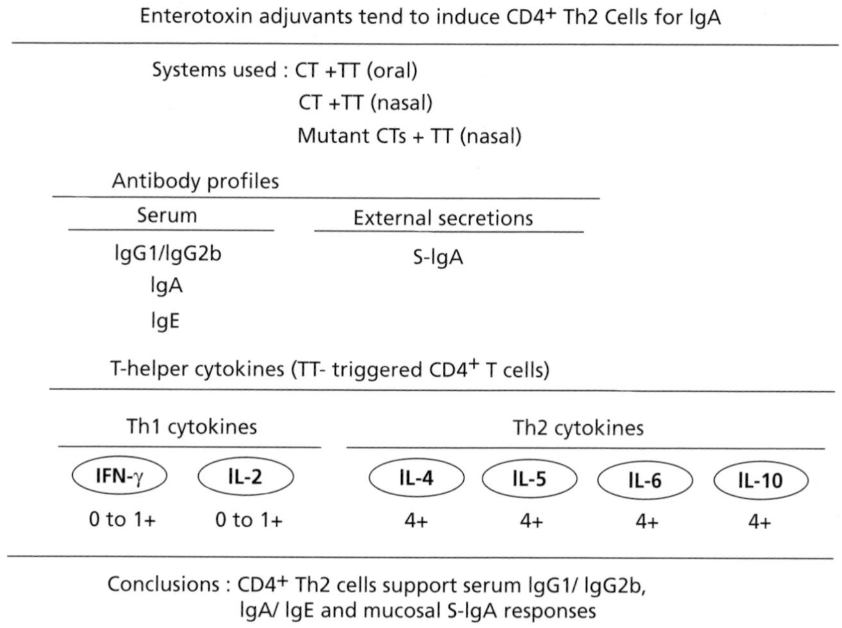

Figure 28.11 *T-helper 2 (Th2) cells for IgA responses. Th2-type cytokines mediate S-IgA Ab response induction. Use of native cholera toxin (CT) or nontoxic mutants of CT with vaccines given orally tend to induce CD4⁺ Th2-type cells with characteristic serum IgG1, IgG2b, IgE, and IgA as well as mucosal S-IgA responses.*

(Okahashi et al. 1996; VanCott et al. 1996). In this section, we have selected studies that illustrate the development of oral and nasal immunization strategies using either mucosal adjuvants or live vectors for mucosal vaccine development.

ORAL IMMUNIZATION

We have purposely selected a small subset of studies to illustrate the nature of murine immune responses which result from oral immunization with microbial vaccines. It is important to emphasize that immune responses vary depending on the nature of antigen used as well as mouse strains selected for study. However, proteins such as tetanus toxoid (TT) or hen egg white lysozyme (HEL) with CT as mucosal adjuvant induce predominantly serum IgG1 and IgE antibodies (Snider et al. 1994; Marinaro et al. 1995) (Figure 28.11). Further, in one study it was shown that systemic challenge of mice orally immunized with HEL and CT led to a fatal anaphylactic response (Snider et al. 1994). Thus, all studies that use CT or its mutant derivatives should be concerned with possible untoward reactions which may occur as a result of induction of IgE Ab responses. Oral immunization of mice with keyhole limpet hemocyanin (KLH) or TT and CT as adjuvant has been shown to induce Ag-specific $CD4^+$ Th cells with a characteristic Th2 phenotype (Wilson et al. 1991; Xu-Amano et al. 1993; Marinaro et al. 1995) (Figure 28.11), e.g. both PP and lamina propria lymphocytes, when restimulated with KLH, produced significant quantities of IL-4 and IL-5, with minimal levels of IFN-γ and IL-2 (Wilson et al. 1991). Thus, several studies now support the notion that oral immunization with soluble proteins and CT as adjuvant induces Th2-type responses, which provide help for characteristic serum IgG1 and IgE as well as mucosal S-IgA Abs. There is evidence that orally co-administered CT can also induce antigen-specific $CD4^+$ Th1-type responses, e.g. mice given a soluble preparation of *Toxoplasma gondii* on three occasions at 10-day intervals harbored splenic *T. gondii*-specific T cells (Bourguin et al. 1993). Further, in vitro restimulation resulted in increased levels of both IFN-γ and IL-2, whereas IL-4 and IL-5 levels were similar to those seen in mice orally immunized with *T. gondii* only (Bourguin et al. 1993).

A more revealing study used the mouse parasite *Trichuris muris* in a soluble form with CT and assessed IFN-γ and IL-5 levels as markers for Th1- or Th2-type responses respectively (Robinson et al. 1995). Interestingly, oral *T. muris* plus CT induced T cells that produced IL-5 before parasite challenge, but which switched to IFN-γ production after *T. muris* infection. This shift suggests that the infection itself results in $CD4^+$ Th1-type responses, even in the presence of a predominant Th2-type response. One study has shown that oral immunization with parasite antigen and CT elicits both serum IgG and mucosal IgA Ab responses (Zhang et al. 1995). This study, which also assessed anti-parasite Abs in bile (where IgA was the predominant isotype), revealed that oral immunization normally induces serum IgA, and in experimental species such as mice, rats, and rabbits, where the serum IgA is predominantly polymeric, the pIgA is transported into the GI tract. Thus, all studies that assess intestinal IgA responses should ensure that the response actually occurs locally and therefore perform assays to detect IgA-producing plasma cells in lamina propria regions of the GI tract.

Attenuated avirulent salmonella strains have received considerable attention as mucosal vaccine delivery vectors for recombinant proteins associated with virulence (Chatfield et al. 1993; Curtiss et al. 1993; Roberts et al. 1994; Doggett and Brown 1996). After oral administration, *Salmonella* spp. replicate directly in the mucosa-associated tissues (e.g. PP) and thereafter disseminate via the MALT to systemic sites (e.g. spleen). This characteristic dissemination pattern of growth in both mucosal and systemic sites allows *Salmonella* spp. to induce broad-based immune responses, including cell-mediated as well as serum IgG and mucosal S-IgA Ab responses. Although a large number of genes from bacteria, viruses, parasites, and mammals have been expressed in attenuated r*Salmonella* spp. (Curtiss et al. 1993; Roberts et al. 1994), few studies have fully characterized both T- and B-cell responses to the expressed protein Ag. In particular, the balance between Ag-specific $CD4^+$ Th1 and Th2 cells, and their subsequent influence on subclass-specific IgG and mucosal IgA responses, have received little attention in these systems. Such clarity is paramount to the development of delivery protocols that will provide the appropriate immune response to a given pathogen.

A pioneering study in this area showed that mice given an oral attenuated *S. typhimurium* (expressing leishmania surface protein gp63) elicited $CD4^+$ T cells that produced IFN-γ and IL-2, but not IL-4 (Yang et al. 1990). The results at first might appear puzzling. As it appears that mucosal S-IgA responses are dependent on Th2 cells and cytokines such as IL-5, IL-6, and IL-10, by what mechanisms do these attenuated r*Salmonella*-expressing foreign protein antigens induce S-IgA responses? Recent studies have addressed this issue by use of r*Salmonella* spp. expressing the *Tox C* gene of TT. Oral administration of r*Salmonella Tox C* resulted in predominant serum IgG2a and IgG2b anti-TT as well as mucosal S-IgA anti-TT Ab responses (VanCott et al. 1996) (Figure 28.12). Further, splenic and PP $CD4^+$ T cells selectively produced IFN-γ and IL-2 as well as the Th2-cytokine IL-10 (VanCott et al. 1996). Also, Mϕs from these mice produced heightened levels of IL-6 (VanCott et al. 1996) (Figure 28.12). Clear verification that IL-4 is not involved was shown by oral immunization of IL-4 knockout ($IL\text{-}4^{-/-}$) mice which produced serum IgG2a and mucosal S-IgA Abs. Interestingly, $CD4^+$ T cells in these mice exhibited two cytokine patterns, a Th1-phenotype as well as T cells that produced IL-6 and IL-10, but not IL-5 (Okahashi et al. 1996) (see Figure 28.11). The latter subset of Th2 cells, which produce only IgA-enhancing cytokines, has been termed 'level 2 Th2-type cells' in contrast to so-called 'level 1 Th2-type cells' producing an array of IL-4, IL-5, IL-6, and IL-10.

NASAL IMMUNIZATION

Nasal antigen plus mucosal adjuvant delivery has emerged as perhaps the most effective route for induction of both peripheral and mucosal immunity. Again, most studies can be divided into those that use soluble vaccine components with mucosal adjuvants such as CT

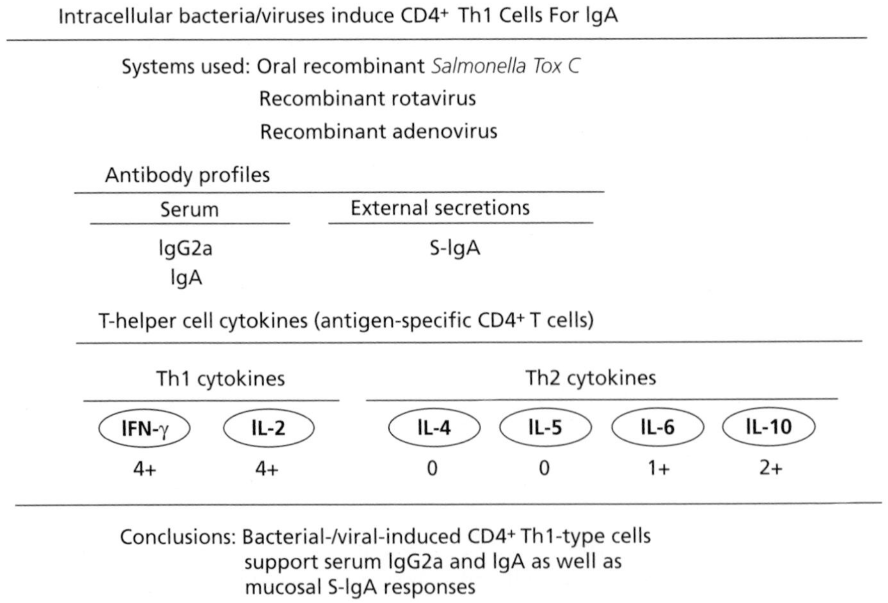

Figure 28.12 *T-helper 1 (Th1) cells for IgA responses: induction of S-IgA Abs via Th1-type responses. Oral administration of recombinant* Salmonella Tox C *resulted in predominant serum IgG2a and IgG2b anti-tetanus toxin (TT) as well as mucosal S-IgA anti-TT Ab responses. Further, splenic and Peyer's patch* $CD4^+$ *T cells selectively produced interferon-γ and interleukin-2 as well as the Th2 cytokine interleukin-10.*

(as well as protein–CT-B conjugates) versus studies with attenuated vectors. A series of extensive studies using the influenza virus model demonstrated that nasal immunization with influenza vaccine provides more effective protective immunity than oral immunization (Hirabayashi et al. 1990; Tamura and Kurata 1996). Nasal immunization with trivalent influenza vaccines in the presence of CT-B containing a trace amount of A subunit provides cross-protection against a broad range of viruses (Tamura et al. 1992). It was also shown that nasal immunization with influenza vaccine together with LT-B (containing a trace amount of the LT) induces antigen-specific immune responses in humans (Hashigucci et al. 1996). These findings show that an appropriate nasal vaccine can provide effective immunity against viral infection.

With regard to vectors, most studies have been limited to respiratory tract viral pathogens, which have been subjected to attenuating mutations or genomic deletions. It is interesting that recombinant adenoviruses (r-Ad), currently used for gene therapy, are also candidates for mucosal delivery of vaccine proteins. In most current protocols, vaccine is instilled into each nostril (usually 10 μg/nostril) and inhaled, resulting in effective delivery of vaccine presumably into NALT. Larger aliquots are subsequently swallowed, resulting in oral immunization. For this reason, any nasal protocol cannot avoid some oral delivery, although most studies of oral immunization employ gastric intubation to avoid potential nasal immunization. It should also be noted that two routes of pulmonary immunization have been used: intratracheal delivery versus nasal instillation. In general, it appears that intratracheal immunization tends to induce responses in the lower lungs and associated cervical and other draining lymph nodes, whereas nasal immunization sensitizes NALT and associated cervical lymph nodes.

Several studies can be used to illustrate principles associated with nasal immunization. In one, nasal administration of inactivated RSV with CT resulted in nasal IgA and serum IgG anti-RSV responses (Reuman et al. 1991). Analysis of IgG subclasses suggests that both IgG1 and IgG2a are induced (Reuman et al. 1991). Interestingly, infection with RSV and subsequent Th1-type responses are characterized by a favorable outcome, whereas Th2-type responses are associated with significant pathology (Graham et al. 1991a, b). Nasal immunization with the C fragment of TT (fragment C) and CT as adjuvant resulted in serum antibody responses characterized by comparable IgG1, IgG2a, and IgG2b anti-fragment C titers, suggesting that the use of CT as an adjuvant with fragment C induces a response characterized by both Th1- and Th2-type responses (Roberts et al. 1995). However, when fragment C is administered nasally with pertussis toxin (PT) or a mutated form of PT known as PT-9K/129G as mucosal adjuvants, anti-fragment C IgG1 predominates, suggesting that an immune response biased toward the Th2-type has been induced (Roberts et al. 1995). Direct comparisons between CT and PT or PT-9K/129 in this study are difficult because the use of CT is associated with much more potent anti-fragment C IgG responses. Further investigation will be needed to determine the role that adjuvants, the vaccine antigen, and the route of immunization play in induction of $CD4^+$ Th1- and Th2-type responses.

Mutants of CT constructed by substitution of serine with phenylalanine at position 61 (mCT-S61F) and glutamate by lysine at position 112 (mCT-E112K) in the ADP-ribosyltransferase activity center of the CT gene from *Vibrio cholerae* 01 strain GP14 display no ADP-ribosyltransferase activity or enterotoxicity (Yamamoto et al. 1997b). These mutants have been studied as potential nasal adjuvants. The levels of antigen-specific serum IgG and S-IgA Abs induced by the mutants are comparable to those induced by wild-type CT and significantly higher than those induced by recombinant CT-B (Yamamoto et al. 1997a, b). Further, the mCT-E112K, like mCT, induces Th2-type responses through a preferential inhibition of Th1-type $CD4^+$ T cells. Mutations in other sites of the CT molecule were reported to induce nontoxic derivatives but the adjuvant activity was also affected.

Mutant LT molecules, whether possessing a residual ADP-ribosyltransferase activity (e.g. LT-72R) or totally devoid of it (e.g. LT-7K and LT-6K3), can function as mucosal adjuvants when intranasally administered to mice together with unrelated antigens (Rappuoli et al. 1999). However, discrepant results were reported when two nontoxic mLTs were tested for their adjuvanticity after oral immunization of mice. Thus, although mutant LT-E112K (bearing a substitution in the active site of the A subunit) was unable to amplify the response to keyhole limpet hemocyanin when both were given orally to C57BL/6 mice, the mutant with a substitution in the protease-sensitive region, LT-R192G, retained the ability to act as a mucosal adjuvant (Dickinson and Clements 1995). Whether the type of the substitution played a role in the reported discrepancies remains to be elucidated. As LT induces a mixed $CD4^+$ Th1-type (i.e. IFN-γ) and Th2-type (i.e. IL-4, IL-5, IL-6, and IL-10) response (Takahashi et al. 1996), one might envision the use of mutants of LT when both Th1- and Th2-type responses are desired.

MUCOSALLY-INDUCED TOLERANCE

Mucosal tolerance

In addition to the beneficial induction of Ag-specific S-IgA and serum IgG Ab responses after mucosal immunization, the mucosal route of Ag delivery can also induce another type of immune response, namely the induction of systemic unresponsiveness (e.g. oral tolerance). Thus, mucosal Ag delivery can either up- or down-regulate systemic immune responses. As discussed above, for the purpose of mucosal vaccine development against infectious diseases, the goal is induction of both mucosal and systemic immunity in order to provide two layers of protection. In contrast, inhibition of Ag-specific immune responses in systemic compartments by mucosal Ag delivery is important for the prevention of over-stimulation of responses and frequently encountered hypersensitivity responses to food proteins and allergens. Further, this system could potentially be applied to the prevention and possibly the treatment of autoimmune diseases by feeding relevant Ags.

Oral administration of a single high-dose or repeated oral delivery of low doses of proteins have been shown to induce systemic unresponsiveness, presumably in the presence of mucosal IgA Ab responses (Challacombe and Tomasi 1980; Tomasi 1980; Mowat 1987; Weiner et al. 1994; Czerkinsky et al. 1999; Garside et al. 1999; Mayer 2000; Fujihashi et al. 2001a) (Figure 28.13). These immunologically distinct responses in mucosa-associated versus systemic-associated lymphoid tissues were originally termed oral tolerance (Tomasi 1980). More recent studies have shown that the nasal administration of proteins also induces systemic unresponsiveness (Hoyne et al. 1993; McMenamin and Holt 1993; Metzler and Wraith 1993; Tian et al. 1996; Higuchi et al. 2000) and has led to the more general term 'mucosal tolerance' to include nasal or oral Ag induction of unresponsiveness.

Mucosal administration of protein Ag is a long-recognized method of inducing peripheral unresponsiveness or tolerance (Wells 1911). This is a unique immune reaction and is characterized by the fact that experimental animals fed large quantities of protein Ag become refractory or have a diminished capability to develop an immune response when re-exposed to that same Ag introduced by the systemic route (e.g. by parenteral injection) (Tomasi 1980; Mowat 1994). This unique response is an important natural physiological mechanism whereby the host presumably avoids development of hypersensitivity reactions to many ingested food proteins and other antigens (Garside et al. 1999). Thus, tolerance (or systemic unresponsiveness) represents the most common response of the host to our environment. The continuous ingestion of several thousand different food proteins is but one important example, whereas tolerance to our indigenous microflora that colonize the large intestine represents another major example. It is also useful to consider that induction of mucosal and systemic immunity by oral immunization is rather difficult and requires use of potent mucosal adjuvants, vectors, or other special delivery systems (see previous section). Further, the development of mucosal tolerance against pollen and dust antigens could also be essential for the inhibition of allergic reactions, including IgE-mediated hypersensitivity.

Most now agree that mucosal tolerance is mediated by T cells which are involved in the generation of active suppression or clonal anergy and/or deletion (Friedman and Weiner 1994), e.g. high doses of antigen given by the oral route induced clonal deletion or anergy (Whitacre et al. 1991; Melamed and Friedman 1993; Chen et al. 1995b) characterized by the absence of T-cell proliferation and diminished IL-2 production, as well as IL-2R expression. Frequently administered, low doses of antigen, however, induced active suppression by $CD4^+$ or $CD8^+$ T cells, which secreted cytokines such as

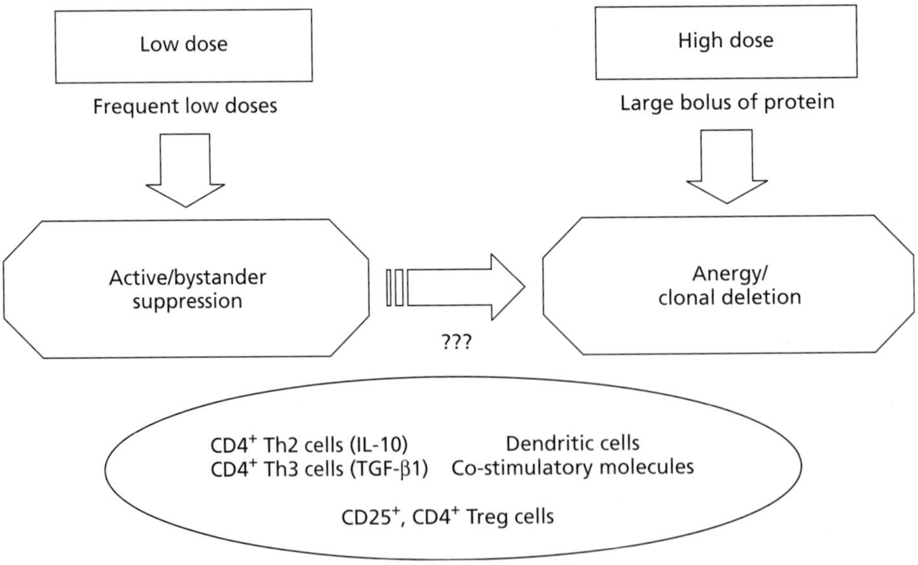

Figure 28.13 *Proposed mechanisms for mucosal tolerance: oral administration of a single high-dose or repeated oral delivery of low doses of proteins have been shown to induce systemic unresponsiveness. High doses of antigen given by the oral route induced clonal deletion or anergy characterized by the absence of T-cell proliferation and diminished interleukin 2 (IL-2) production as well as IL-2 receptor expression. Frequently administered low doses of antigen induced active suppression by $CD4^+$ or $CD8^+$ T cells which secreted cytokines such as transforming growth factor-β, and IL-10.*

TGF-β, IL-4, and IL-10 (Khoury et al. 1992; Chen et al. 1995a) (Figure 28.13). It is interesting to note that the latter scenario involves cytokines that are also known to upregulate IgA production (Czerkinsky and Holmgren 1995) and is thus compatible with the observation that mucosal immune responses and systemic tolerance may develop concomitantly (Asano et al. 1995; McGhee et al. 1999). As oral tolerance is specific for the antigen initially ingested or inhaled, and thus does not influence the development of systemic immune responses against other antigens, its manipulation has become an increasingly attractive strategy for preventing and possibly treating illnesses associated with or resulting from the development of untoward immunological reactions against specific antigens encountered or expressed (autoantigens) in nonmucosal tissues.

Mechanisms to explain oral tolerance

In the late 1970s and early 1980s, mucosal immunologists had already made attempts to investigate the possible mechanisms of oral tolerance at a time when the immune system was not characterized at the cellular and molecular levels (Thomas and Parrott 1974). Although several possible mechanisms (e.g. B-cell tolerance, anti-idiotypic antibody, intestinal antigen-processing events for tolerogen, and APCs) have been shown to be involved in the induction of oral tolerance (Mowat 1994), the most compelling evidence to date suggests that T cells are the major cell type involved in the induction of mucosally induced tolerance. In earlier work, it was shown that systemic unresponsiveness was induced by the adoptive transfer of T cells from rats orally fed bovine serum albumin (Thomas and Parrott 1974). Subsequently, a large number of studies demonstrated that oral immunization of protein antigen induces $CD4^+$ Th cells in mucosa-associated tissues that support IgA responses, whereas suppressor T cells were induced in systemic compartments such as spleen that downregulate Ag-specific IgM, IgG, and IgE responses (Mattingly and Waksman 1978; Ngan and Kind 1978; Kagnoff 1980; Kiyono et al. 1980, 1982b; Richman et al. 1981; Mowat et al. 1988), e.g. oral feeding of ovalbumin to mice led to the generation of Th cells supporting IgA responses and suppressor T cells for IgG and IgE responses in GALT (Mattingly and Waksman 1978; Ngan and Kind 1978; Mowat et al. 1988). Further, the former T cells for IgA responses remained in Peyer's patch, whereas the suppressor T cells migrated into the systemic compartment (e.g. spleen). These observations were considered to be logical explanations for cellular mechanisms of oral tolerance where Peyer's patch-derived $CD4^+$ Th cells supported IgA responses, whereas splenic T-suppressor cells induced systemic unresponsiveness. This must now be re-evaluated, because it has been shown that administration of a large dose of ovalbumin to mice followed by attempts at oral immunization with ovalbumin plus CT resulted in unresponsiveness in both mucosal and peripheral immune compartments (Kato et al. 2001).

A role for αβ T cells in oral tolerance

The αβ TCR^+ T cells appear to be the major players in downregulation of systemic immune responses to orally administered antigens. Most also agree that the status of oral tolerance can be explained by (1) clonal anergy, (2) clonal deletion of T cells, or (3) active suppression by T-regulatory (Treg) cells through the secretion of inhibitory cytokines (Whitacre et al. 1991; Miller et al. 1992; Gregerson et al. 1993; Melamed and Friedman 1993, 1994; Friedman and Weiner 1994; Garside et al. 1995; Hirahara et al. 1995). Low doses of oral antigen tend to favor the latter form of inhibition, whereas higher doses of feeding induce clonal anergy of immunocompetent T cells (Gregerson et al. 1993; Friedman and Weiner 1994; Garside et al. 1995; Hirahara et al. 1995). These two forms of oral tolerance are not mutually exclusive and may occur simultaneously after oral administration of antigens.

T-CELL ANERGY

Anergy is defined as a state of T-cell unresponsiveness characterized by the lack of proliferation and IL-2 synthesis, and by diminished IL-2R expression (Schwartz 1990), a condition reversed by pre-culturing T cells with IL-2 (DeSilva et al. 1991). Oral tolerance to a large dose of ovalbumin Ag-induced anergy in ovalbumin-specific T cells (Melamed and Friedman 1993) (see Figure 28.13). Further, oral myelin basic protein (MBP) diminished IL-2 and IFN-γ synthesis (Whitacre et al. 1991). These findings suggest that Th1-type T cells may be susceptible to the induction of anergy after oral feeding. To support this, it has been shown that Th1-type cells appear to be more sensitive to the induction of tolerance in vitro than Th2-type cells (Williams et al. 1990). In vivo evidence has demonstrated that Th1 cells are likely to be anergized in oral tolerance (Burstein and Abbas 1993). This may be an oversimplification because it has been shown that oral tolerance can be induced in mice defective in Th1 ($STAT4^{-/-}$) or Th2 ($STAT6^{-/-}$) cells (Shi et al. 1999). Further, in order to identify which lymphocyte compartment (e.g. $CD4^+$ versus $CD8^+$ T cells) preferentially mediates the induction of oral tolerance, cell transfer experiments were recently performed using severe combined immunodeficiency (SCID) and *nu/nu* mice (Hirahara et al. 1995). Adoptive transfer of splenic lymphocytes from mice orally tolerized with bovine α-casein resulted in the induction of tolerance in these immunocompromised mice. It was shown that oral tolerance was induced by anergized $CD4^+$ but not $CD8^+$ T cells. Taken together, a form of oral tolerance can be achieved by the induction of anergic $CD4^+$ T cells in the systemic compartment.

AN IMBALANCED TH1/TH2 CYTOKINE NETWORK

The induction of oral tolerance can also be explained by dysregulation of homeostasis between Th1- and Th2-type cells, e.g. preferential activation of Th2 cells may lead to downregulation of Th1 CMI responses by Th2 cytokines such as IL-4 and IL-10 (Burstein and Abbas 1993). In addition, Th1-type cells are much more sensitive to anergy induction after oral administration of protein antigens. These findings suggest that oral tolerance is associated with selective downregulation of Th1 cells by Th2 cells via their respective cytokines in the systemic immune compartment. This possibility is consistent with the fact that oral tolerance has more profound effects on Th1-regulated CMI responses than on Th2-mediated antibody responses. However, recent studies have shown that feeding high doses of ovalbumin inhibited production of both Th1 (IL-2 and IFN-γ) and Th2 (IL-4, IL-5, and IL-10) cytokines and resulted in the reduction of IFN-γ- and IL-4-dependent antigen-specific IgG2a and IgG1 Ab responses, respectively (Garside et al. 1995). These findings indicate that both subsets of Th cells are involved in the induction of oral tolerance and both are downregulated. Oral ovalbumin induced brisk IFN-γ production with inhibition of the IgG-enhancing cytokine IL-4 by Th2 cells, leading to reduced B-cell responses, although no oral tolerance was seen in IFN-γ knockout mice (Kweon et al. 1998). Further, repeated oral administration of high doses of ovalbumin to ovalbumin-specific TCR Tg mice resulted in an IFN-γ-dominated immune responses in the Peyer's patches (Marth et al. 1996). Taken together, the immunological consequences of systemic B-cell tolerance induced by a high dose of oral Ag could be the result of IFN-γ-mediated immune regulation, with significant suppression of Th2-type cells.

T-regulatory cells in oral tolerance

The finding that $CD4^+$ T-cell clones were generated after induction of oral tolerance to MBP clearly led to the description of a new phenotype of regulatory T cells. Clones of $CD4^+$ T cells were MBP specific and, of 48 clones assessed, 42 produced the active form of TGF-β1. Six clones produced high levels of TGF-β1 with essentially no IL-4 or IL-10 (Chen et al. 1994). On the other hand, five clones produced high IL-4 and IL-10, which is of course typical of Th2-type cells. The authors suggested the existence of a TGF-β1-producing, regulatory T cell involved in control of mucosal immune responses and named it Th3 (Chen et al. 1994).

The Treg cells appear to control mucosal immunity, tolerance, and inflammation to a higher degree than comparable Treg cell types in peripheral lymphoid tissues. Generally speaking, Treg cells do not proliferate well in vitro, a characteristic reminiscent of anergic T cells. In fact, cloned anergic T cells can suppress immune response in vivo and this appears to be partly caused by effects on APCs (Taams et al. 1998; Chai et al. 1999; Vendetti et al. 2000). Thus, anergic T cells downregulate DC expression of CD80 and CD86 in a contact-specific fashion (Vendetti et al. 2000). Further, anergic T cells have been shown to produce IL-10, which is a major characteristic of some $CD4^+$ $CD25^+$ Treg cells (Sundstedt et al. 1997; Buer et al. 1998; Sakaguchi 2000; Shevach 2000). Thus, it appears that anergic T cells, through production of IL-10 (and perhaps through other mechanisms), become Treg cells that suppress immune responses to other antigens (Buer et al. 1998), a process sometimes termed 'infectious tolerance' or 'bystander suppression'. Despite their poor proliferative responses to Ag, it has been possible to induce populations of T-cell clones after incubation with IL-10 and alloantigen in humans (Groux et al. 1996) or to ovalbumin peptide in DO11.10 mice (Groux et al. 1997). The T-cell clones obtained had similar properties, including secretion of high levels of IL-10, some production TGF-β1, with no IL-4 synthesis and poor proliferative responses (Maloy and Powrie 2001). Cells with these characteristics are now termed T-regulatory one cells (Tr1). Thus far, Tr1 and Th3 cells have in common the production of TGF-β1 (Th3) or TGF-β1 + IL-10 (Tr1) with suppressive-type properties.

In a hapten-induced model of colitis, it was shown that 2,4,6-trinitrobenzene sulfonic acid (TNBS) coupled to mouse colonic (self) proteins, when given orally, led to oral tolerance to hapten and a failure to induce TNBS colitis (Neurath et al. 1996). Interestingly, both Peyer's patch and lamina propria $CD4^+$ T cells, when stimulated via the TCR, produced high levels of TGF-β1, IL-4, and IL-10, suggesting that Th3 and possibly Tr1 cells regulate this type of tolerance (Neurath et al. 1996). Direct evidence for intestinal tolerance to luminal bacteria in humans was provided by the finding that lamina propria $CD4^+$ T cells responded poorly to *E. coli* proteins, a condition reversed by anti-IL-10 or anti-TGF-β1 mAb treatment (Khoo et al. 1997). The best direct evidence for induction of $CD4^+$ $CD25^+$ Treg cells by oral Ag was provided by an adoptive transfer model of DO11.10 TCR ovalbumin Tg T cells. Transfer followed by either intravenous or oral ovalbumin led to an increase in ovalbumin-specific, $CD4^+$ $CD25^+$ T cells (Thorstenson and Khoruts 2001). It should be emphasized that this last study used 25 mg ovalbumin in drinking water over an 18-h period, suggesting a relatively high oral dose of Ag-induced Treg cells (Thorstenson and Khoruts 2001).

A distinct role for γδ T cells in low-dose oral tolerance

It is well established that mucosal immune compartments such as the intestinal epithelium contain large numbers of γδ T cells in addition to αβ T cells, as does the lamina propria region of the small intestine (Aicher et al. 1992). As γδ T cells are localized in mucosa-associated tissues, we hypothesized that mucosal γδ T cells could be involved in immune responses in the lamina propria of normal mice, e.g. IEL T cells from mice immunized orally with sheep erythrocytes (SRBC) were separated into γδ and αβ T cells. When purified γδ and αβ T cells were adoptively transferred to mice orally tolerized with SRBCs, a conversion of systemic unresponsiveness to IgM, IgG, and IgA anti-SRBC Ab responses was achieved in mice that received γδ but not αβ T cells (Fujihashi et al. 1992). A more recent study has also demonstrated that γδ T cells isolated from mucosa-associated tissues of mice immunized orally with protein vaccine (B subunit of LT from *E. coli* – LT-B) exhibited a similar activity, i.e. IEL γδ T cells from LT-B-fed mice (which were tolerized) abrogated systemic unresponsiveness after adoptive transfer to syngenic mice orally tolerized with LT-B (Takahashi et al. 1995). Thus, γδ T cells appear to be important in the maintenance of mucosal IgA responses and possibly systemic unresponsiveness. In this regard, studies demonstrated that γδ T cells are essential for the induction of oral tolerance using mAb anti-γδ TCR-treated and TCR$\delta^{-/-}$ mice (Ke et al. 1997). Further, a distinct role was suggested for γδ T cells in the induction of high- versus low-dose oral tolerance. Although γδ T cells play a major immunoregulatory role for the induction of low-dose oral tolerance via upregulation of IL-10 synthesis, this T-cell subset is not involved in high-dose oral tolerance (Fujihashi et al. 1999) (see Figure 28.13).

A role for Peyer's patches in oral tolerance

The precise site of Ag uptake in the GIT during oral tolerance induction has not been firmly established. At least three possibilities could be proposed and none is mutually exclusive (Rubas and Grass 1991). First, Ag may be pinocytosed into the epithelial cells themselves and interactions with IELs may influence oral tolerance. Second, Ag may selectively enter the GALT via M cells and lead to APC–T-cell interactions which downregulate T-/B-cell responses. Finally, oral Ag may not perturb the GIT immune system at all, but simply enter and cross the epithelium in a paracellular fashion and reach the bloodstream, where tolerance would be induced. Some investigators have suggested that organized lymphoid tissue in the GIT was not required for oral tolerance to ovalbumin, because B-cell-defective mice, which contain poorly developed Peyer's patches, were fully tolerized at the level of T cells (Alpan et al. 2001). Although the study claimed that GALT was absent, others have shown that some remnants of Peyer's patches are seen in μMT mice (Golovkina et al. 1999). Others have also shown that direct injection of Peyer's patches induced oral tolerance (Chen et al. 2000). The availability of mice without Peyer's patches has allowed reinvestigation of the notion that GALT may be involved in oral tolerance (Figure 28.14). In one study, it was shown that mice lacking GALT but retaining mesenteric lymph nodes (MLN) could be orally tolerized to ovalbumin (Spahn et al. 2001). In other studies, mice lacking Peyer's patches but retaining MLNs were found to be resistant to oral tolerance to protein (Fujihashi et al. 2001b); however, these mice showed normal mucosal S-IgA Ab responses to oral protein given with CT as adjuvant (Yamamoto et al. 2000). One cannot yet conclude whether GALT is a strict requirement for oral tolerance to proteins.

Oral tolerance in humans

Increasing attention is being paid to oral tolerance and the role that it could play in the prevention or treatment of autoimmune diseases, including multiple sclerosis, rheumatoid arthritis, and uveitis, as well as type 1 diabetes and contact hypersensitivity (Weiner 1997). Indeed, humans fed the neoantigen KLH developed systemic unresponsiveness evaluated by delayed-type hypersensitivity and T-cell proliferative responses (Husby et al. 1994). However, B-cell responses were primed in both systemic and mucosal sites (Husby et al. 1994). In more recent studies, humans naturally ingesting the dietary Ags bovine γ-globulin, ovalbumin, and soybean protein developed a T-cell tolerance characterized by anergy (Zivny et al. 2001). Antigen-specific Th3 cells secreting TGF-β have been observed in the blood of multiple sclerosis patients orally treated with a bovine myelin preparation (Fukaura et al. 1996), demonstrating that oral administration of autoantigen can induce autoantigen-specific TGF-β-secreting cells in a human autoimmune disease.

Pilot clinical trials of oral tolerance have been conducted in patients with autoimmune diseases and promising clinical benefits have been reported (Weiner 1997; Czerkinsky et al. 1999). Despite encouraging results that have been reported regarding oral delivery of autoantigens for the prevention and treatment of autoimmune diseases, a follow-up study provides an unfortunate alternative possibility. Oral feeding of autoantigen in mice resulted in the generation of antigen-specific $CD8^+$ CTL responses, which could lead to the aggravation of autoimmune disease (Blanas et al. 1996). Thus, one must also keep in mind that oral administration of autoantigen may induce undesirable $CD8^+$ CTLs that may worsen the disease instead of preventing the development of autoimmune diseases.

Oral desensitization to nickel allergy was reported to reduce nickel-specific T cells and the cutaneous form of eczema (Bagot 1995). Oral Ags had earlier been

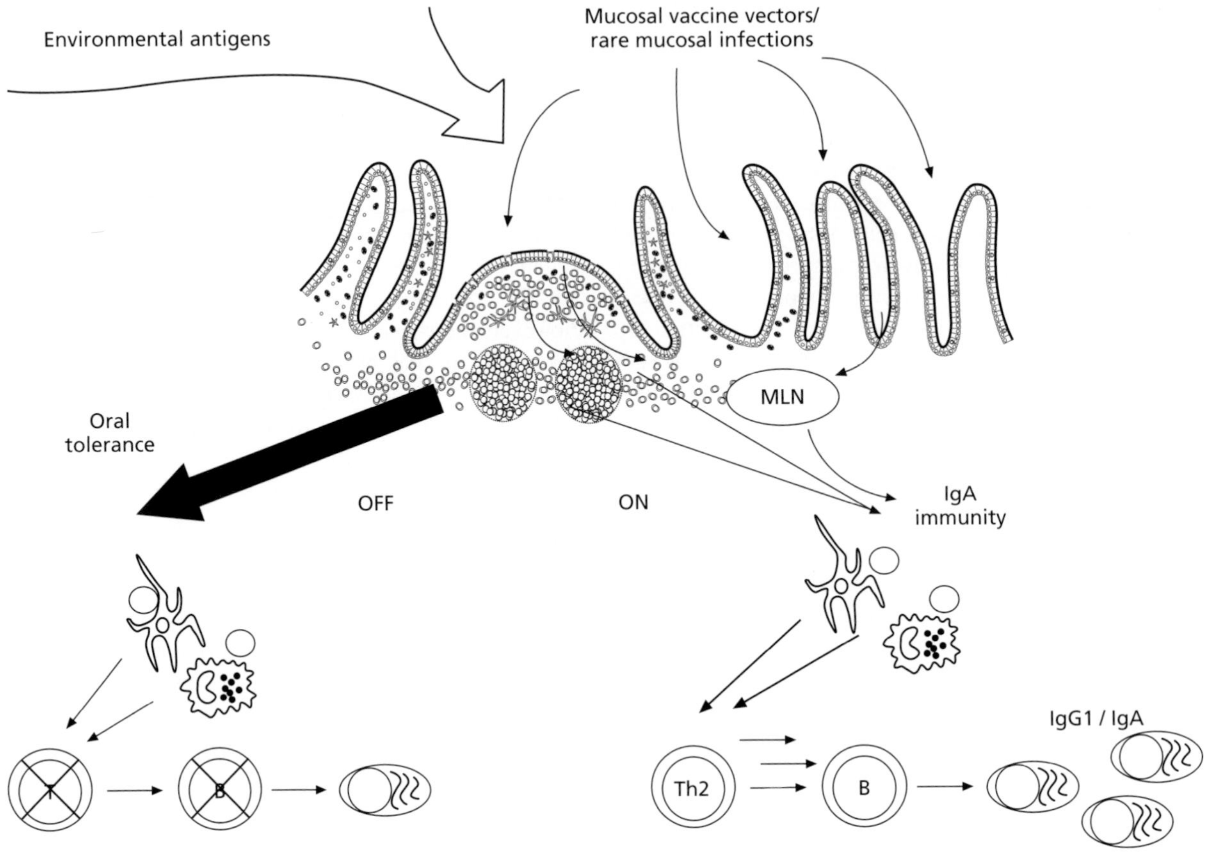

Figure 28.14 *Regulation of mucosal immunity and tolerance: mucosal homeostasis provided by mechanisms of tolerance including oral tolerance may be common and important mucosal immune responses. On the other hand, induction of vaccine-specific IgA responses at mucosal surfaces requires mucosal adjuvants or delivery systems.*

proposed to prevent or even treat allergic reactions to common allergens such as house-dust mite and grass pollens (Wortmann 1977; Rebien et al. 1982). However, this has not yet reached fruition. Thus, the experience of most investigators is that, once an immune response has been induced, it cannot be reversed through mucosal tolerance. Although the above examples indicate that oral tolerance offers promise for inducing antigen-specific immunological tolerance, its therapeutic potential remains limited by practical problems. Indeed, large quantities of orally administered antigens (e.g. milligrams in mice, grams in humans) are required to induce systemic unresponsiveness in experimental animals and humans. Taken together, these initial human trials have shown that oral tolerance, which paralleled results in animal models, could be induced in humans. However, a consistent clinical efficacy remains to be shown in human diseases.

CONCLUSIONS

The mucosal immune system is maintained through well-organized, interactive, innate, and acquired immune compartments. Thus, mucosal surfaces, which cover huge areas, are protected in concert by the two arms of this defense system, respectively. In addition, most studies clearly suggest that the main players in innate immunity serve as a bridge with acquired immunity, e.g. IECs produce antimicrobial peptides such as defensins. Further, an array of cytokines and chemokines is also produced by epithelial cells and these molecular responses subsequently induce expression of MHC I and II as well as co-stimulatory molecules, which are key factors for the APC-directed initiation of acquired mucosal immune responses. In addition, cross-talk by the epithelium to IEL T cells again bridges with acquired immunity. In this regard, IECs and IEL T cells cross-regulate each other in maintaining mucosal homeostasis at the barrier interface.

It is obvious that S-IgA Abs play central roles in mucosal immunity. Thus, large efforts have been made to define how S-IgA Ab responses are regulated. The organized mucosal inductive and effector tissues are essential elements and play key roles in the induction and regulation of S-IgA Ab responses. Inside these tissues, $CD4^+$ T cells and their derived cytokines are essential for B-cell switching to sIgA expression, stimulation, growth, and terminal differentiation into IgA-producing plasma cells. Induction of Ag-specific IgA Ab responses at mucosal surfaces is a rather difficult task (see Figure 28.14). In this regard, potent mucosal adjuvants or former pathogens, including recombinant delivery systems, are essential for mucosal vaccine development, and have been extensively studied. To date, only mucosal immunization (oral, nasal, and rectal routes) successfully induces S-IgA Ab responses. Effective mucosal vaccines provide two layers of defense, the first at mucosal surfaces (S-IgA) and the second in systemic lymphoid sites (plasma IgG). The occurrence of Ag-specific S-IgA Ab responses is a relatively rare type of immune response. Thus, mucosal homeostasis provided by mechanisms of tolerance including oral tolerance may be a more common and important type of mucosal immune response (see Figure 28.14). In summary, the major goals in the past, the present and the future will be to elucidate the cellular and molecular mechanisms involved in the induction and regulation of opposite types of mucosal immune responses, i.e. S-IgA immunity and mucosal tolerance (see Figure 28.14).

ACKNOWLEDGMENTS

We thank Dr Hiroshi Kiyono for extensive discussion of this review and Ms Sheila D. Turner and Ms Kelly Stinson for preparing the manuscript. This work was supported by NIH grants DE 12242, DE 09837, AI 35932, AI 18958, AI 43197, DC 04976, DK 44240, and AI 65299.

REFERENCES

Abreu-Martin, M.T. and Targan, S.R. 1996. Lamina propria lymphocytes: A unique population of mucosal lymphocytes. In: Kagnoff, M.F. and Kiyono, H. (eds), *Essentials of mucosal immunology*. San Diego: Academic Press, 227–45.

Adachi, S., Yoshida, H., et al. 1997. Three distinctive steps in Peyer's patch formation of murine embryo. *Int Immunol*, **9**, 507–14.

Adachi, S., Yoshida, H., et al. 1998. Essential role of IL-7 receptor α in the formation of Peyer's patch anlage. *Int Immunol*, **10**, 1–6.

Agace, W., Hedges, S., et al. 1993. Selective cytokine production by epithelial cells following exposure to *Escherichia coli*. *Infect Immun*, **61**, 602–9.

Aicher, W.K., Fujihashi, K., et al. 1992. Effects of the lpr/lpr mutation on T and B cell populations in the lamina propria of the small intestine, a mucosal effector site. *Int Immunol*, **4**, 959–68.

Akira, S. 2001. Toll-like receptors and innate immunity. *Adv Immunol*, **78**, 1–56.

Alimzhanov, M.B., Kuprash, D.V., et al. 1997. Abnormal development of secondary lymphoid tissues in lymphotoxin β-deficient mice. *Proc Natl Acad Sci USA*, **94**, 9302–7.

Allan, C.H., Mendrick, D.L. and Trier, J.S. 1993. Rat intestinal M cells contain acidic endosomal-lysosomal compartments and express class II major histocompatibility complex determinants. *Gastroenterology*, **104**, 698–708.

Alpan, O., Rudomen, G. and Matzinger, P. 2001. The role of dendritic cells, B cells and M cells in gut-oriented immune responses. *J Immunol*, **166**, 4843–52.

Aradhya, S. and Nelson, D.L. 2001. NF-κB signaling and human disease. *Curr Opin Genet Dev*, **11**, 300–6.

Asai, Y., Ohyama, Y., et al. 2001. Bacterial fimbriae and their peptides activate human gingival epithelial cells through Toll-like receptor 2. *Infect Immun*, **69**, 7387–95.

Asano, S., Kida, K., et al. 1995. A morphologic study of lung secretory leukoprotease inhibitor in pneumonia. *Am J Respir Crit Care Med*, **151**, 1576–81.

Asanuma, H., Inaba, Y., et al. 1995. Characterization of mouse nasal lymphocytes isolated by enzymatic extraction with collagenase. *J Immunol Methods*, **187**, 41–51.

Bagot, M. 1995. Treatment of cutaneous T-cell lymphoma by retinoids and calcitriol. *Lancet*, **346**, 376–7, letter, comment.

Banchereau, J., Bazan, F., et al. 1994. The CD40 antigen and its ligand. *Annu Rev Immunol*, **12**, 881–922.

Barrett, T.A., Gajewski, T.F., et al. 1992. Differential function of intestinal intraepithelial lymphocyte subsets. *J Immunol*, **149**, 1124–30.

Beagley, K.W., Eldridge, J.H., et al. 1988. Recombinant murine IL-5 induces high rate IgA synthesis in cycling IgA-positive Peyer's patch B cells. *J Immunol*, **141**, 2035–42.

Beagley, K.W., Eldridge, J.H., et al. 1989. Interleukins and IgA synthesis. Human and murine IL-6 induce high rate IgA secretion in IgA-committed B cells. *J Exp Med*, **169**, 2133–48.

Bellamy, W., Takase, M., et al. 1992. Antibacterial spectrum of lactoferricin B, a potent bactericidal peptide derived from the N-terminal region of bovine lactoferrin. *J Appl Bacteriol*, **73**, 472–9.

Benson, E.M., Bertolini, J.N. and Brodtmann, M.E. 1990. T cell regulation of immunoglobulin isotypes in health and disease. *Pediatr Infect Dis J*, **9**, S25–35.

Bernstein, J.M. 1992. Mucosal immunology of the upper respiratory tract. *Respiration*, **59**, 3–13.

Bernstein, J.M. 1999. Waldeyer's ring and otitis media: the nasopharyngeal tonsil and otitis media. *Int J Pediatr Otorhinol*, **49**, Suppl. 1, S127–32.

Bienenstock, J., McDermott, M., et al. 1978. A common mucosal immunologic system involving the bronchus, breast and bowel. *Adv Exp Med Biol*, **107**, 53–9.

Bjerke, K., Halstensen, T.S., et al. 1993. Distribution of macrophages and granulocytes expressing L1 protein (calprotectin) in human Peyer's patches compared with normal ileal lamina propria and mesenteric lymph nodes. *Gut*, **34**, 1357–63.

Blanas, E., Carbone, F.R., et al. 1996. Induction of autoimmune diabetes by oral administration of autoantigen. *Science*, **274**, 1707–9.

Blumberg, R.S., Terhorst, C., et al. 1991. Expression of a nonpolymorphic MHC class I-like molecule, CD1d, by human intestinal epithelial cells. *J Immunol*, **147**, 2518–24.

Bockman, D.E. and Cooper, M.D. 1973. Pinocytosis by epithelium associated with lymphoid follicles in the bursa of Fabricius, appendix, and Peyer's patches. *Am J Anat*, **136**, 455–77.

Boismenu, R. and Havran, W.L. 1994. Modulation of epithelial cell growth by intraepithelial γδ T cells. *Science*, **266**, 1253–5.

Bourguin, I., Chardes, T. and Bout, D. 1993. Oral immunization with *Toxoplasma gondii* antigens in association with cholera toxin induces enhanced protective and cell-mediated immunity in C57BL/6 mice. *Infect Immun*, **61**, 2082–8.

Boyaka, P.N., Wright, P.F., et al. 2000. Human nasopharyngeal-associated lymphoreticular tissues. Functional analysis of subepithelial and intraepithelial B and T cells from adenoids and tonsils. *Am J Pathol*, **157**, 2023–35.

Brandeis, J.M., Sayegh, M.H., et al. 1994. Rat intestinal epithelial cells present major histocompatibility complex allopeptides to primed T cells. *Gastroenterology*, **107**, 1537–42.

Brandtzaeg, P. 1974. Presence of J chain in human immunocytes containing various immunoglobulin classes. *Nature*, **252**, 418–20.

Brandtzaeg, P. 1994. Distribution and characteristics of mucosal immunoglobulin-producing cells. In: Ogra, P.L., et al. (eds), *Handbook of mucosal immunology*. San Diego, CA: Academic Press, 251–62.

Brandtzaeg, P. and Farstad, I.N. 1999. The human mucosal B-cell system. In: Ogra, P.L., et al. (eds), *Mucosal immunology*. San Diego, CA: Academic Press, 439–68.

Brandtzaeg, P. and Prydz, H. 1984. Direct evidence for an integrated function of J chain and secretory component in epithelial transport of immunoglobulins. *Nature*, **311**, 71–3.

Brandtzaeg, P., Surjan, L. Jr. and Berdal, P. 1978. Immunoglobulin systems of human tonsils. I. Control subjects of various ages: quantification of Ig-producing cells, tonsillar morphometry and serum Ig concentrations. *Clin Exp Immunol*, **31**, 367–81.

Briere, F., Bridon, J.M., et al. 1994. Interleukin 10 induces B lymphocytes from IgA-deficient patients to secrete IgA. *J Clin Invest*, **94**, 97–104.

Bromander, A.K., Kjerrulf, M., et al. 1993. Cholera toxin enhances alloantigen presentation by cultured intestinal epithelial cells. *Scand J Immunol*, **37**, 452–8.

Buer, J., Lanoue, A., et al. 1998. Interleukin 10 secretion and impaired effector function of major histocompatibility complex class II-restricted T cells anergized in vivo. *J Exp Med*, **187**, 177–83.

Burstein, H.J. and Abbas, A.K. 1993. In vivo role of interleukin 4 in T cell tolerance induced by aqueous protein antigen. *J Exp Med*, **177**, 457–63.

Butcher, E.C., Rouse, R.V., et al. 1982. Surface phenotype of Peyer's patch germinal center cells: implications for the role of germinal centers in B cell differentiation. *J Immunol*, **129**, 2698–707.

Cao, X., Shores, E.W., et al. 1995. Defective lymphoid development in mice lacking expression of the common cytokine receptor γ chain. *Immunity*, **2**, 223–38.

Cario, E., Rosenberg, I.M., et al. 2000. Lipopolysaccharide activates distinct signaling pathways in intestinal epithelial cell lines expressing Toll-like receptors. *J Immunol*, **164**, 966–72.

Chai, J.G., Bartok, I., et al. 1999. Anergic T cells act as suppressor cells in vitro and in vivo. *Eur J Immunol*, **29**, 686–92.

Challacombe, S.J. and Tomasi, T.B. Jr. 1980. Systemic tolerance and secretory immunity after oral immunization. *J Exp Med*, **152**, 1459–1472.

Chatfield, S., Roberts, M., et al. 1993. The development of oral vaccines based on live attenuated *Salmonella* strains. *FEMS Immunol Med Microbiol*, **7**, 1–7.

Chen, Y., Kuchroo, V.K., et al. 1994. Regulatory T cell clones induced by oral tolerance: suppression of autoimmune encephalomyelitis. *Science*, **265**, 1237–40.

Chen, Y., Inobe, J. and Weiner, H.L. 1995a. Induction of oral tolerance to myelin basic protein in CD8-depleted mice: both $CD4^+$ and $CD8^+$ cells mediate active suppression. *J Immunol*, **155**, 910–16.

Chen, Y., Inobe, J., et al. 1995b. Peripheral deletion of antigen-reactive T cells in oral tolerance. *Nature*, **376**, 177–80.

Chen, Y., Song, K. and Eck, S.L. 2000. An intra-Peyer's patch gene transfer model for studying mucosal tolerance: distinct roles of B7 and IL-12 in mucosal T cell tolerance. *J Immunol*, **165**, 3145–53.

Coffman, R.L., Shrader, B., et al. 1987. A mouse T cell product that preferentially enhances IgA production. I. Biologic characterization. *J Immunol*, **139**, 3685–90.

Coffman, R.L., Lebman, D.A. and Schrader, B. 1989. Transforming growth factor β specifically enhances IgA production by lipopolysaccharide-stimulated murine B lymphocytes. *J Exp Med*, **170**, 1039–44.

Crowe, P.T. and Marsh, M.N. 1994. Morphometric analysis of intestinal mucosa. VI: Principals in enumerating intra-epithelial lymphocytes. *Virchow's Arch*, **424**, 301–6.

Crowe, S.E., Alvarez, L., et al. 1995. Expression of interleukin 8 and CD54 by human gastric epithelium after *Helicobacter pylori* infection in vitro. *Gastroenterology*, **108**, 65–74.

Curtiss 3rd, R., Kelley, S.M. and Hassan, J.O. 1993. Live oral avirulent *Salmonella* vaccines. *Vet Microbiol*, **37**, 397–405.

Czerkinsky, C. and Holmgren, J. 1995. The mucosal immune system and prospects for anti-infectious and anti-inflammatory vaccines. *Immunologists*, **3**, 97.

Czerkinsky, C., Anjuere, F., et al. 1999. Mucosal immunity and tolerance: relevance to vaccine development. *Immun Rev*, **170**, 197–222.

De Togni, P., Goellner, J., et al. 1994. Abnormal development of peripheral lymphoid organs in mice deficient in lymphotoxin. *Science*, **264**, 703–7.

DeFrance, T., Vanbervliet, B., et al. 1992. Interleukin 10 and transforming growth factor beta cooperate to induce anti-CD40-activated naive human B cells to secrete immunoglobulin A. *J Exp Med*, **175**, 671–82.

DeSilva, D.R., Urdahl, K.B. and Jenkins, M.K. 1991. Clonal anergy is induced in vitro by T cell receptor occupancy in the absence of proliferation. *J Immunol*, **147**, 3261–7.

Dickinson, B.L. and Clements, J.D. 1995. Dissociation of *Escherichia coli* heat-labile enterotoxin adjuvanticity from ADP-ribosyltransferase activity. *Infect Immun*, **63**, 1617–23.

Dickinson, B.L., Badizadegan, K., et al. 1999. Bidirectional FcRn-dependent IgG transport in a polarized human intestinal epithelial cell line. *J Clin Invest*, **104**, 903–11.

Doggett, T.A. and Brown, P.K. 1996. Attenuated Salmonella as vectors for oral immunization. In: Kiyono, H., et al. (eds), *Mucosal vaccines*. San Diego, CA: Academic Press, 105–8.

Dono, M., Burgio, V.L., et al. 1996a. Subepithelial B cells in the human palatine tonsil. I. Morphologic, cytochemical and phenotypic characterization. *Eur J Immunol*, **26**, 2035–42.

Dono, M., Zupo, S., et al. 1996b. Supepithelial B cells in the human palatine tonsil. II. Functional characterization. *Eur J Immunol*, **26**, 2043–9.

Ebert, E.C. 1994. Effector function of human intraepithelial lymphocytes. In: McGhee, J.R. and Kiyono, H. (eds), *Mucosal immunology: intraepithelial lymphocytes*. New York: Raven Press, 131–7.

Eckmann, L., Kagnoff, M.F. and Fierer, J. 1993a. Epithelial cells secrete the chemokine interleukin-8 in response to bacterial entry. *Infect Immun*, **61**, 4569–74.

Eckmann, L., Jung, H.C., et al. 1993b. Differential cytokine expression by human intestinal epithelial cell lines: regulated expression of interleukin 8. *Gastroenterology*, **105**, 1689–97.

Emoto, M., Neuhaus, O., et al. 1996. Influence of β2-microglobulin expression on gamma interferon secretion and target cell lysis by intraepithelial lymphocytes during intestinal *Listeria monocytogenes* infection. *Infect Immun*, **64**, 569–75.

Ermak, T.H., Dougherty, E.P., et al. 1995. Uptake and transport of copolymer biodegradable microspheres by rabbit Peyer's patch M cells. *Cell Tissue Res*, **279**, 433–6.

Ernst, P.B., Befus, A.D. and Bienenstock, J. 1985. Leukocytes in the intestinal epithelium: an unusual immunological compartment. *Immunol Today*, **6**, 50–5.

Fagarasan, S., Kinoshita, K., et al. 2001. In situ class switching and differentiation to IgA-producing cells in the gut lamina propria. *Nature*, **413**, 639–43.

Farbman, A.I., Brunjes, P.C., et al. 1988. The effect of unilateral naris occlusion on cell dynamics in the developing rat olfactory epithelium. *J Neurosci*, **8**, 3290–5.

Farstad, I.N., Halstensen, T.S., et al. 1994. Heterogeneity of M-cell-associated B and T cells in human Peyer's patches. *Immunology*, **83**, 457–64.

Fearon, D.T. and Locksley, R.M. 1996. The instructive role of innate immunity in the acquired immune response. *Science*, **272**, 50–3.

Ferguson, A. and Parrott, D.M. 1972. The effect of antigen deprivation on thymus-dependent and thymus-independent lymphocytes in the small intestine of the mouse. *Clin Exp Immunol*, **12**, 477–88.

Franken, C., Meijer, C.J. and Dijkman, J.A. 1989. Tissue distribution of antileukoprotesae and lysozyme in humans. *J Histochem Cytochem*, **37**, 493–8.

Friedman, A. and Weiner, H.L. 1994. Induction of anergy or active suppression following oral tolerance is determined by antigen dosage. *Proc Natl Acad Sci USA*, **91**, 6688–92.

Fryksmark, U., Ohlsson, K., et al. 1982. Distribution of antileukoprotease in upper respiratory mucosa. *Ann Otol Rhinol Laryngol*, **91**, 268–71.

Fujihashi, K. and Ernst, P.B. 1999. A mucosal internet: Epithelial cell-immune cell interactions. In: Ogra, P.L., et al. (eds), *Mucosal immunology*. San Diego, CA: Academic Press, 619–30.

Fujihashi, K., McGhee, J.R., et al. 1991. Human appendix B cells naturally express receptors for and respond to interleukin 6 with selective IgA1 and IgA2 synthesis. *J Clin Invest*, **88**, 248–52.

Fujihashi, K., Taguchi, T., et al. 1992. Immunoregulatory functions for murine intraepithelial lymphocytes: γ/δ T cell receptor-positive (TCR^+) T cells abrogate oral tolerance, while α/β TCR^+ T cells provide B cell help. *J Exp Med*, **175**, 695–707.

Fujihashi, K., Yamamoto, M., et al. 1993a. Function of α/β TCR^+ intestinal intraepithelial lymphocytes: Th1-and Th2-type cytokine production by $CD4^+CD8^-$ and $CD4^+CD8^+$ T cells for helper activity. *Int Immunol*, **5**, 1473–81.

Fujihashi, K., Yamamoto, M., et al. 1993b. αβ T cell receptor-positive intraepithelial lymphocytes with $CD4^+$, CD8- and $CD4^+$, $CD8^+$ phenotypes from orally immunized mice provide Th2-like function for B cell responses. *J Immunol*, **151**, 6681–91.

Fujihashi, K., Kawabata, S., et al. 1996a. Interleukin 2 (IL-2) and interleukin 7 (IL-7) reciprocally induce IL-7 and IL-2 receptors on γδ T-cell receptor-positive intraepithelial lymphocytes. *Proc Natl Acad Sci USA*, **93**, 3613–18.

Fujihashi, K., McGhee, J.R., et al. 1996b. γδ T cell-deficient mice have impaired mucosal IgA responses. *J Exp Med*, **183**, 1929–35.

Fujihashi, K., McGhee, J.R., et al. 1997. An interleukin-7 internet for intestinal intraepithelial T cell development: knockout of ligand or receptor reveal differences in the immunodeficient state. *Eur J Immunol*, **27**, 2133–8.

Fujihashi, K., Dohi, T., et al. 1999. γδ T cells regulate mucosally induced tolerance in a dose-dependent fashion. *Int Immunol*, **11**, 1907–16.

Fujihashi, K., Kato, H. and McGhee, J.R. 2001a. A revisit of current dogma for the cellular and molecular basis of oral tolerance. In: Morteau, O. (ed.), *The intestinal mucosa and dietary antigens. Oral tolerance*. Austin, TX: Landes Biosciences, 1–13.

Fujihashi, K., Dohi, T., et al. 2001b. Peyer's patches are required for oral tolerance to proteins. *Proc Natl Acad Sci USA*, **98**, 3310–15.

Fukaura, H., Kent, S.C., et al. 1996. Induction of circulating myelin basic protein and proteolipid protein-specific transforming growth factor-beta 1-secreting Th3 T cells by oral administration of myelin in multiple sclerosis patients. *J Clin Invest*, **98**, 70–7.

Fuleihan, R., Ramesh, N. and Geha, R.S. 1993. Role of $CD40^-CD40^-$ ligand interaction in Ig-isotype switching. *Curr Opin Immunol*, **5**, 963–7.

Futterer, A., Mink, K., et al. 1998. The lymphotoxin β receptor controls organogenesis and affinity maturation in peripheral lymphoid tissues. *Immunity*, **9**, 59–70.

Gapin, L., Cheroutre, H. and Kronenberg, M. 1999. Cutting edge: TCR $\alpha\beta^+$ $CD8\alpha\alpha^+$ T cells are found in intestinal intraepithelial lymphocytes of mice that lack classical MHC class I molecules. *J Immunol*, **163**, 4100–4.

Garside, P., Steel, M., et al. 1995. T helper 2 cells are subject to high dose oral tolerance and are not essential for its induction. *J Immunol*, **154**, 5649–55.

Garside, P., Mowat, A.M. and Khoruts, A. 1999. Oral tolerance in disease. *Gut*, **44**, 137–42.

Garver, R.I. Jr., Goldsmith, K.T., et al. 1994. Strategy for achieving selective killing of carcinomas. *Gene Ther*, **1**, 46–50.

Gebert, A., Rothkötter, H.J. and Pabst, R. 1996. M cells in Peyer's patches of the intestine. *Int Rev Cytol*, **167**, 91–159.

George, A. and Cebra, J.J. 1991. Responses of single germinal-center B cells in T-cell-dependent microculture. *Proc Natl Acad Sci USA*, **88**, 11–15.

Gerard, C. 1998. Bacterial infection. For whom the bell tolls. *Nature*, **395**, 217–19.

Ghosh, D., Porter, E., et al. 2002. Paneth cell trypsin is the processing enzyme for human defensin-5. *Nat Immunol*, **3**, 583–90.

Goldman, A.S., Garza, C., et al. 1982. Immunologic factors in human milk during the first year of lactation. *J Pediatr*, **100**, 563–7.

Golovkina, T.V., Shlomchik, M., et al. 1999. Organogenic role of B lymphocytes in mucosal immunity. *Science*, **286**, 1965–8.

Graham, B.S., Bunton, L.A., et al. 1991a. Role of T lymphocyte subsets in the pathogenesis of primary infection and rechallenge with respiratory syncytial virus in mice. *J Clin Invest*, **88**, 1026–33.

Graham, B.S., Bunton, L.A., et al. 1991b. Respiratory syncytial virus infection in anti-μ treated mice. *J Virol*, **65**, 4936–42.

Gregerson, D.S., Obritsch, W.F. and Donoso, L.A. 1993. Oral tolerance in experimental autoimmune uveoretinitis. Distinct mechanisms of resistance are induced by low dose vs. high dose feeding protocols. *J Immunol*, **151**, 5751–61.

Griebel, P.J. and Hein, W.R. 1996. Expanding the role of Peyer's patches in B-cell ontogeny. *Immunol Today*, **17**, 30–9.

Gropp, R., Frye, M., et al. 1999. Epithelial defensins impair adenoviral infection: implication for adenovirus-mediated gene therapy. *Hum Gene Ther*, **10**, 957–64.

Groux, H., Bigler, M., et al. 1996. Interleukin-10 induces a long-term antigen-specific anergic state in human $CD4^+$ T cells. *J Exp Med*, **184**, 19–29.

Groux, H., O'Garra, A., et al. 1997. A $CD4^+$ T-cell subset inhibits antigen-specific T-cell responses and prevents colitis. *Nature*, **389**, 737–42.

Guy-Grand, D., Malassis-Seris, M., et al. 1991. Cytotoxic differentiation of mouse gut thymodependent and independent intraepithelial T lymphocytes is induced locally. Correlation between functional assays, presence of perforin and granzyme transcripts, and cytoplasmic granules. *J Exp Med*, **173**, 1549–52.

Halstensen, T.S. and Brandtzaeg, P. 1994. Phenotypic characteristics of human intraepithelial lymphocytes. In: McGhee, J.R. and Kiyono, H. (eds), *Mucosal immunology: intraepithelial lymphocytes*. New York: Raven Press, 147–61.

Hamada, H., Hiroi, T., et al. 2002. Identification of multiple isolated lymphoid follicles on the antimesenteric wall of the mouse small intestine. *J Immunol*, **168**, 57–64.

Harriman, G.R., Kunimoto, D.Y., et al. 1988. The role of IL-5 in IgA B cell differentiation. *J Immunol*, **140**, 3033–9.

Hashigucci, K., Ogawa, H., et al. 1996. Antibody responses in volunteers induced by nasal influenza vaccine combined with *Escherichia coli* heat-labile enterotoxin B subunit containing a trace amount of the holotoxin. *Vaccine*, **14**, 113–19.

He, Y.W. and Malek, T.R. 1996. Interleukin-7 receptor α is essential for the development of $\gamma\delta^+$ T cells, but not natural killer cells. *J Exp Med*, **184**, 289–93.

Hedges, S., Svensson, M. and Svanborg, C. 1992. Interleukin-6 response of epithelial cell lines to bacterial stimulation *in vitro*. *Infect Immun*, **60**, 1295–301.

Hendrickson, B.A., Conner, D.A., et al. 1995. Altered hepatic transport of immunoglobulin A in mice lacking the J chain. *J Exp Med*, **182**, 1905–11.

Hendrickson, B.A., Rindisbacher, L., et al. 1996. Lack of association of secretory component with IgA in J chain-deficient mice. *J Immunol*, **157**, 750–4.

Hershberg, R.M., Cho, D.H., et al. 1998. Highly polarized HLA class II antigen processing and presentation by human intestinal epithelial cells. *J Clin Invest*, **102**, 792–803.

Higuchi, K., Kweon, M.N., et al. 2000. Comparison of nasal and oral tolerance for the prevention of collagen induced murine arthritis. *J Rheumatol*, **27**, 1038–44.

Hirabayashi, Y., Kurata, H., et al. 1990. Comparison of intranasal inoculation of influenza HA vaccine combined with cholera toxin B subunit with oral or parenteral vaccination. *Vaccine*, **8**, 243–8.

Hirahara, K., Hisatsune, T., et al. 1995. $CD4^+$ T cells anergized by high dose feeding establish oral tolerance to antibody responses when transferred in SCID and nude mice. *J Immunol*, **154**, 6238–45.

Hirata, I., Austin, L.L., et al. 1986. Immunoelectron microscopic localization of HLA-DR antigen in control small intestine and colon and in inflammatory bowel disease. *Dig Dis Sci*, **31**, 1317–30.

Hiroi, T., Iwatani, K., et al. 1998. Nasal immune system: distinctive Th0 and Th1/Th2 type environments in murine nasal-associated lymphoid tissues and nasal passage, respectively. *Eur J Immunol*, **28**, 3346–53.

Hörnquist, C.E., Ekman, L., et al. 1995. Paradoxical IgA immunity in CD4-deficient mice. Lack of cholera toxin-specific protective immunity despite normal gut mucosal IgA differentiation. *J Immunol*, **155**, 2877–87.

Hoshino, K., Takeuchi, O., et al. 1999. Cutting edge: Toll-like receptor 4 (TLR4)-deficient mice are hyporesponsive to lipopolysaccharide: evidence for TLR4 as the *Lps* gene product. *J Immunol*, **162**, 3749–52.

Hoyne, G.F., O'Hehir, R.E., et al. 1993. Inhibition of T cell and antibody responses to house dust mite allergen by inhalation of the dominant T cell epitope in naive and sensitized mice. *J Exp Med*, **178**, 1783–8.

Huang, F.P., Platt, N., et al. 2000. A discrete subpopulation of dendritic cells transports apoptotic intestinal epithelial cells to T cell areas of mesenteric lymph nodes. *J Exp Med*, **191**, 435–43.

Huang, G.T., Eckmann, L., et al. 1996. Infection of human intestinal epithelial cells with invasive bacteria upregulates apical intercellular adhesion molecule-1 (ICAM-1) expression and neutrophil adhesion. *J Clin Invest*, **98**, 572–83.

Hubbard, R.C. and Crystal, R.G. 1991. Antiprotease. In: Crystal, R.G. and West, J.B. (eds), *The lung: scientific foundation*, Vol. 2. . New York: Raven Press, 1775–88.

Husby, S., Mestecky, J., et al. 1994. Oral tolerance in humans. T cell but not B cell tolerance after antigen feeding. *J Immunol*, **152**, 4663–70.

Inagaki-Ohara, K., Nishimura, H., et al. 1997. Interleukin-15 preferentially promotes the growth of intestinal intraepithelial lymphocytes bearing γδ T cell receptor in mice. *Eur J Immunol*, **27**, 2885–91.

Israel, E.J., Taylor, S., et al. 1997. Expression of the neonatal Fc receptor, FcRn, on human intestinal epithelial cells. *Immunology*, **92**, 69–74.

Iwasaki, A. and Kelsall, B.L. 1999. Freshly isolated Peyer's patch, but not spleen, dendritic cells produce interleukin 10 and induce the differentiation of T helper type 2 cells. *J Exp Med*, **190**, 229–39.

James, S.P., Fiocchi, C., et al. 1986. Phenotypic analysis of lamina propria lymphocytes. Predominance of helper-inducer and cytolytic T-cell phenotypes and deficiency of suppressor-inducer phenotypes in Crohn's disease and control patients. *Gastroenterology*, **91**, 1483–9.

Jones, B.D., Ghori, N. and Falkow, S. 1994. Salmonella typhimurium initiates murine infection by penetrating and destroying the specialized epithelial M cells of the Peyer's patches. *J Exp Med*, **180**, 15–23.

Jung, H.C., Eckmann, L., et al. 1995. A distinct array of proinflammatory cytokines is expressed in human colon epithelial cells in response to bacterial invasion. *J Clin Invest*, **95**, 55–65.

Kagnoff, M.F. 1980. Effects of antigen-feeding on intestinal and systemic immune responses. IV. Similarity between the suppressor factor in mice after erythrocyte-lysate injection and erythrocyte feeding. *Gastroenterology*, **79**, 54–61.

Kanamori, Y., Ishimaru, K., et al. 1996. Identification of novel lymphoid tissues in murine intestinal mucosa where clusters of c-kit$^+$ IL-7R$^+$ Thy1$^+$ lympho-hemopoietic progenitors develop. *J Exp Med*, **184**, 1449–59.

Kang, J.H., Lee, M.K., et al. 1996. Structure-biological activity relationships of 11-residue highly basic peptide segment of bovine lactoferrin. *Int J Pept Prot Res*, **48**, 357–63.

Kato, H., Fujihashi, K., et al. 2001. Oral tolerance revisited: prior oral tolerization abrogates cholera toxin-induced mucosal IgA responses. *J Immunol*, **166**, 3114–21.

Kaufmann, S.H. 1993. Immunity to intracellular bacteria. *Annu Rev Immunol*, **11**, 129–63.

Kawanishi, H., Saltzman, L.E. and Strober, W. 1983a. Mechanisms regulating IgA class-specific immunoglobulin production in murine gut-associated lymphoid tissues I. T cells derived from Peyer's patches that switch sIgM B cells to sIgA B cells in vitro. *J Exp Med*, **157**, 433–50.

Kawanishi, H., Saltzman, L. and Strober, W. 1983b. Mechanisms regulating IgA class-specific immunoglobulin production in murine gut-associated lymphoid tissues. II. Terminal differentiation of postswitch sIgA-bearing Peyer's patch B cells. *J Exp Med*, **158**, 649–69.

Ke, Y., Pearce, K., et al. 1997. γδ T lymphocytes regulate the induction and maintenance of oral tolerance. *J Immunol*, **158**, 3610–18.

Kelsall, B.L. and Strober, W. 1996. Distinct populations of dendritic cells are present in the subepithelial dome and T cell regions of the murine Peyer's patch. *J Exp Med*, **183**, 237–47.

Kennedy, M.K., Glaccum, M., et al. 2000. Reversible defects in natural killer and memory CD8 T cell lineages in interleukin 15-deficient mice. *J Exp Med*, **191**, 771–80.

Kerneis, S., Bogdanova, A., et al. 1997. Conversion by Peyer's patch lymphocytes of human enterocytes into M cells that transport bacteria (see comments). *Science*, **277**, 949–52.

Kerss, S., Allen, A. and Garner, A. 1982. A simple method for measuring thickness of the mucus gel layer adherent to rat, frog and human gastric mucosa: influence of feeding, prostaglandin, *N*-acetylcysteine and other agents. *Clin Sci*, **63**, 187–95.

Khoo, U.Y., Proctor, I.E. and Macpherson, A.J. 1997. CD4$^+$ T cell down-regulation in human intestinal mucosa: evidence for intestinal tolerance to luminal bacterial antigens. *J Immunol*, **158**, 3626–34.

Khoury, S.J., Hancock, W.W. and Weiner, H.L. 1992. Oral tolerance to myelin basic protein and natural recovery from experimental autoimmune encephalomyelitis are associated with downregulation of inflammatory cytokines and differential upregulation of transforming growth factor β, interleukin 4, and prostaglandin E expression in the brain. *J Exp Med*, **176**, 1355–64.

Kilian, M. and Russell, M.W. 1994. Function of mucosal immunoglobulins. In: Ogra, P.L., et al. (eds), *Handbook of mucosal immunology*. San Diego, CA: Academic Press, 127–37.

Kiyono, H., Babb, J.L., et al. 1980. Cellular basis for elevated IgA responses in C3H/HeJ mice. *J Immunol*, **125**, 732–7.

Kiyono, H., McGhee, J.R., et al. 1982a. In vivo immune response to a T-cell-dependent antigen by cultures of disassociated murine Peyer's patch. *Proc Natl Acad Sci USA*, **79**, 596–600.

Kiyono, H., McGhee, J.R., et al. 1982b. Lack of oral tolerance in C3H/HeJ mice. *J Exp Med*, **155**, 605–10.

Kiyono, H., Mosteller-Barnum, L.M., et al. 1985. Isotype-specific immunoregulation: IgA-binding factors produced by Fcα Receptor$^+$ T cell hybridomas regulate IgA responses. *J Exp Med*, **161**, 731–47.

Klimpel, G.R., Chopra, A.K., et al. 1995. A role for stem cell factor and *c-kit* in the murine intestinal tract secretory response to cholera toxin. *J Exp Med*, **182**, 931–42.

Klimpel, G.R., Langley, K.E., et al. 1996. A role for stem cell factor (SCF): *c-kit* interaction(s) in the intestinal tract response to *Salmonella typhimurium* infection. *J Exp Med*, **184**, 271–6.

Kolopp-Sarda, M.N., Bene, M.C., et al. 1994. Immunohistological analysis of macrophages, B-cells and T-cells in the mouse lung. *Anat Rec*, **239**, 150–7.

Komano, H., Fujiura, Y., et al. 1995. Homeostatic regulation of intestinal epithelia by intraepithelial γδ T cells. *Proc Natl Acad Sci USA*, **92**, 6147–51.

Koni, P.A., Sacca, R., et al. 1997. Distinct roles in lymphoid organogenesis for lymphotoxins α and β revealed in lymphotoxin β-deficient mice. *Immunity*, **6**, 491–500.

Krajci, P., Kvale, D., et al. 1992. Molecular cloning and exon-intron mapping of the gene encoding human transmembrane secretory component (the poly-Ig receptor). *Eur J Immunol*, **22**, 2309–15.

Kroese, F.G., Butcher, E.C., et al. 1989. Many of the IgA producing plasma cells in murine gut are derived from self-replenishing precursors in the peritoneal cavity. *Int Immunol*, **1**, 75–84.

Kuper, C.F., Koornstra, P.J., et al. 1992. The role of nasopharyngeal lymphoid tissue. *Immunol Today*, **13**, 219–24.

Kvale, D., Lovhaug, D., et al. 1988. Tumor necrosis factor-α up-regulates expression of secretory component, the epithelial receptor for polymeric Ig. *J Immunol*, **140**, 3086–9.

Kvale, D., Krajci, P. and Brandtzaeg, P. 1992. Expression and regulation of adhesion molecules ICAM-1 (CD54) and LFA-3 (CD58) in human intestinal epithelial cell lines. *Scand J Immunol*, **35**, 669–76.

Kweon, M.N., Fujihashi, K., et al. 1998. Lack of orally induced systemic unresponsiveness in IFN-γ knockout mice. *J Immunol*, **160**, 1687–93.

Labéta, M.O., Vidal, K., et al. 2000. Innate recognition of bacteria in human milk is mediated by a milk-derived highly expressed pattern recognition receptor, soluble CD14. *J Exp Med*, **191**, 1807–12.

Ladel, C.H., Hess, J., et al. 1995. Contribution of α/β and γ/δ T lymphocytes to immunity against Mycobacterium bovis bacillus Calmette Guerin: studies with T cell receptor-deficient mutant mice. *Eur J Immunol*, **25**, 838–46.

Lebman, D.A. and Coffman, R.L. 1988. The effects of IL-4 and IL-5 on the IgA response by murine Peyer's patch B cell subpopulations. *J Immunol*, **141**, 2050–6.

Lebman, D.A., Griffin, P.M. and Cebra, J.J. 1987. Relationship between expression of IgA by Peyer's patch cells and functional IgA memory cells. *J Exp Med*, **166**, 1405–18.

Lebman, D.A., Lee, F.D. and Coffman, R.L. 1990a. Mechanism for transforming growth factor β and IL-2 enhancement of IgA expression in lipopolysaccharide-stimulated B cell cultures. *J Immunol*, **144**, 952–9.

Lebman, D.A., Nomura, D.Y., et al. 1990b. Molecular characterization of germ-line immunoglobulin A transcripts produced during transforming growth factor type β-induced isotype switching. *Proc Natl Acad Sci USA*, **87**, 3962–6.

LeFrançois, L. 1991. Intraepithelial lymphocytes of the intestinal mucosa: curiouser and curiouser. *Semin Immunol*, **3**, 99–108.

LeFrançois, L. and Goodman, T. 1989. In vivo modulation of cytolytic activity and Thy-1 expression in TCR $\gamma\delta^+$ intraepithelial lymphocytes. *Science*, **243**, 1716–18.

Leishman, A.J., Naidenko, O.V., et al. 2001. T cell responses modulated through interaction between CD8αα and the nonclassical MHC class I molecule, TL. *Science*, **294**, 1936–9.

Lodolce, J.P., Boone, D.L., et al. 1998. IL-15 receptor maintains lymphoid homeostasis by supporting lymphocyte homing and proliferation. *Immunity*, **9**, 669–76.

London, S.D., Rubin, D.H. and Cebra, J.J. 1987. Gut mucosal immunization with reovirus serotype 1/L stimulates virus-specific cytotoxic T cell precursors as well as IgA memory cells in Peyer's patches. *J Exp Med*, **165**, 830–47.

London, S.D., Cebra-Thomas, J.A., et al. 1990. CD8 lymphocyte subpopulations in Peyer's patches induced by reovirus serotype 1 infection. *J Immunol*, **144**, 3187–94.

McCormick, B.A., Colgan, S.P., et al. 1993. *Salmonella typhimurium* attachment to human intestinal epithelial monolayers: transcellular signalling to subepithelial neutrophils. *J Cell Biol*, **123**, 895–907.

McGhee, J.R., Mestecky, J., et al. 1989. Regulation of IgA synthesis and immune response by T cells and interleukins. *J Clin Immunol*, **9**, 175–99.

McGhee, J.R., Strober, W., et al. 1994. T cell and cytokine regulation of mucosal antibody responses with emphasis on intraepithelial lymphocytes helper functions. In: McGhee, J.R. and Kiyono, H. (eds), *Mucosal immunology: intraepithelial lymphocytes*. New York: Raven Press, 1–20.

McGhee, J.R., Lamm, M.E. and Strober, W. 1999. Mucosal immune responses: an overview. In: Ogra, P.L., et al. (eds), *Mucosal immunology*. San Diego, CA: Academic Press, 485–506.

MacLennan, I.C. 1994. Germinal centers. *Annu Rev Immunol*, **12**, 117–39.

McMenamin, C. and Holt, P.G. 1993. The natural immune response to inhaled soluble protein antigens involves major histocompatibility complex (MHC) class I-restricted $CD8^+$ T cell-mediated but MHC class II-restricted $CD4^+$ T cell-dependent immune deviation resulting in selective suppression of immunoglobulin E production. *J Exp Med*, **178**, 889–99.

McNeely, T.B., Dealy, M., et al. 1995. Secretory leukocyte protease inhibitor: a human saliva protein exhibiting anti-human immunodeficiency virus 1 activity in vitro. *J Clin Invest*, **96**, 456–64.

Macpherson, A.J., Lamarre, A., et al. 2001. IgA production without μ or δ chain expression in developing B cells. *Nat Immunol*, **2**, 625–31.

McWilliam, A.S., Napoli, S., et al. 1996. Dendritic cells are recruited into the airway epithelium during the inflammatory response to a broad spectrum of stimuli. *J Exp Med*, **184**, 2429–32.

Maki, K., Sunaga, S., et al. 1996. Interleukin 7 receptor-deficient mice lack γδ T cells. *Proc Natl Acad Sci USA*, **93**, 7172–7.

Malizia, G., Trejdosiewicz, L.K., et al. 1985. The microenvironment of coeliac disease: T cell phenotypes and expression of the T2 'T blast' antigen by small bowel lymphocytes. *Clin Exp Immunol*, **60**, 437–46.

Maloy, K.J. and Powrie, F. 2001. Regulatory T cells in the control of immune pathology. *Nat Immunol*, **2**, 816–22.

Marinaro, M., Staats, H.F., et al. 1995. Mucosal adjuvant effect of cholera toxin in mice results from induction of T helper 2 (Th2) cells and IL-4. *J Immunol*, **155**, 4621–9.

Marth, T., Strober, W. and Kelsall, B.L. 1996. High dose oral tolerance in ovalbumin TCR-transgenic mice: systemic neutralization of IL-12 augments TGF-β secretion and T cell apoptosis. *J Immunol*, **157**, 2348.

Maruyama, M., Hay, J.G., et al. 1994. Modulation of secretory leukoprotease inhibitor gene expression in human bronchial epithelial cells by phorbol ester. *J Clin Invest*, **94**, 368–75.

Mathews, M., Jia, H.P., et al. 1999. Production of β-defensin antimicrobial peptides by the oral mucosa and salivary glands. *Infect Immun*, **67**, 2740–5.

Matsuda, J.L., Naidenko, O.V., et al. 2000. Tracking the response of natural killer T cells to a glycolipid antigen using CD1d tetramers. *J Exp Med*, **192**, 741–54.

Mattingly, J.A. and Waksman, B.H. 1978. Immunologic suppression after oral administration of antigen. I. Specific suppressor cells formed in rat Peyer's patches after oral administration of sheep erythrocytes and their systemic migration. *J Immunol*, **121**, 1878–83.

Mayer, L. 2000. Oral tolerance: new approaches, new problems. *Clin Immunol*, **94**, 1–8.

Mayer, L. and Shlien, R. 1987. Evidence for function of Ia molecules on gut epithelial cells in man. *J Exp Med*, **166**, 1471–83.

Mayer, L., Siden, E., et al. 1990. Antigen handling in the intestine mediated by normal enterocytes. In: MacDonald, T., et al. (eds), *Advances in mucosal immunology*. Boston: Kluwer Academic Publishers, 23–33.

Mayer, L., Eisenhardt, D., et al. 1991. Expression of class II molecules on intestinal epithelial cells in humans. Differences between normal and inflammatory bowel disease. *Gastroenterology*, **100**, 3–12.

Medzhitov, R., Preston-Hurlburt, P. and Janeway, C.A. Jr. 1997. A human homologue of the *Drosophila* Toll protein signals activation of adaptive immunity. *Nature*, **388**, 394–7.

Mega, J., Bruce, M.G., et al. 1991. Regulation of mucosal responses by $CD4^+$ T lymphocytes: effects of anti-L3T4 treatment on the gastrointestinal immune system. *Int Immunol*, **3**, 793–805.

Melamed, D. and Friedman, A. 1993. Direct evidence for anergy in T lymphocytes tolerized by oral administration of ovalbumin. *Eur J Immunol*, **23**, 935–42.

Melamed, D. and Friedman, A. 1994. In vivo tolerization of Th1 lymphocytes following a single feeding with ovalbumin: anergy in the absence of suppression. *Eur J Immunol*, **24**, 1974–81.

Mestecky, J. and McGhee, J.R. 1987. Immunoglobulin A (IgA): molecular and cellular interactions involved in IgA biosynthesis and immune response. *Adv Immunol*, **40**, 153–245.

Metzler, B. and Wraith, D.C. 1993. Inhibition of experimental autoimmune encephalomyelitis by inhalation by not oral administration of the encephalitogenic peptide: influence of MHC binding affinity. *Int Immunol*, **5**, 1159–65.

Miller, A., Lider, O., et al. 1992. Suppressor T cells generated by oral tolerization to myelin basic protein suppress both *in vitro* and *in vivo* immune responses by the release of transforming growth factor β after antigen-specific triggering. *Proc Natl Acad Sci USA*, **89**, 421–5.

Miller, K.W., Evans, R.J., et al. 1989. Secretory leukocyte protease inhibitor binding to mRNA and DNA as a possible cause of toxicity to *Escherichia coli*. *J Bacteriol*, **171**, 2166–72.

Mombaerts, P., Arnoldi, J., et al. 1993. Different roles of αβ and γδ T cells in immunity against an intracellular bacterial pathogen. *Nature*, **365**, 53–6.

Moore, T.A., von Freeden-Jeffry, U., et al. 1996. Inhibition of γδ T cell development and early thymocyte maturation in IL-$7^{-/-}$ mice. *J Immunol*, **157**, 2366–73.

Mooren, H.W., Kramps, J.A., et al. 1983. Localisation of a low-molecular-weight bronchial protease inhibitor in the peripheral human lung. *Thorax*, **38**, 180–3.

Mostov, K.E. 1994. Transepithelial transport of immunoglobulins. *Annu Rev Immunol*, **12**, 63–84.

Mostov, K.E., Kraehenbuhl, J.P. and Blobel, G. 1980. Receptor-mediated transcellular transport of immunoglobulin: synthesis of secretory component as multiple and larger transmembrane forms. *Proc Natl Acad Sci USA*, **77**, 7257–61.

Mostov, K.E., Friedlander, M. and Blobel, G. 1984. The receptor for transepithelial transport of IgA and IgM contains multiple immunoglobulin-like domains. *Nature*, **308**, 37–43.

Mowat, A.M. 1987. The regulation of immune responses to dietary protein antigens. *Immunol Today*, **8**, 93.

Mowat, A.M. 1994. Oral tolerance and regulation of immunity to dietary antigens. In: Ogra, P.L., et al. (eds), *Handbook of mucosal immunology*. San Diego, CA: Academic Press, 201, 185, 201.

Mowat, A.M., Lamont, A.G. and Parrott, D.M. 1988. Suppressor T cells, antigen-presenting cells and the role of I-J restriction in oral tolerance to ovalbumin. *Immunology*, **64**, 141–5.

Muramatsu, M., Sankaranand, V.S., et al. 1999. Specific expression of activation induced cytidine deaminase (AID), a novel member of the RNA-editing deaminase family in germinal center B cells. *J Biol Chem*, **274**, 18470–6.

Muramatsu, M., Kinoshita, K., et al. 2000. Class switch recombination and hypermutation require activation-induced cytidine deaminase (AID), a potential RNA editing enzyme. *Cell*, **102**, 553–63.

Murray, P.D., McKenzie, D.T., et al. 1987. Interleukin 5 and interleukin 4 produced by Peyer's patch T cells selectively enhance immunoglobulin A expression. *J Immunol*, **139**, 2669–74.

Neurath, M.F., Fuss, I., et al. 1996. Experimental granulomatous colitis in mice is abrogated by induction of TGF-β mediated oral tolerance. *J Exp Med*, **183**, 2605–16.

Neutra, M.R., Frey, A. and Kraehenbuhl, J.P. 1996. Epithelial M cells: gateways for mucosal infection and immunization. *Cell*, **86**, 345–8.

Ngan, J. and Kind, L.S. 1978. Suppressor T cells for IgE and IgG in Peyer's patches of mice made tolerant by the oral administration of ovalbumin. *J Immunol*, **120**, 861–5.

Nibert, M.L., Furlong, D.B. and Fields, B.N. 1991. Mechanisms of viral pathogenesis. Distinct forms of reoviruses and their roles during replication in cells and host. *J Clin Invest*, **88**, 727–34.

Niles, M.J., Matsuuchi, L. and Koshland, M.E. 1995. Polymer IgM assembly and secretion in lymphoid and nonlymphoid cell lines: evidence that J chain is required for pentamer IgM synthesis. *Proc Natl Acad Sci USA*, **92**, 2884–8.

Nishimura, H., Hiromatsu, K., et al. 1996. IL-15 is a novel growth factor for murine γδ T cells induced by *Salmonella* infection. *J Immunol*, **156**, 663–9.

Noguchi, M., Nakamura, Y., et al. 1993. Interleukin-2 receptor γ chain: a functional component of the interleukin-7 receptor. *Science*, **262**, 1877–80.

Nonoyama, S., Farrington, M., et al. 1993. Activated B cells from patients with common variable immunodeficiency proliferate and synthesize immunoglobulin. *J Clin Invest*, **92**, 1282–7.

Offit, P.A. and Dudzik, K.I. 1989. Rotavirus-specific cytotoxic T lymphocytes appear at the intestinal mucosal surface after rotavirus infection. *J Virol*, **63**, 3507–12.

Ohta, N., Hiroi, T., et al. 2002. IL-15-dependent activation-induced cell death-resistant Th1 type CD8αβ^{+} NK1.1^{+} T cells for the development of small intestinal inflammation. *J Immunol*, **169**, 460–8.

Okahashi, N., Yamamoto, M., et al. 1996. Oral immunization of interleukin-4 (IL-4) knockout mice with a recombinant *Salmonella* strain or cholera toxin reveals that CD4^{+} Th2 cells producing IL-6 and IL-10 are associated with mucosal immunoglobulin A responses. *Infect Immun*, **64**, 1516–25.

Orlic, D. and Lev, R. 1977. An electron microscopic study of intraepithelial lymphocytes in human fetal small intestine. *Lab Invest*, **37**, 554–61.

Ostov, K.E. and Kaetzel, C.S. 1999. Immunoglobulin transport and polymeric immunoglobulin receptor. In: Ogra, P.L., et al. (eds), *Mucosal immunology*. San Diego, CA: Academic Press, 181–211.

Ouellette, A.J. 1997. Paneth cells and innate immunity in the crypt microenvironment. *Gastroenterology*, **113**, 1779–84.

Owen, R. and Nemanic, P. 1978. Antigen processing structures of the mammalian tract: An SEM study of lymphoepithelial organs. In Beecker, R.P. and Johario, O. (eds) *Scanning electron microscopy*, Vol. 11. Scanning Electron Microscopy, Inc., 367.

Owen, R.L. and Jones, A.L. 1974. Epithelial cell specialization within human Peyer's patches: an ultrastructural study of intestinal lymphoid follicles. *Gastroenterology*, **66**, 189–203.

Pabst, R. 1992. Is BALT a major component of the human lung immune system? *Immunol Today*, **13**, 119–22.

Phillips, J.O., Everson, M.P., et al. 1990. Synergistic effect of IL-4 and IFN-γ on the expression of polymeric Ig receptor (secretory component) and IgA binding by human epithelial cells. *J Immunol*, **145**, 1740–4.

Porter, E.M., Liu, L., et al. 1997. Localization of human intestinal defensin 5 in paneth cell granules. *Infect Immun*, **65**, 2389–95.

Pruitt, K.M., Kamau, D.N., et al. 1990. Quantitative, standardized assays for determining the concentrations of bovine lactoperoxidase, human salivary peroxidase, and human myeloperoxidase. *Anal Biochem*, **191**, 278–86.

Pruitt, K.M., Rahemtulla, F., et al. 1991. Peroxidases in human milk. *Adv Exp Med Biol*, **310**, 137–44.

Puddington, L., Olson, S. and LeFrançois, L. 1994. Interactions between stem cell factor and c-Kit are required for intestinal immune system homeostasis. *Immunity*, **1**, 733–9.

Qureshi, S.T., Lariviere, L., et al. 1999. Endotoxin-tolerant mice have mutations in Toll-like receptor 4 (*Tlr4*). *J Exp Med*, **189**, 615–25.

Rappuoli, R., Pizza, M., et al. 1999. Structure and mucosal adjuvanticity of cholera and *Escherichia coli* heat-labile enterotoxins. *Immunol Today*, **20**, 493–500.

Rasmussen, S.J., Eckmann, L., et al. 1997. Secretion of proinflammatory cytokines by epithelial cells in response to *Chlamydia* infection suggests a central role for epithelial cells in chlamydial pathogenesis. *J Clin Invest*, **99**, 77–87.

Rebien, W., Puttonen, E., et al. 1982. Clinical and immunological response to oral and subcutaneous immunotherapy with grass pollen extracts. A prospective study. *Eur J Pediatr*, **138**, 341–4.

Rennert, P.D., Browning, J.L., et al. 1996. Surface lymphotoxin α/β complex is required for the development of peripheral lymphoid organs. *J Exp Med*, **184**, 1999–2006.

Reuman, P.D., Keely, S.P. and Schiff, G.M. 1991. Similar subclass antibody responses after intranasal immunization with UV-inactivated RSV mixed with cholera toxin or live RSV. *J Med Virol*, **35**, 192–7.

Revy, P., Muto, T., et al. 2000. Activation-induced cytidine deaminase (AID) deficiency causes the autosomal recessive form of the hyper-IgM syndrome (HIGM2). *Cell*, **102**, 565–75.

Richman, L.K., Graeff, A.S., et al. 1981. Simultaneous induction of antigen-specific IgA helper T cells and IgG suppressor T cells in the murine Peyer's patch after protein feeding. *J Immunol*, **126**, 2079–83.

Roberts, A.I., Lee, L., et al. 2001. NKG2D receptors induced by IL-15 costimulate CD28-negative effector CTL in the tissue microenvironment. *J Immunol*, **167**, 5527–30.

Roberts, M., Chatfield, S.N. and Dougan, G. 1994. Salmonella as carriers of heterologous antigens. In: O'Hagan, D.T. (ed.), *Novel delivery systems for oral vaccines*. Boca Raton, FL: CRC Press, 27–35.

Roberts, M., Bacon, A., et al. 1995. A mutant pertussis toxin molecule that lacks ADP-ribosyltransferase activity, PT-9K/129G, is an effective mucosal adjuvant for intranasally delivered proteins. *Infect Immun*, **63**, 2100–8.

Roberts, S.J., Smith, A.L., et al. 1996. T-cell $\alpha\beta^+$ and $\gamma\delta^+$ deficient mice display abnormal but distinct phenotypes toward a natural, widespread infection of the intestinal epithelium. *Proc Natl Acad Sci USA*, **93**, 11774–9.

Robinson, K., Bellaby, T. and Wakelin, D. 1995. Efficacy of oral vaccination against the murine intestinal parasite *Trichuris muris* is dependent upon host genetics. *Infect Immun*, **63**, 1762–6.

Roussel, P., Lamblin, G., et al. 1988. The complexity of mucins. *Biochimie*, **70**, 1471–82.

Rubas, W. and Grass, G.M. 1991. Gastrointestinal lymphatic absorption of peptides and proteins. *Adv Drug Del Rev*, **7**, 15–69.

Saito, H., Kanamori, Y., et al. 1998. Generation of intestinal T cells from progenitors residing in gut cryptopatches. *Science*, **280**, 275–8.

Saito, T., Deskin, R.W., et al. 1997. Respiratory syncytial virus induces selective production of the chemokine RANTES by upper airway epithelial cells. *J Infect Dis*, **175**, 497–504.

Sakaguchi, S. 2000. Animal models of autoimmunity and their relevance to human diseases. *Curr Opin Immunol*, **12**, 684–90.

Sandzen, B., Blom, H. and Dahlgren, S. 1988. Gastric mucus gel layer thickness measured by direct light microscopy. An experimental study in the rat. *Scand J Gastroenterol*, **23**, 1160–4.

Schüerer-Maly, C.C., Eckmann, L., et al. 1994. Colonic epithelial cell lines as a source of interleukin-8: stimulation by inflammatory cytokines and bacterial lipopolysaccharide. *Immunology*, **81**, 85–91.

Schwartz, R.H. 1990. A cell culture model for T lymphocyte clonal anergy. *Science*, **248**, 1349–56.

Sharma, S.A., Tummuru, M.K., et al. 1995. Interleukin-8 response of gastric epithelial cell lines to *Helicobacter pylori* stimulation in vitro. *Infect Immun*, **63**, 1681–7.

Shevach, E.M. 2000. Regulatory T cells in autoimmunity. *Annu Rev Immunol*, **18**, 423–49.

Shi, H.N., Grusby, M.J. and Nagler-Anderson, C. 1999. Orally induced peripheral nonresponsiveness is maintained in the absence of functional Th1 or Th2 cells. *J Immunol*, **162**, 5143–8.

Shimazu, R., Akashi, S., et al. 1999. MD-2, a molecule that confers lipopolysaccharide responsiveness on Toll-like receptor 4. *J Exp Med*, **189**, 1777–82.

Shinkura, R., Kitada, K., et al. 1999. Alymphoplasia is caused by a point mutation in the mouse gene encoding Nf-κb-inducing kinase. *Nat Genet*, **22**, 74–7.

Singh, P.K., Jia, H.P., et al. 1998. Production of β-defensins by human airway epithelia. *Proc Natl Acad Sci USA*, **95**, 14961–6.

Sminia, T. and van der Ende, M.B. 1991. Macrophage subsets in the rat gut: an immunohistochemical and enzyme-histochemical study. *Acta Histochem*, **90**, 43–50.

Snider, D.P., Marshall, J.S., et al. 1994. Production of IgE antibody and allergic sensitization of intestinal and peripheral tissues after oral immunization with protein Ag and cholera toxin. *J Immunol*, **153**, 647–57.

Sollid, L.M., Kvale, D., et al. 1987. Interferon-γ enhances expression of secretory component, the epithelial receptor for polymeric immunoglobulins. *J Immunol*, **138**, 4303–6.

Sonoda, E., Matsumoto, R., et al. 1989. Transforming growth factor β induces IgA production and acts additively with interleukin 5 for IgA production. *J Exp Med*, **170**, 1415–20.

Spahn, T.W., Fontana, A., et al. 2001. Induction of oral tolerance to cellular immune responses in the absence of Peyer's patches. *Eur J Immunol*, **31**, 1278–87.

Spalding, D.M., Williamson, S.I., et al. 1984. Preferential induction of polyclonal IgA secretion by murine Peyer's patch dendritic cell-T cell mixtures. *J Exp Med*, **160**, 941–6.

Spencer, J. and MacDonald, T.T. 1994. Development and function of human intraepithelial lymphocytes. In: McGhee, J.R. and Kiyono, H. (eds), *Mucosal immunology: intraepithelial lymphocytes*. New York: Raven Press, 139–46.

Staats, H.F., Jackson, R.J., et al. 1994. Mucosal immunity to infection with implications for vaccine development. *Curr Opin Immunol*, **6**, 572–83.

Stolk, J., Camps, J., et al. 1995. Pulmonary deposition and disappearance of aerosolised secretory leucocyte protease inhibitor. *Thorax*, **50**, 645–50.

Stumbles, P.A., Thomas, J.A., et al. 1998. Resting respiratory tract dendritic cells preferentially stimulate T helper cell type 2 (Th2) responses and require obligatory cytokine signals for induction of Th1 immunity. *J Exp Med*, **188**, 2019–31.

Sundstedt, A., Höidén, I., et al. 1997. Immunoregulatory role of IL-10 during superantigen-induced hyporesponsiveness in vivo. *J Immunol*, **158**, 180–6.

Sydora, B.C., Aranda, R., et al. 1996a. Lymphocyte-epithelial cross-talk in the intestine: Do nonclassical class I molecules have a big part in the dialogue? In: Kagnoff, M.F. and Kiyono, H. (eds), *Essentials of mucosal immunology*. San Diego, CA: Academic Press, 205–26.

Sydora, B.C., Brossay, L., et al. 1996b. TAP-independent selection of $CD8^+$ intestinal intraepithelial lymphocytes. *J Immunol*, **156**, 4209–26.

Taams, L.S., van Rensen, A.J., et al. 1998. Anergic T cells actively suppress T cell responses via the antigen-presenting cell. *Eur J Immunol*, **28**, 2902–12.

Taguchi, T., McGhee, J.R., et al. 1990a. Analysis of Th1 and Th2 cells in murine gut-associated tissues. Frequencies of $CD4^+$ and $CD8^+$ T cells that secrete IFN-γ and IL-5. *J Immunol*, **145**, 68–77.

Taguchi, T., McGhee, J.R., et al. 1990b. Detection of individual mouse splenic T cells producing IFN-γ and IL-5 using the enzyme-linked immunospot (ELISPOT) assay. *J Immunol Methods*, **128**, 65–73.

Takahashi, I., Nakagawa, I., et al. 1995. Mucosal T cells induce systemic anergy for oral tolerance. *Biochem Biophys Res Commun*, **206**, 414–20.

Takahashi, I., Marinaro, M., et al. 1996. Mechanisms for mucosal immunogenicity and adjuvancy of *Escherichia coli* labile enterotoxin. *J Infect Dis*, **173**, 627–35.

Tamura, S., Ito, Y., et al. 1992. Cross-protection against influenza virus infection afforded by trivalent inactivated vaccines inoculated intranasally with cholera toxin B subunit. *J Immunol*, **149**, 981–8.

Tamura, S.I. and Kurata, T. 1996. Intranasal immunization with influenza vaccine. In: Kiyono, H., et al. (eds), *Mucosal vaccines*. San Diego, CA: Academic Press, 425–36.

Teitelbaum, R., Schubert, W., et al. 1999. The M cell as a portal of entry to the lung for the bacterial pathogen *Mycobacterium tuberculosis*. *Immunity*, **10**, 641–50.

Thomas, H.C. and Parrott, M.V. 1974. The induction of tolerance to a soluble protein antigen by oral administration. *Immunology*, **27**, 631–9.

Thompson, R.C. and Ohlsson, K. 1986. Isolation, properties, and complete amino acid sequence of human secretory leukocyte protease inhibitor, a potent inhibitor of leukocyte elastase. *Proc Natl Acad Sci USA*, **83**, 6692–6.

Thorstenson, K.M. and Khoruts, A. 2001. Generation of anergic and potentially immunoregulatory $CD25^+CD4$ T cells in vivo after induction of peripheral tolerance with intravenous or oral antigen. *J Immunol*, **167**, 188–95.

Tian, J., Atkinson, M.A., et al. 1996. Nasal administration of glutamate decarboxylase (GAD65) peptides induces Th2 responses and prevents murine insulin-dependent diabetes. *J Exp Med*, **183**, 1561–7.

Tomasi, T.B. Jr. 1980. Oral tolerance. *Transplantation*, **29**, 353–6.

Toner, P.G. and Ferguson, A. 1971. Intraepithelial cells in the human intestinal mucosa. *J Ultrastruct Res*, **34**, 329–44.

Tsuji, M., Mombaerts, P., et al. 1994. γδ T cells contribute to immunity against the liver stages of malaria in αβ T-cell-deficient mice. *Proc Natl Acad Sci USA*, **91**, 345–9.

van Ginkel, F.W., Wahl, S.M., et al. 1999. Partial IgA-deficiency with increased Th2-type cytokines in TGF-β1 knockout mice. *J Immunol*, **163**, 1951–7.

VanCott, J.L., Staats, H.F., et al. 1996. Regulation of mucosal and systemic antibody responses by T helper cell subsets, macrophages and derived cytokines following oral immunization with live recombinant *Salmonella*. *J Immunol*, **156**, 1504–14.

Vendetti, S., Chai, J.G., et al. 2000. Anergic T cells inhibit the antigen-presenting function of dendritic cells. *J Immunol*, **165**, 1175–81.

Wang, J. and Klein, J.R. 1994. Thymus-neuroendocrine interactions in extrathymic T cell development. *Science*, **265**, 1860–2.

Wang, J. and Klein, J.R. 1995. Hormonal regulation of extrathymic gut T cell development: involvement of thyroid stimulating hormone. *Cell Immunol*, **161**, 299–302.

Wang, J., Whetsell, M. and Klein, J.R. 1997. Local hormone networks and intestinal T cell homeostasis. *Science*, **275**, 1937–9.

Wang, X., Moser, C., et al. 2002. Toll-like receptor 4 mediates innate immune responses to *Haemophilus influenzae* infection in mouse lung. *J Immunol*, **168**, 810–15.

Watanabe, M., Ueno, Y., et al. 1995. Interleukin 7 is produced by human intestinal epithelial cells and regulates the proliferation of intestinal mucosal lymphocytes. *J Clin Invest*, **95**, 2945–53.

Weiner, H.L. 1997. Oral tolerance immune mechanisms and treatment of autoimmune diseases. *Immunol Today*, **18**, 335–43.

Weiner, H.L., Friedman, A., et al. 1994. Oral tolerance: immunologic mechanisms and treatment of animal and human organ-specific autoimmune diseases by oral administration of autoantigens. *Annu Rev Immunol*, **12**, 809–37.

Weinstein, P.D. and Cebra, J.J. 1991. The preference for switching to IgA expression by Peyer's patch germinal center B cells is likely due to the intrinsic influence of their microenvironment. *J Immunol*, **147**, 4126–35.

Weinstein, P.D., Schweitzer, P.A., et al. 1991. Molecular genetic features reflecting the preference for isotype switching to IgA expression by Peyer's patch germinal center B cells. *Int Immunol*, **3**, 1253–63.

Wells, H. 1911. Studies on the chemistry of anaphylaxis III. Experiments with isolated proteins, especially those of hen's egg. *J Infect Dis*, **9**, 147.

Westin, U., Fryksmark, U., et al. 1994. Localisation of secretory leucocyte proteinase inhibitor mRNA in nasal mucosa. *Acta Oto-Laryngol*, **114**, 199–202.

Whitacre, C.C., Gienapp, I.E., et al. 1991. Oral tolerance in experimental autoimmune encephalomyelitis III. Evidence for clonal anergy. *J Immunol*, **147**, 2155–63.

Williams, M.E., Lichtman, A.H. and Abbas, A.K. 1990. Anti-CD3 antibody induces unresponsiveness to IL-2 in Th1 clones but not in Th2 clones. *J Immunol*, **144**, 1208–14.

Wilson, A.D., Bailey, M., et al. 1991. The in vitro production of cytokines by mucosal lymphocytes immunized by oral administration of keyhole limpet hemocyanin using cholera toxin as an adjuvant. *Eur J Immunol*, **21**, 2333–9.

Wilson, C.L., Ouellette, A.J., et al. 1999. Regulation of intestinal α-defensin activation by the metalloproteinase matrilysin in innate host defense. *Science*, **286**, 113–17.

Wolf, J.L. and Bye, W.A. 1984. The membranous epithelial (M) cell and the mucosal immune system. *Annu Rev Med*, **35**, 95–112.

Wolf, J.L., Rubin, D.H., et al. 1981. Intestinal M cells: a pathway for entry of reovirus into the host. *Science*, **212**, 471–2.

Wortmann, F. 1977. Oral hyposensitization of children with pollinosis or house-dust asthma. *Allergol Immunopathol*, **5**, 15–26.

Wu, H.Y., Nguyen, H.H. and Russell, M.W. 1997. Nasal lymphoid tissue (NALT) as a mucosal immune inductive site. *Scand J Immunol*, **46**, 506–13.

Wu, H.Y., Nikolova, E.B., et al. 1996. Induction of antibody-secreting cells and T-helper and memory cells in murine nasal lymphoid tissue. *Immunology*, **88**, 493–500.

Xu-Amano, J., Kiyono, H., et al. 1993. Helper T cell subsets for immunoglobulin A responses: oral immunization with tetanus toxoid and cholera toxin as adjuvant selectively induces Th2 cells in mucosa associated tissues. *J Exp Med*, **178**, 1309–20.

Yamamoto, M., Rennert, P., et al. 2000. Alternate mucosal immune system: organized Peyer's patches are not required for IgA responses in the gastrointestinal tract. *J Immunol*, **164**, 5184–91.

Yamamoto, S., Russ, F., et al. 1993. Listeria monocytogenes-induced gamma interferon secretion by intestinal intraepithelial γδ T lymphocytes. *Infect Immun*, **61**, 2154–61.

Yamamoto, S., Kiyono, H., et al. 1997a. A nontoxic mutant of cholera toxin elicits Th2-type responses for enhanced mucosal immunity. *Proc Natl Acad Sci USA*, **94**, 5267–72.

Yamamoto, S., Takeda, Y., et al. 1997b. Mutants in the ADP-ribosyltransferase cleft of cholera toxin lack diarrheagenicity but retain adjuvanticity. *J Exp Med*, **185**, 1203–10.

Yamanaka, T., Straumfors, A., et al. 2001. M cell pockets of human Peyer's patches are specialized extensions of germinal centers. *Eur J Immunol*, **31**, 107–17.

Yang, D.M., Fairweather, N., et al. 1990. Oral *Salmonella typhimurium* ($AroA^-$) vaccine expressing a major leishmanial surface protein (gp63) preferentially induces T helper 1 cells and protective immunity against leishmaniasis. *J Immunol*, **145**, 2281–5.

Ye, G., Barrera, C., et al. 1997. Expression of B7-1 and B7-2 costimulatory molecules by human gastric epithelial cells: potential role in $CD4^+$ T cell activation during *Helicobacter pylori* infection. *J Clin Invest*, **99**, 1628–36.

Yoshida, H., Honda, K., et al. 1999. IL-7 receptor α^+ $CD3^{(-)}$ cells in the embryonic intestine induces the organizing center of Peyer's patches. *Int Immunol*, **11**, 643–55.

Yoshida, H., Kawamoto, H., et al. 2001. Expression of α(4)β(7) integrin defines a distinct pathway of lymphoid progenitors committed to T cells, fetal intestinal lymphotoxin producer, NK and dendritic cells. *J Immunol*, **167**, 2511–21.

Yoshimura, A., Lien, E., et al. 1999. Cutting edge: recognition of Gram-positive bacterial cell wall components by the innate immune system occurs via Toll-like receptor 2. *J Immunol*, **163**, 1–5.

Zhang, J.R., Mostov, K.E., et al. 2000. The polymeric immunoglobulin receptor translocates pneumococci across human nasopharyngeal epithelial cells. *Cell*, **102**, 827–37.

Zhang, T., Li, E. and Stanley, S.L. Jr. 1995. Oral immunization with the dodecapeptide repeat of the serine-rich *Entamoeba histolytica* protein (SREHP) fused to the cholera toxin B subunit induces a mucosal and systemic anti-SREHP antibody response. *Infect Immun*, **63**, 1349–55.

Zhao, C., Wang, I. and Lehrer, R.I. 1996. Widespread expression of β-defensin hBD-1 in human secretory glands and epithelial cells. *FEBS Lett*, **396**, 319–22.

Zhu, X., Meng, G., et al. 2001. MHC class I-related neonatal Fc receptor of IgG is functionally expressed in monocytes, intestinal macrophages, and dendritic cells. *J Immunol*, **166**, 3266–76.

Zivny, J.H., Moldoveanu, Z., et al. 2001. Mechanisms of immune tolerance to food antigens in humans. *Clin Immunol*, **101**, 158–68.

29

Superantigens

BERNHARD FLEISCHER

'Superantigens' is the designation for a heterogeneous group of proteins that use a common, extremely efficient mechanism of T-lymphocyte stimulation. They bind to MHC class II molecules on antigen-presenting cells and to variable parts of the T-cell receptor on $CD4^+$ and $CD8^+$ T cells, thus mimicking the recognition of specific antigen. The prototype superantigen is the staphylococcal enterotoxin B, member of a family of genetically related pyrogenic exotoxins produced by *Staphylococcus aureus* and *Streptococcus pyogenes*. This principle of T-lymphocyte stimulation has been evolved several times independently by infectious pathogens.

The unusual mechanism of T-lymphocyte stimulation has been explored at a molecular level and it has been shown that the pathogenic effects of these molecules are the result of their ability to stimulate a large fraction of T cells. Consequences of confrontation of the body with superantigenic toxins are:

1 shock, mediated by a massive liberation of cytokines from cells of the immune system;
2 immunosuppression, mainly caused by an uncoordinated activation of the immune system and a massive deletion of T cells;
3 autoimmunity resulting from bypass activation of autoreactive T and B cells.

INTRODUCTION

Antigen recognition by T lymphocytes is one of the most sensitive assays in biology. With its antigen receptor the T cell can respond to only a few antigenic peptides presented by an antigen-presenting cell (APC). This unique sensitivity is provided by a set of molecular mechanisms that intracellularly amplify the initial signal given by one or only a few T-cell receptors (TCR). Superantigens have been adapted in evolution to use the T-cell machinery to become most effective T-cell stimulators. Although there are different types of superantigens that have been independently generated several times in evolution and that are completely unrelated to each other, they all use the same molecular mechanism: they bind to major histocompatibility complex (MHC) class II molecules on APCs and to the TCR, and thus crosslink the TCR to the MHC molecule of the APC. Therefore, by closely mimicking antigen recognition they use most of the amplification mechanisms that the T cell uses normally. Thus, a hallmark of all superantigens is their enormous potency: they are active in concentrations of 10^{-9} mol/l. This means that a few picograms per milliliter can still effectively stimulate T cells in culture. Another characteristic feature of superantigens is their use of variable determinants on molecules of the immune system: all superantigens known so far bind to the variable part of the TCR β chain (Vβ); thus each superantigen stimulates a particular fraction (up to 30 percent) of the T-cell repertoire. On the MHCII molecule there are different binding sites used by different superantigens, some superantigens even involve the antigenic peptide in their binding.

This principle of T-lymphocyte stimulation has evolved several times independently. Infectious pathogens as different as gram-positive cocci, gram-negative rods, a mycoplasma, and retroviruses produce superantigens that are apparently completely unrelated to each other. Obviously, this very special mechanism of

Table 29.1 *Some candidate superantigens produced by microorganisms*

Producing pathogen	Protein	Other activities	Superantigen?
Staphylococcus aureus	SEA-E, SEG-P		Yes
	TSST-1		Yes
	ETA, ETB	Proteases	?
Streptococcus pyogenes	SPEA, C, G–J		Yes
	SSA		Yes
	SMEZ		Yes
	SPEB	Protease	No
	M protein	Receptor	No
	MF ('SPEF')	Nuclease	No
Clostridium perfringens	Enterotoxin[a]	Pore former	No
Pseudomonas aeruginosa	Exotoxin A[b]	ADP-ribosyltransferase	No
Yersinia pseudotuberculosis	YPM		Yes
Yersinia enterocolitica	Undefined[c]		?
Mycobacterium tuberculosis	Undefined[d]		?
Mycoplasma arthritidis	MAS		Yes
Toxoplasma gondii	Undefined[e]		?
MMTV	orf		Yes
HERV	orf		Yes

a) Bowness et al. (1992), McClane (1994), Krakauer et al. (1997).
b) Legaard et al. (1991).
c) Stuart and Woodward (1992).
d) Ohmen et al. (1994).
e) Denkers et al. (1994).

T-cell stimulation has been developed by very different pathogens independently in evolution so it is likely that additional pathogens will also use it. Therefore, in the last few years, there have been a surprisingly large number of reports describing novel superantigens in various viruses, bacteria, or protozoa. With one exception, the lectin *Urtica dioica* agglutinin of the stinging nettle (Saul et al. 2000), all molecules that have been proposed to be superantigens are produced by infectious pathogens. (The lectin has two saccharide-binding sites and its superantigenic properties arise from the simultaneous fixation of glycans on the TCR and MHC molecules.) The long list of candidate superantigens includes a wide range of bacteria, protozoa, and viruses, some of which are listed in Table 29.1. In most cases the evidence is still indirect or the initial report has not been confirmed by an independent study. This review limits the discussion to those superantigens that are beyond any doubt superantigens.

PYROGENIC EXOTOXINS OF *STAPHYLOCOCCUS AUREUS* AND *STREPTOCOCCUS PYOGENES*

Genes and molecules

The pyrogenic exotoxins (PET) produced by these two genera of gram-positive cocci comprise a highly polymorphic family of genetically related toxins consisting of the staphylococcal enterotoxins (SE) and the toxic shock syndrome toxin-1 (TSST-1) produced by *Staphylococcus aureus* and streptococcal pyrogenic exotoxins (SPE) produced by *S. pyogenes*. *S. aureus* is widespread among humans and animals and many of these toxins are also present in *S. aureus* strains from other species. They are heat-stable and protease-resistant molecules of molecular mass 22–28 kDa.

Historically, the staphylococcal enterotoxins were defined by their ability to cause emesis and diarrhea in humans and monkeys. They are a major cause of food poisoning worldwide. Initially, five major serotypes SEA, SEB, SEC, SED, and SEE have been described that were serologically defined by the lack of cross-reaction of specific antisera. TSST-1 was initially designated SEF, but was later renamed TSST-1 because of its association with toxic shock syndrome – and because the initial finding of emetic activity could not be confirmed (Reiser et al. 1983). Currently the staphylococcal enterotoxins include in addition SEG, SEH, SEI, SEJ, SEK, SEL, SEM, SEN, SEO, and SEP (Jarraud et al. 2001; McCormick et al. 2001).

The SPEs are usually discussed separately from the SEs because they are derived from another genus and an enterotoxic activity has not been described. However, as such activity can be detected only in humans or monkeys it is not clear whether this putative difference has been sufficiently investigated. From a genetic point of view the separation of the SPEs from the SEs is not appropriate because some SPEs are more related to SEs than to other

Table 29.2 *Grouping of members of the staphylococcal enterotoxin superfamily according to genetic relatedness (Proft et al. 1999; McCormick et al. 2001)*

Group	Members		Common properties
I	TSST-1	TSST-1 and variants	
II	SEB-like	SEB, $SEC_{(n)}$, SSA, SPEA, SEG	Central cysteine loop
III	SEA-like	SEA, SEE, SEJ, SED, SEH	Central cysteine loop, zinc-binding site
IV	SPEC-like	SPEC, SPEJ, SMEZ, SPEG	Zinc-binding site
V	SPEH-like	SEK, SPEH, SEP, SEI, SEL	Zinc-binding site

Not yet classified: SEM, SEN, SEO (Jarraud et al. 2001).

SPEs. The members of the SE family can be divided into five subgroups (Table 29.2) according to their sequence relatedness (Betley et al. 1992; Munson et al. 1998; Proft et al. 1999, 2001; McCormick et al. 2001).

Homologies vary considerably within the groups. A common feature of all PETs is the overall molecular architecture: globular two-domain proteins of about 22–29 kDa with a long solvent accessible α-helix in the center of the molecule. Although some PETs, such as TSST-1 or SPEC, share little similarity with any other PET, there is sufficient sequence homology among all PETs to suggest that streptococcal and staphylococcal PETs have evolved from a single ancestor gene. This is in line with the finding that staphylococcal and streptococcal toxins are mixed within the different subgroups. Moreover, as other 'accessory proteins' are not required for bacterial growth many of the PETs are encoded on mobile genetic elements – those for SEA, SEE, SPEA, and SPEC are carried within bacteriophage DNA and for SED and SEJ on plasmid DNA (Betley et al. 1992; Johnson and Schlievert 1984; Weeks and Ferretti 1984; Goshorn and Schlievert 1989). Others are encoded within pathogenicity islands on the chromosome, e.g. TSST-1, SEB, or SEC (Novick et al. 2001). The streptococcal superantigen SSA is more related to SEB and SEC than to other streptococcal PETs, suggesting an intergeneric transfer in that it appears to have been acquired by several different clonal lineages of *S. pyogenes* during the twentieth century (Reda et al. 1994).

A characteristic feature of SEs and SPEs is their extensive polymorphism; there are many alleles of some toxins known which differ in only few amino acids, e.g. three subtypes of SEC have been numbered (SEC1–3) and a number of variants of SEC of *S. aureus* strains derived from humans, dogs, cattle, and food have been cloned (Marr et al. 1993). The variants differ only in a few amino acids but may differ in their biological activity (Bohach 1997). Several isolates of SEC3 that are serologically indistinguishable differ in several mutations. SEA and SEE have very high homology and show strong serological crossreaction; thus SEE could even be classified as a variant of SEA. TSST-1 produced by *S. aureus* strains associated with humans has a p*I* of 7.0 whereas *S. aureus* isolates from sheep produce the variant TSST-0 with a p*I* of 8.6 (Ho et al. 1989) which differs in only seven amino acids from TSST-1, but differs dramatically in its biological activity (Murray et al. 1994). Four different variants of SPEA have been described (Nelson et al. 1991) and three variants of SSA (Reda et al. 1994).

A particularly interesting toxin is the streptococcal mitogenic exotoxin Z (SMEZ) of *S. pyogenes* (Kamezawa et al. 1997). It forms a polymorphic family with wide allelic variation leading to significant antigenic variation (Proft et al. 1999, 2000). Currently more than 25 alleles have been identified (Proft et al. 1999, 2000; Gerlach et al. 2000). All SMEZ variants are powerful stimulators of human Vβ4 and Vβ8 T cells and significant production of SMEZ occurs in about 70 percent of all *S. pyogenes* isolates. The gene encoding SMEZ is chromosomal and almost invariably present in all group A streptococci, making it the most common of all PET genes. The extensive degree of variation can be taken as evidence that SMEZ provides an advantage to the producing *S. pyogenes* and that new variants arise as a result of the need to escape neutralizing antibodies (Proft et al. 2000). It is interesting and still unexplained, in spite of this variation, that all SMEZ alleles target Vβ4 and Vβ8 T cells. It has been speculated that these T cells may have a special function in host defense against *S. pyogenes* (Proft et al. 2000). This conserved Vβ specificity is in contrast to, for example, SEA and SEE which in spite of having 85 percent amino acid identity vary in their Vβ specificities (Hudson et al. 1993).

The frequency of enterotoxin producers among clinical *S. aureus* isolates has been determined in several studies (Lehn et al. 1995). Depending on the origin of the isolates approximately 40–65 percent of *S. aureus* strains produce a PET. Most commonly SEA is produced (20–25 percent of strains), followed by TSST-1 (13–23 percent), SEB (7–13 percent), SEC (5–9 percent), SED (3–6 percent), and SEE (>1 percent). Five to 8 percent produce two enterotoxins, usually SEA plus TSST-1 or SEA plus SED, which is a much higher frequency than would have been expected from respective individual frequencies. Isolates producing toxins, e.g. SEG, SEH, or SEI are extremely rare. Data about the production of SPEA and SPEC by *S. pyogenes* strains isolated

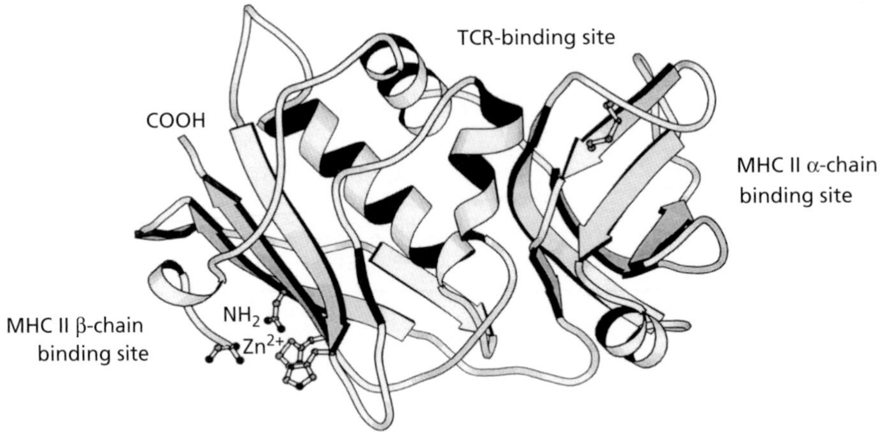

Figure 29.1 *Polypeptide fold of the staphylococcal enterotoxin A molecule. The binding sites for the T-cell receptor TCR Vβ, for the MHCII α chain and the Zn^{2+}-dependent binding site for the MHCII β chain are indicated. The drawing was made according to the published three-dimensional structure of staphylococcal enterotoxin A (Schad et al. 1995).*

from various sources vary considerably, reflecting the variability of clinical sources and the sensitivity of detection, because *S. pyogenes* produces lower amounts of SPE than *S. aureus* of SE. It is remarkable that the *smeZ* and *speG* genes are present in almost all group A streptococci in contrast to the other toxins (Proft et al. 2000). Information about the purification of the natural proteins has been reviewed (Alouf et al. 1991).

For many members of the SE family (the staphylococcal SEA, SEB, SEC2, SED, SEH, and TSST-1, and the streptococcal SPEA, SPEC, SPEH, SMEZ-2, and SSA) crystal structures are now available (Swaminathan et al. 1992; Prasad et al. 1993; Acharya et al. 1994; Papageorgiou et al. 1995; Schad et al. 1995). More recently, the crystal structures of several toxins, e.g. SEB, TSST-1, SEA, complexed with the human MHCII molecule HLA-DR1 have been determined and have – together with a large number of studies using mutated toxins or class II molecules – illustrated the molecular mode of binding of the toxins to the class II molecule (Jardetzky et al. 1994; Kim et al. 1994).

In spite of their low level of overall sequence homology the PETs show a similar overall structure: they are kidney-shaped, tightly packed molecules with a complex tertiary intertwined folding and are composed of two domains both containing β-sheets and α-helical structures (Figure 29.1). An interdomain groove is the TCR-binding site; distinct MHCII-binding sites have been identified. Each toxin has individual surface features explaining the individual mechanism of action and the low or absent serological crossreactivity between toxins.

Fraser et al. first described, for SEA, that some superantigens bind a Zn^{2+} ion by two histidine residues and an aspartate residue; in the case of SEA residues this was His-187, His-225, and Asp-227. This binding of Zn^{2+} is required for binding to MHCII molecules (Fraser et al. 1992; Abrahmsen et al. 1995; Hudson et al. 1995). A similar Zn^{2+}-binding motif is present in SEC but not in SEB and is apparently not related to functional activities (Bohach 1997).

Molecular mechanism of action

BINDING TO MHC CLASS II MOLECULES

A hallmark of superantigens is their requirement for MHCII molecules on presenting cells for optimal stimulation of T cells (Fleischer and Schrezenmeier 1988), reflected by their binding to MHCII molecules (Fischer et al. 1989; Fleischer et al. 1989; Fraser 1989; Scholl et al. 1989). Binding differs from normal presentation of processed peptide antigen because superantigens bind as unprocessed proteins outside the antigen-binding groove of the class II molecule (Jardetzky et al. 1994; Kim et al. 1994). Fixed MHCII-positive cells present superantigens effectively to T cells (Fleischer and Schrezenmeier 1988). However, although this basic mechanism is shared by all superantigens individual members of the PETs have developed unique modes of interaction with the class II molecule. Most intriguing are the many different strategies that various PETs use to accomplish MHC binding. They exhibit different binding sites and binding mechanisms and, by using two different binding sites or by forming homodimers, they can crosslink MHC molecules.

The staphylococcal enterotoxins and the SPEs SSA and SPEA have a generic binding site for the MHC α chain in their N-terminus. The toxins of groups IV and V as well as SEH appear not to use or possess this binding site, but use a high-affinity binding site for the β chain via zinc.

The crystal structures of the complex between HLA-DR1 and SEB or TSST-1 shows that SEB and TSST-1 bind to overlapping regions on the monomorphic α chain. Both toxins use residues of the N-terminal domain for this interaction. SEB binds at the side of the molecule leaving the peptide binding site and the peptide exposed (Jardetzky et al. 1994). This binding is of low affinity and it has been suggested that, in the trimolecular complex of SEB, class II molecule, and TCR, the TCR will interact with the class II molecule to stabilize the complex (Seth et al. 1994). TSST-1, in contrast, binds on the top of the α chain and covers the α chain α-helix peptide-binding site (Kim et al. 1994). Binding to the class II molecule does not change the conformation of TSST-1 (Mitchell et al. 1997). Although the binding sites of SEB and TSST-1 overlap on the class II molecule the two toxins do not compete for binding. This is because the peptide within the antigen-binding groove influences the binding of TSST-1 (von Bonin et al. 1995; Wen et al. 1996). TSST-1 binds only to a subset of class II molecules containing the appropriate peptides to which SEB does not bind. Thus, TSST-1 exploits the extreme variability of the MHC-bound peptides for its superantigenic toxins. The crystal structure of SEH (which does not bind to the α chain) complexed with HLA-DR1 also shows an interaction of the superantigen with the peptide (Petersson et al. 2001). The same may be true for other PETs of this group.

Members of groups III, IV, and V use another binding site at the polymorphic β chain of the class II molecule involving the Zn^{2+}-binding site. This binding is of high affinity and uses a bridge between the Zn^{2+} bound to, for example, SEA (via His-187, His-225, and Asp2-27) and His-81 of the MHCII β chain (Abrahmsen et al. 1995; Hudson et al. 1995). Details of this interaction are described in reviews (Svensson et al. 1997; Papageogiou and Acharya 2000).

Members of the SEA group (except SEH) use this mechanism in addition to the α-chain-binding site. Thus, SEA and similar toxins are able to bind with two distinct binding sites to two different sites on the class II molecule and are, as a consequence, able to crosslink class II molecules on the surface of the presenting cell on its own, in the absence of a T cell. It has been shown that this crosslinking leads to transduction of signals in the cell, resulting in cytokine production in monocytes or costimulation of B cells (Mourad et al. 1990; Fuleihan et al. 1991). SEA competes with SEB and TSST-1 for binding.

Some PETs have the ability to form homodimers and in this way form functionally divalent molecules that are also able to crosslink class II molecules (Papageorgiu and Acharya 2000). The streptococcal SPEC forms a noncovalent homodimer which binds only to the β chain of the class II molecule by a Zn^{2+}-mediated binding. The low-affinity α-chain-binding sites of SPEC are covered by the dimerization (Roussel et al. 1997; Li et al. 1997, 1998). SED has been reported to form a zinc-dependent homodimer (Al-Daccak et al. 1998).

NON-MHC RECEPTORS

Under certain conditions SEs have also been shown to activate T cells in the absence of class II molecules on accessory or target cells. Cytotoxic T cells can, for example, lyse target cells that do not express class II molecules; however, much higher concentrations of SEs are required (Dohlsten et al. 1991; Herrmann et al. 1991). This is not surprising given the fact that PETs can interact directly with the TCR (see below), so a superantigen bound to any surface can in principle activate T cells. Whether there is a second specific receptor or whether the SEs nonspecifically stick to the surface of certain cells is unclear. Additional receptors have also been postulated, e.g. on endothelial cells or on thrombocytes, but have not been characterized (reviewed in Fleischer and Hartwig 1992). It is unclear whether such non-MHC receptors play any physiological role.

INTERACTION WITH THE TCR

The major interaction site on the αβ TCR is the variable part of the β chain (Vβ). Stimulation of murine or human T cells with a given toxin in vitro (Table 29.3), leads to selective expansion of $CD4^+$ and $CD8^+$T cells carrying certain Vβ (Janeway et al. 1989; Kappler et al. 1989; White et al. 1989). A similar preference (for Vγ) was reported for the response of γδ T cells. Transfer of a given Vβ or of an epitope of the hypervariable region 4 of the Vβ, transfers the specific response of the T cell to the recipient T cell (Choi et al. 1990b; Fleischer et al. 1996). The hypervariable region 4 is not involved in peptide-antigen recognition and is located on an exposed lateral region. It is important to note that different Vβs bind to different toxins with different affinities, so T cells with the highest affinity for a given toxin are preferentially expanded in bulk culture. This notion explains that T cells with certain Vβ can respond to a toxin that are not preferentially expanded in such bulk cultures (Fleischer et al. 1991, 1996).

From structural and mutational data a model of the ternary complex of SEB, TCR, and MHCII molecule was hypothesized. The complementarity-determining regions of the TCR are oriented over the MHC peptide-binding site, with the Vβ domain bound to SEB and the Vα domain above the class II β1 domain (Jardetzky et al. 1994). This model is consistent with the findings that the TCR α chain and the polymorphic MHC allotype influence the response of the T cell to some superantigens. In the ternary complex involving SEB the TCR interacts directly with the class II molecule, this is not the case with, for example, SEH (Petersson et al. 2001). Thus individual superantigens vary in the way they crosslink TCR and MHC II.

More recently, a soluble TCR Vβ chain has been used to analyze the binding of PET. The soluble β chain had the same specificity for different PETs as the T cell from which the β chain was derived. Affinities ranged from 0.9 μmol/l to 140 μmol/l, similar to what had been found for the affinities of the TCR to specific peptide/MHC complexes (Li et al. 1998). The three-dimensional structure of the complex between a soluble TCR β chain and

Table 29.3 *Preferential stimulation of human and murine T cells by bacterial toxins*

Toxin	Reported preference for T cells expressing TCR Vβ of: Human T cells	Mouse T cells
SEA	1.1, 5.3, 6.3, 6.4, 6.9, 7.3, 7.4, 9.1, 18	1, 3, 10, 11, 12, 17
SEB	3, 12, 13.1, 13.2, 14, 15, 17, 20	3, 7, 8.1, 8.2, 8.3, 11, 17
SEC1	3, 12, 13.1, 13.2, 14, 15, 17, 20	3, 6.4, 12, 15
SEC2	12, 13.1, 13.2, 14, 15, 17, 20	3, 8.2, 10, 17
SEC3	12, 13.2, 14, 15, 17, 20	3, 5, 12, 13.2
SED	5, 12	3, 8.2, 8.3, 11, 17
SEE	5, 6, 8, 18	11, 15, 17
SEG	3, 12, 13.1, 13.2, 14, 15	
SEH		No stimulation
SEI	1, 5, 6, 9, 23	
SEJ	2, 3, 12, 14, 17	
SEK	5.1, 5.2, 6.7	
SEL		
SEM	6, 7, 8, 9, 18, 21	
SEM		
SEN		
SEO	5, 7, 9, 22	
TSST-1	2	3, 4, 15, 17
SPEA	12, 14, 15	8.2
SPEC	1, 2, 5.1, 10	No stimulation
SPEG	**2.1**, 4.1, 11.2, 19.1, 12, 3	
SPEH	**2.1**, 7.3, 9.1	
SPEI	5.3, 6.9, 9.1, **18.1**, 22	
SPEJ	2, 3, 12, 14, 17 (**2.1**, 8.1)	
SPEK		
SPEL		
SMEZ	4, 8	NA
SSA	1, 3, (5.2), 15	NA
YPMa	3, 9, 13.1, 13.2	7, 8.1, 8.2, 8.3
YPMb	3, 9, 13.1, 13.2	NA
MAS	3.1, 5, 7, 8, 10, 11.1, 12.1, 14, 17.1, 20	5.1, 6, 8.1, 8.2, 8.3

Data are compiled from the literature. Note that determinations have been made in many cases with native and not with recombinant proteins; therefore Vβ specificities of SE and SPE may be affected by contaminations with other toxins, e.g. stimulation of human $V\beta2^+$ and $V\beta8^+$ T cells reported for native SPEA (Abe et al. 1991), and of $V\beta8^+$ T cells reported for native SPEC (Tomai et al. 1992), is not found with recombinant toxins (Braun et al. 1993). Vβ profiles were assayed by polymerase chain reaction or by Vβ-specific antibodies.

SEC3 was determined. The complementarity-determining region (CDR) 2 of the β chain and, to lesser extents, CDR1 and the hypervariable region 4 (HV4) bind in a cleft between the small and large domains of the SE (Fields et al. 1996).

In spite of the requirement for class II molecules in T-cell stimulation, the toxins can also stimulate T cells in the absence of class II molecules. SE-mediated cytotoxicity has been found against several class II-negative target cells (Dohlsten et al. 1991; Herrmann et al. 1991). SEA covalently linked to antibodies against any cell surface molecule can direct lysis of cytotoxic cells to class II-negative target cells (Dohlsten et al. 1991) and toxin bound to plastic can under certain conditions activate T cells (Fleischer et al. 1991). It is noteworthy that some PETs, e.g. SPEC and SPEG and SEH do not stimulate mouse T cells at all, although they do bind to murine MHCII molecules (Proft et al. 1999; Petersson et al. 2001).

The molecular mechanism of T-cell stimulation is thus a multivalent crosslinking of TCR molecules with MHCII molecules on the presenting cell. This crosslinking of the TCR, however, requires – at least at low toxin concentrations – additional adhesion molecules, such as CD2, CD11a, or CD28. The CD4 or CD8 molecules appear not to be required, although in some cases CD4 interaction augments the response (Sekaly et al. 1991). By using this molecular mechanism the superantigen uses the most efficient way to stimulate T lymphocytes. The use of class II molecules as specific receptors restricts the T-cell interaction to the professional APCs, most probably the dendritic cells because macrophages are dispensable to T-cell activation in vivo (Bette et al. 1993).

Biological significance of pyrogenic exotoxins

ROLE OF PYROGENIC EXOTOXINS AS VIRULENCE FACTORS

Although superantigens act on T cells of different species, it appears that they work best in the species that is a natural host for the producing pathogen. The toxins derived from *S. aureus* and *S. pyogenes* (bacteria not found in wild mice) stimulate human T cells much more efficiently than murine T cells, whereas the opposite is true for the mitogen derived from *Mycoplasma arthritidis* (a natural pathogen for rodents) (Fleischer et al. 1991). TSST-1 or SEC produced by ovine strains of *S. aureus* is much more efficient on ovine T cells than on human T cells (Lee et al. 1992; Marr et al. 1993). This suggests that these molecules have been adapted in evolution to the MHC and TCR molecules of the natural host. Acquisition by gene transfer of toxin genes and their subsequent mutation is probably the mechanism of such adaptation, such as transfer of *tst* genes from human to ovine and bovine *S. aureus* strains.

For several reasons it may be expected that the production of a superantigen offers an evolutionary advantage for the respective pathogen. First, the molecular mechanism of action, the crosslinking of TCR Vβ with class II molecules, has evolved several times separately in evolution. Second, the extensive genetic polymorphism of the PETs argues that the presence of multiple forms of a superantigen is advantageous for the producing species. Finally, it appears that superantigens have been adapted by the producing pathogen to the host's immune system, because they have the highest mitogenic potential in the immune system of their respective natural host.

Thus, the evolutionary advantage can be expected to be directly or indirectly linked to the T-cell stimulatory function of superantigens. This has indeed recently been shown for the mouse mammary tumor viruses: T-lymphocyte stimulation is required for effective multiplication and transmission of the virus as discussed below (Held et al. 1994). For the gram-positive cocci there is so far no clear evidence where the advantage of T-cell stimulation lies. The decisive mechanisms against these extracellular bacteria are granulocytes, antibodies, and complement. It is, however, noteworthy that production of a superantigen leads to delayed clearance of *S. aureus* in infected mice (Rott and Fleischer 1994). Moreover, it has been repeatedly shown that humoral and cellular immune responses are diminished if an SE is injected along with a conventional antigen.

ROLE IN PATHOGENICITY

Given the extremely low concentration of picograms per milliliter required for T-cell stimulation and the large amounts of toxin secreted by some strains of staphylococci and streptococci into the culture medium, it is clear that a small focus of bacterial infection can be sufficient to induce a general activation of the immune system and a massive expansion of responding T cells. In patients with toxic shock caused by TSST-1-producing *S. aureus*, $V\beta^+$ cells expand to up to 70 percent of all peripheral blood T cells (Choi et al. 1990a). Consequences of such polyclonal T-cell stimulation can be shock, immunosuppression, and autoimmunity.

The shock-like symptoms induced by these toxins are caused by a massive release of lymphokines (e.g. tumor necrosis factor-α (TNF-α), interferon-γ (IFN-γ), interleukin-2 (IL-2)) and monokines (IL-12). Critical mediators in this shock-like symptom are apparently TNF-α and IFN-γ, both of which are produced by T lymphocytes (Miethke et al. 1992; Bette et al. 1993). The same mediators are involved in the septic shock induced by endotoxin of gram-negative bacteria. It appears that, although distinct cell populations are stimulated in gram-positive and gram-negative shock, a similar cytokine cascade is initiated that ultimately leads to the same terminal events. It is remarkable and still not explained in detail that lipopolysaccharide (LPS) and superantigen potentiate their effects if acting simultaneously in vivo.

Toxic shock syndrome (TSS) is observed during human infections with *S. aureus* and *S. pyogenes*. It is interesting to note that not all SEs have been implicated in such diseases. So far TSST-1 and SEB are almost exclusively involved in staphylococcal toxic shock. Although the gene for TSST-1 is widely distributed among staphylococci, a single *S. aureus* clone accounts for the majority of toxic shock cases in five countries (Musser et al. 1990). This indicates that not the superantigen alone but rather a combination of virulence factors determines pathogenicity. A greater heterogeneity was found with *S. pyogenes* isolates from patients with streptococcal TSS-like syndrome. Here, the ability to cause this syndrome is associated with all of the known SPEs, but SPEA-producing bacteria cause a high proportion of cases. Interestingly, two of four *speA* alleles were present in single bacterial clones that caused the great majority of these cases (Nelson et al. 1991). As a result of the higher invasiveness of *S. pyogenes* streptococcal TSS is associated with higher mortality and certain M types are more strongly associated with TSS than others (reviewed by McCormick et al. 2001).

Immunosuppression can result because stimulation of many T cells will impede the coordinated immune response. Moreover, a toxin can induce anergy and death by apoptosis in those T cells responding to it. After injection of an SE into mice, the initially responding T cells are partially deleted and those remaining in the spleen no longer respond to staphylococcal enterotoxin B or to anti-TCR antibodies. It is also conceivable that activated $CD8^+$ T cells could destroy APCs or B lymphocytes that have toxin molecules bound to their class II antigens.

ASSOCIATION WITH AUTOIMMUNITY

The polyclonal activation of T cells by PETs could bypass the control of autoreactive T cells or helper T cells could be focused on autoreactive B cells and induce autoantibody production. This may be of relevance, e.g. in streptococcal diseases that are associated with autoimmune phenomena. Stimulation of autoreactive B cells by crossreactive epitopes of, for example, M proteins and the generation of help from T cells stimulated by erythrogenic toxins may provide a pathogenic mechanism. The requirement for such an interaction of two different pathogenicity factors of group A streptococci could explain why such poststreptococcal autoimmune diseases are relatively rarely found. In experimental models it was shown that control of autoreactive T cells could be bypassed by injection of a superantigen (Schiffenbauer et al. 1998). An ongoing autoimmune reaction against brain or joint antigens was aggravated by the injection of a superantigen (Cole and Griffiths 1993; Schiffenbauer et al. 1998). Moreover, a resolved experimental allergic encephalomyelitis could be re-exacerbated by injection of a superantigen stimulating the appropriate autoreactive T cells. Moreover in naïve animals a polyclonal T cell activation by a superantigen could prime Vβ-specific T-cell reponses to a selfantigen by a non-Vβ-specific mechanism of 'innocent' bystander activation (Rott et al. 1995).

Interest has been focused on the findings of an increase in $V\beta2^+$ and $V\beta8^+$ T cells in Kawasaki's syndrome, an acute multisystem vasculitis in children. Staphylococci and streptococci producing PETs have been isolated from these patients, their pathogenic relevance is, however, still unclear (Freeman and Shulman 2001).

In patients with atopic dermatitis, a chronic inflammatory skin disease associated with pruritus and elevated serum IgE, persistent colonization with *S. aureus* is a well-known feature. There is evidence that SEs produced by the staphylococci have the potential to trigger the chronic T-cell-mediated skin inflammation (Herz et al. 1998). It is also a common observation that exacerbations of psoriasis are often associated with streptococcal infections and a causal link has been suggested (Ortonne 1996).

THE ENTEROTOXIC ACTIVITY

The staphylococcal enterotoxins are named for their ability to induce a gastrointestinal illness on oral uptake of a few micrograms within 2–4 h in primates. Studies with mutant molecules (Hufnagle et al. 1991; Harris et al. 1993) and with chemically modified SEs (Alber et al. 1990) indicate that the enteropathogenicity of SEs is not caused by an action on T cells. It has been suggested that the symptoms of the gastrointestinal intoxication are caused by leukotrienes and histamine released from mast cells in response to substance P in the mucosa (Alber et al. 1989). The receptors involved are still obscure.

MYCOPLASMA ARTHRITIDIS SUPERANTIGEN

Mycoplasma arthritidis is a pathogen for rodents and induces an acute inflammatory infection in rats and mice. In mice this inflammation is followed by a chronic joint disease. Cell-free supernatants of *M. arthritidis* contain a potent T-cell mitogen, acting on T cells of several species. Although this mitogenic principle has been known of for more than 15 years (Cole and Atkin 1991), only recently has the protein been cloned (Cole et al. 1996). This is a result of the small amounts of M. arthritidis superantigen (MAS) in the mycoplasma culture and of the lability and adhesive property of MAS. MAS is a hydrophobic and basic peptide that is heat labile at 56°C and susceptible to serine proteases. The sequence reveals a protein unrelated to any other superantigen with 153 amino acids and a calculated molecular mass of 25 kDa and a very basic p*I* of 10 (Cole et al. 1996).

Mycoplasma arthritidis superantigen has all the functional properties of superantigens (Matthes et al. 1988; Cole et al. 1990). Its T-cell stimulatory properties are strictly dependent on the presence of H2-IE molecules or HLA-DR molecules on the stimulating cells. MAS stimulates both $CD4^+$ and $CD8^+$ T lymphocytes and responsive γδ T cells have been described. There is a preferential stimulation of mouse T cells expressing Vβ6, 8.1, 8.2, and 8.3, and of human T lymphocytes expressing Vβ17.1 (also designated 19.1). In addition, there are other TCRs that respond to MAS, but with lower affinity (Fleischer et al. 1991).

Injection of MAS into experimental animals induces a mild toxic shock syndrome and pronounced T-cell suppression (Cole and Wells 1990). This is only found in MAS-responsive mouse strains that possess H2-IE molecules. The chronic joint disease is induced only by infection with *Mycoplasma* itself or by intra-articular injection of MAS. The role of the superantigen in the induction of the arthritic disease is still not clear. It is noteworthy that MAS injection induces a flare-up in mice that have recovered from a collagen-induced arthritis. It has been noted that some parameters of the *M. arthritidis*-induced disease can also be found in rheumatoid arthritis and that antibodies to MAS are present in some patients with this disease. An involvement of MAS-like superantigens in the pathophysiology of rheumatoid arthritis has been suspected (Knudtson et al. 1997).

YERSINIA PSEUDOTUBERCULOSIS MITOGEN

The three pathogenic species of *Yersinia*, *Y. enterocolitica*, *Y. pseudotuberculosis*, and *Y. pestis*, produce many virulence factors required for survival in the body. *Y. enterocolitica* and *Y. pseudotuberculosis* have been reported to produce superantigens. Although the putative superantigen of *Y. enterocolitica* still awaits isolation and confirmation, a superantigen designated Y. pseudotuberculosis mitogen (YPM) has been purified and cloned (Ito et al. 1995; Miyoshi-Akiyama et al. 1995). YPM is synthesized as a precursor of 151 amino acids which is cleaved to a mature protein of 14 kDa and 131 amino acids. It has no homology with any other superantigen. The protein has all the characteristics of a superantigen in vitro and in vivo. It is produced by certain serotypes of *Y. pseudotuberculosis* with distinct geographical distribution. The gene encoding YPM was detected in 95 percent of clinical isolates of *Y. pseudotuberculosis* from Japan or the far eastern Russian states but only in 17 percent of European clinical isolates (Yoshino et al. 1995). Recently, a variant YPM was isolated and cloned (Ramamurthy et al. 1997). The two YPMs (designated YPMa and YPMb) have 83 percent homology. A third variant was recently described. This indicates that YPM forms a polymorphic family as the SE.

The infection with *Y. pseudotuberculosis* is characterized by acute mesenteric inflammation and lymphadenopathy and systemic symptoms such as fever and leukocytosis. In patients with *Y. pseudotuberculosis* infections an elevation of Vβ3-bearing T cells has been found (Abe et al. 1997). Several immunopathological diseases can follow an infection with *Y. pseudotuberculosis* such as reactive arthritis or uveitis and erythema nodosum. Moreover, Kawasaki's syndrome has been linked to *Y. pseudotuberculosis* infections. A role of the superantigen YPM in the pathology of this infection is conceivable but still not clear. It has been shown in mice that YPM-deficient *Y. pseudotuberculosis* bacteria have a reduced virulence (Carnoy et al. 2000).

MOUSE MAMMARY TUMOR VIRUSES

The first viral superantigens (vSag) described were those encoded by mouse mammary tumor viruses (MMTV), retroviruses that cause mammary carcinomas in mice. In fact these powerful stimulators were known since 1973 as minor lymphocyte-stimulating antigens (Mls) but remained enigmatic (Janeway 1991) until their association with MMTV was found (reviewed in Acha-Orbea and MacDonald 1995).

The superantigen is encoded in an open reading frame encoding approximately 320 amino acids located adjacent to the 3′ long terminal repeat. As with the bacterial superantigens there is extensive polymorphism. All MMTV superantigens show a high degree of sequence conservation with the exception of the carboxy-terminus which shows extensive polymorphism. This part encodes the putative Vβ-binding part of the molecule. The viral superantigen is synthesized as a glycosylated type II membrane protein with an extracellular carboxy terminus and is then proteolytically processed. In CHO cells the superantigen is cleaved by the endoprotease furin and a carboxy-terminal 18-kDa fragment has been shown to be expressed on the surface. Endoproteases are also possibly able to cleave the superantigen (Denis et al. 2000).

It has been noted that the vSags have functional and structural similarities with the MHCII-associated invariant chain Ii. Both are class II membrane proteins of similar size and both associate with class II molecules inside the cell. Both possess a strong and invariant class II-binding motif, the invariant chain Ii has the CLIP sequence, and the vSag has a class II-binding motif at a location corresponding to CLIP in the Ii (Hsu et al. 2001). This motif is conserved in all MMTV superantigens. A model for the association of vSag with class II molecules implies that vSag competes with Ii for binding to the peptide groove of class II αβ dimers in the endoplasmic reticulum. In the trans-Golgi network the vSag is cleaved by furin, yielding the 18-kDa carboxy-terminal fragment of the superantigen that is bound outside the peptide-binding groove (Hsu et al. 2001). After transport to the cell surface the vSag–class II complex is accessible for T cells. The fate of the remaining portion of the vSag is still unclear.

When taken up by the newborn mouse with the maternal milk, the virus infects naïve B cells and immature dendritic cells (DC) (Vacheron et al. 2002) which express the viral superantigen. Infected B cells stimulate T cells carrying the appropriate Vβs which in turn stimulate infected B cells to proliferate and increase exponentially in number (Held et al. 1993). This allows the virus to persist until the mammary gland has matured. Infected mammary epithelial cells produce virus, allowing the transfer to the newborn mouse. Proviral insertion in epithelial cells can lead to activation of endogenous cellular oncogenes and cell transformation.

Mice harboring integrated endogenous MMTVs or a transgenic superantigen delete T cells carrying the Vβ that has reacted with the vSag of the endogenous MMTV. These mice are protected against infectious MMTV with specificity for the same Vβ (Golovkina et al. 1992). MMTVs in which the vSag has been deleted are still fully infectious but are not able to reach the mammary gland to effect transmission.

HUMAN ENDOGENOUS RETROVIRUSES

After the description of the MMTV superantigen many groups searched for viral superantigens in humans. There were a number of reports that described imbalances in Vβ expression in certain human diseases. However, although they were published in first-class journals they remained either unclear or unconfirmed. Rabies virus (Lafon et al. 1992), HIV (Imberti et al. 1991), cytomegalovirus (CMV) (Dobrescu et al. 1995), or Epstein–Barr virus (EBV) (Sutkowski et al. 1996), for example, were proposed to encode superantigens. However, it was not possible to identify clearly the respective gene in these viruses, e.g. by recombinant expression.

Several groups have also provided indirect evidence for the involvement of superantigens in human diseases. In all these cases an imbalance in the Vβ-composition of T cells from patients has been found, e.g. two groups have demonstrated a selective increase in T cells carrying Vβ14 in the synovial fluid of patients with rheumatoid arthritis (Kotzin et al. 1993). Furthermore, an imbalance in the Vβ repertoire of T cells has repeatedly been reported in patients with AIDS, although not confirmed by all investigators. It is still unclear, however, if this is the result of a superantigen produced by HIV or of secondary infection or a nonsuperantigen-dependent mechanism. Although the idea that superantigens are at work in such diseases is very exciting, one has to bear in mind that preferential stimulation of certain Vβ-bearing T cells can also occur during a normal immune response (Boitel et al. 1992).

More recently, however, compelling evidence has been presented by Conrad et al. (1994) that a human endogenous retrovirus encodes a superantigen. The N-terminal moiety of the envelope gene of a polymorphic and defective provirus originally named IDDMK1,2 encodes an MHCII-dependent Sag. This virus, now designated HERV-K18.1, is one of three alleles of the HERV-K18 family of proviruses, each of which encodes a superantigen with specificity for Vβ7 and Vβ13 T cells.

Conrad et al. (1994) had previously observed that $V\beta7^+$ T cells were selectively expanded among islet-infiltrating T cells in two individuals in the early phase of type 1 diabetes mellitus. Moreover there was evidence of positive selection, after exposure to diabetic islet cell membrane preparations, of $V\beta7^+$ T cells from peripheral blood lymphocytes of individuals who did not have diabetes. They proposed that expression of the superantigen from the HERV-K18.1, induced in professional APCs, leads to β-cell destruction via the systemic activation of autoreactive T cells (Conrad et al. 1997).

Surprisingly, however, several other groups have not been able to find evidence for a superantigen in HERV. Lapatschek et al. (2000) amplified by polymerase chain reaction (PCR) and cloned into open reading frames of eukaryotic expression vectors, which were identical or very similar to IDDMK1,2. Although they were able to demonstrate mRNA expression and protein production in A20 B-lymphoma cells they could not find any evidence that the open reading frame (orf)-stimulated human or murine T cells in a Vβ-specific fashion.

An intriguing observation was that expression of HERV-K18 Sags was inducible by IFN-α and this is sufficient to stimulate Vβ7 T cells to levels comparable to transfectants constitutively expressing HERV-K18 Sags (Stauffer et al. 2001). This link between viral infections and IFN-α-regulated Sag expression could be a mechanism through which environmental factors may cause disease in genetically susceptible individuals. This observation was extended to show that EBV transcriptionally activated the viral superantigen, suggesting that the previously described EBV-associated superantigen activity was caused by the EBV-induced activation of the endogenous retrovirus (Sutkowski et al. 2001).

It has therefore been proposed that the superantigen activity found with several human viruses may not be caused by a viral gene product but by the activation, e.g. via IFN, of endogenous retroviral superantigen expression (Woodland 2002). This could explain the failure to identify molecularly such superantigens in rabies virus, CMV, and EBV. It could also explain the Vβ imbalances found in a number of human autoimmune diseases or HIV infection.

MORE SUPERANTIGENS?

In addition to the members of the PET family, there are other staphylococcal and streptococcal proteins genetically unrelated to the enterotoxins that have been proposed as superantigens, such as the streptococcal M protein, the streptococcal erythrogenic toxin B, and the staphylococcal exfoliative (epidermolytic) toxins. However, the evidence discussed below suggests that these molecules are not superantigens but that their mitogenicity is the result of artifacts (Fleischer et al. 1995).

The staphylococcal exfoliative toxins

The exfoliative toxins A and B of *S. aureus* (ETA and ETB) share a high-sequence homology but are serologically unrelated. They are able to dissociate intercellular adhesion molecules in the skin leading to subgranular epidermolysis. Epidermolytic toxin A is synthesized as a precursor molecule of 31 kDa which is subsequently cleaved to the mature polypeptide of 27 kDa. Both ETA and ETB have an intrinsic esterase activity and are homologous to the staphylococcus V8 protease (Bailey and Redpath 1992). They share the catalytic triad at the protease active center. Mutation of the serine of the active center leads to loss of epidermolytic activity in mice. ETA was reported to be a superantigen stimulating $V\beta2^+$ T cells (Marrack and Kappler 1990).

However, it was subsequently shown that ETA does not bind MHCII molecules (Herrmann et al. 1989) and that recombinant ETA produced in S. aureus had no mitogenic activity toward human peripheral blood mononuclear cells (PBMC) or Vβ2$^+$ T cells (Fleischer and Bailey 1991). More recently, it was described that both ETA and ETB in recombinant form stimulated human Vβ3, -12, -14, -15, and -17 T cells, a profile that is very similar to that of SEB and SEC. MHCII binding was not investigated. In in vivo tests for pyrogenicity only ETB, but not ETB, showed pyrogenic activity (Monday et al. 1999), one of the hallmarks of superantigens. The question if the exfoliative toxins are superantigens (or T-cell-specific mitogens at all) is thus not unequivocally settled.

M proteins and SPEB of *S. pyogenes*

M proteins of *S. pyogenes* are major virulence factors of group A streptococci. They are receptor proteins that show multiple binding to different plasma proteins and protect streptococci against phagocytosis. They form a family of closely related proteins protruding from the cell surface. The variable M-terminal portion of the molecule carries the M-type-specific antigen epitopes. M-protein fragments produced by limited proteolytic digestion of whole streptococci with a molecular mass of 33 kDa (pepM5) have been proposed to be superantigens and to stimulate Vβ2$^+$, 4$^+$, and -8$^+$ human T cells (Tomai et al. 1991, 1992).

If, however, M5 protein or pepM5 is thoroughly purified, it is no longer mitogenic (Fleischer et al. 1992; Degnan et al. 1997). The stimulatory activity for Vβ2$^+$ and Vβ8$^+$ T cells could be separated from each other, suggesting that the superantigenic activity of M protein type 5 could be caused by contamination with at least two different, possibly novel, streptococcal PETs (Schmidt et al. 1995). Recombinant M5 protein or its fragments were not mitogenic (Robinson et al. 1991; Schmidt et al. 1995; Degnan et al. 1997).

Taken together, the available evidence strongly suggests that mitogenicity of M-protein preparations is not the result of an intrinsic activity but of contaminating SPEs, some of them not known at the time of the reports. The Vβ pattern matches well the pattern of SPEC, SPEG, and SMEZ.

The same situation was found with the streptococcal erythrogenic toxin B (SPEB) which is identical to the precursor of the streptococcal protease. It is a molecule of 371 residues with 40 kDa of molecular mass and is successively processed to the mature protease of 253 amino acids and 27 kDa. All group A streptococci have SPEB, and there is only one nonpolymorphic gene for this molecule present in the genome. SPEB has no homologies to any member of the staphylococcal enterotoxin family (Betley et al. 1992). SPEB has been reported to stimulate selectively Vβ8$^+$ human T cells. On proper purification of SPEB, however, it became evident that the superantigenic properties of these molecules are caused by contamination with a novel Vβ8-stimulating PET designated SPEX (Braun et al. 1993) and recombinant SPEB was not mitogenic (Gerlach et al. 1994). The Vβ8-stimulator SPEX is identical to a variant of SMEZ (Kamezawa et al. 1997) and has subsequently been cloned (Gerlach et al. 2000).

The mitogenic factor of *S. pyogenes*

A protein of 26 kDa, the so-called mitogenic factor (MF), or SPEF (Norrby-Teglund et al. 1994), was purified from *S. pyogenes* strain NY5 (the prototype strain from which SPEA, SPEB, SPEC, and SMEZ were originally purified). MF is not polymorphic and is elaborated by all group A streptococci, but not by other streptococci. Interestingly, it has enzymatic activity: it is a nuclease (Iwasaki et al. 1997) and is identical with DNase B. The Vβ profile of the stimulated human T cells was recently described to be Vβ2, -4, -8, -15, and -19, and is surprisingly similar to that of pepM5 (Norrby-Teglund et al. 1994). We have not been able to detect mitogenicity with recombinant MF and have recently shown that SPEC and SMEZ are the contaminants causing mitogenicity of MF (Gerlach et al. 2001).

Taken together, these results raise an important caveat for the work with T-cell mitogens from *S. aureus* and *S. pyogenes*. As SE and SPE are active in concentrations of a few picograms per milliliter, the sensitivity of T cells to these stimulators is several orders of magnitude higher than the sensitivity of any biochemical or serological test and contamination with an SE or SPE is extremely difficult to exclude. Such a contamination can even occur if a recombinant protein is purified on columns previously used for purification of natural enterotoxin. Moreover, given the high polymorphism and unequal distribution of the PET it is surprising that nonpolymorphic proteins, such as SPEB or MF, present in all *S. pyogenes* isolates are superantigens. A number of different proteins of *S. pyogenes* have been purified from culture supernatants and have been found to behave like superantigens (Fleischer et al. 1995). The possibility that *S. pyogenes* has evolved several unrelated superantigens is exciting but we should await the confirmation of their activity using recombinant proteins.

The surprising finding that the unique molecular mechanism of T-cell stimulation has been developed completely independently by infectious agents of four very different classes, gram-positive cocci, gram-negative bacteria, *Mycoplasma*, and retroviruses, has led to the expectation that additional superantigens produced by other infectious pathogens would be found. This expectation together with the appealing designation 'superantigens' has induced a boom in reports of putative novel superantigens, usually in high-impact journals. However, the number of reported candidates exceeds by far the number of superantigens that are likely to exist.

Even a lectin has been reported to act as a superantigen (Saul et al. 2000) but this has not been confirmed by an independent group. For several candidates it is already now reported that attempts to confirm the initial claim have failed or have prompted contradiction. We have, for example, not been able to find any superantigenic activity with purified enterotoxin of *Clostridium perfringens*, both purified from *Clostridium perfringens* cultures and as a recombinant molecule from *Escherichia coli* (Krakauer et al. 1997), and also not with exotoxin A of *Pseudomonas aeruginosa* (unpublished observations). Likewise the initial report on a superantigen in *Toxoplasma gondii* was never confirmed (Denkers et al. 1994), and also one in *M. tuberculosis* (Ohmen et al. 1994).

CONCLUSION

The superantigens described in this chapter constitute the most efficient T-lymphocyte stimulators known. Although their exact benefit as virulence factors for the production of bacteria is not established, it is obvious that their induction of immunosuppression, destruction of APCs, and T-cell anergy should be of advantage to the infecting microorganisms. The manifold mechanisms of interaction with variable target structures of the immune system, the MHCII molecule and the TCR, allow a maximum of biological efficacy combined with a minimum of immunological crossreactivity. This is the basis for the extensive polymorphism of the superantigens that provides the producing species with a multitude of non-crossreacting toxins. The polymorphism is probably maintained and extended by permanent modifications of the superantigen genes through mutations and selection for variants that are optimally stimulatory for the host's immune system.

The determination of the complete genome sequence of *S. aureus* has revealed a cluster of genes called the *sets* (Staphylococcal enterotoxin-like toxins) that are resident in a pathogenicity island SaPIn2 and share structural homology to the SEs and SPEs and in particular to TSST-1 (Williams et al. 2000). They form a highly polymorphic family with more than a dozen members and several members are found within a given *S. aureus* strain. The encoded proteins that are secreted have the three-dimensional structure characteristic of the SEs but do not have the classical functions of superantigens, such as mitogenicity, pyrogenicity or the enhancement of endotoxic shock (Arcus et al. 2002).

Recently, Fraser and coworkers have been able to discover a biological function for an SET. SET1 was found to bind to IgA and to inhibit polyclonal IgA binding to Fc-receptors for IgA on myeloid cells. Moreover, SET1 also binds complement C5 with nanomolar affinity and inhibits complement-mediated lysis (Langley et al. in press). This is an exciting discovery showing that superantigen-related molecules that apparently have evolved from a common ancestor target components of the innate immune system and contribute to virulence and pathogenicity.

REFERENCES

Abe, J., Forrester, J., et al. 1991. Selective stimulation of human T cells with streptococcal erythrogenic toxins A and, B. *J Immunol*, **146**, 3747–50.

Abe, J., Onimaru, M., et al. 1997. Clinical role for a superantigen in *Yersinia pseudotuberculosis* infection. *J Clin Invest*, **99**, 1823–30.

Abrahmsen, L., Dohlsten, M., et al. 1995. Characterization of two distinct MHC class II binding sites in the superantigen staphylococcal enterotoxin, A. *EMBO J*, **14**, 2978–86.

Acha-Orbea, H. and MacDonald, H.R. 1995. Superantigens of mouse mammary tumor virus. *Annu Rev Immunol*, **13**, 459–86.

Acharya, K.R., Passalacqua, E.F., et al. 1994. Structural basis of superantigen action inferred from crystal structure of toxic-shock syndrome toxin-1. *Nature*, **367**, 94–7.

Alber, G., Scheuber, P.H., et al. 1989. Role of substance P in immediate-type skin reactions induced by staphylococcal enterotoxin B in unsensitized monkeys. *J Allergy Clin Immunol*, **84**, 880–5.

Alber, G., Hammer, D.K. and Fleischer, B. 1990. Relationship between enterotoxic and T lymphocyte stimulating activity of staphylococcal enterotoxin B. *J Immunol*, **144**, 4501–6.

Al-Daccak, R., Mehindate, K., et al. 1998. Staphylococcal enterotoxin D is a promiscuous superantigen offering multiple modes of interactions with the MHC class II receptors. *J Immunol*, **160**, 225–32.

Alouf, J.E., Knöll, H. and Köhler, W. 1991. The family of mitogenic, shock-inducing and superantigenic toxins from staphylococci and streptococci. In: Alouf, J.E. and Freer, J.H. (eds), *Sourcebook of bacterial protein toxins*. London: Academic Press, 147–86.

Arcus, V.L., Langley, R., et al. 2002. The three-dimensional structure of a superantigen-like protein, SET3, from a pathogenicity island of the *Staphylococcus aureus* genome. *J Biol Chem*, **277**, 32274–81.

Bailey, C.J. and Redpath, M.B. 1992. The esterolytic activity of epidermolytic toxins. *Biochem J*, **284**, 177–80.

Betley, M.J., Borst, D.W. and Regassa, L.B. 1992. Staphylococcal enterotoxins, toxic shock syndrome toxin and streptococcal pyrogenic exotoxins: a comparative study of their molecular biology. *Chem Immunol*, **55**, 1–35.

Bette, M., Schäfer, M.K., et al. 1993. Distribution and kinetics of superantigen-induced cytokine gene expression in mouse spleen. *J Exp Med*, **178**, 1531–9.

Bohach, G. 1997. Staphylococcal enterotoxins B and C. In: Leung, D.M., Huber, B. and Schlievert, P. (eds), *Superantigens*. New York: Marcel Dekker, 167–98.

Boitel, B., Ermontal, M., et al. 1992. Preferential Vβ gene usage and lack of junctional sequence conservation among human T cell receptors specific for a tetanus toxin-derived peptide: evidence for a dominant role of a germline-encoded V region in antigen/MHC recognition. *J Exp Med*, **175**, 765–78.

Bowness, P., Moss, P.A., et al. 1992. Clostridium perfringens enterotoxin is a superantigen reactive with human T cell receptors Vβ6.9 and Vβ22. *J Exp Med*, **176**, 893–6.

Braun, M.A., Gerlach, D., et al. 1993. Stimulation of human T cells by streptococcal 'superantigens' erythrogenic toxins. Scarlet fever toxins. *J Immunol*, **150**, 2457–67.

Carnoy, C., Muller-Alouf, H., et al. 2000. The superantigenic toxin of Yersinia pseudotuberculosis: a novel virulence factor? *Int J Med Microbiol*, **290**, 477–82.

Choi, Y., Lafferty, J.A., et al. 1990a. Selective expansion of T cells expressing Vβ2 in toxic shock syndrome. *J Exp Med*, **172**, 981–4.

Choi, Y.W., Herman, A., et al. 1990b. Residues of the variable region of the T-cell-receptor β-chain that interact with *S. aureus* toxin superantigens. *Nature*, **346**, 471–3.

Cole, B.C. and Atkin, C.L. 1991. The *Mycoplasma arthritidis* T cell mitogen MAM: a model superantigen. *Immunol Today*, **12**, 271–6.

Cole, B.C. and Griffiths, M.M. 1993. Triggering and exacerbation of autoimmune arthritis by the *Mycoplasma arthritidis* superantigen MAM. *Arthritis Rheum*, **36**, 994–1002.

Cole, B.C. and Wells, D.J. 1990. Immunosuppressive properties of the *Mycoplasma arthritidis* T-cell mitogen in vivo: inhibition of proliferative responses to T-cell mitogens. *Infect Immun*, **58**, 228–36.

Cole, B.C., Kartchner, D.R. and Wells, D.J. 1990. Stimulation of mouse lymphocytes by a mitogen derived from *Mycoplasma arthritidis* (MAM). VIII. Selective activation of T cells expressing distinct Vβ T cell receptors from various strains of mice by the 'superantigen' MAM. *J Immunol*, **144**, 425–31.

Cole, B.C., Knudtson, K.L., et al. 1996. The sequence of the *Mycoplasma arthritidis* superantigen, MAM: identification of functional domains and comparison with microbial superantigens and plant lectin mitogens. *J Exp Med*, **183**, 1105–10.

Conrad, B., Weissmahr, R.N., et al. 1997. A human endogenous retroviral superantigen as candidate autoimmune gene in type I diabetes. *Cell*, **90**, 303–13.

Conrad, B., Weidmann, E., et al. 1994. Evidence for superantigen involvement in insulin-dependent diabetes mellitus aetiology. *Nature*, **371**, 351–5.

Degnan, B., Taylor, J., et al. 1997. Streptococcus pyogenes type 5 M protein is an antigen, not a superantigen, for human T cells. *Hum Immunol*, **53**, 206–15.

Denis, F., Shoukry, N.H., et al. 2000. Alternative proteolytic processing of mouse mammary tumor virus superantigens. *J Virol*, **74**, 3067–73.

Denkers, E.Y., Caspar, P. and Sher, A. 1994. *Toxoplasma gondii* possesses a superantigen activity that selectively expands murine T cell receptor Vβ5-bearing CD8+ lymphocytes. *J Exp Med*, **180**, 985–94.

Dobrescu, D., Ursea, B., et al. 1995. Enhanced HIV-1 replication in V beta 12 T cells due to human cytomegalovirus in monocytes: evidence for a putative herpesvirus superantigen. *Cell*, **82**, 753–63.

Dohlsten, M., Hedlund, G., et al. 1991. Human MHC class II-colon carcinoma cells present staphylococcal superantigens to cytotoxic T lymphocytes: evidence for a novel enterotoxin receptor. *Eur J Immunol*, **121**, 131–5.

Fields, B.A., Malchiodi, E.L., et al. 1996. Crystal structure of a T-cell receptor β-chain complexed with a superantigen. *Nature*, **384**, 188–92.

Fischer, H., Dohlsten, M., et al. 1989. Binding of staphylococcal enterotoxin A to HLA-DR on B cell lines. *J Immunol*, **142**, 3151–7.

Fleischer, B. and Bailey, C.J. 1991. Recombinant epidermolytic. Exfoliative. toxin a of *Staphylococcus aureus* is not a superantigen. *Med Microbiol Immunol*, **180**, 273–8.

Fleischer, B. and Hartwig, U. 1992. T-lymphocyte stimulation by microbial superantigens. *Chem Immunol*, **55**, 36–64.

Fleischer, B. and Schrezenmeier, H. 1988. T cell stimulation by staphylococcal enterotoxins. Clonally variable response and requirement for MHC class II molecules on accessory or target cells. *J Exp Med*, **167**, 1697–708.

Fleischer, B., Schrezenmeier, H. and Conradt, P. 1989. T cell stimulation by staphylococcal enterotoxins. Role of class II molecules and T cell surface structures. *Cell Immunol*, **119**, 92–101.

Fleischer, B., Gerardy-Schahn, R., et al. 1991. A conserved mechanism of T cell stimulation by microbial toxins. Evidence for different affinities of T cell receptor-toxin interaction. *J Immunol*, **146**, 11–17.

Fleischer, B., Schmidt, K.H., et al. 1992. Separation of T cell stimulating activity from streptococcal M protein. *Infect Immun*, **60**, 1767–70.

Fleischer, B., Gerlach, D., et al. 1995. Superantigens and pseudosuperantigens of gram-positive cocci. *Med Microbiol Immunol*, **184**, 1–8.

Fleischer, B., Necker, A., et al. 1996. Reactivity of mouse T cell hybridomas expressing human Vβ gene segments with staphylococcal and streptococcal superantigens. *Infect Immun*, **64**, 987–94.

Fraser, J.D. 1989. High affinity binding of staphylococcal enterotoxins A and B to HLA-DR. *Nature*, **339**, 221–3.

Fraser, J.D., Urban, R.G., et al. 1992. Zinc regulates the function of two superantigens. *Proc Natl Acad Sci USA*, **89**, 5507–11.

Freeman, A.F. and Shulman, S.T. 2001. Recent developments in Kawasaki disease. *Curr Opin Infect Dis*, **14**, 357–61.

Fuleihan, R., Mourad, W., et al. 1991. Engagement of MHC-class II molecules by the staphylococcal exotoxin TSST-1 delivers a progression signal to mitogen activated B cells. *J Immunol*, **146**, 1661–6.

Gerlach, D., Reichardt, W., et al. 1994. Separation of mitogenic and pyrogenic activities from so-called erythrogenic toxin type B: streptococcal proteinase. *Int J Med Microbiol*, **280**, 507–14.

Gerlach, D., Fleischer, B., et al. 2000. Purification and biochemical characterization of a basic superantigen (SPEX/SMEZ$_3$) from *Streptococcus pyogenes*. *FEMS Microbiol Letts*, **188**, 153–63.

Gerlach, D., Schmidt, K.H. and Fleischer, B. 2001. Basic streptococcal superantigens (SPEX/SMEZ or SPEC) are responsible for the mitogenic activity of the so-called mitogenic factor. *FEMS Immunol Med Microbiol*, **30**, 209–16.

Golovkina, T.V., Chervonsky, A., et al. 1992. Transgenic mouse mammary tumor virus superantigen expression prevents viral infection. *Cell*, **15**, 637–65.

Goshorn, S.C. and Schlievert, P.M. 1989. Bacteriophage association of streptococcal pyrogenic exotoxin type, C. *J Bacteriol*, **171**, 3068–73.

Harris, T.O., Grossman, D., et al. 1993. Lack of complete correlation between emetic and T-cell-stimulatory activities of staphylococcal enterotoxins. *Infect Immun*, **61**, 3175–83.

Held, W., Waanders, G.A., et al. 1993. Superantigen-induced immune stimulation amplifies mouse mammary tumor virus infection and allows virus transmission. *Cell*, **74**, 529–40.

Held, W., Acha-Orbea, H., et al. 1994. Superantigens and retroviral infection: insights from mouse mammary tumor virus. *Immunol Today*, **15**, 184–90.

Herrmann, T., Acolla, R.S. and Macdonald, H.R. 1989. Different staphylococcal enterotoxins bind preferentially to distinct MHC class II isotypes. *Eur J Immunol*, **19**, 2171–4.

Herrmann, T., Romero, P., et al. 1991. Staphylococcal enterotoxin-dependent lysis of MHC class II negative target cells by cytolytic T lymphocytes. *J Immunol*, **146**, 2504–12.

Herz, U., Bunikowski, R. and Renz, H. 1998. Role of T cells in atopic dermatitis. New aspects on the dynamics of cytokine production and the contribution of bacterial superantigens. *Int Arch Allergy Immunol*, **115**, 179–90.

Ho, G., Campbell, W.H., et al. 1989. Production of a toxic shock syndrome toxin variant by *Staphylococcus aureus* strains associated with sheep, goats, and cows. *J Clin Microbiol*, **27**, 1946–8.

Hsu, P.N., Wolf Bryant, P., et al. 2001. Association of mouse mammary tumor virus superantigen with MHC class II during biosynthesis. *J Immunol*, **166**, 3309–14.

Hudson, K.R., Robinson, H. and Fraser, J.D. 1993. Two adjacent residues in staphylococcal enterotoxins A and E determine T cell receptor V beta specificity. *J Exp Med*, **177**, 175–84.

Hudson, K.R., Tiedemann, R.E., et al. 1995. Staphylococcal enterotoxin A has two cooperative binding sites on major histocompatibility complex class II. *J Exp Med*, **182**, 711–20.

Hufnagle, W.O., Tremaine, M.T. and Betley, M.J. 1991. The carboxyl-terminal region of staphylococcal enterotoxin type A is required for a fully active molecule. *Infect Immun*, **59**, 2126–34.

Imberti, L., Sottini, A., et al. 1991. Selective depletion in HIV infection of T cells that bear specific T cell receptor V beta sequences. *Science*, **254**, 860–2.

Ito, Y., Abe, J., et al. 1995. Sequence analysis of the gene for a novel superantigen produced by *Yersinia pseudotuberculosis* and expression of the recombinant protein. *J Immunol*, **154**, 5896–906.

Iwasaki, M., Igarashi, H. and Yutsudo, T. 1997. Mitogenic factor secreted by *Streptococcus pyogenes* is a heat-stable nuclease requiring His122 for activity. *Microbiology*, **143**, 2449–55.

Janeway, C. 1991. Immune recognition. Mls: makes a little sense. *Nature*, **349**, 459–61.

Janeway, C.A., Yagi, J., et al. 1989. T cell responses to Mls and to bacterial proteins that mimic its behaviour. *Immunol Rev*, **107**, 61–8.

Jardetzky, T.S., Brown, J.H., et al. 1994. Three-dimensional structure of a human class II histocompatibility molecule complexed with superantigen. *Nature*, **368**, 711–18.

Jarraud, S., Peyrat, M.A., et al. 2001. egc, a highly prevalent operon of enterotoxin gene, forms a putative nursery of superantigens in *Staphylococcus aureus*. Correction. *J Immunol*, **166**, 4260, .

Johnson, L.P. and Schlievert, P.M. 1984. Group A streptococcal phage T12 carries the structural gene for pyrogenic exotoxin type A. *Mol Gen Genet*, **194**, 52–6.

Kamezawa, Y., Nakahara, T., et al. 1997. Streptococcal mitogenic exotoxin, Z., a novel acidic superantigenic toxin produced by a T1 strain of *Streptococcus pyogenes*. *Infect Immun*, **65**, 3828–33.

Kappler, J., Kotzin, B., et al. 1989. Vβ-specific stimulation of human T cells by staphylococcal toxins. *Science*, **244**, 811–14.

Kim, J., Urban, R.G., et al. 1994. Toxic shock syndrome toxin-1 complexed with a class II major histocompatibility molecule HLA-DR1. *Science*, **266**, 1870–4.

Knudtson, K.L., Sawitzke, A.D. and Cole, B.C. 1997. The superantigen Mycoplasma arthritidis mitogen (MAM): Physical properties and immunobiology. In: Leung, D.M., Huber, B. and Schlievert, P. (eds), *Superantigens*. New York: Marcel Dekker, 339–67.

Kotzin, B.L., Leung, D.Y., et al. 1993. Superantigens and their potential role in human disease. *Adv Immunol*, **54**, 99–166.

Krakauer, T., Fleischer, B., et al. 1997. *Clostridium perfringens* enterotoxin lacks superantigenic activity but induces an IL-6 response from human peripheral blood mononuclear cells. *Infect Immun*, **65**, 3485–8.

Lafon, M., Lafage, M., et al. 1992. Evidence for a viral superantigen in humans. *Nature*, **358**, 507–10.

Langley R, Wines B. et al. 2003. The staphyloccal superantigen homologue SET1 binds to IgA and complement C5 and inhibits IgA-FcaRI interaction and complement mediated lysis. *J Exp Med*. in press.

Lapatschek, M., Durr, S., et al. 2000. Functional analysis of the env open reading frame in human endogenous retrovirus IDDMK.1,2.22 encoding superantigen activity. *J Virol*, **74**, 6386–93.

Lee, P.K., Kreiswirth, B.N., et al. 1992. Nucleotide sequences and biologic properties of toxic shock syndrome toxin 1 from ovine- and bovine-associated *Staphylococcus aureus*. *J Infect Dis*, **165**, 1056–63.

Legaard, P.K., Legrand, R.D. and Misfeldt, M.L. 1991. The superantigen Pseudomonas exotoxin A requires additional functions from accessory cells for T lymphocyte proliferation. *Cell Immunol*, **135**, 372–82.

Lehn, N., Schaller, E., et al. 1995. Frequency of toxic shock syndrome toxin- and enterotoxin-producing clinical isolates of *Staphylococcus aureus*. *Eur J Clin Microbiol Infect Dis*, **14**, 43–6.

Li, H., Llera, A. and Mariuzza, R.A. 1998. Structure-function studies of T cell receptor–superantigen interactions. *Immunol Rev*, **163**, 177–86.

Li, P.L., Tiedemann, R.E., et al. 1997. The superantigen streptococcal pyrogenic exotoxin, C.SPE-C. exhibits a novel mode of action. *J Exp Med*, **186**, 375–83.

McClane, B.A. 1994. *Clostridium perfringens* enterotoxin acts by producing small molecule permeability alterations in plasma membranes. *Toxicology*, **87**, 43–67.

McCormick, J.K., Yarwood, J.M. and Schlievert, P.M. 2001. Toxic shock syndrome and bacterial superantigens: an update. *Annu Rev Microbiol*, **55**, 77–104.

Marr, J.C., Lyon, J.D., et al. 1993. Characterization of novel type C staphylococcal enterotoxins: biological and evolutionary implications. *Infect Immun*, **61**, 4254–62.

Marrack, P. and Kappler, J.W. 1990. The staphylococcal enterotoxins and their relatives. *Science*, **248**, 705–11.

Matthes, M., Schrezenmeier, H., et al. 1988. Clonal analysis of human T cell activation by the mycoplasma arthritidis mitogen. *Eur J Immunol*, **18**, 1733–7.

Miethke, T., Wahl, C., et al. 1992. T cell-mediated lethal shock triggered in mice by the superantigen staphylococcal enterotoxin B: critical role of tumor necrosis factor. *J Exp Med*, **175**, 91–8.

Mitchell, D.T., Schlievert, P.M., et al. 1997. Comparison of structures of toxic-shock-syndrome-toxin-1 unbound and bound to a class II MHC molecule. In: Leung, D.M., Huber, B. and Schlievert, P. (eds), *Superantigens*. New York: Marcel Dekker, 167–98.

Miyoshi-Akiyama, T., Abe, A., et al. 1995. DNA sequencing of the gene encoding a bacterial superantigen, *Yersinia pseudotuberculosis*-derived mitogen (YPM), and characterization of the gene product, cloned YPM. *J Immunol*, **154**, 5228–34.

Monday, S.R., Vath, G.M., et al. 1999. Unique superantigen activity of staphylococcal exfoliative toxins. *J Immunol*, **162**, 4550–9.

Mourad, W., Geha, R.S. and Chatila, T. 1990. Engagement of major histocompatibility complex class II molecules induces sustained, LFA-1 dependent cell adhesion. *J Exp Med*, **172**, 1513–16.

Munson, S.H., Tremaine, M.T., et al. 1998. Identification and characterization of staphylococcal enterotoxin types G and I from *Staphylococcus aureus*. *Infect Immun*, **66**, 3337–48.

Murray, D.L., Prasad, G.S., et al. 1994. Immunobiologic and biochemical properties of mutants of toxic shock syndrome toxin-1. *J Immunol*, **152**, 87–95.

Musser, J.M., Schlievert, P.M., et al. 1990. A single clone of *Staphylococcus aureus* causes the majority of cases of toxic shock syndrome. *Proc Natl Acad Sci USA*, **87**, 225–9.

Nelson, K., Schlievert, P.M., et al. 1991. Characterization and clonal distribution of four alleles of the speA gene encoding pyrogenic exotoxin A (scarlet fever toxin) in *Streptococcus pyogenes*. *J Exp Med*, **174**, 1271–4.

Norrby-Teglund, A., Newton, D., et al. 1994. Superantigenic properties of the group A streptococcal exotoxin SpeF (MF). *Infect Immun*, **62**, 5227–33.

Novick, R.P., Schlievert, P.M. and Ruzin, A. 2001. Pathogenicity and resistance islands of staphylococci. *Microb Infect*, **3**, 585–94.

Ohmen, J.D., Barnes, P.F., et al. 1994. Evidence for a superantigen in human tuberculosis. *Immunity*, **1**, 35–43.

Ortonne, J.P. 1996. Aetiology and pathogenesis of psoriasis. *Br J Dermatol*, **135**, 1–5.

Papageogiou, A.C. and Acharya, K.R. 2000. Microbial superantigens: from structure to function. *Trends Microbiol*, **8**, 369–75.

Papageorgiou, A.C., Acharya, K.R., et al. 1995. Crystal structure of the superantigen enterotoxin C2 from *Staphylococcus aureus* reveals a zinc-binding site. *Structure*, **3**, 769–79.

Petersson, K., Hakansson, M., et al. 2001. Crystal structure of a superantigen bound to MHC class II displays zinc and peptide dependence. *EMBO J*, **20**, 3306–12.

Prasad, G.S., Earhart, C.A., et al. 1993. Structure of toxic shock syndrome toxin 1. *Biochemistry*, **32**, 13761–6.

Proft, T., Moffatt, S.L., et al. 1999. Identification and characterization of novel superantigens from *Streptococcus pyogenes*. *J Exp Med*, **189**, 89–102.

Proft, T., Moffatt, S.L., et al. 2000. The streptococcal superantigen SMEZ exhibits wide allelic variation, mosaic structure, and significant antigenic variation. *J Exp Med*, **191**, 1765–76.

Proft, T., Arcus, V.L., et al. 2001. Immunological and biochemical characterization of streptococcal pyrogenic exotoxins I and J (SPE-I and SPE-J) from *Streptococcus pyogenes*. *J Immunol*, **166**, 6711–19.

Ramamurthy, T., Yoshino, K., et al. 1997. Purification, characterization and cloning of a novel variant of the superantigen *Yersinia pseudotuberculosis*-derived mitogen. *FEBS Lett*, **413**, 174–6.

Reda, K.B., Kapur, V., et al. 1994. Molecular characterization and phylogenetic distribution of the streptococcal superantigen gene (SSA) from *Streptococcus pyogenes*. *Infect Immun*, **62**, 1867–74.

Reiser, R.F., Robbins, R.N., et al. 1983. Purification and some physicochemical properties of toxic-shock toxin. *Biochemistry*, **22**, 3907–12.

Robinson, J.H., Atherton, M.C., et al. 1991. Mapping T-cell epitopes in group A streptococcal type 5 M protein. *Infect Immun*, **59**, 4324–31.

Rott, O. and Fleischer, B. 1994. A superantigen as a virulence factor in an acute bacterial infection. *J Infect Dis*, **169**, 1142–6.

Rott, O., Mignon-Godefroy, K., et al. 1995. Superantigens induce primary T cell responses to soluble autoantigens by a non-Vβ-specific mechanism of bystander activation. *Cell Immunol*, **161**, 158–65.

Roussel, A., Anderson, B.F., et al. 1997. Crystal structure of the streptococcal superantigen SPE-C: dimerization and zinc binding suggest a novel mode of interaction with MHC class II molecules. *Nat Struct Biol*, **4**, 635–43.

Saul, F.A., Rovira, P., et al. 2000. Crystal structure of *Urtica dioica* agglutinin, a superantigen presented by MHC molecules of class I and class II. *Structure Fold Des*, **8**, 593–603.

Schad, E.M., Zaitseva, I., et al. 1995. Crystal structure of the superantigen staphylococcal enterotoxin type A. *EMBO J*, **14**, 3292–301.

Schiffenbauer, J., Soos, J. and Johnson, H. 1998. The possible role of bacterial superantigens in the pathogenesis of autoimmune disorders. *Immunol Today*, **19**, 117–20.

Schmidt, K.-H., Gerlach, D., et al. 1995. Mitogenicity of M5-protein extracted from streptococcal cells is due to streptococcal pyrogenic exotoxin C and the mitogenic factor MF. *Infect Immun*, **63**, 4569–75.

Scholl, P., Diez, A., et al. 1989. Toxic shock syndrome toxin-1 binds to class II major histocompatibility molecules. *Proc Natl Acad Sci USA*, **86**, 4210–14.

Sekaly, R.P., Croteau, G., et al. 1991. The CD4 molecule is not always required for the T cell response to bacterial enterotoxins. *J Exp Med*, **173**, 367–71.

Seth, A., Stern, L.J., et al. 1994. Binary and ternary complexes between T-cell receptor, class II MHC and superantigen in vitro. *Nature*, **369**, 324–7.

Stauffer, Y., Marguerat, S., et al. 2001. Interferon-alpha-induced endogenous superantigen. a model linking environment and autoimmunity. *Immunity*, **15**, 591–601.

Stuart, P.M. and Woodward, J.G. 1992. *Yersinia enterocolitica* produces superantigenic activity. *J Immunol*, **148**, 225–33.

Sutkowski, N., Palkama, T., et al. 1996. An Epstein-Barr virus-associated superantigen. *J Exp Med*, **184**, 971–80.

Sutkowski, N., Conrad, B., et al. 2001. Epstein-Barr virus transactivates the human endogenous retrovirus HERV-K18 that encodes a superantigen. *Immunity*, **15**, 579–89.

Svensson, L.A., Schad, E.M., et al. 1997. Staphylococcal enterotoxins A, D and E. Structure and function, including mechanism of T cell superantigenicity. In: Leung, D.M., Huber, B. and Schlievert, P. (eds), *Superantigens*. New York: Marcel Dekker, 199–229.

Swaminathan, S., Furey, W., et al. 1992. Crystal structure of staphylococcal enterotoxin B, a superantigen. *Nature*, **359**, 801–6.

Tomai, M.A., Aelion, J.A., et al. 1991. T cell receptor V gene usage by human T cell stimulated with the superantigen streptococcal M protein. *J Exp Med*, **174**, 285–8.

Tomai, M.A., Schlievert, P.M. and Kotb, M. 1992. Distinct T cell receptor Vβ gene usage by human T lymphocytes stimulated with the streptococcal pyrogenic exotoxins and pepM5 protein. *Infect Immun*, **60**, 701–5.

Vacheron, S., Luther, S.A. and Acha-Orbea, H. 2002. Preferential infection of immature dendritic cells and B cells by mouse mammary tumor virus. *J Immunol*, **168**, 3470–6.

von Bonin, A., Ehrlich, S., et al. 1995. Major histocompatibility complex II-associated peptides determine the binding of the superantigen toxic shock syndrome toxin-1. *Eur J Immunol*, **25**, 2894–8.

Weeks, C.R. and Ferretti, J.J. 1984. The gene for type A streptococcal exotoxin (erythrogenic toxin) is located in bacteriophage T12. *Infect Immun*, **46**, 531–6.

Wen, R., Cole, G.A., et al. 1996. Major histocompatibility complex class II-associated peptides control the presentation of bacterial superantigens to T cells. *J Exp Med*, **183**, 1083–92.

White, J., Herman, A., et al. 1989. The Vβ-specific superantigen staphylococcal enterotoxin B: stimulation of mature T cells and clonal deletion in neonatal mice. *Cell*, **56**, 27–35.

Williams, R.J., Ward, J.M., et al. 2000. Identification of a novel gene cluster encoding staphylococcal exotoxin-like proteins: characterization of the prototypic gene and its protein product, SET1. *Infect Immun*, **68**, 4407–15.

Woodland, D.L. 2002. Immunity and retroviral superantigens in humans. *Trends Immunol*, **23**, 57–8.

Yoshino, K., Ramamurthy, T., et al. 1995. Geographical heterogeneity between Far East and Europe in prevalence of ypm gene encoding the novel superantigen among *Yersinia pseudotuberculosis* strains. *J Clin Microbiol*, **33**, 3356–8.

30

Immunogenetics

MARIE-ANNE SHAW

Knowledge of the human genes involved in determining infectious disease susceptibility will enhance our understanding of the mechanisms of protective immunity and facilitate development of new treatment strategies and prophylactic measures. In some cases, targeting individuals at high risk of chronic manifestations of disease may, where resources are limited, provide a way forward. It is becoming increasingly simp9le to use the multiple polymorphisms available in immune response genes; hence risk prediction will become a realistic possibility in the near future. However, a plethora of small studies appearing in the literature, some of which have little power to reveal minor genetic effects, at present gives an incomplete picture. This chapter concentrates on human rather than murine studies, and common rather than rare genetic variants. It is necessarily a personal view, and does not attempt to list every known gene of interest or every disease investigated. At the start it seems appropriate to highlight the rapid developments not only in human genetics, but also in pathogen sequencing. In the future it will be fruitless to study human or pathogen variation in splendid isolation. Variation in the pathogen may affect virulence and the host immune response. Clearly human and pathogen genetic variations are inextricably linked in determining disease outcome, and their relative importance will vary with disease.

SIMPLE VERSUS COMPLEX INHERITANCE

There are rare single gene disorders that have contributed to understanding of the role of immune response genes and immunological function in infection. Investigations of single gene disorders show that individual mutations may not be the sole determinants of phenotype. Other influences can modify the phenotype, and disease may have a threshold for manifestation. Hence, some disorders that have been regarded as simple Mendelian disorders are now better described as 'complex' traits. A range of mutations, such as seen in the tumor necrosis factor (TNF) receptor gene *TNFRSF1A*, means that some mutations result in immune dysfunction, and others may be low penetrance (i.e. not always expressed) rather than benign mutations (Aksentijevich et al. 2001). Similarly, development of an infectious disease, or position on the disease spectrum, is likely to be caused by an accumulation of predisposing factors, including susceptibility alleles. Most variation in disease susceptibility will be 'multifactorial' i.e. with both genetic and environmental influences. Genetic variation is likely to be polygenic, with many contributing genes and disease resulting from multiple common variants in polymorphic genes, rather than from rare mutations. Examples of genes that were initially shown to have rare deleterious mutations, and are now studied for common nonpathogenic variants, are the interferon receptor genes *IFNGR1* and *IFNGR2* (Gao et al. 1999). It is likely that most variation underlying disease is caused by mildly deleterious alleles. The frequency of susceptibility alleles may be high, and there is likely to be allelic heterogeneity between populations (Pritchard 2001). For immunogenetic studies, assumptions are often made of low allelic heterogeneity within loci, which, when combined with a lack of knowledge of linkage disequilibrium, makes the interpretation of results challenging.

DEFINING CLINICAL PHENOTYPE

One of the key issues for genetic studies is that of defining the clinical phenotype. Most investigations are conducted using qualitative traits, e.g. disease versus absence of disease. However, quantitative traits are also employed, particularly for immune responsiveness in relation to disease. Nongenetic effects, such as routes of infection, age, and sex, must also be accounted for. Although genetic studies have the advantage that DNA may be sampled at any time, and do not require active disease, it is clear that samples pertaining to chronic disease states are more often collected, whether for family or case–control studies. A major problem for an infectious disease is ensuring that disease-free individuals are really resistant, rather than simply not exposed to the infection. For many infections exposure is hard to quantify, although for mycobacterial infections a positive skin test response to crude mycobacterial antigen can be used as an indicator of exposure. Some of the most effective studies do not concern susceptibility to disease itself, but to type of disease, which is often related to the ability to mount an appropriate immune response. Consequently, diseases that have a spectrum of severity, such as mycobacterial and protozoal diseases, have been relatively well studied.

TESTING FOR GENETIC CONTROL

Familial clustering of disease, twin studies, and racial differences may all point to genetic control. Adoptee studies are rare and not appropriate for infectious diseases. A statistic commonly associated with multifactorial conditions is λ_s, the risk to a sibling of an affected case compared with the population prevalence – the higher the value, the larger the role of genetics. However, shared sibling environment makes such estimates unreliable and they are not in common usage for infectious diseases. Nutritional status and co-infections may also be confounding factors. Another statistic is heritability: the proportion of phenotypic variation resulting from genetic causes. It is often used for quantitative traits such as pathogen burden or immune responses. The heritability of immune responses to many pathogen antigens tends to be high, with some of this being the result of non-major histocompatiblity complex (MHC) control.

Segregation analyses are formal tests of the fit of family data to models of inheritance. The occurrence of disease at random in the population is tested using a sporadic model. Rejection of a sporadic model shows a nonrandom distribution of disease. Further models can then be tested, comparing specific modes of inheritance (e.g. single gene control) with polygenic and nongenetic models. Although many segregation analyses for infectious diseases have favored single major gene control, this may reflect the choice of models that have been tested and the limitations of analytical methods.

APPROACHES FOR GENE IDENTIFICATION

Having established that there is genetic control, there are two approaches to gene identification: candidate gene testing and genome scanning. Candidate genes may be genes relevant to the immune response, associated with other similar diseases, implicated in murine model systems or within regions highlighted by genome scans. Genome scanning, as the name implies, covers the entire genome equally in the search for regions controlling susceptibility. Ideally we would like to ascertain not only the number of genes contributing to infectious disease susceptibility but also how they interact – additively or multiplicatively? The relative risk of disease for a particular gene will contribute to the ability to detect its effect. In general methods may loosely be categorized as based on linkage or association, the latter relying on linkage disequilibrium (Ott and Hoh 2000). Whereas linkage is employed for genome scanning, association is often the method of choice for a candidate gene approach. Investigators of other multifactorial conditions, particularly those studying autoimmunity and type 1 diabetes mellitus, pioneered methods of analysis.

LINKAGE

Linkage studies are used to identify broad regions of the genome involved in disease susceptibility. Historically, linkage formed part of a positional cloning strategy. However, with the sequencing of the human genome the necessity for positional cloning has been reduced. Laboratory mice, which can be maintained in environmentally controlled conditions, have been important in linkage mapping and locus identification, because there is much conserved synteny between murine and human genomes (groups of genes in which the order is conserved). Use has been made of recombinant inbred, congenic, and more recently recombinant congenic strains (Fortin et al. 2001b). Recombinant congenic strains are derived from backcrossing of a background strain and a donor strain, followed by brother–sister mating where each resulting strain carries about 10 percent of one parental strain on the genetic background of the other. These strains are used when a limited number of genes have a major effect on phenotype (Malo and Skamene 1994). Transgenic and knock-out mice have been used to confirm findings. Some of the genes identified in mouse models have been catalogued (McLeod et al. 1995), but only selected examples are mentioned in this chapter.

Microsatellite markers, particularly dinucleotide repeats, are usually the polymorphisms of choice for linkage studies. This is because they are highly polymorphic, as measured by polymorphism information content (PIC) or heterozygosity; hence they maximize the information from a given dataset. Haplotypes, using more than a single polymorphic site, can also be used to improve information content. Repeatability of linkage results within a population is essential, and genome scans often adopt a staged approach, with initial results tested in other independent samples. Most genetic markers are expected to be in Hardy–Weinberg equilibrium, and deviations could be indicative of selection or genotyping errors.

There are two methods of linkage analysis: model dependent, where a mode of inheritance must be specified, and model free. The LOD score method is used for parametric, model-dependent analysis and is powerful. A LOD score is the logarithm of odds ratio, where the ratio is the likelihood of the observed results given linkage to a given locus at a recombination fraction of <0.5, over the likelihood under a null hypothesis of no linkage. A maximum likelihood ratio can be expressed as a probability or *p* value (Nyholt 2000). A LOD of 3 has been used as significant evidence of linkage for mendelian traits, and a LOD of −2 as indicative of no linkage. Multipoint analysis, which combines information from multiple loci to localize a disease susceptibility locus on a genetic map, can result in increased power, but such methods are affected by pedigree size and incomplete pedigrees. Use of single large pedigrees, with or without inbreeding, is uncommon for infectious disease (Farrall 1993). Parametric analysis is thought to be sensitive to model misspecification; however, Greenberg et al. (1998) suggested that the critical factor in LOD score analysis is the mode of inheritance for the linked locus, not that of the disease or trait itself. It is easy to examine parent-of-origin effects using parametric methods. This has been employed in studies of asthma and atopy. True combined segregation and linkage analysis, where the mode of inheritance of a disease is assessed at the same time as linkage status of a disease susceptibility locus, is also a parametric method. It is more common for studies to employ a previously ascertained mode of inheritance when assessing linkage. This is simpler but more limited.

Nonparametric methods are not model dependent and often use affected sibling pairs rather than large pedigrees. This use of only affected individuals neatly gets round problems of exposure for infectious disease. Such methods examine alleles or haplotypes from the parents shared by affected sibs (identical by descent (IBD)). Correction may be made for multiple sib-pair comparisons within a family. A contrasting method examines alleles shared by affected relative pairs (identical by state (IBS)). IBS methods have been regarded as less powerful than IBD methods, because they may lose information, although the choice depends on the family structure available. For high relative risk and PIC values distant relatives are better for affected pair methods, whereas for smaller relative risks and PIC values sibs are best (Risch 1990). Attempting to circumvent some of the problems are programs such as GENEHUNTER, which uses all pedigree members in a multipoint approach (Kruglyak et al. 1996). Kruglyak et al. (1996) argue that their nonparametric linkage (NPL) method shows little loss of power compared with parametric methods and is less sensitive to misspecification of allele frequencies, for pedigrees of moderate size.

There are a number of linkage methods appropriate to the study of quantitative traits based on robust regression and powerful variance component methodologies (Sham et al. 2002). In some instances extreme discordant or concordant sibs are selected. Variance component methods are often used, looking at allele-sharing probabilities and the contribution to population variance. Variance may be partitioned into that caused by environmental effects, a major gene, plus other genes, and methods are implemented by programs such as GENEHUNTER (Pratt et al. 2000).

When genome scanning, approximately 300 microsatellite markers are tested for linkage. The amount of correction of the statistical significance of genome scanning results needed to allow for multiple comparisons is controversial; methods are reviewed, and accepted thresholds for genome-wide significance and corrections for multiple testing discussed (Nyholt 2000). Overly cautious approaches will cause loose linkages to be missed; however, enthusiastic reporting will cause confusion. Point-wise and genome-wide significance levels differ (Lander and Kruglyak 1995). Some believe that the degree of type 1 error for claims of linkage and association in complex inheritance is unacceptably high (Morton 1998).

An interesting question arises over the power needed to detect necessary versus susceptibility loci (Greenberg 1993). Whereas linkage is ideal for looking for loci that are necessary if not sufficient, it may be less than ideal for loci that are neither necessary nor sufficient, i.e. susceptibility loci. If the allele confers less than 10 times an increase in risk, as is the case for almost all infectious disease loci, linkage is hard to use. The numbers used for affected sib-pair genome scanning are often in the region of 200 sib-pairs plus parents (800 individuals). Population size and levels of inbreeding affect numbers required for all types of linkage and association studies. In large populations heterogeneity is often addressed by studying large numbers of families; however, in founder populations there is presumed to be decreased heterogeneity and fewer susceptibility alleles (Ober and Cox 1998).

ASSOCIATION

Association methods are often used after linkage studies for fine mapping, or for candidate gene approaches. They rely on linkage disequilibrium – the nonrandom assortment of alleles at adjacent loci within the population. The closer together two loci are, the less likely it is that a particular haplotypic combination will be separated by recombination. Such combinations may also result from admixture, selection, or drift. One cannot assume that the polymorphism under investigation is itself functionally relevant, but rather that it is used as a marker for a small region. As association methods rely on the presence of linkage disequilibrium, they are applicable only over short genetic distances. Many association studies use a case–control design. Typically a chi-squared test is employed, and Fisher's exact test may be required, depending on allele frequencies. It is possible to look at association with alleles (if the Hardy–Weinberg equilibrium holds), genotypes, or carriage (presence versus absence) of a particular allele. Whereas genotypic association is most appropriate for many loci (Sasieni 1997), carriage is appropriate for studies of human leukocyte antigen (HLA). Stratification of data, e.g. by HLA type, to look for more minor genetic influences is often used. Approaches for association mapping, analogous to multipoint linkage mapping, still need to be developed. The degree of linkage disequilibrium will determine the density of markers required to examine a region. Linkage disequilibrium is not uniform over the genome, with estimates ranging from 500 to <50 kb (Abecasis et al. 2001). In addition, linkage disequilibrium appears to be highly structured into discrete blocks, separated by hot spots of recombination (Goldstein 2001). Population size and population history will also affect the degree of linkage disequilibrium. In isolated populations there are limited ancestral haplotypes, and if a mutation is new there will be high linkage disequilibrium. However, results to date suggest that genetic isolates (unlike for linkage) will not prove more useful than larger populations for linkage disequilibrium mapping (Eaves et al. 2000), i.e. levels of linkage disequilibrium are equivalent across populations of varying sizes.

Case–control studies are potentially affected by population stratification; this occurs where the frequencies of both the disease and unlinked alleles vary between populations, and can lead to false-positive or false-negative results. The extent of problems caused by population structure has been questioned, but, to avoid such problems, the transmission disequilibrium test (TDT) is increasingly used to test for association. It is a family-based method, which observes transmission of alleles from heterozygous parents preferably to a single affected child, and is typically implemented in a variety of programs such as ETDT (Sham and Curtis 1995). Transmissions may be from the paternal or maternal side. Although originally described by Spielman et al. (1993) as a test of linkage in the presence of association, the tightness of linkage inferred by this method is debatable (Whittaker et al. 2000); however, as a test of association it avoids problems of population subdivision and admixture (Ewens and Spielman 1995). If parents of affected offspring are not available, deduction of missing parental genotypes can introduce bias, and use of unaffected siblings as controls has been suggested (Curtis 1997; Spielman and Ewens 1998). The haplotype relative risk (HRR) method also gets round population stratification, by using the set of alleles that were not transmitted as controls (Knapp et al. 1993). The TDT, together with the HRR, is the most widely used family-based test for linkage disequilibrium and association (Spielman and Ewens 1996). However, this approach may be less powerful than that of a case–control. TDT can also be performed for quantitative traits (Allison 1997; Rabinowitz 1997; Abecasis et al. 2000).

Association methods are more powerful than linkage, as confirmed by stimulation studies comparing TDT and affected sib-pair methods (Risch and Merikangas 1996). Knapp (1999) gives further consideration to power approximations for the TDT. Sample sizes for TDT have been calculated (Wang and Sun 2000). As for linkage analysis, the need for correction of multiple comparisons when interpreting case–control and family-based association studies has been much discussed. The Bonferroni correction method is most widely used (Bland and Altman 1995) and also the Holm method (Aickin and Gensler 1996). Exactly when to correct has been debated and correction is certainly not uniformly applied (Nyholt 2001). There are now many disease associations in the literature, in many populations. Heterogeneity of findings, even to the extent of positive versus no association in the same population group, is commonplace, and probably reflects both publication bias and the small size of many studies. Recent guidelines for the interpretation of association studies suggest that results should be confirmed with a second study, with $p < 0.001$, similar to the two-stage genome scans for linkage. Meta-analyses are likely to be needed to confirm associations: recent meta-analyses of genetic association studies suggest that only 20–30 percent of association studies are significant and 16 percent of reported associations are supported by further studies (Ioannidis et al. 2001, 2003; Lohmueller et al. 2003). Although not considering specifically infectious disease associations, such studies suggest that many of the reported associations will prove to be false.

The future will bring genome scanning by association using single nucleotide polymorphisms (SNP). It is estimated that there is more than 1 SNP per 1000 basepairs, or more than 3 million in the genome. They may occur in coding sequences and are more stable than microsatellites. Large-scale identification and screening for SNPs is now possible (Wang et al. 1998, see www.ncbi.nlm.nih.gov/SNP/). How polymorphic and densely spaced should SNPs be for a genome scan? One suggestion is that 7–900 moderately polymorphic SNPs, and a map of 1 500–3 000 SNPs, would be superior to the current microsatellite linkage strategy (Kruglyak 1997). Alternatively, a level of linkage disequilibrium of 3 kb would suggest that half a million SNPs are required (Kruglyak 1999)! Use of haplotypes may reduce the number of SNPs required for screening of complex disease (Johnson et al. 2001), as demonstrated by looking at the haplotypic structure of 5q31 (Daly et al. 2001). However, the nonuniformity of linkage disequilibrium in different regions of the genome (Collins et al. 1999) suggests that SNPs for whole genome scanning will have to be suitably chosen region by region.

SINGLE GENE CONTROL OF THE IMMUNE RESPONSE AND BEYOND

It is beyond the scope of this chapter to catalogue primary immunodeficiencies that have been well reviewed elsewhere (Fischer et al. 1997). In general these are rare disorders, in some cases recognized as single gene disorders through pedigree analysis. Many are lethal and some disorders are associated with multiple rare mutations. In other single gene disorders, the gene may be localized but not identified. However, it is worth noting that, according to the defect, infection is likely to be with characteristic pathogens. Some of these opportunistic infections are not usually associated with pathogenicity. Defects of the adaptive immune response include defects in MHC, particularly defects in expression such as bare lymphocyte syndrome (BLS), defects in T-cell development and function, such as the severe combined immunodeficiencies, e.g. X-SCID, and defects in B-cell function with numerous irregularities in immunoglobulin production. Defects also occur in the innate immune response such as those of phagocytic cells, e.g. chronic granulomatous diseases. Somewhat more common are deficiencies in the classic and alternative complement pathways. Whereas defects in classic components tend to result in the autoimmune disorder systemic lupus erythematosus, defects in the membrane attack complex predispose to pyogenic bacteria (Walport 1993). Single gene disorders affecting nonimmune response genes are also associated with particular pathogens. Individuals homozygous for mutations in *CFTR*, resulting in cystic fibrosis, are susceptible to *Pseudomonas aeruginosa*.

Interest in MHC class II expression was the result of expression being inducible by stimuli such as interferon γ (IFN-γ). Cells in BLS have no MHC II molecules. The story of BLS is pleasing for geneticists because heterogeneity in BLS was characterized by classic genetic complementation analysis in culture. There is a defect at the level of transcription, associated with the highly conserved X and Y boxes in the promoters of all class II genes. Complementation group A is caused by the absence of the *trans*-acting factor CIITA (MHC class II transactivator), which is a non-DNA-binding co-activator, necessary for activity of the class II promoter. Complementation groups B and C, on the other hand, are the result of deficiencies in the X-box-binding protein RFX, which is composed of a 75-kDa and a 36-kDa subunit. Failure of RFX to bind to the X box leaves the class II promoter unoccupied, and is associated with change in chromatin structure and the loss of DNase I hypersensitive sites (Reith et al. 1995; DeSandro et al. 1999).

X-linked SCID is the most common form of severe combined immunodeficiency. T and natural killer (NK) cells are affected whereas B-cell function is largely intact. The interleukin-2 (IL-2) receptor is made up of three chains: α, β, and γ (now named 'common γ' or γc). The γc chain is responsible for increasing the binding affinity of the receptor and is involved in intracellular signal transduction; it is also an essential component of other cytokine receptors: IL-4R, IL-7R, IL-9R, and IL-15R. Mutations in the gene for γc result in X-SCID (Sugamura et al. 1996; Cacalano and Johnston 1999). It appears that the primary mechanism of X-SCID is through the absence of the IL-7R necessary for T-cell development (Puel et al. 1998). Mutations in the α chains of both the IL-2R (Sharfe et al. 1997) and the IL-7R (Roifman et al. 2000) also occur. Cytokine receptors are often heterodimers or heterotrimers, and the phenomenon of chain sharing is not uncommon (e.g. the IL-4R chain occurs in both the IL-4 and the IL-13 receptors). This means that their binding specificities may have some overlap, but also that mutation in one chain may have far-reaching consequences. Mutations in signaling molecules, e.g. the Janus kinases, associated with these receptors are responsible for similar phenotypes. A few single gene defects, such as that identified in *IFNGR1*, are described together with the effect of more common variants of the same gene.

Defects in immunoglobulin (Ig) production are characterized by too much or too little of a particular Ig class or subclass. Some of these are caused by failure in class switching. Hyper-IgE syndrome presents as an autosomal dominant disorder with variable expressivity and is rare (Grimbacher et al. 1999a, b). In contrast IgA deficiency is not a single gene disorder and shows some MHC involvement (Vorechovsky et al. 1999). With a prevalence of 1 in 600, such disorders are not likely to be major contributors to disease patterns, but unusual clinical manifestations of an infectious disease may be associated with them. Of more relevance to this chapter are the studies of common variants that control Ig levels. Total IgE levels are the best studied, as a result of involvement in asthma and atopy, and are considered together with the genes on 5q31–q33. A genome scan has been carried out implicating a region of chromosome 13 in control of total IgA levels (Wiltshire et al. 1998).

Aside from investigation of Ig levels, there have been few attempts to examine common genetic control of the immune system, independently of infection. Genetics has a major influence on the variation in peripheral T-cell subset numbers: Hall et al. (2000) reported heritabilities of 65 percent for CD4:CD8 T-cell ratio, about 50 percent for absolute lymphocyte, $CD3^+$ and $CD4^+$, counts, and 56 percent for $CD8^+$ numbers. The human NK-cell repertoire is influenced by variation in *KIR* (coding for killer cell Ig-like receptor) and HLA class I (Shilling et al. 2002). Murine studies have shown that the IgE-suppressive activity of IFN-γ is polymorphic and controlled by a gene outside *H-2* (Matsushita and Katz 1992). Use of an infection-free phenotype, IL-12 responsiveness, and therefore subsequent ability to mount a T-helper 1 (Th1) or T-helper-2 (Th2) response implicated the Th2 gene cluster (Gorham et al. 1996). Examination of the effects of genetic variation on protein production, especially cytokine production, has proved fraught with problems (Nieters et al. 2001). This contrasts with some success in tying in polymorphisms with other immune response phenotypes, and is in part the result of problems associated with laboratory techniques, e.g. use of bulk cultures (Zipp et al. 2001). Proliferative responses to crude and defined antigens such as vaccine candidates, and skin test responsiveness, have been the subjects of limited study in the recent past. As anticipated there is some influence of HLA, but non-MHC genes are also implicated (Jepson et al. 1997a; Blackwell et al. 1999).

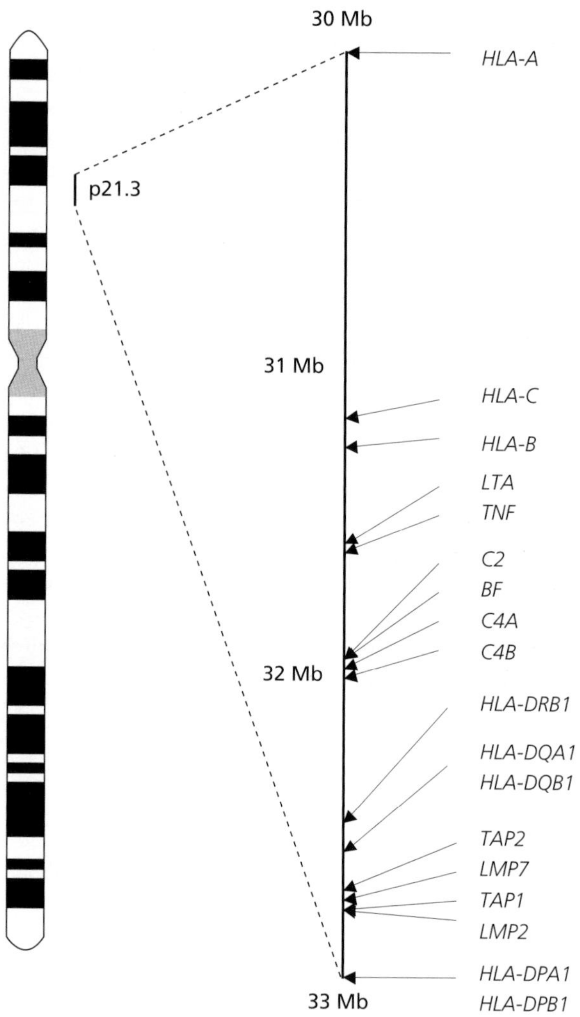

Figure 30.1 *Chromosome 6: the MHC*

COMMONLY INVESTIGATED GENES

Commonly investigated genes for susceptibility/resistance to particular pathogens contribute to both innate and acquired immunity. The genes described below are those most widely investigated and/or genes localized to clusters of immune response genes, which have often arisen through gene duplication.

HLA class I and class II

Classic HLA molecules are particularly relevant to genetic studies through their role in antigen presentation, and consequent influence on responsiveness to infection and immunization. The human MHC, on chromosome 6p21.31, is arguably the most interesting region in immunogenetics because this is the most polymorphic region of the genome, some genes having over 200 allelic variants (Figure 30.1). This multiple allelic diversity contrasts with the mechanisms for generation of diversity in Ig and T-cell receptor molecules, where single proteins are produced from several recombined gene segments. Almost all early immunogenetic studies concerned HLA, and analytically HLA provided the first group of highly polymorphic markers. HLA molecular structure, complexity, and allelic variation are well described (Marsh et al. 2000).

HLA class I was originally investigated genetically through its impact on transplantation, although class II molecules also have significant impact on graft rejection. Typically HLA class I was typed by serological methods, and HLA class II was typed by the mixed lymphocyte reaction. Nowadays, the vast majority of HLA typing is done by polymerase chain reaction (PCR) using sequence-specific primer or sequence-specific oligonucleotide methodology. The improved resolution of DNA-based typing has contributed to the subdivision of previously described HLA alleles, e.g. *HLA-DR2* comprises *HLA-DRB1*15* and *HLA-DRB1*16*, which complicates comparisons across studies. Peptide-binding specificities of alleles have been described. In 1999, ahead of publication of the human genome sequence, a complete sequence and gene map of a human MHC were reported (MHC Sequencing Consortium 1999). At this time there were 224 identified loci, of which it was predicted that 128 were expressed, about half of which had immune function. Many of these genes were identified as a result of the sequencing and many remain of unknown function. As the entire region contains over 200 genes in 3–4 Mb of DNA, the study and use of haplotypes and linkage disequilibrium are very important. HLA associations have been reported for the disease per se, position on the clinical spectra of disease, and ability to respond to crude and defined antigens; both qualitative and quantitative traits. For many infectious diseases, it remains the only region investigated to date.

HLA study design typically uses a case–control approach. Results are expressed as a relative risk of disease when carrying a particular allele. However, there were also early investigations of haplotype sharing among affected siblings, akin to current sib-pair analysis, which tackled the variable penetrance associated with susceptibility genes for complex disease. For the first and best-known HLA association, although more than 90 percent of patients with ankylosing spondylitis have *HLA-B27*, only a small percentage of individuals with *HLA-B27* will get clinical disease. In this way many early disease associations were reported, the most striking being for autoimmune disease. Many such conditions may have infectious triggers, or are more directly linked to known pathogens, such as rheumatoid and reactive arthritis, inflammatory diseases such as Crohn's disease and inflammatory bowel disease, and periodontal disease. HLA associations sometimes differ from other genetic associations because, as a result of the role of the HLA molecules in antigen presentation, a single copy of a particular allele suffices. HLA control of responses to particular antigens is best characterized for the immediate hypersensitivity response to allergens. The influence of HLA on specific IgE responsiveness to a wide variety of allergens has been known for many years, e.g. there are a number of MHC II-restricted epitopes in *Dermatophagoides pteronyssinus* allergen 1 (Higgins et al. 1994) and allergen 2 (Verhoef et al. 1993). However, although there is some evidence for HLA influence on *Der p*-specific IgE responsiveness, other loci are also involved, and genome scanning has implicated several loci (Hizawa et al. 1998a, b).

Although common haplotypes are known to occur, the HLA region is large enough for recombination to be seen and linkage disequilibrium to be incomplete. Linkage disequilibrium mapping, combined with examination of peptide-binding specificities, have been required to ascertain a complete picture. Perhaps the best example is for type 1 diabetes mellitus where a strong *HLA-DR3/DR4* association was known to occur. *HLA-DR3/DR4* alleles were thought to be too common to be disease-susceptibility alleles. In fact these alleles are in linkage disequilibrium with alleles at *HLA-DQB1*, which is the disease locus. Pinpointing disease susceptibility-causing mutations remains a problem in such a complex region.

The MHC has short sequence motifs, which essentially remain unaltered over millions of years. The class I and II regions, unlike the class III region, have many pseudogenes, possibly giving rise to new alleles via gene conversion. Class I and II arose by multiple duplication events (Shiina et al. 1999; Beck and Trowsdale 2000) and further duplication has resulted in differing copy number among haplotypes, which in turn may diverge to new functions. Those for *HLA-DRB* are the best known. How is allelic diversity maintained? The extreme polymorphism observed is likely to be a result of susceptibility/resistance to infectious agents. An excess of heterozygotes has been observed, suggesting balancing selection (Apanius et al. 1997; Jeffrey and Bangham 2000). Two theories are heterozygote advantage, where possession of two different alleles is optimal, and frequency-dependent selection, where low-frequency alleles are an advantage against pathogen-evasion strategies. One possible mechanism for the maintenance of diversity is through odor-mediated mate choice for mates of a different MHC type, hence maintaining heterozygosity. Selection may also promote different combinations of alleles or haplotypes. However, linkage disequilibrium and conservation of haplotypes will be influenced by clustered hot spots of recombination within the MHC (Jeffreys et al. 2001).

Class III genes – *TNF/LTA*

The class III region is the most diverse and gene-dense region, and may be the oldest because the origins of the MHC precede adaptive immunity.

For autoimmune, and later infectious diseases susceptibility, the most investigated cytokine genes are those coding for the macrophage proinflammatory cytokines tumor necrosis factor α (TNF-α) and IL-1. The gene for TNF-α (*TNF*) lies in the class III region between the gene *LTA* coding for lymphotoxin-α (also known as TNF-β) and *LTB* (Figure 30.1). This region is sometimes referred to as the class IV region. There are several polymorphisms in the *TNF* promoter, the best known of which is TNF_{-308}, alleles at which are often simply referred to as *TNF*1* and *TNF*2* (Knight and Kwiatkowski 1999; Ruuls and Sedgwick 1999). There is some confusion in the early literature because the first observed polymorphism, an *NcoI* restriction fragment length polymorphism (RFLP), was assumed to lie within *TNF*, and production of TNF-α appeared to relate to allelic variants. This polymorphism turned out to be in the first intron of *LTA* (Messer et al. 1991): the then described *TNFB*1* resulted in an asparagine at amino acid position 26, whereas *TNFB*2* resulted in a threonine. This variant was reported by Messer et al. (1991) to determine TNF-β rather than TNF-α production. Although TNF_{-308} has been the focus of attention, the *LTA NcoI* RFLP has also been employed as a result of more informative allele frequencies. There is linkage disequilibrium reported between these two polymorphisms in a number of populations: *TNF*1/LTA*1* and *TNF*2/LTA*2* being more common than expected by random assortment.

Many early class I and II associations reported for disease susceptibility could be caused by linkage disequilibrium between these loci and those of the class III region, such as *TNF* and *LTA* (Jacob et al. 1990), e.g. the uncommon allele TNF_{-308}*2, which is often correlated with disease, shows very strong association with *HLA-A1*, *HLA-B8*, and *HLA-DR3* alleles (Wilson et al. 1993). Dissecting genetic effects in the region remains a problem. There have been numerous attempts to correlate particular alleles with function (e.g. Skoog et al. 1999). Many of the problems have related to study design, and the ability to demonstrate stable inter-individual differences in cytokine production is rare (Molvig et al. 1988; Louis and Franchimont 1998). Despite issues over methodology (Kroeger et al. 1999), and diverse results (Brinkman et al. 1996; Wilson et al. 1997), undoubtedly confounded by attempting to examine the effects of a single base change on varied haplotypic backgrounds, TNF_{-308}*2 often shows higher production of TNF-α than TNF_{-308}*1 (Hajeer and Hutchinson 2001). TNF-α binds to two receptors TNF-R1 and TNF-R2, coded for elsewhere in the genome, both of which can be cleaved to release soluble receptors. The receptor genes have received less attention than the cytokine genes themselves, which is perhaps surprising in view of their role in the apoptotic pathway. Other class III genes include several coding for complement components.

The *IL1* gene cluster

The *IL1* gene cluster on chromosome 2q13 comprises *IL1A*, *IL1B*, and *IL1RN*, coding for IL-1α, IL-1β, and the IL-1 receptor antagonist, respectively (Figure 30.2). About 200 kb separates *IL1B* and *IL1RN* (Nicklin et al. 1994). A number of base change, microsatellite, and variable number tandem repeat (VNTR) polymorphisms have been identified in this region (Nothwang et al. 1997). It has been speculated, and occasionally demonstrated, that polymorphisms in each of these three genes may be functional, i.e. influence cytokine production (Pociot et al. 1992; Bailly et al. 1993; Danis et al. 1995). Such studies are difficult with a family of genes that are regulated at transcriptional, translational, and post-translational levels (Arend et al. 1998). The *IL1* gene cluster does show linkage disequilibrium (Cox et al. 1998), e.g. the $IL1B_{-511}$*2/$IL1RNV_{NTR}$*2 haplotype has been observed to be more common than anticipated by random assortment. These two alleles are thought to produce high levels of IL-1β and IL-1RA respectively. Although findings with this gene cluster are not so striking as those for the HLA class III region, *IL1* genes seem to be very important for control of certain infections, e.g. *IL1RN* in susceptibility to *Listeria monocytogenes* (Hirsch et al. 1996).

Some of the genes coding for the family of IL-1 receptors are also to be found on the long arm of chromosome 2, proximal to *IL1A*, *IL1B*, and *IL1RN* (Dale and

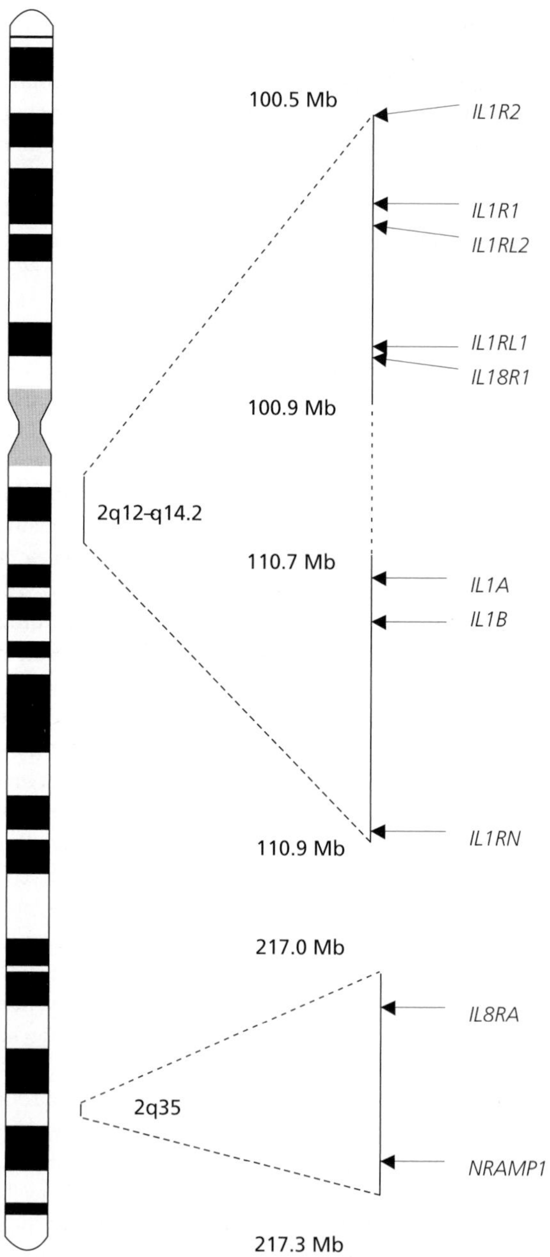

Figure 30.2 *Chromosome 2: the* IL1 *gene cluster and* NRAMP1.

Nicklin 1999). The most investigated are *IL1R1* and *IL1R2*. Another gene, *IL1RL1*, codes for the IL-1 receptor-related protein 1, which is a component of the IL-18 receptor. These genes are part of the larger IL-1 receptor/Toll-like receptor superfamily and additional members are still being described (O'Neill and Dinarello 2000). The proteins have three extracellular Ig-like domains. The soluble part of the type 1 IL-1 receptor has been crystallized together with the IL-1RA (Schreuder and Tardif 1997). As for *TNF*, the receptor genes have received less attention than the cytokine genes themselves, despite early indications that genetic variation of Toll-like receptor 4 may influence risk of gram-negative infections (Agnese et al. 2002). There are polymorphisms available for study, e.g. in the promoter of *IL1R1* (Bergholdt et al. 2000), although association studies with autoimmune conditions have been largely unrewarding. The IL-1 cytokines and receptors necessitate dissection of sometimes small genetic effects in a network of complex regulation and overlapping specificities.

SLC11A1 (*NRAMP1, Lsh/Ity/Bcg*)

SLC11A1, otherwise known as *NRAMP1*, is the best example of a locus that was originally investigated in the context of susceptibility to pathogens, rather than for its role in coding for an immune response protein (Figure 30.2). A number of inbred mouse strains have different susceptibilities to the intracellular macrophage pathogens *Salmonella typhimurium*, *Leishmania donovani*, and *Mycobacterium* spp. This genetic effect is remarkable because there is a clear dichotomy between resistant and susceptible strains, apparently under single gene control, with susceptibility proving recessive. Although the genes were named as *Ity*, *Lsh*, and *Bcg* respectively, following the cloning of *Nramp1* (natural resistance-associated macrophage protein) in 1993 by Vidal et al., it was proven, using a gene knockout and transfection, that the resistance to these intracellular macrophage pathogens was controlled by a single locus (Barton et al. 1995; Vidal et al. 1995). The human gene was named *NRAMP1*, now renamed *SLC11A1*, and lies on chromosome 2q35 near to *IL8R*. *Nramp1* has pleiotropic effects on macrophage function. The murine-resistant allele upregulates production of TNF-α and IL-1 and expression of MHC class II, and hence antigen-presenting capability. *Nramp1* codes for an integral membrane protein, with homology to transporters, and susceptibility is determined by a single nonconservative glycine/asparagine amino acid substitution (Vidal et al. 1993). Although the structure suggests a transport function, and despite identification of *Nramp1* as part of a family of transporter molecules (Cellier et al. 1995), the precise function has proved elusive. Subsequently localized to the late endosomal and lysosomal compartments, the protein is now thought to be an iron transporter (Blackwell and Searle 1999). The murine polymorphism has not been observed in human populations, highlighting potential problems of generalizing across species. However, cloning of the human homolog has been accompanied by identification of a number of other coding and noncoding polymorphisms (Cellier et al. 1994; Blackwell et al. 1995; Liu et al. 1995). One of these, a dinucleotide repeat in the human promoter, has been associated with functional differences in allelic expression (Searle and Blackwell 1998). There have been numerous attempts to demonstrate a clear role for *NRAMP1* in susceptibility to pathogens (Skamene et al. 1998, described below) and fewer studies examining its role in autoimmunity (Shaw et al. 1996; Blackwell and Searle 1999). One allele of the promoter polymorphism shows some association with autoimmune disease susceptibility and another allele with infectious disease susceptibility. However, findings are weak, relative to the murine system. This gene is being examined in other relevant species such as reservoir hosts (Altet et al. 2002).

Mannose-binding lectin and complement genes

Genes for classical, alternative, and membrane attack complex components are distributed throughout the genome. However, they occur in gene clusters, and there is substantial evidence of gene duplication and duplication of particular exons, e.g. those responsible for thioester bond formation, which enable key complement components to attach to the cell surface (Campbell et al. 1988; Schneider and Wurzner 1999). The genes *C2*, *C4A*, and *C4B*, and the gene coding for factor B, lie within the class III region of the MHC (see Figure 30.1). A variety of complement deficiency disorders is known, under single gene control. Unlike many 'single gene disorders', heterozygotes are relatively common, particularly for C2 deficiency: 1–1.5 percent of Caucasians have a *C2* null gene (Colten 1992). As mentioned above, complement deficiencies are associated with the autoimmune disorder systemic lupus erythematosus and infection with pyogenic bacteria (Walport 1993). Of the complement genes that have been investigated, predominantly those in the classical pathway, some, but not all, show polymorphic coding variation (Schneider and Wurzner 1999). As complement receptors, particularly those for C3, can act as receptors for invading microorganisms, and have a significant impact on infections such as HIV-1, it is to be expected that variation in the genes could impact on disease susceptibility (Fearon and Locksley 1996; Speth et al. 1997). However, despite a long history of research into variation in the complement system, these genes remain relatively poorly investigated with respect to infectious disease. There is also strong linkage disequilibrium between complement genes, especially those in the class III region, hence, as for *TNF/LTA* and HLA class II genes, it is difficult to dissect genetic effects. Studies are rarely large enough to establish more than preliminary associations, and reported associations may merely reflect linkage disequilibrium with another nearby gene.

Mannan-binding protein/mannose-binding lectin (MBP/MBL) binds to terminal mannose groups on the surfaces of bacteria and enhances uptake by phagocytes through opsonization. Its structure is like that of C1q and, together with associated proteases, it can initiate the classical pathway in the absence of antibody. As it recognizes a broad range of infectious agents and is part of the early innate immune response, variation in this molecule may be critical in disease susceptibility (Fearon and Locksley 1996; Ezekowitz 1998). Polymorphisms in exon 1 of *MBL* (*MBL2*, chromosome 10q11.2-q21), at codons 52, 54, and 57, lead to low or absent serum MBL. The codon 54 mutation results in an unstable protein that is unable to activate complement. The effects of these mutations are detectable in the heterozygous state. As the frequency of these mutations is high, inevitably this has raised the question of selection. However, no selective advantage has been demonstrated to date (Ezekowitz 1998). There is also variation in the promoter region (Madsen et al. 1998). A number of population studies have attempted to correlate *MBL* haplotypes with varying concentrations of MBL in Old World and New World populations (Madsen et al. 1998; Turner et al. 2000; Boldt and Petzl-Erler 2002). The role of *MBL* variation in susceptibility to infectious disease has received considerable attention (Hill 1998).

The chromosome 5 gene cluster and other genes influencing IgE

The main stimulus for research into genetics of the 5q region has been its connection with the most common group of multifactorial disorders in western populations: asthma and atopy. Looking at linkages for asthma and atopy from the Asthma Gene database, chromosome 5 is most commonly identified (see www.cooke.gsf.de/asthmagen/main.cfm). For asthma/atopy, and latterly for infectious disease susceptibility, studies have concentrated on linkage rather than association. There are many reviews of the genetics of asthma and atopy available (Anderson and Cookson 1999). Genes present in the extended 5q31–q33 region include cytokine genes typically associated with a Th2 response: *IL3*, *IL4* (Arai et al. 1989), *IL5*, *IL9*, *IL13*, and also the gene coding for the p40 subunit of IL-12 (*IL12B*, Sieburth et al. 1992) (Figure 30.3). Other genes of interest include *IRF1* (interferon regulatory factor), *CSF2* (granulocyte–macrophage colony-stimulating factor (GM-CSF)), *CD14* (Goyert et al. 1988), *ADRB2* (β_2-adrenergic receptor), and *CSF1R*. A detailed physical map is available (Frazer et al. 1997). It appears there have been a number of gene duplication events, although some require rapid sequence divergence (van Leeuwen et al. 1989). New genes are being identified for asthma that may have direct links with infectious disease susceptibility. Identification of the *Tim* gene family in the region determining the *Tapr* locus (T-cell and airway phenotype regulator) used mice congenic for the chromosomal region homologous with human 5q23-q35 (McIntire et al. 2001).

The wealth of candidate immune response genes perhaps accounts for why studies either fail to develop beyond linkage approaches or are isolated gene association studies. There are a number of SNP and microsatellite polymorphisms in and between genes in this region (Noguchi et al. 2001). A few have been used extensively in study of disease, some of which are proposed to have functional consequences, such as the IL-13-coding polymorphism (Heinzmann et al. 2000). Where polymorphic sites are sufficiently dense haplotypes have been derived (Drysdale et al. 2000; Graves et al. 2000). Although linkage disequilibrium does occur in this region, unlike for HLA, there have been few attempts to characterize patterns (Takabayashi et al. 1999). There is a potential role of this gene cluster in regulation of Th1/Th2 responses, despite indications that the Th1 versus Th2 split is not controlled by *IL4* directly (Guler et al. 1999). Recent research has centered on control of the genes in this region, in particular the region between *IL4* and *IL13*. By comparing human and mouse sequences, a 401-bp-conserved noncoding sequence CNS-1 immediately downstream of *IL13* has been identified (Loots et al. 2000). Experiments in mice suggested this region as a coordinate regulator of *IL4*, *IL13*, and *IL5* spanning 120 kb. The capacity to develop Th2 cells was compromised in vitro and in vivo in the absence of CNS-1, despite retaining some capacity to produce IL-4 (Mohrs et al. 2001). Chromatin accessibility is likely to be important in cytokine expression (Agarwal et al. 1999; Hural et al. 2000; Guo et al. 2002).

Total IgE has been known to be under genetic control for many years with heritability estimates in excess of 50 percent (Bazaral et al. 1974; Blumenthal et al. 1981). Total IgE is perhaps the best characterized of the multiplicity of asthma/atopy traits. The best linkage known for control of a quantitative immune trait is the linkage of total IgE to the chromosome 5q31 gene cluster, first described by Marsh et al. (1994) in Amish sib-pairs. This linkage has been confirmed in a number of populations (Xu J. et al. 2000) and not detected in a few (Laitinen et al. 1997). In the context of total IgE, *IL4*, *IL13* (Graves et al. 2000; Liu et al. 2000), *CD14* (Baldini et al. 1999), and *ADRB2* (Dewar et al. 1997) have all been studied. There are sufficient data in the literature for meta-analysis, which will hopefully contribute to elucidation of which genes and how many genes are important for disease states in this region (Collins et al. 2000).

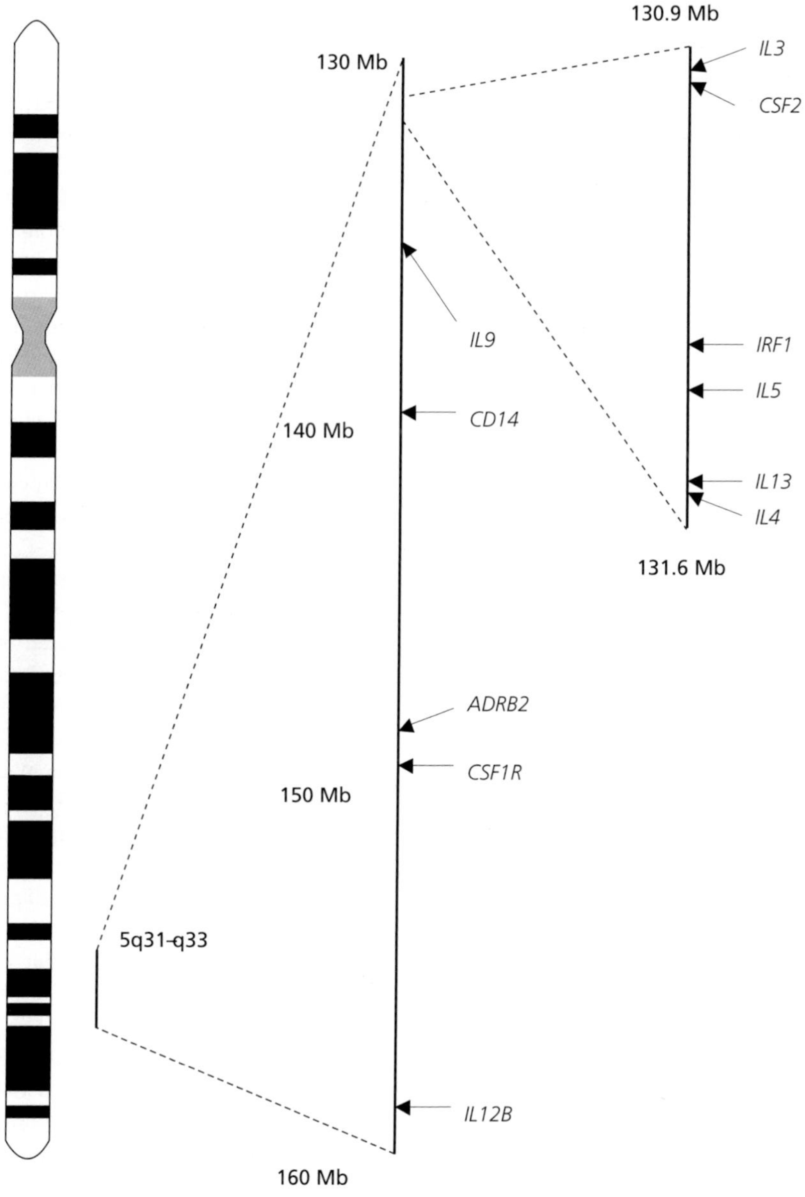

Figure 30.3 *The chromosome 5 gene cluster.*

The 5q cluster is also implicated in a number of inflammatory diseases some of which may have infectious disease etiology. A gene *IBD5* (inflammatory bowel disease 5) confers susceptibility to Crohn's disease and lies in 5q31. Use of a TDT approach gave strong evidence that a common 5q31 haplotype conferred susceptibility to Crohn's disease, although causal mutations remain to be identified (Rioux et al. 2001).

Familial eosinophilia is a rare autosomal dominant disorder. A genome scan provided evidence for linkage of this trait to chromosome 5q31–q35 (Rioux et al. 1998). There were no functional mutations in *IL3*, *IL5*, or *CSF2*, suggesting a defect elsewhere in this region. This may prove comparable to the *IFNGR1* story where there are both rare deleterious mutations and common less or nonpathogenic variants. The region proves to be of interest for helminth infections associated with IgE and eosinophilia.

Variation in receptors for the 5q-encoded cytokines is also implicated in asthma and atopy. The IL-4 and IL-13 receptors are inextricably linked through the sharing of a common IL-4Rα chain and overlapping specificities (IL-4 binding to both receptors) (Callard et al. 1996). The IL-4Rα chain has been extensively investigated in the context of asthma and atopy. There are a number of common coding polymorphisms known, of which the most studied are an extracellular variant Ile50Val (Mitsuyasu et al. 1998, 1999) and a cytoplasmic variant Gln576Arg (Hershey et al. 1997; Grimbacher et al. 1998; Wang et al. 1999). There is some evidence for a functional effect of each polymorphism: Arg576 was associated with increased expression of CD23 after IL-4 stimulation of mononuclear cells, and Ile50-transfected cells showed augmented responses to IL-4, which appeared not to change chain expression but to augment STAT6 activation. However, initial findings have not been entirely supported, and recent studies have suggested that variation at more than one site is necessary for functional effects, e.g. at both positions 50 and 576, or positions 503 and 576 (Kruse et al. 1999). Functional significance of variants within this gene remains topical. In addition, many associations have been reported between alleles at various positions, but with variation between studies. Analysis of *IL4RA* haplotypes has been of some value. The IL-4R story is a good example of confusion through examination of associations, and potential functionality of particular variants, in isolation. However, with more polymorphisms being identified, in both the promoter (Hackstein et al. 2001) and coding (Deichmann et al. 1997) regions, further consideration of haplotypes should prove informative (Risma et al. 2002). Using variants in both *IL13* and *IL4RA* there are early indicators of gene–gene interactions (Howard et al. 2001).

Variants in *IL12B* and receptors for Th1-type cytokines, have been studied primarily in the context of mycobacterial infection and are considered under the appropriate section.

A refined segregation analysis was compatible with more than one gene regulating total IgE (Xu et al. 1995). As total IgE is likely to be a multifactorial trait, a number of other genes have secondarily been implicated, which include *FCER1B*, *IL4RA*, *TNF*, loci on chromosomes 7 (Xu J. et al. 2000) and 12 (Barnes et al. 1996; Nickel et al. 1997; Xu J. et al. 2000), *INFGR1* and *IFNGR2* (Gao et al. 1999), and an *IL18R* splice variant (Watanabe et al. 2002). The gene for the β chain of the high-affinity IgE receptor, *FCER1B*, is on chromosome 11q13, and there is linkage of several asthma/atopy traits to this region in some populations. The original report was notable for its analysis of maternal transmission (Cookson et al. 1992). Three identified coding variants of *FCER1B* have shown some associations, but the precise effect of these polymorphisms is unclear (Furumoto et al. 2000; Hizawa et al. 2000). That results are somewhat mixed for Ile181Leu and Val183Leu, but less so for Glu237Gly, may be indicative of population heterogeneity. There have been very few attempts at haplotype construction across polymorphisms in this region. Other genes in this region, such as *CC16*, may be implicated. Together with the chromosome 5 cluster, 11q13 is the most investigated region in the context of asthma/atopy.

The chromosome 17 genes

Genes on the long arm of chromosome 17 have received less attention than the chromosome 5 cluster (Figures 30.4 and 30.5). However, with increasing interest in chemokines and chemokine receptors, largely stimulated by HIV-1 studies, and the occurrence of multiple candidate genes, it is likely that this region will prove critical in determining susceptibility to infectious disease.

Receiving the most attention to date is *NOS2A*, the gene coding for inducible nitric oxide (NO) synthase. There are three genes coding for nitric oxide synthase, but only the inducible form maps to this region (Marsden et al. 1994; Xu et al. 1994). As NO is a killing mechanism for intracellular macrophage bacteria and protozoa, a rate-limiting enzyme responsible for NO production is clearly important. Several variants in *NOS2A* have been widely investigated in relation to infectious disease susceptibility (Hobbs et al. 2002; Xu W. et al. 2000).

A number of small inducible cytokine genes named '*SCYA*', now renamed as chemokine CC motif ligand 'CCL', also occur in this region. One such molecule is the proinflammatory chemoattractant RANTES (*SCYA5*). Relatively late appearing mRNA transcripts are upregulated in cells stimulated with TNF-α and IL-1β, and TNF-α induces transcriptional activation of *SCYA5*, although regulatory mechanisms may be tissue-specific (Nelson et al. 1993). Also coded in this region are two related C-C chemokines macrophage inflammatory protein 1α(MIP-1α, *SCYA3*) and 1β (MIP-1β, *SCYA4*). The genes are 14 kb apart, arranged in a head-to-head fashion, in keeping with their coordinate regulation. In addition there are reduplicated loci in this region, the presence of which varies between individuals (Irving et al. 1990). Syntenic, but proximal to *SCYA3* and *SCYA4*, between the genes for RANTES and monocyte chemotactic protein-1 (MCP-1) (*SCYA2*), are the genes coding for MCP-2 (*SCYA8*) and MCP-3 (*SCYA7*) (Opdenakker et al. 1994). Breakpoints in the region are associated with several malignancies. It is reasonable to assume, as for C-X-C chemokine genes on chromosome 4q13–q21, C-X-C chemokine receptor genes on chromosome 2q34–q35, and C-C chemokine receptor genes on chromosome 3p21.3, that the origins of these molecules are through gene duplication. This is in keeping with repeat and palindromic sequences in the region (Opdenakker et al. 1994). Another locus in this cluster is eotaxin (*SCYA11*), also stimulated by TNF-α and IL-1α, with eosinophil-specific chemotactic ability and close homology to MCP-4 (*SCYA13*) (Bartels et al. 1996). As for the other genes in this cluster, eotaxin shows polymorphic variation (Miyamasu et al. 2001), in this case associated with plasma eotaxin levels and eosinophil counts, and may account for some of the genetic component proposed to determine eosinophil levels (Holberg et al. 1999).

Other polymorphisms

A number of other immune response genes have been proposed as candidates for resistance/susceptibility to

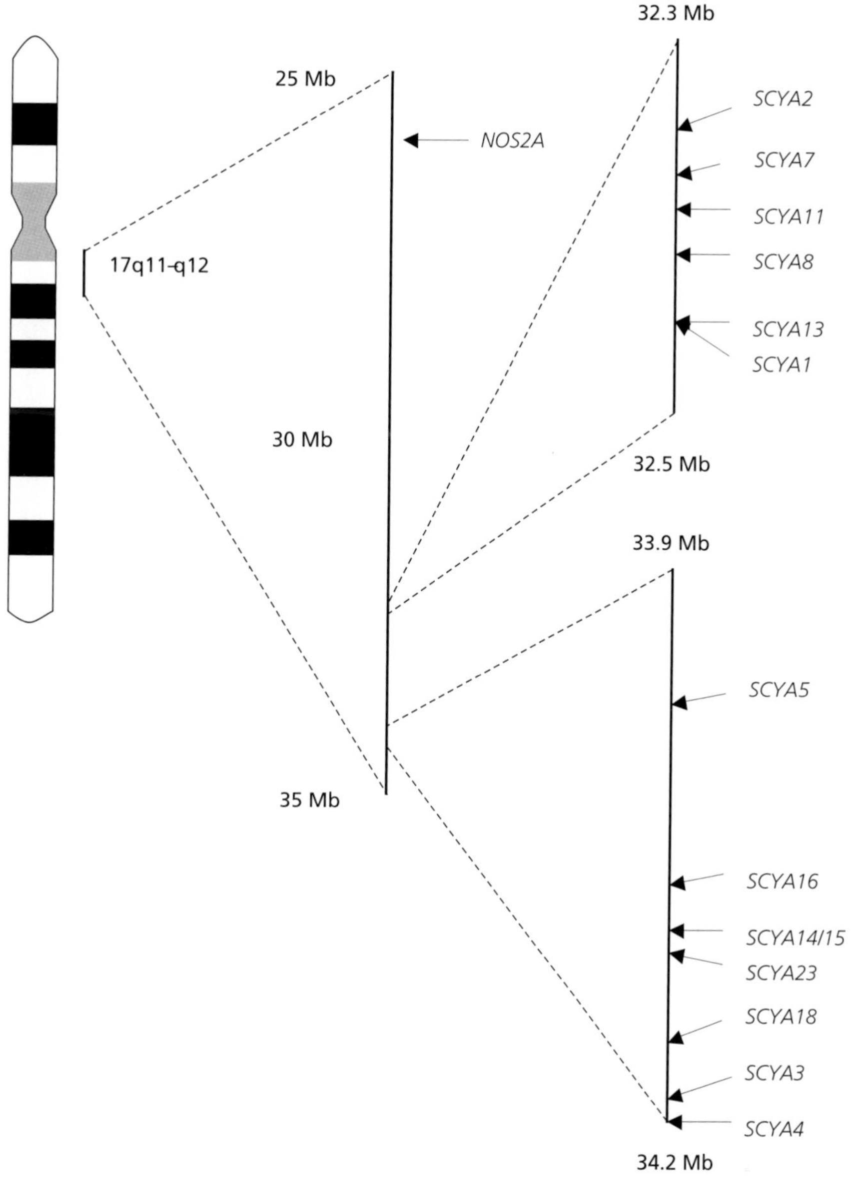

Figure 30.4 *Chromosome 17: genes on the long arm*

infectious disease, although the number of studies to date is limited. These include gene clusters coding for members of the Ig superfamily: Ig gene allotypes, T-cell receptor genes, and Fc receptor genes (including *CD32*) (Figure 30.6). However, the literature on T-cell receptor gene usage outweighs the information on polymorphic diversity. Such gene clusters do not display the high allelic diversity of the MHC. Among the cytokine genes most commonly investigated in an infectious disease context are those coding for IFN-γ (*IFNG*, 12q14), transforming growth factor β (TGF-β1) (*TGFB1*, 19q13), and IL-10 (*IL10*, 1q31–q32). Multiple polymorphic sites allow the construction of haplotypes. There has also been much interest in a variety of receptors, ligands, and adhesion molecules: CTLA-4 (*CTLA4*, 2q33), intercellular adhesion molecule 1 (ICAM-1) (*ICAM1*, 19p13), CD36 (*CD36*, 7q11), DARC (*FY*, 1q21–q22), and the vitamin D receptor (*VDR*, 12q12–q14). All of these, with the exception of *VDR*, have been studied primarily in the context of malaria. The active form of vitamin D is 1,25-dihydroxycholecalciferol, an immunomodulatory molecule, and the *VDR* gene has been considered for several infectious diseases.

Aside from the general web-based databases that catalogue microsatellite and single nucleotide polymorphisms, there are a few more specialized databases. Many of the polymorphisms that have been investigated for multifactorial diseases are in cytokine genes and have been collated (Bidwell et al. 1999a, b; Haukim et al. 2002). This specialist database has the advantage of providing detailed information on functionality and past disease associations. More generally, the On-line

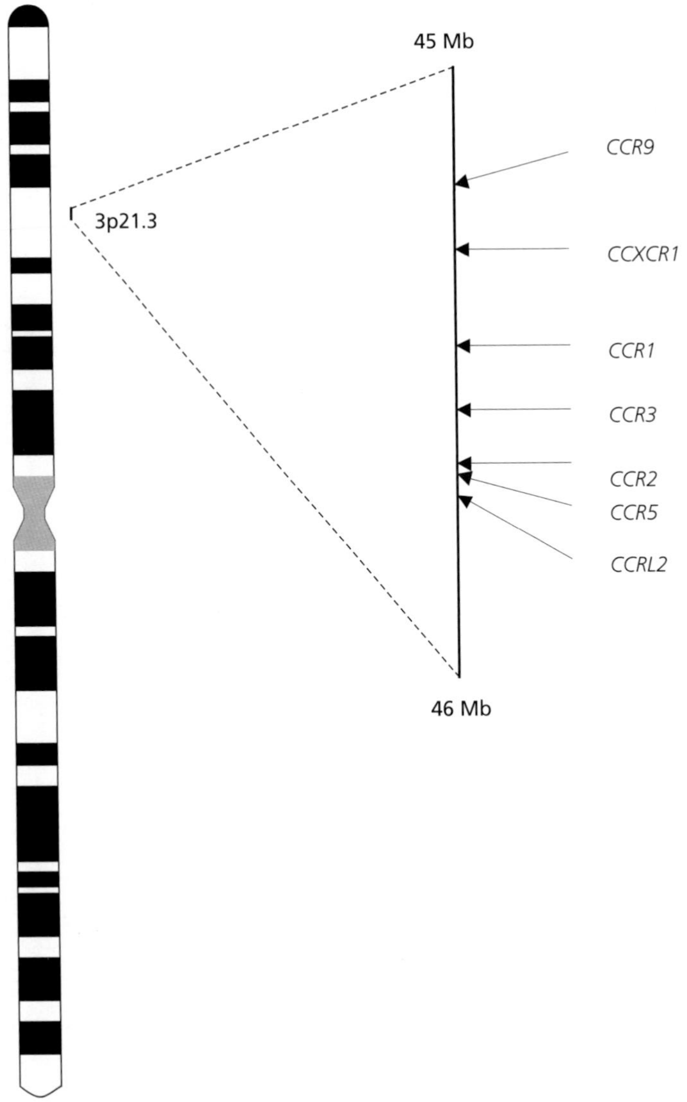

Figure 30.5 *Chromosome 17: genes on the short arm*

Mendelian Inheritance in Man (OMIM) site allows keyword searching and a history of genes and their variants. Whether polymorphisms are of functional relevance is a difficult issue. Clearly polymorphisms in regulatory regions may influence gene expression, and coding variation resulting in amino acid substitutions may affect function. Suffice it to say that there is very little good evidence of functional importance for most polymorphic sites.

Interestingly some cytokine genes, *IL2* and *IL4*, have been shown to be expressed monoallelically in single cells (Matesanz et al. 2000). This phenomenon of allelic exclusion is usually associated with the Ig molecules, where allelic exclusion is clearly necessary if a single cell is to produce a single Ig molecule. The reason for allelic exclusion in cytokine production is less clear. The mechanism appears to be through asynchronous DNA transcription (Mostolavsky et al. 2001).

VIRAL INFECTIONS

The number of human genetic studies on susceptibility to most viral infections is not high. This is surprising because receptor-mediated viral entry provides a number of good candidate genes. Studies are much farther forward in mice, although there are some limitations on simple extrapolation from mouse to humans (Brownstein 1998).

HIV

Human studies have concerned susceptibility to HIV-1 rather than HIV-2. There are a number of reviews available (Rowland-Jones 1998; Kaslow and McNicholl 1999; Michael 1999). Interest is focused in several areas: those individuals who remain seronegative despite

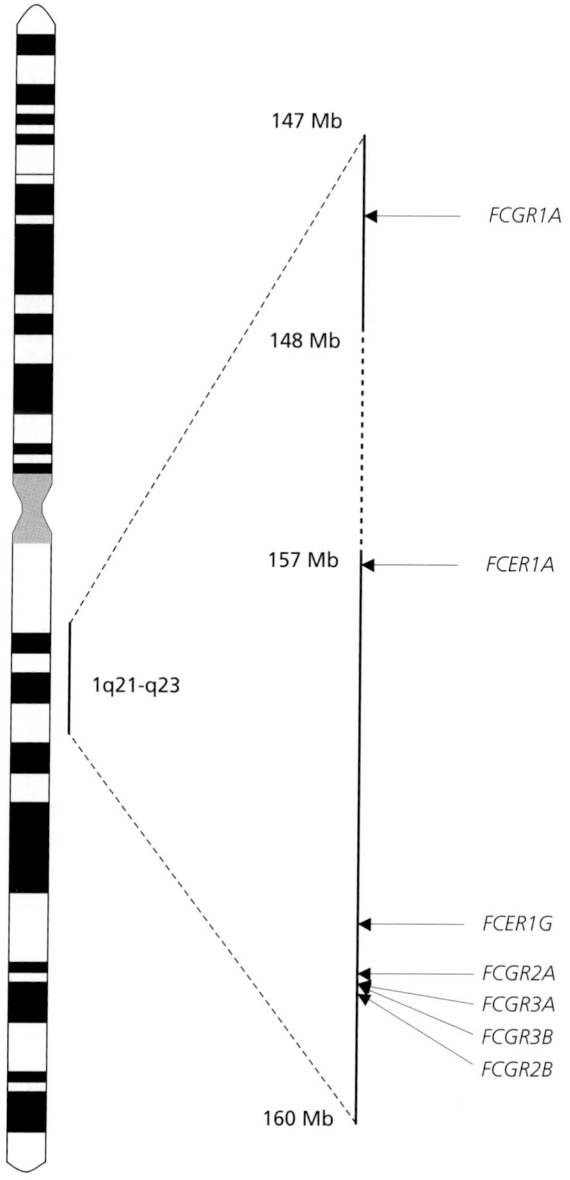

Figure 30.6 *Chromosome 1*

repeated exposure, differences in progression of disease after seroconversion, pediatric infection, and vertical transmission (Matte and Roger 2001), and latterly an interest in susceptibility to the various opportunistic infections. To a limited extent we now have the ability to collect genetic information from patients to give potential indicators as to disease progression (Carrington et al. 2001). HIV-1 uses co-receptors to enter host cells. The first co-receptor identified was CXCR4, then known as fusin, necessary for invasion of syncytium-inducing, T-cell-tropic isolates into $CD4^+$ T cells in the later stages of infection. Recombinant fusin enabled CD4-expressing nonhuman cells to support HIV-1 fusion. Antibodies to fusin blocked cell fusion and infection with normal $CD4^+$ human cells (Feng et al. 1996). CXCR4 is the receptor for stromal-derived factor 1 (SDF-1).

There is a greater literature concerning CCR5, rapidly implicated after CXCR4 (Deng et al. 1996; Dragic et al. 1996), as a necessary co-receptor for entry of nonsyncytium-inducing isolates into macrophages in the early stages of infection. Discovery was followed by description of the mechanism of entry: high-affinity binding of gp120 to CD4 causes conformational changes in gp120, creating a recognition site for CCR5 (Trkola et al. 1996; Wu et al. 1996). CCR5 is the receptor for the CC chemokines MIP-1α, MIP-1β, and RANTES, the genes of which have been studied in relation to HIV-1. Other members of this receptor family, CCR3 (the receptor for eotaxin) and CCR2b, have emerged as potential alternative co-receptors to CCR5.

Samson et al. (1996) showed that a variant 32-bp deletion in *CCR5* makes up about 10 percent of alleles in western Caucasian populations, but was absent from west and central African and Japanese populations. This leads to a truncated protein that is not functionally expressed (Liu et al. 1996). In HIV-infected Caucasians no homozygotes for *CCR5Δ32* were found, and the frequency of heterozygotes was 35 percent lower than in the general population. As primary infections were thought to be with nonsyncytium-inducing strains, initial observations suggested that such homozygotes would be totally refractory. Indeed cells from a homozygous individual were resistant to infection by macrophage tropic viruses. However, a handful of exceptions are now taken to be infection with syncytium-inducing or dual tropic strains utilizing CXCR4. Heterozygotes are not resistant but have slower disease progression, again protection being against nonsyncytium-inducing strains (Michael et al. 1997). Other mutations in *CCR5* occur with lower frequency and, although less is known of their effects, some produce functional alterations. Mutations within the *CCR5* promoter are likely to have less easily detectable effects than those resulting in truncated proteins. The ease with which mutations have been identified in *CCR5* argues for selective pressure favoring these alleles (Blanpain et al. 2000). The *CCR5Δ32*-containing ancestral haplotype has been estimated to be 700 years old, and this recent emergence is consistent with a strong selective event such as a plague epidemic (Stephens et al. 1998). CCR3 and CCR5 are both expressed in microglial cells of the central nervous system (CNS), and are thought to be responsible for transmission of macrophage tropic strains within the CNS (He et al. 1997). *CCR3* also shows several genetic variants (Zimmermann et al. 1998).

A mutation in the gene coding for CCR2b results in a conservative valine-to-isoleucine substitution at codon 64. Although described as affecting HIV progression, this gene is in linkage disequilibrium with *CCR5*, both being on chromosome 3 and only 20 kb apart.

Hence, for these mutations, causal effects can be hard to disentangle. Smith et al. (1997) showed that the *CCR5Δ32* allele is almost in complete linkage disequilibrium with *CCR2-64I*: the two mutations are not found together on the same chromosome. In European populations about 20 percent of the population will carry one of the two mutant alleles (Romano-Spica et al. 2000). However, unlike *CCR5Δ32*, *CCR2-64I* does occur in African populations (Su et al. 1999), where there are slow progressors, despite the much shorter median time from seroconversion to acquired immunodeficiency syndrome (AIDS).

A point mutation in the 3′UTR of the gene coding for SDF-1α, the ligand for CXCR4, *SDF1-3′A* has a recessive protective effect, unlike the effect of *CCR2–64I* which is dominant. Homozygotes make up about 1 percent of Caucasian populations and these people show a much slower disease progression. The frequency of *SDF1-3′A* varies worldwide with high frequencies in Oceanian populations (Su et al. 1999). An *SDF1* heterozygous genotype is one factor implicated in infectivity and hence in mother-to-offspring transmission (John et al. 2000).

Genetic variation has also been studied with respect to other chemokine ligands including MIP-1α, RANTES, and eotaxin (Liu et al. 1999; Modi et al. 2000; Gonzalez et al. 2001). Two polymorphisms in the *SCYA5* promoter at positions −403 and −28 result in GC, AC, and AG haplotypes. The −28G allele, which occurs at a frequency of 17 percent in noninfected Japanese, was associated with reduced $CD4^+$ lymphocyte depletion rates in HIV-1-infected individuals and increased transcription of the RANTES gene (Liu et al. 1999). Homozygosity for the *SCYA5* AC haplotype was associated with increased risk of acquiring HIV-1 as well as accelerated progression in Europeans, but not African–Americans, despite a high prevalence of the haplotype in people of African origin (Gonzalez et al. 2001).

In contrast to the work on chemokines, there has been little consideration of the effects of cytokine polymorphism on HIV-1 infection (Nakayama et al. 2002; Shin et al. 2000). In general findings are weak and concern disease progression. Similarly, there are few studies on the role of genes involved in innate immunity and immunomodulation such as *NRAMP1* (Marquet et al. 1999), *MBL* (Pastinen et al. 1998), and *VDR* (Hill 1998). In a Colombian population four *NRAMP1* genotypes were associated with altered risk of infection. Three genotypes were associated with reduced relative risks (0.24–0.35), but were in strong linkage disequilibrium, and one genotype was associated with an increased relative risk (2.29) (Marquet et al. 1999). Heterozygotes for a *VDR* polymorphism are at reduced risk of infection (Hill 1998).

In contrast there are many observations concerning HIV-1 susceptibility and progression according to HLA type. Findings are variable, which may be in part accounted for by diverse ethnic background (Al Jabri 2002). *HLA-B*35-Cw*04* is associated with rapid progression in white Europeans and, although cytotoxic T lymphocytes (CTL) have been observed to recognize epitopes in the context of *HLA-B*3501*, analysis of subtypes suggests that a single amino acid change may be key (Gao et al. 2001). Lack of alleles *HLA-B*35* and *HLA-Cw*04*, together with full heterozygosity at HLA class I loci, has been associated with extended survival (Carrington et al. 1999). It is interesting in this context that lack of diversity at chimpanzee class I loci has been highlighted in relation to their natural resistance to AIDS: it has been proposed that a selective sweep has occurred as a result of exposure to simian immunodeficiency virus (SIV) or a closely related retrovirus (de Groot et al. 2002). Another well-characterized haplotype, *HLA-A1-B8-DR3*, is associated with rapid progression, and some autoimmune conditions (Candore et al. 1998; Price et al. 1999). Such associations with extended haplotypes raise the possibility of the involvement of class III loci such as *TNF* (Khoo et al. 1997).

Finally, there are some studies concerning the susceptibility to opportunistic infections associated with HIV-1, e.g. inflammatory cytokine and Fc receptor genes have been examined for influence on susceptibility to Kaposi's sarcoma, itself associated with human herpesvirus 8, with some significant associations (Foster et al. 2000; Lehrnbecher et al. 2000).

HTLV-1 and HTLV-2

Human T-cell lymphotropic virus (HTLV)-1 and HTLV-2 are retroviruses where, from rodent models, it may be expected that host genetic background will influence clinical manifestations. HTLV-I causes adult T-cell leukemia/lymphoma (ATL), HTLV-1-associated myelopathy/tropical spastic paraparesis (HAM/TSP), and HTLV-1 uveitis (HU) in a small percentage of infected carriers. Most human genetic studies have been on the MHC. HLA haplotypes have been examined for ATL patients, and a TNF_{-857} allele, associated with enhanced production of TNF-α, correlated with enhanced susceptibility to ATL in Japanese (Tsukasaki et al. 2001). Class II alleles differ among patients developing ATL or HAM/TSP (Manns et al. 1998). An HLA effect for HAM/TSP would be consistent with the suggestion that pathology for this condition is the result of an exaggerated CTL response (Bangham et al. 1999). Concurrence of HAM/TSP and HU is relatively common, but concurrence of either with ATL is rare. *TNF* promoter alleles at positions −1031 and −863 have been proposed as risk factors for HU (Seki et al. 1999). Although many of these studies have considered linkage disequilibrium, elucidation of genetic effects is still in the early stages.

Respiratory syncytial virus

Respiratory syncytial virus infection results in bronchiolitis in a proportion of infected children. Pathology is correlated with neutrophils and IL-8 production. An *IL8* promoter allele was associated with increased IL-8 production in LPS-stimulated blood, and was more frequently transmitted by parents to offspring with bronchiolitis (Hull et al. 2000). This observation has been confirmed and a detailed haplotypic analysis of the region conducted using six SNPs. The putative disease allele resided on two haplotypes, only one of which was implicated in disease, suggesting that the original polymorphism was not functional (Hull et al. 2001). Consistent with observations from other loci, Europeans have few common haplotypes differing at multiple sites whereas Africans show greater haplotypic diversity. There is also some evidence for a role of *IL4* (Choi et al. 2002), and possibly *IL4RA*, in severe bronchiolitis (Hoebee et al. 2003).

In addition to the retroviruses described above, a group of viruses showing latent or asymptomatic infections, with later pathological consequences in a subset of individuals, have been considered for human immunogenetic determinants. These include hepatitis B and hepatitis C, Epstein–Barr virus (EBV), papilloma viruses, cytomegalovirus (CMV), and herpesviruses.

Hepatitis B and hepatitis C

In mice, two non-*H-2*-linked genes have been proposed to determine susceptibility to hepatitis viruses (*Hv1* and *Hv2*; McLeod et al. 1995). Host genetics may be involved in several aspects of infection. Infection may be transmitted from an infected mother to a child perinatally, and there are racial differences in the frequency of perinatal transmission, implicating genetic control. Twin studies in China employed several different markers of hepatitis B (HBV) infection (Lin et al. 1989). No significant difference in the concordance of HBV infection was observed in the monozygotic and dizygotic twins; however, significant differences were seen between twins and controls. Highly significant differences were seen in the concordance of carrier status between monozygotic and dizygotic twins, indicating that genetics may be involved in the persistence of hepatitis B. MHC genotype is a risk factor for developing persistent infection. In addition, the MHC may be involved in nonresponsiveness to immunization. Both carriage of certain MHC alleles and MHC heterozygosity may be important in protection from persistent infection. In a west African population, where 90 percent of adults have been infected and 15 percent have persistent infection, there was some heterozygote advantage for the class II but not for the class I region, as well as a protective association with *HLA-DRB1*1302* (Thursz et al. 1997; Hill 1998). Two further studies have shown this allele or its supertype *HLA-DR6* to be protective. However, in a small Qatari study *HLA-DR2* was associated with clearance and *HLA-DR7* with persistence (Almarri and Batchelor 1994). Heterozygote advantage was confirmed in a study of largely African–American intravenous drug users, which found persistence associated with *HLA-DQA1*0501, DQB1*0301*, and class II homozygosity (Thio et al. 1999). The different allelic associations seen in this study were ascribed to the different age of initial infection. In addition to class II, *TNF* promoter and *VDR* alleles have been associated with HBV clearance (Hill 1998; Bellamy et al. 1999), and in Africans, but not other populations, *MBL* does not appear to influence the risk of HBV persistence (Bellamy et al. 1998b).

A particularly interesting set of questions relates to the chronic persistence of HBV as a risk factor for hepatocellular carcinoma (Wild and Hall 1999). It is possible that even apparently immune individuals are responding to sequestered virus, and risk factors for hepatocellular carcinoma include not only persistent infections such as HBV, but also other lifestyle, environmental, and genetic aspects. It seems likely that HLA determines development of hepatocellular carcinoma in hepatitis B antigen-positive patients (Donaldson et al. 2001). Susceptibility is also reported to be associated with genetic variation in the enzymatic detoxification of aflatoxin B1 (McGlynn et al. 1995), and variation in the gene for cytochrome P450 1A1 (*CYP1A1*), involved in transforming tobacco polycyclic aromatic hydrocarbons into carcinogenic metabolites, affects the risk of hepatocellular carcinoma in smokers (Yu et al. 1999). The complex mechanisms and interactions of these many factors remain to be elucidated.

The more recently described hepatitis C (HCV), like hepatitis B, is successfully cleared only in a minority of individuals. In the persistently infected, some remain asymptomatic whereas others progress to hepatocellular carcinoma. Again the role of HLA has been examined at a number of stages: susceptibility itself, viral clearance, progression to hepatocellular carcinoma, and response to treatment (Donaldson 1999). The first of these questions is dogged by the bugbear of all infectious disease immunogenetics, exposure. The second is the best studied, e.g. in the UK Minton et al. (1998) reported *HLA-DRB1*1101* (a *DR5* allele) and *HLA-DQB1*0301* to be associated with clearance of hepatitis C. This supports a previously observed protective effect of *HLA-DR5* (Zavaglia et al. 1996), although haplotypic analysis suggests *HLA-DQB1*0301* as being key (Alric et al. 1997; Donaldson 1999). However, a number of studies do not fit with such associations (e.g. Lechmann et al. 1999), although some of these studies have relatively small sample sizes. A suggestion that some of the disparities were the result of ethnic diversity (Thio et al. 2001) has stimulated some discussion (Sarmiento et al. 2002). Kuzushita et al. (1998) examined the effects of

HLA on progression to liver damage in HCV-infected subjects and showed that haplotypes that included *HLA-B*54* were associated with liver damage, whereas haplotypes that included *HLA-DRB1*1302-DQB1*0604* were associated with low hepatitis activity. The less frequent alleles of the TNF_{-308} and TNF_{-238} polymorphisms were correlated with development of cirrhosis in hepatitis C carriers (Yee et al. 2000); however, *TNF* has not been studied in conjunction with class I and II alleles. Sustained response to antiviral therapy has been associated with *IL10* but not *TNF* haplotypes (Yee et al. 2001). Outcomes of hepatitis C infection have also been correlated with variation in the gene for the low-density lipoprotein receptor (*LDLR*), apparently through effects on immune function rather than receptor status (Hennig et al. 2002).

Patients with liver–kidney microsomal type 1 antibodies often have detectable hepatitis C. In the presence of hepatitis C, a correlation was seen between the presence of antibodies and *HLA-DR7* in a Spanish study (Jurado et al. 1997), whereas *HLA-DR3* correlated with serum cryoglobulinemia and *HLA-DR4* with serum autoantibodies in a Chinese population (Hwang et al. 2002). The etiologically distinct autoimmune hepatitis, which is not caused or triggered by viral infection, also has well-characterized HLA associations. In addition non-HLA genes may be involved: in studies of *IL1*, *IL10*, *TNF*, and *CTLA4*, susceptibility to type 1 autoimmune hepatitis was associated with *CTLA4* alleles and TNF_{-308}*2 which is interdependent with *HLA-DRB1*0301* (Cookson et al. 1999; Djilali-Saiah et al. 2001).

Other viral infections

A number of other viruses are also associated with specific malignancies. As for hepatitis, there is often evidence for both genetic susceptibility to the virus itself, and genetic susceptibility to malignancy after infection. However, these questions are sometimes difficult to unravel.

Epstein–Barr virus is associated with a variety of malignancies. Interestingly, from a geneticist's point of view, racial groups show clear differences in the type of malignancy, with Burkitt's lymphoma in African populations and nasopharyngeal carcinoma in east Asian populations. It has been proposed that pathogenesis is a result of a failure of EBV-specific immunity (Niedobitek et al. 2001). EBV is ubiquitous and there has been some consideration as to the mechanism by which HLA could control primary infection, either as a co-receptor for viral entry (Haan and Longnecker 2000) or by influencing T-cell precursor frequencies (Toussirot et al. 1999). *IL10* promoter polymorphisms appear to influence susceptibility to primary infection (Helminen et al. 1999, 2001). HLA class I and II, *TNF*, and *IL10* may all play a role in susceptibility to EBV-associated gastric carcinoma (Koriyama et al. 2001; Wu et al. 2002b). *HLA-A*0207*, which is common in Chinese but not Caucasian populations, is associated with nasopharyngeal carcinoma (Hildesheim et al. 2002). *HLA-A*0207* is in linkage disequilibrium with *HLA-B*4601*, a previously identified risk factor, and *HLA-A*1101* is protective. A recent genome scan of Chinese families with nasopharyngeal carcinoma, and using parametric linkage analysis, identified a single region on chromosome 4, with a LOD score of 3.67 to marker D4S405, which was increased by incorporation of information on EBV antibody titer (Feng et al. 2002).

The human papilloma viruses (HPV) infect the squamous epithelial cells of skin, the oral cavity, and the cervix, leading to warts and in some cases cancer. The viral E6 oncoprotein binds to the tumor suppressor p53 and induces degradation. The degradation is affected by a Pro/Arg variation at position 72 in p53, with homozygosity for the Arg variant resulting in increased susceptibility to HPV-16/-18 infection and oral carcinogenesis (Nagpal et al. 2002). Similarly, there is genetic predisposition to cervical cancer (Magnusson and Gyllensten 2000), with MHC involvement, although findings are mixed. *HLA-B53* was found to be at increased frequency in patients with cervical neoplasia and HPV of types other than 16 or 18, whereas *HLA-B55* was increased in HPV-negative neoplasia patients (Krul et al. 1999). MHC II associations have also been reported. In the context of immunization, some HPV-16 E7 oncoprotein epitopes bind to the products of several *HLA-A2* alleles (Ressing et al. 1999).

HLA associations for infection with other human viruses have been identified. HLA restriction of the immune response to dengue virus may affect vaccine development (Loke et al. 2001), and known variation in response to immunization, correlated with HLA restriction, such as in the case of measles, may influence worldwide population vaccine efficacy (Poland 1999). Other genes may influence viral outcome, such as *VDR* and *FCRG2A* in susceptibility to severe dengue hemorrhagic fever (Loke et al. 2002).

In a number of instances, murine studies are well ahead, as with the murine leukemia virus-mapped genes (Malo and Skamene 1994; McLeod et al. 1995). There are at least two regions controlling CMV in mice: the MHC and *Cmv1*. *Cmv1*, an autosomal dominant gene, controls virus replication in the spleen and mediates its effects through NK cells. MHC associations in human CMV infection are also seen and could be caused partly by an effect of the proinflammatory *TNF* gene (Hurme and Helminen 1998). Influenza is controlled by *Mx1* in mice and has been cloned (Malo and Skamene 1994). In susceptible laboratory strains there is a deletion of exons 9–11, or alternatively a point mutation in exon 10, resulting in a stop codon. *Mx1* is controlled by interferons α and β, and has been highly conserved in evolution, being present in all eukaryotes. A gene *Mx2* has also been identified that controls vesicular stomatitis virus in mice. The human homologs will be of interest. Of topical interest is host genetic susceptibility to West Nile Virus, a flavivirus, where a mutation in the gene coding for IFN-γ-inducible 2′,5′-oligoadenylate synthetase is associated with murine susceptibility (Samuel 2002).

Prions

The *PRNP* gene encodes the prion protein (PrP). Classification of prion diseases has been as genetic, infectious, or sporadic; however, all involve modification of PrP (Pruisner and Scott 1997). Approximately 10 percent of prion disease is inherited. There are several mutations in *PRNP* available for study (Kovacs et al. 2002), e.g. the murine equivalent of the PrP P102L mutation, associated with Gerstmann–Straussler syndrome, alters incubation time of transmissible spongiform encephalopathy (Manson et al. 1999). Most notably, all patients to date with variant Creutzfeldt–Jakob disease, and many with sporadic Creutzfeldt–Jakob disease, are homozygous *PRNP* for a methionine at position 129, whereas heterozygotes are protected (Palmer et al. 1991; Windl et al. 1996; Zeidler et al. 1997). The kuru epidemic in New Guinea also preferentially affected individuals with the *PRNP129* M/M genotype, resulting in complete loss of this genotype from affected communities (Lee et al. 2001). Undoubtedly *PRNP* does not act as a sole determinant of disease. Studies in other species, including mice, have searched for additional genetic components. A PrP-like protein, doppel protein, is coded for by *PRND*, close to *PRNP*. Whether variants of *PRND* will influence human prion disease directly, or merely reflect variation in *PRNP*, remains to be established (Peoc'h et al. 2000; Schroder et al. 2001). A recent study implicated HLA in variant Creutzfeldt–Jakob disease, with patients showing a reduced frequency of *HLA-DQB1*0301/4/9* (Jackson et al. 2001). This was an exciting finding, because it was thought to explain why many putatively infected, *PRNP*-susceptible, individuals did not develop disease. However, this finding has not been supported (Laplanche et al. 2003; Partanen 2003; Pepys et al. 2003).

BACTERIAL INFECTIONS

Intracellular bacteria

A number of intracellular bacteria have been investigated for control of infection by host genetic factors. In particular, there have been many studies of bacterial pathogens of macrophages, and these studies may be considered together with those concerning protozoal macrophage parasites such as *Leishmania* spp. Mycobacterial species have been a focus of attention and *Mycobacterium tuberculosis* and *Mycobacterium leprae* are considered separately.

Whereas common genetic variation has been proposed to influence the major infectious diseases, the mycobacteria also provide good examples of rare host deleterious mutations resulting in disease caused by poorly pathogenic bacteria (Ottenhoff et al. 2002). The main infections observed are disseminated *Mycobacterium bovis* BCG and *Mycobacterium avium*, although infections with *Salmonella* spp. also occur (Jouanguy et al. 1999a). The underlying phenotype is of defective bacterial killing resulting from a failure to produce or respond to IFN-γ, and fatal infection is common. Deficiencies may be partial or complete, and inherited in either a recessive or a dominant fashion. These deficiencies are often caused by mutations in cytokine receptor genes, and a variety of mutation types occur (Ottenhoff et al. 2002). The first mutations were identified in Maltese and Tunisian patients (Jouanguy et al. 1996; Newport et al. 1996), where genome scanning for regions of homozygosity in Maltese individuals pinpointed a premature stop codon in *IFNGR1* (Newport et al. 1996). Functional studies confirmed the genetic observations (Newport et al. 1996; Altare et al. 1998b). Later studies identified a deletion hotspot in *IFNGR1* downstream from the mutations first identified (Jouanguy et al. 1999b). These studies were rapidly followed by the identification in other patients of IL-12R deficiency, as a result of premature stop codons in the gene for the β1 subunit of the IL-12R (*IL12RB1*) (Altare et al. 1998a; de Jong et al. 1998). A recent report of complete IL-12Rβ1 deficiency in 41 patients from 17 countries reported a fair prognosis and discussed the redundancy of IL-12 in immunity (Fieschi et al. 2003). To date, mutations have been identified in three further genes, encoding IL-12 p40 (*IL12B*), IFN-γR2 (*IFNGR2*), and STAT1. The p40 subunit of IL-12 principally interacts with the β1 subunit of the IL-12R. Other cytokines and receptors may also have a phenotypic role, such as IL-23, which shares the p40 subunit with IL-12, and IL-23R, which shares IL-12Rβ1 with IL-12R (Ottenhoff et al. 2002). Overlapping cytokine and receptor specificities may account for the appearance of mutations in only a proportion of subunits.

Phenotypic severity in such patients correlates with the degree of impairment of IFN-γ pathways. Complete deficiency of IFN-γR1 and IFN-γR2 are the most severe (Ottenhoff et al. 1998). However, disease phenotype heterogeneity is consistent with involvement of other genetic or environmental factors, in addition to primary mutations (Picard et al. 2002). Indeed such rare deficiencies may be regarded as being at one end of a continuous spectrum of disease severity, with common variation contributing to responses to more pathogenic organisms at the other end of the spectrum. Unlike variation in proinflammatory cytokine genes, and type 2 cytokine and receptor genes, there is little evidence that common variation in type 1 cytokine pathways plays a significant role in noninfectious disease susceptibility.

Studies of common variation in other candidate genes for the less common mycobacterial pathogens, such as *NRAMP1* in *Mycobacterium avium-intracellulare* infections, sometimes associated with HIV, and *Mycobacterium ulcerans* infections, not known to be HIV associated, have not shown allelic associations (Huang et al. 1998; Stienstra et al. 2001).

Leprosy

The clearly defined spectrum of clinical disease in leprosy, from lepromatous to tuberculoid forms, and the slow progression of disease, has long attracted the interest of geneticists. There is also evidence that the incidence of leprosy infection is much higher than the incidence of clinical leprosy, with 95 percent of those infected proposed to have persistent or self-curing subclinical infection (Fine 1983). A genetic predisposition to leprosy has been speculated upon for more than 50 years (Fine 1981; Schurr et al. 1991), with observations of racial differences and familial clustering, although it has been difficult to differentiate between genetic effects and shared environment. Further support for the role of genetics was obtained using twin studies, where concordance in monozygotic twins is consistently higher than in dizygotic twins (Schurr et al. 1991). Studies implicate genetic predisposition to position on the leprosy spectrum as well as to the disease itself. More formal proof has been obtained from family studies, using a variety of methods including complex segregation analyses, carried out on a number of American and Asian populations (Haile et al. 1985; Shields et al. 1987; Abel and Demenais 1988; Wagener et al. 1988; Abel et al. 1992b; Feitosa et al. 1995; Shaw et al. 2001). All studies have demonstrated the importance of host genetics, but, whereas some results suggest major gene control of susceptibility to leprosy itself, there has been no consensus as to the precise mode of inheritance, or to genetic control of severity. Such mixed results may be accounted for in part by limitations of the methods employed, partly by population heterogeneity and partly by strong environmental confounding factors (Feitosa et al. 1995), e.g. segregation analyses rely on liability classes, which should be derived from accurate epidemiological information. Early papers tested only single gene and multifactorial models, whereas a later study used the program COMDS which allowed testing of an oligogenic model (major gene plus additional genetic effects, Shaw et al. 2001). In this study, data from 76 Brazilian multicase leprosy pedigrees supported a two-locus model as the best fit: a recessive major gene plus a recessive modifier gene.

There has been a single recent human genome scan for susceptibility to leprosy (Siddiqui et al. 2001). This study was carried out using 245 affected sib-pairs from an Indian population where leprosy was predominantly tuberculoid. Significant linkage was obtained for a single chromosomal region, 10p13. Surprisingly, there was no linkage to HLA. Further evaluation with 140 additional families, for a region that had shown weak evidence of linkage in the genome scan, identified linkage to a second region at 20p12 in families from Tamil Nadu, but not Andhra Pradesh (Tosh et al. 2002). Transmission disequilibrium testing was employed for fine mapping of the chromosome 20 region, and showed that a marker, D20S835, was associated with protection against leprosy, and presumably lies close to the susceptibility locus. Neither 10p13 nor 20p12 contains obvious candidate genes. These results remain to be investigated in other populations.

The earliest linkage studies of HLA and leprosy involved the observation of nonrandom segregation of parental HLA haplotypes (de Vries et al. 1976; Fine et al. 1979), whereas later studies have also employed parametric linkage approaches (Haile et al. 1985; Dessoukey and El-Shiemy 1996; Shaw et al. 2001), in some instances using information on mode of inheritance derived from the same population. Linkage to the HLA region has been observed in Surinamese, Indian, Egyptian, and Brazilian families. Maximum LOD scores are found at a recombination fraction of 0, directly implicating the MHC (Shaw et al. 2001). Evidence for HLA control has often been found using tuberculoid siblings, but, as this is often the most common type of leprosy, further conclusions on the role of HLA are difficult. A 1976 study reported an increase in haplotype sharing between siblings with similar leprosy type, whereas siblings with different types of leprosy shared haplotypes less often than expected (de Vries et al. 1976). This led to the suggestion that two HLA genes were involved, determining susceptibility to leprosy itself and severity of leprosy, respectively, an idea that remains to be confirmed or refuted.

Some of the many HLA association studies have been reviewed (Todd et al. 1990; Meyer et al. 1998). Results have been variable, and such inconsistencies may reflect the lack of power of studies, variable selection of controls, and statistical false positives, in addition to population heterogeneity. HLA class I associations have not been highly reproducible, and perhaps the only study of note is an *HLA-A11* association which has been reported with erythema nodosum leprosum, seen in some multibacillary patients (Agrewala et al. 1989). The clearest associations, found in several ethnic groups, are for MHC class II: *HLA-DR2* is often associated with both lepromatous and tuberculoid leprosy, and *HLA-DR3* is associated with tuberculoid leprosy. *HLA-DQw1* may also be a susceptibility allele (Jawinska and Serjeantson 1988; Todd et al. 1990). Further resolution of susceptibility and resistance class II haplotypes has been achieved in later studies, and some HLA influence, at least on disease severity, seems certain.

A number of studies have also been performed on HLA control of in vitro immune responsiveness, usually using crude mycobacterial antigens. However, HLA-restricted mycobacterial epitopes might be expected to elicit protective or suppressive immune responses. Although little is known about the nature of such epitopes (Meyer et al. 1998), potential leprogenic motifs are suggested from the observation that arginine residues in the peptide-binding groove of *HLA-DRB1* at codons 13 or 70–71 in pocket 4 conferred a relative risk for tuberculoid leprosy of 8.8 in Indian leprosy patients compared with healthy controls (Zerva et al. 1996). Eleven *HLA-DRB1* motifs positively associated with leprosy in a Nigerian population tended to have basic residues at codons 13, 70, 71, 74, and 86, resulting in a net positive charge, whereas five negatively associated motifs were characterized by acidic residues and a net negative charge (Uko et al. 1999).

It is still possible that observed associations are merely a reflection of linkage disequilibrium occurring within the HLA region, such as with the *TAP2* locus within the class II region showing allelic association with tuberculoid leprosy (Rajalingam et al. 1997). However, studies on *TNF* in the class III region suggest that there may be multiple susceptibility genes in the HLA region. In a study of Indian leprosy patients TNF_{-308}*2 was found at increased frequency in lepromatous but not tuberculoid patients (Roy et al. 1997), an allele commonly thought to be associated with high TNF-α production. In contrast, use of the transmission disequilibrium test for Brazilian leprosy families revealed an association of TNF_{-308}*1 for all types of leprosy (Shaw et al. 2001). Two-locus transmission disequilibrium testing for the class III region identified *TNF*1/LTA*2* as a susceptibility haplotype, *TNF*2/LTA*2* as a resistance haplotype, and *TNF*1/LTA*1* as not associated with leprosy. This confirms that the TNF_{-308} polymorphism is not the whole story. The complex influence of such haplotypes is in accordance with studies on other infectious diseases and this region. *TNF* is also an excellent candidate gene for nerve damage and leprosy reactions, commonly associated with high levels of circulating TNF-α, although no convincing associations have been shown to date (Sarno et al. 2000). There have been no association studies for the other proinflammatory cytokine IL-1. A recent study of Toll-like receptor 2 suggests a promising avenue for exploration (Kang and Chae 2001).

NRAMP1 might be expected to play a role in human susceptibility to leprosy, because susceptibility to *M. lepraemurium* is determined by a single amino acid change in *Nramp1* in inbred mouse strains. Analysis of *NRAMP1* haplotype sharing in predominantly Vietnamese leprosy families, containing both lepromatous and tuberculoid patients, showed significantly nonrandom sharing (Abel et al. 1998), conflicting with two earlier small studies that failed to find evidence of linkage (Shaw et al. 1993; Levee et al. 1994). However, parametric LOD score analysis, on an extended haplotype, showed only very weak evidence for linkage, and no specific allelic associations were identified. A Malian association study found that, for one *NRAMP1* polymorphism, in the 3′UTR, heterozygotes were more common in lepromatous than tuberculoid patients (Meisner et al. 2001). This finding was not reproduced in Indian patients (Roy et al. 1999). No associations were found for leprosy as such. From limited information, it does not appear that *NRAMP1* is a major player in human susceptibility to *M. leprae*. An investigation of skin test responsiveness to lepromin, using the predominantly Vietnamese families, showed linkage of positive Mitsuda reaction to *NRAMP1* (Alcais et al. 2000), building on the observation of familial aggregation of positive Mitsuda reaction in Brazilians (Feitosa et al. 1996). Although linkage was independent of leprosy status, the suggestion that a Mitsuda reaction can be used as a predictor of susceptibility to lepromatous disease makes precise interpretation of these findings difficult.

The *VDR* codon 352 polymorphism has also been examined in Indian leprosy patients (Roy et al. 1999). The homozygous genotype previously associated with low bone mineral density, enhanced clearance of hepatitis B and resistance to pulmonary tuberculosis (TB) was more common in tuberculoid patients than in controls. In contrast, homozygosity for the opposing allele was more common in lepromatous patients than in controls.

Tuberculosis

Studies of genetic susceptibility to *M. tuberculosis* are somewhat fewer than those for *M. leprae*. This may be the result of a less marked contribution of HLA, problems of ensuring reliable diagnosis, and a less polarized spectrum of disease. Almost all genetic studies concern pulmonary TB, and other disease manifestations have been sadly neglected. Twin studies do suggest genetic control of pulmonary TB, with concordance in monozygotic twins being substantially higher than in dizygotic twins (Comstock 1978; Fine 1981; Bellamy and Hill 1998). However, estimates of heritability vary widely. There is a single formal study of genetic control of susceptibility to TB, where complex segregation analysis pointed to oligogenic control of TB in a Brazilian population (Shaw et al. 1997). The lack of more formal proof is surprising in view of efforts expended in gene identification.

The majority of gene studies have employed a candidate gene approach, with HLA, including *TNF*, the *IL1* gene cluster, *NRAMP1*, *MBL*, and *VDR*, all receiving attention. In particular, investigation of *NRAMP1* was triggered by the observations of single gene control of mycobacterial species made in mice more than 20 years ago. Recently, a genome scan in mice has suggested further regions (Lavebratt et al. 1999). However, although murine genome scan results on mycobacterial and leishmanial species are correlated, there is no obvious correlation with patterns seen in humans. A human genome scan using Gambian and South African sib-pairs, and a derivation of homozygosity mapping, dependent on common ancestry, showed suggestive evidence for linkage of TB to chromosomes 15q and Xq (Bellamy et al. 2000). Fine mapping of the 15q11–13 region implicated a gene *UBE3A* coding for ubiquitin protein ligase E3A, or a close flanking gene (Cervino et al. 2002). It remains to be seen whether regions identified from genome scans prove to be more important than previously studied candidate genes, or whether such regions turn out to be study-specific.

As for many infectious diseases HLA has been a candidate region for control of susceptibility. In the case of TB this has been supported by murine studies. However, fewer human studies have been conducted than for leprosy. Most studies have been carried out in association with pulmonary TB and, although results are not consistent between small population groups and there are potential problems of population stratification, a number of studies have reported an association with *HLA-DR2* (later *HLA-DRB1*1501*, reviewed in Meyer et al. 1998). Studies in Indian populations have genotyped additional loci within the class II region (*HLA-DQA1*, *-DQB1*, and *-DPB1*), in an effort to determine susceptibility haplotypes (Mehra et al. 1995; Ravikumar et al. 1999). Consideration of *TAP* genes, also within the class II region, points to a complex picture of haplotypes contributing to disease susceptibility (Rajalingam et al. 1997). TB is a common opportunistic infection in immunosuppressed patients and it is likely that HLA associations in nonimmunosuppressed and immunosuppressed cases will differ. Whereas *HLA-DQA1*0101*, *HLA-DQB1*0501*, and *HLA-DRB1*1501* were risk factors for TB in nonimmunosuppressed Mexican patients, *HLA-DRB1*1101* appeared to influence disease in HIV-infected patients (Teran-Escandon et al. 1999). Unlike several other infectious diseases, including leprosy, limited attempts to find linkage or association to *TNF* in the class III region have often proved negative (Shaw et al. 1997; Goldfeld et al. 1998; Selvaraj et al. 2001). As linkage disequilibrium between class II and III regions is rarely considered, and rarely formally tested, the relative contributions of distinct loci are sometimes hard to unravel. At a minimum, *TNF* is not a major contributor to disease susceptibility.

A few studies have tested the effect of HLA on immune response phenotypes. Most, but not all, concern cellular responsiveness (Bothamley et al. 1989; Jepson et al. 1997b). Selection of active, cured, or relapsed patients may account for some of the discrepancies in the literature. In a small study of Mexican–Americans, where *HLA-DR3* was at a reduced frequency in TB patients, there was an indication of an HLA effect in patients for in vitro proliferation to purified protein derivative (PPD) (*HLA-A9-B40* in strong responders and *HLA-B14-DR1* in weak responders), but not skin test responsiveness (Cox et al. 1988). These findings contrasted with several earlier studies. In a much later study, patients carrying *HLA-DR2* showed an increased proliferative response to *M. tuberculosis* culture filtrate antigens to patients who were *HLA-DR2* negative, whereas low responsiveness to antigen and mitogens was seen in *HLA-DR3*-positive compared with negative healthy individuals (Uma et al. 1999). However, a twin study in The Gambia suggested that non-HLA genes were more important than HLA in determining immune responses to PPD (Jepson et al. 1997b).

Studies in Gambian TB patients showed weak association with the *IL1* gene cluster, *IL1RN*2* of the 86-bp repeat in intron 2 being less common in Gambian TB patients than in controls (Bellamy et al. 1998a). A study on Gujarati TB patients in the UK also implicated the *IL1* gene cluster; however, evidence remains weak (Wilkinson et al. 1999). IL-1Ra and IL-1β induced by *M. tuberculosis* varied according to *IL1RN* and *IL1B* genotype. Although there was no association between genotype and disease, haplotypic associations were seen with tuberculous pleurisy and Mantoux responsiveness.

Polymorphisms in *NRAMP1* were originally identified with a view to ascertaining the role of this macrophage function gene in susceptibility to TB (Liu et al. 1995; Searle and Blackwell 1998). Linkage to the 2q35 region was weak (Shaw et al. 1997), but some association studies have been positive in African, Asian, and later Caucasian populations (Bellamy et al. 1998c; Cervino et al. 2000; Gao et al. 2000; Ryu et al. 2000; Ma et al. 2002). Polymorphic sites, the extent of linkage disequilibrium between these sites, and the degree of association with disease appear to vary between populations. As for HLA, associations may be influenced by fine differences in disease status such as HIV co-infection (Ma et al. 2002) and disease severity (Soborg et al. 2002). A 5′ repeat polymorphism has received attention as a result of its proposed functionality (Gao et al. 2000; Awomoyi et al. 2002), with allele 2 associated with TB and LPS-induced IL-10 production by macrophages (Awomoyi et al. 2002). Monocytes from TB patients also showed high IL-10 production, suggesting that the influence of *NRAMP1* on susceptibility to TB is, at least in part, mediated by IL-10. Roles for TNF-α and IL-1β, regulated by *NRAMP1*, were not shown in this instance. One of the most interesting recent papers shows linkage of TB to 2q35, but not to the MHC, in an extended Aboriginal Canadian family (Greenwood et al. 2000). This was unusual because linkage was conducted using a parametric approach with an autosomal dominant mode of inheritance. Individuals were assigned to liability classes, including information on tuberculin skin test responsiveness, yielding a LOD score of 3.81 with a close marker, D2S424. This emphasized both the power of parametric approaches and the need to be mindful of confounding factors such as immunization status. Despite the identification of *NRAMP1* as a candidate gene through murine studies, and apparent major gene control in this family, differences in the role of *NRAMP1* in TB between mice and humans are evident. Studies of *MBL* have also been mixed with little association seen with TB in Gambians (Bellamy et al. 1998b), but stronger evidence for a role in Indians, independent of association of pulmonary TB with *HLA-DR2* (Selvaraj et al. 1999).

A *VDR* codon 352 genotype, associated with osteoporosis and high levels of circulating 1,25-dihydroxyvitamin D_3 (1,25-D_3), which has widespread effects on cellular immunity, showed a slightly reduced frequency in TB patients (Bellamy et al. 1999). This supports an old observation that vitamin D may be beneficial in treatment of TB, and in vitro observations that 1,25-D_3 enhance the ability of monocytes to restrict growth of *M. tuberculosis* (Bellamy and Hill 1998). More recently three *VDR* polymorphisms were studied in UK Gujaratis, in whom phenotypic vitamin D deficiency was associated with active TB. Although there was no clear association between *VDR* genotype and TB, combination of particular genotypes and vitamin D status is consistent with a contributory role of host genotype (Wilkinson et al. 2000).

Exposure to TB has been suggested to reduce the risk of developing asthma (von Mutius et al. 2000). It is highly likely that such effects are in part influenced by human genotype, particularly through cytokine genes. However, studies are limited on the role of genes such as those in the chromosome 5 cluster and susceptibility to TB. The largely non-MHC control for cellular and humoral responses to PPD also remains to be elucidated (Jepson et al. 1997b), although candidate genes already implicated in susceptibility to TB are implicated in control of lymphocyte responsiveness and tuberculin reactivity (Selvaraj et al. 2000). Overall, TB is a well-studied disease; however, candidate gene associations to date have been weak and inconsistent, with substantial differences between populations (reviewed by Delgado et al. 2002), leaving much scope for identification of further genetic effects.

Salmonellosis

Infection with *Salmonella* spp. is interesting for geneticists on a number of counts. As cited above, rare deleterious mutations in genes such as *IL12B* and *IL12RB1* result in failure to produce IFN-γ, hence the failure in granuloma formation and susceptibility to non-typhi *Salmonella* spp. (Jouanguy et al. 1999a; Lammas et al. 2002). The tiny number of studies in human populations doubtless reflects the difficulties of collecting good patient groups for an acute disease. In contrast, work on mice and chickens spans several decades. Murine infection with *Salmonella typhimurium* is controlled by *Ity* (*NRAMP1*) and *Lps*, involved in innate immunity and macrophage function, and *xid* which modulates humoral immune responses by preventing the production of antibodies against polysaccharides. *Xid* is homologous with the human gene *XLA*, which causes X-linked agammaglobulinemia, and results from mutations in Bruton's tyrosine kinase (Malo and Skamene 1994). A recent genome scan for clearance of *S. enteritidis* in mice identified three regions; one was likely to be *Nramp1* and two were previously unknown (Caron et al. 2002). However, no common variants of human *NRAMP1* were associated with susceptibility to typhoid fever in Vietnamese patients (Dunstan et al. 2001a). In the same Vietnamese population, HLA class II and *TNF* associations were identified (Dunstan et al. 2001b): haplotypes that were protective (TNF_{-308}*1-*DRB1*04*) or predisposed individuals to typhoid fever ($TNF-_{-308}$*2-*DRB1*0301*) were determined.

The second most common single gene disorder prevalent in western Caucasian populations is cystic fibrosis. Homozygosity for mutant alleles has had a massive impact on reproductive fitness. The gene determining cystic fibrosis, *CFTR*, the cystic fibrosis transmembrane conductance regulator, codes for a transmembrane Cl^- channel. About 1 in 23 people are heterozygous carriers for a mutant allele, about 70 percent of which are the ΔF508 mutation, resulting in loss of a single phenylalanine and no protein expression at the cell surface. It has long been supposed that there must be heterozygote advantage in order to maintain mutant alleles at such high frequency. One suggestion is that such an advantage might be an increased resistance of heterozygotes to fluid loss caused by response to toxins from enteric pathogens such as *Vibrio cholerae*. Alternatively it has been proposed that *S. typhi*, but not *S. typhimurium*, uses the *CFTR* to enter intestinal epithelial cells, with ΔF508 cells being partially refractory, potentially decreasing the susceptibility of heterozygous carriers to typhoid fever (Pier et al. 1998). At present there is insufficient evidence for firm conclusions (Guggino 1999).

Immunogenetic studies concerning a number of other human bacterial pathogens appear in the literature. Many are in the context of mouse model systems, where variation in disease outcome between inbred strains, associated with variation in genetic background, is suggestive of genetic control. Use of transgenic and knockout mice has given clues as to immunological mechanisms and potential candidate genes. In some instances mouse susceptibility loci have been mapped, but potentially difficult studies in humans have not followed, e.g. the *Lgn1* gene on mouse chromosome 13 controls susceptibility to *Legionella pneumophila* (Beckers et al. 1997; Diez et al. 2003) and for *Rickettsia tsutsugamushi* a single murine gene has been mapped (Malo and Skamene 1994). In some instances there are HLA association studies, although these are looking for an effect of HLA on immune environment rather than specific phenotypes. *Pseudomonas aeruginosa* susceptibility genes are *Pscr1* and *Pscr2* in mice (listed in McLeod et al. 1995); however, in humans, the effect of HLA on pulmonary phenotype as the site of infection for *P. aeruginosa* in cystic fibrosis patients has been examined (Aron et al. 1999). Genetic studies in humans are found mainly for pathogens associated with particular pathologies of interest. These pathologies may be associated with more than a single pathogen. In some cases the bacteria are intracellular and consequent inflammatory responses are involved.

Meningococcal meningitis

The best-known infection associated with deficiency of the terminal complement components C6–C9 is *Neisseria meningitides*. Although such deficiencies are not necessarily polymorphic, but strictly speaking are rare variants, and studies are usually on individual families, they are still relatively common. Deficiencies of particular components may be the result of a variety of mutations and certain deficiencies are prevalent in certain communities (O'Hara et al. 1998). The genes *C6*, *C7*, and *C9* form a gene cluster on chromosome 5 (Alvarez et al. 1995), and linkage disequilibrium occurs between common variants and the deficiencies (Wurzner et al. 1992).

There have also been multiple studies on the role of FcγR genes in susceptibility to infection and severity of meningococcal meningitis. FcγR polymorphic forms are associated with different functional activities (van der Pol et al. 2001). The FcγRIIA (CD32) R/R131 allotype, which binds IgG2 poorly, was more common in children who had survived fulminant meningococcal septic shock than healthy controls (Bredius et al. 1994). In some cases allotypes have been reported to be similar in patients versus controls; however, the R/R131 allotype is at an increased frequency in the more severe forms of disease such as fulminant meningococcal disease and meningococcemia without meningitis (Domingo et al. 2002). R/R131 homozygous polymorphonuclear leukocytes (PMN) have reduced ability to internalize IgG2 opsonized meningococci (Fijen et al. 2000). Some of the studies have considered extended haplotypes in the FcγR gene cluster on chromosome 1.

Further genetic observations concern molecules involved in inflammation. Homozygosity for a deletion in the gene coding for angiotensin-converting enzyme (ACE), associated with higher tissue ACE, is correlated with increased disease severity (Harding et al. 2002). However, findings on *TNF* and *IL1* cluster genes have been variable. Although some resistance to a fatal outcome was found for $IL1B_{-511}$ heterozygotes, the same survey found no effect of variation in *TNF* (Read et al. 2000). In other studies, the frequency of *IL1RN*A2*, probably in linkage disequilibrium with the *IL1B* locus, and associated with increased IL-1Ra, was the same in cases and controls (Carrol et al. 2002), and the TNF_{-308} polymorphism influenced mortality as a result of meningococcal meningitis (Nadel et al. 1996). Studying first-degree relatives of meningococcal disease patients, families with low TNF-α and high IL-10 production were associated with increased risk of fatal outcome. Whereas TNF-α and IL-10 production were shown to be highly heritable, there was no difference in TNF_{-308} and TNF_{-238} genotype in relatives of survivors versus nonsurvivors (Westendorp et al. 1997).

Helicobacter pylori and gastric cancer

A twin study for infection with *H. pylori* demonstrated a heritability of 57 percent (Malatay et al. 1994). However, the greatest interest in *H. pylori* is a result of infection being a risk factor for gastric cancer. The extent of gastritis in response to *H. pylori* influences risk of cancer, with hypochlorhydria being a precursor. Gastric cancer and duodenal ulceration are mutually exclusive outcomes. Although *HLA-DQB1*0602* is increased and *HLA-DQB1*0301* decreased with different gastric cancer-associated phenotypes in Taiwanese (Wu et al. 2002a), and *HLA-DQA1*0102* associated with resistance in Japanese (Azuma et al. 1998), more complete study of the HLA class II region suggests that the limited associations observed to date are not strong enough to stand correction for multiple comparisons (Yoshitake et al. 1999). A study of three polymorphisms within *IL1B* and the $IL1RNV_{NTR}$ polymorphism demonstrated that haplotypes putatively associated with upregulation of IL-1β had an increased frequency in cases of hypochlorhydria induced by *H. pylori* and of gastric cancer (El-Omar et al. 2000). Most recently, a genome scan of Senegalese siblings used the quantitative trait of specific IgG for *H. pylori*. Linkage analysis followed by transmission disequilibrium testing pinpointed a single gene: *IFNGR1* (Thye et al. 2003). Three variants at positions −56, 318, and 450 were associated with high antibody concentrations, and were more common in Africans than Europeans, perhaps explaining the relatively low pathogenicity in Africans.

Spondyloarthropathies

Both genetic predisposition and a number of bacterial pathogens are implicated in spondyloarthropathies; in particular bacteria are triggers for reactive arthritis, e.g. *Salmonella enteritidis* (see above), *Listeria monocytogenes*, *Yersinia enterocolitica*, *Chlamydia trachomatis*, and *Borrelia burgdorferi* (Lyme disease). A well-known HLA association is that of *HLA-B27* with ankylosing spondylitis. In fact the *HLA-B27* association is with a broad range of spondyloarthropathies, for both development and chronicity of disease. The mechanism of predisposition is unclear but could involve use of HLA-B27 as an antigen-presenting molecule or, alternatively, class II-mediated presentation of B27-derived peptides (Lopez de Castro 1998). Undoubtedly, other molecules involved in immune responsiveness for pathogens will prove to be involved (Pacheco-Tena et al. 2002). For some of the pathogens implicated in reactive arthritis, genetic studies are largely confined to mouse models, e.g. *L. monocytogenes* with a single gene identified, *Lsr1* (Malo and Skamene 1994). For others there are a handful of human studies. For *C. trachomatis* infection, which stimulates an inflammatory response, often resulting in tissue scarring, the less common alleles TNF_{-308}*2 and TNF_{-238}*2 are associated with scarring trachoma (Conway et al. 1997). TNF-α was detected more frequently in tear fluid in patients than in controls, in line with indications that the less common alleles determine higher levels of TNF-α. This is independent of an *HLA-A*6802* association with scarring trachoma. *IL4*, *IL10*, and *MBL* are not strongly implicated (Mozzato-Chamay et al. 2000). In humans, *C. trachomatis* is also known to be a cause of pelvic inflammatory disease and infertility, but there have been no genetic studies to date. In mice, susceptibility to chlamydial salpingitis and subsequent infertility is under genetic control, with both H-2 and non-H-2 genes involved (Tuffrey et al. 1992).

Periodontitis

Oral gingivitis and the more severe periodontitis are the result of mixed microbial infections. Colonizing nonpathogenic bacteria generate the conditions required for secondary species, which tend to be gram-negative anaerobes. The outcome depends both on the species of bacteria and on the human inflammatory response. Hence the multitude of genetic studies often concern the inflammatory responses and consequent pathology, not necessarily susceptibility to bacterial species as such. Bacteria associated with gingivitis include *Streptococcus*, *Actinomyces*, *Haemophilus*, and *Capnocytophaga* spp. whereas tissue-damaging species associated with chronic periodontitis include *Porphyromonas gingivalis*, *Prevotella intermedia*, and *Bacteroides forsythus*, and with aggressive periodontitis *Actinobacillus actinomycetemcomitans*. There are case–control studies for candidate genes. In many instances the studies are small and cross-sectional, and use few polymorphic sites. One problem of drawing together findings is the range of phenotypes and severity criteria used for analysis. Bacterial species are not usually identified. Candidate genes have included *IL2*, *IL4*, *IL10*, *TGFB1*, *TNF*, *LTA*, *ACE*, and *VDR*. Although many polymorphisms show no association, some are weakly associated, and further analysis suggests both gene–gene and gene–environment interactions (Holla et al. 2001), e.g. the gene for plasminogen activator-inhibitor I is a risk factor for periodontitis, particularly in nonsmokers (Holla et al. 2002). Perhaps the most surprising result is a consistent failure to show an effect of variation in *TNF* on susceptibility or severity, even when several polymorphisms are employed (Craandijk et al. 2002).

However, the vast majority of studies concern the *IL1* and *FCGR* gene clusters. A number of investigations have highlighted association between allele 2 of $IL1A_{+4845}$ and $IL1B_{+3954}$ and disease, which may relate to the role of IL-1 as a stimulator of bone resorption. Based on the two *IL1* associations, a predictive test has been developed. However, the usefulness of this test has been questioned (Greenstein and Hart 2002), and population differences in allele frequencies may render the test inappropriate outside western Europeans (Armitage et al. 2000). In the context of IL-1, smoking is an important risk factor, although the nature of this interaction is unclear (Lang et al. 2000; Parkhill et al. 2000; Cullinan et al. 2001; Laine et al. 2001; Meisel et al. 2002). Only a few studies have attempted to correlate *IL1* genotype with protein production in vivo or in vitro (Mark et al. 2000; Shirodaria et al. 2000). Similarly, only a few studies have sought to identify the bacterial species present (Laine et al. 2001; Cullinan et al. 2001), although *IL1* genotype may well influence bacterial flora (Socransky et al. 2000).

The genes *FCGR2A*, *FCGR3A*, and *FCGR3B* have also been widely studied. A *FCGR3B* allele has been reported to influence disease in diverse population groups: elevated in African–Americans with aggressive periodontitis (Fu et al. 2002) and, together with an *FCGR3A* allele, associated with severity of chronic periodontitis in Japanese (Kobayashi et al. 2001). *FCGR3A* is in linkage disequilibrium with *FCGR3B*. In general, allotypes with low activity have been shown to be risk factors for disease. Cells carrying the periodontitis-associated *FCGR3B* allele are less efficient at both phagocytosing and inducing an oxidative burst, in response to IgG1- and IgG3-opsonized *P. gingivalis* (Kobayashi et al. 2000). However, in a group of Caucasian patients there was no significant difference in allele frequencies between mild and severe cases of periodontitis, although the severity of bone loss was correlated with the *FCGR3A* genotype coding for a high affinity receptor (Meisel et al. 2001).

FUNGAL INFECTIONS

There have been surprisingly few studies of genetic susceptibility to fungal infections, because there are many parallels with nonfungal infections. In several respects they provide interesting features. In many cases exposure is widespread with only a few individuals contracting clinical disease. In some instances the fungi are opportunistic infections on backgrounds as diverse as the single gene disorders, such as cystic fibrosis, to acquired immunodeficiency. Immune responses may involve macrophages (*Pneumocystis carinii* – Ezekowitz et al. 1991), *Candida albicans* – Ashman and Papadimitriou 1995), allergic immediate hypersensitivity (aspergillosis – Chauhan et al. 2000), and granuloma formation (blastomycosis, coccidioidomycosis, and histoplasmosis), granulomas themselves being a potential source of pathology. These often chronic infections are likely to be influenced by MHC genes and other genes associated with macrophage function and allergic responses (Taylor et al. 1997; Chauhan et al. 2000).

PROTOZOAL INFECTIONS

Leishmaniasis

There are a number of species of Old and New World *Leishmania*, which are transmitted by sandflies and cause visceral leishmaniasis (VL) or cutaneous leishmaniasis (CL). All are obligate intracellular macrophage pathogens. There is also intraspecific pathogen diversity, although, in a single study, *L. aethiopica* variation was not associated with clinical phenotype in humans (Schonian et al. 2000). However, the *L. infantum* zymodeme MON-1 has been associated with both VL and CL, whereas MON-24 is a common agent of CL (Belhadj et al. 2003). As for mycobacterial disease, infection can be subclinical. In some individuals with the visceral parasite *L. donovani*, post kala-azar dermal leishmaniasis (PKDL) may occur after cure of the initial disease. Similarly, in a proportion of individuals, localized cutaneous lesions are followed by severe and disfiguring mucocutaneous lesions (MCL), sometimes many years after the initial lesion. MCL is economically the most important form of CL, requiring prolonged and expensive antimonial therapy. Particular zymodemes of *L. braziliensis* may have long evolution times and high frequency of involvement in mucosal disease (Saravia et al. 1998). Other species can cause diffuse CL in rare instances. In most instances, cure is dependent on macrophage activation by IFN-γ and production of IL-4, IL-5, and IL-10 is detrimental, although roles vary according to infecting species. The proinflammatory cytokines have protective roles, with NO as a mediator of parasite killing. MCL is characterized by a hyperreactive cellular immune responses with high production of both IFN-γ and IL-4/IL-5. Rare diffuse CL patients have poor cellular immunity and produce ineffectual antibodies in a situation analogous to lepromatous leprosy. The use of *Leishmania* spp. in murine models of immune responsiveness has provided a plethora of candidate genes for study, although there is no good mouse model for MCL. However, the paucity of studies in humans is noticeable.

It is clear from murine studies that different genes may control susceptibility to different *Leishmania* spp. In some murine strains, susceptibility to the visceral parasite *L. donovani* is under single gene control, with susceptibility being recessive, caused by *Nramp1* (see earlier). *Nramp1* also affects visceralization and metastasis of the cutaneous parasite *L. mexicana* (Roberts et al. 1989), but is not involved in *L. major* infection. Findings for cutaneous parasites have been more diverse. A gene controlling chronic *L. major* lesion expansion has been mapped to a region homologous with the human 5q cluster (Roberts et al. 1993; Guler et al. 1996). As well as many candidate cytokine genes, this region is also rich in receptor genes such as that coding for the glucocorticoid receptor, which has been shown to play a role in response to *M. bovis* BCG infection in congenic mouse strains (Brown et al. 1993). Another gene, *Scl-1*, which controls healing of *L. major* lesions, has been mapped to a region of conserved synteny with human chromosome 17 (Mock et al. 1993; Roberts et al. 1993), encoding members of the cc intercrine family as inflammatory agents produced by macrophages and *NOS2A* encoding inducible NO synthase (iNOS). *Scl-2* controlling a sex-related no-lesion growth phenotype for *L. mexicana* is provisionally mapped to a region encoding IFN-α and IFN-β and Janus kinases (Roberts et al. 1990). In 1997, two murine genome scans for susceptibility to *L. major* found H-2 (chromosome 17) and a new region on mouse chromosome 9 (Roberts et al. 1997), and six regions on chromosomes 6, 7, 10, 11, 15, and 16, to be involved in susceptibility (Beebe et al. 1997). Analysis indicates some epistatic interactions between these murine loci (Roberts et al. 1999). Further studies using immunological phenotypes have identified more loci (Lipoldova et al. 2000). Many of these murine loci are unconfirmed and nomenclature is becoming a problem.

Observations on human populations have shown that the proportion of subclinical infections, the proportion of localized CL cases progressing to MCL, and the severity of MCL, vary markedly between racial groups and families (Walton and Valverde 1979). This is likely to reflect genetic variation between populations of both host and parasite. Segregation analysis and initial examination of candidate immune response genes support the role of host genetics in control of human CL. Segregation analysis of more than 2000 individuals, from a total cross-sectional survey of LCL caused by *L. peruviana* in six Andean valleys, supported a two-locus model with a major gene plus a 'modifier' locus (Shaw et al. 1995). A later study of LCL caused by *L. braziliensis* in Bolivia concluded that, in some families, a recessive major gene controlled susceptibility to the primary cutaneous lesion, but did not consider MCL (Alcais et al. 1997). High levels of serum TNF-α are found in MCL patients, and in a small Venezuelan case–control study, a high risk of mucocutaneous disease was observed in individuals carrying $TNF_{-308}*2$ or *LTA*2*, particularly for females (Cabrera et al. 1995). The only other studies of American CL were three studies, which found variable associations with HLA (Barbier et al. 1987; Lara et al. 1991; Petzl-Erler et al. 1991). These associations may not be primary risk factors for disease but reflect strong linkage disequilibrium.

There have been very few studies of human genetics in VL. Segregation analysis has provided support for genetic control of susceptibility, although differentiation between genetic models was poor (Peacock et al. 2001). Confounding factors, such as nutritional status, are difficult to account for in genetic studies. HLA associations with VL are weak or negative (Blackwell 1998; Meddeb-Garnaoui et al. 2001; Peacock et al. 2002). Most notably, Faghiri et al. (1995) reported a 13-fold increase in risk for VL in Iranian *HLA-A26* carriers. There is an effect of variation in *TNF* in some populations (Meddeb-Garnaoui et al. 2001; Karplus et al. 2002), with haplotypes containing $TNF_{-308}*2\ 2$ associated with symptomatic VL by transmission disequilibrium testing in a Brazilian population. Despite absence of a role for *NRAMP1* in a Brazilian population (Blackwell 1998), in a Sudanese population *NRAMP1* influences susceptibility to VL/PKDL (Blackwell et al. 2003).

Toxoplasmosis

The prevalence of *Toxoplasma gondii* infection is high compared with many other pathogens, with seroprevalence varying from 20 percent to over 80 percent. The pathogenesis of disease varies: acute infection causes transient flu-like symptoms, whereas reactivation can lead to serious eye disease in immunocompetent individuals and fatal toxoplasmic encephalitis (TE) in immunosuppressed individuals. Up to 50 percent of AIDS patients who are seropositive for *Toxoplasma* spp. eventually develop TE. Progressive ocular toxoplasmosis, leading to blindness, has a sporadic distribution in most populations; however, clusters of cases occur in South America. *T. gondii* is also a major cause of congenital disease, and twin studies of human congenital infections suggest a genetic component for transplacental transmission (McLeod et al. 1995). There is relatively little variation in *T. gondii*, with a clear distinction between a subset of strains (type 1), which are regarded as acute virulent, and remaining isolates (type 2 and 3) (Howe and Sibley 1995). The majority of clinical disease in humans is caused by type 2 isolates. Limited information is available on human genetic susceptibility to phenotypes caused by *T. gondii*; however, macrophage-mediated mechanisms are of key importance in disease limitation and prevention of reactivation. There are studies of murine toxoplasmosis of phenotypes including cyst numbers in the brain and resistance to, and survival of, encephalitis. Effects of MHC class I and II genes are well established (Brown et al. 1995; Johnson et al. 2002). Other genes implicated will have substantial overlap with loci implicated in control of murine leishmaniasis, with different genes operating in acute versus chronic disease.

Trypanosomiasis

There is very little known about genetic susceptibility to African or American trypanosomes in humans. African trypanosomiasis, caused by *Trypanosoma brucei* subspecies, causes fatal sleeping sickness in humans, and is also an important cause of disease in domestic livestock such as cattle. Resistant cattle breeds are known and genome scans are being performed. Control of susceptibility to *T. congolense* in mice was largely accounted for by genes on chromosomes 1, 5, and 17 (Kemp et al. 1997). Although *H-2* on chromosome 17 is implicated, responses to challenge with trypanosomes other than *T. congolense* suggest that the MHC is not involved in murine resistance. American trypanosomiasis (Chagas' disease) is caused by *T. cruzi*, with cardiomyopathy seen in approximately 30 percent of patients. *T. cruzi* seropositivity showed a heritability of 56 percent, with an additional 23 percent of variation caused by shared household environment, in a Brazilian population (Williams-Blangero et al. 1997a). Whereas an *HLA-DRB1*14-DQB1*0301* haplotype was correlated with protection against *T. cruzi* infection in an endemic area of Peru, no HLA associations were detected for disease severity (Nieto et al. 2000). Similarly, *HLA-A30* conferred susceptibility to Chagas' disease, irrespective of the clinical presentation in Brazilian patients (Deghaide et al. 1998). As for *Leishmania* and *Toxoplasma* spp., *NRAMP1* is a good candidate gene for resistance to *T. cruzi*; however, variation in *NRAMP1* has not been shown to influence *T. cruzi* infection or cardiomyopathy to date (Calzada et al. 2001).

Malaria

There has been a large amount of work on genetic susceptibility to malaria. Aside from the long history of research on the Duffy blood group, which determines resistance to *Plasmodium vivax*, the majority of studies concern *P. falciparum* infection. Genetic factors clearly play a role in infection, development of clinical disease, and prognosis. The single gene variation associated with the red cell hemoglobinopathies is not covered in this text, nor the red cell enzyme glucose-6-phosphate dehydrogenase, or the roles of the glycophorins or band 3. This work stimulated major interest in malaria as a selective force. Malaria remains the only human infectious disease with strong evidence for selective effects, most commonly by selection of otherwise deleterious alleles through heterozygote advantage. Perhaps because of the long history of research into genetic susceptibility and malaria, there have been few formal segregation analyses. Three west African ethnic groups living under similar conditions showed differences in a number of malarial parameters including antibody response, suggestive of genetic involvement (Modiano et al. 1996). A twin study in The Gambia suggested that risk of disease rather than infection was under genetic control (Jepson et al. 1995). Three segregation analyses are all consistent with genetic control of *P. falciparum* parasitemia in west African populations (Abel et al. 1992a; Garcia et al. 1998a; Rihet et al. 1998a) and of incidence and clinical infection in a Sri Lankan mixed *P. falciparum* and *P. vivax* area (Mackinnon et al. 2000). There are also familial correlations for some *P. falciparum*-specific cellular and antibody responses (Stirnadel et al. 1999b; Aucan et al. 2001).

It has been known for a number of years that resistance to *P. chabaudi* in mice, primarily looking at levels of parasitemia and survival, is controlled by multiple genes (Malo and Skamene 1994). More recently genome-wide approaches have identified several quantitative trait loci, named '*Char*' for chabaudi resistance (reviewed in Fortin et al. 2002). *Char1* on mouse chromosome 9 and *Char2* on chromosome 8 (Foote et al. 1997) were described at the same time as the same chromosome 8 locus and a chromosome 5 locus by a second group (Fortin et al. 1997). A third H-2-linked locus on chromosome 17 controlled parasite clearance in females (*Char3* – Burt et al. 1999). Use of recombinant congenic strains, created from strains with susceptibility alleles at *Char1* and *Char2*, identified a fourth locus on chromosome 4 (*Char4* – Fortin et al. 2001a). The genes involved have not yet been identified.

Recent human studies have concentrated on candidate genes involved in immune responsiveness and particularly severe pathology. Surprisingly, there have been few linkage studies and no genome scans.

HLA-B5301, common in sub-Saharan African populations, has been associated with resistance to severe malaria (cerebral malaria and severe malarial anemia) in Gambians (Hill et al. 1991). This observation was followed by elution of peptides from B53 and screening of candidate *P. falciparum* epitopes. HLA-B53-restricted CTLs recognized a conserved nonamer from liver stage-specific antigen 1 (LSA-1) (Hill et al. 1992). Such observations have clear implications for vaccine design and, subsequent to identification of restricted epitopes in LSA-1 for $CD8^+$ cytotoxic T cells, IFN-γ production by CTLs in response to LSA-1 peptide was correlated with protection in a Papua New Guinea (PNG) population (Bucci et al. 2000). Furthermore, the *HLA-DRB1*1302-HLA-DQB1*0501* haplotype was associated with resistance to severe malarial anemia (Hill et al. 1991). This haplotype was more common than the anticipated haplotypic association of *HLA-DRB1*1302* with *HLA-DQB1*0604* seen in Caucasian populations. In Kenyans, however, different associations were seen, with a protective effect for *HLA-DRB1*0101*, but not *HLA-B5301* or *HLA-DRB1*1302*, suggesting significant heterogeneity (Hill 1998, 1999). In a study of variants of circumsporozoite protein CTL epitopes for *HLA-B*3501*, recognition differed significantly between individuals with and those without *B*3501*, with reciprocal antagonism between variants (Gilbert et al. 1998; Hill 1998). This is one of very few studies attempting to identify directly associations between parasite and host genetics reflecting co-evolution.

However, comparison of three ethnic groups in Burkina Faso suggests that susceptibility to malaria may be correlated with immunogenetic differences other than HLA-B53 or hemoglobin S (HbS) (Modiano et al. 2001). This appears particularly true for T-cell help and antibody phenotypes (Riley 1996). Jepson found linkage of mild malaria to HLA using Gambian dizygotic twins as affected sib-pairs (Jepson et al. 1997b), and also looked at twin effects for immune responses, including those to malarial antigens and PPD. Control appeared to be largely non-MHC for cellular and humoral responses (Jepson et al. 1997a). Observation of concordance of antibodies produced in response to Pf155/RESA in monozygotic and dizygotic twins has provided evidence of genetic control, but not within the HLA class II region (Sjoberg et al. 1992). In a PNG population there were no class I or II associations for immune responsiveness to the antigens RESA and MSA-2 (Stirnadel et al. 1999a), although IgG2 against MSP2 was partly explained by class II haplotype sharing (Stirnadel et al. 2000). A strong negative association was found between antibody responses to the synthetic malaria vaccine SPf66 and *DRB1*15* (Beck et al. 1995).

The observation published in 1994 by McGuire et al. that Gambian children homozygous for $TNF_{-308}*2$ have a seven fold relative risk for death or severe neurological sequelae from cerebral malaria was the first of many studies of this polymorphism. This association was independent of HLA class I and II effects; however, association was with the uncommon homozygous genotype. This was followed some years later by the observation that the less common allele of another *TNF* promoter polymorphism (−238) was associated with severe malarial anemia (McGuire et al. 1999). Strangely this allele was in positive linkage disequilibrium with the protective *HLA-B53*, although in negative linkage disequilibrium with the protective *HLA-DRB1*1302*. Logistic regression analysis indicated another independent genetic effect on susceptibility to cerebral malaria caused by a polymorphism determining the transcription factor OCT-1-binding site at position −376 (Knight et al. 1999). This allele was not in linkage disequilibrium with *HLA-B53* but was in negative linkage disequilibrium with TNF_{-308}*2, and positive linkage disequilibrium with TNF_{-238}*2, in Gambians. A contrasting Kenyan dataset showed similar findings for *TNF–376* and *TNF–308*, but a decreased susceptibility to cerebral malaria associated with TNF_{-238}*2 (Knight et al. 1999). TNF_{-376}*2 occurs only in individuals carrying TNF_{-238}*2, hence this haplotype is associated with susceptibility to cerebral malaria in Gambians, but has no effect in Kenyans. A haplotypic analysis of five *TNF* promoter SNPs in patients with cerebral malaria from Myanmar showed an effect of *TNF*-promoter diversity but not at positions –308 or –238 (Ubalee et al. 2001). Preliminary analyses of *TNF*-promoter polymorphism in other African populations have not always indicated an obvious effect (Stirnadel et al. 1999b), and in other instances only relatively mild effects on reinfection patterns (Meyer et al. 2002) and antibody responsiveness (Migot-Nabais et al. 2000). The unraveling of the complex evolutionary history of the *TNF*-promoter region has undoubtedly some way to go.

Two studies on west Africans have shown some evidence for linkage of blood parasitemia to the chromosome 5q31–q33 cluster (Garcia et al. 1998b; Rihet et al. 1998b). Although this trait remains relatively unexplored, the difficulties of getting good quantitative phenotypic information and the limited number of loci selected for testing to date leave many possibilities for further investigation. Investigation of this region in relation to anti-malarial antibody responsiveness is perhaps more tractable (Luoni et al. 2001).

NO is important in malarial pathology. In Gambians the short allele of the *NOS2A* microsatellite was associated with fatal cerebral malaria (Burgner et al. 1998). In contrast, in a longitudinal Gabonese study, the *NOS2A-954* polymorphism protected against severe malaria in the heterozygous state, and stimulated cells from heterozygous carriers showed sevenfold enhancement of iNOS activity (Kun et al. 2001). Whereas an early study suggested an inverse relationship between disease severity and NO production in Tanzanian children, these polymorphisms were not associated with disease severity, *NOS2A* expression, or NO production (Levesque et al. 1999). However, a recent study identified a new polymorphism at position –1173 (Hobbs et al. 2002). The less common allele was significantly associated with protection from symptomatic malaria in Tanzanian children and severe malarial anemia in Kenyan children. The protective allele was associated with increased fasting urine and plasma NO metabolite concentrations, in support of a protective role for NO.

There are few studies on other genes relating to IFN-γ and NO production. Consistent with a potential role of IFN-γ in susceptibility to malaria (Gourley et al. 2002), a study of *IFNGR1*-promoter polymorphisms in Gambian children showed preliminary evidence of associations with cerebral malaria in Mandinkas (Koch et al. 2002). In addition, homozygotes for an *IL12B*-promoter polymorphism showed decreased production of iNOS as reflected in urinary NO, and homozygosity was associated with fatal cerebral malaria in Tanzanian, but not severe malaria in Kenyan, children (Morohan et al. 2002).

The Duffy blood group gene (*FY*) was one of the first loci mapped on human chromosome 1, and was one of the first identified blood group systems (reviewed in Hadley and Peiper 1997). Red cells of most white Europeans are recognized by one or both anti-Fya and anti-Fyb, according to the presence of *FY*A* and *FY*B* allelic specificities. However, the null phenotype Fy(a^-b^-) is common in Africa, particularly west Africa where it is close to fixation. Fy(a^-b^-) red cells fail to be recognized by the rare anti-Fy3 which recognizes a specificity common to both Fy(a^+b^-) and Fy(a^-b^+) individuals. Fy(a^-b^-) red cells are totally refractory to invasion by *P. vivax*, making Duffy the most common immunogenetic variation resulting in an absolute effect on infectious disease susceptibility. However, the molecular basis of the Duffy system was not unraveled until the 1990s. *FY* codes for the Duffy antigen receptor for chemokines (DARC), present on the red cell surface and elsewhere, which binds to molecules such as IL-8 and RANTES. A Duffy binding ligand has been identified in the parasite. The Fy(a^-b^-) phenotype in west Africans arises from a T-to-C substitution at position –46 of an *FY*B* allele (Tournamille et al. 1995). This mutation disrupts the binding of the GATA1 erythroid transcription factor and reduces expression. More recently this same mutation has been discovered on a *FY*A* background in a PNG population, showing it to have arisen independently in at least two places, and more recently in PNG (Zimmerman et al. 1999).

ICAM-1 is thought to be involved in sequestration of parasitized red cells to the vascular endothelium. A series of observations suggests some role for ICAM-1 in malaria pathology, although, at the time of writing, the story is both complex and incomplete. A base change at position 179 results in a lysine-for-methionine substitution at amino acid 29 ($ICAM1_{Kilifi}$) (Fernandez-Reyes et al. 1997). Homozygotes had a relative risk of 2 for cerebral malaria versus nonsevere malaria in a Kenyan study, although this effect was not seen in a Gambian population (Hill 1999). The mutant allele is at a frequency of about 0.3 in Africa, which would be surprisingly high for an allele predisposing to cerebral malaria. However, comparing severe and mild malaria in a Gabonese population, $ICAM1_{Kilifi}$ appeared to be associated with protection against severe malaria (Kun et al. 1999). Functional studies have shown that $ICAM\text{-}1_{Kilifi}$ causes loss of fibrinogen binding and reduction of LFA-1 binding, suggesting a complex scenario with respect to effects of selection (Craig et al. 2000).

Another molecule thought to be involved in sequestration of parasitized red cells is CD36. *CD36* is highly polymorphic, with a number of diverse mutations resulting in CD36 deficiency. Such mutations are relatively common in Africa. However, different mutations are present in Asian populations, and as, unexpectedly, African mutations were initially shown to be associated with susceptibility to severe malaria, it was suggested that selection pressures other than malaria were operating (Aitman et al. 2000). However, a later study of a single polymorphism in African children showed the rare allele to be associated with protection from severe malaria (Pain et al. 2001). A detailed investigation, considering common haplotypes and patterns of linkage disequilibrium, of multiple *CD36* polymorphisms in Thais concluded some protection from cerebral malaria, for mutations coding for lack of production of CD36 (Omi et al. 2003). The above investigations on *ICAM1* and *CD36*, with conflicting results, have stimulated some discussion on the importance of these molecules for malarial infection, the complexity of selection pressures operating on different populations, and whether significance levels from multiple statistical comparisons are valid (Craig et al. 2001). Although it seems likely that diversity in these two genes will prove relevant, the detail is likely to prove as complex as the story developing for the *TNF*-promoter region.

Many other genes have been investigated. Some are adhesion molecules such as *CD31* (Casals-Pascual et al. 2001; Kikuchi et al. 2001); others are receptors such as Ig receptors (Shi et al. 2001; Omi et al. 2002). However, there is no large body of work on such genes and findings are variable in different populations. There is scope for invoking malaria as a selective force in multiple populations, but it is unfortunate that other major diseases have received less consideration from evolutionary biologists.

HELMINTH INFECTION

Immune responses in helminth infection are characterized by high levels of total and specific IgE and eosinophilia, upregulated by Th2 cytokines such as IL-4, IL-5, IL-9, and IL-13. Th2 responses are protective in murine models, and there is accumulating evidence for Th2-mediated protection in human infection. Similar Th2 upregulation is seen in asthma and atopy, which are under strong genetic control. Obvious candidate genes for susceptibility to helminth infection and disease are thus those thought to be involved in the control of Th2 responses in asthma, such as the Th2 cytokine cluster on 5q, *FCER1B*, and *IL4RA*. There is evidence of genetic control of helminth infection from mouse model infections, the most commonly used being *Heligmosomoides polygyrus* and *Trichuris muris* (Wakelin and Blackwell 1988). The first genome scan for a murine parasitic nematode has just been completed for *Angiostrongylus costaricensis* (Ohno et al. 2002), with another for *H. polygyrus* in progress (Behnke et al. 2000). There is also increasing interest in sheep genes controlling gastrointestinal nematode infection.

Gastrointestinal and filarial nematodes

There is evidence for genetic control of worm burden in human populations, with heritabilities of 23–44 percent for *Ascaris lumbricoides*, *Necator americanus*, and *Trichuris trichuria* loads reported (Williams-Blangero et al. 1997b, 1999, 2002a). In contrast, studies of *A. lumbricoides* together with *T. trichuria* in Malaysians and *Strongyloides fuelleborni kellyi* in PNG did not support genetic control of worm burdens (Chan et al. 1994; Smith et al. 1991). Partitioning variance for helminth infections can be problematic, particularly partitioning genetic and household effects, and some differences may be accounted for by study design. Consideration of eosinophil rates among Brazilians infected with intestinal worms with an extra-digestive cycle, supported genetic susceptibility to helminths through influence on eosinophils (Conti et al. 1999). This finding fits well with current views on genetic control of eosinophilic inflammation (Brodie et al. 1999), and with the chromosome 5q cluster implicated in control of asthma/atopy and known to determine autosomal dominant familial eosinophilia (Rioux et al. 1998). There is less information on filarial nematode infection. A study of *Loa loa* in The Cameroons was consistent with some genetic control of microfilaremia, and a dominant major gene model was suggested (Garcia et al. 1999). Similarly genetic effects were compatible with distribution of *Brugia malayi* microfilariae, and possibly anti-filarial IgG4, in an Indonesian population (Terhell et al. 2000). However, maternal infection with *Wuchereria bancrofti* is known to be a risk factor for infection in children (Lammie et al. 1991), perhaps through early induction of immunological tolerance, which highlights potential confounding factors to genetic control. *Onchocerca volvulus*, one of the better-studied parasites for candidate genes, has not been the subject of a heritability study.

There are few small case–control studies suggesting a role for HLA in susceptibility and responsiveness to gastrointestinal nematodes (Holland et al. 1992; Satoh et al. 1999). In Venezuelan children associations were found between homozygosity for Arg16 at *ADRB2* and *A. lumbricoides* specific phenotypes, although other candidate genes on 5q33 were not investigated (Ramsay et al. 1999). This was followed by the only human genome scan for a nematode infection. Williams-Blangero et al. (2002b) genotyped 444 Nepalese, with ascaris worm burdens assessed by egg count. Quantitative trait nonparametric linkage was carried out by variance components methods and significant linkage was found to regions on chromosomes 1 and 13. The chromosome 13 region contains a candidate gene *TNFSF13B* (*BlyS*), and was also found to influence serum IgE levels. There are no obvious effects of HLA on lymphatic filariasis, either Indonesian brugian filariasis by association (Yazdanbakhsh et al. 1995, 1997) or Polynesian bancroftian filariasis by linkage (Ottesen et al. 1981). In contrast, a small study in India suggested associations with *CHIT1* (coding for a phagocyte-specific chitotriosidase) and *MBL2* (Choi et al. 2001). It is notable that the choice of candidate genes in this study varied from those typically used for other infectious diseases. For *O. volvulus HLA-DQA1*0501-DQB1*0301* occurred at an increased frequency in putatively immune versus diseased individuals (Meyer et al. 1994). *HLA-DQA1*0101-DQB1*0501*, and independently *HLA-DQB1*0201*, occurred at increased frequency in individuals with generalized disease compared with localized disease and putatively immune individuals (Meyer and Kremsner 1996). In general, findings for localized disease lay between those for putatively immune and generalized disease. A follow-up study also implicated *HLA-DPA1*, with *HLA-DPA1*02011/2* having increased frequency among the putatively immune and *HLA-DPA1*0301* being associated with localized disease (Meyer et al. 1996). A methionine at position 11 of DPα1 conferred a relative risk of disease of 3.3. A later study comparing patients who had cutaneous depigmentation with patients with high microfilarial loads broadly implicated the same haplotypes (Murdoch et al. 1997). A comparison of generalized onchocercal disease versus patients with low microfilarial numbers and strong IgE responsiveness suggested some association with the Gln110Arg *IL13* polymorphism, which has also been associated with several asthma/atopy phenotypes (Hoerauf et al. 2002).

Schistosomiasis

In 1991, Abel et al. reported a segregation analysis of Brazilian families with major gene (*SM1*) control of intensity of infection by *Schistosoma mansoni*, although there has been debate over the relative role of genetics and exposure (Woolhouse 1992). The same group also suggested major gene control of IL-5 production in the Brazilian *S. mansoni*-infected population (Rodrigues et al. 1996), although whether this is the same gene as that controlling infection intensity remains unclear. A later proposal of a polygenic model would seem more realistic (Bethony et al. 2002). The first genome scan for a human parasitic disease was carried out on the intensity of *S. mansoni* infection using parametric linkage analysis with the model of inheritance defined by segregation analysis of the same population (Marquet et al. 1996). There was strong evidence for linkage to the chromosome cluster at 5q31–q33, with a multipoint LOD score of 5.45. The nearest locus was *CSF1R*. Finding a single region in a genome scan indicates the limitations of this parametric approach and re-analysis of these data using model-free linkage analysis found suggestive evidence for linkage to two further regions on 1p21–q23 and 6p21–q21 (Zinn-Justin et al. 2001). Confirmation of the importance of 5q31–q33 has come from another linkage study of a Senegalese population (Muller-Myhsok et al. 1997). There is less evidence of genetic control of hepatic morbidity resulting from infection with *S. mansoni* (Kariuki et al. 2001); however, this may partly result from variable definitions of severe disease, and pedigree clustering has been observed (Mohamed-Ali et al. 1999). Segregation analysis indicated a co-dominant major gene (*SM2*) controlling advanced hepatic periportal fibrosis in Sudanese *S. mansoni*-infected patients (Dessein et al. 1999). Examination of four candidate loci found evidence of linkage (multipoint LOD score 3.12) to *IFNGR1* at 6q22–q23 (Dessein et al. 1999).

A number of studies have been carried out on HLA control of infection or disease in schistosomiasis. Many of the studies are small and there is some lack of consistency in allelic associations. Early studies concerned HLA control of proliferative responses to *S. japonicum* antigens (Ohta et al. 1982; Hirayama et al. 1987). These were accompanied by an observed increase in *HLA-B40* in high responders to schistosomal antigens and hepatosplenic patients (Ohta et al. 1987). Recent studies on *S. japonicum* are devoted to HLA class II associations and advanced disease/fibrosis (Hirayama et al. 1998, 1999; Waine et al. 1998; McManus et al. 2001). Despite some inconsistencies, one interesting suggestion, from an examination of class II haplotypic associations, is that *HLA-DR* and *HLA-DQ* loci may influence early liver changes, whereas the *HLA-DP* locus may be more important in the later phase (Hirayama et al. 1999). HLA class I associations for hepatosplenic disease, caused by *S. mansoni*, in Egyptian populations vary (Abdel-Salam et al. 1986; Hafez et al. 1991). *HLA-DQB1*0201* was positively associated with hepatosplenic disease in Brazilian patients aged over 15 years (Secor et al. 1996), but not in an Egyptian population (Hafez et al. 1991). A study specifically examining the role of *HLA-DP* showed *HLA-DPA1*0301* to be associated with schistosomiasis and a high re-infection rate after treatment (May et al. 1998).

CONCLUSION

At the time of writing, there is good evidence for genetic control of major viral, bacterial, protozoal, and helminth infections. There are indications of some of the regions involved from linkage studies, in particular from genome scans for several major infections. There are many more association studies for candidate genes, a good proportion of which concern the MHC. The scope of studies is often limited, with insufficient sample sizes and limited polymorphisms investigated. Many findings remain to be replicated, which suggests that there may be many false positives or considerable population heterogeneity. It will be interesting to include information on pathogen diversity in future studies. Moreover there is little understanding of the impact of genetic diversity on immune function. In this respect, knowledge of complex haplotypes in relation to disease susceptibility and immune function is an immediate goal.

ACKNOWLEDGMENTS

Thanks to Rupert Quinnell for use of his brain.

REFERENCES

Abdel-Salam, E., Khalik, A.A., et al. 1986. Association of HLA class I antigens (A1, B5, B8 and CW2) with disease manifestations and infection in human schistosomiasis mansoni in Egypt. *Tissue Antigens*, **27**, 142–6.

Abecasis, G.R., Cardon, L.R. and Cookson, W.O.C. 2000. A general test of association for quantitative traits in nuclear families. *Am J Hum Genet*, **66**, 279–92.

Abecasis, G.R., Noguchi, E., et al. 2001. Extent and distribution of linkage disequilibrium in three genomic regions. *Am J Hum Genet*, **68**, 191–7.

Abel, L. and Demenais, F. 1988. Detection of major genes for susceptibility to leprosy and its subtypes in a Caribbean island: Desirade Island. *Am J Hum Genet*, **42**, 256–66.

Abel, L., Demenais, F., et al. 1991. Evidence for the segregation of a major gene in human susceptibility/resistance to infection by *Schistosoma mansoni*. *Am J Hum Genet*, **48**, 959–70.

Abel, L., Cot, M., et al. 1992a. Segregation analysis detects a major gene controlling blood infection levels in human malaria. *Am J Hum Genet*, **50**, 1308–17.

Abel, L., Lap, V.D., et al. 1992b. Complex segregation analysis of leprosy in Southern Vietnam. *Genet Epidemiol*, **12**, 63–82.

Abel, L., Sanchez, F.O., et al. 1998. Susceptibility to leprosy is linked to the human *NRAMP1* gene. *J Infect Dis*, **177**, 133–45.

Agarwal, S., Viola, J.P.B. and Roa, A. 1999. Chromatin-based regulatory mechanisms governing cytokine gene transcription. *J Allergy Clin Immunol*, **103**, 990–9.

Agnese, D.M., Calvano, J.E., et al. 2002. Human toll-like receptor 4 mutations but not CD14 polymorphisms are associated with an increased risk of Gram-negative infections. *J Infect Dis*, **186**, 1522–5.

Agrewala, J.N., Ghei, S.K., et al. 1989. HLA antigens and erythema-nodosum leprosum (ENL). *Tissue Antigens*, **33**, 486–7.

Aickin, M. and Gensler, H. 1996. Adjusting for multiple testing when reporting research results: the Bonferroni vs Holm methods. *Am J Public Health*, **86**, 726–8.

Aitman, T.J., Cooper, L.D., et al. 2000. Malaria susceptibility and *CD36* mutation. *Nature*, **405**, 1015–16.

Aksentijevich, I., Galon, J., et al. 2001. The tumor-necrosis-factor receptor-associated periodic syndrome: new mutations in *TNFRSF1A*, ancestral origins, genotype-phenotype studies, and evidence for further genetic heterogeneity of periodic fevers. *Am J Hum Genet*, **69**, 301–14.

Al Jabri, A.A. 2002. HLA and in vitro susceptibility to HIV infection. *Mol Immunol*, **38**, 959–67.

Alcais, A., Abel, L., et al. 1997. Evidence for a major gene controlling susceptibility to tegumentary leishmaniasis in a recently exposed Bolivian population. *Am J Hum Genet*, **61**, 968–79.

Alcais, A., Sanchez, F.O., et al. 2000. Granulomatous reaction to intradermal injection of lepromin (Mitsuda reaction) is linked to the human *NRAMP1* gene in Vietnamese leprosy sibships. *J Infect Dis*, **181**, 302–8.

Allison, D.B. 1997. Transmission-disequilibrium tests for quantitative traits. *Am J Hum Genet*, **60**, 676–90.

Almarri, A. and Batchelor, J.R. 1994. HLA and hepatitis-B infection. *Lancet*, **344**, 1194–5.

Alric, L., Fort, M., et al. 1997. Genes of the major histocompatibility complex II influence the outcome of hepatitis C virus infection. *Gastroenterology*, **113**, 1675–81.

Altare, F., Durandy, A., et al. 1998a. Impairment of mycobacterial immunity in human interleukin-12 receptor deficiency. *Science*, **280**, 1432–4.

Altare, F., Jouanguy, E., et al. 1998b. A causative relationship between mutant IFNγR1 alleles and impaired cellular response to IFNγ in a compound heterozygous child. *Am J Hum Genet*, **62**, 723–6.

Altet, L., Francino, O., et al. 2002. Mapping and sequencing of the canine *NRAMP1* gene and identification of mutations in leishmaniasis-susceptible dogs. *Infect Immun*, **70**, 2763–71.

Alvarez, V., Coto, E., et al. 1995. Genetic detection of the silent allele (*-Q0) in hereditary deficiencies of the human complement C6, C7 and C9 components. *Am J Med Genet*, **55**, 408–13.

Anderson, G.G. and Cookson, W.O.C.M. 1999. Recent advances in the genetics of allergy and asthma. *Mol Med Today*, **5**, 264–73.

Apanius, V., Penn, D., et al. 1997. The nature of selection on the major histocompatibility complex. *Crit Rev Immunol*, **17**, 179–224.

Arai, N., Nomura, D., et al. 1989. Complete nucleotide sequence of the chromosomal gene for human IL-4 and its expression. *J Immunol*, **142**, 274–82.

Arend, W.P., Malyak, M., et al. 1998. Interleukin-1 receptor antagonist: role in biology. *Annu Rev Immunol*, **16**, 27–55.

Armitage, G.C., Wu, Y.F., et al. 2000. Low prevalence of a periodontitis-associated interleukin-1 composite genotype in individuals of Chinese heritage. *J Periodontol*, **71**, 164–71.

Aron, Y., Polla, B.S., et al. 1999. HLA class II polymorphism in cystic fibrosis - a possible modifier of pulmonary phenotype. *Am J Respir Crit Care Med*, **159**, 1464–8.

Ashman, R.B. and Papadimitriou, J.M. 1995. Production and function of cytokines in natural and acquired immunity to *Candida albicans* infection. *Microbiol Rev*, **59**, 646.

Aucan, C., Traore, Y., et al. 2001. Familial correlation of immunoglobulin G subclass responses to *Plasmodium falciparum* antigens in Burkina Faso. *Infect Immun*, **69**, 996–1001.

Awomoyi, A.A., Marchant, A., et al. 2002. Interleukin-10 polymorphism in *SLC11A1* (formerly *NRAMP1*), and susceptibility to tuberculosis. *J Infect Dis*, **186**, 1808–14.

Azuma, T., Ito, S., et al. 1998. The role of the HLA-DQA1 gene in resistance to atrophic gastritis and gastric adenocarcinoma induced by *Helicobacter pylori* infection. *Cancer*, **82**, 1013–18.

Bailly, S., di Giovine, F.S., et al. 1993. Genetic polymorphism of human interleukin-1α. *Eur J Immunol*, **23**, 1240–5.

Baldini, M., Lohman, I.C., et al. 1999. A polymorphism in the 5′ flanking region of the *CD14* gene is associated with circulating soluble CD14 levels and with total serum immunoglobulin E. *Am J Respir Crit Care Med*, **20**, 976–83.

Bangham, C.R.M., Hall, S.E., et al. 1999. Genetic control and dynamics of the cellular immune response to the human T-cell leukemia virus, HTLV-1. *Phil Trans R Soc Lond B*, **354**, 691–700.

Barbier, D., Demenais, F., et al. 1987. Susceptibility to human cutaneous leishmaniasis and HLA, Gm, Km markers. *Tissue Antigens*, **30**, 63–7.

Barnes, K.C., Neely, J.D., et al. 1996. Linkage of asthma and total serum IgE concentrations to markers on chromosome 12q: evidence from Afro-Caribbean and Caucasian populations. *Genomics*, **37**, 41–50.

Bartels, J., Schluter, C., et al. 1996. Human dermal fibroblasts express eotaxin: molecular cloning, mRNA expression and identification of eotaxin sequence variants. *Biochem Biophys Res Commun*, **225**, 1045–51.

Barton, C.H., Whitehead, S.H. and Blackwell, J.M. 1995. Nramp transfection transfers *Ity/Lsh/Bcg*-related pleiotropic effects on macrophage activation: influence on oxidative burst and nitric oxide pathways. *Mol Med*, **1**, 267–79.

Bazaral, M., Orgel, H.A. and Hamburger, R.N. 1974. Genetics of IgE and allergy: serum IgE levels in twins. *J Allergy Clin Immunol*, **54**, 288–304.

Beck, H.P., Felger, I., et al. 1995. Evidence of HLA class II association with antibody response against the malaria vaccine SPF66 in a naturally exposed population. *Am J Trop Med Hygiene*, **53**, 284–8.

Beck, S. and Trowsdale, J. 2000. The human major histocompatibility complex: lessons from the DNA sequence. *Annu Rev Genomics Hum Genet*, **1**, 117–37.

Beckers, M.C., Ernst, E., et al. 1997. High resolution linkage map of mouse chromosome 13 in the vicinity of the host resistance locus Lgn1. *Genomics*, **39**, 254–63.

Beebe, A.M., Mauze, S., et al. 1997. Serial backcross mapping of multiple loci associated with resistance to *Leishmania major* in mice. *Immunology*, **6**, 551–7.

Behnke, J.M., Lowe, A., et al. 2000. Mapping genes for resistance to gastrointestinal nematodes. *Acta Parasitol*, **45**, 1–13.

Belhadj, S., Pratlong, F., et al. 2003. Human cutaneous leishmaniasis due to *Leishmania infantum* in the Sidi Bourouis focus (Northern Tunisia): epidemiological study and isoenzymatic characterization of the parasites. *Acta Trop*, **85**, 83–6.

Bellamy, R.J. and Hill, A.V.S. 1998. Genetics and tuberculosis. *Novartis Foundation Symposium*, **217**, 3–23.

Bellamy, R., Ruwende, C., et al. 1998a. Assessment of the interleukin 1 gene cluster and other candidate gene polymorphisms in host susceptibility to tuberculosis. *Tubercle Lung Disease*, **79**, 83–9.

Bellamy, R., Ruwende, C., et al. 1998b. Mannose binding protein deficiency is not associated with malaria, hepatitis B carriage nor tuberculosis in Africans. *Q J Med*, **91**, 13–18.

Bellamy, R., Ruwende, C., et al. 1998c. Variations in the *NRAMP1* gene and susceptibility to tuberculosis in West Africans. *N Engl J Med*, **338**, 640–4.

Bellamy, R., Ruwende, C., et al. 1999. Tuberculosis and chronic hepatitis B virus infection in Africans and variation in the vitamin D receptor gene. *J Infect Dis*, **179**, 721–4.

Bellamy, R., Beyers, N., et al. 2000. Genetic susceptibility to tuberculosis in Africans: a genome-wide scan. *Proc Natl Acad Sci USA*, **97**, 8005–9.

Bergholdt, R., Larsen, Z.M., et al. 2000. Characterization of new polymorphisms in the 5′UTR of the human interleukin-1 receptor type 1 (*IL1R1*) gene: linkage to type 1 diabetes and correlation to IL-1R1 plasma level. *Genes Immun*, **1**, 495–500.

Bethony, J., Williams, J.T., et al. 2002. Additive host genetic factors influence fecal egg excretion rates during *Schistosoma mansoni* infection in a rural area in Brazil. *Am J Trop Med Hygiene*, **67**, 336–43.

Bidwell, J., Keen, L., et al. 1999a. Cytokine polymorphism in human disease: on-line database. *Genes Immun*, **1**, 3–19.

Bidwell, J.L., Wood, N.A.P., et al. 1999b. Human cytokine gene nucleotide sequence alignments: supplement 1. *Eur J Immunogenet*, **26**, 135–223.

Blackwell, J.M. 1998. Genetics of host resistance and susceptibility to intramacrophage pathogens: a study of multicase families of tuberculosis, leprosy and leishmaniasis in north-eastern Brazil. *Int J Parasitol*, **28**, 21–8.

Blackwell, J.M. and Searle, S. 1999. Genetic regulation of macrophage activation: understanding the function of *Nramp1* (*=Ity/Lsh/Bcg*). *Immunol Lett*, **65**, 73–80.

Blackwell, J.M., Barton, C.H., et al. 1995. Genomic organization and sequence of the human *NRAMP* gene: identification and mapping of a promoter region polymorphism. *Mol Med*, **1**, 194–205.

Blackwell, J.M., Black, G.F., et al. 1999. Role of *Nramp1*, HLA, and a gene(s) in allelic association with IL-4, in determining T helper subset differentiation. *Microbes Infect*, **1**, 95–102.

Blackwell, J.M., Searle, S., et al. 2003. Divalent cation transport and susceptibility to infectious and autoimmune disease: continuation of the *Ity/Lsh/Bcg/Nramp1/Slc11a1* gene story. *Immunol Lett*, **85**, 197–203.

Bland, J.M. and Altman, D.G. 1995. Multiple significance tests: the Bonferroni method. *Br Med J*, **310**, 170.

Blanpain, C., Lee, B., et al. 2000. Multiple nonfunctional alleles of *CCR5* are frequent in various human populations. *Blood*, **96**, 1638–45.

Blumenthal, M.N., Namboodiri, K., et al. 1981. Genetic transmission of serum IgE levels. *Am J Med Genet*, **10**, 219–28.

Boldt, A.B.W. and Petzl-Erler, M.L. 2002. A new strategy for mannose-binding lectin gene haplotyping. *Hum Mutat*, **19**, 296–306.

Bothamley, G.H., Swanson Beck, J., et al. 1989. Association of tuberculosis and *M. tuberculosis*-specific antibody levels with HLA. *J Infect Dis*, **159**, 549–55.

Bredius, R.G.M., Derkx, B.H.F., et al. 1994. Fc-gamma receptor IIA (CD32) polymorphisms in fulminant meningococcal septic shock in children. *J Infect Dis*, **170**, 848–53.

Brinkman, B.M.N., Zuijdgeest, D., et al. 1996. Relevance of the tumor necrosis factor alpha (TNFα)-308 promoter polymorphisms in TNFα gene regulation. *J Inflammation*, **46**, 32–41.

Brodie, D.H., Hoffman, H. and Sriramarao, P. 1999. Genes that regulate eosinophilic inflammation. *Am J Hum Genet*, **65**, 302–7.

Brown, C.R., Hunter, C.A., et al. 1995. Definitive identification of a gene that confers resistance against *Toxoplasma* cyst burden and encephalitis. *Immunology*, **85**, 419–28.

Brown, D.H., Sheridan, J., et al. 1993. Regulation of mycobacterial growth by the hypothalamus-pituitary-adrenal axis: differential responses of *Mycobacterium bovis Bcg* resistant and *Bcg* susceptible mice. *Infect Immun*, **61**, 4793–800.

Brownstein, D.G. 1998. Comparative genetics of resistance to viruses. *Am J Hum Genet*, **62**, 211–14.

Bucci, K., Kastens, W., et al. 2000. Influence of age and HLA heterozygosity on IFN-γ responses to a naturally occurring polymorphic epitope of *Plasmodium falciparum* Liver Stage Antigen-1 (LSA-1). *Clin Exp Immunol*, **122**, 94–100.

Burgner, D., Xu, W.M., et al. 1998. Inducible nitric oxide synthase polymorphism and fatal cerebral malaria. *Lancet*, **352**, 1193–4.

Burt, R.A., Baldwin, T.M., et al. 1999. Temporal expression of an H2-linked locus in host response to mouse malaria. *Immunogenetics*, **50**, 278–85.

Cabrera, M., Shaw, M.-A., et al. 1995. Polymorphism in tumor necrosis factor genes associated with mucocutaneous leishmaniasis. *J Exp Med*, **182**, 1259–64.

Cacalano, N.A. and Johnston, J.A. 1999. Interleukin-2 signaling and inherited immunodeficiency. *Am J Hum Genet*, **65**, 287–93.

Callard, R.E., Matthews, D.J. and Hibbert, L. 1996. IL-4 and IL-13 receptors: are they one and the same? *Immunol Today*, **17**, 108–10.

Calzada, J.E., Nieto, A., et al. 2001. Lack of association between *NRAMP1* gene polymorphisms and *Trypanosoma cruzi* infection. *Tissue Antigens*, **57**, 353–7.

Campbell, R.D., Law, S.K.A., et al. 1988. Structure, organization, and regulation of the complement genes. *Annu Rev Immunol*, **6**, 161–95.

Candore, G., Romano, G.C., et al. 1998. Biological basis of the HLA-B8, DR3-associated progression of acquired immunodeficiency syndrome. *Pathobiology*, **66**, 33–7.

Caron, J., Loredo-Osti, J.C., et al. 2002. Identification of genetic loci controlling bacterial clearance in experimental *Salmonellas enteritidis* infection: an unexpected role of *Nramp1* (*Slc11a1*) in the persistence of infection in mice. *Genes Immun*, **3**, 196–204.

Carrington, M., Nelson, G.W., et al. 1999. HLA and HIV-1: heterozygote advantage and *B*35-Cw*04* disadvantage. *Science*, **283**, 1748–52.

Carrington, M., Nelson, G. and O'Brien, S.J. 2001. Considering genetic profiles in functional studies of immune responsiveness to HIV-1. *Immunol Lett*, **79**, 131–40.

Carrol, E.D., Mobbs, K.J., et al. 2002. Variable number tandem repeat polymorphism of the interleukin-1 receptor antagonist gene in meningococcal disease. *Clin Infect Dis*, **35**, 495–7.

Casals-Pascual, C., Allen, S., et al. 2001. Short report: codon 125 polymorphism of *CD31* and susceptibility to malaria. *Am J Trop Med Hygiene*, **65**, 736–7.

Cellier, M., Govoni, G., et al. 1994. Human natural resistance-associated macrophage protein: cDNA cloning, chromosomal mapping, genomic organization, and tissue specific expression. *J Exp Med*, **180**, 1741–52.

Cellier, M., Prive, G., et al. 1995. Nramp defines a family of membrane proteins. *Proc Natl Acad Sci USA*, **92**, 10089–93.

Cervino, A.C.L., Lakiss, S., et al. 2000. Allelic association between the *NRAMP1* gene and susceptibility to tuberculosis in Guinea-Conakry. *Ann Hum Genet*, **64**, 507–12.

Cervino, A.C.L., Lakiss, S., et al. 2002. Fine mapping of a putative tuberculosis-susceptibility locus on chromosome 15q11-13 in African families. *Hum Mol Genet*, **11**, 1599–603.

Chan, L., Bundy, D.A.P. and Kan, S.P. 1994. Genetic relatedness as a determinant of predisposition to *Ascaris lumbricoides* and *Trichuris trichuria* infection. *Parasitology*, **108**, 77–80.

Chauhan, B., Santiago, L., et al. 2000. Evidence for the involvement of two different MHC class II regions in susceptibility or protection in allergic bronchopulmonary aspergillosis. *J Allergy Clin Immunol*, **106**, 723–9.

Choi, E.H., Zimmerman, P.A., et al. 2001. Genetic polymorphisms in molecules of innate immunity and susceptibility to infection with *Wuchereria bancrofti* in South India. *Genes Immun*, **2**, 248–53.

Choi, E.H., Lee, H.J., et al. 2002. A common haplotype of interleukin-4 gene *IL4* is associated with severe respiratory syncytial virus disease in Korean children. *J Infect Dis*, **186**, 1207–11.

Collins, A., Lonjou, C. and Morton, N.E. 1999. Genetic epidemiology of single-nucleotide polymorphisms. *Proc Natl Acad Sci USA*, **96**, 15173–7.

Collins, A., Ennis, S., et al. 2000. Mapping oligogenes for atopy and asthma by meta-analysis. *Genet Mol Biol*, **23**, 1–10.

Colten, H.R. 1992. Complement deficiencies. *Annu Rev Immunol*, **10**, 809–34.

Comstock, G.W. 1978. Tuberculosis in twins: a re-analysis of the Prophit study. *Am Rev Respir Dis*, **117**, 621–4.

Conti, F., Dal, G.M.D., et al. 1999. Evidence for biological inheritance of the eosinophil response to internal parasites in southeastern Brazil. *Genet Mol Biol*, **22**, 481–5.

Conway, D.J., Holland, M.J., et al. 1997. Scarring trachoma is associated with polymorphism in the tumor necrosis factor alpha (TNF-α) gene promoter and with elevated TNF-α levels in tear fluid. *Infect Immun*, **65**, 1003–6.

Cookson, S., Constantini, P.K., et al. 1999. Frequency and nature of cytokine gene polymorphisms in type 1 autoimmune hepatitis. *Hepatology*, **30**, 851–6.

Cookson, W.O.C.M., Young, R.P., et al. 1992. Maternal inheritance of atopic IgE responsiveness on chromosome 11q. *Lancet*, **340**, 381–4.

Cox, A., Camp, N.J., et al. 1998. An analysis of linkage disequilibrium in the interleukin-1 gene cluster, using a novel grouping method for multiallelic markers. *Am J Hum Genet*, **62**, 1180–8.

Cox, R.A., Downs, M., et al. 1988. Immunogenetic analysis of human tuberculosis. *J Infect Dis*, **158**, 1302–8.

Craandijk, J., van Krugten, M.V., et al. 2002. Tumor necrosis factor-alpha gene polymorphisms in relation to periodontitis. *J Clin Periodontol*, **29**, 28–34.

Craig, A., Fernandez-Reyes, D., et al. 2000. A functional analysis of a natural variant of intracellular adhesion molecule-1 (ICAM-1^{KILIFI}). *Hum Mol Genet*, **9**, 525–30.

Craig, A., Hastings, I., et al. 2001. Genetics and malaria – more questions than answers. *Trends Parasitol*, **17**, 55–6.

Cullinan, M.P., Westerman, B., et al. 2001. A longitudinal study of interleukin-1 gene polymorphisms and periodontal disease in a general adult population. *J Clin Periodontol*, **28**, 1137–44.

Curtis, D. 1997. Use of siblings as controls in case-control association studies. *Ann Hum Genet*, **61**, 319–33.

Dale, M. and Nicklin, M.J.H. 1999. Interleukin-1 receptor cluster: gene organization of IL1R2, IL1R1, IL1RL2 (IL-1Rrp2), IL1RL1 (T1/ST2) and IL18R1 (IL-1Rrp) on human chromosome 2q. *Genomics*, **57**, 177–9.

Daly, M.J., Rioux, J.D., et al. 2001. High-resolution haplotype structure in the human genome. *Nat Genet*, **29**, 229–32.

Danis, V.A., Millington, M., et al. 1995. Cytokine production by normal human monocytes: inter-subject variation and relationship to an IL-1 receptor antagonist (IL-1Ra) gene polymorphism. *Clin Exp Immunol*, **99**, 303–10.

de Groot, N.G., Otting, N., et al. 2002. Evidence for an ancient selective sweep in the MHC class I gene repertoire of chimpanzees. *Proc Natl Acad Sci USA*, **99**, 11748–53.

de Jong, R., Altare, F., et al. 1998. Severe mycobacterial and Salmonella infections in interleukin-12 receptor deficient patients. *Science*, **280**, 1435–8.

de Vries, R.R.P., Nijenhuis, L.E., et al. 1976. HLA-linked genetic control of host response to *Mycobacterium leprae*. *Lancet*, **ii**, 1328–30.

Deghaide, N.H.S., Dantas, R.O. and Donadi, E.A. 1998. HLA class I and II profiles of patients presenting with Chagas' disease. *Dig Dis Sci*, **43**, 246–52.

Deichmann, K., Bardutzky, J., et al. 1997. Common polymorphisms in the coding part of the IL-4 receptor gene. *Biochem Biophys Res Commun*, **231**, 696–7.

Delgado, J.C., Baena, A., et al. 2002. Ethnic-specific genetic associations with pulmonary tuberculosis. *J Infect Dis*, **186**, 1463–8.

Deng, H.K., Liu, R., et al. 1996. Identification of a major co-receptor for primary isolates of HIV-1. *Nature*, **381**, 661–6.

DeSandro, A., Nagarajan, U.M. and Boss, J.M. 1999. The bare lymphocyte syndrome: molecular clues to the transcriptional regulation of major histocompatibility complex class II genes. *Am J Hum Genet*, **65**, 279–86.

Dessein, A.J., Hillaire, D., et al. 1999. Severe hepatic fibrosis in *Schistosoma mansoni* infection is controlled by a major locus that is closely linked to the interferon-γ receptor gene. *Am J Hum Genet*, **65**, 709–21.

Dessoukey, M.W. and El-Shiemy, S. 1996. HLA and leprosy: segregation and linkage study. *Int J Dermatol*, **35**, 257–64.

Dewar, J.C., Wilkinson, J., et al. 1997. The glutamine 27 β2-adrenoceptor polymorphism is associated with elevated IgE levels in asthmatic families. *J Allergy Clin Immunol*, **100**, 261–5.

Diez, E., Lee, S.-H., et al. 2003. Bircle is the gene within the *Lgn1* locus associated with resistance to *Legionella pneumophila*. *Nature*, **33**, 55–60.

Djilali-Saiah, I., Ouellette, P., et al. 2001. CTLA-4/CD28 region polymorphisms in children from families with autoimmune hepatitis. *Hum Immunol*, **62**, 1356–62.

Domingo, P., Muniz-Diaz, E., et al. 2002. Associations between Fc gamma receptor IIA polymorphisms and the risk and prognosis of meningococcal disease. *Am J Med*, **112**, 19–25.

Donaldson, P.T. 1999. The interrelationship between hepatitis C virus and HLA. *Eur J Clin Invest*, **29**, 280–3.

Donaldson, P.T., Ho, S., et al. 2001. HLA class II alleles in Chinese patients with hepatocellular carcinoma. *Liver*, **21**, 143–8.

Dragic, T., Litwin, V., et al. 1996. HIV-1 entry into CD4(+) cells is mediated by the chemokine receptor CC-CKR-5. *Nature*, **381**, 667–73.

Drysdale, C.M., McGraw, D.W., et al. 2000. Complex promoter and coding region β2-adrenergic receptor haplotypes alter receptor expression and predict in vivo responsiveness. *Proc Natl Acad Sci USA*, **97**, 10483–8.

Dunstan, S.J., Ho, V.A., et al. 2001a. Typhoid fever and genetic polymorphisms at the natural resistance-associated macrophage protein 1. *J Infect Dis*, **183**, 1156–60.

Dunstan, S.J., Stephens, H.A., et al. 2001b. Genes of the class II and class III major histocompatibility complex are associated with typhoid fever in Vietnam. *J Infect Dis*, **183**, 261–8.

Eaves, I.A., Merriman, T.R., et al. 2000. The genetically isolated populations of Finland and Sardinia may not be a panacea for linkage disequilibrium mapping of common disease genes. *Nat Genet*, **25**, 320–3.

El-Omar, E.M., Carrington, M., et al. 2000. Interleukin-1 polymorphisms associated with increased risk of gastric cancer. *Nature*, **404**, 398–402.

Ewens, W.J. and Spielman, R.S. 1995. The transmission/disequilibrium test: history, subdivision, and admixture. *Am J Hum Genet*, **57**, 455–64.

Ezekowitz, R., Williams, D.J., et al. 1991. Uptake of *Pneumocystis carinii* mediated by the macrophage mannose receptor. *Nature*, **351**, 155–8.

Ezekowitz, R.A.B. 1998. Genetic heterogeneity of mannose binding proteins: the Jekyll and Hyde of innate immunity? *Am J Hum Genet*, **62**, 6–9.

Faghiri, Z., Tabei, S.Z. and Taheri, F. 1995. Study of the association of HLA class I antigens with kala-azar. *Hum Hered*, **45**, 258–61.

Farrall, M. 1993. Homozygosity mapping: familiarity breeds debility. *Nat Genet*, **5**, 107–8.

Fearon, D.T. and Locksley, R.M. 1996. The instructive role of innate immunity in the acquired immune response. *Science*, **272**, 50–3.

Feitosa, F., Borecki, I., et al. 1995. The genetic epidemiology of leprosy in a Brazilian population. *Am J Hum Genet*, **56**, 1179–85.

Feitosa, M., Krieger, H., et al. 1996. Genetic epidemiology of the Mitsuda reaction in leprosy. *Hum Hered*, **46**, 32–5.

Feng, B.J., Huang, W., et al. 2002. Genome-wide scan for familial nasopharyngeal carcinoma reveals evidence of linkage to chromosome 4. *Nat Genet*, **31**, 395–9.

Feng, Y., Broder, C.C., et al. 1996. HIV-1 entry cofactor: functional cDNA cloning of a seven-transmembrane, G protein-coupled receptor. *Science*, **272**, 872–6.

Fernandez-Reyes, D., Criag, A.G., et al. 1997. A high frequency African coding polymorphism in the N-terminal domain of ICAM-1 predisposing to cerebral malaria in Kenya. *Hum Mol Genet*, **6**, 1357–60.

Fieschi, C., Dupuis, S., et al. 2003. Low penetrance, broad resistance, and favourable outcome of interleukin 12 receptor β1 deficiency: medical and immunological implications. *J Exp Med*, **197**, 527–35.

Fijen, C.A.P., Bredius, R.G.M., et al. 2000. The role of Fc gamma receptor polymorphisms and C3 in the immune defense against *Neisseria meningitidis* in complement-deficient individuals. *Clin Exp Immunol*, **120**, 338–45.

Fine, P.E.M. 1981. Immunogenetics of susceptibility to leprosy, tuberculosis and leishmaniasis. An epidemiological perspective. *Int J Leprosy*, **49**, 437–54.

Fine, P.E.M. 1983. Natural history of leprosy – aspects relevant to a leprosy vaccine. *Int J Leprosy*, **51**, 553–5.

Fine, P.E.M., Wolf, E., et al. 1979. HLA-linked genes and leprosy: a family study in Karigiri, South India. *J Infect Dis*, **140**, 152–61.

Fischer, A., Cavazzana-Calvo, M., et al. 1997. Naturally occurring primary deficiencies of the immune system. *Annu Rev Immunol*, **15**, 93–124.

Foote, S.J., Burt, R.A., et al. 1997. Mouse loci for malaria-induced mortality and the control of parasitaemia. *Nat Genet*, **17**, 380–1.

Fortin, A., Belouchi, A., et al. 1997. Genetic control of blood parasitaemia in mouse malaria maps to chromosome 8. *Nat Genet*, **17**, 382–3.

Fortin, A., Cardon, L.R., et al. 2001a. Identification of a new malaria susceptibility locus (Char4) in recombinant congenic strains of mice. *Proc Natl Acad Sci USA*, **98**, 10793–8.

Fortin, A., Diez, E., et al. 2001b. Recombinant congenic strains derived from A/J and C57BL/6J: a tool for genetic dissection of complex traits. *Genomics*, **74**, 21–35.

Fortin, A., Stevenson, M.M. and Gros, P. 2002. Susceptibility to malaria as a complex trait: big pressure from a tiny creature. *Hum Mol Genet*, **11**, 2469–78.

Foster, C.B., Lehrnbecher, T., et al. 2000. An *IL6* promoter polymorphism is associated with a lifetime risk of development of Kaposi sarcoma in men infected with human immunodeficiency virus. *Blood*, **96**, 2562–7.

Frazer, K.A., Ueda, Y., et al. 1997. Computational and biological analysis of 680kb of DNA sequence from the human 5q31 cytokine gene cluster region. *Genome Res*, **7**, 495–512.

Fu, Y.L., Korostoff, J.M., et al. 2002. Fc gamma receptor genes as risk markers for localized aggressive periodontitis in African-Americans. *J Periodontol*, **73**, 517–23.

Furumoto, Y., Hiraoka, S., et al. 2000. Polymorphisms in FceRIB chain do not affect IgE-mediated mast cell activation. *Biochem Biophys Res Commun*, **273**, 765–71.

Gao, P.S., Mao, X.Q., et al. 1999. Nonpathogenic common variants of *IFNGR1* and *IFNGR2* in association with total serum IgE levels. *Biochem Biophys Res Commun*, **263**, 425–9.

Gao, P.-S., Fujishima, S., et al. 2000. Genetic variants of *NRAMP1* and active tuberculosis in Japanese populations. *Clin Genet*, **58**, 74–6.

Gao, X.J., Nelson, G.W., et al. 2001. Effect of a single amino acid change in MHC class I molecules on the rate of progression to AIDS. *N Engl J Med*, **344**, 1668–75.

Garcia, A., Cot, M., et al. 1998a. Genetic control of blood infection levels in human malaria: evidence for a complex genetic model. *Am J Trop Med Hygiene*, **58**, 480–8.

Garcia, A., Marquet, S., et al. 1998b. Linkage analysis of blood *Plasmodium falciparum* levels: interest of the 5q31-q33 chromosome region. *Am J Trop Med Hygiene*, **58**, 705–9.

Garcia, A., Abel, L., et al. 1999. Genetic epidemiology of host predisposition microfilaraemia in human loiasis. *Trop Med Int Health*, **4**, 565–74.

Gilbert, S.C., Plebanski, M., et al. 1998. Association of malaria parasite population structure, HLA and immunological antagonism. *Science*, **279**, 1173–7.

Goldfeld, A.E., Delgado, J.C., et al. 1998. Association of an HLA-DQ allele with clinical tuberculosis. *JAMA*, **279**, 226–8.

Goldstein, D.B. 2001. Islands of linkage disequilibrium. *Nat Genet*, **29**, 109–11.

Gonzalez, E., Dhanda, R., et al. 2001. Global survey of genetic variation in CCR5, RANTES and MIP-1 alpha: impact on the epidemiology of the HIV-1 pandemic. *Proc Natl Acad Sci USA*, **98**, 5199–204.

Gorham, J.D., Guler, M.L., et al. 1996. Genetic mapping of a murine locus controlling development of T helper 1/T helper 2 type responses. *Proc Natl Acad Sci USA*, **93**, 12467–72.

Gourley, I.S., Kurtis, J.D., et al. 2002. Profound bias in interferon-γ and interleukin-6 allele frequencies in Western Kenya, where severe malaria is common in children. *J Infect Dis*, **186**, 1007–12.

Goyert, S.M., Ferrero, E., et al. 1988. The CD14 monocyte differentiation antigen maps to a region encoding growth factors and receptors. *Science*, **239**, 497–500.

Graves, P.E., Kabesch, M., et al. 2000. A cluster of seven tightly linked polymorphisms in the IL-13 gene is associated with total serum IgE levels in three populations of white children. *J Allergy Clin Immunol*, **105**, 506–13.

Greenberg, D.A. 1993. Linkage analysis of 'necessary' disease loci versus 'susceptibility' loci. *Am J Hum Genet*, **52**, 135–43.

Greenberg, D.A., Abreu, P. and Hodge, S.E. 1998. The power to detect linkage in complex disease by means of simple LOD-score analyses. *Am J Hum Genet*, **63**, 870–9.

Greenstein, G. and Hart, T.C. 2002. Clinical utility of a genetic susceptibility test for severe chronic periodontitis – a critical evaluation. *J Am Dental Assoc*, **133**, 452–9.

Greenwood, C.M.T., Fujiwara, M., et al. 2000. Linkage of tuberculosis to chromosome 2q35 loci, including *NRAMP1*, in a large Aboriginal Canadian family. *Am J Hum Genet*, **67**, 405–16.

Grimbacher, B., Holland, S.M. and Puck, J.M. 1998. The interleukin-4 receptor variant Q576R in hyper-IgE syndrome. *N Engl J Med*, **338**, 1073–4.

Grimbacher, B., Holland, S.M., et al. 1999a. Hyper Ig-E syndrome with recurrent infections – an autosomal dominant multisystem disorder. *N Engl J Med*, **340**, 692–702.

Grimbacher, B., Schaffer, A.A., et al. 1999b. Genetic linkage of hyper-IgE syndrome to chromosome 4. *Am J Hum Genet*, **65**, 735–44.

Guggino, S.E. 1999. Evolution of the ΔF508 CFTR mutation. *Trends Microbiol*, **7**, 55–6.

Guler, M.L., Gorham, J.D., et al. 1996. Genetic susceptibility to *Leishmania*: IL-12 responsiveness in TH1 cell development. *Science*, **271**, 984–90.

Guler, M.L., Gorham, J.D., et al. 1999. Tpm1, a locus controlling IL-12 responsiveness, acts by a cell-autonomous mechanism. *J Immunol*, **162**, 1339–47.

Guo, L., Hu-Li, J., et al. 2002. In TH2 cells the IL4 gene has a series of accessibility states associated with distinctive probabilities of IL-4 production. *Proc Natl Acad Sci USA*, **99**, 10623–8.

Haan, K.M. and Longnecker, R. 2000. Coreceptor restriction within the HLA-DQ locus for Epstein–Barr virus infection. *Proc Natl Acad Sci USA*, **97**, 9252–7.

Hackstein, H., Hecker, M., et al. 2001. A novel polymorphism in the 5′ promoter region of the human interleukin-4 receptor α-chain gene is associated with decreased soluble interleukin-4 receptor protein levels. *Immunogenetics*, **53**, 264–9.

Hadley, T.J. and Peiper, S.C. 1997. From malaria to chemokine receptor: the emerging physiologic role of the Duffy blood group antigen. *Blood*, **89**, 3077–91.

Hafez, M., Aboul Hassan, S., et al. 1991. Immunogenetic susceptibility for post-schistosomal hepatic fibrosis. *Am J Trop Med Hygiene*, **44**, 424–33.

Haile, R.W.C., Iselius, L., et al. 1985. Segregation and linkage analyses of 72 leprosy pedigrees. *Hum Hered*, **35**, 43–52.

Hajeer, A.H. and Hutchinson, I.V. 2001. Influence of TNFα gene polymorphisms on TNFα production and disease. *Hum Immunol*, **62**, 1191–9.

Hall, M.A., Ahmadi, K.R., et al. 2000. Genetic influence on peripheral blood T lymphocyte levels. *Genes Immun*, **1**, 423–7.

Harding, D., Baines, P.B., et al. 2002. Severity of meningococcal disease in children and the angiotensin-converting enzyme insertion/deletion polymorphism. *Am J Respir Crit Care Med*, **165**, 1103–6.

Haukim, N., Bidwell, J.L., et al. 2002. Cytokine gene polymorphism in human disease: on-line databases, supplement 2. *Genes Immun*, **3**, 313–30.

He, J., Chen, Y., et al. 1997. CCR3 and CCR5 are co-receptors for HIV-1 infection of microglia. *Nature*, **385**, 645–9.

Heinzmann, A., Mao, X.Q., et al. 2000. Genetic variants of IL-13 signaling and human asthma and atopy. *Hum Mol Genet*, **9**, 549–59.

Helminen, M., Lahdenpohja, N. and Hurme, M. 1999. Polymorphism of the interleukin-10 gene is associated with susceptibility to Epstein–Barr virus infection. *J Infect Dis*, **180**, 496–9.

Helminen, M.E., Kilpinen, S., et al. 2001. Susceptibility to primary Epstein–Barr infection is associated with interleukin-10 gene promoter polymorphism. *J Infect Dis*, **184**, 777–80.

Hennig, B.J.W., Hellier, S., et al. 2002. Association of low-density lipoprotein receptor polymorphisms and outcome of hepatitis C infection. *Genes Immun*, **3**, 359–67.

Hershey, G.K.K., Frierich, M.F., et al. 1997. The association of atopy with a gain of function mutation in the α subunit of the interleukin-4 receptor. *N Engl J Med*, **337**, 1720–5.

Higgins, J.A., Thorpe, C.J., et al. 1994. Overlapping T-cell epitopes in the group I allergen of Dermatophagoides species restricted by HLA-DP and HLA-DR class II molecules. *J Allergy Clin Immunol*, **93**, 891–9.

Hildesheim, A., Apple, R.J., et al. 2002. Association of HLA class I and II alleles and extended haplotypes with nasopharyngeal carcinoma in Taiwan. *J Natl Cancer Inst*, **94**, 1780–9.

Hill, A.V.S. 1998. The immunogenetics of human infectious diseases. *Annu Rev Immunol*, **16**, 593–617.

Hill, A.V.S. 1999. Genetics and genomics of infectious disease susceptibility. *Br Med Bull*, **55**, 401–13.

Hill, A.V.S., Allsopp, C.E.M., et al. 1991. Common West African HLA antigens are associated with protection from severe malaria. *Nature*, **352**, 595–600.

Hill, A.V.S., Elvin, J., et al. 1992. Molecular analysis of the association of *HLA-B53* and resistance to severe malaria. *Nature*, **360**, 434–9.

Hirayama, K., Matsushita, S., et al. 1987. HLA-DQ is epistatic to HLA-DR in controlling the immune response to schistosomal antigen in humans. *Nature*, **327**, 426–30.

Hirayama, K., Chen, H., et al. 1998. Glycine-valine dimorphism at the 86th amino acid of HLA-DRB1 influenced the prognosis of postschistosomal hepatic fibrosis. *J Infect Dis*, **177**, 1682–6.

Hirayama, K., Chen, H., et al. 1999. HLA-DR-DQ alleles and HLA-DP alleles are independently associated with susceptibility to different stages of post-schistosomal hepatic fibrosis in the Chinese population. *Tissue Antigens*, **53**, 269–74.

Hirsch, E., Irikura, V.M., et al. 1996. Functions of interleukin 1 receptor antagonist in gene knockout and overproducing mice. *Proc Natl Acad Sci USA*, **93**, 11008–13.

Hizawa, N., Collins, G., et al. 1998a. Linkage analysis of *Dermatophagoides pteronyssinus*-specific IgE responsiveness with polymorphic markers on chromosome 6p21 (HLA-D region) in Caucasian families by the transmission/disequilibrium test. *J Allergy Clin Immunol*, **102**, 443–8.

Hizawa, N., Freidhoff, L.R., et al. 1998b. Genetic regulation of *Dermatophagoides pteronyssinus*-specific IgE responsiveness: a genome-wide multipoint linkage analysis in families recruited through 2 asthmatic sibs. *J Allergy Clin Immunol*, **102**, 436–42.

Hizawa, N., Yamaguchi, E., et al. 2000. A common *FCERIB* gene promoter polymorphism influences total serum IgE levels in a Japanese population. *Am J Respir Crit Care Med*, **161**, 906–9.

Hobbs, M.R., Udhayakumar, V., et al. 2002. A new *NOS2* promoter polymorphism associated with increased nitric oxide production and protection from severe malaria in Tanzanian and Kenyan children. *Lancet*, **360**, 1468–75.

Hoebee, B., Rietveld, E., et al. 2003. Association of severe respiratory syncytial virus bronchiolitis with interleukin-4 and interleukin 4 receptor α polymorphisms. *J Infect Dis*, **187**, 2–11.

Hoerauf, A., Kruse, S., et al. 2002. The variant Arg110Gln of human IL-13 is associated with an immunologically hyper-reactive form of onchocerciasis (sowda). *Microbes Infect*, **4**, 37–42.

Holberg, C.J., Halonen, M., et al. 1999. Familial aggregation and segregation analysis of eosinophil levels. *Am J Respir Crit Care Med*, **160**, 1604–10.

Holla, L.I., Fassmann, A., et al. 2001. Interactions of lymphotoxin alpha (TNF-beta), angiotensin-converting enzyme (ACE), and endothelin-1 (ET-1) gene polymorphisms in adult periodontitis. *J Periodontol*, **72**, 85–9.

Holla, L.I., Buckova, D., et al. 2002. Plasminogen-activator-inhibitor-1 promoter polymorphism as a risk factor for adult periodontitis in non-smokers. *Genes Immun*, **3**, 292–4.

Holland, C.V., Crompton, D.W.T., et al. 1992. A possible genetic factor influencing protection from infection with *Ascaris lumbricoides* in Nigerian children. *J Parasitol*, **78**, 915–16.

Howard, T.D., Koppelman, G.H., et al. 2001. Gene-gene interaction in asthma: *IL4RA* and *IL13* in a Dutch population with asthma. *Am J Hum Genet*, **70**, 230–6.

Howe, D.K. and Sibley, L.D. 1995. *Toxoplasma gondii* comprises 3 clonal lineages – correlation of parasite genotype with human disease. *J Infect Dis*, **172**, 1561–6.

Huang, J.H., Oefner, P.J., et al. 1998. Analyses of the NRAMP1 and IFN-gamma R1 genes in women with *Mycobacterium avium-intracellulare* pulmonary disease. *Am J Respir Crit Care Med*, **157**, 377–81.

Hull, J., Thomson, A. and Kwiatkowski, D. 2000. Association of respiratory syncytial virus bronchiolitis with the interleukin 8 gene region in UK families. *Thorax*, **55**, 1023–7.

Hull, J., Ackerman, H., et al. 2001. Unusual haplotypic structure of *IL8*, a susceptibility locus for a common respiratory virus. *Am J Hum Genet*, **69**, 413–19.

Hural, J.A., Kwan, M., et al. 2000. An intron transcriptional enhancer element regulates IL-4 gene locus accessibility in mast cells. *J Immunol*, **165**, 3239–49.

Hurme, M. and Helminen, M. 1998. Resistance to human cytomegalovirus infection may be influenced by genetic polymorphisms of the tumour necrosis factor-alpha and interleukin-1 receptor antagonist genes. *Scand J Infect Dis*, **30**, 447–9.

Hwang, S.J., Chu, C.W., et al. 2002. Genetic predispositions for the presence of cryoglobulinemia and serum autoantibodies in Chinese patients with chronic hepatitis C. *Tissue Antigens*, **59**, 31–7.

Ioannidis, J.P.A., Ntzani, E.E., et al. 2001. Replication validity of genetic association studies. *Nat Genet*, **29**, 306–9.

Ioannidis, J.P.A., Trikalinos, T.A., et al. 2003. Genetic associations in large versus small studies: an empirical assessment. *Lancet*, **361**, 567–71.

Irving, S.G., Zipfel, P.F., et al. 1990. Two inflammatory mediator cytokine genes are closely linked and variably amplified on chromosome 17q. *Nucleic Acids Res*, **18**, 3261–70.

Jackson, G.S., Beck, J.A., et al. 2001. HLA-DQ7 antigen and resistance to variant CJD. *Nature*, **414**, 269.

Jacob, C.O., Fronek, Z., et al. 1990. Heritable major histocompatibility complex class II-associated differences in production of tumor necrosis factor a: relevance to genetic predisposition to systemic lupus erythematosus. *Proc Natl Acad Sci USA*, **87**, 1233–7.

Jawinska, E.C. and Serjeantson, S.W. 1988. HLA-DR, -DQ DNA genotyping and T-cell receptor RFLPs in leprosy. *Dis Markers*, **6**, 173–83.

Jeffrey, K.J.M. and Bangham, C.R.M. 2000. Do infectious diseases drive MHC diversity? *Microbes Infect*, **2**, 1335–41.

Jeffreys, A.J., Kauppi, L. and Neumann, R. 2001. Intensely punctate meiotic recombination in the class II region of the major histocompatibility complex. *Nat Genet*, **29**, 217–22.

Jepson, A.P., Banya, W.A., et al. 1995. Genetic regulation of fever in *Plasmodium falciparum* malaria in Gambian twin children. *J Infect Dis*, **172**, 316–19.

Jepson, A., Banya, W., et al. 1997a. Quantification of the relative contribution of major histocompatibility complex (MHC) and non-MHC genes to human immune responses to foreign antigens. *Infect Immun*, **65**, 872–6.

Jepson, A., Sisay-Joof, F., et al. 1997b. Genetic linkage of mild malaria to the major histocompatibility complex in Gambian children: study of affected sibling pairs. *Br Med J*, **315**, 96–7.

John, G.C., Rousseau, C., et al. 2000. Maternal SDF1 3′A polymorphism is associated with increased perinatal human immunodeficiency virus type 1 transmission. *J Virol*, **74**, 5736–9.

Johnson, G.C.L., Esposito, L., et al. 2001. Haplotype tagging for the identification of common disease genes. *Nat Genet*, **29**, 233–7.

Johnson, J., Suzuki, Y., et al. 2002. Genetic analysis of influences on survival following *Toxoplasma gondii* infection. *Int J Parasitol*, **32**, 179–85.

Jouanguy, E., Altare, F., et al. 1996. Interferon gamma receptor deficiency in an infant with fatal bacille Calmette-Guerin infection. *N Engl J Med*, **335**, 1956–61.

Jouanguy, E., Doffinger, R., et al. 1999a. IL-12 and IFN-γ in host defense against mycobacteria and salmonella in mice and men. *Curr Opin Immunol*, **11**, 346–51.

Jouanguy, E., Lamhamedi-Cherradi, S., et al. 1999b. A human *IFNGR1* small deletion hotspot associated with dominant susceptibility to mycobacterial infection. *Nat Genet*, **21**, 370–8.

Jurado, A., Cardaba, B., et al. 1997. Autoimmune hepatitis type 2 and hepatitis C virus infection: study of HLA antigens. *J Hepatol*, **26**, 983–91.

Kang, T.J. and Chae, G.T. 2001. Detection of Toll-like receptor 2 (TLR2) mutation in lepromatous leprosy patients. *FEMS Immunol Med Microbiol*, **31**, 53–8.

Kariuki, H.C., Mbugua, G., et al. 2001. Prevalence and familial aggregation of schistosomal liver morbidity in Kenya: evaluation by new ultrasound criteria. *J Infect Dis*, **183**, 960–6.

Karplus, T.M., Jeronimo, S.M.B., et al. 2002. Association between the tumor necrosis factor locus and the clinical outcome of *Leishmania chagasi* infection. *Infect Immun*, **70**, 6919–25.

Kaslow, R.A. and McNicholl, J.M. 1999. Genetic determinants of HIV-1 infection and its manifestations. *Proc Assoc Am Physns*, **111**, 299–307.

Kemp, S.J., Iraqi, F., et al. 1997. Localization of genes controlling resistance to trypanosomiasis in mice. *Nat Genet*, **16**, 194–6.

Khoo, S.H., Pepper, L., et al. 1997. Tumour necrosis factor c2 microsatellite allele is associated with the rate of HIV disease progression. *AIDS*, **11**, 423–8.

Kikuchi, M., Looareesuwan, S., et al. 2001. Association of adhesion molecule PECAM-1/CD31 polymorphism with susceptibility to cerebral malaria in Thais. *Parasitol Int*, **50**, 235–9.

Knapp, M. 1999. A note on power approximations for the transmission/disequilibrium test. *Am J Hum Genet*, **64**, 1177–85.

Knapp, M., Seucchter, S.A. and Baur, M.P. 1993. The haplotype-relative-risk (HRR) method for analysis of association in nuclear families. *Am J Hum Genet*, **52**, 1085–93.

Knight, J.C. and Kwiatkowski, D. 1999. Inherited variability of tumor necrosis factor production and susceptibility to infectious disease. *Proc Assoc Am Physns*, **111**, 290–8.

Knight, J.C., Udalova, I., et al. 1999. A polymorphism that affects OCT-1 binding to the *TNF* promoter region is associated with severe malaria. *Nat Genet*, **22**, 145–50.

Kobayashi, T., van der Pol, W.L., et al. 2000. Relevance of IgG receptor IIIb (CD16) polymorphism to handling of *Porphyromonas gingivalis*: implications for the pathogenesis of adult periodontitis. *J Periodontol Res*, **35**, 65–73.

Kobayashi, T., Yamamoto, K., et al. 2001. The Fc gamma receptor genotype as a severity factor for chronic periodontitis in Japanese patients. *J Periodontol*, **72**, 1324–31.

Koch, O., Awomoyi, A., et al. 2002. IFNGR1 gene promoter polymorphisms and susceptibility to cerebral malaria. *J Infect Dis*, **185**, 1684–7.

Koriyama, C., Shinkura, R., et al. 2001. Human leukocyte antigens related to Epstein–Barr virus-associated gastric carcinoma in Japanese patients. *Eur J Cancer*, **10**, 69–75.

Kovacs, G.G., Trabattoni, G., et al. 2002. Mutations of the prion protein gene – phenotypic spectrum. *J Neurol*, **249**, 1567–82.

Kroeger, K.M., Steer, J.H., et al. 1999. Effects of stimulus and cell type on the expression of the −308 tumour necrosis factor promoter polymorphism. *Cytokine*, **12**, 110–19.

Kruglyak, L. 1997. The use of a genetic map of biallelic markers in linkage studies. *Nat Genet*, **17**, 21–4.

Kruglyak, L. 1999. Prospects for whole-genome linkage disequilibrium mapping of common disease genes. *Nat Genet*, **22**, 139–44.

Kruglyak, L., Daly, M.J., et al. 1996. Parametric and nonparametric linkage analysis: a unified multipoint approach. *Am J Hum Genet*, **58**, 1347–63.

Krul, E.T.J., Schipper, R.F., et al. 1999. HLA and susceptibility to cervical neoplasia. *Hum Immunol*, **60**, 337–42.

Kruse, S., Japha, T., et al. 1999. The polymorphisms S503P and Q576R in the interleukin-4 receptor α gene are associated with atopy and influence the signal transduction. *Immunology*, **96**, 365–71.

Kun, J.F.J., Klabunde, J., et al. 1999. Association of the ICAM-1_{KILIFI} mutation with protection against severe malaria in Lambarene Gabon. *Am J Trop Med Hygiene*, **61**, 776–9.

Kun, J.F., Mordmuller, B., et al. 2001. Nitric oxide synthase 2 Lambarene (G-954C), increased nitric oxide production and protection against malaria. *J Infect Dis*, **184**, 330–6.

Kuzushita, N., Hayashi, N., et al. 1998. Influence of HLA haplotypes on the clinical courses of individuals infected with hepatitis C virus. *Hepatology*, **27**, 240–4.

Laine, M.L., Farre, M.A., et al. 2001. Polymorphisms of the interleukin-1 gene family, oral microbial pathogens, and smoking in adult periodontitis. *J Dent Res*, **80**, 1695–9.

Laitinen, T., Kauppi, P., et al. 1997. Genetic control of serum IgE levels and asthma: linkage and linkage disequilibrium studies in an isolated population. *Hum Mol Genet*, **6**, 2069–76.

Lammas, D.A., de Heer, E., et al. 2002. Heterogeneity in the granulomatous response to mycobacterial infection in patients with defined genetic mutations in the interleukin 12-dependent interferon-gamma production pathway. *Int J Exp Pathol*, **83**, 1–20.

Lammie, P.J., Hitch, W.L., et al. 1991. Maternal filarial infection as risk factor for infection in children. *Lancet*, **337**, 1005–6.

Lander, E. and Kruglyak, L. 1995. Genetic dissection of complex traits: guidelines for interpreting and reporting linkage results. *Nat Genet*, **11**, 241–7.

Lang, N.P., Tonetti, M.S., et al. 2000. Effect of interleukin-1 gene polymorphisms on gingival inflammation assessed by bleeding on probing in a periodontal maintenance population. *J Periodontol Res*, **35**, 102–7.

Laplanche, J.-L., Lepage, V., et al. 2003. HLA in French patients with variant Creuztfeldt-Jakob disease. *Lancet*, **361**, 531–2.

Lara, M.L., Layrisse, Z., et al. 1991. Immunogenetics of human American cutaneous leishmaniasis: study of HLA haplotypes in 24 families from Venezuela. *Hum Immunol*, **30**, 129–35.

Lavebratt, C., Apt, A.S., et al. 1999. Severity to tuberculosis in mice is linked to distal chromosome 3 and proximal chromosome 9. *J Infect Dis*, **180**, 150–5.

Lechmann, M., Schneider, E.M., et al. 1999. Increased frequency of the HLA-DR15 (BI*15011) allele in German patients with self-limited hepatitis C virus infection. *Eur J Clin Invest*, **29**, 337–43.

Lee, H.-S., Brown, P., et al. 2001. Increased susceptibility to kuru of carriers of the PRNP methionine/methionine genotype. *J Infect Dis*, **183**, 192–6.

Lehrnbecher, T., Foster, C.B., et al. 2000. Variant genotypes of Fc gamma RIIIA influence the development of Kaposi's sarcoma in HIV-infected men. *Blood*, **95**, 2386–90.

Levee, G., Liu, J., et al. 1994. Genetic control of susceptibility to leprosy in French Polynesia: no evidence for linkage with markers on telomeric human chromosome 2. *Int J Leprosy*, **62**, 499–511.

Levesque, M.C., Hobbs, M.R., et al. 1999. Nitric oxide synthase type 2 promoter polymorphisms, nitric oxide production and disease severity in Tanzanian children with malaria. *J Infect Dis*, **180**, 1994–2002.

Lin, T.M., Chen, C.J., et al. 1989. Hepatitis B virus markers in Chinese twins. *Anticancer Res*, **9**, 737–42.

Lipoldova, M., Svobodova, M., et al. 2000. Susceptibility to *Leishmania major* infection in mice: multiple loci and heterogeneity of immunopathological phenotypes. *Genes Immun*, **1**, 200–6.

Liu, H., Chao, D., et al. 1999. Polymorphisms in RANTES chemokine promoter affects HIV-1 disease progression. *Proc Natl Acad Sci USA*, **96**, 4581–5.

Liu, J., Fujiwara, M., et al. 1995. Identification of polymorphisms and sequence variants in the human natural resistance-associated macrophage protein (*NRAMP*) gene, a candidate gene for susceptibility to tuberculosis. *Am J Hum Genet*, **56**, 845–53.

Liu, R., Paxton, W.A., et al. 1996. Homozygous defect in HIV-1 coreceptor accounts for resistance of some multiply-exposed individuals to HIV-1 infection. *Cell*, **86**, 367–77.

Liu, X., Nickel, R., et al. 2000. An *IL13* coding region variant is associated with a high total serum IgE level and atopic dermatitis in the German Multicenter Atopy Study (MAS-90). *J Allergy Clin Immunol*, **106**, 167–70.

Lohmueller, K.E., Pearce, C.L., et al. 2003. Meta-analysis of genetic association studies supports a contribution of common variants to susceptibility to common disease. *Nat Genet*, **33**, 177–82.

Loke, H., Bethell, D.B., et al. 2001. Strong HLA class I-restricted T cell responses in dengue hemorrhagic fever: a double-edged sword? *Infect Dis*, **184**, 1369–73.

Loke, H., Bethell, D., et al. 2002. Susceptibility to dengue hemorrhagic fever in Vietnam: evidence of an association with variation in the vitamin D receptor and FC gamma receptor IIA genes. *Am J Trop Med Hygiene*, **67**, 102–6.

Loots, G.G., Locksley, R.M., et al. 2000. Identification of a coordinate regulator of interleukins 4, 13, and 5 by cross-species sequence comparisons. *Science*, **288**, 136–40.

Lopez de Castro, J.A. 1998. The pathogenetic role of *HLA-B27* in chronic arthritis. *Curr Opin Immunol*, **10**, 59–66.

Louis, E. and Franchimont, D. 1998. Tumour necrosis factor (TNF) gene polymorphism influences TNF-α production in lipopolysaccharide (LPS)-stimulated whole blood cell culture in healthy humans. *Clin Exp Immunol*, **113**, 401–6.

Luoni, G., Verra, F., et al. 2001. Antimalarial antibody levels and *IL4* polymorphism in the Fulani of West Africa. *Genes Immun*, **2**, 411–14.

Ma, X., Dou, S., et al. 2002. 5′ dinucleotide repeat polymorphism of *NRAMP1* and susceptibility to tuberculosis among Caucasian patients in Houston, Texas. *Int J Tuberculosis Lung Dis*, **6**, 818–23.

McGlynn, K.A., Rosvold, E.A., et al. 1995. Susceptibility to hepatocellular carcinoma is associated with genetic variation in the enzymatic detoxification of aflatoxin B1. *Proc Natl Acad Sci USA*, **92**, 2384–7.

McGuire, W., Hill, A.V.S., et al. 1994. Variation in the TNF-alpha promoter region associated with susceptibility to cerebral malaria. *Nature*, **371**, 508–11.

McGuire, W., Knight, J.C., et al. 1999. Severe malarial anemia and cerebral malaria are associated with different tumor necrosis factor promoter alleles. *J Infect Dis*, **179**, 287–90.

McIntire, J.J., Umetsu, S.E., et al. 2001. Identification of *Tapr* (an airway hyperreactivity regulator locus) and the linked *Tim* gene family. *Nat Immunol*, **2**, 1109–16.

Mackinnon, M.J., Gunawardena, D.M., et al. 2000. Quantifying genetic and nongenetic contributions to malarial infection in a Sri Lankan population. *Proc Natl Acad Sci USA*, **97**, 12661–6.

McLeod, R., Buschman, E., et al. 1995. Immunogenetics in the analysis of resistance to intracellular pathogens. *Curr Opin Immunol*, **7**, 539–52.

McManus, D.P., Ross, A.G.P., et al. 2001. HLA class II antigens positively and negatively associated with hepatosplenic schistosomiasis in a Chinese population. *Int J Parasitol*, **31**, 674–80.

Madsen, H.O., Satz, M.L., et al. 1998. Different molecular events result in low protein levels of mannan-binding lectin in populations from Southeast Africa and South America. *J Immunol*, **161**, 3169–75.

Magnusson, P.K.E. and Gyllensten, U.B. 2000. Cervical cancer risk: is there a genetic component? *Mol Med Today*, **6**, 145–8.

Malatay, H.M., Engstrand, L., et al. 1994. *Helicobacter pylori* infection: genetic and environmental influences. A study of twins. *Ann Intern Med*, **120**, 982–6.

Malo, D. and Skamene, E. 1994. Genetic control of host resistance to infection. *Trends Genet*, **10**, 365–71.

Manns, A., Hanchard, B., et al. 1998. Human leukocyte antigen class II alleles associated with human T-cell lymphotropic virus type I infection and adult T-cell leukemia/lymphoma in a black population. *J Natl Cancer Instit*, **90**, 617–22.

Manson, J.C., Jamieson, E., et al. 1999. A single amino acid alteration (101L) introduced into murine PrP dramatically alters incubation time of transmissible spongiform encephalopathy. *EMBO J*, **18**, 6855–64.

Mark, L.L., Haffajee, A.D., et al. 2000. Effect of the interleukin-1 genotype on monocyte IL-1 beta expression in subjects with adult periodontitis. *J Periodontol Res*, **35**, 172–7.

Marquet, S., Abel, L., et al. 1996. Genetic localization of a locus controlling the intensity of infection by *Schistosoma mansoni* on chromosome 5q31-q33. *Nat Genet*, **14**, 181–4.

Marquet, S., Sanchez, F.O., et al. 1999. Variants of the human *NRAMP1* gene and altered human immunodeficiency virus infection susceptibility. *J Infect Dis*, **180**, 1521–5.

Marsden, P.A., Heng, H.H.Q., et al. 1994. Localization of the human gene for inducible nitric oxide synthase (*NOS2*) to chromosome 17q11.2-q12. *Genomics*, **19**, 183–5.

Marsh, D.G., Neely, J.D., et al. 1994. Linkage analysis of *IL4* and other chromosome 5q31.1 markers and total serum immunoglobulin E concentrations. *Science*, **264**, 1152–6.

Marsh, S.G.E., Parham, P. and Barber, L.D. 2000. *The HLA facts book*. London: Academic Press.

Matesanz, F., Delgado, C., et al. 2000. Allelic selection of human IL-2 gene. *Eur J Immunol*, **30**, 3516–21.

Matsushita, S. and Katz, D.H. 1992. B cell sensitivity to IgE suppressive activity of IFN-γ is polymorphic and controlled by a non-H-2-linked gene. *Cell Immunol*, **143**, 212–19.

Matte, C. and Roger, M. 2001. Genetic determinants of pediatric HIV-1 infection: vertical transmission and disease progression among children. *Mol Med*, **7**, 583–9.

May, J., Kremsner, P.G., et al. 1998. HLA-DP control of human *Schistosoma haematobium* infection. *Am J Trop Med Hygiene*, **59**, 302–6.

Meddeb-Garnaoui, A., Gritli, S., et al. 2001. Association analysis of HLA-class II and class III gene polymorphisms in the susceptibility to Mediterranean visceral leishmaniasis. *Hum Immunol*, **62**, 509–17.

Mehra, N.K., Rajalingam, R., et al. 1995. Variants of HLA-DR2/DR51 group haplotypes and susceptibility to tuberculoid leprosy and pulmonary tuberculosis in Asian Indians. *Int J Leprosy*, **63**, 241–8.

Meisel, P., Carlsson, L.E., et al. 2001. Polymorphisms of Fc gamma-receptors RIIa, RIIIa and RIIIb in patients with adult periodontal diseases. *Genes Immun*, **2**, 258–62.

Meisel, P., Siegemund, A., et al. 2002. Smoking and polymorphisms of the interleukin-1 gene cluster (IL-1 alpha, IL-1 beta and IL-1RN) in patients with periodontal disease. *J Periodontol*, **73**, 27–32.

Meisner, S.J., Mucklow, S., et al. 2001. Association of *NRAMP1* polymorphism with leprosy type but not susceptibility to leprosy per se in West Africans. *Am J Trop Med Hygiene*, **65**, 733–5.

Messer, G., Spengler, U., et al. 1991. Polymorphic structure of the tumor necrosis factor (TNF) locus: an NcoI polymorphism in the first intron of the human TNF-β gene correlates with a variant amino acid in position 26 and a reduced level of TNF-β production. *J Exp Med*, **173**, 209–19.

Meyer, C.G. and Kremsner, P.G. 1996. Malaria and onchocerciasis: on HLA and related matters. *Parasitol Today*, **12**, 179–86.

Meyer, C.G., Gallin, M., et al. 1994. HLA-D alleles associated with generalized disease, localized disease, and putative immunity in Onchocerca volvulus infection. *Proc Natl Acad Sci USA*, **91**, 7515–19.

Meyer, C.G., Schnittger, L. and May, J. 1996. Met-11 of HLA class II Dpal first domain associated with onchocerciasis. *Exp Clin Immunogenet*, **13**, 12–19.

Meyer, C.G., May, J. and Stark, K. 1998. Human leukocyte antigens in tuberculosis and leprosy. *Trends Microbiol*, **6**, 148–54.

Meyer, C.G., May, J., et al. 2002. TNFa(-308A) associated with shorter intervals of *Plasmodium falciparum* reinfections. *Tissue Antigens*, **59**, 287–92.

MHC Sequencing Consortium. 1999. Complete sequence and gene map of a human major histocompatibility complex. *Nature*, 401, 921–3.

Michael, N.L. 1999. Host genetic influences on HIV-1 pathogenesis. *Curr Opin Immunol*, **11**, 466–74.

Michael, N.L., Chang, G., et al. 1997. The role of viral phenotype and CCR-5 gene defects in HIV-1 transmission and disease progression. *Nat Med*, **3**, 338–40.

Migot-Nabias, F., Mombo, L.E., et al. 2000. Human genetic factors related to susceptibility to mild malaria in Gabon. *Genes Immun*, **1**, 435–41.

Minton, E.J., Smillie, D., et al. 1998. Association between MHC class II alleles and clearance of circulating hepatitis C virus. *J Infect Dis*, **178**, 39–44.

Mitsuyasu, H., Izuhara, K., et al. 1998. Ile50Val variant of IL4Rα upregulates IgE synthesis and associates with atopic asthma. *Nat Genet*, **19**, 119–20.

Mitsuyasu, H., Yanagihara, Y., et al. 1999. Cutting edge: dominant effect of Ile50Val variant of the human IL-4 receptor α-chain in IgE synthesis. *J Immunol*, **162**, 1227–31.

Miyamasu, M., Sekiya, T., et al. 2001. Variations in the human CC chemokine eotaxin gene. *Genes Immun*, **2**, 461–3.

Mock, B., Blackwell, J., et al. 1993. Genetic control of *Leishmania major* infection in congenic, recombinant inbred and F2 populations of mice. *Eur J Immunogenet*, **20**, 335–48.

Modi, W.S., Goedert, J.J., et al. 2000. A promoter allele in the eotaxin chemokine gene protects against HIV-1 infection. *Am J Hum Genet*, **67**, Suppl. 2, 221, abstract.

Modiano, D., Petrarca, V., et al. 1996. Different response to *Plasmodium falciparum* malaria in West African sympatric ethnic groups. *Proc Natl Acad Sci USA*, **93**, 13206–111.

Modiano, D., Luoni, G., et al. 2001. The lower susceptibility to *Plasmodium falciparum* malaria of Fulani of Burkina Faso (West Africa) is associated with low frequencies of classic malaria-resistance genes. *Trans R Soc Trop Med Hygiene*, **95**, 149–52.

Mohamed-Ali, Q., Elwali, N.E.M.A., et al. 1999. Susceptibility to periportal (Symmers) fibrosis in human *Schistosoma mansoni* infections: evidence that intensity and duration of infection, gender and inherited factors are critical in disease progression. *J Infect Dis*, **180**, 1298–306.

Mohrs, M., Blankespoor, C.M., et al. 2001. Deletion of a coordinate regulator of type 2 cytokine expression in mice. *Nat Immunol*, **2**, 842–7.

Molvig, J., Baek, L., et al. 1988. Endotoxin-stimulated human monocyte secretion of interleukin 1, tumour necrosis factor alpha, and prostaglandin E2 shows stable interindividual differences. *Scand J Immunol*, **27**, 705–16.

Morohan, G., Boutlis, C.S., et al. 2002. A promoter polymorphism in the gene encoding interleukin-12p40 (*IL12B*) is associated with mortality from cerebral malaria and with reduced nitric oxide production. *Genes Immun*, **3**, 414–18.

Morton, N.E. 1998. Significance levels in complex inheritance. *Am J Hum Genet*, **62**, 690–7.

Mostolavsky, R., Singh, N., et al. 2001. Asynchronous replication and allelic exclusion in the immune system. *Nature*, **414**, 221–5.

Mozzato-Chamay, N., Mahdi, O.S.M., et al. 2000. Polymorphisms in candidate genes and risk of scarring trachoma in a *Chlamydia trachomatis*-endemic population. *J Infect Dis*, **182**, 1545–8.

Muller-Myhsok, B., Stelma, F.F., et al. 1997. Further evidence suggesting the presence of a locus on human chromosome 5q31-q33 influencing the intensity of infection with *Schistosoma mansoni*. *Am J Hum Genet*, **61**, 452–4.

Murdoch, M.E., Payton, A., et al. 1997. HLA-DQ alleles associate with cutaneous features of onchocerciasis. *Hum Immunol*, **55**, 46–52.

Nadel, S., Newport, M.J., et al. 1996. Variation in the tumor necrosis factor alpha gene promoter region may be associated with death from meningococcal disease. *J Infect Dis*, **174**, 878–80.

Nagpal, J.K., Patnaik, S. and Das, B.R. 2002. Prevalence of high-risk human papilloma virus types and its association with p53 codon 72 polymorphism in tobacco addicted oral squamous cell carcinoma (OSCC) patients of eastern India. *Int J Cancer*, **97**, 649–53.

Nakayama, E.E., Meyer, L., et al. 2002. Protective effect of interleukin-4 -589T polymorphism on human immunodeficiency virus type 1 disease progression: relationship with virus load. *J Infect Dis*, **185**, 1183–6.

Nelson, P.J., Kim, H.T., et al. 1993. Genomic organization and transcriptional regulation of the *RANTES* chemokine gene. *J Immunol*, **151**, 2601–12.

Newport, M.J., Huxley, C.M., et al. 1996. A mutation in the interferon-γ-receptor gene and susceptibility to mycobacterial infection. *N Engl J Med*, **335**, 1941–9.

Nickel, R., Wahn, U., et al. 1997. Evidence for linkage of chromosome 12q15-q24.1 markers to high total serum IgE concentrations in children of the German Multicenter Allergy Study. *Genomics*, **46**, 159–62.

Nicklin, M.J.H., Weith, A. and Duff, G.W. 1994. A physical map of the region encompassing the human interleukin-1α, interleukin-1β, and interleukin-1 receptor antagonist genes. *Genomics*, **19**, 382–4.

Niedobitek, G., Meru, N. and Delecluse, H.J. 2001. Epstein–Barr virus infection and human malignancies. *Int J Exp Pathol*, **82**, 149–70.

Nieters, A., Brems, S. and Becker, N. 2001. Cross-sectional study of cytokine polymorphisms, cytokine production after T-cell stimulation and clinical parameters in a random sample of a German population. *Hum Genet*, **108**, 241–8.

Nieto, A., Beraun, Y., et al. 2000. HLA haplotypes are associated with differential susceptibility to *Trypanosoma cruzi* infection. *Tissue Antigens*, **55**, 195–8.

Noguchi, E., Nukaga-Nishio, Y., et al. 2001. Haplotypes of the 5′ region of the IL-4 gene and SNPs in the intergene sequence between the IL-4 and IL-13 genes are associated with atopic asthma. *Hum Immunol*, **62**, 1251–7.

Nothwang, H.G., Strahm, B., et al. 1997. Molecular cloning of the interleukin-1 gene cluster: construction of an integrated YAC/PAC contig and a partial transcriptional map in the region of chromosome 2q13. *Genomics*, **41**, 370–8.

Nyholt, D.R. 2000. All LODs are not created equal. *Am J Hum Genet*, **67**, 282–8.

Nyholt, D.R. 2001. Genetic case-control association studies – correcting for multiple testing. *Hum Genet*, **109**, 564–5.

O'Hara, A.M., Fernie, B.A., et al. 1998. C7 deficiency in an Irish family: a deletion defect which is predominant in the Irish. *Clin Exp Immunol*, **114**, 355–61.

Ober, C. and Cox, N.J. 1998. Mapping genes for complex traits in founder populations. *Clin Exp Allergy*, **28**, S101–5.

Ohno, T., Ishih, A., et al. 2002. Chromosomal mapping of host susceptibility loci to *Angiostrongylus costaricensis* nematode infection in mice. *Immunogenetics*, **53**, 925–9.

Ohta, N., Nishimura, Y.K., et al. 1982. Immunogenetic analysis of patients with post-schistosomal liver cirrhosis in man. *Clin Exp Immunol*, **49**, 493–9.

Ohta, N., Hayashi, M., et al. 1987. Immunogenetic factors involved in the pathogenesis of distinct clinical manifestations of *Schistosomiasis japonica* in the Philippine population. *Trans R Soc Trop Med Hygiene*, **81**, 292–6.

Omi, K., Ohashi, J., et al. 2002. Fcγ receptor IIA and IIIB polymorphisms are associated with susceptibility to cerebral malaria. *Parasitol Int*, **51**, 361–6.

Omi, K., Ohashi, J., et al. 2003. CD36 polymorphism is associated with protection from cerebral malaria. *Am J Hum Genet*, **72**, 364–74.

O'Neill, L.A.J. and Dinarello, C.A. 2000. The IL-1 receptor/toll-like receptor superfamily: crucial receptors for inflammation and host defense. *Trends Immunol*, **21**, 206–9.

Opdenakker, G., Fiten, P., et al. 1994. The human MCP-3 gene (*SCYA7*): cloning, sequence analysis, and assignment to the C-C chemokine gene cluster on chromosome 17q11.2-q12. *Genomics*, **21**, 403–8.

Ott, J. and Hoh, J. 2000. Statistical approaches to gene mapping. *Am J Hum Genet*, **67**, 289–94.

Ottenhoff, T.H.M., Kumararatne, D. and Casanova, J.-L. 1998. Novel human immunodeficiencies reveal the essential role of type-1 cytokines in immunity to intracellular bacteria. *Immunol Today*, **11**, 491–4.

Ottenhoff, T.H.M., Verreck, F.A.W., et al. 2002. Genetics, cytokines and human infectious disease: lessons from weakly pathogenic mycobacteria and salmonellae. *Nat Genet*, **32**, 97–105.

Ottesen, E.A., Mendell, N.R., et al. 1981. Familial predisposition to filarial infection – not linked to HLA-A or -B locus specificities. *Acta Tropica*, **38**, 205–16.

Pacheco-Tena, C., Zhang, X., et al. 2002. Innate immunity in host-microbial interactions: beyond B27 in the spondyloarthropathies. *Curr Opin Rheumatol*, **14**, 373–82.

Pain, A., Urban, B.C., et al. 2001. A non-sense mutation in CD36 gene is associated with protection from severe malaria. *Lancet*, **357**, 1502–3.

Palmer, M.S., Dryden, A.J., et al. 1991. Homozygous prion protein genotype predisposes to sporadic Creutzfeldt-Jakob disease. *Nature*, **352**, 340–2.

Parkhill, J.M., Hennig, B.J.W., et al. 2000. Association of interleukin-1 gene polymorphisms with early-expression in subjects with adult periodontitis. *J Periodontol Res*, **35**, 172–7.

Partanen, J. 2003. Genetic susceptibility to variant Creutzfeldt-Jakob disease. *Lancet*, **361**, 447–8.

Pastinen, T., Liitsola, K., et al. 1998. Contribution of the *CCR5* and MBL genes to susceptibility to HIV type 1 infection in the Finnish population. *AIDS Res Hum Retroviruses*, **14**, 695–8.

Peacock, C.S., Collins, A., et al. 2001. Genetic epidemiology of visceral leishmaniasis in northeastern Brazil. *Genet Epidemiol*, **20**, 383–96.

Peacock, C., Sanjeevi, C., et al. 2002. Genetic analysis of multicase families of visceral leishmaniasis in northeastern Brazil: no major role for class II or class III regions of HLA. *Genes Immun*, **3**, 350–8.

Peoc'h, K., Guerin, C., et al. 2000. First report of polymorphisms in the prion-like protein gene (*PRND*): implications for human prion diseases. *Neurosci Lett*, **286**, 144–8.

Pepys, M.B., Bybee, A., et al. 2003. MHC typing in variant Creutzfeldt-Jakob disease. *Lancet*, **361**, 487–9.

Petzl-Erler, M.L., Belich, M.P. and Queiroz-Telles, F. 1991. Association of mucosal leishmaniasis with HLA. *Hum Immunol*, **32**, 254–60.

Picard, C., Fieschi, C., et al. 2002. Inherited interleukin-12 deficiency: *IL12B* genotype and clinical phenotype of 13 patients from six kindreds. *Am J Hum Genet*, **70**, 336–48.

Pier, G.B., Grout, M., et al. 1998. Salmonella typhi uses CFTR to enter intestinal epithelial cells. *Nature*, **393**, 79–82.

Pociot, F., Molvig, J., et al. 1992. A TaqI polymorphisms in the human interleukin-1β (IL-1β) gene correlates with IL-1β secretion in vitro. *Eur J Clin Invest*, **22**, 396–402.

Poland, G.A. 1999. Immunogenetic mechanisms of antibody response to measles vaccine: the role of the HLA genes. *Vaccine*, **17**, 1719–25.

Pratt, S.C., Daly, M.J. and Kruglyak, L. 2000. Exact multipoint quantitative-trait linkage analysis in pedigrees by variance components. *Am J Hum Genet*, **66**, 1153–7.

Price, P., Witt, C., et al. 1999. The genetic basis for the association of the 8.1 ancestral haplotype (A1, B8, DR3) with multiple immunopathological diseases. *Immunol Rev*, **167**, 257–74.

Pritchard, J.K. 2001. Are rare variants responsible for susceptibility to complex disease? *Am J Hum Genet*, **69**, 124–37.

Pruisner, S.B. and Scott, M.R. 1997. Genetics of prions. *Annu Rev Genet*, **31**, 139–75.

Puel, A., Ziegler, S.F., et al. 1998. Defective IL7R expression in T-B+NK+ severe combined immunodeficiency. *Nat Genet*, **20**, 394–7.

Rabinowitz, D. 1997. A transmission disequilibrium test for quantitative trait loci. *Hum Hered*, **47**, 342–50.

Rajalingam, R., Singal, D.P. and Mehra, N.K. 1997. Transporter associated with antigen-processing (TAP) genes and susceptibility to tuberculoid leprosy and pulmonary tuberculosis. *Tissue Antigens*, **49**, 168–72.

Ramsay, C.E., Hayden, C.M., et al. 1999. Association of polymorphisms in the β2-adrenoreceptor gene with higher levels of parasitic infection. *Hum Genet*, **104**, 269–74.

Ravikumar, M., Dheenadhayalan, V., et al. 1999. Associations of HLA-DRB1, DQB1 and DPB1 alleles with pulmonary tuberculosis in south India. *Tubercle Lung Dis*, **79**, 309–17.

Read, R.C., Camp, N.J., et al. 2000. An interleukin-1 genotype is associated with fatal outcome of meningococcal disease. *J Infect Dis*, **182**, 1557–60.

Reith, W., Steimle, V. and Mach, B. 1995. Molecular defects in the bare lymphocyte syndrome and regulation of MHC class II genes. *Immunol Today*, **16**, 539–46.

Ressing, M.E., de Jong, J.H., et al. 1999. Differential binding of viral peptides to HLA-A2 alleles. *Eur J Immunol*, **29**, 1292–303.

Rihet, P., Abel, L., et al. 1998a. Human malaria: segregation analysis of blood infection levels in a suburban area and a rural area in Burkino Faso. *Genet Epidemiol*, **15**, 435–50.

Rihet, P., Traore, Y., et al. 1998b. Malaria in humans: *Plasmodium falciparum* blood infection levels are linked to chromosome 5q31-q33. *Am J Hum Genet*, **63**, 498–505.

Riley, E.M. 1996. The role of MHC- and non-MHC-associated genes in determining the human immune response to malaria antigens. *Parasitology*, **112**, S39–51.

Rioux, J.D., Stone, V.A., et al. 1998. Familial eosinophilia maps to the cytokine gene cluster on human chromosomal region 5q31-q33. *Am J Hum Genet*, **63**, 1086–94.

Rioux, J.D., Daly, M.J., et al. 2001. Genetic variation in the 5q31 cytokine gene cluster confers susceptibility to Crohn disease. *Nat Genet*, **29**, 223–8.

Risch, N. 1990. Linkage strategies for genetically complex traits. III The effect of marker polymorphism on analysis of affected relative pairs. *Am J Hum Genet*, **46**, 242–53.

Risch, N. and Merikangas, K. 1996. The future of genetic studies of complex human diseases. *Science*, **272**, 1516–17.

Risma, K.A., Wang, N., et al. 2002. V75R576 IL-4 receptor α is associated with allergic asthma and enhanced IL-4 receptor function. *J Immunol*, **169**, 1604–10.

Roberts, L.J., Baldwin, T.M., et al. 1997. Resistance to *Leishmania major* is linked to the H2 region on chromosome 17 and to chromosome 9. *J Exp Med*, **185**, 1705–10.

Roberts, L.J., Baldwin, T.M., et al. 1999. Chromosomes X, 9, and the H2 locus interact epistatically to control *Leishmania major* infection. *Eur J Immunol*, **29**, 3047–50.

Roberts, M., Alexander, J. and Blackwell, J.M. 1989. Influence of Lsh, H-2, and an H-11-linked gene on visceralization and metastasis associated with *Leishmania mexicana* infection in mice. *Infect Immun*, **57**, 875–81.

Roberts, M., Alexander, J. and Blackwell, J.M. 1990. Genetic analysis of *Leishmania mexicana* infection in mice: single gene (*Scl-2*) controlled predisposition to cutaneous lesion development. *J Immunogenet*, **17**, 89–100.

Roberts, M., Mock, B.A. and Blackwell, J.M. 1993. Mapping of genes controlling *Leishmania major* infection in CXS recombinant mice. *Eur J Immunogene*, **20**, 349–62.

Rodrigues, V., Abel, L., et al. 1996. Segregation analysis indicates a major gene in the control of interleukine-5 production in humans infected with *Schistosoma mansoni*. *Am J Hum Genet*, **59**, 453–61.

Roifman, C.M., Zhang, J., et al. 2000. A partial deficiency of interleukin-7Rα is sufficient to abrogate T-cell development and cause severe combined immunodeficiency. *Immunobiology*, **96**, 2803–7.

Romano-Spica, V., Ianni, A., et al. 2000. Allelic distribution of *CCR5* and *CCR2* genes in an Italian population sample. *AIDS Res Hum Retroviruses*, **16**, 99–101.

Rowland-Jones, S.L. 1998. Survival with HIV infection: good luck or good breeding? *Trends Genet*, **14**, 343–5.

Roy, S., McGuire, W., et al. 1997. Tumor necrosis factor promoter polymorphisms and susceptibility to lepromatous leprosy. *J Infect Dis*, **176**, 530–2.

Roy, S., Frodsham, A., et al. 1999. Association of vitamin D receptor genotype with leprosy type. *J Infect Dis*, **179**, 187–91.

Ruuls, S.R. and Sedgwick, J.D. 1999. Unlinking tumor necrosis factor biology from the major histocompatibility complex: lessons from human genetics and animal models. *Am J Hum Genet*, **65**, 294–301.

Ryu, S., Park, Y.K., et al. 2000. 3′UTR polymorphisms in the *NRAMP1* gene are associated with susceptibility to tuberculosis in Koreans. *Int J Tuberculosis Lung Dis*, **4**, 577–80.

Samson, M., Libert, F., et al. 1996. Resistance to HIV-1 infection in Caucasian individuals bearing mutant alleles of the CCR-5 chemokine receptor genes. *Nature*, **383**, 722–5.

Samuel, C.E. 2002. Host genetic variability and West Nile virus susceptibility. *Proc Natl Acad Sci USA*, **99**, 11555–7.

Saravia, N.G., Segura, I., et al. 1998. Epidemiologic, genetic and clinical associations among phenotypically distinct populations of *Leishmania (Viannia)* in Colombia. *Am J Trop Med Hygiene*, **59**, 86–94.

Sarmiento, O.L., Ford, C.L., et al. 2002. The importance of assessing effect modification when asserting racial differences in associations between human leukocyte antigen class II alleles and hepatitis C virus outcomes. *J Infect Dis*, **185**, 266–7.

Sarno, E.N., Santos, A.R., et al. 2000. Pathogenesis of nerve damage in leprosy: genetic polymorphism regulates the production of TNF alpha. *Leprosy Rev*, **71**, S154–8.

Sasieni, P.D. 1997. From genotypes to genes: doubling the sample size. *Biometrics*, **53**, 1253–61.

Satoh, M., Toma, H., et al. 1999. Production of a high level of IgG4 antibody associated with resistance to albendazole treatment in *HLA-DRB1*0901* positive patients with strongyloidiasis. *Am J Trop Med Hygiene*, **61**, 668–71.

Schneider, P.M. and Wurzner, R. 1999. Complement genetics: biological implications of polymorphisms and deficiencies. *Immunol Today*, **20**, 2–4.

Schonian, G., Akuffo, H., et al. 2000. Genetic variability within the species *Leishmania aethiopica* does not correlate with clinical variations of cutaneous leishmaniasis. *Mol Biochem Parasitol*, **106**, 239–48.

Schreuder, H. and Tardif, C. 1997. A new cytokine-receptor binding mode revealed by the crystal structure of the IL-1 receptor with an antagonist. *Nature*, **386**, 194–200.

Schroder, B., Franz, B., et al. 2001. Polymorphisms within the prion-like protein gene (*Prnd*) and their implications in human prion diseases, Alzheimer's disease and other neurological disorders. *Hum Genet*, **109**, 319–25.

Schurr, E., Morgan, K., et al. 1991. Genetics of leprosy. *Am J Trop Med Hygiene*, **44**, Suppl., 4–11.

Searle, S. and Blackwell, J.M. 1998. Evidence for a functional repeat polymorphism in the promoter of the human *NRAMP1* gene that correlates with autoimmune versus infectious disease susceptibility. *J Med Genet*, **36**, 295–9.

Secor, W.E., del Corral, H., et al. 1996. Association of hepatosplenic schistosomiasis with *HLA-DQB1*0201*. *J Infect Dis*, **174**, 1131–5.

Seki, N., Yamaguchi, K., et al. 1999. Polymorphism of the 5′-flanking region of the tumor necrosis factor (TNF)-α gene and susceptibility to human T-cell lymphotropic virus type I (HTLV-I) uveitis. *J Infect Dis*, **180**, 880–3.

Selvaraj, P., Kurian, S.M., et al. 2000. Influence of non-MHC genes on lymphocyte response to *Mycobacterium tuberculosis* antigens and tuberculin reactive status in pulmonary tuberculosis. *Ind J Med Res*, **112**, 86–92.

Selvaraj, P., Narayanan, P.R. and Reetha, A.M. 1999. Association of functional mutant homozygotes of the mannose binding protein gene with susceptibility to pulmonary tuberculosis in India. *Tubercle Lung Dis*, **79**, 221–7.

Selvaraj, P., Sriram, U., et al. 2001. Tumour necrosis factor alpha (−238 and −308) and beta gene polymorphisms in pulmonary tuberculosis: haplotype analysis with HLA- A, B and DR genes. *Tuberculosis*, **81**, 335–41.

Sham, P.C. and Curtis, D. 1995. An extended transmission/disequilibrium test (TDT) for multi-allele marker loci. *Ann Hum Genet*, **59**, 323–36.

Sham, P.C., Purcell, S., et al. 2002. Powerful regression-based quantitative-trait linkage analysis of general pedigrees. *Am J Hum Genet*, **71**, 238–53.

Sharfe, N., Dadi, H.K., et al. 1997. Human immune disorder arising from mutation of the α chain of the interleukin-2 receptor. *Proc Natl Acad Sci USA*, **94**, 3168–71.

Shaw, M.-A., Atkinson, S., et al. 1993. An RFLP map for 2q33-q37 from multicase mycobacterial and leishmanial disease families: no evidence for an *Lsh/Ity/Bcg* gene homologue influencing susceptibility to leprosy. *Ann Hum Genet*, **57**, 251–71.

Shaw, M.-A., Davies, C.R., et al. 1995. Human genetic susceptibility and infection with *Leishmania peruviana*. *Am J Hum Genet*, **57**, 1159–68.

Shaw, M.-A., Clayton, D., et al. 1996. Linkage of rheumatoid arthritis to the candidate gene *NRAMP1* on 2q35. *J Med Genet*, **33**, 1–6.

Shaw, M.-A., Collins, A., et al. 1997. Evidence that genetic susceptibility to *Mycobacterium tuberculosis* in a Brazilian population is under oligogenic control: linkage study of the candidate genes NRAMP1 and TNFA. *Tubercle Lung Dis*, **78**, 35–45.

Shaw, M.-A., Donaldson, I.J., et al. 2001. Association and linkage of leprosy phenotypes with HLA class II and tumour necrosis factor genes. *Genes Immun*, **2**, 196–204.

Shi, Y.P., Nahleen, B.L., et al. 2001. Fcγ receptor IIa (CD32) polymorphism is associated with protection of infants against high-density *Plasmodium falciparum* infection VII Asembo Bay cohort project. *J Infect Dis*, **184**, 107–11.

Shields, E.D., Russell, D.A. and Pericak-Vance, M.A. 1987. Genetic epidemiology of the susceptibility to leprosy. *J Clin Invest*, **79**, 1139–43.

Shiina, T., Tamiya, G., et al. 1999. Molecular dynamics of MHC genesis unravelled by sequence analysis of the 1,796,938-bp HLA class I region. *Proc Natl Acad Sci USA*, **96**, 113282–7.

Shilling, H.G., Young, N., et al. 2002. Genetic control of human NK cell repertoire. *J Immunol*, **169**, 239–47.

Shin, H.D., Winkler, C., et al. 2000. Genetic restriction of HIV-1 pathogenesis to AIDS by promoter alleles of IL-10. *Proc Natl Acad Sci USA*, **97**, 14467–72.

Shirodaria, S., Smith, J., et al. 2000. Polymorphisms in the IL-1A gene are correlated with levels of interleukin-1 alpha protein in gingival crevicular fluid of teeth with severe periodontal disease. *J Dent Res*, **79**, 1864–9.

Siddiqui, M.R., Meisner, S., et al. 2001. A major susceptibility locus for leprosy in India maps to chromosome 10p13. *Nat Genet*, **27**, 439–41.

Sieburth, D., Jabs, E.W., et al. 1992. Assignment of genes encoding a unique cytokine (IL12) composed of two unrelated subunits to chromosomes 3 and 5. *Genomics*, **14**, 59–62.

Sjoberg, K., Lepers, J.P., et al. 1992. Genetic regulation of human anti-malarial antibodies in twins. *Proc Natl Acad Sci USA*, **89**, 2101–4.

Skamene, E., Schurr, E. and Gros, P. 1998. Infection genomics: *Nramp1* as a major determinant of natural resistance to intracellular infections. *Annu Rev Med*, **49**, 275–87.

Skoog, T., van't Hooft, F.M., et al. 1999. A common functional polymorphism (C-A substitution at position -863) in the promoter region of the tumour necrosis factor-α (TNF-α) gene associated with reduced circulating levels of TNF-α. *Hum Mol Genet*, **8**, 1443–9.

Smith, M.W., Dean, M., et al. 1997. Contrasting genetic influence of *CCR2* and *CCR5* variants on HIV-1 infection and disease progression. *Science*, **277**, 959–65.

Smith, T., Bhatia, K., et al. 1991. Host genetic factors do not account for variation in parasite loads in *Strongyloides fulleborni kellyi*. *Ann Trop Med Parasitol*, **85**, 533–7.

Soborg, C., Anderson, A.B., et al. 2002. Natural resistance-associated macrophage protein 1 polymorphisms are associated with microscopy-positive tuberculosis. *J Infect Dis*, **186**, 517–21.

Socransky, S.S., Haffajee, A.D., et al. 2000. Microbiological parameters associated with IL-1 gene polymorphisms in periodontitis patients. *J Clin Periodontol*, **27**, 810–18.

Speth, C., Kacani, L. and Dierich, M.P. 1997. Complement receptors in HIV infection. *Immunol Rev*, **159**, 49–67.

Spielman, R.S. and Ewens, W.J. 1996. The TDT and other family-based tests for linkage disequilibrium and association. *Am J Hum Genet*, **59**, 983–9.

Spielman, R.S. and Ewens, W.J. 1998. A sibship test for linkage in the presence of association: the sib transmission/disequilibrium test. *Am J Hum Genet*, **62**, 450–8.

Spielman, R.S., McGinnis, R.E. and Ewens, W.J. 1993. Transmission test for linkage disequilibrium: the insulin gene region and insulin-dependent diabetes mellitus (IDDM). *Am J Hum Genet*, **52**, 506–16.

Stephens, J.C., Reich, D.E., et al. 1998. Dating the origin of the CCR5-Delta 32 AIDS-resistance allele by the coalescence of haplotypes. *Am J Hum Genet*, **62**, 1507–15.

Stienstra, Y., van der Graaf, W.T.A., et al. 2001. Susceptibility to development of *Mycobacterium ulcerans* disease: review of possible risk factors. *Trop Med Int Health*, **6**, 554–62.

Stirnadel, H.A., Beck, H.P., et al. 1999a. Heritability and segregation analysis of immune responses to specific malaria antigens in Papua New Guinea. *Genet Epidemiol*, **17**, 16–34.

Stirnadel, H.A., Stockle, M., et al. 1999b. Malaria infection and morbidity in infants in relation to genetic polymorphisms in Tanzania. *Trop Med Int Health*, **4**, 187–93.

Stirnadel, H.A., Beck, H.P., et al. 2000. Genetic analysis of IgG subclass responses against RESA and MSP2 of *Plasmodium falciparum* in adults in Papua New Guinea. *Epidemiol Infect*, **124**, 153–62.

Su, B., Jin, L., et al. 1999. Distribution of two HIV-1-resistant polymorphisms (SDF1-3′A and CCR2-64I) in east Asian and world populations and its implication in AIDS epidemiology. *Am J Hum Genet*, **65**, 1047–53.

Sugamura, K., Asao, H., et al. 1996. The interleukin-2 receptor γ chain: its role in the multiple cytokine receptor complexes and T cell development in SCID. *Annu Rev Immunol*, **14**, 179–205.

Takabayashi, A., Ihara, K., et al. 1999. Novel polymorphism in the 5′-untranslated region of the interleukin-4 gene. *J Hum Genet*, **44**, 352–3.

Taylor, M.L., Perez-Mejia, A., et al. 1997. Immunologic, genetic and social human risk factors associated to histoplasmosis: studies in the state of Guerrero, Mexico. *Mycopathologia*, **138**, 137–41.

Teran-Escandon, D., Teran-Ortiz, L., et al. 1999. Human leukocyte antigen-associated susceptibility to pulmonary tuberculosis. *Chest*, **115**, 428–33.

Terhell, A.J., Houwing, J.J., et al. 2000. Clustering of *Brugia malayi* infection in a community in South-Sulawesi, Indonesia. *Parasitology*, **120**, 23–9.

Thio, C.L., Carrington, M., et al. 1999. Class II HLA alleles and hepatitis B virus persistence in African Americans. *J Infect Dis*, **179**, 1004–6.

Thio, C.L., Thomas, D.L., et al. 2001. Racial differences in HLA class II associations with hepatitis C virus outcomes. *J Infect Dis*, **184**, 16–21.

Thursz, M.R., Thomas, H.C., et al. 1997. Heterozygote advantage for HLA class-II type in hepatitis B virus infection. *Nat Genet*, **17**, 11–12.

Thye, T., Burchard, G.D., et al. 2003. Genomewide linkage analysis identifies polymorphism in the human interferon-γ receptor affecting *Helicobacter pylori* infection. *Am J Hum Genet*, **72**, 448–53.

Todd, J.R., Burton, C., et al. 1990. Human leukocyte antigen and leprosy: study in northern Louisiana and review. *Rev Infect Dis*, **12**, 63–74.

Tosh, K., Meisner, S., et al. 2002. A region of chromosome 20 is linked to susceptibility in a South Indian population. *J Infect Dis*, **186**, 1190–3.

Tournamille, C., Colin, Y., et al. 1995. Disruption of a GATA motif in the Duffy gene promoter abolishes erythroid gene expression in Duffy-negative individuals. *Nat Genet*, **10**, 224–8.

Toussirot, E., Auger, I., et al. 1999. HLA-DR polymorphism influences T-cell precursor frequencies to Epstein–Barr virus (EBV) gp110: implications for the association of HLA-DR antigens with rheumatoid arthritis. *Tissue Antigens*, **54**, 146–52.

Trkola, A., Dragic, T., et al. 1996. CD4-dependent antibody-sensitive interactions between HIV-1 and its co-receptor CCR-5. *Nature*, **384**, 184–7.

Tsukasaki, K., Miller, C.W., et al. 2001. Tumor necrosis factor alpha polymorphism associated with increased susceptibility to development of adult T-cell leukemia/lymphoma in human T-lymphotropic virus type 1 carriers. *Cancer Res*, **61**, 3770–4.

Tuffrey, M., Alexander, F., et al. 1992. Genetic susceptibility to chlamydial salpingitis and subsequent infertility in mice. *J Reprod Fertil*, **95**, 31–8.

Turner, M.W., Dinan, L., et al. 2000. Restricted polymorphism of the mannose-binding lectin gene of indigenous Australians. *Hum Mol Genet*, **9**, 1481–6.

Ubalee, R., Suzuki, F., et al. 2001. Strong association of a tumor necrosis factor-α promoter allele with cerebral malaria in Myanmar. *Tissue Antigens*, **58**, 407–10.

Uko, G.P., Lu, L.-Y., et al. 1999. HLA-DRB1 leprogenic motifs in Nigerian population groups. *Clin Exp Immunol*, **118**, 56–62.

Uma, H., Selvaraj, P., et al. 1999. Influence of HLA-DR antigens on lymphocyte response to *Mycobacterium tuberculosis* culture filtrate antigens and mitogens in pulmonary tuberculosis. *Tubercle Lung Dis*, **79**, 199–206.

van der Pol, W.L., Huizinga, T.W.J., et al. 2001. Relevance of Fc gamma receptor and interleukin-10 polymorphisms for meningococcal disease. *J Infect Dis*, **184**, 1548–55.

van Leeuwen, B.H., Martinson, M.E., et al. 1989. Molecular organization of the cytokine gene cluster, involving the human IL-3, IL-4, IL-5 and GM-CSF genes, on human chromosome 5. *Blood*, **73**, 1142–8.

Verhoef, A., Higgins, J.A., et al. 1993. Clonal analysis of the atopic immune response to the group II allergen of *Dermatophagoides spp*: identification of HLA-DR and -DQ restricted T cell epitopes. *Int Immunol*, **5**, 1589–97.

Vidal, S.M., Malo, D., et al. 1993. Natural resistance to infection with intracellular parasites: isolation of a candidate for Bcg. *Cell*, **73**, 469–85.

Vidal, S., Tremblay, M.L., et al. 1995. The *Ity/Lsh/Bcg* locus: natural resistance to infection with intracellular parasites is abrogated by disruption of the *Nramp1* gene. *J Exp Med*, **182**, 655–66.

von Mutius, E., Pearce, N., et al. 2000. International patterns of tuberculosis and the prevalence of symptoms of asthma, rhinitis, and eczema. *Thorax*, **55**, 449–53.

Vorechovsky, I., Webster, A.D.B., et al. 1999. Genetic linkage of IgA deficiency to the major histocompatibility complex: evidence for allele segregation distortion, parent-of origin penetrance differences, and the role of anti-IgA antibodies in disease predisposition. *Am J Hum Genet*, **64**, 1096–109.

Wagener, D.K., Schauf, V., et al. 1988. Segregation analysis of leprosy in families of northern Thailand. *Genet Epidemiol*, **5**, 95–105.

Waine, G.J., Ross, A.G.P., et al. 1998. HLA class II antigens are associated with resistance or susceptibility to hepatosplenic disease in a Chinese population infected with *Schistosoma japonicum*. *Int J Parasitol*, **28**, 537–42.

Wakelin, D. and Blackwell, J.M. (eds) 1988. *Genetics resistance to bacterial parasitic infection*. London: Taylor & Francis.

Walport, M.J. 1993. Inherited complement deficiency – clues to the physiological activity of complement in vivo. *Q J Med*, **86**, 355–8.

Walton, B.C. and Valverde, L. 1979. Racial differences in espundia. *Ann Trop Med Parasitol*, **73**, 23–9.

Wang, D. and Sun, F. 2000. Sample sizes for the transmission disequilibrium tests: TDT S-TDT and 1-TDT. *Communications in Statistics - Theory Methods*, **29**, 1129–42.

Wang, D.G., Fan, J.B., et al. 1998. Large-scale identification, mapping, and genotyping of single-nucleotide polymorphisms in the human genome. *Science*, **280**, 1077–82.

Wang, H.Y., Shelburne, C.P., et al. 1999. Cutting edge: effects of an allergy-associated mutation in the human IL-4Rα (Q576R) on human IL-4-induced signal transduction. *J Immunol*, **162**, 4385–9.

Watanabe, M., Kaneko, H., et al. 2002. Predominant expression of 950delCAG of IL-18Rα chain cDNA is associated with reduced IFN-γ production and high serum IgE levels in atopic Japanese children. *J Allergy Clin Immunol*, **109**, 669–75.

Westendorp, R.G.J., Langermans, J.A.M., et al. 1997. Genetic influence on cytokine production and fatal meningococcal disease. *Lancet*, **349**, 170–3.

Whittaker, J.C., Denham, M.C. and Morris, A.P. 2000. The problems of using the transmission/disequilibrium test to infer tight linkage. *Am J Hum Genet*, **67**, 523–6.

Wild, C.P. and Hall, A.J. 1999. Hepatitis B virus and liver cancer: unanswered questions. *Cancer Surv*, **33**, 35–54.

Wilkinson, R.J., Patel, P., et al. 1999. Influence of polymorphism in the genes for the interleukin (IL)-1 receptor antagonist and IL-1beta on tuberculosis. *J Exp Med*, **189**, 1863–74.

Wilkinson, R.J., Llewelyn, M., et al. 2000. Influence of vitamin D deficiency and vitamin D receptor polymorphisms on tuberculosis among Gujarati Asians in west London: a case control study. *Lancet*, **355**, 618–21.

Williams-Blangero, S., Vandeberg, J.L., et al. 1997a. Genetic epidemiology of seropositivity for *Trypanosoma cruzi* infection in rural Goias, Brazil. *Am J Trop Med Hygiene*, **57**, 538–43.

Williams-Blangero, S., Blangero, J. and Bradley, M. 1997b. Quantitative genetic analysis of susceptibility to hookworm infection in a population from rural Zimbabwe. *Hum Biol*, **69**, 201–8.

Williams-Blangero, S., Subedi, J., et al. 1999. Genetic analysis of susceptibility to infection with *Ascaris lumbricoides*. *Am J Trop Med Hygiene*, **60**, 921–6.

Williams-Blangero, S., McGarvey, S.T., et al. 2002a. Genetic component to susceptibility to *Trichuris trichuria*: evidence from two Asian populations. *Genet Epidemiol*, **22**, 254–64.

Williams-Blangero, S., VandeBerg, J.L., et al. 2002b. Genes on chromosomes 1 and 13 have significant effects on Ascaris infection. *Proc Natl Acad Sci USA*, **99**, 5533–8.

Wilson, A.G., de Vries, N., et al. 1993. An allelic polymorphism within the human tumor necrosis factor a promoter region is strongly associated with HLA A1, B8 and DR3 alleles. *J Exp Med*, **177**, 557–60.

Wilson, A.G., Symons, J.A., et al. 1997. Effects of a polymorphism in the human tumor necrosis factor a promoter on transcriptional activation. *Proc Natl Acad Sci USA*, **94**, 3195–9.

Wiltshire, S., Bhattacharyya, S., et al. 1998. A genome scan for loci influencing total serum immunoglobulin levels: possible linkage of IgA to the chromosome 13 atopy locus. *Hum Mol Genet*, **7**, 27–31.

Windl, O., Dempster, M., et al. 1996. Genetic basis of Creutzfeldt-Jakob disease in the United Kingdom: a systematic analysis of predisposing mutations and allelic variation in the *PRNP* gene. *Hum Genet*, **98**, 259–64.

Woolhouse, M.E.J. 1992. Evidence for genetic factors for resistance/ susceptibility to schistosome infection. *Am J Hum Genet*, **51**, 206–7.

Wu, L., Gerard, N.P., et al. 1996. CD4-induced interaction of primary HIV-1 gp120 glycoproteins with the chemokine receptor CCR-5. *Nature*, **384**, 179–83.

Wu, M.S., Hsieh, R.P., et al. 2002a. Association of *HLA-DQB1*0301* and *HLA-DQB1*0602* with different subtypes of gastric cancer in Taiwan. *Jpn J Cancer Res*, **93**, 404–10.

Wu, M.S., Huang, S.P., et al. 2002b. Tumor necrosis factor-alpha and interleukin-10 promoter polymorphisms in Epstein–Barr virus-associated gastric carcinoma. *J Infect Dis*, **185**, 106–9.

Wurzner, R., Rance, N., et al. 1992. C7 M/N protein polymorphisms typing applied to inherited deficiencies of human complement proteins C6 and C7. *Clin Exp Immunol*, **89**, 485–9.

Xu, J., Levitt, R.C., et al. 1995. Evidence for two unlinked loci regulating total serum IgE levels. *Am J Hum Genet*, **57**, 425–30.

Xu, J., Postma, D.S., et al. 2000. Major genes regulating total serum immunoglobulin E levels in families with asthma. *Am J Hum Genet*, **67**, 1163–73.

Xu, W., Charles, I.G., et al. 1994. Mapping of the genes encoding human inducible and endothelial nitric oxide synthase (*NOS2* and *NOS3*) to the pericentric region of chromosome 17 and to chromosome 7 respectively. *Genomics*, **21**, 419–22.

Xu, W., Humphries, S., et al. 2000. Survey of the allelic frequency of a *NOS2A* promoter microsatellite in human populations: assessment of the *NOS2A* gene and predisposition to infectious disease. *Nitric Oxide*, **4**, 379–83.

Yazdanbakhsh, M., Sartono, E., et al. 1995. HLA and elephantiasis in lymphatic filariasis. *Hum Immunol*, **44**, 58–61.

Yazdanbakhsh, M., Abadi, K., et al. 1997. HLA and elephantiasis revisited. *Eur J Immunogenet*, **24**, 439–42.

Yee, L.J., Tang, J., et al. 2000. Tumor necrosis factor gene polymorphisms in patients with cirrhosis from chronic hepatitis C virus infection. *Genes Immun*, **1**, 386–90.

Yee, L.J., Tang, Y.M., et al. 2001. Interleukin 10 polymorphisms as predictors of sustained response in antiviral therapy for chronic hepatitis C infection. *Hepatology*, **33**, 708–12.

Yoshitake, S., Okada, M., et al. 1999. Contribution of major histocompatibility complex genes to susceptibility and resistance in *Helicobacter pylori* related diseases. *Eur J Gastroenterol Hepatol*, **11**, 875–80.

Yu, M.W., Chiu, Y.H., et al. 1999. Cytochrome P450 1A1 genetic polymorphisms and risk of hepatocellular carcinoma among chronic hepatitis B carriers. *Br J Cancer*, **80**, 598–603.

Zavaglia, C., Bortolon, C., et al. 1996. HLA typing in chronic type B, D and C hepatitis. *J Hepatol*, **24**, 658–65.

Zeidler, M., Stewart, G., et al. 1997. Codon 129 genotype and new variant CJD. *Lancet*, **350**, 668.

Zerva, L., Cizman, B., et al. 1996. Arginine at positions 13 or 70-71 in pocket 4 of HLA-DRB1 alleles is associated with susceptibility to tuberculoid leprosy. *J Exp Med*, **183**, 829–36.

Zimmermann, N., Bernstein, J.A. and Rothenberg, M.E. 1998. Polymorphisms in the human CC chemokine receptor-3 gene. *Biochim Biophys Acta*, **1442**, 170–6.

Zimmerman, P.A., Woolley, I., et al. 1999. Emergence of a FY*Anull in a *Plasmodium vivax*-endemic region of Papua New Guinea. *Proc Natl Acad Sci USA*, **96**, 13973–17.

Zinn-Justin, A., Marquet, S., et al. 2001. Genome search for additional human loci controlling infection levels by *Schistosoma mansoni. Am J Trop Med Hygiene*, **65**, 754–8.

Zipp, F., Windemuth, C., et al. 2001. Peripheral blood cell bulk cultures are not suitable for the analysis of the genetic control of T-cell cytokine function. *Immunol Lett*, **78**, 21–7.

PART V

INFECTION AND IMMUNITY

31

Viral interference with the host immune response

ANTONIO ALCAMI, ANN B. HILL, AND ULRICH H. KOSZINOWSKI

INTRODUCTION

The clearance of viruses from infected tissues requires a coordinated scenario of multiple effector functions. The immune response with its two arms of innate and adaptive immune responses represents the system by which the organism controls, preserves, and restores integrity. Clearing of the infection can often cause a substantial loss of cells with little functional impairment as a result of cellular regeneration. In the absence of cellular regeneration, e.g. in the central nervous system (CNS), the same loss may already result in considerable functional defects. Whether or not the immunological clearing of a virus infection protects tissues or causes pathology is defined by the speed and amount of virus replication, the strength of the immune response, and the properties of the infected tissues. Therefore, the outcome of either immunoprotection or immunopathology is defined by properties of the virus, the strength of the immune response and by the regenerative activity of the tissues (Levine 2002). Remarkably, viral immune evasion mechanisms target and modulate all aspects of the innate and the adaptive immune response. To discuss the functional relevance of the different viral function it should be recollected that host defense against viruses occurs in a series of waves.

Cells monitor their normal state and many of the effects of viruses on the intracellular milieu tend to activate the process of apoptosis or programmed cell death. This 'suicide' response can be considered a form of host defense, and most viruses seem to need to interfere with this response in order to be able to replicate. The innate immune response starts with the release of soluble mediators of inflammation. These mediators comprise, among others, the interferons, cytokines, chemokines, complement fragments, prostaglandins, and nitric oxide. These key regulators control cell trafficking and cell recruitment to inflamed sites, cell adhesion, and cell activation, but also induce apoptosis. Different cells produce different mediators. Usually, the organism seeks to eliminate the virus completely and the antiviral activities of some soluble mediators are very potent. However, the life cycle of some viruses, in particular those that establish persistent infections, is more complex and for them the evasion of innate immunity is important to reach the target tissues from which the virus cannot be cleared. Among other viruses the well-known hepatitis viruses B and C, human immunodeficiency virus (HIV), and herpesviruses share this property.

In the temporal scenario of the immune response natural killer (NK) cells form the second line of defense. NK cells play a major role in the early defense to viruses. They do not require prior sensitization to recognize and to kill virus-infected cells. The response is induced within hours of infection and usually peaks around 3 days. Herpesviruses, for example, are very sensitive to the control by NK cells and the molecules by which these viruses defend themselves against this strong effector mechanism of innate immunity today are the subject of active research.

The third wave includes adaptive immune responses which comprise cellular and humoral effector arms. Important cellular effectors are CD8 and CD4 T cells: these are first detectable at days 3–4, and usually peak at about 7 days. CD8 T cells play the critical role and in most cases are able to eliminate the virus. It was noticed first that viruses manage to escape the control of T cells by various molecular principles and this area of research has brought several interesting findings that reshape our understanding of the virus–host balance.

In the antibody response initially immunoglobulin IgM appears about 10 days postinfection, followed by IgG. Antibody plays some role in controlling primary infection but its main role is to prevent reinfection (by neutralization). Antibody effects can be mediated by complement activation. Even the antibody response and complement are diverted by some viruses to their profit.

EFFECTS ON MOLECULES THAT SIGNAL BETWEEN CELLS

Modulation of interferon functions

Interferons (IFN) were discovered because of their ability to protect cells from viral infection. The key role of both type I (α and β) and type II (γ) IFN as one of the first antiviral defense mechanisms is highlighted by the fact that anti-IFN strategies are present in most viruses (Figure 31.1).

Interferons are produced in response to viral infection, secreted from cells, and bind specific receptors that trigger intracellular events through Janus kinase (JAK) and signal transducers and activators of transcription (STAT) pathways (Goodbourn et al. 2000). These signaling events result in the upregulation of cellular proteins that limit viral replication in several ways. Some of the genes upregulated by IFN are the low-molecular-weight protein (LMP)-2 and LMP-7 subunits of the proteasome, involved in the generation of viral peptides

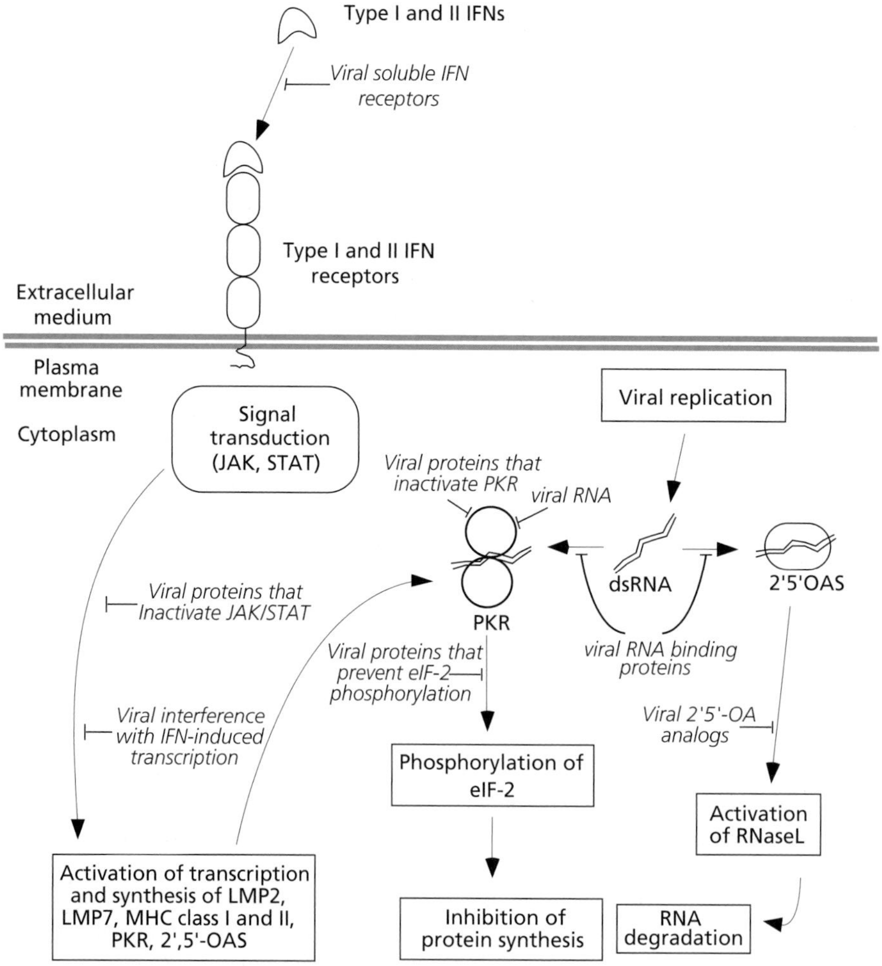

Figure 31.1 *Viral inhibition of interferon activity. See text for abbreviations.*

for the major histocompatibility complex (MHC) class I and class II molecules, the molecules that present viral peptides to T cells. Two major pathways that induce an antiviral state in cells are also upregulated by IFN: the double-stranded ribonucleic acid (RNA) (dsRNA)-dependent protein kinase (PKR) and the 2′,5′-oligoadenylate system (2′,5′-OAS) that activates RNase L. In addition, IFNs have immunomodulatory activity that can influence the type of immune response mounted as a reaction to infection.

Viruses block the activity of IFNs at three different levels: (1) blockade of IFN binding to specific receptors; (2) inhibition of signal transduction pathways induced by IFNs; and (3) inhibition of antiviral effector functions induced by IFNs (see Figure 31.1).

SECRETED VIRAL IFN RECEPTORS AND IFN-BINDING PROTEINS

Poxviruses encode proteins that are secreted from infected cells and bind with high affinity type I or II IFN (McFadden and Murphy 2000; Alcami 2003). These proteins prevent the interaction of IFNs with their receptors and the initiation of biological effects that lead to an antiviral state in the cell. Soluble cytokine receptors or binding proteins for other cytokines have been identified, mainly in the poxvirus family, and examples are discussed below.

The viral IFN-γ receptor (vIFN-γR) was first identified in myxoma virus (MV) and later in other members of the poxvirus family including vaccinia virus (VV) and cowpox virus (CV) (Upton et al. 1992; Alcami and Smith 1995; Mossman et al. 1995). The vIFN-γR has sequence similarity to the IFN-binding domain of the cellular IFN-γ receptor. In addition, VV and other poxviruses also encode a secreted IFN-α/β receptor or binding protein (vIFN-α/βBP) that has very limited sequence similarity to the cellular counterparts (Colamonici et al. 1995; Symons et al. 1995). The vIFN-α/βR has the unique property of binding to the cell surface after secretion (Alcami et al. 2000). This property allows the vIFN-α/βR to cover infected tissues with decoy receptors that prevent in a very efficient way the activation of IFN-mediated pathways. The role of vIFN-γR and vIFN-α/βBP during viral infection has been demonstrated by the attenuated phenotype of VV and MV mutants lacking these IFN inhibitors (Symons et al. 1995; Mossman et al. 1996).

INTERFERENCE WITH IFN SIGNALING

Some viral proteins interfere with the signaling cascade initiated in cells by the interaction of IFN with their receptors, and prevent the activation of antiviral mechanisms that limit viral replication (Goodbourn et al. 2000), e.g. the T antigen of murine polyoma virus binds to and inactivates JAK1 (Weihua et al. 1998), whereas protein V from simian virus 5 interacts with STAT1 and induces its degradation by the proteasome (Didcock et al. 1999). A different mechanism is used by Kaposi's sarcoma-associated herpesvirus (KSHV), a virus that encodes a homolog of the IFN-regulatory factor (IRF) which represses the IFN-mediated transcriptional activation of host genes (Zimring et al. 1998).

VIRAL MODULATION OF IFN EFFECTOR FUNCTIONS

One of the major antiviral effects of IFNs is the induction of the dsRNA-dependent PKR and 2′,5′-OAS pathways which lead to the blockade of gene expression in the cell and prevent the formation of infectious virus particles (Goodbourn et al. 2000). The replication and transcription of viral genomes can lead to the formation of double-stranded RNA (dsRNA) that activates PKR, which phosphorylates the translation initiation factor 2α (eIF-2α), causing its inactivation and the subsequent arrest of protein synthesis in infected cells. Viruses use several strategies to inhibit the activity of PKR (Gale and Katze 1998; Katze et al. 2002). Some viruses encode proteins that bind dsRNA and prevent activation of PKR, such as the VV E3L and reovirus σ3 proteins. Adenovirus and HIV encode RNAs that bind PKR but do not activate the enzyme, whereas herpes simplex virus (HSV) US11 and HIV Tat bind directly to PKR and inactivate the enzyme. An alternate strategy to block the PKR pathway is to prevent the phosphorylation of eIF-2α. This can be achieved by the expression of an eIF-2α homolog, the K3L protein of VV, which acts as a substrate of PKR, or by HSV IC34.5 protein-activating protein phosphatase 1α which removes the phosphate groups from eIF-2α. The formation of dsRNA during viral replication also activates the enzyme 2′,5′-OAS, producing 2′,5′-OA which in turn activates RNase L and the degradation of RNA within the infected cell, causing the blockade of viral replication. The synthesis of analogs of 2′,5′-OA by HSV, which bind RNase L, inhibits this pathway (Goodbourn et al. 2000). The proteins σ3 from reovirus and E3L from VV bind dsRNA and thus inhibit the activation of 2′,5′-OAS as well as PKR (see above).

Modulation of cytokine networks

Cytokines constitute a numerous family of molecules that play an important role in the initiation and regulation of the immune response. Cytokines are normally secreted from cells, although some are expressed at the cell surface, and bind to specific receptors on other cells. In this way, cytokines are used by the immune system to communicate among cells and to send signals that drive the immune response in a particular direction. In addition, some cytokines such as IFN and tumor necrosis factor (TNF) may act directly on infected cells and restrict virus replication.

The importance of cytokines in antiviral defense is highlighted by the number of mechanisms that viruses encode to block the activity of cytokines. The viral anticytokine strategies will normally result in down-regulation of immune responses. However, there are examples in which these viral mechanisms increase viral replication. Large DNA viruses such as poxviruses and herpesviruses have captured in their genomes genes that encode host cytokines and cytokine receptors (McFadden and Murphy 2000; Alcami 2003). This strategy enables these viruses to interfere with or to exploit cytokine pathways for their own benefit (Figure 31.2).

VIRAL CYTOKINES

The first viral cytokine identified was the VV epidermal growth factor homologue (VGF). This viral protein activates cell growth and favors viral replication, but an immune-related function has not been ascribed to it (McFadden and Murphy 2000). The first cytokine with immunomodulatory activity found in viruses is the IL-10 homolog (vIL-10) encoded by Epstein–Barr virus (EBV) (Hsu et al. 1990). Genes encoding IL-10 homologs have also been identified in other viruses. It has been shown that the EBV vIL-10 suppresses cellular immunity by inhibiting the production of IFN-γ, but has lost the immunostimulatory properties of the host counterpart. Other viral cytokines are the IL-6 homolog (vIL-6) encoded by KSHV (Moore et al. 1996) and the IL-17 homolog (vIL-17) encoded by herpesvirus Saimiri (HVS) (Yao et al. 1995). These cytokines may have immunomodulatory activity but vIL-6 and vIL-17 may also promote the proliferation of B and T cells, respectively, which represent the major host cell types for these viruses.

The identification of semaphorin homologs (vSEMA) in poxvirus and herpesvirus genomes was somehow surprising because semaphorins were described as chemoattractants and chemorepellents involved in axonal guidance during nervous system development, and only CD100 had been identified as a semaphorin involved in the immune system (Spriggs 1999). The characterization of vSEMA encoded by VV and ectromelia virus (EV) uncovered a specific receptor in macrophages and its proinflammatory activity, which was observed in mice infected with a VV expressing an active vSEMA protein. The precise role of vSEMA in immune modulation during viral infection remains to be determined.

SECRETED VIRAL CYTOKINE RECEPTORS

Viral genes encoding soluble cytokine receptors have been identified mainly in the poxvirus family. These cytokine receptors lack the transmembrane and cytoplasmic domains of the host counterparts, are secreted in large quantities from infected cells, and have the ability to bind with high affinity the cognate cytokine and block its activity. The poxvirus soluble cytokine receptors were initially identified because of their sequence similarity to the extracellular binding domain of their host counterparts. A second class of cytokine receptors, known as binding proteins, have very limited sequence similarity to the host cytokine receptors and were identified in cytokine binding or activity assays.

The first viral cytokine receptor identified was the viral TNF receptor (vTNFR) M-T2 encoded by MV (Smith et al. 1991). Subsequent studies identified four different genes encoding vTNFR in poxviruses such as CPV, VV, and EV, and were designated cytokine response modifier B (CrmB), CrmC, CrmD, and CrmE (Hu et al. 1994; Smith et al. 1996; Loparev et al. 1998; Saraiva and Alcami 2001). CrmB is equivalent to MV M-T2 but the other proteins are distinct with respect to binding properties and molecular size, and are produced at different times during viral replication. The reasons for such a variety of proteins apparently targeting the

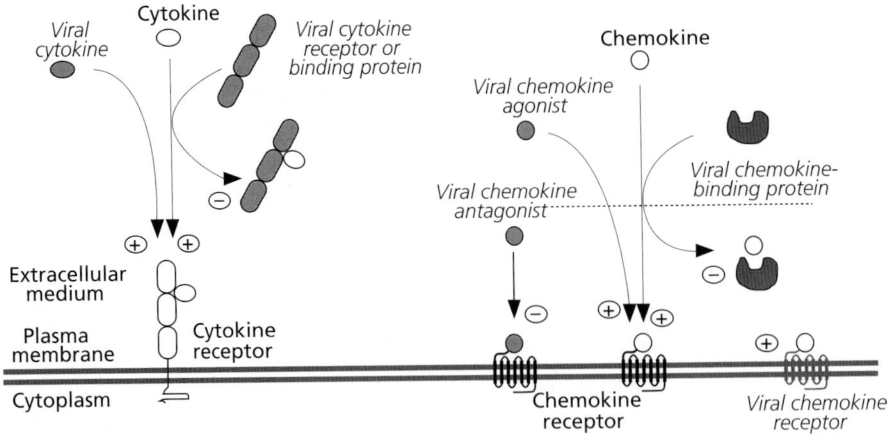

Figure 31.2 *Viral mimicry of cytokines, chemokines, and their receptors.*

same ligand are unknown. Clinical isolates of human cytomegalovirus (HCMV), but not laboratory strains, encode a membrane TNFR homolog related to herpesvirus entry mediator (HVEM) which is retained intracellularly (Benedict et al. 1999). No ligand has been identified for this protein and its function remains to be determined. More recently, another member of the TNFR superfamily has been identified in CPV and EV. In this case, the viral protein is a secreted and shorter version of human and mouse CD30 (Panus et al. 2002; Saraiva et al. 2002). Viral cytokine receptors function as decoy receptors neutralizing the activity of cytokines and, accordingly, vCD30 blocks the interaction of CD30 to CD30 ligand (CD30L). However, in this case the ligand is expressed only at the cell surface and vCD30 induces reverse signaling in CD30L-expressing cells. The function of vCD30 in the context of infection has not been elucidated, but administration of vCD30 to mice has been shown to downregulate type 1 cytokine-mediated inflammatory responses, a property that may help the virus to escape an efficient antiviral response (Saraiva et al. 2002).

The viral IL-1β receptor (vIL-1βR) is related to the human type II IL-1R and also acts as a decoy receptor (Alcami and Smith 1992; Spriggs et al. 1992). In contrast to the membrane IL-1Rs encoded by the host, the viral protein is specific for IL-1β and does not bind IL-1α or IL-1 receptor antagonist. Deletion of this gene in VV causes attenuation when the virus is administered intracranially (Spriggs et al. 1992), but leads to enhanced virulence associated with fever and accelerated death in mice infected through the respiratory route, a natural route of poxvirus transmission (Alcami and Smith 1992, 1996). The enhanced virulence observed after deletion of the vIL-1βR from VV illustrates that the role of some viral immunomodulatory proteins may be to reduce pathology induced by excess production of cytokines, in this case IL-1β, during infection rather than to cause immunosuppression.

VIRAL CYTOKINE-BINDING PROTEINS

IL-18 is a proinflammatory cytokine that is required, together with IL-12, for induction of IFN-γ and the generation of an efficient cellular response against viral infection. The poxvirus-encoded IL-18 binding protein (vIL-18BP) is a homolog of the human IL-18BP but has no sequence similarity to membrane IL-18 receptors. The vIL-18BP is an effective scavenger of IL-18, and downregulates IFN-γ production and NK responses in EV-infected mice (Born et al. 2000; Smith et al. 2000). Interestingly, the vIL-18BP is also expressed by molluscum contagiosum virus (MCV), a poxvirus that causes benign skin tumors and persists in the skin for months without inducing an inflammatory response (Xiang and Moss 1999; Smith et al. 2000). The vIL-18BP is the only cytokine receptor encoded by MCV and may be responsible in part for the lack of inflammation in MCV lesions.

The only soluble cytokine-binding protein identified in herpesvirus is encoded by EBV and binds colony-stimulating factor (vCSF-1BP) (Strockbine et al. 1998). This protein has limited sequence similarity to the cellular receptor and may modulate the response of macrophages during infection. Another example of a viral cytokine-binding protein that binds ligands using different host receptors is a secreted protein that binds granulocyte–macrophage-CSF and IL-2 encoded by orf virus, a virus that causes skin lesions in sheep, goats, and humans (Deane et al. 2000).

Modulation of chemokine networks

Chemokines are a family of small-molecular-size cytokines that induce cell migration and other biological effects, such as cell differentiation and angiogenesis, and play a critical role in the regulation of cells of the immune system throughout the body. There are more than 40 chemokines identified that can be structurally classified as CC, CXC, C, or CX3C, and mediate their biological response by binding and signaling through G-protein-coupled receptors, proteins that have seven-transmembrane domains. More than 20 chemokine receptors have been identified and their distribution in immune cells determines which type of cell migrates in response to infection or inflammation. There are three structural concepts used by viruses, mainly herpesviruses and poxviruses, to modulate chemokine activity: expression of chemokine homologs, chemokine receptor homologs, and secreted chemokine-binding proteins unrelated to the sequence of known host receptor proteins (McFadden and Murphy 2000; Murphy 2001; Alcami 2003)

VIRAL CHEMOKINE HOMOLOGS

The virus-encoded chemokine homologs are secreted from infected cells and function as agonists or antagonists. Chemokine antagonists such as vMIP-II from KSHV and MC148 from MCV, bind to chemokine receptors but do not transduce signals (Boshoff et al. 1997; Kledal et al. 1997; Krathwohl et al. 1997; Damon et al. 1998). These antagonists function as inhibitors of specific chemokine pathways and influence the migration of immune cells into infected tissues. By contrast, the viral chemokine agonists induce cell migration into areas of infection, and thus their function may be unrelated to immune evasion. The current thinking is that viral chemokine agonists recruit to areas of infection immune cells that represent good targets for viral replication and enhance viral dissemination. The chemokine encoded by the gene *UL146* from HCMV, known as vCXC-1, induces neutrophil chemotaxis by binding to CXCR2 and may explain the association of neutrophils with HCMV infections (Penfold et al. 1999). Human herpesvirus 6 (HHV-6) U83 induces monocyte migration that may favor the establishment of viral latency and persistence in the infected host (Zou et al. 1999). Another example of chemokine mimetics is the protein Tat from HIV which shows limited sequence similarity to chemokines. HIV Tat is a chemoattractant for monocytes and may enhance replication and spread of HIV in infected individuals (Albini et al. 1998). Direct evidence for a role of viral chemokine agonists in vivo comes from studies with murine cytomegalovirus (MCMV) mutants lacking the chemokine genes *M131/129*. The MCMV chemokine is encoded by the *m131orf* and is expressed as a fusion protein including the *m129 orf*. The isolated synthetic *m131* product attracts activated macrophages by engaging a receptor with structural properties related to human CCR3 (Saederup et al. 1999). The mutant MCMV lacking the function shows reduced spread to salivary glands, indicating that monocyte attraction serves for virus trafficking.

The role of the viral chemokines encoded by KSHV in viral dissemination has not been defined but they may play a role in pathogenesis as a result of their angiogenic properties which may cause the enhanced vascularization observed in Kaposi's sarcoma lesions (Boshoff et al. 1997). In addition, the KSHV chemokines are chemoattractants for Th2-polarized T cells and may influence the type of immune response initiated after viral infection (Sozzani et al. 1998; Dairaghi et al. 1999; Endres et al. 1999; Stine et al. 2000).

An interesting and recent addition to chemokine mimicry by viruses is the finding that glycoprotein G (gG) of respiratory syncytial virus has partial sequence similarity to fractalkine and has chemokine-like activity (Tripp et al. 2001). This property of gG may be used to facilitate virus attachment to infected cells and to modulate the host immune response.

VIRAL CHEMOKINE RECEPTOR HOMOLOGS

There are several examples of chemokine receptor homologs in members of the herpesvirus family and some in the poxvirus family. The function of these receptors in the viral infectious cycle is varied and difficult to demonstrate. Some viral chemokine receptors bind chemokines and transduce signals inside the cell. The ORF74 protein from KSHV is constitutively active and binding of chemokines can modulate the activation status of the receptor (Arvanitakis et al. 1997; Rosenkilde et al. 1999). The receptor has been shown to induce cell proliferation when expressed in cells in culture and its expression in transgenic mice causes the development of Kaposi's sarcoma-like lesions (Arvanitakis et al. 1997; Yang et al. 2000). The possibility that expression of KSHV ORF74 may contribute to neoplasia through a paracrine effect has been proposed, but may be difficult to demonstrate in KSHV-infected individuals. In any case, ORF74 illustrates how such proteins encoded by viruses may have a direct and profound effect on the pathology caused by viral infection. In vivo studies on the homologous ORF 74 encoded by murine γ-herpesvirus 68 (MHV-68) have revealed that the virus uses this receptor for virus reactivation from latently infected mouse splenocytes (Lee et al. 2003). Of the four chemokine receptor homologs encoded by HCMV, UL78, UL33, US27, and US28, US28 is most extensively studied. MCMV encodes the viral chemokine receptor (vCKR) M33 and M78, which are homologous to their counterparts in HCMV. HCMV US28 can modify the chemokine environment of infected cells by sequestering and internalizing chemokines, and depleting them from the medium (Bodaghi et al. 1998). Similarly, HHV-6 UL51 reduces extracellular accumulation of chemokines by sequestration, but also by a novel mechanism of downregulation of CCL5 (RANTES) transcription (Milne et al. 2000). The potential contribution of viral chemokine receptors to pathology is also illustrated by the fact that HCMV US28 expression on the cell surface mediates cell adhesion and vascular smooth muscle cell migration, and it is thought to be related to vascular disease (Streblow et al. 1999). Evidence for a role for viral chemokine receptors in virus replication in vivo was demonstrated first for MCMV M33 (Davis-Poynter et al. 1997).

VIRAL CHEMOKINE-BINDING PROTEINS

The third class of viral chemokine inhibitors are the viral chemokine-binding proteins (vCKBP) that sequester chemokines in solution without apparent sequence similarity to host chemokine receptors. These proteins were initially described in poxviruses, but an example has been identified recently in the herpesvirus family.

The MV M-T7 (vCKBP-1) is a soluble vIFN-γR with sequence similarity to human IFN receptors but was later found to interact with chemokines. MV M-T7 binds a broad spectrum of chemokines and it has been proposed that it prevents the interaction of chemokines with glycosaminoglycans (GAG) and the correct presentation of chemokines to leukocytes (Lalani et al. 1997). There is evidence that the interaction of chemokines with cell-surface GAGs is important for their function in vivo. The protein vCKBP-2 was identified in the medium from cultures infected with MV, VV, or CPV (Graham et al. 1997; Smith et al. 1997; Alcami et al. 1998). In this case, the protein binds CC chemokines with high affinity and neutralizes their effect by preventing the binding of chemokines to specific receptors in leukocytes. The protein M3 (vCKBP-3) encoded by murine MHV-68 was found to bind a broad range of chemokines, including C, CC, CXC, and CX3C chemokines, and to block their interaction with cellular receptors (Parry et al. 2000; van Berkel et al. 2000).

The generation of relevant virus mutants lacking specific vCKBPs and the infection of rabbits or mice suggest that these proteins may block chemokine-mediated leukocyte infiltration into infected areas in vivo (Mossman et al. 1996; Graham et al. 1997; Lalani et al. 1997). In addition, MHV-68 M3 has been proposed to be required by the virus to establish virus latency and to enable persistence of the virus in the host (Bridgeman et al. 2001). Sequestration of chemokines can also prevent the process of dendritic cell (DC) maturation and trafficking (see below).

VIRAL MODULATION OF CYTOKINE EXPRESSION AND ACTIVATION

Other mechanisms that modulate the synthesis of cytokines and the signaling cascade triggered by them have been described. The expression of cytokines mediated by the nuclear factor κB (NF-κB) and nuclear factor-activated T cell (NFAT) transcription factors in macrophages is blocked by an IκB homolog encoded by African swine fever virus (Miskin et al. 1998). The CPV protein CrmA was found to inhibit the IL-1β-converting enzyme (ICE) (or caspase-1), which proteolytically cleaves the precursor form of proinflammatory cytokine IL-1β (pro-IL-1β) to generate mature, active IL-1β (Ray et al. 1992). CPV CrmA may also prevent the maturation of IL-18, which is also proteolytically cleaved by ICE, and is an inhibitor of apoptosis (see below under Viral inhibitors of caspases).

There are several examples of viruses that inhibit cytokine-mediated signaling. Adenoviruses interfere with signaling induced by TNF at different levels (Mahr and Gooding 1999), and some herpesviruses and poxviruses inhibit signaling through death domains that lead to apoptosis (see below under Viral inhibitors of death receptor-mediated apoptosis). The poxvirus VV encodes two intracellular proteins that block signaling mediated by Toll-like and IL-1 receptors by mimicking intracellular regulatory domains of these receptors (Bowie et al. 2000). The Toll-like receptor pathway is important in NF-κB activation and amplification of inflammatory signals.

Lastly, some viruses may subvert cytokine-mediated signaling for their own benefit. The latent membrane protein 1 (LMP1) of EBV recruits components of the TNFR and CD40 transduction machinery and induce biological responses such as cell proliferation that may enhance virus replication (Farrell 1998).

APOPTOSIS

Programmed cell death (apoptosis) is a ubiquitous and evolutionarily conserved mode of cell death. Individual cells are eliminated or removed from the organism in a temporal manner or in response to specific signals without affecting neighboring cells. Apoptosis plays a central role in tissue homeostasis throughout life (Rathmell and Thompson 2002). Apoptosis is characterized by loss of cell volume or cell shrinkage, chromatin condensation, internucleosomal DNA fragmentation, phosphatidylserine exposure, membrane blebbing, and the formation of apoptotic bodies. These stereotypical morphological changes, associated with natural death, are based on a highly regulated genetic program. The activation of a class of cysteine proteases, termed 'caspases', as the central effectors plays an essential role. Caspases are synthesized initially as single polypeptide chains representing latent precursors (zymogens) which undergo proteolytic processing at specific aspartic acid residues to produce two distinct subunits that assemble to the active heterotetrameric protease. In mammalian cells, activation of the caspase zymogens has been reported to occur through at least three independent mechanisms: cleavage by upstream active caspases; cleavage by granzyme B, an aspartate-specific serine protease found in the granules of cytolytic T cells; and autoprocessing of zymogens with assistance from other caspase-interacting proteins that can occur in either a *cis*- or *trans*-acting manner (for reviews, see Salvesen and Dixit 1997; Benedict et al. 2002; Bortner and Cidlowski 2002; Trapani and Smyth 2002)

There are several caspases that are functionally redundant. Once activated, one caspase can activate other caspases in the proteolytic cascade (Stennicke et al. 1998). The trigger of the proteolytic cascade involves the physical association of zymogens via adaptor proteins with protein interaction modules that assemble the receptor signaling complex. The apoptotic program in cells includes mechanisms that activate and those that inhibit apoptosis. There are two main pathways of apoptosis.

Death receptor-initiated activation of caspases

Cells can receive extrinsic signals that instruct them to die. The primary receptor through which death signals are signaled are members of the TNFR family, such as Fas and TNFR-1(19,24). Binding of receptor and ligand on the cell surface results in the formation of the hetero-oligomeric death-inducing signal complex (DISC). The apoptosis-inducing quality of a death receptor ligand system is defined by the death domain (DD) located in the intracellular portion of the death receptor. The DISC is assembled by complex protein interactions. The DDs and death effector domains (DED) carried by different proteins, e.g. caspases, are essential components. DISC proteins interact with other proteins through homotypic interactions of DD and DED contacts. The basis of the interaction is structural motifs of the DD which form six antiparallel helical bundles. Adaptor proteins such as FADD contain both a DD and a DED motif in one polypeptide and provide the bridging between DD domains of receptors with a DED-containing caspase. Among the caspases, mainly the initiator caspases-8 and -10 are recruited to the DISC. It is thought that the conformational properties and local concentrations of different proteins in the DISC complex govern caspase activation by autocatalytic processing (Schmitz et al. 2000; Walczak and Sprick 2001).

Mitochondrial pathway of caspase activation

Independent of the extrinsic death receptor pathway, apoptosis is also controlled intrinsically at the level of mitochondria. Mitochondrial death can result from the loss of extracellular vital signals (death by neglect), and by signals affecting the cell cycle, through activation of p53 and the proapoptotic p53 target genes (Rathmell and Thompson 2002). Changes in nutrient uptake, serum withdrawal, the deprivation of cytokines, and other metabolic events that affect the cellular redox potential, or the ability properly to regulate active oxygen species, lead to apoptosis. An important molecule in mitochondrial apoptosis is cytochrome *c*. Cytochrome *c* resides in the space between the inner and outer membranes of the mitochondria. The release of cytochrome *c* initiates mitochondrial apoptosis at the apoptosome, a protein complex called Apaf-1. It consists of the caspase-activating molecules, which can bind to caspase-9 through homotypic interaction via a domain defined as caspase-recruitment domain (CARD). For activation of caspases, Apaf-1 requires cytochrome *c*. A number of signals control the oligomerization of Apaf-1–caspase-9 complexes. Additional proteins that have CARD domains can have opposing activities on apoptosome formation, either inhibition or enhancement.

Procaspase-8 activation can also occur at sites other than the cell surface. BAP-31, an integral protein of the endoplasmic reticulum, can recruit an isoform of procaspase-8, procaspase-8L, containing an N-terminal extension in response to apoptotic signals. This suggests an additional organelle-specific pathway of cell death (Ng et al. 1997; Nguyen et al. 2000; Breckenridge et al. 2002). This pathway is also regulated by the Bcl-2 proteins discussed below (Figure 31.3).

Cellular regulation of extrinsic apoptosis

The cellular homolog of the viral caspase-8 (FLICE) inhibitory protein (cFLIP) consists of two DED domains and a caspase domain that lacks the enzymatic active site. Therefore, cFLIP can bind but not cleave cellular zymogen substrates. It is spliced in two forms; one form contains only the two DED domains; the other, long form includes the caspase-like domain. In addition, cFLIP may block caspase-8 recruitment to the DISC or may inhibit proteolytic processing of the proenzyme. However, cFLIP can also promote recruitment of caspase-8, which can stimulate autoprocessing to the active form.

REGULATION OF CASPASE ACTIVITY

Regulation of caspase activity is central to the death process (Bortner and Cidlowski 2002). The inhibitor of apoptosis (IAP) family of proteins regulates caspase activation and activity. The first member of the IAP family was found in baculovirus. The cellular proteins with antiapoptotic function share, with the baculovirus protein, the baculoviral IAP repeat (BIR), a domain that consists of about 70 amino acids with conserved spacing of cysteine and histidine residues, which fold into a zinc-binding structure. Through the BIR domain, IAP molecules bind and directly inhibit caspase activation. Several IAPs also contain a ring-finger domain located near the C termini. Through the activity of the ring-finger domains, IAPs can target caspases for ubiquitinylation and degradation. IAPs themselves are again subject to inhibition by other proteins that activate caspases. IAPs can bind to caspases in either the active configuration or the inactive proform state.

REGULATION OF MITOCHONDRIAL APOPTOSIS

The Bcl-2 family of proteins controls the release of proapoptotic proteins from mitochondria. Bcl-2 is present in the outer mitochondrial membrane and Bcl-2-like proteins have pore-forming activities and prevent the release of cytochrome *c*. The Bcl-2 family proteins are characterized by protein domains defined as Bcl-2 homology (BH). Four such domains, BH1–4, have been identified. BCL-2 proteins have up to four BH domains. The α-helical BH3 domain of one protein interacts with a receptor formed by a hydrophobic pocket created by BH1–3 of the other protein. Through BH domains BH2 family members interact with each other and form homo- and heterodimers, which results in the promotion of abrogation of the function of the binding partner. Bcl-2 family members have either proapoptotic or antiapoptotic properties. Many antiapoptotic Bcl-2 family members contain domains BH1, -2, and -4. Proteins that carry only the BH3 domain define a family of proapoptotic proteins. Many death-signaling pathways require one BH3-only protein to activate the Bcl-2 family members BAX and BAK in order to activate the caspase. BAX and BAK are functionally redundant and their overexpression leads to mitochondrial accumulation of the protein and initiation of apoptosis. BAK-type proteins make the mitochondrial membrane permeable so that it releases intermembrane apoptogenic factors.

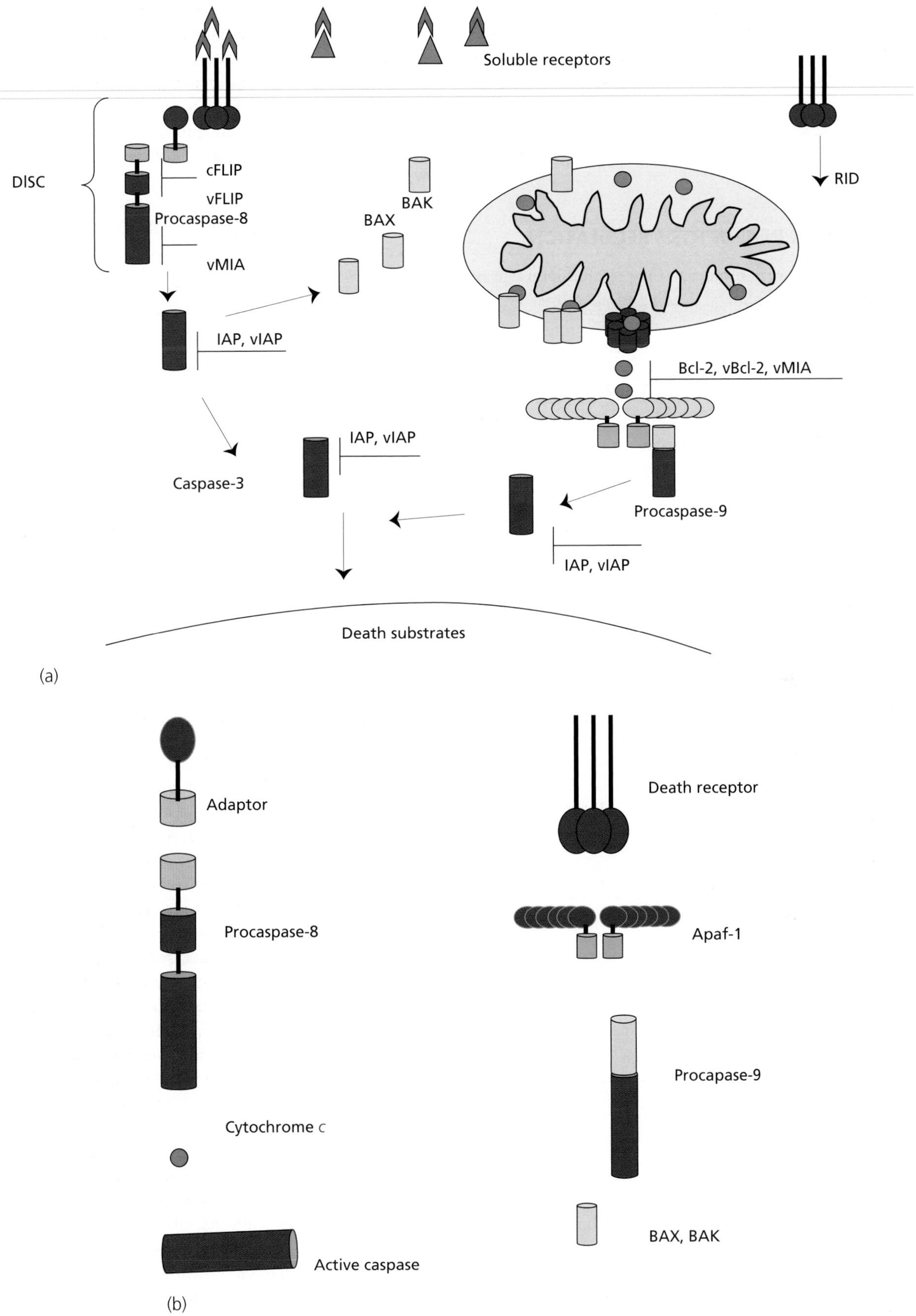

Figure 31.3 *Viral regulation of apoptosis. See text for abbreviations.*

BAX is primarily cytoplasmic but translocates to mitochondria on apoptotic stimuli. Specific conformational alterations of BAX allow mitochondrial docking. Like BAX, BAK has a transmembrane domain and is targeted to mitochondria where it exists as a monomer or in a complex with other Bcl-2 family members. Antiapoptotic Bcl-2 family proteins bind and inhibit the proapoptotic proteins.

CELLS DIFFER IN APOPTOSIS REGULATION

Cell lines differ with respect to the preferential usage of the two signaling pathways leading to apoptosis. Type 1 cells constitutively contain a large amount of caspases at the DISC. Fas triggering results in caspase-8 activation, followed by cleavage of caspase-3 and loss of the mitochondrial transmembrane potential. In type 2 cells, there is little DISC formation and the intrinsic mitochondrial pathway is required as an amplifier to initiate the full apoptosis cascade after Fas activation. Only in type 2 cells can apoptosis triggered by extrinsic signals be blocked by BCL-2 overexpression. Apoptosis in type 2 cells is dependent on the activities of mitochondria, whereas apoptosis in type 1 cells is not. T cells have type 1 and liver cells have type 2 characteristics (Scaffidi et al. 1998).

Chaperones and chaperone-like proteins that support the folding of newly synthesized proteins can also have pro- and antiapoptotic functions. Heat shock protein (HSP) 70-like chaperones inhibit apoptosis, whereas HSP-60 and HSP-10 have proapoptotic functions. Likewise, protein kinases modulate apoptosis. Mitogen-activated kinases (MAPK) control apoptosis through transcription, e.g. the upregulation of cFLIP, and also through transcription-independent mechanisms.

Viral control of apoptosis

Replication for viruses, as obligatory intracellular parasites, is dependent on cellular function. Therefore, for virus replication it is important that apoptosis triggered by soluble mediators of innate immunity via death receptors and caspase cascades is inhibited. The viral replication machinery diverts and exhausts cellular functions. Thus, viral protein synthesis, viral morphogenesis, and viral release must destabilize the homeostasis and integrity of the cell. This results in the activation of the intrinsic pathway of apoptosis. For effective viral progeny generation, it is important to delay this process. Some viruses also have proapoptotic properties, which may contribute to the release of virus particles from the cell that is already depleted from its resources. The execution of a proapoptotic function may also be advantageous, if apoptosis of an infected cell causes phagocytosis by another cell and enables the virus transfer to cells that the virus cannot infect directly. Therefore, it is not surprising that viruses may contain both antiapoptotic and proapoptotic functions. Some of the viral genes controlling apoptosis are derived from the host cell genome; for others there are no known homologs. NK and T-effector cells have two important functions: they kill infected cells through the perforin/granzyme pathway or by engaging fas, and they secrete several cytokines, among which IFN-γ is known to be essential for control of virus in some situations. Both pathways of cytolysis induce apoptosis of targets. The viral antiapoptotic functions may play a role in diminishing effector cell efficacy, but caution is warranted before making this assumption. Virus-infected cells are generally readily lysed by T cells, so long as the T-cell receptor (TCR) is triggered, in spite of the presence of antiapoptotic mechanisms. It is likely that the strength of the death signal imposed, particularly by the perforin/granzyme pathway, is able to overcome most antiapoptotic mechanisms.

VIRAL INHIBITORS OF DEATH RECEPTOR-MEDIATED APOPTOSIS

Poxviruses secrete proteins that bind to cytokines, which in turn activate death receptor-mediated apoptosis. This probably represents the earliest possible defense against apoptosis signals. The expression of the death receptor CD95 is inhibited by viral IFN regulatory factors from HHV-8 that inhibit the binding of IFN-γ induced IFN regulatory factor 1 (IRF-1) to specific domains in the CD95L promoter (Kirchhoff et al. 2002). The functions of adenovirus interfere with the apoptosis mediated by the TNF receptor superfamily at a very early stage and at various levels (Burgert et al. 2002; McNees and Gooding 2002). Post-translational downregulation of FAS is carried out by the E3/10.4K–E3/14.5K protein complex, also named receptor internalization (RID) and degradation, together with the E3/6.7K protein. The RID complex contains transport motifs in the cytoplasmic tail of the proteins which are recognized by the intracellular transport machinery that directs the CD 95/RID complex to lysosomes. Apart from CD95, the TNF-related apoptosis-inducing ligand (TRAIL) receptor can form a death-inducing signaling complex. In addition TRAIL receptors are downregulated by the E3 proteins of adenovirus.

The DISC is the next target for modulatory viral proteins. It is assembled by protein interaction between DDs and DEDs. Search for proteins carrying homology to DEDs led to the identification of viral proteins with two DEDs (Derfuss and Meinl 2002). These viral proteins block the activation of caspase-8 (FLICE) and were therefore named viral FLICE inhibitor proteins (vFLIPs). These vFLIPs have been detected in poxvirus and several herpesvirus genomes. In addition, vFLIPs regulate the expression of transcription factors for proteins involved in apoptosis regulation. The product of the HCMV gene, *UL36 vICA*, binds procaspase-8 but lacks homology to cFLIP (Goldmacher 2002).

VIRAL INHIBITORS OF CASPASES

The archetypal member of the cellular IAP family was found in baculovirus. Through the BIR, a motif that can be present up to three times, IAP molecules bind and directly inhibit caspase activation. Other caspase inhibitors are the poxvirus serine protease inhibitor CrmA (which targets a number of caspases) and related proteins from other poxviruses and African swine fever virus, and p35 of baculovirus. Interestingly, viral proteins can combine IAP properties with properties of BCL-2 protein functions (Wang et al. 2002b).

VIRAL INHIBITORS OF MITOCHONDRIAL APOPTOSIS

Prevention of mitochondrial permeabilization is essential for the replication of many viruses. Many γ-herpesviruses encode one or more molecular homologs of BCL-2, the cellular antiapoptotic protein family (Cuconati and White 2002). Viral BCL-2 homologs are also found in adenovirus and poxvirus genomes. Viral BCL-2 proteins act as apoptosis inhibitors and their structure is similar to that of the cellular BLC-2 proteins. However, despite the preservation of the overall structure the unstructured loops that encode sites for phosphorylation and proteolysis, and which may be required for regulation, the function of the cellular proteins differs between vBCL-2 and cellular BCL-2 proteins. All vBCL-2s have a BH1 and at least one other BH2 or BH3 region. Mitochondrial apoptosis is a limiting factor in the life cycle of DNA viruses, because in cells deficient in BAX and BAK the onset of cytopathic effects is delayed and more viral replication can occur. In adenovirus the E1-B19K inhibits the formation of the highly oligomeric BAX/BAK complex at the mitochondrial membrane.

The viral mitochondrial localized inhibitor of apoptosis encoded by HCMV (vMIA) also targets mitochondria but acts differently from the viral BCL-2 homologs (Goldmacher 2002). It has no BCL-2 homology domains and has no affinity to BAX. However, vMIA forms a complex with adenine nucleotide translocator (ANT), a component of the mitochondrial transition pore complex, which cooperates with BAX in the mitochondrial control of apoptosis (Marzo et al. 1998).

CELLULAR EFFECTOR CELLS OF INNATE IMMUNITY

Natural killer cells, effector cells of innate immunity

Natural killer cells are large granular lymphocytes that have potent antiviral effector mechanisms: they kill infected cells using the perforin/granzyme pathway, and release copious amounts of IFN-γ. In many virus infections, viral titers start to decline as a result of NK function well before the adaptive CD8 immune response has any effect. Unlike T cells, NK cells do not have clonally expressed antigen receptors with specificity for viral peptides. Instead, they use a series of germline-encoded receptors to detect the consequences of virus infection on cells, irrespective of the antigenic composition of the infecting virus. Some of these receptors are activating, and some are inhibitory. Signals from these receptors are integrated, leading either to killing and release of IFN, or no action.

For NK cells to control virus, they need (1) to be induced, (2) to traffic to the site of virus infection, (3) to be able to detect virus-infected cells, and (4) to perform their effector functions (killing cells and releasing IFN-γ). Discussion of interference with NK cells is usually limited to the third step – NK recognition of infected cells. NK trafficking and effector mechanisms are very similar to those of CD8 T cells, and are discussed below. NK cells are induced by cytokines – particularly type I interferons and IL-12, which are produced by infected tissues, and viral interference with production of those cytokines affects the NK response.

Natural killer cells integrate signals from activating and inhibitory receptors to achieve activation threshold (Colonna et al. 1999; Fong and Cambier 1999; Long 1999; Ravetch and Lanier 2000; Lanier 2001). It is likely that not all of these receptors and their ligands have been identified. Two important activating receptors are known: CD16 is an Fc receptor that enables NK cells to lyse cells with bound antibody, a process known as antibody-dependent cell-mediated cytotoxicity (ADCC) (see below under Inhibition of humoral immunity). ADCC is not generally considered to play a major role in antiviral immunity, and obviously plays no role in the NK control of the first few days of infection.

A second major activating receptor – NKG2D – has recently been described (Bauer et al. 1999; Wu et al. 1999). NKG2D is a C-type lectin that homodimerizes to generate a functional receptor. Most NK cells express NKG2D, making it an important activating receptor. Through a positively charged residue in its transmembrane domain, it interacts with the immunoreceptor tyrosine based activation motif (ITAM)-containing DAP10, to deliver a strong activating signal to the cell. In addition to NK cells, NKG2D is expressed on activated classic CD8 T cells and on γδ T cells: for these cells, it acts as a costimulatory molecule, i.e. signaling through NKG2D is not enough to activate the cell. For NK cells, however, NKG2D signaling is sufficient for activation. The ligands for NKG2D show loose homology to MHC class I. It is not yet clear whether all ligands have been identified, and the main ligands are different for humans and mice. In humans, MICA and MICB are stress-inducible molecules expressed mainly in epithelial tissues, and, interestingly, by most carcinomas (Bauer et al. 1999). MIC expression is induced by HCMV infection (Groh et al. 2001). A second set of receptors are the UL16-binding proteins (ULBP), discovered as the targets for HCMV *UL16* (see below) (McNees and Gooding 2002). The ULBP are homologous to one set of murine ligands for NKG2D – the retinoic acid early inducibles (RAE). The other known murine ligand is H60, a minor histocompatibility antigen expressed in BALB/c mice (Diefenbach et al. 2000)

There are two families of inhibitory receptors for human NK cells: the killer immunoglobulin-like receptors (KIR) and the C-type lectin NKG2A/CD94 paired heterodimer. The KIR are members of the immunoglobulin superfamily, and are encoded in a locus on chromosome 19 (Vilches and Parham 2002). They interact with classical MHC class 1 molecules, different members having different specificities. In particular, important inhibitory KIR recognize a limited polymorphism on HLA-C and HLA-B molecules. KIR are expressed on subsets of NK cells; one theory of NK cell development suggests that during their education NK cells must express at least one inhibitory receptor capable of recognizing self-MHC. NKG2A/CD94 interacts with HLA-E, a nonpolymorphic class I molecule that binds peptides derived from the leader sequence of classic MHCI molecules (Braud et al. 1998a). Murine NK cells also have two families of inhibitory receptors. They share NKG2A/CD94 with humans and the murine homolog of HLA-E is Qa1. The second inhibitory receptor family is Ly49, a family of C-type lectins that also recognize polymorphic class I molecules. All of these inhibitory receptors recognize MHCI and they thus enable the NK cells to monitor the function of the class I pathway. Viruses that interfere with the class I antigen-presenting pathway run the risk of rendering infected cells susceptible to NK lysis.

It is important to note that not all KIR and Ly49 molecules are inhibitory. Some lack cytoplasmic tails with immunoreceptor tyrosine-inhibition motifs (ITIM) and instead pair with adaptor molecules to activate cells. Furthermore, some NKG2 family members that recognize HLA-E molecules have an activating function. The function of the inhibitory members of these families in the control of NK lysis appears plausible; the function of the activating members is less clear (with the exception of Ly49H, discussed below).

VIRAL INTERFERENCE WITH NK RECOGNITION OF INFECTED CELLS

Several viruses have been described to interfere with the ability of NK cells to detect infection; this is summarized in Figure 31.4.

Human cytomegalovirus UL18 is a class I homolog – it shares 25 percent amino acid homology with classic class I, and pairs with host β_2-microglobulin for expression on the surface of infected cells. When it became appreciated that loss of cell surface class I, induced by HCMV infection, would make infected cells vulnerable to NK lysis, the idea that UL18 would engage NK inhibitory receptors and prevent NK lysis became an attractive hypothesis. Indeed Reyburn et al. (1997) used transfected cells expressing UL18 to demonstrate protection from NK lysis in vitro. However, it is controversial whether UL18 functions in this way in vivo. First, cell surface expression of UL18 in infected cells is very low. Second, none of the well-characterized NK inhibitory receptors have been shown to interact with UL18. Third, when a ligand for UL18 was identified (see section The leukocyte immunoglobulin-like receptors below), it was found to be mostly expressed on macrophages, B cells, and DCs, although it is also expressed on some NK cells (Cosman et al. 1997). The ligand, leukocyte immunoglobulin-like receptor 1 (LIR-1), is inhibitory, so it may indeed function to inhibit NK lysis.

Murine CMV also encodes a gene – *m144* – with homology to classic MHCI. The gene *m144* also pairs with β_2-microglobulin to produce a class I-like structure. Mice infected with a virus lacking *m144* control it better than they control wild-type virus (Farrell et al. 1997). The difference in titers is particularly evident 3 days after infection, when NK control is most important. Furthermore, mice depleted of NK cells show no difference in their ability to control wild-type virus or the *m144* deletion mutant. All this suggests that *m144* would inhibit NK recognition of infected cells. However, a direct demonstration that *m144* interacts with NK cells to inhibit their activation is lacking. Although it is clear that *m144* acts somewhere in the NK pathway, the exact site of action remains to be demonstrated. As with UL18, the discovery of other class I-interacting molecules (see The leukocyte immunoglobulin-like receptors below) raises possibilities other than direct interaction with NK inhibitory receptors.

Molluscum contagiosum virus is a poxvirus that establishes persistent infection, unlike other poxviruses. It also encodes an MHCI homolog of unknown function, which complexes with β_2-microglobulin (Senkevich and Moss 1998).

Another MCMV gene – *m152* – has been clearly shown to interfere with NK lysis. The gene *m152* is also loosely related to class I by secondary structure. Its best understood function is interference with antigen presentation to $CD8^+$ T cells (see below under Retention of class I molecules in pre-golgi compartments). However, Krmpotic et al. (2002) found a that a virus lacking *m152* had much lower titers 3 days after infection – a time at which NK cells are the main antiviral mechanism – than wild-type virus. This was surprising because *m152* is known to decrease cell surface expression of classical MHC1, and it was thought that it should therefore make the virus more (not less) vulnerable to

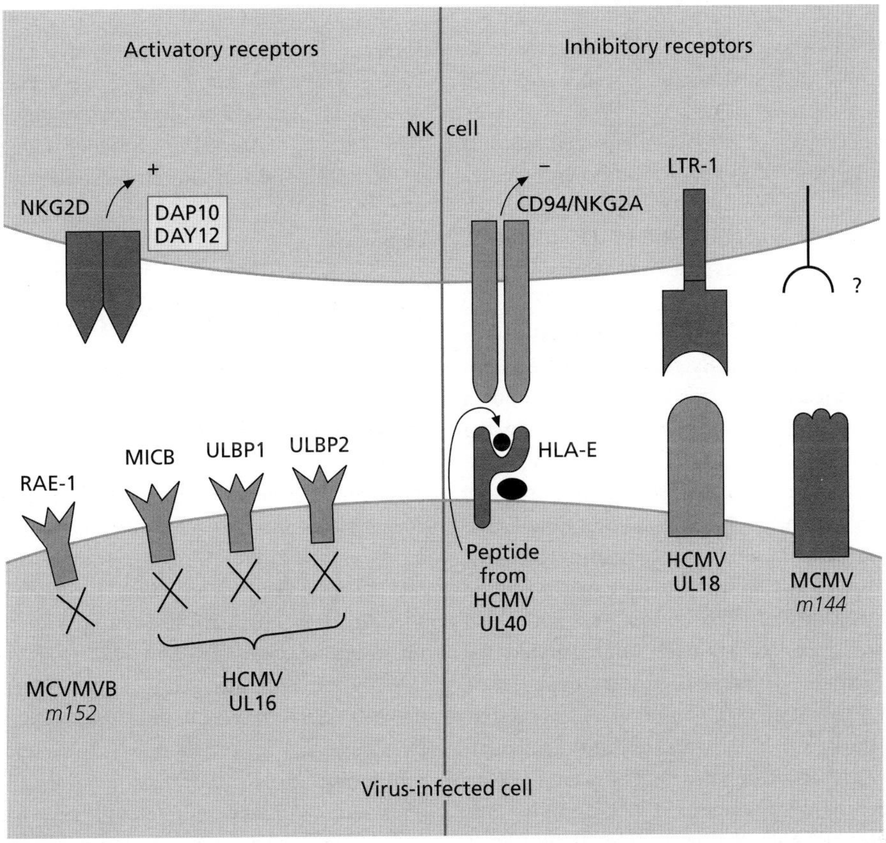

Figure 31.4 *Viral interference with natural killer (NK)-activating receptors and provision of 'decoys' for inhibitory receptors. See text for abbreviations.*

NK control. The riddle was solved when Krmpotic et al. found that *m152* also reduced the level of an NK ligand on the surface of infected cells. As described above, the RAEs and H60 are loosely class I-like molecules, and serve as a ligand for the important NK-activating receptor NKG2D. Cells infected with a virus lacking *m152* had high ligand levels and were more susceptible to NK lysis than those infected with wild-type virus.

In HCMV a soluble form of the *UL16* gene product was found to interact with human ligands for NKG2D: MICB, ULBP1, and ULBP2 (Cosman et al. 2001). The ULBPs were actually identified by their interaction with UL16. UL16 retains MICB, ULBP1, and ULBP2 inside the cell. In fact, HCMV increases the transcription of all NKG2D ligands, and cell surface expression of MICA and ULBP3, the two ligands not targeted by *UL16*, is increased by HCMV infection. How these contradictory effects translate into susceptibility to or protection from NK lysis is still an open question.

Another NK inhibitory effect has been described for HCMV. As described above, NKG2A/CD94 is an important inhibitory receptor on NK cells. NKG2A recognizes the nonpolymorphic HLA class I molecule HLA-E (Braud et al. 1998a). HLA-E binds peptides derived from the leader sequence of classical class I molecules, which must be transported back into the endoplasmic reticulum by transporter associated with antigen processing (TAP) (Braud et al. 1998b). HLA-E cell surface expression is reduced if classical class I is absent or if TAP is impaired. It thus serves to monitor the integrity of the class I pathway. As the HCMV genes *US2* and *US11* cause rapid destruction of newly synthesized class I (see below under Degradation of newly synthesized MHCI molecules) and *US6* blocks the function of TAP, HCMV infection should render cells vulnerable to NK lysis through silencing of NKG2A/CD94 signaling. However, another HCMV protein, UL40, has in its leader sequence a peptide capable of binding to HLA-E (Tomasec et al. 2000). Furthermore, this peptide remains in the endoplasmic reticulum after signal sequence cleavage and is able to bind to HLA-E in the absence of functional TAP. Thus HCMV is able to circumvent the HLA-E pathway. It is still controversial whether the relative effects of either UL40 or class I downregulation dominate the susceptibility of HCMV-infected cells to NK recognition, i.e. whether the final effect is susceptibility or protection (Falk et al. 2002; Wang et al. 2002a). Again, the final outcome may be different in different cell types, times after infection, etc.

HIV does not directly interfere with NK recognition. However, investigators have noted that HIV-nef interference with class I cell surface expression affects HLA-A and -B molecules but not HLA-C (Collins et al.

1998). As HLA-C isoforms are the most important ligands for KIRs, this may prevent HIV-infected cells becoming vulnerable to NK attack as a result of loss of KIR inhibition.

KSHV-K5 is known to downregulate cell surface classic class I molecules. However, it also downregulates intercellular adhesion molecule 1 (ICAM-1) and B7-1, known to be important for NK cell lysis (Ishido et al. 2000). In consequence, K5 expression protects transfected cells from NK lysis.

A viral gene has been reported which, instead of protecting from NK lysis, actually renders infected cells susceptible to a protective NK response. It was known that a gene in the NK locus has a major effect on the susceptibility of different mouse strains to MCMV. Mice from the resistant strains have a more effective NK cell response. It was recently discovered that the gene controlling resistance is *Ly49H* – an activating receptor found on a subset of NK cells. The surprising finding was that the ligand for *Ly49H* is not, as had been presumed, a host-encoded molecule upregulated by infection, but is actually a viral gene product encoded by the gene *m157* (Arase et al. 2002; Smith et al. 2002). The gene *m157* has no known other function and is dispensable for virus replication in vitro and in vivo. It also interacts with an inhibitory receptor, *Ly49C*, and investigators have postulated that this is its true evolutionary function.

THE LEUKOCYTE IMMUNOGLOBULIN-LIKE RECEPTORS

Human CMV encodes a molecule – UL18 – with 25 percent homology to MHCI heavy chain. As described above, it was assumed that UL18 would interact with KIRs and prevent NK lysis of HCMV-infected cells. This idea was supported when it was shown that cells transfected with UL18 were resistant to lysis by some NK cells (Reyburn et al. 1997). However, identification of the ligand for UL18 led to the discovery of an entirely new gene family – the leukocyte immunoglobulin-like receptors (LIR) (Cosman et al. 2001). The LIRs are structurally related to the KIRs and human IgA Fc-receptor, and are encoded in close proximity to those genes on chromosome 19. There are eight LIRs – all but one are membrane glycoproteins; some contain ITIMs, whereas others have an arginine in their transmembrane region which suggests that they pair with another chain and have an activating function (Fanger et al. 1999). The ligand identified for UL18 is LIR-1; its cytoplasmic tail contains ITIMs. It is expressed on most B cells and monocytes and a variable number of T cells and NK cells. In addition to UL18, LIR-1 binds to most HLA-A, -B, and -C molecules. The physiological function of this molecule, and hence what HCMV achieves by encoding a ligand for it, is currently unknown.

Most of the other LIRs are also expressed on monocyte and DCs but not on lymphocytes. LIR-2 also binds class I molecules, but the ligands for the other LIRs are not yet identified. The discovery of this family indicates that the role of MHCI in immunobiology is not yet fully understood, and this should be taken into account when considering the function of viral genes that inhibit class I expression.

EFFECTS ON THE ADAPTIVE IMMUNE RESPONSE

Viral interference with DC functions

The cellular arm of the adaptive immune response consists of CD4 and CD8 T cells. CD8 T cells are the most important effector arm of adaptive antiviral immunity. The effective antiviral T-cell response requires orchestration. Antigen-presenting cells (APC), usually DCs, capture antigen and travel from the site of infection to the draining lymph nodes, where they activate naïve T cells. Naïve T cells that recognize antigen on DCs remain trapped in the lymph node. They start to proliferate for several days, and acquire the effector phenotype. Activated effector T cells can enter tissues. This is essential for CD8 T cells to interact directly with and to lyse virus-infected cells. Infected tissues provide chemokine and cytokine signals that enable T cells to extravasate and direct them to the site of infection. In the tissues, CD8 T cells have two main effector mechanisms that are antiviral: cytolysis of infected cells and release of antiviral cytokines, especially IFN-γ. CD4 T cells can make antiviral cytokines, but also provide critical help for CD8 T cells and for antibody production. Viruses have found several points of intervention within this process. These will now be dealt with individually: first, processes that would affect both CD4 and CD8 T cells, followed by mechanisms specific for each cell type.

Among APCs, mainly DCs are able to activate naïve T cells. DCs are generated in the bone marrow, circulate in the blood, and enter tissues in an immature state. Immature DCs are active in phagocytosis, but are poor APCs as a result of intracellular retention of class I and class II molecules and low expression of costimulatory molecules such as CD80 and CD86. Immature DCs can phagocytose dying cells, cellular debris, immune complexes, and proteins. They can also be infected by many viruses. In the context of adequate mediators produced during infection, they differentiate to mature DCs that are extremely potent APCs and stimulators of T cells. Maturation also triggers their migration into the lymphatics and to the T-cell areas of draining lymph nodes. Maturation signals produced during virus infection include type I IFN from infected cells and TNF-α from tissue macrophages. DCs have two main ways of activating CD8 T cells to initiate the T-cell response to viruses. First, infected DCs can present antigen through the classic endogenous pathway of MHCI-restricted antigen presentation. Second, they can 'crosspresent' antigens that they acquire by phagocytosis of proteins, which are degraded to peptides for loading on to their class I molecules. Sources of material that can be 'crosspresented' include cells dying by either apoptosis or necrosis; cellular debris, immune complexes, and perhaps heat shock proteins from dying cells that have bound viral peptides. Crosspresentation is described in Figure 31.5. The relative importance of the two DC presentation pathways depends on (1) the ability of viruses to directly infect DCs and (2) the extent to which viruses interfere with the direct presentation pathway (Figure 31.5).

For CD4 T cells, crosspresentation is the classical pathway of antigen presentation and is called exogenous presentation. Still controversial is the role of loading of class II molecules with endogenously synthesized viral proteins in infected class II-positive cells. This is discussed further below. Like CD8 T cells, naïve CD4 T cells are found only in blood and secondary lymphoid tissue, and they depend on trafficking of DCs to lymph nodes to be activated. Mature DCs that present viral antigen to naïve T cells are critical for the initiation of a T-cell response. There are three aspects of this with which viruses can interfere:

1 Interference with DC trafficking: DCs enter uninfected tissue, but they enter sites of infection in much greater numbers. Interference with chemokines and cytokines could affect migration.
2 Interference with the ability of DCs to present viral antigen: many viruses interfere with the class I antigen processing and presentation pathway. This would interfere with and perhaps prevent directly infected DCs from activating T cells, but would not interfere with crosspresentation. Although viruses might also be able to interfere with crosspresentation (perhaps via a secreted product), so far no such mechanism has been described.
3 Interference with the ability of immature DCs to mature, which is essential for APC function. The normal response of a DC to virus infection is to mature into an APC. Type I IFNs, induced by most virus infections, are powerful DC maturation stimuli. However, several viruses have been described that do not initiate maturation of DCs, and in fact interfere with the ability of the DCs to mature in response to other stimuli (Figure 31.6).

A well-studied viral interference with DC function occurs during measles virus infection; this infection elicits good protective immunity, including CD8 T cells, and yet is associated with a profound immunosuppression which supports additional infection by other infectious agents. This superinfection contributes to the morbidity and mortality associated with measles. The interaction of measles virus and DCs is complex. Measles virus infects DCs and induces their maturation and IL-12 production (Schnorr et al. 1997). This stimulates virus replication in the infected DCs. However, measles virus-infected DCs inhibit rather than promote proliferation of T cells. A few infected DCs are enough to inhibit the ability of a large number of uninfected

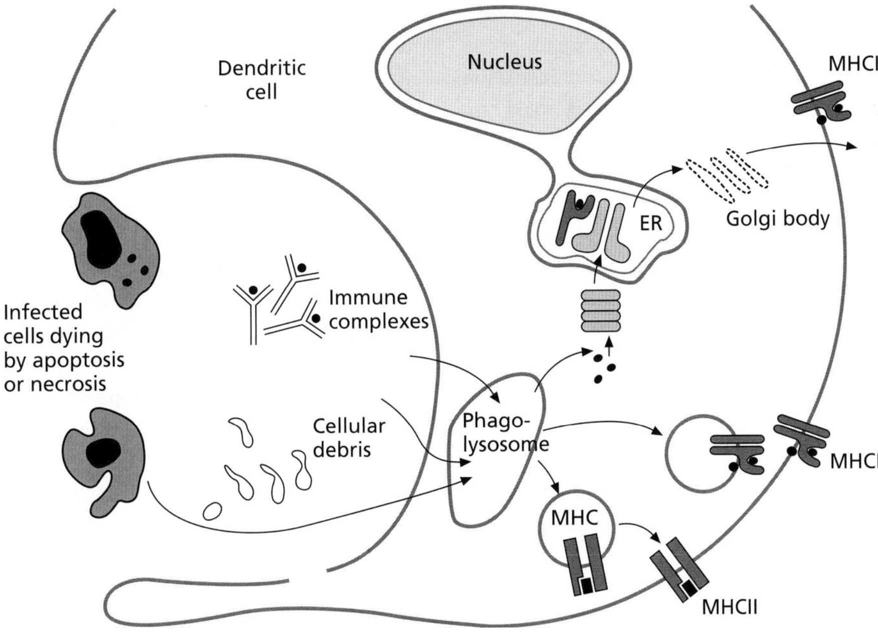

Figure 31.5 *Crosspresentation of viral antigens to CD8 T cells: activation of antiviral T cells despite immune evasion genes. Phagocytosomal material is re-presented on the dendritic cell's MHC molecules. The pathways for crosspresentation via MHCI are still poorly defined.*

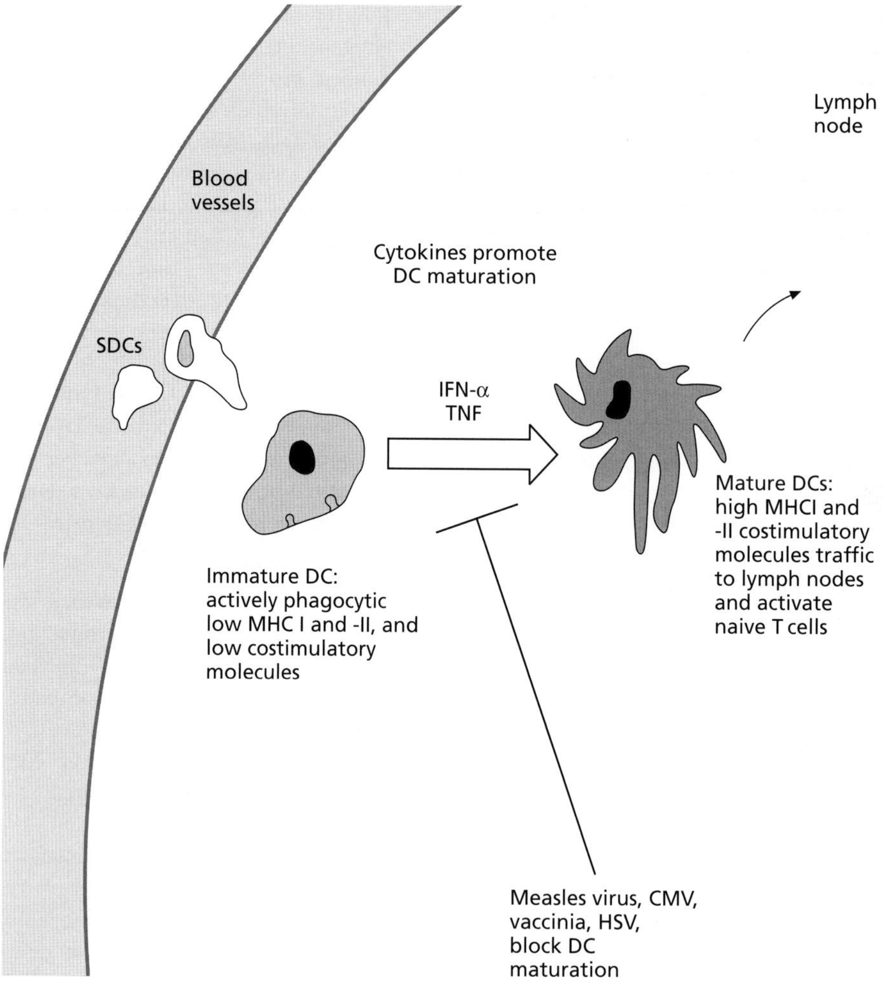

Figure 31.6 *Viral interference with dendritic cell (DC) maturation or function. CMV, cytomegalovirus; IFN-α, interferon α; TNF, tumor necrosis factor.*

DCs to promote T-cell proliferation (Grosjean et al. 1997; Schnorr et al. 1997). Measles virus induces the expression of the apoptosis-inducing ligand TRAIL on DCs (Vidalain et al. 2000); T cells and DCs cocultured with measles virus both undergo apoptosis (Fugier-Vivier et al. 1997; Servet-Delprat et al. 2000). Measles virus interference with DC function is thought to be the major mechanism of the generalized immunosuppression associated with MV infection.

Engelmayer et al. (1999) reported that VV impaired maturation of human DCs, and concluded that this would impair immunity. Drillien et al. (2000) also noted that VV inhibited maturation of human monocyte-derived DCs. However, VV-infected DCs efficiently stimulate memory T cells from infected individuals. In fact, infected DCs have been observed interacting with T cells in vivo (Norbury et al. 2002). Another study in mice concluded that both direct presentation by virus-infected DCs and crosspresentation contribute to CD8 T-cell priming in VV-infected mice (Basta et al. 2002). VV, the vaccine for smallpox, is the poster child of good viral immunogens. If VV does impair DC function, this effect is presumably mild and does not prevent an immune response.

Inhibition of DC maturation has also been reported for HSV (Salio et al. 1999) and MCMV (Andrews et al. 2001). The CD8 T-cell response to MCMV is thought to be largely achieved by crosspresentation (Gold et al. 2002), which suggests that functional DC impairment could play a role. HCMV is also thought to affect DC function. Moutaftsi et al. (2002) reported that HCMV impaired DC maturation. Mature DCs, on the other hand, were reported to increase costimulatory molecules after HCMV infection (Raftery et al. 2001). They also expressed the apoptosis-inducing ligands, FasL and TRAIL, suggesting that they might induce a generalized immunosuppression similar to measles.

Interference with antigen presentation in the MHC class I pathway

The most widely studied and best-appreciated viral immune evasion mechanisms have been found to affect

CD8 T-cell recognition of virus-infected cells. There are two basic strategies: viruses can interfere with the MHCI pathway of antigen presentation, or they can mutate the epitopes that CD8 T cells recognize, forcing the immune system to generate new effectors from naïve precursors.

Several viruses, mostly herpesviruses, have evolved genes that interfere with the MHCI pathway. Immune evasion genes of this type have been called viral genes that interfere with antigen presentation (VIPR) (Yewdell and Hill 2002). The pathway of MHCI-mediated antigen presentation is quite complex, and the past few years have seen a flurry of discoveries of viral gene products that interfere, to varying degrees of specificity, with almost every aspect of this pathway. Some viruses – notably CMV – actually encode several genes that all target this pathway. We begin this section by following the class I antigen presentation pathway and describing the various mechanisms that viruses use to attack it.

ANTIGEN DEGRADATION

The first step in antigen processing for the MHCI pathway is degradation of viral proteins in the cytosol, mostly by the proteasome. Proteasome function is vital for the health of the cells, and few viruses target this aspect. However, the EBNA-1 protein of EBV contains a long segment of repeated glycine and alanine residues, which renders the protein resistant to proteasomal degradation, and peptides for cytotoxic T lymphocyte (CTL) recognition are not generated (Levitskaya et al. 1995). EBNA-1 is the only protein that EBV needs to be expressed during latency, and this mechanism may help to prevent eradication of the latent virus pool.

When HCMV infects a cell the phosphoprotein pp65, a structural protein that has kinase activity, is also introduced. This protein is apparently able to prevent presentation of the immediate early (IE) peptide of the immunodominant IE1 protein, perhaps by phosphorylating IE1 and altering its proteolysis (Gilbert et al. 1996) (Figure 31.7).

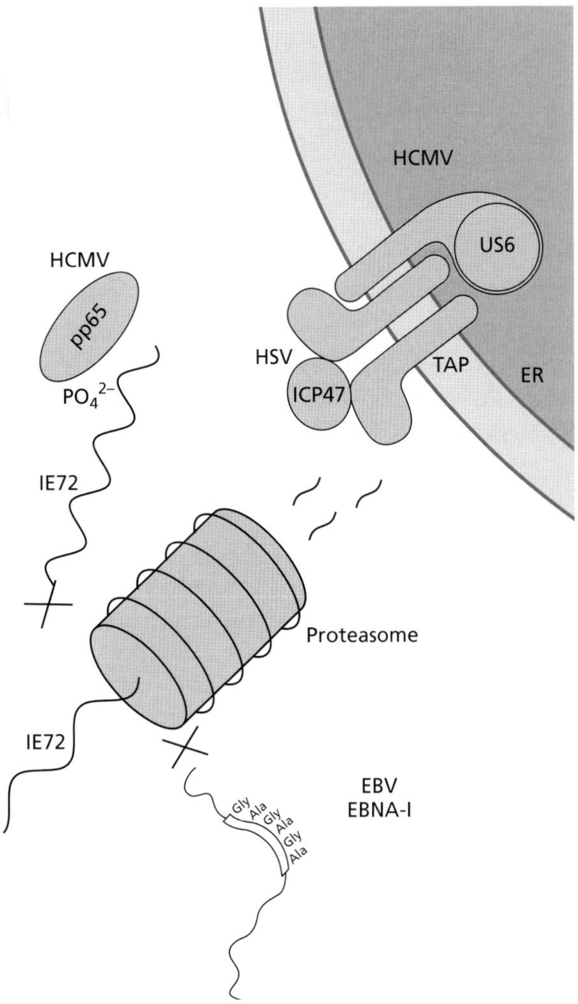

Figure 31.7 Interference with production of peptides and transport into the endoplasmic reticulum (ER). See text for abbreviations.

TRANSPORT OF PEPTIDES BY TAP

Peptides are transported by the TAP from the cytosol into the endoplasmic reticulum where they can bind to class I molecules. TAP is a member of the seven-transmembrane ATP-binding cassette family of transporters, and appears to have no other function. It can thus be incapacitated by viruses without impairing other cellular functions that the virus may need. TAP is specifically targeted by at least two VIPRs. The HSV IE gene *US12* encodes a polypeptide of 87 amino acids, ICP47, which is abundantly expressed in the cytosol (York et al. 1994). It binds to TAP and inhibits peptide transport, with the result that newly synthesized class I molecules are unable to leave the endoplasmic reticulum, and antigen presentation is prevented (Fruh et al. 1995; Hill et al. 1995). Both HSV-1 and HSV-2 encode ICP47; as a result of a frame shift mutation, they are homologous only in their first 35 amino acids, and this region of the molecule is all that is required for inhibition of TAP (Galocha et al. 1997).

The HCMV protein US6 also binds to TAP and inhibits peptide transport, although not as potently as ICP47 (Ahn et al. 1997; Hengel et al. 1997; Lehner et al. 1997). US6 is a transmembrane glycoprotein that binds TAP on the luminal side of the endoplasmic reticulum.

THE PEPTIDE-LOADING COMPLEX

In the endoplasmic reticulum, MHCI molecules associate with TAP as part of a peptide loading complex that also includes tapasin, calreticulin, and a thiol oxidoreductase. This complex not only ensures that class I is in the optimal place to acquire peptides, but also orchestrates peptide loading and provides poorly understood quality control functions. Several VIPRs associate with this complex, but it is not understood whether this is a coincidental consequence of binding their main targets or whether it plays a role in their interference with the pathway. The adenovirus protein Ad5E3 19K binds TAP and interferes with the ability of tapasin to bring class I and TAP together in the peptide-loading complex (Bennett et al. 1999). This function may supplement its ability to retain class I (see below under Retention of class I molecules in pre-golgi compartments).

SYNTHESIS OF MHCI MOLECULES

Many viruses interfere with host gene expression, either globally or selectively. As newly synthesized class I molecules are required for peptide loading, interference with synthesis of MHCI affects antigen presentation. However, the extent to which this mechanism would affect the antiviral efficacy of CTL depends on a number of timing issues: the half-life of class I RNA (if transcription but not RNA stability is affected); the average residence time of MHCI in the endoplasmic reticulum (which varies considerably between class I isoforms); the timing in the viral replication cycle of antigen expression (the earliest expressed proteins and structural viral proteins that can be processed immediately upon viral entry are less affected); and the length of the viral replication cycle (viruses with long replication cycles can gain more from mechanisms that would only impact CTL recognition after a lag time of many hours or days). One virus for which interference with MHCI synthesis has a clear impact on CTL efficacy is HSV. The viral host protein shut off (vhs) factor encoded by HSV UL40 is a virion structural protein. Upon virus entry it strips RNAs from ribosomes, allowing viral transcripts to be translated at the expense of host transcripts. The function is especially potent in HSV-2: within half an hour of virus infection synthesis of host proteins, including MHCI, essentially ceases. HSV UL40 has been shown to affect CTL recognition of infected cells (Tigges et al. 1996).

DEGRADATION OF NEWLY SYNTHESIZED MHCI MOLECULES

One of the most effective VIPR mechanisms is that employed by the HCMV proteins US2 and US11. These proteins bind MHCI in the endoplasmic reticulum and cause it to be transported back through the translocon. In the cytosol, MHCI is ubiquitinylated and destroyed by the proteasome (Wiertz et al. 1996a,b). The process is very potent and in HCMV-infected fibroblasts metabolic labeling reveals very little class I (Beersma et al. 1993). These particular genes have been intensely studied, not just because of their immune evasion function, but also because they have helped to elucidate an important cell biological pathway – the degradation of endoplasmic reticulum proteins. US2 and US11 are both type I membrane glycoproteins, and both bind MHCI via their luminal domains. However, they are not structurally homologous, and show some differences in the way that they achieve MHCI destruction, e.g. the carboxyl end of US2, but not US11, is required for MHCI degradation (Furman et al. 2002). The cytoplasmic tail of MHCI is, however, required (Story et al. 1999). These molecules show a specificity for class I isoforms and degrade HLA-A and -B, but not HLA-C, molecules (Schust et al. 1998). HLA-C can present peptide antigens to CTL, but it also has an important role as ligand for inhibitory KIR receptors on NK cells (see above).

The mouse $\gamma 2$ herpesvirus 68 also causes destruction of class I molecules. The K3 protein of MHV-68 is a ubiquitin ligase: it ubiquitinylates the cytoplasmic tail of endoplasmic reticulum-resident MHCI, targeting it for destruction in the cytosol (Boname and Stevenson 2001). Interestingly, the highly homologous K3 and K5 proteins of KSHV also ubiquitinylate MHCI, but this serves to target cell surface MHCI for degradation (Figure 31.8).

RETENTION OF CLASS I MOLECULES IN PRE-GOLGI COMPARTMENTS

Several VIPRs prevent MHCI from trafficking to the cell surface without causing their destruction. The adenovirus 5 protein E3 19K contains a di-lysine motif in its cytoplasmic tail; this motif binds to coat protein 1 (COP-1), which retrieves vesicles from the Golgi and returns them to the endoplasmic reticulum (Jefferies and Burgert 1990). In fact, this pathway was identified because of the E3 19K protein. The result is that MHC I is retained in the endoplasmic reticulum. Ad5E3 19K does not interact with all MHCI molecules equally, and the result is that some MHCI isoforms are more efficiently retained than others.

The HCMV protein US3 also causes MHCI to be retained in the endoplasmic reticulum. US3 binds to peptide-loaded MHCI molecules. The mechanism of retention is not clear, because US3 does not contain an endoplasmic reticulum retention motif, and is in fact exported (Ahn et al. 1996; Jones et al. 1996). It is thought that the mechanism of retention involves repeated release and rebinding by newly synthesized US3 (Gruhler et al. 2000). As with most of the HCMV VIPRs, US3 has been studied primarily in transfected cells. In infected cells, the destruction of newly synthesized MHCI as a result of US2 and US11 is so rapid that the role of US3 is hard to appreciate. US3 is synthesized earlier in the viral replication cycle than US2 and US11, and it has been hypothesized that it prepares MHCI for destruction by US2 and US11 (Ahn et al. 1996).

Murine CMV also encodes a VIPR that retains class I molecules. The *m152/gp40* causes MHCI to be retained in the endoplasmic reticulum–Golgi intermediate compartment (ERGIC) and, as with US3, the mechanism is unclear (Ziegler et al. 1997). It has quite different efficacy against different MHCI isoforms (Kavanagh et al. 2001). Yet even for isoforms in which retention is not especially impressive (e.g. Kb, which is only 50 percent retained by *m152*), *m152* has a profound

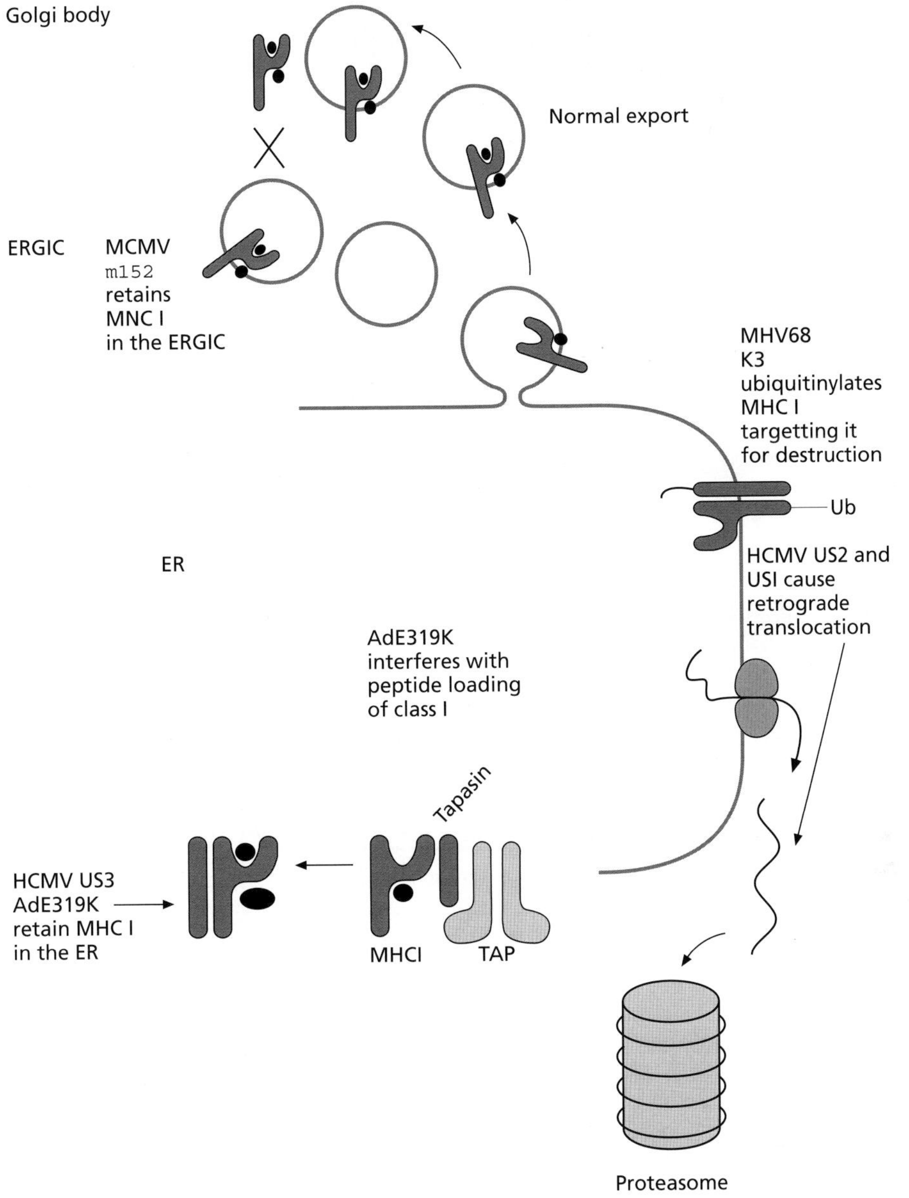

Figure 31.8 *Interference with MHC class I in the endoplasmic reticulum (ER) and endoplasmic reticulum Golgi intermediate compartment (ERGIC).*

effect on antigen presentation. Cells infected with wild-type virus are not detected by CTL, but cells infected with a virus lacking *m152* are readily detected. To prevent recognition of wild-type-infected cells by Kb-restricted CTL, the virus needs the two other MCMV VIPRs – *m4* and *m6* – the mechanisms of which are discussed below. Even so, the importance of *m152* remains enigmatic, and it may indicate that there is more profound synergism in the functions of these genes than is appreciated. Something similar may explain why HCMV needs its four VIPRs. As discussed above, in addition to retaining classical MHCI molecules, *m152* also prevents surface expression of molecules, which activates NK cells (Krmpotic et al. 2002).

REMOVAL OF MHCI MOLECULES FROM THE GOLGI APPARATUS OR THE CELL SURFACE

Several VIPRs remove class I from the cell surface. The KSHV genes *K3* and *K5* both reduce cell-surface MHCI expression. K3 ubiquitinylates MHCI after endoplasmic reticulum export. This signals MHCI internalization from the plasma membrane for endosomal degradation (Hewitt et al. 2002). The MCMV protein m6 contains a di-leucine motif in its cytoplasmic tail, which sorts it to lysosomes. It binds MHCI in the endoplasmic reticulum, and targets MHCI to the lysosome for destruction (Reusch et al. 1999). Of the three MCMV VIPRs, m6 has by far the most profound effect on cell-surface class I; from about 6 h after infection MHCI is rapidly lost

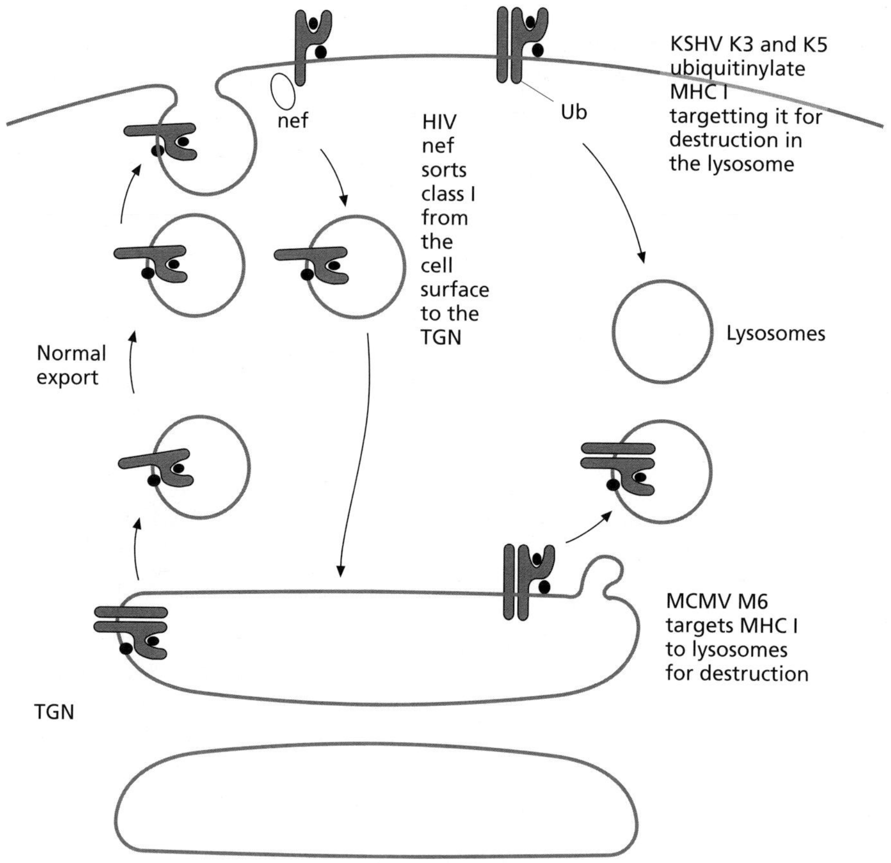

Figure 31.9 *Interference with MHC class I at the Golgi body and cell surface.*

from the cell surface if m6 is present (Wagner et al. 2002).

The HIV (and simian immunodeficiency virus (SIV)) nef protein serves a number of functions. One of them is to remove MHCI from the cell surface and take it to the trans Golgi network (TGN) – an effect that has been shown to impair CTL destruction of HIV-infected cells. The mechanism of action of HIV nef is quite different from that of KSHV-K3. Nef binds to the PACS-1 protein that sorts molecules to the TGN: presumably it acts as a bridge between class I and PACS-1 (Piguet et al. 2000) (Figure 31.9).

The MCMV protein m4/gp34 binds to MHCI both in the endoplasmic reticulum and at the cell surface. m4 is necessary to prevent lysis of infected cells by K^b-restricted CTLs (Kavanagh et al. 2001). The mechanism of action of m4 is not understood, but it is likely that its association with class I at the cell surface prevents the productive engagement of the TCR.

CD8 T-cell epitope variation

With the exception of nef, all the VIPRs described above are encoded by large DNA viruses, the coding capacity of which gives them the luxury of such highly specialized immune evasion devices. Small RNA viruses have also other means of avoiding CTLs. As a result of their rapid mutation rate, they exist in nature as a diverse genetic mix, often referred to as a 'viral swarm'. Mutations in CTL epitopes should allow the selection of escape variants, unless the exact epitope sequence is crucial for viral replicative function. This means that, as CTL clones develop and become immunodominant, virus variants arise that escape detection. Whether CTL escape mutants help the virus to persist in a host has been a matter of debate for some time. However, recent evidence in both monkeys and humans demonstrates that mutants of a particular epitope have a selective advantage in hosts that possess the MHCI molecule capable of binding the epitope, but not in hosts that do not possess that allele (Allen et al. 2000; Goulder et al. 2001).

Significance of viral interference with CD8 function in vivo

Most of the mechanisms reported above have been identified in vitro, and many of them have been described only using cells transfected with an isolated viral gene driven by a strong promoter. Their significance for infected cell recognition by CD8 T cells in vivo remains to be demonstrated. Obviously, true in vivo studies can be carried out only in animal models. The mouse is by far the most useful model for this purpose, although the importance of the HIV epidemic has led to studies of

SIV in infected macaques. As a result of the high degree of variation between the MHCs of different species, and the specificity of VIPRs for MHCI isofoms, studies of immune evasion need to be conducted in the natural virus host. For mice, MCMV is the most useful model, although the vole virus MHV-68 infects laboratory mice well and has provided important insights.

The first VIPR to be studied in vivo was the MCMV gene *m152*. Although wild-type MCMV-infected cells often escape detection by CTLs in vitro, cells infected with viruses lacking *m152* are always readily detected by CTLs. Krmpotic et al. showed that a virus lacking *m152* grew to about a log lower titer at day 7 (the time of peak CTL activity) than wild-type virus, but grew to the same titers in CD8 T-cell-deficient animals (Krmpotic et al. 1999). This effect was modest given the impact that *m152* has on CTL recognition in vitro, and challenges our concept of CD8 T-cell effector function in vivo. It has further been noted that a viral epitope whose presentation is completely abolished by *m152* in vitro is nevertheless equally immunodominant in mice infected with wild-type virus and with virus lacking *m152*, at least during the acute response. This suggests that cross-presentation is the main mode of antigen presentation driving the acute CTL response (Gold et al. 2002). However, viruses lacking *m152*, or indeed all three VIPRs, continue to provoke a very strong CTL response throughout the life of the animal. Therefore, it is unclear how the VIPRs of MCMV modulate the immunobiology of the virus.

MHV-68 K3 downregulates MHCI and prevents CTL recognition of infected cells. MHV-68 has a complex pattern of infection, analogous to EBV (Doherty et al. 2001). After initial replication in the lungs, which is controlled by IFNs and to some extent by CD4 T cells and CD8 T cells, MHV-68 seeds the splenic B cells. These undergo a massive CD4-dependent proliferation, with concomitant amplification of the latent virus load. This situation is brought under control by the immune response, and a truly latent infection is established. Although expression of viral genes is limited during the splenic amplification phase, K3 is expressed. A virus lacking K3 grew to normal titers in the initial lung infection, but did not undergo splenic amplification unless CD8 T cells were removed (Stevenson et al. 2002). Thus this VIPR function is thought to be to prevent CD8 T-cell control of the splenic amplification stage.

The selective advantage of CTL escape mutants in SIV and HIV infection in vivo has been clearly established, as described above under CD8 T-cell epitope variation. There is also evidence that the MHCI downregulating ability of nef is important. As nef has multiple functions, a specific mutant that affected its ability to downregulate MHCI, but not CD4, molecules was made. The mutant and wild-type viruses grew equally well in vitro. However, because the mutation affected a single codon, a mutation back to the wild-type sequence occurred in all four animals infected with the mutant virus within a few weeks (Munch et al. 2001). This suggested a strong selective pressure for the ability to downregulate MHCI.

Modulation of MHCII expression

CD4 T cells play a role in antiviral immunity, but the exact role is controversial. They provide essential help for B cells, and effective CD8 memory also depends on CD4 T cells. Two mechanisms may be involved in CD4 T-cell help for CD8 T cells: secretion of growth-supporting cytokines such as IL-2 and activation of DCs for activation of CD8 T cells. This so-called 'licensing' role requires direct recognition of the DCs by the CD4 T cell. CD4 T cells may also be direct antiviral effectors in their own right. They synthesize antiviral cytokines, especially IFN-γ, and if stimulated by professional APCs in the vicinity of the infection their role in secreting IFN-γ may be significant. Also, some viruses replicate in professional APCs that express MHCII, and many somatic cells are induced to express MHCII by IFN-γ. If these cells express class II loaded with viral antigen, CD4 T cells may have a direct antiviral effect by either killing the infected cell or secretion of cytokines.

Several viruses decrease the cell surface expression of class II by interfering with its synthesis. Most non-hemopoietic cells do not express MHCII, but (at least in humans) can be induced to do so by IFN-γ. Viruses such as herpesviruses and adenoviruses that interfere with IFN-γ signaling pathways will therefore interfere with induction of class II on these cells. MCMV induces the secretion of IL-10 by macrophages, and this leads to a decrease in macrophage MHCII expression (Redpath et al. 1999). Cells infected with HCMV also have decreased cell surface MHCII as a result of transcriptional inhibition of MHCII (Sedmak et al. 1994).

Some of the same HCMV proteins that interfere with MHCI expression have also been shown – in transfected cells – to interfere with MHCII in a similar manner. US2 causes HLA-DRα chains to be re-transported into the cytosol and degraded by the proteasome. Interestingly, it has the same effect on the α chain of HLA-DM, the essential chaperone for peptide loading on to class II (Tomazin et al. 1999). US3 has also been shown to cause intracellular MHCII retention. (Hegde et al. 2002). From the above, it is clear that there may be some advantages to viruses in interfering with MHCII molecules, but in general the functional evidence for interference with presentation of endogenous viral antigens is lacking, and there are no in vivo data. The real significance of these phenomena remains to be demonstrated.

Superantigens

Some viruses manipulate the immune system by stimulating T cells of irrelevant specificity. The B-type retrovirus, mouse mammary tumor virus (MMTV), encodes a superantigen that binds to certain TCR β chains and to MHCII, causing a massive proliferation of all CD4 T cells with the appropriate TCR. These activated T cells provide the necessary stimulation to drive proliferation of virus-infected B cells, which is essential for the infective process (Huber et al. 1994). EBV also has superantigen-like activity. Proliferation of CD4 T cells expressing the V-β13 TCR chain is a feature of EBV infection (Sutkowski et al. 1996). It has recently been shown that EBV activates an endogenous human retrovirus, HERV-K18, the envelope glycoprotein of which has superantigen activity (Sutkowski et al. 2001). Whether this activity plays a role in EBV pathogenesis is unclear but, as EBV undergoes latency in B cells, concomitant B-cell proliferation could aid the establishment of a latent virus pool.

Inhibition of humoral immunity

The production of antibodies specific to viral antigens may neutralize virus particles and thus prevent the infection of susceptible cells. Antibodies bound to viral antigens of cells can be detected by Fc-receptor-carrying effector cells. Viral antigens can activate the complement cascade, directly or in association with antibodies, leading to the destruction of infected cells or enveloped virus particles. Viruses with an RNA genome accumulate mutations caused by the low fidelity of the RNA polymerase. Virus particles with different antigenic properties may evade recognition by specific antibodies. Genetic variability may also generate variant peptide sequences representing new antigens or losing the ability to bind to MHC molecules, thus evading recognition by the cellular immune system as well.

Herpes simples virus and other viruses encode receptors for the Fc domain of IgG to evade the action of antibodies (Johnson and Hill 1998) (Figure 31.10).

In the case of HSV, glycoproteins gE and gI form a heterodimeric Fc receptor that participates in a process termed 'bipolar bridging', in which antibodies bind to their specific HSV antigen and simultaneously interact with gE–gI (Lehner et al. 1975; Frank and Friedman 1989). In this way, the viral Fc receptors inhibit complement-mediated antibody neutralization and antibody-dependent cellular cytotoxicity by cells carrying Fc receptors. HSV gE–gI may also bind other ligands and it has been suggested that it acts as a receptor-binding glycoprotein in the process of cell-to-cell spread.

Several members of the herpesvirus family encode homologs of complement regulatory proteins that block the complement cascade in several ways (Johnson and Hill 1998; Favoreel et al. 2003).

The HSV glycoprotein gC binds the complement factor C3; it protects cell-free virus from complement-mediated neutralization and inhibits the lysis of HSV-infected cells by antibody and complement (Lubinski et al. 1999). HSV gC also functions in virus attachment to cell-surface glycosaminoglycans, especially on the basolateral surfaces of epithelial cells (Sears et al. 1991); thus it has been difficult to interpret the attenuated phenotype of gC virus mutants in vivo (Lubinski et al. 1999). However, in C3 knock-out mice, the disease caused by the gC virus mutant was similar to that of wild-type HSV, suggesting a major role of gC in resistance to complement (Lubinski et al. 1999). HVS, a virus that infects monkeys, encodes a homolog of the

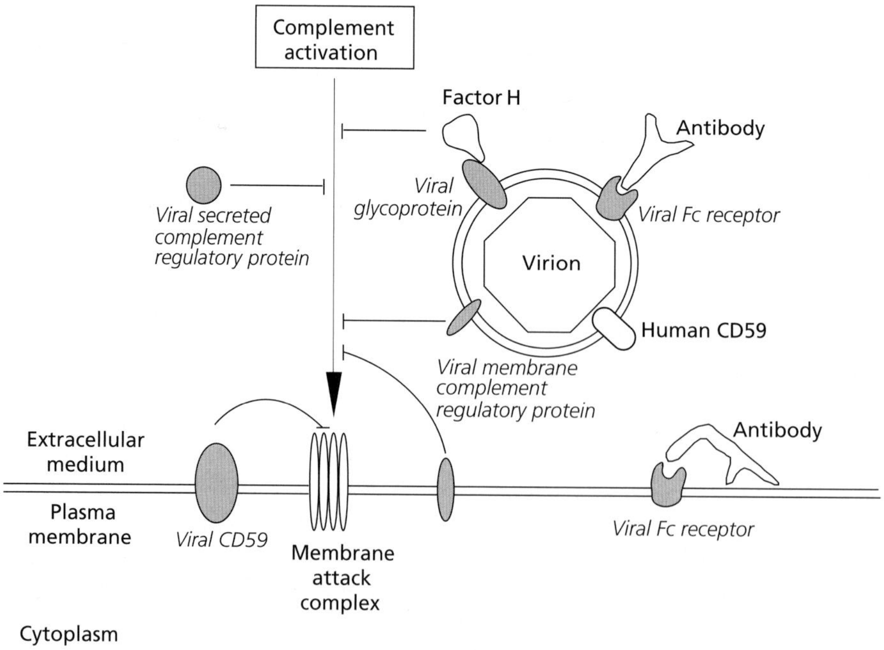

Figure 31.10 *Viral modulation of complement and antibody responses.*

inhibitor of the membrane attack complex CD59, which protects the infected cells from complement-mediated lysis (Rother et al. 1994).

A strategy used by HIV is to recruit the soluble factor H that inhibits complement activation by interacting with the gp120–gp41 complex (Stoiber et al. 1996). Removal of factor H from human serum augments the effect of complement on HIV-infected cells. The poxviruses variola virus (VaV), VV, and CPV encode a secreted protein, known as viral complement control protein (VCP), which blocks the classic and alternate pathways of complement activation (Kotwal et al. 1990; Rosengard et al. 2002). Inactivation of the VCP gene in VV causes virus attenuation in animal models, demonstrating an important role of this protein in preventing host defense mechanisms and a role for complement in antiviral immunity (Isaacs et al. 1992). Interestingly, inactivation of VCP from CPV caused a substantial increase in the inflammatory response in infected mice compared with wild-type CPV infections (Miller et al. 1997). This illustrated that inhibition of the inflammatory response by viral proteins may reduce tissue damage and allow virus replication in host cells that would otherwise be eliminated by the immune response.

Instead of encoding viral homologs of host proteins, HIV, VV, and HCMV, incorporate into the virion envelope complement regulatory proteins, such as CD56 and CD59, which confer complement resistance to the virus particle (Spear et al. 1995; Vanderplasschen et al. 1998)

CONCLUSIONS

A simplistic view of a virus–host interaction is that of a fierce competition between the virus infecting and replicating in a cell until its death, and then spreading to uninfected cells and tissues, whereas the immune system of the host seeks to eliminate all infected cells. This may be true for viruses that are restricted in their growth to mucosal surfaces, those that replicate fast, and those that are directly transmitted. Many viruses replicate slowly and have a tropism only for specific tissues in certain organs to which they have to be transported or disseminated, and often the sites of entry and the sites of release differ. Cell tropism is defined not only by the virus' inability to infect other tissues, but also as a result of the stringent immune control of the host which limits viral spread. Under conditions of immune suppression herpesviruses can infect many tissues, showing that the restriction of the infection to certain sites reflects the virus–host balance of the immunocompetent host. Therefore, the diversity in the biology of closely related viruses has been shaped by evolution, and the biological diversity reflects the function of viral proteins that have been selected to modulate cellular functions.

To describe viral functions as immunoevasive may have been correct for those that directly interfered with antigen processing in the MHCI and MHCII pathways. The reader is cautioned to treat the growing list of viral immune evasion strategies with some skepticism. These strategies are best regarded as modifiers of the immune response, not as immune evasion, e.g. despite the mechanisms described for herpesviruses, they are highly susceptible to NK control in vivo. In fact, recurrent herpesvirus infection is the clinical hallmark of NK deficiency. Later, a host of viral effects on cell functions were also listed as immunoevasive. However, many of these functions affect not only cells of the immune system, e.g. viral functions that affect apoptosis may serve to inhibit proapoptotic molecules released from NK and T cells. However, in the absence of viral anti-apoptotic functions some herpesviruses completely fail to replicate in a number of cell types. Other herpesviruses use functions to keep their host cells in a state of continuous division and to prevent cell death at the same time. Thus, these functions select the viral host cell range and define the biology of a virus.

In a similar vein, the research on viral modulation of chemokine networks has led to hypotheses on Janus-like effects of these viral proteins. A nonfunctional receptor can neutralize the cell-attractive function of a chemokine for cells of the immune system, and thus truly serve an immunoevasive function. On the other hand, there are virus-encoded chemokines that attract host cells. It is thought that these cells serve the virus for reaching target tissues. A remarkable aspect is that some of the cells that provide the 'taxi' service are those that normally would fight the viral infection. Therefore, there is certainly a score that orchestrates the roles of viral chemokines and chemokine receptors in viral dissemination and persistence, but it will take years to understand the music.

Examples of viral proteins that modulate host immune functions presented in this section were mainly taken from viruses with large DNA genomes. In part this is the result of the limited expertise of the authors. Second, many of these functions were first detected in DNA viruses. There is no doubt that several RNA viruses that were not been listed also encode such functions. In general, it appears that viruses need functions to dampen the function of innate immunity and the powerful antiviral functions of the soluble mediators such as the interferons. The analysis of viral functions that affect soluble mediators and/or their subsequent signaling cascades is an area of active research. Another reason for reporting on DNA virus functions is the working hypothesis that in a large virus genome a protein would perhaps serve only one function. There is the tacit belief that the function seen for the isolated gene in vitro also represents the functions that it has in the viral context in vivo. This may probably turn out to be not entirely correct and examples have been mentioned where one protein affects different antiviral principles. If this is true, the pressure for multifunctionality of proteins is even higher in RNA viruses with their smaller genomes.

In apparent contrast to the multifunctionality of proteins is the fact that some viruses encode multiple genes for similar functions, all of which attack the class I pathway. It is not always clear what the purpose of this multiplicity is. One purpose appears to be to deal with MHC polymorphism. MHCI molecules belong to the most polymorphic proteins, as a result of the three class loci – HLA-A, -B, and -C in humans – and to extensive polymorphism at each locus. The length of coevolution of class I and viruses – particularly herpesviruses – makes it likely that some of this polymorphism has evolved to counteract VIPRs. In fact, many VIPRs deal with different class I isoforms with different degrees of efficiency. Thus, the function of some viral proteins are considered complementary. Another function for multiple genes is cooperativity: neither gene is capable of inhibiting antigen presentation alone, but together they function effectively to prevent CTLs recognizing infected cells. A similar multiplicity of genes with related function is also seen with respect to genes controlling apoptosis, and genes controlling chemokine and cytokine networks.

The analysis of the principles evolved by the viruses to target the same mechanism, e.g. the peptide transport or MHCI maturation, indicates that the biological problem – defense against CD8 T-cell control – has been independently addressed by the α and β herpesviruses. Analogous but mechanistically completely different solutions were found. This indicates that the virus subfamilies were already separated before the acquisition of these functions. The primordial immune system fighting the archetype herpesvirus progenitor lacking this function was different as well. There is a strong belief that the constant attack by viruses has shaped both the virus and the mammalian immune system that we know today. Some viral immunomodulatory functions, e.g. some antiapoptotic genes, operate across species barriers, whereas others, e.g. MHCI modulators, often do not. This is explained by the coevolution of viruses with their hosts and could mean that the host-specific functions were acquired at a later stage.

The true function of the immunomodulatory genes can be delineated only by in vivo studies using appropriate combinations of virus mutants and host mutants. Given the plethora of genes, the redundancy of related functions, the multifunctionality and cooperativity of proteins, and the intricate interplay of functions that act differently on different cells at different states of activation and differentiation, and with a different efficacy with respect to the genetic background of the host, it is clear that it will take a long time to test present concepts and to develop a conceptual network of hierarchical functions. This may be of use for modern medicine with its new concepts of treatment that affect immune functions and thus disturb the virus–host balance so carefully tuned by evolution.

ACKNOWLEDGMENTS

ABH was supported by grants from the National Institutes of Health (AI47 206 and AI50099). AA was a Wellcome Senior Research Fellow. UHK was supported by grants of the Deutsche Forschungsgemeinschaft, the Bayerische Forschungsstiftung, and the Verband der Chemischen Industrie.

REFERENCES

Ahn, K., Angulo, A., et al. 1996. Human cytomegalovirus inhibits antigen presentation by a sequential multistep process. *Proc Natl Acad Sci USA*, **93**, 10990–5.

Ahn, K., Gruhler, A., et al. 1997. The ER-luminal domain of the HCMV glycoprotein US6 inhibits peptide translocation by TAP. *Immunity*, **6**, 613–21.

Albini, A., Ferrini, S., et al. 1998. HIV-1 Tat protein mimicry of chemokines. *Proc Natl Acad Sci USA*, **95**, 13153–8.

Alcami, A. 2003. Viral mimicry of cytokines, chemokines and their receptors. *Nature Rev Immunol*, **3**, 36–50.

Alcami, A. and Smith, G.L. 1992. A soluble receptor for interleukin-1 beta encoded by vaccinia virus: a novel mechanism of virus modulation of the host response to infection. *Cell*, **71**, 153–67.

Alcami, A. and Smith, G.L. 1995. Vaccinia, cowpox, and camelpox viruses encode soluble gamma interferon receptors with novel broad species specificity. *J Virol*, **69**, 4633–9.

Alcami, A. and Smith, G.L. 1996. A mechanism for the inhibition of fever by a virus. *Proc Natl Acad Sci USA*, **93**, 11029–34.

Alcami, A., Symons, J.A., et al. 1998. Blockade of chemokine activity by a soluble chemokine binding protein from vaccinia virus. *J Immunol*, **160**, 624–33.

Alcami, A., Symons, J.A. and Smith, G.L. 2000. The vaccinia virus soluble alpha/beta interferon (IFN) receptor binds to the cell surface and protects cells from the antiviral effects of IFN. *J Virol*, **74**, 11230–9.

Allen, T.M., O'Connor, D.H., et al. 2000. Tat-specific cytotoxic T lymphocytes select for SIV escape variants during resolution of primary viraemia. *Nature*, **407**, 386–90.

Andrews, D.M., Andoniou, C.E., et al. 2001. Infection of dendritic cells by murine cytomegalovirus induces functional paralysis. [see comments.]. *Nat Immunol*, **2**, 1077–84.

Arase, H., Mocarski, E.S., et al. 2002. Direct recognition of cytomegalovirus by activating and inhibitory NK cell receptors [see comments.]. *Science*, **296**, 1323–6.

Arvanitakis, L., Geras-Raaka, E., et al. 1997. Human herpesvirus KSHV encodes a constitutively active G-protein-coupled receptor linked to cell proliferation. *Nature*, **385**, 347–50.

Basta, S., Chen, W., et al. 2002. Inhibitory effects of cytomegalovirus proteins US2 and US11 point to contributions from direct priming and cross-priming in induction of vaccinia virus-specific CD8(+) T cells. *J Immunol*, **168**, 5403–8.

Bauer, S., Groh, V., et al. 1999. Activation of NK cells and T cells by NKG2D, a receptor for stress-inducible MICA. *Science*, **285**, 727–9.

Beersma, M.F., Bijlmakers, M.J. and Ploegh, H.L. 1993. Human cytomegalovirus down-regulates HLA class I expression by reducing the stability of class I H chains. *J Immunol*, **151**, 4455–64.

Benedict, C.A., Butrovich, K.D., et al. 1999. Cutting edge: a novel viral TNF receptor superfamily member in virulent strains of human cytomegalovirus. *J Immunol*, **162**, 6967–70.

Benedict, C.A., Norris, P.S. and Ware, C.F. 2002. To kill or be killed: viral evasion of apoptosis. *Nat Immunol*, **3**, 1013–18.

Bennett, E.M., Bennink, J.R., et al. 1999. Cutting edge: adenovirus E 19 has two mechanisms for affecting class I MHC expression. *J Immunol*, **162**, 5049–52.

Bodaghi, B., Jones, T.R., et al. 1998. Chemokine sequestration by viral chemoreceptors as a novel viral escape strategy: withdrawal of chemokines from the environment of cytomegalovirus-infected cells. *J Exp Med*, **188**, 855–66.

Boname, J.M. and Stevenson, P.G. 2001. MHC class I ubiquitination by a viral PHD/LAP finger protein. *Immunity*, **15**, 627–36.

Born, T.L., Morrison, L.A., et al. 2000. A poxvirus protein that binds to and inactivates IL-18, and inhibits NK cell response. *J Immunol*, **164**, 3246–54.

Bortner, C.D. and Cidlowski, J.A. 2002. Cellular mechanisms for the repression of apoptosis. *Annu Rev Pharmacol Toxicol*, **42**, 259–81.

Boshoff, C., Endo, Y., et al. 1997. Angiogenic and HIV-inhibitory functions of KSHV-encoded chemokines. *Science*, **278**, 290–4.

Bowie, A., Kiss-Toth, E., et al. 2000. A46R and A52R from vaccinia virus are antagonists of host IL-1 and toll-like receptor signaling. *Proc Natl Acad Sci USA*, **97**, 10162–7.

Braud, V.M., Allan, D.S., et al. 1998a. HLA-E binds to natural killer cell receptors CD94/NKG2A, B and C [see comments]. *Nature*, **391**, 795–9.

Braud, V.M., Allan, D.S., et al. 1998b. TAP- and tapasin-dependent HLA-E surface expression correlates with the binding of an MHC class I leader peptide. *Curr Biol*, **8**, 1–10.

Breckenridge, D.G., Nguyen, M., et al. 2002. The procaspase-8 isoform, procaspase-8L, recruited to the BAP31 complex at the endoplasmic reticulum. *Proc Natl Acad Sci USA*, **99**, 4331–6.

Bridgeman, A., Stevenson, P.G., et al. 2001. A secreted chemokine binding protein encoded by murine gammaherpesvirus-68 is necessary for the establishment of a normal latent load. *J Exp Med*, **194**, 301–12.

Burgert, H.G., Ruzsics, Z., et al. 2002. Subversion of host defense mechanisms by adenoviruses. *Curr Top Microbiol Immunol*, **269**, 273–318.

Colamonici, O.R., Domanski, P., et al. 1995. Vaccinia virus B18R gene encodes a type I interferon-binding protein that blocks interferon alpha transmembrane signaling. *J Biol Chem*, **270**, 15974–8.

Collins, K.L., Chen, B.K., et al. 1998. HIV-1 Nef protein protects infected primary cells against killing by cytotoxic T lymphocytes. *Nature*, **391**, 397–401.

Colonna, M., Nakajima, H. and Cella, M. 1999. Inhibitory and activating receptors involved in immune surveillance by human NK and myeloid cells. *J Leukoc Biol*, **66**, 718–22.

Cosman, D., Fanger, N., et al. 1997. A novel immunoglobulin superfamily receptor for cellular and viral MHC class I molecules. *Immunity*, **7**, 273–82.

Cosman, D., Mullberg, J., et al. 2001. ULBPs, novel MHC class I-related molecules, bind to CMV glycoprotein UL16 and stimulate NK cytotoxicity through the NKG2D receptor. *Immunity*, **14**, 123–33.

Cuconati, A. and White, E. 2002. Viral homologs of BCL-2: role of apoptosis in the regulation of virus infection. *Genes Dev*, **16**, 2465–78.

Dairaghi, D.J., Fan, R.A., et al. 1999. HHV8-encoded vMIP-I selectively engages chemokine receptor CCR8. Agonist and antagonist profiles of viral chemokines. *J Biol Chem*, **274**, 21569–74.

Damon, I., Murphy, P.M. and Moss, B. 1998. Broad spectrum chemokine antagonistic activity of a human poxvirus chemokine homolog. *Proc Natl Acad Sci USA*, **95**, 6403–7.

Davis-Poynter, N.J., Lynch, D.M., et al. 1997. Identification and characterization of a G protein-coupled receptor homolog encoded by murine cytomegalovirus. *J Virol*, **71**, 1521–9.

Deane, D., McInnes, C.J., et al. 2000. Orf virus encodes a novel secreted protein inhibitor of granulocyte-macrophage colony-stimulating factor and interleukin-2. *J Virol*, **74**, 1313-, 20.

Derfuss, T. and Meinl, E. 2002. Herpesviral proteins regulating apoptosis. *Curr Top Microbiol Immunol*, **269**, 257–72.

Didcock, L., Young, D.F., et al. 1999. The V protein of simian virus 5 inhibits interferon signalling by targeting STAT1 for proteasome-mediated degradation. *J Virol*, **73**, 9928–33.

Diefenbach, A., Jamieson, A.M., et al. 2000. Ligands for the murine NKG2D receptor: expression by tumor cells and activation of NK cells and macrophages. *Nat Immunol*, **1**, 1, 19–26.

Doherty, P.C., Christensen, J.P., et al. 2001. Dissecting the host response to a gamma-herpesvirus. *Phil Trans R Soc Lond, Series B: Biol Sci*, **356**, 581–93.

Drillien, R., Spehner, D., et al. 2000. Vaccinia virus-related events and phenotypic changes after infection of dendritic cells derived from human monocytes. *Virology*, **268**, 471–81.

Endres, M.J., Garlisi, C.G., et al. 1999. The Kaposi's sarcoma-related herpesvirus (KSHV)-encoded chemokine vMIP-I is a specific agonist for the CC chemokine receptor (CCR)8. *J Exp Med*, **189**, 1993–8.

Engelmayer, J., Larsson, M., et al. 1999. Vaccinia virus inhibits the maturation of human dendritic cells: a novel mechanism of immune evasion. *J Immunol*, **163**, 6762–8.

Falk, C.S., Mach, M., et al. 2002. NK cell activity during human cytomegalovirus infection is dominated by US2-11-mediated HLA class I down-regulation. *J Immunol*, **169**, 3257–66.

Fanger, N.A., Borges, L. and Cosman, D. 1999. The leukocyte immunoglobulin-like receptors (LIRs): a new family of immune regulators. *J Leukocyte Biol*, **66**, 231–6.

Farrell, H.E., Vally, H., et al. 1997. Inhibition of natural killer cells by a cytomegalovirus MHC class I homologue in vivo [see comments]. *Nature*, **386**, 510–14.

Farrell, P.J. 1998. Signal transduction from the Epstein-Barr virus LMP-1 transforming protein. *Trends Microbiol*, **6**, 175–7.

Favoreel, H.W., Van de Walle, G.R., et al. 2003. Virus complement evasion strategies. *J Gen Virol*, **84**, 1–15.

Fong, D.C. and Cambier, J.C. 1999. Inhibitory receptors and their modes of action. *Cold Spring Harb Symp Quant Biol*, **64**, 329–34.

Frank, I. and Friedman, H.M. 1989. A novel function of the herpes simplex virus type 1 Fc receptor: participation in bipolar bridging of antiviral immunoglobulin G. *J Virol*, **63**, 4479–88.

Fruh, K., Ahn, K., et al. 1995. A viral inhibitor of peptide transporters for antigen presentation. *Nature*, **375**, 415–18.

Fugier-Vivier, I., Servet-Delprat, C., et al. 1997. Measles virus suppresses cell-mediated immunity by interfering with the survival and functions of dendritic and T cells. *J Exp Med*, **186**, 813–23.

Furman, M.H., Ploegh, H.L. and Tortorella, D. 2002. Membrane-specific, host-derived factors are required for US2- and US11-mediated degradation of major histocompatibility complex class I molecules. *J Biol Chem*, **277**, 3258–67.

Gale, M. Jr. and Katze, M.G. 1998. Molecular mechanisms of interferon resistance mediated by viral-directed inhibition of PKR, the interferon-induced protein kinase. *Pharmacol Ther*, **78**, 29–46.

Galocha, B., Hill, A., et al. 1997. The active site of ICP47, a herpes simplex virus-encoded inhibitor of the major histocompatibility complex (MHC)-encoded peptide transporter associated with antigen processing (TAP), maps to the NH2-terminal 35 residues. *J Exp Med*, **185**, 1565–72.

Gilbert, M.J., Riddell, S.R., et al. 1996. Cytomegalovirus selectively blocks antigen processing and presentation of its immediate-early gene product. *Nature*, **383**, 720–2.

Gold, M.C., Munks, M.W., et al. 2002. The murine cytomegalovirus immunomodulatory gene m152 prevents recognition of infected cells by M45-specific CTL but does not alter the immunodominance of the M45-specific CD8 T cell response in vivo. *J Immunol*, **169**, 359–65.

Goldmacher, V.S. 2002. vMIA, a viral inhibitor of apoptosis targeting mitochondria. *Biochimie*, **84**, 177–85.

Goodbourn, S., Didcock, L. and Randall, R.E. 2000. Interferons: cell signalling, immune modulation, antiviral responses and virus countermeasures. *J Gen Virol*, **81**, 2341–64.

Goulder, P.J., Brander, C., et al. 2001. Evolution and transmission of stable CTL escape mutations in HIV infection. *Nature*, **412**, 334–8.

Graham, K.A., Lalani, A.S., et al. 1997. The T1/35kDa family of poxvirus-secreted proteins bind chemokines and modulate leukocyte influx into virus-infected tissues. *Virology*, **229**, 12–24.

Groh, V., Rhinehart, R., et al. 2001. Costimulation of CD8alphabeta T cells by NKG2D via engagement by MIC induced on virus-infected cells. *Nat Immunol*, **2**, 255–60.

Grosjean, I., Caux, C., et al. 1997. Measles virus infects human dendritic cells and blocks their allostimulatory properties for CD4+ T cells. *J Exp Med*, **186**, 801–12.

Gruhler, A., Peterson, P.A. and Fruh, K. 2000. Human cytomegalovirus immediate early glycoprotein US3 retains MHC class I molecules by transient association. *Traffic*, **1**, 318–25.

Hegde, N.R., Tomazin, R.A., et al. 2002. Inhibition of HLA-DR assembly, transport, and loading by human cytomegalovirus glycoprotein US3: a novel mechanism for evading major histocompatibility complex class II antigen presentation. *J Virol*, **76**, 10929–41.

Hengel, H., Koopmann, J.O., et al. 1997. A viral ER-resident glycoprotein inactivates the MHC-encoded peptide transporter. *Immunity*, **6**, 623–32.

Hewitt, E.W., Duncan, L., et al. 2002. Ubiquitylation of MHC class I by the K3 viral protein signals internalization and TSG101-dependent degradation. *EMBO J*, **21**, 2418–29.

Hill, A., Jugovic, P., et al. 1995. Herpes simplex virus turns off the TAP to evade host immunity. *Nature*, **375**, 411–15.

Hsu, D.H., de Waal Malefyt, R., et al. 1990. Expression of interleukin-10 activity by Epstein-Barr virus protein BCRF1. *Science*, **250**, 830–2.

Hu, F., Smith, C.A. and Pickup, D.J. 1994. Cowpox virus contains two copies of an early gene encoding a soluble secreted form of the type II TNF receptor. *Virology*, **204**, 343–56.

Huber, B.T., Beutner, U. and Subramanyam, M. 1994. The role of superantigens in the immunobiology of retroviruses. *Ciba Found Symp*, **187**, 132–40.

Isaacs, S.N., Kotwal, G.J. and Moss, B. 1992. Vaccinia virus complement-control protein prevents antibody-dependent complement-enhanced neutralization of infectivity and contributes to virulence. *Proc Natl Acad Sci USA*, **89**, 628–32.

Ishido, S., Choi, J.K., et al. 2000. Inhibition of natural killer cell-mediated cytotoxicity by Kaposi's sarcoma-associated herpesvirus K5 protein. *Immunity*, **13**, 365–74.

Jefferies, W.A. and Burgert, H.G. 1990. E3/ 19K from adenovirus 2 is an immunosubversive protein that binds to a structural motif regulating the intracellular transport of major histocompatibility complex class I proteins. *J Exp Med*, **172**, 1653–64.

Johnson, D.C. and Hill, A.B. 1998. Herpesvirus evasion of the immune system. *Curr Top Microbiol Immunol*, **232**, 149–77.

Jones, T.R., Wiertz, E.J., et al. 1996. Human cytomegalovirus US3 impairs transport and maturation of major histocompatibility complex class I heavy chains. *Proc Natl Acad Sci USA*, **93**, 11327–33.

Katze, M.G., He, Y. and Gale, M. Jr. 2002. Viruses and interferon: a fight for supremacy. *Nat Rev Immunol*, **2**, 675–87.

Kavanagh, D.G., Gold, M.C., et al. 2001. The multiple immune-evasion genes of murine cytomegalovirus are not redundant. M4 and m152 inhibit antigen presentation in a complementary and cooperative fashion. *J Exp Med*, **194**, 967–78.

Kirchhoff, S., Sebens, T., et al. 2002. Viral IFN-regulatory factors inhibit activation-induced cell death via two positive regulatory IFN-regulatory factor 1-dependent domains in the CD95 ligand promoter. *J Immunol*, **168**, 1226–34.

Kledal, T.N., Rosenkilde, M.M., et al. 1997. A broad-spectrum chemokine antagonist encoded by Kaposi's sarcoma-associated herpesvirus. *Science*, **277**, 1656–9.

Kotwal, G.J., Isaacs, S.N., et al. 1990. Inhibition of the complement cascade by the major secretory protein of vaccinia virus. *Science*, **250**, 827–30.

Krathwohl, M.D., Hromas, R., et al. 1997. Functional characterization of the C–C chemokine-like molecules encoded by molluscum contagiosum virus types 1 and 2. *Proc Natl Acad Sci USA*, **94**, 9875–80.

Krmpotic, A., Messerle, M., et al. 1999. The immunoevasive function encoded by the mouse cytomegalovirus gene m152 protects the virus against T cell control in vivo. *J Exp Med*, **190**, 1285–96.

Krmpotic, A., Busch, D.H., et al. 2002. MCMV glycoprotein gp40 confers virus resistance to CD8+ T cells and NK cells in vivo [see comments]. *Nat Immunol*, **3**, 529–35.

Lalani, A.S., Graham, K., et al. 1997. The purified myxoma virus gamma interferon receptor homolog M-T7 interacts with the heparin-binding domains of chemokines. *J Virol*, **71**, 4356–63.

Lanier, L.L. 2001. Face off – the interplay between activating and inhibitory immune receptors. *Curr Opin Immunol*, **13**, 326–31.

Lee, B.J., Koszinowski, U.H., et al. 2003. A gammaherpesvirus G protein-coupled receptor homologue is required for increased viral replication in response to chemokines and efficient reactivation from latency. *J Immunol*, **170**, 243–51.

Lehner, P.J., Karttunen, J.T., et al. 1997. The human cytomegalovirus US6 glycoprotein inhibits transporter associated with antigen processing-dependent peptide translocation. *Proc Natl Acad Sci USA*, **94**, 6904–9.

Lehner, T., Wilton, J.M. and Shillitoe, E.J. 1975. Immunological basis for latency, recurrences and putative oncogenicity of herpes simplex virus. *Lancet*, **ii**, 60–2.

Levine, B. 2002. Apoptosis in viral infections of neurons: a protective or pathologic host response? *Curr Top Microbiol Immunol*, **265**, 95–118.

Levitskaya, J., Coram, M., et al. 1995. Inhibition of antigen processing by the internal repeat region of the Epstein–Barr virus nuclear antigen-1. *Nature*, **375**, 685–8.

Long, E.O. 1999. Regulation of immune responses through inhibitory receptors. *Annu Rev Immunol*, **17**, 875–904.

Loparev, V.N., Parsons, J.M., et al. 1998. A third distinct tumor necrosis factor receptor of orthopoxviruses. *Proc Natl Acad Sci USA*, **95**, 3786–91.

Lubinski, J., Wang, L., et al. 1999. In vivo role of complement-interacting domains of herpes simplex virus type 1 glycoprotein gC. *J Exp Med*, **190**, 1637–46.

McFadden, G. and Murphy, P.M. 2000. Host-related immunomodulators encoded by poxviruses and herpesviruses. *Curr Opin Microbiol*, **3**, 371–8.

McNees, A.L. and Gooding, L.R. 2002. Adenoviral inhibitors of apoptotic cell death. *Virus Res*, **88**, 87–101.

Mahr, J.A. and Gooding, L.R. 1999. Immune evasion by adenoviruses. *Immunol Rev*, **168**, 121–30.

Marzo, I., Brenner, C., et al. 1998. Bax and adenine nucleotide translocator cooperate in the mitochondrial control of apoptosis. *Science*, **281**, 2027–31.

Miller, C.G., Shchelkunov, S.N. and Kotwal, G.J. 1997. The cowpox virus-encoded homolog of the vaccinia virus complement control protein is an inflammation modulatory protein. *Virology*, **229**, 126–33.

Milne, R.S., Mattick, C., et al. 2000. RANTES binding and down-regulation by a novel human herpesvirus-6 beta chemokine receptor. *J Immunol*, **164**, 2396–404.

Miskin, J.E., Abrams, C.C., et al. 1998. A viral mechanism for inhibition of the cellular phosphatase calcineurin. *Science*, **281**, 562–5.

Moore, P.S., Boshoff, C., et al. 1996. Molecular mimicry of human cytokine and cytokine response pathway genes by KSHV. *Science*, **274**, 1739–44.

Mossman, K., Upton, C., et al. 1995. Species specificity of ectromelia virus and vaccinia virus interferon-γ binding proteins. *Virology*, **208**, 762–9.

Mossman, K., Nation, P., et al. 1996. Myxoma virus M-T7, a secreted homolog of the interferon-gamma receptor, is a critical virulence factor for the development of myxomatosis in European rabbits. *Virology*, **215**, 17–30.

Moutaftsi, M., Mehl, A.M., et al. 2002. Human cytomegalovirus inhibits maturation and impairs function of monocyte-derived dendritic cells. *Blood*, **99**, 2913–21.

Munch, J., Stolte, N., et al. 2001. Efficient class I major histocompatibility complex down-regulation by simian immunodeficiency virus Nef is associated with a strong selective advantage in infected rhesus macaques. *J Virol*, **75**, 10532–6.

Murphy, P.M. 2001. Viral exploitation and subversion of the immune system through chemokine mimicry. *Nat Immunol*, **2**, 116–22.

Ng, F.W., Nguyen, M., et al. 1997. p28 Bap31, a Bcl-2/Bcl-XL- and procaspase-8-associated protein in the endoplasmic reticulum. *J Cell Biol*, **139**, 327–38.

Nguyen, M., Breckenridge, D.G., et al. 2000. Caspase-resistant BAP31 inhibits fas-mediated apoptotic membrane fragmentation and release of cytochrome c from mitochondria. *Mol Cell Biol*, **20**, 6731–40.

Norbury, C.C., Malide, D., et al. 2002. Visualizing priming of virus-specific CD8+ T cells by infected dendritic cells in vivo. *Nat Immunol*, **3**, 265–71.

Panus, J.F., Smith, C.A., et al. 2002. Cowpox virus encodes a fifth member of the tumor necrosis factor receptor family: A soluble, secreted CD30 homologue. *Proc Natl Acad Sci USA*, **99**, 8348–53.

Parry, C.M., Simas, J.P., et al. 2000. A broad spectrum secreted chemokine binding protein encoded by a herpesvirus. *J Exp Med*, **191**, 573–8.

Penfold, M.E., Dairaghi, D.J., et al. 1999. Cytomegalovirus encodes a potent alpha chemokine. *Proc Natl Acad Sci USA*, **96**, 9839–44.

Piguet, V., Wan, L., et al. 2000. HIV-1 Nef protein binds to the cellular protein PACS-1 to downregulate class I major histocompatibility complexes. *Nat Cell Biol*, **2**, 163–7.

Raftery, M.J., Schwab, M., et al. 2001. Targeting the function of mature dendritic cells by human cytomegalovirus: a multilayered viral defense strategy. *Immunity*, **15**, 997–1009.

Rathmell, J.C. and Thompson, C.B. 2002. Pathways of apoptosis in lymphocyte development, homeostasis, and disease. *Cell*, **109**, suppl, S97–S107.

Ravetch, J.V. and Lanier, L.L. 2000. Immune inhibitory receptors. *Science*, **290**, 84–9.

Ray, C.A., Black, R.A., et al. 1992. Viral inhibition of inflammation: cowpox virus encodes an inhibitor of the interleukin-1 beta converting enzyme. *Cell*, **69**, 597–604.

Redpath, S., Angulo, A., et al. 1999. Murine cytomegalovirus infection down-regulates MHC class II expression on macrophages by induction of IL-10. *J Immunol*, **162**, 6701–7.

Reusch, U., Muranyi, W., et al. 1999. A cytomegalovirus glycoprotein re-routes MHC class I complexes to lysosomes for degradation. *EMBO J*, **18**, 1081–91.

Reyburn, H.T., Mandelboim, O., et al. 1997. The class I MHC homologue of human cytomegalovirus inhibits attack by natural killer cells [see comments]. *Nature*, **386**, 514–17.

Rosengard, A.M., Liu, Y., Nie, Z. and Jimenez, R. 2002. Variola virus immune evasion design: expression of a highly efficient inhibitor of human complement. *Proc Natl Acad Sci USA*, **99**, 8808–13.

Rosenkilde, M.M., Kledal, T.N., Brauner-Osborne, H. and Schwartz, T.W. 1999. Agonists and inverse agonists for the herpesvirus 8-encoded constitutively active seven-transmembrane oncogene product, ORF-74. *J Biol Chem*, **274**, 956–61.

Rother, R.P., Rollins, S.A., et al. 1994. Inhibition of complement-mediated cytolysis by the terminal complement inhibitor of herpesvirus saimiri. *J Virol*, **68**, 730–7.

Saederup, N., Lin, Y.C., et al. 1999. Cytomegalovirus-encoded beta chemokine promotes monocyte-associated viremia in the host. *Proc Natl Acad Sci USA*, **96**, 10881–6.

Salio, M., Cella, M., et al. 1999. Inhibition of dendritic cell maturation by herpes simplex virus. *Eur J Immunol*, **29**, 3245–53.

Salvesen, G.S. and Dixit, V.M. 1997. Caspases: intracellular signaling by proteolysis. *Cell*, **91**, 443–6.

Saraiva, M. and Alcami, A. 2001. CrmE, a novel soluble tumor necrosis factor receptor encoded by poxviruses. *J Virol*, **75**, 226–33.

Saraiva, M., Smith, P., et al. 2002. Inhibition of type 1 cytokine-mediated inflammation by a soluble CD30 homologue encoded by ectromelia (mousepox) virus. *J Exp Med*, **196**, 829–39.

Scaffidi, C., Fulda, S., et al. 1998. Two CD95 (APO-1/Fas) signaling pathways. *EMBO J*, **17**, 1675–87.

Schmitz, I., Kirchhoff, S. and Krammer, P.H. 2000. Regulation of death receptor-mediated apoptosis pathways. *Int J Biochem Cell Biol*, **32**, 1123–36.

Schnorr, J.J., Xanthakos, S., et al. 1997. Induction of maturation of human blood dendritic cell precursors by measles virus is associated with immunosuppression. *Proc Natl Acad Sci USA*, **94**, 5326–31.

Schust, D.J., Tortorella, D., et al. 1998. Trophoblast class I major histocompatibility complex (MHC) products are resistant to rapid degradation imposed by the human cytomegalovirus (HCMV) gene products US2 and US11. *J Exp Med*, **188**, 497–503.

Sears, A.E., McGwire, B.S. and Roizman, B. 1991. Infection of polarized MDCK cells with herpes simplex virus 1: two asymmetrically distributed cell receptors interact with different viral proteins. *Proc Natl Acad Sci USA*, **88**, 5087–91.

Sedmak, D.D., Guglielmo, A.M., et al. 1994. Cytomegalovirus inhibits major histocompatibility class II expression on infected endothelial cells. *Am J Pathol*, **144**, 683–92.

Senkevich, T.G. and Moss, B. 1998. Domain structure, intracellular trafficking, and beta2-microglobulin binding of a major histocompatibility complex class I homolog encoded by molluscum contagiosum virus. *Virology*, **250**, 397–407.

Servet-Delprat, C., Vidalain, P.O., et al. 2000. Consequences of Fas-mediated human dendritic cell apoptosis induced by measles virus. *J Virol*, **74**, 4387–93.

Smith, C.A., Davis, T., et al. 1991. T2 open reading frame from Shope fibroma virus encodes a soluble form of the TNF receptor. *Biochem Biophys Res Commun*, **176**, 335–42.

Smith, C.A., Hu, F.Q., et al. 1996. Cowpox virus genome encodes a second soluble homologue of cellular TNF receptors, distinct from CrmB, that binds TNF but not LT alpha. *Virology*, **223**, 132–47.

Smith, C.A., Smith, T.D., et al. 1997. Poxvirus genomes encode a secreted, soluble protein that preferentially inhibits beta chemokine activity yet lacks sequence homology to known chemokine receptors. *Virology*, **236**, 316–27.

Smith, H.R., Heusel, J.W., et al. 2002. Recognition of a virus-encoded ligand by a natural killer cell activation receptor. *Proc Natl Acad Sci USA*, **99**, 8826–31.

Smith, V.P., Bryant, N.A. and Alcami, A. 2000. Ectromelia, vaccinia and cowpox viruses encode secreted interleukin-18-binding proteins. *J Gen Virol*, **81**, 1223–30.

Sozzani, S., Luini, W., et al. 1998. The viral chemokine macrophage inflammatory protein-II is a selective Th2 chemoattractant. *Blood*, **92**, 4036–9.

Spear, G.T., Lurain, N.S., et al. 1995. Host cell-derived complement control proteins CD55 and CD59 are incorporated into the virions of two unrelated enveloped viruses. Human T cell leukemia/lymphoma virus type I (HTLV-I) and human cytomegalovirus (HCMV). *J Immunol*, **155**, 4376–81.

Spriggs, M.K. 1999. Shared resources between the neural and immune systems: semaphorins join the ranks. *Curr Opin Immunol*, **11**, 387–91.

Spriggs, M.K., Hruby, D.E., et al. 1992. Vaccinia and cowpox viruses encode a novel secreted interleukin-1-binding protein. *Cell*, **71**, 145–52.

Stennicke, H.R., Jurgensmeier, J.M., et al. 1998. Pro-caspase-3 is a major physiologic target of caspase-8. *J Biol Chem*, **273**, 27084–90.

Stevenson, P.G., May, J.S., et al. 2002. K3-mediated evasion of CD8(+) T cells aids amplification of a latent gamma-herpesvirus. *Nat Immunol*, **3**, 733–40.

Stine, J.T., Wood, C., et al. 2000. KSHV-encoded CC chemokine vMIP-III is a CCR4 agonist, stimulates angiogenesis, and selectively chemoattracts TH2 cells. *Blood*, **95**, 1151–7.

Stoiber, H., Pinter, C., et al. 1996. Efficient destruction of human immunodeficiency virus in human serum by inhibiting the protective action of complement factor H and decay accelerating factor (DAF, CD55). *J Exp Med*, **183**, 307–10.

Story, C.M., Furman, M.H. and Ploegh, H.L. 1999. The cytosolic tail of class I MHC heavy chain is required for its dislocation by the human cytomegalovirus US2 and US11 gene products. *Proc Natl Acad Sci USA*, **96**, 8516–21.

Streblow, D.N., Soderberg-Naucler, C., et al. 1999. The human cytomegalovirus chemokine receptor US28 mediates vascular smooth muscle cell migration. *Cell*, **99**, 511–20.

Strockbine, L.D., Cohen, J.I., et al. 1998. The Epstein–Barr virus BARF1 gene encodes a novel, soluble colony-stimulating factor-1 receptor. *J Virol*, **72**, 4015–21.

Sutkowski, N., Palkama, T., et al. 1996. An Epstein–Barr virus-associated superantigen. *J Exp Med*, **184**, 971–80.

Sutkowski, N., Conrad, B., et al. 2001. Epstein–Barr virus transactivates the human endogenous retrovirus HERV-K18 that encodes a superantigen. *Immunity*, **15**, 579–89.

Symons, J.A., Alcami, A. and Smith, G.L. 1995. Vaccinia virus encodes a soluble type I interferon receptor of novel structure and broad species specificity. *Cell*, **81**, 551–60.

Tigges, M.A., Leng, S., et al. 1996. Human herpes simplex virus (HSV)-specific CD8+ CTL clones recognize HSV-2-infected fibroblasts after treatment with IFN-gamma or when virion host shutoff functions are disabled. *J Immunol*, **156**, 3901–10.

Tomasec, P., Braud, V.M., et al. 2000. Surface expression of HLA-E, an inhibitor of natural killer cells, enhanced by human cytomegalovirus gpUL40. *Science*, **287**, 1031.

Tomazin, R., Boname, J., et al. 1999. Cytomegalovirus US2 destroys two components of the MHC class II pathway, preventing recognition by CD4+ T cells. *Nat Med*, **5**, 1039–43.

Trapani, J.A. and Smyth, M.J. 2002. Functional significance of the perforin/granzyme cell death pathway. *Nat Rev Immunol*, **2**, 735–47.

Tripp, R.A., Jones, L.P., et al. 2001. CX3C chemokine mimicry by respiratory syncytial virus G glycoprotein. *Nat Immunol*, **2**, 732–8.

Upton, C., Mossman, K. and McFadden, G. 1992. Encoding of a homolog of IFN-γ receptor by myxoma virus. *Science*, **258**, 1369–72.

van Berkel, V., Barrett, J., et al. 2000. Identification of a gammaherpesvirus selective chemokine binding protein that inhibits chemokine action. *J Virol*, **74**, 6741–7.

Vanderplasschen, A., Mathew, E., et al. 1998. Extracellular enveloped vaccinia virus is resistant to complement because of incorporation of host complement control proteins into its envelope. *Proc Natl Acad Sci USA*, **95**, 7544–9.

Vidalain, P.O., Azocar, O., et al. 2000. Measles virus induces functional TRAIL production by human dendritic cells. *J Virol*, **74**, 556–9.

Vilches, C. and Parham, P. 2002. KIR: diverse, rapidly evolving receptors of innate and adaptive immunity. *Annu Rev Immunol*, **20**, 217–51.

Wagner, M., Gutermann, A., et al. 2002. Major histocompatibility complex class I allele-specific cooperative and competitive interactions between immune evasion proteins of cytomegalovirus. *J Exp Med*, **196**, 805–16.

Walczak, H. and Sprick, M.R. 2001. Biochemistry and function of the DISC. *Trends Biochem Sci*, **26**, 452–3.

Wang, E.C., McSharry, B., et al. 2002a. UL40-mediated NK evasion during productive infection with human cytomegalovirus. *Proc Natl Acad Sci USA*, **99**, 7570–5.

Wang, H.W., Sharp, T.V., et al. 2002b. Characterization of an anti-apoptotic glycoprotein encoded by Kaposi's sarcoma-associated herpesvirus which resembles a spliced variant of human survivin. *EMBO J*, **21**, 2602–15.

Weihua, X., Ramanujam, S., et al. 1998. The polyoma virus T antigen interferes with interferon-inducible gene expression. *Proc Natl Acad Sci USA*, **95**, 1085–90.

Wiertz, E.J., Jones, T.R., et al. 1996a. The human cytomegalovirus US11 gene product dislocates MHC class I heavy chains from the endoplasmic reticulum to the cytosol. *Cell*, **84**, 769–79.

Wiertz, E.J., Tortorella, D., et al. 1996b. Sec61-mediated transfer of a membrane protein from the endoplasmic reticulum to the proteasome for destruction. *Nature*, **384**, 432–8.

Wu, J., Song, Y., et al. 1999. An activating immunoreceptor complex formed by NKG2D and DAP10. *Science*, **285**, 730–2.

Xiang, Y. and Moss, B. 1999. IL-18 binding and inhibition of interferon gamma induction by human poxvirus-encoded proteins. *Proc Natl Acad Sci USA*, **96**, 11537–42.

Yang, T.Y., Chen, S.C., et al. 2000. Transgenic expression of the chemokine receptor encoded by human herpesvirus 8 induces an angioproliferative disease resembling Kaposi's sarcoma. *J Exp Med*, **191**, 445–54.

Yao, Z., Fanslow, W.C., et al. 1995. Herpesvirus Saimiri encodes a new cytokine, IL-17, which binds to a novel cytokine receptor. *Immunity*, **3**, 811–21.

Yewdell, J. and Hill, A.B. 2002. Viral interference with antigen presentation. *Nat Immunol.*

York, I.A., Roop, C., et al. 1994. A cytosolic herpes simplex virus protein inhibits antigen presentation to CD8+ T lymphocytes. *Cell*, **77**, 525–35.

Ziegler, H., Thale, R., et al. 1997. A mouse cytomegalovirus glycoprotein retains MHC class I complexes in the ERGIC/cis-Golgi compartments. *Immunity*, **6**, 57–66.

Zimring, J.C., Goodbourn, S. and Offermann, M.K. 1998. Human herpesvirus 8 encodes an interferon regulatory factor (IRF) homolog that represses IRF-1-mediated transcription. *J Virol*, **72**, 701–7.

Zou, P., Isegawa, Y., et al. 1999. Human herpesvirus 6 open reading frame U83 encodes a functional chemokine. *J Virol*, **73**, 5926–33.

32

Evasion of immune responses by bacteria

KINGSTON H.G. MILLS AND AOIFE P. BOYD

INTRODUCTION

The success of pathogenic microorganisms is dependent on their survival and replication in the face of antimicrobial defense mechanisms, mediated by innate and adaptive responses of the host's immune system. Although the immune system is capable of preventing infection, and eliminating or containing most bacteria, many, if not all, bacterial pathogens have evolved strategies to evade or suppress immune responses to prolong their survival in the host. Ideally, the bacteria should be capable of avoiding or modulating innate and adaptive immunity to such an extent that the host does not succumb to a lethal infection but survives to pass on the organisms to secondary hosts.

Innate immunity

Following infection of host tissue with pathogenic bacteria, tissue macrophages quickly phagocytose and attempt to kill the bacteria (Figure 32.1). This initiates an inflammatory response with the release of cytokines and chemokines and the recruitment of neutrophils, monocytes, and lymphocytes to the site of infection. Binding of conserved secreted or cell-surface bacterial products to molecular structures, called pathogen recognition receptors (PRR), on cells of the innate immune system activates immune response genes, leading to inflammatory cytokine and chemokine production, and enhanced cell surface expression of molecules involved in antigen presentation (Janeway and Medzhitov 2002).

Activation of the alternate complement pathway by bacterial cell wall components results in the production of C3b, which opsonizes bacteria and, together with antibodies, facilitates their phagocytosis by neutrophils and macrophages. Bacteria also activate the classic pathway of complement. The complement membrane attack complex can directly kill certain bacteria and participate in the inflammatory response.

Once inside the phagocytic cells, the bacteria-containing phagosome undergoes a series of fusions with endosomes and lysosomes to form a phagolysosome in which the bacteria are killed by a variety of mechanisms, including reactive oxygen- and nitrogen-dependent mechanisms. However, phagocytic and killing mechanisms of host cells can be overcome by various physical and biochemical evasion strategies evolved by the bacteria. The composition of the bacterial cell wall has a major influence on the ability of phagocytic cells to take up and destroy the bacteria. All bacteria have an inner cell membrane and peptidoglycan layer, which can be attacked by lysozymes and enzymes in the lysosomal vesicles of phagocytic cells. Gram-negative bacteria have an outer lipid bilayer (with lipopolysaccharide), which can be attacked by cationic lipids and complement. Certain bacteria have capsules that prevent phagocytosis or have an extremely complex cell wall (e.g. mycobacteria), which is highly resistant to killing. Bacteria

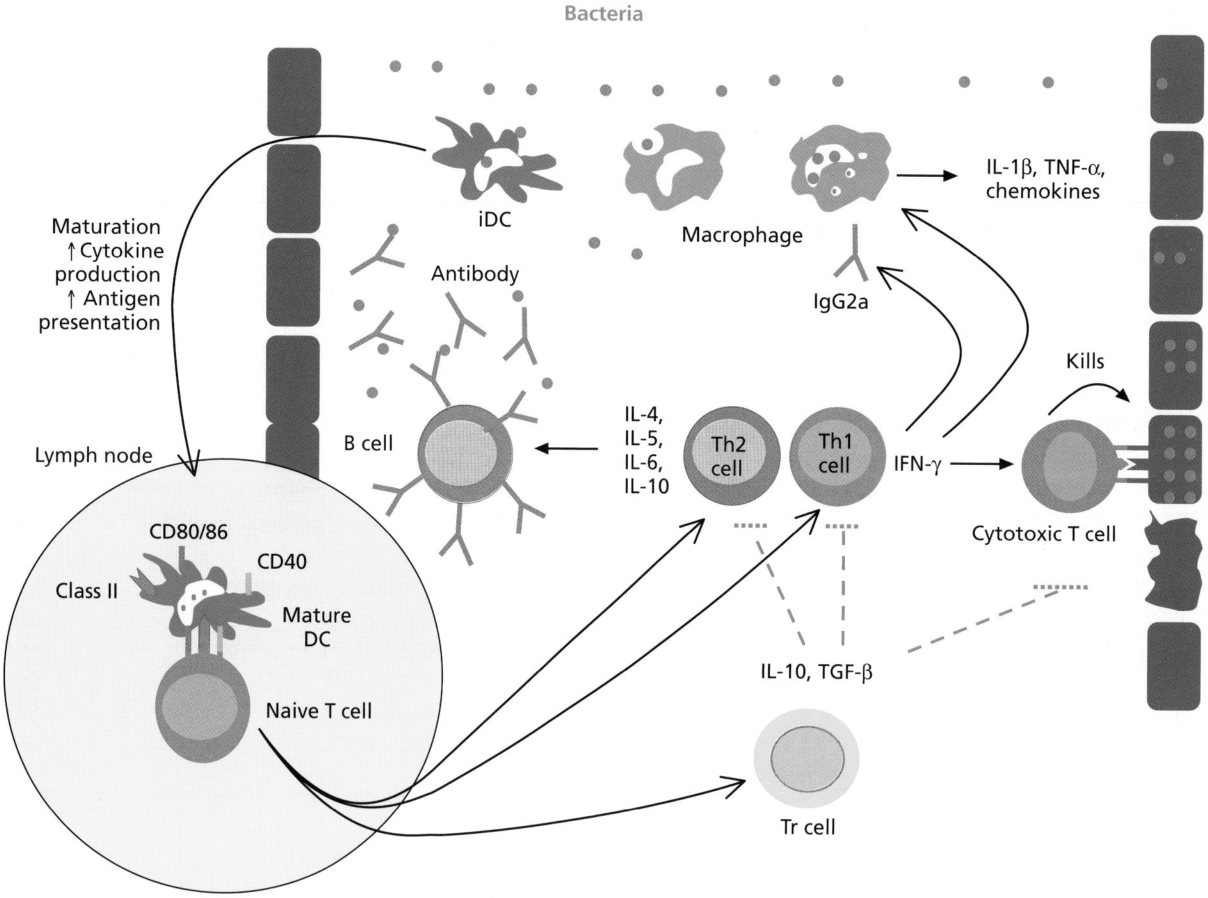

Figure 32.1 *Innate and adaptive immunity to bacteria. Bacteria that enter mucosal tissue, such as the lungs or gastrointestinal tract, are phagocytosed by macrophages and dendritic cells (DCs) of the innate immune system. Immature DCs (iDC) are activated and migrate to the draining lymph node, where they present processed bacterial antigens to naïve T cells. Effector T cells migrate back to the tissues and mediate and regulate the adaptive immune response to the bacteria. T-helper (Th1) cells secrete interferon γ (IFN-γ), which activates macrophages to kill the intracellular bacteria and cytotoxic T lymphocytes (CTL) to kill host cells infected with intracellular bacteria. Th2 and Th1 cells secrete cytokines that activate B-cell antibody production, which prevents bacteria binding to host cells, promotes opsonization, or neutralizes toxins. Finally, Tr cells turn off the adaptive immune response and limit collateral damage to host tissues.*

can also inhibit killing by preventing phagosome–lysosome fusion or by inducing lysosomal discharge into the cytoplasm. Induction of apoptosis in neutrophils, macrophages, and dendritic cells (DC), critical cells in antibacterial host defense and in activating adaptive immunity, is the ultimate subversion strategy evolved by a number of bacterial species to protective immune responses of the host.

Adaptive immunity

Adaptive immune responses are mediated by lymphocytes, called T and B cells. B cells produce antibodies, whereas $CD8^+$ T cells kill host cells infected with intracellular microorganisms and $CD4^+$ T cells provide help for B-cell production of antibody and regulate the immune response to infection (see Figure 32.1). In addition to $CD4^+$ and $CD8^+$ T cells, unconventional T cells, including γδ T cells which recognize phospholigands and CD1-restricted αβ T cells or T cells that express natural killer (NK) markers, termed NKT cells, which recognize glycolipids, also play a role in immunity to intracellular bacteria (Schaible and Kaufmann 2000). Although it takes days rather than hours before the adaptive immune response is effective, unlike the innate immune system, it is able to recall previous encounters with antigen, through the activation of memory T and B cells. Therefore a second or subsequent infection with the bacteria is dealt with more effectively.

After uptake of the bacteria by a macrophage or DC, the professional antigen-presenting cells (APC), process and present peptides of the bacterial antigens to T cells in association with major histocompatibility complex (MHC) molecules on their cell surface. All bacteria, whether they survive intracellularly or extracellularly in the host, can activate MHC class II (MHCII)-restricted $CD4^+$ T-helper (Th) cells. In addition, certain intracellular bacteria can also activate MHCI-restricted $CD8^+$

cytotoxic T lymphocytes (CTL). Induction of MHCII-restricted T cells requires processing by an exogenous route. After binding to specific cell-surface receptors on macrophages and DCs, and uptake into APCs via opsonization, phagocytosis, or receptor-mediated endocytosis, the bacterial antigens are degraded in endosomes or early lysosomes, and digested peptides, 7–20 amino acids long, associate with newly formed or recycled MHCII molecules before being exported to the cell surface. Induction of class I-restricted CTLs is dependent on bacterial antigens entering the endogenous route of antigen processing, usually through their escape from vacuoles/endosomes into the cytoplasm. Many of the intracellular steps of antigen processing are targets of immune evasion by pathogenic bacteria.

Class I-restricted CTLs kill host cells infected with intracellular bacteria, whereas the main function of class II-restricted $CD4^+$ T cells is to release cytokines that activate phagocytosis and killing of bacteria by macrophages, and to provide helper function for antibody production. $CD4^+$ T cells can be divided into a number of functionally distinct subtypes discriminated on the basis of cytokine secretion. Th1 cells secrete interferon-γ (IFN-γ) and tumor necrosis factor-β (TNF-β), activate phagocytosis and killing by macrophages, and provide help for the production of opsonizing (murine IgG2a) antibodies. Th2 cells secrete interleukins IL-4, IL-5, IL-6, IL-9, IL-10, and IL-13 and are considered to be the main helper cells, especially for immunoglobulin (Ig) IgG1, IgA, and IgE. A further subtype of $CD4^+$ T cells, which secrete high levels of IL-10 and/or transforming growth factor (TGF)-β but not IL-4 or IFN-γ, termed regulatory T (Tr) cells, have recently been described during infection with certain pathogens, including bacteria (McGuirk and Mills 2002). Tr cells have suppressive function and may be induced by the host to turn off immune responses, especially Th1 responses, once the bacteria are eliminated and thereby limit immunopathology. Alternately their induction may serve as an evasion strategy by the bacteria to suppress protective Th1 responses.

Although cell-mediated immunity is important in controlling intracellular bacteria, humoral immunity plays a major role in protection against extracellular bacteria. Antibodies help to prevent infection or to eliminate bacteria in a number of ways, and antibodies of different classes and subclasses perform different functions. Extracellular bacteria often bind to epithelial cells in the respiratory or gastrointestinal (GI) tract via adhesins or pili; antibodies against these bacterial virulence factors can help to prevent colonization. The diseases caused by many bacteria are mediated by toxins; antibodies, especially those of the murine IgG1 subclass, can neutralize these toxins and prevent their binding to host target cells, and thereby reduce the severity of disease. Antibodies of the murine IgG2a subclass can promote phagocytosis by opsonizing the bacteria and stimulating complement components C3b and iC3b, which bind complement receptors and further promote phagocytosis. IgA antibodies, induced after bacterial infection of the respiratory tract, GI tract, or other mucosal tissues, function to limit the infection to mucosal surfaces. In an immune individual primed by a selflimiting infection or immunization, antibodies probably play the major role in conferring protective immunity. Almost all bacterial vaccines in use today confer protection by the generation of circulating IgG or memory B cells, which produce an anamnestic antibody response after re-exposure to the bacteria. However, the generation of antibody responses is also dependent on priming of helper T cells, so both T and B cells are critical in the primary as well as the secondary response to bacterial infection. Bacteria have also evolved strategies to circumvent humoral immunity, either by directly cleaving the antibody molecule or by interfering with the functions of B or Th cells.

EVASION OF PHAGOCYTIC KILLING

Phagocytosis provides a specialized mechanism for ingestion and intracellular destruction of microbial pathogens by neutrophils and macrophages (Aderem and Underhill 1999). These include receptors for the opsonic immunoglobulin Fc domain (e.g. FcγR) and the C3b and C3bi complement fragments (e.g. CR3). FcγRs cluster when bound to an IgG-coated bacterium and become phosphorylated by Src tyrosine kinases. Downstream events include activation of the small GTPases, Rac, and Cdc42, which results in polymerization of actin to form an actin cup at the site of bacterial binding to the plasma membrane, followed by the appearance of F-actin-rich membrane ruffles and internalization of the bound particle surrounded by a lipid bilayer membrane and a halo of actin. CR3-mediated phagocytosis is similar to FcγR-mediated phagocytosis in many ways, but uses Rho GTPases instead of Rac and Cdc42. In addition, CR3-mediated phagocytosis does not induce inflammatory mediators.

Together with internalization of the target, intracellular signaling stimulates interaction of the phagosome with the endocytic network, activates the production of reactive oxygen intermediates (ROI) and enhances the expression of specific genes, especially those encoding cytokines (Duclos and Desjardins 2000; Tjelle et al. 2000). The newly formed phagosomes are immature organelles unable to kill or degrade microorganisms and, in order to acquire and exert their microbicidal function, phagosomes must engage in a maturation process referred to as phagolysosome biogenesis. Phagosomes fuse transiently and sequentially with endosomes of increasing age or of increasing maturation level (early endosomes, late endosomes, and lysosomes). The Rab GTPases are associated with different stages in the fusion pathway: Rab5 enables fusion of the phagosome

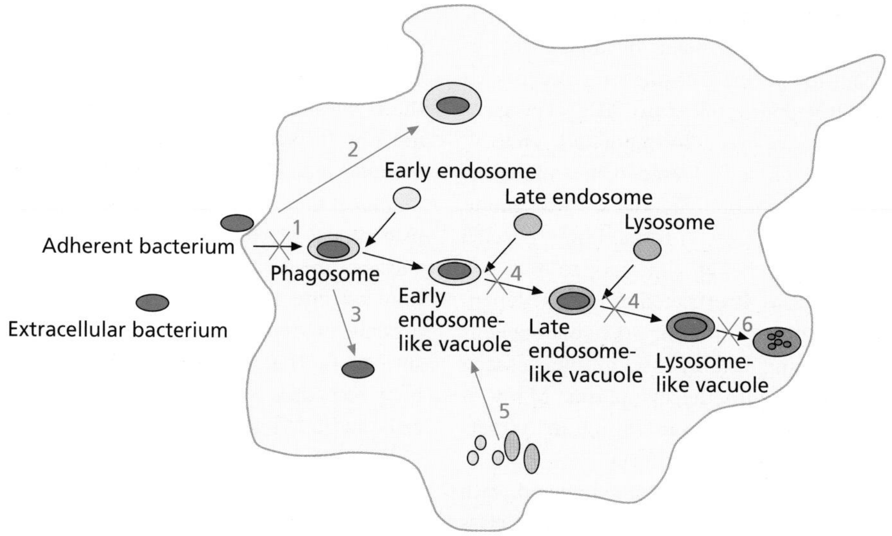

Figure 32.2 *Evasion of phagocytic killing. Phagocytic cell receptors recognize and bind microorganisms on the cell surface. The bacteria are taken up into phagosome vesicles originating from the plasma membrane. Phagosomes mature by fusing transiently and sequentially with endosomes of increasing age and maturation (early endosomes, late endosomes, and lysosomes). Eventually a phagolysosome is formed with an acidic and lytic compartment to kill, degrade, and further process microorganism antigens for presentation at the cell surface. Bacteria have developed a number of strategies to evade killing by phagocytic cells including: (1) inhibition of phagocytic uptake, (2) bacteria-mediated invasion into a nonlysosomal pathway, (3) escape to cytosol, (4) inhibition of endosomal and lysosomal fusion, (5) fusion with nonlysosomal organelles, and (6) resistance to lysosomal killing.*

with early endosomes, whereas Rab7 allows phagosome fusion with late endosomes. During the maturation process phagosomes acquire markers of late endosomes and lysosomes including the proton pump adenosine triphosphatase (ATPase), nicotinamide adenine dinucleotide phosphate (NADPH) oxidase complex, MHCII molecules, various hydrolases including several cathepsins, and specific antimicrobial pore-forming peptides. In addition, maturing phagosomes acquire Nramp1, which transports divalent cations and modulates intraphagosomal iron content. The combination of reactive oxygen and nitrogen, acidic pH, pore-forming peptides, iron imbalance, and hydrolytic enzymes in the final phagolysosome provides a highly effective antimicrobial combination that is capable of killing a wide variety of bacteria, and further degrading and processing the microorganism antigens for presentation at the cell surface. Bacteria have developed a number of strategies to evade killing by phagocytic cells (Figure 32.2).

Inhibition of chemotaxis

Pathogens can prevent killing by neutrophils and macrophages through the inhibition of the migration of these phagocytic cells to the site of infection. Cell chemotaxis is controlled by inflammatory cytokines and chemokines, and complement components, and through the expression of adhesion molecules on the cell surface; each of these regulatory mechanisms can be targeted by a number of pathogens. Pneumolysin, a sulfhydryl-activated toxin produced by *Streptococcus pneumoniae*, can inhibit chemotaxis of human polymorphonuclear cells (Paton and Ferrante 1983). The peptidoglycan fraction of staphylococci induces production of an inhibitory protein by mononuclear cells that inhibits neutrophil chemotaxis and the bacterial peptide *N*-formyl-Met-Leu-Phe inhibits neutrophil migration and killing of *Staphylococcus epidermidis* (Donabedian 1985; Li et al. 2002b).

The AB toxin, pertussis toxin (PT), plays a major role in *Bordetella pertussis* pathogenesis. Binding of the B-oligomer to host cells allows the A subunit to enter the cell, where adenosine diphosphate (ADP)-ribosylation of G_i proteins that transmit inhibitory signals to the adenylyl cyclase complex occurs, resulting in elevated intracellular cyclic adenosine monophosphate (cAMP), which affects signaling pathways in many cell types, including cells of the immune system; this contributes to immune dysfunction. PT has been shown to inhibit macrophage chemotaxis in vivo (Meade et al. 1985) and neutrophil and lymphocyte chemotaxis in vitro by altering intracellular calcium levels (Spangrude et al. 1985). Recent evidence has shown that the leukocytosis induced by PT may result from G-protein-dependent, chemokine-regulated extravasation of leukocytes. PT inhibits the increase in intracellular Ca^{2+} levels in $CD4^+$ and $CD8^+$ T cells, induced by the CC chemokines, macrophage chemoattractant protein 1 (MCP-1), MCP-2, MCP-3, macrophage inflammatory protein 1α (MIP-1α), MIP-1β, and RANTES (Loetscher et al. 1994), Ca^{2+}-mediated activation of neutrophils induced by IL-8 (Schorr et al. 1999), and MCP-1-induced chemotaxis of NK cells (Allavena et al. 1994).

Inhibition of phagocytic uptake

Successful extracellular bacteria have the ability to inhibit uptake by phagocytic cells (Ernst 2000). *Yersinia* spp. share a common mechanism to inhibit phagocytosis by macrophages (Cornelis et al. 1998). These bacteria and a number of other virulent gram-negative animal and plant pathogens possess a dedicated pathogenicity secretion system called a type III secretion system (TTSS), which is responsible for directly delivering effector molecules from the bacterium into the eukaryotic cytosol. These effectors interfere with normal immune cell function, primarily disrupting signal transduction pathways and cytoskeleton arrangements. *Yersinia* spp. express a number of TTSS effectors that inhibit phagocytic uptake, one of which is YopH which after entry into the cell cytoplasm rapidly blocks phagocytosis through Fcγ receptors (Grosdent et al. 2002). YopH is a tyrosine phosphatase that dephosphorylates focal adhesion kinase (FAK) and $p130^{Cas}$. These proteins are found at sites of focal adhesions and are thought to play an important role as adaptor proteins during phagocytosis (Black and Bliska 1997; Persson et al. 1997). A second *yersinia* TTSS effector, YopE, acts together with YopH to inhibit phagocytosis (Rosqvist et al. 1988). YopE is a GTPase-activating protein that selectively increases GTP hydrolysis by RhoA, Rac, and Cdc42, key regulators of actin cytoskeleton dynamics, thereby inactivating them (Von Pawel-Rammingen et al. 2000). The TTSS effector ExoS of *Pseudomonas aeruginosa* acts in a similar manner to disrupt actin filaments and inhibit phagocytosis (Pederson et al. 1999).

Enteropathogenic *Escherichia coli* (EPEC) inhibits FcγR-mediated macrophage phagocytosis but not CR3-mediated phagocytosis via its TTSS (Celli et al. 2001). This is the result of inactivation of phosphatidyl inositol (PI)-3-kinase, leading to inhibition of pseudopod extension and complete phagocytic cup formation. *Helicobacter pylori* expresses another kind of secretion system associated with pathogenic processes – a type IV secretion system. This secretion system also delivers effector molecules into the eukaryotic cell and is responsible for inhibition of bacterial uptake by phagocytic cells (Ramarao et al. 2000). *Mycobacterium tuberculosis* and/or its lipoarabinomannan downregulates macrophage activation, and thereby phagocytosis, by stimulation of SHP-1, a cytosolic protein tyrosine phosphatase (Nandan et al. 2000).

Bacteria-mediated invasion into phagocytic and nonphagocytic cells

Some pathogens survive by living intracellularly in eukaryotic cells. In this way the bacteria avoid recognition by soluble factors, such as complement and antibody, and by immune cells. The bacteria direct their own uptake into nonphagocytic cells and/or phagocytic cells via receptors other than Fc receptors, and in this way bacteria avoid triggering activation of the intracellular bacterial killing mechanisms, so that the bacteria can survive and replicate safely within the cell.

Invasion is initiated by binding of the bacteria to the eukaryotic cell surface. This adhesion is mediated by bacterial adhesins and/or invasins binding to specific receptors on the cell surface. The invasin–receptor interaction then triggers uptake of the bacteria. One set of receptors on eukaryotic cells that is often used by bacteria to enter cells is the integrins (Isberg et al. 2000), which are large heterodimeric transmembrane proteins that are capable of transmitting signals to the cell cytoskeleton after adhesion to substrates. The invasin protein of *Yersinia enterocolitica* uses this receptor to pass through M cells from the gut to the underlying tissue. Bacterial attachment initiates receptor clustering to direct signaling for cytoskeleton rearrangements and entry, a process in which FAK and Rho GTPases are involved. The internalin protein of *Listeria monocytogenes* binds E-cadherin, a cell surface protein involved in cell–cell interactions, and the *Neisseria* family of Opa proteins bind the CD66 family of receptors (Mengaud et al. 1996). Receptors can also be glycosaminoglycans and extracellular matrix proteins such as fibronectin (Joh et al. 1999).

Bacteria can subvert complement for invasion of eukaryotic cells. In contrast to FcγR-induced phagocytosis, complement–induced phagocytosis does not provoke a respiratory burst, nor does it induce inflammatory mediators (Caron and Hall 1998), so the bacteria bypass powerful cellular killing mechanisms, such as H_2O_2 and oxygen free radicals. Deposition of complement on the cell surface allows bacteria, such as *Legionella pneumophila*, to enter host cells via C receptors (Cooper 1991). Alternately, bacteria can enter cells via complement receptors independently of complement itself, such as *E. coli* via Dr adhesins (Pham et al. 1997). Several bacteria use CR3 for intracellular entry, e.g. filamentous hemagglutinin (FHA) of *B. pertussis* (Ishibashi et al. 1994). *M. tuberculosis* binds CR1 and CR3 to enhance its uptake into cells and InlB of *L. monocytogenes* mediates bacterial entry via gC1q-R/p32, a C1q-binding protein (Braun et al. 2000; Schlesinger et al. 1990).

Bacteria can induce their internalization via subversion of actin skeleton arrangements, a process that is often dependent on TTSS effectors (Steele-Mortimer et al. 2000). Entry of *Salmonella* and *Shigella* spp. into eukaryotic cells is determined by actin polymerization at the site of bacterial contact with the cell membrane and, at the peak of extension formation, numerous cytoskeleton proteins are recruited which form the entry foci. The TTSS effectors of *Salmonella* and *Shigella* spp. first interact with specific cytoskeleton proteins to depolymerize actin filaments and microtubules to allow rearrangement of the cytoskeleton components for mediating bacterial entry. The effectors then activate Cdc42 and Rac1 GTPases to induce actin polymerization and stabilize the newly formed cytoskeleton structure to engulf the bacteria.

The mode of entry of the bacteria into the eukaryotic cell will influence their trafficking along the phagolysosomal pathway and the signaling cascades that are activated. Thus, the receptor that mediates particle internalization and the nature of the internalized particle play an important role in phagosome maturation and phagosome–lysomal fusion.

Escape into cytoplasm

Bacteria such as *Listeria* spp., *Rickettsia* spp., enteroinvasive *E. coli*, and *Shigella* spp. lyse the primary phagosome and enter the cytoplasm where they can safely replicate (Goebel and Kuhn 2000). Entry of bacteria into the cytosol is achieved by the action of phospholipases and pore-forming toxins; the mechanism employed by *Listeria* spp. has been studied best. Escape from the phagosome is necessary for intracellular survival and proliferation of *L. monocytogenes*, a process in which the pore-forming cytolysin listeriolysin O (LLO) plays an essential role (Vazquez-Boland et al. 2001). LLO is active only at low pH and thus it specifically lyses the phagosomal membrane when it is released by the bacteria in the phagosome, and not the plasma membrane of the cell, because after vacuole lysis the pH equilibrates and LLO is deactivated (Beauregard et al. 1997). LLO forms holes in the phagosomal membrane allowing access of the bacteria's own phospholipases, or even cellular lipases, to the phagosomal membrane, which result in the subsequent membrane disruption (Smith et al. 1995).

Inhibition of lysosomal fusion

After uptake into the phagosome several bacterial pathogens have the ability to halt maturation of the vacuole, and trafficking to late endosomal and lysosomal compartments by inhibiting endosome–lysome fusion. *Salmonella typhimurium* traffics to an early endosome-like vacuole that does not mature into a lysosome-like vacuole, where the bacteria grow and multiply (Gorvel and Meresse 2001). Direct interaction of the vacuole containing the *Salmonella* with late endosomal compartments is inhibited (Meresse et al. 1999) and TTSS effectors of *Salmonella* are involved in this inhibition of phagosome–lysosome fusion (Uchiya et al. 1999). These effectors are also necessary to prevent the trafficking of the NADPH oxidase complex to the *Salmonella*-containing vacuole (Vazquez-Torres et al. 2000).

Mycobacterium tuberculosis also inhibits lysosomal delivery. The vacuole containing *Mycobacterium* lacks late endosomal markers and retains Rab5, but not Rab7, thus implicating a block between early and late endosomal fusion (Via et al. 1997). A molecule called TACO (coronin 1) is actively retained at the mycobacterial phagosome membrane limiting interaction with endocytic organelles, and allowing *Mycobacterium* to survive within the phagosomes (Ferrari et al. 1999). Phagosomes containing *Mycobacterium* also lack V-ATPase, thereby preventing acidification (Sturgill-Koszycki et al. 1994).

Chlamydia spp. express proteins that modify the vacuole to ensure that trafficking of bacteria is diverted away from the endocytic pathway to the exocytic pathway (Hackstadt et al. 1997; Wyrick 2000). The vacuole interacts with vesicles derived from the trans-Golgi protein trafficking network en route to the cell surface and thus acquires sphingomyelin. It also acquires phosphatidylcholine and PI from the endoplasmic reticulum (ER) and cardiolipin from the mitochondria, so that the vacuole is thus camouflaged and does not interact with lysosomal compartments (Wylie et al. 1997). Chlamydial proteins IncA–G are also incorporated into the vacuole membrane and may be involved in inhibition of vacuole maturation (Scidmore-Carlson et al. 1999).

Transport to nonlysosomal organelles

Instead of trafficking to the endosomal pathway, virulent *Brucella abortus*, *L. pneumophila*, and *Porphymonas gingivalis* traffic to autophagosome-like vacuoles (Dorn et al. 2002). Autophagy is a cellular process for the degradation of organelles and cellular compartments, resulting in breakdown products that are recycled for the synthesis of new components. The nascent autophagosome is a vacuole derived from the rough ER, and contains organelles and undegraded cytoplasmic substances that had been selectively or nonselectively sequestered within the autophagosome. This early autophagosome matures to an acidic late autophagosome lacking hydrolytic enzymes, which then docks and fuses with a lysosome-containing acid proteases. The sequestered cellular components are then degraded and recycled.

Early after infection *Brucella*-containing phagosomes transiently fuse with early endosomes; however, they do not display Rab7 and do not fuse with lysosomes or late endosomal compartments (Pizarro-Cerda et al. 1998). Instead they acquire ER and autophagosomal characteristics, perhaps by fusion with an early autophagosome. Eventually *Brucella* transits from the autophagosome to the ER, where bacterial replication occurs. In this niche the bacteria not only avoid degradation but also obtain a supply of metabolites. The type IV secretion system of *Brucella* sp. is essential for the biogenesis of the autophagosome-like vacuole and for intracellular survival and replication (Comerci et al. 2001). In the absence of a functional type IV secretion system *Brucella* fails to evade the endocytic pathway and is instead targeted to lysosomes for subsequent degradation.

On entry into cells, vacuoles containing *Legionella* sequentially associate with smooth vesicles, mitochondria, and the ER (Horwitz 1983). The vacuoles fail to acquire late endosomal/lysosomal markers, fail to acidify, and are competent for bacterial replication. They are similar to autophagic vacuoles. This process is also controlled by a type IV secretion system, called dot/icm (Roy et al. 1998).

Resistance to lysosomal killing

Pathogenic bacteria have the ability to survive within phagolysosomes. The acidity of these vacuoles is a major obstacle for the bacteria to overcome. Some pathogens can survive in this acidic environment, whereas others attenuate the acidic pH. *Coxiella* spp. survive and multiply in mature lysosomes where they avoid digestion by lysosomal enzymes and actually require the acidic environment to stimulate metabolism and growth (Heinzen et al. 1996). *Bordetella bronchiseptica* can survive the acidic environment in the lysosome and replicate intracellularly, whereas *B. pertussis* cannot (Schneider et al. 2000). In contrast *Mycobacterium* maintain a neutral pH by retaining endosomal Na^+/K^+ ATPase, as do *Chlamydia* (Sturgill-Koszycki et al. 1994; Schramm et al. 1996).

Reactive oxygen species are generated by the respiratory burst in the macrophage vacuoles to kill intracellular bacteria (Hampton et al. 1998; Zahrt and Deretic 2002). The respiratory burst is caused by the NADPH oxidase complex, which assembles at the phagolysosomal membrane. Electrons are transferred from cytoplasmic NADPH to oxygen on the phagosomal side of the membrane, generating superoxide plus a range of other ROIs with toxic bactericidal activity.

Bacteria have many mechanisms for protection against ROIs. Some involve the production of enzymes to inactivate these molecules. *S. typhimurium* expresses superoxide dismutases, enzymes that catalyze the formation of hydrogen peroxide from superoxide anion and which contribute significantly to *Salmonella* virulence (De Groote et al. 1997; Farrant et al. 1997). Superoxide dismutase also protects *M. tuberculosis* from respiratory burst killing (Piddington et al. 2001). Catalases in turn detoxify hydrogen peroxide to water. The *Salmonella* catalase SodC and the *Campylobacter jejuni* KatA enhance survival toward the respiratory burst (De Groote et al. 1997; Day et al. 2000). In addition, several scavenging enzymes including glutathione reductase and thioredoxin reductase use reducing equivalents from NADPH either to generate low-molecular-weight antioxidant species or to repair oxidative lesions. DNA repair enzymes are required for *Salmonella* survival in mice and for resistance to the respiratory burst, because DNA is a critical bacterial target for reactive oxygen (Buchmeier et al. 1993). The production of ROIs can be inhibited by preventing NADPH oxidase complex formation in the vacuole membrane. *Ehrlichia* sp. inhibit superoxide production by downregulating expression of the NADPH oxidase complex component $gp91^{phox}$ (Banerjee et al. 2000) and *L. pneumophila* inhibits protein kinase C which is necessary for the mobilization of cytosolic NADPH phagocyte oxidase components to the membrane (Jacob et al. 1994).

Reactive nitrogen intermediates (RNI) are also formed in the lysosome by inducible nitric oxide synthase (iNOS). Resistance to RNIs can be mediated by the scavenger enzymes that also confer resistance to ROIs (Zahrt and Deretic 2002). It remains unclear whether bacteria have a dedicated RNI resistance mechanism, or whether resistance is the result of coordinated expression of multiple survival-related pathways.

MODULATION OF PRO- AND ANTI-INFLAMMATORY CYTOKINE PRODUCTION

Bacterial activation of cells of the innate immune system

Macrophages, DCs, NK cells, and nonconventional T cells, including NKT cells and γδ T cells, all function in immunity to bacterial infections, either by uptake and killing of the bacteria, lysis of infected host cells, presentation of antigens to T cells, or release of cytokines that activate antibacterial activity of other cells, or by regulating the adaptive immune responses to the bacteria. The immediate inflammatory response to bacterial infection involves the production of proinflammatory cytokines, including TNF-α, IL-1β, IL-12, and IL-18, and chemokines, including MIP-1α MIP-1β, MIP-2, and RANTES, largely by cells of the innate immune system. These cytokines and chemokines recruit leukocytes to the site of infection, activate their antimicrobial function, and in addition regulate the induction of the adaptive response to the bacteria. IL-12 and IL-27 promote the differentiation of Th1 cells, which mediate cellular immunity against intracellular bacteria and also stimulate the production of opsonizing and complement-fixing antibodies. This proinflammatory response is beneficial to the host in eliminating the bacteria, but is also responsible for many undesirable systemic and central effects, including fever and sepsis, which if uncontrolled can cause immunopathological damage to host tissues. The induction of anti-inflammatory cytokines by the bacteria, especially IL-10 and TGF-β, helps to suppress inflammation, but can also be exploited by the bacteria to turn off protective immune responses.

Bacteria stimulate cells of the innate immune system through interaction of conserved bacterial molecules with receptors on the host cells. Whole bacteria and specific bacterial products, termed pathogen-associated molecular patterns (PAMP), including lipopolysaccharide (LPS), CpG motifs in bacterial DNA, and peptidoglycan, bind to PRRs, which include but are not exclusively Toll-like receptors (TLR), expressed on a variety of cells, e.g. macrophages and DCs (Guermonprez et al. 2002). Differential expression of TLRs and other PRRs on distinct DC subtypes determine the response to different PAMPs (Janeway and Medzhitov 2002). Plasmacytoid DCs selectively expressed TLR-7 and TLR-9 and respond to bacterial CpG motifs, whereas myeloid DCs express all TLRs except TLR-7 and TLR-9, and do not respond to CpG, but are stimulated by LPS and peptidoglycan, which bind to TLR-4 and TLR-2, respectively (Jarrossay et al. 2001). Binding to TLRs activates signaling through NF-κB, leading to the production of inflammatory cytokines including IL-12, TNF-α, IL-1β, IL-6, and IL-18, and the increased surface expression of maturation markers on DCs. The same bacteria can also stimulate the production of anti-inflammatory cytokines, IL-10, TGF-β, and IL-1 receptor antagonist (IL-1ra), either using the same or distinct conserved structures, which bind to and activate distinct signaling receptors and pathways.

Suppression of IL-12 and TNF-α production

Suppression of proinflammatory cytokine production, especially IL-12 and TNF-α, either through induction of IL-10 or through interference with steps in the NFκB signaling pathways is a common strategy employed by bacteria to subvert macrophage activation and induction of Th1 responses. *B. pertussis* FHA suppresses IL-12 by macrophages and DCs and the suppression is mediated by the induction of IL-10 production (McGuirk and Mills 2000; McGuirk et al. 2002). Furthermore FHA suppressed IL-12 and IFN-γ production in vivo in response to LPS in a model of septic shock and suppressed influenza virus-specific IFN-γ production when coadministered to mice with influenza virus by the nasal route (McGuirk et al. 2002).

The AB-type toxins cholera toxin (CT) and *E. coli* heat-labile enterotoxin (LT), also modulate the production of regulatory cytokines and chemokines by cells of the innate immune system. CT, LT and the partially toxic mutant LTR72 suppress production of IL-12 and TNF-α and of the inflammatory chemokines, MIP-1α and MIP-1β (Lavelle et al. 2003; Ryan et al. 2000). Furthermore, CT inhibits the production of bioactive IL-12 (p70) and the expression of the β1 and β2 chains of the IL-12 receptor on human monocytes and DCs, leading to a suppression of Th1 cell differentiation and a predominantly Th2-type response (Braun et al. 1999b). Similarly, exposure of human DCs to CT inhibits IL-12p70, TNF-α, but not IL-6, IL-8, or IL-10 secretion in response to LPS or CD40 ligand (Gagliardi et al. 2000). A mutant of LT devoid of ADP-ribosylating activity does not inhibit IL-12 or TNF-α, suggesting that the enzyme activity is responsible for the suppression. Intracellular cAMP induced by active CT and LT appears to affect signaling pathways within the cells involved with IL-12 and TNF-α production. Furthermore, accumulation of intracellular cAMP directly inhibits cytokine production by Th1 cells and enhances Th2 cells (Ryan et al. 2000).

Another ADP-ribosylating toxin, anthrax edema toxin from *Bacillus anthracis*, inhibits LPS-induced TNF-α, and IL-6 production in human monocytes by increasing intracellular cAMP levels (Hoover et al. 1994). Furthermore, exotoxin A from *P. aeruginosa*, which also has ADP-ribosylating activity, inhibits release of TNF-α, TNF-β, IFN-γ, IL-1β, and IL-1α from both macrophages and lymphocytes (Staugas et al. 1992; Braun et al. 1999b). TNF-α production is also suppressed at the site of infection and in Peyer's patches of mice infected with *Y. enterocolitica*; the YopB protein from this bacteria was found to inhibit TNF-α production, but not other inflammatory cytokines, such as IL-1β and IL-6, by murine macrophages in vitro (Beuscher et al. 1995). Suppression of TNF-α production by *Y. enterocolitica* was associated with inhibition of NF-κB activation (Ruckdeschel et al. 1998). High-molecular-weight proteins released by *Brucella suis* inhibit TNF-α production by human macrophages infected with *E. coli* (Caron et al. 1996). Other bacteria, including *M. tuberculosis*, *Lactobacillus reuteri*, and *Histoplasma capsulatum*, suppress macrophage IL-12 production, but the bacterial molecules involved have not been identified (McGuirk and Mills 2002).

Induction of IL-10 and TGF-β production

A number of bacteria, including *Mycobacterium* spp., *L. pneumophilia*, *S. typhimurium*, *L. monocytogenes*, and *Y. enterocolitica*, stimulate IL-10 production by macrophages (Redpath et al. 2001). In a limited number of cases the bacterial molecule responsible has been identified. FHA, an adhesin from *B. pertussis* that binds to CR3 (Ishibashi et al. 1994), induces IL-10 and IL-6 production by macrophages and DCs (McGuirk and Mills 2000; McGuirk et al. 2002). The induction of IL-10 production was linked to suppression of IL-12, induction of Tr cells and suppression of Th1 responses in the lungs and local lymph nodes of *B. pertussis*-infected mice.

The immunosuppression associated with *M. tuberculosis* and the suppressed IFN-γ production in TB-infected individuals has been attributed to IL-10 and TGF-β production by mononuclear cells, including macrophages and DCs. Purified protein derivative (PPD) of *Mycobacterium* induces IL-10 and TGF-β production by human mononuclear cells (Toossi et al. 1995; Othieno et al. 1999) and suppresses the production of IFN-γ, whereas neutralization of IL-10 and TGF-β enhances IFN-γ production (Othieno et al. 1999). Naturally occurring inhibitors of TGF-β (latency-associated peptide and decorin) restored in vitro T-cell responses of patients with TB and decreased growth of the bacteria in vitro and in vivo (Hirsch et al. 1997; Wilkinson et al. 2000). However, in a longitudinal study of TB patients, PPD-specific IL-10 and TGF-β production by peripheral blood mononuclear cells (PBMC) returned to baseline levels after 3 months, although PPD-specific IFN-γ production remained depressed for up to 12 months (Hirsch et al. 1999), suggesting that PPD-specific IL-10 and TGF-β are not the only factors involved in the immunosuppression.

Lipoarabinomannan (LAM), a cell wall component of *M. tuberculosis*, induces IL-10 production from human mononuclear cells (Barnes et al. 1992) and TGF-β from human monocytes (Dahl et al. 1996), and this has also been provided as an explanation for the immunosuppressive effects of the bacteria on antigen-induced T-cell proliferation. However, LAM also stimulated production of granulocyte–macrophage colony-stimulating factor (GM-CSF), IL-1, IL-6. and IL-8 (Barnes et al. 1992), suggesting that it had pro- as well as anti-inflammatory effects. Infection of macrophages with *M. tuberculosis* induces the production of IL-10, IL-1, IL-6, IL-18, and TNF-α, but not IL-12 except in the presence of anti-IL-10 antibody. In contrast, infected DCs secrete IL-12, IFN-α, and TNF-α, but not IL-10 (Giacomini et al. 2001). It was suggested that the differential responses of the cells related to their distinct functions in infection, macrophages establishing inflammation inside granulomas and DCs directing T-cell responses in the draining lymph nodes. It has also been demonstrated that infection of DCs with *M. bovis* BCG induces release of IL-10 and IL-12, and that infected DCs from IL-10-deficient (IL-$10^{-/-}$) mice are more effective at trafficking to the lymph nodes, secrete higher levels of IL-12, and induce higher IFN-γ levels in response to mycobacterial antigens than wild-type DC (Demangel et al. 2002). An analogous finding has been reported for *Chlamydia trachomatis*, where modulation of endogenous IL-10 production by using IL-$10^{-/-}$ mice or antisense IL-10 enhances the ability of APCs to induce *Chlamydia*-specific Th1 responses (Igietseme et al. 2000). This suggests that upregulation of IL-10 production by DCs may serve as a strategy by the pathogen to turn off protective Th1 responses, and that inhibition of IL-10 production by APCs may provide a strategy for therapy or immunization against these diseases.

The virulence of *M. tuberculosis* strains has been linked to their ability to induce IL-10 production, with certain clinical isolates stimulating the highest level of this cytokine from human macrophages (Barnes et al. 1992). Another consequence of monocyte/macrophage IL-10 production by *M. avium* is the induction of soluble TNF receptor 2 (sTNFR2), which can inactivate TNF-α and block TNF-α-induced apoptosis (Balcewicz-Sablinska et al. 1998). Apoptosis of infected cells is a host defense measure to prevent intracellular multiplication of bacteria and this can be circumvented by *M. tuberculosis* and other bacteria (see below under Apoptosis).

There is also evidence from other bacterial species linking virulence to the ability to stimulate IL-10 or TGF-β production. The virulence-associated V antigen (LcrV) of pathogenic *Yersinia* spp. induces IL-10 release from mouse and human macrophages and as a consequence inhibits TNF-α production (Sing et al. 2002). It has been suggested that replication of *Coxiella burnetii* and the development of chronic Q fever may be facilitated by the induction of IL-10 production in macrophages; *C. burnetii* stimulates IL-10 and inhibits TNF-α production by monocytes and bacterial replication is inhibited by neutralizing anti-IL-10 antibodies (Ghigo et al. 2001). Lipidated outer surface protein A (L-OasA) from *Borrelia burgdorferi*, the etiological agent of Lyme disease, induces IL-10 production by human monocytes (Giambartolomei et al. 1998). Inhibition of endogenous IL-10 production with anti-IL-10 inhibits IL-12 and IL-6 antibodies but not IL-1β or TNF-α; this has been explained by a difference in the kinetics of cytokine production by monocytes in response to *B. burgdorferi*, with TNF-α production peaking within 1 h, followed by IL-10 and IL-1β, whereas IL-6 and IL-12 were produced later (Murthy et al. 2000). Inhibition of endogenous or bacteria-stimulated TGF-β2 production in mice infected with *L. monocytogenes* enhances IFN-γ, TNF-α, and IL-12 production and increases survival of the mice (Szalay et al. 1999). Although the source of the TGF-β has not been identified, it has been suggested that it may be derived from γδ T cells, NKT cells, or other cells of the innate immune system. In contrast, injection of anti-TGF-β1 diminishes resistance to *L. monocytogenes*, whereas administration of TGF-β1 protected mice from the infection (Nakane et al. 1996)

Studies in cytokine knock-out mice have provided more definitive evidence of a role for endogenous or bacteria-stimulated IL-10 production on the course of bacterial infections. In certain cases infection is less severe in IL-$10^{-/-}$ mice, confirming that this cytokine may help to subvert protective immunity by suppressing innate and adaptive immune responses, e.g. IL-$10^{-/-}$ mice are highly resistant against infection with *Yersinia* spp. and the bacteria-dependent suppression of TNF-α, mediated by IL-10, was absent in the knock-out mice (Sing et al. 2002). Cell-mediated immunity to *M. bovis* BCG is enhanced in IL-$10^{-/-}$ mice and the knock-out mice eliminate the bacteria faster than wild-type (Jacobs et al. 2000).

However, in other infections, the severity of disease is exacerbated in IL-$10^{-/-}$ mice, suggesting that IL-10 has a protective role, possibly by limiting immune-mediated pathology. IL-$10^{-/-}$ mice succumb to primary and secondary infection with *L. monocytogenes*; the number of cells in the inflammatory infiltrate, the inflammatory cytokine production in the brain and the severity of brain lesions is enhanced in the knock-out mice (Deckert et al. 2001). Although the numbers of bacteria were not significantly different between wild-type and IL-$10^{-/-}$ mice infected with *L. monocytogenes*, there are also examples of bacterial infection in IL-$10^{-/-}$ mice where disease pathology is enhanced or where bacterial clearance is accelerated. Peritonitis and mortality from *E. coli* infection is enhanced in IL-$10^{-/-}$ mice, despite accelerated clearance of the bacteria in knock-out compared with wild-type mice (Sewnath et al. 2001). The colonization of the gastric mucosa by *H. pylori* is reduced in IL-$10^{-/-}$ mice, but the severity of chronic active gastritis is significantly higher than in the wild-type mice (Chen et al. 2001). Similarly, IL-$10^{-/-}$ mice infected with *Helicobacter hepaticus* develop severe inflammation associated with IL-12 production and Th1 responses (Kullberg et al. 2001).

CYTOLYSIS AND APOPTOSIS OF MACROPHAGES, DCS, AND T CELLS

Apoptosis

Apoptosis or programmed cell death is a normal mechanism to remove unwanted cells from the body and plays a critical role in homeostasis in the immune system. After infection, apoptosis of lymphocytes reduces the pool of effector T and B cells, which have recently expanded through stimulation with foreign antigens. The process is carried out and controlled within the cell by a family of cysteine proteases, called caspases, which cleave cellular proteins and activate other caspases, eventually leading to the dismantling of cellular components. Apoptosis is considered to be a mechanism for removing unwanted cells without inducing an inflammatory response. Phagocytic cells bind dying and apoptotic cells, phagocytose them, and prevent release of their intracellular contents.

Induction or inhibition of apoptosis can influence the outcome of infection. Induction of programmed cell death in cells of the immune system, including T and B lymphocytes, macrophages, and DCs, is a common feature of many bacterial infections and serves as a strategy to eliminate cells directly involved in protective immunity. Induction of apoptosis of macrophages infected with intracellular bacteria serves to prolong infection by hindering bacterial killing and promoting the spread of the bacteria. It has also been proposed that bacteria-induced apoptosis may be a mechanism to initiate tissue damage, and evidence has been reported to link apoptosis to acute colitis associated with shigellosis (Zychlinsky and Sansonetti 1997).

Elimination of immune cells can also be achieved via cytolysis. Cytolysins are pore-forming bacterial toxins that lyse cells by cell membrane disruption. As with apoptosis induction, stimulation of this cell death mechanism enhances bacterial survival by killing cells such as leukocytes, monocytes, and neutrophils. These toxins play a crucial role in virulence as judged by in vivo studies and are important components contributing to severe inflammatory disease in response to bacterial infection. In some instances (often dependent on toxin concentration and target cell type) these toxins induce apoptosis.

Bacterial virulence factors can modulate cell death pathways in a variety of ways including:

1 disruption of membrane integrity and leakage of cellular components by pore-forming bacterial toxins
2 inhibition of host cell protein synthesis by bacterial toxins
3 delivery of effector proteins into host cells by bacterial TTSS, some of which can directly interact with caspases
4 deletion of T cells by bacterial superantigens
5 activation of second messengers by a bacterial effector.

Pore-forming toxins

Pore-forming toxins are released from bacteria as monomers, which then assemble into oligomeric pores in the target eukaryotic cell membrane. The pores lead to enhanced membrane permeability to monovalent ions and ATP release and hence cytolysis. Repeat-in-toxin (RTX) toxins (also called α-hemolysins) are one class of pore-forming toxins that are produced by a number of bacterial species and include Lkt of *Pasteurella haemolytica* and α-hemolysin of *E. coli* (Weinrauch and Zychlinsky 1999). Binding of RTX toxins to β_2-integrins results in pore formation, increases in intracellular calcium, and cytolysis (Jeyaseelan et al. 2000; Lally et al. 1997). Both α- and β-hemolysins of *Staphylococcus aureus* and *Clostridium perfringens* β-toxin are β-barrel pore-forming toxins (Menestrina et al. 2001). There are no known receptors for these toxins, which cause cell lysis via release of K^+ and also cause rapid calcium influx by opening of endogenous channels. Thiol-activated cholesterol-binding cytolysins are produced by gram-positive bacteria and include streptolysin O produced by *Streptococcus* spp. and pneumolysin produced by *S. pneumoniae* (Palmer 2001). These toxins are important for virulence of the invasive diseases caused by *Streptococcus* spp. They specifically require cholesterol for membrane insertion and act on any cell type displaying this molecule (Shany et al. 1974; Ohno-Iwashita et al. 1992). The pores formed by these toxins are larger than those formed by hemolysis and permit flow of ions, small metabolites, and macromolecules. Even bacterially secreted proteins such as proteases and nucleases can enter the eukaryotic cells via the pores.

Nucleated animal cells may recover from toxin attack by membrane repair mechanisms, and thus low doses of toxin will affect but not kill target cells. Exposure of immune cells to sublethal doses of pore-forming toxins triggers a variety of proinflammatory reactions such as enhanced cytokine release, cytokine receptor shedding, and nitric oxide generation, as a result of stress activation of NF-κB (Hackett and Stevens 1992; Walev et al. 1996; Braun et al. 1999a).

Pore-forming toxins can also induce apoptosis depending on the toxin structure, toxin concentration, and target cell type. The RTX toxins induce apoptosis by perturbation of mitochondrial structure and function, and by activating caspase-3 and caspase-9 (Guzman et al. 1996; Lally et al. 1997; Korostoff et al. 2000). *L. monocytogenes* kills infected DCs by apoptosis thorough release of listeriolysin O (Guzman et al. 1996). In contrast, *Listeria* spp. do not induce apoptosis in macrophages (Zychlinsky et al. 1992). *B. pertussis* induces apoptosis of macrophages via the activity of adenylyl cyclase hemolysin toxin (AC-Hly) (Khelef et al. 1993; Gueirard et al. 1998). The toxin is a bifunctional protein, with a pore-forming hemolysin domain and an adenylyl cyclase domain that elevates intracellular cAMP. Elevated intracellular cAMP interferes with intracellular signaling in cells of the immune system and modulates a variety of immune effector functions, and also induces apoptosis in macrophages and DCs (Khelef et al. 1993; Gueirard et al. 1998).

Induction of DNA damage and inhibition of host-cell protein synthesis by bacterial toxins

Cytolethal distending toxins (CDT) produced by a variety of bacteria induce apoptosis through DNA damage and it has recently been reported that CDTs from *Haemophilus ducreyi* induce apoptosis in immature, but not mature, DCs (Li et al. 2002a). Apoptosis of HeLa cells by CDTs is associated with phosphorylation of histone H2AX and relocation of the DNA repair Mre11 complex (Li et al. 2002a). Diphtheria toxin (DT) from *Cornyebacterium diphtheria* induces macrophage apoptosis by binding to elongation factor 2 and inhibiting translation; mutant toxins deficient in ADP-ribosylating activity are not cytotoxic (Chang et al. 1989; Morimoto and Bonavida 1992). It has also been suggested that DT has nuclease activity, which may contribute to apoptosis by causing DNA fragmentation (Chang et al. 1989).

CT and LT induce apoptosis in T cells, especially $CD8^+$ T cells. Some reports have suggested that the proapoptotic effect of CT is linked to the ADP-ribosyltransferase activity of the S-1 subunit and increased intracellular cAMP (Yamamoto et al. 1999). However, others have shown that the recombinant B subunit of LT can also induce apoptosis in $CD8^+$ T cells by activating the transcriptional factor c-Myc and caspase-3 via a pathway involving NF-κB (Soriani et al. 2001; Salmond et al. 2002).

Products of type III secretion system interacting with caspases

Shigella spp. induces apoptosis of macrophages but not of other cell types. After phagocytosis of *Shigella* by macrophages it escapes from the phagosome into the cytoplasm, inducing apoptosis (Zychlinsky and Sansonetti 1997). The TTSS effector IpaB of *Shigella* sp. induces apoptosis by binding to and activating caspase-1 (Hilbi et al. 1998). Macrophage apoptosis induced by *Shigella flexneri* is associated with release of IL-1 and IL-18, which require caspase-1 for their activation. Caspase-1-deficient mice do not develop acute inflammation that is normally associated with *Shigella* infection, but they are unable to resolve the infection (Sansonetti et al. 2000). *Salmonella* spp. also induce apoptosis in infected macrophages and the mechanism appears to involve the TTSS and is similar to that described for *Shigella*. Although *Salmonella* sp. does not escape the phagolysosome, the SipB effector protein of *Salmonella* like IpaB of *Shigella*, associates with and activates caspase-1 (Hersh et al. 1999).

The establishment of infection by *Yersinia* spp. is dependent on the TTSS which encodes several Yop effectors; these interfere with the function of cells of the immune system. It has been reported that YopJ/YopP is essential for inducing apoptosis in vivo and in cultured macrophages (Monack et al. 1997, 1998). Induction of apoptosis, together with suppression of TNF-α production, facilitates the establishment of *Yersinia* infection in mice (Beuscher et al. 1995). YopP/YopJ induces apoptosis by impairing NF-κB signaling via binding and inhibiting IKKβ, the NFκB-controlling protein (Ruckdeschel et al. 1998). The inhibition of NF-κB and induction of apoptosis are enhanced by LPS (Ruckdeschel et al. 2001).

Fas-mediated apoptosis

Infection of human alveolar macrophages with *M. tuberculosis* causes apoptosis (Keane et al. 1997). Increased expression of FasL has been shown in macrophages within multibacillary leprosy and tuberculosis granulomas (Mustafa et al. 2001). Fas is a member of the TNF receptor family, which plays an important role in maintaining lymphocyte homeostasis, and activation of Fas in the target cells by FasL is a key mechanism of $CD8^+$ CTL and Th1-mediated killing of target cells. The apoptosis can be rescued by TNF-α, IL-1β, or LPS (Mangan et al. 1991; Mustafa et al. 2001). However, it has also been shown that virulent strains of *M. tuberculosis* induce less macrophage apoptosis than attenuated strains; it was demonstrated that *M. tuberculosis* may evade apoptosis of macrophages through inhibition of TNF-α, and by stimulating release of IL-10 and soluble TNFR2 (Balcewicz-Sablinska et al. 1998).

Survival of *H. pylori* and the manifestation of peptic gastrointestinal diseases has been attributed to the *cag* pathogenicity island (PAI). Products of the *cag* PAI have been linked to the induction of apoptosis in epithelial cells (Wang et al. 2001; Jones et al. 2002). Mice deficient in Fas signaling have reduced epithelial cell apoptosis, impaired Th1 responses, and enhanced disease following *H. pylori* infection (Jones et al. 2002). Furthermore, antibodies to Fas or a caspase-8 inhibitor block the induction of apoptosis by *H. pylori*, whereas inhibition of FasL cleavage with a metalloprotease inhibitor increases apoptosis and this has been linked to products of the *cag* PAI (Wang et al. 2001). Persistent infection with strains expressing the *cag* PAI may be facilitated through negative selection of T cells encountering *H. pylori* antigens. *H. pylori* also induces apoptosis of macrophages and this has been linked to NF-κB-dependent induction of arginase (Gobert et al. 2002).

MODULATION OF DC MATURATION

Dendritic cells are considered to be the primary APCs for driving the differentiation of naïve T cells into distinct T-cell subtypes; therefore they play a key role in establishing immunological memory and in directing different arms of the T-cell response (Guermonprez et al. 2002). Immature DCs (iDC) are found in all lymphoid and many nonlymphoid organs, including mucosal tissues, where they exert a sentinel function, with high phagocytic activity. These iDCs endocytose antigens through a variety of receptors and have high capacity to process antigen for presentation by MHC molecules. Interaction with pathogens, including bacteria or their products, causes maturation of the DCs and migration to the T-cell areas of secondary lymphoid organs. The matured DCs have enhanced surface expression of MHCII costimulatory molecules, CD80 and CD86, and are highly efficient at presenting the processed MHC-bound peptides to T cells.

Infection of DCs with many bacterial species, including *L. monocytogenes*, *Salmonella* spp., *M. tuberculosis*, *M. bovis* BCG, *Treponema pallidum*, *Lactobacillus casei*, *B. pertussis*, *E. coli*, *S. aureus*, *Streptococcus gordonii*, *Mycoplasma catarrhalis*, and *C. trachomatis*, has been shown to activate DC maturation (Reis e Sousa et al. 1999). Maturation with most of these bacteria was associated with enhanced IL-12 secretion. In certain cases the bacterial molecules responsible for DC activation have been identified and many of these bind to TLRs and other PRRs. CpG motifs in bacterial DNA bind to TLR-9, flagellin from *L. monocytogenes* and *S. typhimurium* binds to TLR-5, LPS from gram-negative bacteria binds to CD14 and transduces signals through TLR-4, whereas peptidoglycan and lipoteichoic acid of gram-positive bacteria signal through TLR-2 (Ozinsky et al. 2000; Michelsen et al. 2001; Janeway and Medzhitov 2002). TLR-2 also recognizes lipoproteins derived from *M. tuberculosis*, *B. burgdorferi*, *T. pallidium*, and *Mycoplasma fermantes*, LAM from mycobacteria, glycolipid from *Treponema* spp., and LPS from *Leptospira* and *Porphyromonas* spp. (Akira et al. 2001).

Activation of DCs by different pathogen-derived molecules can influence the differentiation of naïve $CD4^+$ T cells into distinct T-cell subtypes, including Th1, Th2, or Tr cells (Figure 32.3). Binding of microbial molecules to TLRs activates a signaling pathway through NF-κB and MAP kinases, leading to activation of genes coding for inflammatory cytokines, including IL-12. CpG, LPS alone or with PT, can stimulate IL-12 production and activate iDCs into DC1 cells that drive the differentiation of naïve T cells into Th1 cells (Ausiello et al. 2002; de Jong et al. 2002). Stimulation of iDCs with CT or LT activates DC2 cells, which drive the differentiation of Th2 cells (Gagliardi et al. 2000). Finally, CT and *B. pertussis* FHA have been shown to activate DCs into a phenotype, termed DCr, which drives the induction of type 1 Tr cells (Lavelle et al. 2003; McGuirk and Mills 2002).

The induction of Th1 cells in response to infection with intracellular bacteria or the induction of Th2 cells by bacterial toxins or extracellular bacteria is central to the host antibacterial immunological defense mechanism. However, diverting the T-cell response to another nonprotective arm, such as Th2 or Tr1 responses during infection with intracellular bacteria, may be a strategy evolved by the bacteria to subvert protective immunity (see below under Modulation of cellular immunity). Alternately inhibition of maturation of the DCs by bacteria or their products can suppress the development of adaptive immunity to the pathogen. *L. casei* induces IL-12 production and maturation of DCs, whereas *L. reuteri* reduces *L. casei*-induced expression of IL-12 and CD86 (a cell surface costimulatory molecule) (Christensen et al. 2002), and induces a DC phenotype that may favor the induction of Th2 or Tr cells. Stimulation of murine DCs with FHA from *B. pertussis*, as well as activating DCs that drive the induction of Tr1 cells, inhibits the iDCs from maturing into DC1 cells, an effect mediated in part through the induction of IL-10 production (McGuirk et al. 2002).

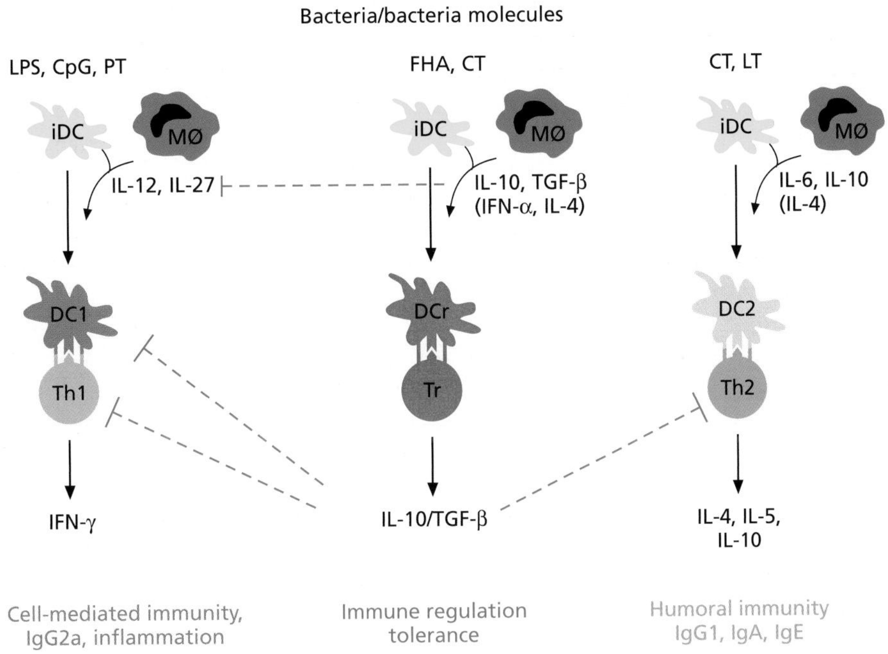

Figure 32.3 *Th cell subtypes in immunity to bacteria. Conserved bacterial structures interact with pathogen recognition receptors (PRRs) and activate maturation of the immature DCs (iDCs) into DC1, DC2, and DCr, which drive the differentiation of naive T-helper cells into Th1, Th2, or Tr cells respectively. Induction of regulatory cytokines by macrophages (Mφs) and DCs in response to conserved bacterial molecules or virulence factors also plays a critical role in the selective development of distinct Th cell subtypes. Protective Th1 or Th2 cells are suppressed either directly or at the level of the antigen-presenting cells, through inhibitory cytokines, IL-10 and TGF-β, secreted by Tr cells. See text for abbreviations.*

MODULATION OF ANTIGEN PROCESSING AND PRESENTATION

Following bacterial uptake, antigens from the bacteria are processed by APCs and degraded peptides are presented in association with MHC molecules to T cells. $CD4^+$ T cells recognize processed antigens in association with MHCII molecules, which have been processed by an exogenous route of antigen processing. In contrast, antigens that are synthesized in host cells or escape from endosomes into the cytoplasm can enter the endogenous route of antigen processing for presentation by MHCI molecules to $CD8^+$ T cells. Finally, glycolipid antigens from bacterial cell walls can be presented by nonpolymorphic class I-like CD1 molecules to $CD8^+$ T cells or $CD4^-CD8^-$ NKT cells. Interference with the intracellular pathways that lead to the production of processed peptides or with the expression of MHC molecules on the surface of the APCs is a common strategy adopted by bacteria to subvert adaptive immune responses (Figure 32.4).

Interference with MHCII processing

Professional APCs, including DCs and macrophages, take up bacteria or their secreted soluble antigens by phagocytosis, macropinocytosis, or receptor-mediated endocytosis. The last occurs through interaction between antibody-coated, or antibody- and complement-coated, bacteria and Fc or complement receptors, or through direct binding of bacterial virulence factors to host cell surface ligands expressed on APCs and exploited by the bacteria for their uptake. Once inside an endosome the bacteria are transferred to late endosomes where they are degraded by lysosomal enzymes. Processed bacterial peptides associate with MHCII molecules after degradation of the invariant chain. Newly synthesized MHCII molecules with associated invariant chain are transported to the endocytic pathway, where an invariant chain-derived peptide class II-associated invariant chain peptide (CLIP) occupies the peptide-binding site in the class II molecule. In the class II-loading compartment CLIP is removed by interaction with HLA-DM and the bacterially-derived peptide is loaded. The stable MHCII-exogenous peptide complex is released to the cell surface where it interacts with the T cell receptor (TCR) of a $CD4^+$ T cell specific for that peptide.

The VacA toxin produced by *H. pylori* interferes with endocytosis in a process that requires Rab7 (Papini et al. 1997) and inhibits antigen processing by interfering with late endocytic membrane trafficking by APCs (Molinari et al. 1998). By lowering the amount of T-cell epitopes generated in the antigen-processing compartments, the toxin is capable of suppressing T-cell activation induced by APCs. Other pathogens have targeted the function of the class II-loading compartment. Patients with Chédiak–Higashai syndrome have a defect in a lyso-

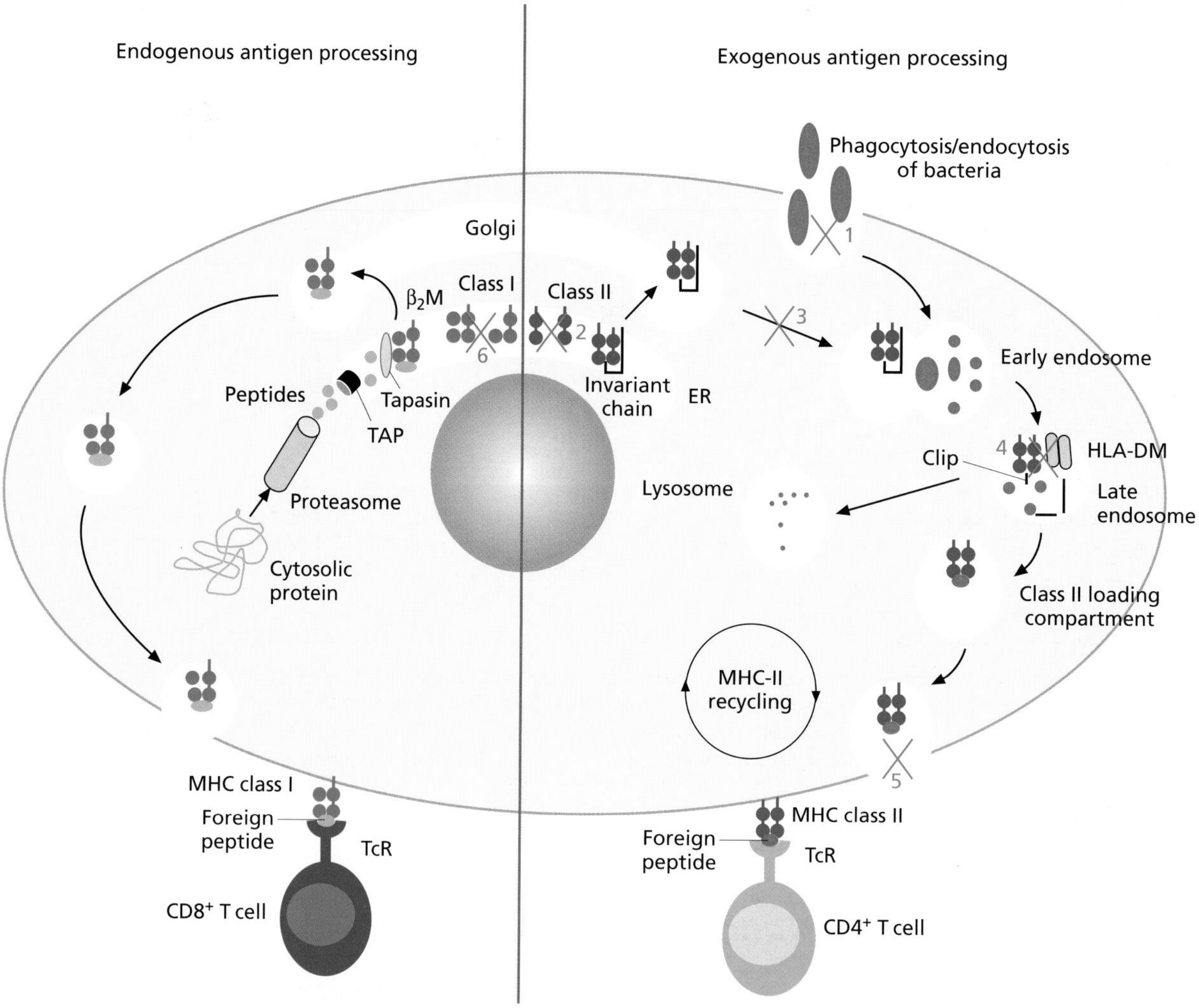

Figure 32.4 *Evasion of antigen processing and presentation. Exogenous antigens, including whole bacteria or bacterial proteins, are taken up by phagocytosis, endocytosis, or pinocytosis, and then degraded by proteolytic enzymes. In the endosome the processed antigen fragments or peptides associate with newly synthesized MHC class II molecules after removal of the invariant chain and the CLIP peptide by HLA-DM. The loaded MHCII molecule is exocytosed and presents the foreign peptide to CD4+ T cells on the surface of the APCs. Endogenous antigens that are synthesized in the host cells, or are released from endosomes into the cytosol, are processed by the proteasomes and TAP, before being loaded onto newly synthesized MHCI molecules in the endoplasmic reticulum. The loaded MHCI–peptide complex is exported to the cells surface, where it activates CD8+ cytoxic T lymphocytes. Bacteria can interfere with class II or I antigen processing and presentation by inhibiting: (1) phagocytosis/endocytosis, (2) class II biosynthesis, (3) export of class II molecules from the Golgi body to endosomes, (4) class II peptide loading, 5) export of the MHCII–peptide complex, or (6) class I biosynthesis. See text for abbreviations.*

somal-trafficking regulator and have enlarged lysosomes; B cells from these patients have altered peptide repertoires and delayed antigen presentation to T cells (Faigle et al. 1998). Enhanced interaction of human leukocyte antigen (HLA)-DR and HLA-DM, and more efficient removal of the CLIP peptide, may explain alterations in the dynamics of peptide loading observed in Chédiak–Higashai syndrome and in cells infected with *C. burnetii*, the rickettsial organism that causes Q fever (Lem et al. 1999).

Intracellular survival of *S. typhimurium* is facilitated by the *phoP* virulence locus, which controls the synthesis of many *Salmonella* proteins required for survival. The products of this locus also appear to affect antigen processing. Macrophages process model antigens expressed by *Salmonella* spp. more efficiently in *phoP-null* than wild-type bacteria (Wick et al. 1995). Furthermore, antigens in bacteria constitutively expressing PhoP are processed less efficiently by macrophages than wild-type bacteria. The *Salmonella phoP* virulence locus has also been found to be responsible for inhibiting antigen presentation in DCs. Although *S. typhimurium* expressing an ovalbumin (OVA) peptide induces maturation of the DCs, the *Salmonella phoP* virulence locus interfered with presentation of the OVA peptide to an OVA-specific T-cell hybridoma (Svensson et al. 2000).

Hemolytic strains of *L. monocytogenes* inhibit MHCII-restricted presentation of antigens to T cells. It has been suggested that listeriolysin, the hemolysin secreted by *L. monocytogenes*, inhibits antigen processing (Cluff et al. 1990). It was later reported that listeriolysin inhibits presentation of native antigens, but not peptides, to T cells; it was suggested that the defect was not caused by inhibition of antigen processing, but may result from irreversible inactivation of T cells that recognize antigen on listeriolysin-treated APCs (Darji et al. 1997).

Antigen processing can be inhibited by the ADP-ribosyltransferase activity of AB toxins; *E. coli*: heat-labile enterotoxin (LT) and cholera toxin (CT), but not the LT B subunit, CT B subunit, or nontoxic LT mutant LT-E112D, suppress intracellular antigen processing in APCs (Matousek et al. 1998). CT and LT inhibited processing of hen egg lysozyme (HEL) expressed in *E. coli* as a HEL fusion protein (containing the HEL 48–61 epitope), but not presentation of pre-existing peptide MHCII complexes to T-cell hybridomas (Matousek et al. 1996, 1998). In contrast, the B subunits of CT or LT or a mutant of LT with reduced enzyme activity do not affect antigen processing, but do enhance antigen presentation (Matousek et al. 1996, 1998). This is consistent with the demonstration that pre-treatment of APCs with wild-type LT or partial inactive mutant LTR72, but not the nontoxic mutant LTK63, suppresses IFN-γ production by a Th1 clone (Ryan et al. 2000). However, APC treatment with LT or LTR72 enhances IL-5 production by a Th2 clone (Ryan et al. 2000).

Yersinia YopH can inhibit activation of B cells by interfering with B-cell antigen-receptor adhesion. Following coincubation with *Yersinia*, B cells are unable to upregulate surface expression of B7-2 (CD86) in response to antigen stimulation (Yao et al. 1999). Downregulation of B7 expression on APCs may also contribute to defective antigen-induced T-cell activation after infection of mice with *M. tuberculosis* (Saha et al. 1994). Delayed-type hypersensitivity responses to crude soluble mycobacterial antigen were suppressed in infected susceptible BALB/c mice, but not in resistant C3H/HeJ mice. The defect appeared to lie in the inability of infected macrophages to provide a costimulatory signal for T cells (Saha et al. 1994).

Modulation of MHCII biosynthesis, intracellular trafficking, and cell surface expression

Different strains of mycobacteria have been shown to have varying abilities to inhibit antigen presentation to T cells by downregulating MHCI and MHCII expression on APCs, and the virulence of the organism has been related to these properties (Weiss et al. 2001). Diminished IFN-γ-induced cell-surface expression of HLA-DR on cells infected with *M. tuberculosis* results from defective transport and processing of class II molecules through the endosomal/lysosomal system (Hmama et al. 1998). Infection of macrophages with *M. bovis* has also been shown to downregulate IFN-γ-induced expression of class II transactivator (CIITA) mRNA, leading to inhibition of induction of MHCII molecules (Wojciechowski et al. 1999). Infection of macrophages with *M. avium* has been shown to arrest phagosome maturation, which limits the intersection of mycobacteria-containing phagosomes with the intracellular trafficking pathways of antigen presentation and results in sequestration of intracellular pools of MHCII and H-2 M molecules (Ullrich et al. 2000).

Phagocytosis of *S. aureus*, *E. coli*, *P. aeruginosa*, or *Salmonella enteritidis* by human monocytes reduces their ability to present an unrelated antigen, purified protein derivative (PPD) to T cells (Pryjma et al. 1994). Although antigen processing is not affected, the infected cells have reduced expression of MHC and accessory molecules, suggesting that the defect is caused by interference with antigen presentation. Phagocytosis of mycobacteria or *E. coli* by monocytes resulted in a failure to process and present antigens to MHCII-restricted T cells as a result of downregulation of MHCII expression, caused by a transient block in the transport of mature class II heterodimers to the surface of the APCs (De Lerma Barbaro et al. 1999). *Chlamydia* spp. can inhibit IFN-γ-induced MHCII expression on epithelial cells, but not IFN-γ-induced expression of the adhesion molecule ICAM-1 or IFN regulatory factor-1 (IRF-1), suggesting that it specifically targets signaling pathways required for MHCII expression (Zhong et al. 1999). The mechanism appears to involve diminished expression of IFN-γ-induced CIITA resulting from degradation of the transcriptional factor, upstream stimulatory factor-1 (USF-1), required for IFN-γ induction of CIITA.

Interference with MHC class I processing and presentation

Unlike viruses, where $CD8^+$ T cells play a major role in limiting infection by killing virally infected cells, MHCI-restricted T cells are induced only against certain intracellular bacteria. Extracellular bacteria do not enter the endogenous route of antigen processing and many intracellular bacteria can survive in intracellular locations distinct from class I processing sites. Therefore strategies for bacterial evasion of class I processing and presentation pathways are more limited. Nevertheless there are a number of reports that demonstrate that certain intracellular bacteria can inhibit expression of MHCI molecules or can bring about changes in the peptide repertoire bound to MHCI molecules.

Infection of murine macrophages with *L. monocytogenes* suppresses constitutive and IFN-γ-induced MHCI gene expression (Schuller et al. 1998). *Chlamydia* spp. can also suppress IFN-γ-induced MHCI expression in infected cells and the mechanism appears to involve degradation of USF-1 and RFX5, an essential downstream transcription factor required for constitutive and IFN-γ-induced MHCI expression (Zhong et al. 2000). *Chlamydia pneumonia* infection of monocytes down-regulates expression of MHCI molecules by inducing the production of IL-10 (Caspar-Bauguil et al. 2000). Thus *C. pneumonia* may suppress $CD8^+$ T-cell responses by inhibiting presentation of bacterial epitopes by MHCI molecules.

Expression of the nonclassic class I molecule, CD1, which presents mycobacterial glycolipids to unconventional T cells, is inhibited after infection of APCs with *M. tuberculosis* (Stenger et al. 1998). The loss of CD1 from the cell surface was associated with complete inhibition of antigen presentation to CD1-restricted T cells.

Invasion of HLA-B27-expressing HeLa cells by *S. typhimurium* enhances expression of IFN-γ-inducible proteasome genes, *LMP*, *MECL*, and *PA28*, and alters the peptide repertoire of HLA-B27 in the infected cell (Maksymowych et al. 1998). The altered peptide repertoire appeared to include peptides of host origin, suggesting that the infection may lead to the generation of autoreactive $CD8^+$ CTLs.

EVASION OF THE HUMORAL RESPONSE

Following activation of the adaptive immune response, B cells produce high concentrations of high-affinity pathogen-specific antibodies, which play a major role in protection against extracellular bacteria. Antibodies directed against adhesins and invasins limit colonization, whereas those directed against bacterial toxins prevent their binding to host target cells and thereby reduce the severity of disease. Murine IgG2a antibodies promote phagocytosis by opsonizing the bacteria and stimulating the complement components C3b and iC3b, which bind complement receptors and further promote phagocytosis. IgA antibodies, induced after bacterial infection of mucosal tissues, function to limit the infection at these sites. In an immune individual primed by a self-limiting infection or immunization, antibodies probably play the major role in conferring protective immunity. Therefore bacteria have evolved strategies to circumvent humoral immunity by evading both complement- and antibody-mediated immune responses (Figure 32.5).

Antigenic variation and phase variation

Most bacteria can vary their surface composition to some extent (Henderson et al. 1999; Hallet 2001). The capacity to vary surface antigens can aid in evasion of complement-mediated killing and opsonophagocytosis, as new antigens are not recognized by existing antibodies and the classic pathway of complement does not become activated. Many of the complement-binding molecules of bacteria undergo phase and/or antigenic variation, giving rise to differences in the levels of serum

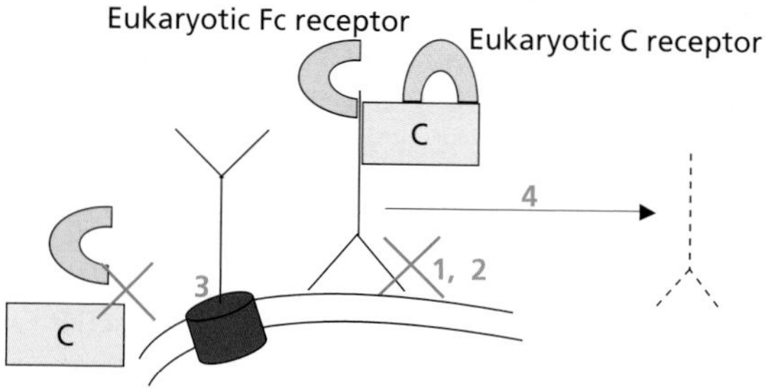

Figure 32.5 *Evasion of antibodies. Specific antibodies bind their cognate ligands on the bacterial surface, recruiting complement factors to the site. The antibodies and complement are recognized by Fc and C receptors on phagocytic cells, which mediate uptake into these cells. The complement cascade is also activated to form membrane attack complexes (MAC) and lyse the bacteria. Evasion of antibodies by bacteria can occur in a number of ways: (1) masking of the bacterial surface from antibody recognition, (2) avoidance of antibody recognition by antigenic and phase variation, (3) binding of antibodies by antibody-binding proteins, and (4) degradation and modification of antibodies.*

resistance in different isolates and strains of the same bacterial species.

Antigenic variation of proteins occurs mainly by spontaneous point mutations in the genes encoding the protein antigen, such that the physical topography of the molecule is altered and antibodies directed against the original antigen do not recognize the altered one. Using phase variation, bacteria frequently and reversibly undergo altered expression of surface molecules resulting from genetic alterations in specific loci of their genomes. These two types of genetic alterations are particularly dominant in two classes of loci: (1) genes encoding surface structures such as LPS, flagella, and fimbriae, and (2) genes encoding virulence factors that modify host cell physiology or protect the bacteria from antimicrobial systems in the host. These surface structures not only affect bacterial virulence but are also key targets of the host immune system, resulting in selective pressure to generate polymorphism in genes coding for antigenic diversity. Varying expression and composition of these molecules allow bacteria not only to counteract the host immune defenses but also to colonize new ecological niches. These variations can be very extensive. In *S. enterica* there are more than 2000 separate serotypes based on differences in carbohydrate structures, such as LPS, and also flagella antigens (Fierer and Guiney 2001). There is enormous variation in the virulence and epidemiology of these serotypes.

CAPSULES

Phase variation can control gene expression in an 'on–off' manner. Genes for the biosynthesis of capsules in *Neisseria meningitidis* and *Haemophilus influenza* undergo this type of regulation (Gilsdorf 1998). The presence of a capsule may be beneficial in some circumstances, e.g. in the formation of biofilms, and a hindrance in others, e.g. for the motile stages of bacterial life. Bacteria growing in biofilms are highly resistant to the immune system of the host. Soluble factors and immune cells have limited access to bacteria in these circumstances as a result of the network of extracellular material surrounding the bacteria. Chronic bacterial infections, such as *P. aeruginosa* infections in the lungs of cystic fibrosis patients and *S. aureus* infections of prostheses, are difficult to treat because of the biofilm nature of growth of the bacteria. However, spread of the bacteria is enhanced when they are released from the biofilm capsule.

LPS AND LIPOOLIGOSACCHARIDE

Bacteria can alter surface molecule composition by controlling expression of genes for LPS and lipooligosaccharide (LOS) biosynthesis and modification (Lerouge and Vanderleyden 2002). LPS variations are mostly caused by differences in the polysaccharide side chains resulting from polymorphisms in the genes that encode the machinery to synthesize these polysaccharides (Liu et al. 1991). Furthermore, the regulation of lipid A modifications by *Salmonella* spp. renders these bacteria more resistant to antimicrobial peptides and renders the LPS less stimulatory for macrophages (Guo et al. 1997). LPS interacts with both antibodies and complement, and much of antibody response to *Salmonella* infection is directed against LPS O-antigens. LPS-specific antibodies play a major role in protecting against *Salmonella* infection and LPS variation allows *Salmonella* spp. to infect hosts that already have antibody directed against a different O-antigen serotype. Variation of LPS during infection may also be advantageous. Changes in *Salmonella* LPS structure result in changes in opsonin binding, in phagocytosis and killing by neutrophils, and in virulence (Jimenez-Lucho et al. 1987; Johnson et al. 1992). Other bacteria that alter their LPS composition include *H. pylori* and *L. pneumophila* (Appelmelk et al. 2000). During the course of an infection, antigens may vary or change with the host response and in *H. pylori* certain LPS structures mimic the eukaryotic Lewis antigens, allowing the bacteria to evade recognition and elimination. *C. jejuni*, *Neisseria gonorrhoeae*, and *H. influenzae* are all capable of altering their LOS structure (Gilsdorf 1998; Harvey et al. 2000; Linton et al. 2000). Acquisition of new LOS epitopes by *H. influenzae* is associated with increased resistance to complement-mediated serum and occurs rapidly among isolates (Kimura and Hansen 1986).

PROTEINS

Outer membrane proteins (OMP) frequently undergo phase and antigenic variation. *N. gonorrhoeae* strains may carry up to 12 phase-variable *opa* genes, encoding OMPs mediating bacterial adhesion and invasion. The expression of these functionally redundant genes is variable, thereby allowing the generation of antigen variants while maintaining and diversifying essential activities. The surface layer protein of *Campylobacter fetus* and OspC of *Borrelia* spp. also undergo antigenic variation (Dworkin and Blaser 1997). Pili and flagella are subject to variation, e.g. *N. gonorrhoea* has 18–19 pilin cassettes with which to make variable type IV pili. *Salmonella* flagella stimulate and activate macrophages and different flagella have varying potencies, suggesting that this flagellar phase variation may be a mechanism to downregulate inflammatory responses (Ciacci-Woolwine et al. 1998).

The *H. influenzae* IgA protease undergoes antigenic variation with over 30 serotypes and, in some cases, these variants result in changes in IgA protease specificity and its antibody inhibition pattern. (Lomholt et al. 1993). A global effect on gene expression can be achieved by variation in expression of a global regulator such as BvgAS of *Bordetella* spp. The acquisition or loss of unstable genetic elements (e.g. in *L. pneumophila*) or pathogenicity islands (e.g. SPI-1 and SPI-2 of *Salmonella* spp.) or pathogenicity plasmids (e.g. pYV plasmids of *Yersinia* spp.) in virulent bacteria can lead to significant changes in the protein composition of the bacterial membrane.

Antigenic variation contributes to the adaptive capacity of the bacterium for new environments and for survival. The ability to rapidly produce and modify specific structures on the cell surface is crucial in the establishment of infection, particularly with respect to the variety of biological niches within the host. Phase variation results in a more versatile and heterogeneous population that can cope better with a variety of different environments. It may result in better colonization as changes arise in structures mediating attachment and invasion of eukaryotic cells. It may lead to better evasion of host defenses as variation allows the bacteria to escape the neutralizing activities of antibodies and thus evade pre-existing host immunity.

Antibody-binding proteins

Several bacteria express immunoglobulin Fc-domain binding proteins, which are associated with the cell surface or released in soluble form from the surface. Binding of immunoglobulins via their Fc portion on the bacterial surface is thought to form a protective covering on the bacteria so that the bacteria are no longer recognized as foreign, and access of complement and specific antibodies to the bacteria is obstructed. Binding of IgG to Fc receptors on bacteria (e.g. SfbI on *Streptococcus pyogenes*) inhibits Fc-mediated phagocytosis by macrophages and antibody-dependent cell-mediated cytotoxicity (Medina et al. 1999). The best-known Ig-binding proteins are protein A of *Staphylococcus* spp. and protein

G of *Streptococcus* spp. (Kronvall 1973; Reis et al. 1984). One of the key events in the elimination of antigen or antigen–antibody complexes (immune complexes) is the covalent binding of C3b. This binding promotes uptake by phagocytic cells via C3 receptors. The two C3b-binding sites on IgG overlap the two regions that are bound by bacterial proteins such as protein A and protein G. Thus, these bacterial proteins directly interfere with C3b binding to the Fc region of IgG (Munoz et al. 1998). The surface-bound, M-protein family of *Streptococcus* spp. is made up of highly characterized, immunoglobulin-binding proteins and in most cases they bind only a single antibody class (Navarre and Schneewind 1999). There is also species specificity in the antibody binding. Binding of both IgG and IgA or IgG alone is found in all-invasive disease, group A streptococcus clinical isolates, whereas it is not so common in septicemia and noninvasive throat isolates (Raeder and Boyle 1995).

Human IgA is abundant in the secretions at mucosal surfaces such as those lining the lungs, gut, and genitourinary tract. These surfaces represent major potential sites of invasion and the immune protection offered by secretory IgA, as the predominant antibody at these sites, serves as a critical initial defense against pathogens. IgA recognizes and binds bacteria and triggers their elimination by interaction of its Fc domain with an Fcα receptor (FcαRI) expressed on neutrophils, eosinophils and macrophages. This interaction stimulates phagocytosis, superoxide generation and release of enzymes and inflammatory mediators. Two *S. pyogenes* IgA Fc-binding proteins, Arp4 and Sir22, both of the M-protein family, are important for virulence (Stenberg et al. 1994; Thern et al. 1998). Arp4 has been shown to inhibit a respiratory burst triggered by the binding of IgA-Fc to FcαRI on neutrophils. B protein of group B *Streptococcus* spp. also binds IgA (Jerlstrom et al. 1991). These three proteins all bind the Cα2-Cα3 interdomain of the IgA Fc domain. This domain is responsible for binding FcαRI and the streptococcal IgA-binding proteins interfere with this interaction (Pleass et al. 2001).

Antibody degradation and modification

Bacteria can degrade immunoglobulins to inactivate them. The degrading proteins are enzymes of broad proteolytic activity, which may also degrade complement and other host factors. IgG is degraded by the *P. gingivalis* PrtH protease, which in addition degrades the complement component C3 (Fletcher et al. 1995). Similar cell-associated proteases are present in *Lactobacillus* and *Streptococcus* spp. (Siezen 1999). IgA1 is degraded by the three leading causes of bacterial meningitis, *H. influenzae*, *N. meningitidis*, and *S. pneumoniae*, important urogenital pathogens, and some members of the oropharyngeal flora. These proteases are important for the ability of bacteria to colonize mucosal membranes in the presence of secretory IgA antibodies and result in a local functional IgA deficiency.

IgA can be inactivated by modification of its immunoglobulin structure. *Streptococcus* and *Veillonella* spp. can remove terminally positioned sialic acid from IgA1. This may have an immune evasion function, because sialic acid protects glycoproteins, including immunoglobulins, from proteolytic enzymes. Deglycosylation of antibodies increases their sensitivity to proteolytic degradation and inhibits the Fc-mediated effector functions that mediate antigen disposal.

EVASION OF COMPLEMENT

The complement system plays a major role in resistance against microbial infections participating in both specific and nonspecific immunity (Rautemaa and Meri 1999). The complement activation pathways comprise a complex set of serum proteins that are activated by antigen–antibody complexes (classic pathway), certain carbohydrates (lectin pathway), or a variety of pathogen surface molecules (alternate pathway). Activation of complement has a number of consequences. Some complement activation products such as C3b, iC3b, C4b, and C1q are opsonins, inducing recognition and phagocytosis of the bacteria by macrophages and polymorphonuclear granulocytes. C3a, C4a, and C5a increase vascular permeability and induce inflammation. The chemotactic C5a also attracts leukocytes to the site of infection and activates them. Membrane attack complexes (MAC), composed of multiple complement factors, form on the surfaces of gram-negative bacteria and cause the collapse of membrane potential, leading to lytic cell death. Microbial activation of the complement system eventually leads to phagocytosis of the target and/or lysis of the bacteria by MACs. Given the dramatic effects of complement activation in the host, the complement system is tightly controlled to protect host cells from complement attack. Both soluble inhibitors, such as factor H, and cell membrane glycoproteins, such as protectin, are critical for regulating complement activation. Protectin regulates MAC insertion into membranes. Factor H inhibits the alternate pathway and C4bp inhibits the classic pathway, by both inhibiting interactions between the complement components and enhancing complement component degradation. Pathogenic bacteria have evolved strategies to evade and inhibit the complement system in order to resist opsonophagocytosis and/or complement-mediated cytolytic damage (Figure 32.6) (Rautemaa and Meri 1999; Wurzner 1999).

Masking the bacterial surface

Pathogens can mask their membrane surfaces to avoid recognition by complement. Prevention of access of

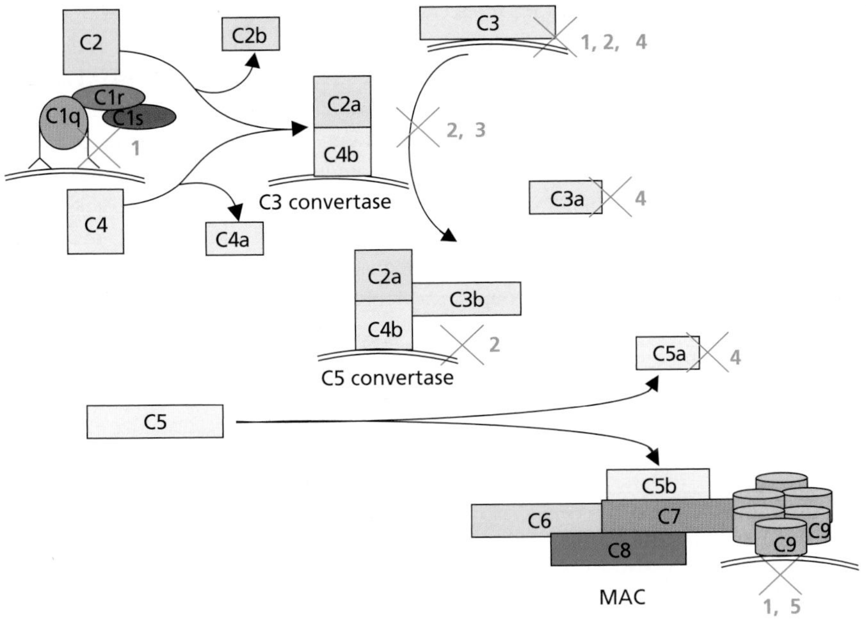

Figure 32.6 *Evasion of complement. In the classic complement cascade antibodies bound to the surface of bacteria recruit C1q, C1r, and C1s. This binding stimulates the cleavage of C2 and C4, releasing C2b and C4a. C2a and C4b associate to form the C3 convertase, which induces cleavage of C3 to C3a and C3b, thus forming a C5 convertase. C1q, C3b, and C4b are opsonins inducing recognition and phagocytosis of the bacteria by macrophages and polymorphonuclear granulocytes, whereas C4a and C5a are anaphylatoxins increasing vascular permeability and inducing inflammation. C5b and the chemotactic C5a are formed from C5, and C5b together with C6, C7, and C8 recruits the assembly of C9 components to form a lytic membrane attack complex (MAC). C3 and C5 convertases and MACs are also generated by the alternate complement pathway. Bacteria use a number of mechanisms to evade complement activation and killing: (1) masking of the bacterial surface, (2) shedding of complement complexes from the bacterial surface, (3) binding of complement inhibition factor H, (4) cleavage of complement components, and (5) inhibition of MAC insertion.*

complement to the cell membrane can by achieved by expression of polysaccharide capsules and/or long and dense LPS by gram-negative bacteria. These structures hinder access of both the initial complement factors and the lytic MACs. The insertion of MACs into the bacterial membrane is inhibited in gram-positive bacteria as a result of the presence of the surrounding peptidoglycan. *S. aureus* capsule expression leads to reduced C3 deposition on the bacterial surface, in turn leading to decreased phagocytic killing in vitro and increased lethality in vivo (Thakker et al. 1998; Cunnion et al. 2001). *S. pneumoniae* capsule expression also leads to decreased C3 deposition and the *H. influenzae* capsule is required for serum resistance and virulence of invasive strains (Brown et al. 1983; Noel et al. 1996). Group B meningococci and group B streptococci express capsular polysaccharides that are rich in sialic acid, which is relatively nonimmunogenic and prevents complement activation (Edwards et al. 1982). LPS composition influences recognition by complement, as in the case of some *Salmonella* spp. which possess LPS with long *O*-polysaccharide side chains that sterically hinder access of complement components such as C1q and MACs to the bacterial membrane and bacterial OMPs (Joiner et al. 1982a, 1982b; Liang-Takasaki et al. 1983). The LPS structure of *Klebsiella pneumoniae*, *C. burnetti*, and *B. abortus* also renders these bacteria more resistant to complement (Vishwanath et al. 1988; Merino et al. 1992; Eisenschenk et al. 1999).

Shedding

Bacterial pathogens can shed strong complement-activating surface molecules and immune complexes from their cell surfaces. Shedding prevents the accumulation of complement factors on the bacterial membrane and also diverts antibodies away from the bacterial surface. *S. aureus* sheds up to 30 percent of the C3 deposited on its surface (Cunnion et al. 2001) and *E. coli* and *S. minnesota* also shed complement factors and/or assembled complement complexes from their cell surfaces (Joiner et al. 1982a; Joiner 1988). Shedding of complement complexes from the surface of *S. pneumoniae* involves the action of the host complement inhibitory factor, protein H (Berge et al. 1997).

Cleavage of complement

Just as bacteria degrade antibodies to inactivate them, bacteria also degrade complement factors to inhibit activation of the complement pathway. *P. aeruginosa* cleaves complement components by extracellular secreted proteases, as do *H. pylori* and *P. gingivalis* (Hong and

Ghebrehiwet 1992; Schenkein et al. 1995; Rokita et al. 1998). *P. aeruginosa* elastase inactivates the anaphylatoxins C3a and C5a, resulting in a reduced inflammatory response. The PrtH protease of *P. gingivalis* is an important virulence factor for the bacterium because it degrades C3, resulting in a reduction of C3b and C3bi on the bacterial surface and inhibition of phagocytosis by neutrophils. *S. pneumonia* degrades C3 by a cell-associated activity that leads to inactivation of C3 and release of C3 from the bacterial surface whereas group A *S. pyogenes* possesses a cell wall-anchored C5a peptidase to inactivate C5a (Wexler et al. 1985; Angel et al. 1994).

Binding complement inhibition proteins

To avoid elimination by complement, microbes can exploit complement regulatory factors of the host. Some bacteria bind proteins, such as factor H or C4bp, that negatively regulate complement activation. The binding of factor H or C4bp confers serum resistance to bacteria and prevents their phagocytosis. Many of these binding molecules undergo phase and/or antigenic variation, giving rise to differences in the levels of serum resistance in different isolates and strains of the same bacterial species. Serum resistance is a major determinant of *N. gonorrhoeae* virulence, because serum-sensitive gonococci predominantly result in symptomatic local inflammation, whereas serum-resistant strains are associated with disseminated infection. The source of complement resistance in these bacteria is sialyation of low-molecular-weight LOS (Ram et al. 1998). Sialic acid-containing structures enhance the interaction between C3b and factor H. Binding of factor H to sialyated LOS leads to rapid conversion of surface-bound C3 to iC3b and to elimination of complement activation components from the cell surface. OMPs are also involved in binding factor H with similar consequences, e.g. *N. gonorrhoeae* Por1A which also binds C4bp and the expression of which correlates with serum resistance and disseminated gonococcal disease (Ram et al. 1998, 2001). Other factor H- and/or C4bp-binding proteins include the majority of the streptococcal M protein family, a family of more than 80 antigenically distinct proteins, most of which have antiphagocytic activity (Horstmann et al. 1988; Johnsson et al. 1996). The M-protein–C4bp interaction is important for serum resistance in these bacteria. In addition, several M-proteins bind immunoglobulins IgG and/or IgA through the constant Fc portion.

Inhibition of MAC insertion

Several gram-negative bacteria can interfere with the assembly of terminal MACs and thereby prevent lethal outer cell membrane damage. The related OMPs, Rck of *S. typhimurium* and Ail of *Y. enterocolitica*, cause a failure in the formation of fully polymerized tubular MACs (Heffernan et al. 1994). The TraT lipoproteins of *Salmonella* spp. and *E. coli* increase resistance to complement killing by interference with the generation of complement factors, and the correct assembly and membrane insertion of MACs (Pramoonjago et al. 1992). The Sic protein of *S. pyogenes* is important for mouse mucosal colonization and inhibits the normal cytolytic effect of MACs (Akesson et al. 1996).

MODULATION OF CELLULAR IMMUNITY

Inhibition of T-cell activation and proliferation

T cells recognize antigens through engagement of the TCR with processed antigenic peptide associated with an MHC molecule expressed on the surface of an APC. However, activation of the T cell is dependent on a second signal provided by interaction of CD28 on the T-cell surface with costimulatory molecules CD80 or CD86, expressed on the surface of activated APCs. In the absence of the second signal, the T cells become anergic and are no longer able to divide or respond to antigen. Engagement of CD3 and CD28 results in redistribution of lipid rafts to the interface between the T cells and APCs. Clustering of TCRs activates the T cell by bringing together tyrosine kinases and permitting their phosphorylation, which initiates a signaling cascade through the CD3 complex and leads to activation of genes required for proliferation and cytokine secretion. Proliferation of T cells with APCs or unpurified PBMCs in vitro, in response to foreign antigen or mitogens, which crosslink surface receptors on the T cells, is often used as a measure of T-cell activation. Alternately, the cytokine secretion pattern is used as an index of activation (or suppression) of distinct T-cell subtypes. Although IL-2 has been used as a marker of Th1 cells, it is now evident that this cytokine can be secreted by precursor T cells as well as by activated Th1 cells. IFN-γ production, without IL-4, IL-5, or IL-10 is a useful marker of Th1 responses, whereas IL-4 and IL-5 without IFN-γ can be used to define Th2 cells. The recently described Tr cells can also be discriminated from Th1 or Th2 cells on the basis of anti-inflammatory cytokines: IL-10 with or without TGF-β but no IL-4 or IFN-γ for Tr1 cells, and TGF-β, with or without IL-10 but no IL-4 or IFN-γ for Th3 cells.

As T-cell activation is an essential step in cellular and humoral immune responses to infectious pathogens, many bacteria have evolved strategies to evade adaptive immunity by suppressing T-cell responses. In a limited number of cases the bacterial molecule and its host cell target have been identified, but most studies on suppressed T-cell responses during bacterial infection have not established the mechanism. Interference with any aspect of antigen uptake processing or presentation by the APCs or signaling in the T cell can inhibit T-cell activation. Furthermore, as activation of distinct T-cell subtypes is regulated by the reciprocal cell populations, factors that strongly promote the induction of one subtype may inhibit the activation of another. Consequently, suppression of T-cell responses or specific T-cell subtypes may reflect subversion of many different aspects of innate as well as adaptive immunity dealt with in other parts in this chapter.

Infection of mice with an attenuated *aroA* strain of *S. typhimurium* results in profound immunosuppression, with inhibition of T- and B-cell proliferation to foreign antigen (al-Ramadi et al. 1991a) and of the T cell's production of IL-2 in response to concanavalin A (Con A) (al-Ramadi et al. 1991b). *H. pylori* suppresses in vitro proliferative responses of human PBMCs to mitogens and antigens and a soluble cytoplasmic fraction of *H. pylori* mediates the suppression by acting on monocytes and directly on the T cells (Knipp et al. 1994). Nitric oxide (NO) was later identified as a soluble macrophage-derived factor capable of mediating *Salmonella*-induced immunosuppression (Gregory et al. 1993; MacFarlane et al. 1999). Treatment of mice with the NO inhibitor, aminoguanidine hemisulfate, blocks the suppressive effect of *Salmonella* infection on T- and B-cell responses, but it also blocks influx of neutrophils and macrophages into the spleen, which was associated with enhanced bacterial load and higher mortality of the mice (MacFarlane et al. 1999), suggesting that NO is involved in host defense as well as immunosuppression. Suppression of T-cell responses by *S. typhimurium* was also found to be mediated by soluble factors released by monocytes/macrophages and was reversed by the addition of IL-4 (al-Ramadi et al. 1991b).

In a limited number of bacterial infections where suppression of T-cell responses has been observed, the immunomodulatory molecules involved have been identified. *Yersinia pseudotuberculosis* can inhibit T- and B-cell activation by interference with T- and B-cell antigen-receptor activation; the effect is mediated by YopH, which has tyrosine phosphatase activity (Yao et al. 1999). Patients with lepromatous leprosy are highly immunosuppressed; their T cells do not respond to *Mycobacterium leprae* antigens and macrophages and $CD8^+$ T cells have been implicated in the suppression (Mehra et al. 1984; Salgame et al. 1984). The *M. leprae* antigen LAM-B, can suppress proliferative responses of PBMCs from lepromatous leprosy patients, tuberculoid leprosy patients, and normal individuals (Kaplan et al. 1987). Lipoglycans from *M. leprae* have also been shown to induce immune suppression in mice, including inhibition of delayed type hypersensitivity (DTH) responses and proliferation of lymph node cells to mitogens (Moura and Mariano 1997).

The OspA protein of *B. burgdorferi* inhibits proliferative responses of human PBMCs to phyohemagglutinin and Con A (Chiao et al. 2000). *B. burgdorferi* infection of disease-susceptible (C3H/HeJ) and disease-resistant (BALB/c) mice results in impaired proliferation of IL-2 and IL-4 production to mitogens (de Souza et al. 1993). More recently it has been suggested that Th1 responses are suppressed whereas Th2 responses are enhanced; *B. burgdorferi* transmission by *Ixodes scapularis* suppressed IL-2 and IFN-γ and enhanced IL-4 production in mice (Zeidner et al. 1997). Similarly, the inhibitory effect of *E. coli* LT on T-cell responses was shown to be specific for Th1 cells and was mediated by the effect of ADP-ribosyltransferase enzyme activity on APCs as well as on T cells (Ryan et al. 2000). Furthermore, it has been reported that *E. coli* LT-treated epithelial cells release soluble factors, probably prostaglandins, that inhibit proliferation of a T-cell hybridoma in vitro (Lopes et al. 2000).

Upsetting Th1/Th2 balance

The demonstration that T cells could be discriminated on the basis of cytokine secretion and function had a considerable impact on our understanding of immunity to infectious diseases. Following the discovery of Th1 and Th2 subtypes of $CD4^+$ T cells in the 1980s, a dogma emerged which stated that Th1 cells secreted IFN-γ and TNF-β and mediated cellular immunity against intracellular pathogens, including viruses and intracellular bacteria, whereas Th2 cells were the true helper cells and mediated humoral immunity against extracellular bacteria and parasites. Furthermore, as Th1 and Th2 responses are crossregulated through IL-4/IL-10 and IFN-γ secreted by the reciprocal subtypes, any upset in the balance of Th1 or Th2 cells could prolong the course of different infections and this could be used as a strategy for pathogens to prolong their survival in the host (see Figure 32.3, p. 657). To a certain extent that still holds; however, it is now full recognized that Th1 cells also provide help for B-cell production of antibody subclasses involved in virus neutralization, opsonization of extracellular bacteria, and complement fixation. Furthermore, other populations of $CD4^+$ T cells with suppressive function, termed 'Tr cells' may also inhibit protective Th1 and possibly Th2 responses to infectious agents.

In the field of bacterial immunity, *M. leprae* provides one of the best examples of the influence of Th1/Th2 responses on the outcome of infection. In patients with lepromatous leprosy, cellular immune responses to many antigens are profoundly depressed and T cells in these patients are also anergized to unrelated antigens. These patients make potent antibody responses to the bacteria but are not protected. In contrast, patients with tuberculoid leprosy have potent cellular immune responses and their macrophages can kill the bacteria. The important distinction between the two diseases states is that the patients with lepromatous leprosy mount Th2 responses, which are not protective, whereas in the tuberculoid leprosy patients Th1 cells are dominant and IFN-γ secreted by these cells activates infected macrophages to kill the bacteria (Sieling and Modlin 1994).

A failure of Th1-cell induction or function has also been shown to result in increased susceptibility to other bacterial infections. Development of *B. burgdorferi* infection after transmission by *I. scapularis*, in disease-susceptible C3H/HeJ mice, is associated with the development of Th2 responses, but not in disease-resistant BALB/c mice (Zeidner et al. 1997). Th1 cells have been implicated in clearance of primary infection and preventing reinfection with *B. pertussis* and mice develop disseminating disease in the absence of functional IFN-γ (Mahon et al. 1997). However, Th1 responses are suppressed in the lungs and draining lymph nodes during acute infection (McGuirk et al. 1998), and this appears to result from a variety of immune subversion strategies by the bacteria, including the induction of *B. pertussis*-specific Tr cells (McGuirk et al. 2002).

Pathogen-specific IL-10/TGF-β secreting Tr cells

$CD4^+$ T cells that constitutively express the IL-2α receptor (CD25) in vivo have been shown to have immunosuppressive properties and to be capable of preventing autoimmune diseases mediated by Th1 cells. Suppressor $CD4^+$ T cells that secrete TGF-β were termed 'Th3 cells' (Chen et al. 1994) and suppressor T-cell clones that secreted high levels of IL-10 and IL-5, but not IFN-γ or IL-4, were termed 'Tr1 cells' (Groux et al. 1997). It was suggested that the primary function of these Tr cells is to maintain immunological homeostasis and tolerance to selfantigens. However, recent evidence suggests that these cells can also be generated against foreign antigen on infectious pathogens.

The first report on Tr cell clones specific for a bacterial antigen were murine Tr1 cells specific for the *B. pertussis* antigens FHA and pertactin from the lungs of *B. pertussis*-infected mice (McGuirk et al. 2002). Human Tr1 or Th3 clones have also been generated against the filarial parasite *Onchocerca volvulus* (Doetze et al. 2000) and the hepatitis C virus core protein (MacDonald et al. 2002). Functional studies on the *B. pertussis*-specific Tr1 clones demonstrated that they were capable of suppressing IFN-γ production by Th1 responses against the same or an unrelated influenza virus antigen in vitro, and also suppressed protective Th1 responses against the bacteria in vivo (McGuirk et al. 1998). The induction of Tr cells against a pathogen may be a means for the host to control or terminate Th1 responses in vivo and thereby limit immunopathology and collateral damage to host tissue. However, it may represent a novel evasion strategy adopted by bacteria to subvert protective cell-mediated immunity. It is interesting that local Th1 responses are suppressed in the lungs and draining lymph nodes during acute infection of mice with *B. pertussis* (McGuirk et al. 1998). Furthermore, in infants and young children the disease is very protracted, with secondary infection in the lung.

In addition to the chronic viral and parasitic diseases, there are a number of other bacterial infections that are either persistent or associated with immunosuppression in vivo. Although there are a variety of explanations, including bacterial interference with antigen processing and presentation or production of anti-inflammatory cytokines by innate cells, the induction of Tr cells by the pathogen may also contribute to this immunosuppression. With the exception of the *B. pertussis* study, bacteria-specific Tr cells have not been cloned or specifically identified at the polyclonal level. However, there is indirect evidence of suppressor, anergic, or IL-10- or TGF-β-secreting T cells in a number of bacterial infections, including infections with *Mycobacteria*, *Pneumocystis*, *Helicobacter*, and *Lactobacillus* spp.

A proportion of patients with active pulmonary TB have defective DTH responses to mycobacterial antigens (i.e. they do not mount a skin test response to PPD) and have a poor clinical outcome. T cells from these anergic patients secreted IL-10, but not IFN-γ, after in vitro stimulation with PPD, whereas PPD skin test-reactive patients secreted IL-10 and IFN-γ; IFN-γ production is augmented in T cells from anergic patients by the addition of anti-IL-10 (Boussiotis et al. 2000). Defective phosphorylation of TCRζ and defective activation of ζ-associated protein (ZAP)-70 and the mitogen-activated protein (MAP) kinase extracellular regulated kinase (ERK) was also demonstrated in the anergic T cells stimulated with anti-CD3 and anti-CD28 (Boussiotis et al. 2000). Furthermore treatment of mice with killed *Mycobacterium vaccae* induces allergen-specific $CD4^+CD45RB^{Lo}$ Tr cells which are capable of protecting against airways inflammation, through an IL-10- and TGF-β-dependent mechanism (Zuany-Amorim et al. 2002). In a study of *Pneumocystis carinii*-infected mice, it was demonstrated that Tr cells may function to control the Th1 response, which are responsible for eliminating the bacteria and mediating lung immunopathology. Adoptive transfer of $CD4^+CD25^+$ T cells delays bacterial clearance, but also prevents development of lethal pneumonia by $CD4^+CD25^-$ T cells (Hori et al. 2002). $CD4^+$ T cells from *Helicobacter hepaticus*-infected mice block colitis in recombinant activation genes $RAG^{-/-}$ of mice induced by transfer of *H. hepaticus*-specific T cells from IL-$10^{-/-}$ mice; suppression was mediated by IL-10 and has been attributed to *H. hepaticus*-induced Tr cells (Kullberg et al. 2002). *Lactobacillus paracasei* has been shown to induce IL-10 and

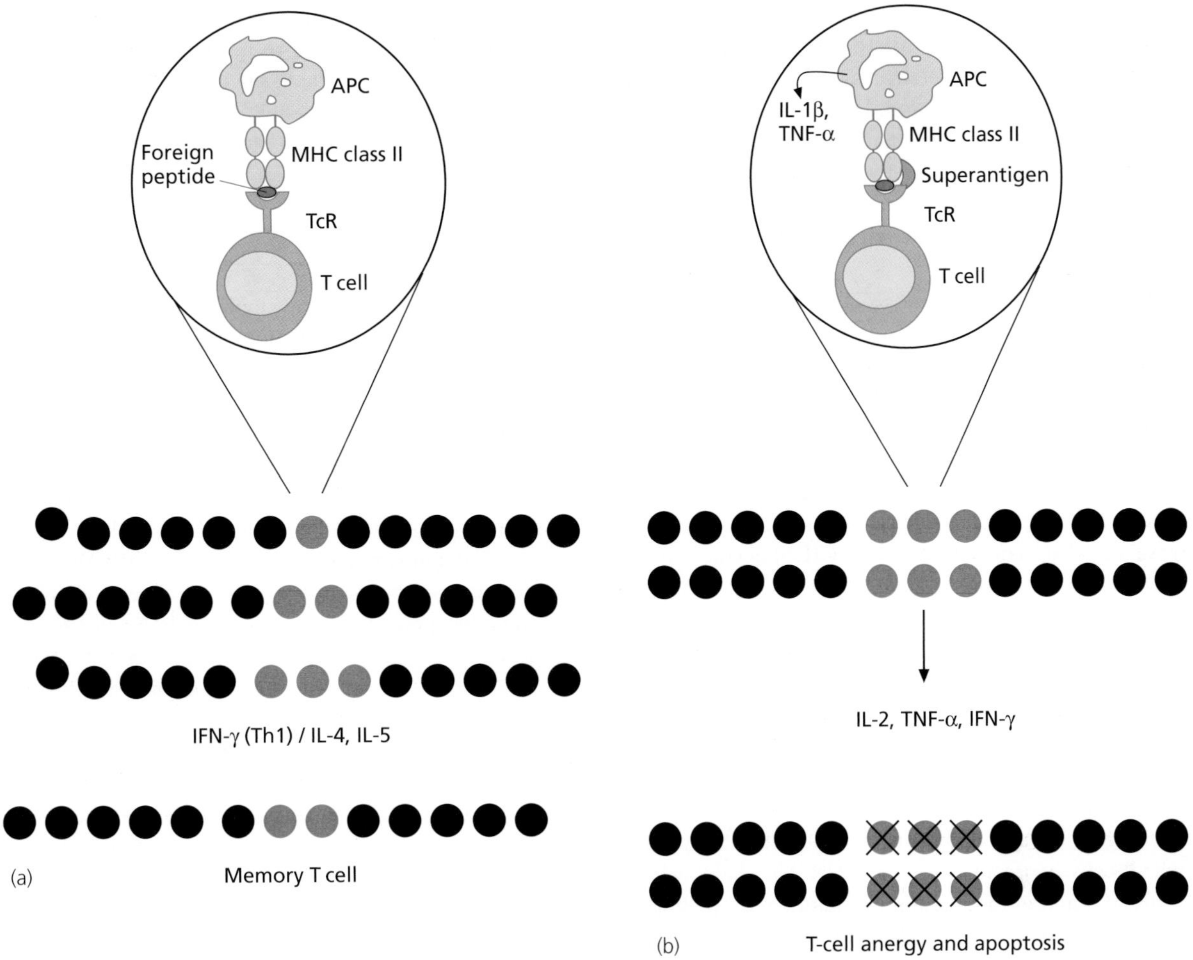

Figure 32.7 *Superantigen versus conventional antigen activation of T cells.* **(a)** *Conventional foreign antigens are processed by antigen-presenting cells (APCs) and peptide fragments associate with variable regions in the groove of the MHC class II molecule, and interact with variable regions of the T-cell receptor (TCR). Only a low frequency of T cells specific for the peptide MHC complex are activated. Activated T cells proliferate and secrete cytokines, and then a proportion goes on to become memory T cells.* **(b)** *Bacterial superantigens bind as intact proteins to MHCII molecules outside the foreign peptide binding groove and crosslink with the variable region of the TCR β chain on T cells. Following this encounter the APC produces proinflammatory cytokines, including interleukin IL-1β and tumor necrosis factor α (TNF-α) and all T cells bearing that Vβ element are activated to produce Th1-type cytokines IL-2, TNF-α, and interferon γ (IFN-γ), and then undergo apoptosis. This results in massive secretion of proinflammatory cytokines and deletion of the T cells expressing that particular TCR Vβ chain.*

IL-12 production by murine spleen cells, and addition of bacteria to cultures of $CD4^+$ T cells stimulated with alloantigens suppresses IFN-γ, IL-4, and IL-5 production and expands a population of Tr-type cells that secreted IL-10 and TGF-β (von der Weid et al. 2001).

Although there is evidence that iDCs drive the induction of anergic or Tr cells, there is growing evidence that differentiation of Tr cell from naïve precursor T cells appears to require DCs in a particular activation status distinct from that required to drive Th1 or Th2 cells. A number of bacterial products that bind to PRRs on macrophages and DCs have been shown to activate DC1 and DC2 in subtypes that direct naïve T cells into Th1 or Th2 respectively (see Figure 32.3, p. 657). It has now been reported that FHA from *B. pertussis* may drive a third population of DCs, termed 'DCr', that drive the induction of Tr1 cells (McGuirk and Mills 2002). IL-10 and IFN-α have been shown to function in differentiation of Tr1 cells, whereas TGF-β and IL-4 have been implicated in the differentiation of Th3 cells. FHA stimulates macrophages and DCs to secrete IL-10 and experiments with TCR transgenic mice demonstrated that FHA-stimulated DCs drove induction of Tr1 cells and this was switched to a Th1 phenotype in the presence of anti-IL-10 antibody. A number of bacteria have been shown to stimulate IL-10 production by macrophages and DCs and, although this may directly contribute to their anti-inflammatory and immunosuppressive effects, it may also create the appropriate cytokine milieu for the induction of Tr cells in vivo. There is also evidence that DCs or other innate cells in the lungs (Akbari et al. 2001), Peyer's patch (Iwasaki and Kelsall 1999), and liver (Khanna et al. 2000) have a propensity either to secrete IL-10 or to promote the induction of anergic T cells. This may facilitate the induction of Tr cells at mucosal surface, where they may play major roles in maintaining tolerance against inhaled antigen, food antigens, and commensal. However, these DCs may be exploited for the induction of antigen-specific Tr cells by many pathogenic bacteria, viruses, and parasites that invade the body through the respiratory tract, gastrointestinal tract, or other mucosal surfaces.

Superantigens

Superantigens are microbial toxins with potent immunomodulatory properties, altering normal immune responses to foreign antigens and promoting autoimmune diseases. Unlike conventional T cells where the TCR binds to processed peptide antigens in the groove of an MHC molecule, superantigens bind outside the grove of MHC and crosslink MHCII molecules with a variable region of the β chain of the TCR, forming a trimolecular complex that activates a much larger number of resting T cells than does conventional antigen (Figure 32.7). Furthermore, superantigens are presented to T cells by MHC molecules usually without the need for antigen processing. Superantigens activate proliferation, secretion of cytokines, including TNF-α, IFN-γ, and IL-2 by 20–25 percent of resting T cells, eventually resulting in anergy, apoptosis, and depletion of peripheral T cells expressing specific TCR Vβ chain, with a resultant immunosuppression. A number of pathogens including *S. aureus*, *S. pyogenes*, *Mycoplasma arthritidis*, *Y. enterocolitica*, *C. perfringens*, and *M. tuberculosis* secrete toxins, which act as superantigens (Fraser et al. 2000; McKay 2001). The best-studied superantigens include the families of staphylococcal enterotoxins and streptococcal pyrogenic exotoxins. These toxins cause food poisoning and toxic shock-like syndrome, and may contribute to autoimmune diseases by breaking tolerance to selfantigens (Fraser et al. 2000).

The enhancement of autoimmune diseases by superantigens appears to be related to enhancement of proinflammatory cytokine production. *M. arthritidis* mitogen (MAM), a superantigen secreted by *M. arthritidis*, induces type 1 cytokine secretion (IL-12, IFN-γ, and TNF-γ, but no IL-4 or IL-10) in arthritis-susceptible C3H/HeJ mice, but Th2 responses in arthritis-resistant BALB/c mice (Mu et al. 2000). In contrast, it has also been demonstrated that repetitive injection of staphylococcus enterotoxin induces a state of unresponsiveness characterized by lack of secretion of the type 1 cytokines IL-2 and IFN-γ. Unresponsive animals were found to have IL-10-secreting $CD4^+$ Tr cells capable of suppressing bacterial superantigen-reactive T cells (Noel et al. 2001). Conversely, it has been demonstrated that natural $CD4^+$ $CD25^+$ Tr cells (Pontoux et al. 2002) can control superantigen-induced proinflammatory cytokine production. Activation of T cells with superantigens in vivo can indirectly induce maturation of DCs into a phenotype distinct from LPS-matured DCs, with high MHCII and CD40 expression but low-to-moderate expression of CD80 and CD86 (Muraille et al. 2002). This DC phenotype is distinct from DC1 cells, suggesting that superantigens may not necessarily favor the induction of Th1 cells.

CONCLUSIONS

The immune system has developed highly sophisticated mechanisms for combating infectious diseases and is capable of eliminating most pathogenic bacteria that invade the host. However, many of these bacteria can cause severe disease, especially in naïve and immunocompromised individuals. This is largely a reflection of the success of pathogenic bacteria in evading or subverting protective immune responses. This chapter has detailed some, but by no means all, of the strategies adapted by bacteria to target different aspects of innate and adaptive immunity. Indeed this may be just the tip of the iceberg and, as a periodic review of the current literature on the immunology of infectious diseases will reveal, there is rapidly expanding knowledge of the interplay between pathogens and their host. We still have a great deal to learn about our own immune system by studying how pathogens have evolved to evade it.

ACKNOWLEDGMENTS

Kingston Mills and Aoife P. Boyd are supported by Science Foundation Ireland. We thank Olive Leavy for reading the manuscript.

REFERENCES

Aderem, A. and Underhill, D.M. 1999. Mechanisms of phagocytosis in macrophages. *Annu Rev Immunol*, **17**, 593–623.

Akbari, O., DeKruyff, R.H. and Umetsu, D.T. 2001. Pulmonary dendritic cells producing IL-10 mediate tolerance induced by respiratory exposure to antigen. *Nat Immunol*, **2**, 725–31.

Akesson, P., Sjoholm, A.G. and Bjorck, L. 1996. Protein SIC, a novel extracellular protein of *S. pyogenes* interfering with complement function. *J Biol Chem*, **271**, 1081–8.

Akira, S., Takeda, K. and Kaisho, T. 2001. Toll-like receptors: critical proteins linking innate and acquired immunity. *Nat Immunol*, **2**, 675–80.

Allavena, P., Bianchi, G., et al. 1994. Induction of natural killer cell migration by monocyte chemotactic protein-1, -2 and -3. *Eur J Immunol*, **24**, 3233–6.

al-Ramadi, B.K., Brodkin, M.A., et al. 1991a. Immunosuppression induced by attenuated *Salmonella*. Evidence for mediation by macrophage precursors. *J Immunol*, **146**, 2737–46.

al-Ramadi, B.K., Chen, Y.W., et al. 1991b. Immunosuppression induced by attenuated *Salmonella*. Reversal by IL-4. *J Immunol*, **147**, 1954–61.

Angel, C.S., Ruzek, M. and Hostetter, M.K. 1994. Degradation of C3 by *S. pneumoniae*. *J Infect Dis*, **170**, 600–8.

Appelmelk, B.J., Martino, M.C., et al. 2000. Phase variation in H type I and Lewis a epitopes of *Helicobacter pylori* lipopolysaccharide. *Infect Immun*, **68**, 5928–32.

Ausiello, C.M., Fedele, G., et al. 2002. Native and genetically inactivated pertussis toxins induce human dendritic cell maturation and synergize with lipopolysaccharide in promoting T helper type 1 responses. *J Infect Dis*, **186**, 351–60.

Balcewicz-Sablinska, M.K., Keane, J., et al. 1998. Pathogenic *Mycobacterium tuberculosis* evades apoptosis of host macrophages by release of TNF-R2, resulting in inactivation of TNF-α. *J Immunol*, **161**, 2636–41.

Banerjee, R., Anguita, J., et al. 2000. Cutting edge: infection by the agent of human granulocytic ehrlichiosis prevents the respiratory burst by down-regulating $gp91^{phox}$. *J Immunol*, **164**, 3946–9.

Barnes, P.F., Chatterjee, D., et al. 1992. Cytokine production induced by *Mycobacterium tuberculosis* lipoarabinomannan. Relationship to chemical structure. *J Immunol*, **149**, 541–7.

Beauregard, K.E., Lee, K.D., Collier, R.J. and Swanson, J.A. 1997. pH-dependent perforation of macrophage phagosomes by listeriolysin O from *Listeria monocytogenes*. *J Exp Med*, **186**, 1159–63.

Berge, A., Kihlberg, B.M., et al. 1997. Streptococcal protein H forms soluble complement-activating complexes with IgG, but inhibits complement activation by IgG-coated targets. *J Biol Chem*, **272**, 20774–81.

Beuscher, H.U., Rodel, F., et al. 1995. Bacterial evasion of host immune defense: *Y. enterocolitica* encodes a suppressor for tumor necrosis factor alpha expression. *Infect Immun*, **63**, 1270–7.

Black, D.S. and Bliska, J.B. 1997. Identification of p130Cas as a substrate of *Yersinia YopH* (Yop51), a bacterial protein tyrosine phosphatase that translocates into mammalian cells and targets focal adhesions. *EMBO J*, **16**, 2730–44.

Boussiotis, V.A., Tsai, E.Y., et al. 2000. IL-10-producing T cells suppress immune responses in anergic tuberculosis patients. *J Clin Invest*, **105**, 1317–25.

Braun, J.S., Novak, R., et al. 1999a. Pneumolysin, a protein toxin of *S. pneumoniae*, induces nitric oxide production from macrophages. *Infect Immun*, **67**, 3750–6.

Braun, M.C., He, J., et al. 1999b. Cholera toxin suppresses interleukin (IL)-12 production and IL-12 receptor β1 and β2 chain expression. *J Exp Med*, **189**, 541–52.

Braun, L., Ghebrehiwet, B. and Cossart, P. 2000. gC1q-R/p32, a C1q-binding protein, is a receptor for the InlB invasion protein of *Listeria monocytogenes*. *EMBO J*, **19**, 1458–66.

Brown, G.V., Anders, R.F. and Knowles, G. 1983. Differential effect of immunoglobulin on the in vitro growth of several isolates of *Plasmodium falciparum*. *Infect Immun*, **39**, 1228–35.

Buchmeier, N.A., Lipps, C.J., et al. 1993. Recombination-deficient mutants of *Salmonella typhimurium* are avirulent and sensitive to the oxidative burst of macrophages. *Mol Microbiol*, **7**, 933–6.

Caron, E. and Hall, A. 1998. Identification of two distinct mechanisms of phagocytosis controlled by different Rho GTPases. *Science*, **282**, 1717–21.

Caron, E., Gross, A., et al. 1996. *Brucella* species release a specific, protease-sensitive, inhibitor of TNF-α expression, active on human macrophage-like cells. *J Immunol*, **156**, 2885–93.

Caspar-Bauguil, S., Puissant, B., et al. 2000. *Chlamydia pneumoniae* induces interleukin-10 production that down-regulates major histocompatibility complex class I expression. *J Infect Dis*, **182**, 1394–401.

Celli, J., Olivier, M. and Finlay, B.B. 2001. Enteropathogenic *Escherichia coli* mediates antiphagocytosis through the inhibition of PI3-kinase-dependent pathways. *EMBO J*, **20**, 1245–58.

Chang, M.P., Baldwin, R.L., et al. 1989. Second cytotoxic pathway of diphtheria toxin suggested by nuclease activity. *Science*, **246**, 1165–8.

Chen, W., Shu, D. and Chadwick, V.S. 2001. *Helicobacter pylori* infection: mechanism of colonization and functional dyspepsia. Reduced colonization of gastric mucosa by *Helicobacter pylori* in mice deficient in interleukin-10. *J Gastroenterol Hepatol*, **16**, 377–83.

Chen, Y., Kuchroo, V.K., et al. 1994. Regulatory T cell clones induced by oral tolerance: suppression of autoimmune encephalomyelitis. *Science*, **265**, 1237–40.

Chiao, J.W., Villalon, P., et al. 2000. Modulation of lymphocyte proliferative responses by a canine Lyme disease vaccine of recombinant outer surface protein A (OspA). *FEMS Immunol Med Microbiol*, **28**, 193–6.

Christensen, H.R., Frokiaer, H. and Pestka, J.J. 2002. Lactobacilli differentially modulate expression of cytokines and maturation surface markers in murine dendritic cells. *J Immunol*, **168**, 171–8.

Ciacci-Woolwine, F., Blomfield, I.C., et al. 1998. *Salmonella* flagellin induces tumor necrosis factor alpha in a human promonocytic cell line. *Infect Immun*, **66**, 1127–34.

Cluff, C.W., Garcia, M. and Ziegler, H.K. 1990. Intracellular hemolysin-producing *Listeria monocytogenes* strains inhibit macrophage-mediated antigen processing. *Infect Immun*, **58**, 3601–12.

Comerci, D.J., Martinez-Lorenzo, M.J., et al. 2001. Essential role of the VirB machinery in the maturation of the *Brucella abortus*-containing vacuole. *Cell Microbiol*, **3**, 159–68.

Cooper, N.R. 1991. Complement evasion strategies of microorganisms. *Immunol Today*, **12**, 327–31.

Cornelis, G.R., Boland, A., et al. 1998. The virulence plasmid of *Yersinia*, an antihost genome. *Microbiol Mol Biol Rev*, **62**, 1315–52.

Cunnion, K.M., Lee, J.C. and Frank, M.M. 2001. Capsule production and growth phase influence binding of complement to *Staphylococcus aureus*. *Infect Immun*, **69**, 6796–803.

Dahl, K.E., Shiratsuchi, H., et al. 1996. Selective induction of transforming growth factor beta in human monocytes by lipoarabinomannan of *Mycobacterium tuberculosis*. *Infect Immun*, **64**, 399–405.

Darji, A., Stockinger, B., et al. 1997. Antigen-specific T cell receptor antagonism by antigen-presenting cells treated with the hemolysin of *Listeria monocytogenes*: a novel type of immune escape. *Eur J Immunol*, **27**, 1696–703.

Day, W.A. Jr., Sajecki, J.L., et al. 2000. Role of catalase in *Campylobacter jejuni* intracellular survival. *Infect Immun*, **68**, 6337–45.

de Jong, E.C., Vieira, P.L., et al. 2002. Microbial compounds selectively induce Th1 cell-promoting or Th2 cell-promoting dendritic cells in vitro with diverse Th cell-polarizing signals. *J Immunol*, **168**, 1704–9.

De Groote, M.A., Ochsner, U.A., et al. 1997. Periplasmic superoxide dismutase protects *Salmonella* from products of phagocyte NADPH-oxidase and nitric oxide synthase. *Proc Natl Acad Sci USA*, **94**, 13997–4001.

De Lerma Barbaro, A., Tosi, G., et al. 1999. Distinct regulation of HLA class II and class I cell surface expression in the THP-1 macrophage cell line after bacterial phagocytosis. *Eur J Immunol*, **29**, 499–511.

de Souza, M.S., Smith, A.L., et al. 1993. Long-term study of cell-mediated responses to *Borrelia burgdorferi* in the laboratory mouse. *Infect Immun*, **61**, 1814–22.

Deckert, M., Soltek, S., et al. 2001. Endogenous interleukin-10 is required for prevention of a hyperinflammatory intracerebral immune response in *Listeria monocytogenes* meningoencephalitis. *Infect Immun*, **69**, 4561–71.

Demangel, C., Bertolino, P. and Britton, W.J. 2002. Autocrine IL-10 impairs dendritic cell (DC)-derived immune responses to mycobacterial infection by suppressing DC trafficking to draining lymph nodes and local IL-12 production. *Eur J Immunol*, **32**, 994–1002.

Doetze, A., Satoguina, J., et al. 2000. Antigen-specific cellular hyporesponsiveness in a chronic human helminth infection is mediated by T(h)3/T(r)1-type cytokines IL-10 and transforming growth factor-beta but not by a Th1 to Th2 shift. *Int Immunol*, **12**, 623–30.

Donabedian, H. 1985. Human mononuclear cells exposed to staphylococci rapidly produce an inhibitor of neutrophil chemotaxis. *J Infect Dis*, **152**, 24–32.

Dorn, B.R., Dunn, W.A. Jr. and Progulske-Fox, A. 2002. Bacterial interactions with the autophagic pathway. *Cell Microbiol*, **4**, 1–10.

Duclos, S. and Desjardins, M. 2000. Subversion of a young phagosome: the survival strategies of intracellular pathogens. *Cell Microbiol*, **2**, 365–77.

Dworkin, J. and Blaser, M.J. 1997. Molecular mechanisms of *Campylobacter fetus* surface layer protein expression. *Mol Microbiol*, **26**, 433–40.

Edwards, K.M., Gewurz, H., et al. 1982. A role for C-reactive protein in the complement-mediated stimulation of human neutrophils by type 27 *S. pneumoniae*. *J Immunol*, **128**, 2493–6.

Eisenschenk, F.C., Houle, J.J. and Hoffmann, E.M. 1999. Mechanism of serum resistance among *Brucella abortus* isolates. *Vet Microbiol*, **68**, 235–44.

Ernst, J.D. 2000. Bacterial inhibition of phagocytosis. *Cell Microbiol*, **2**, 379–86.

Faigle, W., Raposo, G., et al. 1998. Deficient peptide loading and MHC class II endosomal sorting in a human genetic immunodeficiency disease: the Chediak–Higashi syndrome. *J Cell Biol*, **141**, 1121–34.

Farrant, J.L., Sansone, A., et al. 1997. Bacterial copper- and zinc-cofactored superoxide dismutase contributes to the pathogenesis of systemic Salmonellosis. *Mol Microbiol*, **25**, 785–96.

Ferrari, G., Langen, H., et al. 1999. A coat protein on phagosomes involved in the intracellular survival of mycobacteria. *Cell*, **97**, 435–47.

Fierer, J. and Guiney, D.G. 2001. Diverse virulence traits underlying different clinical outcomes of *Salmonella* infection. *J Clin Invest*, **107**, 775–80.

Fletcher, H.M., Schenkein, H.A., et al. 1995. Virulence of a *Porphyromonas gingivalis* W83 mutant defective in the *prtH* gene. *Infect Immun*, **63**, 1521–8.

Fraser, J., Arcus, V., et al. 2000. Superantigens – powerful modifiers of the immune system. *Mol Med Today*, **6**, 125–32.

Gagliardi, M.C., Sallusto, F., et al. 2000. Cholera toxin induces maturation of human dendritic cells and licences them for Th2 priming. *Eur J Immunol*, **30**, 2394–403.

Ghigo, E., Capo, C., Raoult, D. and Mege, J.L. 2001. Interleukin-10 stimulates *Coxiella burnetii* replication in human monocytes through tumor necrosis factor down-modulation: role in microbicidal defect of Q fever. *Infect Immun*, **69**, 2345–52.

Giacomini, E., Iona, E., et al. 2001. Infection of human macrophages and dendritic cells with *Mycobacterium tuberculosis* induces a differential cytokine gene expression that modulates T cell response. *J Immunol*, **166**, 7033–41.

Giambartolomei, G.H., Dennis, V.A. and Philipp, M.T. 1998. *Borrelia burgdorferi* stimulates the production of interleukin-10 in peripheral blood mononuclear cells from uninfected humans and rhesus monkeys. *Infect Immun*, **66**, 2691–7.

Gilsdorf, J.R. 1998. Antigenic diversity and gene polymorphisms in *Haemophilus influenzae*. *Infect Immun*, **66**, 5053–9.

Gobert, A.P., Cheng, Y., et al. 2002. *Helicobacter pylori* induces macrophage apoptosis by activation of arginase II. *J Immunol*, **168**, 4692–700.

Goebel, W. and Kuhn, M. 2000. Bacterial replication in the host cell cytosol. *Curr Opin Microbiol*, **3**, 49–53.

Gorvel, J.P. and Meresse, S. 2001. Maturation steps of the *Salmonella*-containing vacuole. *Microbes Infect*, **3**, 1299–303.

Gregory, S.H., Wing, E.J., Hoffman, R.A. and Simmons, R.L. 1993. Reactive nitrogen intermediates suppress the primary immunologic response to *Listeria*. *J Immunol*, **150**, 2901–9.

Grosdent, N., Maridonneau-Parini, I., et al. 2002. Role of Yops and adhesins in resistance of *Yersinia enterocolitica* to phagocytosis. *Infect Immun*, **70**, 4165–76.

Groux, H., O'Garra, A., et al. 1997. A CD4+ T-cell subset inhibits antigen-specific T-cell responses and prevents colitis. *Nature*, **389**, 737–42.

Gueirard, P., Druilhe, A., et al. 1998. Role of adenylate cyclase-hemolysin in alveolar macrophage apoptosis during *Bordetella pertussis* infection in vivo. *Infect Immun*, **66**, 1718–25.

Guermonprez, P., Valladeau, J., et al. 2002. Antigen presentation and T cell stimulation by dendritic cells. *Annu Rev Immunol*, **20**, 621–67.

Guo, H.F., The, I., et al. 1997. Requirement of Drosophila NF1 for activation of adenylyl cyclase by PACAP38-like neuropeptides. *Science*, **276**, 795–8.

Guzman, C.A., Domann, E., et al. 1996. Apoptosis of mouse dendritic cells is triggered by listeriolysin, the major virulence determinant of *Listeria monocytogenes*. *Mol Microbiol*, **20**, 119–26.

Hackett, S.P. and Stevens, D.L. 1992. Streptococcal toxic shock syndrome: synthesis of tumor necrosis factor and interleukin-1 by monocytes stimulated with pyrogenic exotoxin A and streptolysin O. *J Infect Dis*, **165**, 879–85.

Hackstadt, T., Fischer, E.R., et al. 1997. Origins and functions of the chlamydial inclusion. *Trends Microbiol*, **5**, 288–93.

Hallet, B. 2001. Playing Dr Jekyll and Mr Hyde: combined mechanisms of phase variation in bacteria. *Curr Opin Microbiol*, **4**, 570–81.

Hampton, M.B., Kettle, A.J. and Winterbourn, C.C. 1998. Inside the neutrophil phagosome: oxidants, myeloperoxidase, and bacterial killing. *Blood*, **92**, 3007–17.

Harvey, H.A., Porat, N., et al. 2000. Gonococcal lipooligosaccharide is a ligand for the asialoglycoprotein receptor on human sperm. *Molecular Microbiology*, **36**, 1059–70.

Heffernan, E.J., Wu, L., et al. 1994. Specificity of the complement resistance and cell association phenotypes encoded by the outer membrane protein genes rck from *Salmonella typhimurium* and ail from *Yersinia enterocolitica*. *Infect Immun*, **62**, 5183–6.

Heinzen, R.A., Scidmore, M.A., et al. 1996. Differential interaction with endocytic and exocytic pathways distinguish parasitophorous vacuoles of *Coxiella burnetii* and *Chlamydia trachomatis*. *Infect Immun*, **64**, 796–809.

Henderson, I.R., Owen, P. and Nataro, J.P. 1999. Molecular switches – the ON and OFF of bacterial phase variation. *Mol Microbiol*, **33**, 919–32.

Hersh, D., Monack, D.M., et al. 1999. The *Salmonella* invasin SipB induces macrophage apoptosis by binding to caspase-1. *Proc Natl Acad Sci USA*, **96**, 2396–401.

Hilbi, H., Moss, J.E., et al. 1998. *Shigella*-induced apoptosis is dependent on caspase-1 which binds to IpaB. *J Biol Chem*, **273**, 32895–900.

Hirsch, C.S., Ellner, J.J., et al. 1997. In vitro restoration of T cell responses in tuberculosis and augmentation of monocyte effector function against *Mycobacterium tuberculosis* by natural inhibitors of transforming growth factor beta. *Proc Natl Acad Sci USA*, **94**, 3926–31.

Hirsch, C.S., Toossi, Z., et al. 1999. Depressed T-cell interferon-gamma responses in pulmonary tuberculosis: analysis of underlying mechanisms and modulation with therapy. *J Infect Dis*, **180**, 2069–73.

Hmama, Z., Gabathuler, R., et al. 1998. Attenuation of HLA-DR expression by mononuclear phagocytes infected with *Mycobacterium tuberculosis* is related to intracellular sequestration of immature class II heterodimers. *J Immunol*, **161**, 4882–93.

Hong, Y.Q. and Ghebrehiwet, B. 1992. Effect of *P. aeruginosa* elastase and alkaline protease on serum complement and isolated components C1q and C3. *Clin Immunol Immunopathol*, **62**, 133–8.

Hoover, D.L., Friedlander, A.M., et al. 1994. Anthrax edema toxin differentially regulates lipopolysaccharide-induced monocyte production of tumor necrosis factor alpha and interleukin-6 by increasing intracellular cyclic AMP. *Infect Immun*, **62**, 4432–9.

Hori, S., Carvalho, T.L. and Demengeot, J. 2002. $CD25^{+}CD4^{+}$ regulatory T cells suppress $CD4^{+}$ T cell-mediated pulmonary hyperinflammation driven by *Pneumocystis carinii* in immunodeficient mice. *Eur J Immunol*, **32**, 1282–91.

Horstmann, R.D., Sievertsen, H.J., et al. 1988. Antiphagocytic activity of streptococcal M protein: selective binding of complement control protein factor H. *Proc Natl Acad Sci USA*, **85**, 1657–61.

Horwitz, M.A. 1983. The Legionnaires' disease bacterium (*Legionella pneumophila*) inhibits phagosome-lysosome fusion in human monocytes. *J Exp Med*, **158**, 2108–26.

Igietseme, J.U., Ananaba, G.A., et al. 2000. Suppression of endogenous IL-10 gene expression in dendritic cells enhances antigen presentation for specific Th1 induction: potential for cellular vaccine development. *J Immunol*, **164**, 4212–19.

Isberg, R.R., Hamburger, Z. and Dersch, P. 2000. Signaling and invasin-promoted uptake via integrin receptors. *Microbes Infect*, **2**, 793–801.

Ishibashi, Y., Claus, S. and Relman, D.A. 1994. *Bordetella pertussis* filamentous hemagglutinin interacts with a leukocyte signal transduction complex and stimulates bacterial adherence to monocyte CR3 (CD11b/CD18). *J Exp Med*, **180**, 1225–33.

Iwasaki, A. and Kelsall, B.L. 1999. Freshly isolated Peyer's patch, but not spleen, dendritic cells produce interleukin 10 and induce the differentiation of T helper type 2 cells. *J Exp Med*, **190**, 229–39.

Jacob, T., Escallier, J.C., et al. 1994. *Legionella pneumophila* inhibits superoxide generation in human monocytes via the down-modulation of α and β protein kinase C isotypes. *J Leukoc Biol*, **55**, 310–12.

Jacobs, M., Brown, N., et al. 2000. Increased resistance to mycobacterial infection in the absence of interleukin-10. *Immunology*, **100**, 494–501.

Janeway, C.A. Jr. and Medzhitov, R. 2002. Innate immune recognition. *Annu Rev Immunol*, **20**, 197–216.

Jarrossay, D., Napolitani, G., et al. 2001. Specialization and complementarity in microbial molecule recognition by human myeloid and plasmacytoid dendritic cells. *Eur J Immunol*, **31**, 3388–93.

Jerlstrom, P.G., Chhatwal, G.S. and Timmis, K.N. 1991. The IgA-binding beta antigen of the c protein complex of Group B streptococci: sequence determination of its gene and detection of two binding regions. *Mol Microbiol*, **5**, 843–9.

Jeyaseelan, S., Hsuan, S.L., et al. 2000. Lymphocyte function-associated antigen 1 is a receptor for *Pasteurella haemolytica* leukotoxin in bovine leukocytes. *Infect Immun*, **68**, 72–9.

Jimenez-Lucho, V.E., Joiner, K.A., et al. 1987. C3b generation is affected by the structure of the O-antigen polysaccharide in lipopolysaccharide from Salmonellae. *J Immunol*, **139**, 1253–9.

Joh, D., Wann, E.R., et al. 1999. Role of fibronectin-binding MSCRAMMs in bacterial adherence and entry into mammalian cells. *Matrix Biol*, **18**, 211–23.

Johnson, B.N., Weintraub, A., et al. 1992. Construction of *Salmonella* strains with both antigen O4 (of group B) and antigen O9 (of group D). *J Bacteriol*, **174**, 1911–15.

Johnsson, E., Thern, A., et al. 1996. A highly variable region in members of the Streptococcal M protein family binds the human complement regulator C4BP. *J Immunol*, **157**, 3021–9.

Joiner, K.A. 1988. Complement evasion by bacteria and parasites. *Annu Rev Microbiol*, **42**, 201–30.

Joiner, K.A., Hammer, C.H., et al. 1982a. Studies on the mechanism of bacterial resistance to complement-mediated killing. I. Terminal complement components are deposited and released from *Salmonella minnesota* S218 without causing bacterial death. *J Exp Med*, **155**, 797–808.

Joiner, K.A., Hammer, C.H., Brown, E.J. and Frank, M.M. 1982b. Studies on the mechanism of bacterial resistance to complement-mediated killing. II. C8 and C9 release C5b67 from the surface of *Salmonella minnesota* S218 because the terminal complex does not insert into the bacterial outer membrane. *J Exp Med*, **155**, 809–19.

Jones, N.L., Day, A.S., et al. 2002. Enhanced disease severity in *Helicobacter pylori*-infected mice deficient in Fas signaling. *Infect Immun*, **70**, 2591–7.

Kaplan, G., Gandhi, R.R., et al. 1987. *Mycobacterium leprae* antigen-induced suppression of T cell proliferation in vitro. *J Immunol*, **138**, 3028–34.

Keane, J., Balcewicz-Sablinska, M.K., et al. 1997. Infection by *Mycobacterium tuberculosis* promotes human alveolar macrophage apoptosis. *Infect Immun*, **65**, 298–304.

Khanna, A., Morelli, A.E., et al. 2000. Effects of liver-derived dendritic cell progenitors on Th1- and Th2-like cytokine responses in vitro and in vivo. *J Immunol*, **164**, 1346–54.

Khelef, N., Zychlinsky, A. and Guiso, N. 1993. *Bordetella pertussis* induces apoptosis in macrophages: role of adenylate cyclase-hemolysin. *Infect Immun*, **61**, 4064–71.

Kimura, A. and Hansen, E.J. 1986. Antigenic and phenotypic variations of *Haemophilus influenzae* type b lipopolysaccharide and their relationship to virulence. *Infect Immun*, **51**, 69–79.

Knipp, U., Birkholz, S., et al. 1994. Suppression of human mononuclear cell response by *Helicobacter pylori*: effects on isolated monocytes and lymphocytes. *FEMS Immunol Med Microbiol*, **8**, 157–66.

Korostoff, J., Yamaguchi, N., et al. 2000. Perturbation of mitochondrial structure and function plays a central role in *Actinobacillus actinomycetemcomitans* leukotoxin-induced apoptosis. *Microb Pathog*, **29**, 267–78.

Kronvall, G. 1973. A surface component in group A, C and G streptococci with non-immune reactivity for immunoglobulin G. *J Immunol*, **111**, 1401–6.

Kullberg, M.C., Jankovic, D., et al. 2002. Bacteria-triggered CD4(+) T regulatory cells suppress *Helicobacter hepaticus*-induced colitis. *J Exp Med*, **196**, 505–15.

Kullberg, M.C., Rothfuchs, A.G., et al. 2001. *Helicobacter hepaticus*-induced colitis in interleukin-10-deficient mice: cytokine requirements for the induction and maintenance of intestinal inflammation. *Infect Immun*, **69**, 4232–41.

Lally, E.T., Kieba, I.R., et al. 1997. RTX toxins recognize a beta2 integrin on the surface of human target cells. *J Biol Chem*, **272**, 30463–9.

Lavelle, E., McNeela, E., et al. 2003. Cholera toxin promotes the induction of regulatory T cells by modulation dendritic cell activation. *J Immunol*, **171**, 2384–92.

Lem, L., Riethof, D.A., et al. 1999. Enhanced interaction of HLA-DM with HLA-DR in enlarged vacuoles of hereditary and infectious lysosomal diseases. *J Immunol*, **162**, 523–32.

Lerouge, I. and Vanderleyden, J.U. 2002. O-antigen structural variation: mechanisms and possible roles in animal/plant-microbe interactions. *FEMS Microbiol Rev*, **26**, 17–47.

Li, L., Sharipo, A., et al. 2002a. The *Haemophilus ducreyi* cytolethal distending toxin activates sensors of DNA damage and repair complexes in proliferating and non-proliferating cells. *Cell Microbiol*, **4**, 87–99.

Li, Y., Loike, J.D., et al. 2002b. The bacterial peptide N-formyl-Met-Leu-Phe inhibits killing of *Staphylococcus epidermidis* by human neutrophils in fibrin gels. *J Immunol*, **168**, 816–24.

Liang-Takasaki, C.J., Saxen, H., Makela, P.H. and Leive, L. 1983. Complement activation by polysaccharide of lipopolysaccharide: an important virulence determinant of Salmonellae. *Infect Immun*, **41**, 563–9.

Linton, D., Gilbert, M., et al. 2000. Phase variation of a beta-1,3 galactosyltransferase involved in generation of the ganglioside GM1-like lipo-oligosaccharide of *Campylobacter jejuni*. *Mol Microbiol*, **37**, 501–14.

Liu, D., Verma, N.K., et al. 1991. Relationships among the rfb regions of *Salmonella* serovars A, B and D. *J Bacteriol*, **173**, 4814–19.

Loetscher, P., Seitz, M., et al. 1994. Monocyte chemotactic proteins MCP-1, MCP-2, and MCP-3 are major attractants for human $CD4^+$ and $CD8^+$ T lymphocytes. *FASEB J*, **8**, 1055–60.

Lomholt, H., van Alphen, L. and Kilian, M. 1993. Antigenic variation of immunoglobulin A1 proteases among sequential isolates of *Haemophilus influenzae* from healthy children and patients with chronic obstructive pulmonary disease. *Infect Immun*, **61**, 4575–81.

Lopes, L.M., Maroof, A., et al. 2000. Inhibition of T-cell response by *Escherichia coli* heat-labile enterotoxin-treated epithelial cells. *Infect Immun*, **68**, 6891–5.

MacDonald, A.J., Duffy, M., et al. 2002. CD4 T helper type 1 and regulatory T cells induced against the same epitopes on the core protein in hepatitis C virus-infected persons. *J Infect Dis*, **185**, 720–7.

MacFarlane, A.S., Schwacha, M.G. and Eisenstein, T.K. 1999. In vivo blockage of nitric oxide with aminoguanidine inhibits immunosuppression induced by an attenuated strain of *Salmonella typhimurium*, potentiates *Salmonella* infection, and inhibits macrophage and polymorphonuclear leukocyte influx into the spleen. *Infect Immun*, **67**, 891–8.

McKay, D.M. 2001. Bacterial superantigens: provocateurs of gut dysfunction and inflammation? *Trends Immunol*, **22**, 497–501.

McGuirk, P. and Mills, K.H.G. 2000. Direct anti-inflammatory effect of a bacterial virulence factor: IL-10-dependent suppression of IL-12 production by filamentous hemagglutinin from *Bordetella pertussis*. *Eur J Immunol*, **30**, 415–22.

McGuirk, P. and Mills, K.H.G. 2002. Pathogen-specific regulatory T cells provoke a shift in the Th1/Th2 paradigm in immunity to infectious diseases. *Trends Immunol*, **23**, 450.

McGuirk, P., Mahon, B.P., Griffin, F. and Mills, K.H.G. 1998. Compartmentalization of T cell responses following respiratory infection with *Bordetella pertussis*: hyporesponsiveness of lung T cells is associated with modulated expression of the co-stimulatory molecule CD28. *Eur J Immunol*, **28**, 153–63.

McGuirk, P., McCann, C. and Mills, K.H.G. 2002. Pathogen-specific T regulatory 1 cells induced in the respiratory tract by a bacterial molecule that stimulates interleukin 10 production by dendritic cells: a novel strategy for evasion of protective T helper type 1 responses by *Bordetella pertussis*. *J Exp Med*, **195**, 221–31.

Mahon, B.P., Sheahan, B.J., et al. 1997. Atypical disease after *Bordetella pertussis* respiratory infection of mice with targeted disruptions of interferon-γ receptor or immunoglobulin mu chain genes. *J Exp Med*, **186**, 1843–51.

Maksymowych, W.P., Ikawa, T., et al. 1998. Invasion by *Salmonella typhimurium* induces increased expression of the LMP, MECL and PA28 proteasome genes and changes in the peptide repertoire of HLA-B27. *Infect Immun*, **66**, 4624–32.

Mangan, D.F., Welch, G.R. and Wahl, S.M. 1991. Lipopolysaccharide, tumor necrosis factor-alpha and IL-1β prevent programmed cell death (apoptosis) in human peripheral blood monocytes. *J Immunol*, **146**, 1541–6.

Matousek, M.P., Nedrud, J.G., et al. 1998. Inhibition of class II major histocompatibility complex antigen processing by *Escherichia coli* heat-labile enterotoxin requires an enzymatically active A subunit. *Infect Immun*, **66**, 3480–4.

Matousek, M.P., Nedrud, J.G. and Harding, C.V. 1996. Distinct effects of recombinant cholera toxin B subunit and holotoxin on different stages of class II MHC antigen processing and presentation by macrophages. *J Immunol*, **156**, 4137–45.

Meade, B.D., Kind, P.D. and Manclark, C.R. 1985. Altered mononuclear phagocyte function in mice treated with the lymphocytosis promoting factor of *Bordetella pertussis*. *Dev Biol Stand*, **61**, 63–74.

Medina, E., Molinari, G., et al. 1999. Fc-mediated nonspecific binding between fibronectin-binding protein I of *S. pyogenes* and human immunoglobulins. *J Immunol*, **163**, 3396–402.

Mehra, V., Brennan, P.J., et al. 1984. Lymphocyte suppression in leprosy induced by unique *M. leprae* glycolipid. *Nature*, **308**, 194–6.

Menestrina, G., Dalla Serra, M. and Prevost, G.U. 2001. Mode of action of β-barrel pore-forming toxins of the staphylococcal α-hemolysin family. *Toxicon*, **39**, 1661–72.

Mengaud, J., Ohayon, H., et al. 1996. E-cadherin is the receptor for internalin, a surface protein required for entry of *L. monocytogenes* into epithelial cells. *Cell*, **84**, 923–32.

Meresse, S., Steele-Mortimer, O., et al. 1999. The rab7 GTPase controls the maturation of *Salmonella typhimurium*-containing vacuoles in HeLa cells. *EMBO J*, **18**, 4394–403.

Merino, S., Camprubi, S. and Tomas, J.M. 1992. Effect of growth temperature on outer membrane components and virulence of *Aeromonas hydrophila* strains of serotype O:34. *Infect Immun*, **60**, 4343–9.

Michelsen, K.S., Aicher, A., et al. 2001. The role of toll-like receptors (TLRs) in bacteria-induced maturation of murine dendritic cells (DCs). Peptidoglycan and lipoteichoic acid are inducers of DC maturation and require TLR2. *J Biol Chem*, **276**, 25680–6.

Molinari, M., Salio, M., et al. 1998. Selective inhibition of Ii-dependent antigen presentation by *Helicobacter pylori* toxin VacA. *J Exp Med*, **187**, 135–40.

Monack, D.M., Mecsas, J., et al. 1997. *Yersinia* signals macrophages to undergo apoptosis and YopJ is necessary for this cell death. *Proc Natl Acad Sci USA*, **94**, 10385–90.

Monack, D.M., Mecsas, J., et al. 1998. *Yersinia*-induced apoptosis in vivo aids in the establishment of a systemic infection of mice. *J Exp Med*, **188**, 2127–37.

Morimoto, H. and Bonavida, B. 1992. Diphtheria toxin- and *Pseudomonas A* toxin-mediated apoptosis. ADP ribosylation of elongation factor-2 is required for DNA fragmentation and cell lysis and synergy with tumor necrosis factor-alpha. *J Immunol*, **149**, 2089–94.

Moura, A.C. and Mariano, M. 1997. Lipids from *Mycobacterium leprae* cell wall suppress T-cell activation in vivo and in vitro. *Immunology*, **92**, 429–36.

Mu, H.H., Sawitzke, A.D. and Cole, B.C. 2000. Modulation of cytokine profiles by the Mycoplasma superantigen *Mycoplasma arthritidis* mitogen parallels susceptibility to arthritis induced by *M. arthritidis*. *Infect Immun*, **68**, 1142–9.

Munoz, E., Vidarte, L., et al. 1998. A small domain (6.5 kDa) of bacterial protein G inhibits C3 covalent binding to the Fc region of IgG immune complexes. *Eur J Immunol*, **28**, 2591–7.

Muraille, E., De Trez, C., et al. 2002. T cell-dependent maturation of dendritic cells in response to bacterial superantigens. *J Immunol*, **168**, 4352–60.

Murthy, P.K., Dennis, V.A., et al. 2000. Interleukin-10 modulates proinflammatory cytokines in the human monocytic cell line THP-1 stimulated with *Borrelia burgdorferi* lipoproteins. *Infect Immun*, **68**, 6663–9.

Mustafa, T., Bjune, T.G., et al. 2001. Increased expression of Fas ligand in human tuberculosis and leprosy lesions: a potential novel mechanism of immune evasion in mycobacterial infection. *Scand J Immunol*, **54**, 630–9.

Nakane, A., Asano, M., et al. 1996. Transforming growth factor beta is protective in host resistance against *Listeria monocytogenes* infection in mice. *Infect Immun*, **64**, 3901–4.

Nandan, D., Knutson, K.L., et al. 2000. Exploitation of host cell signaling machinery: activation of macrophage phosphotyrosine phosphatases as a novel mechanism of molecular microbial pathogenesis. *J Leukoc Biol*, **67**, 464–70.

Navarre, W.W. and Schneewind, O. 1999. Surface proteins of gram-positive bacteria and mechanisms of their targeting to the cell wall envelope. *Microbiol Mol Biol Rev*, **63**, 174–229.

Noel, C., Florquin, S., et al. 2001. Chronic exposure to superantigen induces regulatory $CD4^+$ T cells with IL-10-mediated suppressive activity. *Int Immunol*, **13**, 431–9.

Noel, G., Brittingham, A., et al. 1996. Effect of amplification of the Cap b locus on complement-mediated bacteriolysis and opsonization of type b *Haemophilus influenzae*. *Infect Immun*, **64**, 4769–75.

Ohno-Iwashita, Y., Iwamoto, M., et al. 1992. Effect of lipidic factors on membrane cholesterol topology – mode of binding of theta-toxin to cholesterol in liposomes. *Biochim Biophys Acta*, **1109**, 81–90.

Othieno, C., Hirsch, C.S., et al. 1999. Interaction of *Mycobacterium tuberculosis*-induced transforming growth factor-β1 and interleukin-10. *Infect Immun*, **67**, 5730–5.

Ozinsky, A., Underhill, D.M., et al. 2000. The repertoire for pattern recognition of pathogens by the innate immune system is defined by cooperation between toll-like receptors. *Proc Natl Acad Sci USA*, **97**, 13766–71.

Palmer, M. 2001. The family of thiol-activated, cholesterol-binding cytolysins. *Toxicon*, **39**, 1681–9.

Papini, E., Satin, B., et al. 1997. The small GTP binding protein rab7 is essential for cellular vacuolation induced by *Helicobacter pylori* cytotoxin. *EMBO J*, **16**, 15–24.

Paton, J.C. and Ferrante, A. 1983. Inhibition of human polymorphonuclear leukocyte respiratory burst, bactericidal activity, and migration by pneumolysin. *Infect Immun*, **41**, 1212–16.

Pederson, K.J., Vallis, A.J., et al. 1999. The amino-terminal domain of *Pseudomonas aeruginosa* ExoS disrupts actin filaments via small-molecular-weight GTP-binding proteins. *Mol Microbiol*, **32**, 393–401.

Persson, C., Carballeira, N., et al. 1997. The PTPase YopH inhibits uptake of *Yersinia*, tyrosine phosphorylation of p130Cas and FAK, and the associated accumulation of these proteins in peripheral focal adhesions. *EMBO J*, **16**, 2307–18.

Pham, T.Q., Goluszko, P., et al. 1997. Molecular cloning and characterization of Dr-II, a nonfimbrial adhesin-I-like adhesin isolated from gestational pyelonephritis-associated *Escherichia coli* that binds to decay-accelerating factor. *Infect Immun*, **65**, 4309–18.

Piddington, D.L., Fang, F.C., et al. 2001. Cu, Zn superoxide dismutase of *Mycobacterium tuberculosis* contributes to survival in activated macrophages that are generating an oxidative burst. *Infect Immun*, **69**, 4980–7.

Pizarro-Cerda, J., Meresse, S., et al. 1998. *Brucella abortus* transits through the autophagic pathway and replicates in the endoplasmic reticulum of nonprofessional phagocytes. *Infect Immun*, **66**, 5711–24.

Pleass, R.J., Areschoug, T., et al. 2001. Streptococcal IgA-binding proteins bind in the Cα2-Cα3 interdomain region and inhibit binding of IgA to human CD89. *J Biol Chem*, **276**, 8197–204.

Pontoux, C., Banz, A. and Papiernik, M. 2002. Natural CD4 $CD25^+$ regulatory T cells control the burst of superantigen-induced cytokine production: the role of IL-10. *Int Immunol*, **14**, 233–9.

Pramoonjago, P., Kaneko, M., et al. 1992. Role of TraT protein, an anticomplementary protein produced in *Escherichia coli* by R100 factor, in serum resistance. *J Immunol*, **148**, 827–36.

Pryjma, J., Baran, J., et al. 1994. Altered antigen-presenting capacity of human monocytes after phagocytosis of bacteria. *Infect Immun*, **62**, 1961–7.

Raeder, R. and Boyle, M.D. 1995. Analysis of immunoglobulin G-binding-protein expression by invasive isolates of *S. pyogenes*. *Clin Diagn Lab Immunol*, **2**, 484–6.

Ram, S., Cullinane, M., et al. 2001. Binding of C4b-binding protein to porin: a molecular mechanism of serum resistance of *Neisseria gonorrhoeae*. *J Exp Med*, **193**, 281–95.

Ram, S., Sharma, A.K., et al. 1998. A novel sialic acid binding site on factor H mediates serum resistance of sialylated *Neisseria gonorrhoeae*. *J Exp Med*, **187**, 743–52.

Ramarao, N., Gray-Owen, S.D., et al. 2000. *Helicobacter pylori* inhibits phagocytosis by professional phagocytes involving type IV secretion components. *Mol Microbiol*, **37**, 1389–404.

Rautemaa, R. and Meri, S. 1999. Complement-resistance mechanisms of bacteria. *Microbes Infect*, **1**, 785–94.

Redpath, S., Ghazal, P. and Gascoigne, N.R. 2001. Hijacking and exploitation of IL-10 by intracellular pathogens. *Trends Microbiol*, **9**, 86–92.

Reis, K.J., Ayoub, E.M. and Boyle, M.D. 1984. Streptococcal Fc receptors. II. Comparison of the reactivity of a receptor from a group C *Streptococcus* with staphylococcal protein A. *J Immunol*, **132**, 3098–102.

Reis e Sousa, C., Sher, A. and Kaye, P. 1999. The role of dendritic cells in the induction and regulation of immunity to microbial infection. *Curr Opin Immunol*, **11**, 392–9.

Rokita, E., Makristathis, A., et al. 1998. *Helicobacter pylori* urease significantly reduces opsonization by human complement. *J Infect Dis*, **178**, 1521–5.

Rosqvist, R., Bolin, I. and Wolf-Watz, H. 1988. Inhibition of phagocytosis in *Yersinia pseudotuberculosis*: a virulence plasmid-encoded ability involving the Yop2b protein. *Infect Immun*, **56**, 2139–43.

Roy, C.R., Berger, K.H. and Isberg, R.R. 1998. *Legionella pneumophila* DotA protein is required for early phagosome trafficking decisions that occur within minutes of bacterial uptake. *Mol Microbiol*, **28**, 663–74.

Ruckdeschel, K., Harb, S., et al. 1998. *Yersinia enterocolitica* impairs activation of transcription factor NF-κB: involvement in the induction of programmed cell death and in the suppression of the macrophage tumor necrosis factor alpha production. *J Exp Med*, **187**, 1069–79.

Ruckdeschel, K., Mannel, O., et al. 2001. *Yersinia* outer protein P of *Yersinia enterocolitica* simultaneously blocks the nuclear factor-κB pathway and exploits lipopolysaccharide signaling to trigger apoptosis in macrophages. *J Immunol*, **166**, 1823–31.

Ryan, E.J., McNeela, E., et al. 2000. Modulation of innate and acquired immune responses by *Escherichia coli* heat-labile toxin: distinct pro- and anti-inflammatory effects of the nontoxic AB complex and the enzyme activity. *J Immunol*, **165**, 5750–9.

Saha, B., Das, G., et al. 1994. Macrophage-T cell interaction in experimental mycobacterial infection. Selective regulation of co-stimulatory molecules on *Mycobacterium*-infected macrophages and its implication in the suppression of cell-mediated immune response. *Eur J Immunol*, **24**, 2618–24.

Salgame, P.R., Birdi, T.J., et al. 1984. Mechanism of immunosuppression in leprosy – macrophage membrane alterations. *J Clin Lab Immunol*, **14**, 145–9.

Salmond, R.J., Pitman, R.S., et al. 2002. $CD8^+$ T cell apoptosis induced by *Escherichia coli* heat-labile enterotoxin B subunit occurs via a novel pathway involving NF-κB-dependent caspase activation. *Eur J Immunol*, **32**, 1737–47.

Sansonetti, P.J., Phalipon, A., et al. 2000. Caspase-1 activation of IL-1beta and IL-18 are essential for *Shigella flexneri*-induced inflammation. *Immunity*, **12**, 581–90.

Schaible, U.E. and Kaufmann, S.H. 2000. CD1 molecules and CD1-dependent T cells in bacterial infections: a link from innate to acquired immunity? *Semin Immunol*, **12**, 527–35.

Schenkein, H.A., Fletcher, H.M., et al. 1995. Increased opsonization of a prtH-defective mutant of *Porphyromonas gingivalis* W83 is caused by reduced degradation of complement-derived opsonins. *J Immunol*, **154**, 5331–7.

Schlesinger, L.S., Bellinger-Kawahara, C.G., et al. 1990. Phagocytosis of *Mycobacterium tuberculosis* is mediated by human monocyte complement receptors and complement component C3. *J Immunol*, **144**, 2771–80.

Schneider, B., Gross, R. and Haas, A. 2000. Phagosome acidification has opposite effects on intracellular survival of *Bordetella pertussis* and *B. bronchiseptica*. *Infect Immun*, **68**, 7039–48.

Schorr, W., Swandulla, D. and Zeilhofer, H.U. 1999. Mechanisms of IL-8-induced Ca^{2+} signaling in human neutrophil granulocytes. *Eur J Immunol*, **29**, 897–904.

Schramm, N., Bagnell, C.R. and Wyrick, P.B. 1996. Vesicles containing *Chlamydia trachomatis* serovar L2 remain above pH 6 within HEC-1B cells. *Infect Immun*, **64**, 1208–14.

Schuller, S., Kugler, S. and Goebel, W. 1998. Suppression of major histocompatibility complex class I and class II gene expression in *Listeria monocytogenes*-infected murine macrophages. *FEMS Immunol Med Microbiol*, **20**, 289–99.

Scidmore-Carlson, M.A., Shaw, E.I., et al. 1999. Identification and characterization of a *Chlamydia trachomatis* early operon encoding four novel inclusion membrane proteins. *Mol Microbiol*, **33**, 753–65.

Sewnath, M.E., Olszyna, D.P., et al. 2001. IL-10-deficient mice demonstrate multiple organ failure and increased mortality during *Escherichia coli* peritonitis despite an accelerated bacterial clearance. *J Immunol*, **166**, 6323–31.

Shany, S., Bernheimer, A.W., et al. 1974. Evidence for membrane cholesterol as the common binding site for cereolysin, streptolysin O and saponin. *Mol Cell Biochem*, **3**, 179–86.

Sieling, P.A. and Modlin, R.L. 1994. Cytokine patterns at the site of mycobacterial infection. *Immunobiology*, **191**, 378–87.

Siezen, R.J. 1999. Multi-domain, cell-envelope proteinases of lactic acid bacteria. *Antonie Van Leeuwenhoek*, **76**, 139–55.

Sing, A., Roggenkamp, A., et al. 2002. *Yersinia enterocolitica* evasion of the host innate immune response by V antigen-induced IL-10 production of macrophages is abrogated in IL-10-deficient mice. *J Immunol*, **168**, 1315–21.

Smith, G.A., Marquis, H., et al. 1995. The two distinct phospholipases C of *Listeria monocytogenes* have overlapping roles in escape from a vacuole and cell-to-cell spread. *Infect Immun*, **63**, 4231–7.

Soriani, M., Williams, N.A. and Hirst, T.R. 2001. *Escherichia coli* enterotoxin B subunit triggers apoptosis of $CD8^+$ T cells by activating transcription factor c-myc. *Infect Immun*, **69**, 4923–30.

Spangrude, G.J., Sacchi, F., et al. 1985. Inhibition of lymphocyte and neutrophil chemotaxis by pertussis toxin. *J Immunol*, **135**, 4135–43.

Staugas, R.E., Harvey, D.P., et al. 1992. Induction of tumor necrosis factor (TNF) and interleukin-1 (IL-1) by *Pseudomonas aeruginosa* and exotoxin A-induced suppression of lymphoproliferation and TNF, lymphotoxin, gamma interferon and IL-1 production in human leukocytes. *Infect Immun*, **60**, 3162–8.

Steele-Mortimer, O., Knodler, L.A. and Finlay, B.B. 2000. Poisons, ruffles and rockets: bacterial pathogens and the host cell cytoskeleton. *Traffic*, **1**, 107–18.

Stenberg, L., O'Toole, P.W., et al. 1994. Molecular characterization of protein Sir, a streptococcal cell surface protein that binds both immunoglobulin A and immunoglobulin G. *J Biol Chem*, **269**, 13458–64.

Stenger, S., Niazi, K.R. and Modlin, R.L. 1998. Down-regulation of CD1 on antigen-presenting cells by infection with *Mycobacterium tuberculosis*. *J Immunol*, **161**, 3582–8.

Sturgill-Koszycki, S., Schlesinger, P.H., et al. 1994. Lack of acidification in *Mycobacterium* phagosomes produced by exclusion of the vesicular proton-ATPase. *Science*, **263**, 678–81.

Svensson, M., Johansson, C. and Wick, M.J. 2000. *Salmonella enterica serovar typhimurium*-induced maturation of bone marrow-derived dendritic cells. *Infect Immun*, **68**, 6311–20.

Szalay, G., Ladel, C.H., et al. 1999. Cutting edge: anti-CD1 monoclonal antibody treatment reverses the production patterns of TGF-β2 and Th1 cytokines and ameliorates listeriosis in mice. *J Immunol*, **162**, 6955–8.

Thakker, M., Park, J.S., et al. 1998. *Staphylococcus aureus* serotype 5 capsular polysaccharide is antiphagocytic and enhances bacterial virulence in a murine bacteremia model. *Infect Immun*, **66**, 5183–9.

Thern, A., Wastfelt, M. and Lindahl, G. 1998. Expression of two different antiphagocytic M proteins by *Streptococcus pyogenes* of the OF+ lineage. *J Immunol*, **160**, 860–9.

Tjelle, T.E., Lovdal, T. and Berg, T. 2000. Phagosome dynamics and function. *Bioessays*, **22**, 255–63.

Toossi, Z., Young, T.G., et al. 1995. Induction of transforming growth factor beta 1 by purified protein derivative of *Mycobacterium tuberculosis*. *Infect Immun*, **63**, 224–8.

Uchiya, K., Barbieri, M.A., et al. 1999. A *Salmonella* virulence protein that inhibits cellular trafficking. *EMBO J*, **18**, 3924–33.

Ullrich, H.J., Beatty, W.L. and Russell, D.G. 2000. Interaction of *Mycobacterium avium*-containing phagosomes with the antigen presentation pathway. *J Immunol*, **165**, 6073–80.

Vazquez-Boland, J.A., Kuhn, M., et al. 2001. *Listeria* pathogenesis and molecular virulence determinants. *Clin Microbiol Rev*, **14**, 584–640.

Vazquez-Torres, A., Xu, Y., et al. 2000. *Salmonella* pathogenicity island 2-dependent evasion of the phagocyte NADPH oxidase. *Science*, **287**, 1655–8.

Via, L.E., Deretic, D., et al. 1997. Arrest of mycobacterial phagosome maturation is caused by a block in vesicle fusion between stages controlled by rab5 and rab7. *J Biol Chem*, **272**, 13326–31.

Vishwanath, S., Ramphal, R., et al. 1988. Respiratory-mucin inhibition of the opsonophagocytic killing of *Pseudomonas aeruginosa*. *Infect Immun*, **56**, 2218–22.

von der Weid, T., Bulliard, C. and Schiffrin, E.J. 2001. Induction by a lactic acid bacterium of a population of $CD4^+$ T cells with low proliferative capacity that produce transforming growth factor beta and interleukin-10. *Clin Diagn Lab Immunol*, **8**, 695–701.

Von Pawel-Rammingen, U., Telepnev, M.V., et al. 2000. GAP activity of the *Yersinia* YopE cytotoxin specifically targets the Rho pathway: a mechanism for disruption of actin microfilament structure. *Mol Microbiol*, **36**, 737–48.

Walev, I., Vollmer, P., et al. 1996. Pore-forming toxins trigger shedding of receptors for interleukin 6 and lipopolysaccharide. *Proc Natl Acad Sci USA*, **93**, 7882–7.

Wang, J., Brooks, E.G., et al. 2001. Negative selection of T cells by *Helicobacter pylori* as a model for bacterial strain selection by immune evasion. *J Immunol*, **167**, 926–34.

Weinrauch, Y. and Zychlinsky, A. 1999. The induction of apoptosis by bacterial pathogens. *Annu Rev Microbiol*, **53**, 155–87.

Weiss, D.J., Evanson, O.A., et al. 2001. Regulation of expression of major histocompatibility antigens by bovine macrophages infected with *Mycobacterium avium* subsp. paratuberculosis or *Mycobacterium avium* subsp. avium. *Infect Immun*, **69**, 1002–8.

Wexler, D.E., Chenoweth, D.E. and Cleary, P.P. 1985. Mechanism of action of the group A streptococcal C5a inactivator. *Proc Natl Acad Sci USA*, **82**, 8144–8.

Wick, M.J., Harding, C.V., et al. 1995. The phoP locus influences processing and presentation of *Salmonella typhimurium* antigens by activated macrophages. *Mol Microbiol*, **16**, 465–76.

Wilkinson, K.A., Martin, T.D., et al. 2000. Latency-associated peptide of transforming growth factor beta enhances mycobacteriocidal immunity in the lung during *Mycobacterium bovis* BCG infection in C57BL/6 mice. *Infect Immun*, **68**, 6505–8.

Wojciechowski, W., DeSanctis, J., et al. 1999. Attenuation of MHC class II expression in macrophages infected with *Mycobacterium bovis* bacillus Calmette-Guerin involves class II transactivator and depends on the *Nramp1* gene. *J Immunol*, **163**, 2688–96.

Wurzner, R. 1999. Evasion of pathogens by avoiding recognition or eradication by complement, in part via molecular mimicry. *Mol Immunol*, **36**, 249–60.

Wylie, J.L., Hatch, G.M. and McClarty, G. 1997. Host cell phospholipids are trafficked to and then modified by *Chlamydia trachomatis*. *J Bacteriol*, **179**, 7233–42.

Wyrick, P.B. 2000. Intracellular survival by *Chlamydia*. *Cell Microbiol*, **2**, 275–82.

Yamamoto, M., Kiyono, H., et al. 1999. Direct effects on antigen-presenting cells and T lymphocytes explain the adjuvanticity of a nontoxic cholera toxin mutant. *J Immunol*, **162**, 7015–21.

Yao, T., Mecsas, J., et al. 1999. Suppression of T and B lymphocyte activation by a *Yersinia pseudotuberculosis* virulence factor, YopH. *J Exp Med*, **190**, 1343–50.

Zahrt, T.C. and Deretic, V. 2002. Reactive nitrogen and oxygen intermediates and bacterial defenses: unusual adaptations in *Mycobacterium tuberculosis*. *Antioxid Redox Signal*, **4**, 141–59.

Zeidner, N., Mbow, M.L., et al. 1997. Effects of *Ixodes scapularis* and *Borrelia burgdorferi* on modulation of the host immune response: induction of a TH2 cytokine response in Lyme disease-susceptible (C3H/HeJ) mice but not in disease-resistant (BALB/c) mice. *Infect Immun*, **65**, 3100–6.

Zhong, G., Fan, T. and Liu, L. 1999. *Chlamydia* inhibits interferon gamma-inducible major histocompatibility complex class II expression by degradation of upstream stimulatory factor 1. *J Exp Med*, **189**, 1931–8.

Zhong, G., Liu, L., et al. 2000. Degradation of transcription factor RFX5 during the inhibition of both constitutive and interferon gamma-inducible major histocompatibility complex class I expression in *Chlamydia*-infected cells. *J Exp Med*, **191**, 1525–34.

Zuany-Amorim, C., Sawicka, E., et al. 2002. Suppression of airway eosinophilia by killed *Mycobacterium vaccae*-induced allergen-specific regulatory T-cells. *Nat Med*, **8**, 625–9.

Zychlinsky, A. and Sansonetti, P.J. 1997. Apoptosis as a proinflammatory event: what can we learn from bacteria-induced cell death? *Trends Microbiol*, **5**, 201–4.

Zychlinsky, A., Prevost, M.C. and Sansonetti, P.J. 1992. *Shigella flexneri* induces apoptosis in infected macrophages. *Nature*, **358**, 167–9.

33

Parasite evasion

WERNER SOLBACH AND RICHARD LUCIUS

Parasites (Greek: pará-sitos, i.e. 'eat together') are unicellular (protozoan) or multicellular (metazoan) organisms that live in a close relationship on or within their hosts and are able to affect them adversely by acquisition of nutrients, damage to body surfaces, or penetration into tissues. They continue to be an increasing health problem and create a substantial economic burden, especially in less developed areas within the tropics.

Compared with the 5000 genes found in *Escherichia coli* bacteria, parasites have of the order of 7 000–20 000 protein-encoding genes. This genetic complexity may be required for the organization of the eukaryotic cell apparatus, but it is likely that a substantial number of genes contribute to the maintenance of the very diverse lifestyles that are perfectly adapted to survival in intermediate and definitive hosts with extremely different environmental conditions. Many parasites are more nuisance than danger to humans; some can, however, cause severe disease.

It is a characteristic hallmark of parasitic diseases that they are chronic in nature, with or without an acute onset. Chronicity of disease clearly indicates that either the immune system is unable to eradicate the invading pathogen or the continuous struggle of the immune system to combat the invading organisms leads to a state of immunopathology. Chronicity of disease also implies that the parasites have the ability to subvert or evade the immune response. Protozoan parasites with their smaller genomes usually need a relatively short time to replicate, and therefore evade host immune responses, often through mechanisms based on quick mutational or adaptive changes such as variation of their surface antigenic coat. In contrast, helminths have much longer generation times and therefore employ an array of other evasion mechanisms. For some organisms, such as *Trypanosoma brucei*, and, more recently, for *Plasmodium* spp. the molecular basis for immune evasion is quite well understood, whereas for others, especially helminth infections, the underlying mechanisms are much less clear.

The morphological and genetic complexity and the remarkably divergent lifestyles of parasites make them extremely interesting and, at the same time, difficult to approach for immunological studies. Nevertheless, considerable achievements have been made in the last decade and some of the parasites, e.g. *Leishmania* spp., have become paradigmatic to the understanding of basic immunological principles. This knowledge has helped to disclose some of the many determinants that regulate the type, the course, and the intensity of immune responses. It is also a prerequisite to establish a rational basis for the development of prophylactic and therapeutic immune intervention measures.

PROTOZOA AND THE DISEASES THAT THEY CAUSE IN HUMANS

Among the parasitic protozoa there are five major groups: Apicomplexa, Kinetoplastida, Trichomonadida,

Diplomomnadida, and Amebida. Apicomplexans include *Plasmodium* spp., *Toxoplasma gondii*, and *Cryptosporidium parvum*, *Leishmania* spp., and *Trypanosoma* spp. belong to the kinetoplastid protozoa. *Trichomonas vaginalis* is grouped in the order Trichomonadida, and *Giardia lamblia* belongs to the order Diplomonadida. Pseudopodia-forming organisms such as *Entamboeba histolytica* are allocated to the order Amebida. During evolution apicomplexan parasites have adapted to a life within host cells and have distinct organelles that are important for the invasion process. They infect different but distinct cell types depending on the stage of development. Flagellated organisms live outside (*T. vaginalis*, *G. lamblia*) or inside the body, either extracellularly within the bloodstream or the brain (*T. brucei*) or intracellularly in many different cell types (*T. cruzi*) or restricted to a narrow spectrum of host cells such as granulocytes, macrophages, dendritic cells, or fibroblasts in the case of *Leishmania* spp.

Plasmodium spp.

Four different species of *Plasmodium* are responsible for malaria in humans, i.e. *P. falciparum* (for genome sequence, see Gardner et al. 2002), *P. vivax*, *P. malariae*, and *P. ovale*. During a blood meal of an infected female anopheles mosquito (for genome sequence of *A. gambiae*, see Holt et al. 2002) they enter the bloodstream directly as sporozoites. Within less than an hour the sporozoites invade hepatocytes by recognizing glycosaminoglycans on the liver cells, through binding via a set of surface proteins called circumsporozoite protein (CSP) and thrombospondin-related adhesive protein (TRAP) (Muller et al. 1993; Frevert 1994). Inside the hepatocyte, the parasites divide and release merozoites that bind to different glycoproteins on erythrocytes, e.g. to a distinct region of erythrocytic glycophorin A via surface proteins called erythrocyte-binding antigen (EBA) (175) and merozoite surface proteins (MSP) (Orlandi et al. 1992; Perkins and Rocco 1988) or by ligation of the parasite protein P. falciparum erythrocyte membrane protein 1 (PfEMP1) to the complement receptor CR1 (CD35). Interestingly, the CR1 receptor is increased 40- to 70-fold in malaria-exposed African populations (Krych-Goldberg et al. 2002). Inside the erythrocyte, the parasites start to differentiate and multiply to produce more merozoites, which, after rupture of the red blood cell, are released to infect new erythrocytes. Some parasites differentiate into gametocytes which, after ingestion by a blood-feeding mosquito, fuse to form a zygote; this subsequently gives rise to the development of sporozoites that can infect additional humans.

After a typical incubation time of 1–2 weeks, the key features of acute plasmodial disease comprise sudden fever attacks caused by abrupt release of merozoites together with ruptured erythrocytes and its contents and, more seriously, cerebral coma and multiorgan failure (kidney, liver, lung). The latter results from reduced microcirculatory blood flow caused by structural and functional changes of infected (and uninfected) erythrocytes (Dondorp et al. 2000). Parasitized red blood cells adhere to endothelial cells primarily via PfEMP1 proteins, which are expressed on modified membrane regions called 'knobs' and bind to endothelial CD36, intercellular adhesion molecule (ICAM), thrombospondin, platelet endothelial cell adhesion molecule-1 (PECAM-1), and, especially in the placenta, hyaluronic acid and chondroitin sulfate A. In later stages of the disease, anemia develops together with splenomegaly accompanied by leukopenia and thrombocytopenia.

Protective immunity against *Plasmodium* spp. develops slowly and it may be necessary for a child born in a malaria-endemic area to be exposed to many successive infections for a number of years before developing any resistance; complete protection may never be achieved. The apparent inefficacy of antimalarial immunity may be explained by the parasite subverting or evading the immunological armamentarium by sequestration, poor immunogenicity of its antigens, or antigenic diversity and variation. The recent deciphering of the genome of *P. falciparum* (Gardner et al. 2002) has shown that many genes at the end of the parasite's chromosomes code for the expression of different versions of merozoite proteins on the surface of infected erythrocytes, thus confounding the immune responses that aim to destroy the infected cells.

Toxoplasma gondii

Infection with *T. gondii* is one of the most common parasitic infections of humans, other mammalians, birds, and other vertebrates. It is found worldwide with nearly one-third of the world population being exposed. In immunocompetent people, it does not cause serious illness but can lead to devastating disease in those with immunoincompetence, including fetuses and children born to mothers with primary infection during pregnancy as well as in patients with AIDS.

The definite host for the parasite is primarily the young cat (Dubey et al. 1970; Sibley et al. 1998; Carruthers et al. 2000; Brecht et al. 2001). In cats, the parasite's sexual stage occurs intracellularly in intestinal epithelia, leading to non-infective oocysts that are passed with the cat's feces in feed, water, or soil. After sporulation ('ripening') infective oocysts develop. When ingested by intermediate hosts (humans, livestock animals), the oocysts release tachyzoites. Ubiquitously expressed glycosaminoglycans on the host cells recognize secreted toxoplasmal proteins (MIC1 and MIC2), leading to adherence. Invasion occurs actively through an actin–myosin-based process with which the parasites glide, rotate, and undulate into a vacuole that is created mostly from material secreted by apical organelles

(Sibley et al. 1998; Mordue et al. 1999b; Brecht et al. 2001). Through formation of the vacuolar membrane, it selectively excludes host cell plasma membrane proteins (Mordue et al. 1999a) and thus may fail to induce host cell signaling. Within the cell, *Toxoplasma* spp. remain inside the parasitophorous vacuole by inserting their own proteins into the membrane. This prevents acidification and fusion with the lysosomal contents (Carruthers et al. 2000). The parasites divide until the host cell is filled with parasites and transform into bradyzoites. Neighboring cells may be infected or – especially after the host has acquired immunity – the bradyzoites may build up a cystic membrane with hundreds of parasites that can persist for prolonged periods of time, possibly life-long. When cysts, e.g. in undercooked or raw meat, are eaten by another mammal, the bradyzoites can continue the life cycle. After ingestion by a cat, they can initiate the sexual cycle.

In immunocompetent people, most infections are asymptomatic or show mild clinical signs such as low-grade fever, fatigue, headache, and muscle and joint pain. More common is painful swelling of cervical lymph nodes. In people with impaired cellular immunity, as occurs after HIV infection with CD4 T lymphocytes of less than 50/μl peripheral blood, *Toxoplasma* spp. can cause a life-threatening disease. On liberation of bradyzoites from the cysts, about one-third of AIDS patients develop a necrotizing focal encephalitis with dissemination in various organs, often with lethal consequences. Another extremely susceptible population are unborn children who acquire *T. gondii* from women who experience a primary infection during pregnancy. Depending on the intensity and the time point of infection, stillbirth, hydrocephalus, or intracerebral calcification including the retina can occur.

Encystment of toxoplasma parasites is dependent on a robust acquired immunity involving dendritic cells, CD4 and CD8 lymphocytes, as well as interleukin-12 (IL-12) and interferon-γ (IFN-γ) as the central protective elements (Yap and Sher 1999; Scanga et al. 2002).

Cryptosporidium parvum

Cryptosporidia are apicomplexan parasites that have long been known as pathogens for livestock animals, especially calves. The first case of human cryptosporidiasis was reported only in 1976 (Meisel et al. 1976; Nime et al. 1976). The organism is spread from animals to humans but also from person to person, and is often transmitted by contaminated water. It is distributed throughout the world. Its risk for human health is exemplified by a recent outbreak as a result of failure of appropriate water purification processes in the USA (MacKenzie et al. 1994).

The life cycle of *C. parvum* is confined to the microvillous region of the intestinal epithelia within one definitive host. After ingestion of infective oocytes, sporozoites are released which invade enterocytes and form an intracellular but extracytoplasmic parasitophorous vacuole, which is limited by a four-layer membrane. After multiplication and differentiation, merozoites are released which can infect other enterocytes through autoinfection. Some merozoites develop into sexual stages that produce a thick-walled oocyst after fusion in the parasitophorous vacuole, which is shed through the feces and can infect other individuals.

Infection with *C. parvum* may be without any symptoms or may lead to a self-limiting disease with watery diarrhea, nausea, and abdominal cramping for a few days. In patients with underlying illnesses affecting the adaptive immune system such as those with AIDS or on immunosuppressive therapy, the intensity and duration of gastrointestinal symptoms can be life threatening. In addition to the gastrointestinal tract other epithelia such as those of the respiratory system or the gallbladder can be infected (Chen et al. 2002).

Despite substantial knowledge of the life cycle and excellent morphological evidence, comparatively little is known about the immunobiology of *C. parvum* infection as a result of the lack of an appropriate animal model and the inability to culture sufficient numbers of parasites in vitro. Existing evidence suggests, however, that, very similar to Toxoplasma infection, the adaptive cellular immune system is dominant over the humoral immune system to provide protection. The increasing number of genes or genomic DNA fragments registered in GenBank (www.ncbi.nlm.nih.gov/cgi-bin/genbank?Cryptosporidium) will greatly facilitate our understanding of immunological and basic biology aspects in the near future.

Trypanosoma spp.

TRYPANOSOMA BRUCEI COMPLEX (AFRICAN TRYPANOSOMES)

Based on similarities in geographical distribution, infectivity to humans, life cycle, morphology, and major biochemical features, the *Trypanosoma brucei* complex comprises three subspecies: *T. b. brucei*, *T. b. gambiense*, and *T. b. rhodesiense*. In this chapter they are referred to as *T. brucei*. The parasites are endemic in many countries of sub-Saharan Africa.

Metacyclic forms of *T. brucei* are transmitted by the bite of an infected tsetse fly (*Glossina* spp.) through contaminating saliva. After inoculation, they remain at the infectious site for a short time and induce a local inflammatory response of the subdermal tissue ('chancre'). Subsequently, they are disseminated throughout the body once they have gained access to lymph and blood vessels. They multiply rapidly extracellularly and lead to different waves of parasitemia, which are accompanied by systemic inflammation with perivascular infiltration of leukocytes. In later stages of the disease, they enter the central nervous system (CNS), the heart, and endocrine organs. CNS involvement is associated with a wide array of behavioral changes, ranging from aggressiveness to lethargy, somnolence ('sleeping sickness'), or death.

The way in which *T. brucei* causes disease is unclear, but the success of infection is linked to the parasite's ability to select for the expression of one out of hundreds of genes that code for a major surface coat antigen, the variant surface glycoprotein (VSG) (Donelson et al. 1998; Andrews 2002; Berriman et al. 2002). Each VSG induces a strong and specific antibody response, which clears up to 99 percent of the parasites bearing it during a given wave of parasitemia. A minor population of pre-existing parasites (between 0.000001 and 1 percent) expresses a different VSG and thus is not recognized by the specific antibodies. This population then can outgrow and give rise to the next wave of parasitemia, until the new immune response leads to their demise; this scenario is repeated several times.

TRYPANOSOMA CRUZI (NEW WORLD TRYPANOSOMES)

T. cruzi parasites are endemic in several Central and South American countries and they are the cause of Chagas' disease. Metacyclic trypomastigotes are deposited on the skin through the feces of blood-feeding triatomine bugs. They are motile and have the capacity to penetrate abraded skin or the wound caused by the bite of the bug. They can also cross the conjunctiva or nasal and oral mucosa, if bug feces reach these surfaces. Once inside the host, they enter phagocytic or nonphagocytic cells and convert into replicating amastigotes. The responsible attachment and invasion receptors and ligands are not well defined. Contact of trypomastigotes with the host cells leads to the recruitment of host cell lysosomes to the plasma membrane, where both coalesce and fuse, forming a compartment in which the parasites enter to form a phagosome (Andrews 2002) (www.archive.bmn.com/supp/part/andrews.html). This process is initiated by a parasite oligopeptidase B, which triggers transient elevation of the intracellular calcium level in the host cell (Burleigh 2000) and is dependent on the activation of the transforming growth factor β (TGF-β) signaling pathway. *T. cruzi* resides only transiently within the phagosome, because it releases membrane-dissolving molecules that allow the parasite to enter the cytoplasm. After nine cycles of binary replication, the amastigotes differentiate into trypomastigotes and are released in large numbers into the bloodstream and can infect other cells or a triatomine vector.

T. cruzi leads to a number of clinical manifestations, which include lymphadenopathy, generalized edema, enlargement of the heart with arrhythmias, dysfunctions in the alimentary tract with loss of peristalsis, severe obstipation, and progressive dilation of the gut. These signs result from chronic infection of the respective cells, although chronic autoimmune inflammation has been suggested as an underlying pathogenic principle. In patients with AIDS the organism commonly crosses the blood–brain barrier with fatal meningoencephalitis. Both antibodies and T cells are important antiparasitic effector mechanisms necessary to combat the trypanosomal infection at intra- and extracellular locations (Ouaissi et al. 2002).

Leishmania spp.

Leishmania spp. are parasites that infect humans in all continents except Australia. Eighteen species are known to cause human disease. Some lead to localized cutaneous disease, whereas others cause systemic disease.

Leishmania spp. are transmitted by the bite of sand flies (*Phlebotomus* and *Lutzomyia* spp.). In the gut of the insect they develop as flagellated motile promastigotes, which are highly infective in their metacyclic stage – found in the salivary glands (Sacks 2001). During blood feeding they are deposited, together with the sand fly's saliva, in the epidermal and dermal tissue. Saliva components greatly facilitate the establishment of an infection and reduce the infectious dose required to establish a successful infection (Belkaid et al. 2001; Zer et al. 2001). Promastigotes have a dense layer of a lipophosphoglycan (LPG) and a 63-kDa glycoprotein (gp63) zinc metalloprotease, which both serve as virulence factors (Sacks and Kamhawi 2001; Joshi et al. 2002). The outer portion of the LPG extends from the surface of the parasite to form a glycocalix, which activates host complement and leads to deposition of C3 on the parasite's surface. At the same time the glycocalix and gp63 prevent membrane attack complex (C5–C9) being inserted into the parasite's membrane. The C3-coated promastigotes attach to complement receptors 1 and 3 (CR1, CR3) on macrophages. On reorganization of the actin–myosin cytoskeletal apparatus (May and Machesky 2001) of the host cell membrane, components of the endoplasmic reticulum (ER) are recruited close to the surface of the cell, where they fuse with the plasma membrane, which opens up at the site of parasite contact. The parasite then slides into the open ER, whereas the plasma membrane is resealed and the formation of the phagosomal vacuole is initiated (Gagnon et al. 2002).

At very early stages of infection, *Leishmania* spp. are phagocytosed by neutrophilic polymorphonuclear granulocytes (PNG), which are attracted to the site of infection through a parasite-derived chemotactic factor (Van Zandbergen et al. 2002). Inside the PNGs, they delay the usually rapidly occurring granulocytic apoptosis through inhibition of a caspase 3-related pathway (Aga et al. 2002). Thereby they are shielded from the hostile extracellular host milieu until ingestion by mononuclear cells. Once inside the definitive host cells, *Leishmania* are directed to the lysosomal compartment, where they transform into nonflagellated amastigotes, persist, and replicate. Through various mechanisms they inhibit signaling events that would normally lead to macrophage activation and parasite killing. However, interferon-γ (IFN-γ) is able to activate macrophages to overcome this parasite-induced block and is able to promote parasite killing by inducing inducible nitric oxide (NO) synthase expression and NO production (Bogdan 2001). The murine mouse model of subcutaneous *L. major* infection has become paradigmatic for studying the adaptive immune response with respect to the roles of T-helper 1 (Th1) and T-helper 2 (Th2) lymphocytes in vivo.

In humans, disease develops as a result of incomplete parasite killing. This in turn results in chronic lesions at skin or mucosal sites (*L. major*, *L. amazonensis*, *L. braziliensis*, and *L. chagasi*) or in internal organs rich in macrophages such as the liver, spleen, or bone marrow (*L. donovani*, *L. infantum*, and *L. braziliensis*). In addition, excessive and damaging immune responses to the parasite may cause serious and debilitating disease (mucocutaneous leishmaniasis caused by *L. amazonenis*).

Entamoeba histolytica

Six species of amoebae are commonly found in the human gastrointestinal tract, of which *E. histolytica* is of medical importance. The organism is taken up with contaminated drinking water as an infectious cyst. Intraintestinally, the cyst wall is dissolved and gives rise to trophozoites, which can either form new cysts or occasionally penetrate the mucosa and disseminate to other organs, with serious implications such as amoebic colitis or liver abscesses. *E. histolytica* trophozoites are able to kill epithelial and immune cells rapidly. The killing is contact dependent and mediated by the trophozoite, Gal/GalNac lectin, which recognizes and binds host cell glycoconjugates and is associated with the release of pore-forming proteins (Leippe et al. 1994; Petri et al. 2002). Once lectin-mediated host–parasite contact occurs, the parasite activates host cell caspase 3, resulting in immediate cell death by apoptosis (Huston et al. 2000). Both local and systemic humoral and cellular immunity appear to play a role in protection, which may open up a window for the development of a vaccine (Miller-Sims and Petri 2002).

IMMUNITY, PERSISTENCE, AND EVASION IN INFECTIONS WITH PROTOZOAN PARASITES

As has been outlined so far, protozoan parasites have an extremely diverse array of lifestyles. This poses a challenge to the immune system which goes far beyond what is well understood by using experimental model antigens such as bovine serum albumin or relatively simple organisms such as viruses. Instead, the innate immune response has to recognize, at the same time, a vast variety of molecular patterns at one or different sites in the body. In addition, host defense has to be extremely flexible in tailoring the appropriate adaptive immune response as a result of the developmental stages through which many parasites go. The site of infection (skin, mucosa, conjunctiva, direct inoculation by blood-feeding arthropods with saliva), the number of infecting organisms, the parasitic lifestyle (intracellular or extracellular, within a vacuole or in the cytoplasm, replicative or not, production of antigenically distinct progeny), the overall constitution of the host's immune system (influenced by genetic susceptibility/resistance, age, nutritional status, previous experience with parasitic or other infections) are all determinants for what constitutes a protective immune response.

Paradigmatic experimental work on the analysis of the immune response to *L. major* after experimental subcutaneous syringe infection of different inbred mouse strains has shown the importance of the development of a polarized Th1 or Th2 answer. Animals that are able to mount an adaptive response dominated by Th1 lymphocytes survive and are resistant to re-infection, whereas those with a Th2-biased response are highly susceptible and succumb after exposure (for review, see Solbach and Laskay 2000). From these findings it was expected that, in all parasitic infections, a Th1 response would have protective effects, whereas Th2 responses would be associated with a failure to resist infection. It appeared, however, that this perception was not true. Work on immunity to intestinal helminths showed an exactly opposite pattern of severity of disease and the type of adaptive immune response: Th2-type responses in many cases allowed the resolution of infection, whereas Th1-type responses promoted chronic and nonprotective courses of the disease (MacDonald et al. 2002). This led, for a while, to the simplistic concept that a Th1 response alone might be sufficient for immune control of intracellular protozoa whereas a Th2 response, being responsible for the development of antibodies and the dampening of a potentially overreacting Th1 cellular immune response, was meant to keep extracellular parasites restricted. It soon turned out, however, that a delicate balance between Th1 and Th2 immune responses is responsible for shaping the outcome of most, if not all, parasitic infections. It also became clear that this balance varies considerably over time and controls the production of cytokines such as IFN-γ, the interleukins IL-4, IL-10, and transforming growth factor β (TGF-β). At the same time, T cells by themselves are under the tight control of cytokines which constitute the complex mixture of humoral factors at the infectious site. The result of all these determinants is responsible for activation of the protective antiparasitic effector arms.

The kinetics and magnitude of cytokines produced by T cells is determined by the initial interactions of the parasites with early inflammatory cells such as granulocytes and dendritic cells. They are equipped with an array of pathogen recognition receptors (PRR) on their surface. PRRs are activated by the parasite's pathogen-associated molecular patterns (PAMP) and thus serve as innate 'master regulators' of the ensuing adaptive immune response, e.g. the PAMP-protein Tc52 from *T. cruzi* (which is also crucial for the parasite's survival) binds to the PRR Toll-like receptor 2 (TLR-2) on dendritic cells. This interaction induces host cell maturation and production of inflammatory chemokines, and protects mice from an otherwise lethal infection (Ouaissi et al. 2002).

In contrast to prokaryotes, many infecting eukaryotic parasites undergo a series of developmental changes during their establishment, development, or proliferation within the host. In consequence, although infected with only one given parasite species, the host is exposed to numerous sets of PAMPs as the infectious organism proceeds through its developmental pathway, e.g. infection with *Plasmodium* spp. exposes the host to four different extracellular life-cycle stages – the sporozoite, the merozoite, and the male and female gametocytes – plus the additional forms that live within the hepatocytes or erythrocytes. Although all these life-cycle stages share the expression of a basic set of genes, they also express stage-specific genes that code for the proteins required for successful completion of the life cycle. Thus, primary exposure to malaria leads to a series of immune responses directed to related, but antigenically distinct, organisms. The situation is even more complex in helminthic infections. Here, the larval form is often completely different from the adult worm or its progeny, and thus a whole series of different immune responses are initiated and maintained, e.g. eggs produced by adult schistosomes produce a Th2 response, whereas the worms themselves do not (Pearce and MacDonald 2002).

As a response to the antigenic complexity of parasites, the host creates a similarly complex set of immune responses. The relative contribution of the various immune mechanisms in operation throughout the course of infection is far from being understood, e.g. the early CD8 T-cell response is important in dealing with the hepatocytic stage of the infection with *Plasmodium* spp., but is largely irrelevant once the parasites have entered erythrocytes (Good and Doolan 1999). In contrast, in leishmania infections, CD4 T cells of the Th1 type mediate a protective immune response during the acute stage, whereas, for the induction of immunity with low-dose infections and its maintenance in chronic stages, CD8 T cells may be important (for review, see Solbach and Laskay 2000; Belkaid et al. 2002). Finally, maintenance of multiple effector responses, including antibodies, CD4 Th1 cells, and CD8 T cells, is required for the control of *T. cruzi* infections in both the acute and the chronic stages (Tarleton 2001).

In most parasitic infections the immune system sees and responds to a complex array of antigens, possibly with some exceptions, where a restricted number of antigens is dominant, e.g. *T. brucei* populations express for a brief period a given set of variant surface glycoprotein acronym>VSG, and in *L. major* infection of BALB/c mice the leishmania homolog of the receptor for activated c kinase (LACK) antigen is immunodominant (Schilling and Glaichenhaus 2001). The complexity in the immune responses makes it a challenge to develop an appropriate set of vaccine antigens that will elicit the appropriate protective effector mechanisms at relevant sites of infection, i.e. either in the tissues or at mucosal surfaces.

Most parasites survive within most of their hosts for long periods, thereby causing chronic infection (and in some cases chronic disease) and long-term stimulation of the immune system. From an evolutionary point of view, chronicity of parasitic infections indicates success for both the parasite and the host, because both are able to survive with each other for a long time. Recent experimental and clinical evidence suggests that immune responses induced by chronic helminthic infections during early life via the anti-inflammatory activity of IL-10 may shape the development of the immune system towards a Th1 bias such that it prevents immune dysfunctions that result in diseases such as allergy (van den Biggelaar et al. 2000; Bashir et al. 2002; Yazdanbakhsh et al. 2002).

Antigen variation

Chronicity of infection requires that the parasite must in some way be able to evade the immune attack to avoid its own elimination. Some protozoan parasites evade the immune response by sequential variation of their antigenic coat. African trypanosomes live extracellularly in an environment with high concentrations of antibodies which they induce themselves. They evade immune responses by selecting for the expression of one gene from a repertoire of up to 1000 variant genes through transcriptional activation. These genes encode the monomolecular VSG. VSG is composed of glycosylphosphatidylinositol (GPI)-anchored homodimers that are identically oriented and densely packed (10^7 molecules/cells) on the membrane surface. The repetitive VSG elements are scanned by B cells, which become activated without the help of T lymphocytes to produce a rapid IgM response. Within the parasite population, however, a spontaneous VSG gene switching occurs with one switch in 10^2–10^6 cells (Turner 1997). In consequence, the immune response occurring at a given time is appropriate and successful at killing trypanosomes through antibodies directed against the dominant surface antigens. However, the switch in antigen phenotype of an initially small population of parasites allows their expansion until sufficient antibodies are produced that recognize the new VSG variant. In this situation, the host eventually dies without ever completely eliminating the organisms from the body.

Although VSG-specific antibodies provide an important mechanism for controlling trypanosome numbers in the vasculature, antibodies alone are not sufficient to provide a significant level of host resistance. For control of parasites residing in the tissues, an early Th1 response with IL-12-driven and IFN-γ-dependent activation of macrophages is indispensable. This T-cell response is mainly induced by antigens that stem from an internal subregion of the VSG molecules which are liberated from the surface coat.

Antigenic variation is also employed by malaria parasites to avoid destruction by immune mechanisms (Kyes et al. 2001; Beeson and Brown 2002). Once the parasites have gained entry into the erythrocytes, they modify the infected cells with several proteins, which make them 'sticky' to the endothelium (Smith et al. 2002). One of the principal parasite-induced antigen on the red blood cell (RBC) surface is the PfEMP1 which is encoded by a clonally variant, multicopy, nonallelic family termed '*var*'. Modification of the erythrocyte's surface can be regarded as an important adaptation because it prevents the parasitized RBCs from being swept to the spleen, where they would be removed as a result of the aberrant shape that they acquire when parasitized. This advantage of course bears the risk of being identified by the immune system. In fact, antibodies specific for PfEMP1 can prevent the adhesion of parasitized cells to endothelial cells, thereby facilitating sequestration to the spleen. In response, the parasite selects for expression of one out of about seventy of PfEMP1-encoding genes at a given time, thus confounding the immune responses that aim to destroy the infected cells. Genome-wide analysis has identified more than 200 plasmodial genes which are likely to be involved in immune evasion, most of which are found near the ends of the chromosomes (Gardner et al. 2002).

Immediately after inoculation, plasmodium sporozoites circulate for a short time as extracellular organisms rich in surface circumporozoite protein (CSP). CSP is an antigen with multiple tandem repeats which induces a polyclonal Th cell-independent B-cell response. Plasmodia overcome this response by sloughing off their surface CSP coat, thus withdrawing the targets from the attack of antibodies (Ramasamy 1998).

Antigenic variation has also been observed in infections with the intestinal flagellated parasite *G. lamblia*. During infection, the parasite survives the host's reactions by undergoing continuous antigenic variation of its major variant surface protein (VSP). VSPs from *G. lamblia* are cysteine-rich proteins with considerable heterogeneity in size. In vivo, the VSPs expressed by the parasite population continuously diversify under the selection pressure of IgA antibodies and proteases secreted by intestinal cells (Muller and Gottstein 1998).

Intracellular refuge and its consequences

Intracellular residency of protozoans such as *Trypanosoma cruzi*, *Toxoplasma gondii*, or *Leishmania* spp. protects them from detection by defense systems. This advantage, however, requires mechanisms that assure survival and replication within that shelter. In the initial phase of the infection the host cells in many cases are from the macrophage lineage or granulocytes (Aga et al. 2002). They have the potential to inhibit the replication or to kill the microbes, once they become activated to do so. Many parasites have developed strategies to subvert this cellular activation. Metacyclic forms of *Leishmania* spp., for example, bind different sets of entry ligands that contribute to silent entry. These include binding and uptake via CR1 and CR3 receptors, scavenger receptors, the mannose fucose receptor (Solbach and Laskay 2000), or receptors that recognize phosphatidylserine. The last strategy, which is also employed by helminthic schistosomes, fakes the host cell because it signals (falsely) apoptotic structures that are considered to be dealt with without induction of inflammation (Freire-de-Lima et al. 2000; Freitas Balanco et al. 2001; Luder et al. 2001; Van Der Kleij et al. 2002). Other mechanisms include the generation of a 'safe' compartment inside the cell, e.g. *T. cruzi* parasites secrete a lytic protein that releases the parasites into the cytoplasm, thus escaping fusion of the phagosome with the lysosome and its toxic components. *L. donovani* and *T. gondii* create a parasitophorous vacuole that does not fuse with lysosomes. They can also inhibit the acidification of the vacuole or inhibit toxic proteases within the phagolysosome (Mauel 1996).

Once inside the cell, the parasites can suppress the triggering of the respiratory burst and the production of NO or activating cytokines such as IL-1β or IL-12 (Alexander et al. 1999; Bogdan and Rollinghoff 1999; Bogdan 2001). On the other hand, infected macrophages may be induced to overproduce cytokines such as IL-10 or TGF-β which dampen antimicrobial effector mechanisms exerted by IFN-γ-producing natural killer (NK) cells or T lymphocytes.

Activation of the adaptive immune system requires that the infected cells are ready for peptide processing, for antigen presentation via the class I or class II major histocompatibility complex (MHC) pathway and for expression of co-stimulatory molecules. All of these components are inhibited or deviated in parasitized cells depending on the intracellular lifestyle and the direction of the protein release into the different antigen presentation pathways (reviewed in Bogdan and Rollinghoff 1999). An alternate strategy is employed by parasites such as *T. cruzi* which release many different or related proteins of the *trans*-sialidase family into the class I MHC-processing pathway. Immunogenic peptide fragments from these proteins could lead to suboptimal adaptive immune responses either by competing with each other for MHC binding or by acting as inhibitory altered peptide ligands for each other (Vidal and Allen 1996; Plebanski and Hill 2000).

Intracellular life is not restricted to macrophages or erythrocytes but also includes cells found in muscular tissue (chronically infected with *T. cruzi*) or in the CNS (chronically infected with *T. gondii*). Very little is known about the reasons for this tissue propensity but it is tempting to speculate that factors such as anatomical barriers for immunological scanning, poor antigen-presentation capacity of the host cells, and an 'anti-inflammatory' environment all play a role.

HELMINTHS AND THE DISEASES THEY CAUSE IN HUMANS

Helminths are a major public health problem in economically disadvantaged populations and over 2 billion people are affected worldwide (Crompton 1999).There are three major groups of helminth parasites: trematodes, cestodes, and nematodes. Most helminths dwell in the lumen of the gut, and many live in accessory organs of the gastrointestinal tract. Others are adapted to a life within host tissues such as the blood or connective tissue.

Furthermore, helminths have complex life cycles including adult worms, as well as several larval stages that may penetrate the host skin, migrate through tissues, or have phases of arrested development. Except in very few cases, helminths do not replicate within their hosts, but produce offspring in the form of eggs or larvae. These have to reach a new host either by fecal–oral transmission of eggs, penetration of the skin by larvae, ingestion of larvae with contaminated meat of intermediate hosts, or by transmission through vector arthropods. In many species, adult helminths reach life spans of more than 10 years and thus establish long-lasting chronic infections. The worms are therefore exposed to very different environments in their hosts and have to cope with different local immune responses.

Trematodes

The human pathogenic trematodes can be grouped according to their localization: intestinal flukes (many species), liver flukes (*Opisthorchis*, *Clonorchis*, and *Fasciola* spp. as a potentially human pathogenic parasite), lung flukes (*Paragonimus* spp.), and blood flukes (*Schistosoma* spp.). The most important trematode helminths for human are *Schistosoma mansoni*, *S. japonicum*, and *S. haematobium*. Intermediate hosts are freshwater snails, which release cercariae that, by secreting a broad-spectrum elastase and other proteases, actively penetrate through the exposed skin of humans and migrate via the arterial system to the portal vein of the liver (*S. mansoni* and *S. japonicum*) or the blood vessels around the urinary bladder (*S. haematobium*). At these sites, the parasites mature and mate, and female worms produce hundreds of eggs every day. These traverse the wall of the gut or the bladder, and are released to the exterior, where they can infect the intermediate snail host. As the eggs are deposited in the vasculature, the bloodstream may also carry them into the liver or venous capillaries of the bladder, where they are trapped. Antigens released from eggs induce a vigorous Th2 response that orchestrates the formation of a granuloma, which separates them from the host tissue. The granulomatous lesions resolve after death of the encapsulated eggs, but they leave behind fibrotic scars with IL-13 being of central importance in the development of fibrosis. These pathological changes can give rise to portal hypertension or, in the bladder, they can significantly increase the risk of malignant cancer (Pearce and MacDonald 2002).

Cestodes

The most important cestodes (tapeworms) that infect humans are *Taenia saginata*, *T. solium*, and *Echinococcus* spp. The first two worms lodge in the human intestine in their adult stage and are transmitted through intermediate bovine (*T. saginata*) or porcine (*T. solium*) hosts, respectively. The adults produce eggs that, after release with human feces, are ingested by the intermediate hosts, where the larva (oncosphere) hatches and penetrates the intestinal barrier. It then migrates to muscles and other organs where the metacestode, often called a cysticercus, develops. Transmission to humans occurs by ingestion of undercooked meat; inside the gut; the metacestodes are activated and give rise to the adult tapeworms. If a person swallows eggs of *T. solium*, the larvae will hatch and go on to produce cysticerci in many tissues including the brain, eye, heart, and striated muscles.

The adults of *Echinococcus* spp. live in the intestine of canides such as foxes or dogs. The eggs are passed with the feces and have to infect an intermediate host. Eggs of *E. granulosus*, the dog tapeworm, usually infect ungulates such as sheep or cows, where the metacestode forms large liquid-filled cysts (hydatids), mostly in the liver. The eggs of the fox tapeworm *E. multilocularis* develop in small rodents, where the metacestodes proliferate in the liver in a tumor-like manner. After accidental ingestion of eggs by humans, metacestodes of both species may develop in the liver, lung, or brain, and cause severe disease.

Nematodes

Intestinal nematodes are the most prevalent human parasites on earth. Species such as *Ascaris lumbricoides*, the hookworms *Necator* and *Ancylostoma*, the whipworm *Trichuris*, and, to a lesser extent, parasites such as *Trichinella* and *Strongyloides* are found in more than half of the world's population. Infection mostly occurs through the fecal–oral route, with the exception of hookworms and *Strongyloides* spp. that actively penetrate the host's skin. Most nematodes live exclusively in the intestinal lumen and only have a subtle pathogenicity. However, in association with malnutrition and undernutrition they contribute significantly to poor health in many parts of the world, because malnutrition promotes the establishment, survival, and fecundity of these parasites (Koski and Scott 2001).

More severe pathological changes are caused by filarial nematodes that are transmitted by blood-feeding insects. The adult worms live within the lymphatics or in the skin, and produce thousands of first-stage larvae (microfilariae) per day. *Wuchereria bancrofti* and *Brugia malayi*, the causative agents of lymphatic filariasis, are transmitted by mosquitoes such as *Culex*, *Anopheles*, or *Aedes* spp. The filariae cause severe pathological changes through inflammatory obstruction of the lymphatics, which can lead to swellings of the affected limbs ('elephantiasis'). *Onchocerca volvulus* is transmitted by the bite of black flies (*Simulium* spp.). The adult nematodes live within subcutaneous nodules and inflammatory reactions induced by the skin-dwelling microfilariae lead to alterations of the skin and ocular damage ('river blindness'). Recent research has deciphered that intracellular bacterial endosymbionts (*Wolbachia* spp.) of *Onchocerca* may be a valuable target for antibiotic therapy of human filariasis with doxycycline. This therapy lead to a block in microfilarial embryogenesis and, possibly, to a significant reduction in filarial pathology (Hoerauf and Brattig 2002).

IMMUNITY AND PERSISTENCE IN INFECTIONS WITH HELMINTHIC PARASITES

Most helminthic parasites survive within most of their hosts for long periods, thereby causing chronic infection (and in some cases chronic disease) and long-term stimulation of the immune system. From an evolutionary point of view, chronicity of parasitic infections indicates success for both the parasite and the host, because both are able to survive with each other for long periods. Recent experimental and clinical evidence suggests that immune responses induced by chronic helminthic infections during early life via the anti-inflammatory activity of IL-10 may shape the development of the immune system toward a type of response that prevents immune dysfunctions such as allergy and chronic inflammatory diseases (van den Biggelaar et al. 2000; Bashir et al. 2002; Yazdanbakhsh et al. 2002). In this sense helminth infections were even discussed to have beneficial effects in some circumstances (Pritchard and Brown 2001).

One of the hallmarks of helminths is their longevity, with life spans of more than 10 years not being exceptional. This persistence implies that helminths are able to evade the immune effector mechanisms of their hosts, e.g. by skewing the cytokine network toward a predominance of Th2-like responses. Patients with helminthic infections show abundant circulating T cells with a Th2-like response to parasite antigen, with concurrent pronounced IgG4 and IgE antibodies and a high eosinophilia (Mahanty et al. 1992; Williams et al. 1994). T-cell proliferation in patients is severely downregulated, probably as a consequence of a selective anergy or suppression of the Th1-type cells (Allen and Maizels 1996). Even light infections might have such effects, because, for example, a single experimentally implanted *Brugia malayi* filaria is sufficient to inhibit the proliferation of T lymphocytes (Loke et al. 2000). This type of setting favors the survival of established worms, without preventing the host from defending itself against other pathogens.

The induced changes allow not only the tolerance of established worms, but at the same time also protective immune responses against newly intruding larvae of the same species. The main effector mechanism against the larvae is antibody-dependent cellular cytotoxicity (ADCC) with IgE as the most important antibody and eosinophils as effector cells. This 'concomitant immunity' can be considered as a mechanism for the regulation of parasite density (Cox 2001). Therefore, worm burdens in balanced host–parasite relationships are typically low and are usually tolerated without inducing severe pathological effects. Helminthic diseases are usually associated with high worm burdens and in most cases are a consequence of host immune reactions, rather than being the result of direct effects of the worms.

As a cautionary remark, our understanding of immune responses against helminths and their evasion mechanisms is largely based on studies from animal models that investigate the reactions against human pathogenic parasites. Not all of these data have been substantiated by studies in humans. Unfortunately, animal models for human disease are lacking in many cases and, therefore, one has to resort to the study of animal parasites in their natural hosts and draw indirect conclusions.

With regard to the trematodes, the most complete picture of immune reactions and evasion mechanisms comes from the schistosomes. The invasive stages of schistosomes (schistosomula) activate complement and are the target of ADCC reactions as well as of activated macrophages. Efficient killing of the IgE-opsonized schistosomula seems to be a predominant mechanism of protective immunity, whereas adult schistosomes are resistant to immune attack (Butterworth 1998; Pearce and MacDonald 2002).

Adult cestodes affect their hosts mainly as competitors for nutrients and cause little pathogenicity. As the worms dwell in the gut lumen and the only direct contact with the host is through the attachment of the scolex, immune reactions are of limited importance. Established metacestodes are not eliminated by host immune responses, but their growth is influenced by host responses, as shown by differences of parasite proliferation in various inbred strains of mice (Gottstein and Hemphill 1997). The metacestodes develop from larvae ('oncospheres') which are released from ingested tapeworm eggs. They cross the intestinal wall and migrate through blood vessels to their final location. These oncospheres are highly susceptible to lysis by complement-fixing antibodies, which leads to a limitation of superinfections (Lightowlers and Rickard 1988).

Gut-dwelling nematodes reach the intestines either directly or by migration of the larvae through various host tissues. On their way they can be killed by ADCC and inflammatory reactions, particularly in the lungs. The adult stages in the gut are mainly affected by IgE-sensitized mucosal mast cells. After antigen contact, they release mediators that lead to an immediate overproduction of mucus by goblet cells and to an increase in intestinal motility. In consequence, the worms are rapidly expelled (Ahmad et al. 1991). Protective intestinal immune responses against helminths are entirely dependent on Th2 responses and can be ablated by a reversion of the immune response towards a Th1 type (Else and Finkelman 1998; Finkelman et al. 1999). It is currently not clear whether and to what extent reactions of this type occur in humans.

In infections with filarial nematodes, the immune response and the resulting immunopathology depend on largely unknown factors. A minority of exposed persons is able to prevent infections with as yet unknown mechanisms ('putatively immunes'), whereas another subset of individuals is susceptible to infection. Patients who develop pronounced Th2 responses tolerate microfilariae, whereas others develop ADCC reactions and are able to clear the microfilariae.

Immune evasion mechanisms of helminths

Evolution has matched the host's immune armamentarium with a multitude of strategies by which helminths evade and subvert the immune responses (Maizels et al. 1993). As a result of their large genome (about 10^8 base-pairs) and relative long replication times, helminths cannot outpace the immune system by mechanisms involving mutations and gene rearrangements, such as the antigen variation of protozoan parasites. However, it is conceivable that they invest a similar proportion of genes into other types of immune evasion strategies. As ADCC and inflammatory reactions are the main immune effector mechanisms against helminths, their evasion mechanisms are tailored towards specifically coping with:

- complement activation
- the effect of antibodies
- the cytotoxic effect of phagocytes
- antigen presentation
- skewing of the cytokine network.

The strategies are of different complexity and can be grouped into passive approaches such as immune avoidance and blocking of effector mechanisms, and diversion strategies targeting the balance of the immune system by specifically acting on the cytokine network.

Avoidance strategies

Many immune effector mechanisms, similar to complement activation and ADCC, are directed against the surface of helminths. As has been shown for schistosomes, their surface is perfectly adapted to evade immune effector mechanisms. They are covered with a syncytial tegument that consists of an unusual double membrane complex with an apical plasma membrane and an overlying envelope (Hockley and McLaren 1973). The outer membrane is relatively fluid, ensuring a high lateral mobility of membrane lipids which favors repair after immune attack (Foley et al. 1986). The outer membrane of some stages can be replaced by shedding and incorporation of lipid compounds from tegumental storage vesicles (Kusel et al. 1975). Similar processes have also been observed for the infective larvae and adult worms of *Trichinella spiralis* (Philipp and Rumjaneck 1984) and other helminths (for a review, see Lightowlers and Rickard 1988).

Shortly after infection, the surface of schistosoma larvae is recognized by antiparasite antibodies and activates complement, although it gradually loses this antigenicity, acquiring a state of relative inertness. A part of this effect is ascribed to the incorporation of host molecules into the outer membrane of schistosomes, as a result of 'antigen disguise' (Terry and Smithers 1975). It was shown that schistosomes also incorporate membrane elements of the attacking neutrophils and other cells as well as lipids from host serum into their outer membrane (Pearce and Sher 1987). Indeed, MHC molecules, blood group glycolipids, fibronectin, and antibodies bound to the parasite surface by their Fc portion of host origin have all been detected. It was proposed that the outer schistosome membrane contains more host than parasite antigens (Saunders et al. 1987). This mechanism of antigen disguise seems to be employed also by other helminths, e.g. the surface of microfilariae of *W. bancrofti* contains host albumin as a major component (Maizels et al. 1984) and exposes blood group substances A and B (Ridley and Hedge 1977), whereas metacestodes of *E. granulosus* capture complement proteins from their host (Ferreira et al. 2000).

The fact that nematodes exhibit stage-specific patterns of surface antigens has also been interpreted in terms of immune evasion, e.g. the various larval stages of *Trichinella spiralis* have distinct sets of surface antigens (Philipp et al. 1980). It was suggested that antibodies induced by stage-specific surface antigens of an early larval stage do not recognize the surface of later stages. Each molt should thus provide an advantage, forcing the host to build up new and effective anti-surface antibodies. However, this concept was challenged by the finding that surface antigens crossreact between different stages and species of filariae, in spite of an apparent stage specificity as determined by molecular mass analysis (Maizels et al. 1983). Such shared antigenic determinants dominated the immune response, rendering the role of stage-specific antigens uncertain.

A further avoidance strategy consists of the production of a 'mucosal' glycocalix which serves as a surface coat to build a physical barrier between the worm surface and host effector mechanisms. Most probably, all helminths produce such mucous layers. Larvae of the nematode *Toxocara canis* produce a surface coat of about 10-nm thickness which surrounds the worm like a fuzzy envelope and is composed of mucins of different chain lengths that are secreted by the esophageal and secretory glands (Maizels et al. 2000). In vitro incubation of such larvae in immune sera leads to binding of antibodies that mediate the attachment of eosinophils. Subsequent shedding of the surface coat together with the bound eosinophils prevents intimate contact, and thus reduces the damage to the larvae (Badley et al. 1987). A similar shedding was also observed for juvenile stages of *Fasciola hepatica*. Larvae of this fluke are covered by a continuous layer of IgG after incubation in immune sera, and dispose of it by shedding and then replacing the glycocalix. This active process removes effector cells such as eosinophils and neutrophils and reduces the damaging effect of degranulation (Glauert et al. 1985).

Some helminths stimulate the host to produce layers of connective tissue, serving as a barrier that limits the access of immune cells, e.g. adult *Onchocerca volvulus* nematodes induce fibrous nodules in the skin (onchocercomas). Although the females are firmly embedded in these onchocercomas, the males probably move between nodules to inseminate the female worms (Schulz-Key and Karam 1986), and the microfilariae released by the female worms are also capable of leaving the nodule. The connective tissue of the nodule is infiltrated by neutrophils and eosinophils (Buttner et al. 1988). The influx of eosinophils seems to be triggered by the production of microfilariae by female worms (Wildenburg et al. 1996), whereas neutrophils are attracted by products of endobacteria living in symbiosis with the filarial nematodes (Brattig et al. 2001). In a comparable manner, the larval stages of some gut-dwelling nematodes induce the formation of tissues cysts, which may function to create a niche protected from immune effector mechanism. In infections with *Taenia solium* and *Echinococcus granulosus*, a connective tissue capsule with interspersed inflammatory cells surrounds the metacestodes, and the adults of *Paragonimus westermani* are located in cysts connected to the bronchial airways.

Blocking of complement and antibodies

Helminths can evade the consequences of complement-mediated damage through inhibition of complement action and through increased local consumption of complement factors. Moreover, they are able to inactivate antibodies and to induce the production of blocking antibodies.

Although antigens of many helminths activate the complement system, complement-dependent cytotoxicity is apparently restricted to the attrition of cestode oncospheres, which are destroyed by complement-fixing antibodies (Lightowlers and Gauci 2001). The activation of complement components by helminths without subsequent killing suggests the occurrence of mechanisms that inhibit the complement cascade. Indeed, a number of helminth complement inhibitors have been identified.

Young schistosomal larvae are highly susceptible to complement attack, but acquire resistance by several mechanisms within a few hours of penetrating their host. Shortly after infection, they express and probably secrete paracrystalline 'elongate bodies', which consist of the muscle protein paramyosin (Matsumoto et al. 1988). Through binding of C1q and inhibition of the binding of C4, paramyosin can prevent complement activation and thus protect the parasites (Laclette et al. 1992). In addition, a lipid-anchored 28-kDa protease on the surface of schistosome larvae can cleave C3 and C9 complement components and inhibit complement-mediated, neutrophil-dependent killing (Ghendler et al. 1996). Schistosomes also have a protease inhibitor with similarity to human CD59, which blocks the assembly of the membrane attack complex (Parizade et al. 1994).

Schistosomes and *Echinococcus granulosus* can use host-derived molecules for inactivating complement components. In the case of schistosomes, they incorporate the decay-accelerating factor (DAF) in their outer surface membrane or, in the latter case, 'factor H' in the wall of the cysts (Pearce et al. 1990; Ferreira et al. 2000). Both DAF and factor H inhibit the activation of the complement cascade downstream of the formation of the C3b–Bb complex.

Another way of knocking out disadvantageous complement effects is to 'stick' early complement factors to helminthic mucopolysaccharides. Such factors are found in the cystic bladder fluids of the tapeworm *Taenia taeniaeformis* (Hammerberg and Williams 1978).

Antibodies against surface proteins of helminths opsonize the parasites for recognition and effector activation by eosoinophils, neutrophils, and macrophages. Antibody degradation can therefore lead to the inhibition of these functions. Larvae of schistosomes and newly excysted juveniles of *Fasciola hepatica* secrete proteases that cleave IgG or IgE antibodies. As a consequence, the attachment of eosinophils to the worms is inhibited. The degradation products of the antibodies may serve for camouflage. Moreover, the peptides released during this process may downregulate macrophage activation (Auriault et al. 1981; Carmona et al. 1993; Pleass et al. 2000).

The skewing of immune responses after helminthic infections results in a shift of antibody classes and subclasses, which has profound effects on antibody-dependent effector mechanisms. Many helminths induce the production of high levels of IgG4 and IgE, parasite-specific IgG4 being present in much higher quantities compared with IgE, e.g. in filarial infections (Hussain and Ottesen 1986). The massive amounts of IgG4 are supposed to compete with IgE for epitopes, and may thus block otherwise occurring IgE-mediated cytotoxicity and allergic responses. In a similar way, IgG2 and IgM antibodies block anti-schistosomula granulocyte responses that depend on recognition of other isotypes for ADCC reactions. Furthermore, parasite-specific anti-helminth IgE antibodies occur together with unspecific IgE responses arising from the general elevation of IgE production. This effect would dilute parasite-specific IgEs on mast cells, and thus reduce allergic responses.

Inhibition of effector cell functions

Host effector cells are attracted to the site of infection by a variety of chemoattractants. To reach the parasites, the cells have to adhere to the vascular endothelial lining and to cross it by diapedesis. Helminths interfere with this process by various means. The hookworm *Necator americanus* secretes a protease which rapidly degrades the eosinophil-attracting chemokine eotaxin (Culley et al. 2000), and *Brugia malayi* microfilariae inhibit attraction of mononuclear cells and granulocytes by secretion of a serine protease inhibitor. In addition, this protease can inhibit granulocytic enzymes such as elastase and cathepsin G (Zang and Maizels 2001). The adhesion of granulocytes to vascular endothelial cells is inhibited by a glycoprotein from *Ancylostoma* and by eicosanoids from schistosomes (Nevhutalu et al. 1993; Moyle et al. 1994). Tissue-invading larvae of the lung fluke *Paragonimus westermani* inhibit eosinophils to degranulate and produce reactive oxygen species (ROS) through release of a cysteine protease (Shin et al. 2001) and mast cell degranulation is dampened by excretory/secretory (ES) products from adult *Schistosoma mansoni* worms (Mazingue et al. 1980).

Several species of intestinal nematodes secrete acetylcholinesterase, which can hydrolyze acetylcholine. In consequence, many proinflammatory functions of acetylcholine, such as release of granulocytic lysosomal enzymes, release of histamine, or other anaphylactogenic molecules by mast cells, are reduced and thereby may serve the 'well-being' of the nematodes (Lee 1996).

Defense against reactive oxygen species and detoxification

Activated macrophages, neutrophils, and eosinophils produce a variety of toxic products such as hydrogen peroxide, superoxide anion, and hydroxyl radicals, which are collectively termed ROS. ROS lead to protein oxidation, lipid peroxidation, depolymerization of polysaccharides, and DNA modifications, and thus has important antimicrobial functions. All aerobic organisms require mechanisms that protect cells against ROS produced during their own metabolism. Therefore, parasites have antioxidant enzymes such as superoxide dismutases, glutathione peroxidases, catalases, and peroxiredoxins, as components of their normal metabolism. Secretion of antioxidants by nematodes and their presence on or directly beneath the surface suggest, however, that helminths use antioxidants to block the products of the respiratory burst produced by immune cells (Henkle-Dührsen and Kampkotter 2001). Peroxiredoxins have been described from several filarial species and *Ascaris* spp., and it was shown that these proteins remove H_2O_2 and protect DNA from nicking by hydroxyl radicals in vitro. Glutathione peroxidases were identified as major soluble surface proteins of lymphatic filarial species and may function in the repair of oxidatively damaged membranes and the removal of H_2O_2 (Cookson et al. 1992). Catalases and superoxide dismutases have been described in a large number of nematodes and, although parasite-specific functions have been postulated, they have not yet been conclusively demonstrated (Henkle-Dührsen and Kampkotter 2001).

The glutathione *S*-transferases (GST) are a family of detoxification enzymes that catalyze the conjugation of reduced glutathione to xenobiotic and endogenous compounds. They are involved in the protection of tissues against oxidative damage by detoxification of lipid peroxidation products. Schistosomes have several isoforms of GSTs which are abundant in larval and adult worms. The enzymes are located in the subtegument, and at least transiently at or near the worm surface. Enzyme-blocking antibodies induced by experimental animal immunization with recombinant GSTs affect worm viability and fecundity after infection with *Schistosoma mansoni* or *S. japonicum* (Boulanger et al. 1991; Shuxian et al. 1997; Remoué et al. 2000). Studies in *Onchocerca volvulus* showed that this nematode also possesses and releases GSTs (Liebau et al. 1994) and immunization of cattle with GSTs from *Fasciola hepatica* induced protection against metacercarial infection (Morrison et al. 1996).

Inhibition of lymphocyte proliferation

Helminth infections often lead to diminished proliferation of antigen- or mitogen-stimulated lymphocytes. This reaction is the result of secreted products that can directly inhibit T or B cells, act indirectly through the induction of cytokine responses, or have combined activity.

Phosphorylcholine (PC) is a small component of phospholipids that occurs in a multitude of pathogens such as bacteria, trematodes, cestodes, and nematodes, but it is also present in the inner leaflet of vertebrate membranes. Nematodes are very rich in PC; part of the inhibitory activities of helminth culture supernatants is caused by this component. In-depth structural and functional studies on PC were performed with the rodent filaria *Acanthocheilonema viteae*. In vitro studies using the secreted PC-containing protein ES-62 revealed that the proliferation of activated B and T lymphocytes could be inhibited significantly (Harnett and Harnett 2001). The unresponsiveness of B lymphocytes is caused by PC-mediated uncoupling of the antigen receptor from intracellular proliferation signals such as the phosphoinositide-3-kinase and the Ras mitogen-activating protein kinase pathways (Deehan et al. 1998).

Another modulator of innate immune defenses found in many nematodes is the cysteine protease inhibitor cystatin. Recombinant cystatin from *Onchocerca volvulus* (onchocystatin) suppressed the proliferation of human T cells and the expression of MHC class II and CD86 molecules on monocytes. These findings are in line with studies on cystatins of *Brugia malayi* and of a rodent intestinal nematode that revealed an inhibition of class II MHC-restricted antigen processing (Dainichi et al. 2001; Manoury et al. 2001). At the same time, cystatin induced monocytes to produce enhanced levels of IL-10 and tumor necrosis factor α (TNF-α) and reduced amounts of IL-12 (Schonemeyer et al. 2001). These observations suggest that filarial cystatins shift the activities of macrophages toward an anti-inflammatory phenotype. In vivo studies in a rodent model confirmed the relevance of these observations, showing that application of filarial cystatin via osmotic pumps diminished the antigen-specific proliferation of spleen cells, whereas the antibody production was not suppressed (Pfaff et al. 2002). Not only are protease inhibitors found in nematodes; taenia cestodes secrete an inhibitor (taeniastatin) that is able to inhibit the production of IL-2 by T lymphocytes (Leid et al. 1986).

Immunomodulation by cytokine homologs

Helminths not only use molecules such as PC or protease inhibitors to alter the balance of the cytokine network, but also produce functional cytokine homologs that interact with the immune system. This information was initially gained by data mining of genome projects and represents a new aspect of the relationship between helminths and their hosts. For viruses, the strategy to produce mammalian cytokine or cytokine receptor homologs has long been known. The Epstein–Barr virus releases IL-10 homologs that account for a skewing of the cytokine balance towards Th2 responses (Liu et al. 1997) and the myxoma virus and other poxviruses encode for soluble IFN-γ receptors that bind and inactivate host IFN-γ (Upton et al. 1992; Alcami and Smith 1995).

To date there are two examples of helminth-produced cytokine-like molecules, but more of these proteins are likely to be discovered. A comparison of expressed sequence tags revealed that *Brugia malayi* has two genes with homology to macrophage migration inhibitory factor (MIF) (Pastrana et al. 1998). The gene of *B. malayi* MIF has an identity of 40–42 percent with vertebrate MIFs, and genomic homologs have been identified in *Onchocerca volvulus*, *Wuchereria bancrofti*, and also the free-living nematode *Caenorhabditis elegans*. In mammals this cytokine, secreted by T cells, macrophages, and eosinophils, induces macrophage kinesis and is associated with proinflammatory activities. Functionally, recombinant *B. malayi* MIF led to an upregulation of mediator production of macrophages with an ensuing marked eosinophil recruitment (Falcone et al. 2001). Thus, filarial MIF reveals an important link between macrophages and eosinophils during helminth infections. The MIF gene of *B. malayi* is transcribed in microfilariae and adult worms and is secreted in the vicinity of the worms, but it is also present in the hypodermis of adult worms and in the reproductive organs of females. Possibly, the continuous secretion of MIF induces a counterinflammatory phenotype of macrophages and contributes to the generation of 'alternately activated macrophages' that exert counterinflammatory activities (Loke et al. 2000).

In addition to MIF *B. malayi*, microfilariae and adult worms have genes to produce and secrete TGF-β-like proteins that bind to mammalian TGF-β receptors (Maizels et al. 2001). As TGF-β is involved in many downregulatory mechanisms, it is conceivable that this protein has a role in reducing inflammatory host responses.

OUTLOOK

In many areas of the world, individuals experience one or more parasitic infections. Despite considerable progress in controlling parasitic diseases, the threat to human health is increasing. Drug-resistant malaria has re-emerged as one of the most prevalent and dangerous diseases. Sleeping sickness is again epidemic in several countries in central and north-eastern Africa. Schistosomiasis cases do not decline despite available drug therapy.

Pathogens such as cryptosporidia or cyclospora are recognized increasingly as risk factors in food or water.

Understanding of the multiple effects of parasitic infections on the immune system is of increasing interest. Today there is no licensed vaccine for any human parasitic infection. This reflects the complexity of defining and directing of the correct protective immune response. Recent full-sequencing of the *P. falciparum* and *P. yoelii* genome, as well as ongoing efforts to sequence the genomes of *Trypanosoma brucei*, *T. cruzi*, *Toxoplasma gondii*, *Trichomonas vaginalis*, *Entamoeba histolytica*, *Schistosoma mansoni*, or *Brugia malayi*, provide the library from which vaccine candidates will be selected and creates considerable expectations for successful new vaccines. New technologies such as DNA immunization, expression library immunization, prime-boost regimens, or recombinant viruses will aid in the development and delivery of new vaccines. DNA-micro-array technology will help to identify genes that are expressed at particular stages of the infectious process, at the site of both the parasite and the host. In vivo assays to induce or block the organ-specific expression of proteins will help to predict their contribution to immune control. In this context, it will be of prime importance to consider the immune escape mechanisms of protozoan and helminth parasites. Furthermore, parasites are a source of molecules with immunomodulatory activity, because evolution forged these parasites to become specialists in immunomodulation. Knowledge of the mechanisms of parasite immune evasion will thus add to our understanding of immune regulation in general and might at the same time provide concepts and molecules for the management of undesired immune responses.

ACKNOWLEDGMENTS

The authors would like to thank the numerous colleagues who contributed with their ideas and comments, especially Sonja Lotz, Inga Wilde, and Sebastian Schrader for critical reading of the mansuscript. Own work cited was funded by the Deutsche Forschungsgemeinschaft (SFB 367 (B10), GRK 288, So 220/5–3, SPP 1089, Lu 325/8–1, SFB 618 (C2)) Lehrstuhl für Molekulare Parasitologie, Humboldt-Universität zu Berlin, Berlin, Germany.

REFERENCES

Aga, E., Katschinski, D.M., et al. 2002. Inhibition of the spontaneous apoptosis of neutrophil granulocytes by the intracellular parasite *Leishmania major*. *J Immunol*, **169**, 898–905.

Ahmad, A., Wang, C.H. and Bell, R.G. 1991. A role for IgE in intestinal immunity. Expression of rapid expulsion of *Trichinella spiralis* in rats transfused with IgE and thoracic duct lymphocytes. *J Immunol*, **146**, 3563–70.

Alcami, A. and Smith, G.L. 1995. Vaccinia, cowpox, and camelpox viruses encode soluble gamma interferon receptors with novel broad species specificity. *J Virol*, **69**, 4633–9.

Alexander, J., Satoskar, A.R. and Russell, D.G. 1999. Leishmania species: models of intracellular parasitism. *J Cell Sci*, **112**, Pt 18, 2993–3002.

Allen, J.E. and Maizels, R.M. 1996. Immunology of human helminth infection. *Int Arch Allergy Immunol*, **109**, 3–10.

Andrews, N.W. 2002. Lysosomes and the plasma membrane: trypanosomes reveal a secret relationship. *J Cell Biol*, **158**, 389–94.

Auriault, C., Ouaissi, M.A., et al. 1981. Proteolytic cleavage of IgG bound to the Fc receptor of *Schistosoma mansoni schistosomula*. *Parasite Immunol*, **3**, 33–44.

Badley, J.E., Grieve, R.B., et al. 1987. Immune-mediated adherence of eosinophils to *Toxocara canis* infective larvae: the role of excretory-secretory antigens. *Parasite Immunol*, **9**, 133–43.

Bashir, M.E., Andersen, P., et al. 2002. An enteric helminth infection protects against an allergic response to dietary antigen. *J Immunol*, **169**, 3284–92.

Beeson, J.G. and Brown, G.V. 2002. Pathogenesis of *Plasmodium falciparum* malaria: the roles of parasite adhesion and antigenic variation. *Cell Mol Life Sci*, **59**, 258–71.

Belkaid, Y., Hoffmann, K.F., et al. 2001. The role of interleukin (IL)-10 in the persistence of *Leishmania major* in the skin after healing and the therapeutic potential of anti-IL-10 receptor antibody for sterile cure. *J Exp Med*, **194**, 1497–506.

Belkaid, Y., von Stebut, E., et al. 2002. CD8+ T cells are required for primary immunity in C57BL/6 mice following low-dose, intradermal challenge with *Leishmania major*. *J Immunol*, **168**, 3992–4000.

Berriman, M., Hall, N., et al. 2002. The architecture of variant surface glycoprotein gene expression sites in *Trypanosoma brucei*. *Mol Biochem Parasitol*, **122**, 131–40.

Bogdan, C. 2001. Nitric oxide and the immune response. *Nat Immunol*, **2**, 907–16.

Bogdan, C. and Rollinghoff, M. 1999. How do protozoan parasites survive inside macrophages? *Parasitol Today*, **15**, 22–8.

Boulanger, D., Reid, G.D., et al. 1991. Immunization of mice and baboons with the recombinant Sm28GST affects both worm viability and fecundity after experimental infection with *Schistosoma mansoni*. *Parasite Immunol*, **13**, 473–90.

Brattig, N.W., Buttner, D.W. and Hoerauf, A. 2001. Neutrophil accumulation around *Onchocerca* worms and chemotaxis of neutrophils are dependent on *Wolbachia* endobacteria. *Microbes Infect*, **3**, 439–46.

Brecht, S., Carruthers, V.B., et al. 2001. The toxoplasma micronemal protein MIC4 is an adhesin composed of six conserved apple domains. *J Biol Chem*, **276**, 4119–27.

Burleigh, B.A. 2000. Lysosome exocytosis and invasion of non-phagocytic host cells by *Trypanosoma cruzi*. In: Tschudi, C. and Pearce, E.J. (eds), *Biology of Parasitism*. Boston, MA: Kluwer Academic, 195–212.

Butterworth, A.E. 1998. Immunological aspects of human schistosomiasis. *Br Med Bull*, **54**, 357–68.

Buttner, D.W., Albiez, E.J., et al. 1988. Histological examination of adult *Onchocerca volvulus* and comparison with the collagenase technique. *Trop Med Parasitol*, **39**, Suppl 4, 390–417.

Carmona, C., Dowd, A.J., et al. 1993. Cathepsin L proteinase secreted by *Fasciola hepatica* in vitro prevents antibody-mediated eosinophil attachment to newly excysted juveniles. *Mol Biochem Parasitol*, **62**, 9–17.

Carruthers, V.B., Hakansson, S., et al. 2000. *Toxoplasma gondii* uses sulfated proteoglycans for substrate and host cell attachment. *Infect Immun*, **68**, 4005–11.

Chen, X.M., Keithly, J.S., et al. 2002. Cryptosporidiosis. *N Engl J Med*, **346**, 1723–31.

Cookson, E., Blaxter, M.L. and Selkirk, M.E. 1992. Identification of the major soluble cuticular glycoprotein of lymphatic filarial nematode parasites (gp29) as a secretory homolog of glutathione peroxidase. *Proc Natl Acad Sci USA*, **89**, 5837–41.

Cox, F.E. 2001. Concomitant infections, parasites and immune responses. *Parasitology*, **122**, Suppl, S23–38.

Crompton, D.W. 1999. How much human helminthiasis is there in the world? *J Parasitol*, **85**, 397–403.

Culley, F.J., Brown, A., et al. 2000. Eotaxin is specifically cleaved by hookworm metalloproteases preventing its action in vitro and in vivo. *J Immunol*, **165**, 6447–53.

Dainichi, T., Maekawa, Y., et al. 2001. Nippocystatin, a cysteine protease inhibitor from *Nippostrongylus brasiliensis*, inhibits antigen processing and modulates antigen-specific immune response. *Infect Immun*, **69**, 7380–6.

Deehan, M.R., Frame, M.J., et al. 1998. A phosphorylcholine-containing filarial nematode-secreted product disrupts B lymphocyte activation by targeting key proliferative signaling pathways. *J Immunol*, **160**, 2692–9.

Dondorp, A.M., Kager, P.A., et al. 2000. Abnormal blood flow and red blood cell deformability in severe malaria. *Parasitol Today*, **16**, 228–32.

Donelson, J.E., Hill, K.L. and El Sayed, N.M. 1998. Multiple mechanisms of immune evasion by African trypanosomes. *Mol Biochem Parasitol*, **91**, 51–66.

Dubey, J.P., Miller, N.L. and Frenkel, J.K. 1970. The *Toxoplasma gondii* oocyst from cat feces. *J Exp Med*, **132**, 636–62.

Else, K.J. and Finkelman, F.D. 1998. Intestinal nematode parasites, cytokines and effector mechanisms. *Int J Parasitol*, **28**, 1145–58.

Falcone, F.H., Loke, P., et al. 2001. A *Brugia malayi* homolog of macrophage migration inhibitory factor reveals an important link between macrophages and eosinophil recruitment during nematode infection. *J Immunol*, **167**, 5348–54.

Ferreira, A.M., Irigoin, F., et al. 2000. How *Echinococcus granulosus* deals with complement. *Parasitol Today*, **16**, 168–72.

Finkelman, F.D., Wynn, T.A., et al. 1999. The role of IL-13 in helminth-induced inflammation and protective immunity against nematode infections. *Curr Opin Immunol*, **11**, 420–6.

Foley, M., MacGregor, A.N., et al. 1986. The lateral diffusion of lipid probes in the surface membrane of *Schistosoma mansoni*. *J Cell Biol*, **103**, 807–18.

Freire-de-Lima, C.G., Nascimento, D.O., et al. 2000. Uptake of apoptotic cells drives the growth of a pathogenic trypanosome in macrophages. *Nature*, **403**, 199–203.

Freitas Balanco, J.M., Moreira, M.E., et al. 2001. Apoptotic mimicry by an obligate intracellular parasite downregulates macrophage microbicidal activity. *Curr Biol*, **11**, 1870–3.

Frevert, U. 1994. Malaria sporozoite–hepatocyte interactions. *Exp Parasitol*, **79**, 206–10.

Gagnon, E., Duclos, S., et al. 2002. Endoplasmic reticulum-mediated phagocytosis is a mechanism of entry into macrophages. *Cell*, **110**, 119–31.

Gardner, M.J., Hall, N., et al. 2002. Genome sequence of the human malaria parasite *Plasmodium falciparum*. *Nature*, **419**, 498–511.

Ghendler, Y., Parizade, M., et al. 1996. *Schistosoma mansoni*: evidence for a 28-kDa membrane-anchored protease on schistosomula. *Exp Parasitol*, **83**, 73–82.

Glauert, A.M., Lammas, D.A. and Duffus, W.P. 1985. Ultrastructural observations on the interaction in vitro between bovine eosinophils and juvenile *Fasciola hepatica*. *Parasitology*, **91**, Pt 3, 459–70.

Good, M.F. and Doolan, D.L. 1999. Immune effector mechanisms in malaria. *Curr Opin Immunol*, **11**, 412–19.

Gottstein, B. and Hemphill, A. 1997. Immunopathology of echinococcosis. *Chem Immunol*, **66**, 177–208.

Hammerberg, B. and Williams, J.F. 1978. Interaction between *Taenia taeniaeformis* and the complement system. *J Immunol*, **120**, 1033–8.

Harnett, M.M. and Harnett, W. 2001. Antigen receptor signaling is subverted by an immunomodulatory product secreted by a filarial nematode. *Arch Immunol Ther Exp (Warsz)*, **49**, 263–9.

Henkle-Dührsen, K. and Kampkotter, A. 2001. Antioxidant enzyme families in parasitic nematodes. *Mol Biochem Parasitol*, **114**, 129–42.

Hockley, D.J. and McLaren, D.J. 1973. *Schistosoma mansoni*: changes in the outer membrane of the tegument during development from cercaria to adult worm. *Int J Parasitol*, **3**, 13–25.

Hoerauf, A. and Brattig, N. 2002. Resistance and susceptibility in human onchocerciasis – beyond Th1 vs. Th2. *Trends Parasitol*, **18**, 25–31.

Holt, R.A., Subramanian, G.M., et al. 2002. The genome sequence of the malaria mosquito *Anopheles gambiae*. *Science*, **298**, 129–49.

Hussain, R. and Ottesen, E.A. 1986. IgE responses in human filariasis. IV. Parallel antigen recognition by IgE and IgG4 subclass antibodies. *J Immunol*, **136**, 1859–63.

Huston, C.D., Houpt, E.R., et al. 2000. Caspase 3-dependent killing of host cells by the parasite *Entamoeba histolytica*. *Cell Microbiol*, **2**, 617–25.

Joshi, P.B., Kelly, B.L., et al. 2002. Targeted gene deletion in *Leishmania major* identifies leishmanolysin (GP63) as a virulence factor. *Mol Biochem Parasitol*, **120**, 33–40.

Koski, K.G. and Scott, M.E. 2001. Gastrointestinal nematodes, nutrition and immunity: breaking the negative spiral. *Annu Rev Nutr*, **21**, 297–321.

Krych-Goldberg, M., Moulds, J.M. and Atkinson, J.P. 2002. Human complement receptor type 1 (CR1) binds to a major malarial adhesin. *Trends Mol Med*, **8**, 531–7.

Kusel, J.R., Mackenzie, P.E. and McLaren, D.J. 1975. The release of membrane antigens into culture by adult *Schistosoma mansoni*. *Parasitology*, **71**, 247–59.

Kyes, S., Horrocks, P. and Newbold, C. 2001. Antigenic variation at the infected red cell surface in malaria. *Annu Rev Microbiol*, **55**, 673–707.

Laclette, J.P., Shoemaker, C.B., et al. 1992. Paramyosin inhibits complement C1. *J Immunol*, **148**, 124–8.

Lee, D.L. 1996. Why do some nematode parasites of the alimentary tract secrete acetylcholinesterase? *Int J Parasitol*, **26**, 499–508.

Leid, R.W., Suquet, C.M., et al. 1986. Interleukin inhibition by a parasite proteinase inhibitor, taeniaestatin. *J Immunol*, **137**, 2700–2.

Leippe, M., Andra, J., et al. 1994. Amoebapores, a family of membranolytic peptides from cytoplasmic granules of *Entamoeba histolytica*: isolation, primary structure, and pore formation in bacterial cytoplasmic membranes. *Mol Microbiol*, **14**, 895–904.

Liebau, E., Wildenburg, G., et al. 1994. A novel type of glutathione S-transferase in *Onchocerca volvulus*. *Infect Immun*, **62**, 4762–7.

Lightowlers, M.W. and Gauci, C.G. 2001. Vaccines against cysticercosis and hydatidosis. *Vet Parasitol*, **101**, 337–52.

Lightowlers, M.W. and Rickard, M.D. 1988. Excretory-secretory products of helminth parasites: effects on host immune responses. *Parasitology*, **96**, Suppl, S123–66.

Liu, Y., de Waal Malefyt, R., et al. 1997. The EBV IL-10 homologue is a selective agonist with impaired binding to the IL-10 receptor. *J Immunol*, **158**, 604–13.

Loke, P., MacDonald, A.S., et al. 2000. Alternatively activated macrophages induced by nematode infection inhibit proliferation via cell-to-cell contact. *Eur J Immunol*, **30**, 2669–78.

Luder, C.G., Gross, U. and Lopes, M.F. 2001. Intracellular protozoan parasites and apoptosis: diverse strategies to modulate parasite–host interactions. *Trends Parasitol*, **17**, 480–6.

Mac Kenzie, W.R., Hoxie, N.J., et al. 1994. A massive outbreak in Milwaukee of cryptosporidium infection transmitted through the public water supply. *N Engl J Med*, **331**, 161–7.

MacDonald, A.S., Araujo, M.I. and Pearce, E.J. 2002. Immunology of parasitic helminth infections. *Infect Immun*, **70**, 427–33.

Mahanty, S., Abrams, J.S., et al. 1992. Parallel regulation of IL-4 and IL-5 in human helminth infections. *J Immunol*, **148**, 3567–71.

Maizels, R.M., Partono, F., et al. 1983. Cross-reactive surface antigens on three stages of *Brugia malayi*, *B. pahangi* and *B. timori*. *Parasitology*, **87**, Pt 2, 249–63.

Maizels, R.M., Philipp, M., et al. 1984. Human serum albumin is a major component on the surface of microfilariae of *Wuchereria bancrofti*. *Parasite Immunol*, **6**, 185–90.

Maizels, R.M., Bundy, D.A., et al. 1993. Immunological modulation and evasion by helminth parasites in human populations. *Nature*, **365**, 797–805.

Maizels, R.M., Tetteh, K.K. and Loukas, A. 2000. *Toxocara canis*: genes expressed by the arrested infective larval stage of a parasitic nematode. *Int J Parasitol*, **30**, 495–508.

Maizels, R.M., Gomez-Escobar, N., et al. 2001. Immune evasion genes from filarial nematodes. *Int J Parasitol*, **31**, 889–98.

Manoury, B., Gregory, W.F., et al. 2001. Bm-CPI-2, a cystatin homolog secreted by the filarial parasite *Brugia malayi*, inhibits class II MHC-restricted antigen processing. *Curr Biol*, **11**, 447–51.

Matsumoto, Y., Perry, G., et al. 1988. Paramyosin and actin in schistosomal teguments. *Nature*, **333**, 76–8.

Mauel, J. 1996. Intracellular survival of protozoan parasites with special reference to *Leishmania* spp., *Toxoplasma gondii* and *Trypanosoma cruzi*. *Adv Parasitol*, **38**, 1–51.

May, R.C. and Machesky, L.M. 2001. Phagocytosis and the actin cytoskeleton. *J Cell Sci*, **114**, 1061–77.

Mazingue, C., Camus, D., et al. 1980. In vitro and in vivo inhibition of mast cell degranulation by a factor from *Schistosoma mansoni*. *Int Arch Allergy Appl Immunol*, **63**, 178–89.

Meisel, J.L., Perera, D.R., et al. 1976. Overwhelming watery diarrhea associated with a cryptosporidium in an immunosuppressed patient. *Gastroenterology*, **70**, 1156–60.

Miller-Sims, V. and Petri, W. 2002. Opportunities and obstacles in developing a vaccine for *Entamoeba histolytica*. *Curr Opin Immunol*, **14**, 549.

Mordue, D.G., Desai, N., et al. 1999a. Invasion by *Toxoplasma gondii* establishes a moving junction that selectively excludes host cell plasma membrane proteins on the basis of their membrane anchoring. *J Exp Med*, **190**, 1783–92.

Mordue, D.G., Hakansson, S., et al. 1999b. *Toxoplasma gondii* resides in a vacuole that avoids fusion with host cell endocytic and exocytic vesicular trafficking pathways. *Exp Parasitol*, **92**, 87–99.

Morrison, C.A., Colin, T., et al. 1996. Protection of cattle against Fasciola hepatica infection by vaccination with glutathione S-transferase. *Vaccine*, **14**, 1603–12.

Moyle, M., Foster, D.L., et al. 1994. A hookworm glycoprotein that inhibits neutrophil function is a ligand of the integrin CD11b/CD18. *J Biol Chem*, **269**, 10008–15.

Muller, H.M., Reckmann, I., et al. 1993. Thrombospondin related anonymous protein (TRAP) of *Plasmodium falciparum* binds specifically to sulfated glycoconjugates and to HepG2 hepatoma cells suggesting a role for this molecule in sporozoite invasion of hepatocytes. *EMBO J*, **12**, 2881–9.

Muller, N. and Gottstein, B. 1998. Antigenic variation and the murine immune response to *Giardia lamblia*. *Int J Parasitol*, **28**, 1829–39.

Nevhutalu, P.A., Salafsky, B., et al. 1993. *Schistosoma mansoni* and *Trichobilharzia ocellata*: comparison of secreted cercarial eicosanoids. *J Parasitol*, **79**, 130–3.

Nime, F.A., Burek, J.D., et al. 1976. Acute enterocolitis in a human being infected with the protozoan *Cryptosporidium*. *Gastroenterology*, **70**, 592–8.

Orlandi, P.A., Klotz, F.W. and Haynes, J.D. 1992. A malaria invasion receptor, the 175-kilodalton erythrocyte binding antigen of *Plasmodium falciparum* recognizes the terminal Neu5Ac(alpha 2-3)Gal- sequences of glycophorin A. *J Cell Biol*, **116**, 901–9.

Ouaissi, A., Guilvard, E., et al. 2002. The *Trypanosoma cruzi* Tc52-released protein induces human dendritic cell maturation, signals via Toll-like receptor 2, and confers protection against lethal infection. *J Immunol*, **168**, 6366–74.

Parizade, M., Arnon, R., et al. 1994. Functional and antigenic similarities between a 94-kD protein of *Schistosoma mansoni* (SCIP-1) and human CD59. *J Exp Med*, **179**, 1625–36.

Pastrana, D.V., Raghavan, N., et al. 1998. Filarial nematode parasites secrete a homologue of the human cytokine macrophage migration inhibitory factor. *Infect Immun*, **66**, 5955–63.

Pearce, E.J. and MacDonald, A.S. 2002. The immunobiology of schistosomiasis. *Nat Rev Immunol*, **2**, 499–511.

Pearce, E.J. and Sher, A. 1987. Mechanisms of immune evasion in schistosomiasis. *Contrib Microbiol Immunol*, **8**, 219–32.

Pearce, E.J., Hall, B.F. and Sher, A. 1990. Host-specific evasion of the alternative complement pathway by schistosomes correlates with the presence of a phospholipase C-sensitive surface molecule resembling human decay accelerating factor. *J Immunol*, **144**, 2751–6.

Perkins, M.E. and Rocco, L.J. 1988. Sialic-acid dependent binding of *Plasmodium falciparum* merozoite surface antigen, Pf200, to human erythrocytes. *J Immunol*, **141**, 3190–6.

Petri, W.A. Jr., Haque, R. and Mann, B.J. 2002. The bittersweet interface of parasite and host: lectin-carbohydrate interactions during human invasion by the parasite *Entamoeba histolytica*. *Annu Rev Microbiol*, **56**, 39–64.

Pfaff, A.W., Schulz-Key, H., et al. 2002. *Litomosoides sigmodontis* cystatin acts as an immunomodulator during experimental filariasis. *Int J Parasitol*, **32**, 171–8.

Philipp, M., Parkhouse, R.M. and Ogilvie, B.M. 1980. Changing proteins on the surface of a parasitic nematode. *Nature*, **287**, 538–40.

Philipp, M. and Rumjaneck, F.D. 1984. Antigenic and dynamic properties of helminth surface structures. *Mol Biochem Parasitol*, **10**, 245–68.

Pleass, R.J., Kusel, J.R. and Woof, J.M. 2000. Cleavage of human IgE mediated by *Schistosoma mansoni*. *Int Arch Allergy Immunol*, **121**, 194–204.

Plebanski, M. and Hill, A.V. 2000. The immunology of malaria infection. *Curr Opin Immunol*, **12**, 437–41.

Pritchard, D.I. and Brown, A. 2001. Is *Necator americanus* approaching a mutualistic symbiotic relationship with humans? *Trends Parasitol*, **17**, 169–72.

Ramasamy, R. 1998. Molecular basis for evasion of host immunity and pathogenesis in malaria. *Biochim Biophys Acta*, **1406**, 10–27.

Remoué, M.F., Rogerie, F., et al. 2000. Sex-dependent neutralizing humoral response to *Schistosoma mansoni* 28GST antigen in infected human populations. *J Infect Dis*, **181**, 1855–9.

Ridley, D.S. and Hedge, E.C. 1977. Immunofluorescent reactions with microfilariae. 2. Bearing on host–parasite relations. *Trans R Soc Trop Med Hyg*, **71**, 522–5.

Sacks, D. and Kamhawi, S. 2001. Molecular aspects of parasite-vector and vector–host interactions in leishmaniasis. *Annu Rev Microbiol*, **55**, 453–83.

Sacks, D.L. 2001. *Leishmania*–sand fly interactions controlling species-specific vector competence. *Cell Microbiol*, **3**, 189–96.

Saunders, N., Wilson, R.A. and Coulson, P.S. 1987. The outer bilayer of the adult schistosome tegument surface has a low turnover rate in vitro and in vivo. *Mol Biochem Parasitol*, **25**, 123–31.

Scanga, C.A., Aliberti, J., et al. 2002. Cutting edge: MyD88 is required for resistance to Toxoplasma gondii infection and regulates parasite-induced IL-12 production by dendritic cells. *J Immunol*, **168**, 5997–6001.

Schilling, S. and Glaichenhaus, N. 2001. T cells that react to the immunodominant *Leishmania major* LACK antigen prevent early dissemination of the parasite in susceptible BALB/c mice. *Infect Immun*, **69**, 1212–14.

Schonemeyer, A., Lucius, R., et al. 2001. Modulation of human T cell responses and macrophage functions by onchocystatin, a secreted protein of the filarial nematode *Onchocerca volvulus*. *J Immunol*, **167**, 3207–15.

Schulz-Key, H. and Karam, M. 1986. Periodic reproduction of *Onchocerca volvulus*. *Parasitol Today*, **2**, 284–6.

Shin, M.H., Kita, H., et al. 2001. Cysteine protease secreted by *Paragonimus westermani* attenuates effector functions of human eosinophils stimulated with immunoglobulin G. *Infect Immun*, **69**, 1599–604.

Shuxian, L., Yongkang, H., et al. 1997. Anti-fecundity immunity to *Schistosoma japonicum* induced in Chinese water buffaloes (*Bos buffelus*) after vaccination with recombinant 26 kDa glutathione-S-transferase (reSjc26GST). *Vet Parasitol*, **69**, 39–47.

Sibley, L.D., Hakansson, S. and Carruthers, V.B. 1998. Gliding motility: an efficient mechanism for cell penetration. *Curr Biol*, **8**, R12–14.

Smith, B.O., Mallin, R.L., et al. 2002. Structure of the C3b binding site of CR1 (CD35), the immune adherence receptor. *Cell*, **108**, 769–80.

Solbach, W. and Laskay, T. 2000. The host response to *Leishmania* infection. *Adv Immunol*, **74**, 275–317.

Tarleton, R.L. 2001. Parasite persistence in the aetiology of Chagas disease. *Int J Parasitol*, **31**, 550–4.

Terry, R.J. and Smithers, S.R. 1975. Evasion of the immune response by parasites. *Symp Soc Exp Biol*, **29**, 453–65.

Turner, C.M. 1997. The rate of antigenic variation in fly-transmitted and syringe-passaged infections of *Trypanosoma brucei*. *FEMS Microbiol Lett*, **153**, 227–31.

Upton, C., Mossman, K. and McFadden, G. 1992. Encoding of a homolog of the IFN-gamma receptor by myxoma virus. *Science*, **258**, 1369–72.

van den Biggelaar, A.H., van Ree, R., et al. 2000. Decreased atopy in children infected with *Schistosoma haematobium*: a role for parasite-induced interleukin-10. *Lancet*, **356**, 1723–7.

Van Der Kleij, D., Latz, E., et al. 2002. A novel host-parasite lipid cross talk: schistosomal lyso-phosphatidylserine activates toll-like receptor-2 and affects immune polarization. *J Biol Chem*, **277**, 50, 48122–9.

Van Zandbergen, G., Hermann, N., et al. 2002. *Leishmania* promastigotes release a granulocyte chemotactic factor and induce interleukin-8 release but inhibit gamma interferon-inducible protein 10 production by neutrophil granulocytes. *Infect Immun*, **70**, 4177–84.

Vidal, K. and Allen, P.M. 1996. The effect of endogenous altered peptide ligands on peripheral T-cell responses. *Semin Immunol*, **8**, 117–22.

Wildenburg, G., Kromer, M. and Buttner, D.W. 1996. Dependence of eosinophil granulocyte infiltration into nodules on the presence of microfilariae producing *Onchocerca volvulus*. *Parasitol Res*, **82**, 117–24.

Williams, M.E., Montenegro, S., et al. 1994. Leukocytes of patients with *Schistosoma mansoni* respond with a Th2 pattern of cytokine production to mitogen or egg antigens but with a Th0 pattern to worm antigens. *J Infect Dis*, **170**, 946–54.

Yap, G.S. and Sher, A. 1999. Cell-mediated immunity to *Toxoplasma gondii*: initiation, regulation and effector function. *Immunobiology*, **201**, 240–7.

Yazdanbakhsh, M., Kremsner, P.G. and van Ree, R. 2002. Allergy, parasites, and the hygiene hypothesis. *Science*, **296**, 490–4.

Zang, X. and Maizels, R.M. 2001. Serine proteinase inhibitors from nematodes and the arms race between host and pathogen. *Trends Biochem Sci*, **26**, 191–7.

Zer, R., Yaroslavski, I., et al. 2001. Effect of sand fly saliva on *Leishmania* uptake by murine macrophages. *Int J Parasitol*, **31**, 810–14.

PART VI

IMMUNOPATHOLOGY AND IMMUNODEFICIENCY

34

Shock/sepsis

DANIELA N. MÄNNEL

INTRODUCTION

Despite considerable advances in treating the primary causes of sepsis and shock, high rates of morbidity and mortality still remain associated with these conditions. The eradication of the septic focus, killing of invading microorganisms, and the support of blood circulation should allow a full recovery of the body's homeostasis. Unfortunately, this is not always achieved. Microorganisms and their products activate systemic host defense systems, which comprise both humoral (complement and coagulation cascade) and cellular components (monocyte/macrophage, neutrophils, and endothelial cells). Activated cells, in turn, release a vast array of mediators (cytokines, such as tumor necrosis factor (TNF) and interleukin 1 (IL-1), arachidonic acid metabolites, and nitric oxide) that amplify the inflammatory response. Circulatory failure, leading to inadequate oxygen supply to tissues, and direct cytotoxic effects of various mediators released in the course of the generalized inflammatory process may result. As a result of the extremely complex biochemical events that are involved in the pathophysiology of shock after severe sepsis, endogenous factors may contribute to prolongation and aggravation of the exogenous insult leading to a life-threatening autodestructive and selfsustaining perpetuation of inflammation.

DEFINITIONS

Many bacterial and nonbacterial factors may cause inflammation. Sepsis describes a systemic inflammatory response to a documented infection (Balk 2000). The local inflammatory process can cause an exaggerated systemic response, with inflammatory damage to otherwise healthy cells and organs distant to the primary site of the insult. For patients with such a deleterious systemic response without any detectable bacterial focus, the term systemic inflammatory response syndrome (SIRS) is used (Bone et al. 1992). Severe sepsis is sepsis associated with organ dysfunction, hypoperfusion, and hypotension. Multiple organ failure (MOF) has been defined as sequential failure of two or more organ systems in patients with clinical signs of sepsis (Baue 1975). Patients with severe sepsis and sepsis-induced hypotension despite adequate fluid resuscitation, along with the presence of perfusion abnormalities such as lactic acidosis, oligurea, or an acute alteration in mental status, are considered to be in septic shock. Sepsis and organ failure accompanied by (micro)circulatory failure can lead to impaired tissue oxygen supply and refractory shock. Septic shock refers to an acute event induced by bacteria and/or their products and is the most severe case of severe sepsis (Figure 34.1).

MEDIATORS OF IMMUNE REACTIONS

Sensing of pathogen-specific molecular patterns

In addition to microbial toxins and superantigens (which directly affect and modulate the hosts' immune response), a variety of constitutive microbial cell compo-

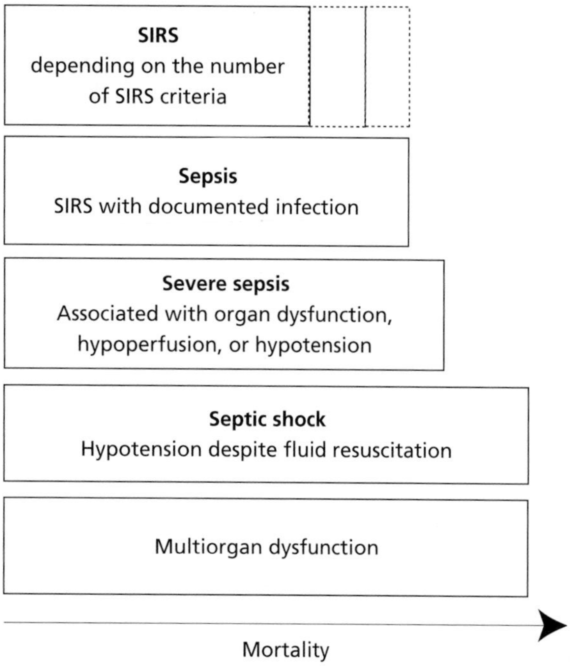

Figure 34.1 *Mortality in the systemic inflammatory response syndrome (SIRS). A progressively higher mortality of patients admitted to intensive care units can be observed as more severe inflammatory response criteria are met.*

nents induce inflammatory reactions. Although, for decades, studies concerning sepsis and shock dealt with gram-negative bacteria, infections with gram-positive bacteria, e.g. *Staphyloccus aureus* and enterococci, are recognized more and more to be of similar clinical relevance. The pathophysiological consequences of the systemic effects of infection are determined by a combination of factors derived from the infecting agent and responses of the host organism to the infection. Invading microorganisms such as bacteria, mycoplasmas, fungi, protozoa, or viruses and products thereof are immediately sensed by either serum proteins or membrane-bound proteins with predefined specificities. In recent years, a large number of so-called 'pathogen-specific pattern recognition molecules' have been described both as plasma components and as cell-surface receptors.

Characteristically, such pathogen-specific pattern recognition molecules specifically bind to repetitive carbohydrate structures on the surface of microorganisms or to an increasing number of defined molecules of microbial origin such as bacterial lipopolysaccharide (LPS), lipoteichoic acid (LTA), or bacterial DNA with cytidine phosphate-guanosine dinucleotide (CpG) motifs, now often referred to as pathogen-associated molecular patterns (PAMP) (Medzhitov and Janeway 1997).

Bacterial LPS, a constituent of the outer cell membrane of gram-negative bacteria, has been extensively studied for many years and represents the endotoxic principle of gram-negative bacteria (Rietschel et al. 1996). In the infected host, LPS is sensed by a specific LPS-binding protein (LBP) which in turn supports the interaction of LPS with either soluble or membrane-associated CD14. LPS-mediated cellular signaling, however, is dependent on a specific cell-surface receptor for LPS, now known as Toll-like receptor 4 (TLR-4) which cooperates with MD-2 (Beutler 2000; Alexander and Rietschel 2001; Heinrich et al. 2001) (Figure 34.2). TLR-4 signaling induces the release of proinflammatory mediators such as TNF (Jack et al. 1997) and initiates a pleiotropic cascade of events, including activation of the coagulation system, recruitment of phagocytes, and localization of the septic focus (Echtenacher et al. 1996). Similarly, LTA (which could be considered as a marker molecule of gram-positive bacteria) triggers the innate immune response using another member of the Toll-like receptor family, i.e. TLR-2, as a signal-transducing membrane receptor (Morath et al. 2002). Likewise, bacterial DNA containing immune stimulatory CpG motifs binds and signals through another member of the Toll-like receptor (TLR) family, i.e. TLR-9 (Krieg 2002).

ACTIVATION OF THE CELLULAR SYSTEM

Toll-like receptors

On the cell surface the Toll-like receptors (TLR) are crucial in transmitting the signal from structures commonly found on or in microorganisms (nonself) but absent on eukaryotic cells (self) into cells (Janeway 1992). A plethora of structures additional to LPS, LTA, and CpG are recognized by members of the TLR family including peptidoglycan (PGN), bacterial or mycobacterial lipoproteins, lipoarabinomannan, yeast cell wall components, or bacterial flagellin. By recognition of and response to a broad spectrum of diverse microbial patterns, the innate immune system orchestrates an inflammatory response to microbial invasion and triggers secretion and increased biosynthesis of key components in the inflammatory process. These genes include those encoding cytokines (TNF, interleukins IL-1, IL-6, and IL-12), chemokines (MIP-1α, IL-8), adhesion molecules, intercellular adhesion molecule 1 (ICAM-1), endothelial leukocyte adhesion molecule 1 (ELAM), inducible nitric oxide synthase (iNOS), and antimicrobial peptides, all of which contribute to the early host response against the invading pathogen (Jefferies and O'Neill 2002). The intracellular signaling cascade after activation of TLR-4 and TLR-2 is well characterized and uses common intracellular signaling intermediates MyD88, IRAK, and TRAF-6, resulting in activation of the nuclear factor κ B (NF-κB), mitogen-activated protein kinase (MAPK), and c-Jun N-terminal kinase (JNK) pathway activation which initiates the transcription of proinflammatory cytokines (Takeuchi and Akira 2001) (see Figure 34.2).

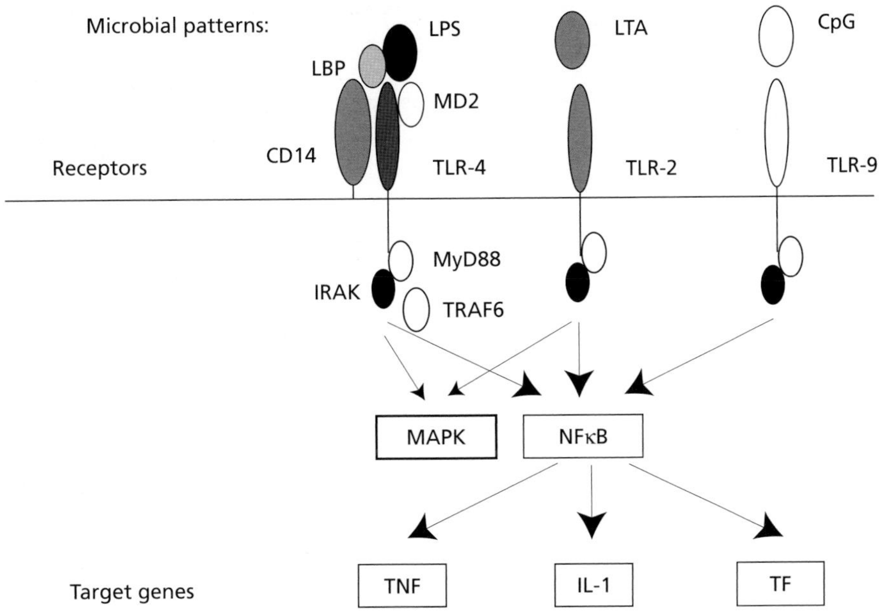

Figure 34.2 *The signaling pathway of Toll-like receptor 4 (TLR-4) after recognition of bacterial lipopolysaccharide (LPS) is mediated by LPS-binding protein (LBP), and CD14, TLR-4, and MD2. IRAK, IL-1 receptor-associated kinase; LTA, lipoteichoic acid; MAPK, mitogen-activated protein kinase; NF-κB, nuclear factor κ B; TNF, tumor necrosis factor; TRAF6, TNF receptor-associated factor 6; TF, tissue factor.*

Inflammatory cytokines

Among the proinflammatory cytokines, TNF and IL-1, are regarded as key players because their biosynthesis is quick and immensely efficient and their biological activities very powerful in starting off a cascade of additional proinflammatory mediators, e.g. via activation of NF-κB. TNF in particular appears to be the most potent mediator of the pathophysiology of the sepsis syndrome (Männel and Echtenacher 2000; Beutler 2002; Knuefermann et al. 2002). In combination with bacterial products or with IL-1, TNF rapidly leads to death with all symptoms of severe sepsis and shock in experimental settings (Okusawa et al. 1988a; Rothstein and Schreiber 1988; Waage and Espevik 1988). Effects on tissue metabolism, cardiac function, and vascular tone are three major mechanisms for the damage exerted by a concerted action of TNF with other mediators through the induction of effector molecules such as NO (Parrillo 1993). Serum TNF as well as IL-1 levels positively correlate with severity of infection (Calandra et al. 1990; Marks et al. 1990). Nuclear extracts from peripheral blood mononuclear cells from patients who succumbed to sepsis showed a significant increase in the nuclear binding activity of NF-κB compared with those of survivors. This supports the view that inflammatory cytokines such as TNF and IL-1 are central regulators of the inflammatory process in sepsis (Bohrer et al. 1997). Elevated levels of macrophage migration inhibitory factor (MIF) – yet another proinflammatory mediator that overrides the anti-inflammatory and immunosuppressive effects of glucocorticoids – can be detected in patients with severe sepsis and septic shock and enhanced survival is achieved by blocking MIF in experimental models of sepsis (Calandra et al. 2000). This gives further emphasis to the causal relationship of an exaggerated inflammatory immune status with sepsis and shock.

Although activation of cells of the innate immune system, e.g. macrophages for production of proinflammatory cytokines and antimicrobial molecules, is essential during the early phase of the infection, upregulation of costimulatory molecules and activation of dendritic cells leads to the instruction of the adaptive immune system. As professional antigen-presenting cells, dendritic cells bridge the gap between the innate and the adaptive immune response. Thus, TLRs can be considered as adjuvant receptors linking innate and adaptive immunity throughout the entire course of the host response to the infection (Kaisho and Akira 2002).

ACTIVATION OF HUMORAL SYSTEMS

Complement

The complement system is an integral part of the innate defense against infection and mediates many cellular and humoral interactions within the immune response, including chemotaxis, phagocytosis, and cell adhesion. Complement may be activated via three different routes: the classical pathway, the lectin pathway, and the alternative pathway (Figure 34.3). The classic activation pathway is initiated by immune complexes, whereas the lectin pathway and the alternative pathway activation

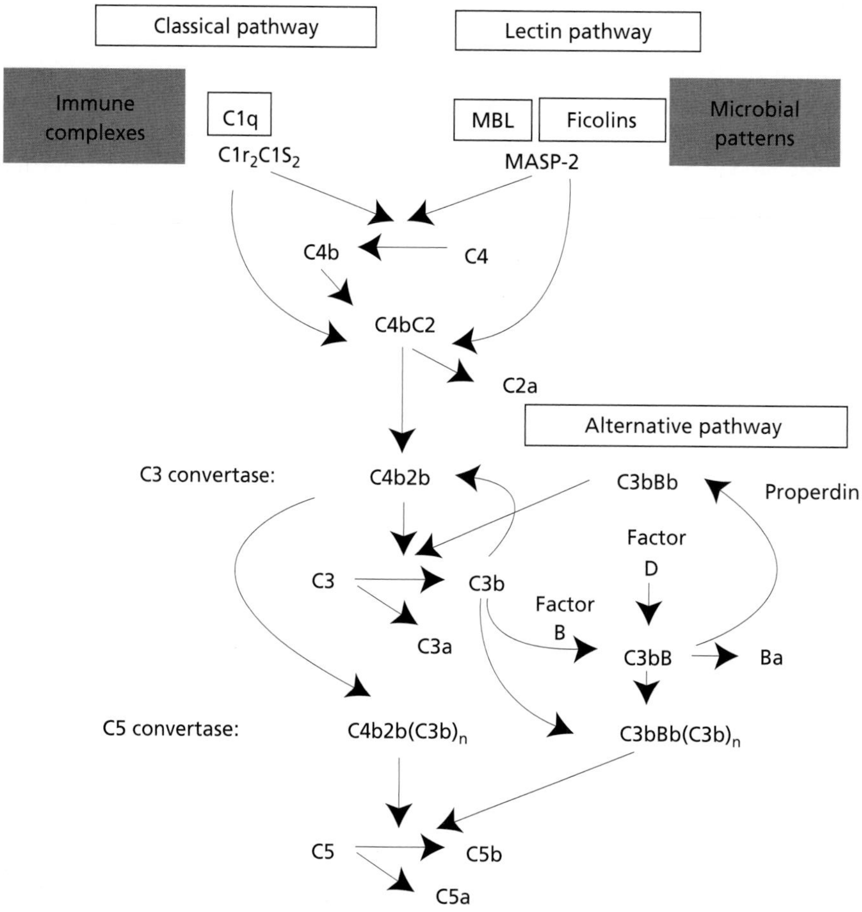

Figure 34.3 *The complement system is activated via the classic pathway initiated by immune complexes or via the lectin pathway initiated by pathogen-specific pattern recognition molecules such as the serum mannan-binding lectin (MBL) or ficolins leading to the activation of MBL-associated serine proteases (MASP). The alternate complement pathway stabilizes the C3 and C5 convertases, leading to generation of the anaphylatoxins C3a and C5a.*

can be initiated in the absence of immunoglobulins. Lectin pathway specific recognition molecules such as mannan-binding lectin (MBL) and the ficolins typically bind repetitive carbohydrate structures present on the surface of microbial organisms and translate this recognition into enzymatic activation of serine proteases associated with these recognition molecules (Neth et al. 2000; Petersen et al. 2001). The first PAMP recognition molecule identified to initiate the lectin pathway activation route of complement was the serum lectin MBL. Three lectin pathway-specific serine proteases have been identified so far and were termed MBL-associated serine proteases (MASP) (Thiel et al. 1997; Vorup-Jensen et al. 2000). As with MBL, ficolins were shown to form multimolecular serum complexes capable of activating complement after binding to microbial carbohydrate structures using MASP. MBL and the ficolins differ in their binding affinity to certain surface carbohydrate residues and thereby broaden the spectrum of potential triggers for lectin pathway activation.

Initiation of the lectin pathway activates the complement factors C4 and C2 to form C4b2b, a central enzymatic complex, which is able to cleave the abundant serum protein C3, thus generating C3 convertase which is common to both the classic and the lectin activation pathways of complement. As a result of complement activation pathway formation of the C3 and C5 convertases, the anaphylatoxins C3a and C5a are generated which increase plasma exudation and polymorphonuclear neutrophil chemotaxis.

The inherently labile C3 and C5 convertase complexes are stabilized by an amplification loop provided by the activation of the alternative complement pathway. A central component of this pathway is properdin; this is a positive regulator of complement activation and is rapidly released from polymorphonuclear neutrophils (PMN) in response to a variety of inflammatory stimuli such as LPS, TNF, or the anaphylatoxin C5a (Wirthmueller et al. 1997; Schwaeble and Reid 1999). Thus, in sites of inflammation where cytokines are secreted and complement is activated, secretion of properdin will amplify the complement cascade. A detailed discussion of the role of complement in infections is given in Chapter 9, Complement).

Inappropriate or excessive complement activation has been associated with septic shock. In plasma of patients with sepsis, complement activation products, especially anaphylatoxins, can be found (Nakae et al. 1996). High concentrations of the anaphylatoxins C3a and C5a and terminal C5b–9 complement complexes seem to correlate with development of MOF and circulatory shock (Hack et al. 1989; Smedegard et al. 1989). Complement will directly promote procoagulant activity and indirectly induce cytokine production (Okusawa et al. 1988b; Scholz et al. 1990). The membrane-bound C5b–9 membrane attack complex and the anaphylatoxins induce tissue factor expression on endothelial cells and monocytes, thereby contributing to increased vascular permeability (Carson and Johnson 1990). Of the anaphylatoxins, C5a in particular is highly chemotactic for PMNs and induces the secretion of lysosomal enzymes from neutrophils and macrophages (Bengtsson et al. 1993). C5a seems to be a key mediator in inflammatory reactions, leading to vascular leakage by inducing TNF and endothelial P-selectin expression, and adhesion, migration, and aggregation of PMNs (Strachan et al. 2000). The receptor for C5a (C5aR) is found to be upregulated in sepsis on a variety of cells such as neutrophils, phagocytes, endothelial cells, and mast cells (Riedemann et al. 2002). Improved survival rates as well as attenuated inflammatory cytokine serum levels after blockade of the C5aR in sepsis models demonstrates the importance of the C5a receptor activation.

Coagulation

Activated humoral protease systems, i.e. coagulation, fibrinolysis, and the plasma kallikrein–kinin system, characterize severe infection and sepsis. Systemic activation of coagulation generates the deposition of fibrin in small blood vessels and microvascular thrombosis in critical organs, leading to organ failure. This occurs as consequence of the cellular activation during infection and of the release of inflammatory cytokines such as TNF and IL-1 (van der Poll et al. 1990). In addition, release of proteases from circulating cells has been suggested as an important factor in developing endothelial damage, leading to extensive permeability changes in various organs (Aasen and Buo 1993).

Tissue factor

A variety of mediators such as LPS and other bacterial products, various cytokines, among others particularly TNF, antigen–antibody complexes, and activated complement components are inducers of monocyte tissue factor (TF). Such mediators of inflammation as LPS, TNF, and IL-1 elicit concurrent changes in expression of leukocyte adhesion molecules on endothelial cells. Endothelial activation can be considered as a coordinated pathophysiological response to inflammation (Pober and Cotran 1990). The adherence of monocytes to P-selectin, an adhesion molecule expressed on the surface of activated platelets and endothelial cells, also induces TF expression. The transcription of the TF gene is mediated by both NF-κB and AP-1 sites located within the TF gene promoter (Mackman et al. 1991). During gram-negative sepsis circulating monocytes express significant levels of TF activity. TF is considered to be the primary triggering agent for the coagulation cascade and by far the most potent procoagulant substance known. Therefore, pathological expression of TF in monocytes and endothelial cells certainly contributes to the enhanced thrombogenesis in sepsis patients.

Platelets

Activated platelets that adhere and aggregate in large numbers at sites of vascular injury rapidly generate high local concentrations of thrombin (Morrissey and Drake 2002). Activation of platelets can also occur by complement components such as C5a and the C5b–9 complex (Rinder et al. 1995). Local activation of the coagulation cascade is immediately countered by anticoagulant systems such as the expression of thrombomodulin, antithrombin, production of TF pathway inhibitor, and protein C. Considering the prominent role of microvascular coagulation in sepsis and of activated protein C in hemostasis, antithrombotic and anticoagulant therapy seemed a reasonable attempt to prevent multiple organ dysfunction syndrome in severe sepsis (Aasen and Buo 1993).

Platelet-activating factor

Platelet-activating factor (PAF), a potent mediator implicated particularly in inflammatory conditions, is an alkylphospholipid produced by, and acting on, a variety of different cell types including PMNs, eosinophils, monocytes, macrophages, platelets, and endothelial cells (Ayala and Chaudry 1996). PAF is a potent chemotactic agent for neutrophils, inducing superoxide release, aggregation, and degranulation. Selfgenerating positive feedback cycles of PAF and various cytokines have become established. Synergistic effects of LPS and TNF with PAF on neutrophils may be crucial in initiating vascular damage in the very early phases of sepsis and shock. Impairment and retraction of endothelial cells by PAF has been observed in experimental systems in vitro.

CIRCULATORY FAILURE AND DIRECT CYTOTOXIC EFFECTS

A new understanding of sepsis pathophysiology has emerged, focused on the tight interplay and coupling of inflammation, microvascular coagulation, and endothelial cell dysfunction (Joyce and Grinnell 2002). In the early events leading to severe sepsis, the host response results in the activation of a number of systems aimed at ridding the host of the infection. After activation of the humoral systems, i.e. the complement cascades, coagulation, fibrinolysis, and the kallikrein–kinin system, cells such as neutrophils, platelets, and mast cells also become involved. Circulating neutrophilic leukocytes are activated and adhere to the endothelium of the blood vessels. Such margination of PMNs and leukostasis provoke massive release of proteases, radicals, and phospholipid derivatives. Infiltrating neutrophils trigger the release of a second wave of chemoattractants/cytokines which amplify the recruitment of additional phagocytes. Margination and activation of neutrophils as a result of the action of inflammatory cytokines can trigger pulmonary vascular endothelial injury and lead to the adult respiratory distress syndrome (ARDS). Sequestration of activated leukocytes may also affect the intestine, leading to translocation of bacteria, and their toxins, leading to further recruitment and activation of monocytes/macrophages, neutrophils, and endothelial cells, respectively.

Microcirculation

The activation of the humoral and cellular inflammatory systems affects the endothelial barrier function and vasoregulation and leads to sepsis-induced dysregulation of the microcirculation at the level of resistance arterioles, nutritional capillary perfusion, and/or postcapillary venules (Lehr et al. 2000). The microcirculation constitutes a functionally highly active system which dynamically interacts with circulatory and tissue-associated cells such as leukocytes, platelets, neutrophils, and mast cells, produces mediators, and contributes to the regulation of the vascular tone. Consequences of microcirculatory dysfunction are the breakdown of endothelial and epithelial barrier function, vasodysregulation, and disturbance of oxygen transport.

A characteristic of septic (hyperdynamic) shock is the increased cardiac output and the loss of peripheral resistance resulting in increased transport of blood into the periphery (Lehr et al. 2000). With the inadequate peripheral resistance which is probably caused by sepsis-induced overproduction of NO and the resultant massive peripheral vasodilatation, the cardiac output is redistributed with compensatory hypoperfusion of visceral organs.

As a consequence of leukocyte activation in sepsis and disseminated intravascular coagulation (DIC) the microcirculation becomes overburdened with inflammatory cells. Endothelial cell swelling, leukocyte sequestration, and microthrombus formation are signs of endothelial cell activation and characterize the state of microcirculation in sepsis. In agreement with clinical observations in septic patients, sequestration of activated leukocytes has been shown to contribute to subsequent tissue injury in animal models.

Neutrophils, macrophages, and other phagocytic cells are capable of generating large amounts of highly toxic molecules such as reactive oxygen intermediates and reactive nitrogen intermediates (Bogdan et al. 2000). Besides their antimicrobial activity, these reactive intermediates are powerful immunoregulators. By inhibition of lymphocyte proliferation they may also serve to control inflammatory processes and to account for the immunosuppressed state in certain infections. Important signaling pathways regulating cytokine production and responses, cell survival, and tissue damage are influenced by reactive oxygen and nitrogen intermediates.

Tissue damage, and in particular endothelial cell damage mediated by free radical production, seems to be of considerable importance in sepsis and shock. The crucial cells for free radical production are PMNs (Nussler et al. 1999). In the inflammatory environment these cells become recruited and activated, and they adhere to the endothelial surface and release lysosomal proteases as described above. Activated neutrophils also produce superoxide by undergoing a respiratory burst. Superoxide is rapidly converted to hydrogen peroxide and toxic free radicals which can damage the endothelium (Ayala and Chaudry 1996). Endothelial membrane injury then leads to increased vascular permeability.

Septic shock is characterized by hypotension, vascular collapse, and multiorgan dysfunction. In sepsis, cardiac dysfunction and altered vascular tone, the loss of vascular homeostasis, and diffuse endothelial cell injury all increase microvascular permeability and favor the development of zones of ischemia. NO released by endothelial cells is a major endogenous arteriolar vasodilator. Thus, the large amounts of NO produced in the vascular wall by the cytokine-inducible NO synthase is considered to play an important role in septic shock (Li and Forstermann 2000). As with many important mediators of the host response to infection, the multifaceted actions of NO generate a picture of beneficial as well as detrimental effects. NO has both anti-inflammatory and proinflammatory properties depending on the type and phase of the inflammatory reaction. NO has a vasoprotective function by inhibiting platelet aggregation and adhesion to the cell wall, thus activating antithrombotic and anti-inflammatory effects by downregulation of NF-κB activation. However, NO is proadhesive for PMNs and can also be seen as an indirect toxic effector substance via the formation of reactive nitrogen species or as a mitochondrial inhibitor (Feihl et al. 2001). A correlation between NO-induced mitochondrial dysfunction and the severity and outcome of septic shock suggested that bioenergetic failure could be an important pathophysiological mechanism for MOF (Brealey et al. 2002).

Endothelial cell damage

The endothelial interface plays a central role in coordinating the microcirculatory system and promoting tissue perfusion and oxygen supply. Endothelial cells serve a number of metabolic and regulatory functions, e.g. production of vasoactive compounds such as prostacyclin, thromboxane, and NO, control of hemostasis, blood coagulation, and fibrinolysis, platelet and leukocyte interactions with the vessel wall, and regulation of the vascular tone and blood pressure. The release of inflammatory mediators such as TNF in the early phase of sepsis initiates endothelial cell-surface activation affecting a number of pathways, e.g. oxidation, adhesion, cytokine release, apoptosis, and NO production. In addition, TNF production contributes to further inflammation through thrombin-induced activation of endothelial cells, platelets, and vascular smooth muscle. These responses can directly damage the vascular endothelium by inducing enhanced microvascular coagulation, endothelial dysfunction, and apoptosis of endothelial cells. However, so far there are no data documenting any role for endothelial cell apoptosis in the pathogenesis of sepsis (Hotchkiss et al. 2002).

As a result of DIC and microvascular thrombosis, decreased tissue perfusion, and hypoxemia organ dysfunction, organ failure, and shock can ensue (Figure 34.4). Therefore, endothelial dysfunction resulting from the cascades of successive activation events is considered to play a central role in modulating the tightly linked and interdependent inflammatory and thrombotic responses that characterize the pathophysiology of systemic inflammation. In patients, various markers for an activated endothelium such as ICAM, vascular cell adhesion molecule (VCAM), and E-selectin are found to correlate with the severity of sepsis (Reinhart et al. 2002). The breakdown of normal vascular homeostasis, combined with depressed myocardial function, alterations in peripheral vasculature, and failure of oxygen exchange, will finally lead to tissue hypoxia and organ failure.

IMPLICATIONS FOR THERAPIES

An infectious insult results in stimulation of the immune system. This response is normally advantageous, but, when uncontrolled or excessive, it becomes deleterious for the host. This is the situation in septic shock.

Management of coagulopathy

The importance of the coagulation system resulting in, and exacerbating, the blockade of microvascular flow, and thus tissue oxygenation in sepsis, has suggested antithrombotic strategies as promising therapeutic approaches. A number of clinical sepsis trials with antithrombin or tissue factor pathway inhibitor have, however, shown that correcting the coagulation defect alone in sepsis was not sufficient to prevent mortality. Besides prevention of DIC by antithrombotic treatment, e.g. with activated protein C, it also seemed important to inhibit the thrombin-induced proinflammatory effects such as activation of platelets and endothelial cells,

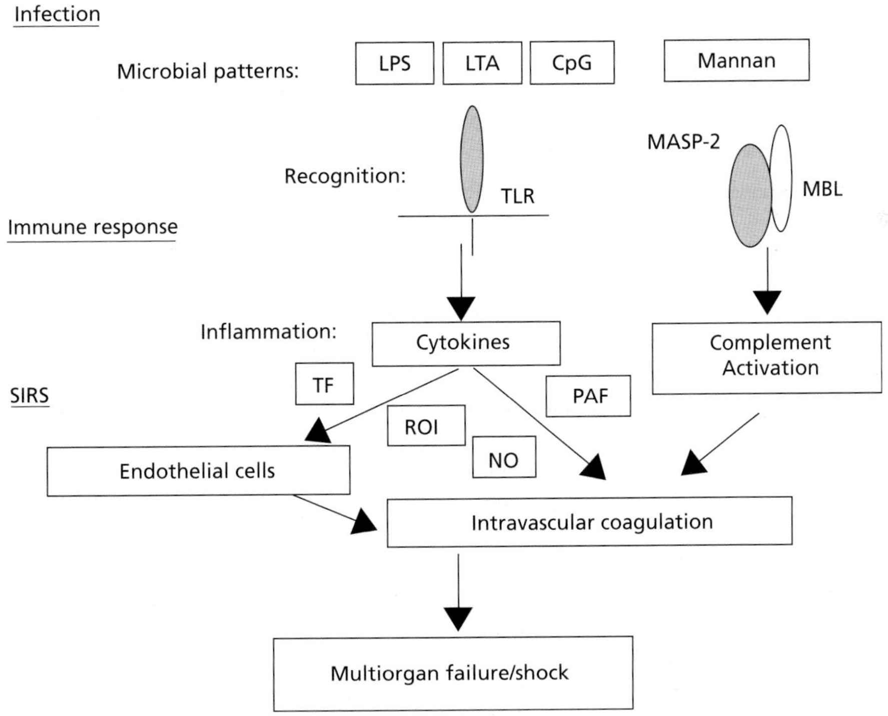

Figure 34.4 *Schematic overview of the pathogenesis of the systemic inflammatory response syndrome (SIRS) developing after infection and leading to severe sepsis and shock. LPS, lipopolysaccharide; LTA, lipoteichoic acid; MASP, MBL-associated serine protease; MBL, mannan-binding lectin; NO, nitric oxide; PAF, platelet-activating factor; ROI, reactive oxygen intermediates; TLR, Toll-like receptor; TF, tissue factor.*

NF-κB-dependent cytokine production, and adhesion molecule expression (Bernard et al. 2001). In addition, direct thrombin-independent anti-inflammatory effects of activated protein C, such as reduced NF-κB-dependent gene activation, may also result in protection of endothelial cells from apoptosis and promote cell survival and therefore may be important in restoring endothelial and mononuclear cell function.

Counterregulation of inflammation

The immune system has evolved potent anti-inflammatory programs to terminate and counterbalance inflammation because homeostasis requires compensatory mechanisms to maintain the internal milieu. A number of anti-inflammatory mediators such as IL-4, IL-10, IL-13, TGF-β, soluble TNF receptors, and IL-1 receptor antagonist are released for downregulating the immune response. In addition to these extracellular molecules, the integral nature of apoptosis provides a means of regulation of immune responses at the cellular level (Mahidhara and Billiar 2000). Delayed apoptosis of neutrophils (correlating with an upregulated inflammatory response), as well as increased lymphocyte apoptosis (possibly implicating immunosuppression), have been observed in patients with severe sepsis.

Endogenous corticosteroids downregulating the inflammatory response play a very important role in infections in general and are essential for the host to survive septic shock. Apart from modulating the immune system, corticosteroids have an important role in modulation of blood pressure and expression of adrenergic receptors. Steroid use in septic shock makes some sense but has conflicting support in the literature (Ritacca et al. 2002). A beneficial effect of corticosteroids in the treatment of sepsis may be a matter of dose, timing, duration of treatment, and patient selection (Spijkstra and Girbes 2000). The observations of beneficial effects of corticosteroids at doses that are close to the levels measured in stress situations support the idea of endocrine effects influencing the inflammatory responses in sepsis.

The theory of uncontrolled inflammation ultimately causing system-wide effects, shock, and end-organ failure, and the understanding of the importance of counterregulation lead to many therapeutic strategies aimed at blocking the early mediators of the proinflammatory response in sepsis. Among others, neutralization of bacterial products (LPS), inhibition of neutrophil recruitment, priming and activation by inhibition of chemoattractants (C3a, C5a), neutralization of chemokines, inhibition of rolling (selectin mediated), sticking (integrin mediated), and adherence, modulation of inflammatory mediators (C5a, TNF, IL-1, MIF, PAF), blockade of NO, arachidonic metabolites, reactive oxygen metabolites, and interference with signal transduction (NF-κB) activity have been tried in many experimental as well as clinical settings. Even though data from good animal models have conclusively demonstrated the importance of these mediators in the pathogenesis of the dysregulation in septic shock, the results of anti-inflammatory therapeutic strategies in the clinic were disappointing.

However, one has to keep in mind that the imminent problem in sepsis therapy is based on the fact that as yet no good parameters are available to evaluate the immunological status of the patients. After infection, patients go through an early inflammatory phase characterized by immediate responses of the innate immune system. In addition to the innate immune response, the adaptive immune response is recruited via, among others, activation of dendritic cells. This activation of the immune system provokes a counterregulatory anti-inflammatory or hypoinflammatory phase. For some time an overlap of the hyperinflammatory and hypoinflammatory phases may be present in the same infected organism, depending on the type of infection and the cell type, organ, or location under investigation. Although at the same time the presence of inflammatory mediators is required for antimicrobial action, anti-inflammatory mechanisms are essential for protection of tissue and organs. In such situations, the application of granulocyte colony-stimulating factor (G-CSF) might be a solution because transiently activated PMNs will be recruited with potent antimicrobial activity and – by an unknown mechanism – G-CSF acts in an anti-inflammatory manner (Boneberg and Hartung 2002).

There are some indications that careful patient stratification based on immunological characteristics that determine the timing for intervention might improve the outcome, as illustrated in the sepsis trial with TNF inhibition (Abraham et al. 1997; Grau and Männel 1997). As global tissue hypoxia is a key development preceding MOF and death, early goal-oriented manipulations of cardiac overload, afterload, and contractility to achieve balance between systemic oxygen delivery and oxygen demand seems to be a more definitive and effective resuscitation strategy (Rivers et al. 2001).

At least of equal importance is the notion that microcirculatory dysfunction during sepsis is not the consequence of one single mediator but of complex cascades of mediator systems, with these mediators having a striking redundancy in their modes of action. Evidently, inhibition of one mediator, even if it is an important one, might not be sufficient to get the dysregulated system back to homeostasis (Lehr et al. 2000). This is suggested by the relatively successful clinical trial with activated protein C where antithrombotic and anti-inflammatory effects are combined (Bernard et al. 2001). The combination of the divergent as well as the redundant effects of the different mediators, the difficulty of obtaining clear parameters to determine the immune status of the patient, as well as the detrimental synergistic positive feedback actions of the inflammatory pathways involved, will continue to make it extremely difficult to find a successful and safe therapeutic strategy for severe sepsis and shock.

ACKNOWLEDGMENTS

The author would like to thank B. Beutler, C. Stover, W. Schwaeble, and T. Glueck for helpful discussions and critical reading of the manuscript.

REFERENCES

Aasen, A.O. and Buo, L. 1993. Activation of humoral systems: coagulation, fibrinolysis, and plasma kallikrein-kinin systems. In: Schlag, G. and Redl, H. (eds), *Pathophysiology of shock, sepsis, and organ failure*. Berlin: Springer Verlag, 456–67.

Abraham, E., Glauser, M.P., et al. 1997. p55 Tumor necrosis factor receptor fusion protein in the treatment of patients with severe sepsis and septic shock. A randomized controlled multicenter trial. Ro 45-2081 Study Group. *JAMA*, **277**, 1531–8.

Alexander, C. and Rietschel, E.T. 2001. Bacterial lipopolysaccharides and innate immunity. *J Endotoxin Res*, **7**, 167–202.

Ayala, A. and Chaudry, I.H. 1996. Platelet activating factor and its role in trauma, shock, and sepsis. *New Horiz*, **4**, 265–75.

Balk, R.A. 2000. Severe sepsis and septic shock. Definitions, epidemiology, and clinical manifestations. *Crit Care Clin*, **16**, 179–92.

Baue, A.E. 1975. Multiple, progressive, or sequential systems failure. A syndrome of the 1970s. *Arch Surg*, **110**, 779–81.

Bengtsson, A., Redl, H. and Schlag, G. 1993. Complement in sepsis. In: Schlag, G. and Redl, H. (eds), *Pathophysiology of shock, sepsis, and organ failure*. Berlin: Springer Verlag, 447–58.

Bernard, G.R., Vincent, J.L., et al. 2001. Efficacy and safety of recombinant human activated protein C for severe sepsis. *N Engl J Med*, **344**, 699–709.

Beutler, B. 2000. Endotoxin, toll-like receptor 4, and the afferent limb of innate immunity. *Curr Opin Microbiol*, **3**, 23–8.

Beutler, B. 2002. *Tumor necrosis factors. The molecules and their emerging role in medicine*. New York: Raven Press.

Bogdan, C., Rollinghoff, M. and Diefenbach, A. 2000. Reactive oxygen and reactive nitrogen intermediates in innate and specific immunity. *Curr Opin Immunol*, **12**, 64–76.

Bohrer, H., Qiu, F., et al. 1997. Role of NFkappaB in the mortality of sepsis. *J Clin Invest*, **100**, 972–85.

Bone, R.C., Balk, R.A., et al. 1992. Definitions for sepsis and organ failure and guidelines for the use of innovative therapies in sepsis. The ACCP/SCCM Consensus Conference Committee. American College of Chest Physicians/Society of Critical Care Medicine. *Chest*, **101**, 1644–55.

Boneberg, E.M. and Hartung, T. 2002. Granulocyte colony-stimulating factor attenuates LPS-stimulated IL-1beta release via suppressed processing of proIL-1beta, whereas TNF-alpha release is inhibited on the level of proTNF-alpha formation. *Eur J Immunol*, **32**, 1717–25.

Brealey, D., Brand, M., et al. 2002. Association between mitochondrial dysfunction and severity and outcome of septic shock. *Lancet*, **360**, 219–23.

Calandra, T., Baumgartner, J.D., et al. 1990. Prognostic values of tumor necrosis factor/cachectin, interleukin-1, interferon-alpha, and interferon-gamma in the serum of patients with septic shock. Swiss-Dutch J5 Immunoglobulin Study Group. *J Infect Dis*, **161**, 982–7.

Calandra, T., Echtenacher, B., et al. 2000. Protection from septic shock by neutralization of macrophage migration inhibitory factor. *Nat Med*, **6**, 164–70.

Carson, S.D. and Johnson, D.R. 1990. Consecutive enzyme cascades: complement activation at the cell surface triggers increased tissue factor activity. *Blood*, **76**, 361–7.

Echtenacher, B., Männel, D.N. and Hültner, L. 1996. Critical protective role of mast cells in a model of acute septic peritonitis. *Nature*, **381**, 75–7.

Feihl, F., Waeber, B. and Liaudet, L. 2001. Is nitric oxide overproduction the target of choice for the management of septic shock? *Pharmacol Ther*, **91**, 179–213.

Grau, G.E. and Männel, D.N. 1997. TNF inhibition and sepsis - sounding a cautionary note. *Nat Med*, **3**, 1193–5.

Hack, C.E., Nuijens, J.H., et al. 1989. Elevated plasma levels of the anaphylatoxins C3a and C4a are associated with a fatal outcome in sepsis. *Am J Med*, **86**, 20–6.

Heinrich, J.M., Bernheiden, M., et al. 2001. The essential role of lipopolysaccharide-binding protein in protection of mice against a peritoneal Salmonella infection involves the rapid induction of an inflammatory response. *J Immunol*, **167**, 1624–8.

Hotchkiss, R.S., Tinsley, K.W., et al. 2002. Endothelial cell apoptosis in sepsis. *Crit Care Med*, **30**, S225–8.

Jack, R.S., Fan, X., et al. 1997. Lipopolysaccharide-binding protein is required to combat a murine gram-negative bacterial infection. *Nature*, **389**, 742–5.

Janeway, C.A. Jr. 1992. The immune system evolved to discriminate infectious nonself from noninfectious self. *Immunol Today*, **13**, 11–16.

Jefferies, C. and O'Neill, L.A.J. 2002. Signal transduction pathway activated by Toll-like receptors. *Mod Asp Immunobiol*, **2**, 169–75.

Joyce, D.E. and Grinnell, B.W. 2002. Recombinant human activated protein C attenuates the inflammatory response in endothelium and monocytes by modulating nuclear factor-kappaB. *Crit Care Med*, **30**, S288–93.

Kaisho, T. and Akira, S. 2002. Toll-like receptors as adjuvant receptors. *Biochim Biophys Acta*, **1589**, 1–13.

Knuefermann, P., Nemoto, S., et al. 2002. Cardiac inflammation and innate immunity in septic shock: is there a role for toll-like receptors? *Chest*, **121**, 1329–36.

Krieg, A.M. 2002. CpG motifs in bacterial DNA and their immune effects. *Annu Rev Immunol*, **20**, 709–60.

Lehr, H.A., Bittinger, F. and Kirkpatrick, C.J. 2000. Microcirculatory dysfunction in sepsis: a pathogenetic basis for therapy? *J Pathol*, **190**, 373–86.

Li, H. and Forstermann, U. 2000. Nitric oxide in the pathogenesis of vascular disease. *J Pathol*, **190**, 244–54.

Mackman, N., Brand, K. and Edgington, T.S. 1991. Lipopolysaccharide-mediated transcriptional activation of the human tissue factor gene in THP-1 monocytic cells requires both activator protein 1 and nuclear factor kappa B binding sites. *J Exp Med*, **174**, 1517–26.

Mahidhara, R. and Billiar, T.R. 2000. Apoptosis in sepsis. *Crit Care Med*, **28**, N105–13.

Männel, D.N. and Echtenacher, B. 2000. TNF in the inflammatory response. *Chem Immunol*, **74**, 141–61.

Marks, J.D., Marks, C.B., et al. 1990. Plasma tumor necrosis factor in patients with septic shock. Mortality rate, incidence of adult respiratory distress syndrome, and effects of methylprednisolone administration. *Am Rev Respir Dis*, **141**, 94–7.

Medzhitov, R. and Janeway, C.A. Jr. 1997. Innate immunity: the virtues of a nonclonal system of recognition. *Cell*, **91**, 295–8.

Morath, S., Stadelmaier, A., et al. 2002. Synthetic lipoteichoic acid from Staphylococcus aureus is a potent stimulus of cytokine release. *J Exp Med*, **195**, 1635–40.

Morrissey, J.H. and Drake, T.A. 2002. Procoagulant response of the endothelium and monocytes. In: Schlag, G. and Redl, H. (eds), *Pathophysiology of shock, sepsis, and organ failure*. Berlin: Springer Verlag, 564–74.

Nakae, H., Endo, S., et al. 1996. Chronological changes in the complement system in sepsis. *Surg Today*, **26**, 225–9.

Neth, O., Jack, D.L., et al. 2000. Mannose-binding lectin binds to a range of clinically relevant microorganisms and promotes complement deposition. *Infect Immun*, **68**, 688–93.

Nussler, A.K., Wittel, U.A., et al. 1999. Leukocytes, the Janus cells in inflammatory disease. *Langenbecks Arch Surg*, **384**, 222–32.

Okusawa, S., Gelfand, J.A., et al. 1988a. Interleukin 1 induces a shock-like state in rabbits. Synergism with tumor necrosis factor and the effect of cyclooxygenase inhibition. *J Clin Invest*, **81**, 1162–72.

Okusawa, S., Yancey, K.B., et al. 1988b. C5a stimulates secretion of tumor necrosis factor from human mononuclear cells in vitro. Comparison with secretion of interleukin 1 beta and interleukin 1 alpha. *J Exp Med*, **168**, 443–8.

Parrillo, J.E. 1993. Pathogenetic mechanisms of septic shock. *N Engl J Med*, **328**, 1471–7.

Petersen, S.V., Thiel, S. and Jensenius, J.C. 2001. The mannan-binding lectin pathway of complement activation: biology and disease association. *Mol Immunol*, **38**, 133–49.

Pober, J.S. and Cotran, R.S. 1990. Cytokines and endothelial cell biology. *Physiol Rev*, **70**, 427–51.

Reinhart, K., Bayer, O., et al. 2002. Markers of endothelial damage in organ dysfunction and sepsis. *Crit Care Med*, **30**, S302–12.

Riedemann, N.C., Guo, R.F., et al. 2002. Increased C5a receptor expression in sepsis. *J Clin Invest*, **110**, 101–8.

Rietschel, E.T., Brade, H., et al. 1996. Bacterial endotoxin: Chemical constitution, biological recognition, host response, and immunological detoxification. *Curr Top Microbiol Immunol*, **216**, 39–81.

Rinder, C.S., Rinder, H.M., et al. 1995. Blockade of C5a and C5b-9 generation inhibits leukocyte and platelet activation during extracorporeal circulation. *J Clin Invest*, **96**, 1564–72.

Ritacca, F.V., Simone, C., et al. 2002. Pro/con clinical debate: are steroids useful in the management of patients with septic shock? *Crit Care*, **6**, 113–16.

Rivers, E., Nguyen, B., et al. 2001. Early goal-directed therapy in the treatment of severe sepsis and septic shock. *N Engl J Med*, **345**, 1368–77.

Rothstein, J.L. and Schreiber, H. 1988. Synergy between tumor necrosis factor and bacterial products causes hemorrhagic necrosis and lethal shock in normal mice. *Proc Natl Acad Sci USA*, **85**, 607–11.

Scholz, W., McClurg, M.R., et al. 1990. C5a-mediated release of interleukin 6 by human monocytes. *Clin Immunol Immunopathol*, **57**, 297–307.

Schwaeble, W.J. and Reid, K.B. 1999. Does properdin crosslink the cellular and the humoral immune response? *Immunol Today*, **20**, 17–21.

Smedegard, G., Cui, L.X. and Hugli, T.E. 1989. Endotoxin-induced shock in the rat. A role for C5a. *Am J Pathol*, **135**, 489–97.

Spijkstra, J.J. and Girbes, A.R. 2000. The continuing story of corticosteroids in the treatment of septic shock. *Intens Care Med*, **26**, 496–500.

Strachan, A.J., Woodruff, T.M., et al. 2000. A new small molecule C5a receptor antagonist inhibits the reverse-passive Arthus reaction and endotoxic shock in rats. *J Immunol*, **164**, 6560–5.

Takeuchi, O. and Akira, S. 2001. Toll-like receptors; their physiological role and signal transduction system. *Int Immunopharmacol*, **1**, 625–35.

Thiel, S., Vorup-Jensen, T., et al. 1997. A second serine protease associated with mannan-binding lectin that activates complement. *Nature*, **386**, 506–10.

van der Poll, T., Buller, H.R., et al. 1990. Activation of coagulation after administration of tumor necrosis factor to normal subjects. *N Engl J Med*, **322**, 1622–7.

Vorup-Jensen, T., Petersen, S.V., et al. 2000. Distinct pathways of mannan-binding lectin (MBL)-and C1-complex autoactivation revealed by reconstitution of MBL with recombinant MBL-associated serine protease-2. *J Immunol*, **165**, 2093–100.

Waage, A. and Espevik, T. 1988. Interleukin 1 potentiates the lethal effect of tumor necrosis factor alpha/cachectin in mice. *J Exp Med*, **167**, 1987–92.

Wirthmueller, U., Dewald, B., et al. 1997. Properdin, a positive regulator of complement activation, is released from secondary granules of stimulated peripheral blood neutrophils. *J Immunol*, **158**, 4444–51.

35

DTH-associated pathology

STEFAN EHLERS AND CHRISTOPH HÖLSCHER

INTRODUCTION

A number of microorganisms have the capacity to remain viable within the host although the latter mounts an adequate immune response against them. This gives rise to a T-cell-mediated chronic inflammatory response aimed at restraining the harmful effects of the persisting microorganism. This response follows a characteristic pathophysiological pattern (granuloma formation) and often entails significant tissue damage in the form of necrosis or fibrosis. A major driving force in current inflammation research is the molecular dissociation of protection and pathology associated with this type of chronic inflammatory response. It remains a challenging therapeutic goal to manipulate, at will, the pathological sequelae of inflammation without impairing antimicrobially active immune defenses expressed concomitantly. This chapter outlines the salient features of immunopathology associated with T-cell-mediated delayed-type hypersensitivity (DTH) and discusses some strategies to prevent them.

DELAYED-TYPE HYPERSENSITIVITY

Definition

Delayed-type hypersensitivity is a highly dynamic, T-cell-mediated inflammatory response to persisting antigen. It is a typical immunological reaction to a variety of facultative intracellular bacteria, fungi, and parasites (Table 35.1) (Zumla and James 1996). Contact sensitivity to some chemical agents, experimental allergic encephalomyelitis, and graft rejection are other prototypes of DTH reactions induced by nonmicrobial stimuli.

The best known example of a DTH reaction is the response of a sensitized individual to intradermal injection of a purified protein derivative (PPD) of the causative agent of tuberculosis, *Mycobacterium tuberculosis*. The DTH reaction to PPD starts with reddening and induration at the site of antigen deposition after about 12 h. This delayed reaction peaks after 48–72 h and slowly wanes thereafter (Figure 35.1). Morphologically, the DTH skin reaction is characterized by the perivascular accumulation of predominantly mononuclear cells in the subcutaneous tissue and dermis. The majority of infiltrating lymphocytes are of the $CD4^+$ subtype. Over time, activated monocytes differentiate into epithelioid macrophages. As microvascular permeability is also increased, there is dermal edema and deposition of fibrin in the interstitium. The induration characteristic of a skin DTH reaction is a consequence of both the persistent infiltration of mononuclear cells and a limited amount of inflammatory fibrosis.

DTH and granuloma formation

Granulomas are defined as focal accumulations of mononuclear cells in response to a chronic antigenic

Table 35.1 *Selected bacteria, fungi and parasites causing DTH reactions and granulomatous disease*

Gram-positive bacteria	Gram-negative bacteria	Fungi	Parasites
Listeria monocytogenes	*Yersinia enterocolitica/ pseudotuberculosis/pestis*	*Cryptococcus neoformans*	*Toxocara canis/cati*
Rhodococcus equi	*Salmonella typhi/paratyphi*	*Blastomyces dermatitidis*	*Leishmania major/donovani*
Nocardia asteroides	*Francisella tularensis*	*Sporothrix schenckii*	*Trypanosoma cruzi*
Treponema pallidum	*Chlamydia trachomatis*	*Coccidioides immitis*	*Schistosoma mansoni/ japonicum*
Mycobacterium tuberculosis	*Bartonella henselae/bacilliformis*	*Paracoccidioides brasiliensis*	
Mycobacterium avium/ leprae	*Rickettsia prowazeki/conori*	*Histoplasma capsulatum*	
	Coxiella burnetii		
	Tropheryma whippelii		
	Calymmatobacterium granulomatis		
	Burkholderia pseudomallei		
	Brucella abortus		

stimulus. Thus, the skin DTH reaction may alternatively be termed a 'mini-granuloma' of the skin. Vice versa, antigen-specific granulomas in visceral organs in most instances fulfill all criteria of a DTH reaction and may therefore be viewed simply as tissue correlates of a DTH reaction.

Histopathologically, granulomas are characterized by aggregates of epithelioid cells with indistinct cell boundaries, which often seem to fuse into one another. The nucleus of activated macrophages is less dense than that of the surrounding lymphocytes ($CD4^+$, $CD8^+$ T cells and B cells), is oval or elongate ('shoe imprint' morphology), and has prominent nucleoli (Figure 35.2). Older granulomas are surrounded by a collar of fibroblasts and connective tissue, e.g. collagen fibers. Depending on the eliciting microorganism, neutrophil

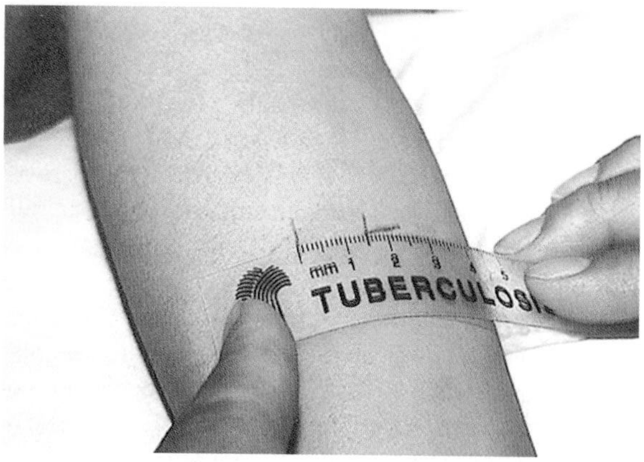

Figure 35.1 *Delayed-type hypersensitivity skin reaction to intracutaneous injection of purified protein derivative of* Mycobacterium tuberculosis. *Within 48–72 h, a positive tuberculosis (TB) skin test is marked by an area of reddish induration greater than 10 mm. It is the palpable induration that determines the size, not the area of redness. (Photograph reproduced with permission from the Saskatchewan Tuberculosis Control Guide (http:\\www.lung.ca/tb/images/full_archive/ 102_tuberculin_wheal.jpg) copyright 2002.)*

and eosinophil granulocytes are also present. Frequently, epithelioid cells fuse to form multinucleated giant cells, which may become as large as 50 μm in diameter, and show either an ordered peripheral arrangement of nuclei (Langhans-type giant cell; Figure 35.2) or a haphazard distribution of nuclei (foreign body-type giant cell).

In contrast to foreign body granulomas, which occur independently of T cells and are characterized by little cellular turnover, T-cell-mediated (DTH-type) granulomas are highly dynamic: in addition to local proliferation of T cells, new mononuclear cells are constantly recruited into the lesion by virtue of mediators secreted by activated, antigen-specific T cells.

Mechanisms of granulomatous inflammation

In the course of a primary immune response, $CD4^+$ cells are sensitized to digested antigen presented in the context of major histocompatibility complex (MHC) class II and appropriate costimulatory molecules, such as CD80 or CD86 on the surface of antigen-presenting cells, e.g. dendritic cells (Jankovic et al. 2001). The nature of the cytokine environment present during this priming phase ultimately determines the differentiation of the $CD4^+$ effector cell subtype: the presence of interleukin (IL) 12 and interferon γ (IFN-γ) will promote the development of T-helper (Th) 1 cells, which are capable of secreting IL-2, IFN-γ, and lymphotoxin α (LT-α), whereas the predominance of IL-4 and IL-10 will favor the differentiation of Th2 cells which preferentially produce IL-4, IL-5, IL-6, IL-9, IL-10, and IL-13 (Chtanova and Mackay 2001). Some of these differentiated cells will become long-lived memory cells. Antigen-specific effector and memory T cells recirculate in the bloodstream and can enter sites of antigen deposition where they subsequently produce cytokines for further amplification of the type 1 and 2 immune reaction patterns, respectively.

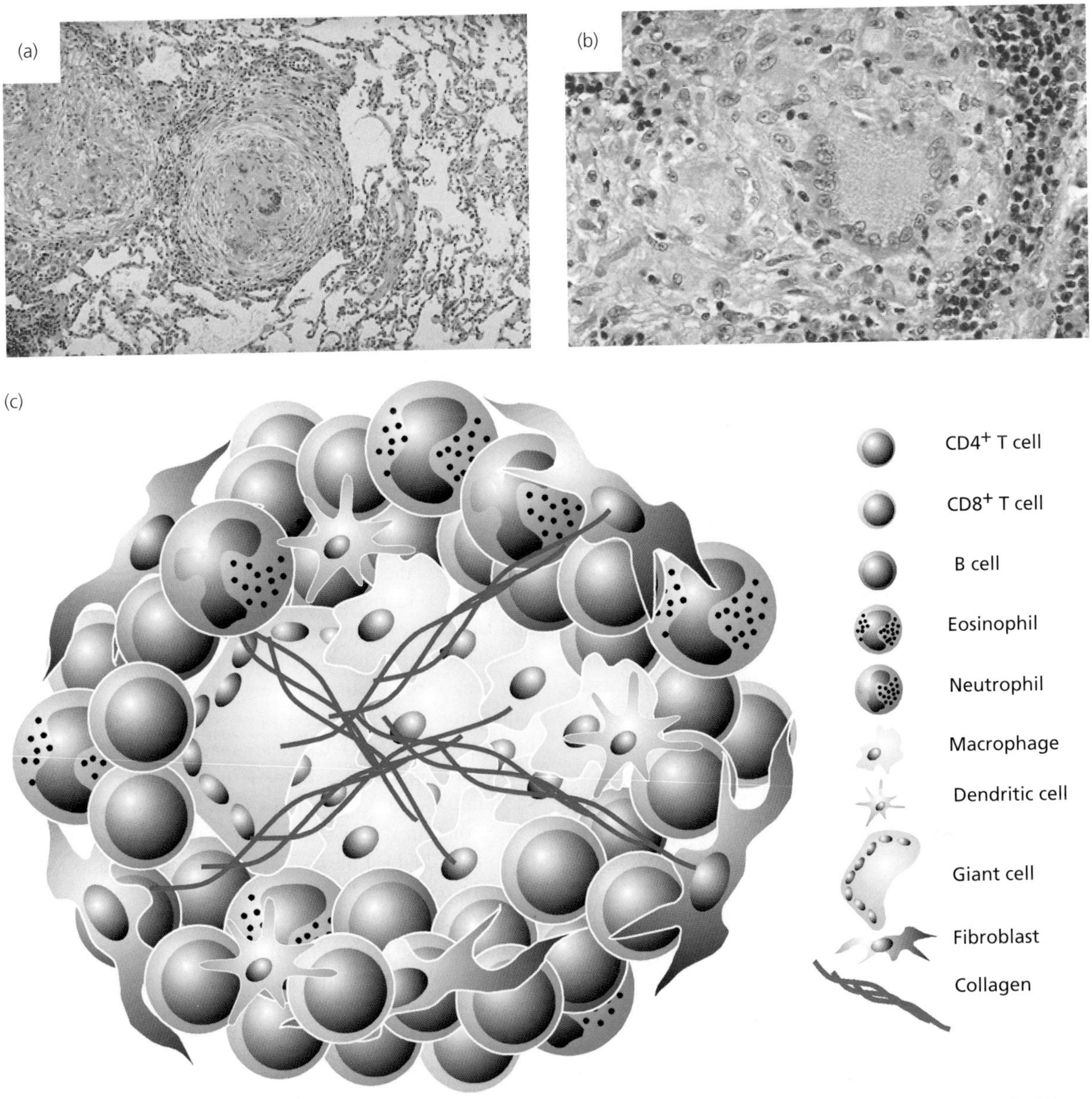

Figure 35.2 *Granulomatous inflammation:* **(a)** *medium power microscopic view of two pulmonary granulomas with giant cells;* **(b)** *high power microscopic view of well-structured granuloma with epithelioid macrophages and Langhans giant cell; and* **(c)** *schematic drawing of cells organized within the granuloma structure. (Photographs* **(a)** *and* **(b)** *reproduced with permission from Webpath, Version 7, 14 March, 2002, copyright 2002, Edward C. Klatt, MD.)*

The recruitment of effector $CD4^+$ cells into inflammatory lesions requires interaction with adhesion molecules as well as the sensing of a gradient of chemoattractant molecules by specific receptors. The course of events is initiated by activated complement components (e.g. C5a), vasoactive amines, bradykinin, leukotriene B_4, platelet-activating factor, and small amounts of IL-1 and tumor necrosis factor (TNF) produced at the site of insult. The last two cytokines upregulate the expression and increase the avidity of selectin and integrin receptors on the surface of the endothelium, thereby facilitating extravasation of leukocytes from the bloodstream (Shikama et al. 1989; Issekutz 1993a,b; Lukacs et al. 1994b).

To produce a manifest DTH, further amplification of this initial inflammatory reaction is necessary. The subsequent quality of the DTH response therefore largely depends on the cytokines produced by the $CD4^+$ effector cells of either Th1 or Th2 subtype initially recruited to the lesion, and the chemokine cascade that they initiate. It is convenient at this point to distinguish between type 1 and type 2 DTH and granuloma formation, depending on the T-helper cell subset mediating the monocytic inflammation. Although for the most part this chapter summarizes data obtained from in vivo infection models, many of the results reviewed in this section are based on an in vivo model of hypersensitivity granuloma elicitation in which presensitized mice are challenged with beads coated with PPD of *Mycobacterium bovis* (Th1-induced type 1 granulomas) or soluble *Schistosoma mansoni* egg antigens (Th2-induced type 2 granulomas) (Kunkel et al. 1996, 1998).

T-helper 1 cells secrete copious quantities of TNF and IFN-γ capable of attracting additional monocytes and T cells into the lesions, mostly by increasing the binding of these cells to inflamed endothelium (Springer 1994). In particular, TNF and IFN-γ were shown to upregulate intercellular adhesion molecule (ICAM) expression on endothelial cells (Lukacs et al. 1994b), a molecule expressing binding sites for lymphocyte function-associated antigen 1 (LFA-1) (present on lymphocytes) and for complement receptor 3 (present on monocytes). The essential role of TNF and IFN-γ for granuloma initiation and maintenance has been amply demonstrated in many models of infection in which neutralization of TNF and IFN-γ effectively abrogates granuloma formation, or converts it to a Th2 pattern with increased eosinophil infiltration and fibrotic degeneration (Kindler et al. 1989; Amiri et al. 1992; Mastroeni et al. 1992; Joseph and Boros 1993; Chensue et al. 1997b; Smith et al. 1997). The injection of IFN-γ alone is able to induce a lymphocytic and monocytic infiltration (Nathan et al. 1986; Issekutz and Issekutz 1993), and TNF and IFN-γ act synergistically in this respect.

Lymphotoxin (LT), another member of the TNF superfamily synthesized by activated lymphocytes, occurs in a homotrimeric form ($LT\alpha_3$) or a heterotrimeric form ($LT\alpha_1\beta_2$), the latter being membrane bound. While the heterotrimer is probably involved in the direct activation of macrophages (Ehlers et al. 2003), $LT\alpha_3$ is necessary for establishing the proper architecture of the granuloma, because, in the absence of $LT\alpha_3$, T cells do not migrate into the granulomatous lesion, but only accumulate in perivascular cuffs (Roach et al. 2001).

The structural organization of type 1 granulomas involves elaboration of specific chemokines and induction of specific chemokine receptors on target cells. TNF and $LT\alpha_3$ orchestrate the early induction of chemokines necessary for initial leukocyte recruitment and thus facilitate granuloma initiation (Roach et al. 2001, 2002), e.g. TNF and lymphotoxins are major inducers of the chemokine CCL5, and IFN-γ and TNF synergize in eliciting CCL5 from endothelial cells (Marfaing-Koka et al. 1995). CCL5 attracts activated or memory Th1 cells, bearing the cognate receptor CCR5, into inflammatory lesions. IFN-γ induces the chemokines CXCL9, CXCL10, and CXCL11, which in turn attract effector Th1 cells bearing the common receptor for these chemokines, CXCR3 (Matsukawa et al. 2001). When newly recruited monocytes become activated and differentiate into epithelioid cells, they are also capable of secreting chemokines, e.g. CCL2, that further attract and activate monocytes (Matsushima et al. 1988; Zachariae et al. 1990). Therefore, when the receptor for CCL2 (CCR2) is absent, type-1 granuloma formation is impaired (Boring et al. 1997). Multinucleated giant cells probably also participate in amplifying the type 1 granulomatous response, because transcripts for TNF, IL-1β, IL-6 were detected in single cells generated in vitro (Seitzer et al. 1997) or analyzed in vivo (Myatt et al. 1994).

Nitric oxide (NO) is probably involved in the termination of the Th1 granulomatous response: NO, produced by the IFN-γ-inducible enzyme nitric oxide synthase (2NOS-2), inhibits type 1 granuloma size and cellularity, particularly with respect to eosinophils and neutrophils, by modulating chemokine (CCL2, CCL3, CXCL10) as well as TNF and IFN-γ expression (Hogaboam et al. 1997; Ehlers et al. 1999).

T-helper 2 cells orchestrate the development of a different kind of granuloma. IL-4 leads to a significant increase in cellularity, size, procollagen type III expression, and accumulation of eosinophils (even in preexisting Th1 granulomas). In addition, endothelial cells may become activated by IL-4 and secrete CCL7 which also induces the recruitment of eosinophils (Shang et al. 2002). IL-4, in the presence of TNF, can induce CCL2 and CCR2 expression in fibroblasts. CCL2 is involved in fibrosis through the regulation of profibrotic cytokines, e.g. transforming growth factor β (TGF-β), and the generation and deposition of a collagen matrix (Hogaboam et al. 1999). Fibroblasts from type 2 granulomas generate more CCL2 than Th1 fibroblasts. Generally speaking, CCL2, CCL7, and CCL8 are more involved in type 2 than in type 1 inflammation (Chensue et al. 1996; Qiu et al. 2001). Likewise, CCL11 (eotaxin) and CCR3 (eotaxin receptor) levels are higher in Th2 than in Th1 granulomas. CCR8 (the receptor for CCL1, CCL4, and CCL17 also found predominantly in type 2 granulomas) is exclusively expressed on Th2 cells and contributes to a functional Th2 granuloma, because, in its absence, there is impaired IL-5 production and eosinophil recruitment (Chensue et al. 2001).

Whereas NOS-2 dominates Th1 immune reactions, arginase is predominantly expressed in Th2 responses and is responsible for fibrosis in type 2 granulomas (Hesse et al. 2001). Arginase production is mediated by IL-13 and regulated by substrate depletion through Th1-induced NOS-2 activity (Rutschman et al. 2001).

It is already obvious from the above that there is extensive opportunity for crossregulation between these two pathways of granuloma formation (Matsukawa et al. 2001), e.g. Th2 cells may – via the secretion of IL-10, IL-4, and IL-13 – effectively diminish a Th1 response by downregulating IL-12, IFN-γ, TNF, and chemokine production in Th1 cells (Ruth et al. 2000). In contrast, the type 1 cytokine IL-12 dramatically reduces type 2 lesion size, primarily curtailing eosinophil recruitment (Chensue et al. 1997a). In the absence of IL-4, type 1 inflammation is exacerbated, but an established Th2 granuloma will not convert to a Th1 granuloma, because persistent expression of IL-13, IL-5, and CCL7 can compensate for the defect (Chensue et al. 1997a). CCL5 promotes the Th1 response and mediates crossregulatory inhibition of type 2 granulomas (Chensue et al. 1999). However, chemokines influence granuloma formation not only through a direct effect on leukocyte chemotaxis, but also through altering the Th1/Th2 cytokine balance, e.g. CCL2 promotes IL-4 production by T cells and inhibits IFN-γ production by Th1 cells (Hogaboam et al. 1998, 1999), and CCL5 downregulates IL-4, IL-5, IL-10, and IL-13 production by Th2 cells (Chensue et al. 1999).

It is a hallmark of the T-cell-mediated granulomatous inflammation that it is qualitatively different from an acute inflammatory reaction, particularly in terms of its dependence on adhesion co-receptors, for example, although the acute myelomonocytic infiltrate that occurs in response to infection with *Listeria monocytogenes* (an intracellular bacterium causing granulomatosis infantiseptica) can be experimentally abrogated by administration of monoclonal antibodies to CD11b (an integrin, part of the complement receptor 3 complex), T-cell-mediated granuloma formation is completely independent of this molecule (Mielke et al. 1989, 1997). Certain tissue selectivities also exist, e.g. recruitment of Th1 cells into the skin is dependent on E- and P-selectin ligands on T cells, whereas this probably does not hold true for homing into other organs (Smithson et al. 2001; Erdmann et al. 2002).

Some textbooks include, among DTH reactions, a form that is mediated by $CD8^+$ cytotoxic cells. These cells are induced during a primary immune response by MHCI presentation of proteasome-processed antigens derived from the cytosol. During the effector phase, these specific $CD8^+$ cells are capable of lysing infected cells, thereby causing tissue damage. As a result of this, and because these cells produce limited amounts of IFN-γ in response to antigen stimulation, they have also been defined as TC1 $CD8^+$ cells (Sad et al. 1995). Although these cells may contribute to the extent of DTH, the overwhelming evidence suggests that no skin DTH, and indeed no T-cell-dependent granuloma formation can occur without the active participation of $CD4^+$ cells, and that specific $CD8^+$ cells alone are incapable of initiating a granulomatous response (Mielke et al. 1988, 1992), at least in response to bacterial infections. TC1 cells clearly represent an important mechanism in combating viral infections and can be associated with significant T-cell-mediated tissue damage, but this takes the form of direct tissue cytotoxicity with subsequent extravasation of granulocytes to clear the debris, rather than the form of classic DTH described above with predominantly mononuclear cell infiltration and fibrin deposition.

Functions of granulomatous inflammation

Extracellular bacteria are ingested and killed by polymorphonuclear leukocytes, leading to abscess formation. Microorganisms that can survive intracellularly require a different strategy for their elimination or containment. The structure of a granuloma, with microbe-bearing macrophages at the center surrounded by T cells, affords a close cooperation of these specialized cells. T cells, by secreting macrophage-activating molecules such as IFN-γ or TNF, or via contact-dependent mechanisms such as granule exocytosis, reprogram the macrophage for bactericidal and bacteriostatic functions (Stenger and Modlin 1999; Ehrt et al. 2001). Conversely, macrophages and dendritic cells secreting cytokines and presenting antigens stimulate and select the type of T cell that ultimately decides the fate of the infectious lesion. Microorganisms may cause macrophage death by apoptosis or necrosis, and the removal of dead and dying cells and their replacement with freshly activated macrophages is a dynamic process guaranteed by the antigen-stimulated T cells in close proximity (Adams 1976).

In addition, the concept of physically walling off the offending organisms within a granuloma appears attractive, particularly when large parasites are involved. According to this view, granulomas would serve to contain microorganisms within a separate compartment, the perigranulomatous fibrotic reaction sealing off indigestible bacteria or parasites and preventing dissemination when macrophages burst or decay. In this secluded compartment, cytotoxic T cells may even lyse exhausted or ineffective macrophages in order to release bacteria that may subsequently be engulfed by newly recruited, activated macrophages, the granulomatous capsule preventing leakage into lymphatic or blood vessels (Kaufmann 1988; Saunders and Cooper 2000; Collins and Kaufmann 2001b). The granuloma is thus viewed as a local inflammatory reaction to prevent systemic sequelae of immune activation. Although this hypothesis has its merits, granulomas – like other tissues – are vascularized and may therefore not have the formidable barrier function ascribed to them. However, when a granuloma becomes entirely fibrotic or calcifies, complete sequestration of enclosed microorganisms is probably achieved.

DTH and pathology

Granulomatous inflammation, although necessary for containment of the infectious burden, displaces parenchymal tissue, thereby impairing organ function, such as pulmonary compliance and hepatic blood circulation. The extent of this damage depends on the size and exact location of the granulomas, and may remain undetected for long periods of time, e.g. when present in the mesenteric lymph nodes, yet cause rapid neurological defects when affecting the spinal cord.

One of the most severe forms of pathology associated with DTH is known as the Koch phenomenon, i.e. T-cell-mediated granuloma necrosis in response to mycobacterial antigens. When Robert Koch injected *M. tuberculosis*-infected guinea-pigs with a crude extract of *M.*

tuberculosis (old tuberculin) intradermally, he noted sloughing of the skin at the injection site as well as necrosis at original sites of *M. tuberculosis* implantation in the lung (Koch 1890). Tuberculin in non-sensitized guinea-pigs did not cause this pathology. Koch immediately proposed that this finding be put to clinical use in the diagnosis and therapy of tuberculosis (TB). The former is still in use today in the form of the diagnostic DTH reaction with appropriate doses of more purified protein extracts of *M. tuberculosis* cultures (see Figure 35.1, p. 706); the latter dismally failed when inappropriately high amounts were applied in severe cases of pulmonary TB, effectively killing patients because of the hyperinflammatory tissue necrosis that was induced. As pulmonary granuloma caseation and cavitation represent the detrimental outcome of a type 1 DTH reaction, we have termed this 'type 1 DTH-associated pathology' (Figure 35.3).

Another typical form of T-cell-mediated tissue damage caused by DTH is granuloma fibrosis. In chronic schistosomiasis, it is the vigorous granulomatous response, aggravated by fibrosis, rather than any toxicity of the parasite itself, that is responsible for the severe hepatic scarification and liver malfunction characteristic of this disease. As unrestrained granuloma fibrosis represents the detrimental outcome of a type 2 DTH reaction, we have termed this 'type 2 DTH-associated-pathology' (Figure 35.3). These two prototype pathological sequelae of a specific T-cell response are now described in more detail in terms of the cells and mediators involved. It should be noted, however, that these two types of pathology can overlap to a considerable extent, and that the complete dissociation as described below is merely an idealization for didactic purposes.

TYPE 1 DTH-ASSOCIATED PATHOLOGY: GRANULOMA NECROSIS DURING TUBERCULOSIS

Clinical manifestations of tuberculosis

Approximately one-third of the world population is infected with the causative agent of TB, *Mycobacterium tuberculosis*. Of infected individuals 90 percent will not develop any overt signs of disease throughout their lifetime, attesting to the potency of innate resistance and acquired immunity against TB. Five percent of those infected will come down with primary progressive TB within months of infection, and another 5 percent of those infected will develop post-primary, reactivating disease after a long period of 'latency', i.e. disease-free

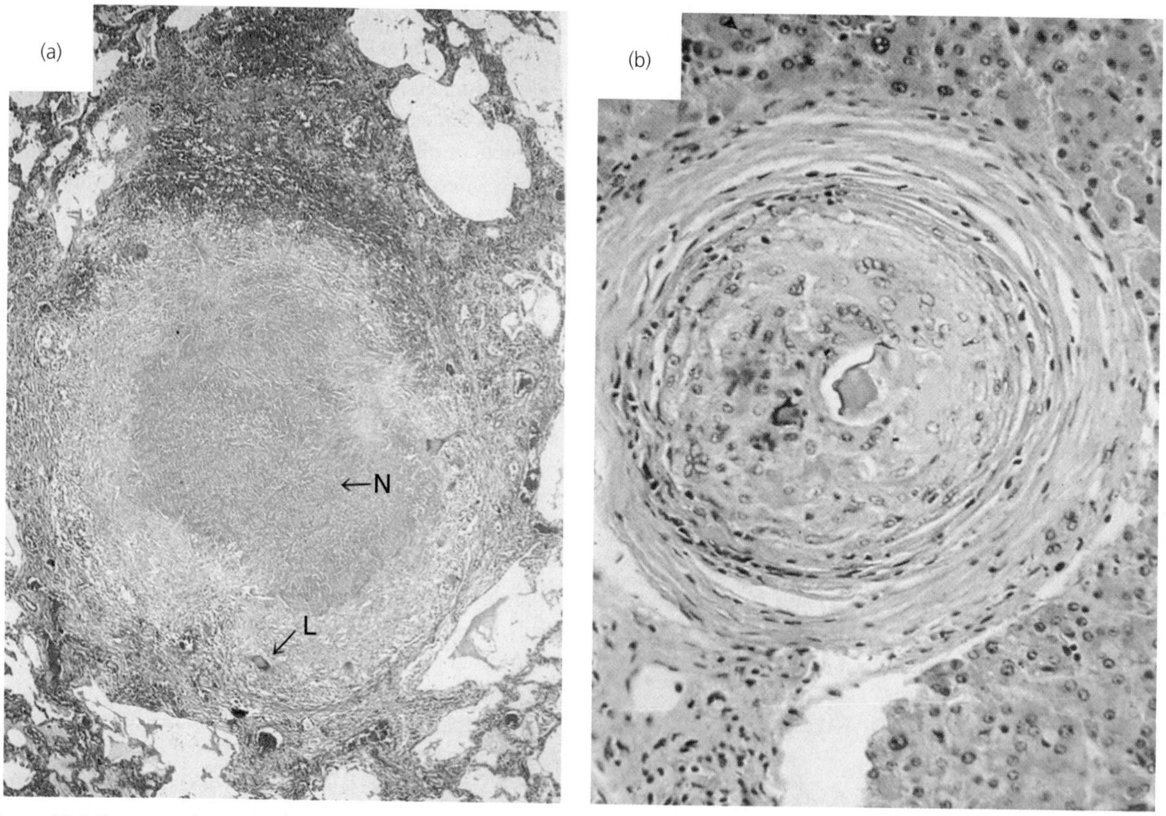

Figure 35.3 *Type 1 and type 2 DTH-associated pathology:* **(a)** *necrotizing granuloma in the lung of* Mycobacterium tuberculosis*-infected patient (type 1 pathology); N, necrosis; L, Langhans' giant cell;* **(b)** *fibrotic granuloma surrounding parasite egg in the liver of* Schistosoma mansoni*-infected patient (type 2 pathology). (Photographs reproduced with permission from C. Thomas et al. (eds),* Infektionskrankheiten, *copyright 1991, Schattauer Verlag.)*

persistence of primary foci containing viable, nonreplicating mycobacteria. Each year, there are approximately 8 million new cases of TB world wide, and 1.8 million individuals will succumb to the disease, making TB the most deadly bacterial infection (World Health Organization 2002).

Tuberculosis is a systemic disease that becomes manifest most prominently in the lung. Prolonged episodes of fever, night sweats, chest or pleuritic pain, and pleural effusions are the most common initial symptoms of disease. Polymorphous pulmonary infiltrates appear soon after infection, are frequently restricted to one lung lobe, and are often associated with hilar lymphadenopathy. Progressive primary TB occurs when the initial inflammatory focus is unable to contain mycobacterial replication and the disease spreads to other parts of the lung, most often to the lower lung fields. Cough with variable amounts of sputum is the typical symptom, but dyspnea, chest discomfort, fever, chills, and weight loss also occur. Lung consolidation on chest radiographs is confluent and extensive, and single cavities may develop.

Post-primary disease develops when a lesion containing a previously 'dormant' organism reactivates. This organism may have been implanted years before during a primary infection that was successfully contained by the host's immune defenses. Reactivation is a consequence of a perturbed immune status of the host, i.e. old age, suboptimal nutrition, or therapy with immunosuppressive drugs. Disease onset is insidious and accompanied by cough and purulent sputum. Symptoms may range from weight loss, fatigue, and low-grade temperature to acute onset with fever, night sweats, and productive cough. Purulent-appearing sputum is produced whenever granuloma necrosis occurs. Some patients may present with hemoptysis, i.e. coughing of blood as a result of ulceration of granulation tissue or cavity vessels.

During primary infection, small numbers of *M. tuberculosis* invariably gain access to the circulation via the lymphatics and embolize to the capillary beds of most organ systems, e.g. liver, spleen, marrow, and brain. Almost always these metastatic foci heal by granulomatous encapsulation, sometimes with calcification, and with little tissue necrosis. Reactivation later in life may lead to localized extrapulmonary TB.

Miliary TB (so termed because of the gross appearance of the affected organ, 'covered with firm small white corpuscles, of the size of millet seeds' – Manget 1700) represents the unchecked hematogenous dissemination, either during primary infection or after reactivation of a latent focus of *M. tuberculosis*. This is most often seen in hosts with highly impaired cellular immunity.

Immunology and pathogenesis of disease

Mycobacterium tuberculosis is a slowly replicating acid-fast rod. Infection occurs after inhalation of droplet nuclei of 5 μm or less in diameter coughed up by an infected individual. These nuclei, containing 1–10 bacteria, are deposited in the alveoli where they are ingested by alveolar macrophages. Depending on the genetic resistance of an individual, either no further replication occurs or unchecked growth ensues until the incompetent macrophage is lysed, seeding bacteria to secondary sites and leading to local mediator release (TNF, IL-1, prostaglandins, vasoactive amines) and development of a small inflammatory focus. Digested fragments of mycobacteria are taken up by dendritic cells and transported to the local lymph node, where a specific immune response is initiated (Figure 35.4). TNF, IL-1, IL-6, IL-12, IL-18, and IL-27 are important soluble cofactors in the priming of naïve T cells, and costimulatory accessory molecules on the surface of antigen-presenting cells, such as CD80, direct the development of Th1 effector cells (Swain 2001; Colombo and Trinchieri 2002; Heath et al. 2002; Pflanz et al. 2002; Robinson and O'Garra 2002). Proliferation of T cells is dependent on IL-2, and further maintenance of long-lived memory cells requires IL-15 and IL-23, particularly in the case of $CD8^+$ cells (Umemura et al. 2001; Frucht 2002).

Circulating antigen-specific T cells home to sites of antigen deposition where $CD4^+$ cells cause granuloma formation. These 'tubercles' (literally: little hard nodes) are the hallmark of all mycobacterial infections (Figure 35.5). At this stage, depending on the bacterial load and the magnitude of the acquired immune response, either infection may be contained or growth and spreading of mycobacteria continue. In most cases, macrophages become sufficiently activated to kill mycobacteria, and tubercles undergo fibrosis and calcification, effectively sealing off the few remaining viable mycobacteria, usually for the lifetime of the host.

Protective immunity involves the secretion of IFN-γ by effector T cells which activates macrophages for bacteriostatic and bactericidal functions (Flynn and Ernst 2000; Shtrichman and Samuel 2001). These include the maturation and acidification of the phagolysosome, the deprivation of nutrients, as well as the generation of oxygen and nitrogen radicals, but the ultimate mechanisms of killing mycobacteria are poorly understood. This is particularly true for human macrophages in which even activation by TNF and IFN-γ results, at best, in bacteriostasis. Alternate mechanisms have therefore been invoked, such as T-cell-induced apoptosis of macrophages, the granule-mediated lysis of macrophages by T cells and killing of mycobacteria by granulysin contained in the granules, and the requirement for additional costimuli, such as CD40 ligand engagement or vitamin D_3 (Mazzaccaro et al. 1998; Stenger et al. 1999; Cho et al. 2000; Collins and Kaufmann 2001b; Hogan et al. 2001). On the other hand, TGF-β (produced in significant quantities within tuberculous lesions) undermines host immune responses, because it promotes T-cell suppression, macrophage deactivation, and tissue

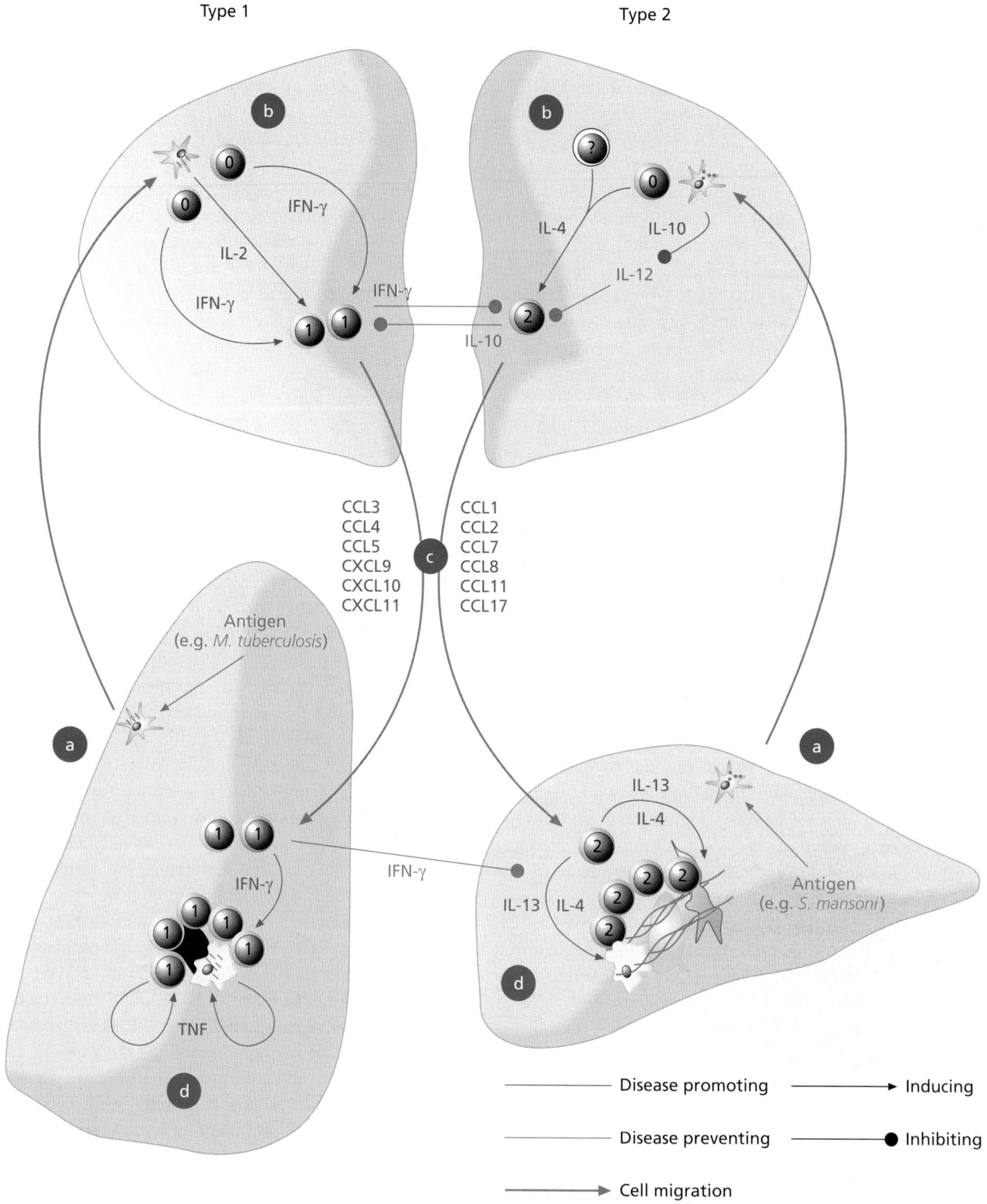

Figure 35.4 *Mechanisms of granuloma formation:* **(a)** *antigen uptake and activation of dendritic cells in infected tissue, e.g. lung or liver;* **(b)** *priming of specific T cells in draining lymph node;* **(c)** *cell recruitment of specific T cells into infected tissue by chemokines; and* **(d)** *granuloma formation and effector response of T cells in infected tissue. 0=Th0, 1=Th1, 2=Th2. For details, see text.*

destruction (Toossi and Ellner 1998). In the absence of significant immunity, i.e. in infants and immunodeficient adults, there is progressive spread with tuberculous pneumonia or miliary TB.

In the face of developing immunity and high antigenic load, there is frequently necrosis of macrophages at the center of the granulomas. Within these necrotic areas, mycobacteria are located extracellularly and do not replicate well. When the necrotic center of a granuloma liquefies, a cavity is formed and multiplication of *M. tuberculosis* resumes. When bronchial erosion occurs, the infective material may disseminate through the

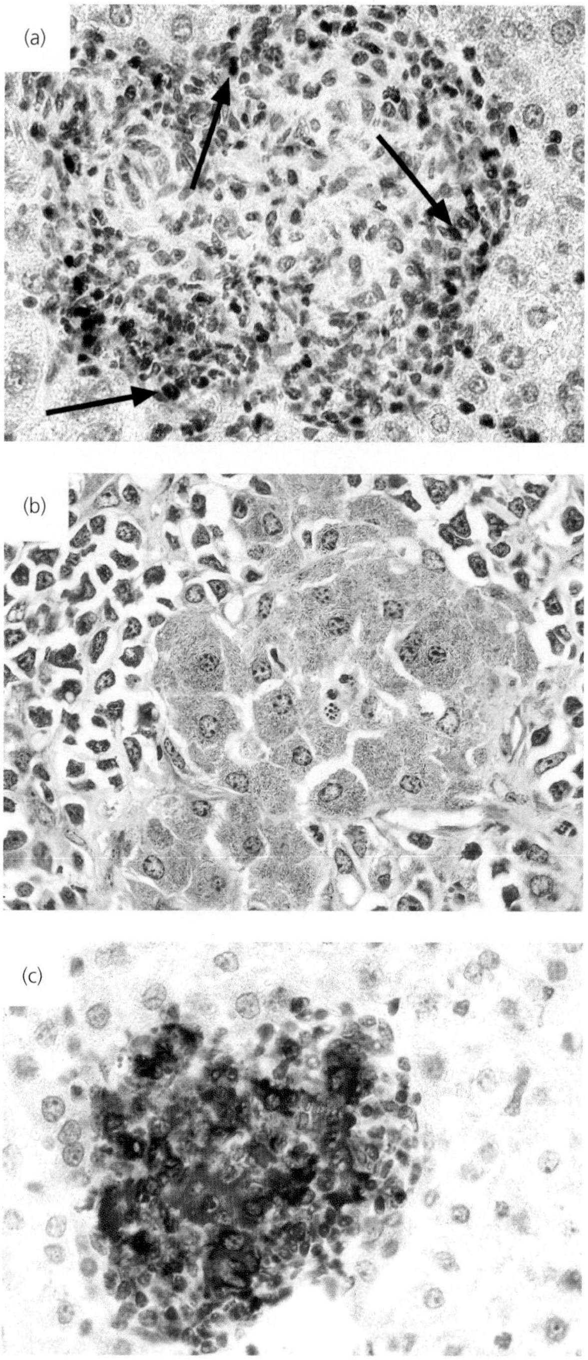

Figure 35.5 *Immunohistopathology of a* mycobacteria-*induced granuloma.* **(a)** *CD3⁺ (T) cells (in dark brown, arrows) at the periphery of an epithelioid granuloma;* **(b)** *acid-fast bacteria (red rods) located exclusively within macrophages at the center of a granuloma, surrounded by lymphocytes with a dense nucleus; and* **(c)** *NOS-2⁺ cells (macrophages, in brown) at the center of an epithelioid granuloma.*

airways to other sites in the lung or may be coughed up, creating infectious aerosols.

In those cases in which T-cell immunity is grossly impaired (e.g. in patients with AIDS), rapid growth of mycobacteria results in widespread tissue necrosis without granulomatous encapsulation. This form of nondemarcated tissue necrosis is probably a consequence of the inherent cytotoxic nature of *M. tuberculosis* and must be clearly differentiated from the typical form of granuloma caseation brought about by specific T cells.

Morphology of type 1 DTH-associated pathology

A typical tuberculous lesion is composed of coalescent granulomas, containing epithelioid cells surrounded by a zone of fibroblasts and lymphocytes. In mice, most of the T lymphocytes are of the $CD4^+$ subtype, but in the periphery $CD8^+$ cells also exist (Gonzalez-Juarrero et al. 2001). There is a considerable number of B cells, often arranged as lymphoid follicles, present in mature granulomas. A study using in situ hybridization and immunohistology to analyze cytokines present in human tuberculous lesions showed that granulomas usually stain positive for IL-12p40, IFN-γ, and TNF transcripts and protein, with a minority also showing IL-4 expression (Fenhalls et al. 2000, 2002). IL-4 positive granulomas were always concomitantly positive for IFN-γ, and necrotic granulomas were always positive for TNF.

As a result of macrophage necrosis within the granuloma, caseation is usually present in the centers of these tubercles – so called because of the cheesy appearance when cut by a pathologist's knife (Figure 35.6). Adjacent to the caseous center, a large number of neutrophils are often found. In addition to 'necrosis' as judged by light microscopic evaluation, there is significant apoptosis of both T cells and macrophages in mature granulomas (Fayyazi et al. 2000).

As the lesions progress, more tubercles coalesce to create a confluent area of consolidation. At this stage, the entire area may be converted to a fibrocalcific scar, or the residual caseous debris may become walled off by collagenous connective tissue. However, when the tubercle erodes into a bronchus, drainage transforms it into a cavity (Figure 35.6). Cavitary fibrocaseous TB may affect one, many, or all lobes of both lungs in the form of isolated small tubercles, confluent caseous foci, or large areas of caseation necrosis (Kobzik and Schoen 1994).

Delayed-type hypersensitivity-associated pathology in the form of granuloma necrosis is therefore not only potentially hazardous to the diseased individual, aggravating tissue damage and organ malfunction, but also epidemiologically relevant, because necrosis, liquefaction, and bronchial erosion ultimately favor the spread of viable mycobacteria into the environment in an aerosolized form.

Mechanisms of granuloma necrosis

In order to dissect a process as complex as T-cell-mediated tissue injury, it is imperative to have a reproducible animal model that mimics the pathology occurring in

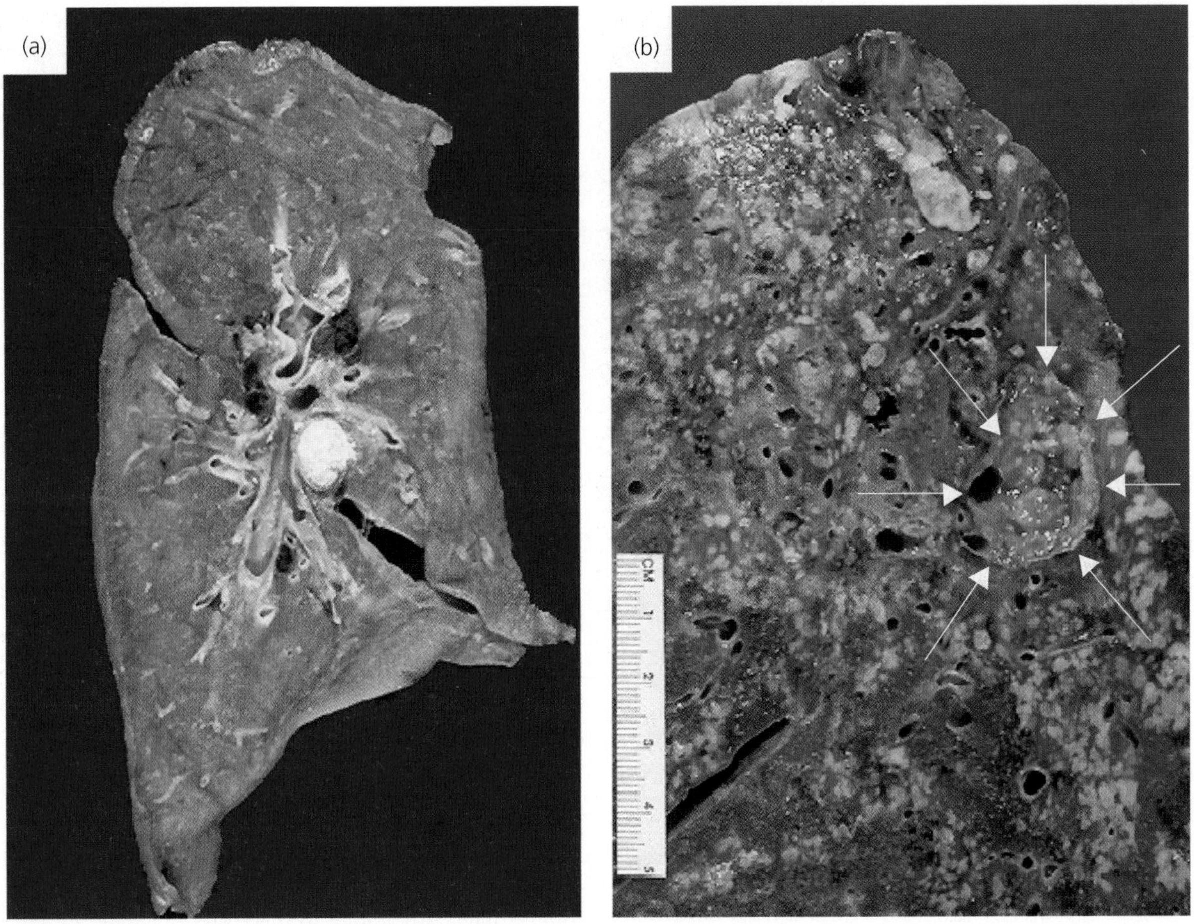

Figure 35.6 *Type 1 pathology: caseous necrosis and cavity formation in the lungs of tuberculosis patients.* **(a)** *Caseating granulomatous lesion in a hilar lymph node.* **(b)** *Extensive caseous necrosis throughout the lung with prominent cavitation (area demarcated by arrows). (Photographs reproduced with permission from Webpath, Version 7, 14 March, 2002, copyright 2002, Edward C. Klatt, MD.)*

humans and allows for a mechanistic study of the factors involved (McMurray et al. 1996).

Aerogenic infections in rabbits faithfully reproduce the pathology present in humans, including liquefaction of caseous necrosis and subsequent cavity formation (Figure 35.7). However, most studies have remained purely descriptive of this phenomenon because immunological reagents are missing to dissect, at the molecular level, the processes underlying granuloma necrosis. A few studies demonstrated that activated macrophages surrounding the caseous center stain positive for β-galactosidase, acid phosphatase, and cathepsin D which may implicate lysosomal enzymes such as proteases, lipases, or nucleases in the liquefaction process (Dannenberg 1968; Dannenberg and Sugimoto 1976; Suga et al. 1980; Converse et al. 1996). Moreover, the endothelial adhesion molecules ICAM-1 and VCAM were found to be preferentially expressed during the chronic stage of infection suggesting their involvement in the granulomatous, rather than acute inflammatory, response (Abe et al. 1996). Aerogenic infections in guinea-pigs also induce caseous necrosis in developing pulmonary granulomas. This is associated with a marked DTH skin response. Again, mechanistic studies on the molecular mediators of tissue necrosis have been lacking because of a paucity of immunological reagents to measure them.

Aerogenic infection in laboratory mice with *M. tuberculosis* is not followed by granuloma necrosis, but is rather associated with chronic interstitial fibrosis (North 1995; Rhoades et al. 1997). However, when mice deficient in the γδ T-cell-receptor (TCR)-positive cell subset are infected, they develop a purulent form of granuloma with many neutrophils infiltrating necrotic areas at the center of the granuloma (D'Souza et al. 1997). Infection with *Listeria monocytogenes* also results in centrally necrotic and purulent granulomas (Mombaerts et al. 1993). These data suggest that γδ T cells perhaps play an important role by influencing local cellular traffic, promoting the influx of lymphocytes and monocytes, and limiting the access of inflammatory cells that do not contribute to protection but may cause tissue damage. Alternately, γδ T cells may produce cytokines and/or chemokines that regulate the potentially harmful effect

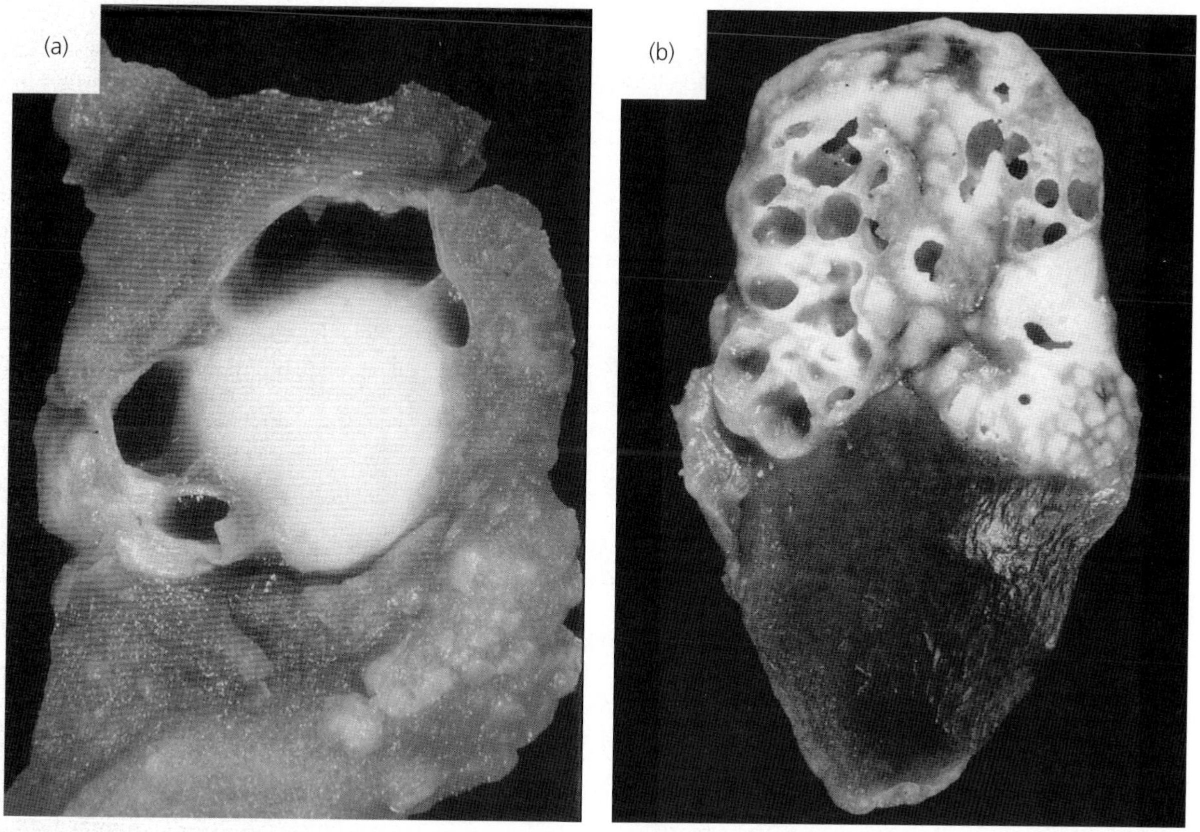

Figure 35.7 *Type 1 pathology in rabbits.* **(a)** *Caseous tubercle at the bifurcation of a bronchus near the hilus in a rabbit after low-dose aerosol infection with* Mycobacterium bovis. **(b)** *Multiloculated cavities in the lungs of aerosol-infected rabbits. (Photographs reproduced with permission from Converse et al. 1996; copyright 1996, The American Society for Microbiology.)*

of a hyperinflammatory Th1 reaction initiated by αβ-TCR$^+$ CD4$^+$ T cells.

Fortuitously, aerogenic infection in mice with a highly virulent strain of *M. avium* (the causative organism of avian TB) results in progressive granuloma caseation with perigranulomatous fibrosis, strongly resembling the pathology occurring in human TB patients (Benini et al. 1999). This model is therefore perfectly suited for the molecular analysis of granuloma necrosis, because immunological tools, such as knock-out mice, may be applied. Using this model, αβ-TCR$^+$ T cells of the CD4$^+$ subset are found to be necessary for granuloma necrosis, whereas γδ-TCR$^+$ cells and CD8$^+$ cells do not contribute (Figure 35.8) (Ehlers et al. 2001). Perforin and apoptotic mechanisms are not required for necrosis in this model (Florido et al. 2002). However, IL-12 and IFN-γ are essential for granuloma necrosis, and in the absence of IL-10 granuloma necrosis is slightly accelerated (Ehlers et al. 2001; Florido et al. 2002). Most interestingly, the absence of NOS-2 does not impact on granuloma necrosis, revealing that IFN-γ-induced mechanisms mostly associated with antibacterial protection (such as induction of NOS-2) need not necessarily coincide with mechanisms that lead to tissue destruction (Ehlers et al. 2001). It was hypothesized that IFN-γ may preferentially induce a variety of chemokines with anti-angiogenic effects, and that reduced vascularization may then lead to granuloma hypoxia and subsequent necrosis, similar to a scenario previously demonstrated in infection-associated tumor regression (Hunter et al. 2001).

Tumor necrosis factor has long been postulated to be directly involved in caseation necrosis, because infection of cells with *M. tuberculosis* rendered them highly sensitive to killing by TNF in vitro (Filley et al. 1992). Moreover, DTH sites were particularly necrosis prone after TNF injection, when small amounts of IL-4 were also present (Hernandez-Pando and Rook 1994; Rook and Zumla 2001). Finally, treatment of *M. tuberculosis*-infected mice with recombinant TNF resulted in increased inflammation in the lungs and accelerated mortality (Moreira et al. 2002).

Studies in *M. tuberculosis*-infected TNF- and TNFRp55-deficient mice are more difficult to interpret, because TNF is necessary for granuloma initiation and maintenance as well as antibacterial protection. TNF-deficient mice will therefore succumb to excessive bacterial loads in a completely necrotic lung, a scenario more reflective of primary progressive TB in immuno-

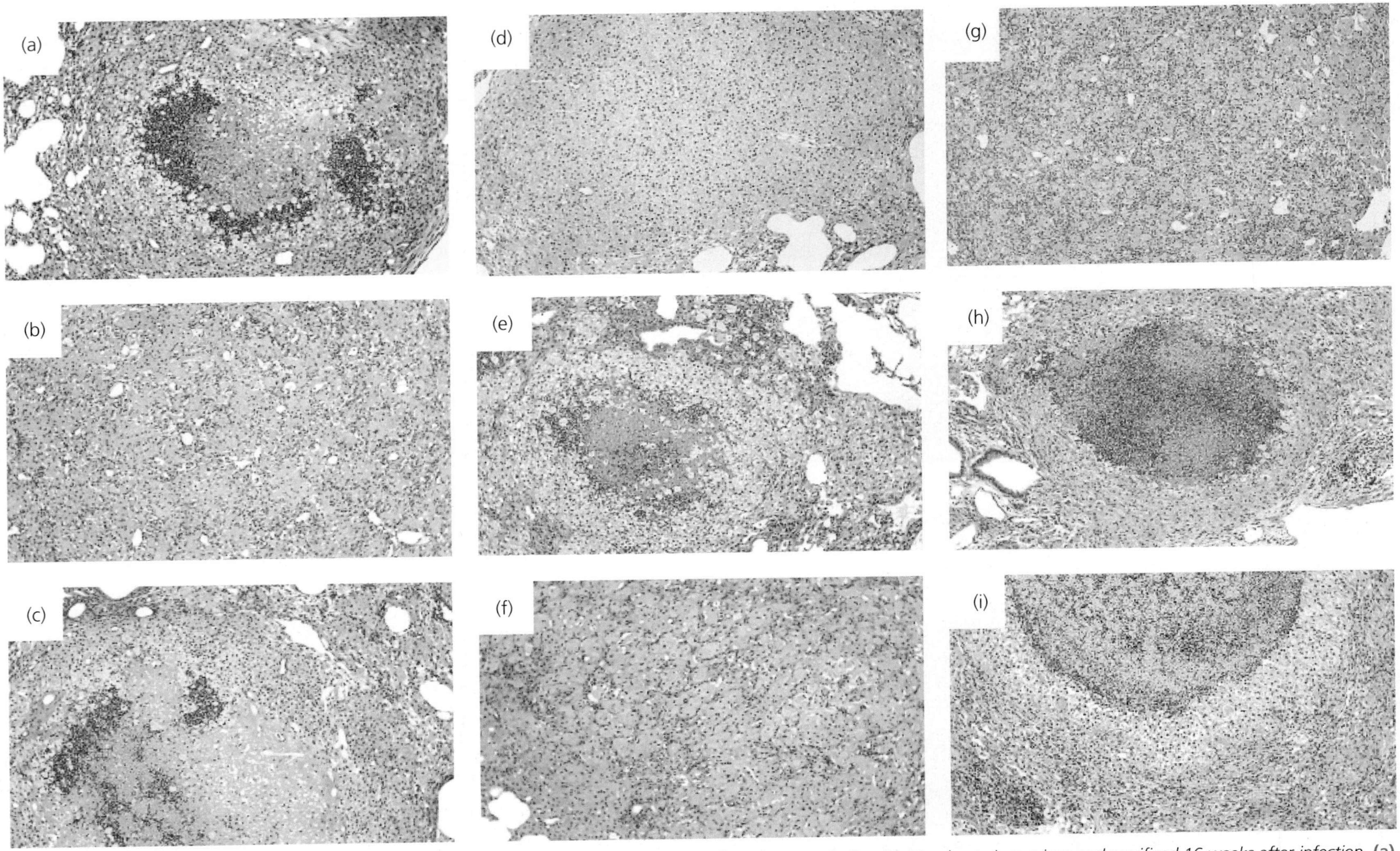

Figure 35.8 *Mechanisms of granuloma necrosis in a mouse model of type 1 pathology. Mice were infected aerogenically with* Mycobacterium avium *and sacrificed 16 weeks after infection.* **(a)** *Centrally necrotizing granulomatous lesion in wild-type mice;* **(b)** *absence of granuloma necrosis in $\alpha\beta$TCR-deficient mice;* **(c)** *centrally necrotizing granuloma in $\gamma\delta$TCR -deficient mice;* **(d)** *absence of granuloma necrosis in MHC class II-deficient mice;* **(e)** *central granuloma necrosis in β_2-microglobulin-deficient mice;* **(f)** *absence of granuloma necrosis in IL-12p40-deficient mice;* **(g)** *absence of centrally necrotizing lesions in IFN-γ-deficient mice;* **(h)** *central granuloma necrosis in IL-10-deficient mice; and* **(i)** *central granuloma necrosis in NOS-2-deficient mice. (Low power micrographs reproduced with permission from Ehlers et al. 2001; copyright 2001, The Rockefeller University Press.)*

deficient individuals (Flynn et al. 1995). Further studies using different microbial challenges, such as *M. avium* and *Corynebacterium parvum*, established that the absence of TNF signaling is associated with an excessive inflammatory response, and (as in the aerosol model of necrosis) is dependent on T cells and IL-12, probably reflecting dysregulated inflammation (Marino et al. 1997; Benini et al. 1999; Ehlers et al. 2000). TNF (and also IFN-γ), possibly via the induction of NOS-2, therefore also serve to downregulate an exacerbated inflammatory response, in part by inducing apoptosis of effector T cells (Kanaly et al. 1999; Chu et al. 2000; Dalton et al. 2000; Cooper et al. 2002).

The frequent presence of granulocytes close to the necrotic center of granulomas is intriguing. It is possible that they act merely as scavengers clearing the debris, but they may also be the source of cytokines and chemokines (such as CXCL9 and CXCL10), amplifying the tissue-damaging loop by recruiting more T cells (Gasperini et al. 1999). Granulocytes may also degranulate, contributing to tissue destruction by a similar mechanism to that postulated for activated macrophages, i.e. the release of aggressive lysosomal proteases and other hydrolyzing enzymes (Dannenberg and Sugimoto 1976).

TGF-β has been implicated in the pathogenesis of many diseases that are associated with tissue destruction and fibrosis (Border and Noble 1994). It promotes the production and deposition of a collagen matrix, but it also increases the production of macrophage collagenases (Wahl et al. 1993). As it is a strong chemotactic molecule for monocytes and polymorphonuclear cells, both of which are rich sources of metalloproteases, TGF-β may be particularly involved in tissue remodeling, with a potential bias towards tissue destruction and scarring (Wahl et al. 1987; Toossi and Ellner 1998).

Finally, degradation of collagen and other matrix proteins is achieved by a family of metalloproteases, which are dependent on zinc ions for their activity (Parks and Shapiro 2001; Brinckerhoff and Matrisian 2002). Metalloproteases comprise: (1) interstitial collagenases, which cleave the fibrillar collagen types I, II, and III; (2) gelatinases, which degrade amorphous collagen as well as fibronectin; (3) stromelysins, which act on a variety of matrix components, including proteoglycans, laminin, fibronectin, and amorphous collagens; and (4) matrilysin, which plays a role in innate immunity of epithelial barriers. These enzymes are produced by several cell types (fibroblasts, macrophages, neutrophils, epithelial cells), and their secretion is induced by many stimuli, including growth factors platelet-derived growth factor (PDGF), fibroblast growth factor (FGF)), cytokines (IL-1, TNF, TGF-β), and phagocytosis. They are elaborated in a latent form that can be activated by oxygen radicals and proteases produced during inflammation, and can be inhibited by specific tissue inhibitors of metalloproteases (TIMP). Degrading collagen is essential in wound repair, and metalloproteases may therefore not only promote, but also alleviate tissue destruction in DTH-associated pathology, depending on the stage of disease (Parks and Shapiro 2001; Winkler and Fowlkes 2002). Macrophage metalloelastase, by cleaving elastin, generates fragments that are chemotactic for monocytes, and may perpetuate macrophage accumulation, leading to progressive and chronic lung destruction (Senior et al. 1980). Table 35.2 summarizes some of the mediators and mechanisms that contribute to granuloma necrosis.

Strategies to reduce granuloma necrosis: Implications for vaccine development

The importance of defining the molecular pathways ultimately causing type 1 DTH-associated pathology is highlighted by the results of recent immunization studies in guinea-pigs. Animals that received a DNA vaccine encoding heat shock protein 60 of *M. tuberculosis* – published as highly efficacious as a therapeutic vaccine (Lowrie et al. 1999) – succumbed to infection significantly earlier than controls showing widespread caseation necrosis in their lungs (Turner et al. 2000). Thus, more immunogenic vaccines simply triggering more of the mediators common to antibacterial protection and granuloma necrosis will inevitably result in more tissue damage, effectively rendering them useless. The trick will be to inhibit, or modulate the pathways involved in DTH-associated pathology while, at the same time, boosting the mechanisms involved in antibacterial protection.

Some investigators have suggested that this may be possible with a careful selection of the antigens in vaccine preparations, i.e. the use of antigens common to all mycobacterial species and avoidance of the species-specific *M. tuberculosis* antigens (Rook and Hernandez-Pando 1996; Rook et al. 2001). Thus far, vaccine and immunotherapy trials have not produced convincing proof of this hypothesis (Durban Immunotherapy Trial Group 1999).

A different strategy is specifically to target $CD8^+$ cells in a vaccine protocol, reducing $CD4^+$ T cell-mediated DTH while possibly exploiting granule-mediated pathways of antibacterial protection (Kaufmann 2000; Stenger and Modlin 1998; Stenger et al. 1998; Collins and Kaufmann 2001a). Given the uncertainty concerning the true level of protection $CD8^+$ T cells afford in vivo against *M. tuberculosis* challenge, this approach may be only part of the solution (Sousa et al. 2000; Mogues et al. 2001). If it turns out that the distinction between antibacterial protection and tissue damage (in terms of mediators required) is more of a quantitative rather than of a qualitative nature, 'differential vaccination' may be altogether out of reach.

Table 35.2 *Some cellular and molecular mediators of type 1 DTH-associated pathology in tuberculosis*

Cells and molecules	Effect on granuloma necrosis	Putative mechanisms regulating necrosis	Reference
$CD4^+$ T cells	+	Production of IFN-γ	Ehlers et al. (2001); Florido et al. (2002)
$CD8^+$ T cells	?/+	Lysis of infected macrophages	Kaufmann (1988); Stenger and Modlin (1999)
γδ-TCR^+ cells	–	Promoting cellular influx preventing necrosis	D'Souza et al. (1997)
	–	Harnessing αβ-TCR^+ cells	Mombaerts et al. (1993)
CD40	+	Costimulation of T cells	Florido et al. (2002)
IL-12	+	inducing IFN-γ production	Ehlers et al. (2001); Florido et al. (2002)
IL-10	0/–	Inhibiting IFN-γ production	Ehlers et al. (2001); Florido et al. (2002)
IFN-γ	+	Chemokine induction	Ehlers et al. (2001)
	–	Limiting T-cell responses	Dalton et al. (2000)
TNF	+	Apoptosis of sensitized cells	Filley et al. (1992); Rook et al. (2001)
	–	Regulating T-cell responses	Kanaly et al. (1999); Ehlers et al. (2000)
IP-10, MIG	?/+	Antiangiogenic effect	Hunter et al. (2001)
MCP-1	?/+	Recruitment of monocytes	Orme and Cooper (1999)
Nitric oxide	0	No direct effect	Ehlers et al. (2001)
	–	Regulating T-cell responses	Dalton et al. (2000); Cooper et al. (2002)
Lysosomal enzymes	+	Tissue digestion	Dannenberg and Sugimoto (1976)
Metalloproteases	+	Breakdown of connective matrix	Matyszak and Perry (1996)
	–	Repair and fibrosis	Parks and Shapiro (2001)

+, inducing; –, limiting; 0, no effect, ?, effect unknown.
For abbreviations see the text.

TYPE 2 DTH-ASSOCIATED PATHOLOGY: GRANULOMA FIBROSIS IN SCHISTOSOMIASIS

Manifestations of clinical schistosomiasis

Schistosomiasis is a disease of the tropical world. According to the World Health Organization, the disease is endemic in 74 countries, affecting about 200 million people (Pearce and MacDonald 2002). The causative agents are digenic trematode worms, also called blood flukes. Three species are important causes of human infection: *Schistosoma mansoni*, *S. japonicum*, and *S. haematobium*. The adult forms of *S. mansoni* and *S. japonicum* live in the portal and mesenteric veins; *S. haematobium* inhabits the vesical plexus of the bladder. Humans are the principal definitive host during the life cycle of these three species of schistosomes and adult worms live in the venous systems of the intestine. The female worm inhabits a groove in the lateral edge of the male's body and produces from 300 (*S. mansoni*) to 3000 (*S. japonicum*) eggs every day. These eggs pass through the venule walls, cross the intestinal mucosa, find their way into the lumen of the bowel, and are excreted with the feces (Figure 35.9). In fresh water, the eggs hatch and release motile ciliated miracidia which penetrate the body of the intermediate host, usually a snail of the genus *Biomphalaria* (*S. mansoni*) or *Oncomelania* (*S. japonicum*). The miracidia multiply asexually inside the snail; within a few weeks, hundreds of motile fork-tailed cercariae emerge. When the cercariae encounter human skin they penetrate it, lose their tails, and change into schistosomula forms, which migrate to the lungs and liver. In approximately 6 weeks they mature into adult worms and pass through the venous system to their final habitat. The life span of the worm is 5–10 years, and by a variety of mechanisms it is capable of evading the host immune response. The worms feed on host erythrocytes and body solutes, and their presence is innocuous to the host. Some of the eggs deposited by the females into the bloodstream are excreted with the feces. However, eggs that do not reach the intestinal lumen are swept into the portal circulation and are trapped in the intestinal wall, the liver, or the lung. This continuous egg deposition induces a chronic granulomatous response in the host that is responsible for the major disease syndrome of chronic schistosomiasis.

The two main clinical conditions, acute and chronic schistosomiasis, are associated with different immune responses. Acute schistosomiasis in humans is a debilitating febrile illness that can occur before the appearance of schistosoma eggs in the feces and which peaks

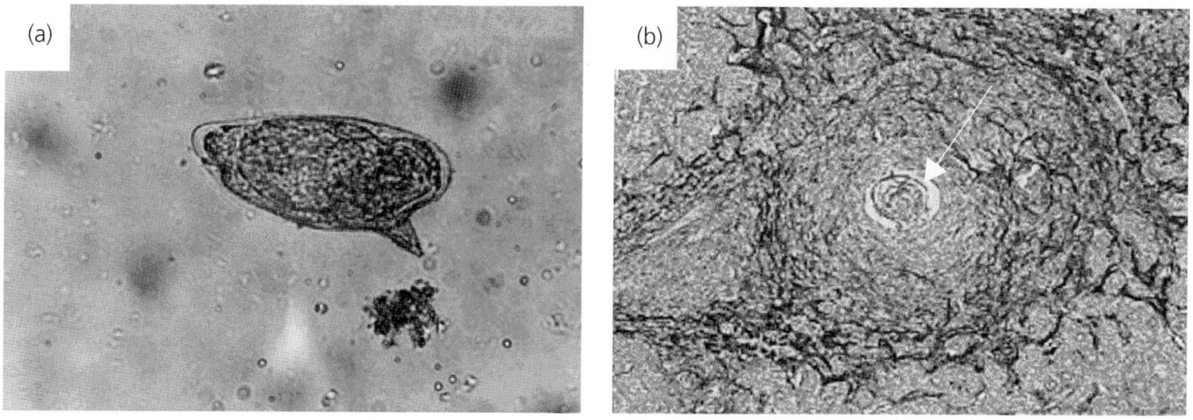

Figure 35.9 *Type 2 pathology:* Schistosoma mansoni-*induced hepatic fibrosis.* **(a)** S. mansoni *egg isolated from hepatic granulomas.* **(b)** *Hepatic granuloma surrounding deposited egg (arrow). Fibrosis in liver section is detected by aniline blue staining. (Micrograph in* **(a)** *reproduced with permission from the Microbiology Laboratory Reference Center Homepage, UT Southwestern Medical Center Dallas, Texas, USA, copyright 2002, Jerry Y. Niederkorn, PhD; micrograph in* **(b)** *reproduced with permission from the Laboratory of Parasitic Diseases Homepage, NIAID, Bethesda, Maryland, USA, copyright 2002, Alan Sher, PhD.)*

generally between 6 and 8 weeks after infection (Rabello 1995). In chronic schistosomiasis, there is a progressive increase in egg burden which affects primarily the intestines and liver. Antigenic properties of the parasite induce a strong immune response resulting in granuloma formation and fibrosis around the eggs in these organs (Figure 35.9). This may result in portal hypertension, massive splenomegaly, and gastrointestinal bleeding from esophageal varices. Patients experience fatigue, abdominal pain, and diarrhea, and in the most severe cases jaundice and liver failure. Occasionally eggs may bypass the liver via the portosystemic collateral circulation and give rise to granulomas in the lung, with pulmonary hypertension and cor pulmonale, or lesions in the brain or spinal cord, which may present as space-occupying lesions, generalized encephalopathy, or transverse myelitis. The severity of the disease directly correlates with the number of eggs present in the tissues. The liver sustains the most severe damage in chronic schistosomiasis, because the chronic granulomatous inflammation results in severe fibrosis which accumulates over the long period of the disease.

Immunology and pathogenesis of schistosomiasis

Schistosomiasis causes a range of illnesses, the development of which is influenced to a large extent by the nature of the induced immune response and its effects on granuloma formation and associated pathologies in target organs (Boros 1999; Dunne and Pearce 1999; Cheever et al. 2000). Host genetics, parasite burden, and sensitization to schistosoma antigens all influence the development of the immune response and, thus, disease severity.

In contrast to early studies showing the participation of eosinophils and IgE in in vitro killing of *S. mansoni* larvae in antibody-dependent cellular cytotoxicity (ADCC) reactions (Romagnani 1996), in vivo studies employing mouse models argue against a function of IgE and eosinophils and support a role for Th1 responses in protection against *S. mansoni* (de Andres et al. 1997; King et al. 1997). During the larval migration and maturation period, resistance is dependent on $CD4^+$ T cells and is associated with a Th1 cytokine response (Vignali et al. 1989; Sher et al. 1990). In particular, IL-12-induced IFN-γ is mandatory for resistance after immunization with irradiated parasites (Smythies et al. 1992; Wilson et al. 1996; Anderson et al. 1998). IFN-γ-activated macrophages and endothelial cells kill larval schistosomes in vitro via an arginine-dependent mechanism involving NO production (James and Glaven 1989; Oswald et al. 1994). In vivo, most parasites are eliminated as they traverse the lungs of immunized mice (Dean and Mangold 1992; Wilson et al. 1996) and NOS-2 can be identified in the pulmonary inflammatory foci around the migrating larvae (Wynn et al. 1994). Moreover, larvacidal properties of NO represent an important effector mechanism because NOS-2-deficient mice display a reduced resistance to *S. mansoni* challenge (James et al. 1998).

Some Th2 effector mechanisms, however, also contribute to protection against *S. mansoni*. In particular, IL-4Rα-mediated signaling by IL-4 and IL-13 participates in the development of immunity. In immunization studies, the defective Th2-type antibody response (i.e. no IgG1 or IgE) in IL-4Rα-deficient mice was associated with increased parasite loads which could be partially prevented by serum transfer (Mountford et al. 2001). As IgE has no protective role against challenge with *S. mansoni* (King et al. 1997; de Andres et al. 1997), protection is probably associated with the IgG1 antibody subclass.

In chronic schistosomiasis, the pathology is predominantly caused by the host reaction to parasite eggs, which are laid in the portal venous system and subsequently trapped in the liver and intestine (Cheever

1972). Although Th2 responses have a beneficial role in modulating potentially life-threatening disease during the initial stages of schistosomiasis, prolonged Th2 responses are responsible for the development of egg-induced hepatic fibrosis and chronic morbidity (Cheever et al. 2000). Even though IL-4 is the primary cytokine driving the differentiation of $CD4^+$ T cells into the Th2 subset, fibrotic pathology in schistosomiasis is not ameliorated in IL-4-deficient mice (Wynn et al. 1993; Cheever et al. 1994; Metwali et al. 1996; Pearce et al. 1996; Chensue et al. 1997b). However, granuloma formation and fibrosis do depend on IL-4Rα-mediated signaling (Kaplan et al. 1996, 1998). As IL-4 and IL-13 share the IL-4Rα as a common receptor component and both activate the Stat6 signaling pathway (Brombacher 2000; Hölscher 2003), pathology in chronic schistosomiasis is a result of IL-13-mediated mechanisms. *Schistosoma*-infected mice in which IL-13 is either neutralized by treatment with soluble IL-13Rα_2-Fc (Chiaramonte et al. 1999a) or absent (IL-13-deficient mice) (Fallon et al. 2000) fail to develop the severe hepatic fibrosis – marked by extensive collagen deposition – that normally occurs during infection, and survive longer (Figure 35.10). Th2 responses are maintained in IL-13-deficient animals, and blocking IL-13 in IL-4-deficient mice does not perturb the Th1/Th2 cytokine balance (Chiaramonte et al. 1999a; Fallon et al. 2000). However, fibrosis is maximally reduced in these mice, again emphasizing the important role played by IL-13 in fibrogenesis.

Given its critical role in fibrosis, differences in the expression of IL-13 could provide a simple explanation for the different degrees of fibrosis that different inbred mouse strains develop after infection with *S. mansoni* (Cheever et al. 1987). However, there is no correlation between the expression of IL-13 and the severity of fibrosis in these strains (Chiaramonte et al. 2001). On the other hand, IFN-γ and IL-10 are key regulatory cytokines in fibrosis (Czaja et al. 1989; Hoffmann et al. 2000; Louis et al. 2000; Nelson et al. 2000; Chiaramonte et al. 2001). In schistosomiasis, the antifibrotic effects of the Th1 cytokine IFN-γ are well documented (Czaja et al. 1989; Wynn et al. 1995). IFN-γ directly downregulates the synthesis of extracellular matrix components (Stephenson et al. 1985), and the IL-13:IFN-γ ratio is predictive of the magnitude of fibrosis (Chiaramonte et al. 2001). In humans, severe hepatic fibrosis correlates with a mutation in the IFN-γR1 (Dessein et al. 1999), and can be explained by the lack of effective suppression of fibrogenesis by IFN-γ. High IL-13 and low IL-10 levels are also predictive of severe fibrosis in inbred mice, whereas inbred mice displaying a low IL-13:IL-10 ratio tend to develop a more modest degree of fibrosis after infection with *S. mansoni* (Chiaramonte et al. 2001). In summary, the magnitude of fibrosis is controlled by the profibrogenic activities of IL-13 and antifibrotic effects of IFN-γ and IL-10.

Morphology of type 2 pathology

Histological examination of lesions from chronically infected individuals with type 2 pathology shows granulomas to be composed mainly of lymphocytes, macrophages, and eosinophils, exhibiting a wide range of granuloma size around deposited eggs from *S. mansoni* (Boros 1989). The cellular constituents of murine liver granulomas also comprise lymphocytes, plasma cells, macrophages, epithelioid and giant cells, eosinophils, neutrophils, mast cells, and fibroblasts (Stenger et al. 1967; Smith 1977). In particular eosinophils and mast cells produce several Th2-associated cytokines (Sabin et al. 1996; Woerly et al. 1999) and are often described as important effector cells in a variety of Th2-mediated pathological disorders. However, there is no correlation between the magnitude of hepatic fibrosis and the cellular composition of the lesions (Chiaramonte et al. 2001).

In general, the development of fibrous tissue is part of the normal process of healing after injury. Nevertheless, in schistosomiasis, fibrosis enhances the disease pathology and greatly contributes to the mortality after infection with *S. mansoni* (Friedman et al. 2000). Fibrotic changes are ranked on the basis of ultrasound patterns that provide a quantitative tool for assessing the severity of disease (Hatz 2001). After infection with *S. mansoni*, the fibrotic reaction is characterized by collagen deposition and collagen synthesis in fibrotic livers increases up to 40-fold over that of normal livers (Dunn and Kamel 1981). Consequently, type I, type III, and B collagens are found in portal spaces, fibrous septa, and granulomas (Biempica et al. 1983). Hepatic fibrosis is mostly associated with circumoval granulomas (see Figure 35.3b, p. 710, and 35.9) and follows the granulomatous inflammatory response occurring at the site of egg deposition (Dunn et al. 1977; Dunn and Kamel 1981). Total liver collagen production positively correlates with egg load (Cheever et al. 1983), but there is no direct relationship between granuloma size and the degree of fibrosis (Hood and Boros 1980).

In *S. mansoni* infection, cells within hepatic granulomas are potentially harmful to adjacent parenchymal cells, because they are in a metabolically activated state, capable of secreting a number of tissue-destroying substances. During phagocytosis, cell activation, or cell death, these mediators diffuse from the granulomas and damage tissue parenchymal cells. Potential tissue-damaging agents that are released in granulomas are lysozyme, β-glucuronidase, collagenase, elastase, proteases, prostaglandins, leukotrienes, superoxide anions, IL-1, and type 1 interferons (James and Glaven 1989). Indeed, healed granulomas usually leave behind scar tissue in their vicinity, indicating focal damage and repair (Von Lichtenberg 1975).

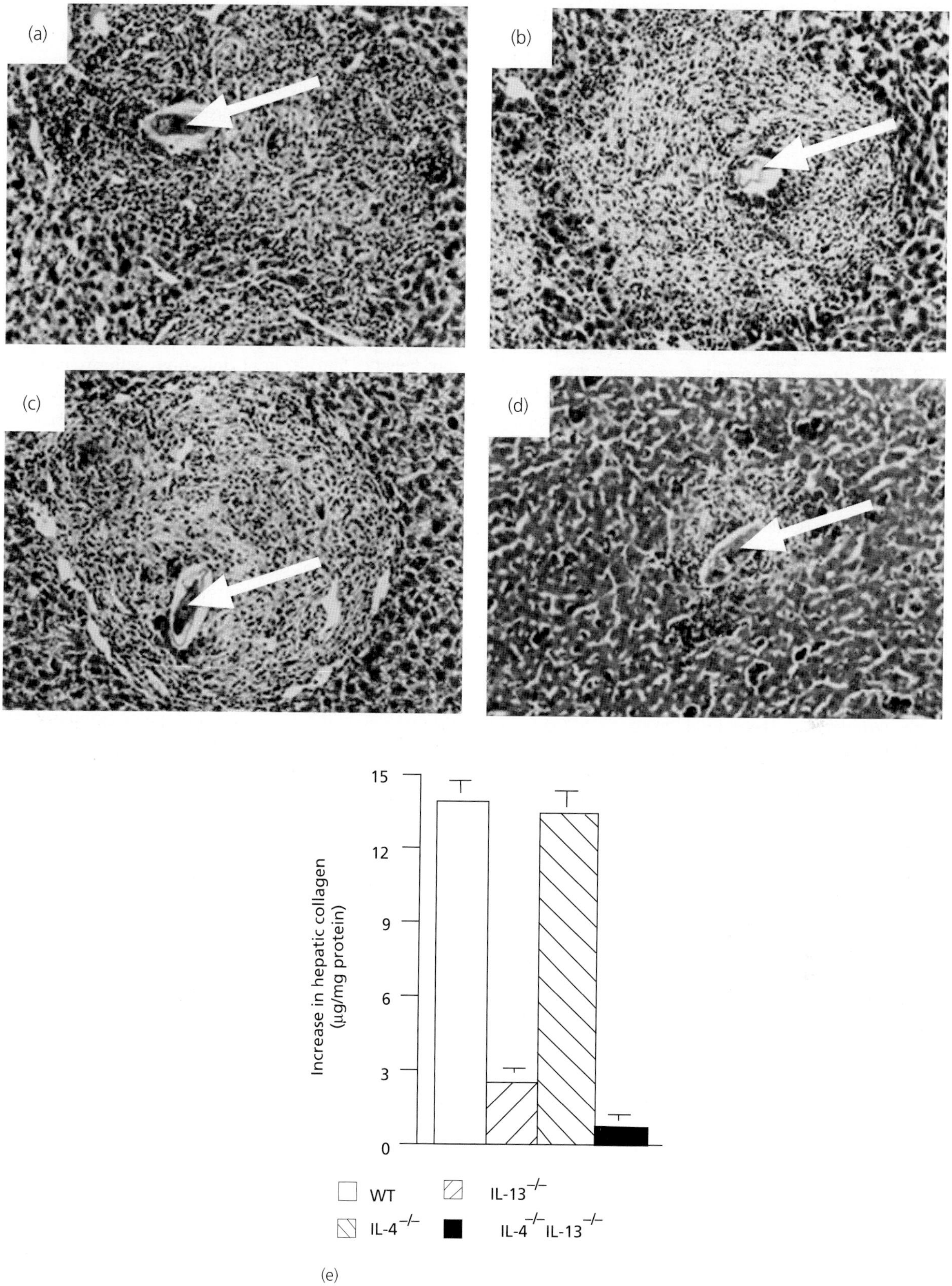

Figure 35.10 *IL-13-mediated type 2 pathology. Mice were infected with* Schistosoma mansoni *and analyzed for hepatic pathology induced by deposited egg (arrow).* **(a)** *Hepatic granuloma in wild-type mice;* **(b)** *hepatic granuloma in IL-4-deficient mice;* **(c)** *hepatic granuloma in IL-13-deficient mice;* **(d)** *reduced granuloma formation in IL-4/IL-13-deficient mice; and* **(e)** *decreased collagen deposition in the absence of IL-13 (tissue collagen in the livers of uninfected and infected mice was quantified and expressed as the increase in hepatic collagen in micrograms of collagen per milligram of protein). (High power micrographs reproduced with permission from Fallon et al. 2000; copyright 2000, The American Association of Immunologists.)*

Mechanisms of granuloma fibrosis in schistosomiasis

The effects of IL-13 on fibrosis are direct and are not dependent on induction of other profibrotic mediators (Lee et al. 2001) or perturbations in the Th1/Th2 cytokine response (Wynn et al. 1995). IL-13 receptors are expressed on fibroblasts (Murata et al. 1998) and IL-13 increases adhesion molecule and inflammatory cytokine expression (Doucet et al. 1998). Moreover, fibroblasts of different origin are able to respond to IL-13 with collagen production (Chiaramonte et al. 1999a; Oriente et al. 2000). Although IL-13 and IL-4 are both capable of promoting collagen production in fibroblasts (Oriente et al. 2000) after infection with *S. mansoni*, expression of IL-13 largely exceeds that of IL-4 (Chiaramonte et al. 1999a). In the pulmonary granuloma model IL-4 is more transiently expressed after egg exposure, whereas expression of IL-13 is much more sustained over time and is observed at greater levels than IL-4 in the granulomatous tissues (Chiaramonte et al. 1999b).

Hepatic fibrosis can be reduced when the *S. mansoni* egg-specific response is directed into a Th1- rather than a Th2-dominated reaction. This is accomplished by sensitization to schistosome egg antigens in the presence of IL-12 or CpG oligonucleotides (Wynn et al. 1995). Several Th1-associated mediators are believed to be involved in preventing the fibrotic response (Hoffmann et al. 1998), particularly NOS-2 (Hesse et al. 2000). NOS-2-deficient mice that have been sensitized with schistosome egg antigen and IL-12 develop a Th1-dominated response, but fail to control the granulomatous inflammation and display a marked exacerbation of hepatic fibrosis. Therefore, the critical downstream component that controls fibrosis in a Th1-dominated response is the functional activity of NOS-2-expressing cells.

As NOS-2 shares L-arginine as a substrate with arginase, substrate depletion by either enzyme is a key regulatory mechanism (Rutschman et al. 2001) and the differential expression of NOS-2 and the hepatic isoform of arginase (Arg-1) is important for regulating or promoting fibrosis. Macrophages are a prominent participant in *S. mansoni* egg-induced granuloma and are the primary producers of NOS-2 and Arg-1. Although it is not yet known which cells, besides macrophages, express Arg-1 after infection with *S. mansoni*, granuloma formation correlates with high arginase activity (Hesse et al. 2001). The Th1 cytokines IFN-γ and TNF activate NOS-2 production in 'classically activated' macrophages, thus regulating hepatic fibrosis by substrate depletion for Arg-1. On the other hand, the profibrotic Th2 cytokine IL-13 induces Arg-1 activity in 'alternately activated' macrophages (Modolell et al. 1995), and Th2-driven arginase expression and activity are the critical component in the development of type 2 pathology (Hesse et al. 2001) (Figure 35.11).

Arg-1 is an essential enzyme of the urea cycle and is expressed at high levels in hepatocytes. The enzyme hydrolyses L-arginine to urea and L-ornithine; therefore, its main function in the liver is the detoxification of ammonia. As L-ornithine, a product of arginase activity, is a necessary metabolite for the production of prolines which in turn control collagen production, arginase activity is linked to hepatic fibrosis after *S. mansoni* infection. The direct involvement of the arginase biosynthetic pathway in type 2 pathology was tested by blocking the L-ornithine-dependent synthesis of polyamines. After blocking ornithine carbamoyltransferase (ODC), competition between ODC and ornithine aminotransferase (OAT) for L-ornithine is eliminated and hepatic fibrosis after infection with *S. mansoni* increases (Hesse et al. 2001). Thus, the utilization of L-ornithine by OAT, which increases the synthesis of prolines (the basic building block of collagen), could explain the enhanced collagen deposition. An earlier study of schistosomiasis had already shown that fibrosis is directly controlled by the availability of proline (Dunn et al. 1981). As IL-4/IL-13-activated macrophages are an important source of proline (Hesse et al. 2001), macrophages act as important controllers of type 2 pathology. However, recently established macrophage-specific IL-4R-α-deficient mice (Herbert et al. 2004), carrying a defective receptor for IL-4 and IL-13 only on macrophages revealed that other cell types such as fibroblast are involved in the development of type 2 pathology.

Biochemically, collagen synthesis occurs by conversion of proline into hydroxyproline. The endogenous proline used for collagen synthesis diffuses into hepatic granulomas and is hydroxylated by prolylhydroxylase, an enzyme that is greatly elevated within granulomatous livers (Dunn et al. 1979). At the peak of granuloma formation, vigorous collagen production is coincident with maximal lesion size after which synthesis declines. However, at this time the collagen content remains maximal because enzymatic degradation of the connective tissue matrix is inhibited and collagen accumulates in hepatic lesions (Dunn et al. 1979). Intragranulomatous protease inhibitors were identified as α_2-macroglobulin and α_1-antiprotease (Truden and Boros 1988). The net effect of synthesis versus degradation results in remodeling of the affected tissues.

Fibroblasts, macrophages, and smooth-muscle cells have all been identified as initiators of hepatic granuloma fibrosis (Boros 1989; Hesse et al. 2001). Granuloma fibroblasts produce CCL2 and CCL3 and are implicated in promoting leukocyte recruitment, granuloma growth, and maintenance of the granulomatous lesion (Lukacs et al. 1994a). Migration of fibroblasts to the site of injury and their subsequent proliferation are triggered by growth factors, such as PDGF, epidermal growth factor (EGF), FGF, and TGF-β, and fibrogenic cytokines derived in part from inflammatory macrophages (Mornex et al. 1994). Some of these growth factors also stimulate synth-

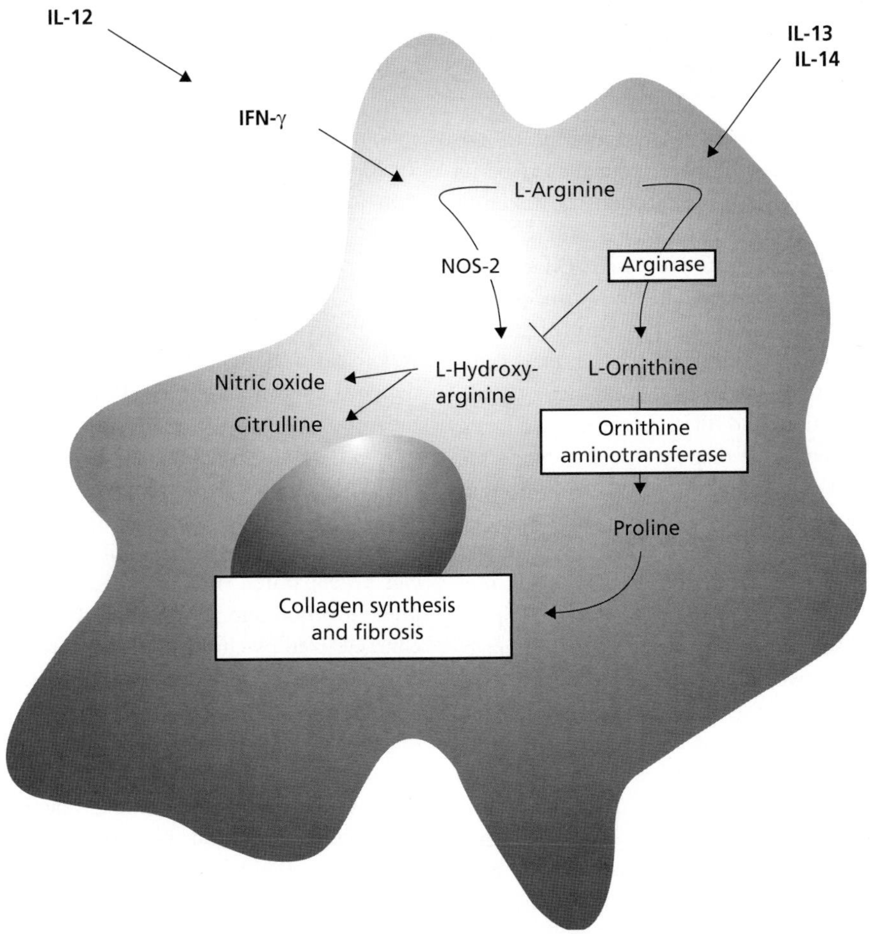

Figure 35.11 *Mechanisms of granuloma fibrosis in type 2 pathology. For details, see the text.*

esis of collagen and other connective tissue molecules and modulate the synthesis and activation of metalloproteases, enzymes that serve to degrade these extracellular matrix components (Winkler and Fowlkes 2002). Mice overexpressing TGF-β in the liver develop multiple tissue lesions including hepatic fibrosis and hepatocyte apoptosis (Sanderson et al. 1995). The inhibition of TGF-β action by the administration of agents that bind TGF-β or block TGF-β expression is effective in experimental models, but its efficacy and safety in human liver fibrosis remain unknown (Gressner et al. 2002).

Strategies to prevent granuloma fibrosis: implications for immunotherapy

Findings from experimental schistosomiasis clearly point to IL-13 as a central and indispensable mediator of fibrosis. Therefore, development of an IL-13 antagonist might be a strategy to treat established and progressive disease. Treatment with soluble IL-13Rα_2 has no influence on egg deposition and granuloma formation, but prevents progression of fibrosis (Chiaramonte et al. 2001). In future studies, it will be interesting to combine the beneficial action of IL-13 antagonists with the chemotherapeutic elimination of the parasite for further acceleration of the healing process.

In this context, molecules that inhibit Th2 responses by favoring Th1 development and modulating IL-13 production might also impact on strategies to treat hepatic fibrosis, for example, the chemokine CCL5 has been implicated in contributing to Th1 immune responses while limiting Th2 responses (Chensue et al. 1999). Treatment with recombinant CCL5 reduced type 2 granuloma size by one-third. Therefore, CCL5 may have therapeutic potential in the treatment of established type 2 hypersensitivity.

Another approach focuses on preventing granuloma fibrosis by immunization. Immunization with irradiated larval stages is followed by a protective Th1 immune response that disturbs the migration of the larvae through the lung (Wilson et al. 1999). Sensitization with eggs in the presence of IL-12 dramatically reduces the tissue fibrosis induced by subsequent infection with *S. mansoni* without affecting protective responses (Wynn et al. 1995). This strategy is an example of an immunization that acts by preventing type 2 pathology rather than infection itself.

THE RELATIONSHIP BETWEEN CELL-MEDIATED IMMUNITY AND DELAYED-TYPE HYPERSENSITIVITY

When Mackaness first introduced the concept of the activated macrophage, the temporal coincidence of its appearance with that of the DTH reaction was taken to imply that both were merely two manifestations of the same cellular and molecular processes (Mackaness 1962, 1964) – hence the frequent description of protective immunity as a 'double-edged sword'. Later, it became apparent that, in some instances, acquired resistance could be maintained even in the absence of granulomatous inflammation and that, in other instances, severe DTH-mediated tissue damage could occur in the virtual absence of antibacterial protection. It thus became necessary conceptually to distinguish between protective cell-mediated immunity (CMI) and tissue-damaging DTH. Today, most investigators hold that separate entities (cells and/or mediators) are responsible for macrophage activation versus tissue damage, although the level at which the respective mechanisms are thought to dissociate is open to debate (Table 35.3). An opposing opinion argues that the cellular and molecular bases of both CMI and DTH are mostly identical, but are regulated differentially in space and time, particularly in terms of the quantities of cytokines/chemokines secreted and of homing capacities of the cells involved, for example, mice lacking the signature structure on ICAM-1 that allows monocytes to migrate into inflamed lesions were still able to contain mycobacterial growth, but showed significantly reduced granulomatous inflammation early during infection (Johnson et al. 1998). However, when the long-term outcome of infection in ICAM-deficient mice was analyzed, they were found to succumb to elevated bacterial loads because they lacked organized granulomas (Saunders et al. 1999).

Table 35.3 *Mediators of protection and pathology in Th1 and Th2 responses*

Granuloma type	Cells and mediators	Protection	Pathology
Necrotic (type 1)	$CD4^+$ T cells	+	+
	$CD8^+$ T cells	+	?/+
	$\gamma\delta$-TCR^+ cells	?/+	?/–
	TNF	+	?/+
	IFN-γ	+	+
	IL-10	–	–
	NOS-2	+	0/–
	MCP-1	0	?/+
	RANTES	?/0	?/+
	MIG	0	?/+
Fibrotic (type 2)	Th1 $CD4^+$	+	–
	Th2 $CD4^+$	0/–	+
	IFN-γ	+	–
	TNF	+	?/0
	IL-4	0/-	0
	IL-10	–	–
	IL-12	+	–
	IL-13	0	+
	NOS-2	+	–
	Arginase	?/0	+
	RANTES	+	–

+, inducing; –, limiting; 0, no effect; ?, effect uncertain.
For abbreviations see the text.

In experimental infections with *L. monocytogenes*, it was clearly demonstrated that granuloma formation depends entirely on the $CD4^+$ T-cell subset, whereas the most potent antibacterial protection is conferred by $CD8^+$ T cells, revealing that pathology and protection could be completely dissociated at the level of effector T cells (Mielke et al. 1988, 1992).

In schistosomiasis, the course of immune responses can be separated into a protective Th1 response early after infection and a pathological Th2 immune response characterized by chronic hepatic fibrosis. With respect to crossregulatory mechanisms, promotion of protective Th1 development results in preventing pathological Th2 responses as demonstrated in IL-12-modulated immunization studies (Lukacs et al. 2001). Treatment of an already established Th2 immune reaction reduces granuloma fibrosis without negatively affecting protection. Therefore, IL-13 antagonists represent a promising strategy to treat already established and progressive type 2 DTH-associated pathology.

In *M. tuberculosis* infection, no equally discriminatory basis for macrophage-activating and tissue-damaging pathways has been identified (Ehlers 1999). Rather, the most powerful antibacterially active T cells are of the $CD4^+$ subtype and secrete IFN-γ, as are the most potent DTH-conferring T cells. Similarly, TNF is involved in both antibacterial defense mechanisms and is pivotal during the inflammatory response. It has even been argued that type 1 DTH-associated pathology can have beneficial effects, because it deprives mycobacteria of their intramacrophage habitat and exposes them to life in a hostile environment, i.e. hypoxia, acid pH, and coagulation necrosis (Dannenberg 1968). According to this view, granuloma necrosis would be the ultimate form of antibacterial protection if macrophage activation fails (Dannenberg 1991).

In an attempt at revitalizing the conceptual dissociation of CMI and DTH in TB, it has been proposed that cytokines, such as IFN-γ, might be viewed as mostly involved in protection, whereas chemokines, such as CCL2 or CXCL10, might be considered as mostly associated with the DTH response (Orme and Cooper 1999). Although it is true that chemokines, in their majority, are not known directly to contribute to antibacterial effector mechanisms, cytokines are clearly major players in granuloma formation (TNF, IFN-γ), somewhat invalidating this hypothesis. It is, however, possible that the amplification of the inflammatory response, and therefore the excess of inflammation leading to tissue damage, is mostly the result of chemokine secretion. As outlined above, it is becoming increasingly apparent that dissociation between macrophage activation and DTH-associated pathology may exist beyond the level of IFN-γ production. Protective mechanisms induced by IFN-γ (e.g. NOS-2) can clearly be dissociated from necrosis-inducing processes that are IFN-γ dependent, but NOS-2 independent, and that may involve certain chemokines. The latter therefore represent attractive targets for therapeutic immunointervention aimed at harnessing tissue-damaging pathways without compromising antibacterial protection.

ACKNOWLEDGMENTS

Work in the authors' laboratory is funded in part by DFG grants SFB 367/C9, SFB 415/C7, SFB 470/CG HO2145/2-1, the German Federal Ministry of Health, the German National Genome Research Network, the Special Research Focus on Host Immunity at Lubeck University, and the German–Israeli Foundation for Scientific Research and Development.

REFERENCES

Abe, Y., Sugisaki, K. and Dannenberg, A.M. Jr. 1996. Rabbit vascular endothelial adhesion molecules: ELAM-1 is most elevated in acute inflammation, whereas VCAM-1 and ICAM-1 predominate in chronic inflammation. *J Leukoc Biol*, **60**, 692–703.

Adams, D.O. 1976. The granulomatous inflammatory response. A review. *Am J Pathol*, **84**, 164–91.

Amiri, P., Locksley, R.M., et al. 1992. Tumour necrosis factor alpha restores granulomas and induces parasite egg-laying in schistosome-infected SCID mice. *Nature*, **356**, 604–7.

Anderson, S., Shires, V.L., et al. 1998. In the absence of IL-12, the induction of Th1-mediated protective immunity by the attenuated schistosome vaccine is impaired, revealing an alternative pathway with Th2-type characteristics. *Eur J Immunol*, **28**, 2827–38.

Benini, J., Ehlers, E.M. and Ehlers, S. 1999. Different types of pulmonary granuloma necrosis in immunocompetent vs. TNFRp55-gene-deficient mice aerogenically infected with highly virulent *Mycobacterium avium*. *J Pathol*, **189**, 127–37.

Biempica, L., Dunn, M.A., et al. 1983. Liver collagen-type characterization in human schistosomiasis. A histological, ultrastructural, and immunocytochemical correlation. *Am J Trop Med Hyg*, **32**, 316–25.

Border, W.A. and Noble, N.A. 1994. Transforming growth factor beta in tissue fibrosis. *N Engl J Med*, **331**, 1286–90.

Boring, L., Gosling, J., et al. 1997. Impaired monocyte migration and reduced type 1 (Th1) cytokine responses in C-C chemokine receptor 2 knockout mice. *J Clin Invest*, **100**, 2552–61.

Boros, D.L. 1989. Immunopathology of *Schistosoma mansoni* infection. *Clin Microbiol Rev*, **2**, 250–69.

Boros, D.L. 1999. T helper cell populations, cytokine dynamics, and pathology of the schistosome egg granuloma. *Microbes Infect*, **1**, 511–16.

Brinckerhoff, C.E. and Matrisian, L.M. 2002. Matrix metalloproteinases: a tail of a frog that became a prince. *Nat Rev Mol Cell Biol*, **3**, 207–14.

Brombacher, F. 2000. The role of interleukin-13 in infectious diseases and allergy. *Bioessays*, **22**, 646–56.

Cheever, A.W. 1972. Pipe-stem fibrosis of the liver. *Trans R Soc Trop Med Hyg*, **66**, 947–8.

Cheever, A.W., Dunn, M.A., et al. 1983. Differences in hepatic fibrosis in ICR, C3H and C57BL/6 mice infected with *Schistosoma mansoni*. *Am J Trop Med Hyg*, **32**, 1364–19.

Cheever, A.W., Duvall, R.H., et al. 1987. Variation of hepatic fibrosis and granuloma size among mouse strains infected with *Schistosoma mansoni*. *Am J Trop Med Hyg*, **37**, 85–97.

Cheever, A.W., Williams, M.E., et al. 1994. Anti-IL-4 treatment of *Schistosoma mansoni*-infected mice inhibits development of T cells and non-B, non-T cells expressing Th2 cytokines while decreasing egg-induced hepatic fibrosis. *J Immunol*, **153**, 753–9.

Cheever, A.W., Hoffmann, K.F. and Wynn, T.A. 2000. Immunopathology of *schistosomiasis mansoni* in mice and men. *Immunol Today*, **21**, 465–6.

Chensue, S.W., Warmington, K.S., et al. 1996. Role of monocyte chemoattractant protein-1 (MCP-1) in Th1 (mycobacterial) and Th2 (schistosomal) antigen-induced granuloma formation: relationship to local inflammation, Th cell expression and IL-12 production. *J Immunol*, **157**, 4602–8.

Chensue, S.W., Warmington, K., et al. 1997a. Effect of slow release IL-12 and IL-10 on inflammation, local macrophage function and the regional lymphoid response during mycobacterial (Th1) and schistosomal (Th2) antigen-elicited pulmonary granuloma formation. *Inflamm Res*, **46**, 86–92.

Chensue, S.W., Warmington, K., et al. 1997b. Mycobacterial and schistosomal antigen-elicited granuloma formation in IFN-gamma and IL-4 knockout mice: analysis of local and regional cytokine and chemokine networks. *J Immunol*, **159**, 3565–73.

Chensue, S.W., Warmington, K.S., et al. 1999. Differential expression and cross-regulatory function of RANTES during mycobacterial (type 1) and schistosomal (type 2) antigen-elicited granulomatous inflammation. *J Immunol*, **163**, 165–73.

Chensue, S.W., Lukacs, N.W., et al. 2001. Aberrant in vivo T helper type 2 cell response and impaired eosinophil recruitment in CC chemokine receptor 8 knockout mice. *J Exp Med*, **193**, 573–84.

Chiaramonte, M.G., Donaldson, D.D., et al. 1999a. An IL-13 inhibitor blocks the development of hepatic fibrosis during a T-helper type 2-dominated inflammatory response. *J Clin Invest*, **104**, 777–85.

Chiaramonte, M.G., Schopf, L.R., et al. 1999b. IL-13 is a key regulatory cytokine for Th2 cell-mediated pulmonary granuloma formation and IgE responses induced by *Schistosoma mansoni* eggs. *J Immunol*, **162**, 920–30.

Chiaramonte, M.G., Cheever, A.W., et al. 2001. Studies of murine schistosomiasis reveal interleukin-13 blockade as a treatment for established and progressive liver fibrosis. *Hepatology*, **34**, 273–82.

Cho, S., Mehra, V., et al. 2000. Antimicrobial activity of MHC class I-restricted $CD8^+$ T cells in human tuberculosis. *Proc Natl Acad Sci USA*, **97**, 12210–15.

Chtanova, T. and Mackay, C.R. 2001. T cell effector subsets: extending the Th1/Th2 paradigm. *Adv Immunol*, **78**, 233–66.

Chu, C.Q., Wittmer, S. and Dalton, D.K. 2000. Failure to suppress the expansion of the activated CD4 T cell population in interferon gamma-deficient mice leads to exacerbation of experimental autoimmune encephalomyelitis. *J Exp Med*, **192**, 123–8.

Collins, H.L. and Kaufmann, S.H. 2001a. Prospects for better tuberculosis vaccines. *Lancet Infect Dis*, **1**, 21–8.

Collins, H.L. and Kaufmann, S.H. 2001b. The many faces of host responses to tuberculosis. *Immunology*, **103**, 1–9.

Colombo, M.P. and Trinchieri, G. 2002. Interleukin-12 in anti-tumor immunity and immunotherapy. *Cytokine Growth Factor Rev*, **13**, 155–68.

Converse, P.J., Dannenberg, A.M. Jr., et al. 1996. Cavitary tuberculosis produced in rabbits by aerosolized virulent tubercle bacilli. *Infect Immun*, **64**, 4776–87.

Cooper, A.M., Adams, L.B., et al. 2002. IFN-gamma and NO in mycobacterial disease: new jobs for old hands. *Trends Microbiol*, **10**, 221–6.

Czaja, M.J., Weiner, F.R., et al. 1989. Gamma-interferon treatment inhibits collagen deposition in murine schistosomiasis. *Hepatology*, **10**, 795–800.

Dalton, D.K., Haynes, L., et al. 2000. Interferon gamma eliminates responding CD4 T cells during mycobacterial infection by inducing apoptosis of activated CD4 T cells. *J Exp Med*, **192**, 117–22.

Dannenberg, A.M. Jr. 1968. Cellular hypersensitivity and cellular immunity in the pathogenesis of tuberculosis: specificity, systemic and local nature, and associated macrophage enzymes. *Bacteriol Rev*, **32**, 85–102.

Dannenberg, A.M. Jr. 1991. Delayed-type hypersensitivity and cell-mediated immunity in the pathogenesis of tuberculosis. *Immunol Today*, **12**, 228–33.

Dannenberg, A.M. Jr. and Sugimoto, M. 1976. Liquefaction of caseous foci in tuberculosis. *Am Rev Respir Dis*, **113**, 257–9.

de Andres, B., Rakasz, E., et al. 1997. Lack of Fc-epsilon receptors on murine eosinophils: implications for the functional significance of elevated IgE and eosinophils in parasitic infections. *Blood*, **89**, 3826–336.

Dean, D.A. and Mangold, B.L. 1992. Evidence that both normal and immune elimination of *Schistosoma mansoni* take place at the lung stage of migration prior to parasite death. *Am J Trop Med Hyg*, **47**, 238–48.

Dessein, A.J., Hillaire, D., et al. 1999. Severe hepatic fibrosis in *Schistosoma mansoni* infection is controlled by a major locus that is closely linked to the interferon-gamma receptor gene. *Am J Hum Genet*, **65**, 709–21.

Doucet, C., Brouty-Boye, D., et al. 1998. IL-4 and IL-13 specifically increase adhesion molecule and inflammatory cytokine expression in human lung fibroblasts. *Int Immunol*, **10**, 1421–33.

D'Souza, C.D., Cooper, A.M., et al. 1997. An anti-inflammatory role for gamma delta T lymphocytes in acquired immunity to *Mycobacterium tuberculosis*. *J Immunol*, **158**, 1217–21.

Dunn, M.A. and Kamel, R. 1981. Hepatic schistosomiasis. *Hepatology*, **1**, 653–61.

Dunn, M.A., Rojkind, M., et al. 1977. Liver collagen synthesis in murine schistosomiasis. *J Clin Invest*, **59**, 666–74.

Dunn, M.A., Kamel, R., et al. 1979. Liver collagen synthesis in *schistosomiasis mansoni*. *Gastroenterology*, **76**, 978–82.

Dunn, M.A., Seifter, S. and Hait, P.K. 1981. Proline trapping in granulomas, the site of collagen biosynthesis in murine schistosomiasis. *Hepatology*, **1**, 28–32.

Dunne, D.W. and Pearce, E.J. 1999. Immunology of hepatosplenic *schistosomiasis mansoni*: a human perspective. *Microbes Infect*, **1**, 553–60.

Durban Immunotherapy Trial Group. 1999. Immunotherapy with *Mycobacterium vaccae* in patients with newly diagnosed pulmonary tuberculosis: a randomised controlled trial. *Lancet*, **354**, 116–19.

Ehlers, S. 1999. Immunity to tuberculosis: a delicate balance between protection and pathology. *FEMS Immunol Med Microbiol*, **23**, 149–58.

Ehlers, S., Kutsch, S., et al. 1999. NOS-2-derived nitric oxide regulates the size, quantity and quality of granuloma formation in *Mycobacterium avium*-infected mice without affecting bacterial loads. *Immunology*, **98**, 313–23.

Ehlers, S., Kutsch, S., et al. 2000. Lethal granuloma disintegration in mycobacteria-infected TNFRp55-/- mice is dependent on T cells and IL-12. *J Immunol*, **165**, 483–92.

Ehlers, S., Benini, J., et al. 2001. Alphabeta T cell receptor-positive cells and interferon-gamma, but not inducible nitric oxide synthase, are critical for granuloma necrosis in a mouse model of mycobacteria-induced pulmonary immunopathology. *J Exp Med*, **194**, 1847–59.

Ehlers, S., Hölscher, C., et al. 2003. The lymphotoxin beta receptor is critically involved in controlling infections with the intracellular pathogens *Mycobacterium tuberculosis* and *Listeria monocytogenes*. *J Immunol*, **170**, 5210–18.

Ehrt, S., Schnappinger, D., et al. 2001. Reprogramming of the macrophage transcriptome in response to interferon-gamma and *Mycobacterium tuberculosis*: signaling roles of nitric oxide synthase-2 and phagocyte oxidase. *J Exp Med*, **194**, 1123–40.

Erdmann, I., Scheidegger, E.P., et al. 2002. Fucosyltransferase VII-deficient mice with defective E-, P- and L-selectin ligands show impaired $CD4^+$ and $CD8^+$ T cell migration into the skin, but normal extravasation into visceral organs. *J Immunol*, **168**, 2139–46.

Fallon, P.G., Richardson, E.J., et al. 2000. Schistosome infection of transgenic mice defines distinct and contrasting pathogenic roles for IL-4 and IL-13: IL-13 is a profibrotic agent. *J Immunol*, **164**, 2585–91.

Fayyazi, A., Eichmeyer, B., et al. 2000. Apoptosis of macrophages and T cells in tuberculosis associated caseous necrosis. *J Pathol*, **191**, 417–25.

Fenhalls, G., Wong, A., et al. 2000. In situ production of gamma interferon, interleukin-4, and tumor necrosis factor alpha mRNA in human lung tuberculous granulomas. *Infect Immun*, **68**, 2827–36.

Fenhalls, G., Stevens, L., et al. 2002. Distribution of IFN-gamma, IL-4 and TNF-alpha protein and CD8 T cells producing IL-12p40 mRNA in human lung tuberculous granulomas. *Immunology*, **105**, 325–35.

Filley, E.A., Bull, H.A., et al. 1992. The effect of *Mycobacterium tuberculosis* on the susceptibility of human cells to the stimulatory and toxic effects of tumour necrosis factor. *Immunology*, **77**, 505–9.

Florido, M., Cooper, A.M. and Appelberg, R. 2002. Immunological basis of the development of necrotic lesions following *Mycobacterium avium* infection. *Immunology*, **106**, 590–601.

Flynn, J.L. and Ernst, J.D. 2000. Immune responses in tuberculosis. *Curr Opin Immunol*, **12**, 432–6.

Flynn, J.L., Goldstein, M.M., et al. 1995. Tumor necrosis factor-alpha is required in the protective immune response against *Mycobacterium tuberculosis* in mice. *Immunity*, **2**, 561–72.

Friedman, S.L., Maher, J.J. and Bissell, D.M. 2000. Mechanisms and therapy of hepatic fibrosis: report of the AASLD Single Topic Basic Research Conference. *Hepatology*, **32**, 1403–8.

Frucht, D.M. 2002. IL-23: a cytokine that acts on memory T cells. *Sci STKE*, 114, RE1.

Gasperini, S., Marchi, M., et al. 1999. Gene expression and production of the monokine induced by IFN-gamma (MIG), IFN-inducible T cell alpha chemoattractant (I-TAC) and IFN-gamma-inducible protein-10 (IP-10) chemokines by human neutrophils. *J Immunol*, **162**, 4928–37.

Gonzalez-Juarrero, M., Turner, O.C., et al. 2001. Temporal and spatial arrangement of lymphocytes within lung granulomas induced by aerosol infection with *Mycobacterium tuberculosis*. *Infect Immun*, **69**, 1722–8.

Gressner, A.M., Weiskirchen, R., et al. 2002. Roles of TGF-beta in hepatic fibrosis. *Front Biosci*, **7**, 793–807.

Hatz, C.F. 2001. The use of ultrasound in schistosomiasis. *Adv Parasitol*, **48**, 225–84.

Heath, V.L., Kurata, H., et al. 2002. Checkpoints in the regulation of T helper 1 responses. *Curr Top Microbiol Immunol*, **266**, 23–39.

Herbert, D.R., Hölscher, C., et al. 2004. IL-4/IL-13-activated alternative macrophages are essential for downmodulation of T-helper 2 responses, immunopathology and survival during schistomiasis. *Immunity*, in press.

Hernandez-Pando, R. and Rook, G.A. 1994. The role of TNF-alpha in T-cell-mediated inflammation depends on the Th1/Th2 cytokine balance. *Immunology*, **82**, 591–5.

Hesse, M., Cheever, A.W., et al. 2000. NOS-2 mediates the protective anti-inflammatory and antifibrotic effects of the Th1-inducing adjuvant, IL-12, in a Th2 model of granulomatous disease. *Am J Pathol*, **157**, 945–55.

Hesse, M., Modolell, M., et al. 2001. Differential regulation of nitric oxide synthase-2 and arginase-1 by type 1/type 2 cytokines in vivo: granulomatous pathology is shaped by the pattern of L-arginine metabolism. *J Immunol*, **167**, 6533–44.

Hoffmann, K.F., Caspar, P., et al. 1998. IFN-gamma, IL-12 and TNF-alpha are required to maintain reduced liver pathology in mice vaccinated with *Schistosoma mansoni* eggs and IL-12. *J Immunol*, **161**, 4201–10.

Hoffmann, K.F., Cheever, A.W. and Wynn, T.A. 2000. IL-10 and the dangers of immune polarization: excessive type 1 and type 2 cytokine responses induce distinct forms of lethal immunopathology in murine schistosomiasis. *J Immunol*, **164**, 6406–16.

Hogaboam, C.M., Chensue, S.W., et al. 1997. Alteration of the cytokine phenotype in an experimental lung granuloma model by inhibiting nitric oxide. *J Immunol*, **159**, 5585–93.

Hogaboam, C.M., Lukacs, N.W., et al. 1998. Monocyte chemoattractant protein-1 synthesis by murine lung fibroblasts modulates $CD4^+$ T cell activation. *J Immunol*, **160**, 4606–14.

Hogaboam, C.M., Bone-Larson, C.L., et al. 1999. Differential monocyte chemoattractant protein-1 and chemokine receptor 2 expression by murine lung fibroblasts derived from Th1- and Th2-type pulmonary granuloma models. *J Immunol*, **163**, 2193–201.

Hogan, L.H., Markofski, W., et al. 2001. *Mycobacterium bovis* BCG-induced granuloma formation depends on gamma interferon and CD40 ligand but does not require CD28. *Infect Immun*, **69**, 2596–603.

Hölscher, C. 2003. Interleukin, 13, genes, receptors and signal transduction. In: Brombacher, F. (ed.), *Interleukin 13*. Georgetown: Landes Bioscience, 1–12.

Hood, A.T. and Boros, D.L. 1980. The effect of splenectomy on the pathophysiology and egg-specific immune response of *Schistosoma mansoni*-infected mice. *Am J Trop Med Hyg*, **29**, 586–91.

Hunter, C.A., Yu, D., et al. 2001. Cutting edge: systemic inhibition of angiogenesis underlies resistance to tumors during acute toxoplasmosis. *J Immunol*, **166**, 5878–81.

Issekutz, T.B. 1993a. Dual inhibition of VLA-4 and LFA-1 maximally inhibits cutaneous delayed-type hypersensitivity-induced inflammation. *Am J Pathol*, **143**, 1286–93.

Issekutz, T.B. 1993b. The contributions of integrins to leukocyte infiltration in inflamed tissues. *Curr Top Microbiol Immunol*, **184**, 177–85.

Issekutz, A.C. and Issekutz, T.B. 1993. Quantitation and kinetics of blood monocyte migration to acute inflammatory reactions and IL-1 alpha, tumor necrosis factor-alpha and IFN-gamma. *J Immunol*, **151**, 2105–15.

James, S.L. and Glaven, J. 1989. Macrophage cytotoxicity against schistosomula of *Schistosoma mansoni* involves arginine-dependent production of reactive nitrogen intermediates. *J Immunol*, **143**, 4208–12.

James, S.L., Cheever, A.W., et al. 1998. Inducible nitric oxide synthase-deficient mice develop enhanced type 1 cytokine-associated cellular and humoral immune responses after vaccination with attenuated *Schistosoma mansoni* cercariae but display partially reduced resistance. *Infect Immun*, **66**, 3510–18.

Jankovic, D., Liu, Z. and Gause, W.C. 2001. Th1- and Th2-cell commitment during infectious disease: asymmetry in divergent pathways. *Trends Immunol*, **22**, 450–7.

Johnson, C.M., Cooper, A.M., et al. 1998. Adequate expression of protective immunity in the absence of granuloma formation in *Mycobacterium tuberculosis*-infected mice with a disruption in the intracellular adhesion molecule 1 gene. *Infect Immun*, **66**, 1666–70.

Joseph, A.L. and Boros, D.L. 1993. Tumor necrosis factor plays a role in *Schistosoma mansoni* egg-induced granulomatous inflammation. *J Immunol*, **151**, 5461–71.

Kanaly, S.T., Nashleanas, M., et al. 1999. TNF receptor p55 is required for elimination of inflammatory cells following control of intracellular pathogens. *J Immunol*, **163**, 3883–9.

Kaplan, M.H., Schindler, U., et al. 1996. Stat6 is required for mediating responses to IL-4 and for development of Th2 cells. *Immunity*, **4**, 313–19.

Kaplan, M.H., Whitfield, J.R., et al. 1998. Th2 cells are required for the *Schistosoma mansoni* egg-induced granulomatous response. *J Immunol*, **160**, 1850–6.

Kaufmann, S.H. 1988. $CD8^+$ T lymphocytes in intracellular microbial infections. *Immunol Today*, **9**, 168–74.

Kaufmann, S.H. 2000. Is the development of a new tuberculosis vaccine possible? *Nat Med*, **6**, 955–60.

Kindler, V., Sappino, A.P., et al. 1989. The inducing role of tumor necrosis factor in the development of bactericidal granulomas during BCG infection. *Cell*, **56**, 731–40.

King, C.L., Xianli, J., et al. 1997. Mice with a targeted deletion of the IgE gene have increased worm burdens and reduced granulomatous inflammation following primary infection with *Schistosoma mansoni*. *J Immunol*, **158**, 294–300.

Kobzik, L. and Schoen, F.J. 1994. The lung. In: Cotran, R.S., Kumar, V. and Robbins, S.L. (eds), *Pathologic basis of disease*. Philadelphia, PA: W.B. Saunders Co, 702–3.

Koch, R. 1890. Weitere Mitteilungen über ein Heilmittel gegen Tuberkulose. *Dtsche Med Wochenschr*, **16**, 1029–32.

Kunkel, S.L., Lukacs, N.W., et al. 1996. Th1 and Th2 responses regulate experimental lung granuloma development. *Sarcoidosis Vasc Diffuse Lung Dis*, **13**, 120–8.

Kunkel, S.L., Lukacs, N.W., et al. 1998. Animal models of granulomatous inflammation. *Semin Respir Infect*, **13**, 221–8.

Lee, C.G., Homer, R.J., et al. 2001. Interleukin-13 induces tissue fibrosis by selectively stimulating and activating transforming growth factor beta(1). *J Exp Med*, **194**, 809–21.

Louis, H., Le Moine, A., et al. 2000. Repeated concanavalin A challenge in mice induces an interleukin 10-producing phenotype and liver fibrosis. *Hepatology*, **31**, 381–90.

Lowrie, D.B., Tascon, R.E., et al. 1999. Therapy of tuberculosis in mice by DNA vaccination. *Nature*, **400**, 269–71.

Lukacs, N.W., Chensue, S.W., et al. 1994a. Production of monocyte chemoattractant protein-1 and macrophage inflammatory protein-1 alpha by inflammatory granuloma fibroblasts. *Am J Pathol*, **144**, 711–18.

Lukacs, N.W., Chensue, S.W., et al. 1994b. Inflammatory granuloma formation is mediated by TNF-alpha-inducible intercellular adhesion molecule-1. *J Immunol*, **152**, 5883–9.

Lukacs, N.W., Hogaboam, C., et al. 2001. Type 1/type 2 cytokine paradigm and the progression of pulmonary fibrosis. *Chest*, **120**, S5–8.

Mackaness, G.B. 1962. Cellular resistance to infection. *J Exp Med*, **116**, 381–406.

Mackaness, G.B. 1964. The immunological basis of acquired cellular resistance. *J Exp Med*, **120**, 105–20.

McMurray, D.N., Collins, F.M., et al. 1996. Pathogenesis of experimental tuberculosis in animal models. *Curr Top Microbiol Immunol*, **215**, 157–79.

Manget, J.J. 1700. *Observatio XLVII. Sepulchretum sive anatomia practica, vol. 1*. London: Cramer & Perachon.

Marfaing-Koka, A., Devergne, O., et al. 1995. Regulation of the production of the RANTES chemokine by endothelial cells. Synergistic induction by IFN-gamma plus TNF-alpha and inhibition by IL-4 and IL-13. *J Immunol*, **154**, 1870–8.

Marino, M.W., Dunn, A., et al. 1997. Characterization of tumor necrosis factor-deficient mice. *Proc Natl Acad Sci USA*, **94**, 8093–8.

Mastroeni, P., Villarreal-Ramos, B. and Hormaeche, C.E. 1992. Role of T cells, TNF alpha and IFN gamma in recall of immunity to oral challenge with virulent salmonellae in mice vaccinated with live attenuated aro-Salmonella vaccines. *Microb Pathog*, **13**, 477–91.

Matsukawa, A., Lukacs, N.W., et al. 2001. III. Chemokines and other mediators, 8. Chemokines and their receptors in cell-mediated immune responses in the lung. *Microsc Res Tech*, **53**, 298–306.

Matsushima, K., Morishita, K., et al. 1988. Molecular cloning of a human monocyte-derived neutrophil chemotactic factor (MDNCF) and the induction of MDNCF mRNA by interleukin 1 and tumor necrosis factor. *J Exp Med*, **167**, 1883–93.

Matyszak, M.K. and Perry, V.H. 1996. Delayed-type hypersensitivity lesions in the central nervous system are prevented by inhibitors of matrix metalloproteinases. *J Neuroimmunol*, **69**, 141–9.

Mazzaccaro, R.J., Stenger, S., et al. 1998. Cytotoxic T lymphocytes in resistance to tuberculosis. *Adv Exp Med Biol*, **452**, 85–101.

Metwali, A., Elliott, D., et al. 1996. The granulomatous response in murine *Schistosomiasis mansoni* does not switch to Th1 in IL-4-deficient C57BL/6 mice. *J Immunol*, **157**, 4546–53.

Mielke, M.E., Ehlers, S. and Hahn, H. 1988. T-cell subsets in delayed-type hypersensitivity, protection, and granuloma formation in primary and secondary *Listeria* infection in mice: superior role of Lyt-2^+ cells in acquired immunity. *Infect Immun*, **56**, 1920–5.

Mielke, M.E., Niedobitek, G., et al. 1989. Acquired resistance to *Listeria monocytogenes* is mediated by Lyt-2^+ T cells independently of the influx of monocytes into granulomatous lesions. *J Exp Med*, **170**, 589–94.

Mielke, M.E., Rosen, H., et al. 1992. Protective immunity and granuloma formation are mediated by two distinct tumor necrosis factor alpha- and gamma interferon-dependent T cell-phagocyte interactions in murine listeriosis: dissociation on the basis of phagocyte adhesion mechanisms. *Infect Immun*, **60**, 1875–82.

Mielke, M.E., Peters, C. and Hahn, H. 1997. Cytokines in the induction and expression of T-cell-mediated granuloma formation and protection in the murine model of listeriosis. *Immunol Rev*, **158**, 79–93.

Modolell, M., Corraliza, I.M., et al. 1995. Reciprocal regulation of the nitric oxide synthase/arginase balance in mouse bone marrow-derived macrophages by Th1 and Th2 cytokines. *Eur J Immunol*, **25**, 1101–4.

Mogues, T., Goodrich, M.E., et al. 2001. The relative importance of T cell subsets in immunity and immunopathology of airborne *Mycobacterium tuberculosis* infection in mice. *J Exp Med*, **193**, 271–80.

Mombaerts, P., Arnoldi, J., et al. 1993. Different roles of alpha beta and gamma delta T cells in immunity against an intracellular bacterial pathogen. *Nature*, **365**, 53–6.

Moreira, A.L., Tsenova, L., et al. 2002. Mycobacterial antigens exacerbate disease manifestations in *Mycobacterium tuberculosis*-infected mice. *Infect Immun*, **70**, 2100–7.

Mornex, J.F., Leroux, C., et al. 1994. From granuloma to fibrosis in interstitial lung diseases: molecular and cellular interactions. *Eur Respir J*, **7**, 779–85.

Mountford, A.P., Hogg, K.G., et al. 2001. Signaling via interleukin-4 receptor alpha chain is required for successful vaccination against schistosomiasis in BALB/c mice. *Infect Immun*, **69**, 228–36.

Murata, T., Husain, S.R., et al. 1998. Two different IL-13 receptor chains are expressed in normal human skin fibroblasts and IL-4 and IL-13 mediate signal transduction through a common pathway. *Int Immunol*, **10**, 1103–10.

Myatt, N., Coghill, G., et al. 1994. Detection of tumour necrosis factor alpha in sarcoidosis and tuberculosis granulomas using in situ hybridisation. *J Clin Pathol*, **47**, 423–6.

Nathan, C.F., Kaplan, G., et al. 1986. Local and systemic effects of intradermal recombinant interferon-gamma in patients with lepromatous leprosy. *N Engl J Med*, **315**, 6–15.

Nelson, D.R., Lauwers, G.Y., et al. 2000. Interleukin-10 treatment reduces fibrosis in patients with chronic hepatitis C: a pilot trial of interferon nonresponders. *Gastroenterology*, **118**, 655–60.

North, R.J. 1995. *Mycobacterium tuberculosis* is strikingly more virulent for mice when given via the respiratory than via the intravenous route. *J Infect Dis*, **172**, 1550–3.

Oriente, A., Fedarko, N.S., et al. 2000. Interleukin-13 modulates collagen homeostasis in human skin and keloid fibroblasts. *J Pharmacol Exp Ther*, **292**, 988–94.

Orme, I.M. and Cooper, A.M. 1999. Cytokine/chemokine cascades in immunity to tuberculosis. *Immunol Today*, **20**, 307–12.

Oswald, I.P., Eltoum, I., et al. 1994. Endothelial cells are activated by cytokine treatment to kill an intravascular parasite, *Schistosoma mansoni*, through the production of nitric oxide. *Proc Natl Acad Sci USA*, **91**, 999–1003.

Parks, W.C. and Shapiro, S.D. 2001. Matrix metalloproteinases in lung biology. *Respir Res*, **2**, 10–19.

Pearce, E.J., Cheever, A., et al. 1996. *Schistosoma mansoni* in IL-4-deficient mice. *Int Immunol*, **8**, 435–44.

Pearce, E.J. and MacDonald, A.S. 2002. The immunobiology of schistosomiasis. *Nat Rev Immunol*, **2**, 499–511.

Pflanz, S., Timans, J.C., et al. 2002. IL-27, a heterodimeric cytokine composed of EBI3 and p28 protein, induces proliferation of naive CD4($^+$) T cells. *Immunity*, **16**, 779–90.

Qiu, B., Frait, K.A., et al. 2001. Chemokine expression dynamics in mycobacterial (type-1) and schistosomal (type-2) antigen-elicited pulmonary granuloma formation. *Am J Pathol*, **158**, 1503–15.

Rabello, A. 1995. Acute human *schistosomiasis mansoni. Mem Inst Oswaldo Cruz*, **90**, 277–80.

Rhoades, E.R., Frank, A.A. and Orme, I.M. 1997. Progression of chronic pulmonary tuberculosis in mice aerogenically infected with virulent *Mycobacterium tuberculosis. Tuber Lung Dis*, **78**, 57–66.

Roach, D.R., Briscoe, H., et al. 2001. Secreted lymphotoxin-alpha is essential for the control of an intracellular bacterial infection. *J Exp Med*, **193**, 239–46.

Roach, D.R., Bean, A.G., et al. 2002. TNF regulates chemokine induction essential for cell recruitment, granuloma formation, and clearance of mycobacterial infection. *J Immunol*, **168**, 4620–7.

Robinson, D.S. and O'Garra, A. 2002. Further checkpoints in Th1 development. *Immunity*, **16**, 755–8.

Romagnani, S. 1996. *The Th1/Th2 paradigm in disease*. Heidelberg: Springer Verlag.

Rook, G.A. and Hernandez-Pando, R. 1996. The pathogenesis of tuberculosis. *Annu Rev Microbiol*, **50**, 259–84.

Rook, G.A., Seah, G. and Ustianowski, A. 2001. *M. tuberculosis*: immunology and vaccination. *Eur Respir J*, **17**, 537–57.

Rook, G.A. and Zumla, A. 2001. Advances in the immunopathogenesis of pulmonary tuberculosis. *Curr Opin Pulm Med*, **7**, 116–23.

Ruth, J.H., Warmington, K.S., et al. 2000. Interleukin 4 and 13 participation in mycobacterial (type-1) and schistosomal (type-2) antigen-elicited pulmonary granuloma formation: multiparameter analysis of cellular recruitment, chemokine expression and cytokine networks. *Cytokine*, **12**, 432–44.

Rutschman, R., Lang, R., et al. 2001. Cutting edge: Stat6-dependent substrate depletion regulates nitric oxide production. *J Immunol*, **166**, 2173–7.

Sabin, E.A., Kopf, M.A. and Pearce, E.J. 1996. *Schistosoma mansoni* egg-induced early IL-4 production is dependent upon IL-5 and eosinophils. *J Exp Med*, **184**, 1871–8.

Sad, S., Marcotte, R. and Mosmann, T.R. 1995. Cytokine-induced differentiation of precursor mouse $CD8^+$ T cells into cytotoxic $CD8^+$ T cells secreting Th1 or Th2 cytokines. *Immunity*, **2**, 271–9.

Sanderson, N., Factor, V., et al. 1995. Hepatic expression of mature transforming growth factor beta 1 in transgenic mice results in multiple tissue lesions. *Proc Natl Acad Sci USA*, **92**, 2572–6.

Saunders, B.M. and Cooper, A.M. 2000. Restraining mycobacteria: role of granulomas in mycobacterial infections. *Immunol Cell Biol*, **78**, 334–41.

Saunders, B.M., Frank, A.A. and Orme, I.M. 1999. Granuloma formation is required to contain bacillus growth and delay mortality in mice chronically infected with *Mycobacterium tuberculosis. Immunology*, **98**, 324–8.

Seitzer, U., Scheel-Toellner, D., et al. 1997. Properties of multinucleated giant cells in a new in vitro model for human granuloma formation. *J Pathol*, **182**, 99–105.

Senior, R.M., Griffin, G.L. and Mecham, R.P. 1980. Chemotactic activity of elastin-derived peptides. *J Clin Invest*, **66**, 859–62.

Shang, X.Z., Chiu, B.C., et al. 2002. Eosinophil recruitment in type-2 hypersensitivity pulmonary granulomas: source and contribution of monocyte chemotactic protein-3 (CCL7). *Am J Pathol*, **161**, 257–66.

Sher, A., Coffman, R.L., et al. 1990. Ablation of eosinophil and IgE responses with anti-IL-5 or anti-IL-4 antibodies fails to affect immunity against *Schistosoma mansoni* in the mouse. *J Immunol*, **145**, 3911–16.

Shikama, Y., Kobayashi, K., et al. 1989. Granuloma formation by artificial microparticles in vitro. Macrophages and monokines play a critical role in granuloma formation. *Am J Pathol*, **134**, 1189–99.

Shtrichman, R. and Samuel, C.E. 2001. The role of gamma interferon in antimicrobial immunity. *Curr Opin Microbiol*, **4**, 251–9.

Smith, D., Hansch, H., et al. 1997. T-cell-independent granuloma formation in response to *Mycobacterium avium*: role of tumour necrosis factor-alpha and interferon-gamma. *Immunology*, **92**, 413–21.

Smith, M.D. 1977. The ultrastructural development of the schistosome egg granuloma in mice. *Parasitology*, **75**, 119–23.

Smithson, G., Rogers, C.E., et al. 2001. Fuc-TVII is required for T helper 1 and T cytotoxic 1 lymphocyte selectin ligand expression and recruitment in inflammation, and together with Fuc-TIV regulates naive T cell trafficking to lymph nodes. *J Exp Med*, **194**, 601–14.

Smythies, L.E., Coulson, P.S. and Wilson, R.A. 1992. Monoclonal antibody to IFN-gamma modifies pulmonary inflammatory responses and abrogates immunity to *Schistosoma mansoni* in mice vaccinated with attenuated cercariae. *J Immunol*, **14**, 3654–8.

Sousa, A.O., Mazzaccaro, R.J., et al. 2000. Relative contributions of distinct MHC class I-dependent cell populations in protection to tuberculosis infection in mice. *Proc Natl Acad Sci USA*, **97**, 4204–8.

Springer, T.A. 1994. Traffic signals for lymphocyte recirculation and leukocyte emigration: the multistep paradigm. *Cell*, **76**, 301–14.

Stenger, R.J., Warren, K.S. and Johnson, E.A. 1967. An ultrastructural study of hepatic granulomas and schistosome egg shells in murine hepatosplenic *schistosomiasis mansoni*. *Exp Mol Pathol*, **7**, 116–32.

Stenger, S. and Modlin, R.L. 1998. Cytotoxic T cell responses to intracellular pathogens. *Curr Opin Immunol*, **10**, 471–7.

Stenger, S. and Modlin, R.L. 1999. T cell-mediated immunity to *Mycobacterium tuberculosis*. *Curr Opin Microbiol*, **2**, 89–93.

Stenger, S., Hanson, D.A., et al. 1998. An antimicrobial activity of cytolytic T cells mediated by granulysin. *Science*, **282**, 121–5.

Stenger, S., Rosat, J.P., et al. 1999. Granulysin: a lethal weapon of cytolytic T cells. *Immunol Today*, **20**, 390–4.

Stephenson, M.L., Krane, S.M., et al. 1985. Immune interferon inhibits collagen synthesis by rheumatoid synovial cells associated with decreased levels of the procollagen mRNAs. *FEBS Lett*, **180**, 43–50.

Suga, M., Dannenberg, A.M. Jr. and Higuchi, S. 1980. Macrophage functional heterogeneity in vivo. Macrolocal and microlocal macrophage activation, identified by double-staining tissue sections of BCG granulomas for pairs of enzymes. *Am J Pathol*, **99**, 305–23.

Swain, S.L. 2001. Interleukin, 18, tipping the balance towards a T helper cell 1 response. *J Exp Med*, **194**, F11–14.

Thomas, C., et al. 1991. *Infektionskrankheiten*. Stuttgart: Schattauer Verlag.

Toossi, Z. and Ellner, J.J. 1998. The role of TGFβ in the pathogenesis of human tuberculosis. *Clin Immunol Immunopathol*, **87**, 107–14.

Truden, J.L. and Boros, D.L. 1988. Detection of alpha 2-macroglobulin, alpha 1-protease inhibitor, and neutral protease-antiprotease complexes within liver granulomas of *Schistosoma mansoni*-infected mice. *Am J Pathol*, **130**, 281–8.

Turner, O.C., Roberts, A.D., et al. 2000. Lack of protection in mice and necrotizing bronchointerstitial pneumonia with bronchiolitis in guinea pigs immunized with vaccines directed against the hsp60 molecule of *Mycobacterium tuberculosis*. *Infect Immun*, **68**, 3674–9.

Umemura, M., Nishimura, H., et al. 2001. Overexpression of IL-15 in vivo enhances protection against *Mycobacterium bovis* bacillus Calmette-Guerin infection via augmentation of NK and T cytotoxic 1 responses. *J Immunol*, **167**, 946–56.

Vignali, D.A., Crocker, P., et al. 1989. A role for $CD4^+$ but not $CD8^+$ T cells in immunity to *Schistosoma mansoni* induced by 20 krad-irradiated and Ro 11-3128-terminated infections. *Immunology*, **67**, 466–72.

Von Lichtenberg, F. 1975. Schistosomiasis as a worldwide problem: pathology. *J Toxicol Environ Health*, **1**, 175–84.

Wahl, S.M., Hunt, D.A., et al. 1987. Transforming growth factor type beta induces monocyte chemotaxis and growth factor production. *Proc Natl Acad Sci USA*, **84**, 5788–93.

Wahl, S.M., Allen, J.B., et al. 1993. Transforming growth factor beta enhances integrin expression and type IV collagenase secretion in human monocytes. *Proc Natl Acad Sci USA*, **90**, 4577–81.

Wilson, R.A., Coulson, P.S., et al. 1996. Impaired immunity and altered pulmonary responses in mice with a disrupted interferon-gamma receptor gene exposed to the irradiated *Schistosoma mansoni* vaccine. *Immunology*, **87**, 275–82.

Wilson, R.A., Coulson, P.S. and Mountford, A.P. 1999. Immune responses to the radiation-attenuated schistosome vaccine: what can we learn from knock-out mice? *Immunol Lett*, **65**, 117–23.

Winkler, M.K. and Fowlkes, J.L. 2002. Metalloproteinase and growth factor interactions: do they play a role in pulmonary fibrosis? *Am J Physiol Lung Cell Mol Physiol*, **283**, L1–L11.

Woerly, G., Roger, N., et al. 1999. Expression of Th1 and Th2 immunoregulatory cytokines by human eosinophils. *Int Arch Allergy Immunol*, **118**, 95–7.

World Health Organization. 2002. WHO Report: Gobal Tuberculosis Control. http://www.who.int/gtb/publications/globrep02/index.html

Wynn, T.A., Eltoum, I., et al. 1993. Analysis of cytokine mRNA expression during primary granuloma formation induced by eggs of *Schistosoma mansoni*. *J Immunol*, **151**, 1430–40.

Wynn, T.A., Oswald, I.P., et al. 1994. Elevated expression of Th1 cytokines and nitric oxide synthase in the lungs of vaccinated mice after challenge infection with *Schistosoma mansoni*. *J Immunol*, **153**, 5200–9.

Wynn, T.A., Cheever, A.W., et al. 1995. An IL-12-based vaccination method for preventing fibrosis induced by schistosome infection. *Nature*, **376**, 594–6.

Zachariae, C.O., Anderson, A.O., et al. 1990. Properties of monocyte chemotactic and activating factor (MCAF) purified from a human fibrosarcoma cell line. *J Exp Med*, **171**, 2177–82.

Zumla, A. and James, D.G. 1996. Granulomatous infections: etiology and classification. *Clin Infect Dis*, **23**, 146–58.

36

Airway hypersensitivity

ELIZABETH R. JARMAN AND JONATHAN R. LAMB

INTRODUCTION

Airway hyperresponsiveness is a prominent feature of a variety of pulmonary diseases, although it is most often associated with asthma. Asthma is a complex disease of the airways associated with bronchial inflammation, reversible airway obstruction, mucus hypersecretion, and hypersensitivity (increased bronchial reactivity to nonspecific spasmogenic stimuli), defined as airway hyperresponsiveness (AHR). In people with chronic asthma these processes culminate in irreversible changes in airway physiology. There has been a marked increase in the prevalence of asthma in the last few decades. Although there is undoubtedly a genetic component underlying the predisposition toward onset of disease, the scale of the increase in the developed world suggests that environmental factors associated with changes in lifestyle and an improvement in the standard of living must also play a role. Asthma is polygenic and multifactoral in origin and is often classified as intrinsic (antigen independent) or extrinsic (allergic) asthma. Allergic asthma is triggered by antigen-specific exposure to common environmental aeroallergens, such as those present in grass or tree pollen, animal dander, or house dust mites. The aim of this chapter is to review our current understanding of the immunological mechanisms underlying asthma and AHR in the light of recent studies that suggest that the increasing prevalence of asthma may be the result of a loss of inherent immunoregulatory mechanisms.

Airway hyperreactivity

The mechanisms underlying the development of AHR are not fully understood. It is thought to arise as a result of successive inflammatory processes in the airway mucosa triggered by respiratory infections or repeated exposure of susceptible individuals to aeroallergens, resulting in the induction of T-helper (Th)2 cytokines, which play both a direct role in the induction of AHR, as well as an indirect role associated with tissue damage caused by the release of inflammatory mediators from effector cells such as eosinophils recruited into the airways after allergen exposure (Holt et al. 1999). Pathophysiological changes in the airways resulting from chronic inflammation, compounded by altered neural regulation of airway tone, are thought to contribute toward AHR. Increased deposition of extracellular matrix (ECM) proteins in the airway submucosa, increased vascularity, and tissue edema, as well as an increase in airway smooth muscle mass (ASM), lead to thickening of the airway wall and exaggerated airway narrowing in response to various stimuli. A number of mediators released during the inflammatory response are though to contribute toward increased ASM. Histamine, platelet-activating factor (PAF), and the leukotrienes (LT), released from mast cells and eosinophils, are potent inducers of increased bronchial permeability, thereby contributing directly to bronchial edema. The injured airway epithelial cell (AEC) is also a potent source of a number of cytokines, chemokines, and inflammatory mediators, thereby contributing toward AHR and airway remodeling (Holgate 1998).

Early acute phase response

Mast cells are essential for the IgE-dependent, immediate hypersensitivity acute phase reaction to aeroallergens. Within minutes of allergen exposure, cross-linking by multivalent allergen of preformed IgE bound to the high-affinity IgE receptor (FcϵRI) on mast cells results in an immediate hypersensitivity reaction, characterized by the release of the preformed mediators histamine and the proteases (tryptase and chymase), cytokine transcription, and the de novo synthesis and secretion of the cyclooxygenase and lipoxygenase metabolites of arachidonic acid, prostaglandin D_2 (PGD_2), and leukotriene C_4 (LTC_4). These inflammatory mediators activate inflammatory effector cells, and cause mucus secretion, smooth muscle constriction, and increased vascular permeability, thereby potentiating airway inflammation and AHR.

Late phase response

The late phase response (LHR) is associated with the eosinophil recruitment, activation and release of the eosinophil-derived inflammatory mediators, eosinophil cationic protein (ECP), major basic protein (MBP), and eosinophil derived neurotoxin (EDN), in addition to leukotrienes, prostaglandins, particularly PGD_2, and PAF. Eosinophils are also a source of a number of cytokines, including the eosinophil activation and survival factor, IL-5, as well as the profibrotic factor transforming growth factor β (TGF-β). There is a close association between pulmonary eosinophilia and AHR in both extrinsic and intrinsic (nonatopic) asthma. Elevated levels of ECP and MBP have been detected in the bronchoalveolar lavage (BAL) of patients with asthma. These proteins can induce AHR as a direct consequence of their damaging effect on the airway epithelium (Wardlow et al. 1988).

Airway remodeling

Airway remodeling and the resulting structural changes are features of chronic asthma, observed in both atopic and nonatopic individuals. Although the inflammatory response associated with both forms of asthma is characterized by the presence of Th2 cytokines, the existence of a specific IgE is not a prerequisite for the development of asthma, which suggests that abnormalities in the airway epithelium, which forms a barrier to the external environment, results in sensitization to allergens and subsequent development of the asthmatic phenotype. This process may be facilitated by exposure to pathogens such as respiratory viruses, or irritants, which further damage the epithelium. In chronic asthma, structural changes in the bronchial epithelium arise as a result of increased collagen deposition beneath the basal lamina with thickening of the basement membrane, goblet cell hyperplasia, and increased mucin production. These changes eventually lead to irreversible airway obstruction, and a reduction in airway function associated with increased bronchial hyperresponsiveness. Increases in mucus production and goblet cell hyperplasia are common features in cases of fatal asthma (Aikawa et al. 1992).

In asthma, products released by mast cells and eosinophils are directly responsible for damage to the epithelium. The interleukin cytokines IL-4, IL-5, IL-9, and IL-13 released by Th2 effector cells are responsible for many of the features of airway remodeling. Goblet cell metaplasia and mucus production are associated with IL-4- and IL-13-induced increases in expression of the genes *muc5ac*, *muc2*, and *muc4* which are detected in bronchial biopsies obtained from people with asthma. Overproduction of IL-4 in the lung induces *muc5ac* gene expression and mucus secretion by airway epithelial cells expressing the common IL-4Rα chain (Temann et al. 1997), and is dependent on STAT6 signaling (Kuperman et al. 1998). The immunoregulatory molecules TGF-β, and more recently IL-10, have been shown in independent studies to induce subepithelial fibrosis, suggesting that certain aspects of airway remodeling may be an undesirable consequence of an attempt to downregulate chronic inflammatory responses (Elias et al. 1999; Lee et al. 2002)

IMMUNOLOGICAL MECHANISMS UNDERLYING THE ASTHMATIC PHENOTYPE

IgE-mediated pathology in asthma and AHR

Genetic linkage studies have identified an association between chromosome 5q and two of the principal features of allergic asthma: total serum IgE levels and bronchial hyperresponsiveness (Marsh et al. 1994; Postma et al. 1995). A number of clinical studies have demonstrated that elevated specific IgE levels in sera are associated with asthma. Whether this reflects the location on chromosome 5q of the cytokines IL-4 and IL-13, which are directly responsible for increased airway hyperresponsiveness, as well as the switch to ϵ germline transcription and IgE synthesis by B cells (Oettgen and Geha 2001), or an essential role for IgE in the initiation of asthmatic responses is disputed. A recent study carried out on a cohort of Australian families concluded that, of the multiple genetic traits that were found to contribute toward the pathophysiology of asthma, the two dominant traits, namely increased serum IgE levels and AHR, were clearly independently inherited (Palmer et al. 2000). Numerous clinical studies have demonstrated that increased serum IgE, although associated with allergic disease, does not necessarily predispose toward development of asthma and AHR (Sunyer et al. 1995). Most studies in murine models of allergic asthma have shown that AHR can be induced in the absence of B cells or specific IgE antibodies (Mehlhop et al. 1997; Hogan et al. 1997; Hamelmann et al. 1997, 1999).

Nevertheless, allergic sensitization to allergens and IgE-mediated responses play a significant role in the development of asthma in a large number of patients. Specific IgE contributes towards the clinical phenotype by inducing mast cell degranulation and release of inflammatory mediators, following crosslinking of the high-affinity FcϵR. Mediators released from mast cells trigger a cascade of events which culminate in asthma and increased AHR. Recently, completed phase II clinical trials have shown that patients with severe asthma, who are known to respond poorly to steroid treatment, demonstrated a marked improvement in symptoms after treatment with a humanized anti-IgE monoclonal antibodies (McAbs). Anti-IgE McAbs are thought to act by binding to and neutralizing circulating IgE antibodies, thereby preventing them from binding to FcϵRs (Bush 2002; Lemanske et al. 2002).

Mechanisms of CD4$^+$ Th2 cytokine-induced pathology in asthma and AHR

Asthma is a chronic inflammatory disorder that can eventually lead to structural changes in the airways, arising as a result of increased collagen deposition, smooth muscle proliferation, and mucus hyperplasia which cause bronchial hyperresponsiveness and variable airflow obstruction. In both allergic and intrinsic asthma, the inflammatory response is associated with the recruitment of activated CD4$^+$ T lymphocytes expressing a Th2 cytokine profile (Ying et al. 1997a), and an influx of eosinophils. The interleukins, IL-4, IL-5, IL-9, and IL-13, expressed by activated CD4$^+$ Th2 cells which are the dominant cell type in bronchoscopic biopsies and BAL samples obtained from patients with asthma, are thought to play a central role in the pathophysiology of asthma (Robinson et al. 1992).

Genetic linkage studies identified an association with asthma and related traits in the region of chromosome 5q, in which the IL-4, IL-5, IL-9, and IL-13 genes are clustered (Marsh et al. 1994; Postma et al. 1995), and a region of chromosome 16p12 in which the gene encoding the IL-4Rα chain is located (Hershey et al. 1997). Multiple polymorphisms have been identified within the IL-13 gene and IL-4R gene complex, which reassociated with asthma (Heinzmann et al. 2000; Ober et al. 2000).

There is considerable functional redundancy among these pleiotropic Th2-derived cytokines in asthma. For this reason, their relative importance in the development of AHR is still not fully defined. Temporal differences in the kinetics of cytokine expression and in the distribution of their receptor molecules will determine the contribution of these cytokines toward the asthmatic response. It has proved difficult to establish the respective roles of the Th2-derived cytokines IL-4 and IL-13. These cytokines exhibit partially overlapping effector profiles as a result of their common use of the IL-4 receptor α chain (IL-4Rα) as the signaling component within the multimeric IL-4 and IL-13 receptor complexes. The IL-4 R consists of the IL-4Rα chain and the common γ chain (of the IL-2 receptor). The functional IL-13 receptor complex is a heterodimer consisting of the IL-13Rα1 chain which interacts with either the IL-4Rα chain or the IL-13Rα2 chain. Signaling through the IL-4Rα chain leads to activation of the Janus kinase family of tyrosine kinases, resulting in the recruitment, phosphorylation, and nuclear translocation of the transcription factor signal transducer and activator of transcription 6 (STAT6) (Shirakawa et al. 2000). The importance of the STAT6 signaling pathway in the induction of airway eosinophilia and increased AHR was demonstrated in STAT6-deficient mice. These mice failed to develop specific IgE antibodies, airway eosinophilia, or AHR on exposure to methylcholine, after sensitization and challenge of the airways with allergens. Mucus production was significantly reduced compared with wild-type animals (Akimoto et al. 1998; Kuperman et al. 1998).

Using selected lines of Th2 cytokine-deficient mice, deficient in single or multiple cytokine genes, it has been possible to demonstrate that, although IL-5, IL-9, and IL-13 all contribute toward the magnitude of the inflammatory response, IL-4 is essential for initial activation of Th2 effector functions (Fallon et al. 2002). IL-4 is critical for the induction of Th2 responses to allergen, but is not essential for the development of late-phase airway inflammation and AHR. AHR can be induced in naïve mice after adaptive transfer of antigen-specific CD4$^+$ Th2 cells obtained from IL-4-deficient mice (Coyle et al. 1995; Cohn et al. 1998). Although not essential, IL-4 enhances a number of STAT6-dependent responses in the airways which contribute toward AHR. These include enhanced mucus production through the induction of *muc5ac* gene expression by epithelial cells in the airways, release of the eosinophil chemoattractant eotaxin, and upregulation of VCAM-1 expression on endothelial cells, thereby promoting increased recruitment of lymphocytes and eosinophils (Nakajima et al. 1994; Rankin et al. 1996; Temann et al. 1997; Mocjizuki et al. 1998).

The pleiotrophic Th2-derived interleukin IL-13 is now recognized as being largely responsible for initiating and maintaining many of the functions associated with the late-phase inflammatory response, which result in altered airway physiology and remodeling, including goblet cell hyperplasia with mucus hypersecretion and AHR. Notably, both these features of the asthmatic response are commonly associated with asphyxiation (Aikawa et al. 1992). IL-13 also exhibits a number of effects that are responsible for enhancing the IgE-mediated acute phase response, including induction of IgE production by B cells and upregulation of CD23 (FcεRII) expression on B cells, and the upregulation of the expression of the integrin vascular adhesion molecule VCAM-1 on endothelial cells (Zurawski and de Vries 1994; Bochner et al. 1995; Emson et al. 1998). Instillation of IL-13 into the lungs of naïve mice was sufficient to induce many of the features of asthma, including elevated serum IgE, airway eosinophilia, increased mucus production, and AHR. The central role of IL-13 as a mediator in asthma was demonstrated by inhibiting its activity through the administration of the soluble IL-13Rα$_2$-IgGFc fusion protein, to sensitized and challenged mice, before secondary exposure to allergen via the airways. These mice exhibited attenuated goblet cell hyperplasia, mucus production, and AHR on challenge with a spasmogenic agent, despite detectable airway eosinophilia and normal IgE levels (Wills-Karp et al. 1998).

The independence of IL-13-mediated AHR in the airways on T-cell-driven airway inflammation and IgE production was demonstrated in RAG-1$^{-/-}$-deficient mice, which lack T and B lymphocytes, indicating that IL-13 mediates its effects though direct activation of cells in the airways (Grunig et al. 1998). This view was confirmed in subsequent studies, which demonstrated that IL-13 is not only necessary but also sufficient for the induction of AHR. The failure of mice deficient in either IL-13 or IL-4 and IL-13 to develop AHR in spite of increases in IL-5-mediated airway eosinophilia, after sensitization and challenge with allergen, could be reversed by the instillation of recombinant IL-13 alone into the airways (Walter et al. 2001). Chronic expression of IL-13 in the airways was sufficient to cause enhanced recruitment of lymphocytes, eosinophils, and macrophages into the airways, together with subepithelial fibrosis, upregulation of mucin (*Muc5ac*) gene expression, and mucus hypersecretion and increased AHR (Zhu et al. 1999). Increases in both mucus hypersecretion and AHR were mediated by IL-13 through STAT6-dependent mechanisms (Kuperman et al. 2002). However, increases in AHR were also observed in IL-4Rα chain-deficient mice constitutively expressing IL-13 in the airways, or after transfer of IL-13-producing, antigen-specific, CD4$^+$ T cells, indicating that separate components of the STAT6-dependent signaling pathway were involved (Mattes et al. 2001). In addition to its direct effect on airway epithelial cells, IL-13 may influence AHR through direct effects on airway smooth muscle and activation of fibroblasts, resulting in altered deposition of matrix proteins.

IL-13-mediated recruitment and activation of CD4$^+$ Th2 lymphocyte and eosinophils in the airways during the inflammatory response also contribute toward AHR. The coordinated temporal and site-directed expression of chemokines and chemokine receptors is central to the complex pathophysiology of asthma. Elevated levels of the CC chemokines, eotaxin, eotaxin-2, RANTES (monocyte chemotactic protein (MCP)-1, -3. and -4 and the chemokine receptor CCR3 expressed on mast cells, basophils, and eosinophilis, as well as CD4$^+$ Th2 lymphocytes and myeloid dendritic cells (DC), have been observed in the lungs of patients with allergic asthma (Ying et al. 1999). IL-13 is a potent inducer of a number of chemokines involved in the development of the asthmatic phenotype. Levels of mRNA for these chemokines were increased in the lungs of CC10-IL-13 transgenic mice, which selectively overexpress the IL-13 transgene in the airways. Many of the inflammatory and profibrotic effects of IL-13 are mediated through the induction of chemokines responsible for the recruitment of inflammatory cells into the airways. IL-13 is a potent inducer of eotaxin expression by airway epithelial cells (Li et al. 1999), which is a principal chemoattractant for eosinophils, and CCR3 expressing CD4$^+$ Th2 lymphocytes during the initiation of airway inflammation. IL-13-induced increases in production of monocyte-derived chemokine (MDC) and MCP-1, the respective ligands for CCR4 expressed on activated CD4$^+$ Th2 cells and CCR2 expressed on macrophages, are thought to enhance recruitment of these cells into the airways. The importance of the coordinated expression of these chemokines in the induction of airway inflammation and remodeling that results in AHR has been demonstrated in murine models of asthma. Neutralization of MDC activity by the use of specific antibodies lead to reductions in CD4$^+$ T lymphocytes recruited from the airway lumen into the lung, which correlated with attenuated AHR (Gonzalo et al. 1999). The enhanced airway inflammation and tissue fibrosis, observed in CC10-IL-13 transgenic mice, were greatly reduced in mice deficient in CCR2 (Zhou et al. 2002). By inducing increased production of MCP-1, the ligand for CCR2, IL-13 drives the recruitment of macrophages into the airways, where they are though to initiate subepithelial fibrosis, through production of the profibrotic factor TGF-β$_1$ (Lee et al. 2001). These studies indicate that IL-13, through the induction of eotaxin, MDC, and MCP-1, indirectly regulate Th2-mediated airway inflammation, eosinophilia, and tissue fibrosis, respectively.

The central role played by IL-13 in the pathology associated with pulmonary inflammation and fibrosis is not restricted to asthma, and has been observed in a number of respiratory diseases including respiratory syncytial virus infection, fungal pneumonitis, and chronic obstructive pulmonary disease (Lukacs et al. 2001; Blease et al. 2000). Alveolar macrophages in the airways may be the initial source of IL-13 in pulmonary inflammatory disease (Prieto et al. 2000), with relative levels of IL-12 and IL-13 production by macrophages in the airways during primary antigen challenge influencing the phenotype of effector T cells.

Levels of the Th2-derived cytokine IL-9 and expression of the IL-9R are elevated in the lungs of patients with allergic asthma (Shimbara et al. 2000). IL-9 stimulates a number of different cell types, including B cells, mast cells, eosinophils, and airway epithelial cells, leading to the development of a number of features that are characteristic of asthma and AHR (Petit-Frere et al. 1993; Longphre et al. 1999; Gounni et al. 2000; Louahed et al. 2001). Transgenic mice exhibiting either constitutive or inducible IL-9 expression in the lung have many of the features associated with asthma, including eosinophilic and lymphocytic infiltration of the airways, mucus hypersecretion, subepithelial fibrosis, mast cell hyperplasia, and AHR (Tenmann et al. 1998). The effects mediated by IL-9 may be the result of increased expression of the Th2 cytokines IL-4, IL-5, and IL-13 in the lungs of IL-9 transgenic mice. Neutralization of IL-13 completely abolished both lung inflammation and mucus production (Tenmann et al. 2002), indicating that expression of IL-9 alone is insufficient to induce pathological changes associated with asthma and that these cytokines are required to act in combination in order to achieve optimal stimulation. The unique role of IL-13 in the induction of AHR is most probably the result of its direct effects on airway epithelial cells, mediated independently of the common IL-4Rα chain.

The role of mast cells in the induction of AHR

Mast cells are important in initiating and amplifying the IgE-mediated acute hypersensitivity response to allergens. Crosslinking of FcϵRs by IgE–allergen complexes causes degranulation and release of inflammatory mediators such as histamine, prostaglandin (PGD_2) and the leukotrienes (LTC_4) which trigger bronchoconstriction in the asthmatic lung (Metcalf et al. 1997; Matsuoka et al. 2000). As a major primary source of IL-4 in the lungs, mast cells and tissue basophils may also play an important role in priming Th2 responses in the airways (Nouri et al. 2001). A number of cytokines (TNF-γ, IL-1, IL-3, granulocyte–macrophage colony-stimulating factor (GM-CSF), IL-4, IL-5, IL-6, and IL-8) and chemokines (MCP-1, macrophage inflammatory protein 1α [MIP-1α], MIP-1β, and eotaxin), expressed by mast cells are important for the recruitment and activation of effector cells, including eosinophilis, which are involved in the late phase response (Das et al. 1998). Nevertheless, studies in mast cell-deficient Kit^{W}/Kit^{W-v} mice indicate that many features of the late phase response, including eosinophilia and AHR, can occur in the absence of mast cells, suggesting that there is considerable redundancy in the mechanisms contributing toward the allergic response (Takeda et al. 1997). Studies in animal models of asthma indicate that, at low concentrations of allergen exposure, mast cells play a prominent role in the induction of IgE-mediated AHR (Kobayashi et al. 2000). Binding of IgE to the FcϵRI on mast cells induces the upregulation of FcϵRI, thereby enhancing IgE-dependent release of inflammatory mediators even at low levels of allergen exposure (Yamaguchi et al. 1999). Furthermore, binding of monomeric IgE to the FcϵRI on mast cells inhibits apoptotic signals, thereby enhancing survival of mast cells in the airways and leading to further amplification of the asthmatic response (Asai et al. 2001).

The role of eosinophils in the induction of AHR

Eosinophils are considered to be the major effector cells in the pathogenesis of the late phase asthmatic response and consequently of AHR. Inflammatory mediators released from their granules, in particular the leukotrienes, can lead to damage of the airway epithelium resulting in AHR (Gleich et al. 1993). Some, but not all clinical studies (McFadden 1994) have observed a correlation between eosinophil levels in BAL and bronchial biopsies obtained from allergic patients, and disease severity as assessed by AHR (Wardlow et al. 1988). There are considerable clinical data that support the view that disease severity in asthma directly correlates with IL-5 and eosinophil levels (Bentley et al. 1993; Sur et al. 1995). The Th2-derived cytokine IL-5 is a key regulator of airway eosinophilia, acting as both a growth factor and a chemoattractant to induce differentiation, activation, recruitment, and survival at sites of allergen exposure (Lopez et al. 1988). Nevertheless, the role of IL-5-dependent airway eosinophilia in the induction of AHR has not been fully clarified. A recent clinical trial performed using a humanized McAb raised against IL-5 revealed that, despite attenuating eosinophil recruitment into the airways, there was no resolution of AHR in patients (Leckie et al. 2000).

Animal models of pulmonary inflammation have provided some insight into the role of eosinophils in the induction of AHR. Increased levels of eosinophils in the airways are associated with AHR (Tomkinson et al. 1999) and AHR can occur independently of the presence of both IL-5 and eosinophils (Corry et al. 1996). However, treatment of sensitized mice with anti-IL-5-neutralizing antibodies before allergen challenge of the airways, while having no effect on early acute phase responses, abolished late-phase inflammatory responses, with a loss of both airway inflammation and AHR (Foster et al. 1996; Hamelmann et al. 1999). STAT6 is essential for many IL-4- and IL-13-mediated responses which impact on the levels of AHR (Kaplan et al. 1996).

Therefore, the ability to induce not only airway eosinophilia, but also AHR on exposure of STAT6-deficient mice to allergen by reconstitution with IL-5 indicates that eosinophilis are sufficient to induce AHR in the absence of specific IgE, mucus production, or Th2 effector cells (Tomkinson et al. 1999). These discrepancies in the data may partially reflect genetic differences between the inbred strains of mice used, which could influence susceptibility to AHR (Wilder et al. 1999; Ewart et al. 2000).

Data obtained from animal models of disease have been interpreted on the assumption that IL-5 is principally responsible for airway eosinophilia. For this reason, studies investigating the role of eosinophils in the induction of AHR have focused primarily on the use of IL-5-deficient mice or IL-5-neutralizing antibodies and have indicated that neutralization of IL-5 is insufficient to abrogate airway eosinophilia. In addition to IL-5, the chemokine eotaxin acts as a major chemoattractant not only for eosinophils, but also for activated $CD4^+$ Th2 cells expressing the CCR3 chemokine receptor (Sallusto et al. 1997). CCR3 is the receptor for a number of chemokines associated with Th2-mediated airway inflammation in asthma, including eotaxin, and appears to be essential for the recruitment of both eosinophils and $CD4^+$ Th2 cells and in the induction of AHR (Lloyd et al. 2000; Ma et al. 2002). Analysis of bronchial biopsies from patients with asthma revealed that the intensity of eotaxin and CCR3 mRNA expression correlated with increased AHR (Ying et al. 1997b). Interestingly, the Th2-derived cytokine IL-13 can also upregulate eotaxin production by residual cells in the airways, including smooth muscle, fibroblasts, and airway epithelial cells, thereby contributing indirectly to tissue eosinophilia (Matsukura et al. 2001; Hirst et al. 2002; Wenzel et al. 2002). Binding of the very-late-activating antigen 4 (VLA-4), expressed on both eosinophils and T cells, to VCAM-1 expressed on the surface of endothelial cells is essential for cellular recruitment into the airways. Attenuation of both airway eosinophilia and AHR, by administration of neutralizing antibodies raised against IL-5 or VLA-4 to sensitized mice immediately before challenge of the airways with allergen, suggests a potentially independent role for $CD4^+$ Th2 effector cells and eosinophils in the induction of AHR (Tomkinson et al. 2001).

Although eosinophils undoubtedly play a prominent role in contributing toward bronchial hyperreactivity, there is considerable evidence that AHR can be induced in their absence. Th2 cells are not only responsible for initiating airway inflammation and eosinophilia but are also directly responsible for inducing AHR through production of cytokines, notably IL-13. This has been clearly demonstrated in STAT6-deficient mice in which the transfer of $CD4^+$ T cells from sensitized mice was sufficient to induce AHR on challenge of the airways with allergen, even in the absence of eosinophilia (Tomkinson et al. 2002). Nevertheless, it is likely that eosinophils contribute toward the induction of AHR, not only as effector cells through their ability to release inflammatory mediators, but also through the induction of Th2 responses. Studies by Mattes et al. (2002) have demonstrated that mice deficient in both IL-5 and eotaxin failed to develop airway eosinophilia and AHR on allergen exposure, and furthermore that $CD4^+$ Th2 cells isolated from these mice were impaired in their ability to produce IL-13, which is directly responsible for the induction of AHR. Transfer of eosinophils from wild-type mice was sufficient to re-establish IL-13 production by $CD4^+$ Th2 effector cells, supporting evidence that eosinophils, acting as antigen-presenting cells, have the potential to promote Th2-dependent responses in the asthmatic airways. Eosinophils isolated from the airways of patients with allergic asthma exhibited elevated levels of MHC class II and the costimulatory molecules CD80 and CD86 (MacKenzie et al. 2001). Furthermore, on exposure to allergen, eosinophils migrate from the airways to the T-cell-rich paracortical zones of draining lymph nodes, where antigen presentation takes place (Shi et al. 2000). It is likely that multiple factors acting either independently or in concert contribute toward AHR. $CD4^+$ Th2 cells are central for the induction of airway inflammation and eosinophilia, and it is therefore likely that they contribute, through the cytokines that they release, both directly and indirectly to AHR. As a major source of both IL-5 and IL-13 (Schmid-Grendelmeier et al. 2002), eosinophils may play a role in amplifying the inflammatory response, leading to chronic airway inflammation, enhanced bronchoconstriction, and AHR.

Antigen-presenting cells in the mucosal surfaces of the airways and their role in the induction of asthma

Dendritic cells are professional antigen-presenting cells that form a dense network in the airways lining the nasal and bronchial mucosa and lung interstitium (Holt et al. 1989). These cells are, therefore, ideally placed to sample antigen, which is then processed and presented to naïve T cells, following migration of DCs to the lymph nodes draining the airways (Vermaelen et al. 2001). Studies in animal models demonstrate that DCs play a critical role not only in the induction of $CD4^+$ Th2 cell-mediated responses and IgE synthesis, but also in maintaining late phase responses in sensitized animals, including airway eosinophilia and goblet cell hyperplasia (Lambrecht et al. 1988). Studies in patients with allergic asthma showed that $CD11c^+$ $HLA\text{-}DR^+$ DCs are rapidly recruited to the airways within hours of allergen exposure (Jahnsen et al. 2001). Independent studies have reported that the number of circulating $CD33^+$ DCs in the peripheral blood of patients with asthma is reduced after allergen exposure (Upham et al. 2002). Evidence for expression of the receptor for the chemokine eotaxin, CCR3, by $CD34^+$ human DCs of the myeloid lineage suggests that these cells are recruited into the airways of people with asthma after upregulation of eotaxin, where they may play a role in maintaining Th2-mediated inflammatory responses (Beaulieu et al. 2002). Recent studies demonstrated that $CD11c^+$ $CD11b^+$ myeloid DCs in the airways are capable of retaining antigen for prolonged periods of time and, furthermore, that these cells are primarily responsible for presenting antigen to effector T cells in the lung (Julia et al. 2002). The presence of specific IgE bound to the high-affinity FcεRI on DCs in the periphery and the bronchial mucosa could potentially lower the activation threshold, thereby increasing responsiveness at low levels of allergen exposure (Tunon de Lara et al. 1996; Holloway et al. 2001). These data suggest that DCs are essential not only for initiating the T-cell-mediated, late phase response to allergens, but also for maintaining low levels of chronic inflammation, which could ultimately lead to airway remodeling.

The airway mucosa is continually exposed to common nonpathogenic environmental antigens. It is, therefore, likely that mechanisms have evolved for maintaining homeostasis, thereby preventing the induction of inappropriate inflammatory responses in the airways. The dramatic increase in the incidence of atopic asthma in the developed world, which has coincided with an increase in auotoimmune diseases, may reflect a loss of inherent immunoregulatory mechanisms. IL-10 is an immunoregulatory cytokine that is produced by a number of cell types and has a wide range of immunosuppressive effects including inhibition of DC maturation and macrophage activation, downregulation of leukocyte adhesion molecule expression, and suppression of T-cell proliferation and Th1 cytokine production (Moore et al. 2001). IL-10 has recently been described as a growth factor for a subset of $CD4^+$ $CD25^+$ T-regulatory cells, which are thought to be central to the induction and maintenance of immunological tolerance to selfantigens, thereby preventing the onset of autoimmune disease (Groux et al. 1997).

Dendritic cells in the airways, through their role in sampling antigen from the environment and their unique ability to prime naïve T-cell responses, may play a determining role in the induction of tolerance and immune regulation on exposure to allergens. In the absence of infection or inflammatory stimuli, DCs retain an immature phenotype. The presentation of antigen to naïve T cells by immature DCs would hypothetically result in T-cell-receptor ligation in the absence of costimulation, leading to the induction of a state of tolerance (Mueller et al. 1989). A direct role for pulmonary DCs in the induction of mucosal tolerance to inhaled antigen has been demonstrated in vivo. DCs isolated from the bronchial lymph nodes draining the lungs of mice exposed via the nasal mucosa to soluble antigen, in the absence of inflammatory stimuli, were able to adoptively transfer a state of antigen-specific tolerance to naïve mice. By repeating these studies in IL-10 knock-out mice, the authors were able to demonstrate that the expression of a tolerogenic pheonotype by DCs was dependent on the presence of IL-10. Furthermore, they found that, by culturing antigen-specific $CD4^+$ T cells with these IL-10-producing pulmonary DCs, they were able to induce a $CD4^+$ T regulatory cell-like phenotype as associated with IL-10 production (Akbari et al. 2001).

In the presence of pathogen-derived inflammatory stimuli, DCs undergo maturation and upregulation of the chemokine receptor CCR7, which facilitates migration to lymph nodes where DCs, which have acquired potent antigen-presenting capacity afer upregulation of MHCII molecules and the costimulatory molecules CD80 and CD86, prime T-cell responses. In vitro studies have demonstrated that autocrine IL-10 can suppress DC maturation in response to stimulation with lipopolysaccharide (LPS), or soluble CD40 ligand, thereby inducing a tolerogenic phenotype (Corinti et al. 2001; Steinbrink et al. 1997). Furthermore, the ability of IL-10 to inhibit upregulation of the chemokine receptor CCR7 on stimulated DCs could prevent DCs from migrating to the draining lymph nodes, where antigen presentation and T-cell priming would normally take place (D'Amico et al. 2000). Studies using labeled T cells demonstrated that primed effector T cells that had migrated to the airways, although being capable of producing cytokines and inducing eosinophilia, failed to proliferate on exposure to antigen (Harris et al. 2002). As effector $CD4^+$ T cells have lost their capacity to migrate out of peripheral tissues, continued priming of effector memory T-cell populations by DCs in the lymph nodes may be necessary in order to maintain a chronic asthmatic state. Production of IL-10 within the airways at the time of allergen challenge may play a role in limiting the inflammatory asthmatic response.

ASSOCIATION BETWEEN INNATE AND ADAPTIVE IMMUNITY IN THE INDUCTION OF AHR

Immunoregulatory mechanisms of γδ T cells in maintaining homeostasis in the airways

Intraepithelial γδ T cells, which are located in the mucosal surfaces of the airways, may be involved in maintaining homeostasis on exposure to inflammatory stimuli, thus protecting against pathological processes culminating in bronchoconstriction and AHR. Mice genetically deficient in γδ T cells (T-cell receptor (TCR)-$\delta^{-/-}$) exhibited elevated levels of AHR on exposure to methylcholine following sensitization and challenge with allergen. No increases in immunoglobulins, Th2-derived cytokines, or eosinophil levels were observed, indicating that $\gamma\delta$ T cells exert their regulatory function through antigen-independent mechanisms, most probably involving a direct interaction with neighboring airway epithelial cells, thereby inhibiting the release of proinflammatory cytokines and chemokines (Lahn et al. 1999). By promoting clearance of necrotic tissue in the airways, $\gamma\delta$ T cells may also play a role in limiting pulmonary injury (King et al. 1999).

Complement factors

Epidemiological studies indicate an association between exposure to particulate matter in air pollutants and exacerbation of bronchoconstriction, leading to increased AHR (Dockery and Pope 1994). This view is supported by data obtained from animal studies, demonstrating an increase in AHR on exposure to particulate matter in diesel fumes (Ohta et al. 1999). Activation of the complement pathway, resulting in cleavage of complement factors C3 and C5 and release of the anaphylotoxins C3a and C5a, is an integral part of the innate immune response to mucosal infection. Their receptors, C5aR and C3aR, are constitutively expressed on bronchial epithelial cells, AECs, smooth muscle cells, and vascular endothelial cells (Drouin et al. 2001). Many of the features of asthma, including smooth muscle contraction, mucus secretion, increased vascular permeability, as well as the recruitment and activation of inflammatory cells, can be mediated by the actions of these anaphylotoxins. C3a is a chemoattractant and activation factor for mast cells and eosinophils. Patients with allergic asthma exhibit increased levels of C3 in the BAL fluid and upregulated expression of C3aR on airway smooth muscle cells shortly after exposure to allergen. Furthermore, mice deficient in C3 or the C3aR fail to develop AHR on sensitization and exposure to allergen, despite exhibiting Th2-mediated airway eosinophilia and increased IgE production (Humbles et al. 2000). Exposure to particulate matter was sufficient to induce AHR in wild-type, but not C3-deficient, mice (Walters et al. 2002). Increases in air pollution may, therefore, account for the rise in both extrinsic and intrinsic asthma, assuming that the complement pathway acts as an antigen-independent link between the innate and adaptive immune response. Interestingly, the gene-encoding complement factor 5 (C5) has been identified as a susceptibility locus for allergen-induced AHR in mice. Studies suggest that C5-mediated responses may protect against the development of Th2-dependent increases in AHR. Blockage of C5a receptor-mediated signaling using a C5aR antagonist inhibited the production of the Th1-promoting cytokine IL-12 by human monocytes stimulated with *Staphylococcus aureus* and furthermore reversed IFN-γ-mediated suppression of IL-10 production (Karp et al. 2000).

IMMUNOREGULATORY NETWORKS

The immunological basis for the hygiene hypothesis

There is increasing evidence that the development of allergic asthma after sensitization to allergen is a consequence of the interaction between environmental factors and the genetic background of that individual. The prevalence of asthma has increased most markedly in the developed world. Although increased pollution and exposure to indoor allergens were originally proposed to account for this increase, epidemiological studies found that asthma prevalence was lower in former East Germany, in spite of high levels of pollution, than in the cleaner more affluent former West Germany (Nicolai and von Mutius 1997). In contrast, epidemiological and immunological data appear to support the 'hygiene hypothesis', which proposes that the increase in the prevalence of asthma is the result of a reduction in childhood infections. The study performed by von Mutius is of particular interest, because it draws attention to the possible role of the bacterial product endotoxin, a LPS found in the outer wall of gram-negative bacteria, in shaping the immune response. This study demonstrated that children raised in rural areas and heavily exposed to farm animals were less likely to develop allergy and asthma than children who had grown up in the same environment but were not exposed to farm animals. Natural exposure to environmental endotoxins in the stables appeared to protect children from developing allergies (Von Mutius et al. 2000). Epidemiological studies provide some support for this hypothesis. An inverse correlation was observed between positive DTH responses to tuberculin and the development of atopy (Shirakawa et al. 1997). Separate studies indicate that early immunization with mycobacteria BCG protects against the development of allergic disease (Aaby et al. 2000).

Studies in animal models of allergic asthma have demonstrated that pretreatment with the BCG before sensitization protects against the subsequent induction of Th2-mediated IgE production, airway eosinophilia, and increased AHR. Protection correlated with increased antigen-specific Th1 immunity and IFN-γ production (Erb et al. 1998; Hertz et al. 1998). Furthermore, administration of mycobacterial antigens to previously sensitized animals attenuated the late phase inflammatory responses and AHR, although IgE levels in serum and early acute phase reactions were not affected (Hopfenspirger and Agrawal 2002). The protective effect of mycobacteria is thought to arise through the induction of IL-12 and IFN-γ resulting in enhanced Th1 immunity, which counterbalances the Th2 response to allergens. Mucosal gene transfer of IFN-γ directly into the airways of sensitized mice significantly inhibits the induction of Th2-mediated airway eosinophilia and AHR on exposure to allergen (Li et al. 1996). Nevertheless, data obtained from a number of independent studies indicates that IFN-γ-dependent Th1 responses may not only fail to counterbalance Th2-mediated immunity, but may also actually exacerbate the ongoing inflammatory response (Hansen et al. 1999).

Mycobacteria may protect against the induction of the Th2-mediated inflammatory response to allergens, by initiating a number of immunoregulatory mechanisms. Mycobacteria are known to stimulate the innate immune response, leading to enhanced levels of IL-12 and IFN-γ production by antigen-presenting cells including DCs, macrophages, and natural killer (NK) cells. Mycobacterially derived heat shock proteins have been shown to protect against the induction of allergen-induced AHR by triggering increased production of both IL-10 and the Th1-derived cytokine, IFN-γ. Recent studies indicate that this protective effect is dependent on γδ T cells, possibly activated through antigen-independent mechanisms such as increases in TNF-α production by DCs and macrophages, after uptake of mycobacteria. γδ T cells may exert their immunoregulatory effects by acting directly on airway epithelial cells to inhibit the release of factors that, either directly or indirectly through stimulation of Th2-mediated inflammatory responses, result in AHR (Kanehiro et al. 2001; Rha et al. 2002).

Lipopolysaccharide/endotoxin, a major constituent of bacterial cells walls, also appears to downregulate Th2 responses by stimulating production of the immunosuppressive and anti-inflammatory cytokine IL-10. Studies in rodent models have shown that exposure to LPS either before or during allergen provocation can protect against the induction of Th2-mediated airway inflammatory responses and eosinophilia, but failed to protect against the development of AHR (Gerhold et al. 2002). Furthermore, once airway inflammation has been established, exposure to LPS exacerbates the inflammatory response (Tulic et al. 2000).

LPS also induces secretion of IL-10 by a number of cell types, including DCs, which are critical for priming T-cell responses to allergens. This has led to speculation that LPS may protect against the development of asthma by the induction of immunoregulatory mechanisms rather than, or in addition to, protecting against Th2 immunity. A number of pathogens appear to trigger IL-10 production. Epidemiological studies have identified a disassociation between helminth infection and allergic disease. The induction of IL-10 production by parasites was associated with reduced skin test reactivity to aeroallergens (van den Biggelaar et al. 2000). This has led to the hypothesis that the immune system may have evolved mechanisms, such as the production of IL-10, for limiting the extent of the inflammatory response to microbial pathogens. The decrease in exposure to parasites or infectious agents, which has occurred in the western world over the last few decades, may account for a reduction in inherent immunoregulatory mechanisms. This may also explain the increasing incidence of autoimmune diseases, which have paralleled the rise in incidents of allergic asthma. Notably, animal studies have demonstrated that IL-10 knock-out mice are highly susceptible to both Th1- and Th2-mediated inflammatory diseases (Hoffmann et al. 2000). Furthermore, mucosal tolerance, which is thought to depend on IL-10 production, cannot be readily induced in animals kept in germ-free conditions, suggesting a minimal requirement for nonpathogenic gut microflora (Sudo et al. 1997). Epidemiological studies have found a significant correlation between the use of antibiotics during the first year of life and the subsequent development of allergic diseases (Wickens et al. 1999). The frequent use of antibiotics may have resulted in a reduction in the gut microflora.

The potential importance of IL-10 in regulating the asthmatic phenotype was revealed in comparative studies, which showed a marked reduction in IL-10 protein levels in BAL fluid of patients with allergic asthma and in cultures of peripheral blood cells on stimulation with LPS, suggestive of an inherent defect in IL-10 production (Borish et al. 1996). Nevertheless, it is highly likely that, in addition to IL-10, a number of other factors, including TGF-β and the activity of $CD4^+CD25^+$ regulatory T cells, contribute to the regulation of immunopathological processes that are involved in bronchoconstriction and AHR. Furthermore IL-10, although exhibiting protective properties during the induction and effector phase of asthma, can also under certain circumstances contribute toward increased AHR.

Immunoregulatory and pathogenic roles of IL-10 in AHR

The role of IL-10 in the development of AHR remains disputed. Evidence for an association between elevated IgE levels and polymorphisms in the promoter region of the IL-10 gene (Hobbs et al. 1998) is backed by clinical studies that have revealed reduced levels of IL-10 transcripts and protein levels in BAL fluid obtained from patients with allergic asthma (Borish et al. 1996). Furthermore, successful standard immunotherapy to insect venom, as assessed by reductions in clinical symptoms on allergen exposure, correlated with an increase in IL-10 production by allergen-reactive T cells in the periphery (Akdis et al. 1998). Animal models have been used in an attempt to evaluate the role of IL-10 in the pathogenesis of asthma and AHR. These studies suggest that, although generally considered as a regulatory and anti-inflammatory cytokine, IL-10 can also contribute toward the pathophysiology of AHR in asthma. Zuany-

Amorim demonstrated that administration of IL-10 into the airways of mice at the time of antigen challenge, but not later, caused a marked reduction in IL-5 production and airway eosinophilia, suggesting that IL-10 may inhibit localized priming of Th2 responses (Zuany-Amorim et al. 1995; Yang et al. 2000). A role for endogenous IL-10 in regulating T-cell-mediated inflammatory responses was confirmed using IL-10 gene knock-out mice (Grunig et al. 1997). An independent study revealed that, in spite of developing pronounced airway inflammation associated with increased levels of the Th2 cytokines IL-5 and IL-13 in BAL, eosinophilia, and mucus production, IL-10-deficient mice failed to develop AHR. Transfer of the IL-10 gene before allergen challenge of the airways was sufficient to reconstitute AHR in sensitized mice, indicating that IL-10 is an important cofactor for induction of AHR (Makela et al. 2000; Justice et al. 2001). However, in the absence of prior sensitization and challenge of the airways with allergen, IL-10 alone is insufficient to induce AHR (Van Scott et al. 2000). In view of the various studies performed to date, it is likely that the role played by IL-10 in the induction of AHR is indirect and not unique. Studies have shown that AHR could be induced after respiratory syncytial virus (RSV) infection of IL-10-deficient mice exhibiting allergen-induced airway inflammation. Furthermore, reductions in airway eosinophilia following treatment of RSV-infected mice with anti-IL-5 neutralizing antibody significantly reduced AHR following allergen exposure, indicating a potential role for eosinophil-derived factors in AHR (Makela et al. 2002). Previous studies indicated that the Th2 cytokines, IL-5 and IL-13, contribute directly toward AHR, suggesting that factors released during airway inflammation are also required for induction of AHR (Foster et al. 1996; Garlisi et al. 1997; Grunig et al. 1998; Hogan et al. 1998; Wills-Karp et al. 1998). Recent studies have shown that eosinophils derived from patients with asthma express IL-13, and furthermore that IL-13. Furthermore, following stimulation with IL-5, IL-13 can be induced in eosophinols obtained from non-asthmatic controls. These data suggest that in an allergic Th2 cytokine-driven asthmatic response, eosinophils, by acting as a source of IL-13, may contribute indirectly towards the induction of AHR (Schmid-Grendelmeier et al. 2002). Most probably elevated levels of IL-13, arising as a result of IL-10-mediated suppression of Th1 cytokine responses, may be a compounding factor in the onset of AHR, because many of the factors known to contribute toward AHR, including mucus metaplasia, are IL-13 dependent.

Immunoregulatory role of IL-12

Allergic asthma and AHR is associated with skewed Th2 cytokine production. It has been proposed that the balance between IL-12-induced Th1 responses and levels of Th2 cytokines, notably IL-4 and IL-13 in the airways, or responsiveness to these cytokines could influence development of an allergic asthmatic phenotype. Interestingly, the genes encoding the Th2 cytokines (IL-4, IL-5, IL-9, and IL-13), as well as the p40 subunit of IL-12, are located within chromosome 5q (Marsh et al. 1994). Identification of rare polymorphisms in the promoter region of the IL-12 subunit genes (Pravica et al. 2000) and their association with disease severity (Morahan et al. 2002) has led to speculation that a failure to suppress aberrant Th2-mediated responses to common aeroallergens in genetically predisposed individuals results in the development of allergic diseases. IL-12, produced by antigen-presenting cells including DCs and macrophages after stimulation with microbial pathogens, is critical for the development of a Th1 phenotype (Trinchieri 1994). Signaling through the IL-12 Rβ_2 subunit is required for Th1 differentiation after STAT4 nuclear translocation and IFN-γ gene transcription. Notably, cells expressing a Th2 phenotype have lost IL-12Rβ_2 expression and therefore their ability to respond to IL-12 (Szabo et al. 1995).

There is increasing evidence from clinical studies that a deregulated IL-12 response may contribute toward the development of an asthmatic phenotype. Bronchial biopsy specimens taken from patients with allergic asthma were found to contain lower levels of IL-12 p40 mRNA than healthy controls (Naseer et al. 1997). The immunoregulatory cytokines TGF-β and IL-10 as well as a number of factors associated with the allergic inflammatory response, in particular IL-4, IL-13, and the inflammatory mediators PGE_2 and histamine, can down-regulate IL-12 production, thereby further amplifying the allergic response (Van der Pouw Kraan et al. 1995; Meyaard et al. 1996; Elenkov et al. 1998). An increase in IL-12 and decrease in IL-13 levels after steroid treatment were observed only in those patients who responded to therapy. Failure to respond to steroid treatment may be linked to reduced levels of IL-12Rβ_2 chain expression (Matsui et al. 1999; Wright et al. 1999).

Studies in murine models of allergic disease have demonstrated the importance of IL-12 in regulating pathogenic Th2 responses. IL-12 appears to play a critical role in protecting against the initial induction of allergic responses. Blockage of endogenous IL-12 in the unresponsive C3H/HeJ strain resulted in development of Th2-mediated responses on allergen exposure with elevated serum IgE levels, eosinophilic infiltration of the airways, and enhanced AHR (Keane-Myers et al. 1998). IL-12 knock-out mice showed enhanced levels of eosinophils in bone marrow and BAL following antigen challenge, compared with wild-type controls (Zhao et al. 2000). Administration of IL-12 during either sensitization or allergen challenge markedly reduced AHR (Kips et al. 1996; Sur et al. 1996; Schwarze et al. 1998). Suppression of Th2-mediated airway responses was associated with a Th1 shift in cytokine responses. Nevertheless, studies in IFN-γR knock-out mice revealed that, although the initial inhibition of IgE production by IL-12 was IFN-γ dependent, suppression of airway eosinophilia and AHR was only partially dependent on IFN-γ, suggesting that other mechanisms are involved in mediating late phase inflammatory responses and AHR (Brusselle et al. 1997). A clinical study demonstrated that subcutaneous administration of recombinant IL-12 had no effect on the late phase airway hyperresponsiveness to allergen challenge, despite a significant reduction in eosinophil numbers and an improvement in the immediate acute hypersensitivity response (Bryan et al. 2000).

CONCLUSIONS

Asthma is a disease of the airways associated with pulmonary inflammation, eosinophilia, mucus hypersecretion, and increased AHR. Although both polygenic and multifactoral in origin, the recent rise in prevalence of asthma in the developed world has increased interest in the immunological mechanisms underlying the pathophysiology of disease. Asthma is associated with recruitment of activated $CD4^+$ Th2 cells producing IL-4, IL-5, IL-9, and IL-13. These cytokines exhibit considerable functional redundancy and only recently, through the use of animal models, has it been possible to establish their role in the asthmatic response. Whereas IL-4 is essential for the induction of Th2 responses, IL-13 appears to be essential for the late phase response associated with AHR. Through the induction of chemokines, IL-13 mediates the recruitment and activation of $CD4^+$ Th2 lymphocytes and eosinophils involved in airway inflammation. In addition, IL-13, through its direct effects on resident airway epithelial cells, fibroblasts, and smooth muscle cells, mediates mucus hypersecretion, tissue fibrosis, and AHR.

The correlation between the rise in incidence of asthma and reduced exposure to bacterial and parasitic infections, which has arisen as a result of improved living standards, has led to speculation that anti-inflammatory responses induced by these agents may protect against the development of aberrant Th2 immune responses to environmental allergens. Immunoregulatory mechanisms, which include IL-10 production by DCs, are also involved in mucosal tolerance induction on exposure of the airways to allergen.

REFERENCES

Aaby, P., Shaheen, S.O., et al. 2000. Early BCG vaccination and reduction in atopy in Guinea-Bissau. *Clin Exp Allergy*, **30**, 644–50.

Aikawa, T., Shimura, S.M., et al. 1992. Marked goblet cell hyperplasia with mucus accumulation in the airways of patients who died of severe acute asthma attack. *Chest*, **101**, 916–21.

Akbari, O., DeKruyff, R.H. and Umetsu, D.T. 2001. Pulmonary dendritic cells producing IL-10 mediate tolerance induced by respiratory exposure to antigen. *Nature Immunol*, **2**, 725–31.

Akdis, C.A., Blesken, T., et al. 1998. Role of interleukin 10 in specific immunotherapy. *J Clin Invest*, **102**, 98–106.

Akimoto, T., Numata, F., et al. 1998. Abrogation of bronchial eosinophilic inflammation and airway hyperreactivity in signal transducers and activators of transcription (STAT) 6-deficient mice. *J Exp Med*, **187**, 1537–42.

Asai, K., Kitaura, J., et al. 2001. Regulation of mast cell survival by IgE. *Immunity*, **14**, 791–800.

Beaulieu, S., Robbiani, D.F., et al. 2002. Expression of a functional exotaxin (CC Chemokine Ligand 11) receptor CCR3 by human dendritic cells. *J Immunol*, **169**, 2925–36.

Bentley, A.M., Meng, Q., et al. 1993. Increases in activated T lymphocytes, eosinophils and cytokine mRNA expression for interleukin-5 and granulocyte/macrophage colony stimulating factor in bronchial biopsies after allergen inhalation challenge in atopic asthmatics. *Am J Respir Cell Mol Biol*, **8**, 35–42.

Blease, K., Mehrad, B., et al. 2000. Enhanced pulmonary allergic responses to *Aspergillus* in CCR2-/- mice. *J Immunol*, **165**, 2603–11.

Bochner, B.S., Klunk, D.A., et al. 1995. IL-13 selectively induces vascular adhesion molecule-1 expression in human endothelial cells. *J Immunol*, **154**, 799–803.

Borish, L., Aarons, A., et al. 1996. Interleukin-10 regulation in normal subjects and patients with asthma. *J Allergy Clin Immunol*, **97**, 1288–96.

Bush, R.K. 2002. The use of anti-IgE in the treatment of allergic asthma. *Med Clin North Am*, **86**, 1113–29.

Brusselle, G.G., Kips, J.C., et al. 1997. Role of IFN-gamma in the inhibition of the allergic airway inflammation caused by IL-12. *Am J Respir Cell Mol Biol*, **17**, 767–71.

Bryan, S.A., O'Connor, B.J., et al. 2000. Effects of recombinant human interleukin-12 on eosinophils, airway hyper-responsiveness and the late asthmatic response. *Lancet*, **356**, 2149–53.

Cohn, L., Tepper, J.S. and Bottomly, K. 1998. IL-4 independent induction of airway hyperresponsiveness by Th2, but not Th1 cells. *J Immunol*, **161**, 3813–16.

Corinti, S., Albanesi, C., et al. 2001. Regulatory activity of autocrine IL-10 on dendritic cell functions. *J Immunol*, **166**, 4312–18.

Coyle, A.J., LeGross, G., et al. 1995. Interleukin-4 is required for the induction of lung Th2 mucosal immunity. *Am J Respir Cell Mol Biol*, **13**, 54–9.

Corry, D.H., Folkesson, M., et al. 1996. Interleukin 4, but not interleukin 5 or eosinophils is required in a murine model of acute airway hyperreactivity. *J Exp Med*, **183**, 109–17.

D'Amico, G., Frascaroli, G., et al. 2000. Uncoupling of inflammatory chemokine receptors by IL-10: generation of functional decoys. *Nat Immunol*, **1**, 387–91.

Das, A.M., Flower, R.J. and Perretti, M. 1998. Resident mast cells are important for eotaxin/induced eosinophil accumulation in vivo. *J Leukoc Biol*, **64**, 156–62.

Dockery, D.W. and Pope, C.A. 1994. Acute respiratory effects of particulate air pollution. *Annu Review Public Health*, **15**, 107–32.

Drouin, S.M., Kildsgaard, J., et al. 2001. Expression of the complement anaphylotoxin C3a and C5a receptors on bronchial epithelial and smooth muscle cells in models of sepsis and asthma. *J Immunol*, **166**, 2025–32.

Elenkov, I.J., Webster, E., et al. 1998. Histamine potently suppresses human IL-12 and stimulates IL-10 production via H2 receptors. *J Immunol*, **161**, 2586–93.

Elias, J.A., Zhu, Z., et al. 1999. Airway remodelling in asthma. *J Clin Invest*, **104**, 1011-, 6.

Emson, C.L., Bell, S.E., et al. 1998. Interleukin (IL)-4-independent induction of immunoglobulin (Ig) E and perturbation of T cell development in transgenic mice expressing IL-13. *J Exp Med*, **188**, 399–404.

Erb, K.J., Holloway, J.W., et al. 1998. Infection of mice with *Mycobacterium bovis*-Bacillus Calmette-Guerin (BCG) suppresses allergen-induced airway eosinophilia. *J Exp Med*, **187**, 561–9.

Ewart, S.L., Kuperman, D., et al. 2000. Quantitative trait loci controlling allergen induced airway hyperresponsiveness in inbreed mice. *Am J Respir Cell Mol Biol*, **23**, 537–45.

Fallon, P.G., Jolin, H.E., et al. 2002. IL-4 induces characteristic Th2 responses even in the combined absence of IL-5, IL-9 and IL-13. *Immunity*, **17**, 7–17.

Foster, P.S., Hogan, A., et al. 1996. Interleukin 5 deficiency abolishes eosinophilia, airway hyperreactivity and lung damage in a mouse model. *J Exp Med*, **183**, 195–201.

Garlisi, C.G., Falcone, A., et al. 1997. Airway eosinophils, T cells, Th2-type cytokine mRNA and hyperreactivity in response to aerosol challenge of allergic mice with previously established pulmonary inflammation. *Am J Respir Cell Mol Biol*, **17**, 642–51.

Gerhold, K., Blumchen, K., et al. 2002. Endotoxins prevent murine IgE production, Th2 immune responses, and development of airway eosinophilia but not hyperreactivity. *J Allergy Clin Immunol*, **110**, 110–16.

Gleich, G.J., Adolphson, C.R. and Leiferman, K.M. 1993. The biology of the eosinophilic leukocyte. *Annu Rev Med*, **44**, 85–101.

Gonzalo, J.A., Pan, Y., et al. 1999. Mouse monocyte-derived chemokine is involved in airway hyperreactivity and lung inflammation. *J Immunol*, **163**, 403-1, 1.

Gounni, A.S., Gregory, E., et al. 2000. Interleukin-9 enhances interleukin-5 receptor expression, differentiation and survival of human eosinophils. *Blood*, **96**, 2163-7, 1.

Grunig, G., Corry, D.B., et al. 1997. Interleukin-10 is a natural suppressor of cytokine production and inflammation in a murine model of allergic bronchopulmonary aspergillosis. *J Exp Med*, **185**, 1089–99.

Grunig, G., Warnock, M., et al. 1998. Requirement for IL-13 independently of IL-4 in experimental asthma. *Science*, **282**, 2261–2.

Groux, H., Bigler, M., et al. 1997. A CD4+ T-cell subset inhibits antigen-specific T cell responses and prevents colitis. *Nature*, **389**, 737–41.

Hamelmann, E., Vella, A.T., et al. 1997. Allergic airway sensitisation induces T cell activation but not airway hyperresponsiveness in B cell deficient mice. *Proc Natl Acad Sci USA*, **94**, 1350–5.

Hamelmann, E., Cieslewicz, G., et al. 1999. Anti-interleukin 5 but not anti-IgE prevents inflammation and airway hyperresponsiveness. *Am J Respir Crit Care Med*, **160**, 934–41.

Hansen, G., Berry, G., et al. 1999. Allergen specific Th1 cells fail to counterbalance Th2 induced airway hyperreactivity but cause severe airway inflammation. *J Clin Invest*, **103**, 175–83.

Harris, N.L., Watt, V., et al. 2002. Differential T cell function and fate in lymph node and nonlymphoid tissues. *J Exp Med*, **195**, 317–26.

Heinzmann, A., Mao, X.Q., et al. 2000. Genetic variants of IL-13 signalling and human asthma and atopy. *Hum Mol Genet*, **9**, 549–59.

Hershey, G.K.K., Friederich, M.F. and Esswein, L.A. 1997. The association of atopy with a gain of function mutation in the α subunit of the interleukin-4 receptor. *N Engl J Med*, **337**, 1720–5.

Hertz, U., Gerhold, K., et al. 1998. BCG infection suppresses allergic sensitization and development of increased airway reactivity in an animal model. *J Allergy Clin Immunol*, **102**, 867–74.

Hirst, S.J., Hallsworth, M.P., et al. 2002. Selective induction of eotaxin release by interleukin-13 or interleukin-4 in human airway smooth muscle cells is synergistic with interleukin-1beta and is mediated by the interleukin-4 receptor alpha-chain. *Am J Respir Crit Care Med*, **165**, 1161–71.

Hobbs, K., Negri, J., et al. 1998. Interleukin-10 and transforming growth factor-β promoter polymorphisms in allergies and asthma. *Am J Respir Crit Care Med*, **158**, 1958–62.

Hoffmann, K.F., Cheever, A.W. and Wynn, T.A. 2000. IL-10 and the dangers of immune polarization: excessive type 1 and type 2 cytokine responses induce distinct forms of lethal immunopathology in murine schistosomiasis. *J Immunol*, **164**, 6404–16.

Hogan, S.P., Mould, A., et al. 1997. Aeroallergen-induced eosinophilic inflammation, lung damage and airway hyperreactivity in mice can occur independently of IL-4 and allergen specific immunoglobulins. *J Clin Invest*, **99**, 1329–39.

Hogan, S.P., Koskinen, A., et al. 1998. Interleukin-5-producing CD4+ T cells play a pivotal role in aeroallergen-induced eosinophilia, bronchial hyperreactivity and lung damage in mice. *Am J Respir Crit Care Med*, **157**, 210–18.

Holgate, S.T. 1998. The inflammation-repair cycle in asthma: the pivotal role of the airway epithelium. *Clin Exp Allergy*, **28**, 97–103.

Holloway, J.A., Holgate, S.T. and Semper, A.E. 2001. Expression of the high affinity IgE receptor on peripheral blood dendritic cells. Differential binding of IgE in atopic asthma. *J Allergy Clin Immunol*, **107**, 1009–18.

Holt, P.G., Schon-Hegrad, M.A., et al. 1989. Ia-positive dendritic cells form a tightly meshed network within the human airway epithelium. *Clin Exp Allergy*, **19**, 597–601.

Holt, P.G., Macaubas, C., et al. 1999. The role of allergy in the development of asthma. *Nature*, **402**, suppl, B12–17.

Hopfenspirger, M.T. and Agrawal, D.K. 2002. Airway hyperresponsiveness, late allergic responses and eosinophilia are reversed with mycrobacterial antigens in ovalbumin-presensitised mice. *J Immunol*, **168**, 2516–22.

Humbles, A.A., Lu, B., et al. 2000. A role of the C3a anaphylotoxin receptor in the effector phase of asthma. *Nature*, **406**, 998–1001.

Jahnsen, F.L., Moloney, E.D., et al. 2001. Rapid dendritic cell recruitment to the bronchial mucosa of patients with atopic asthma in response to local allergen challenge. *Thorax*, **56**, 823–6.

Julia, V., Hessel, E.M., et al. 2002. A restricted subset of dendritic cells capture airborne antigens and remain able to activate specific T cells long after antigen exposure. *Immunity*, **16**, 271–83.

Justice, J.P., Shibata, Y., et al. 2001. IL-10 gene knockout attenuates allergen-induced airway hyperresponsiveness in C57 BL/6 mice. *Am J Physiol Lung Cell Mol Physiol*, **280**, L363–8.

Kanehiro, A., Lahn, M., et al. 2001. Tumour necrosis factor (TNF)-α negatively regulates airway hyperresponsiveness through γδ T cells. *Am J Respir Crit Care Med*, **164**, 2229.

Kaplan, M.H., Schindler, U., et al. 1996. Stat6 is required for mediating responses to IL-4 and for the development of Th2 cells. *Immunity*, **4**, 313–19.

Karp, C.L., Grupe, A., et al. 2000. Identification of complement factor 5 as a susceptibility locus for experimental allergic asthma. *Nat Immunol*, **1**, 221–6.

Keane-Myers, A., Wysocka, M., et al. 1998. Resistance to antigen-induced airway hyperresponsiveness requires endogenous production of IL-12. *J Immunol*, **161**, 919–26.

King, D.P., Hyde, D.M., et al. 1999. Cutting edge: Protective response to pulmonary injury requires γδ T lymphocytes. *J Immunol*, **162**, 5033–6.

Kips, J.C., Brusselle, G.J., et al. 1996. Interleukin-12 inhibits antigen-induced airway hyperresponsiveness in mice. *Am J Respir Crit Care Med*, **153**, 535–9.

Kobayashi, T., Miura, T., et al. 2000. An essential role of mast cells in the development of airway hyperresponsiveness in a murine asthma model. *J Immunol*, **164**, 3855–61.

Kuperman, D., Schofield, B., et al. 1998. Signal transducer and activator of transcription factor 6 (stat6) deficient mice are protected from antigen induced airway hyperresponsiveness and mucus production. *J Exp Med*, **187**, 939–48.

Kuperman, D.A., Huang, X. and Koth, L.L. 2002. Direct effects of interleukin-13 on epithelial cells cause airway hyperreactivity and mucus overproduction in asthma. *Nat Med*, **8**, 885–9.

Lahn, M., Kanehio, A., et al. 1999. Negative regulation of airway responsivenss that is dependent on γδ T cells and independent of αβ T cells. *Nat Med*, **5**, 1150–6.

Lambrecht, B.N., Salomon, B., et al. 1988. Dendritic cells are required for the development of chronic eosinophilic airway inflammation in response to inhaled antigen in sensitised mice. *J Immunol*, **160**, 4090–7.

Leckie, M.J., ten Brinke, A., et al. 2000. Effects of an interleukin-5 blocking monoclonal antibody on eosinophils, airway hyper-responsiveness and the late asthmatic response. *Lancet*, **356**, 2144–8.

Lee, C.G., Homer, R.J., et al. 2001. Interleukin-13 induces tissue fibrosis by selectively stimulating and activating transforming growth factor β1. *J Exp Med*, **194**, 809–21.

Lee, C.G., Homer, R.J., et al. 2002. Transgenic overexpression of interleukin (IL) 10 in the lung causes mucus metaplasia, tissue inflammation and airway remodelling via IL-13 dependent and independent pathways. *J Biol Chem*, **277**, 35466–74.

Lemanske, R.F., Nayak, A., et al. 2002. Omalizumab improves asthma-related quality of life in children with allergic asthma. *Pediatrics*, **110**, e55.

Lloyd, C.M., Delaney, T., et al. 2000. CC chemokine receptor (CCR)3/ eotaxin is followed by CCR4/ monocyte-derived chemokine in mediating pulmonary T helper lymphocyte type 2 recruitment after serial antigen challenge in vivo. *J Exp Med*, **191**, 265–73.

Li, X.-M., Chopra, R.K., et al. 1996. Mucosal IFN-γ gene transfer inhibits pulmonary allergic responses in mice. *J Immunol*, **157**, 3216–19.

Li, L., Xia, Y., et al. 1999. Effects of Th2 cytokines on chemokine expressing in the lung: IL-13 potently induces eotaxin expression by airway epithelial cells. *J Immunol*, **162**, 2477–87.

Longphre, M., Li, D., et al. 1999. Allergen induced IL-9 directly stimulates mucin transcription in respiratory epithelial cells. *J Clin Invest*, **104**, 1375–82.

Lopez, A., Sanderson, J., et al. 1988. Recombinant human interleukin-5 is a selective activator of human eosinophil function. *J Exp Med*, **167**, 219–24.

Louahed, J., Zhou, Y., et al. 2001. Interleukin 9 promotes influx and local maturation of eosinophils. *Blood*, **97**, 1035–42.

Lukacs, N.W., Tekkanat, K.K., et al. 2001. Respiratory syncytial virus predisposes mice to augmented allergic airway responses via IL-13 mediated mechanisms. *J Immunol*, **167**, 1060–5.

Ma, W., Bryce, P.J., et al. 2002. CCR3 is essential for skin eosinophilia and airway hyperresponsiveness in a murine model of allergic skin inflammation. *J Clin Invest*, **109**, 621–8.

McFadden, E.R. 1994. Asthma: morphologic–physiologic interactions. *Am J Respir Crit Care Med*, **150**, S23–6.

MacKenzie, J.R., Mattes, J., et al. 2001. Eosinophils promote allergic disease of the lung by regulating CD4+ Th2 lymphocyte function. *J Immunol*, **167**, 3146–55.

Marsh, D.G., Neely, J.D., et al. 1994. Linkage analysis of IL-4 and other chromosome 5q31.1 markers and total serum immunoglobulin E concentrations. *Science*, **264**, 1152–6.

Makela, M.J., Kanehiro, A., et al. 2000. IL-10 is necessary for the expression of airway hyperresponsiveness but not pulmonary inflammation after allergic sensitisation. *Proc Natl Acad Sci USA*, **97**, 6007–12.

Makela, M.J., Kanehiro, A., et al. 2002. The failure of interleukin-10-deficient mice to develop airway hyperresponsiveness is overcome by respiratory syncytial virus infection in allergen-sensitized/challenged mice. *Am J Respir Crit Care Med*, **165**, 824–31.

Matsui, E., Kaneko, H., et al. 1999. Mutations of the IL-12 receptor beta 2 chain gene in atopic subjects. *Biochem Biophys Res Commun*, **266**, 551–5.

Matsuoka, T., Hirata, M., et al. 2000. Prostaglandin D2 as a mediator of allergic asthma. *Science*, **287**, 2013–17.

Matsukura, S., Stellato, C., et al. 2001. Interleukin-13 upregulates eotaxin expression in airway epithelial cells by a STAT6-dependent mechanism. *Am J Respir Cell Mol Biol*, **24**, 755–61.

Mattes, J., Yang, M., et al. 2001. IL-13 induces airway hyperreactivity independently of the IL-4Rα chain in the allergic lung. *J Immunol*, **167**, 1683–92.

Mattes, J., Yang, M., et al. 2002. Intrinsic defect in T cell production of Interleukin (IL)-13 in the absence of both IL-5 and eotaxin precludes the development of eosinophilia and airway hyperreactivity in experimental asthma. *J Exp Med*, **195**, 1433–44.

Mehlhop, P.D., van de Rijn, M., et al. 1997. Allergen-induced bronchial hyperreactivity and eosinophilic inflammation occur in the absence of IgE in a mouse model of asthma. *Proc Natl Acad Sci USA*, **94**, 1344–9.

Metcalf, D.D., Baram, Y. and Mekori, Y.A. 1997. Mast cells. *Physiol Rev*, **77**, 1033–79.

Meyaard, L., Hovenkamp, E., et al. 1996. IL-12 induced IL-10 production by human T cells as a negative feedback for IL-12 induced immune responses. *J Immunol*, **156**, 2776–82.

Mocjizuki, M., Bartels, J., et al. 1998. IL-4 induces eotaxin: a possible mechanism of selective eosinophil recruitment in helminth infection and atopy. *J Immunol*, **160**, 60–8.

Moore, K.W., de Waal Malefyt, R., et al. 2001. Interleukin-10 and the interleukin-10 receptor. *Annu Rev Immunol*, **19**, 683–765.

Morahan, G., Huang, D., et al. 2002. Association of IL-12B promoter polymorphism with severity of atopic and non-atopic asthma in children. *Lancet*, **360**, 422–3.

Mueller, D.L., Jenkins, M.K. and Schwartz, R.H. 1989. Clonal expansion versus functional inactivation: a co-stimulatory signalling pathway determines the outcome of T cell antigen receptor occupancy. *Annu Rev Immunol*, **7**, 445–80.

Nakajima, H., Sano, H., et al. 1994. Role of vascular cell adhesion molecules 1/very late activation antigen 4 and intercellular adhesion molecule 1/lymphocyte function-associated antigen 1 interactions in antigen-induced eosinophil and T cell recruitment into the tissue. *J Exp Med*, **179**, 1145–54.

Naseer, T., Minshall, E.M., et al. 1997. Expression of IL-12 and IL-13 mRNA in asthma and their modulation in response to steroid therapy. *Am J Respir Crit Care Med*, **155**, 845–51.

Nicolai, T. and von Mutius, E. 1997. Pollution and the development of allergy: the East and West German story. *Arch Toxicol Suppl*, **19**, 201–6.

Nouri, A., Irani, A.-M., et al. 2001. Basophils are recruited and express IL-4 during human allergen-induced asthma. *J Allergy Clin Immunol*, **108**, 205–11.

Ober, C., Leavitt, S.A., et al. 2000. Variation in the interleukin 4-receptor alpha gene confers susceptibility to asthma and atopy in ethnically diverse populations. *Am J Hum Genet*, **66**, 517–526.

Oettgen, H.C. and Geha, R.S. 2001. IgE regulation and roles in asthma pathogenesis. *J Allergy Clin Immunol*, **107**, 429–40.

Ohta, K., Yamashita, N., et al. 1999. Diesel exhaust particulate induces airway hyperresponsiveness in a murine model: essential role of GM-CSF. *J Allergy Clin Immunol*, **104**, 1024–30.

Palmer, L.J., Burton, P.R., et al. 2000. Independent inheritance of serum immunoglobulin E concentration and airway responsiveness. *Am J Respir Crit Care Med*, **161**, 1836–43.

Petit-Frere, C., Dugas, B., et al. 1993. Interleukin-9 potentiates the interlukin-4 induced IgE and IgG1 release form murine B lymphocytes. *Immunology*, **79**, 146–51.

Postma, D.S., Bleecker, E.R., et al. 1995. Genetic susceptibility to asthma-bronchial hyperresponsiveness coinherited with a major gene for atopy. *N Engl J Med*, **333**, 894–900.

Pravica, V., Brogan, I.J. and Hutchinson, I.V. 2000. Rare polymporphsisms in the promoter regions of the human interleukin-12 p35 and interleukin-12 p40 subunit genes. *Eur J Immunogenet*, **27**, 35–6.

Prieto, L., Lensmar, C., et al. 2000. Increased interleukin-13 mRNA expression in bronchoalveolar lavage cells of atopic patients with mild asthma after repeated low-dose allergen provocations. *Respir Med*, **94**, 806–14.

Rankin, J.A., Picarella, D.E., et al. 1996. Phenotypic and physiologic characerization of transgenic mice overexpressing interleukin 4 in the lung: lymphocytic and eosinophilic inflammation without airway hyperreactivity. *Proc Natl Acad Sci USA*, **23**, 7821–5.

Rha, Y.-H., Taube, C., et al. 2002. Effect of microbial heat shock proteins on airway inflammation and hyperresponsiveness. *J Immunol*, **169**, 5300–7.

Robinson, D.S., Hamid, Q., et al. 1992. Predominant Th2 like bronchoalveolar T-lymphocyte population in atopic asthma. *N Engl J Med*, **326**, 298–304.

Sallusto, F., Mackay, C.R. and Lanzavecchia, A. 1997. Selective expression of the eotaxin receptor CCR3 by human T helper 2 cells. *Science*, **277**, 2005–7.

Schmid-Grendelmeier, P., Altznauer, F., et al. 2002. Eosinophil express functional IL-13 in eosinophilic inflammatory diseases. *J Immunol*, **169**, 1021–7.

Schwarze, J., Hamelmann, E., et al. 1998. Local treatment with IL-12 is and effective inhibitor of airway hyperresponsiveness and lung eosinophilia after airway challenge in sensitised mice. *J Allergy Clin Immunol*, **102**, 86–93.

Shi, H.-Z., Humbles, A., et al. 2000. Lymph node trafficking and antigen presentation by endobronchial eosinophils. *J Clin Invest*, **105**, 945–53.

Shimbara, A., Christodoulopoulos, P., et al. 2000. IL-9 and its receptor in allergic and non-allergic lung disease: increased expression in asthma. *J Allergy Clin Immunol*, **105**, 108–15.

Shirakawa, T., Enomoto, T., et al. 1997. The inverse association between tuberculin responses and atopic disorder. *Science*, **275**, 77–9.

Shirakawa, T., Deichmann, K., et al. 2000. Atopy and asthma: genetic variants of IL-4 and IL-13 signaling. *Immunol Today*, **21**, 60–4.

Steinbrink, K., Wolf, M., et al. 1997. Induction of tolerance by IL-10 treated dendritic cells. *J Immunol*, **159**, 4772–80.

Sudo, N., Sawamura, S., et al. 1997. The requirement for intestinal bacterial flora for the development of an IgE production system fully susceptible to oral tolerance induction. *J Immunol*, **159**, 1739–45.

Sunyer, J., Anto, J.M., et al. 1995. Relationship between serum IgE and airway responsiveness in adults with asthma. *J Allergy Clin Immunol*, **95**, 699-70, 6.

Sur, S., Gleich, G.J., et al. 1995. Eosinophilic inflammation is associated with elevation of interleukin 5 in the airways of patients with spontaneous symptomatic asthma. *J Allergy Clin Immunol*, **96**, 661–8.

Sur, S., Lam, J., et al. 1996. Immunomodulatory effects of IL-12 on allergic lung inflammation depend on timing of doses. *J Immunol*, **157**, 4173–80.

Szabo, S.J., Jackson, N.G., et al. 1995. Developmental commitment to the Th2 lineage by extinction of IL-12 signaling. *Immunity*, **2**, 665–75.

Takeda, K., Hamelmann, E., et al. 1997. Development of eosinophilic airway inflammation and airway hyperresponsiveness in mast cell deficient mice. *J Exp Med*, **186**, 449–54.

Temann, U.A., Prasad, B., et al. 1997. A novel role for IL-4 in vivo: induction of MUC5AC gene expression and mucin hypersecretion. *Am J Respir Cell Mol Biol*, **16**, 471–8.

Tenmann, U.A., Geba, G.P., et al. 1998. Expression of interleukin 9 in the lungs of transgenic mice causes airway inflammation, mast cell hyperplasia and bronchial hyperresponsiveness. *J Exp Med*, **188**, 1307–20.

Tenmann, U.A., Ray, P. and Flavell, R.A. 2002. Pulmonary overexpression of IL-9 induces Th2 expression, leading to immune pathology. *J Clin Invest*, **109**, 29-3, 9.

Tomkinson, A., Kanehiro, A., et al. 1999. The failure of STAT6-deficient mice to develop airway eosinophilia and airway hyperresponsiveness is overcome by interleukin-5. *Am J Respir Crit Care Med*, **160**, 1283–91.

Tomkinson, A., Cieslewicz, G., et al. 2001. Temporal association between airway hyperresponsivneness and airway eosinophilia in ovalbumin sensitized mice. *Am J Respir Crit Care Med*, **163**, 721.

Tomkinson, A., Duez, C., et al. 2002. Adoptive transfer of T cells induces airway hyperresponsiveness independently of airway eosinophilia but in a signal transducer and activator of transcription 6-dependent manner. *J Allergy Clin Immunol*, **109**, 810–16.

Trinchieri, G. 1994. Interleukin-12: a cytokine produced by antigen presenting cells with immunoregulatory functions in the generation of T-helper cells type 1 and cytotoxic lymphocytes. *Blood*, **84**, 4008–27.

Tulic, M.K., Wale, J.L., et al. 2000. Modification of the inflammatory response to allergen challenge after exposure to bacterial lipoplysaccharide. *Am J Respir Cell Mol Biol*, **22**, 604–12.

Tunon de Lara, J.M., Redington, A.E., et al. 1996. Dendritic cells in normal and asthmatic airways: expression of the alfa subunit of the high affinity immunoglobulin E receptor. *Clin Exp Allergy*, **26**, 648–55.

Upham, J.W., Denburg, J.A. and O'Byrne, P.M. 2002. Rapid response of circulating myeloid dendritic cells to inhaled allergen in asthmatic subjects. *Clin Exp Allergy*, **32**, 818–23.

van den Biggelaar, A.H., van Ree, R., et al. 2000. Decreased atopy in children infected with *Schistosoma haematobium*: a role for parasite-induced interleukin-10. *Lancet*, **356**, 1723–7.

Van der Pouw Kraan, T.C.T.M.J., Boeije, L.C.M., et al. 1995. Prostaglandin-E2 is a potent inhibitor of human interleukin-12 production. *J Exp Med*, **181**, 775–9.

Van Scott, M.R., Justice, J.P., et al. 2000. IL-10 reduces Th2 cytokine production and eosinophilia but augments airway reactivity in allergic mice. *Am J Physiol Lung Cell Mol Physiol*, **278**, L667–74.

Vermaelen, K.Y., Carro-Muino, I., et al. 2001. Specific migratory dendritic cells rapidly transport antigen from the airways to the thoracic lymph nodes. *J Exp Med*, **193**, 51–60.

Von Mutius, E., Braun-Fahrlander, C., et al. 2000. Exposure to endotoxin or other bacterial components might protect against the development of atopy. *Clin Exp Allergy*, **30**, 1230–4.

Walter, D.M., McIntire, J.J., et al. 2001. Critical role for IL-13 in the development of allergen-induced airway hyperreactivity. *J Immunol*, **167**, 4668–75.

Walters, D.M., Breysse, P.N., et al. 2002. Complement factor 3 mediates particulate matter-induced hyperresponsiveness. *Am J Respir Cell Mol Biol*, **27**, 413–18.

Wardlow, A.J., Dunnette, S., et al. 1988. Eosinophils and mast cells in bronchoalveolar fluid in subjects with asthma: relationship to bronchial hyperreactivity. *Am Rev Respir Dis*, **137**, 62–9.

Wenzel, S.E., Trudeau, J.B., et al. 2002. TGF-beta and IL-13 synergistically increase eotaxin-1 production in human airway fibroblasts. *J Immunol*, **169**, 4613–19.

Wickens, K., Pearce, N., et al. 1999. Antibiotic use in early childhood and the development of asthma. *Clin Exp Allergy*, **6**, 766–71.

Wilder, J.A., Collie, D.S., et al. 1999. Dissociation of airway hyperresponsiveness form immunoglobulin E and airway eosinophilia in a murine model of allergic asthma. *Am J Respir Cell Mol Biol*, **20**, 1326–34.

Wills-Karp, M., Luyimbazi, J., et al. 1998. Interleukin-13: Central mediator of allergic asthma. *Science*, **282**, 2258–61.

Wright, E.D., Christodoulopoulos, P., et al. 1999. Expression of interleukin (IL)-12 (p40) and IL-12 (beta 2) receptors in allergic rhinitis and chronic sinusitis. *Clin Exp Allergy*, **29**, 1320–5.

Yamaguchi, M., Sayama, K., et al. 1999. IgE enhances Fcε receptor I expression and IgE dependent release of histamine and lipid mediators from human umbilical cord blood-derived receptor I expression and mediator release. *J Immunol*, **162**, 5455–65.

Yang, X., Wang, S., et al. 2000. IL-10 deficiency prevents IL-5 overproduction and eosinophil inflammation in a murine model of asthma-like reaction. *Eur J Immunol*, **30**, 382–91.

Ying, S., Humbert, M., et al. 1997a. Expression of IL-4 and IL-5 mRNA and protein product by CD4+ and CD8+ T cells, eosinophils and mast cells in bronchial biopsies obtained from atopic and nonatopic (intrinsic) asthmatics. *J Immunol*, **158**, 3539-4, 4.

Ying, S., Robinson, D.S., et al. 1997b. Enhanced expression of eotaxin and CCR3 mRNA and protein in atopic asthma. Association with airway hyperresponsiveness and predominant co-localization of eotaxin mRNA to bronchial epithelial and endothelial cells. *Eur J Immunol*, **27**, 3507–16.

Ying, S., Meng, K., et al. 1999. Eosinophil chemotactic chemokines (eotaxin, eotaxin-2, RANTES, monocyte chemoattractant protein (MCP)-3 and MCP-4 and C-C chemokine receptor-3 expression in bronchial biopsies from atopic and nonatopic (intrinsic) asthmatics. *J Immunol*, **163**, 632, 1.

Zhao, L.L., Linden, A., et al. 2000. IL-12 regulates bone marrow eosinophilia and airway eotaxin levels induced by airway allergen exposure. *Allergy*, **55**, 749–56.

Zhou, Z., Ma, B., et al. 2002. IL-13 induced chemokine responses in the lung: role of CCR2 in the pathogenesis of IL-13 induced inflammation and remodelling. *J Immunol*, **168**, 2953–62.

Zhu, Z., Homer, R.J., et al. 1999. Pulmonary expression of interleukin-13 causes inflammation, mucus hypersecretion, subepithelial fibrosis, physiologic abnormalities and eotaxin production. *J Clin Invest*, **103**, 779–88.

Zuany-Amorim, C., Haile, S., et al. 1995. Interleukin-10 inhibits antigen induced cellular recruitment into the airways of sensitized mice. *J Clin Invest*, **95**, 2644–51.

Zurawski, G. and de Vries, J.E. 1994. Interleukin-13 an interleukin-4-like cytokine that acts on monocytes and B cells, but not on T cells. *Immunol Today*, **15**, 19–26.

37

Autoimmunity

HELENA CROWLEY AND BRIGITTE T. HUBER

DEFINING AUTOIMMUNITY AND AUTOIMMUNE DISEASE

Autoimmunity is defined as activation of an immune response against self-tissue (Ermann and Fathman 2001). A degree of autoimmunity, or self-reactivity, is a phenomenon that occurs even in healthy individuals. Alternatively, autoimmune disease is an 'attack', which may afflict patients with conditions that are debilitating, even life threatening. Autoimmune disease is marked by the presence of pathogenic antibodies and/or lymphocytes that target self-antigens and mediate tissue destruction. A multitude of factors influence one's susceptibility to autoimmune disease, including host genetics, environmental factors, and immune disregulation (Ermann and Fathman 2001) (Figure 37.1).

The subject of autoimmune disease encompasses a broad spectrum of illnesses of ambiguous etiology and pathogenesis. Despite the uncertainty underscoring any discussion of autoimmune disease, unambiguous evidence demonstrates that self-tolerance has been corrupted. The main function of the immune system is to protect self from nonself. For this purpose, it must operate by its ability to discriminate between what is self and what is not, a paradigm first described by Burnet in

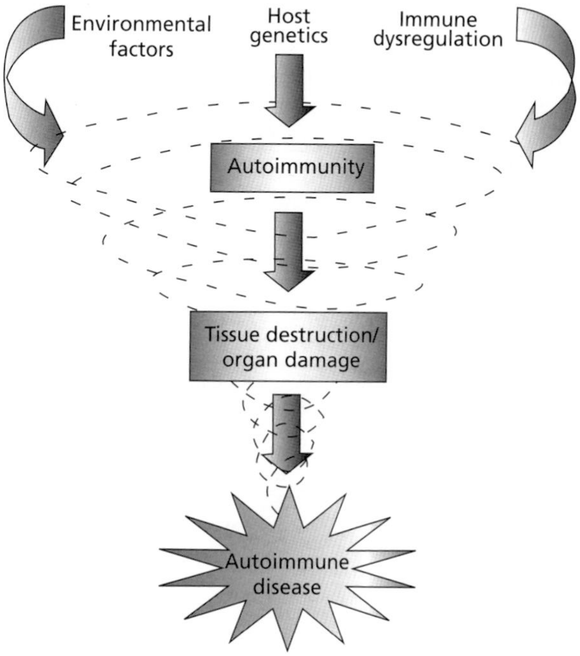

Figure 37.1 *Etiology of autoimmune disease: with several factors underlying its etiology, the development of an autoimmune response is a downward spiral, resulting in tissue destruction, organ damage, and autoimmune disease.*

1959. 'Survival requires both the ability to mount a destructive immune response against non-self and the inability to mount a destructive response against self' (Huston 1997). With a break in self-tolerance, the immune system proceeds to attack itself with the same vigor as it would to eliminate an infectious organism. Ultimately, the dangerous cascade of an autoimmune disease may compromise survival.

Autoimmune diseases affect approximately 5 percent of the global population (Jacobson et al. 1997). In the USA, roughly 14 million people are afflicted with various autoimmune diseases. Women are disproportionately affected, because they represent 75 percent of autoimmune disease patients. To date, over 80 distinct types of autoimmune diseases have been identified. Diseases may be categorized into one of two groups: organ-specific or systemic autoimmune disease (Table 37.1). In organ-specific autoimmune diseases, including Graves' disease (Weetman 2001) and type 1 diabetes (Wucherpfennig and Eisenbarth 2001), the targeted self-antigen is expressed only in the affected organ, whereas, in systemic autoimmune diseases, the self-antigen is expressed throughout the host eliciting tissue damage systemically. Systemic lupus erythematosus (SLE) and rheumatoid arthritis (RA) are two systemic autoimmune diseases with a high prevalence in the USA (Jacobson et al. 1997).

THE DISCOVERY AND REDISCOVERY OF AUTOIMMUNITY

The study of autoimmunity has a controversial, albeit intriguing, history (Silverstein 2001). In 1901, Paul Ehrlich, famed immunologist, adamantly denounced the existence of autoimmune disease or what he dubbed as *horror autotoxicus*. Ehrlich declared that it would be against the design of nature for an organism to jeopardize itself by producing pathogenic autoantibodies. Shortly thereafter, investigators Julius Donath and Karl Landsteiner published findings regarding the pathogenesis of paroxysmal cold hemoglobinuria (PKH). PKH is an unusual disease whereby patients develop acute intravascular red blood cell destruction and subsequent hemoglobinuria following exposure to the cold. In 1904, they proposed that this rare disease is autoimmune in origin, citing their demonstration of a pathogenic autoantibody that reacts with its target cell in the cold. Suffice it to say, Ehrlich and his colleagues disputed these findings and maintained their stance that autoimmune disease did not exist, thereby influencing generations of immunologists to come.

The concept of autoimmunity as a disease model reappeared in the 1950s. Ernest Witebsky published a report demonstrating the induction of autoimmunity in an animal model of chronic thyroiditis (Witebsky and Rose 1956). Indeed, Witebsky was an unlikely candidate to reintroduce the concept of autoimmunity, because he was a faithful disciple of Ehrlich and his campaign to refute autoimmunity. Despite the initial resistance of Ehrlich, Witebsky, and other investigators to acknowledge the existence of autoimmunity, today it is recognized as a major societal burden. Intensive investigative efforts are focused on uncovering the etiology, mechanisms, and treatments for many autoimmune diseases.

MECHANISMS OF TOLERANCE

The ability of the immune system to protect the body against challenge from innumerable exogenous pathogens is conferred in part by a diverse lymphocyte repertoire. In fact, the total diversity of the αβ T-cell receptor (TCR) and B-cell immunoglobulin (Ig) repertoires is estimated at 10^{18} and 10^{14}, respectively (Janeway et al. 2001). This diverse repertoire supports B- and T-cell recognition of a broad range of antigens. The tremendous degree of diversity is further enhanced by the 'plasticity' or cross-reactivity of the receptors (Mason 1998). This flexibility has been attributed to conformational changes in the TCR that occur during engagement of the major histocompatiblity complex (MHC) (Garcia et al. 1998). Given the capacity to recognize countless

Table 37.1 *Prevalence of autoimmune diseases: top ten autoimmune diseases in order of decreasing prevalence*

Disease	Prevalence (%)	Category	Target
Graves' disease	1.1	Organ specific	Thyroid
Rheumatoid arthritis	0.9	Systemic	Joints, lungs, heart, etc.
Hashimoto's thyroiditis	0.8	Organ specific	Thyroid
Vitiligo	0.4	Organ specific	Melanocytes
Type 1 diabetes	0.2	Organ specific	Pancreatic β cells
Pernicious anemia	0.15	Organ specific	Gastric mucosa
Multiple sclerosis	<0.1	Organ specific	Brain (spinal cord)
Glomerulonephritis	<0.1	Organ specific	Kidney
Systemic lupus	<0.1	Systemic	Skin, joints, kidney, brain, blood, lungs, etc.
Sjögren's syndrome	<0.1	Organ specific	Lacrimal and salivary glands

(Jacobson et al. 1997)

antigens, it is not surprising that lymphocytes may inadvertently recognize self-antigens and mount an autoimmune response.

Two criteria underlie the mechanisms by which the immune system protects the body against autoimmunity: self-recognition and self-tolerance. At the initiation of an immune response, self-recognition, or the ability to discriminate between what is self and what is nonself or foreign, is intrinsic to the goal of targeting only foreign antigens. As an immune response is maintained, self-tolerance, or the ability to silence self-reactivity, is an essential component for halting autoimmunity. One of the most effective mechanisms to ensure both self-recognition and self-tolerance is positive and negative selection during T-cell maturation. This occurs centrally in the thymus from the perinatal period until puberty. Later in development, other critical mechanisms of tolerance induction occur in the periphery, including the suppression or elimination of autoreactive lymphocytes.

Establishing self-tolerance in the central lymphoid organs

The first and most effective route for eliminating autoreactive lymphocytes occurs during central tolerance induction in the bone marrow and thymus. After the rearrangement and expression of Ig and TCR genes, B and T cells express antigen-specific receptors. These receptors may have specificity for either self or nonself antigens. Although T cells with high avidity for self-determinants are clonally deleted in the thymus on encounter of self-antigens in association with self-MHC, self-reactive B cells in the bone marrow may escape deletion and modify their Ig by receptor editing (Tiegs et al. 1993).

Central tolerance is an insufficient route for eliminating the entire autoreactive T- and B-lymphocyte population. An analysis of multiple sclerosis (MS) patients demonstrated that autoreactive T cells specific for myelin basic protein (MBP) escape deletion during thymic selection (Ota et al. 1990). Upon activation in the periphery, perhaps during a viral infection, these cells may initiate the destruction of the central nervous system. Self-reactive lymphocytes may escape deletion for several reasons. In the thymus, some self-antigens may not be expressed at sufficient levels to mediate deletion or, perhaps, some self-antigens are not present at all.

Maintaining self-tolerance in the periphery

In the periphery, autoreactive T cells are held in check by tolerance mechanisms that may be characterized as T-cell intrinsic or T-cell extrinsic mechanisms (Walker and Abbas 2002). T-cell intrinsic mechanisms act directly on the T cell, whereas T-cell extrinsic mechanisms involve the tolerogenic functions of additional cells.

T-CELL INTRINSIC MECHANISMS OF PERIPHERAL TOLERANCE

Intrinsic mechanisms include the following: ignorance, anergy, phenotypic skewing, and apoptosis (Walker and Abbas 2002).

T-cell ignorance

This is the process by which autoreactive T cells (or B cells) are unresponsive to antigen. The T cells may ignore the self-antigen because either it binds the TCR with low affinity or it is present at a low concentration (Janeway et al. 2001). Kurts et al. (1999) experimentally documented this state by transferring ovalbumin-specific lymphocytes to mice expressing low levels of pancreatic ovalbumin. The T cells remained ignorant of the ovalbumin antigen at low doses, but were responsive to the antigen at high doses. Interestingly, tissue-specific antigens, such as insulin in the pancreas, are expressed at high concentrations at specific sites. These antigens often have a higher association with autoreactivity (Janeway et al. 2001).

Some T cells remain ignorant because they are never exposed to inaccessible self-antigens, e.g. intraocular proteins are sequestered in the eye, an immunologically privileged site. Unless these proteins are released, autoreactive T cells specific for these proteins are never activated.

T-cell anergy

The state of anergy occurs when lymphocytes do not respond to antigen stimulation. In vivo, T-cell inactivation resulting from anergy induction is dependent on the recognition of the B7 molecule by CTLA-4 (Perez et al. 1997). In mice, the significance of anergy induction is demonstrated by CTLA-4 deficiency that results in severe lymphoproliferation and early death (Waterhouse et al. 1995). The association between CTLA-4 and autoimmune diseases is discussed.

Phenotypic skewing

The induction of tolerance via phenotypic skewing is dependent on which cytokine and chemokine profile is elicited after T-cell activation by a self-antigen. A self-antigen alone may only be able to induce a T-helper type 2 (Th2) response, which is associated with dampening autoimmunity. A self-antigen in association with additional adjuvants, such as the case with bacterial lipopolysaccharide (LPS), may induce a shift towards a T-helper type 1 (Th1) response. The proinflammatory Th1 response is associated with perpetuating an autoimmune response.

Apoptosis

Apoptosis via activation-induced cell death (AICD) is a mechanism for eliminating self-reactive B and T cells in the periphery. The process of apoptotic cell death promotes an anti-inflammatory environment via two routes: (1) inhibition of proinflammatory cytokines by monocytes and macrophages and (2) inducing the release of immunosuppressive cytokines, including IL-10 and transforming growth factor β (TGF-β) (Savill et al. 2002).

Self-reactive, immature B cells expressing surface IgM are eliminated by apoptosis (Janeway et al. 2001). In the case of self-reactive T cells, Walker and Abbas (2002) postulate that the repetitive engagement of TCR by ubiquitous self-antigens may induce the upregulation of the cell-death Fas ligand, thereby initiating AICD. The significance of Fas-mediated apoptosis as an immunoregulatory mechanism to eliminate autoreactive lymphocytes is demonstrated in humans with autoimmune lymphoproliferative syndrome (ALPS). These patients have deleterious defects in the Fas pathway that result in expanded lymphocyte populations and compromised peripheral self-tolerance (Fisher et al. 1995).

T-CELL EXTRINSIC MECHANISMS OF PERIPHERAL TOLERANCE

Extrinsic tolerance mechanisms evoke the functions of dendritic cells (DC) and regulatory T cells (Walker and Abbas 2002). Although it is apparent that both DCs and regulatory T cells play a role in determining whether an immune response is enhanced or suppressed, the precise mechanism of action of these cell types remains to be determined.

Dendritic cells

The DC is a powerful antigen-presenting cell (APC) located in the skin, blood, and lymphatic network (Steinman and Nussenzweig 2002). Immature DCs capture and process antigens, whereas mature DCs, in the presence of infection, present these antigens in association with MHC to T cells (Yewdell and Tscharke 2002) (Figure 37.2). Immature DCs are associated with T-cell tolerance, whereas mature ones are associated with T-cell activation. As DC maturation plays a crucial role in initiating and modulating the immune response, it is subject to regulation, e.g. the maturation and presentation of antigen by DCs is inhibited upon the uptake of dying, apoptotic cells in an effort to maintain tolerance and suppress autoimmunity (Savill et al. 2002). In addition, the maturation of DCs is inhibited by the anti-inflammatory cytokine, interleukin (IL)-10 (Haase et al. 2002).

Dendritic cells also play a role in providing signals to distinguish between an appropriate antigen, as in the case of a pathogen, or an inappropriate antigen, such as a self-antigen. In 1992, Janeway postulated that DCs have pattern-recognition receptors that are specific for motifs associated with microorganisms. The engagement of these receptors triggers an immune response. This

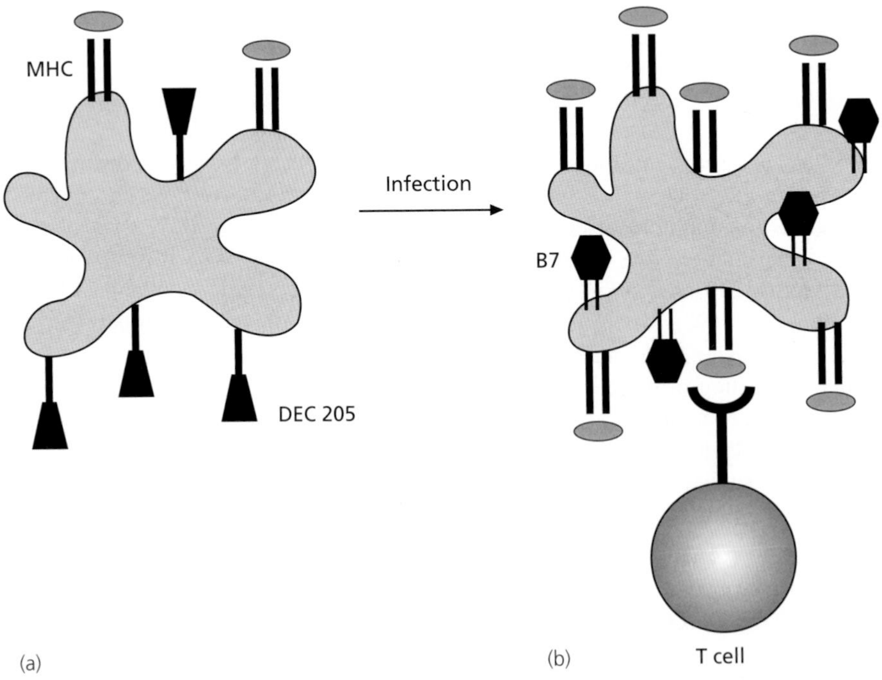

Figure 37.2 (a) *Immature and* **(b)** *mature dendritic cell phenotypes: immature dendritic cells are located in the surface epithelia and solid organs. They express low levels of major histocompatiblity complex (MHC) molecules, as well as the DEC 205 molecule, an antigen-phagocytosing receptor. During infection, immature dendritic cells migrate to lymphoid tissue. These mature dendritic cells increase expression of MHC and B7, a co-stimulatory molecule (Janeway et al. 2001).*

theory was substantiated in 1997 with the identification of Toll-like receptors (TLR) (Medzhitov et al. 1997). TLRs, on the recognition of molecular patterns present on microorganisms, induce an immune response that includes the expression of co-stimulatory molecules and the release of cytokines (Gordon 2002).

Regulatory T cells

Regulatory or suppressor T cells that co-express CD4 and CD25 (the interleukin IL-2 receptor α chain) represent less than 5 percent of the T cells in the blood. These 'sentinel' T cells have the capacity to monitor immune responses by suppressing both $CD4^+$ and $CD8^+$ T cells (Steinman and Nussenzweig 2002). The mechanism of suppression has not yet been elucidated, although it is associated with decreased levels of IL-2 transcription (Thornton and Shevach 1998). The critical role of regulatory T cells in tolerance is demonstrated in a mouse model where a reduced level of regulatory T cells is associated with autoimmune disease (Asano et al. 1996).

Regulatory cells are also subject to immunoregulation. IL-10, a suppressor cytokine, may trigger the generation of regulatory cells. In addition, the presence of immature DCs may generate regulatory T cells (Shevach 2002). DCs mature in the presence of TLR signaling; the absence of mature DCs may be a marker for the absence of an invading pathogen, favoring the suppression of a potential autoimmune response.

GENETICS AS A FACTOR IN AUTOIMMUNE DISEASE SUSCEPTIBILITY

A role for genetic predisposition in autoimmune disease development was suspected, given the propensity for familial aggregation of certain autoimmune diseases. The association was positively identified by a study of the disease concordance rates in monozygotic twins. The disease concordance rates for certain autoimmune diseases, such as type 1 diabetes and SLE, were quite high, 50 and 57 percent, respectively (Jarvinen et al. 1992; Kumar et al. 1993; Redondo et al. 1999). By comparison, the incidence for diabetes and SLE in the general population is significantly less, 0.4 and 0.2 percent, respectively, suggesting an underlying genetic component to disease development.

Today, at the forefront of the search for autoimmune disease genes, there are powerful tools, including linkage analysis, animal models, and gene chip microarrays (Wanstrat and Wakeland 2001). Despite these advantages, the search for genes affecting autoimmune disease is complicated by several factors, including genetic heterogeneity. Genetic heterogeneity, or the various combinations of genes that contribute to a certain phenotype, underlies the genetic predisposition to most autoimmune diseases (Wanstrat and Wakeland 2001). A clear characterization of the role of genetic predisposition in autoimmune disease development is further obscured by epistatic interactions between 'susceptibility genes' and 'resistance genes' (Ermann and Fathman 2001). Fortunately, completion of the Human and Murine Genome Projects offer valuable maps of the mammalian genome that will probably facilitate groundbreaking discoveries in the search for autoimmune disease genes.

The effects of MHC genes on autoimmune disease development

The most intensely studied genes associated with autoimmune disease development are the alleles of the MHC. These genes encode cell-surface molecules on APCs that bind peptides for presentation to antigen-specific T lymphocytes. Some hypothesize that the association between MHC and autoimmune disease susceptibility originates during T-cell development. During this period, the signals resulting from the TCR and MHC molecule–peptide complexes shape the thymic T-cell repertoire and may potentiate the escape of autoreactive T cells. Particular class II MHC molecules may select for autoreactive T cells by increasing positive selection or decreasing negative selection (Marrack et al. 2001), e.g. the MHC II molecule, I-A^{g7}, in the nonobese diabetic (NOD) mouse model, binds peptides very poorly (Carrasco-Marin et al. 1996). If self-peptides are inadequately presented by I-A^{g7} during selection, self-reactive T cells will not be eliminated. Others speculate that the linkage between MHC and autoimmunity is a simple scenario whereby disease susceptibility is determined by the varying degree to which different MHC alleles present self-peptides to autoreactive T cells (Janeway et al. 2001). In the periphery, certain disease-associated MHC II molecules predispose to autoimmunity by presenting self-peptides to autoreactive $CD4^+$ T cells.

The MHC and autoimmune disease linkages are identified by comparing the frequency of certain alleles in patients to the frequency of those alleles in the normal population (Janeway et al. 2001). One of the earliest links between autoimmunity and MHC was noted in the 1970s (Feldmann 2001). HLA-DR (human leukocyte antigen DR) allele subtypes were associated with RA via a 'shared epitope', a six amino acid sequence occurring in the peptide-binding groove of the DR alleles of 70–80 percent of RA patients. Currently, the HLA-DR alleles, HLA-DRB1*0401 and -*0404, are recognized as the most significant contributors to genetic susceptibility to RA (Nepom 1998).

Multiple sclerosis is also associated with particular alleles of HLA-DR, specifically HLA-DR2, as well as alleles of HLA-DQ. However, a comprehensive linkage

Table 37.2 *Examples of some MHC/autoimmune disease associations*

Disease	Association: Class I MHC	Class II MHC
Reactive arthritis	HLA-B27	
Ankylosing spondylitis	HLA-B27	
Multiple sclerosis		HLA-DR2
Treatment-resistant Lyme arthritis		HLA-DR4, HLA-DR1
Rheumatoid arthritis		HLA-DR1, HLA-DR4
Type 1 diabetes		HLA-DQ8, HLA-DQ2

(Wucherpfennig, 2001)

analysis determined that disease development was probably the result of multiple environmental and genetic factors, as opposed to a single disease gene (Haines et al. 1996).

The HLA-DR and HLA-DQ alleles are also strongly associated with type 1 diabetes (Wucherpfennig and Eisenbarth 2001). Interestingly, the complexity arising from the interaction between 'disease-causing genes' and 'disease-modifying genes' is evident in a transgenic mouse model of type 1 diabetes. Mice transgenic for HLA-DQ8 develop spontaneous disease, but the frequency of disease is lower when the mice co-express HLA-DR4 and HLA-DQ8, suggesting a protective role for HLA-DR4 allele (Wucherpfennig and Eisenbarth 2001). In humans, the HLA-DR2–DQ6 haplotype, representing a linkage disequilibrium, is associated with dominant protection from type 1 diabetes (Nepom and Erlich 1991).

The vast majority of MHC and autoimmune disease associations are linked to class II molecules (Table 37.2), although there are exceptions. Ankylosing spondylitis and reactive arthritis are two examples; both diseases are strongly associated with the MHC I molecule, HLA-B27 (Levitin et al. 1976; Pasternack and Tiilikainen 1977).

The effects of non-MHC genes on autoimmune disease development

Genetic mapping studies have identified individual genes on various chromosomes associated with susceptibility towards certain autoimmune diseases. These non-MHC genes are involved in regulating the recognition, presentation, and concentration of autoantigens (Marrack et al. 2001). A polymorphism in the gene that encodes the CTLA-4 is linked to the development of type 1 diabetes, celiac disease, Graves' disease, and autoimmune hypothyroidism (Nistico et al. 1996; Djilali-Saiah et al. 1998). CTLA-4 is a surface T-cell molecule that negatively controls T-cell activation (Linsley et al. 1992). Another polymorphism in the gene encoding IL-2 is associated with NOD mice and experimental autoimmune encephalomyelitis (EAE) animal models (Encinas et al. 1999). IL-2 stimulates the proliferation of T lymphocytes *and* keeps lymphoid growth in check; this example underscores the significance of IL-2 in maintaining peripheral tolerance. A deficiency of C1q in certain strains of mice, as well as in humans, results in a lupus-like disease characterized by autoantibodies to double-stranded DNA or nuclear components (Slingsby et al. 1996; Botto et al. 1998). C1q, a component of the classic complement pathway, aids in the clearance of apoptotic cellular debris including potential nuclear autoantigens. Two mutations that encode transcription factors of unknown function have been implicated in type 1 diabetes, one on chromosome 21 and another on the X chromosome. The former, an autosomal recessive mutation, results in autoimmune polyendocrine syndrome type 1 (APS-1) (Nagamine et al. 1997), and the latter causes X-linked autoimmunity-allergic disregulation syndrome (XLAAD) (Chatila et al. 2000). Mice deficient in IL-10 develop chronic enterocolitis, a disease that is pathologically similar to inflammatory bowel disease (IBD) in humans (Kuhn et al. 1993). Clearly, many non-MHC genetic abnormalities have been associated with autoimmunity.

ENVIRONMENTAL FACTORS AND AUTOIMMUNE DISEASE

An individual's predisposition towards acquiring an autoimmune disease is influenced not only by genetic susceptibility, but also by the environment. In humans, incomplete autoimmune disease concordance rates in monozygotic twins suggest an underlying environmental component to autoimmune disease development. In identical twin pairs, less than 50 percent of the siblings of affected twins will acquire an autoimmune disease (Ermann and Fathman 2001). An intriguing epidemiological study of the incidence of MS in a migrant population revealed that migrants acquired the MS risk of the region to which they relocated (Weinshenker 1996). In animals, inbred strains susceptible to the spontaneous development of SLE and diabetes display incomplete disease penetrance (Wanstrat and Wakeland 2001). In NOD mice, the incidence of diabetes drops dramatically with bacterial infection (Todd 1991).

The association between infectious agents and autoimmune disease has been the subject of intense investigation over the course of the last two decades. Even since its earliest description, autoimmune disease has been linked with infection. In the aforementioned research on PKH, the collaborators Donath and Landsteiner were struck by the correlation between PKH and a pre-existing syphilis infection (Silverstein 2001). To date, contemporary researchers have added considerably to the number of autoimmune diseases linked with pathogens (Table 37.3). The classic examples include: β-hemolytic streptococci and rheumatic fever (Benoist and Mathis 1998); *Trypanosoma cruzi* and Chagas' disease

Table 37.3 *Pathogens and autoimmunity: some common examples of autoimmune diseases linked with pathogens*

Disease	Pathogen	Host self-antigen
Rheumatic fever	Group A streptococci	Cardiac myosin
Guillain–Barré syndrome	*Campylobacter jejuni*	Peripheral nerve ganglioside proteins
Treatment-resistant Lyme arthritis	*Borrelia burgdorferi*	LFA-1
Myocarditis	Group B Coxsackie virus	Cardiac antigens
Chagas' disease	*Trypanosoma cruzi*	Cardiac myosin heavy chain
Herpetic stromal keratitis	Herpes simplex virus	Cornal antigen and IgG2a
Type 1 diabetes	Group B Coxsackie virus	Glutamate decarboxylase
Myasthenia gravis	Herpes simplex virus	Acetylcholine receptor
Multiple sclerosis	Epstein Barr virus	Myelin basic protein

Benoist and Mathis (2001), Regner and Lambert (2001), Marrack et al. (2001).

(Khoury and Fields 1980); and *Borrelia burgdorferi* and Lyme arthritis (Gross et al. 1998). Animal models in which microbial infection directly triggers certain autoimmune diseases further support this link between infection and autoimmunity. In one such model, particular strains of mice develop an autoimmune response against a corneal antigen after ocular infection with herpes simplex virus 1 (Panoutsakopoulou et al. 2001). The mice develop herpetic stromal keratitis (HSK), a leading cause of blindness in humans (Streilein 1997).

Despite the pathogen and autoimmune disease correlations in both humans and mice, the exact mechanisms whereby an infection leads to autoimmune disease have not yet been resolved. In fact, it remains unclear as to whether the pathogen directly or indirectly contributes to autoimmune disease development. Possibly, cross-reactive immune responses against the pathogen and self-molecules closely resembling the pathogen produce disease. Or, perhaps, the inflammation provoked by the pathogen at the site of infection causes a disregulated immune response that disturbs self-tolerance. The etiology of an autoimmune disease triggered by infection may be multifactorial, implicating several mechanisms in pathogenesis that may be relevant at different disease stages (Wucherpfennig 2001).

Mechanisms for pathogen-induced autoimmunity

Several mechanisms have been proposed to account for the post-infectious activation of the immune response against self-targets (Wucherpfennig 2001). Mechanisms may be categorized into two groups: antigen-specific and antigen nonspecific. In the first group, the pathogen directly induces autoimmunity through an antigen-specific response involving a microbial product; molecular mimicry is a well-characterized example. In molecular mimicry, the immune response to a microbial antigen cross-reacts with a host antigen. In the second group, the response is antigen nonspecific; autoimmunity is a product of the pathogen-induced inflammatory environment, e.g. inflammation might prompt the expansion of previously activated T cells, a mechanism known as bystander activation (Wucherpfennig 2001).

ANTIGEN-SPECIFIC MECHANISMS FOR PATHOGEN-INDUCED AUTOIMMUNITY

Molecular mimicry

The theory of molecular mimicry argues that a viral or bacterial pathogen expresses an antigenic determinant on one of its proteins that is sufficiently similar in sequence or structure to a self-peptide (Fujinami and Oldstone 1985). During an infection, the microbial determinant, a linear sequence of 8–15 amino acids, may be presented in the context of a particular MHC molecule to the TCR of an autoreactive T cell. As a result, naïve autoreactive T cells are activated and expanded.

An animal model of EAE provided early evidence for molecular mimicry. Rabbits were immunized with a hepatitis B virus polymerase peptide which shared a six amino acid sequence similarity with the encephalitogenic region of rabbit MBP. After immunization with the peptide, T-cell reactivity to MBP could be demonstrated. Some of the animals also developed EAE as determined by histology (Fujinami and Oldstone 1985).

Autoimmune disease that is MHC I dependent was demonstrated in a mouse model of IBD. Intestinal inflammation was induced by transferring $CD8^+$ T cells, which recognize both mycobacterial and murine heat shock proteins (hsp) in TCR $\beta^{-/-}$ mice. The T-cell infiltrates into the small intestine and the liver resulted in lesions. The results could be reproduced in germ-free mice, implicating host hsp as a target for the $CD8^+$ T cells (Steinhoff et al. 1999).

A highly cited case for the role of molecular mimicry as a mechanism of autoimmune disease is in the pathogenesis of treatment-resistant Lyme arthritis (TRLA). Lyme disease is a multisystem illness caused by the tick-borne spirochete *Borrelia burgdorferi* (Steere et al. 1983). The Lyme disease pathogen expresses numerous antigens, including outer surface protein A (OspA) both on its surface and in its periplasmic space (Barbour and Hayes 1986). The clinical course of the disease begins within days of the blood meal of the *Ixodes scapularis* tick. The characteristic rash, erythema migrans, occurs initially and is followed by cardiac, neurological, and musculoskeletal impairments, including joint inflammation (Steere 1989). A course of antibiotics typically resolves the illness. However, the arthritis never resolves in approximately 10 percent of patients despite extensive antibiotic therapy (Steere et al. 1984). These TRLA patients, who have no detectable spirochetal DNA in joint fluid or synovial tissue, are often HLA-DRB1*0401$^+$ and HLA-DRB1*0101$^+$, the same alleles associated with RA. Furthermore, during arthritic episodes, spiking titers of anti-OspA IgG are detectable in the patient serum (Kalish et al. 1993). These immune responses correlate with the severity and duration of the arthritis. Collectively, this evidence supports the hypothesis that TRLA is an autoimmune disease (Gross et al. 1998).

With molecular mimicry implicated as a mechanism for TRLA, the identification of the immunodominant epitope of OspA, as well as the search for a potential autoantigen, followed suit (Gross et al. 1998). Using an algorithm developed for the identification of peptides binding to HLA-DRB1*0401 (Hammer et al. 1994), $OspA_{165–173}$ was calculated to have the highest score for possible association with this class II molecule. To confirm that this was indeed the immunodominant epitope, HLA-DRB1*0401 transgenic mice were immunized with OspA and their immune T cells were tested in vitro for reactivity with an overlapping OspA peptide library. $OspA_{165–173}$ elicited the strongest recall response in these cells, a result that was confirmed by the response pattern of human T cells isolated from the synovial fluid of DRB1*0401$^+$ TRLA patients. A Genbank Database search for a human autoantigen with a similar amino acid sequence as seen in $OspA_{165–173}$ led to the identification of a stretch of amino acids from 332 to 340 in human leukocyte function antigen-1α (LFA-1α). T cells from the synovial fluid of TRLA patients were also responsive to human LFA-1α (Gross et al. 1998). According to the algorithm of Hammer et al. (1994), LFA-$1\alpha_{332–340}$ was predicted to be effectively bound by HLA-DRB1*0401.

With the identification of the candidate autoantigen, human LFA-1α, a model for autoimmunity as a mechanism for TRLA may be proposed. Following infection with *Borrelia burgdorferi*, the spirochete disseminates systemically to many locations, including the joint. After a period of varying duration, perhaps several months, the inflammatory immune response begins in the joint. The nine-residue peptide $OspA_{165–173}$ is presented in the context of HLA-DRB1*0401, resulting in activation and expansion of $OspA_{165–173}$-specific T cells and an inflammatory Th1 response, characterized by secretion of interferon γ (IFN-γ). The inflammatory milieu in the joint results in the upregulation of MHC II on APCs, as well as the upregulation of LFA-1α on leukocytes and synoviocytes. Despite the eradication of the spirochete by antibiotic treatment, the $OspA_{165–173}$-specific Th1 cells in the joint continue to be activated via cross-reaction with the self-peptide LFA-$1\alpha_{332–340}$, thus propagating the joint arthritis (Figure 37.3).

Superantigen activation

Viral or bacterial superantigens activate T cells expressing particular Vβ genes segments. Superantigens have

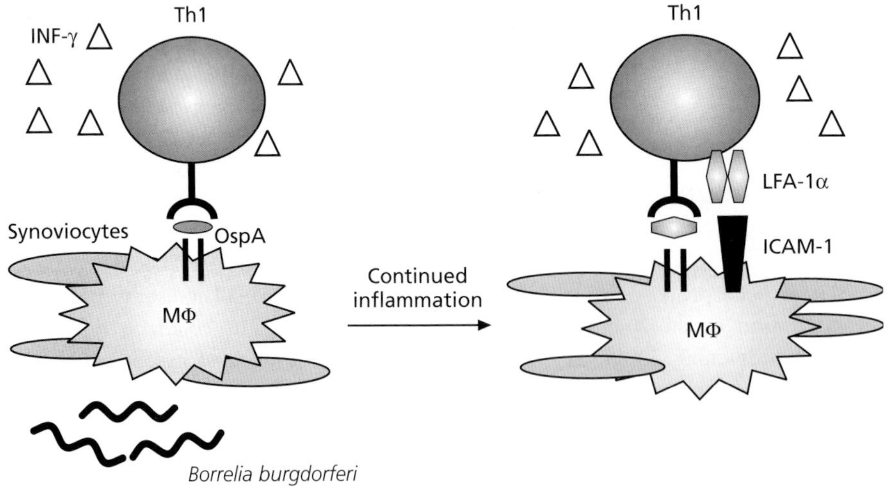

Figure 37.3 *Model for induction of autoimmunity in treatment-resistant Lyme arthritis (TRLA). Following infection with* Borrelia burgdorferi, *the spirochete disseminates systemically to many locations, including the joint. Macrophages (Mφs) and dendritic cells present the outer surface protein $OspA_{165–173}$ to T cells. These activated T cells secrete interferon γ (INF-γ). The inflammatory milieu in the joint results in the upregulation of MHC II on antigen-presenting cells (APCs), as well as the upregulation of human leukocyte function antigen-1α (LFA-1α) on leukocytes and synoviocytes. Despite the eradication of the spirochete by antibiotic treatment, the cross-reactive T cells in the joint continue to be activated via the presentation of self-peptides derived from LFA-1α, propagating the joint arthritis. ICAM, intercellular adhesion molecule.*

the capacity to cause aberrant activation of large numbers of T cells, regardless of their peptide specificity. A subset of these superantigen T cells may be specific for a self-antigen and, thus, could mount an autoimmune response (Wucherpfennig 2001).

Superantigens may also exacerbate an autoimmune process or induce a relapse. In EAE, a murine model of MS, episodes of relapsing paralysis can be induced in PL/J mice with the bacterial superantigen staphylococcal enterotoxin B (SEB). In these mice, EAE is elicited by immunization with the amino-terminal peptide of MBP, Ac_{1-11}. Following an initial paralysis and clinical remission, administration of SEB can induce another episode of paralysis in these mice. The autoreactive T cells specific for the Ac_{1-11} epitope express Vβ8 and are reactivated by the SEB superantigen (Brocke et al. 1993).

ANTIGEN-NONSPECIFIC MECHANISMS FOR PATHOGEN-INDUCED AUTOIMMUNITY

Bystander activation

The inflammatory milieu resulting from a microbial infection may result in the expansion of autoreactive T cells in the absence of antigenic specificity. Activated T cells have a lower threshold for activation than resting T cells and, thus, may target self-antigens (Benoist and Mathis 1998). Microbial products, including LPS, can be potent adjuvants activating the innate immune response and eliciting an increase in proinflammatory cytokines. In this inflammatory environment, APCs enhance antigen processing, increase cell surface MHC II expression and upregulate co-stimulatory molecules such as B7-2 (Vella et al. 1997). Adjuvants may also sustain the antigen-specific T-cell population by inhibiting the AICD death of antigen-specific T cells (Kearney et al. 1994; Vella et al. 1997).

Another possible effect elicited by an inflammatory environment is a shift towards a Th1 T-cell population (Marrack et al. 2001). $CD4^+$ helper T cells differentiate into either Th1 or Th2 cells (Figure 37.4). Typically, microbial infections are associated with a Th-cell commitment to a Th1 cell (Yazdanbakhsh et al. 2002). This subset of cells is associated with the proinflammatory cytokine, INF-γ, and cell-mediated immunity. Th1 cells are also associated with many autoimmune diseases, including RA, Crohn's disease, type 1 diabetes, and MS. Comparatively, Th2 cells produce IL-4 and IL-5 and are associated with allergic and anti-helminth responses. After a microbial infection, the T-cell population may shift towards the Th1 subset, thereby priming an individual for an autoimmune disease. This theory remains hotly contested for a

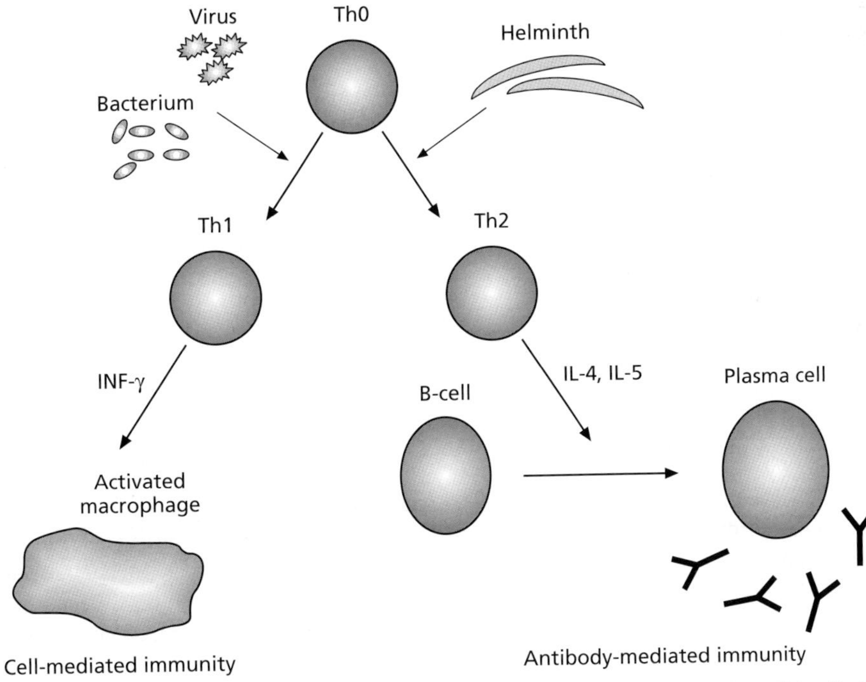

Figure 37.4 *T-helper 1 or 2 (Th1/Th2) cell phenotypes. $CD4^+$ Th cells differentiate into either Th1 cells or Th2 cells. The commitment to a Th1 or a Th2 cell fate is largely determined by transcriptional mechanisms induced by the interleukins IL-12 and IL-4, respectively (Murphy and Reiner 2002). In Th1 cell development, the T-box transcription factor T-bet is responsive to IL-12 and responsible for inducing the production of interferon α (INF-γ). During the commitment of Th cells to Th2 cells, IL-4 promotes the increased expression of the zinc finger transcription factor GATA3 which, in turn, enables the remodeling of the IL-4 locus. Typically, microbial and viral infections are associated with $CD4^+$ T-helper cell differentiation into Th1 cells (Lucey et al. 1996). This subset of cells is associated with activated macrophages secreting the proinflammatory cytokine, INF-γ, as well as cell-mediated immunity. Alternatively, Th2 cells produce IL-4 and IL-5 and are associated with allergic and anti-helminth responses. Th2 cells are associated with antibody-mediated immunity driven by plasma cells. (Adapted from Murphy and Reiner 2002 and Janeway et al. 2001.)*

variety of reasons, including the argument that cytokines have the dual capacity both to heighten and to constrain autoimmune responses. Furthermore, two common autoimmune diseases, ulcerative colitis and SLE, are associated with Th2 responses (O'Shea et al. 2002).

Epitope spreading

During chronic autoimmune disease, the T-cell response may acquire additional epitope specificities, shifting from a dominant epitope to subdominant epitopes on the self or foreign protein (Lehmann et al. 1992). 'Intramolecular spreading' refers to new epitopes on the same protein and 'intermolecular spreading' refers to epitopes on other proteins, perhaps other antigens in the same tissue (Vanderlugt and Miller 2002).

The earliest demonstration of this diversification of the T-cell response was shown in the murine model of EAE (Lehmann et al. 1992). After immunization with either whole MBP or only the N-terminal peptide of MBP (Ac_{1-11}), the T-cell response undergoes intramolecular epitope spreading, shifting reactivity from the original immunodominant peptide to different epitopes of the MBP protein. Evidence of intermolecular epitope spreading is depicted in a murine model of a chronic demyelinating disease mediated by $CD4^+$ T cells. Following infection with Theiler's picornavirus, mice develop a chronic progressive course of encephalomyelitis that resembles MS. The course of the disease appears biphasic. At the onset of clinical symptoms, T-cell responses to the virus are detected. Then, later in the course of the disease, responses to central nervous system antigens are seen, including determinants on the encephalitogenic proteolipid protein (PLP), MBP, and myelin oligodendrocyte glycoprotein (MOG).

Nonmicrobial environmental factors and autoimmunity

The evidence supporting a role for nonmicrobial environmental factors in the development of autoimmune disease is often based on epidemiological studies. Excessive intake of dietary iodide, a component of thyroid hormone, is a risk factor for autoimmune thyroid disease (Bagchi et al. 1985). Other studies correlate stressful life events with the development of Graves' disease (Matos-Santos et al. 2001). A recent study demonstrates that women who breast-feed have a decreased risk of developing SLE, a trend that is correlated with the number of babies breast-fed and the duration of breast-feeding (Cooper et al. 2002). Some literature cites occupational exposure to silica dust as a risk factor for the development of RA, lupus, scleroderma, and glomerulonephritis (Parks et al. 2002). In most cases, further studies are necessary to substantiate a role for nonmicrobial environmental factors in autoimmunity. However, in the case of sympathetic ophthalmia, there is unequivocal proof that trauma to one eye leads to an autoimmune-mediated attack of the other (Jakobiec et al. 1984). The eye is a well-defined immunoprivileged site, complete with T-cell infiltration barriers, and immunosuppressive cytokines, including TGF-β. When injury at this isolated site occurs, previously sequestered self-antigens are available for immunoreactivity.

THE EFFECTS OF IMMUNE DISREGULATION ON AUTOIMMUNE DISEASE DEVELOPMENT

Many of the immune regulation abnormalities identified in autoimmune disease are inextricably linked to genetic mutations, e.g. severe impairment of the AICD pathway results from mutations in the death receptor Fas (CD95) or Fas ligand (FasL or CD178). This pathway plays a critical role in maintaining peripheral tolerance via elimination of autoreactive cells. The absence of Fas or FasL in either *lpr* or *gld* mice, respectively, results in a severe autoimmune phenotype, an SLE-like disorder, marked by lymphadenopathy, autoantibody production, and nephritis (O'Shea et al. 2002). In humans, mutations in Fas result in ALPS. These patients present with lymphadenopathy, hepatosplenomegaly, and hypersplenism (Straus et al. 1999).

Other aberrant immunoregulatory mechanisms have not yet been linked to a single genetic defect, e.g. the T-cell response in active RA patients is dampened, perhaps as a result of aberrant calcium signaling and abnormal ξ chain expression by the TCR. These abnormalities may be a result of the overexpression of tumor necrosis factor α (TNF-α) in RA synovial tissue. These same abnormalities can be reproduced in vitro by chronic stimulation of T cells with TNF-α (Feldmann 2001).

Systemic lupus erythematosus may be the archetypal disease of immune disregulation. SLE, a systemic autoimmune disease, is defined by the production of autoantibodies. The disease has an enormous range of clinical manifestations that may involve the skin, joints, kidneys, and heart. SLE is associated with various abnormalities in lymphocytes at the cellular and molecular level that include antigen-receptor signaling events and cytokine production. In humans, abnormal, hyperreactive B-cell responses have been characterized. They include an increased expression of the CD40 ligand and a co-stimulatory molecule, as well as an increased production of the B-cell-stimulatory cytokines, IL-6 and IL-10 (Lipsky 2001). Altered T-cell signaling may result from the abnormal expression of the TCR ξ chain as well as decreased levels of p65-Rel A protein (Tsokos et al. 2000). The nuclear translocation of the p65-Rel A protein is associated with the activity of the transcription factor, nuclear factor-κB (NF-κB), which in turn is responsible for the activation of IL-2.

MECHANISMS OF TISSUE DESTRUCTION AND ORGAN DAMAGE IN AUTOIMMUNE DISEASES

The 'initiation phase' of an autoimmune disease is mediated by several factors: genetic predisposition, environmental influence, and immune disregulation (Ermann and Fathman 2001). Over time, a chronic autoimmune response invariably results in an 'effector phase' of the disease. During the effector phase, tissues and/or organs sustain damage imparted by destructive cells and cellular products. The effector phase of certain autoimmune diseases may be the product of both immune and nonimmune mechanisms (Ermann and Fathman 2001).

Demyelination and axonal loss in MS

Multiple sclerosis occurs in early adulthood and is the most common demyelinating disease in adults. The disease is characterized by relapsing and remitting episodes of neurological impairment. MS appears to be an autoimmune response targeting various proteins of the myelin sheath, including MBP, MOG, PLP, and αβ crystallin. Lymphocytes are initially activated by a microbial infection or a self-antigen, and then they are essentially 'pulled through' the blood–brain barrier by integrin and adhesion molecule interactions. After the degradation of the extracellular matrix by matrix metalloproteases (MMP), lymphocytes can access the white matter of the central nervous system, resulting in autoantibody production to myelin proteins by B cells and lymphotoxin-α (LT-α) and TNF-α cytokine secretion by T cells. These responses prompt the release of the free radical nitric oxide (NO) and the T-cell stimulator osteopontin (OPN) by macrophages, microglial cells, and astrocytes. The end result of this effector phase cascade is multifocal demyelination and axonal loss in the spinal cord, ultimately resulting in paralysis (Steinman 2001).

Immune complex deposition in SLE

Systemic lupus erythematosus is a systemic autoimmune disease that frequently strikes women during their reproductive years. In humans, this disease has an enormous range of clinical presentations which may include skin lesions, arthritis, serositis, nephritis, and hematological disorders. In fact, renal involvement is the most life-threatening complication of SLE. The immediate precursor to renal tissue destruction and kidney damage in SLE is the IgG autoantibodies to double-stranded DNA. Serum titers of these antibodies correlate with glomerulonephritis in humans and mice (Pearson and Lightfoot 1981). Other autoantibodies are also associated with the tissue destruction found in SLE, including anticardiolipin antibodies and thrombosis, as well as anti-Ro antibodies and congenital heart block (Lipsky 2001). Autoantibodies are the direct mediators of tissue injury in SLE. After the deposition of antigen–antibody immune complexes and the fixation of complement, tissue damage occurs in the manner of a type III hypersensitivity reaction.

Cartilage destruction and bone loss in RA

Another autoimmune disease, RA, afflicts about 1 in 100 people with chronic inflammation of the synovial joints. This chronic immune response ultimately destroys cartilage and bone, rendering the affected joints immobile. Although activated T cells specific for a joint antigen appear to be critical in the initiation of the disease process; cartilage and bone loss are also the products of nonimmune mediators. Enzymes play a critical role in cartilage destruction. Cartilage, an intricate matrix of type II collagen and aggrecan, is degraded by the activity of MMPs, as well as two aggrecanases or ADAMTS (a disintegrin or metalloproteinase with thrombospondin type I motif) (Feldmann 2001). Bone lesions are the product of the destructive osteoclast cell. Inflammation favors bone loss because osteoclastic precursors are induced to differentiate into osteoclasts by proinflammatory cytokines TNF-α and IL-1.

Thyroid-associated ophthalmopathy in autoimmune thyroid disease

Thyroid-associated ophthalmopathy (TAO) is a serious complication of autoimmune thyroid disease. The pathogenesis of TAO includes the deposit of excess connective tissue and fat in the orbital cavity, as well as edema. The clinical outcome is exophthalmos, corneal damage, and, on a rare occasion, loss of sight. The effector phase of TAO begins when the inflammatory cell infiltrate penetrates the extraocular muscles. These T cells mount a response against an orbital autoantigen that is similar enough to a thyroid autoantigen, inciting a cross-reaction. With the release of cytokines, including IL-1, TNF, and INF-γ, and the concomitant activation of fibroblasts, two mediators of edema are released by the fibroblasts: hydrophilic glycosaminoglycan hyaluronate and chondroitin sulfate (Weetman 2001). Interestingly, a subset of these orbital fibroblasts may differentiate into fat cells, explaining the excess orbital fat in TAO. Although the pathology of TAO is unraveling, the identity of the cross-reactive autoantigen remains at large.

EXPERIMENTAL ANIMAL MODELS OF AUTOIMMUNITY

The use of animal models has played a pivotal role in furthering our understanding of autoimmunity. Animal models are implemented to investigate the etiology, pathogenesis, and therapeutic strategies associated with many of the 80 autoimmune diseases that collectively affect roughly 5 percent of the world's population. An animal model offers a wealth of information, far exceeding what can be gleaned from most in vitro experiments; however, it is never an exact replica of a human autoimmune disease. First, studying a human disease in a highly inbred mouse model is not an ideal scenario because humans are outbred relative to mice. Thus, the study of an inbred mouse strain is roughly the equivalent of a 'single case study' in humans (Atkinson and Leiter 1999). Second, and to an even greater extent, extrapolating from an animal model to a human disease is dubious because of the genetic differences between species. There are inherent limitations in extracting pathogenic mechanisms from an animal model of disease as a result of the underlying genus- and species-specific differences that occur between an animal and a human. Under circumstances of critical importance, such as the testing of gene therapy, a species closer to humans, such as primates, may be a better candidate to serve as an experimental surrogate.

The NOD mouse as a model of human type 1 diabetes mellitus

The NOD mouse was first identified in 1980 as a useful model for investigating insulin-dependent human diabetes (Makino et al. 1980). Although the predecessor to the NOD mouse, the biobreeding (BB) rat, was identified several years earlier (Nakhooda et al. 1978), the NOD mouse gained favor and is currently the model of choice for type 1 diabetes researchers. In fact, mice are generally preferable to rats, because their genome is more familiar and analytical reagents, such as monoclonal antibodies, are more readily available (Atkinson and Leiter 1999).

Human type 1 or insulin-dependent diabetes mellitus is a $CD4^+$ and $CD8^+$ T-cell-mediated autoimmune disease that results in the targeted destruction of the insulin-secreting β cells of the pancreatic islets. Diabetic NOD mice display the biochemical and pathological characteristics of diabetes, including a lymphocyte infiltration into the pancreatic islets. Diabetes in NOD mice is heterogeneous, because its development is determined by more than 19 loci (Wucherpfennig and Eisenbarth 2001). In humans, many genetic loci are also responsible for the development of diabetes. Both NOD mice and humans have autoimmune responses to glutamic acid decarboxylase (GAD), insulin, and insulinoma-associated protein 2 (Ia2) (Taneja and David 2001).

A recent breakthrough in the study of the etiology of type 1 diabetes occurred from a comparative analysis between humans and NOD mice. Lee et al. (2001) determined that susceptibility to diabetes is conferred by a mutation in the P9 peptide-binding pocket of the MHC II molecules HLA-DQ8 and $I\text{-}A^{g7}$ in humans and NOD mice, respectively. Using X-ray crystallography, this group was able to characterize the three-dimensional structures of these molecules and determine that they lacked an aspartic acid residue at position 57 of the β chain, resulting in a net positive charge for these molecules. Functionally, the mutation in these MHC II molecules enables them to bind a different repertoire of peptides, including the immunodominant T-cell epitopes of islet antigen peptides in NOD mice (Yu et al. 2000). These results infer that type 1 diabetes in mice and humans may stem from the same antigen-presenting events. They further demonstrate the significance of the NOD mouse as an animal model of type 1 diabetes.

THE NEW ZEALAND BLACK/WHITE MOUSE AS A MODEL OF HUMAN SLE

Systemic lupus erythematosus is a systemic autoimmune disease associated with pathogenic autoantibodies. Some of these pathogenic autoantibodies include anti-DNA in glomerulonephritis, anticardiolipin in thrombosis, and anti-Ro in heart block (Lipsky 2001). The disease has been linked with several MHC genes. In fact, certain MHC alleles have been associated with the occurrence of particular autoantibodies, including HLA-DR2 and HLA-DR3 with anti-Ro and anti-La antibodies, as well as HLA-DR4 and HLA-DQ3 with anti-Sm and anti-RNP antibodies (Chernajovsky et al. 2000). Complement deficiencies, involving the complement molecules C1q, C2, and C4, have also been sited in SLE, as well as a host of other immunoregulatory defects.

The F1 hybrid cross between New Zealand black (NZB) and New Zealand white (NZW) mice generates the NZB/W mouse that is recognized as the best murine model of SLE (Drake et al. 1995). In these mice, the disease develops spontaneously and is characterized by high titers of IgG anti-DNA antibodies. Death in these animals occurs by a progressive, severe glomerulonephritis, similar to the renal destruction seen in human SLE. The development of both human and murine SLE is strongly linked with particular MHC alleles.

The NZB/W mouse model has been used to identify a myriad of abnormalities associated with the autoimmune disease SLE. This animal model was used to identify B-cell hyperreactivity as an immunoregulatory defect in SLE. On T-cell stimulation, resting B cells from these mice display increased proliferation, IgM secretion, and upregulation of co-stimulatory molecules (Jongstra-Bilen et al. 1997). Genetic loci on chromosome 1 in both parental strains NZB and NZW have been implicated in this B-cell hyperreactivity (Vyse et al. 1997; Sobel et al. 1999). This model was also used to delineate a role for cytokines in SLE pathogenesis. The F1 hybrid mouse inherits a dominant gene from the NZW parent that correlates with reduced levels of TNF-α production. The administration of replacement TNF-α delayed the onset of lupus nephritis (Jacob and McDevitt 1988).

This model has also been used to identify multiple genetic susceptibility loci for SLE. Breeding of NZW and NZB strains has yielded a variety of strains called NZM. Using genetic mapping techniques, the analysis of these NZM strains has enabled researchers to identify susceptibility loci for SLE in this model. The analysis of congenic strains with these loci is enabling researchers to determine the functional role that these loci may have in SLE disease pathogenesis.

Strain K/BxN: a spontaneous mouse model of rheumatoid arthritis

In autoimmune disease research, an animal model can often be the framework supporting a new theory in the pathogenesis of an autoimmune disease. Occasionally, an animal model provides evidence to challenge an existing theory, such as in the case of rheumatoid arthritis (RA). RA is a chronic, inflammatory joint disease, characterized by synovial thickening and lymphocyte infiltration, as well as cartilage and bone destruction in the joint. Given the association of this disease with certain MHC II alleles, contemporary researchers believe that $CD4^+$ T cells play a crucial role in the pathogenesis of RA. Therapeutic trials were conducted with antibodies to CD4, but they were not very successful (Feldmann 2001).

Kouskoff et al. (1996) uncovered an intriguing new animal model of arthritis. This group crossed the TCR transgenic line KRNxC57BL/6 (the TCR recognizes a bovine ribonuclease peptide in the context of $I\text{-}A^k$), with the NOD strain. The resulting strain, K/BxN, has a TCR that recognizes a peptide of glucose-6-phosphate isomerase (GPI) in the context of the NOD-derived $I\text{-}A^{g7}$ (Matsumoto et al. 1999). GPI is a ubiquitously expressed protein that catalyzes reactions in glycolysis and gluconeogenesis. All of the K/BxN offspring develop a spontaneous arthritis that is strikingly similar to human RA. Although arthritis is initiated by T-cell activation in this model, joint-specific pathology is mediated by anti-GPI antibodies. In fact, transfer of antibodies can reproduce disease. This model suggests that antibodies may not merely be a phenomenon in RA; they may in fact be the primary mediators of disease.

Rodent EAE as a model of human MS

In the aforementioned animal models, disease develops spontaneously. In contrast, the rodent model of EAE is an induced model of disease. Induced models are advantageous because the onset and progression of the disease can be carefully monitored (Taneja and David 2001). The EAE rodent model is used extensively as a model for human MS. EAE can be induced with a variety of autoantigens, including MBP, PLP, and MOG, e.g. in PL/J mice, EAE is induced with the N-terminal peptide of MBP (Ac1-11). Histologically, the EAE pathology is similar to MS, although the degree of demyelination and the distribution of the lesions are different (Taneja and David 2001). In rodents, predisposition to EAE is also associated with II MHC alleles, similar to MS in humans.

The rodent model of EAE has been a powerful tool for examining important mechanisms in autoimmune disease pathology. Experiments in this model revealed that superantigens could induce relapses or exacerbate autoimmune disease (Brocke et al. 1993). This model was also used to demonstrate the concept of 'epitope spreading', as previously discussed.

Furthermore, the EAE model will invariably play an instrumental role in identifying candidate therapies for human MS, e.g. the injection of a herpes simplex virus vector driving the human fibroblast growth factor gene is reversing the pathological signs of EAE in C57BL/6 mice (Ruffini et al. 2001). Recently, Youssef et al. (2002) have identified a role for atorvastatin, a drug currently given to reduce high cholesterol, in ameliorating the disease severity in three different mouse models of EAE. On repeated administration of atorvastatin, investigators noted increased levels of anti-inflammatory cytokines, including IL-4, IL-10, and TGF-β. The EAE mouse model has also been used to test a therapeutic strategy involving the blockade of very late activated antigen-4 (VLA-4), a T-cell antigen that aids T cells in penetrating the blood–brain barrier. The results of the trial were promising because they demonstrated a reversal of paralysis and eliminated relapses in treated mice. Clinical trials are currently under way with a human antibody to VLA-4 (Steinman 2001).

AUTOIMMUNITY THROUGH IMMUNIZATION

The associations between infection and autoimmunity have accumulated rapidly in the scientific literature since the initial connection between the two was observed in the mid-1960s (Puxeddu et al. 1965). Precisely how an immune response to a pathogen evolves into an autoimmune disease remains unknown. Nevertheless, if an immune response to a pathogen may incite an autoimmune disease, perhaps an immune response to a vaccine may also elicit an autoimmune disease. Given the potential cross-reactivity between an autoantigen and a microbial antigen, could a vaccine pose the threat of priming for autoimmune disease in genetically susceptible individuals? Or could a potent vaccine adjuvant alter immunoreactivity, favoring a break in self-tolerance?

At a recent conference organized by the Fondation Merieux, Schoenfeld and Pless reported their conclusions with hesitancy (Regner and Lambert 2001). They concluded that, despite the lack of data to make a careful assessment, it appears that the connection between immunization and autoimmune disease is weak. Furthermore, they stated that the benefits of immunization far exceed the risks (Regner and Lambert 2001). The initial assessments regarding the safety of the Lyme disease vaccine demonstrated that there were no long-term adverse effects from immunization (Poland and Jacobson 2001; Sikand et al. 2001). In another investigation, immunizing infants with a recombinant hepatitis B virus vaccine did not result in an increase in autoantibody production at a 6-year follow-up study (Belloni et al. 2002). Given the slight possibility for vaccine-induced immunization, the implications for future vaccine design are evident, e.g. a modified vaccine design may include mutating a cross-reactive epitope to preclude molecular mimicry-based autoimmunity.

TREATMENT STRATEGIES FOR AUTOIMMUNE DISEASE

Treating a patient with an autoimmune disease is an inordinately complex task. Treatment is complicated because of the heterogeneous nature of these diseases. At the cellular and molecular level, neither the etiology nor the pathogenesis of autoimmune disease is well defined. Furthermore, for a physician, autoimmune diseases may be vexing for the following reasons: they are chronic; the course of the disease may vacillate between periods of relapse and periods of remission; patients may be affected differently by the same disease; and patients often present when the disease has already progressed to tissue and organ damage (Chernajovsky et al. 2000). Treatment is initiated to reinstate 'immune homeostasis' in the autoimmune disease patient.

Autoimmune diseases are wildly diverse. Although they span the gamut of clinical manifestations, the current management of most autoimmune diseases relies on immunosuppression, including the use of corticosteroids such as prednisone, e.g. patients with RA are administered methotrexate which acts via adenosine to suppress inflammation (Chan and Cronstein 2002). The current treatment strategy for MS includes synthetic glatiramer acetate, an agent that reportedly acts by shifting the T-cell phenotype to Th2 cells (Gran et al. 2000). Generally, immunosuppression has had limited success and is often used for lack of a better alternative (Persidis 1999).

In the case of some autoimmune diseases, recent approaches to modifying the immune system have demonstrated promising clinical improvements. Sustained therapy with TNF-α blockers has been successful in arresting RA (Pisetsky 2000) and Crohn's disease (Podolsky 2002). Patients with relapsing–remitting MS have been responsive to INF-β treatment, a drug administered to inhibit lymphocyte migration to the brain (Mehindate et al. 2001; Steinman 2001). These therapeutic strategies involve immunomodulation with cytokines and cytokine antagonists. Anti-T-cell monoclonal antibodies, signal transduction blockers, and pharmacological agents have also been implemented (Tsokos and Nepom 2000).

Gene therapy is employed by researchers to develop revolutionary treatments for autoimmune disease. This cutting-edge technology is the process of inserting and expressing foreign genes into the host cell genome. Many systems utilize viral vectors as a vehicle to insert genes by transduction. Successful animal trials with gene therapy have included the treatment of RA, MS, diabetes, and lupus (Tarner and Fathman 2001). These successes have supported the clinical trial of gene therapy in humans. With an estimated disease burden of $US65 billion (Persidis 1999), arthritis has featured prominently in human gene therapy investigations. In a recent study, a gene encoding the IL-1 receptor antagonist was transferred to the metacarpophalangeal joints of patients with advanced RA (Evans et al. 1996). Synoviocytes were injected ex vivo with a retroviral vector and reimplanted into the joint. The successful completion of this trial shows promise for the further application of gene therapy (Gouze et al. 2001; Horwood et al. 2002).

CONCLUSION

Autoimmunity constitutes the sustained 'attack' of self-tissue mediated by pathogenic, self-reactive antibodies and/or lymphocytes. Autoimmune diseases are a heterogeneous collection of about 80 distinct illnesses representing a broad range of pathology. The enormous complexity associated with the etiology, mechanisms, and pathogenesis of autoimmune disease is not rivaled by any other human disease.

Autoimmunity and autoimmune disease make up a topic teeming with discrepancies: decades ago, scientists refuted the existence of a disease that is today recognized as a serious societal burden. Autoimmune disease is the erroneous attempt of an organism to protect itself as it attacks itself. The present treatment of autoimmune disease relies on immunosuppression, rendering the patient susceptible to infection and illness.

Despite the complicated, and often contradictory, nature of autoimmune disease, scientists are deftly using valuable tools to unravel autoimmunity, including experimental animal models and gene therapy. With these efforts, scientists seek to understand, as well as to reinstate, the 'immune homeostasis' that has been lost in the autoimmune response.

REFERENCES

Asano, M., Toda, M., et al. 1996. Autoimmune disease as a consequence of developmental abnormality of a T cell subpopulation. *J Exp Med*, **184**, 387–96.

Atkinson, M.A. and Leiter, E.H. 1999. The NOD mouse model of type 1 diabetes: as good as it gets? *Nat Med*, **5**, 601–4.

Bagchi, N., Brown, T.R., et al. 1985. Induction of autoimmune thyroiditis in chickens by dietary iodine. *Science*, **230**, 325–7.

Barbour, A.G. and Hayes, S.F. 1986. Biology of *Borrelia* species. *Microbiol Rev*, **50**, 381–400.

Belloni, C., Avanzini, M.A., et al. 2002. No evidence of autoimmunity in 6-year-old children immunized at birth with recombinant hepatitis B vaccine. *Pediatrics*, **110**, e4.

Benoist, C. and Mathis, D. 1998. Autoimmunity. The pathogen connection. *Nature*, **394**, 227–8.

Benoist, C. and Mathis, D. 2001. Autoimmunity provoked by infection: how good is the case for T cell epitope mimicry? *Nat Immunol*, **2**, 797–801.

Botto, M., Dell'Agnola, C., et al. 1998. Homozygous C1q deficiency causes glomerulonephritis associated with multiple apoptotic bodies. *Nat Genet*, **19**, 56–9.

Brocke, S., Gaur, A., et al. 1993. Induction of relapsing paralysis in experimental autoimmune encephalomyelitis by bacterial superantigen. *Nature*, **365**, 642–4.

Burnet, F.M. 1959. *The clonal selection theory of acquired immunity*. London: Cambridge University Press.

Carrasco-Marin, E., Shimizu, J., et al. 1996. The class II MHC I-Ag7 molecules from non-obese diabetic mice are poor peptide binders. *J Immunol*, **156**, 450–8.

Chan, E.S. and Cronstein, B.N. 2002. Molecular action of methotrexate in inflammatory diseases. *Arthritis Res*, **4**, 266–73.

Chatila, T.A., Blaeser, F., et al. 2000. JM2, encoding a fork head-related protein, is mutated in X-linked autoimmunity-allergic disregulation syndrome. *J Clin Invest*, **106**, R75–81.

Chernajovsky, Y., Dreja, H., et al. 2000. Immuno- and genetic therapy in autoimmune diseases. *Genes Immun*, **1**, 295–307.

Cooper, G.S., Dooley, M.A., et al. 2002. Hormonal and reproductive risk factors for development of systemic lupus erythematosus: results of a population-based, case-control study. *Arthritis Rheum*, **46**, 1830–9.

Djilali-Saiah, I., Schmitz, J., et al. 1998. CTLA-4 gene polymorphism is associated with predisposition to coeliac disease. *Gut*, **43**, 187–9.

Drake, C.G., Rozzo, S.J., et al. 1995. Analysis of the New Zealand Black contribution to lupus-like renal disease. Multiple genes that operate in a threshold manner. *J Immunol*, **154**, 2441–7.

Encinas, J.A., Wicker, L.S., et al. 1999. QTL influencing autoimmune diabetes and encephalomyelitis map to a 0.15-cM region containing Il-2. *Nat Genet*, **21**, 158–60.

Ermann, J. and Fathman, C.G. 2001. Autoimmune diseases: genes, bugs and failed regulation. *Nat Immunol*, **2**, 759–61.

Evans, C.H., Robbins, P.D., et al. 1996. Clinical trial to assess the safety, feasibility, and efficacy of transferring a potentially anti-arthritic cytokine gene to human joints with rheumatoid arthritis. *Hum Gene Ther*, **7**, 1261–80.

Feldmann, M. 2001. Pathogenesis of arthritis: recent research progress. *Nat Immunol*, **2**, 771–3.

Fisher, G.H., Rosenberg, F.J., et al. 1995. Dominant interfering Fas gene mutations impair apoptosis in a human autoimmune lymphoproliferative syndrome. *Cell*, **81**, 935–46.

Fujinami, R.S. and Oldstone, M.B. 1985. Amino acid homology between the encephalitogenic site of myelin basic protein and virus: mechanism for autoimmunity. *Science*, **230**, 1043–5.

Garcia, K.C., Degano, M., et al. 1998. Structural basis of plasticity in T cell receptor recognition of a self peptide-MHC antigen. *Science*, **279**, 1166–72.

Gordon, S. 2002. Pattern recognition receptors: doubling up for the innate immune response. *Cell*, **111**, 927–30.

Gouze, J.N., Ghivizzani, S.C., et al. 2001. Gene therapy for rheumatoid arthritis. *Hand Surg*, **6**, 211–19.

Gran, B., Tranquill, L.R., et al. 2000. Mechanisms of immunomodulation by glatiramer acetate. *Neurology*, **55**, 1704–14.

Gross, D.M., Forsthuber, T., et al. 1998. Identification of LFA-1 as a candidate autoantigen in treatment-resistant Lyme arthritis. *Science*, **281**, 703–6.

Haase, C., Jorgensen, T.N. and Michelsen, B.K. 2002. Both exogenous and endogenous interleukin-10 affects the maturation of bone-marrow-derived dendritic cells in vitro and strongly influences T-cell priming in vivo. *Immunology*, **107**, 489–99.

Haines, J.L., Ter-Minassian, M., The Multiple Sclerosis Genetics Group, et al. 1996. A complete genomic screen for multiple sclerosis underscores a role for the major histocompatibility complex. *Nat Genet*, **13**, 469–71.

Hammer, J., Bono, E., et al. 1994. Precise prediction of major histocompatibility complex class II-peptide interaction based on peptide side chain scanning. *J Exp Med*, **180**, 2353–8.

Horwood, N.J., Smith, C., et al. 2002. High-efficiency gene transfer into nontransformed cells: utility for studying gene regulation and analysis of potential therapeutic targets. *Arthritis Res*, **4**, S215–25.

Huston, D.P. 1997. The biology of the immune system. *JAMA*, **278**, 1804–14.

Jacob, C.O. and McDevitt, H.O. 1988. Tumour necrosis factor-alpha in murine autoimmune 'lupus' nephritis. *Nature*, **331**, 356–8.

Jacobson, D.L., Gange, S.J., et al. 1997. Epidemiology and estimated population burden of selected autoimmune diseases in the United States. *Clin Immunol Immunopathol*, **84**, 223–43.

Jakobiec, F.A., Lefkowitch, J. and Knowles 2nd, D.M. 1984. B- and T-lymphocytes in ocular disease. *Ophthalmology*, **91**, 635–54.

Janeway, C.A. 1992. The immune system evolved to discriminate infectious nonself from noninfectious self. *Immunol Today*, **13**, 11–16.

Janeway, C.A., Travers, P., et al. 2001. *Immunobiology: the immune system in health and disease*. New York: Garland Publishing.

Jarvinen, P., Kaprio, J., et al. 1992. Systemic lupus erythematosus and related systemic diseases in a nationwide twin cohort: an increased prevalence of disease in MZ twins and concordance of disease features. *J Intern Med*, **231**, 67–72.

Jongstra-Bilen, J., Vukusic, B., et al. 1997. Resting B cells from autoimmune lupus-prone New Zealand Black and (New Zealand Black × New Zealand White) F1 mice are hyper-responsive to T cell-derived stimuli. *J Immunol*, **159**, 5810–20.

Kalish, R.A., Leong, J.M. and Steere, A.C. 1993. Association of treatment-resistant chronic Lyme arthritis with HLA-DR4 and antibody reactivity to OspA and OspB of *Borrelia burgdorferi*. *Infect Immun*, **61**, 2774–9.

Kearney, E.R., Pape, K.A., et al. 1994. Visualization of peptide-specific T cell immunity and peripheral tolerance induction in vivo. *Immunity*, **1**, 327–39.

Khoury, E.L. and Fields, K.L. 1980. Chagas' disease and autoimmunity. *Lancet*, **i**, 1088.

Kouskoff, V., Korganow, A.S., et al. 1996. Organ-specific disease provoked by systemic autoimmunity. *Cell*, **87**, 811–22.

Kuhn, R., Lohler, J., et al. 1993. Interleukin-10-deficient mice develop chronic enterocolitis. *Cell*, **75**, 263–74.

Kumar, D., Gemayel, N.S., et al. 1993. North-American twins with IDDM. Genetic, etiological, and clinical significance of disease concordance according to age, zygosity, and the interval after diagnosis in first twin. *Diabetes*, **42**, 1351–63.

Kurts, C., Sutherland, R.M., et al. 1999. CD8 T cell ignorance or tolerance to islet antigens depends on antigen dose. *Proc Natl Acad Sci USA*, **96**, 12703–7.

Lee, K.H., Wucherpfennig, K.W. and Wiley, D.C. 2001. Structure of a human insulin peptide-HLA-DQ8 complex and susceptibility to type 1 diabetes. *Nat Immunol*, **2**, 501–7.

Lehmann, P.V., Forsthuber, T., et al. 1992. Spreading of T-cell autoimmunity to cryptic determinants of an autoantigen. *Nature*, **358**, 155–7.

Levitin, P.M., Gough, W.W. and Davis, J.St. 1976. HLA-B27 antigen in women with ankylosing spondylitis. *JAMA*, **235**, 2621–2.

Linsley, P.S., Wallace, P.M., et al. 1992. Immunosuppression in vivo by a soluble form of the CTLA-4 T cell activation molecule. *Science*, **257**, 792–5.

Lipsky, P.E. 2001. Systemic lupus erythematosus: an autoimmune disease of B cell hyperactivity. *Nat Immunol*, **2**, 764–6.

Lucey, D.R., Clerici, M. and Shearer, G.M. 1996. Type 1 and type 2 cytokine dysregulation in human infectious, neoplastic, and inflammatory diseases. *Microbiol Rev*, **4**, 532–62.

Makino, S., Kunimoto, K., et al. 1980. Breeding of a non-obese, diabetic strain of mice. *Jikken Dobutsu*, **29**, 1–13.

Marrack, P., Kappler, J. and Kotzin, B.L. 2001. Autoimmune disease: why and where it occurs. *Nat Med*, **7**, 899–905.

Mason, D. 1998. A very high level of crossreactivity is an essential feature of the T-cell receptor. *Immunol Today*, **19**, 395–404.

Matos-Santos, A., Nobre, E.L., et al. 2001. Relationship between the number and impact of stressful life events and the onset of Graves' disease and toxic nodular goiter. *Clin Endocrinol*, **55**, 15–19.

Matsumoto, I., Staub, A., et al. 1999. Arthritis provoked by linked T and B cell recognition of a glycolytic enzyme. *Science*, **286**, 1732–5.

Medzhitov, R., Preston-Hurlburt, P. and Janeway, C.A. Jr. 1997. A human homologue of the *Drosophila* Toll protein signals activation of adaptive immunity. *Nature*, **388**, 394–7.

Mehindate, K., Sahlas, D.J., et al. 2001. Proinflammatory cytokines promote glial heme oxygenase-1 expression and mitochondrial iron deposition: implications for multiple sclerosis. *J Neurochem*, **77**, 1386–95.

Murphy, K.M. and Reiner, S.L. 2002. The lineage decisions of helper T cells. *Nat Rev Immunol*, **2**, 933–44.

Nagamine, K., Peterson, P., et al. 1997. Positional cloning of the APECED gene. *Nat Genet*, **17**, 393–8.

Nakhooda, A.F., Wei, C.N., et al. 1978. The spontaneously diabetic Wistar rat (the 'BB' rat): the significance of transient glycosuria. *Diabetes Metab*, **4**, 255–9.

Nepom, G.T. 1998. Major histocompatibility complex-directed susceptibility to rheumatoid arthritis. *Adv Immunol*, **68**, 315–32.

Nepom, G.T. and Erlich, H. 1991. MHC class-II molecules and autoimmunity. *Annu Rev Immunol*, **9**, 493–525.

Nistico, L., Buzzetti, R., Belgian Diabetes Registry, et al. 1996. The CTLA-4 gene region of chromosome 2q33 is linked to, and associated with, type 1 diabetes. *Hum Mol Genet*, **5**, 1075–80.

O'Shea, J.J., Ma, A. and Lipsky, P. 2002. Cytokines and autoimmunity. *Nat Rev Immunol*, **2**, 37–45.

Ota, K., Matsui, M., et al. 1990. T-cell recognition of an immunodominant myelin basic protein epitope in multiple sclerosis. *Nature*, **346**, 183–7.

Panoutsakopoulou, V., Sanchirico, M.E., et al. 2001. Analysis of the relationship between viral infection and autoimmune disease. *Immunity*, **15**, 137–47.

Parks, C.G., Cooper, G.S., et al. 2002. Occupational exposure to crystalline silica and risk of systemic lupus erythematosus: a population-based, case-control study in the southeastern United States. *Arthritis Rheum*, **46**, 1840–50.

Pasternack, A. and Tiilikainen, A. 1977. HLA-B27 in rheumatoid arthritis and amyloidosis. *Tissue Antigens*, **9**, 80–9.

Pearson, L. and Lightfoot, R.W. Jr. 1981. Correlation of DNA-anti-DNA association rates with clinical activity in systemic lupus erythematosus (SLE). *J Immunol*, **126**, 16–19.

Perez, V.L., Van Parijs, L., et al. 1997. Induction of peripheral T cell tolerance in vivo requires CTLA-4 engagement. *Immunity*, **6**, 411–17.

Persidis, A. 1999. Arthritis drug discovery. *Nat Biotechnol*, **17**, 726–8.

Pisetsky, D.S. 2000. Tumor necrosis factor blockers in rheumatoid arthritis. *N Engl J Med*, **342**, 810–11.

Podolsky, D.K. 2002. Inflammatory bowel disease. *N Engl J Med*, **347**, 417–29.

Poland, G.A. and Jacobson, R.M. 2001. The prevention of Lyme disease with vaccine. *Vaccine*, **19**, 2303–8.

Puxeddu, A., Colonna, A., et al. 1965. On a rare case of hemolytic anemia autoimmune caused by influenza B virus. *Haematologica*, **50**, 1073–92.

Redondo, M.J., Rewers, M., et al. 1999. Genetic determination of islet cell autoimmunity in monozygotic twin, dizygotic twin, and non-twin siblings of patients with type 1 diabetes: prospective twin study. *Br Med J*, **318**, 698–702.

Regner, M. and Lambert, P.H. 2001. Autoimmunity through infection or immunization? *Nat Immunol*, **2**, 185–8.

Ruffini, F., Furlan, R., et al. 2001. Fibroblast growth factor-II gene therapy reverts the clinical course and the pathological signs of chronic experimental autoimmune encephalomyelitis in C57BL/6 mice. *Gene Ther*, **8**, 1207–13.

Savill, J., Dransfield, I., et al. 2002. A blast from the past: clearance of apoptotic cells regulates immune responses. *Nat Rev Immunol*, **2**, 965–75.

Shevach, E.M. 2002. $CD4^+$ $CD25^+$ suppressor T cells: more questions than answers. *Nat Rev Immunol*, **2**, 389–400.

Sikand, V.K., Halsey, N., et al. 2001. Safety and immunogenicity of a recombinant *Borrelia burgdorferi* outer surface protein A vaccine against Lyme disease in healthy children and adolescents: a randomized controlled trial. *Pediatrics*, **108**, 123–8.

Silverstein, A.M. 2001. Autoimmunity versus horror autotoxicus: the struggle for recognition. *Nat Immunol*, **2**, 279–81.

Slingsby, J.H., Norsworthy, P., et al. 1996. Homozygous hereditary C1q deficiency and systemic lupus erythematosus. A new family and the molecular basis of C1q deficiency in three families. *Arthritis Rheum*, **39**, 663–70.

Sobel, E.S., Mohan, C., et al. 1999. Genetic dissection of SLE pathogenesis: adoptive transfer of Sle1 mediates the loss of tolerance by bone marrow-derived B cells. *J Immunol*, **162**, 2415–21.

Steere, A.C. 1989. Lyme disease. *N Engl J Med*, **321**, 586–96.

Steere, A.C., Grodzicki, R.L., et al. 1983. The spirochetal etiology of Lyme disease. *N Engl J Med*, **308**, 733–40.

Steere, A.C., Malawista, S.E., et al. 1984. The clinical spectrum and treatment of Lyme disease. *Yale J Biol Med*, **57**, 453–64.

Steinhoff, U., Brinkmann, V., et al. 1999. Autoimmune intestinal pathology induced by hsp60-specific CD8 T cells. *Immunity*, **11**, 349–58.

Steinman, L. 2001. Multiple sclerosis: a two-stage disease. *Nat Immunol*, **2**, 762–4.

Steinman, R.M. and Nussenzweig, M.C. 2002. Avoiding horror autotoxicus: the importance of dendritic cells in peripheral T cell tolerance. *Proc Natl Acad Sci USA*, **99**, 351–8.

Straus, S.E., Sneller, M., et al. 1999. An inherited disorder of lymphocyte apoptosis: the autoimmune lymphoproliferative syndrome. *Ann Intern Med*, **130**, 591–601.

Streilein, J.W. 1997. Regulation of ocular immune responses. *Eye*, **11**, 171–5.

Taneja, V. and David, C.S. 2001. Lessons from animal models for human autoimmune diseases. *Nat Immunol*, **2**, 781–4.

Tarner, I.H. and Fathman, C.G. 2001. Gene therapy in autoimmune disease. *Curr Opin Immunol*, **13**, 676–82.

Thornton, A.M. and Shevach, E.M. 1998. $CD4^+CD25^+$ immunoregulatory T cells suppress polyclonal T cell activation in vitro by inhibiting interleukin 2 production. *J Exp Med*, **188**, 287–96.

Tiegs, S.L., Russell, D.M. and Nemazee, D. 1993. Receptor editing in self-reactive bone marrow B cells. *J Exp Med*, **177**, 1009–20.

Todd, J.A. 1991. A protective role of the environment in the development of type 1 diabetes? *Diabetes Med*, **8**, 906–10.

Tsokos, G.C. and Nepom, G.T. 2000. Genre therapy in the treatment of autoimmune diseases. *J Clin Invest*, **106**, 181–3.

Tsokos, G.C., Wong, H.K., et al. 2000. Immune cell signaling in lupus. *Curr Opin Rheumatol*, **12**, 355–63.

Vanderlugt, C.L. and Miller, S.D. 2002. Epitope spreading in immune-mediated diseases: implications for immunotherapy. *Nat Rev Immunol*, **2**, 85–95.

Vella, A.T., Mitchell, T., et al. 1997. CD28 engagement and proinflammatory cytokines contribute to T cell expansion and long-term survival in vivo. *J Immunol*, **158**, 4714–20.

Vyse, T.J., Rozzo, S.J., et al. 1997. Control of multiple autoantibodies linked with a lupus nephritis susceptibility locus in New Zealand black mice. *J Immunol*, **158**, 5566–74.

Walker, L.S. and Abbas, A.K. 2002. The enemy within: keeping self-reactive T cells at bay in the periphery. *Nat Rev Immunol*, **2**, 11–19.

Wanstrat, A. and Wakeland, E. 2001. The genetics of complex autoimmune diseases: non-MHC susceptibility genes. *Nat Immunol*, **2**, 802–9.

Waterhouse, P., Penninger, J.M., et al. 1995. Lymphoproliferative disorders with early lethality in mice deficient in Ctla-4. *Science*, **270**, 985–8.

Weetman, A.P. 2001. Determinants of autoimmune thyroid disease. *Nat Immunol*, **2**, 769–70.

Weinshenker, B.G. 1996. Epidemiology of multiple sclerosis. *Neurol Clin*, **14**, 291–308.

Witebsky, E. and Rose, N.R. 1956. Chronic thyroiditis and autoimmunization. *J Immunol*, **76**, 408–14.

Wucherpfennig, K.W. 2001. Mechanisms for the induction of autoimmunity by infectious agents. *J Clin Invest*, **108**, 1097–104.

Wucherpfennig, K.W. and Eisenbarth, G.S. 2001. Type 1 diabetes. *Nat Immunol*, **2**, 767–8.

Yazdanbakhsh, M., Kremsner, P.G. and van Ree, R. 2002. Allergy, parasites, and the hygiene hypothesis. *Science*, **296**, 490–4.

Yewdell, J.W. and Tscharke, D.C. 2002. Immunology: Inside the professionals. *Nature*, **418**, 923–4.

Youssef, S., Stuve, O., et al. 2002. The HMG-CoA reductase inhibitor, atorvastatin, promotes a Th2 bias and reverses paralysis in central nervous system autoimmune disease. *Nature*, **420**, 78–84.

Yu, B., Gauthier, L., et al. 2000. Binding of conserved islet peptides by human and murine MHC class II molecules associated with susceptibility to type I diabetes. *Eur J Immunol*, **30**, 2497–2506.

38

The immunocompromised host

ALAIN FISCHER

There are more than 100 recognized diseases that are genetically determined and compromise immune defenses against microorganism invasions. Mutations of 86 genes (Table 38.1) have so far been identified in association with as many immunodeficient conditions. Advances in genomics have helped enormously in identifying these genes. Today, the understanding of how their products contribute to the many complex reactions of different cells involved in immune defense (both innate and adaptive) contributes to a better knowledge of our immune system. This chapter reviews what we know about these conditions.

GENETIC DISORDERS OF INNATE IMMUNITY

Deficiency in granulocyte production

Inherited severe congenital neutropenia (SCN) was reported more than 40 years ago as Kostmann's syndrome (Kostmann 1956). Since then, various forms of inherited neutropenias have been described (Figure 38.1). When neutrophil counts are <200/mm^3 of blood, neutropenia exposes the patient to severe bacterial and fungal infections, which can spread throughout the bloodstream and cause death in the absence of appropriate treatment. The usual sites of infections are located at the interface between body cavities and the outside environment. In addition, chronic severe periodontitis is a hallmark of severe neutropenia. In most cases, Kostmann's syndrome is associated with a block in granulocyte differentiation at the promyelocyte stage. Both autosomal dominant (with variable penetrance) and autosomal recessive patterns of inheritance have been described. In recent years, it has been found that most patients with SCN carry mutations of the neutrophil elastase-2 gene (*ELA-2*) (Dale et al. 2000). The physiopathology of defective neutrophil production is still unclear, although it is thought that mutations of the elastase gene result in a premature apoptosis of neutrophil precursors (Aprikyan et al. 2001). Interestingly, cyclic neutropenia, a condition characterized by regular 21-day cycles of neutrophil counts oscillating between 0 and normal values, is also caused by mutations of ELA-2 with an autosomal dominant inheritance (Horwitz et al. 1999; Dale et al. 2000). The mechanism underlying cyclic hemopoiesis is not understood.

Recently it has been proposed that susceptibility to infections in SCN is the consequence not only of the absence of mobile phagocytic cells migrating to infected tissues, but also of defective release of antibacterial peptides such as α defensins (Putsep et al. 2002).

Other complex conditions can cause severe congenital neutropenia such as Shwachman's syndrome, which is characterized by exocrine pancreas insufficiency, and metaphyseal dysplasia with an autosomal recessive inheritance. The molecular mechanism is presently unknown, although it has recently been shown that Shwachman's syndrome is caused by mutations of the *SBDS* gene (Kyono and Coates 2002; Boocock et al. 2003). Neutropenia is also a feature of glycogenosis Ib (Kyono and Coates 2002). A gain of a function mutation

Table 38.1 Genetically characterized primary immunodeficiencies

Gene/product	Expression	Disease
Immunodeficiencies of neutrophils		
Elastase	Neutrophils	Agranulocytosis cyclic neutropenia
SBDS	Neutrophils	Shwachmann's syndrome
WASP (activating mutation)	Leukocytes	Agranulocytosis
β_2-Integrin	Leukocytes	LAD-I
GDP fucose transporter	Leukocytes/endothelial cells	LAD-II
β-A	Neutrophils	Neutrophil actin dysfunction
Rac-2	Neutrophils	LAD variant
C/EBPε	Neutrophils	Specific granule deficiency
CyBB (gp91 cytochrome *b*)	Phagocytic cells	XL CGD
CyBA (gp22 cytochrome *b*)	Phagocytic cells	AR CGD
NFC1 $p47^{phox}$	Phagocytic cells	AR CGD
NFC2 $p67^{phox}$	Phagocytic cells	AR CGD
G6PD	Phagocytic cells	CGD-like syndrome
Cathepsin C	Neutrophils (?)	Papillon–Lefèvre syndrome
Plasma proteins		
Classic pathway, of complement C1q, -r, -s, C4, C2	Plasma	Infections by encapsulated bacteria
Alternate pathway: B, D,	Plasma	Infections by encapsulated bacteria
Alternate pathway: properdin	Plasma	Neisseria infections
Lectin pathway, MBL	Plasma	?
C3	Plasma	Infections by encapsulated bacteria
C3 regulators: H, I	Plasma	Infections by encapsulated bacteria
Membrane attack complex C5, -6, -7, -8, -9?	Plasma	Neisseria infections
Spleen		
Connexin 43	Spleen	Situs abnormality (asplenia)
ZIC3	Spleen	Situs abnormality (asplenia)
Interface innate/adaptive immunity		
NEMO (IKKγ)	Leukocytes	Anhidrotic ectodermic dysplasia with immunodeficiency
EVER-1, -2	Keratinocytes?	Epidermodysplasia verruciformis
IL-12B (p40)	T, NK cells	
IL-12RB1	T, NK cells	
IFNγR1	Dendritic cells/macrophages	Mendelian susceptibility to mycobacterial infections
IFNγR2	Dendritic cells/macrophages	
STAT-1	Dendritic cells/macrophages	
T lymphocytes	Lymphocyte precursors	
Adenosine deaminase		SCID
γc	T, NK lymphocyte precursors	XL SCID
JAK-3	T, NK lymphocyte precursors	AR SCID
Rag-1	T-, B-lymphocyte precursors V(D)J	AR SCID
Rag-2	T-, B-lymphocyte precursors V(D)J	AR SCID
Artemis	T-, B-lymphocyte precursors V(D)J	AR SCID
IL-7Rα	T-lymphocyte precursors	SCID
CD45	T-, (B)-lymphocyte precursors	SCID
WHN	Epithelial cells	Nude phenotype
Purine nucleotide phosphorylase	T lymphocytes	T-cell deficiency
CD3γ, ε	T lymphocytes	T-cell deficiency
ZAP-70 kinase	T lymphocytes	T-cell deficiency
IL-2Rα	T lymphocytes	T-cell deficiency
Caspase 8	Lymphocytes	Partial mixed deficiency
CIITA	Antigen-presenting cells	

(*Continued over*)

Table 38.1 *Genetically characterized primary immunodeficiencies (Continued)*

Gene/product	Expression	Disease
RFXANK/B	Antigen-presenting cells	HLA-II deficiency
RFX 5	Antigen-presenting cells	
RFX AP	Antigen-presenting cells	
TAP-1	Antigen-presenting cells	HLA-I deficiency
TAP-2	Antigen-presenting cells	
Immunodeficiencies with genomic instability		
DNA ligase IV	Lymphocytes	Combined immunodeficiency
DNA ligase I	Lymphocytes	Combined immunodeficiency
ATM	Lymphocytes	Ataxia telangiectasia (AT)
MRE-11	Lymphocytes	AT-like disorder
NBS I/Nibrin	Lymphocytes	Nijmegen breakage syndrome
DNMT 3B	Lymphocytes	ICF syndrome
BLM	Ubiquitous	Bloom syndrome
Immunodeficiencies with bone disease		
RMRP	?	Cartilage hair hypoplasia
SMARCAL	?	Schimke immuno-osseous dysplasia
Other immunodeficiencies		
WASP	Hemopoietic cells	Wiskott–Aldrich syndrome
CD40L	T lymphocytes	Hyper-IgM syndrome type 1
CD40	B lymphocytes, dendritic cells	Hyper-IgM syndrome type 3
T/NK cytolytic deficiencies		
Perforin	T/NK cytolytic cells	Lymphohistiocytosis
LYST	Ubiquitous	Chédiak–Higashi syndrome
RAB27a	Cytolytic cells, melanocytes	Griscelli's syndrome
SAP/SH2DIA	Lymphocytes	XLP–Purtilo syndrome
Miscellaneous		
AIRE	Thymic epithelial cells	APECED (candidiasis/autoimmunity)
B-cell immunodeficiencies		
μ Heavy chain	B-cell precursors	
Igα	B-cell precursors	
λ5	B-cell precursors	AR agammaglobulinemia
BLNK	B-cell precursors	
BTK	B-cell precursors	XL agammaglobulinemia
AID	B cells (germinal centers)	Hyper-IgM syndrome type 2
IgHγ1	B cells	IgG1 deficiency
IgLK	B cells	IgK deficiency

APECED, polyendocrinopathy–candidiasis–ectodermal dystrophy; AR, autosomal recessive; AT, ataxia telangiectasia; CGD, chronic granulomatosis disease; G6PD, glucose-6-phosphate dehydrogenase; ICF, immunodeficiency centromeric facial; IL, interleukin; LAD, leukocyte adhesion deficiency; MBL, mannose-binding lectin; NK, natural killer; SCID, severe combined immunodeficiency; XL, X-linked.

of the *WASP* gene is causing an X-linked form of SCN (Devriendt et al. 2001). Therapy by administration of granulocyte colony-stimulating factor (G-CSF) is efficient in most forms of SCN (Devriendt et al. 2001). Kostmann's syndrome as well as Schwachman's syndrome predispose to myeloid leukemia. In the former setting, leukemia is often associated with the acquisition of somatic mutations of the intracellular region of the G-CSF receptor (Dale et al. 1993; Tidow et al. 1997; Devriendt et al. 2001). The mechanism of this predisposition is unknown. It is, however, suspected that enhanced precursor proliferation caused by premature daughter cell death could favor secondary genetic alterations.

Disorders of neutrophil function

MIGRATION: LEUKOCYTE ADHESION DEFICIENCY

Neutrophils migrate to tissues from blood vessels upon appropriate inflammatory signaling. Molecules involved in the process of adhesion and migration have now been characterized in part because natural mutants of neutrophil adhesion/migration have been described. These are called leukocyte adhesion deficiency (LAD).

LAD-I, a rare autosomal recessive disorder, is characterized by accumulation of neutrophils in the bloodstream whereas infection sites are devoid of pus. Severe,

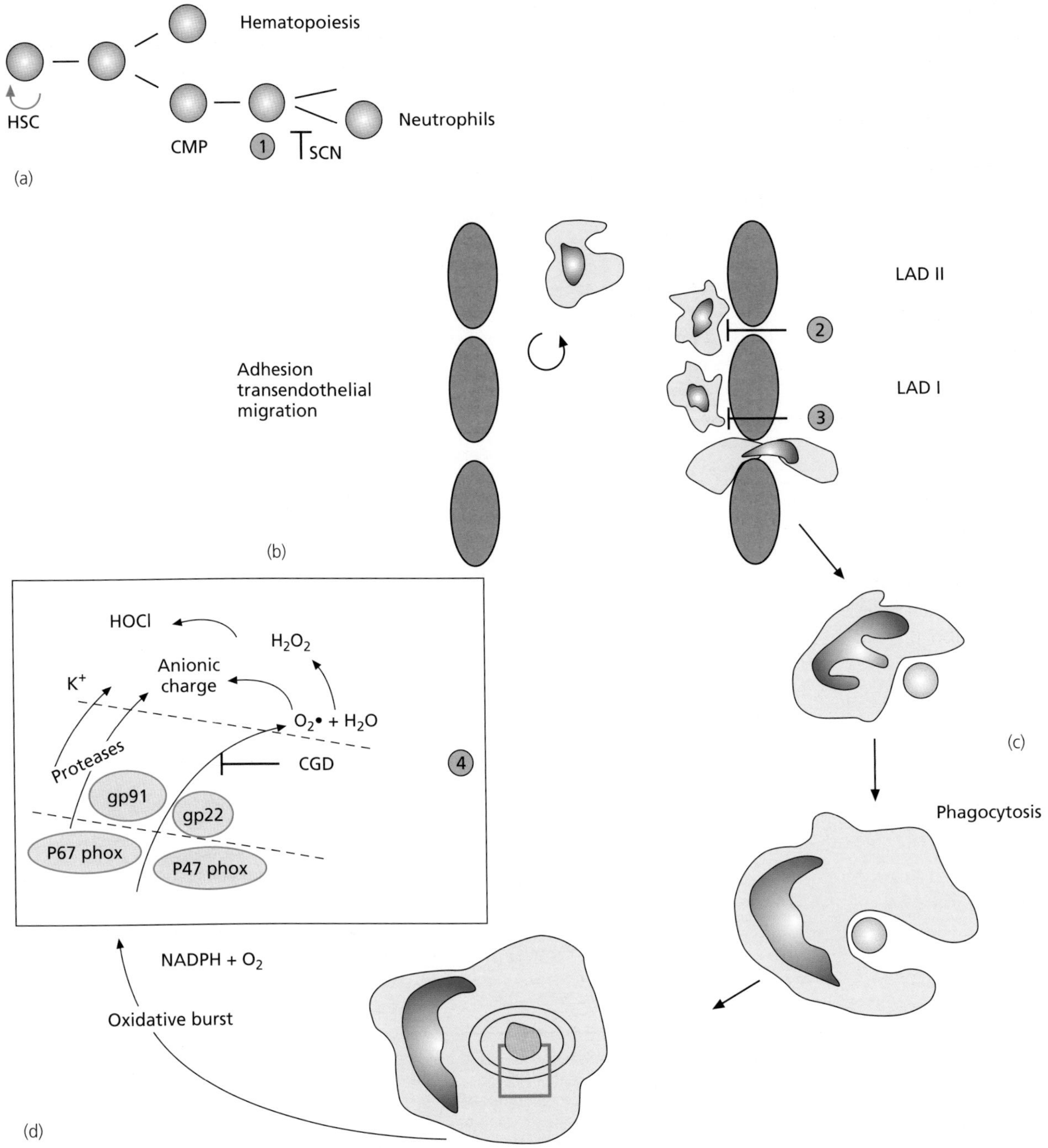

Figure 38.1 *Main phagocytic cell disorders.* **(a)** *Hemopoiesis. HSC, hemopoietic stem cells with self-renewal capacity; common myeloid progenitors. Neutrophil development from myeloid progenitors is impaired in severe congenital neutropenia (SCN) and cyclic neutropenia (CN) caused by elastase mutations (1).* **(b)** *Adhesion to endothelial cells and transendothelial migration of neutrophils. Rolling of neutrophils is abrogated in leukocyte adhesion deficiency II (LAD-II) (2). β_2-integrin-mediated adhesion and transendothelial migrations are blocked in LAD-I (3).* **(c)** *Phagocytosis.* **(d)** *Oxidative burst (magnification in inset). Once microorganisms are phagocytosed, activation of membrane NADPH oxidase composed of four subunits leads to superoxide production, then H_2O_2 after superdismutase action and HOCl (chlorination). In addition, the induced anionic charge triggers a K^+ influx and bacteriolytic protease release into the phagolysosome. Deficiency in any component of NADPH oxidase causes a chronic granulomatous disease (CGD) (4). CMP, common myeloid progenitor.*

unabated, bacterial infections, mostly of soft tissues, ensue, lead to extensive necrosis (Anderson et al. 1985; Fischer et al. 1988). LAD-I is also often associated at birth with delayed loss of the umbilical cord and omphalitis. The absence of pus and leukocytosis led to the suspicion that neutrophils were unable to adhere to and/or migrate along a chemotactic gradient. This was indeed proved to be the case in vitro and in vivo. It was recognized that expression of heterodimeric molecule complexes was defective at leukocyte membranes, i.e.

β_2-integrins including $\alpha_L\beta_2$ (LFA-1), $\alpha_M\beta_2$ (MAC-1), and $\alpha_x\beta_2$ (p150, 95) molecules. Mutations of the gene encoding the β_2-integrin subunit cause this disorder (Kishimoto et al. 1987). Null mutations result in severe life-threatening leukocyte adhesion deficiency whereas missense mutations enabling residual β_2-integrin expression and function are compatible with life, although severe bacterial infections can occur. β_2-integrins are involved in leukocyte adhesion to the endothelial wall and then transendothelial migration after activation of β_2-integrins by chemokines. β_2-integrins bind to intercellular adhesion molecule 1 (ICAM-1) at endothelial surfaces and also iC3b on bacterial surfaces. It is thought that this condition is primarily a neutrophil dysfunction because other leukocytes such as monocytes can use the $\alpha_4\beta_1$-integrin not expressed by neutrophils to compensate for the β_2-integrin deficiency.

Variants characterized by the presence of a nonfunctional β_2-integrin have been described. In these cases, inside-out signaling leading to β_2-integrin activation was shown to be impaired (Kuijpers et al. 1997; Harris et al. 2001). More recently, a third similar case has been reported (Mcdowall et al. 2003). In the latter not only β_2- but also β_1- and β_3-integrins were disabled despite normal structure and expression of these molecules. A bleeding disorder was therefore also present because β_3-integrin is involved in platelet aggregation. The molecular basis of this impaired β-integrin activation is unknown. However, these findings point remarkably to the role of inside-out signaling in driving neutrophil activation to adhere to and migrate toward infectious zones.

LAD-II

Etzioni et al. (1992) have reported a similar condition associated with a dysmorphic syndrome, failure to thrive, and learning disability. This autosomal recessive condition has been found in a very small number of patients so far. There is a lack of expression of the H antigen by erythrocytes (Bombay phenotype) and a defect of leukocytes to migrate from blood. This condition is the consequence of a fucosylation defect (Luhn et al. 2001), which leads to a defective formation of the sialyl Lewis X (sLe^x) carbohydrate, the selectin ligand (L-, E-, and P-selectins). Therefore, the rolling process mediated by repeated short interactions between leukocytes and endothelial cells does not occur properly, impairing the further step of adhesion.

NEUTROPHIL ACTIN DYSFUNCTION

A small number of patients have been reported with a condition characterized by recurrent bacterial and fungal infections associated with abnormal neutrophil movement, whereas β_2-integrins are normally expressed (Luhn et al. 2001). There is decreased actin polymerization in neutrophils in one case, associated with a decrease in a 89-kDa protein expression and an increased expression in leufactin, a protein interacting with F-actin (Coates et al. 1991). A dominant β-actin mutant has been found in another child with a similar syndrome (Nunoi et al. 1999).

RAC-2 DEFICIENCY

In two patients with severe bacterial infections, poor wound healing, and leukocytosis, neutrophils were found to be unable to move along a chemotactic gradient, and also unable to produce superoxide anion when stimulated with the bacterial peptide flmp. These patients were shown to exhibit Rac-2 gene mutation. Rac-2 is a Rho guanosine triphosphatase (GTPase) involved in induction of actin polymerization, integrin complex formation, and activation (Ambruso et al. 2000; Williams et al. 2000).

SPECIFIC GRANULE DEFICIENCY

This rare condition results from the combination of defective chemotaxis with a deficiency in lysosomal proteins such as defensins and lactoferrin. Clinical phenotype is characterized by recurrent bacterial and fungal infections. Specific granules are lacking in neutrophils. Mutations of the transcription factor (CCAAT) enhancer-binding protein (C/EBPϵ), which controls granule protein synthesis, are causing this condition (Lekstrom-Himes and Xanthopoulos 1999).

OXIDATIVE BURST: CHRONIC GRANULOMATOUS DISEASE

Phagocytic cells generate reactive oxygen species by the enzyme nicotinamide adenine dinucleotide phosphate (NADPH) oxidase. The enzyme catalyzes the oxygen reduction to superoxide which can be further transformed to H_2O_2 and, by the myeloperoxidase, to HOCl. These reactive oxygen species (ROS) generated in the membrane of phagolysosomes on activation are thought to play a major role in the killing of engulfed bacteria and fungi by neutrophils and macrophages. This is best demonstrated by chronic granulomatous disease (CGD) in which this generation of ROS is defective. Its incidence is estimated at 1:250 000 live births (Winkelstein et al. 2000). Four molecular defects have been characterized (Segal et al. 2000):

1. deficiency in gp91, a membrane cytochrome *b* component encoded by an X-linked gene (*CYBB*) which is defective in 70 percent of cases
2. deficiency in gp22, a second subunit of cytochrome (CYBA) accounting for 5 percent of CGD
3. $p47^{phox}$ (*NFC1* gene), a cytosolic protein that associates to the cytochrome on neutrophil stimulation; its deficiency accounts for about 20 percent of CGD
4. the $p67^{phox}$ (*NFC2* gene), another cytosolic component binding the cytochrome on activation (5 percent of CGD).

Patients with autosomal recessive CGD tend to have a slightly milder phenotype. CGD is characterized by bacterial infections, mostly as abscesses located in lymph nodes, liver, lung, and bones – all tissues or organs rich in macrophages. Typically, catalase-positive bacteria (which destroy endogenously produced H_2O_2), *Staphylococcus aureus*, *Serratia marcescens*, *Burkholderia cepacia*, and fungi (*Aspergillus* species) are the most frequently encountered pathogens. Of note, non-infectious granuloma can develop in various sites associated with varyingly severe consequences, such as bladder obstruction, pyloric stenosis, colitis, or chronic interstitial pneumonitis. Infections result in a 2.5–5 percent death toll/year of affected patients (autosomal recessive and X-linked form, respectively) (Winkelstein et al. 2000).

The physiopathology concept of this condition has been challenged by Segal and coworkers who proposed, as based on mouse models, that ROS generation is creating an increased anionic charge compensated by entry in a pH-dependent manner of K^+ ions. The rise in ionic strength is stimulating release of proteases, which are possibly responsible for the killing of microorganisms and degradation of debris (Reeves et al. 2002). The same authors have recently shown that catalase-positive and -negative strains of *S. aureus* are equally virulent in CGD mice models, further suggesting that H_2O_2 and chlorinated reagents might not be the primary killer effectors (Messina et al. 2002), thus challenging previous views.

Myeloperoxidase deficiency is a fairly frequent condition, which results in impaired production of chlorinated reagents within phagolysosomes (Nauseef 1990). Interestingly enough, it is mostly an asymptomatic setting except in individuals with diabetes who are prone to candida abscesses (Cech et al. 1979), an observation perhaps further reinforcing Segal's view on how phagocytes kill microorganisms.

NEUTROPHIL GLUCOSE-6-PHOSPHATASE DEHYDROGENASE DEFICIENCY

In very rare patients, the most severe glucose-6-phosphatase dehydrogenase (G6PD) deficiencies lead not only to hemolytic anemia but also to a CGD-like phenotype because G6PD (Mamlok et al. 1987) catalyses the production of NADPH, the required substrate of NADPH oxidase.

The above-mentioned Rac-2 deficiency can also be regarded as an oxidative burst deficiency because Rac-2 is involved in the activation of oxidase activity.

PAPILLON–LEFÈVRE SYNDROME

Papillon–Lefèvre syndrome is characterized by a palmoplantar keratosis associated with a severe periodontopathy and, sometimes, pyogenic liver abscesses. This autosomal recessive disorder is caused by mutations in the cathepsin C gene (Toomes et al. 1999). Cathepsin C processes other proteases, such as granzymes, and may be required in the maturation of proteases necessary to bacterial killing.

A DEFICIENCY OF UNKNOWN MECHANISM: THE HYPER-IGE SYNDROME

The hyper-IgE syndrome (HIES) or Job's syndrome is a rare condition with autosomal dominant inheritance characterized by the association of a dysmorphic syndrome (coarse facies), tooth abnormalities, osteoporosis, and a unique phenotype of susceptibility to infections (Grimbacher et al. 1999a).

These patients suffer from childhood with lung abscesses, and skin, soft tissue, and bone infections associated with very mild inflammatory reaction ('cold abscesses'). *S. aureus* and fungi are the most frequently encountered microorganisms. In the lungs, pneumatoceles are formed as both sequelae and sites of new infections. In most textbooks, HIES is classified as a neutrophil disorder because it has been shown that there is a mild neutrophil chemotaxis disorder in this condition. It is far from clear that this poorly reliable finding contributes to the understanding of HIES physiopathology. There is an HIES locus on chromosome 4 and, so far, almost nothing is known about disease mechanisms (Grimbacher et al. 1999b). The biological hallmark of HIES is an elevated IgE serum level which can be very high in young children (>40 000 IU/ml) and tend to diminish with age, although susceptibility to infections persists. It is thus not known whether hyper-IgE is involved in pathogenesis or is just a surrogate marker. Mystery has been further reinforced by the observation that allogeneic hemopoietic stem-cell transplantation does not cure the disease (Gennery et al. 2000), a finding that suggests that abnormal cells are not of hemopoietic origin. It is thus highly likely that HIES should not in the future be classified within the neutrophil dysfunction chapter!

Disorders of plasmatic proteins

The complement cascade (Figure 38.2) plays an important role in the early steps of defense against pathogens (preimmune step) as well as in immunized individuals. Actually, most of our understanding of the role of the complement system relies on the identification of the natural defects of almost every one of its components (Walport 2001a, 2001b). The complement system can be activated by three mechanisms, i.e. the classic pathway usually triggered by antigen–antibody complexes, mediated by C1q, -r, -s, and C4 and C2, the alternate pathway triggered by microbial surfaces, mediated by C3, B, and D factors and properdin, and the lectin pathway induced by the mannose-binding lectin (MBL). All three result in C3 activation by cleavage into the C3b opsonin. Also, C3b triggers the formation of the membrane attack complex (MAC) formed by C5–9 components. Deficiencies of C3 activation inhibitors (H and I, which cause a C3 depletion), as well as of the classic and the alternate pathway,

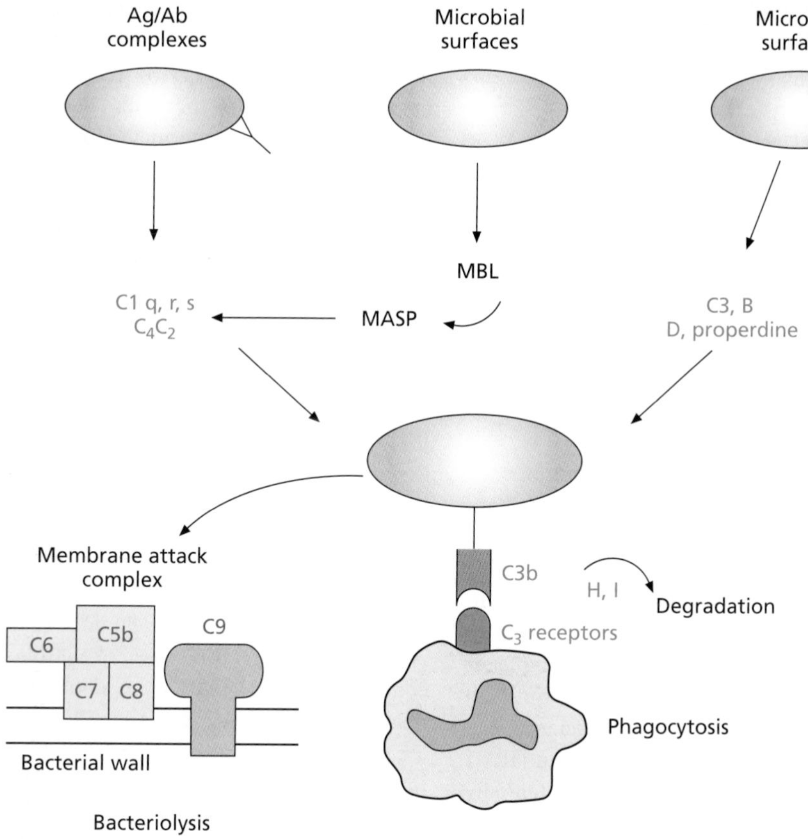

Figure 38.2 *The complement system. C1q, -r, -s and C4, C2, H, I, C3, B, D: encapsulated bacteria; C5, C6, C7, C8, C9: gram-negative bacteria,* Neisseria meningitis.

except for properdin deficiency, all result in infections by encapsulated bacteria such as *Streptococcus pneumoniae*, *S. pyogenes*, and *Haemophilus influenzae*. Infection can be blood borne or localized to the respiratory tract. These findings underline the role of C3b in facilitating opsonization of encapsulated bacteria. C3 deficiency tends to have more severe consequences given its central role. X-linked properdin deficiency is a very rare condition leading in most cases to fulminant meningitis caused by *Neiserria meningitidis* from the unusual strains y and w135. MBL deficiency may be a susceptibility factor for bacterial and candida infections, although this is still debated (Summerfield et al. 1995). Deficiencies from factors of the MAC lead to susceptibility to infection by *Neisseria* spp., particularly *N. meningitidis*, emphasizing the role of MAC-mediated bacteriolysis in the control of this class of bacteria.

Complement deficiencies are also associated with autoimmune manifestations (systemic lupus erythematosus, vasculitis, glomerulonephritis) because of the role of the complement system in the clearance of antigen–antibody complexes and apoptotic bodies.

Congenital asplenia

Congenital absence of spleen can be rarely observed either as one of the manifestations of situs abnormalities – Ivemark syndrome caused by mutations of the Connexin 43 gene (Britz-Cunningham et al. 1995) or the X-linked *ZIC3* gene (Gebbia et al. 1997) – or as an isolated condition with an autosomal dominant inheritance and variable penetrance. Its cause is still unknown. This condition exposes the individual to fulminant, blood-borne infections caused by encapsulated bacteria, mostly *S. pneumoniae*, thought to be the consequence of the defective splenic macrophage filter.

Undescribed deficiencies of innate immunity

It has now been well established that receptors for structures not expressed by eukaryotes are present in phagocytic and other cells. Toll-like receptors are the most salient example. They serve to signal dangers, induce innate immune response mostly through activation of the factor NFκB, and link innate to adaptive immunity (Barton and Medzhitov 2002). A mouse natural mutant of Toll-R4 has been described and characterized by an absence of response to lipopolysaccharide (LPS), its main ligand (Poltorak et al. 1998). A number of knockout (KO) mice in which a given Toll receptor or associated signaling molecule is absent have been engineered and found to be susceptible to different classes of pathogens. Surprisingly, no human counterpart has yet been described. It is not known whether this can be explained by unexpected redundancy between receptors and/or associated signaling pathways, or whether they are very rare conditions.

Nevertheless, Galin et al. reported a single case of a patient with defective cytokine production on bacterial challenge associated with bacterial infections and limited inflammatory response (Kuhns et al. 1997). This syndrome, not yet molecularly characterized to our knowledge, is a good candidate to represent a first example of a Toll receptor pathway deficiency.

NEMO/IKKγ deficiency

NEMO deficiency results in a complex syndrome in which both innate and adaptive immune responses are defective (Zonana et al. 2000; Doffinger et al. 2001; Jain et al. 2001). NEMO is a regulatory element, which forms, together with IKKα and -β, the kinase required to phosphorylate and therefore induced ubiquitinylation of NFκB inhibitors (IκBα), thus enabling NFκB complexes to migrate to the nucleus and exert their transcriptional activity (Courtois et al. 2001). NEMO deficiency can impair responses to cytokines such as interleukin (IL) 1 and tumor necrosis factor (TNF) and also potentially some of the Toll-like receptors. This is, however, a more complex syndrome because NFκB is, for instance, also involved in mediating CD40-induced signals in B lymphocytes; thus NEMO deficiency can result in impaired antibody production. These patients present predisposition to infections with encapsulated bacteria but also mycobacteria in more severe cases. It is thus difficult to distinguish which pathway perturbation is responsible for a given type of infection. There is heterogeneity in the consequences of mutations of the NEMO gene (knowing that null mutations are lethal), which adds to the complexity of the analysis.

As NFκB is also involved in signaling from cells outside the immune system, patients may variably present with anhidrotic ectodermal dysplasia, lymphedema, and osteopetrosis.

Natural killer cells

Natural killer (NK) cell function lies at the border of innate and adaptive immunity. The role of NK cell-mediated defense against infections is not yet well known although recent evidence for a role in resistance to cytomegalovirus (CMV) associated with the Ly-49H molecule in mice has been provided (Brown et al. 2001). No such information has yet been obtained from studies on human immunodeficiencies. A single case of NK cell deficiency has been reported. It has been found associated with recurrent infections of the herpes virus group (Biron et al. 1989). However, no molecular mechanism has been described. In addition, recurrent infections, notably with herpes simplex virus, have been described associated with decreased blood NK cell counts and a modified FcγRIIIA (CD16) receptor. Relationship to pathogenesis has not, however, been firmly established (de Vries et al. 1996; Jawahar et al. 1996). Of note, NK cell cytotoxicity impairment, found in patients with perforin deficiency (together with cytolytic T-cell function impairment), is associated with an entirely distinct phenotype (see below).

Susceptibility to human papilloma virusinfection

In rare families, mutations of either of two genes, *EVER-1* and *EVER-2*, have been reported to predispose to infection, with an autosomal recessive inheritance to epidermodysplasia verruciformis (EV). EV consists of chronic skin infection caused by certain strains of human papilloma virus (HPV), e.g. HPV-5, and predisposing to squamous cell carcinomas (Ramoz et al. 1999, 2002). This is a rather unique setting, because these conditions do not create a susceptibility status for other microorganisms. *EVER-1* and *EVER-2* gene products are expressed among other cells in keratinocytes – the target cell of HPV – and could thus probably interfere locally with viral persistence. This is a privileged setting to analyze further local immunity to HPV. It stresses that the genetic susceptibility factor for infections may not be associated with the classic arms of the immune system.

GENETIC DISORDERS AT THE INTERFACE BETWEEN INNATE AND ADAPTIVE IMMUNITY

Susceptibility to mycobacterial infections

In recent years, it has been determined that several conditions are associated with a Mendelian susceptibility to nonpathogenic mycobacterial infection and to some extent to salmonella infections (Casanova and Abel 2002; Ottenhoff et al. 2002). It turned out that all of them impair the IL-12/interferon-γ (IFN-γ) pathway known to be a major inducer and effector of so-called T-helper 1 responses (Figure 38.3). In about 100 such patients, it was determined that deleterious mutations of IL-12B (IL-12 p40 subunit) (Altare et al. 1998b), IL-12RB1 (IL-12 receptor β subunit) (Altare et al. 1998a), interferon γ receptor β_1 subunit (IFNGR1) (Jouanguy et al. 1996; Newport et al. 1996), IFNGR2 (interferon γ receptor β_2 subunit) (Dorman and Holland 1998), or STAT-1 (transcription factor mediating interferon-induced signaling) (Dupuis et al. 2001) were found.

Clinical severity varies according to several parameters, i.e. type of mutated genes, type of mutations

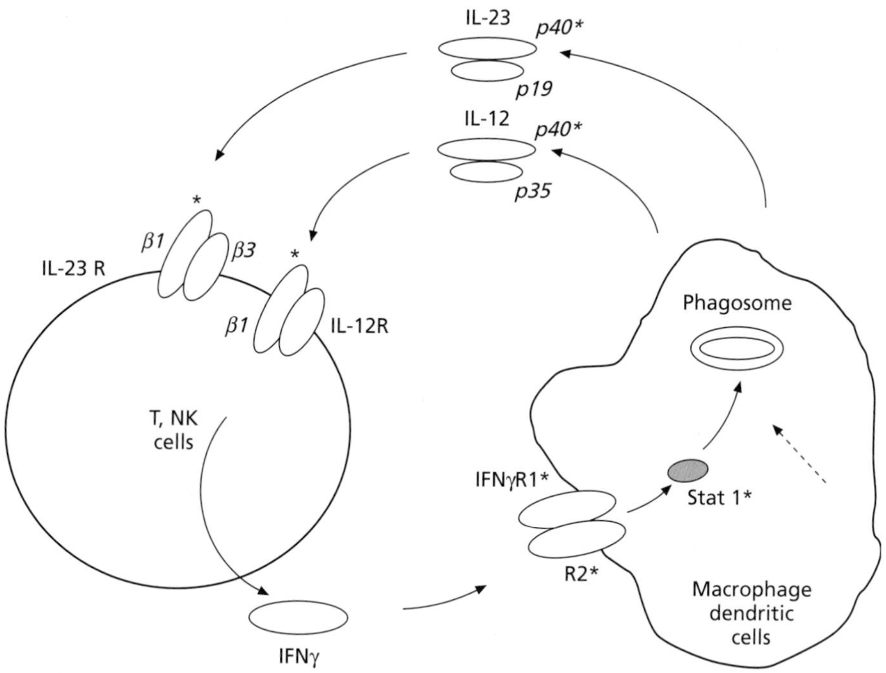

Figure 38.3 *The interleukin 12/interferon γ (IL-12/IFNγ) axis and its defects. *Described deficiencies. Other elements of the pathway are not shown for sake of simplification. The dotted arrow in the macrophage indicates other components of antimycobacterial immunity unrelated to IFNγ.*

from null to missense mutations, and probability to be infected with nonpathogenic mycobacteria. Associated genetic susceptibility factors could potentially also be involved. Both autosomal recessive and dominant (IFNGR1, STAT-1) inheritance patterns have been described. There are some differences in clinical presentation according to the affected genes. Complete IL-12 and IL-12RB1 mutations tend to lead to less severe mycobacterial infections with a reduced lethality compared with complete IFNGR1 deficiency. In the latter case, there is a heavy toll of early mortality caused by disseminated nonpathogenic mycobacterial infections (BCG or environmental) with a characteristic feature of the absence of typical granulomas around infected macrophages (Pierre-Audigier et al. 1997). It is possible that in the IL-12 axis deficiency, a partial IFN-γ production is preserved, accounting for a milder phenotype. In contrast, deficiency of the IL-12RB1 predisposes not only to mycobacterial infections but also to infection with *Salmonella* spp., a rather uncommon finding in IFNγR1/2 deficiencies. This suggests an additional role of IL-12 in immunity toward *Salmonella*.

A surprising hallmark of these syndromes is the rarity of infections caused by other opportunistic infections such as *Pneumocystis carinii* or *Toxoplasma gondii* and of viral infections, which were observed in only two cases. This contrasts sharply with the known susceptibility of IFNγ-deficient mice to virus challenges. No good explanation can as yet be proposed to account for this apparent discrepancy. Study of Mendelian susceptibility to mycobacterial infections has been determinant in pointing to the major and somewhat selective role of the IL-12/IFNγ pathway in the control of mycobacterial infections in humans. As this condition has also been found in a number of patients without defects in IL-12/IFNγ cytokine/receptor, more remains to be learnt about it. It is also not known whether mutations of these genes with milder consequences, could represent susceptibility elements in multifactorial risk factors for *M. tuberculosis* or *M. leprae*, in addition to the few described such as HLA-II, NRAMP1, and as yet undefined loci (Cooke and Hill 2001; Casanova and Abel 2002; Ottenhoff et al. 2002). In other words, do these Mendelian conditions represent the extreme of a more common spectrum of susceptibility?

GENETIC DISORDERS OF ADAPTIVE IMMUNITY

T lymphocytes

Since the 1960s, the central role of T lymphocytes in adaptive immunity has been recognized. The observation of patients in whom no thymus could be detected (Good 2002) brought a significant contribution to that understanding. Since then, a number of rare conditions characterized by defective T-cell development have been described, including intrinsic abnormalities defined as severe combined immunodeficiency (SCID) and environmental abnormalities related to thymic defects.

SEVERE COMBINED IMMUNODEFICIENCY

Strictly defined, SCID represents a group of rare conditions (about 1:10^5 births) characterized by a complete absence of mature T cells. The presence of circulating maternal T cells, which cannot be rejected, or the presence of autologous T cells in 'leaky' phenotypes can sometimes be misleading (Buckley 2000; Fischer 2000). Absence of functional T cells is incompatible with life beyond the first year, emphasizing the major role of adaptive immune response in humans living in a normal environment.

Patients, after a 2- to 3-month latency, become prone to fungal infections, multiple viral infections in particular causing protracted diarrhea and infections resulting from opportunistic agents such as *Pneumocystis carinii*. Interstitial pneumonitis caused by *P. carinii* is actually the most frequent infection leading to diagnosis (Buckley et al. 1997). Also, live vaccines such as BCG can lead to an overwhelming infection with lethal consequences (Stephan et al. 1993). As a result of the absence of T cells, B cells, when present, are also nonfunctional. Multiple SCID phenotypes have been described according to associated lymphocytic (NK, B lymphocytes) or myeloid defects, inheritance pattern and, more recently, molecular analysis (see Figure 38.4). They result either from defective signaling through γc-dependent cytokine receptors (γc, JAK-3, and IL-7Rα specific for the IL-7 receptor) blocking T-cell development before T-cell receptor β (TCRβ) gene rearrangement (Sugamura et al. 1995). A purine metabolism pathway deficiency, i.e. adenosine deaminase deficiency (ADA), which leads to dATP accumulation in lymphocyte precursors and premature cell apoptosis (Hershfield and Mitchell 1995), or from defective V(D)J rearrangements of T- and B-cell antigen receptor genes. The lymphoid-specific *Rag-1* or *Rag-2* genes can be mutated as well as the Artemis gene, which encodes a member of the nonhomologous end-joining repair pathway as the DNA-dependent protein kinase, the abnormal element of severe combined immunodeficient mice (Schwarz et al. 1996; Moshous et al. 2001). The other forms of SCID (reticular dysgenesis and CD45 deficiency) are extremely rare. There are no major differences in predisposition to infections according to the different phenotypes.

Atypical forms of SCID have been described as a cause of leaky phenotype related to mutations with milder consequences or, in a few cases of ADA and γc deficiencies, to a spontaneous reverse mutation in a T-cell precursor. Some mutations of the γc gene enable T-cell development whereas T-cell functions are impaired (but not absent). In some cases, responses to certain γc-dependent cytokines are more affected than others. It results in prolonged survival with occurrence of infections usually after 2–5 years of life. Missense mutations of *Rag-1* and *Rag-2* enabling residual recombinatorial activity can result in the emergence of expanded T-cell clones found in the so-called Omenn syndrome (Villa et al. 1998). Although these patients exhibit the same susceptibility pattern to infections as typical SCID, they, in addition, suffer from immunopathological lesions caused by T-cell infiltration of the skin, gut, and other organs. Recently, hypomorphic Artemis mutations were also shown to cause genomic instability predisposing to lymphomas, although the severity of the immunodeficiency is relatively milder compared with typical SCID (Moshous et al. 2003).

THYMIC DEFECTS

DiGeorge syndrome

DiGeorge syndrome consists of an embryopathy variably associating with conotruncal heart malformation, hypoparathyroidy, a dysmorphic syndrome, and an immunodeficiency. The last results from a defective migration of the

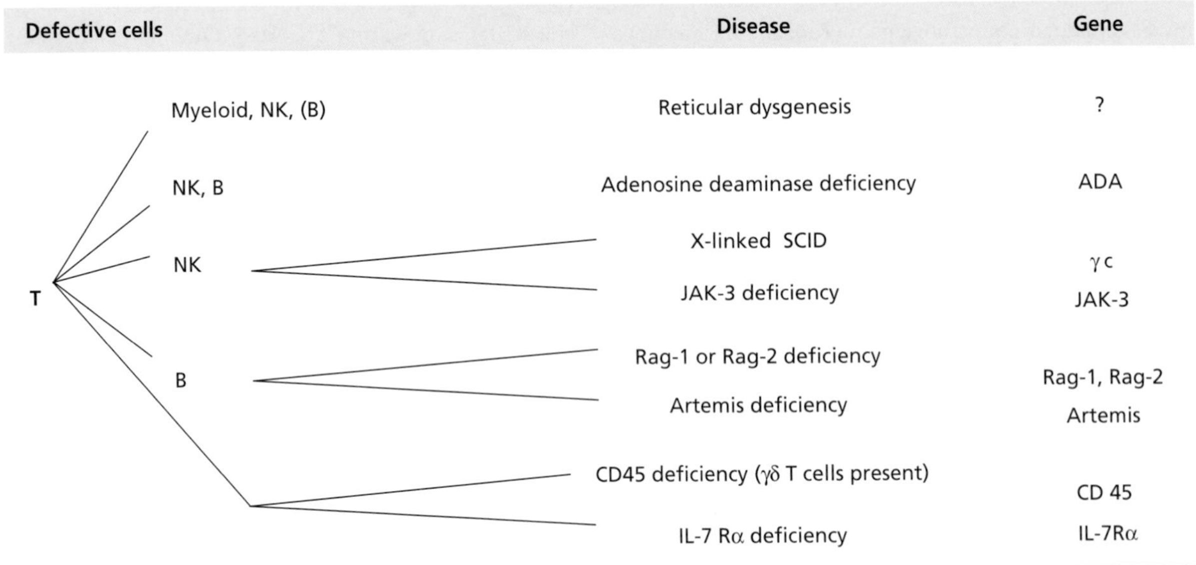

Figure 38.4 *Severe combined immunodeficiencies (SCID). IL, interleukin; NK, natural killer*

third and fourth embryonic branchial arches, which initiate the formation of the thymic gland (Perez and Sullivan 2002). In the rare cases where the thymic defect is complete (about 1 percent of patients with DiGeorge syndrome), patients have virtually no mature T cells in the periphery, showing that extrathymic T-cell differentiation is very limited in humans. Some patients can nevertheless develop oligoclonal T-cell populations in the periphery. In this setting, clinical consequences are as severe as those of SCID conditions. More frequently, T-cell counts are >500/mm^3 of blood and patients are not prone to infections, although late B-cell immunodeficiency and autoimmune manifestations have been occasionally reported (Perez and Sullivan 2002). The most frequent genetic defect found in patients with DiGeorge syndrome consists of hemizygous interstitial deletions of chromosome 22q11 (Carey et al. 1992; Wilson et al. 1992). There is no correlation between phenotype and genotype because some carriers of a same deletion can be very mildly symptomatic whereas others exhibit a full-blown DiGeorge syndrome including profound T-cell lymphocytopenia. There are several candidate genes located within the deletion which usually spans a 250-kb segment of DNA, TBX1, encoding a transcription factor, and *CRKOL* and *UFD1L* genes are expressed in the branchial arches during embryogenesis (Schinke and Izumo 2001). It is nevertheless unclear whether the phenotype can result from deletion of a single gene. Interstitial chromosome 10q deletion has also been rarely reported with DiGeorge syndrome. Interestingly, it has been recently shown that human leukocyte antigen (HLA)-incompatible, newborn thymic transplantation can lead to the development of functional T cells (Markert et al. 1999). These results imply that both positive and negative selection of thymocytes can be mediated by (recipient) bone marrow-derived cells. Also, expansion of HLA-identical peripheral T cells can be of benefit to DiGeorge syndrome patients with severe immune deficiency.

Nude phenotype

In one Italian kindred, a severe T-cell immunodeficiency has been found in association with baldness. This phenotype, highly reminiscent of nude mice, led to the finding of mutations in the *WHN* (winged-helix-nude gene) (Frank et al. 1999). The *WHN* gene is also mutated in the murine counterpart. It encodes a transcription factor expressed in epithelial cells of skin and thymus. Its defect impairs formation of the thymic microenvironment required for T-cell development because *WHN* induces expression of important genes in the program of thymic epithelial cell differentiation.

OTHER T-CELL IMMUNODEFICIENCIES

There are a number of primary immunodeficiencies associated with the detection of T cells in the periphery with variable functional defects. They all create a severe predisposition to infections, particularly to viruses, often associated with inflammatory bowel disease and autoimmune manifestations (Berthet et al. 1994).

Purine nucleoside phosphorylase

Purine nucleoside phosphorylase (PNP) deficiency is a rare cause of immunodeficiency with autosomal recessive inheritance. It is a purine metabolism error preventing conversion of guanine and leading to the toxic accumulation of dGTP in T-cell precursors. The immunodeficiency is often detectable after several years of life. Autoimmunity is a very frequent associated finding, together with a primary neurodevelopmental delay (Aust et al. 1992).

CD3 deficiencies

Four cases from three families with an immunodeficiency related to defect in CD3 components have been described. Although T-cell counts are within normal range, reduced expression of the TCR/CD3 complex was found associated with low CD8 T cell counts in two patients. Proliferation capacity of T cells driven by anti-CD3 antibody was low whereas antigen-induced responses were partially preserved. In one family, heterozygous mutations of the *CD3ε* gene were found whereas, in the other two, distinct mutations of the *CD3γ* gene were identified (Perez-Aciego et al. 1991; Soudais et al. 1993). Patients suffer from variable manifestations from bacterial lung infections to severe autoimmunity.

ZAP-70 deficiency

T-cell activation via the TCR leads to src kinase activation immediately followed by recruitment and activation of the ZAP-70 kinase, which binds to the immunoreceptor tyrosine-based activation (ITAM) motifs of CD3ζ.

A small number of patients with a complete ZAP-70 deficiency have been described (Arpaia et al. 1994; Elder et al. 1994). The clinical phenotype is severe, characterized by early onset of severe opportunistic infections, almost as in SCID patients. Surprisingly, the immunological phenotype is characterized by a selective CD8 T-cell lymphocytopenia. Nevertheless, ZAP-70-deficient CD4 T cells cannot be activated either in vitro or in vivo by antigens.

Other ill-defined severe T-cell deficiencies have been reported, including phenotypes of calcium influx deficiency (Le Deist et al. 1995), functional p56 lck deficiency (Goldman et al. 1998), and defects in cytokine production (Castigli et al. 1993).

IL-2 receptor α chain deficiency

In a single patient, a partial T-cell immunodeficiency has been found in association with lymphoid infiltration in various organs. This immunodeficiency is caused by defective expression of the IL2-Rα chain (Sharfe et al. 1997). It combines inappropriate T-cell response to infectious agents as well as the lymphoproliferative syndrome, possibly related to defective T-lymphocyte apoptosis.

Caspase 8 deficiency

A homozygous caspase 8 deficiency has recently been described in two patients from a single kindred. There is, as expected, a defect in lymphocyte apoptosis and homeostasis, but, surprisingly, there is also an activation deficiency of T, B, and NK lymphocytes (Chun et al. 2002). It resulted in the occurrence of infections, i.e. recurrent herpes simplex virus infections, pneumonia, and chronic diarrhea. This observation reveals an unexpected, yet poorly understood, role of caspase 8 in the early steps of lymphocyte activation.

HLA class II expression deficiencies

These are a rare primary immunodeficiency with autosomal recessive inheritance characterized by defective expression of the HLA-II molecules. It is associated with a severe immunodeficiency. About 100 cases have been reported so far. Infection onset occurs within the first years of life, usually with recurrent pulmonary infections and chronic diarrhea. Chronic cholangitis caused by cryptosporidia is a frequent complication. Viral meningoencephalitis can also occur. Various autoimmune manifestations can be associated. The immunological phenotype is characterized by a CD4 T lymphocytopenia, defective, antigen-specific, HLA-II-restricted, T-cell responses, and defective antibody production (Klein et al. 1993). Detectable CD4 T cells are thought to be the consequence of residual HLA-II expression by thymic epithelial cells. The disease is genetically heterogeneous and four complementation groups have been described. Corresponding genes have been cloned. Their products are all involved in the transcriptional control of HLA-II genes. In group A, a class II transactivator (CIITA), a protein inducible by IFNγ, is defective. It acts as a master control of the binding of proteins to the promoter (Steimle et al. 1993). In groups B, C, and D, respectively, RFX-ANK/RFX-B, RFX5, and RFX-AP were found to be the deficient factors. They are all transcription factors binding to the so-called X box present in HLA-II gene promoters (Steimle et al. 1995; Durand et al. 1997; Masternak et al. 1998; Nagarajan et al. 1999). HLA-II expression cannot occur in the absence of one of them. A variant of the disease with a milder deficiency was recently shown to be a group B variant (Nekrep et al. 2002). There are, however, some variations in phenotype because milder clinical and immunological expressions were described in a small number of kindreds without clear evidence of a leakiness of HLA-II expression (Wiszniewski et al. 2001). HLA-II expression deficiency is instrumental in demonstrating the in vivo central role of CD4 T cells in the generation of efficient immune responses in humans (Villard et al. 2001).

TAP deficiencies

About 10 cases of either TAP-1 or TAP-2 deficiencies have been reported (de la Salle et al. 1994, 1998). TAP-1/TAP-2 make up the HLA-I-associated peptide transporter that goes from the cytosol into the endoplasmic reticulum. Their deficiencies lead to reduced HLA-I expression, inconstantly associated with CD8 T and NK cell lymphopenia.

Clinical consequences are rather unexpected and consist of chronic bronchopneumonitis and in some patients severe vasculitis possibly caused by NK cell aggression to endothelial cells that weakly express HLA-I (Moins-Teisserenc et al. 1999). No clear susceptibility to viral infections has been shown.

Immunodeficiencies with genomic instability

A number of primary immunodeficiencies have been found to be associated with lymphocytic cytogenetic abnormalities, which were later found to correspond to a genomic instability syndrome. They usually provoke a combined T- and B-cell immunodeficiency of increasing severity with age as a result of progressive lymphocytopenia. They are variably associated with a risk of malignancies, particularly lymphomas.

DNA LIGASE 4 DEFICIENCY

DNA ligase 4 deficiency has first been retrospectively found in a child who developed unexpected severe complications of chemotherapy received as treatment for leukemia. It was then found that missense mutations of DNA ligase 4 cause a complex syndrome associating microcephaly, mild learning disability, dysmorphic syndrome, and a combined T- and B-cell immunodeficiency of variable intensity (O'Driscoll et al. 2001). DNA ligase 4 is involved in the ligation of coding ends in the nonhomologous end-joining (NHEJ) process used for V(D)J rearrangements of TCR and B-cell receptor (BCR) genes. It is thus understandable that hypomorphic mutations lead to a partial T- and B-cell immunodeficiency as also found for Artemis deficiency (see above). A case of DNA ligase 1 deficiency has been described in a patient with growth failure, sensitivity to ultraviolet light, severe combined immunodeficiency, and lymphoma (Barnes et al. 1992).

ATAXIA TELANGIECTASIA

Ataxia telangiectasia (AT) is a condition with autosomal recessive inheritance and a 1:40 000 incidence, associating progressive cerebellar ataxia with degeneration of Purkinje cells, oculocutaneous telangiectasias, and an immunodeficiency. The last, in most cases, consists of severe IgA, IgG2, and IgE deficiencies causing recurrent sinopulmonary infections. A progressive reduction in T-cell counts is also observed, although usually there is no susceptibility to opportunistic infections. A hallmark of the disease is illegitimate recombination of BCR and TCR genes inducing chromosomal translocations or inversions. It is the consequence of a genomic instability syndrome marked by a loss in the cell cycle checkpoints because AT cells exhibit radio-resistant DNA synthesis (Gatti et al. 1991; Shiloh 1997). These patients are at very high risk for lymphomas and also mucosal carcinomas. The AT gene has been cloned by Shiloh's group. The *ATM* gene encodes a 350-kDa protein of the phosphatidylinositol-3-phosphate kinase family (Savitsky et al. 1995). It acts as a sensor of DNA lesions together with the MRE 11/Nbs-1/Rad50 complex (see below) and activates a number of metabolic pathways involved in DNA repair or inducing cell apoptosis (Shiloh and Kastan 2001).

A minority of patients with a similar phenotype (AT-like disorder or ATLD) carries mutations of the *MRE-11* gene, part of a complex with Nbs-1 and Rad-50 involved in DNA break sensing and repair (Stewart et al. 1999).

NIGMEGEN BREAKAGE SYNDROME

Nigmegen breakage syndrome (NBS) shares some common findings with AT, i.e. abnormal chromosomal rearrangements, immunodeficiency (although more severe in NBS), and predisposition to lymphomas (Weemaes et al. 1981). There are, however, neither ataxia nor telangiectasias. In contrast, NBS patients present with microcephaly and learning disability. There is a profound T-cell lymphocytopenia in NBS with very poor survival. The NBS gene encodes nibrin or nbs-1, a member of the MRE-11/Rad-50/NBS-1 complex, which is activated by *ATM*, binds to DNA double-stranded breaks, and is involved in DNA repair (Carney et al. 1998; Varon et al. 1998).

IMMUNODEFICIENCY, CENTROMERIC INSTABILITY, AND FACIAL ANOMALIES

This rare syndrome with autosomal recessive inheritance associates a facial dysmorphic syndrome and an immunodeficiency. The latter varies from mild hypogammaglobulinemia to severe T-cell immunodeficiency with severe chronic diarrhea (Brown et al. 1995). There is a typical cytogenetic feature consisting of multibranched chromosomal configurations caused by elongation of secondary constrictions. This abnormality results from defective DNA methylation caused by recessive mutations of the DNA methyl transferase *DNMT3B* gene (Ellis et al. 1995; Xu et al. 1999). The relationship between DNA methylation and immunodeficiency is presently unclear.

BLOOM SYNDROME

This is a rare entity characterized by short stature, light-induced skin lesions, and predisposition to cancer. An immunodeficiency, mostly hypogammaglobulinemia, is often found. This condition is caused by deficiency in the Bloom mutant BLM, a DNA helicase (Xu et al. 1999).

Immunodeficiency with bone abnormalities

Short limb dwarfism or cartilage hair hypoplasia (CHH) is an autosomal recessive disorder associating a short stature with metaphyseal chondrodysplasia, hypoplastic hair, and a T-cell immunodeficiency. This condition is rare and has been mostly described in Finnish and Amish populations, although cases have been found worldwide. The T-cell immunodeficiency varies from a severe T lymphopenia with predispositions to classic infections to a mild, almost asymptomatic immunodeficiency (Makitie and Kaitila 1993). Associated features such as erythroblastopenia, cancer, and Hirschsprung's disease are not uncommon. The CHH-related gene has been recently identified. It encodes an untranslated RNA molecule, which forms part of an RNase ribonuclease mitochondrial RNA processing gene (RMRP) gene complex with endoribonuclease activity. Multiple mutations have been found (Ridanpaa et al. 2001). The physiopathology so far remains obscure.

A severe T-cell immunodeficiency has also been described in association with spondyloepiphyseal dysplasia, nephropathy, cortical blindness, and pigmentary skin changes. This very rare 'Schimke immuno-osseous dysplasia' has recently been shown to be caused by mutations of the *Smarcal* gene (Boerkoel et al. 2002).

Wiskott–Aldrich syndrome

Wiskott–Aldrich syndrome (WAS) is a well-known X-linked inherited condition characterized by the association of a complex immunodeficiency with a bleeding disorder and eczema (Ochs and Rosen 1998). Its incidence is around 1:250 000 live births. There is a spectrum of severity of the disease from isolated thrombocytopenia to a severe immunodeficiency with autoimmune manifestations, which include diffuse vasculitis (McCluggage et al. 1999) and a risk of lymphomas. Patients are prone to infections by encapsulated bacteria, essentially because IgM production is reduced. There is also a susceptibility to viral infections (herpes group particularly) possibly because of a gradual loss in T lymphocytes with age (Ochs and Rosen 1998). The *WASP* gene encodes the *WASP* protein, which is expressed by hemopoietic cells (Derry et al. 1994). *WASP* has multiple interaction sites for protein–protein interactions. In T lymphocytes, *WASP* is involved in rearrangement of the actin cytoskeleton on activation.

WASP-deficient lymphocytes lack surface microvilli and do not normally form filopodal and lamellipodal extensions (Remold-O'Donnell et al. 1996). Polarization of TCR-activated T cells is abnormal (Dupre et al. 2002). It is likely that *WASP* defects impair complex processes involved in activation, migration (in particular response to chemokines), and possibly survival of lymphocytes. There is apparently some degree of correlation between *WASP* genotypes and severity of the phenotypes (Ochs and Rosen 1998). Of note, female cases with WAS have been described in relation either to an abnormal X-chromosome inactivation pattern (predominant inactivation of the X chromosome carrying a normal *WASP* allele) (Parolini et al. 1998) or possibly to an unrelated disease.

Hyper-IgM syndrome: conditions predisposing to opportunistic infections

A 'classic' form of B-cell immunodeficiency is characterized by defective immunoglobulin class switch recombination (CSR) resulting in normal to high levels of serum IgM with very low production of IgG, IgA, and IgE. It is termed the hyper-IgM syndrome (HIgM). Genetic and clinical heterogeneities were noticed a long time ago because there are both X-linked and autosomal recessive forms of HIgM and some patients are prone to opportunistic infections not seen in B-cell immunodeficiencies. These observations led to a progressive delineation of very distinct conditions within the HIgM entity. In this section, only HIgM conditions leading to opportunistic infections are described.

X-LINKED HIGM-CD40L DEFICIENCY

B lymphocytes from X-linked HIgM patients can be induced to switch in vitro to the production of the different Ig isotypes, provided appropriate stimuli are present. This X-linked condition is caused by mutations of the gene encoding the CD40 ligand (CD40L) protein (Notarangelo and Hayward 2000). The latter is expressed at the surface of activated T cells; it is a member of the TNF family. By interacting with CD40 at the B-cell surface, CD40L delivers an essential (but not sufficient) signal for inducing Ig CSR and germinal center formation. However, several patients with CD40L deficiency not only are at risk for bacterial infections of the respiratory tract, as observed in other B-cell immunodeficiencies (see below), but also develop infections related to other mechanisms (Levy et al. 1997). Infected oral ulcerations can be a consequence of neutropenia, frequently found during the course of an infection and probably explained by a CD40-mediated, stress-induced granulopoiesis. More striking is the high risk of CD40L-deficient patients developing infections caused by pathogens that can invaginate in the membrane of epithelial cells, i.e. *P. carinii* and *Cryptosporidium parvum*, causing respectively interstitial pneumonitis and chronic diarrhea. In addition, chronic infections by *Toxoplasma gondii* have been reported. These infections are life-threatening in this setting, e.g. chronic *C. parvum* infection can lead to cholangitis and eventually liver cirrhosis caused by chronic inefficient TNF-mediated inflammation (Ponnuraj and Hayward 2002). These observations stress the role of CD40L in immunity to such pathogens. Mechanism(s) by which CD40L mediates effector functions is not precisely known. It has been shown in mice that CD40-expressing cells of hemopoietic origin are required for efficient immunity to *C. parvum* (Hayward et al. 2001). It could be that CD40L on activated T cells triggers cytokine production, such as IL-12, by CD40-expressing macrophages and/or that CD40-expressing cells trigger an unknown T-cell function. The former mechanism cannot be considered as sufficient because IL-12-deficient patients have a different spectrum of predisposition to infections (see above).

CD40 DEFICIENCY

A small number of patients with autosomal recessive HIgM exhibit a similar spectrum of infections as a consequence of recessive mutations of the CD40 gene, impairing its expression at the surface of B and other cells (Ferrari et al. 2001).

Deficiencies of the perforin-dependent cytolytic pathway

The study of the so-called hemophagocytic syndrome (HPS), which can be a genetically determined condition, has led to the understanding that impairment of the T- and NK cell cytolytic pathway carries rather unexpected consequences. HPS is characterized by polyvisceral infiltration by activated polyclonal T lymphocytes, mostly CD8, associated with macrophage activation (with hemophagocytosis) and massive release of proinflammatory cytokines (IFNγ, IL-1, IL-6, TNFα) (Henter et al. 1991; de Saint Basile and Fischer 2001). HPS occurrence is usually driven by an infection, very frequently by a herpes group infection, among which Epstein–Barr virus plays an important role. There are four known genetic conditions that can induce this HPS. Three of these conditions clearly share an identical immunological phenotype, i.e. defective T and NK cytotoxic activities. These are familial hemophagocytic lymphohistiocytosis (FHL) caused by perforin deficiency (Stepp et al. 1999), Chédiak–Higashi syndrome (CHS) caused by deficiency in the cytolytic lyst protein (Barbosa et al. 1996), and Griscelli's syndrome caused by a deficiency in the small G protein Rab27a (Menasche et al. 2000).

In the first condition, a major cytolytic component – perforin – is missing. In the next two, the intracellular transport of lysosomal secretory granules is defective leading to impaired exocytosis of cytolytic granules (Stinchcombe et al. 2001). It is striking to note that cytolytic T-/NK cell deficiency is not primarily a condition of high susceptibility to viral infections (as severe T-cell deficiencies are) but rather a disease of faulty contraction of expanded CD8 T cells after antigen stimulation (viral infection). This is a similar picture to the one observed in otherwise phenotype-free perforin$^{-/-}$ mice, once infected with the lymphocytic choriomeningitis virus (Matloubian et al. 1999).

A fourth condition is inherited with an X-linked pattern – X-linked proliferative syndrome (XLP) or Purtilo's syndrome. Affected males can develop a similar HPS syndrome usually once infected by Epstein–Barr virus (EBV), although some others can develop lymphomas and/or hypogammaglobulinemia (Morra et al. 2001). XLP is the consequence of mutations of the *SAP/SH2DIA* gene, which is expressed by T and NK cells and is involved in signaling by membrane molecules of the SLAM family (SLAM and 2B4 particularly) (Latour et al. 2001). SLAM–SLAM homologous interaction, and possibly 2B4 interaction with CD48 at the surface of EBV-infected B cells triggers fyn tyrosine kinase activation (Morra et al. 2001). It is unclear yet what the roles of these signaling pathways are. They have been shown to control T-helper 2 T-cell immune response. Interestingly, in the absence of SLAM-associated protein (SAP), the 2B4 NK cell co-receptor triggers inhibitory signals for cytotoxicity (Parolini et al. 1998). It is thus plausible that HPS as observed in XLP usually driven by an EBV infection is also the consequence of defective cytotoxic T lymphocyte (CTL)/NK cytolytic activity. Much remains to be done to understand its mechanism fully. Of note, there are more genetically determined HPS conditions that have not yet been molecularly characterized.

Other T-cell immunodeficiencies

CHRONIC MUCOCUTANEOUS CANDIDIASIS

Some patients exhibit an exquisite sensitivity to infections by candida species. This condition is known as chronic mucocutaneous candidiasis (Kirkpatrick 1994; Lilic 2002). It can persist as a strictly specific predisposition to candida infections of nails, skin, and mucosae associated with a specific deficiency in T-cell response to *Candida*, or become associated later in life with variable Ig isotype deficiencies. Several patterns of inheritance have been described. Cerebral aneurysms can complicate this condition, possibly as a consequence of a vascular fungal infection (Loeys et al. 1999). A locus has been mapped to chromosome 2 (Atkinson et al. 2001), but so far there is no hint about the molecular mechanism underlying this unique infection predisposition. In some cases, chronic candida infection is associated with autoimmune manifestations particularly targeting endocrine glands. This syndrome is known as autoimmune polyendocrinopathy–candidiasis–ectodermal dystrophy (APECED) Ahonen et al., 1990; Finnish–German APECED Consortium 1997). This rare condition is caused by mutations of the gene encoding the AIRE protein, a transcription factor expressed by thymic medullary epithelial cells (TEC) (Nagamine et al. 1997). It has been recently shown that in AIRE$^{-/-}$ mice, which also exhibit autoimmune polyendocrinopathy, AIRE-deficient TEC cells do not express proteins from mature organs, thus preventing a negative selection of autoimmune T-cell clones (Anderson et al. 2002). This work does not, however, provide an explanation on the mechanism of susceptibility to candida infections.

IDIOPATHIC CD4 LYMPHOCYTOPENIA

This condition resembles AIDS, because it is marked by a profound (<300/mm^3) CD4 T-cell lymphocytopenia, but is not caused by HIV, or by any other known environmental trigger (Smith et al. 1993). Opportunistic infections occur as a consequence of this syndrome frequently associated with inflammatory or autoimmune diseases. No etiology is known. The mechanism of CD4 T-cell lymphocytopenia (premature apoptosis?) remains elusive.

B lymphocytes

Genetic disorders of B lymphocytes predominate by far, because they represent 70 percent of primary immunodeficiency disorders (Figure 38.5). Bruton (1952) made the very first description of an immunodeficiency in 1952, X-linked agammaglobulinemia. Since then, several syndromes have been described and, accordingly, the role of the different Ig isotypes in infectious immunity has been better understood. Still, the molecular mechanism of the most frequent form(s) of B-cell immunodeficiency, i.e. common variable immunodeficiency and IgA deficiency, remains elusive (see below).

AGAMMAGLOBULINEMIA

Prototypic B-cell immunodeficiency consists of genetic defects impairing B-cell development. Four such conditions have been described leading to the autosomal recessive form of agammaglobulinemia (Gaspar and Conley 2000). An early block in B-cell development results in a complete absence of mature B cells and thus of Ig production whereas the other cells of the immune system are spared. They thus do provide a 'pure' model to study consequences in humans of an absence of B-cell-mediated immunity. Onset of infections occurs in the first year of life after a few months' delay because of the transient protection provided by maternally transmitted IgG. The most frequent sites of infection are the upper respiratory tract, the lower respiratory tract, the

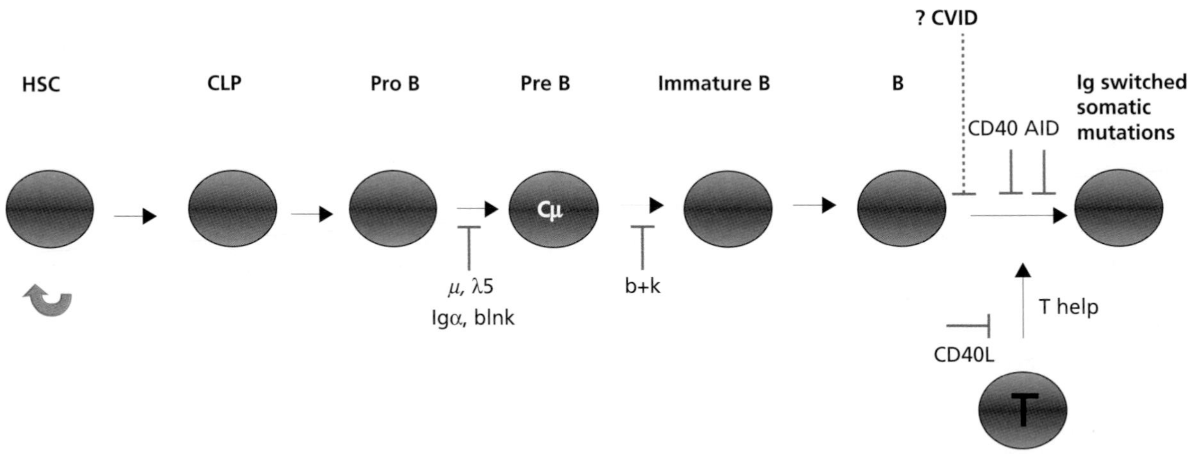

Figure 38.5 *B-cell immunodeficiencies. HSCs (hemopoietic stem cells) differentiate into putative CLPs (common lymphocyte progenitors), giving rise among other lineages to the B-lymphocyte lineage. There is a block in B-cell development (see text for explanation). CVID, common variable immunodeficiency.*

gut, the skin joints, the eyes, and the central nervous system, and sepsis also occurs (Smith and Witte 1998).

Upper and lower respiratory tract infections are recurrent, progressively leading to chronic infectious lesions of the sinuses and bronchi. Bronchiectasis develops which can lead in the absence of treatment to pulmonary insufficiency (Quartier et al. 1999; Conley and Howard 2002; Lopez Granados et al. 2002). The most frequently encountered microorganisms are *H. influenzae*, *S. pneumoniae*, gram-negative bacilli such as *Pseudomonas aeruginosa*, i.e. encapsulated bacteria. In the gut, *Giardia lamblia* causing a chronic parasitic infection can occur. Chronic mycoplasma infections of the joints have also been described. Agammaglobulinemic patients are not prone to viral infections with a single important exception. Chronic enteroviral infections are indeed not uncommon in this setting. Live attenuated polioviruses can induce a severe chronic neurological disease. Chronic enteroviral infections have a large spectrum of expression from chronic diarrhea, failure to thrive, arthritis, hepatitis, pseudo-dermatomyositis osteomyeolitis, to more commonly meningoencephalitis (Quartier et al. 1999; Conley and Howard 2002; Lopez Granados et al. 2002). It remains by far the most severe infectious complication in B-cell-deficient patients. Enteroviral infection can occur in an otherwise well-treated patient. It is difficult to control. It is still unknown how agammaglobulinemic patients exhibit such a high susceptibility to enteroviral infections despite the normality of their T-cell compartments. Some specificity of enterovirus–host interaction remains obviously unknown.

It is interesting to note that IgG substitution by intravenous or subcutaneous route is highly efficient in preventing most of bacterial infections (unless bronchiectasis or a chronic sinusitis is present) suggesting that IgG can essentially substitute the IgA function at mucosal surfaces. Although it is unclear how IgG diffuses at mucosal surface, this observation may help to understand that many IgA-deficient patients are not particularly susceptible to infections.

AUTOSOMAL RECESSIVE AGAMMMAGLOBULINEMIA

There are four conditions characterized by a complete absence of mature B cells because of a block in B-cell differentiation at the pro-B-cell level (Yel et al. 1996; Minegishi et al. 1998, 1999a, 1999b). Mutations in the μ heavy chain gene, the λ5 surrogate light chain gene, the Igα, or the BLNK genes all result in the same phenotype. The faulty expression of a pre-B-cell receptor (Ig μ heavy chain/surrogate light chain) or of the associated signaling apparatus (Igα/CD89a or blnk) prevents further progression in the B-cell development pathway. These are rare conditions, but other autosomal recessive inherited agammaglobulinemias have not yet reached molecular understanding.

X-LINKED AGAMMAGLOBULINEMIA (BRUTON'S DISEASE)

X-linked agammaglobulinemia (XLA) accounts for about 80 percent of the cases of 'agammaglobulinemia'. It is caused by mutations of the Bruton tyrosine kinase gene (*btk*) (Vetrie et al. 1993; Tsukada et al. 1993). However, in most cases, B-cell development block is not as complete as it is in autosomal recessive agammaglobulinemia. Patients tend to have low but variably detectable serum concentrations of the different Ig isotypes. Peripheral B cells can in some cases be detected in the periphery. Typically, bone marrow B-cell differentiation is blocked at the pre-B-cell level (B cells expressing the μ/pseudo light chain complex at the surface). Therefore, the clinical consequence, although very similar to those of autosomal recessive agammaglobulinemia, tends to have a slightly later onset and be slightly less severe (Lopez Granados et al. 2002).

Phenotypic variability is unexpectedly high because several patients with *btk* mutations exhibit a phenotypic picture reminiscent of common variable immunodeficiency (CVID) (see below), i.e. B cells are detectable in periphery (up to 5 percent lymphocytes) with serum IgG concentration up to 2–3 g/l. This variability is independent of the genotype as observed within affected kindreds (Smith and Witte 1998). The extreme of the spectrum has been described as a pure deficiency in antibody response to polysaccharide antigens (Wood et al. 2001). This is actually reminiscent of the *btk*-deficient murine model, either natural (CBA/N-XID strain) or obtained by *btk* gene inactivation, which essentially exhibits a defect in antibody response toward type 2 T-independent antigens (Rawlings et al. 1993). It is possible that modifier genes (with or without environmental factors) modulate the phenotypic expression of XLA.

The btk kinase belongs to the Itk/Tec tyrosine kinase family. It is expressed by hemopoietic cells but seems essential in B-cell and possibly mastocyte development/function. Mutations affecting essentially all domains of the molecules (PH, TH, SH_3, SH_2, and kinase) have been described; *btk* appears as an essential component for signal transduction from several B-cell receptors (BCR) including surface Ig (antigen-specific BCRs), CD40, and cytokine receptors for IL-5, -6 and -10 (Smith and Witte 1998). Calcium flux after phospholipase C γ (PLCγ) phosphorylation, an essential event in BCR-triggered B-cell activation, is dependent on *btk* integrity.

HYPER-IGM SYNDROMES

As described above, HIgM syndromes are the in vivo consequences of defective Ig class switch recombinant (CSR). Besides CD40L–CD40 deficiencies, there are pure HIgM B-cell immunodeficiency conditions. Defective IgG and IgA production is associated with typical susceptibility to bacterial infections in the respiratory and gastrointestinal tracts (Conley et al. 1994). This is most often accompanied by lymph node enlargement as a consequence of hypertrophic germinal centers, full of proliferating B cells. Further phenotypic characterization of this syndrome has revealed that there is also a defect in IgV region somatic hypermutations (SHM). This condition, called HIgM2 syndrome, has been ascribed to activation-induced deaminase (AID) gene recessive mutations (Revy et al. 2000). AID is selectively expressed in germinal centers. It belongs to an RNA-editing enzyme family. AID is thus necessary for both events of somatic Ig gene rearrangements and somatic mutations required for antigen-driven antibody maturation. It is still not known whether AID indeed edits mARN-encoding protein(s) involved in CSR and SHMs or directly modifies DNA as recently suggested (Petersen-Mahrt et al. 2002). There are still HIgM syndromes that are not accounted for by AID gene mutations. Their study might contribute to a further description of the molecular pathways involved in CSR and SHMs.

COMMON VARIABLE IMMUNODEFICIENCY AND IGA DEFICIENCY

IgA deficiency is the most common form of primary immunodeficiencies but it is frequently an asymptomatic condition. Common variable immunodeficiency (CVID) occurs in 1:25 000 individuals, with onset of symptoms usually during the second or the third decade of life (Hammarstrom et al. 2000). It is characterized by a variably decreased concentration of all Ig isotypes. Patients with CVID and symptomatic IgA deficiency are prone to infections similar to the ones encountered in agammaglobulinemic patients. In addition, however, these patients, during adulthood, become at risk of developing granulomatous lesions, inflammatory bowel disease, autoimmune diseases, and cancer. Inheritance pattern of CVID and IgA deficiency is not entirely clear but it is often compatible with an autosomal dominant pattern with variable penetrance. Both conditions can be found in the same kindred or subsequently in the same individual, suggesting that these two conditions are allelic.

Despite intensive research, there is still very little known about the physiopathology of CVID and IgA deficiency. B-cell counts in blood can be diminished (with a trend to decline). There are variable B-cell phenotype abnormalities, which have led to CVID subclassification (Warnatz et al. 2002). It is not known, however, whether this corresponds to potentially distinct disease mechanisms. In some of the patients, functional T-cell defects have also been observed. It is also not known whether there are primary or secondary T-cell abnormalities. Patients with IgA deficiency very often have anti-IgA antibodies. It has been suggested that anti-IgA antibodies could play a causative role because women transmitting the disease have a higher prevalence of anti-IgA antibodies that could induce IgA deficiencies in offspring (Vorechovsky et al. 1999, 2000). Genetic linkage between CVID and IgA deficiency and the HLA locus has been demonstrated. There is a debate about whether the HLA-III region (between the C4b and the C2 genes) and/or the HLA-II region (HLA-DQ locus) is involved (Schroeder et al. 1998; Vorechovsky et al. 1999).

Of note, drug-induced Ig deficiencies (IgA deficiency or CVID) have been described without known mechanisms. IgA deficiency has been also described in patients with aberrations of chromosome 18.

IGG ISOTYPES DEFICIENCIES

Variable IgG isotypes deficiencies have been reported, as either, very rarely, the consequence of autosomal recessive deletions of IgH genes (IgG1 deficiency) or selective IgG2 and -4 (often with IgA) deficiency without abnormality of IgH genes (Oxelius et al. 1981). In the last case, there is a selective antibody production deficiency toward the polysaccharide wall of *S. pneumoniae*, *H. influenzae*, and *P. aeruginosa*, which make these patients very susceptible to infections by these bacteria. The relationship between the $\gamma 2$ gene and specificity of IgG2 antibodies remains puzzling. The physiopathology is unknown. There are family cases suggestive of autosomal recessive inheritance.

Selective antibody production deficiency to polysaccharides without diminution in serum Ig isotypes levels has also been described in a few cases. It has been proposed that such deficiency could reflect a defect in T-independent B1 cell function, but this remains highly hypothetical.

REFERENCES

Ahonen, P., Myllarniemi, S., et al. 1990. Clinical variation of autoimmune polyendocrinopathy-candidiasis-ectodermal dystrophy (APECED) in a series of 68 patients. *N Engl J Med*, **322**, 1829–36.

Altare, F., Durandy, A., et al. 1998a. Impairment of mycobacterial immunity in human interleukin-12 receptor deficiency. *Science*, **280**, 1432–5.

Altare, F., Lammas, D., et al. 1998b. Inherited interleukin 12 deficiency in a child with bacille Calmette-Guerin and *Salmonella enteritidis* disseminated infection. *J Clin Invest*, **102**, 2035–40.

Ambruso, D.R., Knall, C., et al. 2000. Human neutrophil immunodeficiency syndrome is associated with an inhibitory Rac2 mutation. *Proc Natl Acad Sci USA*, **97**, 4654–9.

Anderson, D.C., Schmalsteig, F.C., et al. 1985. The severe and moderate phenotypes of heritable Mac-1, LFA-1 deficiency: their quantitative definition and relation to leukocyte dysfunction and clinical features. *J Infect Dis*, **152**, 668–89.

Anderson, M.S., Venanzi, E.S., et al. 2002. Projection of an immunological self shadow within the thymus by the aire protein. *Science*, **298**, 1395–401.

Aprikyan, A.A., Liles, W.C., et al. 2001. Impaired survival of bone marrow hematopoietic progenitor cells in cyclic neutropenia. *Blood*, **97**, 147–53.

Arpaia, E., Shahar, M., et al. 1994. Defective T cell receptor signaling and CD8+ thymic selection in humans lacking zap-70 kinase. *Cell*, **76**, 947–58.

Atkinson, T.P., Schaffer, A.A., et al. 2001. An immune defect causing dominant chronic mucocutaneous candidiasis and thyroid disease maps to chromosome 2p in a single family. *Am J Hum Genet*, **69**, 791–803.

Aust, M.R., Andrews, L.G., et al. 1992. Molecular analysis of mutations in a patient with purine nucleoside phosphorylase deficiency. *Am J Hum Genet*, **51**, 763–72.

Barbosa, M.D., Nguyen, Q.A., et al. 1996. Identification of the homologous beige and Chediak-Higashi syndrome genes. *Nature*, **382**, 262–5.

Barnes, D.E., Tomkinson, A.E., et al. 1992. Mutations in the DNA ligase I gene of an individual with immunodeficiencies and cellular hypersensitivity to DNA-damaging agents. *Cell*, **69**, 495–503.

Barton, G.M. and Medzhitov, R. 2002. Control of adaptive immune responses by Toll-like receptors. *Curr Opin Immunol*, **14**, 380–3.

Berthet, F., Le Deist, F., et al. 1994. Clinical consequences and treatment of primary immunodeficiency syndromes characterized by functional T and B lymphocyte anomalies (combined immune deficiency). *Pediatrics*, **93**, 265–70.

Biron, C.A., Byron, K.S. and Sullivan, J.L. 1989. Severe herpesvirus infections in an adolescent without natural killer cells. *N Engl J Med*, **320**, 1731–5.

Boerkoel, C.F., Takashima, H., et al. 2002. Mutant chromatin remodeling protein SMARCAL1 causes Schimke immuno-osseous dysplasia. *Nat Genet*, **30**, 215–20.

Boocock, G.R., Morrison, J.A., et al. 2003. Mutations in SBDS are associated with Shwachman–Diamond syndrome. *Nat Genet*, **33**, 97–101.

Britz-Cunningham, S.H., Shah, M.M., et al. 1995. Mutations of the Connexin 43 gap-junction gene in patients with heart malformations and defects of laterality. *N Engl J Med*, **332**, 1323–9.

Brown, D.C., Grace, E., et al. 1995. ICF syndrome (immunodeficiency, centromeric instability and facial anomalies): investigation of heterochromatin abnormalities and review of clinical outcome. *Hum Genet*, **96**, 411–16.

Brown, M.G., Dokun, A.O., et al. 2001. Vital involvement of a natural killer cell activation receptor in resistance to viral infection. *Science*, **292**, 934–7.

Bruton, O.C. 1952. Agammaglobulinemia. *Pediatrics*, **9**, 722–7.

Buckley, R.H. 2000. Advances in immunology: primary immunodeficiency diseases due to defects in lymphocytes. *N Engl J Med*, **343**, 1313–24.

Buckley, R.H., Schiff, R.I., et al. 1997. Human severe combined immunodeficiency: genetic, phenotypic, and functional diversity in one hundred eight infants. *J Pediatr*, **130**, 378–87.

Carey, A.H., Kelly, D., et al. 1992. Molecular genetic study of the frequency of monosomy 22q11 in DiGeorge syndrome. *Am J Hum Genet*, **51**, 964–70.

Carney, J.P., Maser, R.S., et al. 1998. The hMre11/hRad50 protein complex and Nijmegen breakage syndrome: linkage of double-strand break repair to the cellular DNA damage response. *Cell*, **93**, 477–86.

Casanova, J.L. and Abel, L. 2002. Genetic dissection of immunity to mycobacteria: the human model. *Annu Rev Immunol*, **20**, 581–620.

Castigli, E., Pahwa, R., et al. 1993. Molecular basis of a multiple lymphokine deficiency in a patient with severe combined immunodeficiency. *Proc Natl Acad Sci USA*, **90**, 4728–32.

Cech, P., Stalder, H., et al. 1979. Leukocyte myeloperoxidase deficiency and diabetes mellitus associated with *Candida albicans* liver abscess. *Am J Med*, **66**, 149–53.

Chun, H.J., Zheng, L., et al. 2002. Pleiotropic defects in lymphocyte activation caused by caspase-8 mutations lead to human immunodeficiency. *Nature*, **419**, 395–9.

Coates, T.D., Torkildson, J.C., et al. 1991. An inherited defect of neutrophil motility and microfilamentous cytoskeleton associated with abnormalities in 47-Kd and 89-Kd proteins. *Blood*, **78**, 1338–46.

Conley, M.E. and Howard, V. 2002. Clinical findings leading to the diagnosis of X-linked agammaglobulinemia. *J Pediatr*, **141**, 566–71.

Conley, M.E., Larche, M., et al. 1994. Hyper IgM syndrome associated with defective CD40-mediated B cell activation. *J Clin Invest*, **94**, 1404–9.

Cooke, G.S. and Hill, A.V. 2001. Genetics of susceptibility to human infectious disease. *Nat Rev Genet*, **2**, 967–77.

Courtois, G., Smahi, A. and Israel, A. 2001. NEMO/IKK gamma: linking NF-kappa B to human disease. *Trends Mol Med*, **7**, 427–30.

Dale, D.C., Bonilla, M.A., et al. 1993. A randomized controlled phase III trial of recombinant human granulocyte colony-stimulating factor (filgrastim) for treatment of severe chronic neutropenia. *Blood*, **81**, 2496–502.

Dale, D.C., Person, R.E., et al. 2000. Mutations in the gene encoding neutrophil elastase in congenital and cyclic neutropenia. *Blood*, **96**, 2317–22.

de la Salle, H. 1998. In Ochs, H.O., Smith, C.I.E. and Puck, J.M. (eds), *Primary immunodeficiency diseases*. New York: Oxford University Press, 181–8.

de la Salle, H., Hanau, D., et al. 1994. Homozygous human TAP peptide transporter mutation in HLA class I deficiency. *Science*, **265**, 237–41.

de Saint Basile, G. and Fischer, A. 2001. The role of cytotoxicity in lymphocyte homeostasis. *Curr Opin Immunol*, **13**, 549–54.

de Vries, E., Koene, H.R., et al. 1996. Identification of an unusual Fc gamma receptor IIIa (CD16) on natural killer cells in a patient with recurrent infections. *Blood*, **88**, 3022–7.

Derry, J.M., Ochs, H.D. and Francke, U. 1994. Isolation of a novel gene mutated in Wiskott–Aldrich syndrome. *Cell*, **78**, 635–44.

Devriendt, K., Kim, A.S., et al. 2001. Constitutively activating mutation in WASP causes X-linked severe congenital neutropenia. *Nat Genet*, **27**, 313–17.

Doffinger, R., Smahi, A., et al. 2001. X-linked anhidrotic ectodermal dysplasia with immunodeficiency is caused by impaired NF-kappaB signaling. *Nat Genet*, **27**, 277–85.

Dorman, S.E. and Holland, S.M. 1998. Mutation in the signal-transducing chain of the interferon-gamma receptor and susceptibility to mycobacterial infection. *J Clin Invest*, **101**, 2364–9.

Dupre, L., Aiuti, A., et al. 2002. Wiskott–Aldrich syndrome protein regulates lipid raft dynamics during immunological synapse formation. *Immunity*, **17**, 157–66.

Dupuis, S., Dargemont, C., et al. 2001. Impairment of mycobacterial but not viral immunity by a germline human STAT1 mutation. *Science*, **293**, 300–3.

Durand, B., Sperisen, P., et al. 1997. RFXAP, a novel subunit of the RFX DNA binding complex is mutated in MHC class II deficiency. *EMBO J*, **16**, 1045–55.

Elder, M.E., Lin, D., et al. 1994. Human severe combined immunodeficiency due to a defect in ZAP-70, a T cell tyrosine kinase. *Science*, **264**, 1596–9.

Ellis, N.A., Groden, J., et al. 1995. The Bloom's syndrome gene product is homologous to RecQ helicases. *Cell*, **83**, 655–66.

Etzioni, A., Frydman, M., et al. 1992. Brief report: recurrent severe infections caused by a novel leukocyte adhesion deficiency. *N Engl J Med*, **327**, 1789–92.

Ferrari, S., Giliani, S., et al. 2001. Mutations of CD40 gene cause an autosomal recessive form of immunodeficiency with hyper IgM. *Proc Natl Acad Sci USA*, **98**, 12614–19.

Finnish–German APECED Consortium. 1997. An autoimmune disease, APECED, caused by mutations in a novel gene featuring two PHD-type zinc-finger domains, autoimmune polyendocrinopathy-candidiasis-ectodermal dystrophy. *Nat Genet*, **17**, 399–403.

Fischer, A. 2000. Severe combined immunodeficiencies (SCID). *Clin Exp Immunol*, **122**, 143–9.

Fischer, A., Lisowska-Grospierre, B., et al. 1988. Leukocyte adhesion deficiency: molecular basis and functional consequences. *Immunodefic Rev*, **1**, 39–54.

Frank, J., Pignata, C., et al. 1999. Exposing the human nude phenotype. *Nature*, **398**, 473–4.

Gaspar, H.B. and Conley, M.E. 2000. Early B cell defects. *Clin Exp Immunol*, **119**, 383–9.

Gatti, R.A., Boder, E., et al. 1991. Ataxia-telangiectasia: an interdisciplinary approach to pathogenesis. *Medicine (Balt)*, **70**, 99–117.

Gebbia, M., Ferrero, G.B., et al. 1997. X-linked situs abnormalities result from mutations in ZIC3. *Nat Genet*, **17**, 305–8.

Gennery, A.R., Flood, T.J., et al. 2000. Bone marrow transplantation does not correct the hyper IgE syndrome. *Bone Marrow Transplant*, **25**, 1303–5.

Goldman, F.D., Ballas, Z.K., et al. 1998. Defective expression of p56lck in an infant with severe combined immunodeficiency. *J Clin Invest*, **102**, 421–9.

Good, R.A. 2002. Cellular immunology in a historical perspective. *Immunol Rev*, **185**, 136–58.

Grimbacher, B., Holland, S.M., et al. 1999a. Hyper-IgE syndrome with recurrent infections – an autosomal dominant multisystem disorder. *N Engl J Med*, **340**, 692–702.

Grimbacher, B., Schaffer, A.A., et al. 1999b. Genetic linkage of hyper-IgE syndrome to chromosome 4. *Am J Hum Genet*, **65**, 735–44.

Hammarstrom, L., Vorechovsky, I. and Webster, D. 2000. Selective IgA deficiency (SIgAD) and common variable immunodeficiency (CVID). *Clin Exp Immunol*, **120**, 225–31.

Harris, E.S., Shigeoka, A.O., et al. 2001. A novel syndrome of variant leukocyte adhesion deficiency involving defects in adhesion mediated by beta1 and beta2 integrins. *Blood*, **97**, 767–76.

Hayward, A.R., Cosyns, M., et al. 2001. Marrow-derived CD40-positive cells are required for mice to clear *Cryptosporidium parvum* infection. *Infect Immun*, **69**, 1630–4.

Henter, J.I., Elinder, G., et al. 1991. Hypercytokinemia in familial hemophagocytic lymphohistiocytosis. *Blood*, **78**, 2918–22.

Hershfield, M. and Mitchell, B. 1995. In: Scriver, C., Beaudet, A., et al. (eds), *Metabolic basis of inherited disease*. New York: McGraw Hill, 1725–68.

Horwitz, M., Benson, K.F., et al. 1999. Mutations in ELA2, encoding neutrophil elastase, define a 21-day biological clock in cyclic haematopoiesis. *Nat Genet*, **23**, 433–6.

Jain, A., Ma, C.A., et al. 2001. Specific missense mutations in NEMO result in hyper-IgM syndrome with hypohydrotic ectodermal dysplasia. *Nat Immunol*, **2**, 223–8.

Jawahar, S., Moody, C., et al. 1996. Natural killer (NK) cell deficiency associated with an epitope-deficient Fc receptor type IIIA (CD16-II). *Clin Exp Immunol*, **103**, 408–13.

Jouanguy, E., Altare, F., et al. 1996. Interferon-gamma-receptor deficiency in an infant with fatal bacille Calmette–Guerin infection. *N Engl J Med*, **335**, 1956–61.

Kirkpatrick, C.H. 1994. Chronic mucocutaneous candidiasis. *J Am Acad Dermatol*, **31**, S14–17.

Kishimoto, T.K., Hollander, N., et al. 1987. Heterogeneous mutations in the beta subunit common to the LFA-1, Mac-1, and p150,95 glycoproteins cause leukocyte adhesion deficiency. *Cell*, **50**, 193–202.

Klein, C., Lisowska-Grospierre, B., et al. 1993. Major histocompatibility complex class II deficiency: clinical manifestations, immunologic features, and outcome. *J Pediatr*, **123**, 921–8.

Kostmann, R. 1956. Infantile genetic aganulocytosis. *Acta Paediatr Scand Suppl*, **1456**, 1.

Kuhns, D.B., Long Priel, D.A. and Gallin, J.I. 1997. Endotoxin and IL-1 hyporesponsiveness in a patient with recurrent bacterial infections. *J Immunol*, **158**, 3959–64.

Kuijpers, T.W., Van Lier, R.A., et al. 1997. Leukocyte adhesion deficiency type 1 (LAD-1)/variant. A novel immunodeficiency syndrome characterized by dysfunctional beta2 integrins. *J Clin Invest*, **100**, 1725–33.

Kyono, W. and Coates, T.D. 2002. A practical approach to neutrophil disorders. *Pediatr Clin North Am*, **49**, 929–71, viii.

Latour, S., Gish, G., et al. 2001. Regulation of SLAM-mediated signal transduction by SAP, the X-linked lymphoproliferative gene product. *Nat Immunol*, **2**, 681–90.

Le Deist, F., Hivroz, C., et al. 1995. A primary T-cell immunodeficiency associated with defective transmembrane calcium influx. *Blood*, **85**, 1053–62.

Lekstrom-Himes, J. and Xanthopoulos, K.G. 1999. CCAAT/enhancer binding protein epsilon is critical for effective neutrophil-mediated response to inflammatory challenge. *Blood*, **93**, 3096–105.

Levy, J., Espanol-Boren, T., et al. 1997. Clinical spectrum of X-linked hyper-IgM syndrome. *J Pediatr*, **131**, 47–54.

Lilic, D. 2002. New perspectives on the immunology of chronic mucocutaneous candidiasis. *Curr Opin Infect Dis*, **15**, 143–7.

Loeys, B.L., Van Coster, R.N., et al. 1999. Fungal intracranial aneurysm in a child with familial chronic mucocutaneous candidiasis. *Eur J Pediatr*, **158**, 650–2.

Lopez Granados, E., Porpiglia, A.S., et al. 2002. Clinical and molecular analysis of patients with defects in micro heavy chain gene. *J Clin Invest*, **110**, 1029–35.

Luhn, K., Wild, M.K., et al. 2001. The gene defective in leukocyte adhesion deficiency II encodes a putative GDP-fucose transporter. *Nat Genet*, **28**, 69–72.

McCluggage, W.G., Alderdice, J.M. and Walsh, M.Y. 1999. Polypoid uterine lesions mimicking endometrial stromal sarcoma. *J Clin Pathol*, **52**, 543–6.

Mcdowall, A., Inwald, D., et al. 2003. A novel form of integrin dysfunction involving beta1, beta2, and beta3 integrins. *J Clin Invest*, **111**, 51–60.

Makitie, O. and Kaitila, I. 1993. Cartilage-hair hypoplasia: clinical manifestations in 108 Finnish patients. *Eur J Pediatr*, **152**, 211–17.

Mamlok, R.J., Mamlok, V., et al. 1987. Glucose-6-phosphate dehydrogenase deficiency, neutrophil dysfunction and *Chromobacterium violaceum* sepsis. *J Pediatr*, **111**, 852–4.

Markert, M.L., Boeck, A., et al. 1999. Transplantation of thymus tissue in complete DiGeorge syndrome. *N Engl J Med*, **341**, 1180–9.

Masternak, K., Barras, E., et al. 1998. A gene encoding a novel RFX-associated transactivator is mutated in the majority of MHC class II deficiency patients. *Nat Genet*, **20**, 273–7.

Matloubian, M., Suresh, M., et al. 1999. A role for perforin in downregulating T-cell responses during chronic viral infection. *J Virol*, **73**, 2527–36.

Menasche, G., Pastural, E., et al. 2000. Mutations in RAB27A cause Griscelli syndrome associated with haemophagocytic syndrome. *Nat Genet*, **25**, 173–6.

Messina, C.G., Reeves, E.P., et al. 2002. Catalase negative *Staphylococcus aureus* retain virulence in mouse model of chronic granulomatous disease. *FEBS Lett*, **518**, 107–10.

Minegishi, Y., Coustan-Smith, E., et al. 1998. Mutations in the human lambda5/14.1 gene result in B cell deficiency and agammaglobulinemia. *J Exp Med*, **187**, 71–7.

Minegishi, Y., Coustan-Smith, E., et al. 1999a. Mutations in Igalpha (CD79a) result in a complete block in B-cell development. *J Clin Invest*, **104**, 1115–21.

Minegishi, Y., Rohrer, J., et al. 1999b. An essential role for BLNK in human B cell development. *Science*, **286**, 1954–7.

Moins-Teisserenc, H.T., Gadola, S.D., et al. 1999. Association of a syndrome resembling Wegener's granulomatosis with low surface expression of HLA class-I molecules. *Lancet*, **354**, 1598–603.

Morra, M., Howie, D., et al. 2001. X-linked lymphoproliferative disease: a progressive immunodeficiency. *Annu Rev Immunol*, **19**, 657–82.

Moshous, D., Callebaut, R., et al. 2001. ARTEMIS, a novel DNA double-strand break repair/V(D)J recombination protein is mutated in Human Severe Combined Immune Deficiency with increased radiosensitivity (RS-SCID). *Cell*, **105**, 177–86.

Moshous, D., Pannetier, C., et al. 2003. Partial T and B lymphocyte immunodeficiency and predisposition to lymphoma in patients with hypomorphic mutations in Artemis. *J Clin Invest*, **111**, 381–7.

Nagamine, K., Peterson, P., et al. 1997. Positional cloning of the APECED gene. *Nat Genet*, **17**, 393–8.

Nagarajan, U.M., Louis-Plence, P., et al. 1999. RFX-B is the gene responsible for the most common cause of the bare lymphocyte syndrome, an MHC class II immunodeficiency. *Immunity*, **10**, 153–62.

Nauseef, W.M. 1990. Myeloperoxidase deficiency. *Hematol Pathol*, **4**, 165–78.

Nekrep, N., Jabrane-Ferrat, N., et al. 2002. Mutation in a winged-helix DNA-binding motif causes atypical bare lymphocyte syndrome. *Nat Immunol*, **3**, 1075–81.

Newport, M.J., Huxley, C.M., et al. 1996. A mutation in the interferon-gamma-receptor gene and susceptibility to mycobacterial infection. *N Engl J Med*, **335**, 1941–9.

Notarangelo, L.D. and Hayward, A.R. 2000. X-linked immunodeficiency with hyper-IgM (XHIM). *Clin Exp Immunol*, **120**, 399–405.

Nunoi, H., Yamazaki, T., et al. 1999. A heterozygous mutation of beta-actin associated with neutrophil dysfunction and recurrent infection. *Proc Natl Acad Sci USA*, **96**, 8693–8.

O'Driscoll, M., Cerosaletti, K.M., et al. 2001. DNA ligase IV mutations identified in patients exhibiting developmental delay and immunodeficiency. *Mol Cell*, **8**, 1175–85.

Ochs, H. and Rosen, F.S. 1998. The Wiskott Aldrich syndrome. In: Ochs, H.O., Smith, C.I.E. and Puck, J.M. (eds), *Primary immunodeficiency diseases*. New York: Oxford Press, 292–305.

Ottenhoff, T.H., Verreck, F.A., et al. 2002. Genetics, cytokines and human infectious disease: lessons from weakly pathogenic mycobacteria and salmonellae. *Nat Genet*, **32**, 97–105.

Oxelius, V.A., Laurell, A.B., et al. 1981. IgG subclasses in selective IgA deficiency: importance of IgG2-IgA deficiency. *N Engl J Med*, **304**, 1476–7.

Parolini, O., Ressmann, G., et al. 1998. X-linked Wiskott–Aldrich syndrome in a girl. *N Engl J Med*, **338**, 291–5.

Perez, E. and Sullivan, K.E. 2002. Chromosome 22q11.2 deletion syndrome (DiGeorge and velocardiofacial syndromes). *Curr Opin Pediatr*, **14**, 678–83.

Perez-Aciego, P., Alarcon, B., et al. 1991. Expression and function of a variant T cell receptor complex lacking CD3-gamma. *J Exp Med*, **174**, 319–26.

Petersen-Mahrt, S.K., Harris, R.S. and Neuberger, M.S. 2002. AID mutates *E. coli* suggesting a DNA deamination mechanism for antibody diversification. *Nature*, **418**, 99–103.

Pierre-Audigier, C., Jouanguy, E., et al. 1997. Fatal disseminated *Mycobacterium smegmatis* infection in a child with inherited interferon gamma receptor deficiency. *Clin Infect Dis*, **24**, 982–4.

Poltorak, A., He, X., et al. 1998. Defective LPS signaling in C3H/HeJ and C57BL/10ScCr mice: mutations in Tlr4 gene. *Science*, **282**, 2085–8.

Ponnuraj, E.M. and Hayward, A.R. 2002. Requirement for TNF-Tnfrsf1 signalling for sclerosing cholangitis in mice chronically infected by *Cryptosporidium parvum*. *Clin Exp Immunol*, **128**, 416–20.

Putsep, K., Carlsson, G., et al. 2002. Deficiency of antibacterial peptides in patients with morbus Kostmann: an observation study. *Lancet*, **360**, 1144–9.

Quartier, P., Debre, M., et al. 1999. Early and prolonged intravenous immunoglobulin replacement therapy in childhood agammaglobulinemia: a retrospective survey of 31 patients. *J Pediatr*, **134**, 589–96.

Ramoz, N., Rueda, L.A., et al. 1999. A susceptibility locus for epidermodysplasia verruciformis, an abnormal predisposition to infection with the oncogenic human papillomavirus type 5, maps to chromosome 17qter in a region containing a psoriasis locus. *J Invest Dermatol*, **112**, 259–63.

Ramoz, N., Rueda, L.A., et al. 2002. Mutations in two adjacent novel genes are associated with epidermodysplasia verruciformis. *Nat Genet*, **32**, 579–81.

Rawlings, D.J., Saffran, D.C., et al. 1993. Mutation of unique region of Bruton's tyrosine kinase in immunodeficient XID mice. *Science*, **261**, 358–61.

Reeves, E.P., Lu, H., et al. 2002. Killing activity of neutrophils is mediated through activation of proteases by K^+ flux. *Nature*, **416**, 291–7.

Remold-O'Donnell, E., Rosen, F.S. and Kenney, D.M. 1996. Defects in Wiskott–Aldrich syndrome blood cells. *Blood*, **87**, 2621–31.

Revy, P., Muto, T., et al. 2000. Activation-induced cytidine deaminase (AID) deficiency causes the autosomal recessive form of the Hyper-IgM syndrome (HIGM2). *Cell*, **102**, 565–75.

Ridanpaa, M., Van Eenennaam, H., et al. 2001. Mutations in the RNA component of RNase MRP cause a pleiotropic human disease, cartilage-hair hypoplasia. *Cell*, **104**, 195–203.

Savitsky, K., Bar-Shira, A., et al. 1995. A single ataxia telangiectasia gene with a product similar to PI-3 kinase. *Science*, **268**, 1749–53.

Schinke, M. and Izumo, S. 2001. Deconstructing DiGeorge syndrome. *Nat Genet*, **27**, 238–40.

Schroeder, H.W. Jr., Zhu, Z.B., et al. 1998. Susceptibility locus for IgA deficiency and common variable immunodeficiency in the HLA-DR3, -B8, -A1 haplotypes. *Mol Med*, **4**, 72–86.

Schwarz, K., Gauss, G.H., et al. 1996. RAG mutations in human B cell-negative SCID. *Science*, **274**, 97–9.

Segal, B.H., Leto, T.L., et al. 2000. Genetic, biochemical, and clinical features of chronic granulomatous disease. *Medicine (Balt)*, **79**, 170–200.

Sharfe, N., Dadi, H.K., et al. 1997. Human immune disorder arising from mutation of the alpha chain of the interleukin-2 receptor. *Proc Natl Acad Sci USA*, **94**, 3168–71.

Shiloh, Y. 1997. Ataxia-telangiectasia and the Nijmegen breakage syndrome: related disorders but genes apart. *Annu Rev Genet*, **31**, 635–62.

Shiloh, Y. and Kastan, M.B. 2001. ATM: genome stability, neuronal development, and cancer cross paths. *Adv Cancer Res*, **83**, 209–54.

Smith, C.I.E. and Witte, O.N. 1998. X-linked agammaglobulinemia: a disease of Btk tyrosine kinase. In: Ochs, H.O., Smith, C.I.E. and Puck, J.M. (eds), *Primary immunodeficiency diseases*. New York: Oxford University Press, 263–84.

Smith, D.K., Neal, J.J. and Holmberg, S.D. 1993. Unexplained opportunistic infections and CD4+ T-lymphocytopenia without HIV infection. An investigation of cases in the United States. The Centers for Disease Control Idiopathic CD4+ T-lymphocytopenia Task Force. *N Engl J Med*, **328**, 373–9.

Soudais, C., De Villartay, J.P., et al. 1993. Independent mutations of the human CD3-epsilon gene resulting in a T cell receptor/CD3 complex immunodeficiency. *Nat Genet*, **3**, 77–81.

Steimle, V., Otten, L.A., et al. 1993. Complementation cloning of an MHC class II transactivator mutated in hereditary MHC class II deficiency (or bare lymphocyte syndrome). *Cell*, **75**, 135–46.

Steimle, V., Durand, B., et al. 1995. A novel DNA-binding regulatory factor is mutated in primary MHC class II deficiency (bare lymphocyte syndrome). *Genes Dev*, **9**, 1021–32.

Stephan, J.L., Vlekova, V., et al. 1993. Severe combined immunodeficiency: a retrospective single-center study of clinical presentation and outcome in 117 patients. *J Pediatr*, **123**, 564–72.

Stepp, S.E., Dufourcq-Lagelouse, R., et al. 1999. Perforin gene defects in familial hemophagocytic lymphohistiocytosis. *Science*, **286**, 1957–9.

Stewart, G.S., Maser, R.S., et al. 1999. The DNA double-strand break repair gene hMRE11 is mutated in individuals with an ataxia-telangiectasia-like disorder. *Cell*, **99**, 577–87.

Stinchcombe, J.C., Bossi, G., et al. 2001. The immunological synapse of CTL contains a secretory domain and membrane bridges. *Immunity*, **15**, 751–61.

Sugamura, K., Asao, H., et al. 1995. The common gamma-chain for multiple cytokine receptors. *Adv Immunol*, **59**, 225–77.

Summerfield, J.A., Ryder, S., et al. 1995. Mannose binding protein gene mutations associated with unusual and severe infections in adults. *Lancet*, **345**, 886–9.

Tidow, N., Pilz, C., et al. 1997. Clinical relevance of point mutations in the cytoplasmic domain of the granulocyte colony-stimulating factor receptor gene in patients with severe congenital neutropenia. *Blood*, **89**, 2369–75.

Toomes, C., James, J., et al. 1999. Loss-of-function mutations in the cathepsin C gene result in periodontal disease and palmoplantar keratosis. *Nat Genet*, **23**, 421–4.

Tsukada, S., Saffran, D.C., et al. 1993. Deficient expression of a B cell cytoplasmic tyrosine kinase in human X-linked agammaglobulinemia. *Cell*, **72**, 279–90.

Varon, R., Vissinga, C., et al. 1998. Nibrin, a novel DNA double-strand break repair protein, is mutated in Nijmegen breakage syndrome. *Cell*, **93**, 467–76, in process citation.

Vetrie, D., Vorechovsky, I., et al. 1993. The gene involved in X-linked agammaglobulinaemia is a member of the src family of protein-tyrosine kinases. *Nature*, **361**, 226–33.

Villa, A., Santagata, S., et al. 1998. Partial V(D)J recombination activity leads to Omenn syndrome. *Cell*, **93**, 885–96.

Villard, J., Masternak, K., et al. 2001. MHC class II deficiency: a disease of gene regulation. *Medicine (Balt)*, **80**, 405–18.

Vorechovsky, I., Webster, A.D., et al. 1999. Genetic linkage of IgA deficiency to the major histocompatibility complex: evidence for allele segregation distortion, parent-of-origin penetrance differences, and the role of anti-IgA antibodies in disease predisposition. *Am J Hum Genet*, **64**, 1096–109.

Vorechovsky, I., Cullen, M., et al. 2000. Fine mapping of IGAD1 in IgA deficiency and common variable immunodeficiency: identification and characterization of haplotypes shared by affected members of 101 multiple-case families. *J Immunol*, **164**, 4408–16.

Walport, M.J. 2001a. Complement. I. *N Engl J Med*, **344**, 1058–66.

Walport, M.J. 2001b. Complement. II. *N Engl J Med*, **344**, 1140–4.

Warnatz, K., Denz, A., et al. 2002. Severe deficiency of switched memory B cells (CD27(+)IgM(−)IgD(−)) in subgroups of patients with common variable immunodeficiency: a new approach to classify a heterogeneous disease. *Blood*, **99**, 1544–51.

Weemaes, C.M., Hustinx, T.W., et al. 1981. A new chromosomal instability disorder: the Nijmegen breakage syndrome. *Acta Paediatr Scand*, **70**, 557–64.

Williams, D.A., Tao, W., et al. 2000. Dominant negative mutation of the hematopoietic-specific Rho GTPase, Rac2, is associated with a human phagocyte immunodeficiency. *Blood*, **96**, 1646–54.

Wilson, D.I., Cross, I.E., et al. 1992. A prospective cytogenetic study of 36 cases of DiGeorge syndrome. *Am J Hum Genet*, **51**, 957–63.

Winkelstein, J.A., Marino, M.C., et al. 2000. Chronic granulomatous disease. Report on a national registry of 368 patients. *Medicine (Balt)*, **79**, 155–69.

Wiszniewski, W., Fondaneche, M.C., et al. 2001. Mutation in the class II trans-activator leading to a mild immunodeficiency. *J Immunol*, **167**, 1787–94.

Wood, P.M., Mayne, A., et al. 2001. A mutation in Bruton's tyrosine kinase as a cause of selective anti-polysaccharide antibody deficiency. *J Pediatr*, **139**, 148–51.

Xu, G.L., Bestor, T.H., et al. 1999. Chromosome instability and immunodeficiency syndrome caused by mutations in a DNA methyltransferase gene. *Nature*, **402**, 187–91.

Yel, L., Minegishi, Y., et al. 1996. Mutations in the mu heavy-chain gene in patients with agammaglobulinemia. *N Engl J Med*, **335**, 1486–93.

Zonana, J., Elder, M.E., et al. 2000. A novel X-linked disorder of immune deficiency and hypohidrotic ectodermal dysplasia is allelic to incontinentia pigmenti and due to mutations in IKK-gamma (NEMO). *Am J Hum Genet*, **67**, 1555–62.

39

Acquired immunodeficiencies

RALF IGNATIUS AND THOMAS SCHNEIDER

INTRODUCTION

Acquired immunodeficiency represents an emerging medical challenge, the major medical causes of which are summarized in Table 39.1. In contrast to primary immune deficiencies, which are rare and at constant numbers over the last decades, the numbers of patients with acquired immunodeficiency are dramatically increasing. This is the result not only of the pandemic spread of the human immunodeficiency virus (HIV) (Clinton 2003) but also of rising numbers of patients on immunosuppressive therapy or who have diabetes, leukemia, Hodgkin's disease, or rheumatic disorders, or who are alcohol abusers (Murray and Lopez 1997; Singer and McCune 1999; Mossad et al. 2001; Simon and Fleischhack 2001; Messingham et al. 2002). In addition, older age is a well-known condition of acquired immunodeficiency (immunosenescence), and the numbers of older individuals have been continuously increasing in developed countries (Gavazzi and Krause 2002). In some regions of the world, e.g. Australia, the increasing ultraviolet radiation may also exert immunosuppressive effects (Staples et al. 2003).

Importantly, malnutrition of children in developing countries is still an unsolved problem, leading in these children to immunodeficiency, which considerably increases their susceptibility to the leading infectious causes of death world wide: enteric and pulmonary infections (reviewed by Bhaskaram 2002). It may come as a surprise to many that malnutrition in childhood is less often the result of lack of food than of the enormous burden of infectious diseases, notably diarrheal diseases, that commonly afflicts children in the developing world. Infective diarrhea reduces food intake and increases the loss of important nutrients from the body. After a single infection the child can recover rapidly and may suffer from only a brief period of accelerated height and weight velocity called 'catch-up' growth. In the developing world, however, repetitive episodes of diarrhea are often seen in children, thus greatly impairing their chances of regaining lost growth. The accumulative effect of such episodes greatly influences the growth and mental development of these children, and at the same time also has a profound impact on their immunological defense mechanisms (reviewed by Keusch 1982, 2003).

In addition to the aforementioned causes for acquired immunodeficiency, phases of immunosuppression may also occur in the context of various infectious diseases. Infections with HIV, human T-cell lymphotropic virus 1 (HTLV-1), and measles virus all induce suppression of cellular immune responses, leading to clinically apparent secondary infections and/or tumors. These diseases are of varying epidemiological importance. The horrendous spread of the HIV-1 pandemic is well recognized and the World Health Organization (WHO) has estimated that there were 40 million infections worldwide at the end of 2001, whereas HTLV-1 infection possesses rather regional interest. Sadly, despite the opportunity to prevent measles through effective immunization, about 1.1 million children died in 1990, mostly in developing countries, from measles-related events (Murray and Lopez 1997), and in 1999 the number of deaths caused by measles was estimated as 700 000 (Duke and Mgone 2003). In most cases, secondary infections, such as bacterial pneumonia, often combined with malnutrition, but not measles itself, were the cause of death (reviewed in Schneider-Schaulies and ter Meulen 2002).

Table 39.1 *Causes of acquired immunodeficiency*

Disease	Suspected immune defect	Frequent infectious diseases
Infection		
HIV	Loss of $CD4^+$ T cells, MHC I downregulation	PCP, toxoplasmosis, CMV infections, microsporidiosis, and others
HTLV-1	Impaired T- and B-cell function	Strongyloidiasis, cryptococal meningitis, PCP
Measles	Transient lymphopenia, transient reduced Th1 response	Bacterial pneumonia, otitis media, sinusitis
Neoplasms		
Hodgkin's disease	Impaired T-cell function	Infections with intracellular bacteria: TBC, listeriosis, salmonellosis
Multiple myeloma	Hypogammaglobulinemia	Bacterial pneumonia and meningitis
Chronic lymphocytic leukemia	Hypogammaglobulinemia	Bacterial pneumonia and meningitis
Acute myelocytic or lymphocytic leukemia	Granulocytopenia	Infections with extracellular gram-positive and gram-negative bacteria, fungal infections
Other conditions		
Diabetes	Impaired cell-mediated immunity and phagocyte function	Fungal infections (candidiasis, mucormycosis), urinary tract and soft tissue infections
Alcoholism	Impaired cell-mediated immunity and phagocyte function	TBC, soft tissue infections, osteomyelitis
Old age (elderly)	Impaired T- and B-cell function	Bacterial pneumonia, TBC, urinary tract and soft tissue infections, viral diarrhea, *Clostridium difficile* toxin-induced colitis
Splenectomy[a]	Reduced immune response against bacteria	Bacterial pneumonia, bacterial meningitis, babesiosis
Iatrogen (therapy-induced immune suppression)		
Drugs frequently used in autoimmune diseases		
Glucocorticoids	Impaired monocyte and T-cell activation	Fungal infection, bacterial pneumonia
Cyclophosphamide[b]	Reduces antigen driven T- and B-cell response	Bacterial and fungal infection, PCP, CMV infections
Methotrexate[b]	Inhibition of antibody production, lymphopenia, monocytopenia	Bacterial and fungal infection, PCP, CMV infections
Anti-TNF-α[c]	Suppression of inflammatory response, reduces granulocyte and macrophage activation	Reactivation of TBC, bacterial and fungal infections
Drugs frequently used in organ transplant recipients		
Ciclosporine, FK-506 (tacrolimus), rapamycin	Inhibition of T-cell activation (inhibition of IL-2 gene activation)	Reactivated viral infections (especially herpesvirus group), infections with respiratory syncytial virus, adenovirus, and parvovirus B19
Azathioprine	Inhibition of antibody production, lymphopenia, monocytopenia	Bacterial and fungal infections
Anti-CD3, anti-CD4, anti-IL2	Inhibition of T-cell activation	PCP, reactivated viral infections (especially herpesvirus group), infections with respiratory syncytial virus, adenovirus, and parvovirus B19
Drugs and methods frequently used in tumor therapy		
Cytostatic therapy	Reducing the number of B cells, T cells, macrophages, and granulocytes	CMV infections, progressive multifocal leukencephalitis (JC virus infection), PCP
Radiation	Suppression of number and function of T and B cells	CMV infections, progressive multifocal leukencephalitis (JC virus infection), PCP

CMV, cytomegalovirus; IL, interleukin; MHC, major histocompatibility complex; PCP, *Pneumocystis carinii* pneumonia; TBC, tuberculosis; TNF, tumor necrosis factor.

a) If splenectomy can be planned patients should receive haemophilus, meningococcal, and pneumococcal immunization before.

b) Patients who are treated with this immunosuppressive drug (either cyclophosphamide or methotrexate) in combination with glucocorticoids should receive trimethoprim–sulfamethoxazole as prophylaxis against PCP.

c) Patients with positive tuberculin test or TBC in their history treated with anti- TNF-α should receive isoniazid as prophylaxis against TBC reactivation.

The scope of this chapter is to concentrate on these three viral infections which have various similarities but also significant differences with respect to their effects on cellular immune functions. Importantly, HIV and HTLV-1 are retroviruses and integrate via a provirus in the human genome; thereby they can persist and potentially cause life-long damage to the immune system. In contrast, effective immune responses are usually induced against measles virus; these lead to viral clearance, and immunosuppression lasts for only a limited period of time.

HIV INFECTION

The virus

In 1983 scientists from the Pasteur Institute in Paris recovered the causal agent of acquired immune deficiency syndrome (AIDS) from lymph nodes of an asymptomatic individual with generalized lymphadenopathy (Barré-Sinoussi et al. 1983). This new retrovirus was finally named HIV-1. HIV-1 belongs to the lentiviruses in the taxonomic classification of retroviruses (Gelderblom et al. 1985). The lentiviruses are complex spherical viruses characterized by a unique virion morphology with cylindrical or conical cores (Gelderblom et al. 1987). The proviral genome of HIV-1 encodes *gag*, *pol*, and *env* genes characteristic of all known retroviruses. Both ends of the proviral genome are flanked by noncoding direct-repeat sequences called long terminal repeats (LTR). LTRs mediate proviral integration and contain *cis*-acting regulatory elements important for viral transcription, viral mRNA processing, and reverse transcription. The LTRs of HIV-1 also contain the binding site for NF-κB, which is present in the nuclei of activated human T lymphocytes and can stimulate both basal and Tat-induced levels of HIV-1 replication (Nabel and Baltimore 1987). The genome structure of human pathogenic retroviruses is more complex than that of other retroviruses, containing several additional open reading frames encoding for nonstructural regulatory or accessory proteins. Some of these viral proteins may contribute to immunosuppression.

Tat is an indispensable viral protein, which increases the steady-state levels of viral RNA by a multiplication factor of around several hundred (Dayton et al. 1986). Tat seems to be involved in T-cell activation that results in an increased viral transcription in two ways: increasing the concentration of cellular factors CDK9 and cyclin T1 for Tat activation and increasing the activation of NF-κB. Tat may also inhibit antigen-induced, but not mitogen-induced, proliferation of peripheral blood mononuclear cells (PBMC) and therefore play a role in immunosuppression (Viscidi et al. 1989).

Nef seems to have a positive influence on the progression to AIDS in vivo (Kestler et al. 1991). It may ensure survival of HIV-1 through distinct mechanisms of immune evasion and antiapoptosis (for a review, see Fackler and Baur 2002). In vitro, several functions of Nef have been described:

- Nef downregulates the cell surface expression of CD4 (Garcia and Miller 1991). Studies with HIV-Nef mutants in severe combined immunodeficiency (SCID) mice implanted with human fetal thymus revealed that the functional domain that is required for CD4 downregulation correlates with Nef-mediated enhancement of viral pathogenesis (Stoddart et al. 2003). The ability of Nef to downregulate CD4 may influence the function of T-helper cells and contribute to acquired immunosuppression of HIV-infected patients.
- Nef downregulates the cell surface expression of major histocompatibility complex (MHC) class I molecules (Schwartz et al. 1996). This MHC I downregulation may limit the ability of cytotoxic T lymphocytes (CTL) to recognize and eliminate HIV-infected cells and may be one way that the virus escapes the host's immune response (Collins et al. 1998). More sophisticated Nef selectively downregulates certain MHC I molecules, avoiding downregulation of those (HLA-C and HLA-E), that would induce attack by natural killer (NK) cells (Cohen et al. 1999).
- One important function of Nef may be the activation of lymphocytes (Luo and Peterlin 1997). A natural occurring mutant simian immunodeficiency virus (SIV) nef allele induces extensive T-cell activation and proliferation (Du et al. 1995). This mutant is only an arginine-to-tyrosine mutation in the *nef* gene, which results in a sequence reminiscent of an immunoreceptor tyrosine-based activation motif (ITAM). Such motifs in the cytoplasmic tails of T- and B-cell receptors are essential for lymphocyte activation. The SIV *nef* mutant seems to activate T-cell signaling (Luo and Peterlin 1997). Macaques infected with this SIV strain rapidly develop a fatal disease, leading to the death of the animals because of severe gastrointestinal symptoms (Du et al. 1995). Nef expression in macrophages induces expression and secretion of the chemokines macrophage inflammatory protein (MIP) MIP-1α and MIP-1β, which are capable of activating lymphocytes (Swingler et al. 1999).

Natural course of HIV infection

The course of HIV-1 infection is usually divided into three phases: (1) the primary HIV-1 infection, (2) the chronic asymptomatic phase and (3) AIDS; the individual pattern and course of the disease may, however, be highly variable.

THE PRIMARY HIV-1 INFECTION

Primary HIV-1 infection (PHI) is rarely diagnosed and represents a self-limited disease. However, recognition of this early phase of HIV-1 infection is important for two major reasons. First, the severity of PHI predicts progression to AIDS; it is therefore thought that treatment of PHI may prevent or retard progression to AIDS. Second, from the public health perspective the diagnosis of PHI is important because these patients are highly infectious and early diagnosis will prevent the spread of disease to the patients' sexual partners. The severity of symptoms during PHI is highly variable; about 12 percent of seroconverting patients are hospitalized (for a review, see Apoola et al. 2002).

At the beginning of PHI, patients are usually seronegative for anti-HIV antibodies; the p24 antigen-capture assay and polymerase chain reaction (PCR) for the HIV genome are positive. Viremia levels reach extremely high values, and high titers of infectious virus can be isolated from the blood. During the first 5–10 days of PHI, the patients show a characteristic lymphopenia which affects both $CD4^+$ and $CD8^+$ T cells. In this phase, $CD4^+$ T cells may drop to levels as low as those observed in AIDS, and in vitro tests of both B and T cells show impairment. Nevertheless opportunistic infections in this short period are rare (for a review, see Apoola et al. 2002).

During PHI the virus spreads to several organs of the body including the lymph nodes, central nervous system, skin, and mucosa. Therefore, patients with PHI may present variable symptoms. Cutaneous manifestations are frequent and include the classic maculopapular rash or ulcers, which may occur at genital, oral, and esophageal mucosae (Cooper et al. 1985; Schacker et al. 1996). Ulcerations in other parts of the gastrointestinal mucosa are more rarely observed. A common feature of PHI is the so-called 'mononucleosis-like illness', which is characterized by fever, pharyngitis, arthralgia, myalgia, and lymphadenopathy (for a review, see Apoola et al. 2002).

THE CHRONIC ASYMPTOMATIC PHASE

The primary HIV-1 infection is followed by a long-lasting phase of clinical latency of about 8–12 years with a median time of 9.8 years (Bacchetti and Moss 1989). However, 10–20 percent of HIV-infected individuals progress more rapidly to the final stage of the disease in about 5 years (Phair et al. 1992). This group is called 'rapid progressors'. At the other extreme, 5–15 percent of HIV-infected people, called 'slow progressors', will remain in this stage of the disease for about 15 years (Sheppard et al. 1993). This wide variability of the natural course of the disease implicates different driving forces, including genetic factors of the host as well as virological factors (Fauci 1996). In this chronic phase of HIV infection no symptoms are present. Virus replication and $CD4^+$ T cells remain relatively stable during this time. Virus replication and the accumulation of virus trapped by follicular dendritic cells occur in lymph nodes, however, where a progressive structural and functional deterioration takes place, resulting in an impairment of specific immune response over time (Pantaleo et al. 1993). Finally, there is steady decrease of $CD4^+$ T cells with an increasing risk of developing infections (Figure 39.1). Acquiring an AIDS-defining opportunistic infection leads to the transfer to the end-stage of the disease.

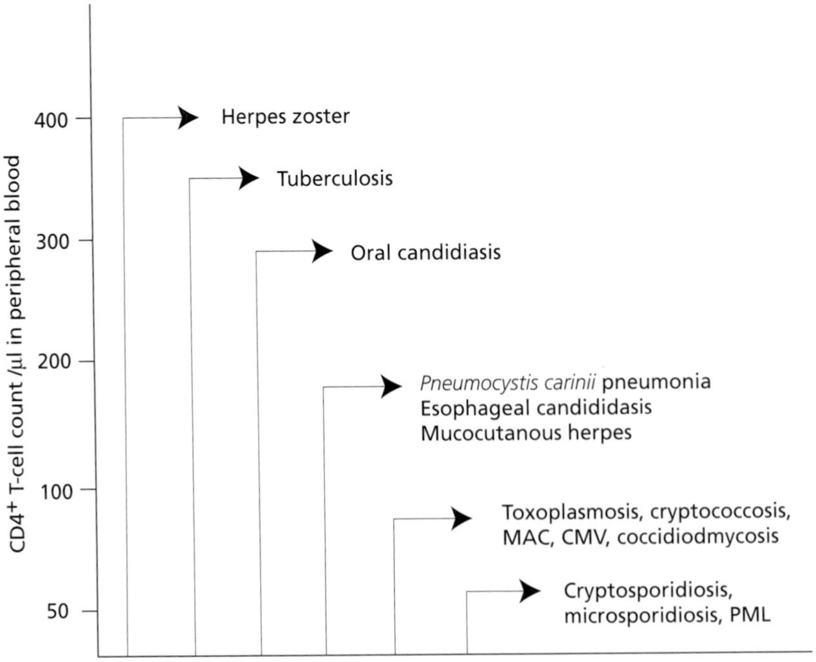

Figure 39.1 *Association between opportunistic infections and $CD4^+$ T-cell count. CMV, cytomegalovirus; MAC,* Mycobacterium avium *complex; PML, progressive multifocal leukoencephalopathy.*

AIDS

AIDS defines the end-stage of HIV-1 infection. Before the introduction of highly active antiretroviral therapy (HAART), this phase of the disease leads to death within 1–2 years (Bacchetti et al. 1988). The major causes of death are opportunistic infections resulting from a breakdown of the immune system. The hallmark of the disease is a steady decline in the number of $CD4^+$ T cells, which correlates with an increasing number of certain opportunistic infections (Figure 39.1). Fortunately, the introduction of HAART has significantly decreased morbidity and mortality of HIV-1 infection (Palella et al. 1998).

Immune dysfunctions

$CD4^+$ T LYMPHOCYTES

The progressive loss of peripheral $CD4^+$ T lymphocytes is a hallmark of HIV infection, coinciding with the failure of the immune control toward a variety of infectious pathogens including HIV-1 itself. The underlying mechanisms, however, are still a matter of controversial debate. The increased proliferation and loss of CD4 cells were interpreted as the death of virally infected cells being succeeded by a homeostatic proliferation of new T cells (Ho et al. 1995; Wei et al. 1995). Nevertheless, these conclusions have been questioned based on the observations that (1) relatively small numbers of T cells are actually productively or latently infected in vivo (Haase 1999), (2) significant numbers of uninfected cells apparently die (Finkel et al. 1995), and (3) the decline of CD4 cells in the peripheral blood is not necessarily paralleled by similar changes in the lymphoid tissues (Rosok et al. 1996). As a result, a different scenario was proposed where a general activation of the immune system leads to dysregulated homeostatic processes.

Different T-cell labeling techniques in vivo and mathematical models have been applied to investigate whether the T-cell proliferation is the immunological response to previous T-cell death, or whether cell death is the result of previous activation and proliferation, and T-cell loss is exclusively caused by continuous destruction or additional to impaired production (Douek et al. 2003). The data, however, are inconclusive, indicating complex processes influenced by various host and viral factors, e.g. CD4 T-cell dysfunctions, viral cytopathicity, cytotoxicity, apoptosis, activation-induced cell death (AICD), altered T-cell migration patterns, and impaired T-cell production.

$CD4^+$ T-cell dysfunction

Cytokine production by $CD4^+$ T cells is profoundly perturbed in HIV-1 infection leading to qualitatively and quantitatively different cytokine secretion patterns (see section on Cytokines). In addition, proliferation to alloantigens, e.g. tetanus toxoid and purified protein derivative, and importantly also to HIV antigens is decreased, which is the result of a progressive loss of memory CD4 T cells (Miedema et al. 1988; Clerici et al. 1989; Meyaard et al. 1994). In fact, HIV-specific $CD4^+$ T cells in the peripheral blood are easier to detect by intracellular cytokine staining than by proliferation (Pitcher et al. 1999). The reduced responsiveness of $CD4^+$ T cells in HIV-1 infection correlates with a decreased expression of CD28 and CD40 ligand (Borthwick et al. 1994; Chirmule et al. 1995), as well as changes in the $CD4^+$ T-cell receptor repertoire (Connors et al. 1997; Gea-Banacloche et al. 1998). Notably, patients with long-term non-progressing (LTNP) disease exhibit strong antigen-specific proliferative responses (Rosenberg et al. 1997).

Cytopathicity

HIV-1 preferentially infects rapidly expanding, activated, naïve (HIV-1 specific) CD4 T cells (Douek et al. 2002), and kills the cells by apoptosis independently of the expression of Fas (Gandhi et al. 1998), although necrotic cell death of HIV-1-infected T cells has recently been reported (Lenardo et al. 2002). Additional cytopathic effects involving viral gp120 and CD4 can lead to giant cells (syncytia) that can contain uninfected T cells (Lifson et al. 1986; Sodroski et al. 1986). In vivo this mechanism may be of less importance except for the central nervous system where giant cell formation is more frequently seen in the context of HIV-1 infection (Williams and Hickey 2002). Although viral burden in lymphoid tissue is greater than in peripheral blood where only small numbers of infected cells are usually seen, virus-mediated killing alone most probably does not account for the decline of peripheral CD4 T cells and the development of AIDS.

Cytotoxicity

Death of HIV-infected cells may also be caused by cytotoxic immune responses. There is an early and strong induction of HIV-1-specific CTL responses, and antibody-dependent cellular cytotoxicity (ADCC) may contribute to the reduction of HIV-1 infected cells. Nevertheless, as most of these immune responses are also, at least to some extent, impaired in chronic HIV-1 infection, they most probably do not primarily drive the depletion of $CD4^+$ T cells. Interestingly, lysis of uninfected $CD4^+$ T cells by $\gamma\delta$ T cells has recently been described, thus suggesting a role for this subset in the CD4 T-cell decline in HIV-1 patients (Sindhu et al. 2003).

Apoptosis

In vitro, T cells from HIV-1 infected individuals die of spontaneous apoptosis, which is further enhanced on stimulation (Groux et al. 1992; Meyaard et al. 1992), whereas spontaneous T-cell apoptosis is reduced in cells from LTNPs (Liegler et al. 1998). In vivo, apoptosis of infected, and to a greater extent of uninfected, bystander CD4 T cells has been noted (Finkel et al. 1995) and attributed to direct, e.g. virus-induced apoptosis of infected cells, and indirect, e.g. macrophage-mediated, apoptosis of uninfected CD4 T cells (Herbein et al. 1998).

Fas (CD95) expression on T cells from HIV-1-infected individuals is increased and its ligation induces apoptosis (Kobayashi et al. 1990; Katsikis et al. 1995). After the interaction of Nef with the T-cell receptor ζ chain, HIV also induces Fas ligand expression on T cells (Xu et al. 1999), whereas Fas ligand expression is increased on macrophages in the lymphoid tissue from HIV patients (Dockrell et al. 1998). Apoptosis of uninfected T cells can occur on interaction with Fas and secretion of tumor necrosis factor (TNF) α (Badley et al. 1997).

Moreover, cross-linking of CD4 with gp120 efficiently primes CD4 T cells for Fas-mediated apoptosis (Banda et al. 1992). Monocytes can bind immune-complexed gp120 via CD16, and thereby interact with CD4 on T cells and induce Fas-dependent apoptosis (Orlikowsky et al. 1997; Oyaizu et al. 1997). Importantly, various HIV proteins, e.g. Nef and Vpu, can downregulate CD4, thus avoiding death of infected $CD4^+$ T cells through this mechanism (Willey et al. 1992; Salghetti et al. 1995). Fas-independent mechanisms might contribute to accelerated T-cell apoptosis (Badley et al. 2000; Gougeon 2003). Thus, increased apoptosis of uninfected (and infected) T cells may critically add to the HIV-induced immunopathogenesis. Regulation of apoptosis in HIV-1 infection seems, however, to be complex, because various HIV gene products have been attributed to pro- as well as antiapoptotic functions (Badley et al. 2000; Gougeon 2003).

Activation-induced cell death

There is increasing evidence for a critical role of activation of the immune system and the induction of T-cell proliferation and, as its physiological consequence, AICD of uninfected cells in the immunopathogenesis of HIV infection. A prerequisite for AICD is the interaction of Fas and its ligand, and the expression of both molecules is significantly increased in HIV-1 infection, as discussed above.

Studies in HIV-1 patients before and after antiretroviral therapy suggested that T-cell proliferation is mainly driven by immune activation, suggesting AICD as an additional mechanism of CD4 cell depletion besides virus-mediated killing (Hazenberg et al. 2000). This immune activation is primarily the result of antigenic stimulation by HIV-1 itself, as well as opportunistic infections (Orendi et al. 1998; Cohen Stuart et al. 2000), correlating both with apoptosis and better with disease progression than plasma viral burden (Gougeon et al. 1996; Giorgi et al. 1999). Consistent with these findings are data obtained from HIV-2 infected patients. Here, lower levels of T-cell activation and apoptosis correlate with a better clinical prognosis, whereas HIV-2 patients with a similar level of immune activation as seen in HIV-1 infection also suffer from CD4 T-cell depletion despite significantly lower viral loads (Michel et al. 2000; Sousa et al. 2002). Similarly, both rhesus macaques and sooty mangabeys develop high viremia after SIV infection, but, although the macaques ultimately succumb to simian AIDS, mangabeys do not develop immunodeficiency correlating with differences in cellular and humoral immune responses (Kaur et al. 1998). It is interesting that the numbers of $CD25^+CD4^+$ T lymphocytes (regulatory T cells?) increase in infected mangabeys, whereas this cell population declines in macaques. Finally, although chimpanzees can be infected with HIV-1 but rarely develop immunodeficiency, increased levels of apoptosis and immune hyperactivation were seen in two animals who did develop a progressive loss of $CD4^+$ T cells after HIV-1 infection (Davis et al. 1998). The critical impact of immune activation on T-cell homeostasis was recently demonstrated in a murine study using CD70 transgenic mice where severe T-cell depletion, induced by chronic activation of CD27, led to lethal *Pneumocystis carinii* infections (Tesselaar et al. 2003).

Reciprocally, in chronic HIV-1 infection, the activation of latently infected cells favors the local transmission of virus in the lymphoid tissue, thereby supporting the viral life cycle (Grossman et al. 1998).

Altered T-cell migration patterns

Exposure of resting $CD4^+$ T lymphocytes to HIV-1 upregulated the homing receptor CD62L (L-selectin) on the cellular surface, thereby supporting the migration of these cells to the lymphoid tissue of SCID mice (Wang et al. 1997). Interestingly, signaling through these homing receptors (but not through other surface molecules) led to apoptotic cell death of immigrated CD4 T cells (Wang et al. 1999). Likewise, reinfused $CD4^+$ blood T lymphocytes of HIV-1 patients rapidly migrated and homed to lymph nodes and bone marrow at increased levels (Chen et al. 2002). Therefore, HIV-induced alterations of T-cell migration and homing may add to the decline of peripheral CD4 T cells in HIV-1 infection.

Impaired T-cell production

Regenerative dysfunction or failure of the bone marrow is commonly seen in late-stage HIV-1 patients, leading to suppressed hemopoiesis. Its origin, however, is often multifactorial, i.e. besides HIV-1 infection itself, opportunistic infections and the application of myelosuppressive drugs may considerably contribute to this development (Moses et al. 1998). As infection of $CD34^+$ hemopoietic progenitor cells is apparently rather low,

HIV-1-induced alterations of bone marrow functions are mostly the result of infected auxiliary cells and perturbations of cytokine secretion. In addition, dysfunction of the thymus caused by HIV-1 infection has been attributed to impaired T-cell production (McCune 2001).

In summary, HIV-1-induced immune activation and changes in T-cell homeostasis most probably lead to increased T-cell proliferation to maintain sufficient numbers of infectable CD4 T cells at the principal sites of viral replication, i.e. the lymphoid tissues, followed by cell death of infected and uninfected cells. Various mechanisms appear to contribute synergistically to the development of $CD4^+$ T-cell immunodeficiency that is paralleled by the decline of these cells in the periphery. The impact of these mechanisms on HIV-1 immunopathogenesis may vary in different populations of infected individuals, e.g. neonates and adults.

$CD8^+$ T LYMPHOCYTES

Specific $CD8^+$ CTLs combat HIV-1 infection by both lysis of target cells via the granule exocytosis pathway and the secretion of β-chemokines, i.e. RANTES (regulated on activation, normal T cell expressed and secreted, CCL5), MIP-1α (CCL3), and MIP-1β (CCL4), which block viral entry at the site of the co-receptor (Gandhi and Walker 2002). Other crucial soluble mediators secreted by CTLs and involved in inhibition of viral replication include the interleukin (IL)-16 (Baier et al. 1995) (see section on Cytokines) and α-defensins (Zhang et al. 2002).

An effective viral strategy to avoid lysis of infected cells is the emergence of escape mutants where changes in the epitopes interfere with peptide binding to the MHC molecule, leading to unrecognized target cells (Johnson and Desrosiers 2002). In addition, the phenotype and function of $CD8^+$ T cells can be altered and impaired at multiple levels. More sensitive in vitro assays have been developed for better detection of antigen-specific interferon (IFN)-γ-secreting cells in the blood or lymphoid tissues, because monitoring of tetramer-positive, HIV-specific cells does not necessarily provide information on the functional status of the cells. On application of these methods, significant numbers of HIV-specific CTLs unable to produce IFN-γ indicated impaired cellular functions (Goepfert et al. 2000; Shankar et al. 2000), whereas opposing results were found by others (Appay et al. 2000; Goulder et al. 2000). Recent data suggest a better correlation between tetramer staining and IFN-γ secretion early after infection, compared with later stages of the infection (Kostense et al. 2002). In addition, the impaired cytolytic capacity of $CD8^+$ T cells has been related to significantly lower levels of perforin in CTLs in the blood and lymphoid tissues from HIV-1 patients (Andersson et al. 1999; Appay et al. 2000).

Defects in $CD8^+$ T-cell-mediated immune responses in HIV-1 infection have also been detected at the level of antigen presentation. The viral protein Nef can downmodulate MHC I molecules on infected cells, resulting in reduced peptide presentation and thereby protection against killing by CTLs (Schwartz et al. 1996; Collins et al. 1998). In addition, downmodulation of the CD3 ζ chain expression and decreased expression of the protein tyrosine kinases and the signal-transducing molecules Lck, Fyn, and ZAP-70 in peripheral CD8 cells from HIV-infected individuals contributes to impaired T-cell receptor (TCR) signaling and is associated with disease progression (Stefanova et al. 1996; Trimble and Lieberman 1998). At the same time, the co-stimulatory molecule CD28 is downregulated on these cells (Vingerhoets et al. 1995; Trimble et al. 2000).

Other phenotypic distinctions of HIV-1-specific CD8 T cells are a persistent CD27 expression suggesting impaired maturation of the cells (Appay et al. 2000), and an enhanced expression of the activation markers HLA-DR and CD38 (Giorgi et al. 1994). The expression of CD38 correlates with rapid CD4 depletion whereas the presence of $HLA\text{-}DR^+CD38^-$ cells is associated with a better disease prognosis. Of additional importance may be the expression of HLA-class I-specific inhibitory receptors (iNKR) (De Maria and Moretta 2000). Similar to NK cells, $CD8^+$ T lymphocytes can express molecules from different families of receptors that can downmodulate T-cell functions, e.g. cytolytic activity, upon MHC I binding. In HIV-1-infection, increased expression of killer cell Ig-like receptors (KIR), as well as receptors from the lectin-type CD94/NKG2 family, has been shown for $CD8^+$ T cells. These $CD8^+iNKR^+$ T cells may further contribute to the HIV-1-induced impairment of cellular immune functions by enhanced secretion of IL-4 and IL-5 (De Maria et al. 2000). Notably, $CD8^+$ T cells from LTNPs express similar levels of iNKR as $CD8^+$ T cells from uninfected controls (Costa et al. 2003).

$CD8^+$ T cell homeostatic defects in HIV-1 infection comprise alterations in migration, proliferation, and cell death. Effector CTLs accumulate at considerably lower numbers in lymphoid tissues, the sites of the predominant viral replication (Pantaleo et al. 1997), and these migratory defects could be caused by a reduced expression of homing receptors to lymphoid tissue, e.g. CCR7 (Chen et al. 2001). A high turnover of CTLs has been observed in HIV-1-infected individuals, ultimately leading to the decline of HIV-1-specific and -unspecific CD8 cells (Sachsenberg et al. 1998; Kovacs et al. 2001). Death of CTLs has been attributed to lymphocyte-reactive autoantibodies or apoptosis induced by FasL-expressing HIV-infected cells (Wang et al. 1998; Mueller et al. 2001). Remarkably, HIV-1-specific $CD57^+CD8^+$ T lymphocytes were unable to proliferate on antigenic stimulation, but died of activation-induced apoptotic death (Brenchley et al. 2003).

The loss of CD4 help caused by the decline of CD4 T cells in the course of the disease might have a significant impact on the failure of CD8-mediated HIV-1 control (Altfeld and Rosenberg 2000). HIV-1-specific proliferative responses correlate with levels of CTLs and inversely correlate with plasma viral load. In late stages of HIV-1 infection and in the absence of HIV-1-specific CD4 T cells, despite larger numbers of HIV-1-specific CTLs, the effector activity of these CTLs is markedly reduced (Spiegel et al. 2000). In vertically infected children, impaired CTL functions were seen in those with low CD4 counts but also in children younger than 3 years, indicating that the development of effective CD8 T-cell responses may take years (Sandberg et al. 2003). In summary, the data suggest considerably impaired (mainly HIV-1-specific) effector functions of $CD8^+$ T lymphocytes in HIV-1-infected individuals.

DENDRITIC CELLS

Dendritic cells (DC) can be subdivided into two phenotypically and functionally distinct populations, i.e. myeloid dendritic cells (mDC) and plasmacytoid dendritic cells (pDC). Myeloid DCs comprise most of the DC subsets characterized to date; potent antigen-presenting cells (APC) in the blood and peripheral tissues from where they migrate via the afferent lymphatics to the lymph nodes. In contrast, pDCs represent a unique cell population, able to secrete large amounts of type I interferons on stimulation and found only in the blood and lymphoid tissue, to which they migrate via the high endothelial venules. Both DC populations are of particular interest in the context of HIV-1 infection for their potent immunostimulatory capacities, although direct effects of HIV-1 on both subsets might significantly promote HIV-1-induced immunosuppression (Weissman and Fauci 1997; Siegal and Spear 2001; Frank and Pope 2002).

Myeloid DCs are probably the first cells that encounter HIV-1 during mucosal transmission of the virus (Steinman et al. 2003). Immature mDCs, such as Langerhans' cells (LC) in the epidermis, are located in the periphery directly under the epithelial layers and express the receptors required for viral entry, i.e. CD4 and chemokine receptors, at an immature state of differentiation, mainly CCR5 (Zaitseva et al. 1997). In addition, DC-SIGN (CD209), a recently identified C-type lectin receptor on the cell surface, can bind HIV-1 envelope glycoprotein gp120 and transfer the virus to T cells (Geijtenbeek et al. 2000). Its in vivo relevance remains controversial, however, because vaginal, but not rectal, epithelial mDCs are $CD209^-$ (Soilleux and Coleman 2001; Jameson et al. 2002), and, at least in the SIV macaque model, monocyte-derived DCs can transmit the virus independently of CD209 (Wu et al. 1999). Other lectins, such as langerin, might therefore primarily serve as HIV-1-binding sites on epithelial mDCs whereas emigrated DCs and pDCs may predominantly bind gp120 via CD4 (Turville et al. 2002). After binding and/or internalization of HIV-1, mDCs can hand over the virus to the $CD4^+$ T-lymphocyte compartment, thereby readily initiating viral replication in these cells either at the site of infection or in the draining lymph nodes. Viral replication in mDCs themselves is inhibited on maturation of the cells (Bakri et al. 2001). After the establishment of infection, only low numbers of infected mDCs, compared with $CD4^+$ T cells, can be found in the tissue and lymphoid organs (Steinman et al. 2003).

Although pDCs might significantly contribute to the early immune activation in HIV-1 infection, particularly through the secretion of IFN-α (Ferbas et al. 1994), they also co-express CD4 and various chemokine receptors (Penna et al. 2001), can be infected with HIV-1 in vitro (Patterson et al. 2001), and are therefore also possible targets of direct HIV-1 infection. Although the literature is controversial on this subject, both mDCs and pDCs may be impaired in numbers and/or functions in chronically HIV-1-infected individuals (Chehimi et al. 2002; Barron et al. 2003), and proviral DNA was recently detected in both mDC and pDC subsets in vivo (Donaghy et al. 2003). Thus, although both antigen-presenting mDCs and IFN-α-secreting pDCs are most probably involved in the innate and adaptive immune responses against HIV, dysfunctions of these cells may contribute to the immune suppression during HIV-1 infection, in particular in later stages of the disease.

MONOCYTES AND MACROPHAGES

Monocytes and macrophages express CD4 and, depending on their stage of differentiation, various chemokine receptors, and therefore serve as potential targets for HIV-1. Only low numbers (< 1 percent) of HIV-1-infected monocytes can be detected in the peripheral blood and bone marrow of HIV-1 patients (Kedzierska et al. 2003). Likewise, the in vitro infectibility of freshly isolated monocytes is limited and considerably less than in macrophages. In vitro culture and activation/differentiation of monocytes, however, allow a productive, yet noncytopathic, infection. There are conflicting data about whether macrophages contain increased amounts of HIV-1 as such compared with monocytes in HIV-1-infected patients. However, tissue macrophages can become a source of vigorous viral production in the context of opportunistic infections (Orenstein et al. 1997). Moreover, monocytes from HIV-1-infected patients produce high amounts of various proinflammatory cytokines, such as IL-1, IL-6, and TNF-α, which have been shown to promote replication of HIV-1 in vitro (Poli et al. 1990a, b).

A decline in chemotaxis and the in vitro survival of monocytes isolated from the peripheral blood of HIV-1 patients has been noted early (Smith et al. 1984; Muller et al. 1990b). Similarly, a decreased oxidative burst activity of monocytes and monocyte-derived macrophages was found (Muller et al. 1990a, b; Spear et al. 1990). Monocytes from HIV-1 patients also express fewer co-stimulatory molecules than cells from uninfected controls, coinciding with impaired T-cell-stimulatory capacity (Miedema et al. 1988; Dudhane et al. 1996). Recent flow cytometry studies from whole blood obtained from HIV-1-infected patients indicated an activated phenotype of monocytes in vivo (increased CD11b and decreased CD62L, L-selectin, expression, as well as increased actin polymerization), enhanced H_2O_2 production, and decreased expression of the adhesion molecules sialyl-Lewis X and CD31 related to the disease stage of the patients (Elbim et al. 1999; Pillet et al. 1999).

Phagocytosis of *Staphylococcus aureus* by monocytes from AIDS patients was decreased (Pos et al. 1992), and ADCC and cytotoxic activity, via CD4 against gp120/41-expressing cells by HIV-1-infected macrophages, and monocytes from HIV-1-infected individuals, were reduced (Baldwin et al. 1990; Ahmad and Menezes 1996). How ever, normal or increased chemotaxis, phagocytosis, and superoxide anion release by monocytes from HIV-1 patients (Nielsen et al. 1986; Bandres et al. 1993), as well as normal or increased phagocytosis by alveolar macrophages, have also been reported (Musher et al. 1990; Gordon et al. 2001).

The macrophage mannose receptor (MMR), a pattern recognition molecule and C-type lectin, is involved in recognition and binding of *Pneumocystis carinii* (now known as *P. jiroveci*), an opportunistic pathogen frequently seen in AIDS patients. Consequently, the downregulation of the MMR in alveolar macrophages isolated from HIV-1-infected patients, which has been related to a Tat-mediated reduction of the receptor promoter activity, interferes with these functions (Wehle et al. 1993; Koziel et al. 1998; Caldwell et al. 2000). The additionally impaired oxidative burst response and an altered cytokine secretion by these cells in response to *P. carinii* may critically contribute to patients' increased susceptibility to *P. carinii* pneumonia (Kandil et al. 1994; Koziel et al. 2000). Further defects of macrophage antifungal activity may exist against *Histoplasma capsulatum*, *Aspergillus fumigatus*, and *Candida* spp. (Baldwin et al. 1990; Kedzierska et al. 2003).

Similarly, HIV-1-infected macrophages and monocyte(s)-derived macrophages isolated from AIDS patients displayed defects in phagocytosis and intracellular killing, together with reduced H_2O_2 production, of opsonized *Toxoplasma gondii*, another opportunistic infectious agent in HIV-1 patients (Delemarre et al. 1994; Biggs et al. 1995). Phagocytosis of opsonized *T. gondii* has been shown to be Fc receptor (FcR) dependent, and FcRs as well as complement receptors are actually decreased on macrophages on in vitro infection with HIV-1 and on monocytes from HIV-1-infected individuals, possibly related to changes in intracellular tyrosine phosphorylation (Kedzierska et al. 2003).

In summary, various HIV-1-related alterations of monocyte/macrophage phenotype and functions have been reported. Methodological problems may arise, however, from the evaluation of functions of primary tissue cells, such as macrophages, after in vitro generation, differentiation, and infection. These problems, as well as different experimental approaches and additional effects on monocyte/macrophage functions, e.g. by drug treatment, may account for some conflicting results.

B LYMPHOCYTES

HIV-1 infection exerts profound effects on the B-lymphocyte compartment, i.e. polyclonal B-cell activation with spontaneous secretion of HIV-1-specific as well as HIV-1-nonspecific antibodies, leading to hypergammaglobulinemia, accompanied by decreased B-cell responses to mitogens in vitro (Lane et al. 1983; Shirai et al. 1992). These in vivo and in vitro effects have been attributed to a newly appearing B-cell subpopulation expressing reduced levels of CD21 (Moir et al. 2001).

Viral gp120 has been shown to bind to B cells expressing immunoglobulin VH3 gene products and activate these as a superantigen (Berberian et al. 1993). This is followed by a decrease of this cell subset with changes being more prominent in activated 'memory' rather than resting B cells. It may contribute to impaired responses to bacterial infections and partly explain the frequency of pneumococcal infections in which B cells expressing VH3 genes are important for the antibody repertoire against polysaccharides (Janoff et al. 1992; Scamurra et al. 2000). In addition to viral components, membrane-bound TNF-α on HIV-1-infected $CD4^+$ T lymphocytes may critically be involved in these B-cell perturbations (Macchia et al. 1993).

Immaturity and activation of peripheral B cells in HIV-1 infection coincide with a loss of $CD27^+$ memory B cells (Martinez-Maza et al. 1987; De Milito et al. 2001) and elevated serum levels of soluble CD27 (Widney et al. 1999). This could be the result of an enhanced expression of the CD27 ligand CD70 by activated T lymphocytes, thereby stimulating memory B cells and driving their differentiation to Ig-secreting plasma cells resulting in hypergammaglobulinemia (Nagase et al. 2001). Virions bound to follicular DCs in lymph nodes might significantly contribute to the observed B-cell activation (Zamarchi et al. 2002), whereas activated B cells themselves can promote viral expression in T cells by TNF-α and IL-6 secretion (Rieckmann et al. 1991). Further, alterations in the B-cell compartment of HIV-1-infected individuals comprise significantly less IgA secretion at mucosal sites (Kotler et al. 1987), elevated IgE levels (Wright et al. 1990), and reduced HLA-DR expression by B cells (Ginaldi et al. 1998).

The chronic B-cell activation and concomitant loss of T-cell function promote the genesis of B-cell lymphoma in AIDS patients, and cytokine homologues encoded by additional viral pathogens, such as vIL-10 by Epstein–Barr virus and vIL-6 by the human herpesvirus 8 might significantly contribute to this development

(Martinez-Maza and Breen 2002). Thus, in HIV-1-infected patients several functional abnormalities of B lymphocytes and Ig production are seen that often precede the characteristic decline of peripheral $CD4^+$ T cells.

NEUTROPHIL GRANULOCYTES

Several studies have demonstrated altered neutrophil functions in HIV-1 patients. Increased oxidative burst activity was detected in neutrophils from HIV-1 patients (Murphy et al. 1988; Bandres et al. 1993), whereas others reported on unchanged or even decreased production of reactive oxygen intermediates, possibly resulting from previous activation in vivo (Nielsen et al. 1986; Roilides et al. 1990; Chen et al. 1993; Pitrak et al. 1993; Flo et al. 1994; Wenisch et al. 1996). Similarly, increased phagocytosis of *Staphylococcus aureus*, *Escherichia coli*, and *Candida* spp. (Bandres et al. 1993; Wenisch et al. 1996), but also a reduction in phagocytosis of bacterial and fungal pathogens, were reported (Pos et al. 1992; Gabrilovich et al. 1994). Several studies suggested considerably decreased intracellular killing of bacteria or fungi by neutrophils from HIV-1-infected individuals (Ellis et al. 1988; Murphy et al. 1988; Roilides et al. 1993; Wenisch et al. 1996), whereas two groups reported on unaltered killing of *S. aureus* and *Candida* spp. (Pos et al. 1992; Cassone et al. 1997). Further defects in neutrophils from HIV-1-infected individuals include reduced chemotaxis (Valone et al. 1984), accelerated neutrophil apoptosis (Pitrak et al. 1996), and a reduced 5-lipoxygenase metabolism, leading to lower leukotriene production (Coffey et al. 1998). Remarkably, a soluble factor in the serum of HIV-1 patients reduced the ability of neutrophils to opsonize bacterial pathogens (Ellis et al. 1988). Beside some neutrophil dysfunctions, HIV-1-patients may have neutropenia which occurs either induced by infection or, more often, as a result from myelosuppressive therapies.

In conclusion, the literature on potential dysfunctions of neutrophil granulocytes in HIV-1 patients is inconclusive, most probably the result of methodological differences. In addition, the patients included in these studies may not have been comparable over the stages of disease and pharmacological treatments with possible side effects on neutrophil functions. Nevertheless, non-neutropenic HIV-1-infected individuals apparently do not have invasive mycoses, such as aspergillosis or candidemia, to the same extent as patients who are neutropenic as a result of chemotherapy.

INNATE CYTOTOXIC CELLS (NK CELLS AND γδ T CELLS)

Natural killer cells are critically important in the early combat of viral infections. In HIV-1 infection NK cell-mediated direct lysis of infected target cells, ADCC, and cytokine secretion (especially of IFN-γ and TNF-α) represent important mechanisms that interfere with viral replication. Similar to NK cells, T lymphocytes bearing the γδ TCR are cytotoxic and can release proinflammatory cytokines. These cells constitute a small proportion (up to 10 percent) of peripheral $CD3^+$ T cells, and, in contrast to other immune cells, they recognize phosphorylated nonpeptidic microbial metabolites and alkylamines. Both ID="12332"NK and γδ T cells can additionally interfere with HIV-1 replication by the secretion of chemokines; in the case of NK cells an inverse relationship between this function and the level of viremia has been described (Malkovsky et al. 2000; Levy 2001; Kottilil et al. 2003).

There are various studies demonstrating increasingly impaired NK cell functions in HIV-1-infected individuals correlating with disease progression. Qualitative defects in cytotoxicity of NK and lymphokine-activated killer (LAK) cells in HIV-1-infected patients appear early during HIV-1 infection and are accompanied by a low NK cell responsiveness to IFN-α (Brenner et al. 1993; Ullum et al. 1995, 1999). A deficiency of tubulin rearrangement may significantly contribute to the reduced potency of the cells to kill target cells (Sirianni et al. 1988).

Binding of Ig to the FcγRIII (CD16) on NK cells initiates ADCC. A loss of cytolytic $CD16^+$ NK cells in the peripheral blood was described early, however (Brenner et al. 1989), and explains the profound defects of ADCC found in HIV-1-infected individuals (Brenner et al. 1991; Ahmad et al. 1994). Essential signaling molecules involved in the CD16-dependent cytolysis, i.e. ζ molecules, were found to be decreased in NK cells from HIV-1 patients (Geertsma et al. 1999). Moreover, a selective depletion of primarily cytotoxic, mature, $CD56^{dim}$ NK cells without major changes in the cytokine-secreting $CD56^{bright}$ population correlates with reduced NK cell activity (Hu et al. 1995; Tarazona et al. 2002). Simultaneously increased numbers of a more immature $CD16^+CD56^-$ NK cell subset may indicate a defective differentiation of NK cells in HIV-1 infection.

An important strategy of HIV-1 to escape NK cell-mediated lysis is the selective downregulation of HLA-A and -B, leaving HLA-C and -E on the cellular surface, thereby avoiding NK cell cytotoxicity (Cohen et al. 1999). Further phenotypic changes involve the expression of inhibitory cellular receptors on NK cells which can dampen their function on binding to MHC I molecules. C-type lectin receptors of the CD94/NKG2 family are upregulated on NK cells in HIV-1 infection whereas the results regarding KIR expression are controversial (Andre et al. 1999; Galiani et al. 1999).

Alterations also occur on the level of γδ T cells in HIV-1 infection. The majority (60–95 percent) of peripheral γδ T cells in healthy individuals express the Vγ9 and Vδ2 TCR chains and inhibitory NK cell receptors, mostly of the CD94/NKG2 complex, but lack both CD4 and CD8 molecules. In HIV-1 infection, this subset is considerably diminished and displays serious functional defects, including reduced secretion of IFN-γ and TNF-α, which may contribute to the increased susceptibility of HIV-1 patients to opportunistic infections (Poccia et al. 1996; Wallace et al. 1997). At the same time, $V\delta1^+$ cells are significantly expanded in both bone marrow and peripheral blood of HIV-1-infected individuals (De Paoli et al. 1991; De Maria et al. 1992; Rossol et al. 1998). These cells represent an activated, potentially cytotoxic population, fully capable of proinflammatory cytokine secretion (Boullier et al. 1997), and a recent study suggests that these cells may contribute to HIV-1-associated immunopathogenesis through depletion of uninfected $CD4^+$ T lymphocytes (Sindhu et al. 2003). An inverse correlation of cytotoxicity with CD4 counts has also been reported for NK cells (Ahmad et al. 2001). Thus, alterations of subpopulations and/or functions of NK and γδ T cells may contribute to the overall immunosuppression observed in HIV-1 patients.

CYTOKINES

The secretion of IL-2, IL-12, and IFN-γ has been associated with protective immune responses to HIV-1; however, secretion of IL-2 is significantly reduced in HIV-1 patients, possibly as a result of the increased susceptibility of IL-2-producing Th1 cells to apoptosis (Clerici and Shearer 1994; Ledru et al. 1998). Similarly, IL-12 is produced in PBMCs significantly less from HIV-1 patients (Chehimi et al. 1994). The percentages and absolute numbers of Gag-specific $IFN\text{-}\gamma^+IL\text{-}2^+CD4^+$ T lymphocytes in the blood correlate inversely with viral loads in LTNPs (Boaz et al. 2002), and low IFN-γ secretion (by $CD8^+$ T cells and others) was related to disease progression (Ullum et al. 1997). Restoration of immune functions under antiretroviral therapy of HIV-1-infected infants is associated with increased IFN-γ and IL-2 secretion (Reuben et al. 2002).

The loss of the previously discussed cytokines and/or increased levels of IL-4 and/or IL-10 may favor disease progression in both HIV-1-infected infants and adults. In particular, IL-10 secretion has been attributed to T-cell dysfunction, disease progression, and poor prognosis in HIV-1 infection (Clerici and Shearer 1994). Notably, whole blood cultures recently revealed a reduced secretion of IL-10 as well as of TNF-α, IFN-γ, IL-1, IL-12, and IL-2 on stimulation with lipopolysaccharide (LPS) and phytohaemagglutinin (PHA), correlating with progression of HIV-1 (Ostrowski et al. 2003).

In HIV-1 infection altered secretion is also seen for other cytokines. Levels of IL-7 are increased, most probably as part of a homeostatic mechanism in response to T-cell depletion, and a reduced expression of its receptor (CD127) was found on $CD8^+$ T lymphocytes from HIV-1-infected individuals (Fry et al. 2001; MacPherson et al. 2001; Napolitano et al. 2001). Although IL-15 could potentially exert some beneficial effects on functions of various immune cells in HIV-1 infection (Waldmann and Tagaya 1999), it also stimulated the expression of inhibitory NK cell receptors on $CD8^+$ T and NK cells (Mingari et al. 1997, 1998). In addition, high IL-15 serum levels in HIV patients, which correlate with the extent of hypergammaglobulinemia, point towards a role for IL-15 in the pathogenesis of HIV infection (Waldmann and Tagaya 1999).

Levels of IL-16 are increased during the asymptomatic phase of HIV-1 infection, followed by a significant decline of IL-16 serum concentrations in disease progression (Amiel et al. 1999). IL-16 is secreted by CD8 cells and capable of inhibiting HIV-1 infection in CD4 T cells by repressing the HIV-1 promoter activity (Baier et al. 1995; Maciaszek et al. 1997). The reduction of activation-induced cell death of lymphocytes by IL-16 may contribute to a suggested protective role in HIV infection (Idziorek et al. 1998). T-cell clones from LTNPs produce significantly larger amounts of IL-16 than cell clones from asymptomatic or AIDS patients (Scala et al. 1997).

Both IFN-α and IFN-β possess similar in vitro activity against HIV-1. Paradoxically, high levels of IFN-α and IFN-inducible protein 10 are detected in HIV patients, associated with advanced disease (Stylianou et al. 2000). In addition, an acid-labile form of IFN-α with reduced antiviral activity in vitro and associated with poor disease prognosis has been described (DeStefano et al. 1982; Gendelman et al. 1992). Therefore, these data indicate that the altered production of various cytokines may add to the observed defects in cellular immune responses in HIV-1 patients.

Particular immune dysfunctions in distinct immune compartments

LYMPH NODES

One of the characteristic clinical signs of HIV infection is the development of generalized lymphadenopathy. Studies on lymph node biopsies revealed at least three distinct histological patterns: follicular hyperplasia, follicular involution, and lymphocyte depletion (Tenner-Racz et al. 1985; Biberfeld et al. 1987; Racz et al. 1991). Similar changes were found in the spleen (Falk et al. 1988). It must be emphasized that the changes described in lymph nodes from HIV-infected patients are not specific because follicular hyperplasia and follicular involution, in particular, can also be found in other pathological conditions such as bacterial infections, and in rheumatoid arthritis (Ewing et al. 1985; Stanley and Frizzera 1986). Changes in lymph nodes, however, mirror the progression of the disease, with implications for the pathogenesis of AIDS (Pantaleo et al. 1993).

Immunpathogenesis

HIV reaches the lymph nodes during PHI. The virus is trapped by follicular DCs and replicates in $CD4^+$ T cells.

HIV particles can be demonstrated in the germinal centers of lymph nodes by electron microscopy and immunohistology (for a review, see Pantaleo et al. 1993). Adhesion of HIV virions to the follicular DC network in lymph nodes and germinal centers may contribute to the B-cell activation observed during HIV infection. It could be further demonstrated that lymph nodes are the major reservoir for HIV in the human body (for a review, see Pantaleo et al. 1993). Indeed, in the early stage of HIV infection, levels of viral burden and replication are far greater in lymph nodes compared with peripheral blood. During this time about 25 percent of $CD4^+$ T cells in germinal centers are infected with HIV (for a review, see Pantaleo et al. 1993). In the early and intermediate stages of the disease viral particles in lymph nodes are restricted to germinal centers with follicular DCs. HIV accumulates in germinal centers complexed with Ig and complement trapped by the follicular DCs, in agreement with their role in antigen clearance and presentation (for a review, see Pantaleo et al. 1993). Follicular DCs in germinal centers induce increased expression of the HIV-1 co-receptor CXCR4 on surrounding $CD4^+$ T cells, thereby facilitating infection of these cells by HIV. In contrast to their central role in induction of protective immune response in other infections, follicular DCs in HIV infection promote and enhance the spread and replication of HIV by presenting the replication-competent virus to susceptible cells such as $CD4^+$ T cells and macrophages (for a review, see Pantaleo et al. 1993).

As antigen-activated lymphocytes migrate into and through lymph nodes, they may come into contact with HIV immune complexes on the surface of follicular DCs and infect themselves. This may explain the slow but steady decrease of $CD4^+$ T cells in the peripheral blood (for a review, see Pantaleo et al. 1993). In late stages of the disease germinal centers involute and the network of follicular DCs is destroyed. Thus, the virus is no longer trapped in the lymph nodes and can quickly spread unchecked, resulting in viremia, characteristic of late-stage disease – AIDS. Furthermore, the absence of an intact network of follicular DCs in the germinal centers of lymph nodes results in an impaired immune response toward other infections by an inadequate antigen presentation necessary for the maintenance of T- and B-memory responses (for a review, see Pantaleo et al. 1993). Besides the direct reduction in the number of follicular DCs in the germinal centers of lymph nodes during infection with HIV/SIV, a reduced chemokine production and a reduced expression of markers that are involved in the trafficking of follicular DCs may further contribute to progressing systemic immunodeficiency in the course of HIV/SIV infection (Choi et al. 2003).

THYMUS

The thymus is not necessary for normal T-lymphocyte function in adults because a subset of mature post-thymic peripheral T lymphocytes is self-renewing (Stutman 1978). However, when the normal T-lymphocyte pool is destroyed by infection with HIV, the thymus may be necessary for complete regeneration of T lymphocytes. In late stages of HIV-1 infection, pronounced lymphocyte depletion and destruction of the thymus are observed (Schnittmann et al. 1990). Work on CD45 isoform expression by the T-cell subset has provided evidence for defective thymopoiesis in AIDS because peripheral $CD4^+$ T cells, which appear after HAART in AIDS patients, are derived from a regeneration of peripheral, post-thymic, $CD45RO^+$, memory T lymphocytes and not from $CD45RA^+$, naïve T cells produced in the thymus (Ho et al. 1995).

As in lymph nodes, three different histopathological patterns were determined.

Thymitis

HIV-induced thymitis is characterized by irregularly shaped follicles, $CD8^+$ T-cell infiltration of the follicles, and the start of follicular DC network fragmentation (Prevot et al. 1992). Thymic epithelial cells are injured early in infection as seen in HIV-infected humans (Seemayer et al. 1984). The degree of thymic hyperplasia in early HIV-1 infection may be variable, but can lead to an abnormally enlarged thymus (Prevot et al. 1992).

Precocious involution

As with lymph nodes, the thymus of patients in the intermediate and late stages of HIV infection shows a thymic involution (Seemayer et al. 1984). This stage of the disease may be accompanied by the infiltration of plasma cells (Seemayer et al. 1984) and macrophages (Papiernik et al. 1992) in the fat adjacent to the cord of the involved thymus.

Thymic dysplasia

This is the final stage of thymus changes during HIV infection, characterized by epithelial rosette formation (Seemayer et al. 1984) and calcification or loss of Hassall's bodies (Seemayer et al. 1984).

HIV target cells in the thymus

Not only $CD4^+$ thymocytes but also immature triple-negative thymocytes, which express CD4 but at very low levels, are susceptible to HIV-1 infection (Schnittmann et al. 1990). A further separation of these triple-negative cells revealed that only $CD1a^+$, but not $CD1a^-$, triple negative thymocytes (presumably the most immature subset) can be infected by HIV-1 (Valentin et al. 1994). Interestingly, protease inhibitor-resistant HIV-1 strains, which develop in some patients treated with protease inhibitors, are impaired in their capability to replicate in thymus tissue (Stoddart et al. 2001). This would explain why patients with increasing viral load resulting from protease-resistance do not have a fall in their $CD4^+$ T-cell count.

Immune reconstitution of the thymus in HIV-infected patients

Neither thymic transplantation (Ciobanu et al. 1985; Dwyer et al. 1987) nor substitution of thymus-derived hormones (Hermans and Clumeck 1989) in HIV-infected patients leads to convincing evidence of immune reconstitution. The introduction of an effective antiretroviral therapy – HAART – clearly has a beneficial effect on the immune reconstitution of the thymus, however (Sempowski and Haynes 2002). The restoration of thymic function during HAART could be better monitored by the development and introduction of a new assay of thymus function in adults (the measurement of T-cell receptor excition circles (TREC)) (Ye et al. 2003). Measurement of TRECs revealed a loss of TREC levels within naïve $CD4^+$ T cells, indicating reduced thymic output during HIV infection (Douek et al. 2001). Poor $CD4^+$ T-cell increase in patients with good virological response to HAART seems to be caused by low thymic output (Teixeira et al. 2001). Fortunately, most HIV-1 infected patients, adults (Franco et al. 2002) and children (Correa and Munoz-Fernandez 2002), show an increased thymic output of $CD4^+$ T cells, which seems to correlate with an increase in thymic size in adults during the treatment with HAART (Franco et al. 2002).

HIV AND THE GASTROINTESTINAL MUCOSA

The gastrointestinal tract is not only a potential portal for HIV entry, but also an organ that plays a central role in pathogenesis and secondary opportunistic infections (for review see Schneider et al. 1997a). During the course of HIV infection, most of the patients develop gastrointestinal symptoms. The intestinal immune system, represented by specialized local immune system termed gut-associated lymphoid tissue (GALT), has special features which seem to be involved during HIV/SIV infection (for a review, see Schneider et al. 1997a).

HIV infection of the gastrointestinal tract

As lamina propria lymphocytes (LPL) belong to the effector compartment, most of them are already activated and represent a memory phenotype which makes these cells susceptible to HIV infection without prior stimulation (Lapenta et al. 1999). The increased state of activation seems to be the major factor in increased HIV-1 replication in lamina propria $CD4^+$ T lymphocytes (Sheriff et al. 2004). The increased susceptibility to HIV infection of intestinal $CD4^+$ T cells may also result from the expression of a higher amount of the chemokine receptors CCR5 and CXCR4 (Anton et al. 2000). Indeed, independent of the route of infection, HIV/SIV can even be found early after infection in the lamina propria of the intestinal tract (Veazey et al. 1998; Kewenig et al. 1999). The virus content seems to be higher in the intestinal mucosa compared with the peripheral blood (Kotler et al. 1991; Fackler et al. 1998; Veazey et al. 1998; Kewenig et al. 1999), and this higher mucosal virus load seems to result from an increased replication or translation (Fackler et al. 1998). The major target cells in the lamina propria of the intestine are $CD4^+$ T cells and not macrophages (Meng et al. 2000). Experimental infection of rhesus macaques by atraumatic application of pathogenic SIV to the tonsils, a mucosa-associated lymphoid organ, leads to primary infection of $CD4^+$ T lymphocytes and not to infection of the DC-rich squamous epithelium (Stahl-Hennig et al. 1999). The epithelial cells of the intestinal mucosa are not productively infected but serve as virus transmitters (Bomsel 1997). The transepithelial transport of HIV-1 by epithelial and M cells is mediated by the same receptors: the galactosyl cerebroside molecule and the chemokine receptors CCR5 and CXCR4 (Yahi et al. 1992; Fotopoulos et al. 2002). There is in vitro evidence that HIV can be transported via M cells (Amerongen et al. 1991). It is interesting that primary intestinal epithelial cells selectively transfer R5 HIV-1 to $CCR5^+$ $CD4^+$ T cells of the lamina propria (Meng et al. 2002).

HIV-induced immune activation and the consequences for the gastrointestinal mucosa

The mucosal infection with HIV-1 induces a primary T-cell activation which may lead to ulcers – the so-called 'giant ulcer' – in some patients (R. Ignatius and T. Schneider unpublished data). An initial mucosal immune activation with high production of cytokines (R. Ignatius and T. Schneider unpublished data) may induce a hyperproliferative villus atrophy in the small intestine, as seen in HIV-infected patients and even in very early stages of SIV infection (Kotler et al. 1984; Kewenig et al. 1999). The massive immune activation with secretion of proinflammatory cytokines such as TNF-α will affect the barrier function, inducing a leak flux that may further contribute to diarrhea without the presence of secondary opportunistic enteric pathogens (Schafer et al. 2002; Schmitz et al. 2002). Mucosal inflammation in HIV-infected patients may reach levels comparable to those of patients with inflammatory bowel disease (Olsson et al. 2000).

Mucosal immunodeficiency

- $CD4^+$ T cells: the course of mucosal HIV/SIV infection is further characterized by a rapid and nearly complete loss of $CD4^+$ T LPLs (Lim et al. 1993a; Schneider et al. 1995), which occurs in the SIV model within 2 weeks after infection (Veazey et al. 1998; Kewenig et al. 1999). The decline of $CD4^+$ T cells in the intestinal mucosa is more pronounced, especially in the early stages of the disease than in the peripheral blood (Figure 39.2) (Schneider et al. 1995). As measurements of $CD4^+$ T LPLs in this compartment are thus far based on percentages, it is not yet completely clear whether this reflects a real loss of $CD4^+$ T LPLs or is the result of a massive increase of $CD8^+$ T LPLs with a relative decrease of $CD4^+$ T lymphocytes, as is the case for other body compartments (Sopper et al. 2003). There is a preferential decrease of $CCR5^+CD4^+$ T cells, which express the mucosa-homing receptor $\alpha4\beta7$ (CD103) in the peripheral blood of HIV-infected patients (Krzysiek et al. 2001). However, a selective reduction of $CD103^+CD4^+$ LPLs could not be found in late stages of the disease (Schneider et al. 1994).

- $CD8^+$ T cells: in the lamina propria, the percentage of $CD8^+$ LPLs is increased, which seems to be caused by an increase of activated $HLADR^+CD8^+$ LPLs and cytotoxic $CD11a^+CD8^+$ LPLs (Schneider et al. 1994). These activated cytotoxic $CD8^+$ LPLs may recognize HIV antigens and play a role in the control of HIV infection (Couedel-Courteille et al. 1997), but they could also be harmful by damaging the intestinal epithelium as in HIV-associated alveolitis (Autran et al. 1988).
- Natural killer cells: NK cells that can eliminate virus-infected and tumor cells were found to be reduced in the intestinal mucosa of AIDS patients, which may further facilitate infections and malignancies in the intestine (Schneider et al. 1994).
- Intraepithelial lymphocytes: the percentage of $\gamma\delta$ receptor-positive intraepithelial lymphocytes (IEL) in the intestine of AIDS patients seems to be altered. Interestingly, reduced numbers of $\gamma\delta$ IELs in the duodenum in late stages of the disease were associated with short survival expectancy (Nilssen et al. 1996).
- Macrophages: macrophages of the intestinal mucosa in HIV-infected patients are also impaired because the antigen-presenting subset is reduced (Lim et al. 1993b).
- B cells and mucosal humoral immunity: insufficient helper function of $CD4^+$ T LPLs is also indicated by the reduced proportion of IgA plasma cells in the large intestine of AIDS patients because terminal IgA B-cell differentiation is $CD4^+$ T-cell dependent (for a review, see Schneider et al. 1997b). Most investigators found a reduced IgA production in the intestine of HIV-infected patients and SIV-infected macaques (Kotler et al. 1987; Schafer et al. 2002). More impressive, however, is an increase in the production of the normally not predominant intestinal IgG (Janoff et al. 1994; Schneider et al. 1998; Schafer et al. 2002). As only secretory IgA exhibits the full protective immune function at mucosal surfaces (for a review, see Brandtzaeg et al. 1985; Mazanec et al. 1993) by immunoexclusion (Stokes et al. 1975), and even intracellular neutralization of viruses within epithelial cells (Bomsel et al. 1998), a predominance of IgG and a lack or decrease of IgA may reflect a breakdown of the mucosal immune effector arm. Indeed, a lack of or restricted secretory HIV/SIV-specific IgA production is found in HIV-infected humans and SIV-infected macaques (Janoff et al. 1994; Schneider et al. 1997a; Schafer et al. 2002). This local immune deficiency may further contribute to a rapid and massive spread of HIV/SIV in the intestinal mucosa (Kotler et al. 1991; Fackler et al. 1998; Veazey et al. 1998; Kewenig et al. 1999).

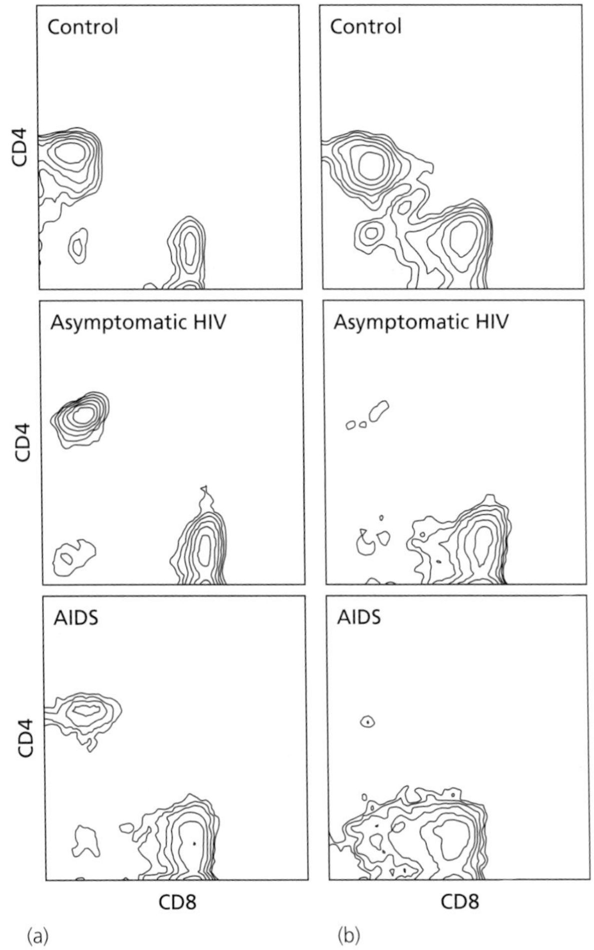

Figure 39.2 *Pronounced loss of $CD4^+$ T cells in duodenal mucosa compared with the peripheral blood. Contour blots of two-color immunofluorescence profile of gated $CD3^+$ T cells isolated from* **(a)** *the peripheral blood and* **(b)** *the duodenum of a control patient, of an asymptomatic HIV-1-infected patient, and an AIDS patient. Logarithmic intensities for red fluorescence (CD4) and green fluorescence (CD8) are shown on the y axis and x axis, respectively (Schneider et al. 1995).*

Immune reconstitution under HAART

The immune reconstitution currently measured by the increase of $CD4^+$ T cells in the peripheral blood after installation of HAART is, beside the HIV RNA levels, the central parameter in determining the success or failure of treatment (O'Brien et al. 1997). It still remains unclear, however, if all functions and the entire repertoire of $CD4^+$ T cells can be restored after prolonged infection with HIV (Connors et al. 1997). A three-phase T-cell reconstitution is generally seen after initiating HAART: (1) an early rise of memory $CD4^+$ cells, (2) a reduction in T-cell activation correlated to the decreasing retroviral activity, together with an improved $CD4^+$ T-cell reactivity to recall antigens, and (3) a late rise of naïve $CD4^+$ lymphocytes while $CD8^+$ T cells decline (Autran et al. 1997). In one study 20 patients treated with HAART were followed up for 12 months, and CD4 cell proliferative responses to cytomegalovirus and tuberculin antigens were monitored. The investigators were able to demonstrate that HAART can induce sustained recovery of CD4 T-cell reactivity against opportunistic pathogens in severely immunosuppressed patients (Li et al. 1998). The restoration of cytomegalovirus-specific $CD4^+$ T-cell response in HIV-infected patients treated with HAART could be further confirmed by more specific techniques (Komanduri et al. 1998). Immune recovery under HAART could also be observed for other opportunistic pathogens such as *Toxoplasma gondii* (Fournier et al. 2001). Nevertheless, there is lack of functional reconstitution of HIV-specific, CD4-mediated immune response after HAART. Only in some patients can an increase in HIV-specific neutralizing antibodies be detected (Kim et al. 2001). A stringent consequence of the immune recovery of HIV-infected patients under HAART is the impressive decrease in the incidence of opportunistic infections and Kaposi's sarcoma in HIV-infected patients since the introduction of HAART (Palella et al. 1998). Fortunately, immune reconstitution can also be achieved in HIV-infected children, even in those with late stage disease, with HAART (Ometto et al. 2002). One problem of the immune reconstitution under HAART is, in rare cases, the immune reconstitution inflammatory syndrome, which is characterized by an exuberant inflammatory response towards previously present opportunistic pathogens (Shelburne and Hamill 2003).

HTLV-1 INFECTION

HTLV-1 and disease

Human T-cell lymphotropic virus type 1 was the first recognized human retrovirus (Poiesz et al. 1980). The best-known disease linked to HTLV-1 infection is the adult T-cell leukemia/lymphoma (ATL) (Uchiyama et al. 1977). In 1985 a group of patients with a neurological disease known as tropical spastic paraparesis (TSP) was found to be seropositive for HTLV-1 (Gessain et al. 1985). Subsequently, a report from Japan described a neurological disorder as HTLV-1-associated myelopathy, now considered to be identical to TSP (Osame et al. 1986).

Chronic inflammatory arthropathy and uveitis seems to be a rare complication in HTLV-1-infected individuals (Sato et al. 1991; Mochizuki et al. 1996). Beside these diseases patients with ATL or carriers of HTLV-1 show impairment of cellular immune responses (Cappell and Chow 1987).

Epidemiology

The three major reported routes of transmission are sexual intercourse, administration of blood products, and mother-to-child transfer. In endemic areas seropositive persons are clustered around the families, reflecting the predominance of mother-to-child transmission. It is estimated that approximately 10–20 million people are infected by HTLV-1 (Franchini 1995).

HTLV-1 infection is present in widely scattered populations in the world. The best-studied areas are the islands of southwestern Japan, where approximately 20 percent of the adults are seropositive (Hinuma et al. 1982), and the Caribbean basin, which includes the West Indies, northern South America, and the southeastern USA, where 2–5 percent of black adults are seropositive (Schupbach et al. 1983). Other hot spots of HTLV-1 infections have also been reported from west and central Africa, Melanesia, India, the Middle East, and parts of South America (Ifthikharuddin and Rosenblatt 2000).

The virus

HTLV-1 virions are spherical, 100 nm in diameter, and composed of an internal core of structural proteins (p15, p24, and p19) surrounding the viral RNA and polymerase, and an outer layer of viral envelope glycoproteins (gp46 and gp21) anchored in a lipid membrane (Wong-Staal and Gallo 1985). The proviral genome of HTLV-1 encodes *gag*, *pol*, and *env* genes characteristic of all known retroviruses. Both ends of the proviral genome are flanked by noncoding direct-repeat sequences called LTRs. LTRs mediate proviral integration and contain *cis*-acting regulatory elements important for viral transcription, viral mRNA processing, and reverse transcription. Beside the genes for the structural proteins, HTLV-1 has additional open reading frames, which encode for the important regulatory proteins such as Tax and Rex (Franchini 1995).

HTLV-1 Tax is a 40-kDa protein essential for the viral life cycle and transformation of human T lymphocytes (Slamon et al. 1984). It usually localizes in the nucleus of infected cells, here it is capable of activating several cellular transcription factors resulting in an enhanced trancription of cellular genes such as the interleukins IL-1, IL-2, IL-3, IL-6, granulocyte–macrophage colony-stimulating factor (GM-CSF), c-*fos*, c-*cis*, c-*myc*, vimetin, parathyroid hormone-related protein (PTHrP), transforming growth factor β1 (TGF-β1), MHC I, NF-κB, nerve growth factor, and TNF-β (Franchini 1995). Tax is also capable of transactivating the adhesion molecule ICAM-1 (Tanaka et al. 1996). Such promiscuous transactivation of numerous genes by Tax is thought to play a crucial role in neoplastic transformation of T cells and may also be of central importance for the development of T-cell deficiency in HTLV-I infection.

The 27-kDa regulatory protein Rex plays an important role in regulating viral mRNA processing and is essential for export of full-length *gag/pol* and single-spliced *env* mRNA from nucleus to cytoplasm (Hanly et al. 1989). Furthermore, Rex enhances the expression of the IL-2Rα-chain (Kanamori et al. 1990), whereas p12, another regulatory protein of HTLV-1, seems to downregulate the β and γ_c chains of IL-2R (Mulloy et al. 1996). The modification of the IL-2 receptor of HTLV-1-infected T cells by regulatory proteins may influence T-cell function and T-cell transformation in HTLV-1 infection.

HTLV usually infects T cells. However, the cellular receptor for this virus is unknown so far. Experiments with the HTLV-1 surface glycoprotein revealed binding on T and B cells, NK cells, and macrophages (Nath et al. 2003). The putative HTLV-1 receptor seems to be upregulated by T-cell activation (Manel et al. 2003; Nath et al. 2003), especially during early activation (Manel et al. 2003). Moreover, the amount of HTLV-1-infected cells in HTLV-1 carriers seems to be increased during inflammation of infectious diseases (Nishimura et al. 2003). For the spread of HTLV-1 between cells and between individuals, cell contact is required because naturally infected lymphocytes produce virtually no cell-free infectious HTLV-1 particles. After contact between an infected and uninfected T cell, a polarization of the cytoskeleton of the infected cell to the cell–cell junction is induced (Igakura et al. 2003). HTLV-1 core complexes and the HTLV-1 genome accumulate at the cell–cell junction and are then transferred to the uninfected cell (Igakura et al. 2003).

Natural course of HTLV-1 infection

ADULT T-CELL LEUKEMIA/LYMPHOMA

Adult T-cell leukemia/lymphoma is a proliferative disorder of T cells characterized by lymphadenopathy, hypercalcemia, lytic bone lesions, skin involvement, and hepatosplenomegaly (Takatsuki et al. 1985). The skin lesions of HTLV-1 infection are manifold, including diffuse papules, nodules, plaques, erythematous patches, and diffuse erythroderma. In the blood abnormal lymphocytes with convoluted nuclei – so-called flower cells – are found. The malignant T cells in ATL are mature $CD4^+/CD8^-$ and have increased IL-2R α chain (CD25) expression (Hattori et al. 1981). The lifetime risk of developing ATL in HTLV-1 patients is estimated at 1–4 percent (Tajima and Kuroishi 1985). The latent phase from infection to actual development of disease is estimated to be 30–50 years (Tajima and Kuroishi 1985; Murphy et al. 1989). This long incubation period implies that most adult persons developing ATL were infected during early childhood. The most frequent mode of HTLV-1 transmission during this time is breast-feeding by HTLV-1-positive mothers. After manifestation of ATL the prognosis is poor and depends on the disease subtype, which can be distinguished based on clinical criteria (Shimoyama 1991). One of the major reasons for death in ATL patients is the development of opportunistic infections because of the acquired immunodeficiency.

TROPICAL SPASTIC PARAPARESIS

Tropical spastic paraparesis is also is a chronic progressive demyelinating disease affecting the spinal cord and the white matter of the central nervous system (CNS) (Bhigjee et al. 1991). The lifetime incidence of TSP in HTLV-1-infected patients is less than 5 percent (Kaplan et al. 1990). The disease appears usually in the fourth decade of life and women are about twice as likely to be affected as men (Vernant et al. 1987). TSP and ATL rarely occur in the same patient (Kawai et al. 1989). Similar to acute disseminated encephalomyelitis in measles, an autoimmune process is thought to play a key role in the pathogenesis of TSP. Myelin and axon destruction is accompanied by infiltrating $CD8^+$ T cells (Bhigjee et al. 1991), and a high frequency of cytolytic T cells with specificity against the HTLV-1 regulatory protein Tax was found in TSP patients (Koenig et al. 1993). Recently, a cross-reactive epitope between Tax and human neurons was described (Levin et al. 2002). The progression from asymptomatic to symptomatic HTLV-1 infection seems to be triggered by the increasing production of proinflammatory cytokines such as IFN-γ and TNF-α by Tax-expressing cells (Furukawa et al. 2003). For both diseases, ATL and TSP, until now no effective treatment exists.

Immunosuppression

Patients with ATL are immunocompromised and at increased risk of dying as a result of opportunistic infections. The median survival time of patients with acute ATL is only 10 months (Shimoyama et al. 1991). Most deaths in patients with symptomatic HTLV-1 disease are caused by opportunistic infections (White et al. 1995). As in HIV-infected patients, in HTLV-1-infected ATL patients *P. carinii* pneumonia, cryptococcal meningitis, and other disseminated fungal infections are seen (Bunn et al. 1983), which indicate an impaired Th-cell function. In addition, herpesvirus co-infection such as cytomegalovirus, herpes zoster, and generalized herpes simplex virus infection is frequent in ATL patients (Bunn et al. 1983).

In particular, hyperinfection with *Strongyloides stercoralis* is a common problem in ATL patients (Nakada et al. 1987; Sato and Shiroma 1989; Newton et al. 1992; Plumelle et al. 1997). This phenomenon may indicate a selective immune defect (Newton et al. 1992). A Japanese study showed that 58 percent of the patients with *S. stercoralis* infection are HTLV-1 positive and, of these, 67 percent had a monoclonal integration of HTLV-1 proviral DNA in their blood lymphocytes (Nakada et al. 1987). This leads to speculation that strongyloides infection may be a co-factor for the development of ATL. Leukemic cells of ATL patients suppress B-cell immunoglobulin secretion by a complex mechanism involving induction of suppressor cells after activation of normal suppressor cell precursors (Waldmann et al. 1984).

Immunity in HTLV-1-infected patients seems to be impaired even before diseases like ATL or TSP become apparent. Fungal and bacterial skin infections occur frequently (Kawano et al. 1985; LaGrenade et al. 1990) and may be a marker for the HTLV-1 infection in endemic regions (LaGrenade et al. 1990). Delayed-type hypersensitivity is suppressed in HTLV-1 carriers (Murai et al. 1990).

Double infections with HIV-1 and HTLV-1 have been reported, but it is not clear so far if this accelerates progression to AIDS (Bartholomew et al. 1987; Cleghorn and Blattner 1992; Gotuzzo et al. 1992).

MEASLES

Measles is a highly contagious viral disease. After a prodromal stage with fever, coryza, cough, and conjunctivitis, a generalized maculopapular rash appears. Introduction of measles into virgin populations, as well as endemic transmission in populations lacking access to adequate medical care, is associated with high mortality (Griffin 2001; Duke and Mgone 2003). Despite the successful development of a live attenuated vaccine, measles remains a major cause of mortality in children of developing countries, accounting for 1 100 000 deaths annually (Murray and Lopez 1997; Duke and Mgone 2003).

The virus

Morbilliviruses are distinct from other paramyxoviruses in that they form intranuclear inclusion bodies. Virions are pleomorphic and range in size from 100 to 300 nm. The envelope carries two viral proteins: transmembrane hemagglutinin and fusion glycoproteins. The nucleocapsid is packed within the envelope in the form of an asymmetrical coil. Nonstructural proteins encoded by the measles virus include the C and the V proteins. Both are dispensable for viral replication in vitro, but may play a role in viral pathogenesis in vivo (for a review, see Griffin 2001).

RECEPTOR USAGE

CD46 (membrane co-factor protein (MCP)) is expressed on human nucleated cells and was the first cellular receptor identified for the measles virus. An extended binding site within CD46, spanning the two short conserved domains, SCR1 and SCR2, most distal to the membrane, interacts with the measles virus transmembrane hemagglutinin protein; the binding sites for the natural ligands, the C3b/C4b complement components, map in SCR3 and SCR4. However, more recent studies have questioned the role that CD46 plays for measles virus not passaged in vitro. These and all other measles virus strains tested so far use CD150 (signaling lymphocyte activation molecule (SLAM)) as an entry receptor. The expression of CD150 on activated T and B cells, memory cells, and immature thymocytes seems to be compatible with the well-recognized tropism of measles virus for the cells of the lymphoid compartment (for a review, see Schneider-Schaulies and Ter Meulen 2002).

NATURAL COURSE OF MEASLES INFECTION

Immunopathology

Measles is typically a childhood infection spread by the respiratory route. Virus replication takes place first in tracheal and bronchial epithelial cells (Sherman and Ruckle 1958). There is evidence that the virus is acquired from the basolateral side of epithelial cells by tissue-resident macrophages and DCs (Mrkic et al. 2000). The virus is probably transported by these cells to local lymph nodes, where the measles virus replicates and spreads by cell-associated viremia to a variety of organs (Ruckle and Rogers 1957; Forthal et al. 1992). The primary target cell in the blood is the monocyte (Esolen et al. 1993), and the viremia is accompanied by leukopenia (Sergiev et al. 1960). Lymphoid organs and tissues such as the thymus, spleen, lymph nodes, appendix, and tonsils are prominent sites of virus replication (Hall et al. 1971). Infection of thymocytes with the measles virus leads to apoptosis of these cells and a prolonged decrease in the size of the thymic cortex (White and Boyd 1973). Measles virus spreads to numerous other organs, including the skin, kidney, lung, gastrointestinal tract, genital mucosa, and liver. In these organs the virus replicates primarily in endothelial and epithelial cells. Endothelial cell infection is accompanied by vascular dilatation, increased vascular permeability, mononuclear cell infiltration, and infection of surrounding tissue (Denton 1925). Bright-red spots with a bluish center, the so-called Koplik's spots, appear on the oral mucosa 1–3 days before the skin rash, are pathologically similar to it, and involve the submucous glands (Denton 1925).

Clinical course

The clinical picture of measles develops after an incubation period of 10–14 days. The first prodromal symptoms are fever, malaise, cough, and coryza. This prodrome usually lasts 2–3 days during which the Koplik's spots appear on the oral mucosa. The typical maculopapular rash then appears, first on the face and behind the ears, from where it spreads centrifugally to the trunk and extremities. The rash fades 3–4 days from the start. During this time lymphadenopathy, mild splenomegaly, and appendicitis may be present. Clinical recovery begins soon after the appearance of the rash (Figure 39.3).

COMPLICATIONS

Predictors of poor outcome are severe lymphopenia (Coovadia et al. 1978) and poor antibody response (Wesley et al. 1982). Mortality in infection with measles is more frequent at the extremes of age. Most of the fatal outcomes observed in measles occur in children in developing countries. Malnutrition increases mortality caused by measles, and measles in turn worsens malnutrition (Dossetor et al. 1977). Death is most often the consequence of secondary infections or the reactivation of persistent infections such as tuberculosis (Duke and Mgone 2003). Most of the severe life-threatening pneumonia observed during measles is the result of secondary bacterial and viral infections (Beckford et al. 1985; Quiambao et al. 1998). The reactivation and exacerbation of tuberculosis were already mentioned in medical textbooks of the nineteenth century, and in 1908 von Pirquet reported the disappearance of delayed-type hypersensitivity skin responses to tuberculin during a measles outbreak. More recently, the reactivation and spread of herpesvirus infections, especially in the respiratory tract, has been reported (Orren et al. 1981; Suga et al. 1992). Importantly, young children in developing countries frequently develop diarrhea as a result of secondary bacterial and protozoal infections, worsening the precarious nutritional status of these children during infection with measles (Greenberg et al. 1991). Secondary and reactivated infections complicate the natural course of measles and are often the cause of fatal outcomes, underlining the importance of immune suppression during infection with the measles virus.

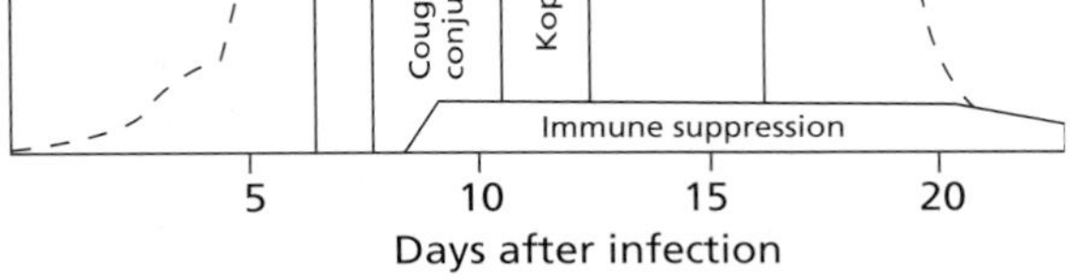

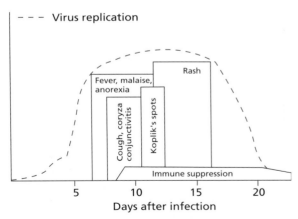

Figure 39.3 *Natural course of* measles virus *infection. Note that immune suppression begins usually 8–10 days after infection and before Koplik's spots and the skin rash appear. The duration of immune suppression exceeds that of clinical symptoms and may last up to 4 weeks after the rash has disappeared.*

Immunosuppression

Although the measles virus was the first pathogen recognized to cause immunosuppression, it was only recently that the underlying mechanisms were partially revealed. In vivo, delayed-type hypersensitivity skin test responses to recall antigens, such as tuberculin, are suppressed before the rash and for several weeks after apparent clinical recovery from measles infection (Figure 39.4) (Von Pirquet 1908; Tamashiro et al. 1987). Furthermore, cellular and humoral immune responses to new antigens during infection with measles are impaired (Coovadia et al. 1974). Isolated peripheral blood lymphocytes from patients with measles respond with reduced proliferation (Figure 39.5) and impaired cytokine production after stimulation with mitogens (Hirsch et al. 1984; Ward et al. 1991).

MONOCYTES AND DCS

Monocyte function is impaired by several mechanisms during measles. Both measles virus receptors, CD46 and CD150, are downregulated on the cell surface after contact with measles virus (for a review, see Schneider-Schaulies and ter Meulen 2002). The downregulation of CD46 may trigger lysis of uninfected lymphocytes by activating complement, as shown in vitro, and so may contribute to enhanced immune suppression. There is some evidence that CD46 can function, together with CD3, as a co-stimulatory molecule in the induction of T-cell proliferation and T-cell activation, which could as a consequence be blocked by measles-induced

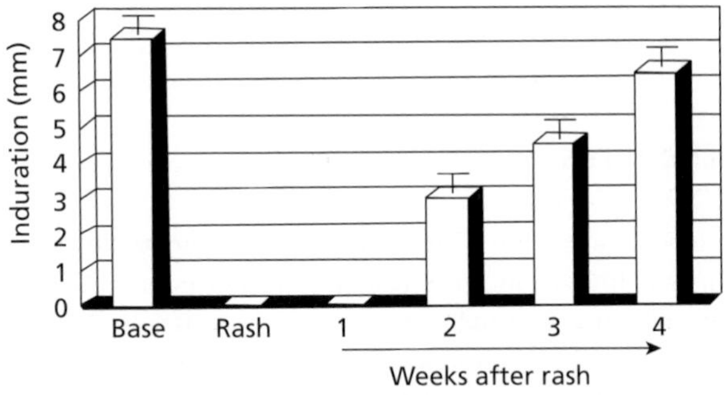

Figure 39.4 *Immune suppression during measles infection: changes in tuberculin-induced delayed-type hypersensitivity (DTH) skin test responses in children with measles who had previously been immunized against tuberculosis. (Modified after Tamashiro et al. 1987 and Griffin 2001, with permission.)*

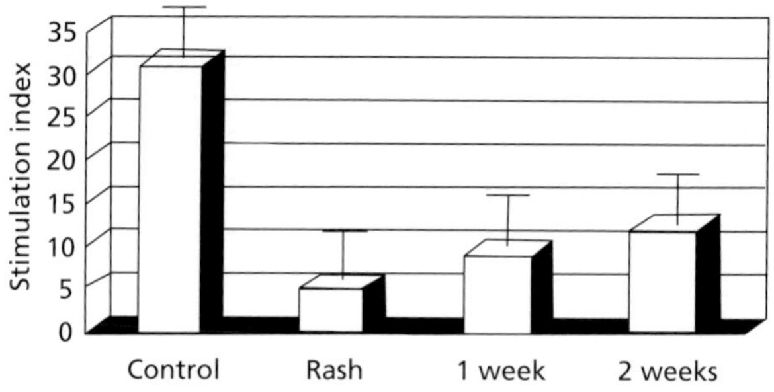

Figure 39.5 *Immune suppression during measles infection. Changes in proliferation of peripheral blood mononuclear cells to the mitogen phytohemagglutinin. (Modified after Hirsch et al. 1984, and Griffin 2001).*

downregulation. The downregulation of CD46 on monocytes infected with the measles virus results in a decreased IL-12 production (for a review, see Schneider-Schaulies and Ter Meulen 2002). The measles virus nucleocapsid protein inhibits IL-12 release from mouse monocytes. These observations are further supported by in vivo data showing a prolonged impairment of IL-12 production by monocytes from patients after natural measles infection. A decrease of IL-12 production by macrophages and monocytes may result in a decreased IFN-γ production by T cells. Furthermore, as stimulation of macrophages via CD46 seems to be involved in the response of macrophages to IFN-γ which stimulates the production of nitric oxide (NO) (for a review, see Schneider-Schaulies and Ter Meulen 2002). The downregulation of CD46 may result in a reduced production of NO and an altered immune response to intracellular pathogens such as mycobacteria.

The measles virus hemagglutinin seems to be responsible for CD150 downregulation (Tanaka et al. 2002). Recently, it could be demonstrated in an animal model that wild-type measles virus strains, which in contrast to vaccine virus induce strong immune suppression, exclusively used the CD150 and not the CD46 receptor (Pfeuffer et al. 2003). After infection and downregulation of CD105 on T cells, cell division and proliferation of these cells are inhibited (Hahm et al. 2003). Signaling events triggered after binding to this receptor are complex and can result not only in activation but also in cellular apoptosis (Sidorenko and Clark 1993). The IFN-γ production of $CD4^+$ T cells can be upregulated by ligation to the CD150 receptor (Aversa et al. 1997). Thus, downregulation of this molecule after infection with measles virus may impair Th1 responses toward intracellular pathogens, as seen in humans with measles (Griffin 1995). This hypothesis is further supported by recent experiments in transgenic mice expressing the measles virus receptor CD46. After infection with measles virus these animals were more susceptible to infection with *Listeria monocytogenes* as a result of the reduced number of macrophages and substantial defects in IFN-γ-producing $CD4^+$ T cells (Slifka et al. 2003). IFN-γ production is important for the defense of intracellular bacteria (Kaufmann 1992) and impairment in this pathway explains the observed increased bacterial infections during and after infection with measles. TNF-α production by monocytes is reduced during acute infection and recovery (Griffin et al. 1987). In vitro experiments with monocytic cell lines show a decrease in TNF-α production after infection with the measles virus (Leopardi et al. 1992).

The effect of the measles virus on DCs has not been clear until now. DCs isolated from peripheral blood showed normal release of IL-12 after stimulation with bacterial cell wall components; DCs generated in vitro, however, showed impaired production of IL-12 (for a review, see Schneider-Schaulies and Ter Meulen 2002). The reduced IL-12 production by DCs and monocytes may have consequences affecting the quality of T-cell responses and could explain an inadequate Th1 response during measles infection (Griffin et al. 1989; Ward and Griffin 1993). In fact measles virus-infected DCs are unable to stimulate allogenic T-cell proliferation, and even actively suppress in vitro-stimulation of T-cell proliferation (for a review, see Schneider-Schaulies and Ter Meulen 2002).

LYMPHOCYTES

A lymphopenia affecting both CD4 and CD8 cells is observed during infection with measles (Okada et al. 2000). Although the CD4:CD8 T-cell ratio normally remains unaltered (Arneborn and Biberfeld 1983), a greater decrease of $CD4^+$ T cells with decreased CD4:CD8 ratios has been found in children with malnutrition (Ryon et al. 2002). The mechanism responsible for the lymphopenia is thought to be measles-induced apoptosis of uninfected lymphocytes (Okada et al. 2000; Ryon et al. 2002). A selective loss of peripheral lymphocyte function-associated antigen ($LFA\text{-}1^{high}$)-expressing T cells was observed in the course of measles virus infection, and this could reflect aberrant lymphocyte trafficking by random homing to tissues (Nanan et al. 1999). This may also contribute to leukopenia. The role of leukopenia for measles virus-induced immunosuppression is unclear, because the duration of immune function impairment clearly exceeds the panlymphopenic phase of the disease (Okada et al. 2000).

One reason for the reduced T-cell proliferation in vitro to mitogens during measles infection and during the first weeks of convalescence is inadequate IL-2 production. Addition of recombinant IL-2 to lymphocyte cultures from patients with measles restores lymphocyte proliferation ability (Griffin et al. 1986; Ward and Griffin 1993). Investigation of other T-cell cytokines revealed low IFN-γ release and high IL-4 production compared with controls (Ward et al. 1991; Griffin and Ward 1993). In vitro neutralization of IL-4 with antibodies also improves lymphocyte proliferation (Griffin and Ward 1993). This T-cell cytokine profile suggests a shift toward a Th2-type response and may explain the suppression of delayed-type hypersensitivity during and after the first weeks of infection.

In contrast to natural infection with measles virus, measles virus immunization does not result in a reduced IL-12 and IFN-γ production. Measles virus glycoprotein seems directly to block the proliferative response of lymphocytes to mitogens in vitro, whereas anti-measles virus antibodies and genetic exchange of measles glycoprotein abolish such inhibition of proliferation (for a review, see Schneider-Schaulies and Ter Meulen 2002). Direct in vitro infection of T cells results in a reduced proliferative response to mitogens and soluble antigens as well as in an impaired cytotoxic function (for a review, see Schneider-Schaulies and Ter Meulen 2002). IFN-α production is important to limit viral infections and infections with secondary viral infections, especially herpesvirus infections, which are frequently observed during and after measles virus infection (for a review, see Schneider-Schaulies and Ter Meulen 2002). In agreement with this clinical observation is the experimental finding that, after in vitro infection with measles virus, a suppression in the IFN-α-signaling pathway was documented (Yokota et al. 2003). Infection with the measles virus resulted in a suppression of Jak1 phosphorylation and association of the viral accessory proteins C and V with the IFN-α receptor complex (Yokota et al. 2003).

Infection of B cells in vitro with the measles virus reduces Ig production (Casali et al. 1984; Tishon et al. 1996). Measles virus nucleocapsid protein binds to activated B cells and reduces antibody production in vitro (Ravanel et al. 1997). However, in vivo experimental measles virus infection revealed an impaired T-cell function but no B-cell defect (Niewiesk et al. 2000).

Soluble factors such as cytokines and viral proteins account for the immunosuppression of infected and uninfected lymphocytes during and for several weeks after measles infection and seem to be more important than mechanisms directly induced by infection of T and B cells. However, the in vitro effects of infection of leukocytes, macrophages, and B and T cells by measles virus cannot be ruled out, and may also be relevant to the immune suppression observed during natural measles infection.

Impaired function of immunocompetent cells such as macrophages, DCs, and B and T cells can be found at different time points after measles virus infection. There seems to be a dichotomy between the immune response toward measles virus and other pathogens. This dichotomy may be resolved by investigations of a newly discovered regulatory $CD4^{+}CD25^{+}$ T-cell subpopulation. These cells are present after several infections in order to restrict and limit immune responses to certain pathogens, thus avoiding the induction of autoimmune diseases (Belkaid et al. 2002). The following scenario is therefore possible: after measles virus infection, a strong measles virus-specific T-cell and B-cell response is induced, which is capable of clearing the measles virus; after several days this immune response has to be restricted, and regulatory $CD4^{+}CD25^{+}$ T cells appear, which suppress and limit ongoing or newly induced immune responses; these cells may be active for several weeks, during which time the host is vulnerable to secondary infections.

REFERENCES

Ahmad, A. and Menezes, J. 1996. Defective killing activity against gp120/41-expressing human erythroleukaemic K562 cell line by monocytes and natural killer cells from HIV-infected individuals. *AIDS*, **10**, 143–9.

Ahmad, A., Morisset, R., et al. 1994. Evidence for a defect of antibody-dependent cellular cytotoxic (ADCC) effector function and anti-HIV gp120/41-specific ADCC-mediating antibody titres in HIV-infected individuals. *J Acquir Immune Defic Syndr*, **7**, 428–37.

Ahmad, R., Sindhu, S.T., et al. 2001. Modulation of expression of the MHC class I-binding natural killer cell receptors and NK activity in relation to viral load in HIV-infected/*AIDS* patients. *J Med Virol*, **65**, 431–40.

Altfeld, M. and Rosenberg, E.S. 2000. The role of CD4(+) T helper cells in the cytotoxic T lymphocyte response to HIV-1. *Curr Opin Immunol*, **12**, 375–80.

Amerongen, H.M., Weltzin, R., et al. 1991. Transepithelial transport of HIV-1 by intestinal M cells: a mechanism for transmission of *AIDS*. *J Acquir Immune Defic Syndr*, **4**, 760–5.

Amiel, C., Darcissac, E., et al. 1999. Interleukin-16 (IL-16) inhibits human immunodeficiency virus replication in cells from infected subjects, and serum IL-16 levels drop with disease progression. *J Infect Dis*, **179**, 83–91.

Andersson, J., Behbahani, H., et al. 1999. Perforin is not co-expressed with granzyme A within cytotoxic granules in CD8 T lymphocytes present in lymphoid tissue during chronic HIV infection. *AIDS*, **13**, 1295–303.

Andre, P., Brunet, C., et al. 1999. Differential regulation of killer cell Ig-like receptors and CD94 lectin-like dimers on NK and T lymphocytes from HIV-1-infected individuals. *Eur J Immunol*, **29**, 1076–85.

Anton, P.A., Elliott, J., et al. 2000. Enhanced levels of functional HIV-1 co-receptors on human mucosal T cells demonstrated using intestinal biopsy tissue. *AIDS*, **14**, 1761–5.

Apoola, A., Ahmad, S. and Radcliffe, K. 2002. Primary HIV infection. *Int J STD AIDS*, **13**, 71–8.

Appay, V., Nixon, D.F., et al. 2000. HIV-specific CD8(+) T cells produce antiviral cytokines but are impaired in cytolytic function. *J Exp Med*, **192**, 63–75.

Arneborn, P. and Biberfeld, G. 1983. T-lymphocyte subpopulations in relation to immunosuppression in measles and varicella. *Infect Immun*, **39**, 29–37.

Aversa, G., Chang, C.C., et al. 1997. Engagement of the signalling lymphocytic activation molecule (SLAM) on activated T cells results in IL-2-independent, cyclosporin A-sensitive T cell proliferation and IFN-gamma production. *J Immunol*, **158**, 4036–44.

Autran, B., Carcelain, G., et al. 1997. Positive effects of combined antiretroviral therapy on CD4+ T cell homeostasis and function in advanced HIV disease. *Science*, **277**, 112–16.

Autran, B., Mayaud, C.M., et al. 1988. Evidence for a cytotoxic T-lymphocyte alveolitis in human immunodeficiency virus-infected patients. *AIDS*, **2**, 179–83.

Bacchetti, P. and Moss, A.R. 1989. Incubation period of AIDS in San Francisco. *Nature*, **338**, 251–3.

Bacchetti, P., Osmond, D., et al. 1988. Survival patterns of the first, 500 patients with AIDS in San Francisco. *J Infect Dis*, **157**, 1044–7.

Badley, A.D., Dockrell, D., et al. 1997. Macrophage-dependent apoptosis of CD4+ T lymphocytes from HIV-infected individuals is mediated by FasL and tumor necrosis factor. *J Exp Med*, **185**, 55–64.

Badley, A.D., Pilon, A.A., et al. 2000. Mechanisms of HIV-associated lymphocyte apoptosis. *Blood*, **96**, 2951–64.

Baier, M., Werner, A., et al. 1995. HIV suppression by interleukin-16. *Nature*, **378**, 563.

Bakri, Y., Schiffer, C., et al. 2001. The maturation of dendritic cells results in postintegration inhibition of HIV-1 replication. *J Immunol*, **166**, 3780–8.

Baldwin, G.C., Fleischmann, J., et al. 1990. Human immunodeficiency virus causes mononuclear phagocyte dysfunction. *Proc Natl Acad Sci USA*, **87**, 3933–7.

Banda, N.K., Bernier, J., et al. 1992. Crosslinking CD4 by human immunodeficiency virus gp120 primes T cells for activation-induced apoptosis. *J Exp Med*, **176**, 1099–106.

Bandres, J.C., Trial, J., et al. 1993. Increased phagocytosis and generation of reactive oxygen products by neutrophils and monocytes of men with stage 1 human immunodeficiency virus infection. *J Infect Dis*, **168**, 75–83.

Barré-Sinoussi, F., Chermann, J.C., et al. 1983. Isolation of a T-lymphotropic retrovirus from a patient at risk for acquired immune deficiency syndrome (AIDS). *Science*, **220**, 868–70.

Barron, M.A., Blyveis, N., et al. 2003. Influence of plasma viremia on defects in number and immunophenotype of blood dendritic cell subsets in human immunodeficiency virus 1-infected individuals. *J Infect Dis*, **187**, 26–37.

Bartholomew, C., Blattner, W. and Cleghorn, F. 1987. Progression to AIDS in homosexual men co-infected with HIV and HTLV-I in Trinidad. *Lancet*, **ii**, 1469.

Beckford, A.P., Kaschula, R.O.C. and Stephen, C. 1985. Factors associated with fatal cases of measles: A retrospective autopsy study. *S Afr Med J*, **68**, 858–63.

Belkaid, Y., Piccirillo, C.A., et al. 2002. CD4+CD25+ regulatory T cells control *Leishmania* major persistence and immunity. *Nature*, **420**, 502–7.

Berberian, L., Goodglick, L., et al. 1993. Immunoglobulin VH3 gene products: natural ligands for HIV gp120. *Science*, **261**, 1588–91.

Biberfeld, P., Ost, A., et al. 1987. Histopathology and immunohistology of HTLV-III/LAV related lymphadenopathy and AIDS. *Acta Pathol Microbiol Immunol Scand*, **95**, 47–65.

Biggs, B.A., Hewish, M., et al. 1995. HIV-1 infection of human macrophages impairs phagocytosis and killing of *Toxoplasma gondii*. *J Immunol*, **154**, 6132–9.

Bhaskaram, P. 2002. Micronutrient malnutrition, infection, and immunity: an overview. *Nutr Rev*, **60**, S40–45.

Bhigjee, A.I., Wiley, C.A., et al. 1991. HTLV-I-associated myelopathy: Clinicopathologic correlation with localization of provirus to spinal cord. *Neurology*, **41**, 1990–2.

Boaz, M.J., Waters, A., et al. 2002. Presence of HIV-1 Gag-specific IFN-gamma+IL-2+ and CD28+IL-2+ CD4 T cell responses is associated with nonprogression in HIV-1 infection. *J Immunol*, **169**, 6376–85.

Bomsel, M. 1997. Transcytosis of infectious human immunodeficiency virus across a tight human epithelial cell line barrier. *Nat Med*, **3**, 42–7.

Bomsel, M., Heyman, M., et al. 1998. Intracellular neutralization of HIV transcytosis across tight epithelial barriers by anti-HIV envelope protein dIgA or IgM. *Immunity*, **9**, 277–87.

Borthwick, N.J., Bofill, M., et al. 1994. Lymphocyte activation in HIV-1 infection. II. Functional defects of CD28- T cells. *AIDS*, **8**, 431–41.

Boullier, S., Dadaglio, G., et al. 1997. V delta, 1 T cells expanded in the blood throughout HIV infection display a cytotoxic activity and are primed for TNF-alpha and IFN-gamma production but are not selected in lymph nodes. *J Immunol*, **159**, 3629–37.

Brandtzaeg, P., Valnes, K., et al. 1985. The human gastrointestinal secretory immune system in health and disease. *Scand J Gastroenterol Suppl*, **114**, 17–38.

Brenchley, J.M., Karandikar, N.J., et al. 2003. Expression of CD57 defines replicative senescence and antigen-induced apoptotic death of CD8+ T cells. *Blood*, **101**, 2711–20.

Brenner, B.G., Dascal, A., et al. 1989. Natural killer cell function in patients with acquired immunodeficiency syndrome and related diseases. *J Leukoc Biol*, **46**, 75–83.

Brenner, B.G., Gryllis, C. and Wainberg, M.A. 1991. Role of antibody-dependent cellular cytotoxicity and lymphokine-activated killer cells in AIDS and related diseases. *J Leukoc Biol*, **50**, 628–40.

Brenner, B.G., Gryllis, C., et al. 1993. Changes in natural immunity during the course of HIV-1 infection. *Clin Exp Immunol*, **93**, 142–8.

Bunn, P.A. Jr, Schechter, G.P., et al. 1983. Clinical course of retrovirus-associated adult T-cell lymphoma in the United States. *N Engl J Med*, **309**, 257–64.

Caldwell, R.L., Egan, B.S. and Shepherd, V.L. 2000. HIV-1 Tat represses transcription from the mannose receptor promoter. *J Immunol*, **165**, 7035–41.

Cappell, M.S. and Chow, J. 1987. HTLV-I-associated lymphoma involving the entire alimentary tract and presenting with an acquired immune deficiency. *Am J Med*, **82**, 649–54.

Casali, P., Rice, G.P. and Oldstone, M.B. 1984. Viruses disrupt functions of human lymphocytes: Effects of measles virus and influenza virus on lymphocyte-mediated killing and antibody production. *J Exp Med*, **159**, 1322–37.

Cassone, A., Chiani, P., et al. 1997. Possible participation of polymorphonuclear cells stimulated by microbial immunomodulators in the dysregulated cytokine patterns of AIDS patients. *J Leukoc Biol*, **62**, 60–6.

Chehimi, J., Starr, S.E., et al. 1994. Impaired interleukin 12 production in human immunodeficiency virus-infected patients. *J Exp Med*, **179**, 1361–6.

Chehimi, J., Campbell, D.E., et al. 2002. Persistent decreases in blood plasmacytoid dendritic cell number and function despite effective highly active antiretroviral therapy and increased blood myeloid dendritic cells in HIV-infected individuals. *J Immunol*, **168**, 4796–801.

Chen, G., Shankar, P., et al. 2001. CD8 T cells specific for human immunodeficiency virus, Epstein-Barr virus, and cytomegalovirus lack molecules for homing to lymphoid sites of infection. *Blood*, **98**, 156–64.

Chen, J.J., Huang, J.C., et al. 2002. CD4 lymphocytes in the blood of HIV(+) individuals migrate rapidly to lymph nodes and bone marrow: support for homing theory of CD4 cell depletion. *J Leukoc Biol*, **72**, 271–8.

Chen, T.P., Roberts, R.L., et al. 1993. Decreased superoxide anion and hydrogen peroxide production by neutrophils and monocytes in human immunodeficiency virus-infected children and adults. *Pediatr Res*, **34**, 544–50.

Chirmule, N., McCloskey, T.W., et al. 1995. HIV gp120 inhibits T cell activation by interfering with expression of costimulatory molecules CD40 ligand and CD80 (B71). *J Immunol*, **155**, 917–24.

Choi, Y.K., Fallert, B.A., et al. 2003. Simian immunodeficiency virus dramatically alters expression of homeostatic chemokines and dendritc cell markers during infection in vivo. *Blood*, **101**, 1684–91.

Ciobanu, N., Paietta, E., et al. 1985. Thymus fragment transplantation in the acquired immunodeficiency syndrome. *Ann Intern Med*, **103**, 479.

Cleghorn, F.R. and Blattner, W.A. 1992. Does human T-cell lymphotropic virus type I and human immunodeficiency virus type I co-infection accelerate acquired immune deficiency syndrome? *Arch Intern Med*, **152**, 1372–3.

Clerici, M. and Shearer, G.M. 1994. The Th1-Th2 hypothesis of HIV infection: new insights. *Immunol Today*, **15**, 575–81.

Clerici, M., Stocks, N.I., et al. 1989. Detection of three distinct patterns of T helper cell dysfunction in asymptomatic, human immunodeficiency virus-seropositive patients. Independence of CD4+ cell numbers and clinical staging. *J Clin Invest*, **84**, 1892–9.

Clinton, W.J. 2003. Turning the tide on the AIDS pandemic. *N Engl J Med*, **348**, 1800–2.

Coffey, M.J., Phare, S.M., et al. 1998. Granulocyte colony-stimulating factor administration to HIV-infected subjects augments reduced leukotriene synthesis and anticryptococcal activity in neutrophils. *J Clin Invest*, **102**, 663–70.

Cohen, G.B., Gandhi, R.T., et al. 1999. The selective downregulation of class I major histocompatibility complex proteins by HIV-1 protects HIV-infected cells from NK cells. *Immunity*, **10**, 661–71.

Cohen Stuart, J.W., Hazebergh, M.D., et al. 2000. The dominant source of CD4+ and CD8+ T-cell activation in HIV infection is antigenic stimulation. *J Acquir Immune Defic Syndr*, **25**, 203–11.

Collins, K.L., Chen, B.K., et al. 1998. HIV-1 Nef protein protects infected primary cells against killing by cytotoxic T lymphocytes. *Nature*, **391**, 397–401.

Connors, M., Kovacs, J.A., et al. 1997. HIV infection induces changes in CD4+ T-cell phenotype and depletions within the CD4+ T-cell repertoire that are not immediately restored by antiviral or immune-based therapies. *Nat Med*, **3**, 533–40.

Cooper, D.A., Gold, J., et al. 1985. Acute AIDS retrovirus infection. Definition of a clinical illness associated with seroconversion. *Lancet*, **i**, 537–40.

Coovadia, H.M., Parent, M.A., et al. 1974. An evaluation of factors associated with the depression of immunity in malnutrition and in measles. *Am J Clin Nutr*, **27**, 665–9.

Coovadia, H.M., Wessley, A. and Brain, P. 1978. Immunologic events in acute measles influencing outcome. *Arch Dis Child*, **53**, 861–7.

Correa, R. and Munoz-Fernandez, M.A. 2002. Production of new T cells by thymus in children: effect of HIV infection and antiretroviral therapy. *Pediatr Res*, **52**, 207–12.

Costa, P., Rusconi, S., et al. 2003. Low expression of inhibitory natural killer receptors in CD8 cytotoxic T lymphocytes in long-term non-progressor HIV-1-infected patients. *AIDS*, **17**, 257–60.

Couedel-Courteille, A., Le Grand, R., et al. 1997. Direct ex vivo Simian immunodeficiency virus (SIV)-specific cytotoxic activity detected from small intestine intraepithelial lymphocytes of SIV-infected macaques at advanced stage of infection. *J Virol*, **71**, 1052–7.

Davis, I.C., Girard, M. and Fultz, P.N. 1998. Loss of CD4+ T cells in human immunodeficiency virus type 1-infected chimpanzees is associated with increased lymphocyte apoptosis. *J Virol*, **72**, 4623–32.

Dayton, A.I., Sodroski, J.G., et al. 1986. The trans-activator gene of the human T cell lymphotropic virus type III is required for replication. *Cell*, **44**, 941–7.

De Maria, A. and Moretta, L. 2000. HLA-class I-specific inhibitory receptors in HIV-1 infection. *Hum Immunol*, **61**, 74–81.

De Maria, A., Ferrazin, A., et al. 1992. Selective increase of a subset of T cell receptor gamma delta T lymphocytes in the peripheral blood of patients with human immunodeficiency virus type 1 infection. *J Infect Dis*, **165**, 917–19.

De Maria, A., Mavilio, D., et al. 2000. Multiple HLA-class I-specific inhibitory NK receptor expression and IL-4/IL-5 production by CD8+ T-cell clones in HIV-1 infection. *Immunol Lett*, **72**, 179–82.

De Milito, A., Morch, C., et al. 2001. Loss of memory (CD27) B lymphocytes in HIV-1 infection. *AIDS*, **15**, 957–64.

De Paoli, P., Gennari, D., et al. 1991. A subset of gamma delta lymphocytes is increased during HIV-1 infection. *Clin Exp Immunol*, **83**, 187–91.

Delemarre, F.G., Stevenhagen, A., et al. 1994. Effect of IFN-gamma on the proliferation of Toxoplasma gondii in monocytes and monocyte-derived macrophages from AIDS patients. *Immunology*, **83**, 646–50.

Denton, J. 1925. The pathology of fatal measles. *Am J Med Sci*, **169**, 531–43.

DeStefano, E., Friedman, R.M., et al. 1982. Acid-labile human leukocyte interferon in homosexual men with Kaposi's sarcoma and lymphadenopathy. *J Infect Dis*, **146**, 451–9.

Dockrell, D.H., Badley, A.D., et al. 1998. The expression of Fas Ligand by macrophages and its upregulation by human immunodeficiency virus infection. *J Clin Invest*, **101**, 2394–405.

Donaghy, H., Gazzard, B., et al. 2003. Dysfunction and infection of freshly isolated blood myeloid and plasmacytoid dendritic cells in patients infected with HIV-1. *Blood*, **6**, 6.

Dossetor, J., Whittle, H.C. and Greenwood, B.M. 1977. Persistent measles infection in malnourished children. *BMJi*, **i**, 1633–5.

Douek, D.C., Betts, M.R., et al. 2001. Evidence for increased T cell turnover and decreased thymic output in HIV infection. *J Immunol*, **167**, 6663–8.

Douek, D.C., Brenchley, J.M., et al. 2002. HIV preferentially infects HIV-specific CD4+ T cells. *Nature*, **417**, 95–8.

Douek, D.C., Picker, L.J. and Koup, R.A. 2003. T cell dynamics in HIV-1 infection. *Annu Rev Immunol*, **21**, 265–304.

Du, Z., Lang, S.M., et al. 1995. Identification of a nef allele that causes lymphocyte activation and acute disease in Macaque monkeys. *Cell*, **82**, 665–74.

Dudhane, A., Conti, B., et al. 1996. Monocytes in HIV type 1-infected individuals lose expression of costimulatory B7 molecules and acquire cytotoxic activity. *AIDS Res Hum Retroviruses*, **12**, 885–92.

Duke, T. and Mgone, C.S. 2003. Measles: not just another viral exanthem. *Lancet*, **361**, 763–73.

Dwyer, J.M., Wood, C.C., et al. 1987. Transplantation of thymus tissue into patients with *AIDS*: An attempt to reconstitute the immune system. *Arch Intern Med*, **147**, 513–17.

Elbim, C., Pillet, S., et al. 1999. Redox and activation status of monocytes from human immunodeficiency virus-infected patients: relationship with viral load. *J Virol*, **73**, 4561–6.

Ellis, M., Gupta, S., et al. 1988. Impaired neutrophil function in patients with AIDS or AIDS-related complex: a comprehensive evaluation. *J Infect Dis*, **158**, 1268–76.

Esolen, L.M., Ward, B.J., et al. 1993. Infection of monocytes during measles. *J Infect Dis*, **168**, 47–52.

Ewing, E.P., Chandler, R.W., et al. 1985. Primary lymph node pathology in AIDS and AIDS-related lymphadenopathy. *Arch Pathol Lab Med*, **109**, 977–81.

Fackler, O. and Baur, A.S. 2002. Live and let die: Nef functions beyond HIV replication. *Immunity*, **16**, 493–7.

Fackler, O., Schäfer, M., et al. 1998. HIV-1 p24 but not proviral load is increased in the intestinal mucosa compared to the peripheral blood in HIV-infected patients. *AIDS*, **12**, 139–46.

Falk, S., Muller, H. and Stutte, H. 1988. The spleen in acquired immunodeficiency syndrome (*AIDS*). *Pathol Res Oract*, **183**, 425–33.

Fauci, A.S. 1996. Host factors and the pathogenesis of HIV-induced disease. *Nature*, **384**, 529–34.

Ferbas, J.J., Toso, J.F., et al. 1994. CD4+ blood dendritic cells are potent producers of IFN-alpha in response to in vitro HIV-1 infection. *J Immunol*, **152**, 4649–62.

Finkel, T.H., Tudor-Williams, G., et al. 1995. Apoptosis occurs predominantly in bystander cells and not in productively infected cells of HIV- and SIV-infected lymph nodes. *Nat Med*, **1**, 129–34.

Flo, R.W., Naess, A., et al. 1994. A longitudinal study of phagocyte function in HIV-infected patients. *AIDS*, **8**, 771–7.

Forthal, D.N., Aarnaes, S., et al. 1992. Degree and length of viremia in adults with measles. *J Infect Dis*, **166**, 421–4.

Fotopoulos, G., Harai, A., et al. 2002. Transepithelial transport of HIV-1 by M cells is receptor-mediated. *Proc Natl Acad Sci USA*, **99**, 9410–14.

Fournier, S., Rabian, C., et al. 2001. Immune recovery under highly active antiretroviral therapy is associated with restoration of lymphocyte proliferation and interferon-gamma production in the presence of *Toxoplasma gondii* antigens. *J Infect Dis*, **183**, 1586–91.

Franchini, G. 1995. Molecular mechanisms of human T-cell leukemia/lymphotropic virus type I infection. *Blood*, **86**, 3619–39.

Franco, J.M., Rubio, A., et al. 2002. T-cell repopulation and thymic volume in HIV-1-infected adult patients after highly active antiretroviral therapy. *Blood*, **99**, 3702–6.

Frank, I. and Pope, M. 2002. The enigma of dendritic cell-immunodeficiency virus interplay. *Curr Mol Med*, **2**, 229–48.

Fry, T.J., Connick, E., et al. 2001. A potential role for interleukin-7 in T-cell homeostasis. *Blood*, **97**, 2983–90.

Furukawa, Y., Saito, M., et al. 2003. Different cytokine production in Tax-expressing cells between patients with human T cell lymphotropic virus type I (HTLV-I)-associated myelopathy/tropical spastic paraparesis and asymptomatic HTLV-I carriers. *J Infect Dis*, **187**, 1116–25.

Gabrilovich, D., Ivanova, L., et al. 1994. Clinical significance of neutrophil functional activity in HIV infection. *Scand J Infect Dis*, **26**, 41–7.

Galiani, M.D., Aguado, E., et al. 1999. Expression of killer inhibitory receptors on cytotoxic cells from HIV-1-infected individuals. *Clin Exp Immunol*, **115**, 472–6.

Gandhi, R.T. and Walker, B.D. 2002. Immunologic control of HIV-1. *Annu Rev Med*, **53**, 149–72.

Gandhi, R.T., Chen, B.K., et al. 1998. HIV-1 directly kills CD4+ T cells by a Fas-independent mechanism. *J Exp Med*, **187**, 1113–22.

Garcia, J.C. and Miller, A.D. 1991. Serine phosphorylation-independent downregulation of cell-surface CD4 by nef. *Nature*, **350**, 508–11.

Gavazzi, G. and Krause, K.H. 2002. Ageing and infection. *Lancet Infect Dis*, **11**, 659–66.

Gea-Banacloche, J.C., Weiskopf, E.E., et al. 1998. Progression of human immunodeficiency virus disease is associated with increasing disruptions within the CD4+ T cell receptor repertoire. *J Infect Dis*, **177**, 579–85.

Geertsma, M.F., Stevenhagen, A., et al. 1999. Expression of zeta molecules is decreased in NK cells from HIV-infected patients. *FEMS Immunol Med Microbiol*, **26**, 249–57.

Geijtenbeek, T.B., Kwon, D.S., et al. 2000. DC-SIGN, a dendritic cell-specific HIV-1-binding protein that enhances trans-infection of T cells. *Cell*, **100**, 587–97.

Gelderblom, H., Özel, M. and Pauli, G. 1985. T-Zell-spezifische Retroviren des Menschen: Vergleichende morphologische Klassifizierung und mögliche funktionelle Aspekte. *Bundesgesundheitsblatt*, **28**, 161–71.

Gelderblom, H.R., Hausmann, E.H., et al. 1987. Fine structure of human immunodeficiency virus (HIV) and immunolocalization of structural proteins. *Virology*, **156**, 41–60.

Gendelman, H.E., Baca, L.M., et al. 1992. Induction of IFN-alpha in peripheral blood mononuclear cells by HIV-infected monocytes. Restricted antiviral activity of the HIV-induced IFN. *J Immunol*, **148**, 422–9.

Gessain, A., Barin, F., et al. 1985. Antibodies to human T-lymphotropic virus type-I in patients with tropical spastic paralysis. *Lancet*, **ii**, 407–10.

Ginaldi, L., De Martinis, M., et al. 1998. Changes in antigen expression on B lymphocytes during HIV infection. *Pathobiology*, **66**, 17–23.

Giorgi, J.V., Ho, H.N., et al. 1994. CD8+ lymphocyte activation at human immunodeficiency virus type 1 seroconversion: development of HLA-DR+ CD38- CD8+ cells is associated with subsequent stable CD4+ cell levels. The Multicenter AIDS Cohort Study Group. *J Infect Dis*, **170**, 775–81.

Giorgi, J.V., Hultin, L.E., et al. 1999. Shorter survival in advanced human immunodeficiency virus type 1 infection is more closely associated with T lymphocyte activation than with plasma virus burden or virus chemokine coreceptor usage. *J Infect Dis*, **179**, 859–70.

Goepfert, P.A., Bansal, A., et al. 2000. A significant number of human immunodeficiency virus epitope-specific cytotoxic T lymphocytes detected by tetramer binding do not produce gamma interferon. *J Virol*, **74**, 10249–55.

Gordon, S.B., Molyneux, M.E., et al. 2001. Opsonic phagocytosis of *Streptococcus pneumoniae* by alveolar macrophages is not impaired in human immunodeficiency virus-infected Malawian adults. *J Infect Dis*, **184**, 1345–9.

Gotuzzo, E., Escamilla, J., et al. 1992. The impact of human T-lymphotropic virus type I/II infection on the prognosis of sexually acquired cases of acquired immune deficiency syndrome. *Arch Intern Med*, **152**, 1429–32.

Gougeon, M.L. 2003. Cell death and immunity: Apoptosis as an HIV strategy to escape immune attack. *Nat Rev Immunol*, **3**, 392–404.

Gougeon, M.L., Lecoeur, H., et al. 1996. Programmed cell death in peripheral lymphocytes from HIV-infected persons: increased susceptibility to apoptosis of CD4 and CD8 T cells correlates with lymphocyte activation and with disease progression. *J Immunol*, **156**, 3509–20.

Goulder, P.J., Tang, Y., et al. 2000. Functionally inert HIV-specific cytotoxic T lymphocytes do not play a major role in chronically infected adults and children. *J Exp Med*, **192**, 1819–32.

Greenberg, B.L., Sack, R.B., et al. 1991. Measles-associated diarrhea in hospitalized children in Lima, Peru: Pathogenic agents and impact on growth. *J Infect Dis*, **163**, 495–502.

Griffin, D.E. 1995. Immune response during measles virus infections. *Curr Top Microbiol Immunol*, **191**, 117–34.

Griffin, D.E. 2001. Measles virus. In: Bernard, P.M., Fields, N., et al. (eds), *Measles virus*, Vol. 1. 4th edn. Philadelphia, PA: Lippincott, Williams & Wilkins, 1401–41.

Griffin, D.E. and Ward, J.B. 1993. Differential CD4 T cell activation in measles. *J Infect Dis*, **168**, 275–81.

Griffin, D.E., Moench, T.R., et al. 1986. Peripheral blood mononuclear cells during natural measles virus infection: Cell surface phenotypes and evidence for activation. *Clin Immunol Immunopathol*, **40**, 305–12.

Griffin, D.E., Johnson, R.T., et al. 1987. In vitro studies of the role of monocytes in the immunosuppression associated with natural measles virus infections. *Clin Immunol Immunopathol*, **45**, 375–83.

Griffin, D.E., Ward, B.J., et al. 1989. Immune activation in measles. *N Engl J Med*, **320**, 1667–72.

Grossman, Z., Feinberg, M.B. and Paul, W.E. 1998. Multiple modes of cellular activation and virus transmission in HIV infection: a role for chronically and latently infected cells in sustaining viral replication. *Proc Natl Acad Sci USA*, **95**, 6314–19.

Groux, H., Torpier, G., et al. 1992. Activation-induced death by apoptosis in CD4+ T cells from human immunodeficiency virus-infected asymptomatic individuals. *J Exp Med*, **175**, 331–40.

Haase, A.T. 1999. Population biology of HIV-1 infection: viral and CD4+ T cell demographics and dynamics in lymphatic tissues. *Annu Rev Immunol*, **17**, 625–56.

Hahm, B., Arbour, N., et al. 2003. Measles virus infects and suppresses proliferation of T lymphocytes from transgenic mice bearing human signaling lymphocytic activation molecule. *J Virol*, **77**, 3505–15.

Hall, W.C., Kovatch, R.M., et al. 1971. Pathology of measles in rhesus monkeys. *Vet Pathol*, **8**, 307–19.

Hanly, S.M., Rimsky, L.T., et al. 1989. Comparative analysis of the HTLV-1 rex and HIV-1 rev trans-regulatory proteins and their RNA response elements. *Genes Dev*, **3**, 1534–44.

Hattori, T., Uchiyama, T., et al. 1981. Surface phenotype of Japanese adult T-cell leukemia cells characterized by monoclonal antibodies. *Blood*, **58**, 645–7.

Hazenberg, M.D., Hamann, D., et al. 2000. T cell depletion in HIV-1 infection: how CD4+ T cells go out of stock. *Nat Immunol*, **1**, 285–9.

Herbein, G., Van Lint, C., et al. 1998. Distinct mechanisms trigger apoptosis in human immunodeficiency virus type 1-infected and in uninfected bystander T lymphocytes. *J Virol*, **72**, 660–70.

Hermans, P. and Clumeck, N. 1989. Preliminary results on clinical and immunological effects of thymus hormone preparations in AIDS. *Med Oncol Tumor Pharmcother*, **6**, 55–8.

Hinuma, Y., Komoda, H., et al. 1982. Antibodies to adult T-cell leukemia-virus-associated (ATLA) in sera from patients with ATL and controls in Japan: A nation-wide seroepidemiologic study. *Int J Cancer*, **29**, 631–5.

Hirsch, R.L., Griffin, D.E., et al. 1984. Cellular immune responses during complicated and uncomplicated measles virus infections of man. *Clin Immunol Immunopathol*, **31**, 1–12.

Ho, D.D., Neumann, A.U., et al. 1995. Rapid turnover of plasma virions and CD4 lymphocytes in HIV-1 infection. *Nature*, **373**, 123–6.

Hu, P.F., Hultin, L.E., et al. 1995. Natural killer cell immunodeficiency in HIV disease is manifest by profoundly decreased numbers of

CD16+CD56+ cells and expansion of a population of CD16dimCD56– cells with low lytic activity. *J Acquir Immune Defic Syndr Hum Retrovirol*, **10**, 331–40.

Idziorek, T., Khalife, J., et al. 1998. Recombinant human IL-16 inhibits HIV-1 replication and protects against activation-induced cell death (AICD). *Clin Exp Immunol*, **112**, 84–91.

Ifthikharuddin, J.J. and Rosenblatt, J.D. 2000. In Mandell, G.L., Bennett, J.E., and Dolin, R. (eds) *Human T-cell lymphotropic virus types I and II*, Vol. 2, 5th edn. Edinburgh: Churchill Livingstone.

Igakura, T., Stinchcombe, J.C., et al. 2003. Spread of HTLV-1 between lymphocytes by virus-induced polarization of the cytoskeleton. *Science*, **299**, 1713–16.

Jameson, B., Baribaud, F., et al. 2002. Expression of DC-SIGN by dendritic cells of intestinal and genital mucosae in humans and rhesus macaques. *J Virol*, **76**, 1866–75.

Janoff, E.N., Breiman, R.F., et al. 1992. Pneumococcal disease during HIV infection. Epidemiologic, clinical, and immunologic perspectives. *Ann Intern Med*, **117**, 34–24.

Janoff, E.N., Jackson, S., et al. 1994. Intestinal mucosa immunoglobulins during Human Immunodeficiency Virus Type 1 infection. *J Infect Dis*, **170**, 299–307.

Johnson, W.E. and Desrosiers, R.C. 2002. Viral persistence: HIV's strategies of immune system evasion. *Annu Rev Med*, **53**, 499–518.

Kanamori, H., Suzuki, N., et al. 1990. HTLV-I p27rex stabilizes human interleukin-2 receptor alpha chain mRNA. *EMBO J*, **9**, 4161–6.

Kandil, O., Fishman, J.A., et al. 1994. Human immunodeficiency virus type 1 infection of human macrophages modulates the cytokine response to *Pneumocystis carinii*. *Infect Immun*, **62**, 644–50.

Kaplan, J.E., Osame, M., et al. 1990. The risk of development of HTLV-I-associated myelopathy/tropical spastic paraparesis among persons infected with HTLV-I. *J Acquir Immun Defic Syndr*, **3**, 1096–101.

Katsikis, P.D., Wunderlich, E.S., et al. 1995. Fas antigen stimulation induces marked apoptosis of T lymphocytes in human immunodeficiency virus-infected individuals. *J Exp Med*, **181**, 2029–36.

Kaufmann, S.H.E. 1992. Immunity to intracellular bacteria. *Annu Rev Immunol*, **11**, 129–63.

Kaur, A., Grant, R.M., et al. 1998. Diverse host responses and outcomes following simian immunodeficiency virus SIVmac239 infection in sooty mangabeys and rhesus macaques. *J Virol*, **72**, 9597–611.

Kawai, H., Nishida, Y., et al. 1989. HTLV-I associated myelopathy with adult T-cell leukemia. *Neurology*, **39**, 1129–31.

Kawano, F., Yamaguchi, K., et al. 1985. Variation in the clinical courses of adult T-cell leukemia. *Cancer*, **55**, 851–6.

Kedzierska, K., Azzam, R., et al. 2003. Defective phagocytosis by human monocyte/macrophages following HIV-1 infection: underlying mechanisms and modulation by adjunctive cytokine therapy. *J Clin Virol*, **26**, 247–63.

Kestler, H.W., Ringler, D.J., et al. 1991. Importance of the nef gene for maintenance of high virus loads and for the development of AIDS. *Cell*, **65**, 651–62.

Keusch, G.T. 1982. Nutrition and infections. *Compr Ther*, **8**, 7–15.

Keusch, G.T. 2003. The history of nutrition: malnutrition, infection and immunity. *J Nutr*, **133**, S336–40.

Kewenig, S., Schneider, T., et al. 1999. Rapid mucosal CD4+ T cell depletion and enteropathy in Simian Immunodeficiency Virus-infected Rhesus Macaques. *Gastroenterology*, **116**, 1115–23.

Kim, J.H., Mascola, J.R., et al. 2001. Selective increase in HIV-specific neutralizing antibody and partial reconstitution of cellular immune responses during prolonged, successful drug therapy of HIV infection. *AIDS Res Hum Retroviruses*, **17**, 1021–34.

Kobayashi, N., Hamamoto, Y., et al. 1990. Anti-Fas monoclonal antibody is cytocidal to human immunodeficiency virus-infected cells without augmenting viral replication. *Proc Natl Acad Sci USA*, **87**, 9620–4.

Koenig, S., Woods, R.M., et al. 1993. Characterization of MHC class I restricted cytotoxic T cell response to tax in HTLV-1 infected patients with neurological disease. *J Immunol*, **151**, 3874–83.

Komanduri, K.V., Viswanathan, M.N., et al. 1998. Restoration of cytomegalovirus-specific CD4+ T-lymphocyte response after ganciclovir and highly active antiretroviral therapy in individuals infected with HIV-1. *Nat Med*, **4**, 953–6.

Kostense, S., Vandenberghe, K., et al. 2002. Persistent numbers of tetramer+ CD8(+) T cells, but loss of interferon-gamma+ HIV-specific T cells during progression to AIDS. *Blood*, **99**, 2505–11.

Kotler, D.P., Gaetz, H.P., et al. 1984. Enteropathy associated with the acquired immunodeficiency syndrome. *Ann Intern Med*, **101**, 421–8.

Kotler, D.P., Scholes, J.V. and Tierney, A.R. 1987. Intestinal plasma cell alterations in acquired immunodeficiency syndrome. *Dig Dis Sci*, **32**, 129–38.

Kotler, D.P., Reka, S., et al. 1991. Detection, localization and quantitation of HIV-associated antigens in the intestinal biopsies from patients with HIV. *Am J Pathol*, **139**, 823–30.

Kottilil, S., Chun, T.W., et al. 2003. Innate immunity in human immunodeficiency virus infection: effect of viremia on natural killer cell function. *J Infect Dis*, **187**, 1038–45.

Kovacs, J.A., Lempicki, R.A., et al. 2001. Identification of dynamically distinct subpopulations of T lymphocytes that are differentially affected by HIV. *J Exp Med*, **194**, 1731–41.

Koziel, H., Eichbaum, Q., et al. 1998. Reduced binding and phagocytosis of *Pneumocystis carinii* by alveolar macrophages from persons infected with HIV-1 correlates with mannose receptor downregulation. *J Clin Invest*, **102**, 1332–44.

Koziel, H., Li, X., et al. 2000. Alveolar macrophages from human immunodeficiency virus-infected persons demonstrate impaired oxidative burst response to *Pneumocystis carinii* in vitro. *Am J Respir Cell Mol Biol*, **23**, 452–9.

Krzysiek, R., Rudent, A., et al. 2001. Preferential and persistent depletion of CCR5+ T-helper lymphocytes with nonlymphoid homing potential despite early treatment of primary HIV infection. *Blood*, **98**, 3169–71.

LaGrenade, L., Hanchard, B., et al. 1990. Infective dermatitis of Jamaican children: A marker for HTLV-I infection. *Lancet*, **336**, 1345–7.

Lane, H.C., Masur, H., et al. 1983. Abnormalities of B-cell activation and immunoregulation in patients with the acquired immunodeficiency syndrome. *N Engl J Med*, **309**, 453–8.

Lapenta, C., Boirivant, M., et al. 1999. Human intestinal lamina propria lymphocytes are naturally permissive to HIV-1 infection. *Eur J Immunol*, **29**, 1202–8.

Ledru, E., Lecoeur, H., et al. 1998. Differential susceptibility to activation-induced apoptosis among peripheral Th1 subsets: correlation with Bcl-2 expression and consequences for *AIDS* pathogenesis. *J Immunol*, **160**, 3194–206.

Lenardo, M.J., Angleman, S.B., et al. 2002. Cytopathic killing of peripheral blood CD4(+) T lymphocytes by human immunodeficiency virus type 1 appears necrotic rather than apoptotic and does not require env. *J Virol*, **76**, 5082–93.

Leopardi, R., Vainionpaa, R., et al. 1992. Measles virus infection enhances IL-1β but reduces tumor necrosis factor-α expression in human monocytes. *J Immunol*, **149**, 2397–401.

Levin, M.C., Lee, S.M., et al. 2002. Cross-reactivity between immunodominant human T lymphotropic virus type I tax and neurons: implication for molecular mimicry. *J Infect Dis*, **186**, 1514–17.

Levy, J.A. 2001. The importance of the innate immune system in controlling HIV infection and disease. *Trends Immunol*, **22**, 312–16.

Li, T.S., Tubiana, R., et al. 1998. Long-lasting recovery in CD4 T-cell function and viral-load reduction after highly active antiretroviral therapy in advanced HIV-1 disease. *Lancet*, **351**, 1682–6.

Liegler, T.J., Yonemoto, W., et al. 1998. Diminished spontaneous apoptosis in lymphocytes from human immunodeficiency virus-infected long-term nonprogressors. *J Infect Dis*, **178**, 669–79.

Lifson, J.D., Reyes, G.R., et al. 1986. AIDS retrovirus induced cytopathology: giant cell formation and involvement of CD4 antigen. *Science*, **232**, 1123–7.

Lim, S.G., Condez, A., et al. 1993a. Loss of mucosal CD4 lymphocytes is an early feature of HIV infection. *Clin Exp Immunol*, **92**, 448–54.

Lim, S.G., Condez, A. and Poulter, L.W. 1993b. Mucosal macrophage subset of the gut in HIV: decrease in antigen-presenting cell phenotype. *Clin Exp Immunol*, **92**, 442–7.

Luo, W. and Peterlin, B.M. 1997. Activation of the T-cell receptor signaling pathway by Nef from an aggressive strain of simian immunodeficiency virus. *J Virol*, **71**, 9531–7.

Macchia, D., Almerigogna, F., et al. 1993. Membrane tumour necrosis factor-alpha is involved in the polyclonal B-cell activation induced by HIV-infected human T cells. *Nature*, **363**, 464–6.

Maciaszek, J.W., Parada, N.A., et al. 1997. IL-16 represses HIV-1 promoter activity. *J Immunol*, **158**, 5–8.

McCune, J.M. 2001. The dynamics of CD4+ T-cell depletion in HIV disease. *Nature*, **410**, 974–9.

MacPherson, P.A., Fex, C., et al. 2001. Interleukin-7 receptor expression on CD8(+) T cells is reduced in HIV infection and partially restored with effective antiretroviral therapy. *J Acquir Immune Defic Syndr*, **28**, 454–7.

Malkovsky, M., Wallace, M., et al. 2000. Alternative cytotoxic effector mechanisms in infections with immunodeficiency viruses: gammadelta T lymphocytes and natural killer cells. *AIDS*, **14**, S175–86.

Manel, N., Kinet, S., et al. 2003. The HTLV receptor is an early T-cell activation marker whose expression requires de novo protein synthesis. *Blood*, **101**, 1913–18.

Martinez-Maza, O. and Breen, E.C. 2002. B-cell activation and lymphoma in patients with HIV. *Curr Opin Oncol*, **14**, 528–32.

Martinez-Maza, O., Crabb, E., et al. 1987. Infection with the human immunodeficiency virus (HIV) is associated with an in vivo increase in B lymphocyte activation and immaturity. *J Immunol*, **138**, 3720–4.

Mazanec, M.B., Nedrud, J.G., et al. 1993. A three-tiered view of the role of IgA in mucosal defense. *Immunol Today*, **14**, 430–5.

Meng, G., Sellers, M.T., et al. 2000. Lamina propria lymphocytes, not macrophages, express CCR5 and CXCR4 and are the likely target cell for human immunodeficiency virus type 1 in the intestinal mucosa. *J Infect Dis*, **182**, 785–91.

Meng, G., Wei, X., et al. 2002. Primary intestinal epithelial cells selectively transfer R5 HIV-1 to CCR5+ cells. *Nat Med*, **8**, 150–6.

Messingham, K.A., Faunce, D.E. and Kovacs, E.J. 2002. Review article. Alcohol, injury, and cellular immunity. *Alcohol*, **28**, 137–49.

Meyaard, L., Otto, S.A., et al. 1992. Programmed death of T cells in HIV-1 infection. *Science*, **257**, 217–19.

Meyaard, L., Otto, S.A., et al. 1994. Quantitative analysis of CD4+ T cell function in the course of human immunodeficiency virus infection. Gradual decline of both naïve and memory alloreactive T cells. *J Clin Invest*, **94**, 1947–52.

Michel, P., Balde, A.T., et al. 2000. Reduced immune activation and T cell apoptosis in human immunodeficiency virus type 2 compared with type 1: correlation of T cell apoptosis with beta2 microglobulin concentration and disease evolution. *J Infect Dis*, **181**, 64–75.

Miedema, F., Petit, A.J., et al. 1988. Immunological abnormalities in human immunodeficiency virus (HIV)-infected asymptomatic homosexual men. HIV affects the immune system before CD4+ T helper cell depletion occurs. *J Clin Invest*, **82**, 1908–14.

Mingari, M.C., Vitale, C., et al. 1997. Interleukin-15-induced maturation of human natural killer cells from early thymic precursors: selective expression of CD94/NKG2-A as the only HLA class I-specific inhibitory receptor. *Eur J Immunol*, **27**, 1374–80.

Mingari, M.C., Ponte, M., et al. 1998. HLA class I-specific inhibitory receptors in human T lymphocytes: interleukin, 15-induced expression of CD94/NKG2A in superantigen- or alloantigen-activated CD8+ T cells. *Proc Natl Acad Sci USA*, **95**, 1172–7.

Mochizuki, M., Ono, A., et al. 1996. HTLV-I uveitis. *J AIDS Hum Retrovirus*, **13**, suppl, 50–6.

Moir, S., Malaspina, A., et al. 2001. HIV-1 induces phenotypic and functional perturbations of B cells in chronically infected individuals. *Proc Natl Acad Sci USA*, **98**, 10362–7.

Moses, A., Nelson, J. and Bagby, G.C. Jr. 1998. The influence of human immunodeficiency virus-1 on hematopoiesis. *Blood*, **91**, 1479–95.

Mossad, S.B., Avery, R.K., et al. 2001. Infectious complications within the first year after nonmyelablative allogeneic peripheral blood stem cell transplantation. *Bone Marrow Transplant*, **28**, 491–5.

Mrkic, B., Odermatt, B., et al. 2000. Lymphatic dissemination and comparative pathology of recombinant measles viruses in genetically modified mice. *J Virol*, **74**, 1364–72.

Mueller, Y.M., De Rosa, S.C., et al. 2001. Increased CD95/Fas-induced apoptosis of HIV-specific CD8(+) T cells. *Immunity*, **15**, 871–82.

Muller, F., Rollag, H. and Froland, S.S. 1990a. Reduced oxidative burst responses in monocytes and monocyte-derived macrophages from HIV-infected subjects. *Clin Exp Immunol*, **82**, 10–15.

Muller, F., Rollag, H., et al. 1990b. Impaired in vitro survival of monocytes from patients with HIV infection. *Clin Exp Immunol*, **81**, 25–30.

Mulloy, J.C., Crownley, R.W., et al. 1996. The human T-cell leukemia/lymphotropic virus type I p12 protein binds the interleukin-2 receptor β and γ chains and affects their expression on the cell surface. *J Virol*, **70**, 3599–605.

Murai, K., Tachibana, N., et al. 1990. Suppression of delayed-type hypersensitivity to PPD and PHA in elderly HTLV-I carriers. *J Aquir Immune Defic Syndr*, **3**, 1006–9.

Murphy, E.L., Hanchard, B., et al. 1989. Modelling the risk of adult T-cell leukemia/lymphoma in persons infected with human T-lymphotropic virus type I. *Int J Cancer*, **43**, 250–3.

Murphy, P.M., Lane, H.C., et al. 1988. Impairment of neutrophil bactericidal capacity in patients with *AIDS*. *J Infect Dis*, **158**, 627–30.

Murray, C.J. and Lopez, A.D. 1997. Mortality by cause for eight regions of the world: Global burden of disease study. *Lancet*, **349**, 1269–76.

Musher, D.M., Watson, D.A., et al. 1990. The effect of HIV infection on phagocytosis and killing of *Staphylococcus aureus* by human pulmonary alveolar macrophages. *Am J Med Sci*, **299**, 158–63.

Nabel, G. and Baltimore, D. 1987. An inducible transcription factor activates expression of human immunodeficiency virus in T cells. *Nature*, **326**, 711–13.

Nagase, H., Agematsu, K., et al. 2001. Mechanism of hypergammaglobulinemia by HIV infection: circulating memory B-cell reduction with plasmacytosis. *Clin Immunol*, **100**, 250–9.

Nakada, K., Yamaguchi, K., et al. 1987. Monoclonal integration of HTLV-I proviral DNA in patients with strongyloidiasis. *Int J Cancer*, **40**, 145–8.

Nanan, R., Chittka, B., et al. 1999. Measles infection causes transient depletion of activated T cells from peripheral circulation. *J Clin Virol*, **12**, 201–10.

Napolitano, L.A., Grant, R.M., et al. 2001. Increased production of IL-7 accompanies HIV-1-mediated T-cell depletion: implications for T-cell homeostasis. *Nat Med*, **7**, 73–9.

Nath, M.D., Ruscetti, F.W., et al. 2003. Regulation of the cell-surface expression of an HTLV-I binding protein in human T cells during immune activation. *Blood*, **101**, 3085–92.

Newton, R.C., Limpuangthip, P., et al. 1992. *Strongyloides stercoralis* hyperinfection in a carrier of HTLV-I virus with evidence of selective immunosuppression. *Am J Med*, **92**, 202–8.

Nielsen, H., Kharazmi, A. and Faber, V. 1986. Blood monocyte and neutrophil functions in the acquired immune deficiency syndrome. *Scand J Immunol*, **24**, 291–6.

Niewiesk, S., Gotzelmann, M. and ter Meulen, V. 2000. Selective in vivo suppression of T lymphocyte responses in experimental measles virus infection. *Proc Natl Acad Sci USA*, **97**, 4251–5.

Nilssen, D.E., Müller, F., et al. 1996. Intraepithelial γ/δ T cells in duodenal mucosa are related to the immune state and survival time in *AIDS*. *J Virol*, **70**, 3545–50.

Nishimura, M., Maeda, M., et al. 2003. Influence of cytokine and mannose binding protein gene polymorphisms on human T-cell leukemia virus type 1 (HTLV-I) provirus load in HTLV-I asymptomatic carriers. *Hum Immunol*, **64**, 453–7.

O'Brien, W.A., Hartigan, P.M., et al. 1997. Changes in plasma HIV RNA levels and CD4+ lymphocyte counts predict both response to antiretroviral therapy and therapeutic failure. VA Cooperative Study Group on AIDS. *Ann Intern Med*, **126**, 939–44.

Okada, H., Kobune, F., et al. 2000. Extensive leukopenia due to apoptosis of uninfected lymphocytes in acute measles patients. *Arch Virol*, **45**, 905–20.

Olsson, J., Poles, M., et al. 2000. Human immunodeficiency virus type 1 infection is associated with significant mucosal inflammation characterized by increased expression of CCR5, CXCR4 and beta-chemokines. *J Infect Dis*, **182**, 1625–35.

Ometto, L., DeForni, D., et al. 2002. Immune reconstitution in HIV-1-infected children on antiretroviral therapy: role of thymic output and viral fitness. *AIDS*, **16**, 839–49.

Orendi, J.M., Bloem, A.C., et al. 1998. Activation and cell cycle antigens in CD4+ and CD8+ T cells correlate with plasma human immunodeficiency virus (HIV-1) RNA level in HIV-1 infection. *J Infect Dis*, **178**, 1279–87.

Orenstein, J.M., Fox, C. and Wahl, S.M. 1997. Macrophages as a source of HIV during opportunistic infections. *Science*, **276**, 1857–61.

Orlikowsky, T., Wang, Z.Q., et al. 1997. Cytotoxic monocytes in the blood of HIV type 1-infected subjects destroy targeted T cells in a CD95-dependent fashion. *AIDS Res Hum Retroviruses*, **13**, 953–60.

Orren, A., Kipps, A., et al. 1981. Increased susceptibility to herpes simplex virus infections in children with acute measles. *Infect Immun*, **31**, 1–6.

Osame, M., Usuku, K., et al. 1986. HTLV-I associated myelopathy, a new clinical entity. *Lancet*, **i**, 1031–2.

Ostrowski, S.R., Gerstoft, J., et al. 2003. Impaired production of cytokines is an independent predictor of mortality in HIV-1-infected patients. *AIDS*, **17**, 521–30.

Oyaizu, N., Adachi, Y., et al. 1997. Monocytes express Fas ligand upon CD4 cross-linking and induce CD4+ T cells apoptosis: a possible mechanism of bystander cell death in HIV infection. *J Immunol*, **158**, 2456–63.

Palella, F., Delaney, K., et al. 1998. Declining morbidity and mortality among patients with advanced human immunodeficiency virus infection. *N Engl J Med*, **338**, 853–60.

Pantaleo, G., Graziosi, C. and Fauci, A. 1993. New concepts in the immunopathogenesis of human immunodeficiency virus infection. *N Engl J Med*, **328**, 327–35.

Pantaleo, G., Soudeyns, H., et al. 1997. Accumulation of human immunodeficiency virus-specific cytotoxic T lymphocytes away from the predominant site of virus replication during primary infection. *Eur J Immunol*, **27**, 3166–73.

Papiernik, M., Brossard, Y., et al. 1992. Thymic abnormalities in fetuses aborted from human immunodeficiency virus type 1 seropositive women. *Pediatrics*, **89**, 297–301.

Patterson, S., Rae, A., et al. 2001. Plasmacytoid dendritic cells are highly susceptible to human immunodeficiency virus type 1 infection and release infectious virus. *J Virol*, **75**, 6710–13.

Penna, G., Sozzani, S. and Adorini, L. 2001. Cutting edge: selective usage of chemokine receptors by plasmacytoid dendritic cells. *J Immunol*, **167**, 1862–6.

Pfeuffer, J., Puschel, K., et al. 2003. Extent of measles virus spread and immune suppression differentiates between wild-type and vaccine strains in the cotton rat model (*Sigmodon hispidus*). *J Virol*, **77**, 150–8.

Phair, J., Jacobson, L., et al. 1992. Acquired immune deficiency syndrome occurring within, 5 years of infection with human immunodeficiency virus type 1: The Multicenter *AIDS* Cohort Study. *J Acquir Immune Defic Syndr*, **5**, 490–6.

Pillet, S., Prevost, M.H., et al. 1999. Monocyte expression of adhesion molecules in HIV-infected patients: variations according to disease stage and possible pathogenic role. *Lab Invest*, **79**, 815–22.

Pitcher, C.J., Quittner, C., et al. 1999. HIV-1-specific CD4+ T cells are detectable in most individuals with active HIV-1 infection, but decline with prolonged viral suppression. *Nat Med*, **5**, 518–25.

Pitrak, D.L., Bak, P.M., et al. 1993. Depressed neutrophil superoxide production in human immunodeficiency virus infection. *J Infect Dis*, **167**, 1406–10.

Pitrak, D.L., Tsai, H.C., et al. 1996. Accelerated neutrophil apoptosis in the acquired immunodeficiency syndrome. *J Clin Invest*, **98**, 2714–19.

Plumelle, Y., Gonin, C., et al. 1997. Effect of *Strongyloides stercoralis* infection and eosinophilia on age at onset and prognosis of adult T-cell leukemia. *Am J Clin Pathol*, **107**, 81–7.

Poccia, F., Boullier, S., et al. 1996. Peripheral V gamma, 9/V delta, 2 T cell deletion and anergy to nonpeptidic mycobacterial antigens in asymptomatic HIV-1-infected persons. *J Immunol*, **157**, 449–61.

Poiesz, B.J., Ruscetti, F.W., et al. 1980. Detection and isolation of type C retrovirus particles from fresh and cultured lymphocytes of a patient with cutaneous T-cell lymphoma. *Proc Natl Acad Sci USA*, **77**, 7415–19.

Poli, G., Bressler, P., et al. 1990a. Interleukin, 6 induces human immunodeficiency virus expression in infected monocytic cells alone and in synergy with tumor necrosis factor alpha by transcriptional and post-transcriptional mechanisms. *J Exp Med*, **172**, 151–8.

Poli, G., Kinter, A., et al. 1990b. Tumor necrosis factor alpha functions in an autocrine manner in the induction of human immunodeficiency virus expression. *Proc Natl Acad Sci USA*, **87**, 782–5.

Pos, O., Stevenhagen, A., et al. 1992. Impaired phagocytosis of *Staphylococcus aureus* by granulocytes and monocytes of AIDS patients. *Clin Exp Immunol*, **88**, 23–8.

Prevot, S., Audouin, J., et al. 1992. Thymic pseudotumorous enlargement due to follicular hyperplasia in human immunodeficiency virus seropositive patient. *Am J Clin Pathol*, **97**, 420–5.

Quiambao, B.P., Gatchalian, S., et al. 1998. Coinfection is common in measles-associated pneumonia. *Pediatr Infect Dis J*, **17**, 89–93.

Racz, P., Tenner-Racz, K., et al. 1991. Classification of histopathological changes of lymph nodes in HIV-1 infection. Significance of Castleman's disease-like lymph node lesion concerning the diagnosis of HIV-1-related Kaposi's sarcoma. *Antibiot Chemother*, **43**, 201–13.

Ravanel, K., Castelle, C., et al. 1997. Measles virus nucleocapsid protein binds to FcgammaRII and inhibits human B cell antibody production. *J Exp Med*, **186**, 269–78.

Reuben, J.M., Lee, B.N., et al. 2002. Magnitude of IFN-gamma production in HIV-1-infected children is associated with virus suppression. *J Allergy Clin Immunol*, **110**, 255–61.

Rieckmann, P., Poli, G., et al. 1991. Activated B lymphocytes from human immunodeficiency virus-infected individuals induce virus expression in infected T cells and a promonocytic cell line, U1. *J Exp Med*, **173**, 1–5.

Roilides, E., Mertins, S., et al. 1990. Impairment of neutrophil chemotactic and bactericidal function in children infected with human immunodeficiency virus type 1 and partial reversal after in vitro exposure to granulocyte-macrophage colony-stimulating factor. *J Pediatr*, **117**, 531–40.

Roilides, E., Holmes, A., et al. 1993. Impairment of neutrophil antifungal activity against hyphae of *Aspergillus fumigatus* in children infected with human immunodeficiency virus. *J Infect Dis*, **167**, 905–11.

Rosenberg, E.S., Billingsley, J.M., et al. 1997. Vigorous HIV-1-specific CD4+ T cell responses associated with control of viremia (see comments). *Science*, **278**, 1447–50.

Rosok, B.I., Bostad, L., et al. 1996. Reduced CD4 cell counts in blood do not reflect CD4 cell depletion in tonsillar tissue in asymptomatic HIV-1 infection. *AIDS*, **10**, F35–38.

Rossol, R., Dobmeyer, J.M., et al. 1998. Increase in Vdelta1+ gammadelta T cells in the peripheral blood and bone marrow as a selective feature of HIV-1 but not other virus infections. *Br J Haematol*, **100**, 728–34.

Ruckle, G. and Rogers, K.D. 1957. Studies with measles virus. II. Isolation of virus and immunologic studies in persons who have had the natural disease. *J Immunol*, **78**, 341–55.

Ryon, J.J., Moss, W.J., et al. 2002. Functional and phenotypic changes in circulating lymphocytes from hospitalized Zambian children with measles. *Clin Diagn Lab Immunol*, **9**, 994–1003.

Sachsenberg, N., Perelson, A.S., et al. 1998. Turnover of CD4+ and CD8+ T lymphocytes in HIV-1 infection as measured by Ki-67 antigen. *J Exp Med*, **187**, 1295–303.

Salghetti, S., Mariani, R. and Skowronski, J. 1995. Human immunodeficiency virus type 1 Nef and p56lck protein-tyrosine kinase interact with a common element in CD4 cytoplasmic tail. *Proc Natl Acad Sci USA*, **92**, 349–53.

Sandberg, J.K., Fast, N.M., et al. 2003. HIV-specific CD8+ T cell function in children with vertically acquired HIV-1 infection is critically influenced by age and the state of the CD4+ T cell compartment. *J Immunol*, **170**, 4403–10.

Sato, Y. and Shiroma, Y. 1989. Concurrent infections with *Strongyloides* and T-cell leukemia virus and their possible effect on immune responses of host. *Clin Immunol Immunopathol*, **52**, 214–24.

Sato, K., Maruyama, I., et al. 1991. Arthritis in patients infected with human T lymphotropic virus type 1. Clinical and immunopathologic features. *Arthritis Rheum*, **34**, 714–21.

Scala, E., D'Offizi, G., et al. 1997. C-C chemokines, IL-16, and soluble antiviral factor activity are increased in cloned T cells from subjects with long-term nonprogressive HIV infection. *J Immunol*, **158**, 4485–92.

Scamurra, R.W., Miller, D.J., et al. 2000. Impact of HIV-1 infection on VH3 gene repertoire of naïve human B cells. *J Immunol*, **164**, 5482–91.

Schacker, T., Collier, A.C., et al. 1996. Clinical and epidemiologic features of primary HIV infection. *Ann Intern Med*, **125**, 257–64.

Schafer, F., Kewenig, S., et al. 2002. Lack of SIV-specific IgA response in the intestine of SIV-infected rhesus macaques. *Gut*, **50**, 608–14.

Schmitz, H., Rokos, K., et al. 2002. Supernatants of HIV-infected immune cells affect the barrier function of human HT-29/B6 intestinal epithelial cells. *AIDS*, **16**, 983–91.

Schneider, T., Ullrich, R., et al. 1994. Abnormalities in subset distribution, activation, and differentiation of T cells isolated from large intestine biopsies in HIV infection. *Clin Exp Immunol*, **95**, 430–5.

Schneider, T., Jahn, H.-U., et al. 1995. Loss of CD4 T lymphocytes in patients infected with human immunodeficiency virus type 1 is more pronounced in the duodenal mucosa than in the peripheral blood. Berlin Diarrhea/Wasting Syndrome Study Group. *Gut*, **37**, 524–9.

Schneider, T., Ullrich, R. and Zeitz, M. 1997a. Immunopathology of HIV infection in the gastrointestinal tract. *Springer Semin Immun*, **18**, 515–33.

Schneider, T., Zippel, T., et al. 1997b. Abnormal predominance of IgG in HIV-specific antibodies produced by short-term cultured duodenal biopsies from patients infected with HIV. *J Aquir Immunodefic Syndr*, **16**, 333–9.

Schneider, T., Zippel, T., et al. 1998. Increased immunoglobulin G production by short-term cultured duodenal biopsies from HIV-infected patients. *Gut*, **42**, 357–61.

Schneider-Schaulies, S. and Ter Meulen, V. 2002. Modulation of immune functions by measles virus. *Springer Semin Immunopathol*, **24**, 127–48.

Schnittmann, S.M., Denning, S.M., et al. 1990. Evidence for susceptibility of intrathymic T cell precursors and their progeny carrying T cell antigen receptor phenotypes TCRαβ+and TCRγδ+ to human immunodeficiency virus infection: A mechanism for CD4+ (T4) lymphocyte depletion. *Proc Natl Acad Sci USA*, **87**, 7727–31.

Schupbach, J., Kalyanaraman, V.S., et al. 1983. Antibodies against three purified proteins of the human type C retrovirus, human T-cell leukemia-lymphoma virus, in adult T-cell leukemia-lymphoma patients and healthy blacks from the Caribbean. *Cancer Res*, **43**, 886–91.

Schwartz, O., Marechal, V., et al. 1996. Endocytosis of major histocompatibility complex class I molecules is induced by the HIV-1 Nef protein. *Nat Med*, **2**, 338–42.

Seemayer, T.A., Laroche, A.C., et al. 1984. Precocious thymic involution manifest by epithelial injury in the acquired immunodeficiency syndrome. *Hum Pathol*, **15**, 469–74.

Sempowski, G.D. and Haynes, B.F. 2002. Immune reconstitution in patients with HIV infection. *Annu Rev Med*, **53**, 269–84.

Sergiev, P.G., Ryazantseva, N.E. and Shroit, I.G. 1960. The dynamics of pathological processes in experimental measles in monkeys. *Acta Virol*, **4**, 265–73.

Shankar, P., Russo, M., et al. 2000. Impaired function of circulating HIV-specific CD8(+) T cells in chronic human immunodeficiency virus infection. *Blood*, **96**, 3094–101.

Shelburne, S.A. and Hamill, R.J. 2003. The immune reconstitution inflammatory syndrome. *AIDS Rev*, **5**, 67–79.

Sheppard, H.W., Lang, W., et al. 1993. The characteristics of non-progressors: Long term HIV-1 infection with stable CD4+ T-cell levels. *AIDS*, **7**, 1159–66.

Sheriff, A., Fackler, O.T. et al. 2004. Elevated activation status of human lamina propria lymphocytes correlates with preferential replication of HIV-1 in the gastrointestinal tract. *J Acquir Immune Defic Syndr*, in press.

Sherman, F.E. and Ruckle, G. 1958. In vivo and in vitro cellular changes specific for measles. *Arch Pathol*, **65**, 587.

Shimoyama, M. 1991. Diagnostic criteria and classification of clinical subtypes of adult T-cell leukaemia-lymphoma. A report from the Lymphoma Study Group (1984–1987). *Br J Haematol*, **79**, 428–37.

Shimoyama, M., Takatsuki, K., et al. 1991. Major prognostic factors of patients with adult T-cell leukemia/lymphoma: a cooperative study. *Leukemia Res*, **15**, 81–90.

Shirai, A., Cosentino, M., et al. 1992. Human immunodeficiency virus infection induces both polyclonal and virus-specific B cell activation. *J Clin Invest*, **89**, 561–6.

Sidorenko, S.P. and Clark, E.A. 1993. Characterization of a cell surface protein IPO-3, expressed on activated human B and T cells. *J Immunol*, **151**, 4614.

Siegal, F.P. and Spear, G.T. 2001. Innate immunity and HIV. *AIDS*, **15**, S127–37.

Simon, A. and Fleischhack, G. 2001. Surveillance for nosocomial infections in pediatric hematology/oncology patients. *Klin Pädiatr*, **213**, suppl 1, A106–113.

Sindhu, S.T., Ahmad, R., et al. 2003. Peripheral blood cytotoxic gammadelta T lymphocytes from patients with human immunodeficiency virus type 1 infection and AIDS lyse uninfected CD4+ T cells, and their cytocidal potential correlates with viral load. *J Virol*, **77**, 1848–55.

Singer, N.G. and McCune, W.J. 1999. Prevention of infectious complications in rheumatic disease patients: immunization, Pneumocystis carinii prophylaxis, and screening for latent infections. *Curr Opin Rheumatol*, **11**, 173–8.

Sirianni, M.C., Soddu, S., et al. 1988. Mechanism of defective natural killer cell activity in patients with AIDS is associated with defective distribution of tubulin. *J Immunol*, **140**, 2565–8.

Slamon, D.J., Shimotohno, K., et al. 1984. Identification of the putative transforming protein of the human T-cell leukemia viruses HTLV-I and HTLV-II. *Science*, **226**, 61–5.

Slifka, M.K., Homann, D., et al. 2003. Measles virus infection results in suppression of both innate and adaptive immune responses to secondary bacterial infections. *J Clin Invest*, **111**, 805–10.

Smith, P.D., Ohura, K., et al. 1984. Monocyte function in the acquired immune deficiency syndrome. Defective chemotaxis. *J Clin Invest*, **74**, 2121–8.

Sodroski, J., Goh, W.C., et al. 1986. Role of the HTLV-III/LAV envelope in syncytium formation and cytopathicity. *Nature*, **322**, 470–4.

Soilleux, E.J. and Coleman, N. 2001. Langerhans cells and the cells of Langerhans cell histiocytosis do not express DC-SIGN. *Blood*, **98**, 1987–8.

Sopper, S., Nierwetberg, D., et al. 2003. Impact of simian immunodeficiency virus (SIV) infection on lymphocyte numbers and T-cell turnover in different organs of rhesus monkeys. *Blood*, **101**, 1213–19.

Sousa, A.E., Carneiro, J., et al. 2002. CD4 T cell depletion is linked directly to immune activation in the pathogenesis of HIV-1 and HIV-2 but only indirectly to the viral load. *J Immunol*, **169**, 3400–6.

Spear, G.T., Kessler, H.A., et al. 1990. Decreased oxidative burst activity of monocytes from asymptomatic HIV-infected individuals. *Clin Immunol Immunopathol*, **54**, 184–91.

Spiegel, H.M., Ogg, G.S., et al. 2000. Human immunodeficiency virus type 1- and cytomegalovirus-specific cytotoxic T lymphocytes can persist at high frequency for prolonged periods in the absence of circulating peripheral CD4(+) T cells. *J Virol*, **74**, 1018–22.

Stahl-Hennig, C., Steinmann, R.M., et al. 1999. Rapid infection of oral mucosal-associated lymphoid tissue with simian immunodeficiency virus. *Science*, **285**, 1261–5.

Stanley, M.W. and Frizzera, G. 1986. Diagnostic specificity of histologic features in lymph node biopsy specimens from patients at risk for the acquired immunodeficiency syndrome. *Hum Pathol*, **17**, 1231–9.

Staples, J.A., Ponsonby, A.L., et al. 2003. Ecologic analysis of some immune-related disorders, including type 1 diabetes, in Australia: latitude, regional ultraviolet radiation, and disease prevalence. *Environ Health Perspect*, **111**, 518–23.

Stefanova, I., Saville, M.W., et al. 1996. HIV infection-induced posttranslational modification of T cell signaling molecules associated with disease progression. *J Clin Invest*, **98**, 1290–7.

Steinman, R.M., Granelli-Piperno, A., et al. 2003. The interaction of immunodeficiency viruses with dendritic cells. *Curr Top Microbiol Immunol*, **276**, 1–30.

Stoddart, C.A., Liegler, T.J., et al. 2001. Impaired replication of protease inhibitor-resistant HIV-1 in human thymus. *Nat Med*, **6**, 712–18.

Stoddart, C.A., Geleziunas, R., et al. 2003. Human immunodeficiency virus type 1 Nef-mediated downregulation of CD4 correlates with Nef enhancement of viral pathogenesis. *J Virol*, **77**, 2124–33.

Stokes, C.R., Soothill, J.F. and Turner, M.W. 1975. Immune exclusion is a function of IgA. *Nature*, **255**, 745–6.

Stutman, O. 1978. Intrathymic and extrathymic T cell maturation. *Immunol Rev*, **42**, 138–84.

Stylianou, E., Aukrust, P., et al. 2000. Interferons and interferon (IFN)-inducible protein, 10 during highly active anti-retroviral therapy (HAART)-possible immunosuppressive role of IFN-alpha in HIV infection. *Clin Exp Immunol*, **119**, 479–85.

Suga, S., Yoshikawa, T., et al. 1992. Activation of human herpesvirus-6 in children with acute measles. *J Med Virol*, **38**, 278–82.

Swingler, S., Mann, A., et al. 1999. HIV-1 Nef mediates lymphocytes chemotaxis and activation by infected macrophages. *Nat Med*, **5**, 997–10003.

Tajima, K. and Kuroishi, T. 1985. Estimation or rate of incidence of ATL among ATLV (HTLV-I) carriers in Kyushu, Japan. *Jpn J Clin Oncol*, **15**, 423–30.

Takatsuki, K., Yamaguchi, K., et al. 1985. Clinical aspects of adult T-cell leukemia/lymphoma. *Curr Top Microbiolol Immunol*, **115**, 89–97.

Tamashiro, V.G., Perez, H.H. and Griffin, D.E. 1987. Prospective study of the magnitude and duration of changes in tuberculin reactivity during complicated and uncomplicated measles. *Pediatr Infect Dis J*, **6**, 451–4.

Tanaka, K., Minagawa, H., et al. 2002. The measles virus hemagglutinin downregulates the cellular receptor SLAM (CD150). *Arch Virol*, **147**, 195–203.

Tanaka, Y., Hayashi, M., et al. 1996. Differential transactivation of the intercellular adhesion molecule, 1 gene promoter by Tax1 and Tax2 of human T-cell leukemia viruses. *J Virol*, **72**, 8508–17.

Tarazona, R., Casado, J.G., et al. 2002. Selective depletion of CD56(dim) NK cell subsets and maintenance of CD56(bright) NK cells in treatment-naïve HIV-1-seropositive individuals. *J Clin Immunol*, **22**, 176–83.

Teixeira, L., Valdez, H., et al. 2001. Poor CD4 T cell restoration after suppression of HIV-1 replication may reflect lower thymic function. *AIDS*, **15**, 1749–56.

Tenner-Racz, K., Racz, P., et al. 1985. Altered dendritic follicular cells and virus-like particles in AIDS and AIDS-related lymphadenopathy. *Lancet*, **i**, 105–6.

Tesselaar, K., Arens, R., et al. 2003. Lethal T cell immunodeficiency induced by chronic costimulation via CD27-CD70 interactions. *Nat Immunol*, **4**, 49–54.

Tishon, A., Manchester, M., et al. 1996. A model of measles virus-induced immunosuppression: Enhanced susceptibility of neonatal human PBLs. *Nat Med*, **2**, 1250–4.

Trimble, L.A. and Lieberman, J. 1998. Circulating CD8 T lymphocytes in human immunodeficiency virus-infected individuals have impaired function and downmodulate CD3 zeta, the signaling chain of the T-cell receptor complex. *Blood*, **91**, 585–94.

Trimble, L.A., Shankar, P., et al. 2000. Human immunodeficiency virus-specific circulating CD8 T lymphocytes have down-modulated CD3zeta and CD28, key signaling molecules for T-cell activation. *J Virol*, **74**, 7320–30.

Turville, S.G., Cameron, P.U., et al. 2002. Diversity of receptors binding HIV on dendritic cell subsets. *Nat Immunol*, **3**, 975–83.

Uchiyama, T., Yodoi, J., et al. 1977. Adult T-cell leukemia: Clinical and hematologic features of, 16 cases. *Blood*, **50**, 481–92.

Ullum, H., Gotzsche, P.C., et al. 1995. Defective natural immunity: an early manifestation of human immunodeficiency virus infection. *J Exp Med*, **182**, 789–99.

Ullum, H., Cozzi Lepri, A., et al. 1997. Low production of interferon gamma is related to disease progression in HIV infection: evidence from a cohort of 347 HIV-infected individuals. *AIDS Res Hum Retroviruses*, **13**, 1039–46.

Ullum, H., Cozzi Lepri, A., et al. 1999. Natural immunity and HIV disease progression. *AIDS*, **13**, 557–63.

Valentin, H., Nugeyre, M.-T., et al. 1994. Two subpopulations of human triple-negative thymic cells are susceptible to infection by human immunodeficiency virus type in vitro. *J Virol, 68*, **1**, 3041–50.

Valone, F.H., Payan, D.G., et al. 1984. Defective polymorphonuclear leukocyte chemotaxis in homosexual men with persistent lymph node syndrome. *J Infect Dis*, **150**, 267–71.

Veazey, R.S., DeMaria, M., et al. 1998. Gastrointestinal tract as a major site of CD4+ T cell depletion and viral replication in SIV infection. *Science*, **280**, 427–31.

Vernant, J.C., Maurs, L., et al. 1987. Endemic tropical spastic paraparesis associated with human T-lymphotropic virus Type I. *Ann Neurol*, **21**, 123–30.

Vingerhoets, J.H., Vanham, G.L., et al. 1995. Increased cytolytic T lymphocyte activity and decreased B7 responsiveness are associated with CD28 down-regulation on CD8+ T cells from HIV-infected subjects. *Clin Exp Immunol*, **100**, 425–33.

Viscidi, R.P., Mayur, K., et al. 1989. Inhibition of antigen-induced lymphocyte proliferation by Tat protein from HIV-1. *Science*, **246**, 1606–8.

Von Pirquet, C. 1908. Verhalten der kutanen Tuberkulin-Reaktion während der Masern. *Dtsch Med Wochenschr*, **34**, 1297–300.

Waldmann, T.A. and Tagaya, Y. 1999. The multifaceted regulation of interleukin-15 expression and the role of this cytokine in NK cell differentiation and host response to intracellular pathogens. *Annu Rev Immunol*, **17**, 19–49.

Waldmann, T.A., Greene, W.C., et al. 1984. Functional and phenotypic comparison of human T-cell leukemia/lymphoma virus positive adult T-cell leukemia with human T-cell leukemia/lymphoma virus negative Sezary leukemia and their distinction using anti-Tac monoclonal antibody identifying the human receptor for T-cell growth factor. *J Clin Invest*, **73**, 1711–18.

Wallace, M., Scharko, A.M., et al. 1997. Functional gamma delta T-lymphocyte defect associated with human immunodeficiency virus infections. *Mol Med*, **3**, 60–71.

Wang, L., Robb, C.W. and Cloyd, M.W. 1997. HIV induces homing of resting T lymphocytes to lymph nodes. *Virology*, **228**, 141–52.

Wang, L., Chen, J.J., et al. 1999. A novel mechanism of CD4 lymphocyte depletion involves effects of HIV on resting lymphocytes: induction of lymph node homing and apoptosis upon secondary signaling through homing receptors. *J Immunol*, **162**, 268–76.

Wang, Z.Q., Horowitz, H.W., et al. 1998. Lymphocyte-reactive autoantibodies in human immunodeficiency virus type 1-infected persons facilitate the deletion of CD8 T cells by macrophages. *J Infect Dis*, **178**, 404–12.

Ward, B.J. and Griffin, D.E. 1993. Changes in cytokine production after measles virus vaccination: predominant production of IL-4 suggests induction of a Th2 response. *Clin Immunol Immunopathol*, **67**, 171–7.

Ward, B.J., Johnson, R.T. and Vaisberg, A. 1991. Cytokine production in vitro and the lymphoproliferative defect of natural measles virus infection. *Clin Immunol Immunopathol*, **61**, 236–48.

Wehle, K., Schirmer, M., et al. 1993. Quantitative differences in phagocytosis and degradation of *Pneumocystis carinii* by alveolar macrophages in AIDS and non-HIV patients in vivo. *Cytopathology*, **4**, 231–6.

Wei, X., Ghosh, S.K., et al. 1995. Viral dynamics in human immunodeficiency virus type 1 infection. *Nature*, **373**, 117–22.

Weissman, D. and Fauci, A.S. 1997. Role of dendritic cells in immunopathogenesis of human immunodeficiency virus infection. *Clin Microbiol Rev*, **10**, 358–67.

Wenisch, C., Parschalk, B., et al. 1996. Dysregulation of the polymorphonuclear leukocyte – *Candida* spp. interaction in HIV-positive patients. *AIDS*, **10**, 983–7.

Wesley, A.G., Coovadia, H.M. and Kiepiela, P. 1982. Further predictive indices of clinical severity of measles. *S Afr Med J*, **61**, 663–5.

White, J.D., Zaknoen, S.L., et al. 1995. Infectious complications and immunodeficiency in patients with HTLV-1-associated adult T-cell leukemia/lymphoma. *Cancer*, **75**, 1598–607.

White, R.G. and Boyd, J.F. 1973. The effect of measles on the thymus and other lymphoid tissue. *Clin Exp Immunol*, **13**, 343–57.

Widney, D., Gundapp, G., et al. 1999. Aberrant expression of CD27 and soluble CD27 (sCD27) in HIV infection and in AIDS-associated lymphoma. *Clin Immunol*, **93**, 114–23.

Willey, R.L., Maldarelli, F., et al. 1992. Human immunodeficiency virus type 1 Vpu protein induces rapid degradation of CD4. *J Virol*, **66**, 7193–200.

Williams, K.C. and Hickey, W.F. 2002. Central nervous system damage, monocytes and macrophages, and neurological disorders in AIDS. *Annu Rev Neurosci*, **25**, 537–62.

Wong-Staal, F. and Gallo, R.C. 1985. Human T-lymphotropic retrovirus. *Nature*, **317**, 395–403.

Wright, D.N., Nelson, R.P., et al. 1990. Serum IgE and human immunodeficiency virus (HIV) infection. *J Allergy Clin Immunol*, **85**, 445–52.

Wu, Q., Wang, Y., et al. 1999. The requirement of membrane lymphotoxin for the presence of dendritic cells in lymphoid tissues. *J Exp Med*, **190**, 629–38.

Xu, X.N., Laffert, B., et al. 1999. Induction of Fas ligand expression by HIV involves the interaction of Nef with the T cell receptor zeta chain. *J Exp Med*, **189**, 1489–96.

Yahi, N., Baghdiguian, S., et al. 1992. Galactosyl ceramide (or a closely related molecule) is the receptor for human immunodeficiency virus type 1 on human colon epithelial HT29 cells. *J Virol*, **66**, 4848–54.

Ye, P., Kourtis, A.P. and Kirshner, D.E. 2003. Reconstitution of thymic function in HIV-1 patients treated with highly active antiretroviral therapy. *Clin Immunol*, **106**, 95–105.

Yokota, S., Saito, H., et al. 2003. Measles virus suppresses interferon-alpha signaling pathway: suppression of Jak1 phosphorylation and association of viral accessory proteins, C and V, with interferon-alpha receptor complex. *Virology*, **306**, 135–46.

Zaitseva, M., Blauvelt, A., et al. 1997. Expression and function of CCR5 and CXCR4 on human Langerhans cells and macrophages: implications for HIV primary infection (see comments). *Nat Med*, **3**, 1369–75.

Zamarchi, R., Barelli, A., et al. 2002. B cell activation in peripheral blood and lymph nodes during HIV infection. *AIDS*, **16**, 1217–26.

Zhang, L., Yu, W., et al. 2002. Contribution of human alpha-defensin, 1, 2 and 3 to the anti-HIV-1 activity of CD8 antiviral factor. *Science*, **298**, 995–1000.

PART VII

VACCINES

40

New approaches to vaccine delivery

CHARALAMBOS D. PARTIDOS

THE RATIONALE FOR NEEDLE-FREE DELIVERY OF VACCINES

Vaccination has arguably had the greatest impact of any medical intervention on human health. Worldwide immunization/vaccination programs have been successful in significantly reducing the incidence of serious infectious diseases, such as poliomyelitis and measles, and eradicating smallpox. In many industrialized countries, effective immunization campaigns have resulted in a drop in incidence rates of the target diseases to such low levels that adverse reactions to vaccines rather than the diseases themselves have become a new area of awareness for the public (Andre 2001). To this end, public confidence and media coverage play a significant role in vaccine compliance. Participation rates in immunization programs drop rapidly after negative publicity about adverse effects of injecting vaccines (Miller and Pisani 1999). In addition, children normally associate the sight of a needle with pain which could result in a drop of the rate of compliance (Cohen et al. 2001). As an average, an infant receives 20–25 injections for immunization against different childhood infections by 18 months of age, there is considerable pressure to minimize vaccine-related visits by combining antigens and simplifying immunization procedures (Ward 2000; Jacobson et al. 2001). Needle-free immunization practices hold a great deal of promise in changing the public's attitude of 'being forced to get a shot' to seeking out vaccines.

Most vaccines are injectable preparations administered via parenteral routes. As a result, immunization requires needles and syringes and trained medical personnel, is expensive, normally does not induce mucosal immunity, and may lead to injection site reactions. In addition, in many instances, particularly in less developed countries, immunization may lead to infections by blood-borne pathogens as a result of the use of contaminated needles (Kane et al. 1999; Simonsen et al. 1999). Routine immunization programs account for about a billion injections per year (Kane et al. 1999) and such injections are believed to be safer than many nonimmunization injections (therapeutic injections) in most countries. However, the World Health Organization (WHO) has recently estimated that up to one-third of immunization injections are unsafe in four of six regions of the world (Miller and Pisani 1999). Several reports from countries in sub-Saharan Africa, Asia, and the Middle East have estimated that from 31 percent to more than 90 percent of childhood immunizations are unsafe (Simonsen et al. 1999). The main reasons for unsafe injections are: lack of sufficient quantities of syringes and needles, lack of operational sterilization equipment or fuel to operate such equipment, and patient demand for injections (Kane et al. 1999). Furthermore, there is a common misconception that it is safe to reuse syringes between patients if the needle is changed. In some countries, four of five disposable syringes, many of them supplied for immunization, are reused.

Population-based studies from China, India, and former Soviet states have shown unsafe injections to be a major source of hepatitis B virus (HBV) infection (Simonsen et al. 1999). In Egypt, nationwide injection campaigns against schistosomiasis between 1920 and 1980 played a major role in the extensive spread of hepatitis C virus (HCV) leading to the high current prevalence (18 percent) of the virus in the population

(Simonsen et al. 1999). It has been estimated that unsafe injections may cause 8–16 million HBV infections every year, 2.3–4.7 million HCV infections, and 80 000–160 000 HIV/AIDS infections (Kane et al. 1999). The transmission of hepatitis viruses and HIV are by no means the only risks involved with unsafe injections; many outbreaks involving other pathogens, such as Ebola and Lassa virus infections, and malaria have been reported (Simonsen et al. 1999).

With the availability of whole genome sequences, the potential number of candidate vaccine antigens has increased, and it is anticipated that the number of injections will increase further. Therefore, it is not surprising that the development of new approaches for their effective and safer delivery to the immune system ranks high in the WHO's priority list (Jodar et al. 2001). Safety is a major issue because vaccines are administered to prevent disease in healthy people (Clements et al. 1999). To increase compliance, as well as to make the vaccine more economical, vaccines should be effective after a single immunization using needle-free or noninvasive delivery systems.

Ideally, future vaccines should:

- be administered via noninvasive routes, such as the mucosae (436 m^2) and the skin (2 m^2) which cover a large surface area of the human body
- require only a single administration, or at the most two, to elicit protective immune responses
- be capable of immunizing at a very early age
- be available in formulations already combined with either multiple other vaccines or other vaccines at the moment of administration
- exhibit temperature stability to minimize the stringency of cold chain requirements.

New skin and mucosal vaccine delivery options (vaccine patches, nasal sprays, or edible vaccines) are promising to revolutionize the way that vaccines will be delivered in the future. Needle-free vaccine delivery systems will make immunization simpler, more economical, practical, and safer.

SKIN DELIVERY OF VACCINES

The skin barrier

The skin is the largest organ of the body (10 percent of body mass) and represents a readily accessible surface area for absorption (2 m^2 in adult humans). This offers a distinct advantage for exploiting the skin immune system for delivery of vaccines. The skin is made up of the epidermis and the dermis. The dermis (1–2 mm) contains fibroblasts, nerves, and blood vessels. The outermost layer of the epidermis, which constitutes an effective physical and chemical barrier, in the stratum corneum (10–20 μm thick in humans), is composed of keratinocytes anchored in a lipophilic matrix. Keratinocytes undergo terminal differentiation, a specialized form of programmed cell death. As a result, they lose their nuclei and crosslink, becoming resilient rigid corneocytes, and eventually they complex with lipids (Fuchs 1990). This is a well-regulated process required for the maintenance of the physiological thickness of the skin and the preservation of its barrier functions. Ceramides, cholesterol, and free fatty acids seem to play an important role in the corneocyte cohesion, contributing also to the permeability barrier of the skin (Morganti et al. 2001). Thus, the function of the skin is to preclude appreciable exchange of materials between the skin surface and the deep layers, and to protect against ultraviolet light.

Below the stratum corneum are layers of epidermis (50–100 μm) which are made up of keratinocytes at various stages of differentiation (Morganti et al. 2001). The stratum basale, just above the dermis, is the most metabolically active layer of the epidermis with large columnar cells. Interspersed among the basal keratinocytes are other cells, such as melanocytes, Langerhans' cells (LC), and sensory Merkel cells. Once keratinocytes leave the basal layer, they migrate upward via the stratum spinosum and stratum granulosum to the stratum corneum, acquiring the characteristics of fully differentiated corneocytes which are eventually sloughed at the skin surface. During this migration process, keratinocytes undergo morphological and biochemical changes necessary to discard their proliferative functions and adopt new protective roles.

The skin as a site of immune surveillance

As the skin is the principal interface with the external environment, it acts as an immune barrier protecting the host from invading pathogens. For this purpose, it is equipped with a unique set of immunocompetent cells, i.e. keratinocytes, and LCs, strategically located lymph nodes, and subsets of T lymphocytes that constitute the skin-associated lymphoid tissue (SALT) (Streilein 1983; Bos and Kapsenberg 1993). The intraepidermal lymphocytes constitute only about 2 percent of SALT and the majority are CD8$^+$ T cells (De Panfilis 1998; Debenedictis et al. 2001). The predominance of CD8$^+$ epidermal T cells is in contrast to the normal 2:1 ratio of CD4$^+$:CD8$^+$ T cells seen in peripheral blood; therefore, it is apparent that the population of T cells found in the epidermis is a special population of memory cells, which have selectively extravasated into the epidermis (Debenedictis et al. 2001). By contrast, the dermis contains both populations of CD4$^+$ and CD8$^+$ T cells in equivalent ratios (Debenedictis et al. 2001).

Keratinocytes, apart of being responsible for establishing the physical barrier of the skin (the viable epidermis is composed of about 90–95 percent keratinocytes) and guaranteeing the structural integrity of the epidermis, produce a wide range of cytokines on activation by various stimuli. These include interleukins (IL), interferons (IFN), colony-stimulating factor (CSF), tumor necrosis factor (TNF), growth factors, and chemokines (Uchi et al. 2000). Resting keratinocytes synthesize and secrete low levels of cytokines. However, stimuli such as allergens, irritants, ultraviolet light, bacterial products, and physical trauma induce keratinocytes to produce significant amounts of cytokines (Uchi et al. 2000). These cytokines shape the local microenvironment of the skin to help maintain the appropriate balance of skin immune responses, and stimulate the maturation and migration of LCs. In particular, IL-1β and low levels of TNF-α are critically involved in the induction of LC migration from the skin (Wang et al. 1999). Keratinocytes do not just secrete cytokines; they also perform a scavenger function, eliminating foreign material from the intercellular spaces of the epidermis (Wolff and Honigsmann 1971) and responding to cytokines secreted by neighboring cells (Debenedictis et al. 2001). When they are exposed to IFN-γ produced by T cells, keratinocytes upregulate intercellular adhesion molecule 1 (ICAM-1) and class II major histocompatibility complex (MHC) antigens (keratinocytes do not constitutively express MHC class II molecules). This enables them to serve as accessory cells by providing co-stimulatory signals to support a T-cell-mediated response to bacterially derived superantigens, phytohemagglutinin, and anti-CD3 monoclonal antibody (Nickoloff et al. 1993).

LCs are powerful antigen-presenting cells (APC) (up to 1 000 cells/mm^2) that cover almost 20 percent of the surface area through their horizontal orientation and long protrusions (Debenedictis et al. 2001). They are of myeloid lineage, originally migrating to the skin during fetal development. LCs are defined by their dendritic morphology and the presence of a unique intracytoplasmic organelle, the Birbeck granule (Lappin et al. 1996). They are located at the basal layer of the epidermis as immature cells playing a sentinel role in the epidermis. LCs capture and process antigens and, during their migration via the efferent lymphatics to the paracortical T-cell areas of the draining lymph nodes, they mature and present antigenic peptides to naïve T cells. At this stage, they express co-stimulatory molecules of the B7 family, upregulate the surface expression of MHC class I and II molecules bound to peptides, and secrete high levels of proinflammatory cytokines, such as IL-12 and IL-1 (Lappin et al. 1996; Debenedictis et al. 2001).

Percutaneous absorption of antigens

Antigens applied on to bare skin penetrate across the continuous stratum corneum, mainly via the intracellular or intercellular routes (Barry 2001). However, appendages including hair follicles, or sebaceous or sweat glands can also serve as portals of antigen entry (Figure 40.1). The specific pathway that an antigen will follow depends on several parameters, such as its physicochemical characteristics and the method of antigen delivery. As the stratum corneum is lipophilic, antigens of a lipophilic nature would be better accepted (Naik et al. 2000; Barry 2001). Moreover, an antigen must be sufficiently 'mobile' to diffuse across the stratum corneum. Solute diffusivity has been shown to decrease exponentially as molecular volume (and hence molecular weight) increases, imposing a size restriction on favorable transport across the skin (Naik et al. 2000). After antigen diffusion through the stratum corneum, its re-partition into the more aqueous viable epidermis beneath would facilitate its move toward the basal layer, where LCs reside. Therefore, ideally, the antigen should possess both lipoidal and aqueous solubility for effective skin penetration (Naik et al. 2000; Barry 2001).

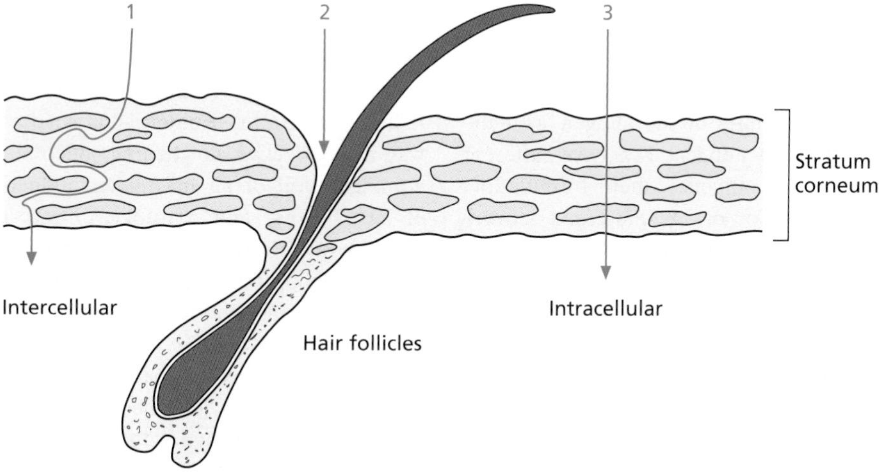

Figure 40.1 *Percutaneous absorption of antigens. Routes that an antigen can follow after application on to bare skin.*

However, when the skin is hydrated, its barrier functions are less pronounced and large molecules can pass through.

Studies on percutaneous absorption of various molecules have shown that the intercellular pathway is mainly favored by liposomes or low-molecular-mass uncharged molecules, whereas molecules delivered by electroporation or gene gun penetrate via the intracellular space (Morganti et al. 2001). Hair follicles could provide a shunt route through which large molecules, such as oligonucleotides, liposome-complexed DNA, or naked plasmid DNA (pDNA), can cross the stratum corneum (Prausnitz 1997; Fan et al. 1999; Morganti et al. 2001).

As stratum corneum lipids limit the transport of most compounds, efforts to increase percutaneous absorption have often focused on altering the lipid bilayer structure. This can be achieved by chemical or physical approaches. The most effective chemical enhancers act by disrupting or fluidizing lipid bilayer structures within the stratum corneum, thereby increasing the diffusion of molecules through the skin (Prausnitz 1997; Faldvari 2000; Barry 2001). Chemical enhancers such as dimethyl sulfoxide, unsaturated fatty acids, or surfactants have been shown to increase percutaneous absorption of small molecules (Prausnitz 1997). However, they frequently cause significant skin irritation and may affect the stability of co-administered molecules. For these reasons they have little practical impact beyond preclinical studies.

Liposomes have been shown to increase topical and transdermal delivery of various low-molecular-mass molecules. In particular, lipid-based biphasic delivery systems are capable of encapsulating compounds such as proteins and DNA and delivering them effectively through the skin, e.g. formulations with recombinant *Pasteurella haemolytica* leukotoxin and hen egg lysozyme can induce strongly polarized, T-helper 2 (Th2)-type, antigen-specific, immune responses after topical application (Baca-Estrada et al. 2000a). Transdermal delivery of lipid-based DNA vaccines can induce both antibody and cytokine responses in mice, although the responses are weak (Baca-Estrada et al. 2000b). When formulating vaccine antigens with liposomes, it is critical to determine the compatibility of the antigen with the liposome because different antigens can have different chemical properties that influence their formulation. Furthermore, the composition of the lipid-based delivery systems can influence their percutaneous absorption (Babiuk et al. 2000). To improve the absorption of topically applied liposomes, ultradeformable liposomes termed 'transferosomes' have been developed (Cevc et al. 1998). These carriers can cross the intact mammalian skin with an efficacy close to 100 percent, and ensure an efficiency of delivery greater than 50 percent. After topical application, they have been shown to increase the immunogenicity of incorporated Gap junctional proteins (Paul et al. 1998). Their mechanism of skin penetration appears to be related to their ability to squeeze through polar channels on hydration gradients (Cevc et al. 1998).

One of the physical enhancement technologies that has been tested for transdermal vaccine delivery is electroporation (Vanbever and Préat 1999). It uses high-voltage, short-duration pulses that induce: (1) a disorganization of the stratum corneum lipid bilayers; (2) an increase of skin hydration; and (3) a decrease of skin resistance. It permeabilizes keratinocytes without affecting skin viability in vivo (Dujardin et al. 2002). Skin electroporation was shown to increase immune responses to a myristilated peptide derived from hepatitis B surface antigen (HBsAg) when administered without adjuvant but not to a larger size antigen, such as diphtheria toxoid (DT) (Misra et al. 1999). This suggests that small antigens can be targeted in sufficient amounts to the LC-rich area of the epidermis, to mount a good immune response. However, there are still limited in vivo data concerning immunogenicity and skin toxicological studies for establishing the clinical value of this method.

A novel technology known as transdermal powder delivery (TPD) represents an alternate physical method for vaccine delivery. This method uses a supersonic flow of gas to accelerate vaccine-coated particles to a sufficiently high speed to enable them to penetrate the outer layers of the skin. The particles are sufficiently hard and robust not to deform significantly or shatter on impact, and penetrate the epidermis and dermis proportional to the product of their velocity, diameter, and density. A single administration of influenza vaccine using a helium-powered device elicited serum antivirus IgG antibody titers that were significantly higher than those induced by either intramuscular or subcutaneous injection. A booster administration resulted in a further increase of antibody titers and 100 percent protection against homologous virus challenge (Chen et al. 2000). Similarly, powderject delivery of DT was increased by 25- and 250-fold when 1 μg DT was co-administered with alum or a CpG motif, respectively. The induced antibodies neutralized the toxin and were long lasting, and their isotype was dependent on the adjuvant used (Chen et al. 2001a). Epidermal powderject immunization was also effective in eliciting mucosal immunity after administration of an inactivated influenza virus (Chen et al. 2001b), and cytotoxic T-cell responses after delivery of HBsAg or a synthetic peptide from influenza virus nucleoprotein (Chen et al. 2001c). The efficacy of this system can be attributed to the fact that it delivers vaccine antigens to LCs.

Another physical approach to vaccine delivery is the use of needle-free jet injectors (JI) that deliver the dose of vaccine at high velocity into dermal and subcutaneous layers with high-pressure fluid. Needle-free injectors have the potential to eliminate the risk of accidental needlestick injuries after injections and during discard of waste. However, vaccine administration with JIs has been associated with higher levels of pain in female recipients, reported at the time of immunization, as well as with the occurrence of local injection site reactions in comparison to vaccine administration with needles and syringes (Jackson et al. 2001). When four types of injectors were tested for their safety, all were found to transmit significant (>10 pl) volumes of blood, although the volumes and frequency of contamination varied with the injector (Hoffman et al. 2001). This raises the risk of transmission of infectious diseases, such as HBV. Also a problem associated with the use of needle-free jet injection devices is that currently they cost several times what less developed countries now pay for conventional syringes and needles. In addition, a healthcare worker is required to administer the vaccine.

Immunization on to bare skin

For a long time it was thought that the skin barrier was impermeable to large molecules, but studies by Glenn et al. (1998a) have demonstrated that topical application of cholera toxin (CT) on to hydrated skin can induce strong systemic and mucosal immune responses and confer protection against lethal mucosal toxin challenge (Glenn et al. 1998b). CT is an exotoxin secreted by *Vibrio cholerae*. It is made up of five identical B subunits that bind with high affinity to G_{M1} gangliosides at cell surfaces and a single A subunit. The latter, after proteolytic cleavage, generates the enzymatically active A1 peptide, which activates adenylyl cyclase (Spangler 1992). A similar effect was demonstrated with another adenosine diphosphate (ADP)-ribosylating exotoxin, the heat-labile enterotoxin (LT) of *Escherichia coli* (Glenn et al. 1999; Beignon et al. 2001). Parallel to their immunogenic potential, these molecules act as adjuvants, potentiating immune responses to topically co-applied antigens, including toxoids (Scharton-Kersten et al. 1999; Hammond et al. 2000), proteins (Glenn et al. 1998a; Scharton-Kersten et al. 1999; Partidos et al. 2001), peptides (Beignon et al. 2001, 2002a), and viruses (El-Ghorr et al. 2000; Hammond et al. 2001a). It is the combination of their binding activity and built-in adjuvanticity that make these molecules powerful immunogens and adjuvants. When recombinant CTB, which is devoid of ADP-ribosylating activity, was used as an adjuvant with DT, anti-DT antibody responses were of a lower magnitude than those of the group in which CT was used. However, when a small amount of CT was added to the recombinant CTB, the adjuvant activity was restored to levels comparable to that of CT (Scharton-Kersten et al. 2000). In another study, pre-incubation of CT with G_{M1} gangliosides before topical application significantly reduced the serum and mucosal anti-CT antibody responses (Beignon et al. 2001).

Following these initial observations, the potential of skin as a noninvasive route for vaccine delivery has been demonstrated with several types of antigens:

- viruses: herpes simplex virus (HSV), adenovirus, inactivated rabies virus, recombinant mengo virus
- parasites: *Dirofilaria immitis*
- plasmid DNA: HBsAg, influenza antigens
- bacterial toxins (CT, LT), toxoids (tetanus toxoid (TT), DT)
- proteins: bovine serum albumin (BSA), β-galactosidase
- peptides: Th, B, cytoxic lymphocyte (CTL) epitopes.

Also, preliminary results from a phase 1 trial conducted in human volunteers (Glenn et al. 2000) have shown that topical application of LT with a patch: (1) does not induce local or systemic adverse reactions – only one volunteer developed a mild dermatitis at the adhesive site; (2) elicits anti-LT IgG responses that were boosted after the second and third topical application of LT; (3) induces long-lasting immunity and detectable anti-LT IgG or IgA antibodies in urine and stools; and (4) visualizes enlarged and rounded LCs using anti-CD1a staining at the site of immunization after 24 and 48 h.

Overall, these findings suggest that the skin barrier is not as highly resistant to permeation by antigenic molecules as previously thought, but rather has variable resistance. However, it should be noted that, in certain instances of skin disease, i.e. atopic dermatitis or psoriasis, as well as in skin wounds and burns, the permeability of the skin is increased as a result of alterations of its lipid content (Morganti et al. 2001).

CHARACTERISTICS AND REQUIREMENTS FOR APPLYING VACCINES ON TO BARE SKIN

Immunization on to bare skin is a needle-free and pain-free immunization procedure, which delivers antigens into the epidermis by simple topical application (Figure 40.2). With the experimental evidence that has been accumulated so far, some general rules can be drawn for vaccine application on to bare skin.

Skin hydration

Hydration of the skin before vaccine application appears to disrupt the barrier function of the stratum corneum to absorption. An increase in hydration of the skin is associated with a swelling of the stratum corneum and a softening of its texture (Barry 2001). Water is the most natural penetration enhancer that strongly binds to the keratin of corneocytes and increases the 'hydrophilic' character of the stratum corneum (Barry 2001). Glycerol has also been evaluated for its potentiating effects on the immune responses to CTB after topical application. Combination of hydration with glycerol enhanced the anti-CTB antibody responses approximately two- to

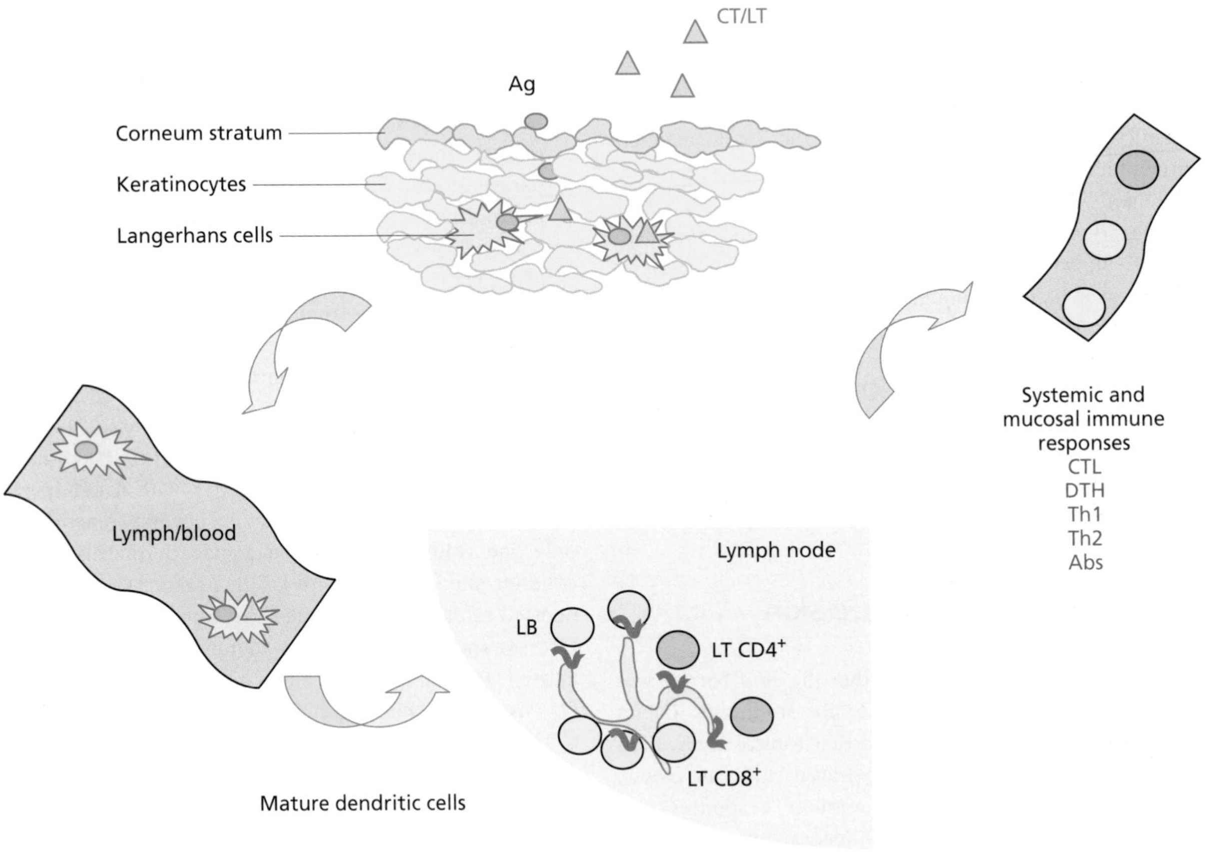

Figure 40.2 *Immunization on to bare skin. After penetration of vaccine formulation across the stratum corneum, the antigen is taken up by Langerhans' cells (LCs) and, in the presence of the co-administered adjuvant, they mature and migrate to the regional lymph nodes, where they present antigenic peptides to naïve T cells. This results in the induction of antigen-specific humoral and cellular responses.*

fourfold in comparison to the responses measured in mice with skin that was not hydrated (Hammond et al. 2001b).

The requirement of an adjuvant

Adjuvants are important to potentiate immune responses to antigens and ADP-ribosylating exotoxins, such as CT and LT, are suitable adjuvants for skin immunization. They enhance the antibody and T-cell responses to the co-administered antigen without signs of toxicity, normally associated with their mucosal delivery (when high doses are used). Furthermore, the anti-toxin antibody response does not interfere with the immune responses to co-administered antigen. Therefore, the same adjuvant can be used for multiple applications. The selection of adjuvant is also critical for the induction of long-lasting immunity and type of Th response. Several other adjuvants have been tested for skin immunization, such as synthetic oligodeoxynucleotides (ODN) containing CpG motifs, lipopolysaccharide (LPS), muramyl dipeptide (MDP), alum, IL-2, and IL-12 (Scharton-Kersten et al. 2000):

- ADP-ribosylating exotoxins (CT, pertussis toxin (PT), LT)
- mutants of ADP-ribosylating toxins (LTK63, LTR72, LTR192G)
- dangerous signals (LPS, CpG motifs, MDP)
- cytokines (IL-1b, IL-2, IL-12, TNF-α, GM-CSF).

Although they enhanced the antibody titers to co-applied antigen, the responses were short-lived and weaker than those induced in the presence of CT or LT.

Both CT and LT elicit predominantly Th2-type responses that might have a detrimental effect in individuals sensitive to allergic reactions. Normally, some adverse reactions to immunization are common and tolerated for the benefit of immunity. In several instances high levels of IgE responses have been noticed with DT vaccines (Mark et al. 1995). Although the exact role of IgE responses remains to be elucidated, there is always the possibility that the presence of high levels of IgE might be associated with high risk of anaphylaxis, particularly in individuals with atopic predisposition (Sakaguchi and Inouye 2000). On the other hand, antigen-specific IgE appears to correlate with protection in diseases such as schistosomiasis (Khalife et al. 2000). Therefore, successful immunization protocols will be needed to induce the appropriate types of immune responses in a selective and reliable way.

Beignon et al. (2002a) have demonstrated the possibility of modulating immune responses to topically applied antigens. Co-application of a promiscuous (non-MHC-restricted) Th epitope from influenza virus hemagglutinin (amino acids 307–319) with CT and an ODN containing a CpG motif on to hydrated bare skin of mice elicited peptide- and virus-specific $CD4^+$ T cells, increased the levels of IFN-γ and IL-6 secretion, and downregulated the total serum IgE antibody levels. CpG motifs have been shown to induce activation and maturation of LCs (Hartmann et al. 1999). Furthermore, their injection into the dermis enhances the expression of MHC and co-stimulatory molecules by LCs, and promotes their migration (Ban et al. 2000). Thus, it appears that CpG motifs can act synergistically with CT to promote a Th1-type of response. The exact series of events that lead to this synergistic effect is not yet clear. Similarly, mutants of LT with no or residual toxicity have been shown to enhance antigen-specific antibody and T-cell responses after topical immunization (Scharton-Kersten et al. 2000; Beignon et al. 2002b). Furthermore, the mutant LTR72, which retains some residual toxicity, was shown preferentially to stimulate the secretion of high levels of IFN-γ whereas the mutant LTK63, which is devoid of toxicity, did not (Beignon et al. 2002b).

Topical application of DNA vaccines

The success of topical application of DNA vaccines on to untreated skin depends on the ability to transfect effectively cells of the epidermis that will subsequently express the encoded antigen in sufficient quantities to elicit an immune response (Shi et al. 1999). It appears that the production of very small amounts of protein in the skin is sufficient to elicit an immune response. LCs and dermal dendritic cells (DC), which are specialized in initiating immune responses, can acquire antigen through direct transfection or through uptake and presentation of antigen synthesized by transfected keratinocytes or other skin cells (Pfutzner and Vogel 2000). The application of pDNA expressing the lacZ and HBsAg on to intact skin resulted in the induction of anti-HBsAg antibody and cellular responses (Fan et al. 1999). The predominant isotype of antibodies was IgG1, suggesting a Th2-type of response. For the HBsAg, the antibody and cellular responses were of the same order of magnitude of those induced after intramuscular injection with the commercially available recombinant HBsAg vaccine (Fan et al. 1999). Finally, in the same study it was demonstrated that efficient uptake of pDNA required the presence of intact hair follicles. Thus, the distal part of the human hair follicle immune system appears to represent a specialized compartment, where interacting intraepithelial T cells and LCs can generate effective immune responses (Christoph et al. 2000). The feasibility of topical genetic immunization has also been demonstrated with chitosan-based nanoparticles containing plasmid DNA (Cui and Mumper 2001). Two types of nanoparticles were investigated: (1) pDNA-condensed chitosan nanoparticles and (2) pDNA coated on preformed cationic chitosan/carboxymethylcellulose (CMC) nanoparticles. After their application on to bare skin, antigen expression was detectable at quantifiable levels in mouse skin after 24 h, and antigen-specific antibodies were measured in serum samples.

Induction of mucosal immunity

Immunization on to bare skin of mice with ADP-ribosylating exotoxins mixed with proteins elicits not only serum antibody responses but also significant levels of IgG and more modest levels of IgA antibodies in serum and multiple mucosal secretions (Glenn et al. 1999; Gockel et al. 2000; Beignon et al. 2001; Yu et al. 2002). Secretory IgA antibodies can decrease the colonization of mucosal surfaces by a number of microorganisms, and can effectively neutralize viruses and bacterial toxins generated within the lumen of the gut. In addition IgG antibodies present in mucosal fluids have recently been demonstrated to neutralize viruses (Baba et al. 2000). Thus, topical immunization provides an effective means to induce both systemic and mucosal immunity.

The exact mechanisms involved in the induction of mucosal immunity are still not clear. Studies by Enioutina et al. (2000) have provided evidence that 1,25-dihydroxy-vitamin D_3 [$1,25(OH)_2D_3$], which is derived from normal circulating 25-hydroxy-vitamin D_3 ($25(OH)D_3$) after its exposure to the enzymatic activity of 1α-hydroxylase, redirects the migration of dendritic cells from the skin into lymphoid organs committed to initiating mucosal immune responses. CT and LT, as a result of their ability to activate adenylyl cyclase, share the capacity to elevate intracellular levels of cAMP (Spangler 1992). Taking into account that the vitamin D_3–1α-hydroxylase gene, encoding the cellular enzyme that converts $25(OH)D_3$ to $1,25(OH)_2D_3$ is under cAMP control (Kong et al. 1999), it could be argued that ADP-ribosylating exotoxins stimulate the induction of mucosal immunity through the stimulation of $25(OH)D_3$–1α-hydroxylase expression (Enioutina et al. 2000).

Variability of immune responses and potential of peptides as immunogens

Data from immunogenicity studies using proteins, toxoids, and viruses suggest that large molecules can penetrate the skin barrier and with the help of an adjuvant elicit immune responses (Hammond et al. 2001b). However, antibody responses to co-applied antigens are normally variable, significantly lower, and with slower onset compared with those induced by co-application

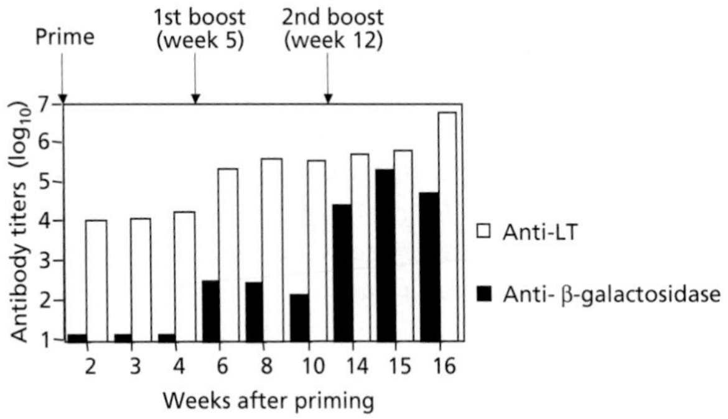

Figure 40.3 *Kinetics of serum anti-heat-labile enterotoxin (LT) and anti-β-galactosidase antibody responses after co-immunization on to bare skin of BALB/C mice (n = 6) with 100 μg LT and 100 μg β-galactosidase. Data represent mean of antibody titers.*

with CT or LT (Figure 40.3). Moreover, in a recent study where the safety and immunogenicity of a prototype enterotoxigenic *E. coli* vaccine was assessed in adult volunteers after topical application, only 68 and 53 percent were found to have serum anti-colonizing factor CS6 IgG and IgA antibodies, respectively (Guerena-Burgueno et al. 2002).

The use of synthetic peptides that normally have a small molecular size could potentially overcome this problem. This view is supported by the observation that most of the commonly used and effective drugs applied to bare skin have a molecular mass of <500 Da. In addition, chemicals that cause allergic contact dermatitis are <700 Da (Bos and Meinardi 2000). Peptide antigens have indeed been reported to induce protective antitumor CTL responses after application on to disrupted (by stripping) skin (Seo et al. 2000). This mechanical intervention removes the stratum corneum and activates LCs (through the stimulation of cytokine secretion by keratinocytes). Therefore, immune responses can be induced without the need of an adjuvant (Katoh et al. 1997); however, this procedure is painful and poorly reproducible. Recent studies have demonstrated that peptides are effective immunogens when co-applied with an ADP-ribosylating exotoxin or mutants of LT on to bare skin, eliciting peptide- and antigen-specific $CD4^+$ T cells (Beignon et al. 2001, 2002a, 2002b). This is particularly important in the context of vaccine design and delivery, because $CD4^+$ T cells produce cytokines that have a direct effect on viruses, help B cells to produce neutralizing and protective antivirus antibodies, and enhance the magnitude of cytotoxic cell responses to clear virus-infected cells.

FUTURE PROSPECTS AND CHALLENGES FOR DELIVERING VACCINES ON TO BARE SKIN

Over the last few years there has been remarkable progress in the field of immunodermatology. More recently, the realization that the skin has a number of characteristic features, such as easy accessibility, the presence of powerful APCs, and cells such as keratinocytes that secrete a wide range of cytokines, makes it an attractive route for vaccine delivery. However, for effective delivery, several variables related to the nature of the antigen and characteristics of the skin barrier must first be overcome, e.g. the diffusion of an antigen through the stratum corneum is dependent on its physicochemical properties and its molecular interactions with skin constituents (Morganti et al. 2001). These variables are:

- variability of percutaneous absorption as a result of the site, disease, age, species differences, and physicochemical characteristics of the vaccine formulation
- dermal metabolism of topically applied antigens
- incomplete understanding of the technologies that may be used to facilitate absorption and mechanisms of immune induction.

This could explain the differences in immunogenicity of several antigens after their application to bare skin. It is also important to stress the fact that the increased immunogenicity of ADP-ribosylating exotoxins depends mainly on their inherent adjuvanticity and ability to bind to cell surface receptors. Furthermore, the skin of humans and animals both pose unique barriers resulting from differences in anatomy and physiology between species, e.g. small laboratory animals always present a skin barrier that is more permeable than that of larger animals, including humans (Wester and Maibach 1987). The primary difference between rodent and human skin is the lipid composition and organization of the stratum corneum (Bond and Barry 1988). For these reasons, all these variables make the task of extrapolating the findings of studies performed in different animal species to the target species difficult. Percutaneous absorption through porcine and monkey skin (squirrel and rhesus) is more closely related to that through human skin (Wester and Maibach 1987). Porcine skin has been shown to be histologically and biochemically similar to human skin and, in addition, has permeability characteristics similar to that of human skin (Wester and Maibach 1987; Dick and Scott 1992); as such, it provides the most suitable experimental model for dermatological research on humans.

In situations of skin disease, eczematous reactions can develop after topical application of protein allergens on the nonlesional skin of atopic dermatitis patients, demonstrating that high-molecular-mass proteins could penetrate through this type of skin and induce an allergen-specific, delayed-type hypersensitivity response (Castelain 1995). This suggests that the skin can be a site of sensitization to environmental protein allergens. Therefore, topical application of vaccines might be an unsuitable option for immunization of individuals with skin disease. The main challenge ahead is the development of approaches to increase the permeability of the skin barrier to various vaccine antigen formulations, and to optimize the induction of long-term mucosal and systemic immune responses.

MUCOSAL DELIVERY OF VACCINES

The mucosal routes offer an attractive alternative to currently used parenteral immunization. This is mainly because vaccines can be easily administered via the nose or orally, and mucosal immunization stimulates the induction of both systemic and local immunity. The latter is of paramount importance because most invading pathogens enter the body via mucosal surfaces. Over the last few years significant progress has been made in understanding the immunological mechanisms involved for maintaining the balance between immunity and tolerance. This has helped in the design and development of new immunization strategies and technologies, promising to deliver future vaccines via the mucosal routes using edible preparations or nasal sprays.

Antigen uptake by the mucosal surfaces

The mucosal surfaces constitute a vast surface area (about 300–400 m^2 in an adult), permanently challenged by numerous exogenous microorganisms associated with infectious diseases. As a consequence, the mucosal epithelium has evolved into a sophisticated physical and immunological barrier, protecting the host from environmental pathogens. Its cellular organization (stratified epithelium versus simple epithelium) and antigen-sampling mechanisms differ, depending on the mucosal site (Table 40.1).

The stratified epithelium is composed of multiple layers of cells that lack tight junctions. However, its barrier function is provided by a glycoprotein that they secrete, which seals the intercellular space and excludes the entry of most infectious agents and vaccines (Neutra et al. 1996). In stratified epithelia, DCs migrate to the outer limit of the epithelium, where they sample antigens for subsequent presentation in local or distant organized lymphoid tissues (McWilliam et al. 1994). Simple mucosal epithelia are made up of a layer of epithelial cells and their barrier function is provided by tight junctions that seal the intercellular space (Neutra et al. 1996). Antigens are sampled by microfold (M) cells that transport them from the lumen to the organized lymphoid tissue within the underlying mucosa. These are specialized epithelial cells located in the dome region of the epithelial layer, known as follicle-associated epithelium (Neutra 1999). Parallel to their sampling function, M cells can also serve as a portal of entry for several microorganisms, including bacteria, viruses, and protozoa (Siebers and Finlay 1996). Adherence to M cells has also been shown greatly to facilitate antigen transport and enhance immunogenicity (Frey and Neutra 1997; Wu et al. 2001).

Mucosa-associated lymphoid tissue and induction of immune responses

The mammalian mucosal immune system has evolved to fulfill several functions, including: (1) the production of secretory IgA (sIgA) antibody responses; (2) the distribution of effector B and T cells to local and distant mucosal sites; and (3) the induction of tolerance. The mucosa-associated lymphoid tissue (MALT) can be divided into two anatomically and functionally distinct compartments or sites: (1) the inductive sites, which are defined lymphoid microcompartments, and (2) the effector sites, which contain diffuse accumulations of large numbers of lymphoid cells that do not associate into apparently organized structures (McGhee et al. 1992). In the upper respiratory tract of rodents and humans, the major inductive sites are the nasal associated lymphoid tissue (NALT), which is organized lymphoid tissue at the base of the nasal cavity and the tonsils, respectively (Kuper et al. 1992). Mucosal inductive sites of the gastrointestinal tract include the Peyer's patches (PP), appendix, and solitary lymphoid nodules, which collectively comprise gut-associated lymphoid tissue (GALT).

The antigen is first encountered in the inductive sites, which contain B and T lymphocytes and APCs, and initial responses are elicited. After sensitization, antigen-specific B and T lymphocytes migrate from the inductive sites to regional lymph nodes and proceed via the lymph into the circulation, from where they 'home' to distant mucosal effector sites, such as the lamina propria of the respiratory, gastrointestinal, and reproductive tracts and

Table 40.1 *Types of mucosal epithelia and antigen-sampling mechanisms*

Type of epithelium	Mucosal site	Antigen-sampling
Stratified epithelia	Lower genital tract Upper digestive tract	APCs migrate to the outermost limit of the epithelium where they sample antigens
Simple epithelia	Lower digestive tract Airways	Migrating APCs can sample antigen
	Upper genital tract	Resident M cells transport antigens across the epithelial barrier

APCs, antigen-presenting cells; M, microfold.

the lacrimal, salivary, and mammary glands where immune responses are expressed. This cell distribution from the inductive sites to the effector sites has been termed the 'common mucosal immune system' (McDermott and Bienenstock 1979) and ensures that all mucosal surfaces are furnished with antigen-specific immunocompetent cells for protection.

Following mucosal immunization, humoral and cellular immune responses can be developed. After the antigen is sampled and passed through endocytic vesicles to the underlying lymphoid cells in the submucosa, antigen processing and presentation occur. This results in the activation of T cells which in turn provide help to B cells to develop into IgA plasma cells. Secretory IgA plays an important role in mucosal defense by providing protection against viruses or bacteria, and neutralizing microbial toxins (McGhee et al. 1992). These functions appear to be facilitated, at least in part, by the high-affinity binding of sIgA to mucus. Intranasal immunization induces sIgA responses to a wider range of mucosal tissues than does oral immunization. This is probably caused by the more promiscuous profile of homing receptors possessed by the circulating IgA-secreting cells that is induced after intranasal immunization (Quiding-Jarbrink et al. 1995).

For the induction of an effective mucosal immune response, the activation of T cells ($CD4^+$ and $CD8^+$) is of paramount importance because they provide help to B cells to become IgA-producing cells. These cells also release cytokines and chemokines that are involved in all aspects of mucosal immunity and, finally, they contribute to clearing viral infections. As $CD4^+$ T cells mature in response to foreign antigens, they take on unique characteristics normally manifested by production of a distinct set of cytokines. The Th1 cells, which result after infection with viruses or intracellular bacteria, produce IL-2, IFN-γ, and IL-12, and the Th2 cells, which are triggered by exogenous antigens, produce IL-4, IL-5, and IL-10 (Mosmann and Coffman 1989). Some of these cytokines regulate the expression of B-cell Ig isotypes and subclasses as well as influence the maturation of B-cell responses through induction of terminal differentiation into plasma cells.

Edible vaccines

The idea of using genetically modified plants to produce and deliver protective antigens via the oral route has several attractive features:

- Edible vaccines can be easily produced at low cost. The cultivation, harvesting, storage, and processing of transgenic crops could use the existing infrastructure and therefore would require relatively little capital investment. In this way, the purchase price of a dose of vaccine can be significantly reduced, increasing the chances of sustainable immunization strategies, particularly in less developed countries where vaccines are still expensive. It has been estimated that the cost of producing recombinant proteins in plants could be 10- to 50-fold lower than producing the same protein in *E. coli* (Kusnadi et al. 1997).
- There is a reduced health risk from pathogen contamination because plants do not harbor human infectious pathogens.
- Edible vaccines have the added advantage of providing natural bioencapsulation to the expressed antigens, protecting them from degradation in the harsh environment of the stomach.
- Edible vaccines induce mucosal immunity that can be advantageous for the control of pathogens entering via the mucosal surfaces and causing enteric, respiratory, and sexually transmitted infections.
- They can be administered easily and have the potential to deliver multiple immunogens, so increasing vaccine compliance.
- They can deliver multiple antigens.

EDIBLE VACCINES EXPRESSING VIRAL ANTIGENS

In 1992, Mason and co-workers successfully integrated the DNA-encoding HBsAg into tobacco plants. The expressed HBsAg retained its capacity for self-association and, more importantly, was structurally and antigenically similar to the HBsAg derived from human serum and recombinant yeast. Subsequent studies have demonstrated that oral immunization of mice with HBsAg expressed in potato tubers with CT as an adjuvant elicited strong serum antibody responses that reached a peak of 103 mIU/ml 4 weeks after the third dose and >10 mIU/ml (level of protective serum anti-HBsAg antibodies) at week 11 (Kong et al. 2001). Oral feeding of potato tubers expressing HBsAg has also resulted in strong memory responses, as assessed by the rise of antibody titers to 3 300 mIU/ml 3 weeks after parenteral immunization with a subimmunogenic dose of alum-absorbed recombinant HBsAg (Kong et al. 2001). Thus, the strategy of combining the oral and parenteral routes of immunization can be advantageous in less developed countries where the logistics of multiple delivery doses of parenteral vaccines have hampered global HBV immunization efforts. In the same study it was demonstrated that cooking the transgenic potatoes (boiling) before feeding mice significantly reduced the immunogenicity of the edible vaccine. An alternate approach to overcome this problem could be the use of transgenic bananas, which are grown extensively throughout the less developed world and, in contrast to potatoes, can be eaten raw.

As degradation of proteins in the stomach limits their bioavailability, much higher concentrations of antigens are normally required for effective oral immunization compared with parenteral immunization. Therefore, increasing the levels of antigen expression in plant tissues would enhance the utility of transgenic plants as a source of recombinant antigen. A systematic study of factors influencing the accumulation of HBsAg in transgenic potatoes has demonstrated a striking improvement of antigen expression. This resulted from alternate polyadenylation signals and fusion protein-targeting signals designed to enhance integration or retention of HBsAg in the ER of plant cells (Richter et al. 2000). However, there is always the risk that a single high dose or repeated low doses of a protein antigen can induce oral tolerance. To overcome this potential problem, mucosal adjuvants that enhance antigen-specific mucosal and systemic immune responses have been used (Mason et al. 1996).

Another example of edible vaccine is the expression of Norwalk virus capsid protein (NVCP) in transgenic plants (Mason et al. 1996). The virus is responsible for an acute gastroenteritis in humans. The expression of recombinant NVCP in transgenic tobacco leaves resulted in self-assembled virus-like particles that were morphologically and physically similar to the recombinant protein produced in insect cells. When extracts of tobacco leaves expressing the NVCP were given orally (50 μg protein with or without 10 μg CT on days 1, 2, 11, and 28) by gavage to mice, both IgG and secretory IgA anti-NVCP antibodies were detected in serum and fecal samples. The presence of CT enhanced antibody levels during the early phases of immunization but, at the final time point (40 days after the first immunization), the titers in mice fed with transgenic tobacco with or without CT were very similar (Mason et al. 1996). In a human clinical trial, ingestion of raw transgenic potatoes constitutively expressing the NVCP induced immune responses in the absence of adjuvant (Tacket et al. 2000). The majority (95 percent) of volunteers had a significant increase in the number of antigen-specific IgA antibody-secreting cells, 20 percent developed antigen-specific serum IgG antibodies, whereas, in 30 percent of the volunteers, antigen-specific IgA antibodies were detected in their stools. In terms of safety, there were few symptoms other than nausea and cramps. More importantly, none of the volunteers had a change in serum anti-potatin (the major protein contained in potatoes) IgG antibodies after ingesting the transgenic potato vaccine (Tacket et al. 2000).

EDIBLE VACCINES EXPRESSING BACTERIAL ANTIGENS

The feasibility of using transgenic plant expression systems for vaccine use has also been documented with bacterial antigens. Mason et al. (1998) have designed and constructed a plant-optimized synthetic gene encoding the *Escherichia coli* heat-labile enterotoxin B subunit (LTB). Expression of LTB gene in potatoes increased antigen expression in leaves and tubers, and LTB molecules were assembled into native pentameric structures that were able to bind to their ganglioside receptors. When mice were fed with raw tuber slices they developed serum and fecal IgA anti-LTB antibodies, and were partially protected against challenge to orally delivered LT (Mason et al. 1998). This edible vaccine was also tested in human volunteers who received 50–100 g raw transgenic potato. Most of the participants (10 of 11 tested) developed serum anti-LTB antibodies (Tacket et al. 1998). Also transgenic potatoes engineered to synthesize CTB pentamers with affinity to G_{M1} gangliosides were immunogenic (inducing serum and intestinal CTB-specific antibodies) when fed to mice (Arakawa et al. 1998a). The serum samples neutralized the activity of CT on Vero cells and the immunized mice were partially protected (60 percent reduction in diarrheal fluid accumulation in the small intestine).

A plant-based multicomponent vaccine has been demonstrated to protect mice from enteric disease (Yu and Langridge 2001). This edible vaccine consisted of two CT fusion genes, one expressing a 22-amino acid immunodominant epitope of the murine rotavirus enterotoxin NSP4 to the CTB subunit (C-terminal fusion) and the other expressing the *E. coli* fimbrial colonization factor CFA/I to the CTA2 subunit (N-terminal fusion). When mice were fed with transgenic potato tuber tissues expressing the CT fusion proteins, antibody responses (serum IgG and intestinal IgG and IgA) against the NSP4, CTB, and CFA/I were detected. Cultured splenocytes from immune mice secreted IL-2 and IFN-γ, and diarrheal symptoms were reduced in severity and duration in passively immunized neonatal mice following rotavirus challenge.

FUTURE PROSPECTS AND CHALLENGES FOR THE DEVELOPMENT OF EDIBLE VACCINES

For almost a decade, research on the development of edible vaccines has focused on viral and bacterial antigens. These studies helped to establish the proof of the concept and the identification of appropriate methods for enhancing protein expression, as well as providing answers to fundamental questions such as the selection of an appropriate crop, the quantity of plant tissue constituting a vaccine dose, and the importance of structural integrity of expressed antigen. Moreover, human clinical trials have demonstrated that edible vaccines are safe and can induce systemic and mucosal immune responses without the aid of an adjuvant. Despite all these positive aspects, the immune responses elicited in this way are still modest and this remains one of the limiting factors for the development of an effective edible vaccine for human use. Furthermore, there is always the risk that induction of immunity after oral immunization may lead to inflammatory or allergic reactions as a result of the breakdown of the physiological tolerance toward food antigens.

By improving our understanding of the basic mechanisms involved in induction of immunity or tolerance, it should be possible to manipulate the GALT. This will allow the preferential stimulation of protective systemic and mucosal immune responses against infectious pathogens or antigen-specific tolerance, which could be advantageous for treating autoimmune diseases or allergic disorders (Arakawa et al. 1998b). Furthermore, the determination of the molecular requirements for directing mucosally primed immunocompetent cells from the inductive sites to the effector sites will help in the design of more effective mucosal vaccines.

Nasal vaccines

Vaccines that can be administered via the nose appear to hold more promise than oral vaccines, because intranasal immunization generally requires a much lower dose of antigen, and elicits more potent immune responses (Table 40.2). There are several advantages to using the nose as a route of immunization and an intense search to develop safe and immunogenic nasal vaccines is currently under way:

- It is easily accessible.
- It is highly vascularized.
- The presence of numerous microvilli covering the nasal epithelium generates a large absorption surface.
- After intranasal immunization both systemic and mucosal immune responses are induced.
- Immune responses can be induced at distant mucosal sites.
- Its a noninvasive route and therefore it does not require needles and syringes.

After intranasal immunization, the balance between active immunity and tolerance would depend greatly on the nature of the antigen and its interaction with the NALT, as well as on the dose, adjuvant, frequency of antigen administration, and genetic background of the host (Kuper et al. 1992). Particulate antigens can be either removed by the mucociliary clearance system or sampled by M cells (which overlay the NALT); they are then transported to the posterior cervical lymph nodes (Kuper et al. 1992). In the case of soluble antigens, these molecules can penetrate the mucosal epithelium and reach the superficial cervical lymph nodes (Kuper et al. 1992). High doses of antigen administered intranasally are likely to reach the intestinal tract (Willoughby and Willoughby 1977) or be taken up directly by the posterior cervical lymph nodes instead of the superficial ones (Kuper et al. 1992). The superficial cervical lymph nodes, which drain the nasal mucosa, appear to be instrumental in the induction of mucosal tolerance (Kuper et al. 1992). Posterior cervical lymph nodes are involved in the generation of sIgA responses (Kuper et al. 1992). This suggests that the lymphocyte composition differs in different lymph nodes as a result of their 'homing' behavior, which underlies the observed divergence in the induction of either tolerance or immunity.

Table 40.2 *Differences between oral and nasal routes of immunization*

	Oral route	Nasal route
Proteolytic activity	High	Moderate
Distance to transport	Long	Small
Dose of antigen	High	Medium
Requirement of adjuvant	Yes	Yes
Antigen uptake	Poor	Good
Targeting requirement	Yes	Not necessary
Humoral responses	Low	High
Cellular responses	Low	High

VACCINE DELIVERY VIA THE NOSE

For the development of safer and better vaccines, much effort has been devoted to defining and producing protective antigens or epitopes from the pathogen of concern. When these antigens are given intranasally, they are weakly immunogenic or induce tolerance. To circumvent these problems, delivery systems and mucosal adjuvants have been developed:

- Use of replicating vectors expressing the antigen (live attenuated viruses or bacteria).
- Use of nonreplicating vectors (liposomes, microparticles, immune-stimulating complexes (ISCOM)).
- Use of recombinant plant viruses expressing antigens (cowpea mosaic virus).
- Use of cold-adapted influenza virus (FluMist vaccine).
- Antigen co-administered with an adjuvant (CT, LT, CpG, cytokines, etc.).
- Antigen adsorbed on bioadhesive polymers (chitosan, microparticles, etc.).

Vectors for delivering antigens via the nose

Replicating delivery systems present the antigen (protein or epitopes) in the context of a genetically modified live attenuated bacterium or virus, which provides a continuous antigenic stimulation and elicits broad humoral or cellular immune responses. It is important that these vectors express adequate amounts of antigen, have a tropism for the mucosal epithelium, and do not revert to the virulent form. As vectored vaccines are live, they are likely to share the same antigen-processing and presentation pathway as the pathogen, and therefore elicit the desired type of immune responses. Among the recombinant vectors that have been widely tested are: *Mycobacterium bovis* (Langermann et al. 1994), *Vibrio cholerae* (Chen et al. 1998), *E. coli* (Turner et al. 2001), *Shigella flexneri* (Anderson et al. 2000), *Salmonella typhi* (Galen et al. 1997), vaccinia virus (Bernstein 2000), adenovirus

(Gallichan and Rosenthal 1996), and poliovirus (Crotty et al. 1999). However, for live attenuated microorganisms, the induction of immunity to the organism used as a carrier could preclude their use for booster immunizations, and reversion to virulence may be a potential problem. As an alternative, plant viruses, which are not infectious to mammals, have been tested with antigenic peptides (Dalsgaard et al. 1997; Durrani et al. 1998; Olszewska and Steward 2001), and commensal lactobacilli (*Lactobacillus plantarum*) have begun to receive attention as safe noninvasive vectors (Shaw et al. 2000).

The intranasal delivery of vaccines using nonreplicating vectors has the advantage that it eliminates one of the major concerns, that of reversion to virulence. For successful intranasal immunization, the nonreplicating vector should: (1) protect the antigen from degradation; (2) allow its transport via the M cells; and (3) promote the appropriate type of immune responses required for protection. Among the various nonreplicating vector systems, particles such as liposomes (Mader et al. 2000), virosomes (Cusi et al. 2000), ISCOMs (Hu et al. 2001), biodegradable microparticles (Vajdy and O'Hagan 2001), biovector systems (Von Hoegen 2001), and proteosomes (Levi et al. 1995) have been extensively studied. The availability of so many different formulations allows the selection of the most appropriate to address the clinical needs, the nature of the antigen, and the type of desired immune responses. However, for some of these vectors there are certain limitations for human use, e.g. toxicity is a major drawback of using ISCOMs as a vaccine delivery system. This is because of the presence of saponins that have strong hemolytic and cytolytic activity even at low doses. For biodegradable microparticles, there are several concerns about the stability of the entrapped antigen during storage, the efficacy of microparticle uptake by the mucosal epithelium, and problems in the production of sterile preparations for human use.

An alternate approach to encapsulation is to adsorb antigens on to the surface of biodegradable polymeric lamellar substrate particles (PLSP). This is a simple procedure that avoids pH changes caused by bulk polymer degradation and the use of solvents and, therefore, should be less damaging to the vaccine. Several antigens such as proteins, peptides, and viral particles have been adsorbed on to PLSPs and tested for immunogenicity after nasal administration (Jabbal-Gill et al. 2001), e.g. adsorbed influenza vaccine induced strong secretory and systemic antibody responses (Jabbal-Gill et al. 2000). Carbohydrate biopolymers have also been tested for their ability to enhance the immunogenicity of adsorbed antigens. In particular, chitosan, which is a cationic polysaccharide and binds strongly to negatively charged cell surfaces and mucus, greatly improves the absorption of antigens from the nasal cavity and augments antigen-specific immune responses (Bacon et al. 2000; Illum et al. 2001).

Adjuvants for intranasal immunization

Administration of antigens via the nose has the potential to induce a wide range of immune responses; the types of response induced in this way can be significantly influenced by the use of adjuvants. In experimental animal models, the most potent mucosal adjuvants are CT and LT. Both are strong mucosal immunogens in their own right and can act as effective adjuvants to intranasally co-administered antigens by enhancing serum and secretory antibody responses and cytotoxic T-cell responses (Imaoka et al. 1988; Rappuoli et al. 1999; Kurono et al. 1999; Partidos et al. 1999). As their enzymatic activity precludes their use in humans, much effort has been devoted to attempting to dissociate their adjuvant properties from their toxicity. Using site-directed mutagenesis, several mutants have been generated with significantly reduced ADP-ribosylating activity and toxicity compared with the holotoxin (Rappuoli et al. 1999; Pizza et al. 2001). These molecules have been shown to exert adjuvant activity to co-administered antigens by increasing serum and secretory antibody responses (Pizza et al. 2001), modulating immune responses as a consequence of their ADP-ribosylating activity (Ryan et al. 2000), and potentiating CTL responses (Partidos et al. 1996). However, there are several concerns about the role of G_{M1}-binding molecules that target neuronal tissues in mucosal immunity. Intranasal delivery of CT targets the main olfactory nerves and epithelium, which is directly connected with the olfactory bulbs, and raises the possibility of the induction of neuronal damage (Van Ginkel et al. 2000). Furthermore, it has been suggested that the use of CT as intranasal adjuvant results in the redirection of vaccine proteins into the CNS (Van Ginkel et al. 2000). However, recent studies in mice have shown that LT mutants are safe and that they do not induce any detectable inflammatory response in any anatomical site (Peppoloni et al. 2003).

Bacterial DNA has potent immunostimulatory properties caused by the presence of unmethylated CpG motifs, which are far more common in bacterial than in vertebrate DNA (Krieg 2002). A similar immunostimulatory effect can be seen with synthetic ODNs containing CpG motifs (ODN-CpG) (Roman et al. 1997). In studies where vaccine antigens were co-delivered with an ODN-CpG via the mucosal routes, strong systemic and mucosal immune responses were detected (McCluskie et al. 2001a). Furthermore, in some instances protective immune responses were enhanced, as demonstrated in mice immunized intranasally with an ODN-CpG and a recombinant glycoprotein of HSV1 (Gallichan et al. 2001) or with an influenza virus peptide representing a mimic of the antigenic site A of hemagglutinin (Partidos et al. 2001). CpG motifs can also modulate the adjuvant effect of CT or mutants of LT when they are co-administered with recombinant proteins or peptides, promoting a Th1-type immune responses (Olszewska et al. 2000; McCluskie et al. 2001b). Therefore, CpG-ODNs are novel mucosal adjuvants, which either alone or in combination with other adjuvants can modulate and enhance humoral and cellular immunity.

An alternate approach to the potentiation of immune responses to intranasally administered antigens is to use cytokines as adjuvants. The cytokine microenvironment at the site of antigen delivery plays a critical role in the induction and regulation of immune responses. Boyaka et al. (1999) and Boyaka and McGhee (2001) have demonstrated that intranasally delivered IL-6 and IL-12 can enhance antigen-specific serum antibody responses to co-administered protein antigen, but only IL-12 is able to trigger antigen-specific secretory IgA responses. Also it has been reported that IL-1α and IL-1β exhibit mucosal adjuvant activity for the induction of serum IgG and mucosal IgA antibody responses when they are nasally co-administered with soluble protein antigens (Staats and Ennis 1999). In addition, it was found that the combination of IL-1α + IL-18, IL-1α + IL-12, and IL-1α + IL-12 + GM-CSF each induced optimal splenocyte anti-HIV CTL responses in mice immunized intranasally (Staats et al. 2001). Despite the mucosal adjuvanticity of certain cytokines it should be noted that they are pleotropic molecules and, therefore, they have complex effects that depend on the state of activation of different immunocompetent cells and the balance of other cytokines.

CONCLUDING REMARKS

This is an exciting time in the field of vaccinology. Thanks to the technological advances in biomedical sciences we now have a wide range of new immunization strategies and vaccine delivery options. More importantly, the widespread administration of vaccines without the use of needles is now a distinct possibility and this is a significant advantage for immunization programs in less developed countries, because such administration would be simple, painless, and economical.

An intranasal vaccine against influenza virus (NasalFlu, containing inactivated virus and LT as an adjuvant) has already been approved in Switzerland. In addition, another influenza vaccine – the FluMist, a live cold-adapted virus – has been developed for delivery in the form of a spray and is close to being licensed for human use. It is certain that more 'needle-free' vaccines will follow.

REFERENCES

Anderson, R.J., Pasetti, M.F., et al. 2000. Attenuated *Shigella flexneri* 2a strain CVD 1204 as a *Shigella* vaccine and as a live mucosal delivery system for fragment C of tetanus toxin. *Vaccine*, **18**, 2193–202.

Andre, F.E. 2001. The future of vaccines, immunisation concepts and practice. *Vaccine*, **19**, 2206–9.

Arakawa, T., Chong, D.K. and Langridge, W.H. 1998a. Efficacy of a food plant-based oral cholera toxin B subunit vaccine. *Nat Biotechnol*, **16**, 292–7.

Arakawa, T., Yu, J., et al. 1998b. A plant-based cholera toxin B subunit-insulin fusion protein protects against the development of autoimmune diabetes. *Nat Biotechnol*, **16**, 934–8.

Baba, T.W., Liska, V., et al. 2000. Human neutralizing monoclonal antibodies of the IgG1 subtype protect against mucosal simian-human immunodeficiency virus infection. *Nat Med*, **6**, 200–6.

Babiuk, S., Baca-Estrada, M., et al. 2000. Cutaneous vaccination: the skin as an immunologically active tissue and the challenge of antigen delivery. *J Control Release*, **66**, 199–214.

Baca-Estrada, M.E., Foldvari, M., et al. 2000a. Effects of IL-12 on immune responses induced by transcutaneous immunization with antigens formulated in a novel lipid-based biphasic delivery system. *Vaccine*, **18**, 1847–54.

Baca-Estrada, M.E., Foldvari, M., et al. 2000b. Vaccine delivery: lipid-based delivery systems. *J Biotechnol*, **83**, 91–104.

Bacon, A., Makin, J., et al. 2000. Carbohydrate biopolymers enhance antibody responses to mucosally delivered vaccine antigens. *Infect Immun*, **68**, 5764–70.

Ban, E., Dupre, L., et al. 2000. CpG motifs induce Langerhans cell migration in vivo. *Int Immunol*, **12**, 737–45.

Barry, B.W. 2001. Novel mechanisms and devices to enable successful transdermal drug delivery. *Eur J Pharm Sci*, **14**, 101–14.

Beignon, A.-S., Briand, J.-P., et al. 2001. Immunization onto bare skin with heat-labile enterotoxin of *Escherichia coli* enhances immune responses to coadministered protein and peptide antigens and protects mice against lethal toxin challenge. *Immunology*, **102**, 344–51.

Beignon, A.-S., Briand, J.-P., et al. 2002a. Immunization onto bare skin with synthetic peptides: immunomodulation with a CpG-containing oligodeoxynucleotide and effective priming of influenza virus-specific CD4+ T cells. *Immunology*, **105**, 204–12.

Beignon, A.-S., Briand, J.-P., et al. 2002b. The LTR72 mutant of heat-labile enterotoxin of *Escherichia coli* enhances the ability of peptide antigens to elicit $CD4^+$ T cells and secrete IFN-γ after co-application onto bare skin. *Infect Immun*, **70**, 3012–19.

Bernstein, D.I. 2000. Effect of route of vaccination with vaccinia virus expressing HSV-2 glycoprotein D on protection from genital HSV-2 infection. *Vaccine*, **18**, 1351–8.

Bond, J. and Barry, B. 1988. Hairless mouse skin is limited as a model for assessing the effects of penetration enhancers in human skin. *J Invest Dermatol*, **90**, 810–13.

Bos, J.D. and Kapsenberg, M.L. 1993. The skin immune system: progress in cutaneous biology. *Immunol Today*, **14**, 75–8.

Bos, J.D. and Meinardi, M.M.H.M. 2000. The 500 Dalton rule for the skin penetration of chemical compounds and drugs. *Exp Dermatol*, **9**, 165–9.

Boyaka, P.N., Marinaro, M., et al. 1999. IL-12 is an effective adjuvant for induction of mucosal immunity. *J Immunol*, **162**, 122–8.

Boyaka, P.N. and McGhee, J.R. 2001. Cytokines as adjuvants for the induction of mucosal immunity. *Adv Drug Deliv Rev*, **51**, 71–9.

Castelain, M. 1995. Atopic dermatitis and delayed hypersensitivity to dust mites. *Clin Rev Allergy Immunol*, **13**, 161–72.

Cevc, G., Gebauer, D., et al. 1998. Ultraflexible vesicles, transfersomes, have an extremely low pore penetration resistance and transport therapeutic amounts of insulin across the intact mammalian skin. *Biochim Biophys Acta*, **1368**, 201–15.

Chen, I., Finn, T.M., et al. 1998. A recombinant live attenuated strain of *Vibrio cholerae* induces immunity against tetanus toxin and *Bordetella pertussis* tracheal colonization factor. *Infect Immun*, **66**, 1648–53.

Chen, D., Endres, R.L., et al. 2000. Epidermal immunization by a needle-free powder delivery technology: immunogenicity of influenza vaccine and protection in mice. *Nat Med*, **6**, 1187–90.

Chen, D., Erickson, C.A., et al. 2001a. Adjuvantation of epidermal powder immunization. *Vaccine*, **19**, 2908–17.

Chen, D., Periwal, S.B., et al. 2001b. Serum and mucosal immune responses to an inactivated influenza virus vaccine induced by epidermal powder immunization. *J Virol*, **75**, 7956–65.

Chen, D., Weis, K.F., et al. 2001c. Epidermal powder immunization induces both cytotoxic T-lymphocyte and antibody responses to protein antigens of influenza and hepatitis B viruses. *J Virol*, **75**, 11630–40.

Christoph, T., Muller-Rover, S., et al. 2000. The human hair follicle immune system: cellular composition and immune privilege. *Br J Dermatol*, **142**, 862–73.

Clements, C.J., Evans, G., et al. 1999. Vaccine safety concerns everyone. *Vaccine*, **17**, S90–4.

Cohen, L.L., Blount, R.L., et al. 2001. Children's expectations and memories of acute distress: short- and long-term efficacy of pain management interventions. *J Pediatr Psychol*, **26**, 367–74.

Crotty, S., Lohman, B.L., et al. 1999. Mucosal immunization of cynomolgus macaques with two serotypes of live poliovirus vectors expressing simian immunodeficiency virus antigens: stimulation of humoral, mucosal, and cellular immunity. *J Virol*, **73**, 9485–95.

Cui, Z. and Mumper, R.J. 2001. Chitosan-based nanoparticles for topical genetic immunization. *J Control Release*, **75**, 409–19.

Cusi, M.G., Zurbriggen, R., et al. 2000. Intranasal immunization with mumps virus DNA vaccine delivered by influenza virosomes elicits mucosal and systemic immunity. *Virology*, **277**, 111–18.

Dalsgaard, K., Uttenthal, A., et al. 1997. Plant-derived vaccine protects target animals against a viral disease. *Nat Biotechnol*, **15**, 248–52.

De Panfilis, G. 1998. $CD8^+$ cytolytic T lymphocytes and the skin. *Exp Dermatol*, **7**, 121–31.

Debenedictis, C., Joubeh, S., et al. 2001. Immune functions of the skin. *Clin Dermatol*, **19**, 573–85.

Dick, I. and Scott, R. 1992. Pig ear skin as an in vitro model for human skin permeability. *J Pharm Pharmacol*, **44**, 641–55.

Dujardin, N., Staes, E., et al. 2002. In vivo assessment of skin electroporation using square wave pulses. *J Control Release*, **79**, 219–27.

Durrani, Z., McInerney, T.L., et al. 1998. Intranasal immunization with a plant virus expressing a peptide from HIV-1 gp41 stimulates better mucosal and systemic HIV-1-specific IgA and IgG than oral immunization. *J Immunol Meth*, **220**, 93–103.

El-Ghorr, A.A., Williams, R.M., et al. 2000. Transcutaneous immunisation with herpes simplex virus stimulates immunity in mice. *FEMS Immunol Med Microbiol*, **29**, 255–61.

Enioutina, E.Y., Visic, D. and Daynes, R.A. 2000. The induction of systemic and mucosal immune responses to antigen-adjuvant compositions administered into the skin: alterations in the migratory properties of dendritic cells appears to be important for stimulating mucosal immunity. *Vaccine*, **18**, 2753–67.

Faldvari, M. 2000. Non-invasive administration of drugs through the skin: challenges in delivery system design. *PSTT*, **3**, 417–25.

Fan, H., Lin, Q., et al. 1999. Immunization via hair follicles by topical application of naked DNA to normal skin. *Nat Biotechnol*, **17**, 870–2.

Frey, A. and Neutra, M.R. 1997. Targeting of mucosal vaccines to Peyer's patch M cells. *Behring Inst Mitt*, **98**, 376–89.

Fuchs, E. 1990. Epidermal differentiation: the bare essentials. *J Cell Biol*, **111**, 2807–14.

Galen, J.E., Gomez-Duarte, O.G., et al. 1997. A murine model of intranasal immunization to assess the immunogenicity of attenuated *Salmonella typhi* live vector vaccines in stimulating serum antibody responses to expressed foreign antigens. *Vaccine*, **15**, 700–8.

Gallichan, W.S. and Rosenthal, K.L. 1996. Long-lived cytotoxic T lymphocyte memory in mucosal tissues after mucosal but not systemic immunization. *J Exp Med*, **184**, 1879–90.

Gallichan, W.S., Woolstencroft, R.N. and Guarasci, T. 2001. Intranasal immunization with CpG oligodeoxynucleotides as an adjuvant dramatically increases IgA and protection against herpes simplex virus-2 in the genital tract. *J Immunol*, **166**, 3451–7.

Glenn, G.M., Rao, M., et al. 1998a. Skin immunization made possible by cholera toxin. *Nature*, **391**, 851.

Glenn, G.M., Scharton-Kersten, T., et al. 1998b. Transcutaneous immunization with cholera toxin protects mice against lethal mucosal toxin challenge. *J Immunol*, **161**, 3211–14.

Glenn, G.M., Scharton-Kersten, T., et al. 1999. Transcutaneous immunization with bacterial ADP-ribosylating exotoxins as antigens and adjuvants. *Infect Immun*, **67**, 1100–6.

Glenn, G.M., Taylor, D.N., et al. 2000. Transcutaneous immunization: a human vaccine delivery strategy using a patch. *Nat Med*, **6**, 1403–6.

Gockel, C.M., Bao, S. and Beagley, K.W. 2000. Transcutaneous immunization induces mucosal and systemic immunity: a potent method for targeting immunity to the female reproductive tract. *Mol Immunol*, **37**, 537–44.

Guerena-Burgueno, F., Hall, E.R., et al. 2002. Safety and immunogenicity of a prototype enterotoxigenic *Escherichia coli* vaccine administered transcutaneously. *Infect Immun*, **70**, 1874–80.

Hammond, S.A., Tsonis, C., et al. 2000. Transcutaneous immunization of domestic animals: opportunities and challenges. *Adv Drug Deliv Rev*, **43**, 45–55.

Hammond, S.A., Walwender, D., et al. 2001a. Transcutaneous immunization: T cell responses and boosting of existing immunity. *Vaccine*, **19**, 2701–7.

Hammond, S.A., Guebre-Xabier, M., et al. 2001b. Transcutaneous immunization: an emerging route of immunization and potent immunostimulation strategy. *Crit Rev Ther Drug Carrier Syst*, **18**, 503–26.

Hartmann, G., Weiner, G.J. and Krieg, A.M. 1999. CpG DNA: a potent signal for growth, activation, and maturation of human dendritic cells. *Proc Natl Acad Sci USA*, **96**, 9305–10.

Hoffman, P.N., Abuknesha, R.A., et al. 2001. A model to assess the infection potential of jet injectors used in mass immunisation. *Vaccine*, **19**, 4020–7.

Hu, K.F., Lovgren-Bengtsson, K. and Morein, B. 2001. Immunostimulating complexes (ISCOMs) for nasal vaccination. *Adv Drug Deliv Rev*, **51**, 149–59.

Illum, L., Jabbal-Gill, I., et al. 2001. Chitosan as a novel nasal delivery system for vaccines. *Adv Drug Deliv Rev*, **51**, 81–96.

Imaoka, K., Miller, C.J., et al. 1988. Nasal immunization of nonhuman primates with simian immunodeficiency virus p55gag and cholera toxin adjuvant induces Th1/Th2 help for virus-specific immune responses in reproductive tissues. *J Immunol*, **161**, 5952–8.

Jabbal-Gill, I., Lin, W., et al. 2000. Potential of polymeric lamellar substrate particles (PLSP) as adjuvants for vaccines. *Vaccine*, **18**, 238–50.

Jabbal-Gill, I., Lin, W., et al. 2001. Polymeric lamellar substrate particles for intranasal vaccination. *Adv Drug Deliv Rev*, **51**, 97–111.

Jacobson, R.M., Swan, A., et al. 2001. Making vaccines more acceptable: methods to prevent and minimize pain and other common adverse events associated with vaccines. *Vaccine*, **19**, 2418–27.

Jackson, L.A., Austin, G., et al. 2001. Safety and immunogenicity of varying dosages of trivalent inactivated influenza vaccine administered by needle-free jet injectors. *Vaccine*, **19**, 4703–9.

Jodar, L., Duclos, P., et al. 2001. Ensuring vaccine safety in immunization programmes – a WHO perspective. *Vaccine*, **19**, 1594–605.

Kane, A., Lloyd, J., et al. 1999. Transmission of hepatitis B, hepatitis C and human immunodeficiency viruses through unsafe injections in the developing world: model-based regional estimates. *Bull World Health Organ*, **77**, 801–7.

Katoh, N., Hirano, S., et al. 1997. Acute cutaneous barrier perturbation induces maturation of Langerhans' cells in hairless mice. *Acta Derm Venereol*, **77**, 365–9.

Khalife, J., Cetre, C., et al. 2000. Mechanisms of resistance to *S. mansoni* infection: the rat model. *Parasitol Int*, **49**, 339–45.

Kong, X.F., Zhu, X.H., et al. 1999. Molecular cloning, characterization, and promoter analysis of the human 25-hydroxyvitamin D3-1alpha-hydroxylase gene. *Proc Natl Acad Sci USA*, **96**, 6988–93.

Kong, Q., Richter, L., et al. 2001. Oral immunization with hepatitis B surface antigen expressed in transgenic plants. *Proc Natl Acad Sci USA*, **98**, 11539–44.

Krieg, A.M. 2002. CpG motifs in bacterial DNA and their immune effects. *Annu Rev Immunol*, **20**, 709–60.

Kuper, C.F., Koornstra, P.J., et al. 1992. The role of nasopharyngeal lymphoid tissue. *Immunol Today*, **13**, 219–24.

Kurono, Y., Yamamoto, M., et al. 1999. Nasal immunization induces *Haemophilus influenzae*-specific Th1 and Th2 responses with mucosal IgA and systemic IgG antibodies for protective immunity. *J Infect Dis*, **180**, 122–32.

Kusnadi, A., Nikolov, Z.L. and Howard, J.A. 1997. Production of recombinant proteins in transgenic plants: practical considerations. *Biotechnol Bioeng*, **56**, 473–84.

Langermann, S., Palaszynski, S., et al. 1994. Systemic and mucosal immunity induced by BCG vector expressing outer-surface protein A of *Borrelia burgdorferi*. *Nature*, **372**, 552–5.

Lappin, M.B., Kimber, I. and Norval, M. 1996. The role of dendritic cells in cutaneous immunity. *Arch Dermatol Res*, **288**, 109–21.

Levi, R., Aboud-Pirak, E., et al. 1995. Intranasal immunization of mice against influenza with synthetic peptides anchored to proteosomes. *Vaccine*, **13**, 1353–9.

McCluskie, M.J., Weeratna, R.D., et al. 2001a. The potential of CpG oligodeoxynucleotides as mucosal adjuvants. *Crit Rev Immunol*, **21**, 103–20.

McCluskie, M.J., Weeratna, R.D., et al. 2001b. Mucosal immunization of mice using CpG DNA and/or mutants of the heat-labile enterotoxin of *Escherichia coli* as adjuvants. *Vaccine*, **19**, 3759–68.

McDermott, M.R. and Bienenstock, J. 1979. Evidence for a common mucosal immunologic system. I. Migration of B immunoblasts into intestinal, respiratory, and genital tissues. *J Immunol*, **122**, 1892–8.

McGhee, J.R., Mestecky, J., et al. 1992. The mucosal immune system: from fundamental concepts to vaccine development. *Vaccine*, **10**, 75–88.

McWilliam, A.S., Nelson, D., et al. 1994. Rapid dendritic cell recruitment is a hallmark of the acute inflammatory response at mucosal surfaces. *J Exp Med*, **179**, 1331–6.

Mader, D., Huang, Y., et al. 2000. Liposome encapsulation of a soluble recombinant fragment of the respiratory syncytial virus (RSV) G protein enhances immune protection and reduces lung eosinophilia associated with virus challenge. *Vaccine*, **18**, 1110–17.

Mark, A., Bjorksten, B. and Granstrom, M. 1995. Immunoglobulin E responses to diphtheria and tetanus toxoids after booster with aluminium-adsorbed and fluid DT-vaccines. *Vaccine*, **13**, 669–73.

Mason, H.S., Lam, D.M. and Arntzen, C.J. 1992. Expression of hepatitis B surface antigen in transgenic plants. *Proc Natl Acad Sci USA*, **89**, 11745–9.

Mason, H.S., Ball, J.M., et al. 1996. Expression of Norwalk virus capsid protein in transgenic tobacco and potato and its oral immunogenicity in mice. *Proc Natl Acad Sci USA*, **93**, 5335–40.

Mason, H.S., Haq, T.A., et al. 1998. Edible vaccine protects mice against *Escherichia coli* heat-labile enterotoxin (LT): potatoes expressing a synthetic LT-B gene. *Vaccine*, **16**, 1336–43.

Miller, M.A. and Pisani, E. 1999. The cost of unsafe injections. *Bull World Health Organ*, **77**, 808–11.

Misra, A., Ganga, S. and Upadhyay, P. 1999. Needle-free, non-adjuvanted skin immunization by electroporation-enhanced transdermal delivery of diphtheria toxoid and a candidate peptide vaccine against hepatitis B virus. *Vaccine*, **18**, 517–23.

Morganti, P., Ruocco, E., et al. 2001. Percutaneous absorption and delivery systems. *Clin Dermatol*, **19**, 489–501.

Mosmann, T.R. and Coffman, R.L. 1989. TH1 and TH2 cells: different patterns of lymphokine secretion lead to different functional properties. *Annu Rev Immunol*, **7**, 145–73.

Naik, A., Kalia, Y.N. and Guy, R.H. 2000. Transdermal drug delivery: overcoming the skin's barrier function. *PSTT*, **3**, 318–26.

Neutra, M.R. 1999. M cells in antigen sampling in mucosal tissues. *Curr Top Microbiol Immunol*, **236**, 17–32.

Neutra, M.R., Pringault, E. and Kraehenbuhl, J.P. 1996. Antigen sampling across epithelial barriers and induction of mucosal immune responses. *Annu Rev Immunol*, **14**, 275–300.

Nickoloff, B.J., Mitra, R.S., et al. 1993. Accessory cell function of keratinocytes for superantigens. Dependence on lymphocyte function-associated antigen-1/intercellular adhesion molecule-1 interaction. *J Immunol*, **150**, 2148–59.

Olszewska, W. and Steward, M.W. 2001. Nasal delivery of epitope-based vaccines. *Adv Drug Deliv Rev*, **51**, 161–71.

Olszewska, W., Partidos, C.D. and Steward, M.W. 2000. Antipeptide antibody responses following intranasal immunization: effectiveness of mucosal adjuvants. *Infect Immun*, **68**, 4923–9.

Partidos, C.D., Pizza, M., et al. 1996. The adjuvant effect of a non-toxic mutant of heat-labile enterotoxin of *Escherichia coli* for the induction of measles virus-specific CTL responses after intranasal co-immunization with a synthetic peptide. *Immunology*, **89**, 483–7.

Partidos, C.D., Salani, B.F., et al. 1999. Heat-labile enterotoxin of *Escherichia coli* and its site-directed mutant LTK63 enhance the proliferative and cytotoxic T-cell responses to intranasally co-immunized synthetic peptides. *Immunol Lett*, **67**, 209–16.

Partidos, C.D., Beignon, A.-S., et al. 2001. The bare skin and the nose as non-invasive routes for administering peptide vaccines. *Vaccine*, **19**, 2708–15.

Paul, A., Cevc, G. and Bachhawat, B.K. 1998. Transdermal immunisation with an integral membrane component, gap junction protein, by means of ultradeformable drug carriers, transferosomes. *Vaccine*, **16**, 188–95.

Peppoloni, S., Ruggiero, P., et al. 2003. Mutants of the *Escherichia coli* heat-labile enterotoxin as safe and strong adjuvants for intranasal delivery of vaccines. *Expert Rev Vaccines*, **2**, 285–93.

Pfutzner, W. and Vogel, J.C. 2000. Advances in skin gene therapy. *Expert Opin Invest Drugs*, **9**, 2069–83.

Pizza, M., Giuliani, M.M., et al. 2001. Mucosal vaccines: non toxic derivatives of LT and CT as mucosal adjuvants. *Vaccine*, **19**, 2534–41.

Prausnitz, M.R. 1997. Reversible skin permeabilization for transdermal delivery of macromolecules. *Crit Rev Ther Drug Carrier Syst*, **14**, 455–83.

Quiding-Jarbrink, M., Lakew, M., et al. 1995. Human circulating specific antibody-forming cells after systemic and mucosal immunizations: differential homing commitments and cell surface differentiation markers. *Eur J Immunol*, **25**, 322–7.

Rappuoli, R., Pizza, M., et al. 1999. Structure and mucosal adjuvanticity of cholera and *Escherichia coli* heat-labile enterotoxins. *Immunol Today*, **20**, 493–500.

Richter, L.J., Thanavala, Y., et al. 2000. Production of hepatitis B surface antigen in transgenic plants for oral immunization. *Nat Biotechnol*, **18**, 1167–71.

Roman, M., Martin-Orozco, E., et al. 1997. Immunostimulatory DNA sequences function as T helper-1-promoting adjuvants. *Nat Med*, **3**, 849–54.

Ryan, E.J., McNeela, E., et al. 2000. Modulation of innate and acquired immune responses by *Escherichia coli* heat-labile toxin: distinct pro- and anti-inflammatory effects of the nontoxic AB complex and the enzyme activity. *J Immunol*, **165**, 5750–9.

Sakaguchi, M. and Inouye, S. 2000. IgE sensitization to gelatin: the probable role of gelatin-containing diphtheria-tetanus-acellular pertussis (DTaP) vaccines. *Vaccine*, **18**, 2055–8.

Scharton-Kersten, T., Glenn, G.M., et al. 1999. Principles of transcutaneous immunization using cholera toxin as an adjuvant. *Vaccine*, **17**, S37–43.

Scharton-Kersten, T., Yu, J., et al. 2000. Transcutaneous immunization with bacterial ADP-ribosylating exotoxins, subunits, and unrelated adjuvants. *Infect Immun*, **68**, 5306–13.

Seo, N., Tokura, Y., et al. 2000. Percutaneous peptide immunization via corneum barrier-disrupted murine skin for experimental tumor immunoprophylaxis. *Proc Natl Acad Sci USA*, **97**, 371–6.

Shaw, D.M., Gaerthe, B., et al. 2000. Engineering the microflora to vaccinate the mucosa: serum immunoglobulin G responses and activated draining cervical lymph nodes following mucosal application of tetanus toxin fragment C-expressing lactobacilli. *Immunology*, **100**, 510–18.

Shi, Z., Curiel, D.T. and Tang, D.C. 1999. DNA-based non-invasive vaccination onto the skin. *Vaccine*, **17**, 2136–41.

Siebers, A. and Finlay, B.B. 1996. M cells and the pathogenesis of mucosal and systemic infections. *Trends Microbiol*, **4**, 22–9.

Simonsen, L., Kane, A., et al. 1999. Unsafe injections in the developing world and transmission of blood-borne pathogens: a review. *Bull World Health Organ*, **77**, 789–800.

Spangler, B.D. 1992. Structure and function of cholera toxin and the related *Escherichia coli* heat-labile enterotoxin. *Microb Rev*, **56**, 622–47.

Staats, H.F. and Ennis, F.A. Jr. 1999. IL-1 is an effective adjuvant for mucosal and systemic immune responses when coadministered with protein immunogens. *J Immunol*, **162**, 6141–7.

Staats, H.F., Bradney, C.P., et al. 2001. Cytokine requirements for induction of systemic and mucosal CTL after nasal immunization. *J Immunol*, **167**, 5386–94.

Streilein, J.W. 1983. Skin-associated lymphoid tissues (SALT): origins and functions. *J Invest Dermatol*, **80**, S12–16.

Tacket, C.O., Mason, H.S., et al. 1998. Immunogenicity in humans of a recombinant bacterial antigen delivered in a transgenic potato. *Nat Med*, **4**, 607–9.

Tacket, C.O., Mason, H.S., et al. 2000. Human immune responses to a novel Norwalk virus vaccine delivered in transgenic potatoes. *J Infect Dis*, **182**, 302–5.

Turner, A.K., Terry, T.D., et al. 2001. Construction and characterization of genetically defined aro omp mutants of enterotoxigenic *Escherichia coli* and preliminary studies of safety and immunogenicity in humans. *Infect Immun*, **69**, 4969–79.

Uchi, H., Terao, H., et al. 2000. Cytokines and chemokines in the epidermis. *J Dermatol Sci*, **24**, S29–38.

Vajdy, M. and O'Hagan, D.T. 2001. Microparticles for intranasal immunization. *Adv Drug Deliv Rev*, **51**, 127–41.

Vanbever, R. and Préat, V. 1999. In vivo efficacy and safety of skin electroporation. *Adv Drug Deliv Rev*, **35**, 77–88.

Van Ginkel, F.W., Jackson, R.J., et al. 2000. Cutting edge: the mucosal adjuvant cholera toxin redirects vaccine proteins into olfactory tissues. *J Immunol*, **165**, 4778–82.

Von Hoegen, P. 2001. Synthetic biomimetic supra molecular biovector (SMBV) particles for nasal vaccine delivery. *Adv Drug Deliv Rev*, **51**, 113–25.

Wang, B., Amerio, P. and Sauder, D.N. 1999. Role of cytokines in epidermal Langerhans cell migration. *J Leukoc Biol*, **66**, 33–9.

Ward, B.J. 2000. Vaccine adverse events in the new millennium: is there reason for concern? *Bull World Health Organ*, **78**, 205–15.

Wester, R.C. and Maibach, H.I. 1987. Animal models for transdermal delivery. In: Kydonieus, A.F. and Berner, B. (eds), *Transdermal delivery of drugs*, Vol. 1. Boca Raton, FL: CRC Press, 61–70.

Willoughby, J.B. and Willoughby, W.F. 1977. In vivo responses to inhaled proteins. I. Quantitative analysis of antigen uptake, fate, and immunogenicity in a rabbit model system. *J Immunol*, **119**, 2137–46.

Wolf, K. and Honigsmann, H. 1971. Permeability of the epidermis and the phagocytic activity of keratinocytes. Ultrastructural studies with thorotrast as a marker. *J Ultrastr Research*, **36**, 176–90.

Wu, Y., Wang, X., et al. 2001. M cell-targeted DNA vaccination. *Proc Natl Acad Sci USA*, **98**, 9318–23.

Yu, J. and Langridge, W.H. 2001. A plant-based multicomponent vaccine protects mice from enteric diseases. *Nat Biotechnol*, **19**, 548–52.

Yu, J., Cassels, F., et al. 2002. Transcutaneous immunization using colonization factor and heat-labile enterotoxin induces correlates of protective immunity for enterotoxigenic *Escherichia coli. Infect Immun*, **70**, 1056–68.

41

New vaccine technologies

JAMES P. NATARO AND MYRON M. LEVINE

Immunization/vaccination remains the most efficient intervention against infectious diseases. However, for many infections the traditional approaches have not yielded safe, effective, convenient or affordable vaccines. For these applications and in the interest of safer and more practical interventions for diseases already covered by traditional vaccines, there remains a need for improved vaccine technologies. In this chapter, we summarize some of the most promising vaccine delivery technologies and evaluate their future promise.

TRANSCUTANEOUS IMMUNIZATION

Transcutaneous immunization (TCI) is the direct application of antigen and adjuvant to intact or slightly abraded skin. Once through the skin, an antigen encounters a dense population of efficient antigen-presenting cells (APC), the Langerhans' cells, which trigger innate and adaptive immune responses to antigens surmounting the integument (Hammond et al. 2001a). The potential advantages of TCI are many. Foremost is the ease of vaccine administration, avoiding the expense, logistics, and risk of needle-based injection. TCI is presumably safer than other parenteral routes, although information about this is still preliminary.

Successful TCI requires delivery of the immunogen through the stratum corneum (SC), the skin's principal barrier to the passage of molecules (Scharton-Kersten et al. 1999). Several strategies have been devised to permit facile penetration of the SC by molecular immunogens. Simple hydration results in significant, but transient, changes in the SC, and may be sufficient to allow penetration of some immunogens (Kaiserlian and Etchart 1999).

Preclinical experience with TCI appears very promising, and has illuminated several prerequisites of this approach. Foremost among these is the need for adjuvant co-administration to enhance immune responsiveness. The adjuvants most frequently employed are the cholera enterotoxin (CT) and the related *E. coli* heat-labile toxin (LT) (Glenn et al. 1998, 1999; Scharton-Kersten et al. 2000; Chen et al. 2002; John et al. 2002; Yu et al. 2002), although other adjuvants may also be effective (Scharton-Kersten et al. 2000). The mixture of CT or LT with tetanus toxoid dramatically increases antibody responses when compared with the administration of the antigens alone (Hammond et al. 2001b). Mice immunized with diphtheria toxoid (DTx) and CT developed excellent immune responses which persisted for over 9 months. Using tetanus toxoid as a model antigen, Hammond et al. (2001b) found that TCI induced both T-helper (Th) 1 and 2 (Th1 and Th2) responses (with a Th2 bias) partly dependent on choice of adjuvant. Several studies have also suggested that TCI can elicit mucosal immune responses (John et al. 2002; Yu et al. 2002) as well as cell-mediated responses (Yu et al. 2002). John et al. (2002) found that TCI of mice with CT resulted in mucosal responses similar to those engendered by a live attenuated cholera vaccine administered orally.

The adjuvant-dependent immunogenicity of a TCI vaccine was demonstrated in volunteers receiving CS6 colonization factor of enterotoxigenic *E. coli* (ETEC). Participants received patches containing 250, 500, 1000, or 2000 μg CS6 alone or with 500 μg LT, dosed at 0, 1, and 3 months (Guerena-Burgueno et al. 2002). In the absence of LT, there were no demonstrable immune responses to the CS6 antigen. In contrast, when CS6 was given with LT, 68 percent and 53 percent had anti-CS6 IgG and IgA, respectively, and 100 percent and 90 percent had anti-LT IgG and IgA, respectively. Fourteen (74 percent) of 19 volunteers developed mild delayed-type hypersensitivity (DTH) skin reactions after the second or third dose; no other adverse events were reported.

Questions that remain to be answered about TCI include the precision of dosing, as well as efficacy and safety in infants and young children, whose skin may be more porous than adults and in whom hypersensitivity may be a concern. In addition, the efficacy of LT/CT as an adjuvant may be limited in immune populations, perhaps precluding its use more than once (see Chapter 40, New approaches to vaccine delivery for further discussion of this aspect of vaccinology).

VIROSOMES

Liposomes, vesicles comprised of membrane-type phospholipids, can act as effective adjuvants for protein antigens that are incorporated into the vesicle membrane (Gregoriadis and Allison 1974; Allison and Gregoriadis 1976, 1990; Tan and Gregoriadis 1990) (Figure 41.1). Liposomes are efficiently taken up by APCs and their contents are processed largely via major histocompatibility complex (MHC) class II-dependent pathways. Liposome uptake can be further facilitated in a number of ways. Coating liposomes with antibodies, for example, can target them to Fcγ receptors on APCs. Liposomes produced by reconstitution of viral glycoproteins and lipids (virosomes) have many of the properties of the parent viruses. Virosomes have been adapted as delivery vehicles for antigens, antigen DNA, drugs, proteins, and water-soluble materials (Bron et al. 1993, 1994).

Virosomes initiate an immune response by binding and fusing with the eukaryotic plasma membrane, thereby discharging their cargo into the cytoplasm. As would therefore be predicted, antigens are chiefly presented in the context of MHC-I molecules. Effective $CD8^+$ cytotoxic T-cell (CTL) responses to virosome-encapsulated antigens are reported (Gregoriadis and Allison 1974; Gregoriadis 1990; Nerome et al. 1990; Miller et al. 1992; Arkema et al. 2000; Gluck et al. 2000). Bungener et al. (2002a, 2002b) have shown that membrane fusion-active virosomes, but not fusion-inactive virosomes, are able to deliver a test antigen to dendritic cells for MHC-I presentation; fusion activity of virosomes was not required for MHC-II presentation of the same antigen. Mucosal application of virosomes can elicit systemic and secretory IgA (sIgA) responses (Cusi et al. 2000, 2002).

Virosome-based influenza vaccines

Influenza virosomes are prepared by detergent purification of influenza surface glycoproteins and reconstitution with a mixture of phosphatidylcholine (70 percent), phosphatidylethanolamine (20 percent), and influenza virus envelope phospholipids (10 percent). This mixture was carefully chosen: egg yolk phosphatidylcholine has an excellent safety record of administration to humans; phosphatidylethanolamine has been shown to stimulate B cells to secrete antibody in the absence of T-cell help (Garcon and Six 1991); and the influenza virus glycoproteins haemagglutinin (HA) and neuraminidase (NA) play key roles in virosome function. HA is the major fusion-promoting protein of the virosome, and also directly mediates binding to APCs.

The influenza virosome vaccine has been tested in humans of all ages and appears to be safe and immunogenic when administered intranasally (Kaji et al. 1992;

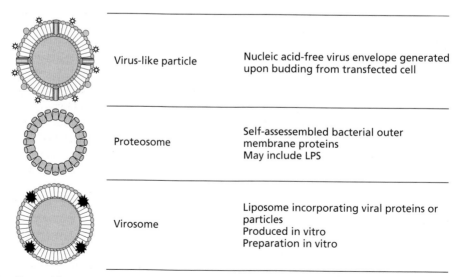

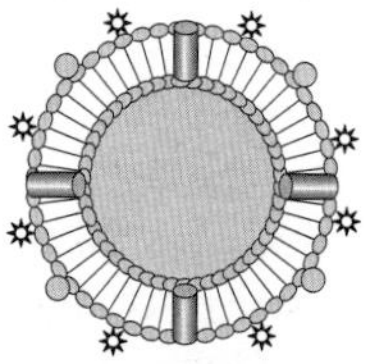	Virus-like particle	Nucleic acid-free virus envelope generated upon budding from transfected cell
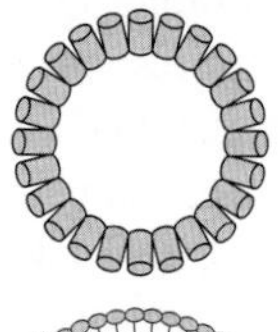	Proteosome	Self-assessembled bacterial outer membrane proteins May include LPS
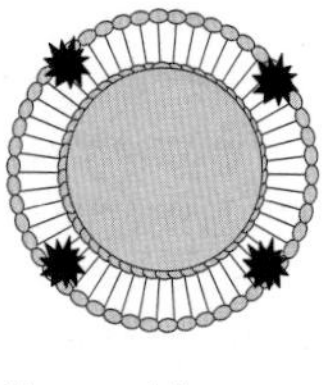	Virosome	Liposome incorporating viral proteins or particles Produced in vitro Preparation in vitro

Figure 41.1 *Virus-like particles, proteosomes, and virosomes are artificial, membrane-bound bodies that are used to deliver antigens to the immune system.*

Gluck et al. 1994, 2000; Conne et al. 1997; Schaad et al. 2000; Herzog et al. 2002). Following the excellent performance of the influenza prototype and the natural versatility of the virosome approach, antigens from other viruses have been incorporated into influenza virosomes. These notably include the F antigen from respiratory syncytial virus (Cusi et al. 2002), the protective core peptide of hepatitis C virus (Hunziker et al. 2002), and the hepatitis A virus vaccine, considered in greater detail below.

Hepatitis virosome vaccines

The first breakthrough in the use of virosomes for delivery of foreign antigen was the generation of a hepatitis A vaccine comprising hepatitis A virus (HAV) strain RG-SB integrated into influenza-derived virosomal particles (Loutan et al. 1994). In phase 3 clinical studies, seroconversion was documented in more than 98 percent of volunteers within 4 weeks of immunization (Argentini et al. 1995; Gluck et al. 1992). Booster injections of the virosomal vaccine 12 months after the initial dose resulted in 100 percent seroconversion, increasing anti-HAV antibody titers by 11- to 40-fold (Loutan et al. 1994).

The nature of virosomes makes them particularly amenable to the integration and presentation of multiple antigens. Hepatitis B surface antigen (HBsAg) has been successfully integrated into HAV-containing virosomes (Mengiardi et al. 1995). In further steps, the diphtheria toxoid, the α-tetanus toxoid, the β-tetanus toxoid, and the inactivated hepatitis A virion were additionally crosslinked to the virosome surface (Gluck 1995). Several such combination vaccines are licensed in Europe and Asia.

Other virosome applications

As virosomes efficiently fuse their contents with the cell cytoplasm, virosomes may be effective vectors for nucleic acid vaccine delivery (Cusi and Gluck 2000; Cusi 2001). They may also increase the uptake of antisense oligonucleotides (ODN), considered as promising therapeutic agents against viral diseases and cancer, or as immunomodulators.

Virosomes were used to deliver synthetic peptide-based malaria vaccine SPf66 (Poltl-Frank et al. 1999). Immunization of mice with two intramuscular doses of the virosome vaccine engendered higher antibody titers to the malaria antigen than when the antigen was administered with alum. An HIV vaccine, based on genetically modified glycoprotein and nonstructural peptides, is also under development (Kaneda 2000).

PROTEOSOMES

The proteosome nomenclature emphasizes the distinctive physical and biological properties of preparations of the outer membrane proteins (OMP) of gram-negative bacteria (Lowell et al. 1988a, 1988b). As membrane proteins, OMPs are highly hydrophobic; when isolated by detergent extraction, hydrophobic protein–protein interactions cause them to self-assemble into multimolecular particles with morphological characteristics of vesicles up to several hundred nanometers in diameter. The typical method of creating a proteosome-based vaccine is to process a mixture of detergent-solubilized OMPs with amphiphilic antigens, in a manner that facilitates noncovalent association of the antigens with the proteins and excludes the detergent (Wetzler et al. 1989, 1992; Wetzler 1994). Proteosomes therefore comprise noncovalent complexes of bacterial OMPs studded with amphiphilic antigen. A nasal proteosome influenza vaccine constructed in this way is currently in clinical trials. A second approach to deriving proteosome vaccines is to formulate a mixture of vaccine antigen with a soluble pre-formed proteosome adjuvant preparation made up of proteosome particles complexed with lipopolysaccharide (LPS). This system (termed 'IVX-908') may either incorporate amphiphilic or entirely hydrophilic molecules, or result from mixing of antigens with the pre-formed LPS-solubilized proteosome particles. IVX-908 possesses immunostimulatory properties in part resulting from its LPS. A proteosome shigella LPS vaccine has been shown to be promising in phase 1 and 2 clinical trials (see below) (Fries et al. 2001).

Proteosome vaccine particles exhibit certain characteristics that improve their safety and immunogenicity. Their surface hydrophobicity may improve uptake and processing by APCs, in particular promoting Th1-type responses. It has also been suggested that the immunogenicity of proteosomes is improved by the interaction of bacterial OMPs (Massari et al. 2002) and LPS (Chow et al. 1999) with the Toll-like receptors (TLR) of APCs. Although interaction with TLRs could cause some concern with inflammatory side effects, experience with the gram-negative OMPs (from *Neisseria meningitidis*) serving as carriers in *Haemophilus influenzae* vaccines has been positive (Heath 1998).

FluINsure, the nasal proteosome-based vaccine for influenza under development by ID Biomedical Corp., has undergone extensive clinical testing, with generally positive results (Plante et al. 2001). Phase 1 or 2 clinical trials of FluINsure using single-dose (15, 30, or 45 μg HA) and two-dose (7.5, 15, or 30 μg HA per dose) regimens in a total of 330 healthy adults have documented a high degree of safety and tolerance, in the presence of serum IgG responses similar to intramuscular vaccines (Treanor et al. 2001; Halperin et al. 2002). In addition, FluINsure recipients exhibited rises in sIgA titers to levels thought to be protective against influenza infection (Plante et al. 2001).

The proteosome shigella vaccine candidate comprises LPS and OMPs of *Shigella sonnei* and *S. flexneri* 2a (Fries et al. 2001). In dose-escalating phase 1 and 2 clinical studies, 111 healthy adults received two intranasal doses of the vaccine 2 weeks apart (Fries et al. 2001; McKenzie et al. 2001). Adverse effects were limited to mild nasal congestion and rhinorrhea in half to two-thirds of vaccinees. More than 90 percent of vaccinees demonstrated significant antibody-secreting cell responses (ASC); 60–90 percent responded with serum antibodies (four-fold geometric mean titer or GMT increases in IgG and IgA were typical at 1-mg doses).

In a challenge study using live *S. flexneri* given less than 48 days after immunization, vaccine efficacy was 36 percent against any diarrhea ($p = 0.04$), 78 percent against fever ($p = 0.003$), and 56 percent against severe symptoms including dysentery ($p = 0.03$) (Durbin et al. 2001). Although this vaccine appears to be well tolerated and fairly immunogenic, the brief duration of immune response after two doses limits its appeal. Nevertheless, the vaccine provides an interesting proof of principle that could be improved on in further iterations of this strategy. The most practical target for intranasal proteosome vaccines is likely to be respiratory viruses, for which a brief period of protection during the peak season would be beneficial. Parenterally administered proteosome vaccines could have broader application, but require additional clinical development.

VIRUS-LIKE PARTICLES

Virus-like particles (VLP) are nonreplicating, recombinant, viral capsids, with a structure similar to that of the virions from which they are derived. VLPs are formed by self-assembly of viral structural protein(s) on synthesis in eukaryotic or prokaryotic expression systems; they therefore present the native conformation of viral antigens but lack viral nucleic acid (Kruger et al. 1999). VLPs are particularly useful when native virions cannot be readily isolated or produced or when a very high degree of vaccine safety is desired (e.g. immunization of immunocompromised patients). They may be made up of single viral capsid proteins (e.g. papillomavirus and hepatitis B core protein) or multiple proteins contributing to a more complex structure (e.g. herpesviruses, rotavirus, and Ebola virus).

The immune response to VLPs is typically balanced to include neutralizing antibodies and cytotoxic T-cell responses, presumably as a result of the presentation of multiple native antigens in each particle (Sedlik et al. 1997, 1999, 2000). The balance of systemic vs mucosal immune responses is determined by the route of administration, as well as by the antigenic characteristics of the VLP itself. Papillomavirus VLPs have been shown to induce strong peripheral IgG responses on parenteral administration, and good sIgA responses when given by the oral route (Gerber et al. 2001). Unlike many other new vaccine delivery approaches, immunogenicity is strong without the need for an additional adjuvant (see below). However, although cytotoxic (Sedlik et al. 1997) and Th1 responses (Lo-Man et al. 1998) are typically robust on VLP administration, responses can be further augmented or modified by co-administration of adjuvant (Siadat-Pajouh and Cai 2001), often approaching that derived from native viral infection.

Manufacture of VLPs has been made possible only by the advent of molecular biotechnology. The fundamental approach entails the cloning of genes encoding viral capsid proteins into a mammalian expression vector or other expression system. Among the many systems successfully adapted are baculovirus (Garnier et al. 1995), *Pichia pastoris* (yeast cells) (Sasnauskas et al. 1999), plant systems (e.g. *Nicotiana*) (O'Brien et al. 2000), and bacterial expression systems (Chen et al. 2001). The expression vector and host cell system typically must be optimized. On protein expression, some VLPs bud from the plasma membrane and self-assemble, whereas others must be post-translationally modified or otherwise manipulated.

The versatility of the VLP approach has proved to be formidable. A partial list of vaccines in various stages of testing include those against rotavirus (O'Neal et al. 1998; Jiang et al. 1999; Coste et al. 2000, 2001; Siadat-Pajouh and Cai 2001), Norwalk virus (Ball et al. 1999), parvovirus (Sedlik et al. 1997, 1999), hepatitis viruses (Li et al. 1997; Lorenzo et al. 2001), papillomavirus (Pumpens et al. 2002; Schiller and Lowy 2001b), calicivirus (Nagesha et al. 1999), HIV (Garnier et al. 1995; Weber et al. 1995; Peters et al. 1997), hantavirus (Koletzki et al. 2000), polyoma virus (Goldmann et al. 1999), and influenza virus (Latham and Galarza 2001; Watanabe et al. 2002).

Some VLPs have progressed to phase 1 or 2 clinical trials (Ball et al. 1999; Zhang et al. 2000; Evans et al. 2001; Schiller and Lowy 2001a). In nearly all such studies, VLPs have fulfilled their promise in providing an excellent safety profile, coupled with good immunogenicity. Evans et al. (2001) reported on a phase 1 study of VLPs comprising the L1 protein of human papilloma viruses (HPV). The vaccine was well tolerated and induced high levels of both binding and neutralizing antibodies. The vaccine induced strong B- and T-cell responses, and T-helper epitopes appear to be conserved across HPV types. Harro et al. (2001) reported the results of a double-masked, placebo-controlled, dose-escalation trial to evaluate the safety and immunogenicity of an HPV type 16 (HPV16) L1 VLP vaccine in healthy adults. Volunteers were given intramuscular injections with placebo or with 10- or 50-μg doses of HPV16 L1 VLP vaccine without adjuvant, or with alum or MF59 as adjuvants at 0, 1, and 4 months. All vaccine formulations were well tolerated, and all participants receiving vaccine seroconverted. With the higher dose, most of the recipients achieved serum antibody titers that were approximately 40-fold higher than what is observed in natural infection. Zhang et al. (2000) administered multiple doses of HPV VLPs (HPV6b) without adjuvant to 33 participants with genital warts. All subjects mounted DTH responses to the vaccine. Complete regression of genital warts was observed in 25 of 33 evaluable participants over the 20-week observation period. The vaccine was well tolerated.

Ball et al. (1999) have conducted trials of a Norwalk virus (NV) VLP made up of a single capsid protein. Twenty adults received two doses of vaccine 3 weeks apart. No side effects were observed or reported by the volunteers. All vaccinees given the highest dose responded with fourfold or more increases in serum IgG antibody titers. Most of the volunteers (83 percent; 15 of 18) responded after the first rNV VLP dose and showed no increase in serum IgG antibody titer after the second dose. Tacket et al. (2003) fed Norwalk VLPs without adjuvant to 36 healthy adult volunteers at doses of 250 μg ($n = 10$), 500 μg ($n = 10$), and 2000 μg ($n = 10$); six volunteers received a single dose of placebo. Of those who received 250 μg 90 percent developed rises in serum anti-VLP IgG antibodies. Higher doses did not produce higher responses. All vaccinees developed significant rises in IgA anti-VLP ASCs, although only 30–40 percent of volunteers developed mucosal anti-VLP IgA antibodies. Lymphoproliferative responses and interferon γ (IFN-γ) production were observed transiently among those who received 250 μg or 500 μg, but not 2000 μg of VLP.

Peters et al. (1997) reported the results of a phase 2 study of the yeast-derived VLP HIV vaccine Ty.p24.VLP (p24-VLP), in HIV-antibody-positive asymptomatic volunteers. Fifteen volunteers, with p24 antibody titers >1/100, p24 antigen <20 pg/l, and CD4 $>350 \times 10^9$/l, were enrolled. Five were immunized with aluminum hydroxide placebo, five with 25 μg, and five with 100 μg p24-VLP in alum adjuvant at weeks 0 and 4 by the intramuscular route. No serious adverse events were observed in any of the groups, although efficacy data have not been provided.

VLPs represent a highly versatile strategy for vaccine delivery. Human trials have thus far borne out the safety and immunogenicity of this immunization strategy, although no VLP vaccine has yet been licensed. One important question about this class of vaccines is the duration and breadth of protection, and the possible requirement for adjuvant has not yet been determined for mucosally administered VLP vaccines.

LIVE ATTENUATED VECTOR VACCINES

The use of attenuated bacterial strains as mucosal live vectors to deliver antigens of unrelated pathogens is a highly promising vaccine strategy for several reasons (Medina and Guzman 2001):

- The mucosal route of administration efficiently induces both systemic and local protective immunity, which is favorable for pathogens and toxins that enter through mucosal surfaces.
- Mucosal delivery is usually associated with low reactogenicity.
- Logistics of vaccine administration are typically easier for mucosal vaccines, especially in the context of mass immunization campaigns.
- As they are perceived as less invasive than parenteral vaccines, oral vaccines have a generally high level of public acceptance and increased compliance.
- Genetic engineering strategies used to construct mucosal vaccines confer a high degree of versatility. Live attenuated enteric vaccines would be expected to have relatively low manufacturing costs compared with many other vaccines.

Live attenuated salmonella vaccines

Attenuated *Salmonella enterica* serovar Typhi vaccines were among the first oral bacterial vaccines, and they remain among the most promising. The great promise of *S. typhi* as a live attenuated vaccine derives from its pathogenic strategy (Kingsley and Baumler 2000; Santos et al. 2003; Zhang et al. 2003). *S. typhi* briefly colonizes the small intestinal mucosa, and invades at the level of the Peyer's patch epithelium (Figure 41.2). On entry into the lymphoid follicles, the organisms are taken up into macrophages, which transport the bacteria throughout the body. Attenuation strategies have been devised that permit the organism to enter the lymphoid tissue but not to persist or circulate via the bloodstream. This modified pathway is ideal for presentation of antigens to the gut-associated lymphoid tissue.

Germanier and Fuer (1975) derived the first attenuated *S. typhi* vaccine (designated Ty21a) by nonspecific chemical mutagenesis of parent strain Ty2. Ty21a harbors a galactose epimerase mutation, does not express the Vi (virulence) capsular polysaccharide, and exhibits many additional mutations that collectively contribute to its attenuation. Although Ty21a has served as a safe and effective typhoid fever vaccine for more than a decade, it has certain shortcomings, chief among these being the requirement for multiple doses to achieve protective efficacy (Levine et al. 1990). The advent of genetic engineering provides an opportunity to exploit specific attenuation strategies, because this organism is genetically tractable.

Several groups have prepared recombinant *S. typhi* vaccine candidates and tested them in phase 1 studies in human volunteers. Four strains proved to be sufficiently well tolerated and immunogenic to stimulate interest in additional clinical trials. These include: Ty800 (attenuated by virtue of mutation in the two-component regulatory system PhoPQ) (Hohmann et al. 1996), χ4372 (inactivated in the CRP transcriptional regulator) (Tacket et al. 1992a), CVD 908-*htrA* (inactivated in aromatic biosynthesis pathway and production of a stress protease) (Tacket et al. 2000b), and ZH9 (inactivated in

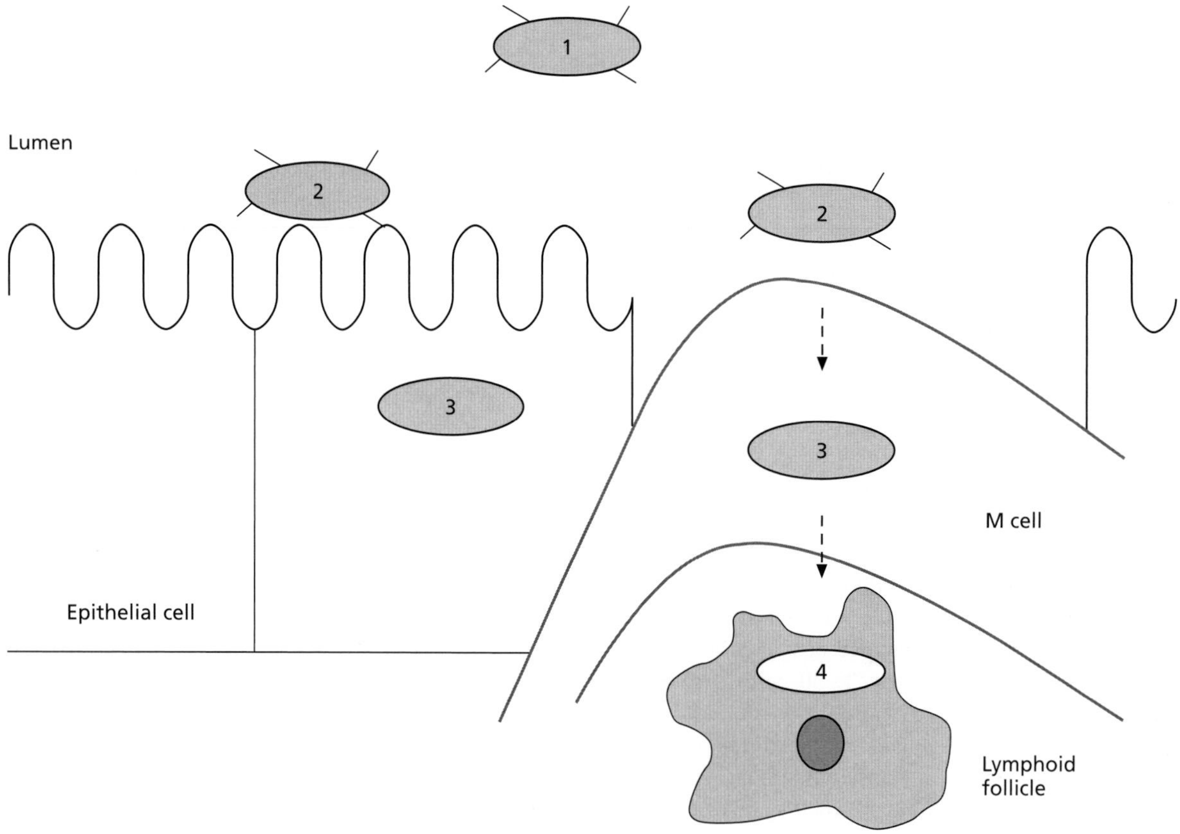

Figure 41.2 *Microanatomical locations of live attenuated vaccine vectors. Nonliving vaccines remain in the lumen of the gastrointestinal tract (1) and can be sampled passively by the gut-associated lymphoid tissue. Some live vaccine vectors, e.g. those derived from* Vibrio cholerae, *actively adhere to the surface of the absorptive epithelium (2) or to the M cells overlying the lymphoid follicles. Invasive bacterial vectors, e.g. strains of* Shigella *and* Listeria *spp., invade the epithelial cells but remain in the cytoplasm (3), whereas vectors such as* Salmonella *translocate through the epithelial layer and access the underlying antigen-presenting cells (4). The focus of live attenuated vector technology is to construct mutants that target the immunogen to one or more of these compartments.*

the aromatic biosynthesis pathway and the salmonella pathogenicity island-2 type III secretion system secreton) (Hindle et al. 2002; Khan et al. 2003).

The immediate predecessor of CVD 908-*htrA* was CVD 908 (Hone et al. 1991), attenuated by virtue of two nonreverting deletion mutations within the chromosomal *aroC* and *aroD* genes. These two genes encode enzymes critical in the biosynthetic pathway leading to synthesis of chorismate, the key precursor required for synthesis of the aromatic amino acids (Hoiseth and Stocker 1981); chorismate is further required for the synthesis of *p*-aminobenzoic acid, which is ultimately converted to the purine nucleotides ATP and GTP. Although immunization of volunteers with CVD 908 is well tolerated and highly immunogenic (Tacket et al. 1992a, p. 216), a silent vaccinemia was detected in 100 percent of volunteers who ingested 5×10^8 colony-forming units (cfu), wherein vaccine organisms were recovered from blood cultures collected between days 4 and 8 after immunization (Levine et al. 1996, 1997). This silent bacteremia was not associated with adverse clinical symptoms and was self-limiting. Nevertheless, further attenuation to obviate vaccinemias was pursued.

CVD 908 was attenuated further by a defined deletion mutation in the *htrA* gene, which encodes a heat shock-induced serine protease responsible for degradation of misfolded periplasmic proteins (Pallen and Wren 1997). As predicted, CVD 908-*htrA* was well tolerated at doses up to 5×10^9 without vaccinemia (Tacket et al. 1997). Volunteers ingesting CVD 908-*htrA* manifested a broad immune response to *S. typhi* antigens, including intestinal sIgA antibodies, serum IgG antibodies, and cellular immune responses.

The versatility of *S. typhi* as a vector to deliver foreign antigens has been demonstrated in both CVD 908 and CVD 908-*htrA* backgrounds. Volunteers receiving two doses of *S. typhi* CVD 908 expressing the *Plasmodium falciparum* circumsporozoite protein (CSP) developed cytotoxic T lymphocytes (CTL) to CSP-transfected target cells (Gonzalez et al. 1994). In a second study, 21 healthy adult volunteers received a single dose of CVD 908-*htrA*-carrying, plasmid-encoded, tetanus toxin fragment C under the control of one or two different promoters induced in vivo (*nirB* and *lpp*) (Tacket et al. 2000a). Neither vaccine induced fever or vaccinemia. Of three seronegative volunteers who received 10^9 cfu CVD

908-*htrA* (pTET*lpp*), a single oral dose of the live vector expressing fragment C seroconverted one of the three and elicited a rise in serum tetanus anti-toxin 43 times above the protective level.

McKenzie et al. (2002) fed CVD 908-*htrA*-expressing *Helicobacter pylori* urease to healthy volunteers at doses up to about 5×10^9 cfu; the vaccine was well tolerated and induced urease-specific IgA and IgG ASCs in 25 percent and 88 percent of the immunized individuals.

With the establishment of the ability of *S. typhi* to deliver foreign antigens, attention has turned to improving the technical aspects of heterologous gene expression (Galen and Levine 2001). Accordingly, genetic tools have been developed to express heterologous antigens from strong in vivo-induced promoters (see above); assure recombinant plasmid replication in the absence of antibiotic selection (Galen et al. 1999); and enable secretion of foreign antigens to the extracellular milieu. With experience and expertise accumulating rapidly, the future of *Salmonella* spp. as a live attenuated vector vaccine appears bright.

Live attenuated shigella vaccines

Similar to *Salmonella*, shigella strains invade the intestinal mucosa and enter the gut-associated lymphoid tissue. Unlike *Salmonella*, *Shigella* spp. are not adapted for long-term persistence in macrophages, and bacteremias are rare. *Shigella* spp. therefore offer some advantages and some disadvantages to use as a live vector. Similar to *Salmonella*, advances in the understanding of shigella pathogenesis allow precise disruption of virulence genes without alteration in the invasive phenotype, which is believed to be required for a protective response. Recently identified attenuating strategies are finally yielding vaccine candidate strains that are immunogenic in humans, yet are well tolerated clinically.

Sansonetti and co-workers (1991) constructed a series of *Shigella flexneri* 5a strains with mutations in the *virG* (*icsA*) gene, which is involved in cell-to-cell spread (Bernardini et al. 1989) but which is not required for invasiveness. Additional mutations were constructed in *ompB* or *iuc*, the latter encoding the siderophore aerobactin (Sansonetti et al. 1991). In animal studies, the *ompB/virG* strain was well tolerated but not fully protective against shigella challenge. In contrast, the *virG/iuc* strain caused mild adverse effects in some animals, but 100 percent protection after challenge (Sansonetti and Arondel 1989). Similarly, a *S. flexneri* 2a strain with the *virG* and *iuc* mutations (SC602) caused symptoms of mild shigellosis in healthy adult volunteers at doses of 10^6 and 10^8 cfu, whereas a dose of 10^4 caused only mild symptoms in a few volunteers (Coster et al. 1999). Importantly, volunteers ingesting a single dose of 10^4 SC602 were protected against challenge with wild-type *S. flexneri* 2a. This experience underscores the dose-related relationship between immune response and reactogenicity; however, doses tolerated by healthy adults may not be so for children or other more vulnerable hosts, and thus a higher level of safety is desirable.

A *virG*-deleted strain of *S. sonnei*, strain WRSS1, has been evaluated in a phase 1 clinical study. A single dose of 10^3, 10^4, 10^5, or 10^6 cfu caused low-grade fever or mild diarrhea in 22 percent of recipients (Kotloff et al. 2002). However, the vaccine was highly immunogenic, generating impressive levels of serum anti-shigella LPS and anti-LPS IgA ASCs (Kotloff et al. 2002).

Work at the CVD has yielded similar experience. Noriega and co-workers (1994) generated *S. flexneri* 2a vaccine candidate CVD 1203, with mutations in *aroA* and *virG*. A single dose of 10^6 CVD 1203 was well tolerated and immunogenic. However, at doses of 10^8 or 10^9 cfu, short-lived adverse reactions, including fever, diarrhea, and/or mild dysentery, were observed (Kotloff et al. 1996). This experience again illustrates the dose-dependent nature of adverse effects and calls for a higher degree of safety in attenuated shigella constructs.

In progress toward achieving the correct balance of immunogenicity and safety, Noriega and co-workers (1994) generate *S. flexneri* 2a strain CVD 1204, harboring a deletion in the *guaBA* operon (Anderson et al. 2000). This mutation, which renders the bacteria auxotrophic for guanine, is more attenuating and virtually nonreactogenic in the guinea-pig model of keratoconjunctivitis. Two further derivatives of CVD 1204 were constructed: CVD 1208 carries additional mutations in the genes encoding shigella enterotoxins 1 and 2 (ShET1 and ShET2, encoded by *set* and *sen*, respectively), and CVD 1207, which harbors a deletion in *virG* in addition to the mutations in *guaBA*, *set*, and *sen* (Kotloff et al. 2000; Levine 2000). Human studies on this series of candidates are under way. Both CVD 1207 and CVD 1208 have proved to be well tolerated but the latter appears to be more immunogenic (Kotloff et al. 2000).

Live attenuated *Vibrio cholerae* vaccines

Vibrio cholerae has many attributes that make it an attractive vaccine delivery vehicle. It is a noninvasive organism which colonizes the human intestinal mucosa and induces potent, long-lived mucosal and systemic humoral responses (Kaper et al. 1995). The lack of invasiveness of *V. cholerae* reduces the likelihood of systemic reactions and theoretically reduces the need for global attenuation of the pathogen. *V. cholerae* has been intensively studied at the molecular level and is genetically tractable.

Several live attenuated *V. cholerae* vaccine constructs are safe and immunogenic in humans (Sack and Albert 1994; Liu et al. 1995; Cohen 1997; Herzog et al. 1997;

Tacket et al. 1999; Yamamoto 2000). CVD 103HgR (*ctxA*−, *hly*−, *recA*, classic Inaba strain 569B) is the first recombinant live attenuated cholera vaccine, and it continues to set the standard for safety and efficacy for cholera vaccines (Levine et al. 1988; Migasena et al. 1989; Cryz et al. 1990; Kotloff et al. 1992; Su-Arehawaratana et al. 1992; Tacket et al. 1992b, 1999; Gotuzzo et al. 1993; Simanjuntak et al. 1993; Sack and Albert 1994; Lagos et al. 1995; Losonsky et al. 1997; Perry et al. 1998; Yamamoto 2000). The organism is principally attenuated via deletion of the CTA subunit, but its parent strain also shows a mild defect in its ability to colonize the human intestine (Levine et al. 1988). CVD 103-HgR has been administered to more than 6000 individuals in placebo-controlled phase 1 and 2 trials, including infants and HIV-infected individuals (Levine et al. 1988; Migasena et al. 1989; Cryz et al. 1990, 1992; Kotloff et al. 1992; Su-Arehawaratana et al. 1992; Suharyono et al. 1992; Tacket et al. 1992b, 1999; Gotuzzo et al. 1993; Losonsky et al. 1993, 1997; Simanjuntak et al. 1993; Lagos et al. 1995, 1999a, b; Perry et al. 1998; Taylor et al. 1999; Richie et al. 2000). In all studies, neither diarrhea nor any other adverse reaction occurred significantly more often in vaccinees than in placebo recipients. CVD 103HgR conferred strong protective immunity in North American volunteers against experimental challenge with wild-type *V. cholerae* strains. In one study, a single dose conferred 100 percent protection against experimental challenge with a toxigenic classic strain when volunteers were challenged only 8 days after immunization; protective immunity was also documented to extend to at least 6 months after immunization, the longest interval tested (Tacket et al. 1992b). In a randomized, double-masked, placebo-controlled, multicenter trial, a single dose of this strain conferred 91 percent protective efficacy against moderate or severe diarrhea after challenge with toxigenic El Tor *V. cholerae* (Tacket et al. 1999). The ability of CVD 103-HgR to provide long-term protection against natural challenge in cholera-endemic countries has not been established. Over 4 years of surveillance during a field trial in Indonesia, only 14 percent efficacy was observed overall (Richie et al. 2000). During the first 6 months of this trial (when protection might be expected to b maximal), few cases of cholera occurred. However, during a post-licensure intervention with CVD 103-HgR carried out under the auspices of the World Health Organization during a cholera outbreak in Micronesia, it was calculated that the vaccine provided 79 percent effectiveness in preventing cholera (Claire-Lise Chaignat, WHO, personal communication). In view of its consistent efficacy in multiple experimental challenge studies in conferring a high level of protection in North American volunteers against both classic and El Tor cholera caused by either Inaba or Ogawa serotypes, and its ability to elicit strong vibriocidal antibody responses, CVD 103-HgR has been licensed in many countries (including Canada, Australia, and Switzerland).

Several other attenuated cholera vaccines have been tested in humans (Levine et al. 1988; Taylor et al. 1994; Kaper et al. 1995; Liu et al. 1995; Sack et al. 1997; Benitez et al. 1999; Valle et al. 2000). A series of nonmotile cholera variants is well tolerated and immunogenic in healthy adults and is undergoing further clinical trials (Taylor et al. 1994).

V. cholerae vector strains have been used to deliver heterologous antigens (Butterton et al. 1995) such as *Shigella sonnei* LPS (Favre et al. 1996), *E. coli* Shiga toxin B subunit (Acheson et al. 1996), enterohemorrhagic *E. coli* intimin (Butterton et al. 1997), tetanus toxin fragment C (Chen et al. 1998), *B. pertussis* tracheal colonization factor (Chen et al. 1998), *Entamoeba histolytica* surface protein (Ryan et al. 1997b), and *Clostridium difficile* toxin A (Ryan et al. 1997a).

BCG-based vector vaccines

The currently licensed bacille Calmette–Guérin (BCG) vaccine is a multiply passaged *Mycobacterium bovis* strain, originally developed in 1908 (Fine 1989). The bacterium is highly attenuated and acceptably safe, but it is only partially protective against tuberculous disease, principally the extrapulmonary forms (Fine 2001). By virtue of its derivation from *M. bovis* and its history of multiple passage, BCG is lacking 16 discrete regions of the *M. tuberculosis* genome. There is therefore no risk of reversion to virulent *M. tuberculosis*. The efficacy of BCG varies among countries, and indeed the BCG vaccines used throughout the world display substantial genetic diversity attributed to its handling over the course of the twentieth century (Fine 1995, 2001; Behr and Small 1997, 1999; Behr et al. 1999; Fine and Vynnycky 1998).

Similar to mycobacteria that naturally infect humans, BCG is taken up into macrophage and dendritic cells and undergo limited replication within the phagolysosome (Inaba et al. 1993). As expected, therefore, BCG presents antigens predominantly in the context of MHC-II (Kaufmann and Ladel 1994; Kaufmann et al. 1995; Ladel et al. 1995a, b); BCG elicits predominantly a CD4-mediated Th1-type response. However, modifications of the route, timing, and dose of administration can elicit more balanced Th1/Th2 immunity (Bretscher 1992, 1994; Power et al. 1998).

BCG has been considered as a vector for delivery of antigens when a Th1 response is desired. As *Listeria monocytogenes* is an intracellular pathogen normally controlled by Th1 responses, several investigators have adapted BCG for use in listeria vaccine development (Hess et al. 1998; Conradt et al. 1999). Hess and colleagues expressed the p60 protective antigen of *L. monocytogenes* in various cellular compartments of the BCG bacterium (Hess 2002). Not unexpectedly, surface display or secretion of p60 provided the strongest responses. The market for a human listeria vaccine is doubtful, but progress in a BCG-derived listeria vaccine development may constitute an important proof of principle.

BCG-derived vaccine candidates have been constructed against various pathogens, including bacteria (e.g. *Borrelia burgdorferi* (Langermann et al. 1994a), *Bordetella pertussis* (Nascimento et al. 2000), and *Streptococcus pneumoniae* (Langermann et al. 1994b; Miyaji et al. 2001)); parasites (*Leishmania* (Connell et al. 1993; Abdelhak et al. 1995) and *Schistosoma* (Kremer et al. 1996)); and viral pathogens (HIV (Aldovini and Young 1990, 1991) and papillomavirus (Jabbar et al. 2000)). Edelman et al. (1999) at the University of Maryland tested a recombinant BCG (rBCG) vaccine expressing the outer surface protein A (OspA) of *B. burgdorferi*. Before human studies, the vaccine had proven highly immunogenic and protective in mice (Stover et al. 1993). Twenty-four adults received one intradermal injection of the rBCG-OspA vaccine containing escalating vaccine doses ranging from 2×10^4 to 2×10^7 cfu (Edelman et al. 1999). Local ulceration was the most common adverse effect; however, 83 percent of recipients of the highest dose developed BCG-positive draining lesions at the immunization site, persisting for up to 70 days (Figure 41.3). Despite these reactions, none of the volunteers at any dose manifested detectable post-immunization OspA antibody titers, although over half of vaccine recipients developed positive purified protein derivative (PPD) responses. These data illustrate the limitations of BCG as a vaccine vector, including limited antibody responses; more importantly, however, the threat of persistent shedding of BCG from cutaneous sites would constitute a potential risk to immunocompromised contacts.

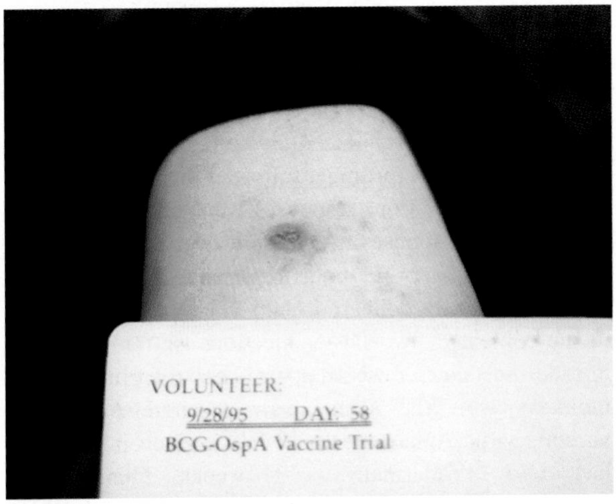

Figure 41.3 *Eschar caused by recombinant* BCG *vaccine. Large ulcerating eschar on the arm of a patient receiving one dose of* BCG*–outer surface protein A (OspA) vaccine 58 days previously. (Courtesy of R. Edelman, University of Maryland Center for Vaccine Development.)*

Live attenuated listeria vaccines

As a prototypical intracellular pathogen amenable to genetic manipulation, *L. monocytogenes* has been proposed as a vaccine vector against infections controlled by CTL and CD8 responses. *L. monocytogenes* pursues a pathogenic strategy similar to that of *Shigella*, in which the organism is engulfed by the eukaryotic cell, lyses the phagosome, and takes up residence in the cytoplasm (Portnoy et al. 2002). From this privileged site, the bacterium is protected from antibody responses, but can be eradicated by strong, cell-mediated, IFN-γ-driven responses (Portnoy et al. 1989; Finelli et al. 1999; Kerksiek and Pamer 1999; O'Riordan et al. 2002).

L. monocytogenes has been exploited for MHC-I presentation of a large number of viral, parasite, and tumor antigens, in either protein or nucleic acid form (Schafer et al. 1992; Dietrich et al. 2000, 2002; Gentschev et al. 2000, 2001, 2002; Spreng et al. 2000). Several of these constructs have proved to be safe and effective vaccines in mouse models (Ikonomidis et al. 1994; Ochsenbein et al. 1999; Dietrich et al. 2002; Soussi et al. 2002). However, as *L. monocytogenes* is a human pathogen, there is justified concern over possible adverse effects, especially in immunocompromised vaccinees. Friedman et al. (2000) have constructed a highly attenuated strain of *L. monocytogenes* that requires D-alanine, which is not available in human tissues. These investigators engineered the bacteria to express the HIV-1 Gag protein, and showed that the recombinant vaccine was as efficient at stimulating Gag-specific human CTLs in vitro as wild-type recombinants. This vaccine is considered to be a candidate for human trials and could serve as an important test case for *Listeria*-based vaccine strategies.

Other vector vaccines

Several other bacteria have been advanced as vector vaccines. Among these are several commensals, which imply a high degree of safety. Medaglini and colleagues (1995) engineered *Streptococcus gordonii*, a normal inhabitant of the human mouth, to express antigens of the M protein of *S. pyogenes*. In preparation for clinical trials of the vectored vaccine, K.L. Kotloff (personal communication) and co-workers evaluated the ability to implant the carrier strain (*S. gordonii*) resistant to streptomycin and 5-fluoro-2-deoxyuridine) into the nose and mouth of volunteers, and then delineated the time to eradication, both spontaneous and antibiotic induced. Inoculation was generally well tolerated. Symptoms reported most often within 4 days of inoculation were stuffy nose (36 percent), headache (30 percent), and sore throat (19 percent). The strain was detected by culture in the mouths of 97 percent of participants. A 5-day course of azithromycin eliminated the strain in all participants. Without antibiotics, 82 percent spontaneously eradicated the implanted strain within 1 week, and all cleared by 1 month. Results of these studies will be used to design future phase I trials to evaluate a *S. gordonii* live vector vaccine expressing, on its surface, the conserved region of *S. pyogenes* M protein.

PRIME-BOOST IMMUNIZATION

Despite the success of vaccine technologies against a plethora of infectious diseases, certain infections have resisted vaccine strategies. Chief among these are HIV, malaria, and to a large extent tuberculosis. These infections have in common a requirement for strong cell-mediated responses, which are difficult to generate using traditional parenteral vaccine delivery strategies. In response to this problem, various innovative strategies have been devised, including some already discussed in this chapter. An additional, highly innovative immunization approach comprises a multiple-dose schedule in which the initial dose(s) prime the immune response, and subsequent doses deliver the same target antigens in the context of a different delivery vehicle, thereby engendering strong responses. This strategy, termed 'heterologous prime boost', has led to vigorous cell-mediated responses not as yet achieved by any other approach.

One of the earliest illustrations of the value of prime boost for generation of protective cell-mediated immunity (CMI) responses was provided by Li and co-workers in 1993. These investigators constructed a recombinant influenza virus expressing a CD8 T-cell epitope from the CSP of *Plasmodium yoelii*. Immunization of mice with the recombinant influenza virus, followed by a recombinant vaccinia virus expressing the entire CSP, induced protective immunity against a live sporozoite challenge. However, immunization with recombinant vaccinia virus first, followed by a booster injection with recombinant influenza virus, failed to induce protection. Subsequent to this promising start, several other groups corroborated the findings in malaria using several different heterologous prime-boost regimens (Hill et al. 2000; Bruna-Romero et al. 2001; Jones et al. 2001; Rogers et al. 2001; Schneider et al. 2001), and the utility of this approach for malaria immunization is being hotly pursued.

Also, in 1993, two separate groups reported highly promising results employing a heterologous prime-boost approach to HIV immunization. Graham et al. (1993) inoculated 12 volunteers with recombinant vaccinia virus expressing HIV gp160 glycoprotein, and then boosted them with recombinant gp160 protein. After booster immunization, the sera of all vaccinees showed strong antibody responses detected by western blot and enzyme-linked immunosorbent assay (ELISA); five blocked binding of CD4 cells to gp120. The prime-boost strategy was more immunogenic than either product alone. The same month, Cooney et al. (1993) independently reported the results of a similar phase 1 study in which 13 participants immunized with recombinant vaccinia virus expressing gp160 were boosted with recombinant gp160. T cell and antibody responses detected after immunization with either vaccine alone were of low magnitude and transient. In contrast, recipients of the combination regimen developed higher, more prolonged, T-cell proliferative responses to gp160.

Since these pioneering studies, the power of the prime-boost phenomenon in HIV immunization has been extended to other targets as well. Evans et al. (1999) have shown that a canarypox vaccine expressing multiple HIV antigens yielded stronger responses in volunteers when accompanied by injection of recombinant gp120. An interesting twist to this study was that the gp120 inoculation produced the same boost when administered simultaneously with the canarypox vaccine.

A great deal of attention has surrounded the phenomenon of priming with a nucleic acid vaccine, followed by parenteral boost with the protein antigen, usually delivered in a viral vector. Kent et al. (1998) evaluated a consecutive immunization strategy in mice involving priming with DNA and boosting with recombinant fowlpox virus vaccines, each encoding Gag and Pol HIV-1 antigens. The heterologous prime-boost approach induced greater HIV-1-specific immunity than either vaccine given alone; mice given the prime-boost regimen were protected from challenge with a recombinant vaccinia virus expressing HIV-1 antigens. In a subsequent experiment using rhesus macaques, a dramatic boosting effect on DNA vaccine-primed HIV-1-specific helper and cytotoxic T-lymphocyte responses was observed, although accompanied by a decline in HIV-1 antibody titers. The prime-boost regimen protected macaques from an intravenous HIV-1 challenge.

Robinson et al. (1999, 2000) compared eight different immunization protocols for their abilities to induce responses to nonpathogenic immunodeficiency virus challenge in rhesus macaque monkeys. The best containment response was induced by a regimen comprising intradermal DNA priming followed by fowlpox virus booster immunization; responses were characterized by strong T-cell responses which were over ten-fold higher than homologous prime-boost regimens. These investigators subsequently delivered Gag, Pol, and Env antigens in the context of two DNA injections (intramuscular or intradermal) given 8 weeks apart. They then boosted the monkeys with the same proteins expressed in the vaccinia virus Ankara vector (MVA), given intramuscularly and intradermally at 24 weeks. This regimen elicited high levels of antigen-specific T cells, of both CD4 and CD8 type. The monkeys were protected from intrarectal viral challenge with the highly pathogenic simian–human immunodeficiency virus 89.6P given 7 months after immunization. Curiously, however, these investigators were later to show that two doses of the MVA vaccine, without DNA vaccine boost, were able to induce significant protection.

Since the initial success with prime boost in malaria and HIV vaccine efforts, this approach has been extended to other vaccines. In sum, this is substantial evidence that mucosal priming followed by parenteral boosting yields augmented, and broadened, immune responses, including TH1, TH2, and SIGA components. The concept of enteral prime/parenteral boost was first suggested by human studies using oral polio vaccine (OPV) and parenteral inactivated polio vaccine (IPV) recipients, boosted with either OPV or IPV (Herremans et al. 1999). In this study, parenteral IPV immunization boosted systemic and mucosal IgA antibody responses in previously OPV-immunized patients, but not in IPV-immunized individuals. Interestingly, IPV immunization of OPV-primed patients, although immunized decades earlier, mounted rapid (by day 7) and vigorous IgG as well as IgA responses in the periphery as well as at the mucosal level. IPV boosting of OPV-primed individuals resulted in broader immune responses which were at least as vigorous in all aspects as those seen in individuals primed and boosted with the parenteral vaccine.

These human data have subsequently been reproduced in mouse models. Using the pertactin protein of *Bordetella pertussis* expressed cytoplasmically in an attenuated salmonella vector, Anderson et al. (1996) demonstrated that effective boosting can occur in the setting of very weak responses to the initial prime (i.e. the mucosa may be primed without exhibiting demonstrable antibody response). Neither mice immunized with pertactin alone nor those immunized just with two doses of recombinant *S. typhimurium* pertactin exhibited anamnestic responses. The investigators also measured anti-pertactin IgG subclasses and found that mice immunized orally with *S. typhimurium* pertactin and boosted with 10 μg purified antigen produced IgG2a and IgG2b, whereas purified pertactin alone induced primarily IgG1. Splenic T-cell proliferation was observed in mice immunized orally with *S. typhimurium* pertactin and boosted with only 0.1 μg pertactin, thus demonstrating not only antibody but also T-cell priming by *S. typhimurium* pertactin. Interestingly, the 0.1 μg parenteral boosting dose of pertactin did not generate an immune response in the absence of priming. Ward et al. (1999) have documented similar findings using *S. typhimurium* expressing the C-terminal domain of *Clostridium difficile* toxin A (cytoplasmically). Using *Salmonella*-expressing antigens from *Streptococcus mutans* (Jespersgaard et al. 2001) and *Helicobacter pylori* (Londono-Arcila et al. 2002), other investigators have demonstrated that mucosal prime/parenteral boost results in boosting of systemic responses with good TH1/TH2 balance and boosting of SIGA. The limitations of enteral prime-parenteral boost are yet to be fully delineated, although the data generated thus far suggest that this is a very promising approach to the development of a strong, balanced response to protein antigens.

The immunological basis of the prime-boost phenomenon remains incompletely understood. The priming antigen apparently induces the maturation of antigen-specific T and B cells, some of which will persist and circulate widely as memory cells when the antigen is no longer present. These memory cells will rapidly expand on re-exposure to the same antigen, even if the antigen is given at a site very distant from the initial exposure. The mechanism behind the apparent synergy of prime-boost responses is harder to explain. One hypothesis states that, as prime-boost presents the dominant epitopes in different backgrounds, the immune response is spared the 'noise' of a large array of low-affinity epitopes. This focused response may be optimally vigorous. A second hypothesis suggests that the heterologous prime-boost approach avoids a secondary response to the vector, which some feel may be inhibitory to maximal antigen-specific boosting. Complete understanding of this phenomenon will be a significant contribution to future vaccine development strategies.

CONCLUSIONS

The science of vaccinology has produced some of the most important breakthroughs in the history of medicine. Yet despite our ability to control and even eradicate infections using immunization, limitations and weaknesses remain. Among these are infections so far recalcitrant to immunization strategies, our inability to engender the most appropriate class of immune response, and the need for ever-increasing levels of vaccine safety. In this chapter, we have highlighted just a few of the many new applications of biotechnology to address these problems. These and many other technologies offer hope in providing economically feasible barriers to control some of our most dangerous enemies.

REFERENCES

Abdelhak, S., Louzir, H., et al. 1995. Recombinant BCG expressing the leishmania surface antigen Gp63 induces protective immunity against *Leishmania major* infection in BALB/c mice. *Microbiology*, **141**, Pt 7, 1585–92.

Acheson, D.W., Levine, M.M., et al. 1996. Protective immunity to Shiga-like toxin I following oral immunization with Shiga-like toxin I B-subunit-producing *Vibrio cholerae* CVD 103-HgR. *Infect Immun*, **64**, 355–7.

Aldovini, A. and Young, R.A. 1990. Development of a BCG recombinant vehicle for candidate AIDS vaccines. *Int Rev Immunol*, **7**, 79–83.

Aldovini, A. and Young, R.A. 1991. Humoral and cell-mediated immune responses to live recombinant BCG-HIV vaccines. *Nature*, **351**, 479–82.

Allison, A.C. and Gregoriadis, G. 1976. Liposomes as immunological adjuvants. *Recent Results Cancer Res*, **56**, 58–64.

Allison, A.C. and Gregoriadis, G. 1990. Vaccines: recent trends and progress. *Immunol Today*, **11**, 427–9.

Anderson, R., Dougan, G. and Roberts, M. 1996. Delivery of the Pertactin/P.69 polypeptide of *Bordetella pertussis* using an attenuated

Salmonella typhimurium vaccine strain: expression levels and immune response. *Vaccine*, **14**, 1384–90.

Anderson, R.J., Pasetti, M.F., et al. 2000. DeltaguaBA attenuated *Shigella flexneri* 2a strain CVD 1204 as a *Shigella* vaccine and as a live mucosal delivery system for fragment C of tetanus toxin. *Vaccine*, **18**, 2193–202.

Argentini, C., D'Ugo, E., et al. 1995. Sequence and phylogenetic analysis of the VP1 gene in two cell culture-adapted HAV strains from a unique pathogenic isolate. *Virus Genes*, **10**, 37–43.

Arkema, A., Huckriede, A., et al. 2000. Induction of cytotoxic T lymphocyte activity by fusion-active peptide-containing virosomes. *Vaccine*, **18**, 1327–33.

Ball, J.M., Graham, D.Y., et al. 1999. Recombinant Norwalk virus-like particles given orally to volunteers: phase I study. *Gastroenterology*, **117**, 40–8.

Behr, M.A. and Small, P.M. 1997. Has BCG attenuated to impotence? *Nature*, **389**, 133–4.

Behr, M.A. and Small, P.M. 1999. A historical and molecular phylogeny of BCG strains. *Vaccine*, **17**, 915–22.

Behr, M.A., Wilson, M.A., et al. 1999. Comparative genomics of BCG vaccines by whole-genome DNA microarray. *Science*, **284**, 1520–3.

Benitez, J.A., Garcia, L., et al. 1999. Preliminary assessment of the safety and immunogenicity of a new CTXPhi-negative, hemagglutinin/protease-defective El Tor strain as a cholera vaccine candidate. *Infect Immun*, **67**, 539–45.

Bernardini, M.L., Mounier, J., et al. 1989. Identification of icsA, a plasmid locus of *Shigella flexneri* that governs bacterial intra- and intercellular spread through interaction with F-actin. *Proc Natl Acad Sci USA*, **86**, 3867–71.

Bretscher, P.A. 1992. A strategy to improve the efficacy of vaccination against tuberculosis and leprosy. *Immunol Today*, **13**, 342–5.

Bretscher, P.A. 1994. Prospects for low dose BCG vaccination against tuberculosis. *Immunobiology*, **191**, 548–54.

Bron, R., Ortiz, A., et al. 1993. Preparation, properties, and applications of reconstituted influenza virus envelopes (virosomes). *Methods Enzymol*, **220**, 313–31.

Bron, R., Ortiz, A. and Wilschut, J. 1994. Cellular cytoplasmic delivery of a polypeptide toxin by reconstituted influenza virus envelopes (virosomes). *Biochemistry*, **33**, 9110–17.

Bruna-Romero, O., Gonzalez-Aseguinolaza, G., et al. 2001. Complete, long-lasting protection against malaria of mice primed and boosted with two distinct viral vectors expressing the same plasmodial antigen. *Proc Natl Acad Sci USA*, **98**, 11491–6.

Bungener, L., Huckriede, A., et al. 2002a. Delivery of protein antigens to the immune system by fusion-active virosomes: a comparison with liposomes and ISCOMs. *Biosci Rep*, **22**, 323–38.

Bungener, L., Serre, K., et al. 2002b. Virosome-mediated delivery of protein antigens to dendritic cells. *Vaccine*, **20**, 2287–95.

Butterton, J.R., Beattie, D.T., et al. 1995. Heterologous antigen expression in *Vibrio cholerae* vector strains. *Infect Immun*, **63**, 2689–96.

Butterton, J.R., Ryan, E.T., et al. 1997. Coexpression of the B subunit of Shiga toxin 1 and EaeA from enterohemorrhagic *Escherichia coli* in *Vibrio cholerae* vaccine strains. *Infect Immun*, **65**, 2127–35.

Chen, D., Colditz, I.G., et al. 2002. Effect of transcutaneous immunization with co-administered antigen and cholera toxin on systemic and mucosal antibody responses in sheep. *Vet Immunol Immunopathol*, **86**, 177–82.

Chen, I., Finn, T.M., et al. 1998. A recombinant live attenuated strain of *Vibrio cholerae* induces immunity against tetanus toxin and *Bordetella pertussis* tracheal colonization factor. *Infect Immun*, **66**, 1648–53.

Chen, X.S., Casini, G., et al. 2001. Papillomavirus capsid protein expression in *Escherichia coli*: purification and assembly of HPV11 and HPV16 L1. *J Mol Biol*, **307**, 173–82.

Chow, J.C., Young, D.W., et al. 1999. Toll-like receptor-4 mediates lipopolysaccharide-induced signal transduction. *J Biol Chem*, **274**, 10689–92.

Cohen, J. 1997. Cholera and typhoid vaccine. The current state of play. *Aust Fam Physician*, **26**, 943–6.

Conne, P., Gauthey, L., et al. 1997. Immunogenicity of trivalent subunit versus virosome-formulated influenza vaccines in geriatric patients. *Vaccine*, **15**, 1675–9.

Connell, N.D., Medina-Acosta, E., et al. 1993. Effective immunization against cutaneous leishmaniasis with recombinant bacille Calmette-Guerin expressing the *Leishmania* surface proteinase gp63. *Proc Natl Acad Sci USA*, **90**, 11473–7.

Conradt, P., Hess, J. and Kaufmann, S.H. 1999. Cytolytic T-cell responses to human dendritic cells and macrophages infected with *Mycobacterium bovis* BCG and recombinant BCG secreting listeriolysin. *Microbes Infect*, **1**, 753–64.

Cooney, E.L., McElrath, M.J., et al. 1993. Enhanced immunity to human immunodeficiency virus (HIV) envelope elicited by a combined vaccine regimen consisting of priming with a vaccinia recombinant expressing HIV envelope and boosting with gp160 protein. *Proc Natl Acad Sci USA*, **90**, 1882–6.

Coste, A., Sirard, J.C., et al. 2000. Nasal immunization of mice with virus-like particles protects offspring against rotavirus diarrhea. *J Virol*, **74**, 8966–71.

Coste, A., Cohen, J., et al. 2001. Nasal immunisation with *Salmonella typhimurium* producing rotavirus VP2 and VP6 antigens stimulates specific antibody response in serum and milk but fails to protect offspring. *Vaccine*, **19**, 4167–74.

Coster, T.S., Hoge, C.W., et al. 1999. Vaccination against shigellosis with attenuated *Shigella flexneri* 2a strain SC602. *Infect Immun*, **67**, 3437–43.

Cryz, S.J. Jr., Levine, M.M., et al. 1990. Randomized double-blind placebo controlled trial to evaluate the safety and immunogenicity of the live oral cholera vaccine strain CVD 103-HgR in Swiss adults. *Vaccine*, **8**, 577–80.

Cryz, S.J. Jr., Levine, M.M., et al. 1992. Safety and immunogenicity of a booster dose of Vibrio cholerae CVD 103-HgR live oral cholera vaccine in Swiss adults. *Infect Immun*, **60**, 3916–17.

Cusi, M.G. 2001. The response to plasmid DNA-virosome vaccination: a role for circulating antibodies? *Trends Immunol*, **22**, 355.

Cusi, M.G. and Gluck, R. 2000. Potential of DNA vaccines delivered by influenza virosomes. *Vaccine*, **18**, 1435.

Cusi, M.G., Lomagistro, M.M., et al. 2000. Immunopotentiating of mucosal and systemic antibody responses in mice by intranasal immunization with HLT-combined influenza virosomal vaccine. *Vaccine*, **18**, 2838–42.

Cusi, M.G., Zurbriggen, R., et al. 2002. Influenza virosomes are an efficient delivery system for respiratory syncytial virus-F antigen inducing humoral and cell-mediated immunity. *Vaccine*, **20**, 3436–42.

Dietrich, G., Spreng, S., et al. 2000. Bacterial systems for the delivery of eukaryotic antigen expression vectors. *Antisense Nucleic Acid Drug Dev*, **10**, 391–9.

Dietrich, G., Gentschev, I. and Goebel, W. 2002. Delivery of protein antigens and DNA vaccines by Listeria monocytogenes. In: Goebel, W. (ed.), *Vaccine delivery strategies*. Wymondham: Horizon Scientific Press, 263–88.

Durbin, A., Bourgeois, A., et al., 2001. Intranasal immunization with proteosome-*Shigella flexneri* 2a LPS vaccine: factors associated with protection in a volunteer challenge model. In 39th Annual Meeting of the Infectious Diseases Society of America. San Francisco, CA.

Edelman, R., Palmer, K., et al. 1999. Safety and immunogenicity of recombinant Bacille Calmette–Guerin (rBCG) expressing *Borrelia burgdorferi* outer surface protein A (OspA) lipoprotein in adult volunteers: a candidate Lyme disease vaccine. *Vaccine*, **17**, 904–14.

Evans, T.G., Keefer, M.C., et al. 1999. A canarypox vaccine expressing multiple human immunodeficiency virus type 1 genes given alone or with rgp120 elicits broad and durable CD8+ cytotoxic T lymphocyte responses in seronegative volunteers. *J Infect Dis*, **180**, 290–8.

Evans, T.G., Bonnez, W., et al. 2001. A Phase 1 study of a recombinant viruslike particle vaccine against human papillomavirus type 11 in healthy adult volunteers. *J Infect Dis*, **183**, 1485–93.

Favre, D., Cryz, S.J. Jr. and Viret, J.F. 1996. Development of *Shigella sonnei* live oral vaccines based on defined rfbInaba deletion mutants of *Vibrio cholerae* expressing the Shigella serotype D O polysaccharide. *Infect Immun*, **64**, 576–84.

Fine, P.E. 1989. The BCG story: lessons from the past and implications for the future. *Rev Infect Dis*, **11**, Suppl 2, 353–9.

Fine, P.E. 1995. Variation in protection by BCG: implications of and for heterologous immunity. *Lancet*, **346**, 1339–45.

Fine, P.E. 2001. BCG: the challenge continues. *Scand J Infect Dis*, **33**, 243–5.

Fine, P.E. and Vynnycky, E. 1998. The effect of heterologous immunity upon the apparent efficacy of (e.g. BCG) vaccines. *Vaccine*, **16**, 1923–8.

Finelli, A., Kerksiek, K.M., et al. 1999. MHC class I restricted T cell responses to *Listeria monocytogenes*, an intracellular bacterial pathogen. *Immunol Res*, **19**, 211–23.

Friedman, R.S., Frankel, F.R., et al. 2000. Induction of human immunodeficiency virus (HIV)-specific CD8 T-cell responses by *Listeria monocytogenes* and a hyperattenuated *Listeria* strain engineered to express HIV antigens. *J Virol*, **74**, 9987–93.

Fries, L.F., Montemarano, A.D., et al. 2001. Safety and immunogenicity of a proteosome-*Shigella flexneri* 2a lipopolysaccharide vaccine administered intranasally to healthy adults. *Infect Immun*, **69**, 4545–53.

Galen, J.E. and Levine, M.M. 2001. Can a 'flawless' live vector vaccine strain be engineered? *Trends Microbiol*, **9**, 372–6.

Galen, J.E., Nair, J., et al. 1999. Optimization of plasmid maintenance in the attenuated live vector vaccine strain *Salmonella typhi* CVD 908-htrA. *Infect Immun*, **67**, 6424–33.

Garcon, N.M. and Six, H.R. 1991. Universal vaccine carrier. Liposomes that provide T-dependent help to weak antigens. *J Immunol*, **146**, 3697–702.

Garnier, L., Ravallec, M., et al. 1995. Incorporation of pseudorabies virus gD into human immunodeficiency virus type, 1 Gag particles produced in baculovirus-infected cells. *J Virol*, **69**, 4060–8.

Gentschev, I., Dietrich, G., et al. 2000. Delivery of protein antigens and DNA by virulence-attenuated strains of *Salmonella typhimurium* and *Listeria monocytogenes*. *J Biotechnol*, **83**, 19–26.

Gentschev, I., Dietrich, G., et al. 2001. Recombinant attenuated bacteria for the delivery of subunit vaccines. *Vaccine*, **19**, 2621–8.

Gentschev, I., Dietrich, G., et al. 2002. Delivery of protein antigens and DNA by attenuated intracellular bacteria. *Int J Med Microbiol*, **291**, 577–82.

Gerber, S., Lane, C., et al. 2001. Human papillomavirus virus-like particles are efficient oral immunogens when coadministered with *Escherichia coli* heat-labile enterotoxin mutant R192G or CpG DNA. *J Virol*, **75**, 4752–60.

Germanier, R. and Fuer, E. 1975. Isolation and characterization of Gal E mutant Ty 21a of *Salmonella typhi*: a candidate strain for a live, oral typhoid vaccine. *J Infect Dis*, **131**, 553–8.

Glenn, G.M., Scharton-Kersten, T., et al. 1998. Transcutaneous immunization with cholera toxin protects mice against lethal mucosal toxin challenge. *J Immunol*, **161**, 3211–14.

Glenn, G.M., Scharton-Kersten, T., et al. 1999. Transcutaneous immunization with bacterial ADP-ribosylating exotoxins as antigens and adjuvants. *Infect Immun*, **67**, 1100–6.

Gluck, R. 1995. Liposomal presentation of antigens for human vaccines. *Pharm Biotechnol*, **6**, 325–45.

Gluck, R., Mischler, R., et al. 1992. Immunopotentiating reconstituted influenza virus virosome vaccine delivery system for immunization against hepatitis A. *J Clin Invest*, **90**, 2491–5.

Gluck, R., Mischler, R., et al. 1994. Immunogenicity of new virosome influenza vaccine in elderly people. *Lancet*, **344**, 160–3.

Gluck, R., Mischler, R., et al. 2000. Safety and immunogenicity of intranasally administered inactivated trivalent virosome-formulated influenza vaccine containing *Escherichia coli* heat-labile toxin as a mucosal adjuvant. *J Infect Dis*, **181**, 1129–32.

Goldmann, C., Petry, H., et al. 1999. Molecular cloning and expression of major structural protein VP1 of the human polyomavirus JC virus: formation of virus-like particles useful for immunological and therapeutic studies. *J Virol*, **73**, 4465–9.

Gonzalez, C., Hone, D., et al. 1994. Salmonella typhi vaccine strain CVD, 908 expressing the circumsporozoite protein of *Plasmodium falciparum*: strain construction and safety and immunogenicity in humans. *J Infect Dis*, **169**, 927–31.

Gotuzzo, E., Butron, B., et al. 1993. Safety, immunogenicity, and excretion pattern of single-dose live oral cholera vaccine CVD 103-HgR in Peruvian adults of high and low socio-economic levels. *Infect Immun*, **61**, 3994–7.

Graham, B.S., Matthews, T.J., et al. 1993. Augmentation of human immunodeficiency virus type, 1 neutralizing antibody by priming with gp160 recombinant vaccinia and boosting with rgp160 in vaccinia-naive adults. The NIAID AIDS Vaccine Clinical Trials Network. *J Infect Dis*, **167**, 533–7.

Gregoriadis, G. 1990. Immunological adjuvants: a role for liposomes. *Immunol Today*, **11**, 89–97.

Gregoriadis, G. and Allison, A.C. 1974. Entrapment of proteins in liposomes prevents allergic reactions in pre-immunised mice. *FEBS Lett*, **45**, 71–4.

Guerena-Burgueno, F., Hall, E.R., et al. 2002. Safety and immunogenicity of a prototype enterotoxigenic *Escherichia coli* vaccine administered transcutaneously. *Infect Immun*, **70**, 1874–80.

Halperin, S., McNeil, S., et al., 2002. Phase 1 safety and immunogenicity of FluINsure, proteosome trivalent influenza vaccine, given nasally to adults. The 42nd Interscience conference on antimicrobial agents and chemotherapy, San Diego, CA.

Hammond, S.A., Guebre-Xabier, M., et al. 2001a. Transcutaneous immunization: an emerging route of immunization and potent immunostimulation strategy. *Crit Rev Ther Drug Carrier Syst*, **18**, 503–26.

Hammond, S.A., Walwender, D., et al. 2001b. Transcutaneous immunization: T cell responses and boosting of existing immunity. *Vaccine*, **19**, 2701–7.

Harro, C.D., Pang, Y.Y., et al. 2001. Safety and immunogenicity trial in adult volunteers of a human papillomavirus 16 L1 virus-like particle vaccine. *J Natl Cancer Inst*, **93**, 284–92.

Heath, P.T. 1998. *Haemophilus influenzae* type b conjugate vaccines: a review of efficacy data. *Pediatr Infect Dis J*, **17**, S117–22.

Herremans, T.M., Reimerink, J.H., et al. 1999. Induction of mucosal immunity by inactivated poliovirus vaccine is dependent on previous mucosal contact with live virus. *J Immunol*, **162**, 5011–18.

Herzog, C., Wegmuller, B. and Cryz, S.J. 1997. Live oral cholera vaccine. *Lancet*, **349**, 1772–3.

Herzog, C., Metcalfe, I.C. and Schaad, U.B. 2002. Virosome influenza vaccine in children. *Vaccine*, **20**, Suppl, B24–8.

Hess, J. 2002. Live mycobacterial vaccine candidates. In: Goebel, W. (ed.), *Vaccine delivery strategies*. Wymondham: Horizon Scientific Press, 245–62.

Hess, J., Miko, D., et al. 1998. Mycobacterium bovis Bacille Calmette–Guerin strains secreting listeriolysin of *Listeria monocytogenes*. *Proc Natl Acad Sci USA*, **95**, 5299–304.

Hill, A.V., Reece, W., et al. 2000. DNA-based vaccines for malaria: a heterologous prime-boost immunisation strategy. *Dev Biol (Basel)*, **104**, 171–9.

Hindle, Z., Chatfield, S.N., et al. 2002. Characterization of *Salmonella enterica* derivatives harboring defined aroC and Salmonella pathogenicity island 2 type III secretion system (ssaV) mutations by immunization of healthy volunteers. *Infect Immun*, **70**, 3457–67.

Hohmann, E.L., Oletta, C.A., et al. 1996. phoP/phoQ-deleted *Salmonella typhi* (Ty800) is a safe and immunogenic single-dose typhoid fever vaccine in volunteers. *J Infect Dis*, **173**, 1408–14.

Hoiseth, S.K. and Stocker, B.A. 1981. Aromatic-dependent *Salmonella typhimurium* are non-virulent and effective as live vaccines. *Nature*, **291**, 238–9.

Hone, D.M., Harris, A.M., et al. 1991. Construction of genetically defined double aro mutants of *Salmonella typhi*. *Vaccine*, **9**, 810–16.

Hunziker, I.P., Grabscheid, B., et al. 2002. In vitro studies of core peptide-bearing immunopotentiating reconstituted influenza virosomes as a non-live prototype vaccine against hepatitis C virus. *Int Immunol*, **14**, 615–26.

Ikonomidis, G., Paterson, Y., et al. 1994. Delivery of a viral antigen to the class I processing and presentation pathway by *Listeria monocytogenes*. *J Exp Med*, **180**, 2209–18.

Inaba, K., Inaba, M., et al. 1993. Dendritic cell progenitors phagocytose particulates, including bacillus Calmette–Guerin organisms, and sensitize mice to mycobacterial antigens in vivo. *J Exp Med*, **178**, 479–88.

Jabbar, I.A., Fernando, G.J., et al. 2000. Immune responses induced by BCG recombinant for human papillomavirus L1 and E7 proteins. *Vaccine*, **18**, 2444–53.

Jespersgaard, C., Zhang, P., et al. 2001. Effect of attenuated *Salmonella enterica* serovar Typhimurium expressing a *Streptococcus mutans* antigen on secondary responses to the cloned protein. *Infect Immun*, **69**, 6604–11.

Jiang, B., Estes, M.K., et al. 1999. Heterotypic protection from rotavirus infection in mice vaccinated with virus-like particles. *Vaccine*, **17**, 1005–13.

John, M., Bridges, E.A., et al. 2002. Comparison of mucosal and systemic humoral immune responses after transcutaneous and oral immunization strategies. *Vaccine*, **20**, 2720–6.

Jones, T.R., Narum, D.L., et al. 2001. Protection of *Aotus* monkeys by *Plasmodium falciparum* EBA-175 region II DNA prime-protein boost immunization regimen. *J Infect Dis*, **183**, 303–12.

Kaiserlian, D. and Etchart, N. 1999. Epicutaneous and transcutaneous immunization using DNA or proteins. *Eur J Dermatol*, **9**, 169–76.

Kaji, M., Kaji, Y., et al. 1992. Phase, 1 clinical tests of influenza MDP-virosome vaccine (KD-5382). *Vaccine*, **10**, 663–7.

Kaneda, Y. 2000. Virosomes: evolution of the liposome as a targeted drug delivery system. *Adv Drug Deliv Rev*, **43**, 197–205.

Kaper, J.B., Morris, J.G. Jr. and Levine, M.M. 1995. Cholera. *Clin Microbiol Rev*, **8**, 48–86.

Kaufmann, S.H. and Ladel, C.H. 1994. Role of T cell subsets in immunity against intracellular bacteria: experimental infections of knock-out mice with *Listeria monocytogenes* and *Mycobacterium bovis* BCG. *Immunobiology*, **191**, 509–19.

Kaufmann, S.H., Ladel, C.H. and Flesch, I.E. 1995. T cells and cytokines in intracellular bacterial infections: experiences with *Mycobacterium bovis* BCG. *Ciba Found Symp*, **195**, 123–32, discussion 132-6.

Kent, S.J., Zhao, A., et al. 1998. Enhanced T-cell immunogenicity and protective efficacy of a human immunodeficiency virus type 1 vaccine regimen consisting of consecutive priming with DNA and boosting with recombinant fowlpox virus. *J Virol*, **72**, 10180–8.

Kerksiek, K.M. and Pamer, E.G. 1999. T cell responses to bacterial infection. *Curr Opin Immunol*, **11**, 400–45.

Khan, S.A., Stratford, R., et al. 2003. *Salmonella typhi* and *S. typhimurium* derivatives harbouring deletions in aromatic biosynthesis and Salmonella Pathogenicity Island-2 (SPI-2) genes as vaccines and vectors. *Vaccine*, **21**, 538–48.

Kingsley, R.A. and Baumler, A.J. 2000. Salmonella interactions with professional phagocytes. *Subcell Biochem*, **33**, 321–42.

Koletzki, D., Lundkvist, A., et al. 2000. Puumala (PUU) hantavirus strain differences and insertion positions in the hepatitis B virus core antigen influence B-cell immunogenicity and protective potential of core-derived particles. *Virology*, **276**, 364–75.

Kotloff, K.L., Wasserman, S.S., et al. 1992. Safety and immunogenicity in North Americans of a single dose of live oral cholera vaccine CVD 103-HgR: results of a randomized, placebo-controlled, double-blind crossover trial. *Infect Immun*, **60**, 4430–2.

Kotloff, K.L., Noriega, F., et al. 1996. Safety, immunogenicity, and transmissibility in humans of CVD 1203, a live oral *Shigella flexneri* 2a vaccine candidate attenuated by deletions in aroA and virG. *Infect Immun*, **64**, 4542–8.

Kotloff, K.L., Noriega, F.R., et al. 2000. *Shigella flexneri* 2a strain CVD, 1207, with specific deletions in virG, sen, set, and guaBA, is highly attenuated in humans. *Infect Immun*, **68**, 1034–9.

Kotloff, K.L., Taylor, D.N., et al. 2002. Phase I evaluation of delta virG *Shigella sonnei* live, attenuated, oral vaccine strain WRSS1 in healthy adults. *Infect Immun*, **70**, 2016–21.

Kremer, L., Riveau, G., et al. 1996. Neutralizing antibody responses elicited in mice immunized with recombinant bacillus Calmette-Guerin producing the *Schistosoma mansoni* glutathione S-transferase. *J Immunol*, **156**, 4309–417.

Kruger, D.H., Ulrich, R. and Gerlich, W.H. 1999. Chimeric virus-like particles as vaccines. *Biol Chem*, **380**, 275–6.

Ladel, C.H., Daugelat, S. and Kaufmann, S.H. 1995a. Immune response to *Mycobacterium bovis* bacille Calmette Guerin infection in major histocompatibility complex class I- and II-deficient knock-out mice: contribution of CD4 and CD8 T cells to acquired resistance. *Eur J Immunol*, **25**, 377–84.

Ladel, C.H., Hess, J., et al. 1995b. Contribution of alpha/beta and gamma/delta T lymphocytes to immunity against *Mycobacterium bovis* bacillus Calmette Guerin: studies with T cell receptor-deficient mutant mice. *Eur J Immunol*, **25**, 838–46.

Lagos, R., Avendano, A., et al. 1995. Attenuated live cholera vaccine strain CVD 103-HgR elicits significantly higher serum vibriocidal antibody titers in persons of blood group O. *Infect Immun*, **63**, 707–9.

Lagos, R., Fasano, A., et al. 1999a. Effect of small bowel bacterial overgrowth on the immunogenicity of single-dose live oral cholera vaccine CVD 103-HgR. *J Infect Dis*, **180**, 1709–12.

Lagos, R., San Martin, O., et al. 1999b. Palatability, reactogenicity and immunogenicity of engineered live oral cholera vaccine CVD 103-HgR in Chilean infants and toddlers. *Pediatr Infect Dis J*, **18**, 624–30.

Langermann, S., Palaszynski, S., et al. 1994a. Systemic and mucosal immunity induced by BCG vector expressing outer-surface protein A of *Borrelia burgdorferi*. *Nature*, **372**, 552–5.

Langermann, S., Palaszynski, S.R., et al. 1994b. Protective humoral response against pneumococcal infection in mice elicited by recombinant bacille Calmette-Guerin vaccines expressing pneumococcal surface protein A. *J Exp Med*, **180**, 2277–86.

Latham, T. and Galarza, J.M. 2001. Formation of wild-type and chimeric influenza virus-like particles following simultaneous expression of only four structural proteins. *J Virol*, **75**, 6154–65.

Levine, M.M. 2000. Immunization against bacterial diseases of the intestine. *J Pediatr Gastroenterol Nutr*, **31**, 336–55.

Levine, M.M., Kaper, J.B., 1988. Safety, immunogenicity, and efficacy of recombinant live oral cholera vaccines, CVD, 103 and CVD, 103-HgR. *Lancet*, **ii**, 467–70.

Levine, M.M., Ferreccio, C., et al. 1990. Comparison of enteric-coated capsules and liquid formulation of Ty21a typhoid vaccine in randomised controlled field trial. *Lancet*, **336**, 891–4.

Levine, M.M., Galen, J., et al. 1996. Attenuated Salmonella as live oral vaccines against typhoid fever and as live vectors. *J Biotechnol*, **44**, 193–6.

Levine, M.M., Galen, J., et al. 1997. Attenuated *Salmonella typhi* and *Shigella* as live oral vaccines and as live vectors. *Behring Inst Mitt*, 120–3.

Li, S., Rodrigues, M., et al. 1993. Priming with recombinant influenza virus followed by administration of recombinant vaccinia virus induces CD8+ T-cell-mediated protective immunity against malaria. *Proc Natl Acad Sci USA*, **90**, 5214–18.

Li, T.C., Yamakawa, Y., et al. 1997. Expression and self-assembly of empty virus-like particles of hepatitis E virus. *J Virol*, **71**, 7207–13.

Liu, Y.Q., Qi, G.M., et al. 1995. A natural vaccine candidate strain against cholera. *Biomed Environ Sci*, **8**, 350–8.

Lo-Man, R., Rueda, P., et al. 1998. A recombinant virus-like particle system derived from parvovirus as an efficient antigen carrier to elicit a polarized Th1 immune response without adjuvant. *Eur J Immunol*, **28**, 1401–7.

Londono-Arcila, P., Freeman, D., et al. 2002. Attenuated *Salmonella enterica* serovar *Typhi* expressing urease effectively immunizes mice against *Helicobacter pylori* challenge as part of a heterologous mucosal priming-parenteral boosting vaccination regimen. *Infect Immun*, **70**, 5096–106.

Lorenzo, L.J., Duenas-Carrera, S., et al. 2001. Assembly of truncated HCV core antigen into virus-like particles in *Escherichia coli*. *Biochem Biophys Res Commun*, **281**, 962–5.

Losonsky, G.A., Tacket, C.O., et al. 1993. Secondary *Vibrio cholerae*-specific cellular antibody responses following wild-type homologous challenge in people vaccinated with CVD, 103-HgR live oral cholera vaccine: changes with time and lack of correlation with protection. *Infect Immun*, **61**, 729–33.

Losonsky, G.A., Lim, Y., et al. 1997. Vibriocidal antibody responses in North American volunteers exposed to wild-type or vaccine *Vibrio cholerae* O139: specificity and relevance to immunity. *Clin Diagn Lab Immunol*, **4**, 264–9.

Loutan, L., Bovier, P., et al. 1994. Inactivated virosome hepatitis A vaccine. *Lancet*, **343**, 322–4.

Lowell, G.H., Ballou, W.R., et al. 1988a. Proteosome-lipopeptide vaccines: enhancement of immunogenicity for malaria CS peptides. *Science*, **240**, 800–2.

Lowell, G.H., Smith, L.F., et al. 1988b. Peptides bound to proteosomes via hydrophobic feet become highly immunogenic without adjuvants. *J Exp Med*, **167**, 658–63.

McKenzie, R., Durbin, A., et al. 2001. Safety and immunogenicity of an intranasal vaccine for *Shigella flexneri*. In 39th Annual Meeting of the Infectious Diseases Society of America. San Francisco, CA.

McKenzie, R., Baqar, S., et al. 2002. A Phase 1 study of the safety and immunogenicity of two attenuated *Salmonella typhi* vectors expressing the urease vaccine antigen of *H. pylori*. In 102nd General Meeting of the American Society for Microbiology, Salt Lake City, UT, E-45.

Massari, P., Henneke, P., et al. 2002. Cutting edge: Immune stimulation by neisserial porins is toll-like receptor 2 and MyD88 dependent. *J Immunol*, **168**, 1533–7.

Medaglini, D., Pozzi, G., et al. 1995. Mucosal and systemic immune responses to a recombinant protein expressed on the surface of the oral commensal bacterium *Streptococcus gordonii* after oral colonization. *Proc Natl Acad Sci SA*, **92**, 6868–72.

Medina, E. and Guzman, C.A. 2001. Use of live bacterial vaccine vectors for antigen delivery: potential and limitations. *Vaccine*, **19**, 1573–80.

Mengiardi, B., Berger, R., et al. 1995. Virosomes as carriers for combined vaccines. *Vaccine*, **13**, 1306–15.

Migasena, S., Pitisuttitham, P., et al. 1989. Preliminary assessment of the safety and immunogenicity of live oral cholera vaccine strain CVD 103-HgR in healthy Thai adults. *Infect Immun*, **57**, 3261–4.

Miller, M.D., Gould-Fogerite, S., et al. 1992. Vaccination of rhesus monkeys with synthetic peptide in a fusogenic proteoliposome elicits simian immunodeficiency virus-specific CD8+ cytotoxic T lymphocytes. *J Exp Med*, **176**, 1739–44.

Miyaji, E.N., Dias, W.O., et al. 2001. PsaA (pneumococcal surface adhesin A) and PspA (pneumococcal surface protein A) DNA vaccines induce humoral and cellular immune responses against *Streptococcus pneumoniae*. *Vaccine*, **20**, 805–12.

Nagesha, H.S., Wang, L.F. and Hyatt, A.D. 1999. Virus-like particles of calicivirus as epitope carriers. *Arch Virol*, **144**, 2429–39.

Nascimento, I.P., Dias, W.O., et al. 2000. Recombinant Mycobacterium bovis BCG expressing pertussis toxin subunit S1 induces protection against an intracerebral challenge with live *Bordetella pertussis* in mice. *Infect Immun*, **68**, 4877–83.

Nerome, K., Yoshioka, Y., et al. 1990. Development of a new type of influenza subunit vaccine made by muramyldipeptide-liposome: enhancement of humoral and cellular immune responses. *Vaccine*, **8**, 503–9.

Noriega, F.R., Wang, J.Y., et al. 1994. Construction and characterization of attenuated delta aroA delta virG *Shigella flexneri* 2a strain CVD 1203, a prototype live oral vaccine. *Infect Immun*, **62**, 5168–72.

O'Brien, G.J., Bryant, C.J., et al. 2000. Rotavirus VP6 expressed by PVX vectors in *Nicotiana benthamiana* coats PVX rods and also assembles into virus-like particles. *Virology*, **270**, 444–53.

Ochsenbein, A.F., Karrer, U., et al. 1999. A comparison of T cell memory against the same antigen induced by virus versus intracellular bacteria. *Proc Natl Acad Sci USA*, **96**, 9293–8.

O'Neal, C.M., Clements, J.D., et al. 1998. Rotavirus 2/6 virus-like particles administered intranasally with cholera toxin, *Escherichia coli* heat-labile toxin (LT) and LT-R192G induce protection from rotavirus challenge. *J Virol*, **72**, 3390–3.

O'Riordan, M., Yi, C.H., et al. 2002. Innate recognition of bacteria by a macrophage cytosolic surveillance pathway. *Proc Natl Acad Sci USA*, **99**, 13861–6.

Pallen, M.J. and Wren, B.W. 1997. The HtrA family of serine proteases. *Mol Microbiol*, **26**, 209–21.

Perry, R.T., Plowe, C.V., et al. 1998. A single dose of live oral cholera vaccine CVD 103-HgR is safe and immunogenic in HIV-infected and HIV-noninfected adults in Mali. *Bull World Health Organ*, **76**, 63–71.

Peters, B.S., Cheingsong-Popov, R., et al. 1997. A pilot phase II study of the safety and immunogenicity of HIV p17/p24:VLP (p24-VLP) in asymptomatic HIV seropositive subjects. *J Infect*, **35**, 231–5.

Plante, M., Jones, T., et al. 2001. Nasal immunization with subunit proteosome influenza vaccines induces serum HAI, mucosal IgA and protection against influenza challenge. *Vaccine*, **20**, 218–25.

Poltl-Frank, F., Zurbriggen, R., et al. 1999. Use of reconstituted influenza virus virosomes as an immunopotentiating delivery system for a peptide-based vaccine. *Clin Exp Immunol*, **117**, 496–503.

Portnoy, D.A., Schreiber, R.D., et al. 1989. Gamma interferon limits access of *Listeria monocytogenes* to the macrophage cytoplasm. *J Exp Med*, **170**, 2141–6.

Portnoy, D.A., Auerbuch, V. and Glomski, I.J. 2002. The cell biology of *Listeria monocytogenes* infection: the intersection of bacterial pathogenesis and cell-mediated immunity. *J Cell Biol*, **158**, 409–14.

Power, C.A., Wei, G. and Bretscher, P.A. 1998. Mycobacterial dose defines the Th1/Th2 nature of the immune response independently of whether immunization is administered by the intravenous, subcutaneous, or intradermal route. *Infect Immun*, **66**, 5743–50.

Pumpens, P., Razanskas, R., et al. 2002. Evaluation of HBs, HBc, and frCP virus-like particles for expression of human papillomavirus 16 E7 oncoprotein epitopes. *Intervirology*, **45**, 24–32.

Richie, E.E., Punjabi, N.H., et al. 2000. Efficacy trial of single-dose live oral cholera vaccine CVD 103-HgR in North Jakarta, Indonesia, a cholera-endemic area. *Vaccine*, **18**, 2399–410.

Robinson, H.L., Montefiori, D.C., et al. 1999. Neutralizing antibody-independent containment of immunodeficiency virus challenges by DNA priming and recombinant pox virus booster immunizations. *Nat Med*, **5**, 526–34.

Robinson, H.L., Montefiori, D.C., et al. 2000. DNA priming and recombinant pox virus boosters for an AIDS vaccine. *Dev Biol (Basel)*, **104**, 93–100.

Rogers, W.O., Baird, J.K., et al. 2001. Multistage multiantigen heterologous prime boost vaccine for *Plasmodium knowlesi* malaria provides partial protection in rhesus macaques. *Infect Immun*, **69**, 5565–72.

Ryan, E.T., Butterton, J.R., et al. 1997a. Protective immunity against *Clostridium difficile* toxin A induced by oral immunization with a live, attenuated *Vibrio cholerae* vector strain. *Infect Immun*, **65**, 2941–9.

Ryan, E.T., Butterton, J.R., et al. 1997b. Oral immunization with attenuated vaccine strains of *Vibrio cholerae* expressing a dodecapeptide repeat of the serine-rich *Entamoeba histolytica* protein fused to the cholera toxin B subunit induces systemic and mucosal antiamebic and anti-*V. cholerae* antibody responses in mice. *Infect Immun*, **65**, 3118–25.

Sack, D.A., Sack, R.B., et al. 1997. Evaluation of Peru-15, a new live oral vaccine for cholera, in volunteers. *J Infect Dis*, **176**, 201–5.

Sack, R.B. and Albert, M.J. 1994. Summary of cholera vaccine workshop. *J Diarrhoeal Dis Res*, **12**, 138–43.

Sansonetti, P.J. and Arondel, J. 1989. Construction and evaluation of a double mutant of *Shigella flexneri* as a candidate for oral vaccination against shigellosis. *Vaccine*, **7**, 443–50.

Sansonetti, P.J., Arondel, J., et al. 1991. OmpB (osmo-regulation) and icsA (cell-to-cell spread) mutants of *Shigella flexneri*: vaccine candidates and probes to study the pathogenesis of shigellosis. *Vaccine*, **9**, 416–22.

Santos, R.L., Tsolis, R.M., et al. 2003. Pathogenesis of *Salmonella*-induced enteritis. *Braz J Med Biol Res*, **36**, 3–12.

Sasnauskas, K., Buzaite, O., et al. 1999. Yeast cells allow high-level expression and formation of polyomavirus-like particles. *Biol Chem*, **380**, 381–6.

Schaad, U.B., Buhlmann, U., et al. 2000. Comparison of immunogenicity and safety of a virosome influenza vaccine with those of a subunit influenza vaccine in pediatric patients with cystic fibrosis. *Antimicrob Agents Chemother*, **44**, 1163–7.

Schafer, R., Portnoy, D.A., et al. 1992. Induction of a cellular immune response to a foreign antigen by a recombinant *Listeria monocytogenes* vaccine. *J Immunol*, **149**, 53–9.

Scharton-Kersten, T., Glenn, G.M., et al. 1999. Principles of transcutaneous immunization using cholera toxin as an adjuvant. *Vaccine*, **17**, Suppl 2, S37–43.

Scharton-Kersten, T., Yu, J., et al. 2000. Transcutaneous immunization with bacterial ADP-ribosylating exotoxins, subunits, and unrelated adjuvants. *Infect Immun*, **68**, 5306–13.

Schiller, J. and Lowy, D. 2001a. Papillomavirus-like particle vaccines. *J Natl Cancer Inst Monogr*, **28**, 50–4.

Schiller, J.T. and Lowy, D.R. 2001b. Papillomavirus-like particle based vaccines: cervical cancer and beyond. *Expert Opin Biol Ther*, **1**, 571–81.

Schneider, J., Langermans, J.A., et al. 2001. A prime-boost immunisation regimen using DNA followed by recombinant modified vaccinia virus Ankara induces strong cellular immune responses against the *Plasmodium falciparum* TRAP antigen in chimpanzees. *Vaccine*, **19**, 4595–602.

Sedlik, C., Saron, M., et al. 1997. Recombinant parvovirus-like particles as an antigen carrier: a novel nonreplicative exogenous antigen to elicit protective antiviral cytotoxic T cells. *Proc Natl Acad Sci USA*, **94**, 7503–8.

Sedlik, C., Dridi, A., et al. 1999. Intranasal delivery of recombinant parvovirus-like particles elicits cytotoxic T-cell and neutralizing antibody responses. *J Virol*, **73**, 2739–44.

Sedlik, C., Dadaglio, G., et al. 2000. In vivo induction of a high-avidity, high-frequency cytotoxic T-lymphocyte response is associated with antiviral protective immunity. *J Virol*, **74**, 5769–75.

Siadat-Pajouh, M. and Cai, L. 2001. Protective efficacy of rotavirus 2/6-virus-like particles combined with CT-E29H, a detoxified cholera toxin adjuvant. *Viral Immunol*, **14**, 31–47.

Simanjuntak, C.H., O'Hanley, P., et al. 1993. Safety, immunogenicity, and transmissibility of single-dose live oral cholera vaccine strain CVD 103-HgR in 24- to 59-month-old Indonesian children. *J Infect Dis*, **168**, 1169–76.

Soussi, N., Saklani-Jusforgues, H., et al. 2002. Effect of intragastric and intraperitoneal immunisation with attenuated and wild-type LACK-expressing *Listeria monocytogenes* on control of murine *Leishmania major* infection. *Vaccine*, **20**, 2702–12.

Spreng, S., Dietrich, G., et al. 2000. Novel bacterial systems for the delivery of recombinant protein or DNA. *FEMS Immunol Med Microbiol*, **27**, 299–304.

Stover, C.K., Bansal, G.P., et al. 1993. Protective immunity elicited by recombinant bacille Calmette–Guerin (BCG) expressing outer surface protein A (OspA) lipoprotein: a candidate Lyme disease vaccine. *J Exp Med*, **178**, 197–209.

Su-Arehawaratana, P., Singharaj, P., et al. 1992. Safety and immunogenicity of different immunization regimens of CVD 103-HgR live oral cholera vaccine in soldiers and civilians in Thailand. *J Infect Dis*, **165**, 1042–8.

Suharyono, Simanjuntak, C., et al. 1992. Safety and immunogenicity of single-dose live oral cholera vaccine CVD 103-HgR in 5–9-year-old Indonesian children. *Lancet*, **340**, 689–94.

Tacket, C.O., Hone, D.M., et al. 1992a. Comparison of the safety and immunogenicity of delta aroC delta aroD and delta cya delta crp *Salmonella typhi* strains in adult volunteers. *Infect Immun*, **60**, 536–41.

Tacket, C.O., Losonsky, G., et al. 1992b. Onset and duration of protective immunity in challenged volunteers after vaccination with live oral cholera vaccine CVD 103-HgR. *J Infect Dis*, **166**, 837–41.

Tacket, C.O., Sztein, M.B., et al. 1997. Safety of live oral *Salmonella typhi* vaccine strains with deletions in htrA and aroC aroD and immune response in humans. *Infect Immun*, **65**, 452–6.

Tacket, C.O., Cohen, M.B., et al. 1999. Randomized, double-blind, placebo-controlled, multicentered trial of the efficacy of a single dose of live oral cholera vaccine CVD 103-HgR in preventing cholera following challenge with *Vibrio cholerae* O1 El tor inaba three months after vaccination. *Infect Immun*, **67**, 6341–5.

Tacket, C.O., Galen, J., et al. 2000a. Safety and immune responses to attenuated *Salmonella enterica* serovar typhi oral live vector vaccines expressing tetanus toxin fragment C. *Clin Immunol*, **97**, 146–53.

Tacket, C.O., Sztein, M.B., et al. 2000b. Phase 2 clinical trial of attenuated *Salmonella enterica* serovar typhi oral live vector vaccine CVD, 908-htrA in U.S. volunteers. *Infect Immun*, **68**, 1196–201.

Tacket, C.O., Sztein, M.B., et al. 2003. Humoral, mucosal, and cellular immune responses to oral Norwalk virus-like particles in volunteers. *Clin Immunol*, **108**, 241–7.

Tan, L.S. and Gregoriadis, G. 1990. A simple method for coating of liposomes with proteins. *Ann Acad Med Sing*, **19**, 827–30.

Taylor, D.N., Killeen, K.P., et al. 1994. Development of a live, oral, attenuated vaccine against El Tor cholera. *J Infect Dis*, **170**, 1518–23.

Taylor, D.N., Sanchez, J.L., et al. 1999. Expanded safety and immunogenicity of a bivalent, oral, attenuated cholera vaccine, CVD 103-HgR plus CVD 111, in United States military personnel stationed in Panama. *Infect Immun*, **67**, 2030–4.

Treanor, J., Burt, D., et al. 2001. Evaluation of an intranasal proteosome-influenza vaccine in health adults. In 4th Annual National Foundation of Infectious Diseases Conference on Vaccine Research, Arlington, VA.

Valle, E., Ledon, T., et al. 2000. Construction and characterization of a nonproliferative El Tor cholera vaccine candidate derived from strain 638. *Infect Immun*, **68**, 6411–18.

Ward, S.J., Douce, G., et al. 1999. Immunogenicity of a *Salmonella typhimurium* aroA aroD vaccine expressing a nontoxic domain of *Clostridium difficile* toxin A. *Infect Immun*, **67**, 2145–52.

Watanabe, T., Watanabe, S., et al. 2002. Immunogenicity and protective efficacy of replication-incompetent influenza virus-like particles. *J Virol*, **76**, 767–73.

Weber, J., Cheinsong-Popov, R., et al. 1995. Immunogenicity of the yeast recombinant p17/p24:Ty virus-like particles (p24-VLP) in healthy volunteers. *Vaccine*, **13**, 831–4.

Wetzler, L.M. 1994. Immunopotentiating ability of neisserial major outer membrane proteins. Use as an adjuvant for poorly immunogenic substances and potential use in vaccines. *Ann NY Acad Sci*, **730**, 367–70.

Wetzler, L.M., Blake, M.S. and Gotschlich, E.C. 1989. Protein I (Por) of *Neisseria gonorrhoeae* as an immunogen: liposomes, proteosomes, and the lack of blocking antibodies. *Trans Assoc Am Physicians*, **102**, 78–90.

Wetzler, L.M., Blake, M.S., et al. 1992. Gonococcal porin vaccine evaluation: comparison of Por proteosomes, liposomes, and blebs isolated from rmp deletion mutants. *J Infect Dis*, **166**, 551–5.

Yamamoto, T. 2000. Current status of cholera and rise of novel mucosal vaccine. *Jpn J Infect Dis*, **53**, 181–8.

Yu, J., Cassels, F., et al. 2002. Transcutaneous immunization using colonization factor and heat-labile enterotoxin induces correlates of protective immunity for enterotoxigenic *Escherichia coli*. *Infect Immun*, **70**, 1056–68.

Zhang, L.F., Zhou, J., et al. 2000. HPV6b virus like particles are potent immunogens without adjuvant in man. *Vaccine*, **18**, 1051–8.

Zhang, S., Kingsley, R.A., et al. 2003. Molecular pathogenesis of *Salmonella enterica* serotype typhimurium-induced diarrhea. *Infect Immun*, **71**, 1–12.

42

Peptide vaccines

CLAUDE P. MULLER AND MIKE M. PUTZ

INTRODUCTION

For several decades synthetic peptides have been extremely valuable tools for dissecting the immune response to complex antigens and pathogens on an epitope level. Peptides as antigens have been extensively reviewed (Van Regenmortel and Muller 1999). Vaccines based on synthetic peptides or defined epitopes have met considerable interest and high expectations. A large number of vaccines have been tested in clinical trials and even more in animal models, but so far none has been licensed. This chapter is an attempt to present the current status of the vast field of experimental or candidate vaccines based on synthetic peptides. Much of what can be said about peptide vaccines applies also to other epitope-based strategies, but these are beyond the scope of this review. We acknowledge that such a review can never be complete and is necessarily biased toward the authors' experience – or the lack of it.

T- AND B-CELL EPITOPES

Sequence and post-translational modifications provide a protein with a unique three-dimensional surface architecture, which is the basis of cognate interactions with its molecular partners. The unique surface structure is exploited by the immune system to recognize antigens and to discriminate between self and nonself. Complementary domains, epitopes, and paratopes of antigens and antibodies are the minimal cognate structures (Jerne 1960), and the basis of the primordial intelligence that drives the teleological choices of the immune system, first at the induction stage and again at the effector stage of the immune response (Muller 2001b). T and B cells recognize epitopes and antigens in fundamentally different ways. Although B cells bind to intact antigens, T cells recognize only processed antigens presented as peptides by molecules of the major histocompatibility complex (MHC) of antigen presenting cells. Over the past years, both T-cell epitopes (TCE) and B-cell epitopes (BCE) have been identified in most antigens. Peptides have been used as minimal surrogate antigens to induce a prophylactic or therapeutic T- and/or B-cell response against pathogens, tumors, and other diseases.

PEPTIDE VACCINES BASED ON B-CELL EPITOPES

Conformational and sequential BCEs

The antibody paratope recognizes the congruent and complementary epitope of the antigen in its native, unprocessed, three-dimensional conformation. Complementary features of epitope and paratope converge to form relatively flat, bumpy surfaces of several square nanometers in size covering only a fraction of the solvent accessible surface of the antigen. Seminal radiological studies with hen egg lysozyme revealed, for instance, that 16 residues interact with 17 amino acids of a monoclonal antibody (reviewed by Bentley 1996). When analyzed by amino acid replacement techniques, antibody binding appears to be mediated by a smaller set of well-defined 'contact' residues plus additional weaker interactions, which are usually more difficult to define but add to the affinity of binding. Mutation of a critical contact residue may abrogate antibody binding, and allow a pathogen to escape neutralization. Usually such contact residues are on distant sequence domains, brought together by protein folding to form conformational, discontinuous, or assembled epitopes. Most neutralizing and protective BCEs are conformational antigenic sites. Occasionally most elements of an epitope are contributed by amino acid residues, which are all within a short stretch of sequence. These continuous, segmental, linear, or sequential epitopes, in contrast to conformational epitopes, can be operationally defined by their ability to be mimicked by synthetic peptides of the same sequence. Despite sometimes-complex conformations such as helices, β sheets, or loops, these can be mimicked by sequence-homologous synthetic peptides (Table 42.1).

Identification of sequential BCEs

C- and N-terminal ends of proteins are frequently surface exposed. As a result of lower structural constraints, termini tend to be more flexible and are more easily mimicked by peptides. Peptides of many antigenic N- or C-terminal epitopes have been used to obtain antibodies against proteins. In some cases the N-terminus carried a protective epitope (Langeveld et al. 1994a). Loops protruding from the antigen surface and surface-accessible helices are also frequent targets of antibodies and sometimes they can be mimicked by short synthetic peptides. In the absence of structural data, the prediction of sequential epitopes is guesswork. Among the numerous strategies that have been utilized to identify *protective* sequential BCEs (Morris 1996), the most straightforward is to screen overlapping peptides covering the whole sequence or at least predicted surface-exposed domains with protective monoclonal antibodies (mAb) by pepscan, multispin assays, or SPOT assays. Larger (e.g. recombinant, tryptic, or other) fragments or peptide libraries (e.g. synthetic or phage displayed) and polyclonal antibodies can serve as second-rate alternatives to define sequential epitopes. Substitution analogs of synthetic peptides (e.g. alanine scan) combined with mAbs are powerful tools to identify contact residues of sequential epitopes. As a result of the many degrees of rotational freedom, the conformation of most peptides is ill-defined. For these reasons, only a limited number of neutralizing or protective sequential epitopes have been identified for some pathogens and none for others (Table 42.1).

Mimotopes mimic conformational BCEs

Conformational epitopes are even more difficult to mimic with small synthetic molecules, referred to as mimotopes. Mimotopes may have no sequence homology with the protein, but the spatial arrangement of their residues provides an array of atoms that resembles those contacted by the paratope in the protein epitope. Among a variety of approaches the most powerful are based on synthetic peptide libraries or (random) peptide libraries expressed by phages. Peptides as mimotopes have been used as surrogate antigens of experimental vaccines against proteins (Steward 2001) and even carbohydrates (reviewed by Monzavi-Karbassi et al. 2002). Many (antigenic) mimotopes that react with (preformed) antibodies have been described, but only a fraction of them also induced antibodies that crossreacted in vivo. When peptide mimotopes are used for immunization, usually few of the highly antigenic peptides induce virus-crossreactive antibodies, reflecting a severe disparity among antigenicity, immunogenicity, and crossreactive immunogenicity (El Kasmi et al. 1999b) with or without neutralizing or protective activity (reviewed by Deroo and Muller 2001) (Table 42.2). Steward and colleagues (Steward et al. 1995; Olszewska et al. 2000) described a remarkable peptide mimotope, which was selected against an mAb of the measles virus fusion protein. Although the mAb did not neutralize the virus in vitro, the mimotope induced antibodies, which protected in a rodent model against a viral challenge. In another study, the same group described a peptide mimotope selected with a combinatorial solid-phase peptide library against a protective mAb of the fusion protein of the respiratory syncytial virus. These mimotopes, presented as multiple antigenic peptides (MAP), induced antibodies, which neutralized the virus in vitro, and reduced the virus load in immunized mice to 1 percent (Chargelegue et al. 1997, 1998).

Peptide vaccines based on BCEs: general features

THE BEGINNING

Chemical synthesis of peptides was developed during the 1960s (Marglin and Merrifield 1970), and thanks to numerous technological advances peptides became increasingly popular in immunology. In 1963, Anderer and colleagues showed for the first time that a C-terminal peptide of the coat protein of tobacco mosaic virus induced virus-neutralizing antibodies. More than 10 years later, Langbeheim et al. (1976) inactivated a bacteriophage by immunizing with a synthetic polymer of its coat protein made of 20 peptides. In the early 1980s protective immunity in the host animal was obtained with a peptide corresponding to the GH loop of the VP1 capsid protein of food-and-mouth disease

Table 42.1 *B-cell immunity peptide vaccines*[a]

Pathogen	Antigen	Delivery system	Host[b]	Activity	References
Viruses					
MV	F protein	Peptide/CFA	Mice	N, P	Obeid et al. (1995); Atabani et al. (1997); Partidos et al. (1997)
		Peptide/CT	Mice	N, P	Hathaway et al. (1995, 1998)
	H protein NE	Peptide/CFA	Mice	N, P	El Kasmi et al. (1998, 1999a)
	H protein HNE	Peptide/CFA	Mice	N, P	El Kasmi et al. (2000)
		DT, TT/alum	Mice	P	Putz et al. (2003b, 2004)
		Recombinant polyepitope/CFA	Mice	N	Bouche et al. (2003)
CDV	F protein	Peptide/CFA	Mice	P	Obeid et al. (1995)
RSV	G protein	MVA	Mice	P	Simard et al. (1995)
		KLH/CFA	Mice	P	Simard et al. (1997)
		Recombinant fd/CFA	Mice	P	Bastien et al. (1997)
		Peptide/CT	Mice	P	Bastien et al. (1999)
Influenza virus	HA	TT/CFA	Mice	N, P	Muller et al. (1982)
		TT/CFA	Mice		Muller et al. (1990)
		BSA, OVA/CFA liposomes	Mice	P	Friede et al. (1994)
FMDV	Site A VP1	KLH/CFA	Mice	N	Strohmaier et al. (1982)
		KLH/alum, CFA	Guinea-pigs	N, P	Bittle et al. (1982); Pfaff et al. (1982)
		KLH, TT/alum liposomes	Guinea-pigs	N	Francis et al. (1985)
		Peptide, KLH/CFA	Guinea-pigs, *cattle*	N, P	DiMarchi et al. (1986)
		Peptide-P3C	Guinea-pigs, *cattle*	P	Wiesmüller et al. (1989); Hohlich et al. (2003)
		MAP/IFA, alum	Guinea-pigs	N	Francis et al. (1991)
		Retro-all-d/KLH/alum	Guinea-pigs	N, P	Briand et al. (1997)
		Peptide/oil adjuvant	*Cattle*	N, P	Taboga et al. (1997)
		Peptide/Montanide	Guinea-pigs, *swine*	N, P	Wang et al. (2001, 2002a)
Poliovirus	VP1	BSA, KLH/CFA	Rabbits	N	Emini et al. (1983); Wimmer et al. (1984); Jameson et al. (1985)
	VP2	BSA/CFA	Rabbits	N	Emini et al. (1984b)
HAV	VP1	BSA/CFA	Rabbits, guinea-pigs	N	Emini et al. (1985)
		KLH, MAP/liposomes	Mice	N	Haro et al. (1995, 2003)
	VP1, VP2, VP3	CFA + liposomes	Mice	N	Bosch et al. (1998)
HCV	HVR1	Recombinant HVR1-CTB via TMV	Mice		Nemchinov et al. (2000)
		KLH/CFA	Mice		Li et al. (2001)
	Multivalent	Recombinant polyepitope/alum	Mice, monkeys		Li et al. (2003)
HIV-1	gp120 V3 loop	MAP/Alum	Guinea-pigs	N	Wang et al. (1991)

(Continued over)

Table 42.1 *B-cell immunity peptide vaccines*[a] *(Continued)*

Pathogen	Antigen	Delivery system	Host[b]	Activity	References
		MAP-P3C/Liposomes	Mice, guinea-pigs, rabbits	N	Defoort et al. (1992a); Nardelli et al. (1992)
		Peptide/CFA	Mice	N	Ahlers et al. (1993)
		fil HA, PPD, toxin A, TT	Guinea-pigs	N	Cryz et al. (1995); Rubinstein et al. (1999)
		Peptide/CT	Mice	N	Staats et al. (1996); Bradney et al. (2002)
		Recombinant rhinovirus	Guinea-pigs	N	Zhang et al. (1999)
		BSA/CFA	Mice	N	Xiao et al. (2000)
		Branched peptide/Alum	*Humans*	N	Gorse et al. (1996); Keefer et al. (1997)
		PPD	*Humans*	N	Rubinstein et al. (1995, 1999)
		MAP/alum	*Humans*	N	Kelleher et al. (1997); Phanuphak et al. (1997); Li et al. (1997)
		MAP/Alum	*Humans*	N	Lambert et al. (2001a)
	gp160	Peptide/Montanide	*Humans*	N	Pinto et al. (1999)
	Multivalent	MAP/CT	Mice	N	Bukawa et al. (1995); Kato et al. (2000)
		BSA/CFA	Rabbits	N	Lu et al. (2000)
HIV-2	gp 125	ISCOMs	Macaques	P	Putkonen et al. (1994)
SIV	gp 120, gp32	Recombinant β-Gal/CFA	Macaques	N, P	Shafferman et al. (1991)
CPV	VP2	KLH/alum + Quil A	*Dogs*	P	Langeveld et al. (1994a)
		KLH/alum + Quil A,CFA	Rabbits	N	Langeveld et al. (1994b)
		CPMV VLP/CFA	*Dogs*	P	Dalsgaard et al. (1997)
		KLH,OVA/CFA	Mice, rabbits	N	Casal et al. (1995); Langeveld et al. (2001a)
MEV	VP2	KLH/ISCOMs	Mink	P	Langeveld et al. (1995)
HBV	HBsAg S region	KLH/CFA	Chimpanzees	P	Gerin et al. (1983)
		KLH/CFA	Chimpanzees	P	Itoh et al. (1986)
		Peptide/CFA	Chimpanzees	P	Emini et al. (1989)
		MAP/CFA	Rabbits		Tam and Lu (1989)
HPV	E7 protein	Polyepitope/CFA, ISCOMs	Mice		Fernando et al. (1995)
		ISCAR/CFA	Mice	P	Tindle et al. (1995)
	L2 capsid protein	BSA/CFA	Mice	N	Kawana et al. (1999)
		Peptide/CT	Mice	N	Kawana et al. (2001)
		Peptide envelope	*Humans*	N	Kawana et al. (2003)
Japanese encephalitis virus	Glycoprotein	OVA/CFA	Mice	N	Dewasthaly et al. (2001)
Bacteria					
Neisseria meningitidis	Class 1 OMP	TT/Alum, Quil A	Mice	B	Hoogerhout et al. (1995)
	PorA	Peptide/CFA	Mice	P	Koroev et al. (2000)
	OpaB	Peptide/CFA	Mice	P	Koroev et al. (2001)

(Continued over)

Table 42.1 *B-cell immunity peptide vaccines*[a] *(Continued)*

Pathogen	Antigen	Delivery system	Host[b]	Activity	References
Streptococcus pyogenes	M protein	Peptide/CFA	Mice, rabbits	P	Beachey et al. (1981, 1986)
	TT/CFA		Mice, rabbits	P	Dale et al. (1983); Beachey et al. (1984)
Group A streptococcus	M protein C region	CTB	Mice	P	Bessen and Fischetti (1988, 1990)
		KLH/CFA or CTB	Rabbits, mice	P	Bronze et al. (1992)
		Peptide/CFA	Mice	B	Pruksakorn et al. (1992)
		LCP	Mice	P	Olive et al. (2002a)
		DT/CTB	Mice	P	Olive et al. (2002b)
		DT/Alum, SBAS2	Mice	B, P	Batzloff et al. (2003)
		Peptide/alum	Mice	P	Bruner et al. (2003)
	Streptolysin S	KLH/CFA	Rabbits	B	Dale et al. (2002)
Porphyromonas gingivalis	Fimbrillin	Peptide/IFA	Guinea-pigs	P	Ogawa (1994)
		BSA/CFA	Mice	P	Deslauriers et al. (1996)
	RgpA-Kgp	DT/IFA	Mice	P	O'Brien-Simpson et al. (2000)
Bacillus anthracis	*B. anthracis* capsule	BSA, rPA, rEPA	Mice		Schneerson et al. (2003)
		KLH/CFA	Mice		Wang et al. (2004)
Staphylococcus aureus	FnBP	CPMV VLP/ISCOM, QS-21	Mice		Brennan et al. (1999a)
Pseudomonas aeruginosa	OMP F	CPMV VLP/alum, CFA	Mice	P	Brennan et al. (1999b)
		Chimeric influenza virus	Mice	P	Staczek et al. (1998)
		TMV VLP/Alum, CFA	Mice	P	Staczek et al. (2000)
	Pilin	TT/Adjuvax	Mice	P	Cachia et al. (1998); Cachia and Hodges (2003)
Nontypable *Haemophilus influenzae*	P5	Peptide/CFA	Chinchilla	P	Bakaletz et al. (1997, 1999)
	Peptide/CFA		Rats	P	Webb and Cripps (2000)
	BSA, KLH/CFA		Chinchilla, rat	P	Kyd et al. (2003)
Vibrio cholerae	TcpA pilin	KLH/CFA	Rabbits, mice	P	Sun et al. (1997)
		Peptides/PCPP, CRL-1005	Mice	P	Wu et al. (2001)
Parasites					
Schistosoma mansoni	9B-antigen	BSA/CFA	Mice	P	Tarrab-Hazdai et al. (1998)
		Recombinant salmonella flagellin	Mice	P	Ben-Yedidia et al. (1999)
	Sm14	MPL-TDL	Mice	P	Vilar et al. (2003)
	Multivalent	Recombinant polyepitope or DNA	Mice		Yang et al. (2000)
	Glyceraldehyde-3-phosphate dehydrogenase	MAP/CFA	Mice	P	Tallima et al. (2003)

(Continued over)

Table 42.1 *B-cell immunity peptide vaccines*[a] *(Continued)*

Pathogen	Antigen	Delivery system	Host[b]	Activity	References
Plasmodium berghei	Pre-erythrocytic stage CSP	TT/CFA	*Mice*, rats	P	Zavala et al. (1987)
		MAP/CFA	*Mice*	P	Tam et al. (1990); Zavala and Chai (1990)
		BSA/RaLPS	*Mice*	P	Reed et al. (1996)
		MAC/RaLPS	*Mice*	P	Reed et al. (1997)
Plasmodium yoelii	Pre-erythrocytic stage CSP	MAC/RaLPS	*Mice*		Reed et al. (1997)
		Recombinant HBcAg	*Mice*	P	Schodel et al. (1997)
Plasmodium vivax	Pre-erythrocytic stage CSP	MAC/alum, RaLPS	Monkeys	P	Yang et al. (1997)
Plasmodium falciparum Pre-erythrocytic stage	CSP	TT/CFA	Rabbits	N	Zavala et al. (1985)
		TT/Alum	*Humans*	P	Herrington et al. (1987); Etlinger et al. (1988)
		MAP/CFA, alum	Mice, monkeys		Moreno et al. (1999)
		MAP/Alum,QS21	*Humans*		Nardin et al. (2000)
		Polyoxime MAP-P3C	*Humans*		Nardin et al. (2001)
		MAP/CFA	Mice	N	Joshi et al. (2001)
		Recombinant HBc/CFA, alum	Mice, monkeys		Birkett et al. (2002)
	LSA-3	Palmitoyl-lipopeptide	Chimpanzees	P	BenMohamed et al. (1997); Daubersies et al. (2000)
Asexual blood stage	MSP-1	BSA, TT/CFA	Rabbits, monkeys	N, P	Cheung et al. (1986)
		MAP/CFA	Monkeys	P	Rivera et al. (2002)
	RESA	Recombinant polyepitope/CFA	Monkeys	P	Collins et al. (1986)
	KLH, TT/CFA		Rabbits	N	Berzins et al. (1986)
	RESA, Pf55, Pf35	BSA/CFA	Monkeys	P	Patarroyo et al. (1987); Rodriguez et al. (1990)
Multistage multivalent	'SPf66'	Polyepitope/CFA	Monkeys	P	Rodriguez et al. (1990); Ruebush et al. (1990)
		Polyepitope/alum	*Humans*	P	Patarroyo et al. (1988); Amador et al. (1992a); Valero et al. (1993)
		Polyepitope/alum	*Humans*	N	Salcedo et al. (1991)
	CDC/NIIMALVAC-1	Recombinant polyepitope/CFA, P1005	Rabbits, Mice	N	Shi et al. (1999, 2000)
				N	Shi et al. (2000)
Taenia solium	KETc7	Peptide, MAP, OVA/CFA	Mice	P	Toledo et al. (1999)
	KETc1, KETc12	Peptide/Saponin	Mice	P	Toledo et al. (2001)
	KETc1, KETc7, KETc12	Peptide/Saponin	*Swine*	P	Huerta et al. (2001)
Toxins					
Vibrio cholerae	Cholera toxin B chain	TT/CFA	Rabbits	P	Jacob et al. (1983, 1986a)
		Recombinant β-Gal/CFA	Rabbits	P	Jacob et al. (1985)
		Peptide-MDP	Rabbits	P	Jacob et al. (1986b)

(Continued over)

Table 42.1 *B-cell immunity peptide vaccines*[a] *(Continued)*

Pathogen	Antigen	Delivery system	Host[b]	Activity	References
Escherichia coli	Heat-labile enterotoxin	TT/CFA	Rabbits	P	Jacob et al. (1986a)
Corynebacterium diphtheriae	Diphtheria toxin	BSA/CFA	Guinea-pigs	P	Audibert et al. (1981)
		Peptide-MDP	Guinea-pigs	P	Audibert et al. (1982)
Shigella dysenteriae	Shiga toxin B chain	pDGDL, TT/CFA	Mice, rabbits, rats	N, P	Harari et al. (1988); Harari and Arnon (1990)
Bungarus multicinctus (Taiwan banded krait)	β_1-Bungarotoxin	Peptide, OVA/CFA	Mice	P	Dolimbek and Atassi (1996)
		BSA/CFA	Mice	P	Yang and Chan (1998)
Contraceptive vaccines					
	hCG	TT/CFA, CGP-11637	*Mice, rabbits,*	C	Stevens et al. (1981a, b)
		TT/CGP-11637	*Baboons, humans*		Jones et al. (1988)
	ZP3	KLH/CFA	*Mice, macaques*	C	Millar et al. (1989); Mahi-Brown and Moran (1995)
		Peptide/CFA	*Mice, macaques*	C	Lou et al. (1995); Bagavant et al. (1997)
		DT/CFA	*Rabbits*		Afzalpurkar et al. (1997a, b)
		Peptide, TT/MDP + Morris	*Marmosets, mice,* primates	C	Paterson et al. (1999, 2002)
	GnRH	KLH/CFA	*Pigs*	C	Meloen et al. (1994); Beekman et al. (1999)
		KLH, OVA/CFA, Specol	*Pigs*	C	Oonk et al. (1998), Zeng et al. (2001)
	LHRH	Peptide/CFA	*Mice*	C	Ghosh and Jackson (1999)
	Sperm antigen LDH-C_4	DT/CGP-11637	*Baboons*	C	O'Hern et al. (1995)
		Peptide/CFA, CGP-11637	*Rabbits, baboons*	C	O'Hern et al. (1997)
	Sperm antigen YLP12	CTB	*Mice*	C	Naz and Chauhan (2002); Naz (2004)
	ZP3, LDH-C_4	Peptide/CFA	*Mice*	C	Sadler et al. (1999)
	RCP	Peptide/CFA	*Rats*	C	Subramanian et al. (2000)
Therapeutic vaccines					
Alzheimer's disease	Amyloid-β peptide	Peptide/CFA	Mice	P	Schenk et al. (1999)
		Peptide/LT	Mice	P	Weiner et al. (2000); Lemere et al. (2001)
		Recombinant fd	Mice	N, P	Frenkel et al. (2001, 2003)
		Polylysine peptide/CFA	Mice	P	Sigurdsson et al. (2001)
		Palmitoylpeptide/liposomes	Mice	P	Nicolau et al. (2002)
		BSA/CFA	Mice		Monsonego et al. (2001)
		Peptide oligomers/CFA	Rabbits	N	Lambert et al. (2001b)
		Peptide/alum	*Humans*		Schenk (2002); Nicoll et al. (2003)
Myasthenia gravis	AChR B-cell ARM	KLH/CFA	Rat	P (EAMG)	Araga et al. (1993)
	AChR T-cell ARM	MAP/CFA	Rat	P (EAMG)	Araga et al. (2000)

(Continued over)

Table 42.1 *B-cell immunity peptide vaccines*[a] *(Continued)*

Pathogen	Antigen	Delivery system	Host[b]	Activity	References
Multiple sclerosis	MBP T-cell ARM	KLH/CFA	Mice	P (EAE)	Zhou and Whitaker (1996)
Guillain–Barré syndrome	Bovine P2 T-cell ARM	KLH/AjuPrime	Mice	P (EAN)	Araga et al. (1999)
AIDS	CD4–CDR2 effector site	Peptide/CFA	Guinea-pigs	N	Wang et al. (2002b)
Tumour vaccines (BCE)					
Adenocarcinoma (breast, ovary)	HER-2	Universal ThB cell epitope-peptide conjugate (44-mer) + squalene/Arlacel A + CRL 1005	Antibodies in 3/5 killing human breast cancer cells in vitro		Dakappagari et al. (2000)
Breast cancer (metastatic)	MUC1	16-mer conjugated to KLH + Detox	Antibody in 3/16. $CD8^+$ in 7/11. No clinical response reported		Reddish et al. (1998)
Adenocarcinoma (various tumors)	MUC1	VNTR (5 repeats, 100-mer) conjugated to mannan	DTH. Antibody in 60% of intraperitoneal injected patients. T-cell responses in 28%. No clinical response		Karanikas et al. (2001)
Adenocarcinoma (breast, colon, stomach)	MUC1	VNTR (5 repeats) conjugated to mannan	MUC1 antibodies in 13/25. CTLs in 2/10. Th in 4/15. No clinical response reported		Karanikas et al. (1997)
Breast cancer	MUC1	VNTR (1.5 repeats, 30-mer) conjugated to KLH +QS-21	Antibody (9/9), no T-cell response. Recurrence of disease in only 2/9 high-risk patients		Gilewski et al. (2000)
Follicular B lymphoma	Idiotype	Peptide-KLH conjugate + DC	2/4 CRs, 1 PR		Hsu et al. (1996)
B lymphoma	Idiotype	Peptide-KLH conjugate + GM-CSF	Tumor-specific T cells in 19/20; 8/11 molecular remission		Bendandi et al. (1999)

a) Abbreviations: AChR, nicotinic acetylcholine receptor; ARM, antigen receptor mimetic; B, bactericidal activity; BCE, B-cell epitope; β-Gal, β-galactosidase fusion protein; BSA, bovine serum albumin conjugate; C, contraception or castration; CDV, canine distemper virus; CFA, complete Freund's adjuvant; CPMV, cowpea mosaic virus; CPV, canine parvovirus; CR, complete remission; CSP, circumsporozoite protein; CT, cholera toxin; CTB, cholera toxin B subunit; CTLE, cytotoxic T lymphocyte epitope; DT, diphtheria toxoid conjugate; EAE, experimental allergic encephalomyelitis; EAMG, experimental autoimmune myasthenia gravis; F, fusion protein; fil HA, filamentous hemagglutinin of *Bordatella pertussis*; FMDV, foot-and-mouth disease virus; FnBP, fibronectin-binding protein; H, measles virus hemagglutinin protein; HA, influenza hemagglutinin protein; HAV, hepatitis A virus; HBsAg, hepatitis B surface antigen; HBV, hepatitis B virus; HCV, hepatitis C virus; HIV, human immunodeficiency virus; HPV, human papillomavirus; HVR, hypervariable region; IFA, incomplete Freund's adjuvant; ISCARs, immunostimulatory carrier; ISCOMs, immunostimulating complexes; gp, glycoprotein; KLH, keyhole limpet hemocyanin conjugate; LCP, lipid core peptide construct; LDH, lactate dehydrogenase; LOS, lipo-oligosaccharide; LT, heat-labile enterotoxin; MAC, multiple-antigen construct; MAP, multiple-antigen peptide; MBP, myelin basic protein; MDP, *N*-acetylmuramyl-l-alanyl-d-isoglutamine; MEV, mink enteritis virus; MPL-TDL, monophosphoryl lipid A/ trehalose dicorynomycolate; MSA, merozoite major surface antigen; MV, measles virus; MVA, recombinant modified vaccinia virus Ankara; N, in vitro neutralization/growth inhibition; OMP, outer membrane protein; OVA, ovalbumin conjugate; P, in vivo protection or reduction of viral load; P3C, tripalmitoyl-*S*-glyceryl-cysteinylserylserine; PCPP, poly-di(carboxyatophenoxy)phosphazene; pDGDL, poly-d-glutamic-acid-d-lysine conjugate; peptide, free synthetic linear or chimeric TCE-BCE peptide; PPD, purified protein derivative of *Mycobacterium tuberculosis*; PR, partial remission; RaLPS, detoxified lipopolysaccharide; RCP, riboflavin carrier protein; rec fd, recombinant filamentous bacteriophage; rEPA, recombinant *Pseudomonas aeruginosa* exotoxin conjugate; RESA, ring-infected erythrocyte surface antigen; rPA, recombinant *B. anthracis* protective antigen conjugate; SIV, simian immunodeficiency virus; TCE, T-cell epitope; ThE, T-helper cell epitope; toxin A, *Pseudomonas aeruginosa* toxin A conjugate; TPI, triose phosphate isomerase; TMV, tobacco mosaic virus; TT, tetanus toxoid conjugate; VLP, virus-like particles.

b) Natural hosts in italic.

Table 42.2 *Examples of neutralizing and protective mimotopes*[a]

Pathogen	BCE	Delivery system	Host	Activity	References
Viruses					
MV	F protein mimotope	Peptide/CFA	Mice	P	Steward et al. (1995); Olszewska et al. (2000)
RSV	F protein mimotope	MAP/CFA	Mice	N, P	Chargelegue et al. (1997, 1998)
	F protein mimotope	MAP, CTLE, ThE	Mice	P	Hsu et al. (1998)
	F protein mimotope	MAP, CTLE, ThE/IFA	Mice	P	Hsu et al. (1999)
Hepatitis C	HVR1 mimotopes	MAPs/CFA	Rabbits		Roccasecca et al. (2001)
Hepatitis B	HbsAg mimotope	Recombinant phage/CFA	Mice		Motti et al. (1994)
Bacteria					
Neisseria meningitidis	Mimotope	Proteosome complex	Mice	P	Westerink et al. (1995); Prinz et al. (2004)
	Polymimotopes	DNA/Alum	Mice	N, P	Westerink et al. (2001); Prinz et al. (2003)
	Mimotope	DT/CFA	Mice		Charalambous and Feavers (2000)
Nontypable *Haemophilus influenzae*	LOS mimotope	KLH/CFA	Rabbits, mice	P	Hou and Gu (2003)
Parasites					
Schistosoma mansoni	9B-antigen mimotope	BSA/CFA	Mice	P	Arnon et al. (2000)
Cryptococcus neoformans glucuronoxylomannan		P13-BSA P13-TT	Mice Mice	Prolonged Survival	Fleuridor et al. 2001
Other					
	IgE mimotope	Peptide	Rabbits	P, N	Rudolf et al. (1998); Stadler et al. (1999)
Fibrosarcoma	Sialyl Lewis X	MAP mimotope	Mice	Inhibition of tumor growth	Kieber-Emmons et al. (1999)
Lymphoma (RAW117-HA)	EDA-alpha		Mice	Inhibits metastasis	Ishikawa et al. (1998)

a) Abbreviations: see Table 42.1.

(DiMarchi et al. 1986). These early studies encouraged many authors to explore immunization strategies based on sequential BCE and synthetic peptides. Peptides corresponding to neutralizing epitopes have been identified in a number of surface proteins of viruses, bacteria, and parasites (see Table 42.1). However, after the initial enthusiasm, it became clear that peptides are far from being ideal antigens. Our own experience taught us that it is a long way from the identification of a neutralizing linear epitope to a protective vaccine (Ziegler et al. 1996; Putz et al. 2004).

CHEMICALLY DEFINED VACCINES

A major advantage of chemically synthesized peptides in comparison to biological products is at the level of production, quality, and safety. Peptides are relatively simple to synthesize in large quantities. They are chemically fully defined, and can be obtained with high purity and minimal batch variations. They are thermostable and have long shelf-lives at room temperature. They do not require cold chains, which are expensive and difficult to maintain in developing countries. In comparison to recombinant products, peptides do not require complex fermenting and downstream-processing capacity. Unlike live vectors, peptides have no infectious potential. Containment requirements are minimal in comparison to those for the production of large quantities of infectious microorganisms. There is no risk of reversion of attenuation.

CONFORMATIONAL STABILITY

Most neutralizing and protective BCEs are conformational and difficult to mimic with linear peptides (see earlier section 'Mimotopes mimic conformational BCEs'). In the case of a sequential epitope, linear peptides may miss some structural features of the native epitope involved in antibody interaction. Furthermore, peptides are highly flexible structures, presenting to the

B-cell repertoire a multitude of different conformations, only some of which may resemble the native epitope and induce antibodies crossreacting with the parent protein (crossreactive immunogenicity).

To overcome problems with peptide flexibility, different strategies have been explored including constraining peptides by chemical or peptidic scaffolds (Valero et al. 2000; Hudecz 2001), e.g. the M protein of the group A streptococci (GAS) contains a sequential epitope targeted by opsonizing and protective antibodies (reviewed by Olive et al. 2004). However, synthetic peptides representing this epitope alone did not display the helical structure of the native protein. Only when flanked by irrelevant yeast-derived GCN4 sequences did the epitope peptide fold into the helical structure and induce protective antibodies (Relf et al. 1996; Hayman et al. 1997). Such strategies reduce conformational diversity but structural similarity may suffer. A poor balance between conformational constraints and conformational similarity of the peptide with the native protein critically determines crossreactive immunogenicity.

IMMUNOGENICITY

Live-attenuated viruses induce a strong immune response, protecting sometimes for decades after a single injection without the need of adjuvants. Recombinant proteins formulated with adjuvants protect after several boosts for 5–10 years. In comparison, synthetic peptides have a weak inherent immunogenicity; normally they are much less immunogenic than their parent proteins even after repeated injections with relatively high doses. They depend on potent adjuvants (Van Regenmortel and Muller 1999), which are not licensed for human use. Most experimental vaccines have been tested by invasive routes using a variety of formulations, adjuvants, and cytokines (see Table 42.1). Adjuvants have been reviewed by Del Giudice and Rappuoli (see Chapter 45, Adjuvants and subunit vaccines). The low immunogenicity, combined with conformational diversity of a peptide antigen, are the major obstacles to the induction of high levels of crossreactive or neutralizing antibodies.

ENZYMATIC DEGRADATION IN VIVO

In vivo, peptides are rapidly degraded by proteases further limiting their immunogenicity. To overcome this drawback numerous attempts have been made to develop more stable peptide derivatives using non-natural amino acids (Chorev and Goodman 1995; Briand et al. 1997; Nargi et al. 1999), analogs with modified peptide bonds (pseudopeptides) (Bianco 1999) and other so-called peptidomimetics (Benkirane et al. 1996a; Stemmer et al. 1999), e.g. a retro-inverso peptide induced protective antibodies against foot-and-mouth disease (Briand et al. 1997) and a pseudopeptide inhibited experimental allergic encephalitis (Jameson et al. 1994).

Requirement for TCEs

A CHOICE OF HELPER TCE

To be immunogenic in the context of a natural population, the BCEs must be combined with a peptide containing a potent T-helper cell epitope, which can be presented by most MHC class II haplotypes or an immunogenic carrier protein. Broadly, MHC II-reactive TCEs have been proposed for this purpose (Table 42.3), including non-natural pan-DR-binding peptides, engineered to bind to a wide range of DR molecules (Panina-Bordignon et al. 1989; Alexander et al. 1994, 1998). The carrier proteins most frequently used in experimental conjugate vaccines include tetanus toxoid (TT), diphtheria toxoid (DT), keyhole limpet hemocyanin, ovalbumin (OVA), and bovine serum albumin

Table 42.3 *Promiscuous T-helper cell epitopes*[a]

Antigen	Sequence	Position	Reference
Tetanus toxoid	NSVDDALINSTKIYSYFPSV	580–599	Ho et al. (1990)
Tetanus toxoid	QYIKANSKFIGITEL	830–844	Demotz et al. (1989)
Tetanus toxoid	PGINGKAIHLVNNESSE	916–932	Ho et al. (1990)
Tetanus toxoid	FNNFTVSFWLRVPKVSASHLE	947–967	Panina-Bordignon et al. (1989)
Tetanus toxoid	GQIGNDPNRDIL	1273–1284	Demotz et al. (1989)
P. falciparum CSP	EKKIAKMEKASSVFNV	380–395	Sinigaglia et al. (1988)
MV F protein	LSEIKGVIVHRLEGV	288–302	Partidos and Steward (1990)
FMDV VP1 protein	ETQVQRRHHTDVGFIMDRFY	21–40	Collen et al. (1991)
HIV gp160	KQIIMNWQEVGKAMYAPPISGQIR	428–451	Berzofsky et al. (1991)
Pan-DR epitope	aK(X)VAAWTLKAa	Non-natural	Alexander et al. (1994)
HAV	NVPDPQVGITTMRDLKG	17–33	Ivanov et al. (1994)
HAV	MSRIAAGDLESSVDDPRSEEDRR	276–298	Ivanov et al. (1994)
HBV envelope protein	WPEANQVGAGAFGPGF	52–67	Doh et al. (2003)
HPV16	DRAHYNI	48–54	Tindle et al. (1991)

a) Abbreviations: see Table 42.1.

(BSA). TT and DT, two highly immunogenic carriers both licensed for human use, have been successfully utilized in experimental peptide conjugate vaccines (Muller et al. 1982; Herrington et al. 1987; Putz et al. 2004). Despite difficulties to obtain efficient loading and homogeneous conjugates, this technology is commonly used in licensed polysaccharide conjugate vaccines against bacteria. Coupling the BCE to a TCE or carrier protein, however, undermines some advantages of peptides including chemical purity, homogeneity, and stability.

DESIGN OF PEPTIDES CONTAINING BOTH T- AND B-CELL EPITOPES

Although in some cases simple mixing of a TCE peptide with a BCE peptide has given satisfactory results (Partidos et al. 1992a; Brons et al. 1996), covalent coupling is generally believed to be required. Co-linear synthesis of the BCE with a peptide containing a (promiscuous) TCE is one option (Partidos et al. 1991). Although the technology to produce peptides of increasing length has made considerable progress (reviewed by Demotz et al. 2001), yield, purity, and production costs are likely to limit peptide length. The longer the peptide, the less competitive the chemical synthesis will be in comparison to production of recombinants.

The need for a conjugated TCE adds several levels of complexity to the design of peptide vaccines: the antigenic peptide may be conjugated C or N terminally to one or several TCE peptides (or a carrier protein). Orientation, number, and structural propensity of the TCE critically determine the conformation of the BCE, and crossreactive immunogenicity with the native protein as well as neutralizing activity of antibodies (Dyrberg and Oldstone 1986; Lipkin et al. 1988; Lu et al. 1991; Partidos et al. 1992b, c; Fernandez et al. 1993; Sharma et al. 1993; El Kasmi et al. 1998, 2000). Although some permutational T–B constructs produced low levels of antibodies without crossreactivity, others containing the same BCE framed differently with the same TCE, or flanked in the same way with different TCE, induced crossreactive antibodies. Although inactive and cross-neutralizing antibody-inducing constructs can be very similar, iterative optimization can be tedious (El Kasmi et al. 1999a). Systematic studies seem to suggest that TCE–TCE–BCE ('TTB') constructs may be the most efficient (Obeid et al. 1995; El Kasmi et al. 1999a). The orientation of co-linear peptides may also influence the immunogenicity of the TCE by activating T cells against neoepitopes which have no resemblance to pathogen-specific TCEs. TCEs and BCEs may also be combined using different chemical conjugation strategies including the formation of thioesters (Defoort et al. 1992b), oxime bonds (Rose 1994), disulfide bonds (Drijfhout and Bloemhoff 1991), thioether bonds (Schnolzer and Kent 1992), thiazolidine bonds (Rao and Tam 1994), and others (Spetzler and Tam 1995; Purcell et al. 2003; reviewed by Jackson et al. 2002). These coupling chemistries differed in conjugation yield, in vivo stability, and immunogenicity (Powell et al. 1993; Fitzmaurice et al. 2000; W. Zeng et al. 2001). In addition to linear coupling strategies, peptides can also be assembled in branched geometries as in MAPs on lysine scaffolds (Tam 1988; Tam et al. 1990; Lu et al. 1991; Ahlborg 1995; Fitzmaurice et al. 1996; reviewed by Nardelli and Tam 1995). In MAPs, the orientation appears to be less critical for immunogenicity, and optimal MAP constructs were shown to contain equimolar amounts of BCEs and TCEs (Tam et al. 1990). Enhanced immunogenicity of branched peptides seems to be the result of a higher resistance of MAPs to enzymatic degradation and more efficient antigen presentation (Fitzmaurice et al. 2000).

IMMUNE RESPONSE TO PEPTIDE-CARRIER CONJUGATES

Conjugation of a (small) BCE to a (bulky) carrier protein tends to divert the immune response to the larger immunogenic carrier protein and away from the (peptide) epitope (Herzenberg and Tokuhisa 1980; Schutze et al. 1985; Etlinger et al. 1988). Pre-existing antibodies against the carrier protein may influence the immunogenicity of the conjugate, although this does not seem to be a major obstacle at least in the case of polysaccharide conjugate vaccines (Eskola et al. 1990; Kurikka et al. 1996). In the case of an experimental peptide-conjugate vaccine considerable differences between the resistance to pre-existing antibodies of TT and DT were observed (Putz et al. 2004). Peptide-specific epitopic suppression was stronger after passive priming with carrier or conjugate antibodies. DT as a carrier was less susceptible to suppression than TT and suppression could be overcome by boosting (Putz et al. 2004), as also shown for polysaccharide conjugates (Sarvas et al. 1992). The ability to provide T-cell help without diverting the immune response is perhaps the major advantage of using a defined T-helper epitope.

ONE OR MORE EPITOPES

Important mutations in the targeted epitopes of pathogens may require the combination of peptides corresponding to several nonoverlapping neutralizing epitopes or a mix of mutated peptides of the same epitope. Vaccines based on single epitopes may favor the development of escape mutants. In this case, the epitope vaccines should include variants of a given epitope (Wang et al. 2001) or more than one BCE. This can be produced by chemical polymerization (Patarroyo et al. 1988), as MAPs (Tam et al. 1990), multiple antigen constructs (Yang et al. 1997), or polyoximes (Nardin et al. 1998), or by genetic fusion (Shi et al. 1999; Theisen et al. 2000; Bouche et al. 2003).

Noninvasive routes of delivery

Some experimental vaccines have also been tested by nasal delivery using cholera toxin (CT) from *Vibrio cholerae* (Bergquist et al. 1998) and heat-labile enterotoxin from *Escherichia coli* (LT, Hathaway et al. 1995; Partidos et al. 1996), or nontoxic mutants as mucosal adjuvants (Di Tommaso et al. 1996; Yamamoto et al. 1998). CpG (reviewed by Krieg 2002) and immunostimulating complexes (ISCOM) (Sjolander et al. 2001) have been proposed as mucosal adjuvants and proteosomes as carrier proteins (Levi et al. 1995; Mallett et al. 1995) for intranasal immunization in humans (Haneberg et al. 1998; Oftung et al. 1999). Studies also seem to suggest that peptides can be delivered through the bare skin when mixed with LT, although the efficiency of this route remains to be demonstrated (Partidos et al. 2001; MM Putz and CP Muller, unpublished data).

Targeting selected epitopes

PROTEINS: A CHOICE OF EPITOPES

All currently licensed vaccines and most of those that are in clinical trials are meant to induce a strong neutralizing and protective immune response against pathogens prone to mutations in genetically diverse human or animal populations. The efficacy of these vaccines, irrespective of genetic variability of the host or pathogen, relies on the ability of the immune system to select from a large number of epitopes (TCEs or BCEs). In prophylactic vaccines, the exact epitopes involved in the response are normally of little clinical interest. With the advent of recombinant technology, we have learned to appreciate the advantages of guiding immune reactions against defined proteins of a pathogen and this is now being exploited in numerous experimental and a few licensed recombinant vaccines. In contrast to protein subunit vaccines, peptides rely on only a few epitopes of an antigen. Relative advantages such as chemical stability, biological safety, and low production costs normally do not outweigh the low (crossreactive) immunogenicity of peptide vaccines in different genetic contexts of hosts and pathogens.

PEPTIDES: AN EPITOPE OF CHOICE

Immunologically, the most important feature of peptide vaccines or other epitope vaccines is their ability to target defined epitopes. It has been proposed, for instance, to use peptides complementary to major antigenic regions of autoantigens to induce anti-idiotype antibodies for the treatment of autoimmune diseases (reviewed by Weathington and Blalock 2003). Peptide-induced anti-idiotype antibodies have also been successfully used to treat B-cell lymphomas (Hsu et al. 1996, Bendandi et al. 1999; Table 42.4). Peptides are also useful to avoid undesired immune responses, such as non-neutralizing antibodies which block neutralizing antibodies, enhancing or tumor-stimulating antibodies, autoimmune responses, or the induction of tolerization or suppressor cells (Aichele et al. 1995; Toes et al. 1996a, b). When the use of whole pathogens or proteins is limited by important constraints, epitope-based vaccines are unrivalled by other approaches. Although peptides may outrun other epitope immunization strategies, alternatives such as DNA minigenes (see Chapter 44, Naked DNA vaccines) or recombinant polyepitopes (reviewed by Suhrbier 2002) should also be considered. Essentially every feature of peptide vaccines has to be evaluated against competing vaccine technologies. There are still only few examples where a vaccine would clearly benefit from selected beneficial BCEs or from excluding detrimental BCEs, but applications are emerging for the treatment of autoimmunity (Weathington and Blalock 2003), allergies, and malignancies (Table 42.4), as well as infectious diseases (see below).

An example of a prophylactic epitope vaccine

The following describes one of the few examples of a prophylactic vaccine strategy against a pathogen where an epitope approach may be specifically justified. Infants are partially protected against measles by transplacentally acquired maternal antibodies. However, many children lose these antibodies within the first months of birth. As a result they become susceptible to measles before they can be immunized with the current live-attenuated vaccine recommended only at 9–15 months of age (Muller 2001a; Putz and Muller 2003). At this age, measles is associated with many complications and a high mortality rate. To close this susceptibility gap in infants, we developed an immunization strategy based on two subdominant sequential epitopes of the measles virus (MV) hemagglutinin protein (Ziegler et al. 1996; Fournier et al. 1997). Peptides corresponding to these sequential epitopes induce neutralizing and protective antibodies against the virus, but are not neutralized themselves by passively acquired antibodies induced by natural measles infection or after immunization with whole virus (El Kasmi et al. 1999a, 2000). Antibodies against measles surface glycoproteins provide full protection even in the absence of a T-cell response. In particular, newborns are solely protected by passively acquired maternal antibodies. Despite immaturity of their immune system, newborns and infants are capable of developing vigorous and protective antibody responses against proteins (e.g. DT and TT). In fact, during their early lives, antibodies are the main mechanisms of vaccine-induced protection of infants.

The generation of protective antibodies against the peptides requires a vigorous T-helper (Th) 2 response.

Table 42.4 *Experimental peptide vaccines against tumor antigens tested in cancer patients*

Tumor	Tumor antigen	Peptide vaccine formulation	Immunological outcome/clinical outcome	Reference
Adenocarcinoma (breast, ovary, colon)	HER-2	CTL epitope (9-mer) + IFA	Peptide-specific CTL in 3/4. No clinical response	Zaks and Rosenberg (1998)
Adenocarcinoma (breast, ovary, lung)	HER-2	3 peptides (15–18-mers) each with overlapping Th and CTL epitopes + GM-CSF	CTLs in 86% of patients. Peptide-specific CTLs kill HER-2 expressing tumor cells. T-helper response against peptide (14/18) and against HER-2 protein (up to 50%). Immune response lasted > 1 year. Tumor not evaluable	Knutson et al. (2001)
Adenocarcinoma (breast, ovary, lung)	HER-2	2 mixtures of 3 Th epitopes (15–18-mers, ICD, ECD) + GM-CSF	T-cell proliferation against peptides (8/8) and protein (6/8). Tumor not evaluable	Disis et al. (1999, 2000); Disis and Cheever (1998)
Adenocarcinoma (breast, ovary, lung)	HER-2/neu	3 mixtures of 3 T-helper epitopes + GM-CSF	T cells to peptides in 92%, 68% to protein	Disis et al. (2002)
Adenocarcinoma (breast, ovary)	HER-2/neu	9-mer CTL epitope + GM-CSF	CTLs in 2/4	Knutson et al. (2002)
Adenocarcinoma (breast, lung)	HER-2/neu	Mixtures of 4 peptide T-helper epitopes	T-cell response in 25% of patients	Salazar et al. (2003)
Adenocarcinoma (breast, ovary, pancreas)	MUC-1	Synthetic mucin polypeptide core (105-mer) with 5 repeated epitopes + BCG	Infiltration of T cells at immunization site in 37/55. Increased CTLs in 7/22. DTH in 3/63. No clinical response.	Goydos et al. (1996)
Adenocarcinoma expressing CEA	CEA	CTL epitope (9-mer) + Detox PC	CTLs secreting low levels of IFN-α in 1/5	Arlen et al. (2000)
Colon, breast, ovary, pancreas	CEA	CAP-1 (9-mer + DC)	No DTH. 1/19 minor clinical response.	Morse et al. (1999)
Thyroid carcinoma	CEA	CAP-1 (9-mer + DC)	1/7 PR	Schott et al. (2001)
Pancreas carcinoma	K-ras	Mononuclear cells pulsed with peptide (17-mer)	$CD4^+$ in 2/5. No clinical response	Gjertsen et al. (1995, 1996a, b)
	K-ras	ras (13-mer) + Detox	$CD4^+$ in 3/10, $CD8^+$ in 3/10 against peptide. No clinical response	Khleif et al. (1999)
	K-Ras	4 peptides (17-mers) with mutated TCE + GM-CSF	Peptide-specific T cells or DTH of 25/43. Significant increase in survival	Gjertsen et al. (2001)
Prostate carcinoma	Prostate acid phosphatase	CTL peptide + GM-CSF	> 50% reduction of PSA in 3/31.	Small et al. (2000)
	PSMA	CTL peptides + DC (PSM-P1, PSM-P2)	DTH, $CD8^+$ response. 19/62 reduction in PSA. 2/25 CRs, 6 PRs	Murphy et al. (1999a); Tjoa et al. (1999); Lodge et al. (2000); Salgaller et al. (1998)
	PSMA	PSM-P1 (LLHETDSAV) ± DC	Specific CTLs in few patients	Murphy et al. (1996)
		PSM-P2 (ALFDIESKV) ± DC	7/51 reduction in PSA	Tjoa et al. (1997)
	PSMA	PSM-P1 peptide, PSM-P2 peptide	DTH, $CD8^+$. No clinical response	Murphy et al. (2000)

(Continued over)

Table 42.4 *Experimental peptide vaccines against tumor antigens tested in cancer patients (Continued)*

Tumor	Tumor antigen	Peptide vaccine formulation	Immunological outcome/clinical outcome	Reference
Bladder cancer	MAGE-3	CTL peptide + DC	1/4 PR	Nishiyama et al. (2001)
HPV-associated carcinomas	E7 of HPV16	86-mer CTL peptide + PADRE + Montanide ISA51	Induction of CTLs. No clinical response	Steller et al. (1998)
	E7 of HPV16	10-mer + 8-mer + PADRE	Response to PADRE (4/12). No CTL response. No clinical response	Van Driel et al. (1999); Ressing et al. (2000)
E7 protein of HPV16		CTL epitope (9-mer) plus a CTL-pan Th (PADRE) lipopeptide conjugate + IFA	Epitope-specific CTL activity in 10/16. No DTH. 3/17 CRs, 9/17 PRs	Muderspach et al. (2000)
Chronic myelogenous leukemia	Bcr-abl fusion protein, p210	5 peptides (9–25-mers) with Th and CTL epitopes + QS21	Peptide-specific T-cell proliferation in 50% of patients. No CTL activity	Pinilla-Ibarz et al. (2000)
Acute myeloid leukemia	WT1	9-mer CTL peptide + KLH + GM-CSF	CR in 1/1	Mailander et al. (2004)
Melanoma (metastatic)	gp100	Modified CTL epitope (9-mer), + IFA + either IL-2, GM-CSF, or IL-12	Tumor regressions in 6/16 patients tested. IFA + IL-2. IFA + GM-CSF: 0/13. IFA + IL-12: 0/14	Rosenberg et al. (1999)
Melanoma	MAGE-3	CTL peptide (9-mer), no adjuvant	No peptide-specific CTLs. 3/25 CRs, 4/25 PRs. 2/25 disease free for 2 years	Marchand et al. (1999)
Melanoma	MAGE-3	CTL peptide (9-mer) with pan class II peptide + IFA	Tumor response not evaluable (*n* = 18)	Weber et al. (1999)
Melanoma	MAGE-3	CTL peptides + DC	8/11 peptide-specific CTLs. 54% tumor response (single metastases)	Thurner et al. (1999)
Melanoma	MAGE-3	CTL peptide	Peptide-specific CTLs in 4/9 responding; in 1/14 non-responding patients. 39% tumor response	Coulie et al. (2002)
Melanoma	MAGE-3	DC pulsed with Th epitope	Majority of patients developed peptide-specific Th cells.	Schuler-Thurner et al. (2002)
Melanoma and others	NY-ESO-1	3 CTL peptides (9–11-mers) ± GM-CSF	4/12 peptide-specific CTLs, 4/12 DTH. 7/12 SD	Jager et al. (2000a)
Melanoma	Tyrosinase	4 CTL peptides (9-mers) + GM-CSF	4/18 peptide-specific CTLs. 1/5 mxR, 2/5 SD	Scheibenbogen et al. (2000)
Melanoma	Tyrosinase	CTL peptides (9-mer) + QS21	0/7 tumor response	Lewis et al. (2000)
Melanoma	gp100	3 CTL peptides (9-mer) + IFA	1/20 tumor response	Salgaller et al. (1996)
Melanoma	gp100$_{209–217}$ 210M	Modified CTL epitope (9-mer) + IFA or +IFA + IL-2	Peptide-specific CTLs in 91%. IFA: 0/11 tumor responses. IFA + IL-2; 1/31 CRs. 12/31 PRs	Rosenberg et al. (1998)
Melanoma	gp100	CTL epitope (9-mer) + 1. QS21 or Montanide ISA-5I2. Tetanus helper peptide + QS21 or Montanide ISA-5I3. Gp100-tetanus 24-mer + QS21 or Montanide ISA-5I	Peptide-specific Th and CTL response in 79% and 14% of patients respectively. Tumor not evaluable (*n* = 20). 75% survival after 4.7 years	Slingluff et al. (2001)
Melanoma	gp100 (210M), tyrosinase	Modified CTL epitope (9-mer) + IFA ± IL-12	37/42 peptide-specific CTLs. Tumor not evaluable. Increased disease-free survival	Lee et al. (2001)
Melanoma	gp100, tyrosinase	4 CTL epitopes (9-mers) + GM-CSF + Montanide ISA-51	CTL responses to peptides in 2–5/5 tumor-specific CTLs (5/5) in vitro	Yamshchikov et al. (2001)
Melanoma	gp100, tyrosinase	CTL peptides ± GM-CSF	37/42 peptide-specific CTLs; improved immunization. Tumor not evaluable	Weber et al. (2003)

(Continued over)

Table 42.4 *Experimental peptide vaccines against tumor antigens tested in cancer patients (Continued)*

Tumor	Tumor antigen	Peptide vaccine formulation	Immunological outcome/clinical outcome	Reference
Melanoma	Melan-A/MART-1_{27-35}	CTL epitope (9-mer) + IFA	7/8 peptide-specific CTLs. 1/18 PRs	Cormier et al. (1997)
Melanoma (resected)	Melan-A/MART-1_{27-35}	CTL epitope (9-mer) + IFA + CRL 1005	IFN-γ-secreting peptide-specific T cells in 12/20. Tumors not evaluable because of resection. Increased disease-free survival correlated with immune response	Wang et al. (1999a)
Melanoma	MART-1	CTL peptide (10-mer) + SB-AS 2 adjuvant/Montanide	Peptide-specific CTLs	Pittet et al. (2001)
Melanoma	MART-1, gp100	CTL peptides + DCs + no adjuvant	1/5 developed peptide-specific CTLs. Tumor response 1/7	Panelli et al. (2000)
Melanoma	Melan-A/MART-1, tyrosinase, gp100/Pmel17	6 CTL epitope (9, 10 mers)	5/6 DTH, 2/6 SD	Jaeger et al. (1996)
Melanoma	MART-1, tyrosinase, gp_{100}	CTL peptides + DC	2/28 CRs, 1/28 PRs	Lotze et al. (2000)
Melanoma	Melan-A/MART-1, tyrosinase, gp100, MAGE-3	CTL peptides + DC	16/18 peptide-specific CTLs. Immunity to peptides correlated with delayed tumor progression. Regression of some metastasis	Banchereau et al. (2001)
Melanoma	Tumor lysate	Peptide cocktail or tumor lysate + DC	DTH reaction to peptide-pulsed DC in 11/16. 31% tumor response	Nestle et al. (1998)
Melanoma	$gp100_{209-217}$210M0	Modified CTL peptide alone or modified CTL peptide + IL-2	Peptide-specific CTLs in 7/7. 0/7 tumor response	Lee et al. (1999)
			Peptide-specific CTLs in 1/11. 5/11 tumor response	
		Modified CTL peptide + IL-12	Peptide-specific CTLs in 4/5. 0% tumor response	
Melanoma	N-ras	ras (25-mer) + GM-CSF	DTH in 8/10, $CD4^+$ in 2/10. Clinical response, not examined	Hunger et al. (2001)
Melanoma	gp100, tyrosinase	4 CTL epitopes + GM-CSF + universal T-helper epitope + Montanide ISA-51	T-cell response in 42% patients.	Slingluff et al. (2003)
Melanoma	gp100 (210 M), MART-1	2 CTL epitopes	T-cell response in 95%. Clinical response in 0/22	Phan et al. (2003)
	gp100 (210 M), MART-1	2 CTL epitopes + 1 helper epitope	T-cell response in 50%. Clinical response in 1/19	
Melanoma	gp100, MART-1, tyrosinase	3 CTL epitopes + IFA + SD-9427	7/10 in ELISPOT essay. 11/12 in MHC-pep-tetramer essay	Pullarkat et al. (2003)
Melanoma	Melan-A	10-mer CTL peptide + rhIL-12	1/24 CRs, 1/24 PRs, 6/24 SD	Cebon et al. (2003)
Melanoma	Melanoma tyrosinase	9-mer CTL peptide + KLH + GM-CSF	T-cell response in 5/9	Scheibenbogen et al. (2003)
Melanoma	Tyrosinase	9-mer CTL peptide + KLH + GM-CSF	T-cell response in 2/2. 2 years disease-free recurred	Scheibenbogen et al. (2002)
Melanoma	MAGE-3	9-mer CTL peptide + KLH + GM-CSF	T-cell response in 2/9. Regression in 5/9	Coulie et al. (2002)

BCG, Bacillus Calmette–Guérin; CEA, carcinoembryonic antigen; IFA, incomplete Freund's adjuvant; MUC, mucin; PSA, peptide-specific antigen; PSMA, peptide-specific membrane antigen; rhIL-12, recombinant interleukin 12; SD, stable disease. See Table 42.1 for other abbreviations.

The induction of MV antibodies is complicated by observations of enhanced atypical disease after immunization with inactivated MV vaccine during the 1960s. This complication is now attributed to priming of nonprotective MV-specific Th2-biased cells (Polack et al. 1999). Thus, it is critical that the Th cells are unrelated to MV. Therefore, the peptides corresponding to the above sequential epitopes were conjugated to (unrelated) carrier proteins such as DT or TT. These peptide conjugates induced high levels of anti-peptide antibodies, which protected against MV utilizing TCEs of the carrier protein (Putz et al. 2004). Thus the risk of priming for measles-specific T cells was avoided and the main cause of atypical measles, i.e. an aberrant measles-specific Th2 priming, was precluded.

In this example the advantage of using a peptide as a protective BCE was a three-fold:

1 The peptide, in contrast to whole virus or viral proteins, was not susceptible to neutralization by pre-existing anti-whole virus antibodies.
2 By limiting the MV sequence to 20 amino acids priming by pathogenic TCEs was essentially avoided.
3 The relatively low immunogenicity and the short duration of an anti-peptide response may prove to be an asset here because protection of limited duration, at least against severe disease (to reduce complication rates and mortality, but not necessarily infection) is required, until the live-attenuated vaccine can be administered.

We have shown that this experimental vaccine is compatible both with pre-existing antibodies against the carrier protein DT and against whole MV, and that subsequent boosting with whole virus is possible (Putz et al. 2004).

CANDIDATE PEPTIDE VACCINES AGAINST BCES

Paramyxoviruses

MEASLES VIRUS

This single-strand, negative-sense RNA virus is the prototype morbillivirus (family of Paramyxoviridae). The current live-attenuated vaccine is poorly immunogenic in early infancy, as a result of the presence of neutralizing maternal antibodies passively acquired through the placenta and the immaturity of the infant immune system. Therefore a number of experimental vaccines based, for example, on recombinant MV proteins, viral and bacterial vectors, or naked DNA, have been developed (reviewed by Putz et al. 2003a). Among these numerous immunization strategies some are based on peptides of the hemagglutinin (H) and fusion (F) protein. MV-neutralizing antibodies are directed against both the F and the H glycoproteins, and sequential epitopes have been identified for both proteins. The rationale of peptides as a vaccine to protect during early infancy against measles is discussed in the previous section.

Steward and colleagues described two adjacent sequential epitopes contained within a short immunodominant region (F388–420) of the F protein (Partidos et al. 1991), crossreacting with sera from African children with acute measles (Atabani et al. 1997). Co-linearly synthesized with one or two copies of a promiscuous TCE (Partidos and Steward 1990), one of these peptides was immunogenic in mice and induced MV-crossreactive and -neutralizing antibodies (Atabani et al. 1997). Passive transfer of anti-peptide serum partially protected mice against a challenge with a neuroadapted MV strain (Obeid et al. 1995; Atabani et al. 1997) and cross-protected against canine distemper virus, a related morbillivirus (Obeid et al. 1995). In addition, intranasal co-immunization with a synthetic peptide containing two copies of a TCE and one copy of a BCE together with cholera toxin B (CTB) induced MV-neutralizing antibodies and conferred protection in the mouse model (Hathaway et al. 1995, 1998). When copies of the BCE (Obeid et al. 1995) and an N protein TCE were fused C terminally to the secretion signal of *E. coli* hemolysin and expressed by the attenuated *S. typhimurium* aroA strain, an MV-specific humoral and cellular immune response was induced after oral immunization which partially protected susceptible mice (Verjans et al. 1995; Spreng et al. 2000).

Two sequential BCEs have been identified on the H protein by screening a panel of neutralizing and protective mAbs against a complete set of overlapping synthetic peptides (Ziegler et al. 1996; Fournier et al. 1997). Several mAbs reacted with peptides defining the neutralizing epitope (NE) (H236–256) and blocked hemolysis of monkey erythrocytes without inhibiting hemagglutination, suggesting that they acted at the functional interface of the H and F protein and did not inhibit virus binding to host cells (Fournier et al. 1997). Co-linear synthesis of this BCE in different orientations and copy numbers with various TCE-generated peptides was capable of inducing antibodies that neutralized MV in vitro (El Kasmi et al. 1998). After passive transfer, these sera were shown to protect young mice against a lethal challenge with the neuroadapted MV strain (El Kasmi et al. 1999a). Interestingly, NE peptides were not recognized by mouse sera generated by immunization with whole virus, and protective levels of passively transferred anti-MV antibodies did not suppress a humoral response against the NE peptide (El Kasmi et al. 1999a). Mimotopes generated against mAbs of this epitope were highly antigenic but induced no neutralizing antibodies (Deroo et al. 1998; El Kasmi et al. 1998, 2000).

Another set of mAbs identified a second sequential epitope of the H protein, the hemagglutinin noose epitope (HNE) (H381–400). This sequence contains three cysteine residues (in positions 381, 386, and 394) which are conserved in all morbilliviruses (Ziegler et al. 1996), and HNE peptides formulated in Complete Freund's adjuvant (CFA) induced MV-crossreactive and -neutralizing sera even in the presence of protective levels of whole virus-specific antibodies (El Kasmi et al. 2000). The HNE domain is a highly conserved, subdominant, antigenic determinant (Putz et al. 2003b) and it was shown that sera of measles in late-convalescent women of child-bearing age do not recognize this peptide (Ziegler et al. 1996). These results suggest that passively acquired maternal antibodies in infants would not interfere with the immune response to this peptide. The protective binding motif of this peptide was revealed using surface plasmon resonance and a shortened, optimized sequence of the HNE, conjugated to immunogenic carrier proteins (DT or TT) and an adjuvant licensed for human use (alum) induced MV-crossreactive and protective antibodies (Putz et al. 2003b, 2004). Co-administration of the HNE conjugates with cholera toxin induced MV-crossreactive and -protective antibodies after intranasal and lower levels of peptide-specific antibodies following transcutaneous immunization (MM Putz and CP Muller, unpublished results).

Transgenic edible plants have been used to express viral antigens and chimeric high-molecular-weight polyepitopes. Such constructs (24.5–45.5 kDa), based on the permutational recombination of multiple paired copies of the HNE and NE sequences with a promiscuous, TT-derived TCE were developed and expressed in transgenic carrots (Bouche et al. 2003). One of these polyepitope proteins was shown to induce high levels of neutralizing antibodies in mice. These sera neutralized a wide range of wild-type MV isolates of different genotypes and from geographic origins (Bouche et al. 2003). Moreover, these sera neutralized all wild-type isolates tested irrespective of mutations in the HNE epitope (unpublished results).

RESPIRATORY SYNCYTIAL VIRUS

This single-strand, negative-sense RNA virus (pneumovirus of the Paramyxoviridae family) causes a severe lower respiratory tract infection in infants and immunosuppressed individuals. Despite decades of research, no vaccine has been licensed to protect against this disease. The numerous experimental vaccines also include a strategy based on synthetic peptides.

Residues 124–203 of the G glycoprotein represent a major immunogenic domain. When mice were immunized with a recombinant vaccinia virus expressing the corresponding peptide, protein G-crossreactive antibodies were induced and viral load in the lungs was significantly reduced following intranasal challenge with live respiratory syncytial virus (RSV) (Simard et al. 1995). Interestingly a short polymer of 14 peptides (amino acids 174–187), derived from this domain and coupled to keyhole limpet hemocyanin (KLH) conjugate, was sufficient to reduce viral load in the lungs of challenged animals (Simard et al. 1997). The same peptide epitope, inserted into the pIII coat protein of a recombinant bacteriophage, also elicited high levels of RSV-specific antibodies which conferred complete resistance to an RSV challenge (Bastien et al. 1997). Intranasal delivery of this peptide epitope mixed with CT also gave complete protection (Bastien et al. 1999).

By screening a random combinatorial octameric peptide library, a number of peptide mimotopes were identified against a neutralizing and protective mAb specific for the RSV F protein (Chargelegue et al. 1997). When mice were immunized with MAP constructs carrying these peptide mimotopes mixed with a promiscuous Th epitope peptide and CFA, virus-crossreactive antibodies were elicited which neutralized RSV in vitro. In vivo a significant decrease of infectious particles was found in the lungs of immunized mice (Chargelegue et al. 1997, 1998). A significant reduction of viral load was also achieved in mice immunized intranasally with cytotoxic T lymphocytes (CTL) epitope peptides (Hsu et al. 1998). When mice were immunized subcutaneously with a cocktail containing the MAP-mimotope construct, and Th and CTL peptides emulsified in incomplete Freund's adjuvant (IFA), an almost 200-fold reduction in the viral load was detected after challenge in comparison to the mice immunized with either of the peptides alone (Hsu et al. 1999). The RSV infection was more effectively cleared by a combined humoral and cellular response induced by the peptide cocktail than either peptide-induced humoral or cellular immunity alone. With the difficulties involved in developing an RSV vaccine by any strategy, the peptide approach is worth pursuing, although it is not clear why an approach based on defined epitopes would be an advantage.

Orthomyxovirus

INFLUENZA A VIRUS

The development of efficient influenza vaccines is complicated by the many subtypes and high mutation rates and of the virus and its reassortment. Thus, this virus is less than ideal for the development of an epitope-based vaccine. None the less, various hemagglutinin-derived peptides, conjugated to TT and immunized with CFA, induced antibodies inhibiting hemagglutination and virus growth in vitro and partially protecting mice against challenge with different influenza strains (Muller et al. 1982; Shapira et al. 1984). Peptides may thus induce a broader crossreactive and protective humoral response than expected. A similar observation was made with a polyepitope consisting of repeats of the MV HNE epitope, which induced antibodies neutralizing several MV strains with mutated critical contact residues in their HNE domain (Bouche et al. 2004).

Protective antibodies against influenza were also elicited using liposome-conjugated peptides even without CFA (Friede et al. 1994), and protective immunogenicity was further improved with cyclic peptides, assuring a better structural mimicry of the viral antigenic determinant (Muller et al. 1990).

Picornaviruses

FOOT-AND-MOUTH DISEASE VIRUS

This member of the aphthoviruses is one of the most infectious veterinary viruses, causing a devastating disease of livestock. Immunization with an inactivated whole virus precludes the possibility of distinguishing between immunized and infected animals. A safe, nonreplicating, subunit vaccine inducing a protective response in cattle and swine, against both disease and infection, and which could be differentiated from natural infection, would be an asset. Among the four structural proteins VP1–VP4, VP1 induces neutralizing antibodies (Pfaff et al. 1982), targeting two dominant antigenic sites (A and C). Synthetic peptides, corresponding to these domains, conjugated to KLH-induced antibodies that crossreacted with foot-and-mouth disease virus (FMDV) particles (Parry et al. 1988), neutralized virus infectivity in vitro, and protected in vivo (Bittle et al. 1982). Protective immunity was achieved in animal models, as well as in the natural host species, i.e. swine and cattle (DiMarchi et al. 1986; Morgan and Moore 1990). Chimeric peptides including epitopes of two different serotypes protected guinea-pigs against both serotypes (Doel et al. 1992). Serotype variability and possibly escape by mutation of this RNA virus may be overcome by the combination of peptides. In larger immunization trials of cattle with peptides derived from site A and C, coupled to a VP1-derived immunodominant TCE (Collen et al. 1991), only 40 percent protection was achieved (Taboga et al. 1997). Protection was undermined by the rapid generation of escape mutants in immunized animals (Taboga et al. 1997). In a more recent study with a vaccine consisting of unconjugated peptides with the built-in adjuvant tripalmitoyl-*S*-glyceryl-cysteinylserylserine (P3C) (Wiesmüller et al. 1989; Hohlich et al. 2003), protection did not correlate with the detection of high levels of antibody. Instead, strong peptide-specific T-cell responses were detected, (Hohlich et al. 2003). Retro-all-d-peptide analogs of site A (Muller et al. 1995; Benkirane et al. 1996b) further improved the immunogenicity and induced high levels of neutralizing and protective antibodies (Briand et al. 1997).

Various different peptide formulations were used. Neutralizing and protective antibodies were obtained by peptides either conjugated to an immunogenic carrier protein (e.g. KLH, TT; Bittle et al. 1982), unconjugated P3C peptides (Wiesmüller et al. 1989; Hohlich et al. 2003) or delivered in liposomes (Francis et al. 1985), as MAP constructs (Francis et al. 1991) or emulsified in oil adjuvants (Taboga et al. 1997; Wang et al. 2001, 2002a). Site A epitope is a highly disordered loop within the VP1 (Acharya et al. 1989). Crossreactive immunogenicity of a synthetic peptide epitope results from the right balance between rigidity and flexibility, and cyclization of site A peptide was shown to produce a more stable immunogenic structure (Camarero et al. 1993; Valero et al. 2000). The peptide was also constrained in recombinant proteins (Benito and Villaverde 1994; Benito and Van Regenmortel 1998) and, if one gave a better mimic of the viral epitope than conjugated synthetic peptides, others did not (Benito and Van Regenmortel 1998).

POLIOVIRUS

At the present, late stage of polio eradication, the development of an effective nonreplicating vaccine becomes an important issue. Although the inactivated Salk vaccine would be suitable, current production capacities are not sufficient. The development of a peptide vaccine is complicated by the three serotypes, each requiring its own neutralizing antibodies. Several VP1- and VP2-derived peptide epitopes were identified and shown to induce virus-neutralizing antibodies in various animal models, including guinea-pigs and rabbits when conjugated to carrier proteins (Emini et al. 1983, 1984a; Jameson et al. 1985). However, crossreactive immunogenicity was modest, as less than 30 percent of the animals developed neutralizing antibodies.

HEPATITIS A VIRUS

A sequential neutralizing epitope has been identified on the VP1 protein by comparison of surface probability profiles between hepatitis A virus (HAV) and poliovirus (Emini et al. 1985), despite minimal homology between their primary and secondary structures. Virus cross-reacting and in vitro neutralizing antibodies were induced with a VP1-peptide BSA (Emini et al. 1985), KLH conjugate, or MAP constructs (Haro et al. 1995). Two other sequential BCEs were reported on the VP2 (Robertson et al. 1989) and VP3 surface proteins (Wheeler et al. 1986). Each of the three VP1, VP2, and VP3 peptides, encapsulated in multilamellar liposomes, induced virus-neutralizing antibodies (Bosch et al. 1998). The best virus-crossreactive/neutralizing antibodies were obtained with VP3-derived peptide (Bosch et al. 1998). However, this strategy would offer no obvious advantage over current vaccines.

Flavivirus

HEPATITIS C VIRUS

This is a major cause of acute and chronic hepatitis with 180 million cases worldwide. The development of an effective vaccine against hepatitis C virus (HCV) has been so far unsuccessful. The hypervariable region 1 (HVR1) of the main E2 envelope protein has been identified as a target of neutralizing antibodies (Farci et al.

1996). A consensus sequence of HVR1 was genetically fused to the C terminus of the B subunit of CTB and expressed in plants using a tobamoviral vector (Nemchinov et al. 2000). Intranasal immunization of mice with a crude plant extract containing the recombinant chimeric HVR1-CTB protein induced antibodies crossreacting with HCV-like particles (Nemchinov et al. 2000). HCV-crossreacting antibodies were also elicited in mice using HVR1-derived peptides conjugated to KLH (Li et al. 2001) or recombinantly expressed polyepitope constructs (Li et al. 2003), and in rabbits with MAPs containing mimotope peptides (Roccasecca et al. 2001).

Retrovirus

HUMAN IMMUNODEFICIENCY VIRUS (HIV)

Despite worldwide efforts, there is no vaccine available against human immunodeficiency viruses 1 and 2 (HIV-1 and HIV-2). The characteristic viral envelope spike is formed by monomers of the two surface glycoproteins gp41 and gp120 and carries several well-characterized BCEs targeted by broadly reactive human neutralizing mAbs (Burton et al. 2004). For safety reasons, vaccine development has principally focused on subunits rather than live attenuated or chemically inactivated virus. The development of an effective vaccine is particularly difficult because there is no natural recovery from infection, which could serve as a model for a protective immune response, but neutralizing antibodies are (again) thought to be important for protection. The situation is further complicated of course by antigenic variability.

Most of the BCE experimental vaccines against HIV are based on the 'principal neutralizing domain', i.e. the third variable domain (V3) of the gp120 glycoprotein of HIV-1. MAPs, derived from this sequence, coupled to the 'built-in' adjuvant tripalmitoyl-*S*-glycerylcysteine (Deres et al. 1989) and formulated in liposomes, induced in laboratory animals gp120-specific antibodies which neutralized virus infectivity in vitro (Defoort et al. 1992b; Nardelli et al. 1992). However, neutralizing antibodies were type specific and crossreactivity in enzyme-linked immunosorbent assay (ELISA) with other strains was weak (Nardelli et al. 1992). 'Cluster peptides', consisting of synthetic peptide constructs of the V3 loop and overlapping multideterminant Th epitopes of gp160, induced V3-specific neutralizing antibodies in several strains of mice (Berzofsky et al. 1991; Ahlers et al. 1993). Intranasal immunization with free V3 loop peptides and the mucosal adjuvant CT generated HIV-1-neutralizing antibody responses in two strains of mice (Staats et al. 1996). In addition to high serum anti-peptide responses, significant vaginal anti-peptide IgG and IgA levels were obtained (Staats et al. 1996). Neutralizing secretory IgA antibodies were also induced after oral delivery of multivalent MAPs mixed with CT (Bukawa et al. 1995; Kato et al. 2000). Systemic and mucosal antibody responses were further improved by co-administration of proinflammatory cytokines, such as the interleukins IL-1α, IL-12, and IL-18, instead of CT (Bradney et al. 2002).

Synthetic peptide vaccines have also been tested in clinical trials with encouraging long-term safety profiles when adjuvants other than IFA were used. Long-lasting, peptide-specific, neutralizing humoral responses were obtained with a purified protein derivative (PPD) conjugate vaccine without the use of an adjuvant (Rubinstein et al. 1995, 1999). HIV-seropositive vaccinees over time exhibited a uniform increase in antibodies capable of neutralizing laboratory-adapted and primary isolates of HIV-1. Highest titers were observed after 12 months in a regimen where the peptide conjugate was inoculated intradermally, monthly for the first 3 months and then at 3-month intervals to 18 months. In three of seven patients, a progressive decline in viral loads occurred (Rubinstein et al. 1999). Although viral mutants with amino acid substitutions within the V3 loop sequence appeared in these three patients during the immunization program, virus loads remained at low levels for several months (Lenz et al. 2001). However, about a year after discontinuation of immunization, in six patients viremia was at preimmunization levels or higher and was paralleled by a loss in V3 loop-specific antibodies (Rubinstein et al. 1999). An unconjugated, octameric, branching, V3 loop peptide adsorbed on alum induced in vitro neutralizing antibodies in eight of ten HIV-1-uninfected, healthy adults after intramuscular administration (Gorse et al. 1996). Whereas the same vaccine formulation displayed a similar high neutralizing efficacy (19 of 20 vaccinees) in a trial in Bangkok, Thailand (Phanuphak et al. 1997), lower seroconversion rates (3 of 13 vaccinees) were observed in a trial in Longchuan County, China (Li et al. 2001). This octameric peptide vaccine was weakly immunogenic (4 of 24 vaccinees seroconverted) when delivered subcutaneously in combination with alum (Kelleher et al. 1997), and after oral administration of peptides encapsulated in biodegradable microspheres no significant humoral, cellular, or mucosal immune responses were found (Lambert et al. 2001a).

However, sterilizing immunity to HIV-1 will most probably be achieved only through a combination of protective antibody and CTL responses. Promising results have been obtained with peptide vaccines eliciting cellular immune responses (Letvin 1998; Suhrbier 2002).

Parvoviruses

CANINE PARVOVIRUS

The use of a peptide vaccine against canine parvovirus (CPV) was among the first to demonstrate the induction of protection in the natural host (Langeveld et al. 1994b). Among the three structural proteins VP1–VP3 of the virus capsid, VP2 is the major immunogen. Immunization with two overlapping peptides of the N-terminal domain of VP2 conjugated to KLH protected dogs against a lethal challenge with CPV, despite the intriguing observation that virus-neutralizing antibodies were not detected in any of the immunized and protected animals before challenge (Langeveld et al. 1994a, b). Protection was attributed to the high flexibility of the epitope and its functional importance for viral replication (Langeveld et al. 1994a). Efficacy of the peptide vaccine was shown to result from two distinct but overlapping epitopes, each of which induced neutralizing antibodies in rabbits (Langeveld et al. 1994b; Casal et al. 1995). Mutation rates are low in this DNA virus (in comparison to RNA viruses) and this N-terminal epitope is conserved in different virus isolates (Parrish et al. 1988), including the three closely related virus species, mink enteritis virus (MEV), feline panleukopenia virus (FPLV), and raccoon parvovirus. Thus, the same epitope could be used in three important animal species: dogs (Langeveld et al. 1994a), cats (Langeveld et al. 2001a), and band minks (Langeveld et al. 1995). Immunization with the CPV-derived peptide conjugated to KLH protected minks against MEV (Langeveld et al. 1995). When the corresponding MEV oligonucleotide coding sequence was inserted into the plant virus, cowpea mosaic virus, the epitope was expressed on the surface of the chimeric virus particles propagated in the black-eyed bean, an edible plant. Subcutaneous injections of minks with recombinant virus-like particles protected against clinical disease and virtually abolished shedding of virus after challenge with virulent MEV (Dalsgaard et al. 1997). Chimeric virus-like particles also protected dogs from a lethal challenge with CPV (Langeveld et al. 2001b). A multivalent vaccine based on peptides of CPV, canine distemper virus (CDV), and *Pseudomonas aeruginosa* could be a commercially viable strategy because they would protect dogs against two important canine diseases and minks against the three major diseases in mink farming.

Hepadnavirus

HEPATITIS B VIRUS

It is estimated that 400 million people are chronically infected worldwide with hepatitis B virus (HBV). Protective antibodies in humans mostly target the hepatitis B virus surface antigen (HBsAG). Several continuous BCEs have been identified on HBsAg (Gerin et al. 1983). When coupled to a carrier protein, such as KLH, some of these peptides induced a weak, but partially protective, humoral response in chimpanzees (Gerin et al. 1983; Itoh et al. 1986). Protective immune responses were also obtained with unconjugated, longer polymers of 55 peptides (Emini et al. 1989). MAPs induced increased antibody responses in rabbits (Tam and Lu 1989). A peptide-based approach using CTL epitopes has also been explored (reviewed by Engler et al. 2001). After initial encouraging results (Vitiello et al. 1995; Livingston et al. 1997, 1999) CTL responses were weak in later human trials (Heathcote et al. 1999).

Papovavirus

HUMAN PAPILLOMAVIRUS

Human papillomavirus (HPV) is a double-stranded, circular DNA virus with more than 100 genotypes. In particular the high-risk genotypes (HPV16, -18, -31, -33, and -45) are found in almost all cervical carcinomas. Experimental preventive and therapeutic vaccines against HPV-mediated cervical cancer were recently reviewed (Fausch et al. 2003; Roden and Wu 2003). A peptide from the E7 protein of HPV16 containing a BCE, a promiscuous T helper, and a CTL epitope were coupled to immunostimulatory carriers (ISCAR) (Tindle et al. 1995) or combined as polymeric conjugates (Fernando et al. 1995) with either CFA or ISCOMs. These constructs induced E7-crossreactive antibodies and E7-specific CTLs with in vitro killing activity (Tindle et al. 1995), and conferred in vivo protection against an E7 gene-transfected tumor cell inoculum (Tindle et al. 1995). Sequential neutralizing BCEs have also been identified of the L1 (major) and L2 (minor) structural proteins using mAbs (Kawana et al. 1998). A BSA-conjugated L2-derived peptide induced antibodies that crossneutralized HPV16 and -6 (Kawana et al. 1999). Intranasal immunization with the same epitope in TCE-containing chimeric peptides, mixed to CT, induced antibodies cross-binding to HPV6, -16 ,and -18, and neutralizing HPV11 authentic virions and HPV16 pseudovirions in vitro (Kawana et al. 1999, 2001). These results suggest that this BCE is shared by other genital HPVs and may induce broadly reactive, cross-neutralizing antibodies. Early safety and immunogenicity trials in humans were promising. Intranasal delivery of a linear polymer of 13 peptides without adjuvant induced antibodies neutralizing HPV15 and -52 (Kawana et al. 2003). Peptide vaccines targeting tumor-specific CTL responses are discussed later in the chapter.

Bacteria

NEISSERIA MENINGITIDIS SEROGROUP C

Most of the infections by *Neisseria meningitidis*, gram-negative encapsulated bacteria, are caused by any of the four prevalent serogroups: A, B, C, and Y. Polysaccharide-conjugate vaccines induce neutralizing antibodies against surface loops of class 1 outer membrane proteins (OMP), which play a major role in protection. TT-based conjugates loaded with cyclic peptides derived from OMP induced mouse antibodies with bactericidal activity in vitro (Hoogerhout et al. 1995). Protective immune responses against experimental challenge were seen in mice with unconjugated, free peptides of the PorA and the OpaB outer membrane proteins (Koroev et al. 2000, 2001). Polysaccharides can be mimicked using peptides or anti-idiotype antibodies as surrogate antigens (reviewed by Monzavi-Karbassi et al. 2002). Immunization with mimotopes conjugated to DT induced antibodies crossreacting with the meningococcal outer-membrane lipo-oligosaccharide (Charalambous and Feavers 2000). Short peptides derived from the CDR sequences of protective anti-idiotype antibodies, and conjugated to proteosomes, induced antibodies protecting mice against a lethal dose of *N. meningitidis* (Westerink et al. 1995; Prinz et al. 2004). Mimotope peptides were also incorporated into DNA constructs. After DNA immunization, significant anti-polysaccharide antibody responses were induced, neutralizing bacterial activity in vitro and protecting against a challenge in vivo (Westerink et al. 2001; Prinz et al. 2003).

Several other peptide-based vaccines have been developed to protect against *Pseudomonas aeruginosa* (reviewed by Cachia and Hodges 2003) and group A streptococcus (reviewed by Olive et al. 2004) and others (see Table 42.1).

Parasites

MALARIA

This is by far the most important parasitic disease in humans, caused by four *Plasmodium* species (*P. falciparum*, *P. malariae*, *P. ovale*, *P. vivax*) and spread by female anopheles mosquitoes. More than 200 species are known to parasitize mammals (e.g. *P. berghei* and *P. yoelii* in mice, *P. knowlesi* in monkeys), birds, and reptiles. The development of a malaria vaccine is a difficult task for various reasons: the life cycle of malaria parasites in humans is complex with morphologically and antigenically distinct stages. There is a high degree of antigenic variation among *Plasmodium* species. Immunity is stage specific. An important part of the population does not respond to particular parasite antigens. Nevertheless, several peptide epitopes inducing neutralizing and protective antibodies have been identified on antigens of the pre-erythrocytic (e.g. circumsporozoite protein (CSP); thrombospondin-related anonymous protein (TRAP); liver stage antigen 3 (LSA-3)) and the asexual blood stage (e.g. major merozoite surface protein (MSP-1); ring-infected erythrocyte surface antigen (RESA)). Malaria vaccine developments have been reviewed by Tsuji and Zavala (2001) and Moorthy et al. (2004).

A synthetic immunodominant repeat sequence, derived from the *P. falciparum* CSP, conjugated to TT, induced antibodies crossreacting with the parasite surface and neutralizing its infectivity in vitro (Zavala et al. 1985). This peptide conjugate proved its safety and immunogenicity in phase I and II clinical trials where the majority of recipients seroconverted. One of three challenged vaccinees was totally protected and in the others the infection was delayed and/or reduced (Herrington et al. 1987). Significant T-cell responses to the coupled peptide were reported which may play a role in priming for protection (Etlinger et al. 1988). In another trial, however, the clinical efficacy of the conjugate was substantially lower and only one of seven vaccinees was protected against a sporozoite challenge (Herrington et al. 1990). MAPs, containing BCEs and TCEs, significantly improved immunogenicity (Tam et al. 1990). MAPs induced higher titers of neutralizing antibodies in mice (Joshi et al. 2001) and, in combination with alum and saponin QS21, in monkeys (Moreno et al. 1999) and humans (Nardin et al. 2000). Novel multi-epitope polyoxime constructs containing the CSP repeat epitope, a CSP-derived universal TCE and the built-in adjuvant P3C, induced high antibody levels in human volunteers of diverse HLA types (Nardin et al. 2001).

A repeat domain epitope derived from *P. berghei* CSP induced high serum titers of protective antibody responses in mice when administered as TT conjugates. In these constructs, the orientation of the conjugated peptide, as well as the peptide:carrier ratio, was critical for protection (Zavala et al. 1987). Only BSA conjugates with a high enough peptide load achieved total protection in animals (Reed et al. 1996). Multiple antigen delivery systems containing *P. berghei* CSP-derived BCEs and TCEs induced protective immune responses in mice when combined with CFA (Tam et al. 1990) or detoxified lipopolysaccharide (RaLPS) (Reed et al. 1997). Despite the presence of a *P. yoelii* CSP-derived BCE in the multiple antigen constructs of Reed et al. (1997), protection was weak against *P. berghei* and negative against *P. yoelii*. However, when delivered in a recombinant HBV nucleocapsid antigen (HBcAg), the *P. yoelii* CSP-derived BCE induced protective immune responses in mice (Schodel et al. 1997) and results were promising in preclinical trials in primates (Birkett et al. 2002).

Multiple antigen constructs (MAC) containing a BCE from the *P. vivax* CSP repeat region and a promiscuous TCE from TT induced a protective immune response in monkeys when administered with alum or RaLPS (Yang et al. 1997).

LSA-3 is a highly conserved pre-erythrocytic antigen and a promising vaccine candidate (Perlaza et al. 2001). A 26-residue sequence of this protein induced strong B, Th cell, and CTL responses in chimpanzees when delivered as palmitoyl-conjugated lipopeptides (BenMohamed et al. 1997). Protective immune responses were achieved with a combination of lipopeptides (Daubersies et al. 2000).

Several peptides derived from the merozoite MSP-1 antigen were included in conjugates using BSA or TT as carriers (Berzins et al. 1986) or, more recently, in 'double dimer constructs' (Rivera et al. 2002). These peptides induce antibodies that partially protected monkeys against a challenge infection. Peptides of another well-characterized asexual blood stage antigen, the RESA protein, coupled to TT or KLH, inhibited merozoite reinvasion of erythrocytes in vitro (Cheung et al. 1986) and gave partial protection in monkeys (Patarroyo et al. 1987). Similarly, peptide conjugates from other merozoite stage antigens, such as Pf55 and Pf35, provided partial protection in monkeys and even complete protection when three conjugates were combined (Patarroyo et al. 1987).

Multicomponent and multistage strategies have been considered in order to induce several lines of defense against the different stages of its life cycle. Patarroyo and colleagues developed a synthetic hybrid polymer, containing the peptide sequences derived from MSP-1, Pf55, and Pf35, and repeat sequences from CSP, which was further polymerized using cysteine residues at its N- and C-terminal ends to result in a high-molecular-weight synthetic protein (150 000) inducing protective immune responses in monkeys (Patarroyo et al. 1988; Rodriguez et al. 1990; Ruebush et al. 1990). Very promising results were initially obtained with this fully synthetic protein termed 'SPf66', in early clinical trials, when administered together with alum as adjuvant: delay or even complete suppression of parasitemia was observed in immunized human volunteers (Patarroyo et al. 1988; Amador et al. 1992a, b; Valero et al. 1993). Antibodies induced in humans markedly inhibited parasite growth in vitro (Salcedo et al. 1991). The vaccine was shown to be highly immunogenic and safe in children aged 1–14 years (Patarroyo et al. 1992). Efficacy of up to 80 percent was observed (Amador et al. 1992b). However, the efficacies reported subsequently in larger field trials were consistently below 40 percent (Valero et al. 1993, 1996) and in a study in northern Thailand, an area with a high *P. falciparum* attack rate, no protection was observed (Nosten et al. 1996). In a different approach Shi and colleagues used a recombinant polyepitope containing twelve BCE, six T-helper epitopes, and three CTL epitopes derived from nine stage-specific *P. falciparum* antigens expressed in the baculovirus system (Shi et al. 1999). This polyepitope induced antibodies cross-reacting with the different stages of the parasite and neutralizing parasite activity in vitro (Shi et al. 1999). Recombinant polyepitope constructs based on CTL epitopes are being further explored with encouraging results (Tsuji and Zavala 2001).

SCHISTOSOMIASIS

Schistosomes are parasitic trematodes causing chronic disease in an estimated 200 million people worldwide. Infections in humans are mostly caused by one of the three helminth species *Schistosoma manson i*, *S. haematobium*, and *S. japonicum*, and candidate vaccines are currently being investigated in clinical trials (Capron et al. 2002). Several antigens or fragments derived from them, e.g. 9B (Tarrab-Hazdai et al. 1998), P28-1 (Wolowczuk et al. 1989), Sm23 (Reynolds et al. 1992), triose phosphate isomerase (TPI) (Reynolds et al. 1994), Sm14 (Tendler et al. 1996), and glutathione-*S*-transferase (Sm28-GST) (Ferru et al. 1997) have been identified as targets of specific B-cell and Th-cell responses. Early work on synthetic peptide vaccines against schistosomiasis has been discussed by Harn et al. (1995). In more recent studies a polymer of 14 peptides derived from the 9B antigen, conjugated to BSA, induced an immune response that was able to reduce significantly the worm burden after challenge in a murine model (Tarrab-Hazdai et al. 1998). Protective immune responses were also observed after intranasal immunization with a recombinant salmonella flagellin protein carrying this 9B epitope sequence (Ben-Yedidia et al. 1999). By screening a solid-phase octamer library against a 9B-specific mAb, four peptide mimotopes were identified, one of which induced a protective immune response (Arnon et al. 2000). It is noteworthy that protection against *S. mansoni* challenge was also obtained after immunization with two unconjugated peptides (derived from the Sm14 antigen) in the presence of the adjuvant system monophosphoryl lipid A/trehalose dicorynomycolate (MPL-TDM) (Vilar et al. 2003). Interestingly, these Sm14-derived epitopes cross-protected mice against a challenge with *Fasciola hepatica*, a helminth affecting sheep and cattle (Vilar et al. 2003). A multiepitope approach, combining 10 different epitopes of various *S. mansoni* antigens, was investigated using DNA and recombinant protein immunization. However, none of the tested constructs induced a protective response (Yang et al. 2000).

CYSTICERCOSIS

Taenia solium, a parasitic tapeworm causing cysticercosis, is highly prevalent in humans and pigs in Latin America, Asia, and Africa, and has serious health and economic consequences. Experimental vaccines for use in pigs, the obligatory intermediate host, are currently under development and include a peptide-based approach (reviewed by Sciutto et al. 2002).

Four recombinant antigens (KETc1, -4, -7, and -12) expressed during the cysticercus stage of both *T. solium* and *T. crassiceps*, a cestode causing murine cysticercosis, confer different levels of protection in immunized mice (Manoutcharian et al. 1996). A synthetic 18-residue peptide GK-1, derived from the KETc7 protein and emulsified in saponin, induces antibodies crossreacting with the cognate antigen without the use of a carrier protein (Toledo et al. 1999). It is noteworthy that this

GK-1 peptide contains at least one TCE, which was demonstrated by its ability to stimulate proliferation of $CD8^+$ and to a lesser extent $CD4^+$ T cells. GK-1-induced immunity only partially protected against a challenge infection with *T. crassiceps* and this did not improve when the peptide was delivered as MAP or coupled to BSA (Toledo et al. 1999). Similarly, two polymeric peptides of 13 and 9 residues, derived from the KETc1 and -12 antigens, induced B-cell and T-cell responses, partially protecting mice against cysticercosis caused by *T. crassiceps* (Toledo et al. 2001). In a controlled field trial, immunization of piglets with a combination of the unconjugated peptides KETc1, -7, and -12 with saponin decreased the total number of viable *T. solium* cysticerci by almost 98 percent and the prevalence of cysticercosis among immunized animals by more than half (Huerta et al. 2001).

Contraception

A vaccine providing safe, inexpensive, and reversible contraception would greatly help to regulate the world's growing population (reviewed by Aitken 2002). A peptide approach would at least be inexpensive, reversible after 1–2 years, and would not require a cold chain.

A C-terminal peptide of human chorionic hormone (hCG), an essential hormone during pregnancy, coupled to TT, induced high titers of antibodies, successfully reducing fertility in female baboons (Stevens et al. 1981a). Further studies in mice, rabbits, and baboons led to the formulation of a vaccine based on the water-soluble synthetic adjuvant, *N*-acetylglucosamine-3-yl-acetyl-l-alanyl-d-isoglutamine (CGP-11637) suitable for use in humans (Stevens et al. 1981b). In clinical trials, hCG-crossreactive antibodies were observed, which were thought to neutralize the biological activity of hCG, but definitive proof of a contraception was not obtained in this study (Jones et al. 1988). The low immunogenicity of this hCG peptide was overcome by immunizing with the entire β-subunit of hCG and prevention of pregnancy was shown in clinical trials (Talwar 1999). The luteinizing hormone-releasing hormone (LHRH) is a short decapeptide hormone secreted by the hypothalamus. Branched peptide constructs containing the LHRH peptide and a T-helper cell epitope (ThCE) induced sterilizing antibodies in female mice (Ghosh and Jackson 1999).

A synthetic BCE of the zona pellucida glycoprotein ZP3, either conjugated to KLH (Millar et al. 1989) or delivered as a chimeric peptide containing a foreign promiscuous TCE (Lou et al. 1995; Sadler et al. 1999), induced antibodies in mice crossreacting with the cognate protein, providing a long-term, but reversible, contraception without impairment of normal ovarian functions. Immunocontraception was also produced in female macaques after administration of conjugates with coupled human and macaque ZP3 peptides (Mahi-Brown and Moran 1995; Mahi-Brown 1996). Antibodies inhibiting human sperm binding to oocytes in vitro were obtained using chimeric TCE–BCE peptides in macaques (Bagavant et al. 1997) and common marmosets, but the antibodies did not reduce fertility in a primate model (Paterson et al. 1999, 2002). Antibodies targeting an epitope located on the human sperm antigen lactate dehydrogenase (LDH)-C_4 have been induced in baboons using peptide conjugates and chimeric peptides (O'Hern et al. 1995, 1997). Fertility in immunized animals was reduced by 70 percent and the contraceptive effect lasted for almost a year. The same epitope in chimeric peptides induced significant contraception in mice (Sadler et al. 1999). Recently, a novel peptide epitope (YLP12) was identified on human sperm, eliciting long-lasting sperm-specific antibodies that assured contraception in female mice when conjugated to CTB and administered intranasally (Naz and Chauhan 2002; Naz 2004). Fertility was fully restored after 10 months when the antibody titers had fallen below a certain threshold.

Immunocastration has been developed as an economical alternative to surgical castration of male pigs to prevent the growth of testes and the production of male sexual steroid hormones, which is associated with an unappealing odor of the meat. Immunocastration was obtained in male pigs after CFA-adjuvanted immunization with peptides derived from gonadotropin-releasing hormone (GnRH) and conjugated to KLH or OVA (Meloen et al. 1994) or ISCOMs (Beekman et al. 1999). Similarly high responding rates were obtained with low doses of conjugated double-dimer peptides mixed with a mild oil adjuvant (Specol; Oonk et al. 1998; X.Y. Zeng et al. 2001). With the encouraging results and the specific advantages of a peptide vaccine, this approach may become a truly inexpensive alternative to current contraceptive drugs.

Alzheimer's disease

Alzheimer's disease, the most common cause of dementing disorders in elderly people, causes progressive loss of central nervous functions. Pathogenesis involves the overproduction of the 42-residue amyloid-β peptide ($A\beta_{42}$) derived from the amyloid precursor protein (APP), progressive accumulation of $A\beta_{42}$ in extracellular plaques within the cerebral cortex and the hippocampus (Reilly et al. 2003), followed by neurodegeneration (Selkoe 1999). The progress of and drawbacks in antibodies as therapeutic agents in Alzheimer's disease have been extensively discussed by Morgan (2003) and Solomon (2002).

Transgenic mouse models have been used to investigate the possibility of therapeutic immunization against Alzheimer's disease (Games et al. 1995). Immunization with the synthetic $A\beta_{42}$-induced $A\beta_{42}$-specific antibodies, which prevented the development of β-amyloid plaque and Alzheimer's disease-type neuropathologies in animals immunized at a young age (Schenk et al. 1999). Moreover, these antibodies greatly reduced progressive degeneration and even cleared pre-existing plaques of $A\beta_{42}$ deposits in older animals (Schenk et al. 1999). Furthermore, $A\beta_{42}$ immunization prevented learning and age-related memory defects normally developing in transgenic mice (Janus et al. 2000; Morgan et al. 2000). Significant decrease in the cerebral β-amyloid plaque burden was also obtained in mice after intranasal administration of synthetic $A\beta_{42}$ using LT as adjuvant (Weiner et al. 2000; Lemere et al. 2001). In vitro studies revealed that mAbs specific for a short $A\beta_{42}$ N-terminal fragment prevented fibrillar aggregation and $A\beta_{42}$-mediated neurotoxicity in a concentration-dependent manner (Solomon et al. 1997). Immunization of mice using a recombinant filamentous phage displaying an N-terminal derived tetramer peptide sequence induced antibodies that exhibited in vitro anti-aggregating properties and neutralizing $A\beta_{42}$-related toxicity (Frenkel et al. 2001, 2003). This phage also markedly reduced the number of plaques in the brain of transgenic mice (Frenkel et al. 2003). Similar protective in vivo effects were obtained after immunization with a modified $A\beta_{42}$-derived, polylysine peptide (Sigurdsson et al. 2001). Furthermore, low antibody titers and self-tolerance were proposed to result primarily from inadequate T-cell help, which could be overcome by using palmitoylated $A\beta_{42}$ reconstituted in liposomes–lipid A (Nicolau et al. 2002) or by conjugating a short $A\beta_{42}$-derived polymer of 15 residues to BSA (Monsonego et al. 2001). However, immunization with conjugated, short, serum amyloid protein-derived peptides did not protect mice against β-amyloid plaque deposits (Schenk et al. 1999). Antibodies against plaque components themselves may not be sufficient to prevent plaque aggregation and antibodies targeting specifically the $A\beta_{42}$ seem to be required for preventing disease.

A phase I study showed that immunization with the synthetic $A\beta_{42}$ was well tolerated and some patients developed $A\beta_{42}$-specific antibodies (Schenk 2002). However, phase IIa trials had to be discontinued because of several reports of inflammatory symptoms of the central nervous system which resembled encephalitis or meningitis (Check 2002). Autopsy of a brain from a treated patient provided astonishing evidence of how anti-$A\beta_{42}$ antibodies efficiently cleared $A\beta_{42}$ deposits in the cerebral cortex (Nicoll et al. 2003). Intriguing parallels between the rare cerebral amyloid angiopathy-associated inflammation and the vaccine-related encephalitis suggests that the vaccine-mediated inflammatory response was directed not only against the $A\beta_{42}$ plaques but also against vascular amyloid (Greenberg et al. 2003; Nicoll et al. 2003; Robinson et al. 2003). With more refined immunotherapeutic approaches, which will avoid autoimmune and acute neuroinflammatory responses (Robinson et al. 2003; Weller and Nicoll 2003), peptide-based immunotherapy against Alzheimer's disease may become a realistic option.

BCE peptide vaccines against cancer

Although most studies with peptide vaccines against tumors target CTLs (see later), interesting results have also been obtained with peptides eliciting anti-tumor antibodies, e.g. Kaumaya and colleagues (Dakappagari et al. 2000) developed a chimeric HER-2 BCE vaccine in mice transgenic for a homolog of human HER-2. These mice developed mammary tumors that resembled human breast cancer. Peptides corresponding to predicted BCEs were co-linearly synthesized with a promiscuous TCE of MV, induced antibodies in rabbits that crossreacted and interrupted the development of mammary tumors in the above transgenic mouse model, and mediated killing of human tumor cells in vitro (Dakappagari et al. 2000). Table 42.1 shows that such antibodies against breast cancer and others have also been elicited in humans by immunization with peptides derived from different tumor-associated antigens (TAA). In the case of B-cell lymphomas, peptides inducing anti-idiotype responses resulted in a clinical response in most patients (Hsu et al. 1996; Bendandi et al. 1999).

PEPTIDE-BASED VACCINES AGAINST TCES

Although peptides have also been used to induce protective CTLs against infectious and other disease, the focus of this section is on CTLs of malignant tumors.

Tumor immunology and peptides

A number of reviews have been published on different aspects of synthetic peptides as cancer vaccines (Mayordomo et al. 1996; Slingluff 1996; Olive et al. 2001; Buteau et al. 2002; Machiels et al. 2002; Parmiani et al. 2002a, b; Sundaram et al. 2002). Some authors have concentrated on certain tumors, or tumor antigens including melanoma (Mocellin et al. 2003), HPV-associated malignancies (Fausch et al. 2003), and Her-2/neu (Correa and Plunkett 2001; Disis et al. 2001; Knutson and Disis 2001; Salit et al. 2002).

Early studies showed that the injection of tumor-derived material in animals or even cancer patients limited tumor growth. With the discovery of TAAs it became possible to investigate the immune response against cancer (reviewed by Herlyn and Koprowski 1988; Schreiber et al. 1988; Urban and Schreiber 1992; Boon et al. 1994). These studies showed that T cells mediate the principal effector mechanisms against tumors, although the humoral response as demonstrated by therapeutic monoclonal antibodies such as trastuzumab (Herceptin, Baselga 2001), rituximab (Rituxan, Davis et al. 1999; Huhn et al. 2001), and peptide-specific antibodies (see Table 42.1) must not be underestimated.

Unlike B cells (see earlier), T cells do not recognize intact proteins but rather MHC-bound antigen-derived peptides. These peptides are generated during antigen processing and are presented by MHC class I or II molecules to $CD8^+$ or $CD4^+$ T cells. Normally CTL epitopes originate from intracellular proteins degraded in the cytosol by the proteasome and carried by specialized transporters (TAPs) into the endoplasmic reticulum, where they bind to MHCI to be taxied to the cell surface for a date with $CD8^+$ T cells. In contrast, $CD4^+$-restricted epitopes originate from exogenous proteins taken up and degraded in phagolysosomes into peptides that co-localize with MHCII, which shuttles them back to the cell surface, where they meet with $CD4^+$ T cells. MHC molecules fix peptides in an extended conformation and synthetic peptides are undistinguishable from natural peptides.

T cells specific for TAAs were found in many cancer patients but also in healthy donors. In healthy individuals, frequencies of such CTLs seem to be lower (Marincola et al. 1996; Altieri et al. 1999; Nagorsen et al. 2000; Andersen et al. 2001) and of a different phenotype. In healthy donors these were of the $CD45RO^+$ naive T-cell subset, whereas in melanoma patients peptide-specific CTL precursors were of the functionally distinct $CD45RO^+$, $CCR7^+$ memory phenotype (D'Souza et al. 1998; Anichini et al. 1999; Dunbar et al. 2000).

In clinical trials in tumor patients, promising results such as full or partial remission have been largely attributed to the induction of $CD8^+$ MHCI-restricted CTLs. Many TAA-derived MHCI-restricted peptides are recognized by tumor-specific CTLs at both the induction and the effector stage (see Table 42.4; Jager et al. 2001). In addition, MHCII-restricted ThCEs of a number of TAAs have been identified (Topalian et al. 1996; Manici et al. 1999; Pieper et al. 1999; Wang et al. 1999b; Chiari et al. 2000; Renkvist et al. 2001). In the first application of a peptide vaccine in humans, HBV-negative volunteers were immunized with a lipopeptide construct containing an HLA-A*0201-restricted peptide, a pan-class II-binding peptide, and palmitic acid tails. CTLs were induced that lysed syngeneic HBV-infected target cells in vitro (Vitiello et al. 1995). Cytotoxic TCEs restricted by some of the more frequent MHCI alleles have been identified for an increasing number of TAAs (reviewed by Maeurer et al. 1996). Peptides derived from a variety of TAAs have sometimes induced vigorous responses against tumors. Regression of primary tumors and metastasis were seen using a variety of different immunization protocols.

However, to measure the success of tumor immunization, the identification of surrogate in vitro read-outs, which correlate and may even predict clinical outcome, is of paramount importance. Besides conventional assays such as CTL and cytokine assays, increasingly sophisticated reagents based on synthetic peptides such as a MHC–tetramer (www.niaid.nih.gov/reposit/tetramer/index.html) and MHC–Streptamer complexes (Knabel et al. 2002, www.iba-go.com) become commercially available to study and even isolate peptide-specific T cells for functional assays.

Identification of CTL epitopes

Synthetic peptides have been powerful tools to identify class II- and I-restricted TCEs by systematic screening in functional assays. MHC-bound peptides eluted directly from tumor material of patients were identified on the basis of their mass and partial sequence by highly sensitive tandem mass spectrometry (Hunt et al. 1992). Increasingly refined prediction algorithms support these studies since the structural basis of MHC-peptide binding became understood (Pamer et al. 1991). Pool sequencing of MHC-eluted peptides (Rotzschke et al. 1990; Falk et al. 1991) has revealed that peptides bind to MHCI via an allele-specific consensus motif of anchor residues. Thus, MHC molecules encoded by different gene loci and different haplotypes bind their own distinct (but sometimes overlapping) family of peptides, usually with eight to ten amino acids (for a review, see Rammensee 1995; Rammensee et al. 1995, 1997). Interactive websites (www.syfpeithi.bmi-heidelberg.com, www.bimas.dcrt.nih.gov/molbio/index.html) identify peptides within a submitted antigen sequence that bind to a given MHC. Other consensus motifs have been identified to predict peptides surviving antigen processing (Nussbaum et al. 1998, 2001; Kuttler et al. 2000) and contributed to interactive websites (www.paproc.de, www.mpiib-berlin.mpg.de/MAPPP) to predict TCEs. In the light of these developments, prediction algorithms based on structural considerations such as amphipathic helices (DeLisi and Berzofsky 1985) must now be considered obsolete.

The rationale of peptide-based vaccines against cancer TCEs

Cancer vaccines can be based on whole cancer cells, TAAs, or peptide fragments of TAAs. Whole tumor cells of a good quality and quantity can be obtained only from large surgical tumors. Early detection of small tumors and tumor regression under conventional therapy severely limits the availability of tumor material. Immunization as an adjuvant therapy against (minimal) residual disease would also suffer from lack of tumor material. Furthermore, the preparation of a vaccine from an ex vivo tumor is laborious and expensive. Although recombinant TAAs may seem like obvious antigens of tumor vaccines, most TAAs are not tumor specific. TAAs often resemble antigen with limited expression in healthy tissues and may succumb to self/nonself discrimination. In some cases, such as Her-2/neu antigen, peptides elicited immunity when whole proteins were unable to do so (Disis et al. 1996). In humans, delivery systems to induce CTL responses such as replicating or nonreplicating viral vectors, DNA, or lipophilic adjuvants are often only poorly immunogenic or are not safe in immunosuppressed tumor patients. Peptides, which can be produced easily and in large quantities, are more than an alternative of convenience; in fact, peptides derived from TAAs are the true antigens recognized by the T cells. In contrast to proteins, peptides can deliver epitopes in high molar concentrations (directly in vivo, or by dendritic cell (DC) pulsing in vitro) to improve MHC loading, although high concentrations have sometimes led to tolerization (Aichele et al. 1995; Toes et al. 1996a, b).

Increasing the immunogenicity of peptide tumor vaccines

Although clinical trials demonstrated that peptides induce CTLs, their immunogenicity in cancer patients is often too low to clear the tumor and even partial tumor regression is unreliable (Marchand et al. 1999). To enhance the immunogenicity of TAA-derived peptides numerous strategies have been developed.

CD4 T-CELL HELP

Activated $CD4^{+}$ T cells help to initiate and amplify the CTL response. Class II-restricted TCEs have been identified from a number of tumor antigens (Jager et al. 2000b; Zarour et al. 2000; G. Zeng et al. 2001). The identification of class II-restricted epitopes is complicated by the open-ended binding groove of MHCII which accommodates peptides that are much less well defined in terms of length (Chicz et al. 1992; Rammensee et al. 1995), anchor positions (Rammensee et al. 1997), and processing (Robinson and Delvig 2002). Some studies have included TAA-derived class II-restricted TCEs in peptide vaccine trials (see Table 42.4). If these may be more efficient, they need to be defined for each TAA and the MHC context of every individual patient. Alternately, it has been proposed to include promiscuous helper TCEs that bind to many class II molecules (see earlier). These TCEs are normally derived from tumor-unrelated antigens such as TT (Kaumaya et al. 1993; Dakappagari et al. 2000; Slingluff et al. 2001) or they are totally artificial such as the broadly reactive PADRE peptide (Weber et al. 1999) (see Table 42.3). Despite some exceptions (Phan et al. 2003), clinical studies seem to suggest that the inclusion of a class II-restricted helper TCE may improve the level and duration of anti-tumor CTL activity, although few systematic studies have been reported.

MODIFIED PEPTIDES

HLA–peptide–T-cell receptor (TCR) complexes can be optimized for improved T-cell activation by peptide modifications (Chen et al. 1996), e.g. modification of MHC-binding anchor residues of peptides of the Melan-A/MART-1(27–35), the gp100 (209–217), Her2/neu, or folate-binding protein resulted in improved peptide–HLA binding and stability (Fisk et al. 1995; Parkhurst et al. 1996; Valmori et al. 1998; Tourdot et al. 2000). By mutating peptide residues of epitopes of Melan-A/MART-1(27–35), carcinoembryonic antigen (CEA) and NY-ESO-1 signaling of TCR and T-cell stimulation was enhanced (Rivoltini et al. 1999; Salazar et al. 2000). Systematic positional scanning with sets of peptide libraries, each containing in each position every amino acid flanked by undefined amino acids, has been performed to improve peptide interactions within the MHC–TCR complex (Fleckenstein et al. 1996; Wiesmüller et al. 2001). Peptide analogs with improved properties have been defined for Melan-A-specific CTL clones (Pinilla et al. 1999, 2001). Other modifications including terminal acetylation or amidation may protect against premature proteolytic degradation in vivo (Brinckerhoff et al. 1999).

PEPTIDE FORMULATIONS

Alum is the only adjuvant licensed for human use, with decades of experience. However, this adjuvant is well known to induce a Th2-biased response, which elicits a humoral rather than a CTL response. More recently virosomes (influenza virus-like particles) have been licensed (Moser et al. 2003) but so far this has not been included in cancer peptide vaccine trials. Thus, peptide vaccine trials used either no adjuvants (see Table 42.4) or experimental adjuvants or cytokines (reviewed by Machiels et al. 2002). Although, in early studies, peptides without adjuvant have led to complete remission of metastatic tumors (Marchand et al. 1995), immunization regimens reinforced with adjuvants and cytokines tend to improve the immune response and, sometimes, the clinical outcome. Some adjuvants (Montanide ISA-51, QS-21) induced specific CTLs in a few high-risk resected melanoma patients associated with a 75 percent 5-year survival rate (Slingluff et al. 2001). The combination of different adjuvant strategies may have some benefit, e.g. low-dose IL-12 improved the immune response of IFA-emulsified peptides, but without clinical improvement (Lee et al. 2001). The modified gp100 peptide g209-2M, combined with IFA and high doses of IL-2 (but not without IFA or with granulocyte–macrophage colony-stimulating factor (GM-CSF)), showed a good clinical response (Rosenberg et al. 1999). Besides soluble or lipophilic adjuvants, other formulations include biodegradable beads targeting peptides to antigen-presenting cells (Frangione-Beebe et al. 2000, 2001). Table 42.4 shows many examples of adjuvants used in clinical trials, but patient groups and interventions are difficult to compare in a systematic way. In these trials side effects were attributed mostly to the adjuvants used (Goydos et al. 1996), rather than the peptides that normally show no or only mild toxicities.

DENDRITIC CELLS-PRESENTED PEPTIDES

Dendritic cells (DC) are the most potent antigen-presenting cells and they effectively induce CTL responses (reviewed by Banchereau et al. 2000; Guermonprez et al. 2002). They can be obtained from the patient's blood or bone marrow and expanded to large numbers in vitro (reviewed by Mayordomo et al. 1997). Peptides can be loaded on to autologous differentiated DCs, which are returned to the patient to induce tumor-specific T cells (for a review, see Parmiani et al. 2002a, b). The route of administration (e.g. intravenously or subcutaneously) of peptide-loaded DCs seemed to be important, perhaps because of differential homing of the DCs into regional lymph nodes or the spleen (Eggert et al. 1999). Co-administration of cytokines such as IL-12 (Grohmann et al. 1997a, b) or pulsing DCs with mixtures of CD4- and CD8-restricted TCEs improved results. Overall, this very fastidious procedure gave mixed and sometimes very encouraging results (Banchereau et al. 2001; Thurner et al. 1999; Nestle et al. 1998; Murphy et al. 1999b; Kugler et al. 2000). TAA-peptide-loaded DC vaccines seem to generate CTL responses, more often and more efficiently, than peptide with or without IFA, but clinical responses remained low. A notable exception was the anti-idiotype vaccine against follicular B-cell lymphoma which gave, in two of four patients, a complete and, in one, a partial clinical response (Hsu et al. 1996). Follow-up studies with GM-CSF as an adjuvant instead of DCs gave a tumor-specific T-cell response and a complete and durable molecular remission in eight of eleven patients with minimal residual disease (Bendandi et al. 1999).

Alternate delivery of peptide vaccines

To improve the immune response in the cancer patient, multiple CTL epitopes of one or several TAAs combined with or without BCEs and aided by vigorous T-helper epitopes may be required. A number of strategies have been proposed to bring together peptides of different epitopes covalently. The synthesis of constructs consisting of longer or multiple peptides rivals recombinant strategies. Numerous strategies based on recombinant viruses, DNA, or RNA have been developed to deliver oligonucleotides encoding peptides directly into host cells via different invasive or noninvasive routes (reviewed by Arnon and Ben-Yedidia 2003). The use of synthetic TCE vaccines consisting of one or a few peptides is limited by MHC polymorphism. To overcome these limitations peptides have been fused genetically to form polyepitopes (reviewed by Suhrbier 2002). These were either produced as recombinant proteins fusing, e.g. a large number of CTL epitopes of Epstein–Barr virus, or as recombinant viral vectors (modified vaccinia Ankara (MVA)), or DNA in the case of HIV (Hanke and McMichael 2000; Wee et al. 2002) and *Plasmodium falciparum* epitopes (Gilbert et al. 1997; Richie and Saul 2002). Polyepitopes were also used to pulse DCs to immunize against malignant melanoma (Smith et al. 2001) and breast cancer (Scardino et al. 2001). A detailed discussion of these recombinant polyepitope strategies is beyond the scope of this review.

Synthetic TCE peptide vaccines against tumor viruses

Prophylactic immunization against viruses with MHC-restricted peptides is not practical for obvious reasons. However, some viruses are responsible for the induction of human cancers, including hepatocellular carcinoma, cervical carcinoma, and others. With the long tradition of immunization against viruses it was logical that the first peptide immunization against cancer was a viral peptide derived from HBV (Vitiello et al. 1995), although most progress has been reported with peptide immunization against HPV (reviewed by Fausch et al. 2003). Early animal studies showed that peptides derived from HPV protected mice against a HPV protein-expressing tumor both prophylactically and curatively (Feltkamp et al. 1993; Zwaveling et al. 2002). With the identification of HLA-A2-restricted HPV16 and HPV18 peptides, which induced CTLs, clinical trials became possible (Feltkamp et al. 1995). These were further encouraged by observations that class II-restricted memory responses against E6 and E7, the only HPV proteins expressed in cervical carcinoma, were found in patients but not in healthy volunteers (Da Silva et al. 2001). In a clinical trial with advanced cancer patients, two HPV-E7 peptides and a T-helper peptide in Montanide ISA51 induced a T-helper response in four of twelve patients but no E7-specific response (Ressing et al. 2000). In another trial with late-stage tumors, a lipidated E7 peptide induced a specific CTL response but no clinical response (Steller et al. 1998). Ten of sixteen patients with high-grade tumors showed CTL responses and partial or complete remission (Muderspach et al. 2000).

Peptides as cancer vaccines: Concluding remarks

The use of synthetic peptides has resulted in significant advances in the understanding of the immune response at the epitope level. They have also been shown to induce vigorous CTL responses, which sometimes correlated with partial or even complete tumor regression. In some cases this response was long lasting. However, a number of challenges must be tackled to turn peptides into effective anti-cancer vaccines (Buteau et al. 2002). Heterogeneity and small numbers of patients, immunization regimens that are difficult to compare, and variability in monitoring clinical and immunological outcome are only some of the factors that complicate comparisons between different clinical trials. Clinical trials comparing different parameters are therefore warranted, each with sufficient numbers of patients. Some authors believe that, before any further progress can be made, the understanding of the mechanisms involved in tumor killing needs to improve (Mocellin et al. 2003), e.g. Rosenberg et al. (1998) observed that co-administration of IL-2 with gp100 peptides dramatically enhanced tumor response but reduced peptide-specific CTL response from 10 of 11 to 3 of 19 (see Table 42.4). This sheds serious doubts on the utility of CTL assays as an objective parameter to monitor tumor cytotoxicity and more appropriate assays may be required for immune monitoring (Machiels et al. 2002). It also seems important to complement in vitro cytotoxicity with a detailed phenotyping of CTLs. More molecular studies are also necessary to understand the mechanism by which the tumor undermines the development of an efficient immune response and escapes effector mechanisms (Marincola et al. 2000).

Mechanisms that lead to epitope-specific T-cell tolerization, instead of T-cell activation, need to be explored (Aichele et al. 1995; Toes et al. 1996a, b). Immunization with certain peptides can lead to tolerance in protocols that induce protection with other peptides (Feltkamp et al. 1993; Mandelboim et al. 1994; Melief and Kast 1994, 1995; Toes et al. 1996b). CTL epitopes have so far been identified for only a few HLA molecules. Although it can be expected that, after proof of the concept, peptides restricted by most MHC molecules would be identified, MHC polymorphism severely limits peptide immunization studies in humans. MHC transgenic mice could help but experimental tumors poorly reflect human tumors. On the other hand, polyepitope vaccines based on (genetically) fused peptides could overcome some of these problems, although some regulatory issues remain unsolved (Suhrbier 2002). With few exceptions clinical response was below 30 percent. Although this seems low, many of the studies were done in patients with advanced stage disease and this response has been obtained with minimal side effects. Peptide immunization is probably more efficient in low-grade tumor patients with an intact immune system. Thus, peptide immunization could be a treatment of choice in the case of minimal residual disease when the immune system has recovered from suppression caused by the tumor and aggressive therapy and when tolerance for side effects is low (Bendandi et al. 1999; Jager et al. 1999). The demonstration of a benefit would, however, take many years of observation. Immunization protocols are far from being optimal and most results need to be confirmed in large prospective clinical trials, to systematically compare different TAAs, epitopes, peptide formulations, adjuvants, and routes.

FINAL COMMENTS: DIFFICULTIES AND MISCONCEPTIONS

The main difficulty in developing a peptide-vaccine based on a BCE is its conformational diversity. Even in the case of a peptide inducing (low) neutralizing antibodies, chemical stabilization of the proper conformation should be considered. In this respect, most peptides are perhaps only lead structures that guide the development of structurally stabilized antigens, rather than being the antigens themselves.

Many of the obstacles to the development of TCE-based peptide vaccines against tumors are inherent to tumor immunology and are not particular to peptide vaccines. In this respect, peptides as tumor vaccines have done very well. With the ease of immunization with peptides and the low levels of side effects, their potential should be more systematically explored in minimal residual disease or in patients in remission with a high risk of relapse.

Peptide vaccines tend to suffer from an inherent contradiction: low cost, biological safety, and chemical and thermal stability are mostly features of prophylactic vaccines, meant to protect healthy vaccinees against pathogens. Such prophylactic vaccines, however, do not normally require an epitope-based approach. In contrast, in therapeutic vaccines, in particular against neoplasms, allergies, and autoimmune disease where epitope-based strategies may be important, features such as low cost, safety, and stability are much less relevant.

To judge the success or failure of experimental peptide vaccines, a comparison with other vaccine strategies is warranted. No peptide vaccine is licensed so far, but also only a few recombinant vaccines had reached the (American) market by 2001 (HBV, cholera, pertussis) without being subsequently withdrawn (*Borrelia*, rotavirus). The US Institute of Medicine estimated that, of the more than 30 new vaccines that will reach the market by 2010, about 25 percent are obtained by recombinant technology, but none will be peptide based (Landry 2002).

ACKNOWLEDGMENTS

Financial support from the Centre de Recherche Public-Santé, the European Union, the Ministère de la Culture, de l'Enseignement Supérieur et de la Recherche (Bourse BFR to MMP) is gratefully acknowledged. We thank Carole Weis for excellent secretarial support.

REFERENCES

Acharya, R., Fry, E., et al. 1989. The three-dimensional structure of foot-and-mouth disease virus at 2.9 A resolution. *Nature*, **337**, 709–16.

Afzalpurkar, A., Sacco, A.G., et al. 1997a. Induction of native protein reactive antibodies by immunization with peptides containing linear B-cell epitopes defined by anti-porcine ZP3 beta monoclonal antibodies. *J Reprod Immunol*, **33**, 113–25.

Afzalpurkar, A., Shibahara, H., et al. 1997b. Immunoreactivity and in-vitro effect on human sperm-egg binding of antibodies against peptides corresponding to bonnet monkey zona pellucida-3 glycoprotein. *Hum Reprod*, **12**, 2664–70.

Ahlborg, N. 1995. Synthesis of a diepitope multiple antigen peptide containing sequences from two malaria antigens using Fmoc chemistry. *J Immunol Methods*, **179**, 269–75.

Ahlers, J.D., Pendleton, C.D., et al. 1993. Construction of an HIV-1 peptide vaccine containing a multideterminant helper peptide linked to a V3 loop peptide 18 inducing strong neutralizing antibody responses in mice of multiple MHC haplotypes after two immunizations. *J Immunol*, **150**, 5647–65.

Aichele, P., Brduscha-Riem, K., et al. 1995. T cell priming versus T cell tolerance induced by synthetic peptides. *J Exp Med*, **182**, 261–6.

Aitken, R.J. 2002. Immunocontraceptive vaccines for human use. *J Reprod Immunol*, **57**, 273–87.

Alexander, J., Sidney, J., et al. 1994. Development of high potency universal DR-restricted helper epitopes by modification of high affinity DR-blocking peptides. *Immunity*, **1**, 751–61.

Alexander, J., Fikes, J., et al. 1998. The optimization of helper T lymphocyte (HTL) function in vaccine development. *Immunol Res*, **18**, 79–92.

Altieri, D.C., Marchisio, P.C. and Marchisio, C. 1999. Surviving apoptosis: an interloper between cell death and cell proliferation in cancer. *Lab Invest*, **79**, 1327–33.

Amador, R., Moreno, A., et al. 1992a. Safety and immunogenicity of the synthetic malaria vaccine SPf66 in a large field trial. *J Infect Dis*, **166**, 139–44.

Amador, R., Moreno, A., et al. 1992b. The first field trials of the chemically synthesized malaria vaccine SPf66: safety, immunogenicity and protectivity. *Vaccine*, **10**, 179–84.

Anderer, F.A. 1963. Recent studies on the structure of tobacco mosaic virus. *Adv Protein Chem*, **18**, 1–35.

Andersen, M.H., Pedersen, L.O., et al. 2001. Identification of a cytotoxic T lymphocyte response to the apoptosis inhibitor protein survivin in cancer patients. *Cancer Res*, **61**, 869–72.

Anichini, A., Molla, A., et al. 1999. An expanded peripheral T cell population to a cytotoxic T lymphocyte (CTL)-defined, melanocyte-specific antigen in metastatic melanoma patients impacts on generation of peptide-specific CTLs but does not overcome tumor escape from immune surveillance in metastatic lesions. *J Exp Med*, **190**, 651–67.

Araga, S., LeBoeuf, R.D. and Blalock, J.E. 1993. Prevention of experimental autoimmune myasthenia gravis by manipulation of the immune network with a complementary peptide for the acetylcholine receptor. *Proc Natl Acad Sci USA*, **90**, 8747–51.

Araga, S., Kishimoto, M., et al. 1999. A complementary peptide vaccine that induces T cell anergy and prevents experimental allergic neuritis in Lewis rats. *J Immunol*, **163**, 476–82.

Araga, S., Xu, L., et al. 2000. A peptide vaccine that prevents experimental autoimmune myasthenia gravis by specifically blocking T cell help. *FASEB J*, **14**, 185–96.

Arlen, P., Tsang, K.Y., et al. 2000. The use of a rapid ELISPOT assay to analyze peptide-specific immune responses in carcinoma patients to peptide vs. recombinant poxvirus vaccines. *Cancer Immunol Immunother*, **49**, 517–29.

Arnon, R. and Ben-Yedidia, T. 2003. Old and new vaccine approaches. *Int Immunopharmacol*, **3**, 1195–204.

Arnon, R., Tarrab-Hazdai, R. and Steward, M. 2000. A mimotope peptide-based vaccine against *Schistosoma mansoni*: synthesis and characterization. *Immunology*, **101**, 555–62.

Atabani, S.F., Obeid, O.E., et al. 1997. Identification of an immunodominant neutralizing and protective epitope from measles virus fusion protein by using human sera from acute infection. *J Virol*, **71**, 7240–5.

Audibert, F., Jolivet, M., et al. 1981. Active antitoxic immunization by a diphtheria toxin synthetic oligopeptide. *Nature*, **289**, 593–4.

Audibert, F., Jolivet, M., et al. 1982. Successful immunization with a totally synthetic diphtheria vaccine. *Proc Natl Acad Sci USA*, **79**, 5042–6.

Bagavant, H., Fusi, F.M., et al. 1997. Immunogenicity and contraceptive potential of a human zona pellucida 3 peptide vaccine. *Biol Reprod*, **56**, 764–70.

Bakaletz, L.O., Leake, E.R., et al. 1997. Relative immunogenicity and efficacy of two synthetic chimeric peptides of fimbrin as vaccinogens against nasopharyngeal colonization by nontypeable *Haemophilus influenzae* in the chinchilla. *Vaccine*, **15**, 955–61.

Bakaletz, L.O., Kennedy, B.J., et al. 1999. Protection against development of otitis media induced by nontypeable *Haemophilus influenzae* by both active and passive immunization in a chinchilla model of virus-bacterium superinfection. *Infect Immun*, **67**, 2746–62.

Banchereau, J., Briere, F., et al. 2000. Immunobiology of dendritic cells. *Annu Rev Immunol*, **18**, 767–811.

Banchereau, J., Palucka, A.K., et al. 2001. Immune and clinical responses in patients with metastatic melanoma to CD34(+) progenitor-derived dendritic cell vaccine. *Cancer Res*, **61**, 6451–8.

Baselga, J. 2001. Phase I and II clinical trials of trastuzumab. *Ann Oncol*, **12**, S49–55.

Bastien, N., Trudel, M. and Simard, C. 1997. Protective immune responses induced by the immunization of mice with a recombinant bacteriophage displaying an epitope of the human respiratory syncytial virus. *Virology*, **234**, 118–22.

Bastien, N., Trudel, M. and Simard, C. 1999. Complete protection of mice from respiratory syncytial virus infection following mucosal delivery of synthetic peptide vaccines. *Vaccine*, **17**, 832–6.

Batzloff, M.R., Hayman, W.A., et al. 2003. Protection against group A streptococcus by immunization with J8-diphtheria toxoid: contribution of J8- and diphtheria toxoid-specific antibodies to protection. *J Infect Dis*, **187**, 1598–608.

Beachey, E.H., Seyer, J.M., et al. 1981. Type-specific protective immunity evoked by synthetic peptide of *Streptococcus pyogenes* M protein. *Nature*, **292**, 457–9.

Beachey, E.H., Tartar, A., et al. 1984. Epitope-specific protective immunogenicity of chemically synthesized 13-, 18-, and 23-residue peptide fragments of streptococcal M protein. *Proc Natl Acad Sci USA*, **81**, 2203–7.

Beachey, E.H., Gras-Masse, H., et al. 1986. Opsonic antibodies evoked by hybrid peptide copies of types 5 and 24 streptococcal M proteins synthesized in tandem. *J Exp Med*, **163**, 1451–8.

Beekman, N.J., Schaaper, W.M., et al. 1999. Highly immunogenic and fully synthetic peptide-carrier constructs targetting GnRH. *Vaccine*, **17**, 2043–50.

Bendandi, M., Gocke, C.D., et al. 1999. Complete molecular remissions induced by patient-specific vaccination plus granulocyte-monocyte colony-stimulating factor against lymphoma. *Nat Med*, **5**, 1171–7.

Benito, A. and Van Regenmortel, M.H. 1998. Biosensor characterization of antigenic site A of foot-and-mouth disease virus presented in different vector systems. *FEMS Immunol Med Microbiol*, **21**, 101–15.

Benito, A. and Villaverde, A. 1994. Insertion of a 27 amino acid viral peptide in different zones of *Escherichia coli* beta-galactosidase: effects on the enzyme activity. *FEMS Microbiol Lett*, **123**, 107–12.

Benkirane, N., Guichard, G., et al. 1996a. Exploration of requirements for peptidomimetic immune recognition. Antigenic and immunogenic properties of reduced peptide bond pseudopeptide analogues of a histone hexapeptide. *J Biol Chem*, **271**, 33218–24.

Benkirane, N., Guichard, G., et al. 1996b. Mimicry of viral epitopes with retro-inverso peptides of increased stability. *Dev Biol Stand*, **87**, 283–91.

BenMohamed, L., Gras-Masse, H., et al. 1997. Lipopeptide immunization without adjuvant induces potent and long-lasting B, T helper, and cytotoxic T lymphocyte responses against a malaria liver stage antigen in mice and chimpanzees. *Eur J Immunol*, **27**, 1242–53.

Bentley, G.A. 1996. The crystal structures of complexes formed between lysozyme and antibody fragments. *Exs*, **75**, 301–19.

Ben-Yedidia, T., Tarrab-Hazdai, R., et al. 1999. Intranasal administration of synthetic recombinant peptide-based vaccine protects mice from infection by *Schistosoma mansoni*. *Infect Immun*, **67**, 4360–6.

Bergquist, C., Lagergard, T. and Holmgren, J. 1998. Antibody responses in serum and lung to intranasal immunization with *Haemophilus influenzae* type b polysaccharide conjugated to cholera toxin B subunit and tetanus toxoid. *Apmis*, **106**, 800–6.

Berzins, K., Perlmann, H., et al. 1986. Rabbit and human antibodies to a repeated amino acid sequence of a *Plasmodium falciparum* antigen, Pf 155, react with the native protein and inhibit merozoite invasion. *Proc Natl Acad Sci USA*, **83**, 1065–9.

Berzofsky, J.A., Pendleton, C.D., et al. 1991. Construction of peptides encompassing multideterminant clusters of human immunodeficiency virus envelope to induce in vitro T cell responses in mice and humans of multiple MHC types. *J Clin Invest*, **88**, 876–84.

Bessen, D. and Fischetti, V.A. 1988. Influence of intranasal immunization with synthetic peptides corresponding to conserved epitopes of M protein on mucosal colonization by group A streptococci. *Infect Immun*, **56**, 2666–72.

Bessen, D. and Fischetti, V.A. 1990. Synthetic peptide vaccine against mucosal colonization by group A streptococci. I. Protection against a heterologous M serotype with shared C repeat region epitopes. *J Immunol*, **145**, 1251–6.

Bianco, A. 1999. Combinatorial synthetic oligomers. In: Jung, G. (ed.), *Combinatorial chemistry: Synthesis, analysis, screening*. Chichester: Wiley.

Birkett, A., Lyons, K., et al. 2002. A modified hepatitis B virus core particle containing multiple epitopes of the *Plasmodium falciparum* circumsporozoite protein provides a highly immunogenic malaria vaccine in preclinical analyses in rodent and primate hosts. *Infect Immun*, **70**, 6860–70.

Bittle, J.L., Houghten, R.A., et al. 1982. Protection against foot-and-mouth disease by immunization with a chemically synthesized peptide predicted from the viral nucleotide sequence. *Nature*, **298**, 30–3.

Boon, T., Cerottini, J.C., et al. 1994. Tumor antigens recognized by T lymphocytes. *Annu Rev Immunol*, **12**, 337–65.

Bosch, A., Gonzalez-Dankaart, J.F., et al. 1998. A new continuous epitope of hepatitis A virus. *J Med Virol*, **54**, 95–102.

Bouche, F.B., Marquet-Blouin, E., et al. 2003. Neutralising immunogenicity of a polyepitope antigen expressed in a transgenic food plant: a novel antigen to protect against measles. *Vaccine*, **21**, 2065–72.

Bouche, F.B., Steinmetz, A., et al. 2004. Induction of broadly neutralizing antibodies against measles virus mutants using a polyepitope vaccine strategy. *Vaccine*, in press.

Bradney, C.P., Sempowski, G.D., et al. 2002. Cytokines as adjuvants for the induction of anti-human immunodeficiency virus peptide immunoglobulin G (IgG) and IgA antibodies in serum and mucosal secretions after nasal immunization. *J Virol*, **76**, 517–24.

Brennan, F.R., Gilleland, L.B., et al. 1999a. A chimaeric plant virus vaccine protects mice against a bacterial infection. *Microbiology*, **145**, Pt 8, 2061–7.

Brennan, F.R., Jones, T.D., et al. 1999b. Immunogenicity of peptides derived from a fibronectin-binding protein of *S. aureus* expressed on two different plant viruses. *Vaccine*, **17**, 1846–57.

Briand, J.P., Benkirane, N., et al. 1997. A retro-inverso peptide corresponding to the GH loop of foot-and-mouth disease virus elicits high levels of long-lasting protective neutralizing antibodies. *Proc Natl Acad Sci USA*, **94**, 12545–50.

Brinckerhoff, L.H., Kalashnikov, V.V., et al. 1999. Terminal modifications inhibit proteolytic degradation of an immunogenic MART-1(27-35) peptide: implications for peptide vaccines. *Int J Cancer*, **83**, 326–34.

Brons, N.H., Blaich, A., et al. 1996. Hierarchic T-cell help to non-linked B-cell epitopes. *Scand J Immunol*, **44**, 478–84.

Bronze, M.S., Courtney, H.S. and Dale, J.B. 1992. Epitopes of group A streptococcal M protein that evoke cross-protective local immune responses. *J Immunol*, **148**, 888–93.

Bruner, M., James, A., et al. 2003. Evaluation of synthetic, M type-specific peptides as antigens in a multivalent group A streptococcal vaccine. *Vaccine*, **21**, 2698–703.

Bukawa, H., Sekigawa, K., et al. 1995. Neutralization of HIV-1 by secretory IgA induced by oral immunization with a new macromolecular multicomponent peptide vaccine candidate. *Nat Med*, **1**, 681–5.

Burton, D.R., Desrosiers, R.C., et al. 2004. HIV vaccine design and the neutralizing antibody problem. *Nat Immunol*, **5**, 233–6.

Buteau, C., Markovic, S.N. and Celis, E. 2002. Challenges in the development of effective peptide vaccines for cancer. *Mayo Clin Proc*, **77**, 339–49.

Cachia, P.J. and Hodges, R.S. 2003. Synthetic peptide vaccine and antibody therapeutic development: prevention and treatment of *Pseudomonas aeruginosa*. *Biopolymers*, **71**, 141–68.

Cachia, P.J., Glasier, L.M., et al. 1998. The use of synthetic peptides in the design of a consensus sequence vaccine for *Pseudomonas aeruginosa*. *J Peptide Res*, **52**, 289–99.

Camarero, J.A., Andreu, D., et al. 1993. Cyclic disulfide model of the major antigenic site of serotype-C foot-and-mouth disease virus. Synthetic, conformational and immunochemical studies. *FEBS Lett*, **328**, 159–64.

Capron, A., Capron, M. and Riveau, G. 2002. Vaccine development against schistosomiasis from concepts to clinical trials. *Br Med Bull*, **62**, 139–48.

Casal, J.I., Langeveld, J.P., et al. 1995. Peptide vaccine against canine parvovirus: identification of two neutralization subsites in the N terminus of VP2 and optimization of the amino acid sequence. *J Virol*, **69**, 7274–7.

Cebon, J., Jager, E., et al. 2003. Two phase I studies of low dose recombinant human IL-12 with Melan-A and influenza peptides in subjects with advanced malignant melanoma. *Cancer Immun*, **3**, 7.

Charalambous, B.M. and Feavers, I.M. 2000. Peptide mimics elicit antibody responses against the outer-membrane lipooligosaccharide of group B *Neisseria meningitidis*. *FEMS Microbiol Lett*, **191**, 45–50.

Chargelegue, D., Obeid, O.E., et al. 1997. Peptide mimics of a conformationally constrained protective epitope of respiratory syncytial virus fusion protein. *Immunol Lett*, **57**, 15–17.

Chargelegue, D., Obeid, O.E., et al. 1998. A peptide mimic of a protective epitope of respiratory syncytial virus selected from a combinatorial library induces virus-neutralizing antibodies and reduces viral load in vivo. *J Virol*, **72**, 2040–6.

Check, E. 2002. Nerve inflammation halts trial for Alzheimer's drug. *Nature*, **415**, 462.

Chen, W., Ede, N.J., et al. 1996. CTL recognition of an altered peptide associated with asparagine bond rearrangement. Implications for immunity and vaccine design. *J Immunol*, **157**, 1000–5.

Cheung, A., Leban, J., et al. 1986. Immunization with synthetic peptides of a *Plasmodium falciparum* surface antigen induces antimerozoite antibodies. *Proc Natl Acad Sci USA*, **83**, 8328–32.

Chiari, R., Hames, G., et al. 2000. Identification of a tumor-specific shared antigen derived from an Eph receptor and presented to CD4 T cells on HLA class II molecules. *Cancer Res*, **60**, 4855–63.

Chicz, R.M., Urban, R.G., et al. 1992. Predominant naturally processed peptides bound to HLA-DR1 are derived from MHC-related molecules and are heterogeneous in size. *Nature*, **358**, 764–8.

Chorev, M. and Goodman, M. 1995. Recent developments in retro peptides and proteins – an ongoing topochemical exploration. *Trends Biotechnol*, **13**, 438–45.

Collen, T., Dimarchi, R. and Doel, T.R. 1991. A T cell epitope in VP1 of foot-and-mouth disease virus is immunodominant for vaccinated cattle. *J Immunol*, **146**, 749–55.

Collins, W.E., Anders, R.F., et al. 1986. Immunization of *Aotus* monkeys with recombinant proteins of an erythrocyte surface antigen of *Plasmodium falciparum*. *Nature*, **323**, 259–62.

Cormier, J.N., Salgaller, M.L., et al. 1997. Enhancement of cellular immunity in melanoma patients immunized with a peptide from MART-1/Melan A. *Cancer J Sci Am*, **3**, 37–44.

Correa, I. and Plunkett, T. 2001. Update on HER-2 as a target for cancer therapy: HER2/neu peptides as tumor vaccines for T cell recognition. *Breast Cancer Res*, **3**, 399–403, Epub 2001 Sep 20.

Coulie, P.G., Karanikas, V., et al. 2002. Cytolytic T-cell responses of cancer patients vaccinated with a MAGE antigen. *Immunol Rev*, **188**, 33–42.

Cryz, S.J. Jr, Goldstein, H., et al. 1995. Human immunodeficiency virus-1 principal neutralizing domain peptide-toxin A conjugate vaccine. *Vaccine*, **13**, 67–71.

Da Silva, D.M., Eiben, G.L., et al. 2001. Cervical cancer vaccines: emerging concepts and developments. *J Cell Physiol*, **186**, 169–82.

Dakappagari, N.K., Douglas, D.B., et al. 2000. Prevention of mammary tumors with a chimeric HER-2 B-cell epitope peptide vaccine. *Cancer Res*, **60**, 3782–9.

Dale, J.B., Seyer, J.M. and Beachey, E.H. 1983. Type-specific immunogenicity of a chemically synthesized peptide fragment of type 5 streptococcal M protein. *J Exp Med*, **158**, 1727–32.

Dale, J.B., Chiang, E.Y., et al. 2002. Antibodies against a synthetic peptide of SagA neutralize the cytolytic activity of streptolysin S from group A streptococci. *Infect Immun*, **70**, 2166–70.

Dalsgaard, K., Uttenthal, A., et al. 1997. Plant-derived vaccine protects target animals against a viral disease. *Nat Biotechnol*, **15**, 248–52.

Daubersies, P., Thomas, A.W., et al. 2000. Protection against *Plasmodium falciparum* malaria in chimpanzees by immunization with the conserved pre-erythrocytic liver-stage antigen 3. *Nat Med*, **6**, 1258–63.

Davis, T.A., White, C.A., et al. 1999. Single-agent monoclonal antibody efficacy in bulky non-Hodgkin's lymphoma: results of a phase II trial of rituximab. *J Clin Oncol*, **17**, 1851–7.

Defoort, J.P., Nardelli, B., et al. 1992a. A rational design of synthetic peptide vaccine with a built-in adjuvant. A modular approach for unambiguity. *Int J Pept Protein Res*, **40**, 214–21.

Defoort, J.P., Nardelli, B., et al. 1992b. Macromolecular assemblage in the design of a synthetic AIDS vaccine. *Proc Natl Acad Sci USA*, **89**, 3879–83.

DeLisi, C. and Berzofsky, J.A. 1985. T-cell antigenic sites tend to be amphipathic structures. *Proc Natl Acad Sci USA*, **82**, 7048–52.

Demotz, S., Lanzavecchia, A., et al. 1989. Delineation of several DR-restricted tetanus toxin T cell epitopes. *J Immunol*, **142**, 394–402.

Demotz, S., Moulon, C., et al. 2001. Native-like, long synthetic peptides as components of sub-unit vaccines: practical and theoretical considerations for their use in humans. *Mol Immunol*, **38**, 415–22.

Deres, K., Schild, H., et al. 1989. In vivo priming of virus-specific cytotoxic T lymphocytes with synthetic lipopeptide vaccine. *Nature*, **342**, 561–4.

Deroo, S. and Muller, C.P. 2001. Antigenic and immunogenic phage displayed mimotopes as substitute antigens: applications and limitations. *Comb Chem High Throughput Screen*, **4**, 75–110.

Deroo, S., El Kasmi, K.C., et al. 1998. Enhanced antigenicity of a four-contact-residue epitope of the measles virus hemagglutinin protein by phage display libraries: evidence of a helical structure in the putative active site. *Mol Immunol*, **35**, 435–43.

Deslauriers, M., Haque, S. and Flood, P.M. 1996. Identification of murine protective epitopes on the *Porphyromonas gingivalis* fimbrillin molecule. *Infect Immun*, **64**, 434–40.

Dewasthaly, S., Ayachit, V.M., et al. 2001. Monoclonal antibody raised against envelope glycoprotein peptide neutralizes Japanese encephalitis virus. *Arch Virol*, **146**, 1427–35.

Di Tommaso, A., Saletti, G., et al. 1996. Induction of antigen-specific antibodies in vaginal secretions by using a nontoxic mutant of heat-labile enterotoxin as a mucosal adjuvant. *Infect Immun*, **64**, 974–9.

DiMarchi, R., Brooke, G., et al. 1986. Protection of cattle against foot-and-mouth disease by a synthetic peptide. *Science*, **232**, 639–41.

Disis, M.L. and Cheever, M.A. 1998. HER-2/neu oncogenic protein: issues in vaccine development. *Crit Rev Immunol*, **18**, 37–45.

Disis, M.L., Gralow, J.R., et al. 1996. Peptide-based, but not whole protein, vaccines elicit immunity to HER-2/neu, oncogenic self-protein. *J Immunol*, **156**, 3151–8.

Disis, M.L., Grabstein, K.H., et al. 1999. Generation of immunity to the HER-2/neu oncogenic protein in patients with breast and ovarian cancer using a peptide-based vaccine. *Clin Cancer Res*, **5**, 1289–97.

Disis, M.L., Schiffman, K., et al. 2000. Delayed-type hypersensitivity response is a predictor of peripheral blood T-cell immunity after HER-2/neu peptide immunization. *Clin Cancer Res*, **6**, 1347–50.

Disis, M.L., Knutson, K.L., et al. 2001. Clinical translation of peptide-based vaccine trials: the HER-2/neu model. *Crit Rev Immunol*, **21**, 263–73.

Disis, M.L., Gooley, T.A., et al. 2002. Generation of T-cell immunity to the HER-2/neu protein after active immunization with HER-2/neu peptide-based vaccines. *J Clin Oncol*, **20**, 2624–32.

Doel, T.R., Doel, C.M., et al. 1992. Cross-reactive and serotype-specific antibodies against foot-and-mouth disease virus generated by different regions of the same synthetic peptide. *J Virol*, **66**, 2187–94.

Doh, H., Roh, S., et al. 2003. Response of primed human PBMC to synthetic peptides derived from hepatitis B virus envelope proteins: a search for promiscuous epitopes. *FEMS Immunol Med Microbiol*, **35**, 77–85.

Dolimbek, B.Z. and Atassi, M.Z. 1996. Protection against alpha-bungarotoxin poisoning by immunization with synthetic toxin peptides. *Mol Immunol*, **33**, 681–9.

Drijfhout, J.W. and Bloemhoff, W. 1991. A new synthetic functionalized antigen carrier. *Int J Pept Protein Res*, **37**, 27–32.

D'Souza, S., Rimoldi, D., et al. 1998. Circulating Melan-A/Mart-1 specific cytolytic T lymphocyte precursors in HLA-A2+ melanoma patients have a memory phenotype. *Int J Cancer*, **78**, 699–706.

Dunbar, P.R., Smith, C.L., et al. 2000. A shift in the phenotype of melan-A-specific CTL identifies melanoma patients with an active tumor-specific immune response. *J Immunol*, **165**, 6644–52.

Dyrberg, T. and Oldstone, M.B. 1986. Peptides as antigens. Importance of orientation. *J Exp Med*, **164**, 1344–9.

Eggert, A.A., Schreurs, M.W., et al. 1999. Biodistribution and vaccine efficiency of murine dendritic cells are dependent on the route of administration. *Cancer Res*, **59**, 3340–5.

El Kasmi, K.C., Theisen, D., et al. 1998. The molecular basis of virus crossreactivity and neutralization after immunisation with optimised chimeric peptides mimicking a putative helical epitope of the measles virus hemagglutinin protein. *Mol Immunol*, **35**, 905–18.

El Kasmi, K.C., Theisen, D., et al. 1999a. A hemagglutinin-derived peptide-vaccine ignored by virus-neutralizing passive antibodies, protects against murine measles encephalitis. *Vaccine*, **17**, 2436–45.

El Kasmi, K.C., Deroo, S., et al. 1999b. Crossreactivity of mimotopes and peptide homologues of a sequential epitope with a monoclonal antibody does not predict crossreactive immunogenicity. *Vaccine*, **18**, 284–90.

El Kasmi, K.C., Fillon, S., et al. 2000. Neutralization of measles virus wild-type isolates after immunization with a synthetic peptide vaccine which is not recognized by neutralizing passive antibodies. *J Gen Virol*, **81**, 729–35.

Emini, E.A., Jameson, B.A. and Wimmer, E. 1983. Priming for and induction of anti-poliovirus neutralizing antibodies by synthetic peptides. *Nature*, **304**, 699–703.

Emini, E.A., Jameson, B.A. and Wimmer, E. 1984a. Identification of a new neutralization antigenic site on poliovirus coat protein VP2. *J Virol*, **52**, 719–21.

Emini, E.A., Wimmer, E., et al. 1984b. Neutralization antigenic sites of poliovirus and peptide induction of neutralizing antibodies. *Ann Sclavo Collana Monogr*, **1**, 139–46.

Emini, E.A., Hughes, J.V., et al. 1985. Induction of hepatitis A virus-neutralizing antibody by a virus-specific synthetic peptide. *J Virol*, **55**, 836–9.

Emini, E.A., Larson, V., et al. 1989. Protective effect of a synthetic peptide comprising the complete preS2 region of the hepatitis B virus surface protein. *J Med Virol*, **28**, 7–12.

Engler, O.B., Dai, W.J., et al. 2001. Peptide vaccines against hepatitis B virus: from animal model to human studies. *Mol Immunol*, **38**, 457–65.

Eskola, J., Kayhty, H., et al. 1990. A randomized, prospective field trial of a conjugate vaccine in the protection of infants and young children against invasive *Haemophilus influenzae* type b disease. *N Engl J Med*, **323**, 1381–7.

Etlinger, H.M., Felix, A.M., et al. 1988. Assessment in humans of a synthetic peptide-based vaccine against the sporozoite stage of the human malaria parasite, Plasmodium falciparum. *J Immunol*, **140**, 626–33.

Falk, K., Rotzschke, O., et al. 1991. Allele-specific motifs revealed by sequencing of self-peptides eluted from MHC molecules. *Nature*, **351**, 290–6.

Farci, P., Shimoda, A., et al. 1996. Prevention of hepatitis C virus infection in chimpanzees by hyperimmune serum against the hypervariable region 1 of the envelope 2 protein. *Proc Natl Acad Sci USA*, **93**, 15394–9.

Fausch, S.C., Da Silva, D.M., et al. 2003. HPV protein/peptide vaccines: from animal models to clinical trials. *Front Biosci*, **8**, S81–91.

Feltkamp, M.C., Smits, H.L., et al. 1993. Vaccination with cytotoxic T lymphocyte epitope-containing peptide protects against a tumor induced by human papillomavirus type 16-transformed cells. *Eur J Immunol*, **23**, 2242–9.

Feltkamp, M.C., Vreugdenhil, G.R., et al. 1995. Cytotoxic T lymphocytes raised against a subdominant epitope offered as a synthetic peptide eradicate human papillomavirus type 16-induced tumors. *Eur J Immunol*, **25**, 2638–42.

Fernandez, I.M., Snijders, A., et al. 1993. Influence of epitope polarity and adjuvants on the immunogenicity and efficacy of a synthetic peptide vaccine against Semliki Forest virus. *J Virol*, **67**, 5843–8.

Fernando, G.J., Stenzel, D.J., et al. 1995. Peptide polymerisation facilitates incorporation into ISCOMs and increases antigen-specific IgG2a production. *Vaccine*, **13**, 1460–7.

Ferru, I., Georges, B., et al. 1997. Analysis of the immune response elicited by a multiple antigen peptide (MAP) composed of two distinct protective antigens derived from the parasite *Schistosoma mansoni*. *Parasite Immunol*, **19**, 1–11.

Fisk, B., Savary, C., et al. 1995. Changes in an HER-2 peptide upregulating HLA-A2 expression affect both conformational epitopes and CTL recognition: implications for optimization of antigen presentation and tumor-specific CTL induction. *J Immunother Emphasis Tumor Immunol*, **18**, 197–209.

Fitzmaurice, C.J., Brown, L.E., et al. 1996. The assembly and immunological properties of non-linear synthetic immunogens containing T-cell and B-cell determinants. *Vaccine*, **14**, 553–60.

Fitzmaurice, C.J., Brown, L.E., et al. 2000. The geometry of synthetic peptide-based immunogens affects the efficiency of T cell stimulation by professional antigen-presenting cells. *Int Immunol*, **12**, 527–35.

Fleckenstein, B., Kalbacher, H., et al. 1996. New ligands binding to the human leukocyte antigen class II molecule DRB1*0101 based on the activity pattern of an undecapeptide library. *Eur J Biochem*, **240**, 71–7.

Fleuridor, R., Lees, A. and Pirofski, L. 2001. A cryptococcal capsular polysaccharide mimotope prolongs the survival of mice with *Cryptococcus neoformans* infection. *J Immunol*, **166**, 1087–96.

Fournier, P., Brons, N.H., et al. 1997. Antibodies to a new linear site at the topographical or functional interface between the haemagglutinin and fusion proteins protect against measles encephalitis. *J Gen Virol*, **78**, 1295–302.

Francis, M.J., Fry, C.M., et al. 1985. Immunological priming with synthetic peptides of foot-and-mouth disease virus. *J Gen Virol*, **66**, Pt 11, 2347–54.

Francis, M.J., Hastings, G.Z., et al. 1991. Immunological evaluation of the multiple antigen peptide (MAP) system using the major immunogenic site of foot-and-mouth disease virus. *Immunology*, **73**, 249–54.

Frangione-Beebe, M., Albrecht, B., et al. 2000. Enhanced immunogenicity of a conformational epitope of human T-lymphotropic virus type 1 using a novel chimeric peptide. *Vaccine*, **19**, 1068–81.

Frangione-Beebe, M., Rose, R.T., et al. 2001. Microencapsulation of a synthetic peptide epitope for HTLV-1 in biodegradable poly(d,l-lactide-co-glycolide) microspheres using a novel encapsulation technique. *J Microencapsul*, **18**, 663–77.

Frenkel, D., Kariv, N. and Solomon, B. 2001. Generation of auto-antibodies towards Alzheimer's disease vaccination. *Vaccine*, **19**, 2615–19.

Frenkel, D., Dewachter, I., et al. 2003. Reduction of beta-amyloid plaques in brain of transgenic mouse model of Alzheimer's disease by EFRH-phage immunization. *Vaccine*, **21**, 1060–5.

Friede, M., Muller, S., et al. 1994. Selective induction of protection against influenza virus infection in mice by a lipid-peptide conjugate delivered in liposomes. *Vaccine*, **12**, 791–7.

Games, D., Adams, D., et al. 1995. Alzheimer-type neuropathology in transgenic mice overexpressing V717F beta-amyloid precursor protein. *Nature*, **373**, 523–7.

Gerin, J.L., Alexander, H., et al. 1983. Chemically synthesized peptides of hepatitis B surface antigen duplicate the d/y specificities and induce subtype-specific antibodies in chimpanzees. *Proc Natl Acad Sci USA*, **80**, 2365–9.

Ghosh, S. and Jackson, D.C. 1999. Antigenic and immunogenic properties of totally synthetic peptide-based anti-fertility vaccines. *Int Immunol*, **11**, 1103–10.

Gilbert, S.C., Plebanski, M., et al. 1997. A protein particle vaccine containing multiple malaria epitopes. *Nat Biotechnol*, **15**, 1280–4.

Gilewski, T., Adluri, S., et al. 2000. Vaccination of high-risk breast cancer patients with mucin-1 (MUC1) keyhole limpet hemocyanin conjugate plus QS-21. *Clin Cancer Res*, **6**, 1693–701.

Gjertsen, M.K., Bakka, A., et al. 1995. Vaccination with mutant ras peptides and induction of T-cell responsiveness in pancreatic carcinoma patients carrying the corresponding RAS mutation. *Lancet*, **346**, 1399–400.

Gjertsen, M.K., Saeterdal, I., et al. 1996a. Characterisation of immune responses in pancreatic carcinoma patients after mutant p21 ras peptide vaccination. *Br J Cancer*, **74**, 1828–33.

Gjertsen, M.K., Bakka, A., et al. 1996b. Ex vivo ras peptide vaccination in patients with advanced pancreatic cancer: results of a phase I/II study. *Int J Cancer*, **65**, 450–3.

Gjertsen, M.K., Buanes, T., et al. 2001. Intradermal ras peptide vaccination with granulocyte-macrophage colony-stimulating factor as adjuvant: Clinical and immunological responses in patients with pancreatic adenocarcinoma. *Int J Cancer*, **92**, 441–50.

Gorse, G.J., Keefer, M.C., et al. 1996. A dose-ranging study of a prototype synthetic HIV-1MN V3 branched peptide vaccine. The National Institute of Allergy and Infectious Diseases AIDS Vaccine Evaluation Group. *J Infect Dis*, **173**, 330–9.

Goydos, J.S., Elder, E., et al. 1996. A phase I trial of a synthetic mucin peptide vaccine. Induction of specific immune reactivity in patients with adenocarcinoma. *J Surg Res*, **63**, 298–304.

Greenberg, S.M., Bacskai, B.J. and Hyman, B.T. 2003. Alzheimer disease's double-edged vaccine. *Nat Med*, **9**, 389–90.

Grohmann, U., Bianchi, R., et al. 1997a. A tumor-associated and self antigen peptide presented by dendritic cells may induce T cell anergy in vivo, but IL-12 can prevent or revert the anergic state. *J Immunol*, **158**, 3593–602.

Grohmann, U., Bianchi, R., et al. 1997b. Dendritic cells and interleukin 12 as adjuvants for tumor-specific vaccines. *Adv Exp Med Biol*, **417**, 579–82.

Guermonprez, P., Valladeau, J., et al. 2002. Antigen presentation and T cell stimulation by dendritic cells. *Annu Rev Immunol*, **20**, 621–67, Epub 2001 Oct 4.

Haneberg, B., Dalseg, R., et al. 1998. Intranasal administration of a meningococcal outer membrane vesicle vaccine induces persistent local mucosal antibodies and serum antibodies with strong bactericidal activity in humans. *Infect Immun*, **66**, 1334–41.

Hanke, T. and McMichael, A.J. 2000. Design and construction of an experimental HIV-1 vaccine for a year-2000 clinical trial in Kenya. *Nat Med*, **6**, 951–5.

Harari, I. and Arnon, R. 1990. Carboxy-terminal peptides from the B subunit of Shiga toxin induce a local and parenteral protective effect. *Mol Immunol*, **27**, 613–21.

Harari, I., Donohue-Rolfe, A., et al. 1988. Synthetic peptides of Shiga toxin B subunit induce antibodies which neutralize its biological activity. *Infect Immun*, **56**, 1618–24.

Harn, D.A., Reynolds, S.R., et al. 1995. Synthetic peptide vaccines for schistosomiasis. *Pharm Biotechnol*, **6**, 891–905.

Haro, I., Pinto, R.M., et al. 1995. Anti-hepatitis A virus antibody response elicited in mice by different forms of a synthetic VP1 peptide. *Microbiol Immunol*, **39**, 485–90.

Haro, I., Perez, S., et al. 2003. Liposome entrapment and immunogenic studies of a synthetic lipophilic multiple antigenic peptide bearing VP1 and VP3 domains of the hepatitis A virus: a robust method for vaccine design. *FEBS Lett*, **540**, 133–40.

Hathaway, L.J., Partidos, C.D., et al. 1995. Induction of systemic immune responses to measles virus synthetic peptides administered intranasally. *Vaccine*, **13**, 1495–500.

Hathaway, L.J., Obeid, O.E. and Steward, M.W. 1998. Protection against measles virus-induced encephalitis by antibodies from mice immunized intranasally with a synthetic peptide immunogen. *Vaccine*, **16**, 135–41.

Hayman, W.A., Brandt, E.R., et al. 1997. Mapping the minimal murine T cell and B cell epitopes within a peptide vaccine candidate from the conserved region of the M protein of group A streptococcus. *Int Immunol*, **9**, 1723–33.

Heathcote, J., McHutchison, J., et al. 1999. A pilot study of the CY-1899 T-cell vaccine in subjects chronically infected with hepatitis B virus. The CY1899 T Cell Vaccine Study Group. *Hepatology*, **30**, 531–6.

Herlyn, M. and Koprowski, H. 1988. Melanoma antigens: immunological and biological characterization and clinical significance. *Annu Rev Immunol*, **6**, 283–308.

Herrington, D.A., Clyde, D.F., et al. 1987. Safety and immunogenicity in man of a synthetic peptide malaria vaccine against *Plasmodium falciparum* sporozoites. *Nature*, **328**, 257–9.

Herrington, D.A., Clyde, D.F., et al. 1990. Human studies with synthetic peptide sporozoite vaccine (NANP)3-TT and immunization with irradiated sporozoites. *Bull World Health Organ*, **68**, suppl, 33–7.

Herzenberg, L.A. and Tokuhisa, T. 1980. Carrier-priming leads to hapten-specific suppression. *Nature*, **285**, 664–7.

Ho, P.C., Mutch, D.A., et al. 1990. Identification of two promiscuous T cell epitopes from tetanus toxin. *Eur J Immunol*, **20**, 477–83.

Hohlich, B.J., Wiesmuller, K.H., et al. 2003. Induction of an antigen-specific immune response and partial protection of cattle against challenge infection with foot-and-mouth disease virus (FMDV) after lipopeptide vaccination with FMDV-specific B-cell epitopes. *J Gen Virol*, **84**, 3315–24.

Hoogerhout, P., Donders, E.M., et al. 1995. Conjugates of synthetic cyclic peptides elicit bactericidal antibodies against a conformational epitope on a class 1 outer membrane protein of *Neisseria meningitidis*. *Infect Immun*, **63**, 3473–8.

Hou, Y. and Gu, X.X. 2003. Development of peptide mimotopes of lipooligosaccharide from nontypeable *Haemophilus influenzae* as vaccine candidates. *J Immunol*, **170**, 4373–9.

Hsu, F.J., Benike, C., et al. 1996. Vaccination of patients with B-cell lymphoma using autologous antigen-pulsed dendritic cells. *Nat Med*, **2**, 52–8.

Hsu, S.C., Chargelegue, D. and Steward, M.W. 1998. Reduction of respiratory syncytial virus titer in the lungs of mice after intranasal immunization with a chimeric peptide consisting of a single CTL epitope linked to a fusion peptide. *Virology*, **240**, 376–81.

Hsu, S.C., Chargelegue, D., et al. 1999. Synergistic effect of immunization with a peptide cocktail inducing antibody, helper and cytotoxic T-cell responses on protection against respiratory syncytial virus. *J Gen Virol*, **80**, Pt 6, 1401–5.

Hudecz, F. 2001. Manipulation of epitope function by modification of peptide structure: a minireview. *Biologicals*, **29**, 197–207.

Huerta, M., de Aluja, A.S., et al. 2001. Synthetic peptide vaccine against *Taenia solium* pig cysticercosis: successful vaccination in a controlled field trial in rural Mexico. *Vaccine*, **20**, 262–6.

Huhn, D., von Schilling, C., et al. 2001. Rituximab therapy of patients with B-cell chronic lymphocytic leukemia. *Blood*, **98**, 1326–31.

Hunger, R.E., Brand, C.U., et al. 2001. Successful induction of immune responses against mutant ras in melanoma patients using intradermal injection of peptides and GM-CSF as adjuvant. *Exp Dermatol*, **10**, 161–7.

Hunt, D.F., Henderson, R.A., et al. 1992. Characterization of peptides bound to the class I MHC molecule HLA-A2.1 by mass spectrometry. *Science*, **255**, 1261–3.

Ishikawa, D., Kikkawa, H., et al. 1998. GD1alpha-replica peptides functionally mimic GD1alpha, an adhesion molecule of metastatic tumor cells, and suppress the tumor metastasis. *FEBS Lett*, **441**, 20–4.

Itoh, Y., Takai, E., et al. 1986. A synthetic peptide vaccine involving the product of the pre-S(2) region of hepatitis B virus DNA: protective efficacy in chimpanzees. *Proc Natl Acad Sci USA*, **83**, 9174–8.

Ivanov, V.S., Kulik, L.N., et al. 1994. Synthetic peptides in the determination of hepatitis A virus T-cell epitopes. *FEBS Lett*, **345**, 159–61.

Jackson, D.C., Purcell, A.W., et al. 2002. The central role played by peptides in the immune response and the design of peptide-based vaccines against infectious diseases and cancer. *Curr Drug Targets*, **3**, 175–96.

Jacob, C.O., Sela, M. and Arnon, R. 1983. Antibodies against synthetic peptides of the B subunit of cholera toxin: crossreaction and neutralization of the toxin. *Proc Natl Acad Sci USA*, **80**, 7611–15.

Jacob, C.O., Leitner, M., et al. 1985. Priming immunization against cholera toxin and *E. coli* heat-labile toxin by a cholera toxin short peptide-beta-galactosidase hybrid synthesized in *E. coli*. *EMBO J*, **4**, 3339–43.

Jacob, C.O., Arnon, R. and Sela, M. 1986a. Anti-cholera response elicited by a completely synthetic antigen with built-in adjuvanticity administered in aqueous solution. *Immunol Lett*, **14**, 43–8.

Jacob, C.O., Arnon, R. and Finkelstein, R.A. 1986b. Immunity to heat-labile enterotoxins of porcine and human *Escherichia coli* strains achieved with synthetic cholera toxin peptides. *Infect Immun*, **52**, 562–7.

Jaeger, E., Bernhard, H., et al. 1996. Generation of cytotoxic T-cell responses with synthetic melanoma-associated peptides in vivo: implications for tumor vaccines with melanoma-associated antigens. *Int J Cancer*, **66**, 162–9.

Jager, D., Jager, E. and Knuth, A. 2001. Immune responses to tumor antigens: implications for antigen specific immunotherapy of cancer. *J Clin Pathol*, **54**, 669–74.

Jager, E., Jager, D. and Knuth, A. 1999. CTL-defined cancer vaccines: perspectives for active immunotherapeutic interventions in minimal residual disease. *Cancer Metastasis Rev*, **18**, 143–50.

Jager, E., Gnjatic, S., et al. 2000a. Induction of primary NY-ESO-1 immunity: CD8+ T lymphocyte and antibody responses in peptide-vaccinated patients with NY-ESO-1+ cancers. *Proc Natl Acad Sci USA*, **97**, 12198–203.

Jager, E., Jager, D., et al. 2000b. Identification of NY-ESO-1 epitopes presented by human histocompatibility antigen (HLA)-DRB4*0101-0103 and recognized by CD4(+) T lymphocytes of patients with NY-ESO-1-expressing melanoma. *J Exp Med*, **191**, 625–30.

Jameson, B.A., Bonin, J., et al. 1985. Natural variants of the Sabin type 1 vaccine strain of poliovirus and correlation with a poliovirus neutralization site. *Virology*, **143**, 337–41.

Jameson, B.A., McDonnell, J.M., et al. 1994. A rationally designed CD4 analogue inhibits experimental allergic encephalomyelitis. *Nature*, **368**, 744–6.

Janus, C., Pearson, J., et al. 2000. A beta peptide immunization reduces behavioural impairment and plaques in a model of Alzheimer's disease. *Nature*, **408**, 979–82.

Jerne, N.K. 1960. Immunological speculations. *Annu Rev Microbiol*, **14**, 341–58.

Jones, W.R., Bradley, J., et al. 1988. Phase I clinical trial of a World Health Organization birth control vaccine. *Lanceti*, **i**, 1295–8.

Joshi, M.B., Gam, A.A., et al. 2001. Immunogenicity of well-characterized synthetic *Plasmodium falciparum* multiple antigen peptide conjugates. *Infect Immun*, **69**, 4884–90.

Karanikas, V., Hwang, L.A., et al. 1997. Antibody and T cell responses of patients with adenocarcinoma immunized with mannan-MUC1 fusion protein. *J Clin Invest*, **100**, 2783–92.

Karanikas, V., Thynne, G., et al. 2001. Mannan mucin-1 peptide immunization: influence of cyclophosphamide and the route of injection. *J Immunother*, **24**, 172–83.

Kato, H., Bukawa, H., et al. 2000. Rectal and vaginal immunization with a macromolecular multicomponent peptide vaccine candidate for HIV-1 infection induces HIV-specific protective immune responses. *Vaccine*, **18**, 1151–60.

Kaumaya, P.T., Kobs-Conrad, S., et al. 1993. Peptide vaccines incorporating a 'promiscuous' T-cell epitope bypass certain haplotype restricted immune responses and provide broad spectrum immunogenicity. *J Mol Recognit*, **6**, 81–94.

Kawana, K., Matsumoto, K., et al. 1998. A surface immunodeterminant of human papillomavirus type 16 minor capsid protein L2. *Virology*, **245**, 353–9.

Kawana, K., Yoshikawa, H., et al. 1999. Common neutralization epitope in minor capsid protein L2 of human papillomavirus types 16 and 6. *J Virol*, **73**, 6188–90.

Kawana, K., Kawana, Y., et al. 2001. Nasal immunization of mice with peptide having a cross-neutralization epitope on minor capsid protein L2 of human papillomavirus type 16 elicit systemic and mucosal antibodies. *Vaccine*, **19**, 1496–502.

Kawana, K., Yasugi, T., et al. 2003. Safety and immunogenicity of a peptide containing the cross-neutralization epitope of HPV16 L2 administered nasally in healthy volunteers. *Vaccine*, **21**, 4256–60.

Keefer, M.C., Wolff, M., et al. 1997. Safety profile of phase I and II preventive HIV type 1 envelope vaccination: experience of the NIAID AIDS Vaccine Evaluation Group. *AIDS Res Hum Retroviruses*, **13**, 1163–77.

Kelleher, A.D., Emery, S., et al. 1997. Safety and immunogenicity of UBI HIV-1MN octameric V3 peptide vaccine administered by subcutaneous injection. *AIDS Res Hum Retroviruses*, **13**, 29–32.

Khleif, S.N., Abrams, S.I., et al. 1999. A phase I vaccine trial with peptides reflecting ras oncogene mutations of solid tumors. *J Immunother*, **22**, 155–65.

Kieber-Emmons, T., Luo, P., et al. 1999. Vaccination with carbohydrate peptide mimotopes promotes anti-tumor responses. *Nat Biotechnol*, **17**, 660–5.

Knabel, M., Franz, T.J., et al. 2002. Reversible MHC multimer staining for functional isolation of T-cell populations and effective adoptive transfer. *Nat Med*, **8**, 631–7.

Knutson, K.L. and Disis, M.L. 2001. Expansion of HER2/neu-specific T cells ex vivo following immunization with a HER2/neu peptide-based vaccine. *Clin Breast Cancer*, **2**, 73–9.

Knutson, K.L., Schiffman, K. and Disis, M.L. 2001. Immunization with a HER-2/neu helper peptide vaccine generates HER-2/neu CD8 T-cell immunity in cancer patients. *J Clin Invest*, **107**, 477–84.

Knutson, K.L., Schiffman, K., et al. 2002. Immunization of cancer patients with a HER-2/neu, HLA-A2 peptide, p369-377, results in short-lived peptide-specific immunity. *Clin Cancer Res*, **8**, 1014–18.

Koroev, D.O., Kotel'nikova, O.V., et al. 2000. [Induction of anti-meningitis immunity using the synthetic peptides. I. The immunoreactive synthetic fragments of porin A from *Neisseria meningitidis*]. *Bioorg Khim*, **26**, 323–9.

Koroev, D.O., Vol'pina, O.M., et al. 2001. [Induction of antimeningitis immunity by synthetic peptides. II. Immunoactive synthetic fragments of OpaB protein from *Neisseria meningitidis*]. *Bioorg Khim*, **27**, 21–6.

Krieg, A.M. 2002. CpG motifs in bacterial DNA and their immune effects. *Annu Rev Immunol*, **20**, 709–60.

Kugler, A., Stuhler, G., et al. 2000. Regression of human metastatic renal cell carcinoma after vaccination with tumor cell-dendritic cell hybrids. *Nat Med*, **6**, 332–6.

Kurikka, S., Kayhty, H., et al. 1996. Comparison of five different vaccination schedules with *Haemophilus influenzae* type b-tetanus toxoid conjugate vaccine. *J Pediatr*, **128**, 524–30.

Kuttler, C., Nussbaum, A.K., et al. 2000. An algorithm for the prediction of proteasomal cleavages. *J Mol Biol*, **298**, 417–29.

Kyd, J.M., Cripps, A.W., et al. 2003. Efficacy of the 26-kilodalton outer membrane protein and two P5 fimbrin-derived immunogens to induce clearance of nontypeable *Haemophilus influenzae* from the rat middle ear and lungs as well as from the chinchilla middle ear and nasopharynx. *Infect Immun*, **71**, 4691–9.

Lambert, J.S., Keefer, M., et al. 2001a. A Phase I safety and immunogenicity trial of UBI microparticulate monovalent HIV-1 MN oral peptide immunogen with parenteral boost in HIV-1 seronegative human subjects. *Vaccine*, **19**, 3033–42.

Lambert, M.P., Viola, K.L., et al. 2001b. Vaccination with soluble Abeta oligomers generates toxicity-neutralizing antibodies. *J Neurochem*, **79**, 595–605.

Langbeheim, H., Arnon, R. and Sela, M. 1976. Antiviral effect on MS-2 coliphage obtained with a synthetic antigen. *Proc Natl Acad Sci USA*, **73**, 4636–40.

Landry, S. (ed.) 2002. *The Jordan Report*. Washington DC: US Department of Health and Human Services.

Langeveld, J.P., Casal, J.I., et al. 1994a. Effective induction of neutralizing antibodies with the amino terminus of VP2 of canine parvovirus as a synthetic peptide. *Vaccine*, **12**, 1473–80.

Langeveld, J.P., Casal, J.I., et al. 1994b. First peptide vaccine providing protection against viral infection in the target animal: studies of canine parvovirus in dogs. *J Virol*, **68**, 4506–13.

Langeveld, J.P., Kamstrup, S., et al. 1995. Full protection in mink against mink enteritis virus with new generation canine parvovirus vaccines based on synthetic peptide or recombinant protein. *Vaccine*, **13**, 1033–7.

Langeveld, J.P., Martinez-Torrecuadrada, J., et al. 2001a. Characterisation of a protective linear B cell epitope against feline parvoviruses. *Vaccine*, **19**, 2352–60.

Langeveld, J.P., Brennan, F.R., et al. 2001b. Inactivated recombinant plant virus protects dogs from a lethal challenge with canine parvovirus. *Vaccine*, **19**, 3661–70.

Lee, K.H., Wang, E., et al. 1999. Increased vaccine-specific T cell frequency after peptide-based vaccination correlates with increased susceptibility to in vitro stimulation but does not lead to tumor regression. *J Immunol*, **163**, 6292–300.

Lee, P., Wang, F., et al. 2001. Effects of interleukin-12 on the immune response to a multipeptide vaccine for resected metastatic melanoma. *J Clin Oncol*, **19**, 3836–47.

Lemere, C.A., Maron, R., et al. 2001. Nasal vaccination with beta-amyloid peptide for the treatment of Alzheimer's disease. *DNA Cell Biol*, **20**, 705–11.

Lenz, J., Su, M., et al. 2001. V3 variation in HIV-seropositive patients receiving a V3- targeted vaccine. *Aids*, **15**, 577–81.

Letvin, N.L. 1998. Progress in the development of an HIV-1 vaccine. *Science*, **280**, 1875–80.

Levi, R., Aboud-Pirak, E., et al. 1995. Intranasal immunization of mice against influenza with synthetic peptides anchored to proteosomes. *Vaccine*, **13**, 1353–9.

Lewis, J.J., Janetzki, S., et al. 2000. Evaluation of CD8(+) T-cell frequencies by the Elispot assay in healthy individuals and in patients with metastatic melanoma immunized with tyrosinase peptide. *Int J Cancer*, **87**, 391–8.

Li, C., Candotti, D. and Allain, J.P. 2001. Production and characterization of monoclonal antibodies specific for a conserved epitope within hepatitis C virus hypervariable region 1. *J Virol*, **75**, 12412–20.

Li, D., Forrest, B.D., et al. 1997. International clinical trials of HIV vaccines: II. Phase I trial of an HIV-1 synthetic peptide vaccine evaluating an accelerated immunization schedule in Yunnan, China. *Asian Pac J Allergy Immunol*, **15**, 105–13.

Li, Q., Dong, C., et al. 2003. Induction of hepatitis C virus-specific humoral and cellular immune responses in mice and rhesus by artificial multiple epitopes sequence. *Viral Immunol*, **16**, 321–33.

Lipkin, W.I., Schwimmbeck, P.L. and Oldstone, M.B. 1988. Antibody to synthetic somatostatin-28(1-12): immunoreactivity with somatostatin in brain is dependent on orientation of immunizing peptide. *J Histochem Cytochem*, **36**, 447–51.

Livingston, B.D., Crimi, C., et al. 1997. The hepatitis B virus-specific CTL responses induced in humans by lipopeptide vaccination are comparable to those elicited by acute viral infection. *J Immunol*, **159**, 1383–92.

Livingston, B.D., Crimi, C., et al. 1999. Immunization with the HBV core 18-27 epitope elicits CTL responses in humans expressing different HLA-A2 supertype molecules. *Hum Immunol*, **60**, 1013–17.

Lodge, P.A., Jones, L.A., et al. 2000. Dendritic cell-based immunotherapy of prostate cancer: immune monitoring of a phase II clinical trial. *Cancer Res*, **60**, 829–33.

Lotze, M.T., Shurin, M., et al. 2000. Interleukin-2: developing additional cytokine gene therapies using fibroblasts or dendritic cells to enhance tumor immunity. *Cancer J Sci Am*, **6**, S61–6.

Lou, Y., Ang, J., et al. 1995. A zona pellucida 3 peptide vaccine induces antibodies and reversible infertility without ovarian pathology. *J Immunol*, **155**, 2715–20.

Lu, Y.A., Clavijo, P., et al. 1991. Chemically unambiguous peptide immunogen: preparation, orientation and antigenicity of purified peptide conjugated to the multiple antigen peptide system. *Mol Immunol*, **28**, 623–30.

Lu, Y., Xiao, Y., et al. 2000. Multiepitope vaccines intensively increased levels of antibodies recognizing three neutralizing epitopes on human immunodeficiency virus-1 envelope protein. *Scand J Immunol*, **51**, 497–501.

Machiels, J.P., van Baren, N. and Marchand, M. 2002. Peptide-based cancer vaccines. *Semin Oncol*, **29**, 494–502.

Maeurer, M.J., Storkus, W.J., et al. 1996. New treatment options for patients with melanoma: review of melanoma-derived T-cell epitope-based peptide vaccines. *Melanoma Res*, **6**, 11–24.

Mahi-Brown, C.A. 1996. Primate response to immunization with a homologous zona pellucida peptide. *J Reprod Fertil Suppl*, **50**, 165–74.

Mahi-Brown, C.A. and Moran, F. 1995. Response of cynomolgus macaques to immunization against a synthetic peptide from the human zona pellucida. *J Med Primatol*, **24**, 258–70.

Mailander, V., Scheibenbogen, C., et al. 2004. Complete remission in a patient with recurrent acute myeloid leukemia induced by vaccination with WT1 peptide in the absence of hematological or renal toxicity. *Leukemia*, **18**, 165–6.

Mallett, C.P., Hale, T.L., et al. 1995. Intranasal or intragastric immunization with proteosome-*Shigella* lipopolysaccharide vaccines protects against lethal pneumonia in a murine model of *Shigella* infection. *Infect Immun*, **63**, 2382–6.

Mandelboim, O., Berke, G., et al. 1994. CTL induction by a tumour-associated antigen octapeptide derived from a murine lung carcinoma. *Nature*, **369**, 67–71.

Manici, S., Sturniolo, T., et al. 1999. Melanoma cells present a MAGE-3 epitope to CD4(+) cytotoxic T cells in association with histocompatibility leukocyte antigen DR11. *J Exp Med*, **189**, 871–6.

Manoutcharian, K., Rosas, G., et al. 1996. Cysticercosis: identification and cloning of protective recombinant antigens. *J Parasitol*, **82**, 250–4.

Marchand, M., Weynants, P., et al. 1995. Tumor regression responses in melanoma patients treated with a peptide encoded by gene MAGE-3. *Int J Cancer*, **63**, 883–5.

Marchand, M., van Baren, N., et al. 1999. Tumor regressions observed in patients with metastatic melanoma treated with an antigenic peptide encoded by gene MAGE-3 and presented by HLA-A1. *Int J Cancer*, **80**, 219–30.

Marglin, A. and Merrifield, R.B. 1970. Chemical synthesis of peptides and proteins. *Annu Rev Biochem*, **39**, 841–66.

Marincola, F.M., Rivoltini, L., et al. 1996. Differential anti-MART-1/MelanA CTL activity in peripheral blood of HLA-A2 melanoma patients in comparison to healthy donors: evidence of in vivo priming by tumor cells. *J Immunother Emphasis Tumor Immunol*, **19**, 266–77.

Marincola, F.M., Jaffee, E.M., et al. 2000. Escape of human solid tumors from T-cell recognition: molecular mechanisms and functional significance. *Adv Immunol*, **74**, 181–273.

Mayordomo, J.I., Loftus, D.J., et al. 1996. Therapy of murine tumors with p53 wild-type and mutant sequence peptide-based vaccines. *J Exp Med*, **183**, 1357–65.

Mayordomo, J.I., Zorina, T., et al. 1997. Bone marrow-derived dendritic cells serve as potent adjuvants for peptide-based antitumor vaccines. *Stem Cells*, **15**, 94–103.

Melief, C.J. and Kast, W.M. 1994. Prospects for T cell immunotherapy of tumours by vaccination with immunodominant and subdominant peptides. *Ciba Found Symp*, **187**, 97–104, discussion 104–12.

Melief, C.J. and Kast, W.M. 1995. T-cell immunotherapy of tumors by adoptive transfer of cytotoxic T lymphocytes and by vaccination with minimal essential epitopes. *Immunol Rev*, **145**, 167–77.

Meloen, R.H., Turkstra, J.A., et al. 1994. Efficient immunocastration of male piglets by immunoneutralization of GnRH using a new GnRH-like peptide. *Vaccine*, **12**, 741–6.

Millar, S.E., Chamow, S.M., et al. 1989. Vaccination with a synthetic zona pellucida peptide produces long-term contraception in female mice. *Science*, **246**, 935–8.

Mocellin, S., Rossi, C.R., et al. 2003. Dissecting tumor responsiveness to immunotherapy: the experience of peptide-based melanoma vaccines. *Biochim Biophys Acta*, **1653**, 61–71.

Monsonego, A., Maron, R., et al. 2001. Immune hyporesponsiveness to amyloid beta-peptide in amyloid precursor protein transgenic mice: implications for the pathogenesis and treatment of Alzheimer's disease. *Proc Natl Acad Sci USA*, **98**, 10273–8.

Monzavi-Karbassi, B., Cunto-Amesty, G., et al. 2002. Peptide mimotopes as surrogate antigens of carbohydrates in vaccine discovery. *Trends Biotechnol*, **20**, 207–14.

Moorthy, V.S., Good, M.F. and Hill, A.V. 2004. Malaria vaccine developments. *Lancet*, **363**, 150–6.

Moreno, C.A., Rodriguez, R., et al. 1999. Preclinical evaluation of a synthetic *Plasmodium falciparum* MAP malaria vaccine in *Aotus* monkeys and mice. *Vaccine*, **18**, 89–99.

Morgan, D. 2003. Antibody therapy for Alzheimer's disease. *Expert Rev Vaccines*, **2**, 53–9.

Morgan, D., Diamond, D.M., et al. 2000. A beta peptide vaccination prevents memory loss in an animal model of Alzheimer's disease. *Nature*, **408**, 982–5.

Morgan, D.O. and Moore, D.M. 1990. Protection of cattle and swine against foot-and-mouth disease, using biosynthetic peptide vaccines. *Am J Vet Res*, **51**, 40–5.

Morris, E.G. 1996. Epitope mapping protocols. *Methods Mol Biol*, **66**, 121–7.

Morse, M.A., Deng, Y., et al. 1999. A Phase I study of active immunotherapy with carcinoembryonic antigen peptide (CAP-1)-pulsed, autologous human cultured dendritic cells in patients with metastatic malignancies expressing carcinoembryonic antigen. *Clin Cancer Res*, **5**, 1331–8.

Moser, C., Metcalfe, I.C. and Viret, J.F. 2003. Virosomal adjuvanted antigen delivery systems. *Expert Rev Vaccines*, **2**, 189–96.

Motti, C., Nuzzo, M., et al. 1994. Recognition by human sera and immunogenicity of HBsAg mimotopes selected from an M13 phage display library. *Gene*, **146**, 191–8.

Muderspach, L., Wilczynski, S., et al. 2000. A phase I trial of a human papillomavirus (HPV) peptide vaccine for women with high-grade cervical and vulvar intraepithelial neoplasia who are HPV 16 positive. *Clin Cancer Res*, **6**, 3406–16.

Muller, C.P. 2001a. Measles elimination: old and new challenges? *Vaccine*, **19**, 2258–61.

Muller, C.P. 2001b. *Epitopes. Encyclopaedia of life sciences*. London: Macmillan Reference Ltd.

Muller, G.M., Shapira, M. and Arnon, R. 1982. Anti-influenza response achieved by immunization with a synthetic conjugate. *Proc Natl Acad Sci USA*, **79**, 569–73.

Muller, S., Plaue, S., et al. 1990. Antigenic properties and protective capacity of a cyclic peptide corresponding to site A of influenza virus haemagglutinin. *Vaccine*, **8**, 308–14.

Muller, S., Guichard, G., et al. 1995. Enhanced immunogenicity and cross-reactivity of retro-inverso peptidomimetics of the major antigenic site of foot-and-mouth disease virus. *Pept Res*, **8**, 138–44.

Murphy, G., Tjoa, B., et al. 1996. Phase I clinical trial: T-cell therapy for prostate cancer using autologous dendritic cells pulsed with HLA-A0201-specific peptides from prostate-specific membrane antigen. *Prostate*, **29**, 371–80.

Murphy, G.P., Tjoa, B.A., et al. 1999a. Infusion of dendritic cells pulsed with HLA-A2-specific prostate-specific membrane antigen peptides: a phase II prostate cancer vaccine trial involving patients with hormone-refractory metastatic disease. *Prostate*, **38**, 73–8.

Murphy, G.P., Tjoa, B.A., et al. 1999b. Phase II prostate cancer vaccine trial: report of a study involving 37 patients with disease recurrence following primary treatment. *Prostate*, **39**, 54–9.

Murphy, G.P., Tjoa, B.A., et al. 2000. Higher-dose and less frequent dendritic cell infusions with PSMA peptides in hormone-refractory metastatic prostate cancer patients. *Prostate*, **43**, 59–62.

Nagorsen, D., Keilholz, U., et al. 2000. Natural T-cell response against MHC class I epitopes of epithelial cell adhesion molecule, her-2/neu, and carcinoembryonic antigen in patients with colorectal cancer. *Cancer Res*, **60**, 4850–4.

Nardelli, B. and Tam, J.P. 1995. The MAP system. A flexible and unambiguous vaccine design of branched peptides. *Pharm Biotechnol*, **6**, 803–19.

Nardelli, B., Lu, Y.A., et al. 1992. A chemically defined synthetic vaccine model for HIV-1. *J Immunol*, **148**, 914–20.

Nardin, E.H., Calvo-Calle, J.M., et al. 1998. *Plasmodium falciparum* polyoximes: highly immunogenic synthetic vaccines constructed by chemoselective ligation of repeat B-cell epitopes and a universal T-cell epitope of CS protein. *Vaccine*, **16**, 590–600.

Nardin, E.H., Oliveira, G.A., et al. 2000. Synthetic malaria peptide vaccine elicits high levels of antibodies in vaccinees of defined HLA genotypes. *J Infect Dis*, **182**, 1486–96.

Nardin, E.H., Calvo-Calle, J.M., et al. 2001. A totally synthetic polyoxime malaria vaccine containing *Plasmodium falciparum* B cell and universal T cell epitopes elicits immune responses in volunteers of diverse HLA types. *J Immunol*, **166**, 481–9.

Nargi, F., Kramer, E., et al. 1999. Protection of swine from foot-and-mouth disease with one dose of an all-D retro peptide. *Vaccine*, **17**, 2888–93.

Naz, R.K. 2004. Human synthetic peptide vaccine for contraception targeting sperm. *Arch Androl*, **50**, 113–19.

Naz, R.K. and Chauhan, S.C. 2002. Human sperm-specific peptide vaccine that causes long-term reversible contraception. *Biol Reprod*, **67**, 674–80.

Nemchinov, L.G., Liang, T.J., et al. 2000. Development of a plant-derived subunit vaccine candidate against hepatitis C virus. *Arch Virol*, **145**, 2557–73.

Nestle, F.O., Alijagic, S., et al. 1998. Vaccination of melanoma patients with peptide- or tumor lysate-pulsed dendritic cells. *Nat Med*, **4**, 328–32.

Nicolau, C., Greferath, R., et al. 2002. A liposome-based therapeutic vaccine against beta-amyloid plaques on the pancreas of transgenic NORBA mice. *Proc Natl Acad Sci USA*, **99**, 2332–7.

Nicoll, J.A., Wilkinson, D., et al. 2003. Neuropathology of human Alzheimer disease after immunization with amyloid-beta peptide: a case report. *Nat Med*, **9**, 448–52.

Nishiyama, T., Tachibana, M., et al. 2001. Immunotherapy of bladder cancer using autologous dendritic cells pulsed with human lymphocyte antigen-A24-specific MAGE-3 peptide. *Clin Cancer Res*, **7**, 23–31.

Nosten, F., Luxemburger, C., et al. 1996. Randomised double-blind placebo-controlled trial of SPf66 malaria vaccine in children in northwestern Thailand. Shoklo SPf66 Malaria Vaccine Trial Group. *Lancet*, **348**, 701–7.

Nussbaum, A.K., Dick, T.P., et al. 1998. Cleavage motifs of the yeast 20S proteasome beta subunits deduced from digests of enolase 1. *Proc Natl Acad Sci USA*, **95**, 12504–9.

Nussbaum, A.K., Kuttler, C., et al. 2001. PAProC: a prediction algorithm for proteasomal cleavages available on the WWW. *Immunogenetics*, **53**, 87–94.

Obeid, O.E., Partidos, C.D., et al. 1995. Protection against morbillivirus-induced encephalitis by immunization with a rationally designed synthetic peptide vaccine containing B- and T-cell epitopes from the fusion protein of measles virus. *J Virol*, **69**, 1420–8.

O'Brien-Simpson, N.M., Paolini, R.A., et al. 2000. RgpA-Kgp peptide-based immunogens provide protection against *Porphyromonas gingivalis* challenge in a murine lesion model. *Infect Immun*, **68**, 4055–63.

Oftung, F., Naess, L.M., et al. 1999. Antigen-specific T-cell responses in humans after intranasal immunization with a meningococcal serogroup B outer membrane vesicle vaccine. *Infect Immun*, **67**, 921–7.

Ogawa, T. 1994. The potential protective immune responses to synthetic peptides containing conserved epitopes of *Porphyromonas gingivalis* fimbrial protein. *J Med Microbiol*, **41**, 349–58.

O'Hern, P.A., Bambra, C.S., et al. 1995. Reversible contraception in female baboons immunized with a synthetic epitope of sperm-specific lactate dehydrogenase. *Biol Reprod*, **52**, 331–9.

O'Hern, P.A., Liang, Z.G., et al. 1997. Colinear synthesis of an antigen-specific B-cell epitope with a 'promiscuous' tetanus toxin T-cell epitope: a synthetic peptide immunocontraceptive. *Vaccine*, **15**, 1761–6.

Olive, C., Toth, I. and Jackson, D. 2001. Technological advances in antigen delivery and synthetic peptide vaccine developmental strategies. *Mini Rev Med Chem*, **1**, 429–38.

Olive, C., Batzloff, M.R., et al. 2002a. A lipid core peptide construct containing a conserved region determinant of the group A streptococcal M protein elicits heterologous opsonic antibodies. *Infect Immun*, **70**, 2734–8.

Olive, C., Clair, T., et al. 2002b. Protection of mice from group A streptococcal infection by intranasal immunisation with a peptide vaccine that contains a conserved M protein B cell epitope and lacks a T cell autoepitope. *Vaccine*, **20**, 2816–25.

Olive, C., Batzloff, M.R. and Toth, I. 2004. Lipid core peptide technology and group A streptococcal vaccine delivery. *Expert Rev Vaccines*, **3**, 43–58.

Olszewska, W., Obeid, O.E. and Steward, M.W. 2000. Protection against measles virus-induced encephalitis by anti-mimotope antibodies: the role of antibody affinity. *Virology*, **272**, 98–105.

Oonk, H.B., Turkstra, J.A., et al. 1998. New GnRH-like peptide construct to optimize efficient immunocastration of male pigs by immunoneutralization of GnRH. *Vaccine*, **16**, 1074–82.

Pamer, E.G., Harty, J.T. and Bevan, M.J. 1991. Precise prediction of a dominant class I MHC-restricted epitope of *Listeria monocytogenes*. *Nature*, **353**, 852–5.

Panelli, M.C., Wunderlich, J., et al. 2000. Phase 1 study in patients with metastatic melanoma of immunization with dendritic cells presenting epitopes derived from the melanoma-associated antigens MART-1 and gp100. *J Immunother*, **23**, 487–98.

Panina-Bordignon, P., Tan, A., et al. 1989. Universally immunogenic T cell epitopes: promiscuous binding to human MHC class II and promiscuous recognition by T cells. *Eur J Immunol*, **19**, 2237–42.

Parkhurst, M.R., Salgaller, M.L., et al. 1996. Improved induction of melanoma-reactive CTL with peptides from the melanoma antigen gp100 modified at HLA-A*0201-binding residues. *J Immunol*, **157**, 2539–48.

Parmiani, G., Castelli, C., et al. 2002a. Cancer immunotherapy with peptide-based vaccines: what have we achieved? Where are we going? *J Natl Cancer Inst*, **94**, 805–18.

Parmiani, G., Sensi, M., et al. 2002b. T-cell response to unique and shared antigens and vaccination of cancer patients. *Cancer Immun*, **2**, 6.

Parrish, C.R., Aquadro, C.F. and Carmichael, L.E. 1988. Canine host range and a specific epitope map along with variant sequences in the capsid protein gene of canine parvovirus and related feline, mink, and raccoon parvoviruses. *Virology*, **166**, 293–307.

Parry, N.R., Syred, A., et al. 1988. A high proportion of anti-peptide antibodies recognize foot-and-mouth disease virus particles. *Immunology*, **64**, 567–72.

Partidos, C.D. and Steward, M.W. 1990. Prediction and identification of a T cell epitope in the fusion protein of measles virus immunodominant in mice and humans. *J Gen Virol*, **71**, 2099–105.

Partidos, C.D., Stanley, C.M. and Steward, M.W. 1991. Immune responses in mice following immunization with chimeric synthetic peptides representing B and T cell epitopes of measles virus proteins. *J Gen Virol*, **72**, 1293–9.

Partidos, C.D., Obeid, O.E. and Steward, M.W. 1992a. Antibody responses to non-immunogenic synthetic peptides induced by co-immunization with immunogenic peptides. *Immunology*, **77**, 262–6.

Partidos, C., Stanley, C. and Steward, M. 1992b. The effect of orientation of epitopes on the immunogenicity of chimeric synthetic peptides representing measles virus protein sequences. *Mol Immunol*, **29**, 651–8.

Partidos, C., Stanley, C. and Steward, M. 1992c. The influence of orientation and number of copies of T and B cell epitopes on the specificity and affinity of antibodies induced by chimeric peptides. *Eur J Immunol*, **22**, 2675–80.

Partidos, C.D., Pizza, M., et al. 1996. The adjuvant effect of a non-toxic mutant of heat-labile enterotoxin of *Escherichia coli* for the induction of measles virus-specific CTL responses after intranasal co-immunization with a synthetic peptide. *Immunology*, **89**, 483–7.

Partidos, C.D., Ripley, J., et al. 1997. Fine specificity of the antibody response to a synthetic peptide from the fusion protein and protection against measles virus-induced encephalitis in a mouse model. *J Gen Virol*, **78**, Pt 12, 3227–32.

Partidos, C.D., Beignon, A.S., et al. 2001. The bare skin and the nose as non-invasive routes for administering peptide vaccines. *Vaccine*, **19**, 2708–15.

Patarroyo, G., Franco, L., et al. 1992. Study of the safety and immunogenicity of the synthetic malaria SPf66 vaccine in children aged 1–14 years. *Vaccine*, **10**, 175–8.

Patarroyo, M.E., Romero, P., et al. 1987. Induction of protective immunity against experimental infection with malaria using synthetic peptides. *Nature*, **328**, 629–32.

Patarroyo, M.E., Amador, R., et al. 1988. A synthetic vaccine protects humans against challenge with asexual blood stages of *Plasmodium falciparum* malaria. *Nature*, **332**, 158–61.

Paterson, M., Wilson, M.R., et al. 1999. Design and evaluation of a ZP3 peptide vaccine in a homologous primate model. *Mol Hum Reprod*, **5**, 342–52.

Paterson, M., Jennings, Z.A., et al. 2002. The contraceptive potential of ZP3 and ZP3 peptides in a primate model. *J Reprod Immunol*, **53**, 99–107.

Perlaza, B.L., Sauzet, J.P., et al. 2001. Long synthetic peptides encompassing the *Plasmodium falciparum* LSA3 are the target of human B and T cells and are potent inducers of B helper, T helper and cytolytic T cell responses in mice. *Eur J Immunol*, **31**, 2200–9.

Pfaff, E., Mussgay, M., et al. 1982. Antibodies against a preselected peptide recognize and neutralize foot and mouth disease virus. *EMBO J*, **1**, 869–74.

Phan, G.Q., Touloukian, C.E., et al. 2003. Immunization of patients with metastatic melanoma using both class I- and class II-restricted peptides from melanoma-associated antigens. *J Immunother*, **26**, 349–56.

Phanuphak, P., Teeratakulpixarn, S., et al. 1997. International clinical trials of HIV vaccines: I. Phase I trial of an HIV-1 synthetic peptide vaccine in Bangkok, Thailand. *Asian Pac J Allergy Immunol*, **15**, 41–8.

Pieper, R., Christian, R.E., et al. 1999. Biochemical identification of a mutated human melanoma antigen recognized by CD4(+) T cells. *J Exp Med*, **189**, 757–66.

Pinilla, C., Martin, R., et al. 1999. Exploring immunological specificity using synthetic peptide combinatorial libraries. *Curr Opin Immunol*, **11**, 193–202.

Pinilla, C., Rubio-Godoy, V., et al. 2001. Combinatorial peptide libraries as an alternative approach to the identification of ligands for tumor-reactive cytolytic T lymphocytes. *Cancer Res*, **61**, 5153–60.

Pinilla-Ibarz, J., Cathcart, K., et al. 2000. Vaccination of patients with chronic myelogenous leukemia with bcr-abl oncogene breakpoint fusion peptides generates specific immune responses. *Blood*, **95**, 1781–7.

Pinto, L.A., Berzofsky, J.A., et al. 1999. HIV-specific immunity following immunization with HIV synthetic envelope peptides in asymptomatic HIV-infected patients. *Aids*, **13**, 2003–12.

Pittet, M.J., Speiser, D.E., et al. 2001. Expansion and functional maturation of human tumor antigen-specific CD8+ T cells after vaccination with antigenic peptide. *Clin Cancer Res*, **7**, 796S-803S.

Polack, F.P., Auwaerter, P.G., et al. 1999. Production of atypical measles in rhesus macaques: evidence for disease mediated by immune complex formation and eosinophils in the presence of fusion-inhibiting antibody. *Nat Med*, **5**, 629–34.

Powell, M.F., Stewart, T., et al. 1993. Peptide stability in drug development. II. Effect of single amino acid substitution and glycosylation on peptide reactivity in human serum. *Pharm Res*, **10**, 1268–73.

Prinz, D.M., Smithson, S.L., et al. 2003. Induction of a protective capsular polysaccharide antibody response to a multiepitope DNA vaccine encoding a peptide mimic of meningococcal serogroup C capsular polysaccharide. *Immunology*, **110**, 242–9.

Prinz, D.M., Smithson, S.L. and Westerink, M.A. 2004. Two different methods result in the selection of peptides that induce a protective antibody response to *Neisseria meningitidis* serogroup C. *J Immunol Methods*, **285**, 1–14.

Pruksakorn, S., Galbraith, A., et al. 1992. Conserved T and B cell epitopes on the M protein of group A streptococci. Induction of bactericidal antibodies. *J Immunol*, **149**, 2729–35.

Pullarkat, V., Lee, P.P., et al. 2003. A phase I trial of SD-9427 (progenipoietin) with a multipeptide vaccine for resected metastatic melanoma. *Clin Cancer Res*, **9**, 1301–12.

Purcell, A.W., Zeng, W., et al. 2003. Dissecting the role of peptides in the immune response: theory, practice and the application to vaccine design. *J Pept Sci*, **9**, 255–81.

Putkonen, P., Bjorling, E., et al. 1994. Long-standing protection of macaques against cell-free HIV-2 with a HIV-2 iscom vaccine. *J Acquir Immune Defic Syndr*, **7**, 551–9.

Pütz, M.M. and Muller, C.P. 2003. The rationale of a peptide-conjugate vaccine against measles. *Vaccine*, **21**, 663–6.

Pütz, M.M., Bouche, F.B., et al. 2003a. Experimental vaccines against measles in a world of changing epidemiology. *Int J Parasitol*, **33**, 525–45.

Pütz, M.M., Hoebeke, J., et al. 2003b. Functional fine-mapping and molecular modeling of a conserved loop epitope of the measles virus hemagglutinin protein. *Eur J Biochem*, **270**, 1515–27.

Pütz, M.M., Ammerlaan, W., et al. 2004. Humoral immune responses to a protective peptide-conjugate against measles after different prime-boost regimens. *Vaccine*, **22**, 4173–82.

Rammensee, H.G. 1995. Chemistry of peptides associated with MHC class I and class II molecules. *Curr Opin Immunol*, **7**, 85–96.

Rammensee, H.G., Friede, T. and Stevanovic, S. 1995. MHC ligands and peptide motifs: first listing. *Immunogenetics*, **41**, 178–228.

Rammensee, H., Bachmann, J. and Stevanovic, S. 1997. *MHC ligands and peptide motifs*. Berlin: Springer.

Rao, C. and Tam, J. 1994. Synthesis of peptide dendrimer. *J Am Chem Soc*, **116**, 6975–6.

Reddish, M., MacLean, G.D., et al. 1998. Anti-MUC1 class I restricted CTLs in metastatic breast cancer patients immunized with a synthetic MUC1 peptide. *Int J Cancer*, **76**, 817–23.

Reed, R.C., Louis-Wileman, V., et al. 1996. Re-investigation of the circumsporozoite protein-based induction of sterile immunity against *Plasmodium berghei* infection. *Vaccine*, **14**, 828–36.

Reed, R.C., Louis-Wileman, V., et al. 1997. Multiple antigen constructs (MACs): induction of sterile immunity against sporozoite stage of rodent malaria parasites, *Plasmodium berghei* and *Plasmodium yoelii*. *Vaccine*, **15**, 482–8.

Reilly, J.F., Games, D., et al. 2003. Amyloid deposition in the hippocampus and entorhinal cortex: quantitative analysis of a transgenic mouse model. *Proc Natl Acad Sci USA*, **100**, 4837–42.

Relf, W.A., Cooper, J., et al. 1996. Mapping a conserved conformational epitope from the M protein of group A streptococci. *Pept Res*, **9**, 12–20.

Renkvist, N., Castelli, C., et al. 2001. A listing of human tumor antigens recognized by T cells. *Cancer Immunol Immunother*, **50**, 3–15.

Ressing, M.E., van Driel, W.J., et al. 2000. Detection of T helper responses, but not of human papillomavirus-specific cytotoxic T lymphocyte responses, after peptide vaccination of patients with cervical carcinoma. *J Immunother*, **23**, 255–66.

Reynolds, S.R., Shoemaker, C.B. and Harn, D.A. 1992. T and B cell epitope mapping of SM23, an integral membrane protein of *Schistosoma mansoni*. *J Immunol*, **149**, 3995–4001.

Reynolds, S.R., Dahl, C.E. and Harn, D.A. 1994. T and B epitope determination and analysis of multiple antigenic peptides for the *Schistosoma mansoni* experimental vaccine triose-phosphate isomerase. *J Immunol*, **152**, 193–200.

Richie, T.L. and Saul, A. 2002. Progress and challenges for malaria vaccines. *Nature*, **415**, 694–701.

Rivera, Z., Granados, G., et al. 2002. Double dimer peptide constructs are immunogenic and protective against *Plasmodium falciparum* in the experimental Aotus monkey model. *J Pept Res*, **59**, 62–70.

Rivoltini, L., Squarcina, P., et al. 1999. A superagonist variant of peptide MART1/Melan A27-35 elicits anti-melanoma CD8+ T cells with enhanced functional characteristics: implication for more effective immunotherapy. *Cancer Res*, **59**, 301–6.

Robertson, B.H., Brown, V.K., et al. 1989. Structure of the hepatitis A virion: identification of potential surface-exposed regions. *Arch Virol*, **104**, 117–28.

Robinson, J.H. and Delvig, A.A. 2002. Diversity in MHC class II antigen presentation. *Immunology*, **105**, 252–62.

Robinson, S.R., Bishop, G.M. and Munch, G. 2003. Alzheimer vaccine: amyloid-beta on trial. *Bioessays*, **25**, 283–8.

Roccasecca, R., Folgori, A., et al. 2001. Mimotopes of the hyper variable region 1 of the hepatitis C virus induce cross-reactive antibodies directed against discontinuous epitopes. *Mol Immunol*, **38**, 485–92.

Roden, R. and Wu, T.C. 2003. Preventative and therapeutic vaccines for cervical cancer. *Expert Rev Vaccines*, **2**, 495–516.

Rodriguez, R., Moreno, A., et al. 1990. Studies in owl monkeys leading to the development of a synthetic vaccine against the asexual blood stages of *Plasmodium falciparum*. *Am J Trop Med Hyg*, **43**, 339–54.

Rose, K. 1994. Facile synthesis of homogeneous artificial proteins. *J Am Chem Soc*, **116**, 30–3.

Rosenberg, S.A., Yang, J.C., et al. 1998. Immunologic and therapeutic evaluation of a synthetic peptide vaccine for the treatment of patients with metastatic melanoma. *Nat Med*, **4**, 321–7.

Rosenberg, S.A., Yang, J.C., et al. 1999. Impact of cytokine administration on the generation of antitumor reactivity in patients with metastatic melanoma receiving a peptide vaccine. *J Immunol*, **163**, 1690–5.

Rotzschke, O., Falk, K., et al. 1990. Isolation and analysis of naturally processed viral peptides as recognized by cytotoxic T cells. *Nature*, **348**, 252–4.

Rubinstein, A., Goldstein, H., et al. 1995. Safety and immunogenicity of a V3 loop synthetic peptide conjugated to purified protein derivative in HIV-seronegative volunteers. *Aids*, **9**, 243–51.

Rubinstein, A., Mizrachi, Y., et al. 1999. Immunologic responses of HIV-1-infected study subjects to immunization with a mixture of peptide protein derivative-V3 loop peptide conjugates. *J Acquir Immune Defic Syndr*, **22**, 467–76.

Rudolf, M.P., Vogel, M., et al. 1998. Epitope-specific antibody response to IgE by mimotope immunization. *J Immunol*, **160**, 3315–21.

Ruebush, T.K., Campbell, G., et al. 1990. Immunization of owl monkeys with a combination of Plasmodium falciparum asexual blood-stage synthetic peptide antigens. *Am J Trop Med Hyg*, **43**, 355–66.

Sadler, K., Bird, P.H., et al. 1999. The antigenic and immunogenic properties of synthetic peptide immunocontraceptive vaccine candidates based on gamete antigens. *Vaccine*, **18**, 416–25.

Salazar, E., Zaremba, S., et al. 2000. Agonist peptide from a cytotoxic t-lymphocyte epitope of human carcinoembryonic antigen stimulates production of tc1-type cytokines and increases tyrosine phosphorylation more efficiently than cognate peptide. *Int J Cancer*, **85**, 829–38.

Salazar, L.G., Fikes, J., et al. 2003. Immunization of cancer patients with HER-2/neu-derived peptides demonstrating high-affinity binding to multiple class II alleles. *Clin Cancer Res*, **9**, 5559–65.

Salcedo, M., Barreto, L., et al. 1991. Studies on the humoral immune response to a synthetic vaccine against *Plasmodium falciparum* malaria. *Clin Exp Immunol*, **84**, 122–8.

Salgaller, M.L., Marincola, F.M., et al. 1996. Immunization against epitopes in the human melanoma antigen gp100 following patient immunization with synthetic peptides. *Cancer Res*, **56**, 4749–57.

Salgaller, M.L., Lodge, P.A., et al. 1998. Report of immune monitoring of prostate cancer patients undergoing T-cell therapy using dendritic cells pulsed with HLA-A2-specific peptides from prostate-specific membrane antigen (PSMA). *Prostate*, **35**, 144–51.

Salit, R.B., Kast, W.M. and Velders, M.P. 2002. Ins and outs of clinical trials with peptide-based vaccines. *Front Biosci*, **7**, E204–213.

Sarvas, H., Kurikka, S., et al. 1992. Maternal antibodies partly inhibit an active antibody response to routine tetanus toxoid immunization in infants. *J Infect Dis*, **165**, 977–9.

Scardino, A., Alves, P., et al. 2001. Identification of HER-2/neu immunogenic epitopes presented by renal cell carcinoma and other human epithelial tumors. *Eur J Immunol*, **31**, 3261–70.

Scheibenbogen, C., Schmittel, A., et al. 2000. Phase 2 trial of vaccination with tyrosinase peptides and granulocyte-macrophage colony-stimulating factor in patients with metastatic melanoma. *J Immunother*, **23**, 275–81.

Scheibenbogen, C., Nagorsen, D., et al. 2002. Long-term freedom from recurrence in 2 stage IV melanoma patients following vaccination with tyrosinase peptides. *Int J Cancer*, **99**, 403–8.

Scheibenbogen, C., Schadendorf, D., et al. 2003. Effects of granulocyte-macrophage colony-stimulating factor and foreign helper protein as immunologic adjuvants on the T-cell response to vaccination with tyrosinase peptides. *Int J Cancer*, **104**, 188–94.

Schenk, D. 2002. Amyloid-beta immunotherapy for Alzheimer's disease: the end of the beginning. *Nat Rev Neurosci*, **3**, 824–8.

Schenk, D., Barbour, R., et al. 1999. Immunization with amyloid-beta attenuates Alzheimer-disease-like pathology in the PDAPP mouse. *Nature*, **400**, 173–7.

Schneerson, R., Kubler-Kielb, J., et al. 2003. Poly(gamma-D-glutamic acid) protein conjugates induce IgG antibodies in mice to the capsule of *Bacillus anthracis*: a potential addition to the anthrax vaccine. *Proc Natl Acad Sci USA*, **100**, 8945–50.

Schnolzer, M. and Kent, S.B. 1992. Constructing proteins by dovetailing unprotected synthetic peptides: backbone-engineered HIV protease. *Science*, **256**, 221–5.

Schodel, F., Peterson, D., et al. 1997. Immunization with hybrid hepatitis B virus core particles carrying circumsporozoite antigen epitopes protects mice against *Plasmodium yoelii* challenge. *Behring Inst Mitt*, **Feb**, 114–19.

Schott, M., Seissler, J., et al. 2001. Immunotherapy for medullary thyroid carcinoma by dendritic cell vaccination. *J Clin Endocrinol Metab*, **86**, 4965–9.

Schreiber, H., Ward, P.L., et al. 1988. Unique tumor-specific antigens. *Annu Rev Immunol*, **6**, 465–83.

Schuler-Thurner, B., Schultz, E.S., et al. 2002. Rapid induction of tumor-specific type 1 T helper cells in metastatic melanoma patients by vaccination with mature, cryopreserved, peptide-loaded monocyte-derived dendritic cells. *J Exp Med*, **195**, 1279–88.

Schutze, M.P., Leclerc, C., et al. 1985. Carrier-induced epitopic suppression, a major issue for future synthetic vaccines. *J Immunol*, **135**, 2319–22.

Sciutto, E., Fragoso, G., et al. 2002. New approaches to improve a peptide vaccine against porcine *Taenia solium* cysticercosis. *Arch Med Res*, **33**, 371–8.

Selkoe, D.J. 1999. Translating cell biology into therapeutic advances in Alzheimer's disease. *Nature*, **399**, A23–31.

Shafferman, A., Jahrling, P.B., et al. 1991. Protection of macaques with a simian immunodeficiency virus envelope peptide vaccine based on conserved human immunodeficiency virus type 1 sequences. *Proc Natl Acad Sci USA*, **88**, 7126–30.

Shapira, M., Jibson, M., et al. 1984. Immunity and protection against influenza virus by synthetic peptide corresponding to antigenic sites of hemagglutinin. *Proc Natl Acad Sci USA*, **81**, 2461–5.

Sharma, P., Kumar, A., et al. 1993. Co-dominant and reciprocal T-helper cell activity of epitopic sequences and formation of junctional B-cell determinants in synthetic T:B chimeric immunogens. *Vaccine*, **11**, 1321–6.

Shi, Y.P., Hasnain, S.E., et al. 1999. Immunogenicity and in vitro protective efficacy of a recombinant multistage *Plasmodium falciparum* candidate vaccine. *Proc Natl Acad Sci USA*, **96**, 1615–20.

Shi, Y.P., Das, P., et al. 2000. Development, expression, and murine testing of a multistage *Plasmodium falciparum* malaria vaccine candidate. *Vaccine*, **18**, 2902–14.

Sigurdsson, E.M., Scholtzova, H., et al. 2001. Immunization with a nontoxic/nonfibrillar amyloid-beta homologous peptide reduces Alzheimer's disease-associated pathology in transgenic mice. *Am J Pathol*, **159**, 439–47.

Simard, C., Nadon, F., et al. 1995. Evidence that the amino acid region 124-203 of glycoprotein G from the respiratory syncytial virus (RSV) constitutes a major part of the polypeptide domain that is involved in the protection against RSV infection. *Antiviral Res*, **28**, 303–15.

Simard, C., Nadon, F., et al. 1997. Subgroup specific protection of mice from respiratory syncytial virus infection with peptides encompassing the amino acid region 174-187 from the G glycoprotein: the role of cysteinyl residues in protection. *Vaccine*, **15**, 423–32.

Sinigaglia, F., Guttinger, M., et al. 1988. A malaria T-cell epitope recognized in association with most mouse and human MHC class II molecules. *Nature*, **336**, 778–80.

Sjolander, A., Drane, D., et al. 2001. Immune responses to ISCOM formulations in animal and primate models. *Vaccine*, **19**, 2661–5.

Slingluff, C.L. Jr. 1996. Tumor antigens and tumor vaccines: peptides as immunogens. *Semin Surg Oncol*, **12**, 446–53.

Slingluff, C.L. Jr, Yamshchikov, G., et al. 2001. Phase I trial of a melanoma vaccine with gp100() peptide and tetanus helper peptide in adjuvant: immunologic and clinical outcomes. *Clin Cancer Res*, **7**, 3012-24, 280–8.

Slingluff, C.L. Jr, Petroni, G.R., et al. 2003. Clinical and immunologic results of a randomized phase II trial of vaccination using four melanoma peptides either administered in granulocyte-macrophage colony-stimulating factor in adjuvant or pulsed on dendritic cells. *J Clin Oncol*, **21**, 4016–26.

Small, E.J., Fratesi, P., et al. 2000. Immunotherapy of hormone-refractory prostate cancer with antigen-loaded dendritic cells. *J Clin Oncol*, **18**, 3894–903.

Smith, S.G., Patel, P.M., et al. 2001. Human dendritic cells genetically engineered to express a melanoma polyepitope DNA vaccine induce multiple cytotoxic T-cell responses. *Clin Cancer Res*, **7**, 4253–61.

Solomon, B. 2002. Immunological approaches as therapy for Alzheimer's disease. *Expert Opin Biol Ther*, **2**, 907–17.

Solomon, B., Koppel, R., et al. 1997. Disaggregation of Alzheimer beta-amyloid by site-directed mAb. *Proc Natl Acad Sci USA*, **94**, 4109–12.

Spetzler, J.C. and Tam, J.P. 1995. Unprotected peptides as building blocks for branched peptides and peptide dendrimers. *Int J Pept Protein Res*, **45**, 78–85.

Spreng, S., Gentschev, I., et al. 2000. Salmonella vaccines secreting measles virus epitopes induce protective immune responses against measles virus encephalitis. *Microbes Infect*, **2**, 1687–92.

Staats, H.F., Nichols, W.G. and Palker, T.J. 1996. Mucosal immunity to HIV-1: systemic and vaginal antibody responses after intranasal immunization with the HIV-1 C4/V3 peptide T1SP10 MN(A). *J Immunol*, **157**, 462–72.

Staczek, J., Gilleland, H.E. Jr, et al. 1998. A chimeric influenza virus expressing an epitope of outer membrane protein F of *Pseudomonas aeruginosa* affords protection against challenge with *P. aeruginosa* in a murine model of chronic pulmonary infection. *Infect Immun*, **66**, 3990–4.

Staczek, J., Bendahmane, M., et al. 2000. Immunization with a chimeric tobacco mosaic virus containing an epitope of outer membrane protein F of *Pseudomonas aeruginosa* provides protection against challenge with *P. aeruginosa*. *Vaccine*, **18**, 2266–74.

Stadler, B.M., Zurcher, A.W., et al. 1999. Mimotope and anti-idiotypic vaccines to induce an anti-IgE response. *Int Arch Allergy Immunol*, **118**, 119–21.

Steller, M.A., Gurski, K.J., et al. 1998. Cell-mediated immunological responses in cervical and vaginal cancer patients immunized with a lipidated epitope of human papillomavirus type 16 E7. *Clin Cancer Res*, **4**, 2103–9.

Stemmer, C., Quesnel, A., et al. 1999. Protection against lymphocytic choriomeningitis virus infection induced by a reduced peptide bond analogue of the H-2Db-restricted CD8(+) T cell epitope GP33. *J Biol Chem*, **274**, 5550–6.

Stevens, V.C., Powell, J.E., et al. 1981a. Antifertility effects of immunization of female baboons with C-terminal peptides of the beta-subunit of human chorionic gonadotropin. *Fertil Steril*, **36**, 98–105.

Stevens, V.C., Cinader, B., et al. 1981b. Preparation and formulation of an HCG anti-fertility vaccine: selection of adjuvant and vehicle. *Am J Reprod Immunol*, **6**, 315–21.

Steward, M.W. 2001. The development of a mimotope-based synthetic peptide vaccine against respiratory syncytial virus. *Biologicals*, **29**, 215–19.

Steward, M.W., Stanley, C.M. and Obeid, O.E. 1995. A mimotope from a solid-phase peptide library induces a measles virus-neutralizing and protective antibody response. *J Virol*, **69**, 7668–73.

Strohmaier, K., Franze, R. and Adam, K.H. 1982. Location and characterization of the antigenic portion of the FMDV immunizing protein. *J Gen Virol*, **59**, 295–306.

Subramanian, S., Karande, A.A. and Adiga, P.R. 2000. Immunocontraceptive potential of major antigenic determinants of chicken riboflavin carrier protein in the female rat. *Vaccine*, **19**, 1172–9.

Suhrbier, A. 2002. Polytope vaccines for the codelivery of multiple CD8 T-cell epitopes. *Expert Rev Vaccines*, **1**, 207–13.

Sun, D., Lafferty, M.J., et al. 1997. Domains within the *Vibrio cholerae* toxin coregulated pilin subunit that mediate bacterial colonization. *Gene*, **192**, 79–85.

Sundaram, R., Dakappagari, N.K. and Kaumaya, P.T. 2002. Synthetic peptides as cancer vaccines. *Biopolymers*, **66**, 200–16.

Taboga, O., Tami, C., et al. 1997. A large-scale evaluation of peptide vaccines against foot-and-mouth disease: lack of solid protection in cattle and isolation of escape mutants. *J Virol*, **71**, 2606–14.

Tallima, H., Montash, M., et al. 2003. Differences in immunogenicity and vaccine potential of peptides from *Schistosoma mansoni* glyceraldehyde 3-phosphate dehydrogenase. *Vaccine*, **21**, 3290–300.

Talwar, G.P. 1999. Vaccines and passive immunological approaches for the control of fertility and hormone-dependent cancers. *Immunol Rev*, **171**, 173–92.

Tam, J.P. 1988. Synthetic peptide vaccine design: synthesis and properties of a high-density multiple antigenic peptide system. *Proc Natl Acad Sci USA*, **85**, 5409–13.

Tam, J.P. and Lu, Y.A. 1989. Vaccine engineering: enhancement of immunogenicity of synthetic peptide vaccines related to hepatitis in chemically defined models consisting of T- and B-cell epitopes. *Proc Natl Acad Sci USA*, **86**, 9084–8.

Tam, J.P., Clavijo, P., et al. 1990. Incorporation of T and B epitopes of the circumsporozoite protein in a chemically defined synthetic vaccine against malaria. *J Exp Med*, **171**, 299–306.

Tarrab-Hazdai, R., Schechtman, D. and Arnon, R. 1998. Synthesis and characterization of a protective peptide-based vaccine against *Schistosoma mansoni*. *Infect Immun*, **66**, 4526–30.

Tendler, M., Brito, C.A., et al. 1996. A *Schistosoma mansoni* fatty acid-binding protein, Sm14, is the potential basis of a dual-purpose anti-helminth vaccine. *Proc Natl Acad Sci USA*, **93**, 269–73.

Theisen, D.M., Bouche, F.B., et al. 2000. Differential antigenicity of recombinant polyepitope-antigens based on loop- and helix-forming B and T cell epitopes. *J Immunol Methods*, **242**, 145–57.

Thurner, B., Haendle, I., et al. 1999. Vaccination with mage-3A1 peptide-pulsed mature, monocyte-derived dendritic cells expands specific cytotoxic T cells and induces regression of some metastases in advanced stage IV melanoma. *J Exp Med*, **190**, 1669–78.

Tindle, R.W., Fernando, G.J., et al. 1991. A 'public' T-helper epitope of the E7 transforming protein of human papillomavirus 16 provides cognate help for several E7 B-cell epitopes from cervical cancer-associated human papillomavirus genotypes. *Proc Natl Acad Sci USA*, **88**, 5887–91.

Tindle, R.W., Croft, S., et al. 1995. A vaccine conjugate of 'ISCAR' immunocarrier and peptide epitopes of the E7 cervical cancer-associated protein of human papillomavirus type 16 elicits specific Th1- and Th2-type responses in immunized mice in the absence of oil-based adjuvants. *Clin Exp Immunol*, **101**, 265–71.

Tjoa, B.A., Erickson, S.J., et al. 1997. Follow-up evaluation of prostate cancer patients infused with autologous dendritic cells pulsed with PSMA peptides. *Prostate*, **32**, 272–8.

Tjoa, B.A., Simmons, S.J., et al. 1999. Follow-up evaluation of a phase II prostate cancer vaccine trial. *Prostate*, **40**, 125–9.

Toes, R.E., Blom, R.J., et al. 1996a. Enhanced tumor outgrowth after peptide vaccination. Functional deletion of tumor-specific CTL induced by peptide vaccination can lead to the inability to reject tumors. *J Immunol*, **156**, 3911–18.

Toes, R.E., Offringa, R., et al. 1996b. Peptide vaccination can lead to enhanced tumor growth through specific T-cell tolerance induction. *Proc Natl Acad Sci USA*, **93**, 7855–60.

Toledo, A., Larralde, C., et al. 1999. Towards a *Taenia solium* cysticercosis vaccine: an epitope shared by *Taenia crassiceps* and *Taenia solium* protects mice against experimental cysticercosis. *Infect Immun*, **67**, 2522–30.

Toledo, A., Fragoso, G., et al. 2001. Two epitopes shared by *Taenia crassiceps* and *Taenia solium* confer protection against murine *T. crassiceps* cysticercosis along with a prominent T1 response. *Infect Immun*, **69**, 1766–73.

Topalian, S.L., Gonzales, M.I., et al. 1996. Melanoma-specific CD4+ T cells recognize nonmutated HLA-DR-restricted tyrosinase epitopes. *J Exp Med*, **183**, 1965–71.

Tourdot, S., Scardino, A., et al. 2000. A general strategy to enhance immunogenicity of low-affinity HLA-A2. 1-associated peptides: implication in the identification of cryptic tumor epitopes. *Eur J Immunol*, **30**, 3411–21.

Tsuji, M. and Zavala, F. 2001. Peptide-based subunit vaccines against pre-erythrocytic stages of malaria parasites. *Mol Immunol*, **38**, 433–42.

Urban, J.L. and Schreiber, H. 1992. Tumor antigens. *Annu Rev Immunol*, **10**, 617–44.

Valero, M.L., Camarero, J.A., et al. 2000. Native-like cyclic peptide models of a viral antigenic site: finding a balance between rigidity and flexibility. *J Mol Recognit*, **13**, 5–13.

Valero, M.V., Amador, L.R., et al. 1993. Vaccination with SPf66, a chemically synthesised vaccine, against *Plasmodium falciparum* malaria in Colombia. *Lancet*, **341**, 705–10.

Valero, M.V., Amador, R., et al. 1996. Evaluation of SPf66 malaria vaccine during a 22-month follow-up field trial in the Pacific coast of Colombia. *Vaccine*, **14**, 1466–70.

Valmori, D., Fonteneau, J.F., et al. 1998. Enhanced generation of specific tumor-reactive CTL in vitro by selected Melan-A/MART-1 immunodominant peptide analogues. *J Immunol*, **160**, 1750–8.

Van Driel, W.J., Ressing, M.E., et al. 1999. Vaccination with HPV16 peptides of patients with advanced cervical carcinoma: clinical evaluation of a phase I-II trial. *Eur J Cancer*, **35**, 946–52.

Van Regenmortel, M.H.V and Muller, S. (eds) 1999. *Synthetic peptides as antigens*. Amsterdam: Elsevier, 1–381.

Verjans, G.M., Janssen, R., et al. 1995. Intracellular processing and presentation of T cell epitopes, expressed by recombinant *Escherichia coli* and *Salmonella typhimurium*, to human T cells. *Eur J Immunol*, **25**, 405–10.

Vilar, M.M., Barrientos, F., et al. 2003. An experimental bivalent peptide vaccine against schistosomiasis and fascioliasis. *Vaccine*, **22**, 137–44.

Vitiello, A., Ishioka, G., et al. 1995. Development of a lipopeptide-based therapeutic vaccine to treat chronic HBV infection. I. Induction of a primary cytotoxic T lymphocyte response in humans. *J Clin Invest*, **95**, 341–9.

Wang, C.Y., Looney, D.J., et al. 1991. Long-term high-titer neutralizing activity induced by octameric synthetic HIV-1 antigen. *Science*, **254**, 285–8.

Wang, C.Y., Chang, T.Y., et al. 2001. Synthetic peptide-based vaccine and diagnostic system for effective control of FMD. *Biologicals*, **29**, 221–8.

Wang, C.Y., Chang, T.Y., et al. 2002a. Effective synthetic peptide vaccine for foot-and-mouth disease in swine. *Vaccine*, **20**, 2603–10.

Wang, C.Y., Shen, M., et al. 2002b. Synthetic AIDS vaccine by targeting HIV receptor. *Vaccine*, **21**, 89–97.

Wang, F., Bade, E., et al. 1999a. Phase I trial of a MART-1 peptide vaccine with incomplete Freund's adjuvant for resected high-risk melanoma. *Clin Cancer Res*, **5**, 2756–65.

Wang, R.F., Wang, X. and Rosenberg, S.A. 1999b. Identification of a novel major histocompatibility complex class II-restricted tumor antigen resulting from a chromosomal rearrangement recognized by CD4(+) T cells. *J Exp Med*, **189**, 1659–68.

Wang, T.T., Fellows, P.F., et al. 2004. Induction of opsonic antibodies to the gamma-D-glutamic acid capsule of *Bacillus anthracis* by immunization with a synthetic peptide-carrier protein conjugate. *FEMS Immunol Med Microbiol*, **40**, 231–7.

Weathington, N.M. and Blalock, J.E. 2003. Rational design of peptide vaccines for autoimmune disease: harnessing molecular recognition to fix a broken network. *Expert Rev Vaccines*, **2**, 61–73.

Webb, D.C. and Cripps, A.W. 2000. A P5 peptide that is homologous to peptide 10 of OprF from *Pseudomonas aeruginosa* enhances clearance of nontypeable *Haemophilus influenzae* from acutely infected rat lung in the absence of detectable peptide-specific antibody. *Infect Immun*, **68**, 377–81.

Weber, J., Sondak, V.K., et al. 2003. Granulocyte-macrophage-colony-stimulating factor added to a multipeptide vaccine for resected Stage II melanoma. *Cancer*, **97**, 186–200.

Weber, J.S., Hua, F.L., et al. 1999. A phase I trial of an HLA-A1 restricted MAGE-3 epitope peptide with incomplete Freund's adjuvant in patients with resected high-risk melanoma. *J Immunother*, **22**, 431–40.

Wee, E.G., Patel, S., et al. 2002. A DNA/MVA-based candidate human immunodeficiency virus vaccine for Kenya induces multi-specific T cell responses in rhesus macaques. *J Gen Virol*, **83**, 75–80.

Weiner, H.L., Lemere, C.A., et al. 2000. Nasal administration of amyloid-beta peptide decreases cerebral amyloid burden in a mouse model of Alzheimer's disease. *Ann Neurol*, **48**, 567–79.

Weller, R.O. and Nicoll, J.A. 2003. Cerebral amyloid angiopathy: pathogenesis and effects on the ageing and Alzheimer brain. *Neurol Res*, **25**, 611–16.

Westerink, M.A., Giardina, P.C., et al. 1995. Peptide mimicry of the meningococcal group C capsular polysaccharide. *Proc Natl Acad Sci USA*, **92**, 4021–5.

Westerink, M.A., Smithson, S.L., et al. 2001. Development and characterization of anti-idiotype-based peptide and DNA vaccines which mimic the capsular polysaccharide of Neisseria meningitidis serogroup C. *Int Rev Immunol*, **20**, 251–61.

Wheeler, C.M., Robertson, B.H., et al. 1986. Structure of the hepatitis A virion: peptide mapping of the capsid region. *J Virol*, **58**, 307–13.

Wiesmüller, K.H., Jung, G. and Hess, G. 1989. Novel low-molecular-weight synthetic vaccine against foot-and-mouth disease containing a potent B-cell and macrophage activator. *Vaccine*, **7**, 29–33.

Wiesmüller, K.H., Fleckenstein, B. and Jung, G. 2001. Peptide vaccines and peptide libraries. *Biol Chem*, **382**, 571–9.

Wimmer, E., Emini, E.A. and Jameson, B.A. 1984. Peptide priming of a poliovirus neutralizing antibody response. *Rev Infect Dis*, **6**, suppl 2, S505–9.

Wolowczuk, I., Auriault, C., et al. 1989. Protective immunity in mice vaccinated with the *Schistosoma mansoni* P-28-1 antigen. *J Immunol*, **142**, 1342–50.

Wu, J.Y., Wade, W.F. and Taylor, R.K. 2001. Evaluation of cholera vaccines formulated with toxin-coregulated pilin peptide plus polymer adjuvant in mice. *Infect Immun*, **69**, 7695–702.

Xiao, Y., Zhao, Y., et al. 2000. Epitope-vaccine induces high levels of ELDKWA-epitope-specific neutralizing antibody. *Immunol Invest*, **29**, 41–50.

Yamamoto, M., Briles, D.E., et al. 1998. A nontoxic adjuvant for mucosal immunity to pneumococcal surface protein A. *J Immunol*, **161**, 4115–21.

Yamshchikov, G.V., Barnd, D.L., et al. 2001. Evaluation of peptide vaccine immunogenicity in draining lymph nodes and peripheral blood of melanoma patients. *Int J Cancer*, **92**, 703–11.

Yang, C., Collins, W.E., et al. 1997. Induction of protective antibodies in Saimiri monkeys by immunization with a multiple antigen construct (MAC) containing the *Plasmodium vivax* circumsporozoite protein repeat region and a universal T helper epitope of tetanus toxin. *Vaccine*, **15**, 377–86.

Yang, C.C. and Chan, H.L. 1998. Neutralizing epitope mapping of six beta1-bungarotoxin monoclonal antibodies and its application in beta1-bungarotoxin peptide vaccine design. *Biochem J*, **330**, Pt 1, 497–503.

Yang, W., Jackson, D.C., et al. 2000. Multi-epitope schistosome vaccine candidates tested for protective immunogenicity in mice. *Vaccine*, **19**, 103–13.

Zaks, T.Z. and Rosenberg, S.A. 1998. Immunization with a peptide epitope (p369-377) from HER-2/neu leads to peptide-specific cytotoxic T lymphocytes that fail to recognize HER-2/neu+ tumors. *Cancer Res*, **58**, 4902–8.

Zarour, H.M., Storkus, W.J., et al. 2000. NY-ESO-1 encodes DRB1*0401-restricted epitopes recognized by melanoma-reactive CD4+ T cells. *Cancer Res*, **60**, 4946–52.

Zavala, F. and Chai, S. 1990. Protective anti-sporozoite antibodies induced by a chemically defined synthetic vaccine. *Immunol Lett*, **25**, 271–4.

Zavala, F., Tam, J.P., et al. 1985. Rationale for development of a synthetic vaccine against *Plasmodium falciparum* malaria. *Science*, **228**, 1436–40.

Zavala, F., Tam, J.P., et al. 1987. Synthetic peptide vaccine confers protection against murine malaria. *J Exp Med*, **166**, 1591–6.

Zeng, G., Wang, X., et al. 2001. CD4(+) T cell recognition of MHC class II-restricted epitopes from NY-ESO-1 presented by a prevalent HLA DP4 allele: association with NY-ESO-1 antibody production. *Proc Natl Acad Sci USA*, **98**, 3964–9.

Zeng, W., Ghosh, S., et al. 2001. Assembly of synthetic peptide vaccines by chemoselective ligation of epitopes: influence of different chemical linkages and epitope orientations on biological activity. *Vaccine*, **19**, 3843–52.

Zeng, X.Y., Turkstra, J.A., et al. 2001. Active immunization against gonadotrophin-releasing hormone in Chinese male pigs. *Reprod Domest Anim*, **36**, 101–5.

Zhang, A., Geisler, S.C., et al. 1999. A disulfide-bound HIV-1 V3 loop sequence on the surface of human rhinovirus 14 induces neutralizing responses against HIV-1. *Biol Chem*, **380**, 365–74.

Zhou, S.R. and Whitaker, J.N. 1996. Active immunization with complementary peptide PBM 9-1: preliminary evidence that it modulates experimental allergic encephalomyelitis in PL/J mice and Lewis rats. *J Neurosci Res*, **45**, 439–46.

Ziegler, D., Fournier, P., et al. 1996. Protection against measles virus encephalitis by monoclonal antibodies binding to a cystine loop domain of the H protein mimicked by peptides which are not recognized by maternal antibodies. *J Gen Virol*, **77**, 2479–89.

Zwaveling, S., Ferreira Mota, S.C., et al. 2002. Established human papillomavirus type 16-expressing tumors are effectively eradicated following vaccination with long peptides. *J Immunol*, **169**, 350–8.

43

Live vaccine carriers

GORDON DOUGAN, RICHARD J. ASPINALL, FRANCES BOWE AND LILJANA PETROVSKA

Since the first recognized vaccinations performed by Edward Jenner the use of live attenuated microorganisms as vaccine components has been a practical option. Live vaccines often offer the advantage over nonliving vaccines of enhanced immunogenicity. In the early days of vaccine development when investigators used essentially empirical approaches, live vaccines were often a favored practical route because there is no requirement for the identification of component protective antigens. Also, dead whole cells were often either reactogenic or nonprotective. Although live approaches were often useful for inducing immunity, old-style live vaccines ran the risk of reversion to virulence to the extent that, over the years, there were many accidents with their use. Over the past few decades our ability to manipulate microorganisms using genetic approaches has opened up the option of rational attenuation. This is the so-called designer approach to live vaccine development. Rational attenuation involves the identification and stable inactivation of genes in pathogens that normally contribute to pathogenesis in the host. By knocking out genes that are essential for virulence, but not for life, it is possible selectively to disable pathogens in terms of their ability to cause disease. Theoretically, combinations of attenuating mutations can be employed to optimize both immunogenicity and safety simultaneously. In practice this can be a difficult goal to achieve, particularly if optimization is first attempted in a model rather than the target host. An alternative to rational attenuation is the complete characterization (total sequence) of the genetic content of well-characterized attenuated vaccine strains. Examples here would include various attenuated viruses such as those derived from polio virus and vaccinia or even bacterial vaccine strains. This sequence information can be used as a platform to quality control vaccine lots or provide a basis for further genetic modifications of the vaccine strain.

It is clear from the above that we are now entering a new era of rational live vaccine development. The aim is to develop live vaccines that are safe (nonreverting and nonreactogenic) in both normal and compromised hosts and which are protective following the administration of single vaccine doses. A further attraction of live vaccination is that with some attenuated microorganisms there is the option of immunizing using alternative (intranasal, oral, rectal, etc.) routes of immunization that could avoid the use of needles while offering the potential of inducing local alongside systemic immune responses (see Chapter 40, New approaches to vaccine delivery).

Our enhanced ability to manipulate microorganisms genetically has opened up further attractive options for vaccine development. Using recombinant DNA approaches, it is now possible to introduce the genes for heterologous protective vaccine antigens into attenuated microorganisms where the foreign antigens can potentially be expressed as components of the normal proteosome of the host vector. The challenge here is to express the foreign antigen in a stable manner that does not compromise the inherent immunogenicity of the vaccine carrier. Taking this approach it is enticing to imagine the development of live vaccine strains which, in a single dose, can be used to immunize simultaneously against more than one pathogen. It might be feasible, for example, to immunize in a single vaccine shot against bacterial and viral infectious agents. In fact this goal has now been achieved on many occasions in model hosts such as the mouse (Chatfield et al. 1989), but this technology is proving more difficult to translate into practical immunization formulations for use in humans or target veterinary species (Mastroeni et al. 2001). Part of the problem is the major differences in the way that the immune systems of different hosts respond to vaccines. In addition, individual pathogen strains are often adapted to favor growth in a particular host. Thus, a formulation can be highly immunogenic in one host but poorly immunogenic even in a closely related species. This means that clinical studies can often be disappointing and we need to learn more about how to transfer technology from one species to another. In other words we need better immune correlates. Nevertheless, despite some early problems there is still a great deal of interest and effort in this area, which is the subject of this chapter.

LIVE VACCINES ARE INHERENTLY IMMUNOGENIC

By learning more about the way that the immune system recognizes infectious agents and discriminates between antigens from dangerous sources, such as pathogens from self, it should be possible to understand why live vaccines are immunogenic. Pathogens harbor or synthesize particular degenerate structures that are distinct to themselves and often not natural components of higher eukaryotic hosts. Examples of such molecules include lipopolysaccharide (LPS), flagellins, and double-stranded RNA (dsRNA). Mammalian cells have evolved a series of ligands and receptors that target these pathogen-specific structures. Perhaps the best characterized of these are the Toll receptors which recognize pathogen-associated molecular patterns (PAMP). Binding of the Toll pathway by pathogen components can lead to the activation of the innate immune system and, ultimately, to the amplification of acquired immunity. In fact we now know that many adjuvants act by activating the innate immune system via these types of pathways and that live vectors have inherent immunogenicity because they incorporate PAMPs.

As we move towards pure nonliving vaccines there is a tendency to remove PAMPs from vaccine formulations and consequently to reduce inherent immunogenicity. Adjuvants then have to be added back. We can take advantage of PAMPs for improving vaccine formulations. Even bacterial DNA has a signature that is distinct from eukaryotic DNA. Consequently, bacterial DNA is targeted by Toll-like receptor 9 (TLR9) in both mice (Hemmi et al. 2000) and humans (Takeshita et al. 2001). The technique of so-called DNA immunization (see Chapter 44, Naked DNA vaccines) has now been extensively studied since the first demonstration that intramuscular injection of bacterially derived plasmid DNA could result in the expression of an encoded protein (Wolff et al. 1990) capable of eliciting humoral immune responses (Tang et al. 1992), as well as priming antigen-specific cytotoxic T lymphocytes (CTL) (Ulmer et al. 1993). DNA vaccines are effective partly because of the immunostimulatory properties of unmethylated cytidine phosphate–guanosine (CpG) dinucleotide sequences that can upregulate expression of interleukins IL-12, IL-6, and interferon γ (IFN-γ) by macrophages and B cells as well as activating dendritic cells (DC) (Jakob et al. 1998). Immunostimulatory CpG motifs are either absent from eukaryotic DNA or modified. Simply cloning an active CpG site in the correct context into an existing DNA vaccine construct can markedly enhance its efficacy (Sato et al. 1996).

Clearly the combination of PAMPs associated with live vectors enhances immunogenicity but live vaccines are normally much more immunogenic than the equivalent dead microbes. Hence, the fact that live organisms colonize the host using the steps normally associated with infection also clearly enhances their immunogenic potential. Live microorganisms will target and colonize host cells, including immune cells, and antigens will be processed along natural intracellular pathways. It is extremely difficult to reproduce such patterns of immunostimulation and antigen processing using dead cell vaccines. Adjuvants are substances incorporated into vaccine formulations to accelerate, enhance, or prolong the specific immune response. Mechanisms of adjuvant action can include increasing the half-life of vaccine antigens in vivo, inducing the production of immunomodulatory cytokines or other immunomodulatory molecules, or improving vaccine delivery to antigen-presenting cells (APC) and enhancing antigen processing or presentation (Vogel 2000). In a sense, live immunization has the potential to meet all of these needs although microorganisms that target APCs and modify their activity could be particularly attractive.

EXAMPLES OF VIRAL AND BACTERIAL VECTORS

Various attenuated vaccine strains have been modified to present heterologous antigens to the immune system. These combined vaccines can be based on attenuated strains, which in their own right can be used as vaccines against a particular disease, e.g. *Salmonella enterica* serovar Typhi (*S. typhi*) strains that have been developed as human oral typhoid vaccines and have been exploited as carriers with the aim of extending the range of protection (Tacket et al. 2000b). In contrast vaccinia viruses, which are the basis of smallpox vaccines, have been exploited with more focus on their simple use as vectors, although the emphasis may change in the future now that smallpox vaccines are back on the agenda (Fauci 2002). Many different pathogens have been engineered as vectors for expression of polypeptides from other pathogens. A list of some of these is provided in Table 43.1 which is not comprehensive but includes some selected examples. The goal of the use of these vectors is to present foreign antigen to the immune system in the context of live vector and thereby develop broad immunity (humoral and cellular) to the corresponding pathogen from which the antigen is derived. The recombinant polypeptide is expressed and either transported to the host cell surface to stimulate antibody production or is broken down into peptides that are transported to the cell surface in the context of major histocompatibility complex (MHC) molecules, where they elicit cellular responses such as CTL responses. In other words, immunity to the heterologous antigen is enhanced through co-delivery with the vector. Clearly, the type of immunity induced will be greatly influenced by the choice of vector for delivery. Also, different antigens may be more suitable for delivery by one vector compared with another, e.g. many viral proteins cannot be easily expressed in a conformationally correct form in bacteria so viral vector delivery might be the best option in these cases. Alternately, *Salmonella* may be more attractive for delivery of an antigen from another enteric bacterium, particularly if mucosal targeting is desired. In this chapter, examples of representative vectored delivery systems are described but there is no attempt to cover all vectors.

Attenuated viral vectors

Attenuated viruses can be modified for use as vaccine carriers by inserting sequences encoding target antigens into their genome. A number of different viruses have been engineered as vectors for expression of 'foreign'

Table 43.1 *Examples of host/vector system*

Vector	Antigen	Reference
BCG	*Borrelia burgdorferi* OspA	Langermann et al. (1994a, 1994b)
	Toxoplasma gondii GRA1	Supply et al. (1999)
	Plasmodium yoelii (MSP-1)	Bruna-Romero et al. (2000)
	SIV Gag, Pol, Env, and Nef	Leung et al. (2000)
	Measles virus N protein	Zhu et al. (1997)
	Schistosoma mansoni Sm28GST	Kremer et al. (1996)
	HIV-1 V3	Kawahara et al. (2002)
	Schistosoma haematobium Sh28GST	Kremer et al. (1998)
	Pertussis toxin subunit S1	Abomoelak et al. (1999)
	Leishmania surface protease gp63	Connell et al. (1993)
Salmonella	*Helicobacter pylori* urease	Londono-Arcila et al. (2002)
	L1 papillomavirus	Revaz et al. (2001)
	Hepatitis B virus core	Schodel et al. (1996)
	Toxin hybrid	Barry et al. (1996)
	Plasmodium falciparum (NANP)	Ruiz-Perez et al. (2002)
	Pneumococcal PspA	Kang et al. (2002)
	Lassa virus nucleocapsid protein	Djavani et al. (2001)
	Tuberculosis ESAT-6	Mollenkopf et al. (2001)
	Leishmania mexicana gp63	Gonzalez et al. (1998)
	Pneumococcal surface protein A	Nayak et al. (1998)
Shigella	(HIV-1) gp120 DNA	Shata and Hone (2001)
	Measles virus DNA	Fennelly et al. (1999)
	HIV DNA	Vecino et al. (2002)
Yersinia	*Brucella abortus* P39 DNA	Al-Mariri et al. (2002)
Bordetella pertusis	*Schistosoma mansoni* Sm28GST	Mielcarek et al. (1998)
	Neiserria meningitidis TbpB	Coppens et al. (2001)
MVA/Vaccinia	SHIV-89.6P	Barouch et al. (2001)
	Herpes simplex virus-2 glycoprotein D	Meseda et al. (2002)
	Leishmania infantum P36/LACK	Gonzalo et al. (2001)
	Plasmodium yoelii (AdPyCS)	Bruna-Romero et al. (2000)
	Mycobacterium tuberculosis Ag85	Malin et al. (2000)
Adenovirus	*Mycobacterium tuberculosis* Mtb39	Lewinsohn et al. (2002)
	Foot-and-mouth disease virus	Grubman and Mason (2002)

For abbreviations see the text.

polypeptides from other pathogens. The goal is to present foreign antigen to the immune system in the context of the live vector, so that the immune system responds to the antigen as a live immunogen and thereby develop broader immunity (humoral and cellular) to the corresponding pathogen. One advantage of this approach is that it is possible to avoid administering viruses such as HIV which could be considered unsafe even in an attenuated form. Recombinant vaccinia and related poxviruses have attracted particular attention as possible vectors for immunization against both infectious disease agents and cancers (Wang et al. 1995). Other viral vectors that have received considerable attention are the adenoviruses, which have also been used extensively for delivering genes as gene therapy vectors (Chen et al. 1996). The advantages of viral vectors include the production of the inevitable cellular damage that occurs during viral infection. Cellular damage could generate danger signals that could be a basis for activating the innate immune system. Viruses also have the potential to directly infect APCs with subsequent processing of viral antigens via the class I pathway.

However, there are obviously potential disadvantages with the use of viruses, particularly with the use of vaccinia vectors where the presence of pre-existing immunity can dampen responses to the heterologous antigen, compromising homologous boosting approaches. In addition, because of our limited repertoire of antiviral agents, there are additional risks from potential enhanced vaccine-associated infection in the immunocompromised.

The prototype viral vaccine vector is vaccinia virus, an animal-derived poxvirus that was used in the immunization program that successfully eradicated smallpox. Poxviruses are among the largest viruses and are almost visible to the naked eye using conventional microscopy. They harbor relatively large genomes and encode a variety of immunomodulatory proteins that can regulate the immune response during infection and potentially immunization. Different vaccinia derivatives harbor distinct repertoires of immunomodulatory genes and differ in their potential to replicate in different mammalian hosts. Hence, it is possible to have both replication-proficient and replication-defective forms of poxvirus vectors. Fowlpoxvirus and canarypox viruses are also being developed as live vectors that can infect human cells, but not produce infectious viral progeny (Moss 1992), thus providing a mechanism for natural attenuation (Fries et al. 1996). This clearly has implications for both immunogenicity and safety.

Many different recombinant polypeptides have been expressed in vaccinia virus, and immunization of animals with such vectors can protect against the pathogen encoding the recombinant polypeptide (Moss 1992; see Table 43.1). This approach has become routine as an experimental system. Some of the recombinant vaccinia viruses, e.g. those expressing influenza virus hemagglutinin and type I herpesvirus glycoprotein D have been shown to be protective in mice against subsequent challenge with the corresponding virulent heterologous viruses (Bennink et al. 1984). Recombinant vaccinia virus immunization has also now been extended to several veterinary target species. However, live recombinant vectors that can replicate in vivo may not be considered sufficiently safe for widespread use as prophylactic vaccines in humans.

To increase the safety of the poxviruses as vaccine vectors, the replication-incompetent strains have been exploited. Modified vaccinia virus Ankara (MVA) is replication impaired in primary human cells (Blanchard et al. 1998) and has been proposed as an alternate safe vaccine for use in smallpox eradication programs. The genome of MVA has also been sequenced and harbors six large deletions resulting in a loss of 31 kb of the genome. Lost genes include those encoding receptors for IFN-γ, tumor necrosis factor α (TNFα), type I IFN, and CC chemokines (Blanchard et al. 1998). Although delivery by MVA can be used to enhanced immunogenicity often this approach alone is not sufficient to induce protection. The potency of MVA/vaccinia immunization can be further enhanced by adopting 'prime-boost' strategies. A particularly fruitful approach has been to use an initial DNA vaccine as a priming agent followed by a recombinant viral vector such as modified vaccinia as a boost (Ramshaw and Ramsay 2000). The ability to induce $CD8^+$ CTL responses can be greatly increased by combining DNA vaccines with attenuated live viral vectors encoding the same or similar antigens (Sutter and Moss 1992; Ramshaw and Ramsay 2000). This prime-boost strategy has been further enhanced by co-administering cytokines such as IL-12, IFN-γ, or granulocyte–macrophage colony-stimulating factor (GM-CSF) (Chow et al. 1998). In the murine malaria model, immunization with DNA or MVA vaccines alone did not induce complete protection against virulent challenge, whereas a heterologous prime-boost strategy of DNA priming followed by MVA boosting was highly effective at inducing $CD8^+$ T cells and conferred complete protection (Schneider et al. 1998). Similar success in enhancing immunogenicity has been obtained with immunization exploiting viral antigens (Degano et al. 1999) and strongly reactive antigen-specific $CD8^+$ CTL responses have been demonstrated in primate models of HIV infection (Allen et al. 2000). Alternate prime-boost strategies, involving initial immunization with DNA or viruses and boosting with the relevant heterologous protein, have generally been poor inducers of CTLs, with specific humoral responses being stronger (Excler and Plotkin 1997).

Clinical trials using the MVA-based approach are under way for several infectious diseases including malaria (Seder and Hill 2000) and there is much interest in determining whether prime-boost methods can enhance the cellular responses to tumor-associated antigens. Animal studies have already shown that heterologous boosting strategies can be useful in increasing the efficacy of recombinant DNA anti-cancer vaccines (Irvine et al. 1997) and early trials in humans appear promising (Bonnet et al. 2000; Oertli et al. 2002).

Many other viruses have been used as carriers of heterologous antigens in immunization experiments. One of the most spectacular projects has been the exploitation of the components of the yellow fever flavivirus genome as a platform for vaccines against several diseases including dengue (Guirakhoo et al. 2001). A yellow fever–dengue live chimeric vaccine has been taking into the clinic with excellent safety and immunogenicity profiles (Monath et al. 2002). This vaccine has the potential to be the first licensed recombinant viral carrier for humans. The use of some viruses such as polio virus as carriers is compromised to some extent by the relatively small capacity of the genomes to incorporate the genes for heterologous antigens but nevertheless some interesting progress has been made (Mandle et al. 2001). Adenoviruses have been extensively exploited as vectors for gene therapy and have also received attention as live vaccine components, particularly in prime-boost immunization (Gilbert et al. 2002). Adenoviruses have the potential to be used as mucosal targeting agents increasing their potential. Other viruses such as herpesviruses (Varghese and Rabkin 2002) have also been tested as experimental live carriers, resulting partly from their ability to infect nondividing cells, potential high expression levels and broad host-range.

Live attenuated bacteria as vaccine vectors

Various bacterial species have been studied for their ability to deliver heterologous antigens, including *Salmonella*, *Shigella* spp., *Escherichia coli*, and *Listeria* spp. (Shata et al. 2000). Bacteria as live vectors have the potential advantage over viruses in that their genomes are theoretically able to harbor many foreign genes, in contrast to viruses, which offer limited capacity to encapsulate foreign DNA. Recent advances in our understanding of the molecular pathogenesis of bacterial infections, particularly the roles of virulence genes and pathogenicity islands (Jones and Falkow 1996; Groisman and Ochman 1996) have encouraged the rational development of attenuated strains for use as vaccines (Levine et al. 1996). The ideal bacterial vaccine vector should retain enough infectivity to invade and target APCs, while eliciting an effective immune response with a minimum of reactogenicity (Raupach and Kaufmann 2001). The most common bacteria used as live vectors are members of the Enterobacteriaceae and the mycobacteria, particularly BCG. *Salmonella* Typhi has been the focus of the many efforts in terms of live vaccine development and clinical testing (Tacket et al. 2000a). *Shigella flexneri* has also been engineered to deliver different heterologous antigens. Interestingly, attenuated *S. flexneri* was used as a prototype strain to delivery antigens encoded on recombinant plasmids capable of driving antigen expression from eukaryotic promoters (as a combined live vector/nucleic acid vaccine) (Sizemore et al. 1995). *S. flexneri* are known to readily escape from intracellular vacuoles into the cell cytoplasm in vivo, possibly facilitating the transfer of DNA from the bacteria to the eukaryotic nucleus or transcription apparatus.

Salmonella as live vectors

Attenuated mutants of *S. enterica* have been extensively exploited for the delivery of heterologous antigens for immunization against bacteria, parasites, and viruses (Chatfield et al. 1989). Also, in recent years, these bacteria have been increasingly used in experimental models of anticancer immunization (Chabalgoity et al. 2002). In contrast to killed bacterial preparations, live attenuated *S. enterica* can induce cellular immune responses to bacterial and heterologous recombinant antigens (Hormaeche et al. 1995). *Salmonella* Typhi also offers the attraction of being deliverable via the mucosal route. After oral ingestion, attenuated *Salmonella* Typhi has the potential to invade or interact with Peyer's patch-associated M cells, enterocytes, macrophages, and DCs. Hence, the combination of mucosal delivery and immune targeting has encouraged research in this area.

Salmonella Typhi is a serovar of *S. enterica*. As *Salmonella* Typhi is human restricted much of the work associated with salmonella vaccine development has focused on *S. enterica* serovar Typhimurium (*Salmonella* Typhimurium) which is adapted to the mouse and consequently is much more convenient to study. By selecting the combination of attenuating mutations carefully, it is possible to design *S. enterica* derivatives with differing potential to replicate to some extent intracellularly or to disseminate to reticuloendothlial tissues in different hosts (Sirard et al. 1999). Thus, not only can the immunogenicity of the strain be modified, but the degree of dissemination in normal or immunocompromised individuals can theoretically be controlled. This has even been shown to be the case in humans where *Salmonella* Typhi *aro* mutants were able to disseminate, whereas similar *Salmonella* Typhi *aro*, *htrA* mutants were not detected in blood of human volunteers (Tacket et al. 1997). Many different attenuated derivatives of *S. enterica* have been constructed and characterized. Among the first defined mutant strains were the *aroA* auxotrophic derivatives of *Salmonella* Typhimurium which are defective in aromatic amino acid biosynthesis and dependent for growth on supplementation of aromatic compounds into their culture medium (Hoiseth and Stocker 1981). *Salmonella* Typhimurium *aroA* (and other single or combination *aro* mutants) retain immunogenicity and favor stimulation of a Th1 response in mice (Dunstan et al. 1998). After oral administration to mice, these salmonella derivatives invade APCs in the gut mucosa and are retained within endocytic vacuoles (Figure 43.1). The subsequent lack of their essential metabolic supplements induces many of the administered bacteria to die within 24–48 h, releasing their contents into the APCs. Compared with extracellular bacteria, antigens carried by *Salmonella* have the enhanced potential to be presented in association with MHC class I molecules by infected macrophages and DCs, clearly a desirable mechanism if protective $CD8^+$ T-cell responses are sought (Wick and Ljunggren 1999). However, it should be noted that repeated experiments have shown that *Salmonella* Typhimurium derivatives are less potent inducers of CTLs than many other adjuvants and delivery systems (Allsop et al. 1996). Nevertheless, the subsequent location of the recombinant antigens within the APCs may influence subsequent immunity. Interestingly some mutations, such as those in the *sifA* gene (Beuzon et al. 2000), increase the level of release of *Salmonella* Typhimurium from the vacuole in APCs and these mutations may have some potential for enhancing or modulating *Salmonella* Typhimurium-associated immune responses (Figure 43.1).

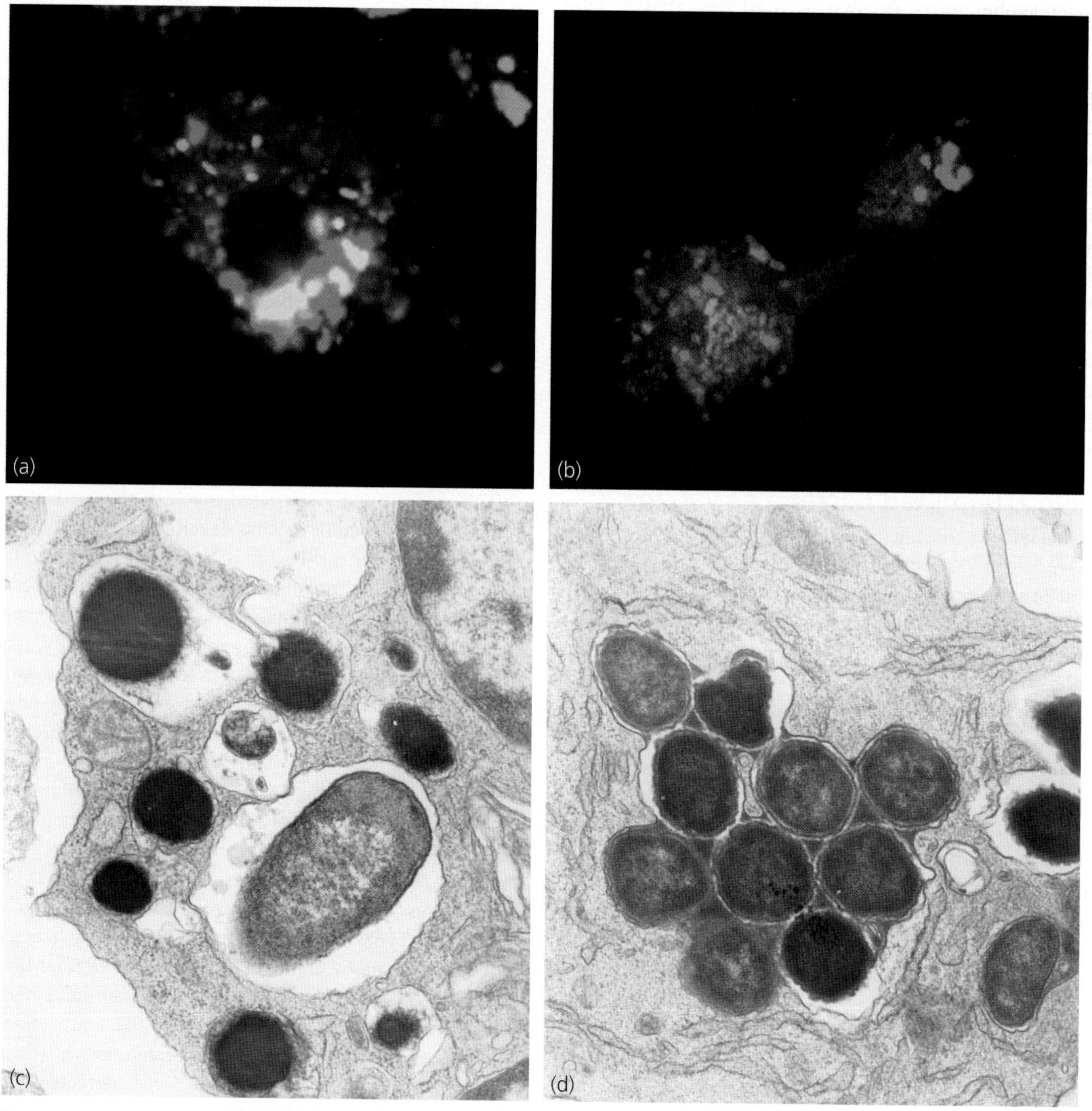

Figure 43.1 *Interaction of green fluorescent protein-positive* Salmonella *with dendritic cells cultured from the bone marrow of a mouse. Note that normal bacteria* **(a)** *interact with MHC molecules (yellow color) whereas sifA mutants* **(b)** *which escape the vacuole do so less well. The equivalent electron micrographs showing sifA mutants escaping the vacuole are shown in* **(c)** *(wild-type* Salmonella*) and* **(d)** *(sifA mutant* Salmonella*).*

The location or distribution of the expressed heterologous antigen within the *Salmonella* Typhimurium carrier cell may influence the subsequent immune response to the antigen. Although antigens expressed in the bacterial cytoplasm can be used to immunize and protect effectively, surface expression or secretion has the potential to enhance immunogenicity to some antigens (Strugnell et al. 1992). Antigen location within the bacterial cell may be critical for the induction of CTL responses which are often poor and efforts have been made to target antigen to or beyond the surface of the bacterial cell (Hess et al. 1996). The subsequent route for processing and presentation of MHC class I-associated salmonella antigens may also differ between APCs (Yrlid et al. 2000). Furthermore, because *Salmonella* Typhimurium invasion of macrophages can induce apoptosis (Monack et al. 1996), membrane 'blebs' containing bacterial antigens (and potentially plasmid DNA) may be taken up and processed by DCs via the MHC-I and -II pathways, resulting in activation of $CD4^+$ and $CD8^+$ T cells (Yrlid and Wick 2000).

The genes that encode heterologous antigens are often introduced into salmonella vaccine strains on plasmids. Plasmids that direct the expression of potentially toxic foreign proteins under the control of unregulated promoters can be rapidly lost from attenuated bacterial vector strains in vivo (Maskell et al. 1987). This gene loss can significantly reduce the level of the immune response to the heterologous antigen. To maintain stable antigen expression and thus enhance vaccine immunogenicity, growth-phase inducible promoters may be required (Dunstan et al. 1999; Marshall et al. 2000). Alternately, the stability of heterologous antigen expression may be enhanced by placing genes encoding heterologous antigens on the bacterial chromosome (Strugnell et al. 1990).

The intracellular life cycle of *Salmonella* also appears well suited to delivering expression plasmids as DNA vaccines. Indeed, many studies of bacterial to mammalian gene transfer have been carried out using *Salmonella* Typhimurium (Weiss and Chakraborty 2001). *Salmonella*-mediated mucosal DNA immunization was effectively demonstrated in mice using *Salmonella* Typhimurium to elicit the expression of ActA and listeriolysin from eukaryotic promoters, encoded on plasmids delivered to eukaryotic cells via these bacterial vectors. The development of protective CTL and antibody responses against the listeria-derived antigens was demonstrated after immunization with live *Salmonella*Typhimurium vectors (Darji et al. 1997). *Salmonella* Typhimurium was also successfully exploited as a vector to induce protection against a murine fibrosarcoma expressing β-galactosidase as a model tumor antigen using both eukaryotic and prokaryotic promoters to drive antigen expression (Paglia et al. 1998; Medina et al. 1999). Interestingly, in a mouse model of melanoma, attenuated *Salmonella* Typhimurium was used to deliver a DNA vaccine construct harboring the murine ubiquitin gene fused to minigenes encoding peptide epitopes gp100(25–33) and TRP-2(181–188). Immunized mice displayed protective anti-tumor immunity (Xiang et al. 2000). Similarly, transgenic mice expressing the tumor antigen carcinoembryonic antigen (CEA) had their peripheral tolerance broken by oral DNA immunization, with *Salmonella* Typhimurium, generating protection against CEA-expressing lung carcinoma cells (Niethammer et al. 2001).

Shigella

A great deal of effort has been made to generate different shigella derivatives for use as live oral vaccines against *Shigella*-associated dysentery. Despite many promising starts many candidate vaccines have floundered because of reactogenicity or poor immunogenicity in volunteers. Consequently, there are no licensed live shigella vaccines. *Shigella* has long been considered as a potential carrier of heterologous antigens. Early nonrecombinant experiments used hybrid genetic crosses between *Shigella* and the genomes of other enteric bacteria as possible extended-spectrum diarrhea vaccines. However, this approach ultimately proved unfruitful. As with *Salmonella*, *Shigella* spp. are also facultative intracellular bacteria but in comparison they have an enhanced ability to escape from the vacuole, become motile within the cytoplasm, and spread directly to adjacent cells (Sansonetti et al. 1986). A number of attenuated shigella mutants are available as experimental vaccines and these have been exploited (Karnell et al. 1995) to carry heterologous antigens (Noriega et al. 1996). An auxotrophic shigella mutant, dependent on supplementation with diaminopimelate (*dap*) for cell wall synthesis, was used for the first demonstration of functional DNA transfer from bacteria to mammalian cells (Sizemore et al. 1995). Since then, several studies have shown the induction of strong $CD8^+$ immune responses against viral antigens delivered as DNA vaccines by *Shigella* (Fennelly et al. 1999; Shata and Hone 2001). In a murine model of DNA immunization against HIV antigens, a *dap*-dependent shigella vector stimulated higher levels of IFN-γ-secreting $CD8^+$ cells compared with either *Salmonella* Typhimurium or *Salmonella* Typhi Ty21a (Vecino et al. 2002).

BCG

BCG is an attenuated live bacteria derived from a virulent *Mycobacterium bovis* by extensive laboratory propagation and is widely used for human and animal immunization. *Mycobacterium* spp. have the capacity to establish persistent infections and in vivo recombinant BCG may provide a continuous and prolonged stimulation of the cellular immune system. Both cellular and humoral immune responses against a number of foreign antigens delivered by BCG have been observed in mice and other species including primates such as the rhesus monkey (Leung et al. 2000). Some of the BCG-based heterologous vaccines have been demonstrated to elicit protection against the corresponding pathogen. BCG expressing the outer surface protein A (OspA) from *Borrelia bugdorferi* induced a long-term protective response after intranasal immunization. Highly sustained levels of anti-OspA and BCG-specific secretory IgA and serum IgG responses were observed (Langermann et al. 1994a, b). As BCG vaccine can be given at birth, without interfering with maternal neutralizing antibodies, the possibility of administering recombinant antigens against childhood diseases such as measles has also been explored in rhesus monkeys. Intranasal administration of recombinant BCG producing the measles virus N nucleoprotein provided protection against subsequent challenge with measles virus. Even though immunization did not prevent systemic infection, immunized monkeys showed a significant reduction of lung inflammation and reduced virus titers in lymph nodes. Nucleoprotein specific T-cell proliferative responses to the measles virus were detected in the absence of anti-N antibody response, suggesting T-cell prevention of virus-induced lung pathology (Zhu et al. 1997). Recombinant BCG vectors can induce humoral and cellular immune response to the major proteins of simian immunodeficiency virus (SIV) polypeptides Gag, Pol, Env, and Nef in rhesus monkeys. A single simultaneous inoculation of all four recombinants elicited SIV-specific IgA and IgG antibodies, as well as cellular immune responses, including CTL and helper T-cell proliferation (Leung et al. 2000). Live BCG secreting a carboxyl terminus of MSP-1 from *Plasmodium yoelii* induced more efficient protective immunity against plasmodium challenge, inducing MSP-1-specific antibodies and IFN-γ (Bruna-Romero et al. 2000).

Other bacterial vectors

Vaccines based on *Escherichia coli* vectors are at a relatively early stage of development. Investigators have concentrated on trying to maximize the targeting of antigens to macrophages and DCs. One approach has been to link heterologous protein expression to the α-haemolysin (HlyA) type I secretory system of uropathogenic *E. coli* to release antigens into the phagosome or cytosol of infected cells (Gentschev et al. 2002). An alternate method of increasing cytosolic antigen delivery (and therefore MHC-I presentation of antigen) is to enable *E. coli* itself to escape from the phagosome. This was demonstrated by transforming an attenuated auxotrophic *E. coli* mutant with a plasmid encoding the *hly* gene from *Listeria monocytogenes*, thereby producing the pore-forming listeriolysin and releasing bacteria and their carried antigens into the cytosol (Higgins et al. 1999). One potential problem with the use of *E. coli* for delivery is that these bacteria normally reside in the lumen of the intestine and consequently may be inherently less immunogenic than the invasive enteric bacteria. DNA delivery using modified *E. coli* strains has been achieved by adapting *E. coli* to express the *invasin* gene from *Yersinia pseudotuberculosis* to enhance the invasion rate of nonphagocytic cells and enhance vacuole escape through the hemolysin (Grillot-Courvalin et al. 1998). The bacterium *L. monocytogenes* can also efficiently escape from intracellular vacuoles, replicate in the cytosol, and spread directly to adjacent cells, albeit at a lower efficiency than *Shigella* (Tilney and Portnoy 1989; Chastellier and Berche 1994). *Listeria* has a powerful ability to stimulate MHC-I-restricted $CD8^+$ cytotoxic immunity to itself and, potentially, carried antigens (Schafer et al. 1992). A number of attenuated listeria mutants have been adapted for heterologous antigen delivery (Dietrich et al. 1998; Thompson et al. 1998). An attenuated listeria mutant was used to induce immune responses against influenza nucleoprotein serving as a model antigen in tumor cells, and protection was induced against challenge with tumor cells expressing this antigen (Pan et al. 1995). The antitumor response involved the stimulation of multiple effector pathways, including $CD4^+$ and $CD8^+$ T cells, DCs, NK cells, and several key cytokines including IL-2, IL-4, IL-12, IFN-γ, and TNF-α (Weiskirch et al. 2001). Attenuated listeria mutants have also been used in several other murine tumor models including immunization against a β-galactosidase-expressing fibrosarcoma (Paglia et al. 1997), E7 protein from the cervical cancer-associated human papillomavirus 16 (HPV16), and a lymphocytic choriomeningitis virus (LCMV) nucleoprotein-expressing glioma (Liau et al. 2002).

ENHANCED TARGETING OF THE IMMUNE SYSTEM WITH LIVE VECTORS

The mechanisms by which the immune system protects against disease are diverse and include the induction of neutralizing antibodies and the generation of T-cell responses, including T-helper cells and CTLs. Antibodies provide protection against some bacteria by recruiting bactericidal mechanisms and neutralizing bacterial toxins. Antibodies also play a pivotal role in protection against some viral diseases, such as polio, by virus neutralization mechanisms and preventing viruses from infecting cells. T cells contribute to resistance to bacterial and viral diseases by producing cytokines and inflammatory molecules, which can stimulate antibody, macrophage activation, and CTL responses. Several strategies have been developed specifically to enhance CTL immune responses and improve antigen presentation on MHC-I molecules. Viral and bacterial vectors that can actively invade cytoplasm of host cells have been introduced into APCs for targeted delivery to the immune system. Live vectors that have been used for this purpose include vaccinia, canarypox virus, adenoviruses, *L. monocytogenes*, *Salmonella*, and BCG.

Based on their biology and ability to present antigens, DCs have been described as 'nature's adjuvant' (Banchereau and Steinman 1998) and this is one of the key reasons why some recent therapeutic strategies have incorporated DCs as an effective way to target carrier vectors to immune sites (Banchereau et al. 2001). While in an immature, sentinel state, DCs effectively take up antigens, and subsequently process them through both the class I and II MHC pathways, a step required for the efficient activation of $CD8^+$ CTL and $CD4^+$ T-helper cells. After exposure to certain infectious agents, inflammatory cytokines, or activation of their CD40 receptors, DCs are mobilized from the site of antigen uptake to the peripheral lymphoid organs, where encounter with antigen-specific T cells can take place. During this migration, DCs mature into cells that are specialized in presenting high numbers of peptide/MHC complexes in a rich co-stimulatory context (Banchereau et al. 2000), necessary for activating T-cell responses. The level of maturation of the DCs may be of critical importance in the nature of immune response to DC-delivered antigen. Recent studies suggested that, in some cases, antigen-loaded mature DCs induce a protective (Th1) immune response, whereas antigen-loaded immature DCs may 'silence' the immune response via expansion of IL-10 producing T cells (Jonuleit et al. 2000; Dhodapkar et al. 2001). The expression pattern of different chemokines and chemokine receptors involved in homing dendritic cells to the lymphoid organs also varies throughout the dendritic cell maturation process (Sallusto et al. 1999). DCs have also been shown efficiently to take up and crosspresent antigens from apoptotic or necrotic cells in their vicinity (Albert et al. 1998). This hallmark has being used as a means to target antigens directly to DCs in vivo. Fas-mediated apoptotic cell death can lead to more efficient delivery of HIV-1 antigens to professional APCs, enhancing the priming of antigen-specific CTLs (Chattergoon et al. 2000).

As DCs are critical for the initiation of a cellular immune response, they have become a focus for many researchers to examine the possibility of inducing protective immunity against intracellular pathogens. DCs can efficiently internalize and process live intact bacteria for presentation by both MHC-I and -II molecules (Yrlid and Wick 2000). The bacterial carriers may function as a natural adjuvant, because they can induce the release of proinflammatory mediators such as TNFα, IFN-γ, and IL-12 and enhance early innate immunity, which creates an inflammatory context that probably induces dendritic maturation and antigen-presenting function (Banchereau and Steinman 1998). Bone marrow-derived DCs pulsed ex vivo with BCG and administered intratracheally can generate activated T cells and IFN-γ-secreting cells in the draining lymph nodes, leading to significant protection against aerosol *M. tuberculosis* infection (Demangel et al. 1999) in mice. Likewise, DCs pulsed ex vivo with killed *Chlamydia* and administered intravenously to mice-primed $CD4^+$ T cells provided protection against genital chlamydial infection equivalent to that obtained after immunization with live organisms. Besides intracellular pathogens, DCs have been successfully used as a vaccine against noninvasive, extracellular bacteria. DCs pulsed ex vivo with *Pseudomonas aeruginosa* and administered intravenously to mice induced a $CD4^+$ T-cell proliferative response and prolonged survival after a lethal pulmonary challenge with *P. aeruginosa* (Worgall et al. 2001). Homologous or even heterologous DCs pulsed with heat-killed *Bordetella pertussis* administered intravenously or intranasally to mice induced protective immune responses associated with strong *B. pertussis*-specific IgG and IgA responses in the lung (George-Chandy et al. 2001).

Monocyte-derived DCs infected with live viral replicative or nonreplicative vectors are being used as an effective means of delivery in HIV-1 vaccine development. Nonreplicative viruses are considered as a safer approach for immunizing human volunteers, but are typically weak immunogens, leading to efforts to target the vaccine to DCs for eliciting effective antivaccine immunity such as expanded CTL production. Immature monocytic DCs infected with vesicular stomatitis virus–pseudotyped HIV-1 presented antigens to $CD4^+$ and $CD8^+$ T cells from HIV-infected individuals as effectively as replicative pox vectors (Granelli-Piperno et al. 2000). Replicative recombinant canarypox (ALVAC) HIV-1 vaccines have been administered to >200 HIV-seronegative individuals with a good safety profile. However, this vaccine elicited antigen-specific CTLs in only a third of the volunteers, and therefore, in an attempt to engineer a better vaccine, monocytic DCs pulsed ex vivo with the vaccine are being considered as a possible delivery route for targeting immune cells. Preclinical data showing that the infected DCs are functional in T-cell stimulation assays performed using cells from HIV-1-infected individuals support the ongoing HIV vaccine trial that is comparing conventional vaccine delivery routes with ex vivo vaccine-loaded autologous DCs.

Adenoviruses are ubiquitous human pathogens and can be used efficiently to transduce a wide range of human cells and tissues, including DCs. With this property in mind, adenoviruses have been considered as a vaccine delivery vector, but a recent report by Roth et al. (2002) suggested that pre-existing antiviral immunity may limit the possibility of their clinical application.

INFLUENCE OF ROUTE OF DELIVERY

The route of delivery of a vaccine can have a major influence on the type of immunity induced. The mucosal route has been an attractive option for avoiding the use of needles and stimulating local mucosal immunity along with systemic responses. The oral route of vaccine administration is particularly attractive, but the ability to elicit mucosal immunity using nonliving antigens involves the use of high doses of antigens and repeated administrations. This results partly from the instability of the antigens in the proteolytic and acidic environment of the stomach, but is also caused by the poor natural mucosal immunogenicity of many antigens at mucosal surfaces. Clearly, live delivery offers potential advantages for oral immunization. However, there are still potential problems. There is potential strong ecological competition for live vectors with resident commensal flora in the gastrointestinal tract. Already problems have been encountered in moving some live vaccines from western volunteers into the field in less developed countries and the normal flora, together with immunological barriers, may be responsible. However, such barriers may not exist for all vaccine vectors.

An attractive alternative to oral delivery is potentially the intranasal route of immunization. Intranasal immunization has the advantage that the respiratory tract is less acidic and also less heavily colonized by microorganisms than the gastrointestinal tract. Less antigen is also needed to induce mucosal immunity via the intranasal compared with the oral route (Douce et al. 1999). Several vectors, including BCG and *Salmonella* Typhi, have been successfully used to deliver heterologous antigens via both the oral and intranasal routes (Langermann et al. 1994a; Hopkins et al. 1995; Corthesy-Theulaz et al. 1998; Kremer et al. 1998). Specific antigen presentation by the resident APCs in the respiratory and gastrointestinal tracts can differ compared with the systemic immune response. When recombinant BCG expressing an intracellular 28-kDa glutathione *S*-transferase from *Schistostoma haematobium* (Sh28GST) was administered intranasally to mice, the vaccine induced high levels of humoral systemic immune responses to Sh28GST, levels similar to responses after intraperitoneal administration of the recombinant antigen. Intranasal delivery also induced a mucosal IgA response against Sh28GST, which was not elicited after intraperitoneal administration. This anti-Sh28GST response was greatly enhanced after a second intranasal immunization that remained high for at least 12 weeks after the boost (Langermann et al. 1994b). When the related 28-kDa glutathione *S*-transferase from *Schistostoma mansoni* (Sm28GST) was administered intraperitoneally, this antigen also induced equivalent levels of anti-glutathione *S*-transferase (anti-GST) antibodies, but, surprisingly, intranasal administration of Sm28GST induced lower levels of anti-GST antibodies than Sh28GST (Kremer et al. 1996).

As transmission of HIV occurs predominantly via mucosal surfaces, immunization targeted to the induction of HIV-specific immune responses at mucosal sites could contain viral replication in the early stages of infection. Many studies have investigated the effect of the route of immunization with recombinant modified vaccinia viruses on eliciting mucosal immune responses. Mucosal immunization of macaques, with MVA-based vectors expressing the simian–human immunodeficiency virus (SHIV) strain SHIV89.6gp160, provided better protection than subcutaneous immunization, after intrarectal exposure to SHIV. These studies suggest that cutaneous or intramuscular immunization generated antigen-specific cells that may not travel to mucosal sites (Kantele et al. 1999; Cromwell et al. 2000). When highly attenuated poxvirus vectors (NYVAC) encoding the SIV_{makow} Gag, Pol, and Env products were introduced intramuscularly into macaques, they provided long-term virus containment after both intravenous or intracellular challenge with SIV_{mac251} (Benson et al. 1998). The results suggested that, even in the absence of priming at mucosal sites, systemic immunization can lead to virus control after mucosal challenge (Benson et al. 1998; Hel et al. 2001). However, a recent study, designed to explore the extent of the mucosal immune responses to a Gag-immunodominant SIV_{mac251} epitope after intramuscular, intranasal, or intracellular route of immunization with highly attenuated poxvirus NYVAC/SIV_{gpe} in macaques, concluded that immunization with live vector vaccine results in the elicitation of $CD8^+$ T-cell responses at mucosal sites even when the vaccine is delivered by nonmucosal routes (Stevceva et al. 2002).

CONCLUSIONS

Live vectors are receiving considerable attention as vehicles for the efficient delivery of antigens via several different routes of immunization and in a number of different target species including humans. In humans, some vectored delivery systems have proved to be less immunogenic than in model animals, e.g. *Salmonella* Typhimurium vectors in mice have consistently proved more efficient at heterologous antigen delivery compared with *Salmonella* Typhi in humans. This could be the result of inherent differences in the immunogenicity of *Salmonella* Typhimurium compared with *Salmonella* Typhi vectors (Hindle et al. 2002) but is equally likely to be the result of the use of poorly optimized expression systems used to drive the expression of the heterologous antigens in the clinical studies. The application of optimized delivery systems together with prime-boost approaches may prove fruitful for the development of a new generation of live human vaccines.

ACKNOWLEDGMENTS

This work was supported by grants from The Wellcome Trust, EU MUCIMM and the Digestive Disorders Foundation.

REFERENCES

Abomoelak, B., Huygen, K., et al. 1999. Humoral and cellular immune responses in mice immunized with recombinant *Mycobacterium bovis*

Bacillus Calmette-Guerin producing a pertussis toxin-tetanus toxin hybrid protein. *Infect Immun*, **67**, 5100–5.

Albert, M.L., Sauter, B. and Bhardwaj, N. 1998. Dendritic cells acquire antigen from apoptotic cells and induce class I-restricted CTLs. *Nature*, **392**, 86–9.

Allen, T.M., Vogel, T.U., et al. 2000. Induction of AIDS virus-specific CTL activity in fresh, unstimulated peripheral blood lymphocytes from rhesus macaques vaccinated with a DNA prime/modified vaccinia virus Ankara boost regimen. *J Immunol*, **164**, 4968–78.

Allsop, C.E.M., Plebanski, M., et al. 1996. Comparison of numerous delivery systems for the induction of cytotoxic T lymphocytes by immunisation. *Eur J Immunol*, **26**, 1951–9.

Al-Mariri, A., Tibor, A., et al. 2002. *Yersinia enterocolitica* as a vehicle for a naked DNA vaccine encoding *Brucella abortus* bacterioferritin or P39 antigen. *Infect Immun*, **70**, 1915–23.

Banchereau, J. and Steinman, R.M. 1998. Dendritic cells and the control of immunity. *Nature*, **92**, 245–52.

Banchereau, J., Briere, F., et al. 2000. Immunobiology of dendritic cells. *Annu Rev Immunol*, **18**, 767–811.

Banchereau, J., Schuler-Thurner, B., et al. 2001. Dendritic cells as vectors for therapy. *Cell*, **106**, 271–4.

Barouch, D.H., Santra, S., et al. 2001. Reduction of simian-human immunodeficiency virus, 89.6P viremia in rhesus monkeys by recombinant modified vaccinia virus Ankara vaccination. *J Virol*, **75**, 5151–8.

Barry, E.M., Gomez-Duarte, O., et al. 1996. Expression and immunogenicity of pertussis toxin S1 subunit-tetanus toxin fragment C fusions in *Salmonella typhi* vaccine strain CVD 908. *Infect Immun*, **64**, 4172–81.

Bennink, J.R., Yewdell, J.W., et al. 1984. Recombinant vaccinia virus primes and stimulates influenza haemagglutinin-specific cytotoxic T cells. *Nature*, **311**, 578–9.

Benson, J., Chougnet, C., et al. 1998. Recombinant vaccine-induced protection against the highly pathogenic simian immunodeficiency virus SIV(mac251): dependence on route of challenge exposure. *J Virol*, **72**, 4170–82.

Beuzon, C.R., Meresse, S., et al. 2000. Salmonella maintains the integrity of its intracellular vacuole through the action of SifA. *EMBO J*, **19**, 3235–49.

Blanchard, T.J., Alcami, A., et al. 1998. Modified vaccinia virus Ankara undergoes limited replication in human cells and lacks several immunomodulatory proteins: implications for use as a human vaccine. *J Gen Virol*, **79**, 1159–67.

Bonnet, M.C., Tartaglia, J., et al. 2000. Recombinant viruses as a tool for therapeutic vaccination against human cancers. *Immunol Lett*, **74**, 11–25.

Bruna-Romero, O., Gonzalez-Aseguinolaza, G., et al. 2000. Complete, long-lasting protection against malaria of mice primed and boosted with two distinct viral vectors expressing the same plasmodial antigen. *Proc Natl Acad Sci USA*, **98**, 11491–6.

Chabalgoity, J.A., Dougan, G., et al. 2002. Live bacteria as the basis for immunotherapies against cancer. *Expert Rev Vaccines*, **1**, 495–505.

Chastellier, C. and Berche, P. 1994. Fate of *Listeria monocytogenes* in murine macrophages: Evidence for simultaneous killing and survival of intracellular bacteria. *Infect Immun*, **62**, 543–53.

Chatfield, S.N., Strugnell, R.A. and Dougan, G. 1989. Live Salmonella as vaccines and carriers of foreign antigenic determinants. *Vaccine*, **7**, 495–8.

Chattergoon, M.A., Kim, J.J., et al. 2000. Targeted antigen delivery to antigen-presenting cells including dendritic cells by engineered Fas-mediated apoptosis. *Nat Biotechnol*, **18**, 974–9.

Chen, P.W., Wang, M., et al. 1996. Therapeutic antitumor response after immunization with a recombinant adenovirus encoding a model tumor-associated antigen. *J Immunol*, **156**, 224–31.

Chow, Y.H., Chiang, B.L., et al. 1998. Development of Th1 and Th2 populations and the nature of immune responses to hepatitis B virus DNA vaccines can be modulated by co-delivery of various cytokine genes. *J Immunol*, **160**, 1320–9.

Connell, N.D., Medina-Acosta, E., et al. 1993. Effective immunization against cutaneous leishmaniasis with recombinant bacille Calmette-Guerin expressing the *Leishmania* surface proteinase gp63. *Proc Natl Acad Sci USA*, **90**, 11473–7.

Coppens, I., Alonso, S., et al. 2001. Production of *Neisseria meningitidis* transferrin-binding protein B by recombinant *Bordetella pertussis*. *Infect Immun*, **69**, 5440–6.

Corthesy-Theulaz, I.E., Hopkins, S., et al. 1998. Mice are protected from *Helicobacter pylori* infection by nasal immunization with attenuated *Salmonella typhimurium* phoPc expressing urease A and B subunits. *Infect Immun*, **66**, 581–6.

Cromwell, M.A., Veazey, R.S., et al. 2000. Induction of mucosal homing virus-specific CD8(+) T lymphocytes by attenuated simian immunodeficiency virus. *J Virol*, **74**, 8762–6.

Darji, A., Guzman, C.A., et al. 1997. Oral somatic transgene vaccination using attenuated *S. typhimurium*. *Cell*, **91**, 765–75.

Degano, P., Schneider, J., et al. 1999. Gene gun intradermal DNA immunization followed by boosting with modified vaccinia virus Ankara: enhanced CD8+ T cell immunogenicity and protective efficacy in the influenza and malaria models. *Vaccine*, **18**, 623–32.

Demangel, C., Bean, A.G., et al. 1999. Protection against aerosol *Mycobacterium tuberculosis* infection using *Mycobacterium bovis* Bacillus Calmette Guerin-infected dendritic cells. *Eur J Immunol*, **29**, 1972–9.

Dhodapkar, M.V., Steinman, R.M., et al. 2001. Antigen-specific inhibition of effector T cell function in humans after injection of immature dendritic cells. *J Exp Med*, **193**, 233–8.

Dietrich, G., Bubert, A., et al. 1998. Delivery of antigen-encoding plasmid DNA into the cytosol of macrophages by attenuated suicide *Listeria monocytogenes*. *Nature Biotechnol*, **1**, 181–5.

Djavani, M., Yin, C., et al. 2001. Mucosal immunization with *Salmonella typhimurium* expressing Lassa virus nucleocapsid protein cross-protects mice from lethal challenge with lymphocytic choriomeningitis virus. *J Human Virol*, **4**, 103–8.

Douce, G., Giannella, V., et al. 1999. Genetically detoxified mutants of heat-labile toxin of *Escherichia coli* are able to act as oral adjuvants. *Infect Immun*, **67**, 4400–6.

Dunstan, S.J., Simmons, C.P. and Strugnell, R.A. 1998. Comparison of the abilities of different attenuated *Salmonella typhimurium* strains to elicit humoral immune responses against a heterologous antigen. *Infect Immun*, **66**, 732–40.

Dunstan, S.J., Simmons, C.P. and Strugnell, R.A. 1999. Use of in vivo-regulated promoters to deliver antigens from attenuated *Salmonella enterica* var. Typhimurium. *Infect Immun*, **67**, 5133–41.

Excler, J.L. and Plotkin, S. 1997. The prime-boost concept applied to HIV preventive vaccines. *AIDS*, **11**, Suppl A, S127–37.

Fauci, A.S. 2002. Smallpox vaccination policy – the need for dialogue. *N Engl J Med*, **346**, 1319–20.

Fennelly, G.J., Khan, S.A., et al. 1999. Mucosal DNA vaccine immunization against measles with a highly attenuated *Shigella flexneri* vector. *J Immunol*, **162**, 1603–10.

Fries, L.F., Tartaglia, J., et al. 1996. Human safety and immunogenicity of a canarypox-rabies glycoprotein recombinant vaccine: an alternative poxvirus vector system. *Vaccine*, **14**, 428–34.

Gentschev, I., Dietrich, G. and Goebel, W. 2002. The *Escherichia coli* alpha-hemolysin secretion system and its use in vaccine development. *Trends Microbiol*, **10**, 39–45.

George-Chandy, A., Mielcarek, N., et al. 2001. Vaccination with *Bordetella pertussis*-pulsed autologous or heterologous dendritic cells induces a mucosal antibody response in vivo and protects against infection. *Infect Immun*, **69**, 4120–4.

Gilbert, S.C., Schneider, J., et al. 2002. Enhanced CD8 T cell immunogenicity and protective efficacy in a mouse malaria model using a recombinant adenoviral vaccine in heterologous prime-boost immunisation regimes. *Vaccine*, **20**, 1039–45.

Gonzalez, C.R., Noriega, F.R., et al. 1998. Immunogenicity of a *Salmonella typhi* CVD 908 candidate vaccine strain expressing the major surface protein gp63 of *Leishmania mexicana*. *Vaccine*, **16**, 1043–52.

Gonzalo, R.M., Rodriguez, J.R., et al. 2001. Protective immune response against cutaneous leishmaniasis by prime/booster immunization regimens with vaccinia virus recombinants expressing *Leishmania infantum* p36/LACK and IL-12 in combination with purified p36. *Microbes Infect*, **3**, 701–11.

Granelli-Piperno, A., Zhong, L., et al. 2000. Dendritic cells, infected with vesicular stomatitis virus-pseudotyped HIV-1, present viral antigens to CD4+ and CD8+ T cells from HIV-1-infected individuals. *J Immunol*, **165**, 6620–6.

Grillot-Courvalin, C., Goussard, S., et al. 1998. Functional gene transfer from intracellular bacteria to mammalian cells. *Nature Biotechnol*, **16**, 862–6.

Groisman, E.A. and Ochman, H. 1996. Pathogenicity islands: bacterial evolution in quantum leaps. *Cell*, **87**, 791–4.

Grubman, M.J. and Mason, P.W. 2002. Prospects, including time-frames, for improved foot and mouth disease vaccines. *Rev Sci Technol*, **21**, 589–600.

Guirakhoo, F., Arroyo, J., et al. 2001. Construction, safety, and immunogenicity in nonhuman primates of a chimeric yellow fever-dengue virus tetravalent vaccine. *J Virol*, **75**, 7290–304.

Hel, Z., Tsai, W.P., et al. 2001. Potentiation of simian immunodeficiency virus (SIV)-specific CD4(+) and CD8(+) T cell responses by a DNA-SIV and NYVAC-SIV prime/boost regimen. *J Immunol*, **167**, 7180–91.

Hemmi, H., Takeuchi, O., et al. 2000. A Toll-like receptor recognizes bacterial DNA. *Nature*, **408**, 740–5.

Hess, J., Gentschev, I., et al. 1996. Superior efficacy of secreted over somatic antigen display in recombinant *Salmonella* vaccine induced protection against listeriosis. *Proc Natl Acad Sci USA*, **93**, 1458–63.

Higgins, D.E., Shastri, N. and Portnoy, D.A. 1999. Delivery of protein to the cytosol of macrophages using *Escherichia coli* K-12. *Mol Microbiol*, **31**, 1631–41.

Hindle, Z., Chatfield, S.N., et al. 2002. Characterization of *Salmonella enterica* derivatives harboring defined *aroC* and Salmonella pathogenicity Island 2 type III secretion system (ssaV) mutations by immunization of healthy volunteers. *Infect Immun*, **70**, 3457–67.

Hoiseth, S.K. and Stocker, B.A.D. 1981. Aromatic-dependent *Salmonella typhimurium* are non-virulent and effective as live vaccines. *Nature*, **29**, 238–9.

Hopkins, S., Kraehenbuhl, J.P., et al. 1995. Recombinant *Salmonella typhimurium* vaccine induces local immunity by four different routes of immunization. *Infect Immun*, **63**, 3279–86.

Hormaeche, C.E., Khan, C.M.A., et al. 1995. Salmonella vaccines: mechanisms of immunity and their use as carriers of recombinant antigens. In: Ala'Aldeen, D.A.A. and Hormaeche, C.E. (eds), *Molecular and clinical aspects of bacterial vaccine development*. Chichester: Wiley & Sons.

Irvine, K.R., Chamberlain, R.S., et al. 1997. Enhancing efficacy of recombinant anticancer vaccines with prime/boost regimens that use two different vectors. *J Natl Cancer Instit*, **89**, 1595–601.

Jakob, T., Walker, P.S., et al. 1998. Activation of cutaneous dendritic cells by CpG-containing oligodeoxynucleotides: a role for dendritic cells in the augmentation of Th1 responses by immunostimulatory DNA. *J Immunol*, **161**, 3042–9.

Jones, B.D. and Falkow, S. 1996. Salmonellosis: host immune responses and bacterial virulence determinants. *Annu Rev Immunol*, **14**, 533–61.

Jonuleit, H., Schmitt, E., et al. 2000. Induction of interleukin 10-producing, non-proliferating CD4(+) T cells with regulatory properties by repetitive stimulation with allogeneic immature human dendritic cells. *J Exp Med*, **192**, 1213–22.

Kang, H.Y., Srinivasan, J. and Curtiss 3rd, R. 2002. Immune responses to recombinant pneumococcal PspA antigen delivered by live attenuated *Salmonella enterica* serovar typhimurium vaccine. *Infect Immun*, **70**, 1739–49.

Kantele, A., Zivny, J., et al. 1999. Differential homing commitments of antigen-specific T cells after oral or parenteral immunization in humans. *J Immunol*, **162**, 5173–7.

Karnell, A., Li, A., et al. 1995. Safety and immunogenicity study of the auxotrophic *Shigella flexneri* 2a vaccine SFL1070 with a deleted *aroD* gene in adult Swedish volunteers. *Vaccine*, **13**, 88–99.

Kawahara, M., Hashimoto, A., et al. 2002. Oral recombinant *Mycobacterium bovis* Bacillus Calmette-Guerin Expressing HIV-1 antigens as a freeze-dried vaccine induces long-term, HIV-specific mucosal and systemic immunity. *Clin Immunol*, **105**, 326–31.

Kremer, L., Riveau, G., et al. 1996. Neutralizing antibody responses elicited in mice immunized with recombinant bacillus Calmette-Guerin producing the *Schistosoma mansoni* glutathione *S*-transferase. *J Immunol*, **156**, 4309–17.

Kremer, L., Dupre, L., et al. 1998. Systemic and mucosal immune responses after intranasal administration of recombinant *Mycobacterium bovis* bacillus Calmette-Guerin expressing glutathione S-transferase from *Schistosoma haematobium*. *Infect Immun*, **66**, 5669–76.

Langermann, S., Palaszynski, S., et al. 1994a. Systemic and mucosal immunity induced by BCG vector expressing outer-surface protein A of *Borrelia burgdorferi*. *Nature*, **372**, 552–5.

Langermann, S., Palaszynski, S.R., et al. 1994b. Protective humoral response against pneumococcal infection in mice elicited by recombinant bacille Calmette-Guerin vaccines expressing pneumococcal surface protein A. *J Exp Med*, **180**, 2277–86.

Leung, N.J., Aldovini, A., et al. 2000. The kinetics of specific immune responses in rhesus monkeys inoculated with live recombinant BCG expressing SIV Gag, Pol, Env and Nef proteins. *Virology*, **268**, 94–103.

Levine, M.M., Galen, J., et al. 1996. Attenuated *Salmonella* as live oral vaccines against typhoid fever and as live vectors. *J Biotechnol*, **44**, 193–6.

Lewinsohn, D.A., Lines, R.A. and Lewinsohn, D.M. 2002. Human dendritic cells presenting adenovirally expressed antigen elicit *Mycobacterium tuberculosis*-specific CD8+ T cells. *Am J Respir Crit Care Med*, **166**, 843–8.

Liau, L.M., Jensen, E.R., et al. 2002. Tumor immunity within the central nervous system stimulated by recombinant *Listeria monocytogenes* vaccination. *Cancer Res*, **62**, 2287–93.

Londono-Arcila, P., Freeman, D., et al. 2002. Attenuated *Salmonella enterica* serovar *Typhi* expressing urease effectively immunizes mice against *Helicobacter pylori* challenge as part of a heterologous mucosal priming-parenteral boosting vaccination regimen. *Infect Immun*, **70**, 5096–106.

Malin, A.S., Huygen, K., et al. 2000. Vaccinia expression of *Mycobacterium tuberculosis*-secreted proteins: tissue plasminogen activator signal sequence enhances expression and immunogenicity of *M. tuberculosis* Ag85. *Microbes Infect*, **2**, 1677–85.

Mandle, S., Hix, L. and Andino, R. 2001. Pre-existing immunity to poliovirus does not impair the efficacy of recombinant poliovirus vaccine vectors. *J Virol*, **75**, 622–7.

Marshall, D., Fowler, R., et al. 2000. Use of the stationary phase inducible promoters, spv and dps, to drive heterologous antigen expression in *Salmonella* vaccine strains. *Vaccine*, **18**, 1298–306.

Maskell, D.J., Sweeney, K.J., et al. 1987. *Salmonella typhimurium* aroA mutants as carriers of the *Escherichia coli* heat-labile enterotoxin B subunit to the murine secretory and systemic immune systems. *Microb Pathogen*, **2**, 211–21.

Mastroeni, P., Chabalgoity, J.A., et al. 2001. Salmonella: immune responses and vaccines. *Vet J*, **161**, 132–64.

Medina, E., Guzman, C.A., et al. 1999. Salmonella vaccine carrier strains: effective delivery system to trigger anti-tumor immunity by oral route. *Eur J Immunol*, **29**, 693–9.

Meseda, C.A., Elkins, K.L., et al. 2002. Prime-boost immunization with DNA and modified vaccinia virus ankara vectors expressing herpes simplex virus-2 glycoprotein D elicits greater specific antibody and cytokine responses than DNA vaccine alone. *J Infect Dis*, **186**, 1065–73.

Mielcarek, N., Riveau, G., et al. 1998. Homologous and heterologous protection after single intranasal administration of live attenuated recombinant *Bordetella pertussis*. *Nature Biotechnol*, **16**, 454–7.

Mollenkopf, H.J., Groine-Triebkorn, D., et al. 2001. Protective efficacy against tuberculosis of ESAT-6 secreted by a live *Salmonella typhimurium* vaccine carrier strain and expressed by naked DNA. *Vaccine*, **19**, 4028–35.

Monack, D.M., Raupach, B., et al. 1996. *Salmonella typhimurium* invasion induces apoptosis in infected macrophages. *Proc Natl Acad Sci USA*, **93**, 9833–8.

Monath, T.P., McCarthy, K., et al. 2002. Clinical proof of principle for ChimeriVax: recombinant live attenuated vaccines against flavivirus infections. *Vaccine*, **20**, 1004–18.

Moss, B. 1992. Vaccinia virus vectors. *Biotechnology*, **20**, 345–62.

Nayak, A.R., Tinge, S.A., et al. 1998. A live recombinant avirulent oral Salmonella vaccine expressing pneumococcal surface protein A induces protective responses against *Streptococcus pneumoniae*. *Infect Immun*, **66**, 3744–51.

Niethammer, A.G., Primus, F.J., et al. 2001. An oral DNA vaccine against human carcinoembryonic antigen (CEA) prevents growth and dissemination of Lewis lung carcinoma in CEA transgenic mice. *Vaccine*, **20**, 421–9.

Noriega, F.R., Losonsky, G., et al. 1996. Further characterization of delta *aroA* delta *virG Shigella flexneri* 2a strain CVD 1203 as a mucosal *Shigella* vaccine and as a live-vector vaccine for delivering antigens of enterotoxigenic *Escherichia coli*. *Infect Immun*, **64**, 23–7.

Oertli, D., Marti, W.R., et al. 2002. Rapid induction of specific cytotoxic T lymphocytes against melanoma-associated antigens by a recombinant vaccinia virus vector expressing multiple immunodominant epitopes and costimulatory molecules in vivo. *Hum Gene Ther*, **13**, 569–75.

Paglia, P., Arioli, I., et al. 1997. The defined attenuated *Listeria monocytogenes* delta mp12 mutant is an effective oral vaccine carrier to trigger a long-lasting immune response against a mouse fibrosarcoma. *Eur J Immunol*, **27**, 1570–5.

Paglia, P., Medina, E., et al. 1998. Gene transfer in dendritic cells, induced by oral DNA vaccination with *Salmonella typhimurium*, results in protective immunity against a murine fibrosarcoma. *Blood*, **92**, 3172–6.

Pan, Z.K., Ikonomidis, G., et al. 1995. A recombinant *Listeria monocytogenes* vaccine expressing a model tumour antigen protects mice against lethal tumour cell challenge and causes regression of established tumours. *Nat Med*, **1**, 471–7.

Ramshaw, I.A. and Ramsay, A.J. 2000. The prime-boost strategy: exciting prospects for improved vaccination. *Immunol Today*, **21**, 163–5.

Raupach, B. and Kaufmann, S.H. 2001. Bacterial virulence, proinflammatory cytokines and host immunity: how to choose the appropriate Salmonella vaccine strain? *Microbes Infect*, **3**, 1261–9.

Revaz, V., Benyacoub, J., et al. 2001. Mucosal vaccination with a recombinant *Salmonella typhimurium* expressing human papillomavirus type 16(HPV16) L1 virus-like particles (VLPs) or HPV16 VLPs purified from insect cells inhibits the growth of HPV16-expressing tumor cells in mice. *Virology*, **279**, 354–60.

Roth, M.D., Cheng, Q., et al. 2002. Helper-dependent adenoviral vectors efficiently express transgenes in human dendritic cells but still stimulate antiviral immune responses. *J Immunol*, **169**, 4651–6.

Ruiz-Perez, F., Leon-Kempis, R., et al. 2002. Expression of the *Plasmodium falciparum* immunodominant epitope (NANP)(4) on the surface of *Salmonella enterica* using the autotransporter MisL. *Infect Immun*, **70**, 3611–20.

Sallusto, F., Palermo, B., et al. 1999. Distinct patterns and kinetics of chemokine production regulate dendritic cell function. *Eur J Immunol*, **29**, 1617–25.

Sansonetti, P.J., Ryter, A. and Clerc, P. 1986. Multiplication of *Shigella flexneri* within HeLa cells: lysis of the phagocytic vacuole and plasmid-mediated contact haemolysis. *Infect Immun*, **51**, 461–9.

Sato, Y., Roman, M., et al. 1996. Immunostimulatory DNA sequences necessary for effective intradermal gene immunization. *Science*, **273**, 352–4.

Schafer, R., Portnoy, D.A., et al. 1992. Induction of a cellular immune response to a foreign antigen by a recombinant *Listeria monocytogenes* vaccine. *J Immunol*, **149**, 53–9.

Schneider, J., Gilbert, S.C., et al. 1998. Enhanced immunogenicity for CD8+ T cell induction and complete protective efficacy of malaria DNA vaccination by boosting with modified vaccinia virus Ankara. *Nat Med*, **4**, 397–402.

Schodel, F., Kelly, S., et al. 1996. Hybrid hepatitis B virus core antigen as a vaccine carrier moiety. II. Expression in avirulent *Salmonella* spp. for mucosal immunization. *Adv Exp Med Biol*, **397**, 15–21.

Seder, R.A. and Hill, A.V.S. 2000. Vaccines against intracellular infections requiring cellular immunity. *Nature*, **406**, 793–8.

Shata, M.T. and Hone, D.M. 2001. Vaccination with a *Shigella* DNA vaccine vector induces antigen-specific CD8(+) T cells and antiviral protective immunity. *J Virol*, **75**, 9665–70.

Shata, M.T., Stevceva, L., et al. 2000. Recent advances with recombinant bacterial vaccine vectors. *Mol Med Today*, **6**, 66–71.

Sirard, J.C., Niedergang, F. and Kraehenbuhl, J.P. 1999. Live attenuated *Salmonella*: a paradigm of mucosal vaccines. *Immunol Rev*, **171**, 5–26.

Sizemore, D.R., Branstrom, A.A. and Sadoff, J.C. 1995. Attenuated *Shigella* as a DNA delivery vehicle for DNA-mediated immunization. *Science*, **270**, 299–302.

Stevceva, L., Alvarez, X., et al. 2002. Both mucosal and systemic routes of immunization with the live, attenuated NYVAC/simian immunodeficiency virus SIV(gpe) recombinant vaccine result in gag-specific CD8(+) T-cell responses in mucosal tissues of macaques. *J Virol*, **76**, 11659–76.

Strugnell, R.A., Maskell, D., et al. 1990. Stable expression of foreign antigens from the chromosome of *Salmonella typhimurium* vaccine strains. *Gene*, **88**, 57–63.

Strugnell, R., Dougan, G., et al. 1992. Characterisation of a *Salmonella typhimurium aro* vaccine strain expressing the P. 69 antigen of *Bordetella pertussis*. *Infect Immun*, **60**, 3994–4002.

Supply, P., Sutton, P., et al. 1999. Immunogenicity of recombinant BCG producing the GRA1 antigen from *Toxoplasma gondii*. *Vaccine*, **17**, 705–14.

Sutter, G. and Moss, B. 1992. Nonreplicating vaccinia vector efficiently expresses recombinant genes. *Proc Natl Acad Sci USA*, **89**, 10847–51.

Tacket, C.O., Sztein, M.B., et al. 1997. Safety and immune response in humans of a live oral *Salmonella typhi* vaccine strain deleted in *htrA* and *aroC*, *aroD* and demonstration in mice of their use as vaccine vectors. *Infect Immun*, **65**, 452–6.

Tacket, C.O., Galen, J., et al. 2000a. Safety and immune responses to attenuated *Salmonella enterica* serovar *Typhi* oral live vector vaccines expressing tetanus toxin fragment C. *Clin Immunol*, **97**, 146–53.

Tacket, C.O., Sztein, M.B., et al. 2000b. Phase 2 clinical trial of attenuated *Salmonella typhi* oral live vector vaccine CVD908-htrA in U.S. volunteers. *Infect Immun*, **68**, 1196–201.

Takeshita, F., Leifer, C.A., et al. 2001. Cutting edge: Role of Toll-like receptor 9 in CpG DNA-induced activation of human cells. *J Immunol*, **167**, 3555–8.

Tang, D.C., DeVit, M. and Johnston, S.A. 1992. Genetic immunization is a simple method for eliciting an immune response. *Nature*, **356**, 152–4.

Thompson, R.J., Bouwer, H.G., et al. 1998. Pathogenicity and immunogenicity of a *Listeria monocytogenes* strain that requires D-alanine for growth. *Infect Immun*, **66**, 3552–61.

Tilney, L.G. and Portnoy, D.A. 1989. Actin filaments and the growth, movement, and spread of the intracellular parasite, *Listeria monocytogenes*. *J Cell Biol*, **109**, 1597–608.

Ulmer, J.B., Donnelly, J.J., et al. 1993. Heterologous protection against influenza by injection of DNA encoding a viral protein. *Science*, **259**, 1745–9.

Varghese, S. and Rabkin, S.D. 2002. Oncolytic herpes simplex virus vectors for cancer virotherapy. *Cancer Gene Therapy*, **9**, 967–78.

Vecino, W.H., Morin, P.M., et al. 2002. Mucosal DNA vaccination with highly attenuated *Shigella* is superior to attenuated *Salmonella* and comparable to intramuscular DNA vaccination for T cells against HIV. *Immunol Lett*, **82**, 197–204.

Vogel, F.R. 2000. Improving vaccine performance with adjuvants. *Clin Infect Dis*, **30**, Suppl 3, S266–70.

Wang, M., Bronte, V., et al. 1995. Active immunotherapy of cancer with a non-replicating recombinant fowlpox virus encoding a model tumor-associated antigen. *J Immunol*, **154**, 4685–92.

Weiskirch, L.M., Pan, Z.K. and Paterson, Y. 2001. The tumor recall response of antitumor immunity primed by a live, recombinant *Listeria monocytogenes* vaccine comprises multiple effector mechanisms. *Clin Immunol*, **98**, 346–57.

Weiss, S. and Chakraborty, T. 2001. Transfer of eukaryotic expression plasmids to mammalian host cells by bacterial carriers. *Curr Opin Biotechnol*, **12**, 467–72.

Wick, M.-J. and Ljunggren, H.G. 1999. Processing of bacterial antigens for peptide presentation on MHC class I molecules. *Immunol Rev*, **172**, 153–62.

Wolff, J.A., Malone, R.W., et al. 1990. Direct gene transfer into mouse muscle in vivo. *Science*, **247**, 1465–8.

Worgall, S., Kikuchi, T., et al. 2001. Protection against pulmonary infection with *Pseudomonas aeruginosa* following immunization with *P. aeruginosa*-pulsed dendritic cells. *Infect Immun*, **69**, 4521–7.

Xiang, R., Lode, H.N., et al. 2000. An autologous oral DNA vaccine protects against murine melanoma. *Proc Natl Acad Sci USA*, **97**, 5492–7.

Yrlid, U. and Wick, M.J. 2000. *Salmonella*-induced apoptosis of infected macrophages results in presentation of a bacteria-encoded antigen after uptake by bystander dendritic cells. *J Exp Med*, **191**, 613–24.

Yrlid, U., Svensson, M., et al. 2000. Salmonella infection of bone marrow-derived macrophages and dendritic cells: influence on antigen presentation and initiating an immune response. *FEMS Immunol Med Microbiol*, **27**, 313–20.

Zhu, Y.D., Fennelly, G., et al. 1997. Recombinant bacille Calmette-Guerin expressing the measles virus nucleoprotein protects infant rhesus macaques from measles virus pneumonia. *J Infect Dis*, **176**, 1445–53.

44

Naked DNA vaccines

LINDA S. KLAVINSKIS

Over the last decade, there has been considerable excitement about the potential of a radically new approach to infectious disease prophylaxis stemming from the development of 'naked' DNA vaccine technology. Although previous vaccine strategies have relied on using a live replicating vector, purified protein, or an attenuated version of the pathogen, DNA vaccines consist of a plasmid DNA expression vector encoding the gene of interest for targeting the immune response. When administered to an animal, cellular uptake of the plasmid DNA results in expression of the encoded antigen in situ, leading to the induction of antigen-specific immunity.

In many ways, DNA vaccines share attributes of live attenuated vaccines, as exemplified by their ability to synthesize native protein for B-cell recognition and generate antigens endogenously, to enter the major histocompatibility complex (MHC) class I processing pathway and stimulate induction of $CD8^+$ cytotoxic T lymphocytes (CTL). However, unlike live vaccine vectors, DNA vaccines are noninfectious (therefore considered safe to administer in immunocompromised individuals), relatively easy to engineer and manufacture, and heat stable, and can easily be lyophilized (therefore without the need for cold storage). Despite the elegance and simplicity of DNA vaccines, the generation of a strong humoral immune response has not been as universally successful as immunization with protein combined with an adjuvant. This may be the result of the small amount of antigen that is produced. Studies with plasmids encoding reporter proteins indicate that only picogram to nanogram amounts of protein are expressed (Wolff et al. 1990; Klavinskis et al. 1999).

This chapter discusses the background to this technology, the architecture of the vectors used for immunization, modes of administration, the immunological basis for the responses elicited by DNA vaccines, current approaches to augment vaccine potency, and considers safety for human use, including findings from early human clinical trials.

HISTORICAL BACKGROUND

The inception of DNA vaccines goes back to a largely unnoticed observation by Ito (1960) who demonstrated the induction of papillomas in rabbit skin by injection of purified nucleic acid extracted from the Shope rabbit papilloma virus. It was not until Wolff et al. (1990) reported that intramuscular injection of plasmid DNA in a simple saline solution could transfect muscle cells in vivo and persist in an episomal form that the potential to induce an immune response against the expressed proteins became appreciated. Tang et al. (1992) were the first to demonstrate induction of antigen-specific antibody from plasmid DNA injected via a 'gene gun' into mice. This was rapidly followed by a consortium from Vical and Merck (Ulmer et al. 1993) who demonstrated that DNA vaccines could protect mice from influenza virus challenge by induction of antibody and CD8$^+$ CTL responses. Since then, the immunogenicity or protective efficacy of DNA vaccines in preclinical models of infectious disease, allergy, and cancer has been established in several animal species, and attests to the simplicity and robustness of the technology.

DESCRIPTION OF DNA EXPRESSION VECTORS

DNA vaccines include the basic elements of a bacterial plasmid (the vector: Figure 44.1): a promoter and enhancer (to enable transcription of the inserted foreign gene), an mRNA transcription termination/polyadenylation signal (for directing expression in mammalian cells), an antibiotic resistance gene (to confer an antibiotic selectable marker for growth in *Escherichia coli*), an origin of replication for growth in *E. coli*, and specific nucleotide sequences, cytidine phosphate–guanosine (referred to as CpG motifs) that are stimulatory for lymphocytes and act as an adjuvant.

Plasmid vector

The essential feature of a plasmid DNA vector for optimal expression in mammalian cells is a strong promoter/enhancer and transcriptional/termination sequence. Most DNA vaccines contain the human cytomegalovirus (CMV) immediate/early (IE) promoter (Boshart et al. 1985), the SV40 early promoter (Moreau et al. 1981), or the Rous sarcoma virus long terminal repeat (LTR) (Gorman et al. 1982) in conjunction with polyadenylation sequences from bovine growth hormone (BGH) or SV40 to stabilize the mRNA (Pfarr et al. 1986). There is some evidence that interferon-γ (IFN-γ), released in situ during the priming of an immune response (as a result of the inflammatory cytokine-inducing properties of bacterial DNA), can suppress transcription from many viral promoters (Harms and Splinter 1995; Romero and Lavine 1996). This in turn can affect the magnitude of the immune response, by limiting antigen production for B- and T-cell priming. Alternatives to virus-derived control elements, based on promoter/enhancer sequences driving expression of MHC class I and II (Xiang et al. 1997; Gebhard et al. 2000), dectin (in Langerhans' cells: Bonkobara et al. 2001) and muscle-specific genes (Barnhart et al. 1998; Kwissa et al. 2000), have been used successfully in DNA vaccines. Tissue and/or cell-specific expression has been achieved by these promoter elements but levels of expression do not exceed those achieved from the human cytomegalovirus (HCMV) immediate early gene (IE) promoter combined with the CMV intron A. Further optimization of expression has been reported by the inclusion of a 'Kozak' translational initiation sequence 5′ to the start codon of the inserted 'foreign' gene.

The ColE1 origin of replication (ori) derived from bacterial pUC plasmids is generally included in DNA vaccine vectors, because it provides an increased copy number in bacteria and high yields of plasmid DNA on purification. Early DNA vaccines studied in mice contained the ampicillin resistance gene (for plasmid selection during bacterial culture); however, this is precluded for use in humans and has been replaced by

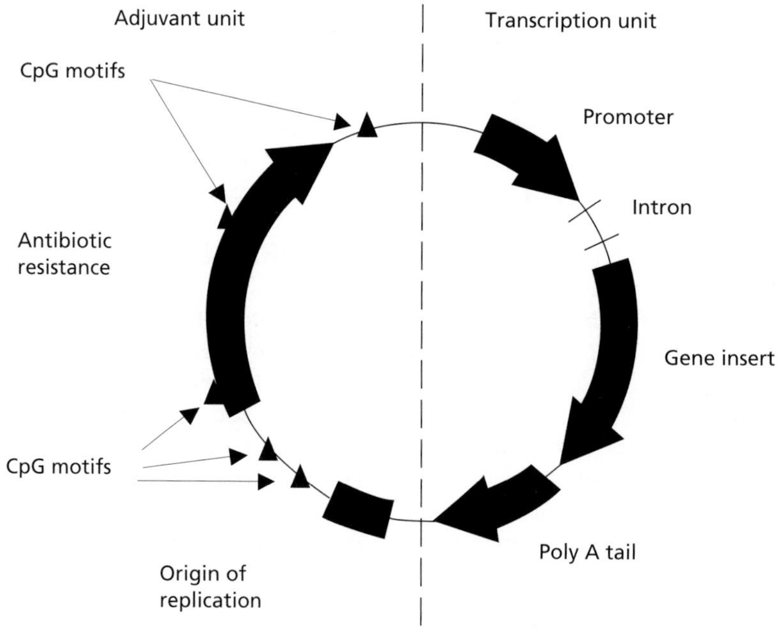

Figure 44.1 *Schematic representation of the basic elements of a plasmid DNA vector. The transcriptional unit consists of a viral promoter (e.g. human cytomegalovirus immediate early promoter), the gene of interest for targeting the immune response and transcription/termination sequences (poly-A tail). The backbone of the vector contains a bacterial origin of replication and an antibiotic resistance gene, which allow for growth and selection in bacteria. These elements of the vector also contain a number of CpG motifs and represent the adjuvant unit of the vector.*

kanamcyin or antibiotic-free approaches for selection of plasmid DNA (Cranenburgh et al. 2001).

CpG motifs of plasmid DNA

Aside from the regulatory elements of the vector concerned with transcription, bacterial plasmid DNA also contains immunostimulatory sequences (ISS) consisting of CpG dinucleotide sequences, usually flanked by two 5′ purines and two 3′ pyrimidines (Sato et al. 1996). Stimulatory bacterial CpGs differ from vertebrate DNA in that they are unmethylated and expressed at the expected frequency (predicted from random base utilization), whereas this frequency is suppressed 20-fold in vertebrate genomes (Bird 1986). These structural differences within bacterial DNA are recognized as 'foreign' by vertebrate immune systems and directly activate the innate immune system to produce multiple proinflammatory cytokines (including tumor necrosis factor α (TNF-α), IL-6, IL-12, IL-18, and IFN-α and -γ (Klinman et al. 1996)) which enhance the ability of antigen-presenting cells (APC) to present antigen and stimulate T-cell activation. This property of bacterial DNA has been described as the 'natural' adjuvant of DNA vaccines. Direct proof of the contribution of CpG DNA to the immunogenicity of DNA vaccines was provided by substitution of a CpG-containing ampR gene for a kanR-selectable marker (containing additional CpG motifs). The modified plasmid DNA was found to induce an enhanced CTL and IgG response compared with the original vector (Sato et al. 1996). This ability of CpG sequences in DNA vaccines to stimulate an immune response is abrogated by in vitro methylation (Pasquini et al. 1999). Co-administration of an empty vector (i.e. without any antigen-coding sequence) may boost the immune response to a DNA vaccine; however, there appears to be an upper limit to the ability of additional CpG motifs to improve the immune response (Krieg et al. 1998). This may reflect saturation of the innate cell-signaling pathway (see discussion below).

IMMUNOSTIMULATORY EFFECTS AND MECHANISMS OF CpG

Recognition of bacterial CpG is mediated by a conserved receptor, Toll-like receptor 9 (TLR9) expressed by macrophages and dendritic cells (DC) (Bauer et al. 2001). Current data suggest that CpG oligonucleotides cross the cell membrane via sequence nonspecific receptor-mediated endocytosis and are recruited to an endosomal compartment where TLR9 co-localizes (Ahmad-Nejad et al. 2002). One possibility is that plasmid-derived CpG oligonucleotides are liberated after degradation of injected plasmid DNA by extracellular nucleases. It appears that endosomal acidification of CpG DNA is required to initiate signaling via the Toll/interleukin 1 receptor (IL-1R) pathway, because specific inhibitors such as chloroquine block the immunostimulatory activity of CpG DNA (Hacker et al. 1998). In macrophages and DCs, CpG-DNA-mediated TLR9 signaling is transduced by a common adapter protein, myeloid differentiation factor 88 (MyD88), which results in the downstream generation of intracellular reactive oxygen species (Yi et al. 1998), and activation of the mitogen-activated kinases (MAPK) and nuclear factor κB (NFκB: Yi and Krieg 1998; Yi et al. 1998). The biological outcome of CpG-driven TLR9 ligation in DCs is secretion of T-helper 1 (Th1) polarizing cytokines (IL-12 and IL-18), upregulation of co-stimulatory molecules (CD40, CD80, and CD86) and functional maturation for antigen presentation (Sparwasser et al. 1998). These observations indicate that the plasmid backbone functions as a Th1-polarizing adjuvant in DNA vaccines and explains the IgG2a antibody and CTL responses seen after intramuscular immunization. CpG DNA also delivers T-independent survival signals to DCs, which are mediated by upregulation of the cellular inhibitor of active caspase (cIAP: Park et al. 2002). This might be a mechanism by which CpG DNA may prolong DC presentation of naked DNA-encoded antigen and compensate for the relatively low levels of antigen produced (compared with replicating vectors). CpG DNA also directly activates monocytes and macrophages to secrete Th1-like cytokines and express increased levels of cell surface co-stimulatory molecules (Schattenberg et al. 2000b). The signaling pathways activated by CpG DNA in B cells stimulate secretion of IL-6, IL-10, and IL-12 and also immunoglobulin in a polyclonal T-independent manner (Krieg et al. 1995). These CpG-mediated effects synergize with signaling through the B-cell antigen receptor by antigen secreted in situ from naked DNA.

Immune recognition of CpG DNA varies between species, with mouse cells expressing a high-responder phenotype and human cells a low-responder phenotype (Bauer et al. 2001). The CpG motifs optimally active in mice are poor stimulators of innate immunity in human peripheral blood mononuclear cells (PBMC: Bauer et al. 2001). Extensive screening assays have identified structurally distinct CpG oligodeoxynucleotide (ODN) sequences, with enhanced stimulation for human cells. K-type CpG ODNs stimulate IL-6 production by monocytes/DCs and B-cell proliferation and IgM production, whereas D-type CpG ODNs preferentially stimulate IFN-γ production by natural killer (NK) cells (Verthelyi et al. 2001). Thus, it may be possible to improve DNA vaccines for human use by the mutagenesis of endogenous plasmid CpG sequences. However, as discussed above, a relative increase in the levels of IFN-γ induced by CpG-DNA will be compensated by IFN-γ-mediated suppression of viral promoter activity, which drives antigen expression. A further level of complexity that is being unraveled is the differential responsiveness of human DC subsets. Human plasmacytoid DCs ($CD11c^{-}$ $CD123^{+}$) are responsive to CpG DNA, but monocyte-derived $CD11^{+}$ DCs lack TLR9 and do not appear to be stimulated (Bauer et al. 2001). Currently, this difference is difficult to rationalize, in view of the front-line defensive location of $CD11c^+$ DCs at body surfaces.

IMMUNOSUPPRESSIVE CpG Motifs

Certain CpG motifs can be inhibitory and abrogate immune activation and cytokine production (Hacker et al. 1998). These motifs termed 'neutralizing' CpG (CpG-N) contain a dinucleotide motif preceded by a cytidine (i.e. CCG) followed by a guanosine (i.e. CGG) or contain CG repeats (CGCGCG). The immunostimulatory (s) activity of a CpG-S oligonucleotide can be blocked by certain suppressive motifs. Removal of the suppressive motifs from the plasmid DNA backbone improved the immunogenicity of the plasmid DNA (Krieg et al. 1998). These observations suggest that the presence or absence of these inhibitory sequences in DNA vaccines may profoundly affect the immunogenicity of the vaccine.

ROUTES AND MODE OF DNA VACCINE DELIVERY

A variety of routes have been used to deliver DNA vaccines. Systemic routes of delivery include intramuscular or intradermal needle injection, transdermal application via occluded patches, or ballistic delivery into the skin. For needle injection, naked plasmid DNA is administered in water, saline, phosphate-buffered saline, or sucrose solution. Ballistic delivery of DNA vaccines involves bombardment of cells with plasmid DNA precipitated onto gold or tungsten microparticles. This is usually achieved by a blast of pressurized gas (generally helium) delivering DNA-coated particles from a gene gun (Feltquate et al. 1997). Topical or aerosol delivery of naked DNA vaccines to mucosal surfaces has also been achieved and is highly desirable, because this provides the possibility of generating immunity both at the sites of pathogen entry and in the systemic compartment. Moreover, needle-free delivery increases patient compliance.

Intramuscular delivery of naked DNA

One of the simplest modes of administering naked DNA is in saline to the quadriceps or tibialis anterior muscle in mice or to the axillary or gluteal muscle in nonhuman primates. Typically 10–50 μg plasmid DNA is required to elicit a response in mice but substantially higher doses (1–5 mg) are required to elicit detectable responses in nonhuman and human primates. Some investigators have reported improved immune responses induced by pretreatment of the muscle tissue with agents including cardiotoxin, local anesthetics such as bupivacaine, or hypertonic solutions (Davis et al. 1993; Coney et al. 1994). Whether or not this effect reflects an increase in plasmid-encoded antigen expression in regenerating muscle cells or an increase in recruitment of APCs to the site of tissue damage is contentious. There is agreement that, after intramuscular injection, plasmid DNA rapidly disseminates throughout the body and persists briefly in highly vascular tissues and in muscle at the site of injection for at least 8 weeks (Parker et al. 1999). The persistence of plasmid DNA, principally in muscle cells, may provide a reservoir of antigen production to sustain (via crosspriming, see 'Processing and presentation of plasmid DNA-encoded antigen' below) the strong CTL responses reported in mice.

The characteristics and quantity of an antigen are known to be important in defining the type of immune response elicited. However, intramuscularly injected DNA vaccines typically, but not exclusively, elicit a Th1 immune response, characterized by IFN-γ production by antigen-restimulated $CD4^+$ T cells, and the predominance of serum IgG2a antibody to the antigen. This profile is attributed to the adjuvant effect of the CpG motifs within the plasmid backbone, which induce IL-12 secretion by APCs.

Intradermal or ballistic delivery of naked DNA

Intradermal or ballistically delivered DNA vaccines target the dermal and epidermal tissues of the skin. Small amounts of DNA, typically 1–10 μg (for needle injection) or sub-microgram amounts (for ballistic delivery), are required to elicit immune responses in mice that are often superior to those elicited at higher concentrations by the intramuscular route. This most probably reflects the higher concentration of APCs, Langerhans' cells, and dermal DCs within the skin and also the cascade of cytokines (IL-1α, IL-1β, TNFα, IL-6, IL-7, IL-10, IL-12, IL-15) and chemokines (macrophage inflammatory protein 1α (MIP-1α), monocyte chemoattractant protein 2 (MCP-2), RANTES, IP-10) that are liberated after needle or ballistic trauma. Initial reports suggested that gene-gun- (or ballistically-) delivered DNA vaccines elicited a predominantly Th2 response and serum IgG1 antibody, whereas intramuscular injection with the same plasmid DNA resulted in Th1 priming for CTLs and predominantly serum IgG2a antibody (Feltquate et al. 1997). Other reports indicate induction of potent Th1 responses after intradermal injection of plasmid DNA (Raz et al. 1994). These differences may be reconciled with the type of plasmid DNA-encoded antigen, the age and type of mouse strain used, and the dose of plasmid DNA (low doses contributing to exclusive Th2 priming), rather than a correlation between injection route and polarization of the immune response. It has been suggested that the adjuvant effect of plasmid DNA operates in priming Th1 responses at a dose range of 20–100 μg/vaccine (Reimann and Schirmbeck 2000), accounting for the preferential priming of Th2 responses by the intradermal or ballistic route. However, priming for Th1 responses can be established at low plasmid DNA doses by co-injection of low concentrations of CpG oligonucleotide at the intradermal site of plasmid DNA delivery (Reimann and Schirmbeck 2000). Other reagents (IFNs, IL-12, IL-18, or poly[I/C]) can also deviate a plasmid DNA-elicited Th2 response to a Th1 type in this system.

Mucosal delivery

Protection against infection at the mucosal epithelia generally requires induction of local immunity, which is optimally elicited by vaccines delivered to mucosal inductive sites (Czerkinsky et al. 1999). To date, the vast majority of DNA vaccines have been delivered by parenteral routes, although data indicating induction of secretory IgA or IgG antibodies by intramuscularly or intradermally administered plasmid DNA have not been compelling (Fynan et al. 1993). A number of studies have reported the induction of weak immune responses by direct topical delivery of naked plasmid DNA to various mucosal surfaces, including the nasal, oral, and vaginal epithelia (Etchart et al. 1997; Wang et al. 1997; Klavinskis et al. 1999). These observations may be the result of the low efficiency of transgene expression achieved at nasal and intestinal epithelia by naked plasmid DNA (Klavinskis et al. 1999; L.S. Klavinskis, C. Barnfield, and P. Hobson, 2000, unpublished observations). This may arise from the presence of physical and chemical barriers impeding transfection in the respiratory and gastrointestinal tract, including endonucleases, mucolytic enzymes, low pH, and turbulence. To increase plasmid DNA uptake and transfection efficiency, several approaches have focused on condensing (or encapsulating) the naked plasmid DNA with either cationic liposomes (Perrie et al. 2001), cytofectins based on cationic lipids (Klavinskis et al. 1999), cationic block co-polymers (Laus et al. 2001), or biodegradable microspheres such as poly (dl-lactide-co-glycolide: Herrmann et al. 1999; Kaneko et al. 2000). Bacterial systems including attenuated *Shigellla flexneri* and *Salmonella typhimurium*, which invade mucosal epithelial cells, have also been developed for oral delivery of DNA vaccines (Darji et al. 2000; Shata and Hone 2001). Detailed discussion of these systems lies outside the focus of this chapter.

GENERATION OF IMMUNE RESPONSES BY NAKED DNA VACCINES

Plasmid DNA uptake

The precise mechanism by which naked plasmid DNA enters cells and is translocated to the nucleus to initiate transcription is not fully understood. Evidence from electron micrographs suggests that plasmid DNA is internalized by electrostatic binding to the cell membrane and endocytosed via clathrin-coated pits (Figure 44.2) (Zabner et al. 1995; Friend et al. 1996). Direct fusion with the cell membrane and/or fluid phase endocytosis (macropinocytosis: Apodaca 2001) may also contribute to cellular uptake of plasmid DNA (Figure 44.2). Endosomal uptake of plasmid DNA can be increased by complexing the DNA with cationic liposomes, cytofectins, or ligands to cell surface receptors (Fasbender et al. 1997; Harbottle et al. 1998; Klavinskis et al. 1999; Perrie et al. 2001). Once plasmid DNA is internalized, rapid escape from the endosome is critical to the efficiency of plasmid-encoded antigen expression. Endosomes mature through various stages of acidification and eventually fuse with lysosomes containing enzymes, which degrade DNA. Release of plasmid DNA from the endolysosome is thought to be a consequence of membrane disruption. Cationic lipids or peptides (e.g. from the hemagglutinin of influenza virus) that fuse with the endosomal membrane have been reported to increase transfection efficiency (Fasbender et al. 1997; Zhang et al. 2001). Despite these modifications, only a fraction of internalized plasmid DNA penetrates the cytoplasm. Plasmid DNA is prone to further degradation by cytosolic nucleases. Thus, only a very small proportion of transfected DNA is available for transport across the nuclear membrane (reviewed by Johnson-Saliba and Jans 2001). The size of plasmid DNA vectors (2–10 MDa) is generally assumed to preclude efficient diffusion across the nuclear pore complex, thus compounding the inefficiency of plasmid DNA transfection. After transcription, mRNA is translated and plasmid-encoded protein within the cytoplasm is accessible to the TAP-dependent MHC-I-processing pathway. The induction of immune responses by DNA vaccines is all the more remarkable in view of the multiple cellular barriers that impede efficient transfection of plasmid DNA and attests to the importance of the adjuvant activity of CpG DNA.

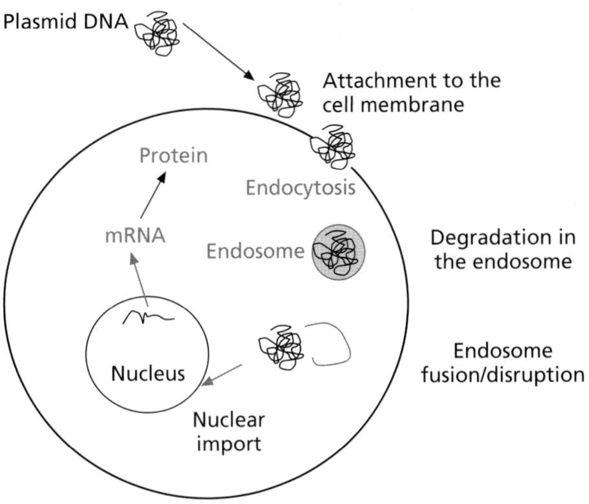

Figure 44.2 *Schematic representation of critical steps in the cytosolic synthesis of plasmid encoded antigen after membrane binding of plasmid DNA.*

Processing and presentation of plasmid DNA-encoded antigen

For the presentation of plasmid DNA-encoded antigen to B cells, it appears that, as long as antigen is accessible to the B-cell receptor, the nature of the transfected cell exporting the plasmid DNA-encoded protein is immaterial (Loirat et al. 1999; Armand et al. 2000). For DNA vaccines expressing purely cytosolic proteins, it had been suggested that antigen release to the extracellular milieu might be effected by CTL lysis of the transfected cell. However, recent data indicated that neither perforin nor $CD8^+$ T-cell-mediated lysis is required for priming $CD4^+$ T-cell or antibody responses (Hassett et al. 1999).

For the priming of $CD8^+$ T-cell responses there are at least three mechanisms by which a plasmid DNA-encoded antigen may be processed and presented. These include: (1) direct transfection and priming by somatic cells (such as myocytes, fibroblast, and keratinocytes); (2) crosspriming, whereby antigen is transferred from transfected somatic cells to professional APCs; or (3) direct transfection of APCs.

DIRECT PRIMING BY SOMATIC CELLS

The seminal observation that intramuscular injection of plasmid DNA-induced protein expression in muscle (Wolff et al. 1990) and elicited strong $CD8^+$ CTL responses in mice (Ulmer et al. 1993) suggested that muscle cells were critically involved in the initiation of CTL responses. In support of this premise, it was shown that adoptive transfer of stably transfected myoblasts expressing influenza nucleoprotein into mice was sufficient to induce $CD8^+$ CTLs and protect from virus challenge (Ulmer et al. 1996). This provided compelling evidence that antigen expression by muscle cells was sufficient to prime for CTL-mediated protection. It was unresolved whether CTL responses were directly induced by myocytes expressing the encoded antigen or they were indirectly induced through antigen transfer from myocytes to professional APCs. A conceptual difficulty with direct priming was that muscle cells do not express co-stimulatory molecules (CD80, CD86) essential to initiate T-cell responses and were therefore unlikely to act as APCs. To resolve the contribution of somatic versus bone-marrow derived APCs in CTL priming, bone-marrow-derived cells were adoptively transferred to irradiated F1 hybrid mice, to create bone marrow chimeras with somatic cells of both F1 MHC haplotypes and APCs of a single MHC haplotype of the donor bone marrow. Peptide-specific CTLs were induced only by immunization of mice with plasmid DNA encoding the peptide presented by the MHC-I molecules found on the donor bone marrow (Fu et al. 1997; Iwasaki et al. 1997). These studies demonstrated that bone-marrow-derived APCs play a dominant role in CTL priming and suggested that either APCs were directly transfected or antigens (or their epitopes) synthesized in somatic cells could be transferred to APCs (by crosspriming, see below) for presentation by MHC-I molecules.

CROSSPRIMING BY DNA VACCINES

Crosspresentation of antigenic material from apoptotic cells to DCs has been established as an important mechanism for the induction of $CD8^+$ CTL responses against tumor or pathogen-derived antigens (Bevan 1976). In vitro studies have established that this mechanism is distinct from the classic endogenous TAP-dependent pathway of MHC class I restricted peptide presentation. Several lines of evidence indicate that crosspriming also occurs after DNA immunization. Loirat et al. (1999) have shown that immunization with a plasmid DNA vector driven by a muscle-specific promoter elicited CTLs, despite expression of antigen restricted to muscle cells, suggesting that crosspresentation of antigen to APCs was involved. Second Corr et al. (1999) demonstrated, using a transactivating plasmid system and bone marrow chimeras, that CTL induction by plasmid DNA was critically dependent on antigen expression by somatic cells and transfer to APCs. However, a complementary mechanism involving direct transfection of APCs could not be excluded (see below). More recently, crosspresentation of antigen to DCs has been facilitated by constructing DNA vaccines, which induce apoptotic death of the antigen-expressing cell. Co-immunization with DNA vaccines that express Fas or a mutated version of a caspase gene that induces the creation of apoptotic bodies has been reported to enhance cell-mediated immunity (Chattergoon et al. 2000; Sasaki et al. 2001). The underlying mechanism by which antigen is transferred from somatic cells to APCs is not fully understood. Chaperones, including heat shock proteins 70 and 73 (hsp70, hsp73), have been implicated in the transfer of immunogenic material from plasmid DNA-transfected macrophages or somatic cells to DCs (Kumaraguru et al. 2000; Kammerer et al. 2002). The precise mechanism by which chaperone-bound peptides are released and cross-presented by DCs remains to be resolved. Candidate mechanisms include either a facilitated exchange or delivery system, whereby chaperone-bound peptide is internalized after receptor-mediated DC binding with peptide exchange between nascent MHC class I molecules and the chaperone (Figure 44.3a). Alternately, chaperone-bound peptide may be directly exchanged with cell-surface MHC class I bound peptide (Figure 44.3a).

DIRECT TRANSFECTION OF APCS BY DNA VACCINES

Although current data provide a compelling case for indirect CTL priming through crosspresentation, other studies provide evidence that APCs are directly transfected after DNA immunization. Removal of muscle (within 10 min) from the injection site of a DNA

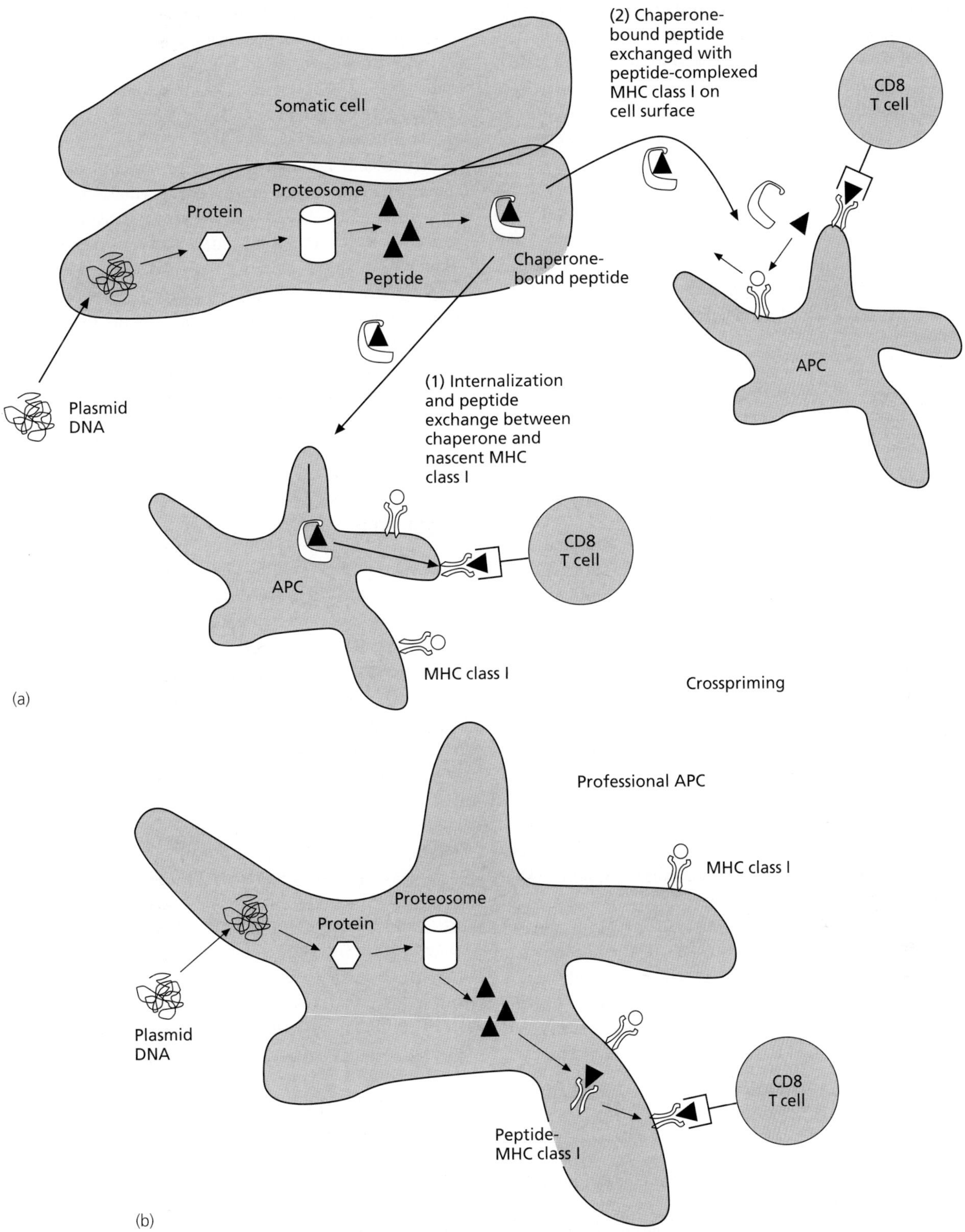

Figure 44.3 *Mechanisms of antigen presentation after DNA immunization.* **(a)** *Crosspresentation of antigenic material from plasmid DNA-transfected somatic cells to antigen-presenting cells (APCs) in vivo. Injection of plasmid DNA leads to transfection of somatic cells (muscle cells, keratinocytes or any MHC class II negative cells). Newly synthesized protein is targeted to proteosomes for proteolytic cleavage and peptide transport across the endoplasmic reticulum (ER). Chaperones, such as heat shock proteins, bind these peptides, which are crosspresented by MHC-I molecules on professional APCs to CD8⁺ T cells. The precise mechanism is unclear but may involve either (1) receptor-mediated internalization of peptide bound chaperone and peptide exchange between the chaperone and newly synthesized MHC class I or (2) peptide exchange between cell surface MHC class I and chaperone-bound peptide.* **(b)** *Direct transfection of bone marrow-derived APCs. Injection of plasmid DNA leads to direct transfection of a small number of dendritic cells. Peptides generated* in situ *are presented by MHC class I molecules to CD8⁺ T cells*

vaccine did not alter the magnitude or quality of the subsequent immune response, suggesting that transfection of cells (possibly APCs) distal to the injection site is sufficient to prime for CTLs (Torres et al. 1997). Antigen and reporter genes have been demonstrated in macrophages, Langerhans' cells, and DCs present both at the site of DNA vaccine delivery and in draining lymph nodes (Chattergoon et al. 1998; Akbari et al. 1999; Barnfield et al. 2000). This suggests that APCs are transfected in situ and migrate to draining lymph nodes or alternately are transfected within lymph nodes after lymphatic drainage of plasmid DNA (Figure 44.3b). Conclusively, plasmid-encoded mRNA has been demonstrated in isolated DCs after either intradermal or mucosal DNA vaccine delivery (Bouloc et al. 1999; Barnfield et al. 2000). Functional studies have demonstrated that DCs isolated from plasmid DNA injected skin or nasal tissue were able to stimulate the proliferation of T-cell responses in vitro (Bouloc et al. 1999; Barnfield et al. 2000). Second, DCs isolated after DNA immunization were shown to prime for CTL responses in naïve mice following adoptive transfer (Bouloc et al. 1999). These reports indicate that different routes of DNA vaccine delivery result in direct transfection of APCs and lead to induction of CTL responses. Current evidence suggests that the efficiency of DC transfection in vivo is very low (Barnfield et al. 2000). However, considering the potent stimulatory activity of DCs (reviewed by Steinman and Poe 2002), large numbers of transfected DCs may not actually be essential to elicit CTL responses. In support of this hypothesis, adoptive transfer of as few as 500–1000 in vitro transfected DCs to mice induced a comparable cellular and humoral immune response to that elicited by gene-gun immunization with the same antigen-encoding plasmid DNA (Timares et al. 1998).

In summary, two major pathways for CTL priming by DNA vaccines have been established. Enhancement of crosspriming has been established by co-delivery of plasmid DNA-encoding apoptotic proteins. Formulations or delivery systems that target APCs directly may also increase plasmid DNA uptake and CTL priming.

AUGMENTING THE IMMUNOGENICITY OF DNA VACCINES

Preclinical studies in several murine models of infectious disease have shown that DNA vaccines effectively elicit cellular and humoral immune responses, which confer protection from pathogen challenge (e.g. Ulmer et al. 1993; Li et al. 1998; Gebhard et al. 2000). Although these observations have been very encouraging, the magnitude of the immune responses induced in human and nonhuman primates by the first generation of naked DNA vaccines has proved lower than that achieved by attenuated or protein adjuvanted vaccines (see MacGregor et al. 1998; Amara et al. 2001). This difference in efficacy of DNA vaccines between species results partly from the higher level of protein expression achieved in mice after intramuscular injection than in other species (Jiao et al. 1992). Second, the dose of plasmid DNA injected in mice per kilogram body weight significantly exceeds the per kilogram dose administered to human and nonhuman primates, so comparisons of immunogenicity are not appropriate. Furthermore, murine cells reportedly demonstrate greater sensitivity than human cells to the adjuvant activity of CpG DNA (Bauer et al. 2001). Thus although naked DNA vaccines on their own may not be adequate to protect against disease in humans, technological developments in vector construction, incorporation of genetic or conventional adjuvants, deployment of novel delivery vehicles, or poxvirus booster inoculations (see below) may lead to the development of effective DNA vaccines.

Modification of the vector

PROMOTER

It is generally believed that the level of gene expression attained in vivo after DNA immunization correlates with the immune response generated. Therefore, approaches to improve gene expression may enhance DNA vaccine potency. Virally-derived promoters, including the most frequently used CMV immediate early enhancer–promoter, provide high levels of gene expression within mammalian cells (Manthorpe et al. 1993). However, these promoters are subject to transcriptional silencing, after CpG DNA-mediated activation of proinflammatory cytokines (Romero and Lavine 1996). Elimination or methylation of CpG motifs within the plasmid backbone reportedly increases the duration of antigen expression (e.g. Yew et al. 2001; Reyes-Sandoral and Ertl 2004). Although this modification may provide the longer-term expression required for gene replacement therapy, it needs to be balanced with the loss of adjuvant activity required for DC maturation and to initiate T-cell priming. Alternate promoters, including cell-specific, tissue-specific, and hybrid CMV promoters, have been evaluated (Xiang et al. 1997; Barnhart et al. 1998; Gebhard et al. 2000; Kwissa et al. 2000; Bonkobara et al. 2001). Plasmid vectors containing the human ubiquitin promoter could be particularly useful. Sustained, high-level gene expression has been achieved with this promoter in the presence of plasmid backbones containing CpG motifs (Yew et al. 2001).

CODON OPTIMIZATION

Optimizing codon usage for eukaryotic cells can also enhance expression of antigens. Codon bias has been observed in several species and may differ from the codons most frequently used by pathogens. Changes in codon usage, which modify RNA structure, have been shown to enhance the expression of HIV *env* and *gag* genes. In mammalian cells the *env* and *gag* genes are made as long unspliced transcripts that contain overlapping reading frames with the small regulatory genes of HIV *rev* and *tat*. These transcripts are retained in the nucleus and are rapidly spliced in the absence of *rev*, thus preventing the transport of full-length message to the endoplasmic reticulum (ER). The transcripts are inhibited from transport to the ER by *rev*-dependent sequences that are themselves part of the structural gene sequence. Structural modification of the RNA through changing codon usage has led to an increase in HIV *envelope* and *gag* expression with an increase in anti-HIV gp160 CTLs and antibody reported (Andre et al. 1998; Vinner et al. 1999).

Modification of the inserted gene

By altering the cellular location where antigen is expressed or by the inclusion of protein sorting or targeting sequences, DNA vaccines have been modified either to increase priming for $CD8^+$ T-cell responses or to enhance B-cell activation. The addition of N-terminal ubiquitin sequences has been reported to lead to an increase in CTL precursor frequency and a reduction in antibody responses (Wu and Kipps 1997; Rodriguez et al. 1998). This is most probably the result of enhanced targeting of *de novo* synthesized cytosolic proteins to the proteosome (an organelle in which the protein is hydrolyzed to short peptides for TAP-dependent entry into the ER and MHC-I presentation). Proteins are thus rapidly processed to short peptides, which precludes or reduces the release of native protein for efficient antibody production. Another approach has been to design vectors that incorporate the E3 leader sequence from adenovirus, which facilitates transport of antigens from the cytosol directly into the ER for binding to MHC-I molecules. The addition of the E3 leader sequence has been reported to increase CTL responses to certain (Ciernik et al. 1996; Iwasaki et al. 1999), but not all (Ciernik et al. 1996), plasmid DNA-encoded antigens. Similarly, immunization with plasmid DNA encoding an antigen fused C terminally to a truncated cytosolic chaperone (heat shock protein 73 or hsp73) has been reported to increase CTL induction by bypassing the normal proteosome/TAP route of peptide entry into the ER (Kammerer et al. 2002). The stable *de novo* expression of antigen with hsp73 in the cytosol from a DNA vector may facilitate crosspresentation of antigen to DCs in vivo.

$CD4^+$ T-cell responses can be augmented by addition of sorting signals from membrane proteins, which are normally targeted to the lysosomal compartment, thereby directing plasmid-encoded proteins toward the MHC-II antigen-presentation pathway (Langlade-Demoyen et al. 2003). The immunological consequence of lysosomal targeting appears variable and depends on the primary sequence of the encoded antigen (Rodriguez et al. 2001). Plasmid DNA-encoded $CD4^+$ T-cell epitopes, which contain cleavage sites for the lysosomal endopeptidase (cathepsin D), were destroyed when targeted to lysosomes.

Humoral immune responses can be enhanced by the addition of a signal sequence fused to the antigen-coding sequence to direct protein transport through the ER and export from the cell surface (Lewis et al. 1999). Thus, synthesized protein bypasses the normal proteosome/TAP route of peptide delivery into the ER and is secreted for B-cell binding. Immune responses in mice immunized with a secreted form of antigen demonstrate an enhanced serum IgG1 response and increased levels of IL-4 by antigen-restimulated lymph node T cells in vitro (Lewis et al. 1999).

DNA delivery

The distribution of plasmid DNA from the site of vaccine delivery and efficiency of cellular uptake are key factors limiting the potency of DNA vaccines. One approach to increase DNA delivery is in vivo electroporation. A low intensity of electric pulses (100–200 V/cm) delivered from electrodes applied to the muscle or skin has resulted in significant enhancement in the cellular and humoral immune responses generated to injected DNA vaccines (Kadowaki et al. 2000; Widera et al. 2000). The wide-scale feasibility, user friendliness, and safety of this immunization approach remains to be established. The potential for DNA integration into host genomes is a concern, because electroporation results in a much larger copy number of copies of plasmid DNA per cell than achieved by injected naked plasmid DNA (Dupuis et al. 2000).

An alternate approach to increase DNA vaccine delivery is through formulations designed to protect plasmid DNA from degradation and to increase the release of plasmid DNA from the endosomal compartment and entry into the nucleus. Various liposomes, cationic lipids, and cationic block polymers (polycations combined with hydrophilic nonionic polymers) were initially developed to enhance therapeutic gene therapy (reviewed by Lechardeur and Lukas 2002). Several groups have since demonstrated that cationic lipid or polymer-complexed plasmid DNA also enhanced the induction of cellular and humoral immune responses (Klavinskis et al. 1999; Hartikka et al. 2001; D'Souza et al. 2002). There is some evidence to indicate that these formulations (or cytofectins) may not only increase plasmid DNA uptake but also synergize with bacterial CpG to activate the innate response and augment T-cell priming by DNA vaccines. Lipid-complexed plasmid DNA has been reported to increase DC activation and increase proinflammatory cytokine (IL-12 and IFN-γ) production at the site of plasmid DNA delivery (Freimark et al. 1998; Barnfield et al. 2000). Lipid-complexed plasmid DNA may (like liposome-complexed antigens) demonstrate preferential uptake by APCs.

Another approach to augmenting the immunogenicity of plasmid DNA-encoded antigens has been the use of biodegradable polymeric microparticles. Plasmid DNA encapsulated by the polymer poly(lactide-co-glycolide) (PLG) can be delivered by systemic and mucosal routes and has been reported to elicit immune responses (Chen et al. 1998; Kaneko et al. 2000) that confer protection in a murine rotavirus challenge model (Chen et al. 1998). Adsorption of plasmid DNA on to pre-formed PLG microparticles has also been shown to prime for both antibody and cellular immune responses (Singh et al. 2000). PLG-mediated vaccine delivery appears to act, in part, by targeting PLG-containing microspheres to APCs, rather than achieving an increase in gene expression (Singh et al. 2000).

Genetic adjuvants for DNA vaccines

Several groups have used plasmid DNA encoding various cytokine, chemokine, or co-stimulatory molecules to enhance or polarize the type of immune response generated by DNA immunization (summarized in Tables 44.1 and 44.2). In some instances the outcome attributed to a particular immunomodulator has been inconclusive or variable depending on the antigen, mouse strain, or plasmid vector used. The variability in response may also reflect the complexity of effects attributed to an immunomodulator and those elicited in response to bacterial components of the vaccine vector (described earlier). Co-immunization with plasmid DNA encoding Th1 cytokines, IL-12, IL-18, IFN-γ, and TNFα or the chemokines granulocyte–macrophage colony-stimulating factor (GM-CSF) or RANTES with antigen-coding DNA vaccine constructs has resulted in enhanced CTL and/or Th-cell proliferative responses (summarized in Tables 44.1 and 44.2). Co-immunization with plasmid DNA encoding IL-12 also appears to prolong the duration of the CTL response (Chattergoon et al. 2004). Conversely, co-immunization with plasmid DNA encoding certain Th2 cytokines (e.g. IL-4, IL-5, IL-6), or IL-2, IL-15, IL-18, or GM-CSF, has been reported to augment humoral immune responses (Table 44.1).

Other investigators have targeted transgene products to lymph nodes or APCs by constructing DNA vaccines encoding secreted fusion proteins that contain CTLA-4, L-selectin, or CD40L, the cognate ligands of which are present on APCs. By targeting secreted antigens for APC uptake, stronger immune responses have been reported (Mendoza et al. 1997; Boyle et al. 1998; Sin et al. 2000). Similarly, expression of plasmid DNA-encoded co-stimulatory molecules (CD80 or CD86) on transfected somatic or APCs can provide critical secondary signals for T-cell activation, through ligation of cognate receptors (CD28/CTLA-4). A number of studies have reported that co-administration of plasmid DNA-encoding antigen and CD80 or CD86 increased T-cell responses without any change in the humoral immune response (Iwasaki et al. 1997; Kim et al. 1997).

Table 44.1 *Modulation of DNA vaccines by co-delivery of cytokines and chemokines*

Cytokine	Antibody	Cellular response	CTLs	Reference
Chemokine				
IL-1	↑ IgG	↑ proliferation	↑ CTLs	Hakim et al. (1996); Kim et al. (1998)
IL-2	↑ IgG	↑ proliferation	↑ CTLs	Kim et al. (1998)
			↑CTLs	Barouch et al. (2000)
IL-4	↑ IgG1	↓ DTH, ↑ IL-4		Geissler et al. (1997)
Il-5	↑ IgG1	± proliferation		Kim et al. (1998)
IL-6	↑ IgG, ↑ IgA	↑ proliferation		Barnfield (2000)
IL-7	↑ IgG2a	↑ IFN-γ		Prayaga et al. (1997)
IL-8	↑ IgG	↑ proliferation		Kim et al. (2000)
	↑ neutrophils			Hengge et al. (1995)
IL-10	↓ IgG2a	↓ proliferation		Daheshia et al. (1997)
IL-12	↑ IgG2a	↑ DTH	↑ CTLs (and memory)	Iwasaki et al. (1997); Okada et al. (1997); Chattergoon et al. (2004)
IL-15	↑ IgG	± ↑ proliferation	↑ CTLs	Kim et al. (1998)
IL-18	↑ IgG	↑ proliferation	↑ CTLs	Kim et al. (1998)
TNF-α	↑ IgG	↑ proliferation	↑ CTLs	Kim et al. (1998)
GM-CSF	↑ IgG	↑ proliferation	↑ CTLs	Iwasaki et al. (1997)
	↑ IgG1	↑ IL-4		Xiang and Ertl (1995)
IFN-γ	↑ IgG	↑ IFN-γ, ↓ IL-5		Xiang and Ertl (1995)
MIP-1α	↑ IgG	↑ proliferation		Kim et al. (2000)
γIP-10	± ↑ IgG	± no effect		Kim et al. (2000)
RANTES	± no effect	↑ proliferation		Sin et al. (2000)
		↑ proliferation	↑ CTLs	Kim et al. (2000)

See text for abbreviations.

Table 44.2 *Modulation of DNA vaccines by co-delivery of co-stimulatory genes*

Co-stimulatory gene	Antibody	Cellular response	CTLs	Reference
CD80			↑ CTLs	Iwasaki et al. (1997) Kim et al. (1997)
CD86		↑ DTH	↑ CTLs	Iwasaki et al. (1997) Kim et al. (1997)
CD40L	↑ IgG2a	↑ IFN-γ	↑ CTLs	Mendoza et al. (1997)
	↑ IgG2a	↑ proliferation, ↑ IFN-γ		Sin et al. (2001)
LFA-3		↑ proliferation, ↑ IFN-γ	↑ CTLs	Kim et al. (1999)
L-Selectin	↑ IgG	↑ proliferation		Boyle et al. (1998)
CTLA-4	↑ IgG (IgG1 > IgG2a)	↑ proliferation		Boyle et al. (1998)

See text for abbreviations.

PRIME-BOOST APPROACHES

The relative lack of effectiveness of DNA vaccines in nonhuman primates has led to the development of heterologous immunization regimens, where the immune response induced by plasmid DNA is enhanced by a boost from a heterologous vector or protein. Strategies have included priming with a DNA vaccine and boosting with a recombinant protein-adjuvanted vaccine. Enhancement in the humoral immune response has been demonstrated with variable protection of nonhuman primates from pathogen challenge (Letvin et al. 1997; Putkonen et al. 1998; Cherpelis et al. 2001). Superior CTL responses in nonhuman primates against antigens from HIV, simian immunodeficiency virus (SIV), Ebola virus, and malaria have been demonstrated where DNA vaccines were used as priming agents and augmented by various viral vectors, such as fowlpox viruses (Kent et al. 1998; Robinson et al. 1999), vaccinia virus (Sedegah et al. 2000), modified vaccinia Ankara (MVA: Scheider et al. 1998; Hanke et al. 1999; Allen et al. 2000; Mwau et al. 2004), or adenovirus (Sullivan et al. 2000; Shiver et al. 2002). The superiority of the DNA prime-viral vector boost approach may reside in the ability of the DNA vaccine component to focus the immune response on to a single antigen, without competition from the myriad of viral vector-encoded antigens. The relative inefficiency of DNA vaccines to boost immune responses primed by viral vectors is most probably the result of the small amount of antigen generated and the weak induction of immunomodulatory cytokines and chemokines required to trigger expansion of antigen-specific memory cells.

SAFETY CONSIDERATIONS FOR VACCINE ADMINISTRATION IN HUMANS

To date, DNA vaccines have been shown to be well tolerated in both preclinical and phase 1 clinical trials (see below). Immunopathological reactions such as inflammation and general immunosuppression have not been observed, although a number of safety concerns remain. These include: (1) the possibility that DNA vaccines could integrate into the host genome, which could result in the activation of oncogenes or the inactivation of tumor suppressor genes; (2) the induction of responses against self-antigens expressed on transfected cells and that initiate autoimmune disease; (3) the induction of tolerance rather than active immunity to plasmid DNA-encoded antigens; and (4) the stimulation and production of antibodies to the injected DNA.

Potential for integration

The primary safety concern of plasmid DNA vaccines is their potential to integrate into the genome of host cells. This could increase the risk of malignancy by causing either the activation of oncogenes or inactivation of tumor suppressor genes. If integration occurs in germline cells, there is also a potential for germline transmission. These concerns stem from the knowledge that plasmids can integrate at a very low level into cellular DNA when transfected into actively dividing cells. However, it is believed that only a small fraction of integration events would alter a gene and prove harmful to a host cell. The probability of integration in vivo is likely to be further reduced by physical–chemical barriers that impede efficient uptake of plasmid DNA in vivo, including exonucleases, interstitial DNA-binding proteins, and a lower rate of cellular proliferation than cells in vitro synchronized for transfection under S-phase conditions. Despite concerns raised, there is no clear evidence to date that naked DNA vaccines can integrate. Gel-purified genomic DNA isolated from many tissues (including germline) following intramuscular injection of plasmid DNA and assayed by polymerase chain reaction (PCR) has produced no evidence of integration to a detection sensitivity of one copy plasmid per microgram of DNA (Ledwith et al. 2000; Schattenberg et al. 2000a). This rate is at least three orders of magnitude lower than the theoretical frequency of spontaneous gene-inactivating mutations (Nicols et al. 1995). Thus, for plasmid DNA vaccines delivered by intramuscular injection, the risk of mutation caused by integration appears to be negligible. Other methods of plasmid DNA delivery (including gene gun or electroporation), or use of novel formulations or adjuvants that increase the efficiency of cell transfection, could potentially influence the integration frequency. Indeed compelling evidence for integration of plasmid DNA following electroporation has recently been reported (Wang et al. 2004).

Potential for induction of immunological tolerance or autoimmunity

Most vaccines intended for human use are administered to infants and young children. As a result of the immaturity of their immune system, there is a potential risk that exposure to DNA vaccines during the neonatal period may induce tolerance rather than immunity. As protein encoded by a DNA vaccine is produced endogenously and expressed in the context of self-MHC, the potential exists for the neonatal immune system to recognize the encoded antigen as 'self', resulting in tolerance rather than immunity. Consistent with this possibility, in one report a plasmid DNA vaccine encoding the circumsporozoite protein (CSP) of malaria induced long-lasting tolerance when administered to newborn but not adult mice (Ichino et al. 1999). Co-administration of plasmid DNA encoding GM-CSF prevented the development of neonatal tolerance in this model (Ishii et al. 1999). The simplest explanation appears to be that, although CpG motifs associated with plasmid DNA are responsible for the activation of DC, additional maturational signals may be required to optimize the response to certain DNA vaccines in neonates. Nevertheless, most studies performed to date in rodents and nonhuman primates have demonstrated induction of significant cellular and humoral immunity in neonates (Manickan et al. 1997; Prince et al. 1997; Sarzotti et al. 1997; Bot et al. 1998). Increasing the content of CpG oligonucleotides or co-administration of plasmid DNA-encoding, Th1-driving cytokines (IL-12 or IFN-γ) has augmented Th1-type responses where additional DC maturational signals were found to be required in neonates (Kovarik et al. 1998). Overall, neonatal DNA vaccines, rather than proving tolerogenic, are substantially more effective in inducing Th1 responses than conventional vaccines.

Another theoretical concern is that autoimmune responses could occur as a result of immune-mediated destruction of plasmid DNA-transfected cells expressing antigen. Cytolysis of antigen-expressing cells would release self-antigens for uptake and presentation by DCs, theoretically capable of initiating autoreactive T- and B-cell responses. However, presentation of self-antigen occurs during normal cell turnover and in the course of viral and bacterial infections, without pathological sequelae. In this respect, it appears unlikely that DNA vaccines would pose any greater risk in initiating organ-specific autoimmunity than conventional viral or bacterial vaccines. A theoretical concern that has not been addressed to date is the ability of DNA vaccines to induce responses to cryptic or subdominant epitopes, which theoretically may crossreact with 'self' and trigger potentially autoreactive T cells.

Potential for induction of anti-DNA antibodies

Concerns that DNA vaccines may promote the development of autoantibodies to double-stranded DNA (dsDNA) (believed to be the hallmark of autoimmune disease such as systemic lupus erythematosus (SLE)) arise from a series of observations. Bacterial DNA has been reported to induce anti-dsDNA antibodies in normal mice and to accelerate the development of autoimmunity in strains genetically predisposed to lupus disease (Gilkeson et al. 1993). Bacterial CpG can also stimulate the production of IL-6, block apoptosis of activated lymphocytes, and block the suppressive effect of regulatory T cells (Krieg et al. 1995; Klinman et al. 1996; Pasare and Medzhitov 2003), mechanisms that may facilitate the persistent activation of B cells and predisposition to the development of SLE. Although an increase in IgG anti-DNA-secreting cells has been reported immediately after repeated immunization of normal mice with plasmid DNA, the increases were small when compared with the spontaneous production of autoantibodies reported in lupus-prone mice (Mor et al. 1997). Furthermore, the transient increase in serum IgG anti-DNA reported did not result in either the development of disease in normal mice or acceleration of disease in lupus-prone strains of mice (Mor et al. 1997). Although the possibility remains that a subset of DNA vaccines encoding determinants crossreactive with self-antigens may stimulate an autoimmue response, current data suggest that the level of anti-DNA antibody induced by plasmid DNA is unlikely to induce systemic autoimmune disease.

CLINICAL TRIALS

The first clinical trials were designed to determine whether DNA vaccines were safe, well tolerated, and immunogenic in normal healthy adults. A naked anti-malaria DNA vaccine administered by the intramuscular route was well tolerated up to a 2.5 mg dose and induced CTLs in 11 of 17 individuals, in the absence of detectable antibody (Wang et al. 1997). Pilot studies with an HIV *env/rev* and an HIV *gag/pol* DNA vaccine administered by the intramuscular route also demonstrated that weak T-cell responses were induced in the absence of adverse local or systemic effects at doses as high as 3 mg (Boyer et al. 2000; Tellez et al. 2000). A candidate HIV-1 clade A (HIVA) DNA vaccine (containing more than 25 HIV CTL epitopes fused in tandem to the HIV *p17* and *p24* gene) has undergone phase 1 clinical trials in the UK and Kenya. The vaccine appears to be well tolerated and CTL responses have been detected in a number of vaccinees (McMichael et al. 2002). Ongoing studies, sponsored by the UK Medical Research Council and the International AIDS Vaccine Initiative (IAVI) are testing an HIVA DNA vaccine augmented by an MVA boost (coding the same HIV epitopes). Data reported from individuals receiving the combination vaccine are encouraging for the prime-boost approach and indicate that eight out of nine volunteers elicited CTL responses after the boost (McMichael et al. 2002; Mwau et al. 2004). Similar findings have been reported from a phase 1 trial of an HIV clade B *gag* DNA vaccine boosted with an adenoviral vector encoding the cognate HIV antigens (Emini 2002).

CONCLUSIONS

DNA vaccines have advanced rapidly in the past 10 years from laboratory phenomena into clinical trials. We now have a broader understanding of how they work and the limitations of the first generation of naked DNA vaccines in nonhuman primates, and have an appreciation of their safety profile. Several promising technologies are under development for increasing DNA vaccine potency. Data from the preliminary phase 1 clinical trials are encouraging and indicate that DNA priming followed by recombinant virus boost works significantly better than naked DNA alone. As newer technologies proceed into the clinic, the true potential of this vaccine technology will be established.

ACKNOWLEDGMENTS

The assistance of Philip Hobson with graphic design is gratefully acknowledged. Parts of this review were based on studies supported by MRC and BBSRC grants to LSK.

REFERENCES

Ahmad-Nejad, P., Hacker, H., et al. 2002. Bacterial CpG-DNA and lipopolysaccharides activate Toll-like receptors at distinct cellular compartments. *Eur J Immunol*, **32**, 1958–68.

Akbari, O., Panjwani, N., et al. 1999. DNA vaccination: transfection and activation of dendritic cells as key events for immunity. *J Exp Med*, **189**, 169–78.

Allen, T.M., Vogel, T.U., et al. 2000. Induction of AIDS virus-specific CTL activity in fresh, unstimulated peripheral blood lymphocytes from rhesus macaques vaccinated with a DNA prime/modified vaccinia virus Ankara boost regimen. *J Immunol*, **164**, 4968–78.

Amara, R.R., Villinger, F., et al. 2001. Control of a mucosal challenge and prevention of AIDS by a multiprotein DNA/MVA vaccine. *Science*, **292**, 69–74.

Andre, S., Seed, B., et al. 1998. Increased immune response elicited by DNA vaccination with a synthetic gp120 sequence with optimized codon usage. *J Virol*, **72**, 1497–503.

Apodaca, G. 2001. Endocytic traffic in polarized epithelial cells: role of the actin and microtubule cytoskeleton. *Traffic*, **2**, 149–51.

Armand, M.A., Grange, M.P., et al. 2000. Targeted expression of HTLV-1 envelope proteins in muscle by DNA immunization of mice. *Vaccine*, **18**, 2212–22.

Barnfield, C. 2000. The cellular basis of immune induction at mucosal surfaces by plasmid DNA cytofectin complexes. PhD thesis, University of London.

Barnfield, C., Brew, R., et al. 2000. The cellular basis of immune induction at mucosal surfaces by DNA vaccination. *Dev Biol (Basel)*, **104**, 159–64.

Barnhart, K.M., Hartikka, J., et al. 1998. Enhancer and promoter chimeras in plasmids designed for intramuscular injection: a comparative *in vivo* and *in vitro* study. *Hum Gene Ther*, **9**, 2545–53.

Barouch, D.H., Santra, S., et al. 2000. Control of viremia and prevention of clinical AIDS in rhesus monkeys by cytokine-augmented DNA vaccination. *Science*, **290**, 486–92.

Bauer, S., Kirschning, C.J., et al. 2001. Human TLR9 confers responsiveness to bacterial DNA via species-specific CpG motif recognition. *Proc Natl Acad Sci USA*, **98**, 9237–42.

Bevan, M.J. 1976. Minor H antigens introduced on H-2 different stimulating cells cross-react at the cytotoxic level during *in vivo* priming. *J Immunol*, **117**, 2233–8.

Bird, A.P. 1986. CpG-rich islands and the function of DNA methylation. *Nature*, **321**, 209–13.

Bonkobara, M., Zukas, P.K., et al. 2001. Epidermal Langerhans' cell-targeted gene expression by a dectin-2 promoter. *J Immunol*, **167**, 6893–900.

Boshart, M., Weber, F., et al. 1985. A very strong enhancer is located upstream of an immediate early gene of human cytomegalovirus. *Cell*, **41**, 521–30.

Bot, A., Bot, S. and Bona, C. 1998. Enhanced protection against influenza virus of mice immunized as newborns with a mixture of plasmids expressing hemagglutinin and nucleoprotein. *Vaccine*, **16**, 1675.

Bouloc, A., Walker, P., et al. 1999. Immunization through dermal delivery of protein-encoding DNA: a role for migratory dendritic cells. *Eur J Immunol*, **29**, 446–54.

Boyer, J.D., Cohen, A.D., et al. 2000. Vaccination of seronegative volunteers with a human immunodeficiency virus type 1 env/rev DNA vaccine induces antigen-specific proliferation and lymphocyte production of beta-chemokines. *J Infect Dis*, **181**, 476–83.

Boyle, J.S., Brady, J.L. and Lew, A.M. 1998. Enhanced responses to a DNA vaccine encoding a fusion antigen that is directed to sites of immune induction. *Nature*, **392**, 408–11.

Chattergoon, M.A., Robinson, T.M., et al. 1998. Specific immune induction following DNA-based immunization through *in vivo* transfection and activation of macrophages/antigen-presenting cells. *J Immunol*, **160**, 5707–18.

Chattergoon, M.A., Kim, J.J., et al. 2000. Targeted antigen delivery to antigen-presenting cells including dendritic cells by engineered Fas-mediated apoptosis. *Nat Biotechnol*, **18**, 974–9.

Chattergoon, M.A., Saulino, V., et al. 2004. Co-immunization with plasmid IL-12 generates a strong T-cell memory response in mice. *Vaccine*, **22**, 1744–50.

Chen, S.C., Jones, D.H., et al. 1998. Protective immunity induced by oral immunization with a rotavirus DNA vaccine encapsulated in microparticles. *J Virol*, **72**, 5757–61.

Cherpelis, S., Shrivastava, I., et al. 2001. DNA vaccination with the human immunodeficiency virus type 1 SF162DeltaV2 envelope elicits immune responses that offer partial protection from simian/human immunodeficiency virus infection to CD8(+) T-cell-depleted rhesus macaques. *J Virol*, **75**, 1547–50.

Ciernik, I.F., Berzofsky, J.A. and Carbone, D.P. 1996. Induction of cytotoxic T lymphocytes and antitumor immunity with DNA vaccines expressing single T cell epitopes. *J Immunol*, **156**, 2369–75.

Coney, L., Wang, B., et al. 1994. Facilitated DNA inoculation induces anti-HIV-1 immunity *in vivo*. *Vaccine*, **12**, 1545–9.

Corr, M., von Damm, A., et al. 1999. In vivo priming by DNA injection occurs predominantly by antigen transfer. *J Immunol*, **163**, 4721–7.

Cranenburgh, R.M., Hanak, J.A., et al. 2001. *Escherichia coli* strains that allow antibiotic-free plasmid selection and maintenance by repressor titration. *Nucleic Acids Res*, **29**, 5, E26.

Czerkinsky, C., Anjuere, F., et al. 1999. Mucosal immunity and tolerance: relevance to vaccine development. *Immunol Rev*, **170**, 197–222.

Darji, A., zur Lage, S., et al. 2000. Oral delivery of DNA vaccines using attenuated *Salmonella typhimurium* as carrier. *FEMS Immunol Med Microbiol*, **27**, 341–9.

Daheshia, M., Kuklin, N., et al. 1997. Suppression of ongoing ocular inflammatory disease by topical administration of plasmid DNA encoding IL-10. *J Immunol*, **159**, 1945–52.

Davis, H.L., Michel, M.L. and Whalen, R.G. 1993. DNA-based immunization induces continuous secretion of hepatitis surface antigen and high levels of circulating antibody. *Hum Mol Genet*, **2**, 1847–51.

D'Souza, S., Rosseels, V., et al. 2002. Improved tuberculosis DNA vaccines by formulation in cationic lipids. *Infect Immun*, **70**, 3681–8.

Dupuis, M., Denis-Mize, K., et al. 2000. Distribution of DNA vaccines determines their immunogenicity after intramuscular injection in mice. *J Immmunol*, **165**, 2850–8.

Emini E. 2002. A potential HIV-1 vaccine using a replication defective adenoviral vector. 9th International Conference on Retrovirus and Opportunistic Infections (www.63.126.3.84/2002/).

Etchart, N., Buckland, R., et al. 1997. Class I-restricted CTL induction by mucosal immunization with naked DNA encoding measles virus haemagglutinin. *J Gen Virol*, **78**, 1577–80.

Fasbender, A., Zabner, J., et al. 1997. Effect of co-lipids in enhancing cationic lipid-mediated gene transfer *in vitro* and *in vivo*. *Hum Gene Ther*, **4**, 716–25.

Feltquate, D.M., Heaney, S., et al. 1997. Different T helper cell types and antibody isotypes generated by saline and gene gun DNA immunization. *J Immunol*, **158**, 2278–84.

Freimark, B.D., Blezinger, H.P., et al. 1998. Cationic lipids enhance cytokine and cell influx levels in the lung following administration of plasmid: cationic lipid complexes. *J Immunol*, **160**, 4580–6.

Friend, D.S., Papahadjopoulos, D. and Debs, R.J. 1996. Endocytosis and intracellular processing accompanying transfection mediated by cationic liposomes. *Biochim Biophys Acta*, **1278**, 41–50.

Fu, T.M., Ulmer, J.B., et al. 1997. Priming of cytotoxic T lymphocytes by DNA vaccines: requirement for professional antigen-presenting cells and evidence for antigen transfer from myocytes. *Mol Med*, **3**, 362–71.

Fynan, E.F., Webster, R.G., et al. 1993. DNA vaccines: protective immunizations by parenteral, mucosal, and gene-gun inoculations. *Proc Natl Acad Sci USA*, **90**, 11478–82.

Gebhard, J.R., Zhu, J., et al. 2000. DNA immunization utilizing a herpes simplex virus type 2 myogenic DNA vaccine protects mice from mortality and prevents genital herpes. *Vaccine*, **18**, 1837–46.

Geissler, M., Gesien, A., et al. 1997. Enhancement of cellular and humoral immune responses to hepatitis C virus core protein using DNA-based vaccines augmented with cytokine-expressing plasmids. *J Immunol*, **158**, 1231–7.

Gilkeson, G.S., Ruiz, P., et al. 1993. Induction of immune-mediated glomerulonephritis in normal mice immunised with bacterial DNA. *Clin Immunol Immunopathol*, **68**, 283–92.

Gorman, C.M., Merlino, G.T., et al. 1982. The Rous sarcoma virus long terminal repeat is a strong promoter when introduced into a variety of eukaryotic cells by DNA-mediated transfection. *Proc Natl Acad Sci USA*, **79**, 6777–81.

Hacker, H., Mischak, H., et al. 1998. CpG-DNA-specific activation of antigen-presenting cells requires stress kinase activity and is preceded by non-specific endocytosis and endosomal maturation. *EMBO J*, **17**, 6230.

Hakim, I., Levy, S. and Levy, R. 1996. A nine-amino acid peptide from IL-1beta augments antitumor immune responses induced by protein and DNA vaccines. *J Immunol*, **157**, 5503–11.

Hanke, T., Samuel, R.V., et al. 1999. Effective induction of simian immunodeficiency virus-specific cytotoxic T lymphocytes in macaques by using a multiepitope gene and DNA prime-modified vaccinia virus Ankara boost vaccination regimen. *J Virol*, **73**, 7524–32.

Harbottle, R.P., Cooper, R.G., et al. 1998. An RGD-oligolysine peptide: a prototype construct for integrin-mediated gene delivery. *Hum Gene Ther*, **9**, 1037–47.

Harms, J.S. and Splinter, G.A. 1995. Interferon-gamma inhibits transgene expression driven by SV-40 or CMV promoters but augments expression driven by mammalian MHC I promoter. *Hum Gene Ther*, **6**, 1291–7.

Hartikka, J., Bozoukova, V., et al. 2001. Vaxfectin enhances the humoral immune response to plasmid DNA-encoded antigens. *Vaccine*, **19**, 1911–12.

Hassett, D.E., Zhang, J. and Whitton, J.L. 1999. Induction of antiviral antibodies by DNA immunization requires neither perforin-mediated nor CD8+ T cell mediated lysis of antigen presenting cells. *J Virol*, **73**, 7870–3.

Hengge, U.R., Chan, E.F., et al. 1995. Cytokine gene expression in epidermis with biological effects following injection of naked DNA. *Nat Genet*, **10**, 161–6.

Herrmann, J.E., Chen, S.C., et al. 1999. Immune responses and protection obtained by oral immunization with rotavirus VP4 and VP7 DNA vaccines encapsulated in microparticles. *Virology*, **259**, 148–53.

Ichino, M., Mor, G., et al. 1999. Factors associated with the development of neonatal tolerance after the administration of a plasmid DNA vaccine. *J Immunol*, **162**, 3814–18.

Ishii, K.J., Weiss, W.R. and Kleinman, D.M. 1999. Prevention of neonatal tolerance by a plasmid encoding granulocyte–macrophage colony stimulating factor. *Vaccine*, **18**, 703–10.

Ito, Y. 1960. A tumor-producing factor extracted by phenol from papillomatous tissue (Shope) of cottontail rabbit. *Virology*, **12**, 596–9.

Iwasaki, A., Torres, C.A., et al. 1997. The dominant role of bone marrow-derived cells in CTL induction following plasmid DNA immunization at different sites. *J Immunol*, **159**, 11–14.

Iwasaki, A., Dela Cruz, C.S., et al. 1999. Epitope-specific cytotoxic T lymphocyte induction by minigene DNA immunization. *Vaccine*, **17**, 2081–8.

Jiao, S., Williams, P., et al. 1992. Direct gene transfer into nonhuman primate myofibres *in vivo*. *Hum Gene Ther*, **3**, 21–33.

Johnson-Saliba, M. and Jans, D.A. 2001. Gene therapy: optimising DNA delivery to the nucleus. *Curr Drug Targets*, **2**, 371–99.

Kadowaki, S., Chen, Z., et al. 2000. Protection against influenza virus infection in mice immunized by administration of hemagglutinin-expressing DNAs with electroporation. *Vaccine*, **18**, 2779–88.

Kammerer, R., Stober, D., et al. 2002. Noncovalent association with stress protein facilitates cross-priming of $CD8^+$ T cells to tumor cell antigens by dendritic cells. *J Immunol*, **168**, 108, 117.

Kaneko, H., Bednarek, I., et al. 2000. Oral DNA vaccination promotes mucosal and systemic immune responses to HIV envelope glycoprotein. *Virology*, **267**, 8–16.

Kent, S.J., Zhao, A. and Best, S.J. 1998. Enhanced T-cell immunogenicity and protective efficacy of a human immunodeficiency virus type 1 vaccine regimen consisting of consecutive priming with DNA and boosting with recombinant fowlpox virus. *J Virol*, **72**, 10180–8.

Kim, J.J., Bagarazzi, M.L., et al. 1997. Engineering of in vivo immune responses to DNA immunization via co-delivery of costimulatory molecule genes. *Nat Biotech*, **15**, 641–6.

Kim, J.J., Trivedi, N.N., et al. 1998. Modulation of amplitude and direction of in vivo immune responses by co-administration of cytokine gene expression cassettes with DNA immunogens. *Eur J Immunol*, **28**, 1089–103.

Kim, J.J., Tsai, A., et al. 1999. Intracellular adhesion molecule-1 modulates beta-chemokines and directly costimulates T cells in vivo. *J Clin Invest*, **103**, 869–77.

Kim, J.J., Yang, J.S., et al. 2000. Chemokine gene adjuvants can modulate immune responses induced by DNA vaccines. *J Interferon Cytokine Res*, **20**, 487–98.

Klavinskis, L.S., Barnfield, C., et al. 1999. Intranasal immunization with plasmid DNA-lipid complexes elicits mucosal immunity in the female genital and rectal tracts. *J Immunol*, **162**, 254–62.

Klinman, D.M., Yi, A.K., et al. 1996. CpG motifs present in bacteria DNA rapidly induce lymphocytes to secrete interleukin 6, interleukin 12, and interferon gamma. *Proc Natl Acad Sci USA*, **93**, 2879–83.

Kovarik, J., Bozzotti, P., et al. 1998. CpG Oligodeoxynucleotides can circumvent the Th2 polarisation of neonatal responses to vaccines but may fail to fully redirect Th2 responses established by neonatal priming. *J Immunol*, **162**, 1611–17.

Krieg, A.M., Yi, A.K., et al. 1995. CpG motifs in bacterial DNA trigger direct B-cell activation. *Nature*, **1374**, 546–9.

Krieg, A.M., Wu, T., et al. 1998. Sequence motifs in adenoviral DNA block immune activation by stimulatory CpG motifs. *Proc Natl Acad Sci USA*, **95**, 12631–6.

Kumaraguru, U., Gierynska, M., et al. 2000. Immunization with chaperone-peptide complex induces low-avidity cytotoxic T lymphocytes providing transient protection against herpes simplex virus infection. *J Virol*, **76**, 136–41.

Kwissa, M., von Kampen, K., et al. 2000. Efficient vaccination by intradermal or intramuscular inoculation of plasmid DNA expressing hepatitis B surface antigen under desmin promoter/enhancer control. *Vaccine*, **18**, 2337–44.

Langlade-Demoyen, P., Garcia-Pons, F., et al. 2003. Role of T cell help and endoplasmic reticulum targeting in protective CTL responses against influenza virus. *Eur J Immunol*, **33**, 720–8.

Laus, M., Sparnacci, K., et al. 2001. Complex associates of plasmid DNA and a novel class of block coploymers with PEG and cationic segments as new vectors for gene delivery. *J Biomater Sci Polymer Edn*, **12**, 209–22.

Lechardeur, D. and Lukas, G.L. 2002. Intracellular barriers to non-viral gene transfer. *Curr Gene Ther*, **2**, 183–94.

Ledwith, B.J., Manam, S., et al. 2000. Plasmid DNA vaccines: assay for integration into host genomic DNA. *Dev Biol (Basel)*, **104**, 33–43.

Letvin, N.L., Montefiori, D.C., et al. 1997. Potent, protective anti-HIV immune responses generated by bimodal HIV envelope DNA plus protein vaccination. *Proc Natl Acad Sci USA*, **94**, 9378–83.

Lewis, P.J., van Drunen, S., et al. 1999. Altering the cellular location of an antigen expressed by a DNA based vaccine modulates the immune response. *J Virol*, **73**, 10214–23.

Li, X., Sambhara, S., et al. 1998. Protection against respiratory syncytial virus infection by DNA immunization. *J Exp Med*, **188**, 681–8.

Loirat, D., Li, Z., et al. 1999. Muscle specific expression of hepatitis B surface antigen: No effect on DNA-raised immune responses. *Virology*, **260**, 74–83.

MacGregor, R.R., Boyer, J.D., et al. 1998. First human trial of a DNA-based vaccine for treatment of human immunodeficiency virus type 1 infection: safety and host response. *J Infect Dis*, **178**, 92–100.

McMichael, A., Mwau, M. and Hanke, T. 2002. Design and tests of an HIV vaccine. *Br Med Bull*, **62**, 87–98.

Manickan, E., Yu, Z. and Rouse, B.T. 1997. DNA immunization of neonates induces immunity despite the presence of maternal antibody. *J Clin Invest*, **100**, 2371.

Manthorpe, M., Cornefert, J.F., et al. 1993. Gene therapy by intramuscular injection of plasmid DNA: Studies on firefly luciferase gene expression. *Hum Gene Ther*, **4**, 419–31.

Mendoza, R.B., Cantwell, M.J. and Kipps, T.J. 1997. Immunostimulatory effects of a plasmid expressing CD40 ligand (CD154) on gene immunization. *J Immunol*, **15**, 5777–81.

Mor, G., Singla, M., et al. 1997. Do DNA vaccines induce autoimmune disease? *Hum Gene Ther*, **8**, 293–300.

Moreau, P., Hen, R., et al. 1981. The SV40 72 base repair repeat has a striking effect on gene expression both in SV40 and other chimeric recombinants. *Nucleic Acids Res*, **9**, 6047–68.

Mwau, M., Cebere, I., et al. 2004. A human immunodeficiency virus 1 (HIV1) clade A vaccine in clinical trials: stimulation of HIV-specific T-cell responses by DNA and recombinant modified vaccine virus Ankara (MVA) vaccines in humans. *J Gen Virol*, **85**, 911–19.

Nicols, W.W., Ledwith, B.J., et al. 1995. Potential DNA vaccine integration into host cell genome. *Ann NY Acad Sci*, **772**, 30–9.

Okada, E., Sasaki, S., et al. 1997. Intranasal immunization of a DNA vaccine with IL-12- and granulocyte macrophage colony-stimulating factor (GM-CSF)-expressing plasmids in liposomes induces strong mucosal and cell-mediated immune responses against HIV-1 antigens. *J Immunol*, **159**, 3638–47.

Park, Y., Lee, S.W. and Sung, Y.C. 2002. CpG DNA inhibits dendritic cell apoptosis by up-regulating cellular inhibitor of apoptosis proteins through the phosphatidylinositide-3′-OH kinase pathway. *J Immunol*, **168**, 5–8.

Parker, S.E., Borellini, F., et al. 1999. Plasmid DNA malaria vaccine: tissue distribution and safety studies in mice and rabbits. *Hum Gene Ther*, **10**, 741–58.

Pasare, C. and Medzhitov, R. 2003. Toll pathway-dependent blockade of $CD4^+$ $CD25^+$ T-cell mediated suppression by dendritic cells. *Science*, **299**, 1033–6.

Pasquini, S., Deng, H., et al. 1999. The effect of CpG sequences on the B cell response to a viral glycoprotein encoded by a plasmid vector. *Gene Ther*, **6**, 1448–55.

Perrie, Y., Frederik, P.M. and Gregoriadis, G. 2001. Vaccine liposome-mediated DNA vaccination: the effect of vesicle composition. *Vaccine*, **19**, 3301–10.

Pfarr, D.S., Rieser, L.A., et al. 1986. Differential effects of polyadenylation regions on gene expression in mammalian cells. *DNA*, **5**, 115–22.

Prayaga, S.K., Ford, M.J., et al. 1997. Manipulation of HIV-1 gp120-specific immune responses elicited via gene gun-based DNA immunization. *Vaccine*, **15**, 1349–52.

Prince, A.M., Whalen, R. and Brotman, B. 1997. Successful nucleic acid-based immunization of newborn chimpanzees against hepatitis B virus. *Vaccine*, **15**, 916.

Putkonen, P., Quesada-Rolander, M., et al. 1998. Immune responses but no protection against SHIV by gene-gun delivery of HIV-1 DNA followed by recombinant subunit protein boosts. *Virology*, **250**, 293–301.

Raz, E., Carson, D.A., et al. 1994. Intradermal gene immunization: the possible role of DNA uptake in the induction of cellular immunity to viruses. *Proc Natl Acad Sci USA*, **91**, 9519–23.

Reimann, J. and Schirmbeck, R. 2000. Modulating specific priming of immune effector functions by DNA-based vaccination strategies. *Dev Biol (Basel)*, **104**, 15–24.

Reyes-Sandoral, A. and Ertl, H.C. 2004. CpG methylation of a plasmid vector results in extended transgene product expression by circumventing induction of immune responses. *Mol Ther*, **9**, 249–261.

Robinson, H.L., Montefiori, D.C., et al. 1999. Neutralizing antibody-independent containment of immunodeficiency virus challenges by DNA priming and recombinant pox virus booster immunizations. *Nat Med*, **5**, 526–34.

Rodriguez, F., An, L.L., et al. 1998. DNA immunization with minigenes: low frequency of memory cytotoxic T lymphocytes and inefficient antiviral protection are rectified by ubiquitination. *J Virol*, **72**, 5174–81.

Rodriguez, F., Harkins, S., et al. 2001. CD4+ T cells induced by a DNA vaccine: immunological consequences of epitope-specific lysosomal targeting. *J Virol*, **75**, 10421–30.

Romero, R. and Lavine, J.E. 1996. Cytokine inhibition of the hepatitis B virus core promoter. *Hepatology*, **23**, 17–23.

Sarzotti, M., Dean, T.A., et al. 1997. Induction of CTL responses in newborn mice by DNA immunization. *Vaccine*, **15**, 795.

Sasaki, S., Amara, R.R., et al. 2001. Apoptosis-mediated enhancement of DNA-raised immune responses by mutant caspases. *Nat Biotechnol*, **19**, 543–7.

Sato, Y., Roman, M., et al. 1996. Immunostimulatory DNA sequences necessary for effective intradermal gene immunization. *Science*, **273**, 352–4.

Schattenberg, D., Ledwith, B.J., et al. 2000a. Plasmid DNA vaccines: assay for integration into host genomic DNA. *Dev Biol (Basle)*, **104**, 33–43.

Schattenberg, D., Schott, M., et al. 2000b. Response of human monocyte-derived dendritic cells to immunostimulatory DNA. *Eur J Immunol*, **30**, 2824–31.

Scheider, J., Gilbert, S.C., et al. 1998. Enhanced immunogenicity for CD8+ T cell induction and complete protective efficacy of malaria DNA vaccination by boosting with modified vaccinia virus Ankara. *Nat Med*, **4**, 397–402.

Sedegah, M., Weiss, W., et al. 2000. Improving protective immunity induced by DNA-based immunization: priming with antigen and GM-CSF-encoding plasmid DNA and boosting with antigen-expressing recombinant poxvirus. *J Immunol*, **164**, 5905–12.

Shata, M. and Hone, D.M. 2001. Vaccination with a *Shigella* DNA vaccine vector induces antigen-specific $CD8^+$ T cells and antiviral protective immunity. *J Virol*, **75**, 9665–70.

Shiver, J.W., Fu, T.M., et al. 2002. Replication-incompetent adenoviral vaccine vector elicits effective anti-immunodeficiency-virus immunity. *Nature*, **415**, 331–5.

Sin, J., Kim, J.J., et al. 2000. DNA vaccines encoding interleukin-8 and RANTES enhance antigen-specific Th1-type CD4(+)T-cell-mediated protective immunity against herpes simplex virus type 2 in vivo. *J Virol*, **74**, 11173–80.

Sin, J.I., Kim, J.J., et al. 2001. Modulation of cellular responses by plasmid CD40L: CD40L plasmid vectors enhance antigen-specific helper T cell type 1 CD4+ T cell-mediated protective immunity against herpes simplex virus type 2 in vivo. *Hum Gene Ther*, **12**, 1091–102.

Singh, M., Briones, M., et al. 2000. Cationic microparticles: a potent delivery system for DNA vaccines. *Proc Natl Acad Sci USA*, **97**, 811–16.

Sparwasser, T., Koch, E.S., et al. 1998. Bacterial DNA and immunostimulatory CpG oligonucleotides trigger maturation and activation of murine dendritic cells. *Eur J Immunol*, **28**, 2045–54.

Steinman, R.M. and Poe, M. 2002. Exploiting dendritic cells to improve vaccine efficiency. *J Clin Invest*, **109**, 1519–26.

Sullivan, N.J., Sanchez, A., et al. 2000. Development of a preventive vaccine for Ebola virus infection in primates. *Nature*, **408**, 527–8.

Tang, D.C., DeVit, M. and Johnston, S.A. 1992. Genetic immunization is a simple method for eliciting an immune response. *Nature*, **356**, 152–4.

Tellez, I., Sabbaj, S., et al. 2000. HIV-1 specific T cell responses in seronegative volunteers immunized with an HIV gag-pol vaccine. 2/2/2000 7th Conference on retroviruses and opportunistic infections, San Francisco, California.

Timares, L., Takashima, A. and Johnston, S.A. 1998. Quantitative analysis of the immmunogenicity of genetically transfected dendritic cells. *Proc Natl Acad Sci USA*, **95**, 13147–52.

Torres, C.A., Iwasaki, A., et al. 1997. Differential dependence on target site tissue for gene gun and intramuscular DNA immunizations. *J Immunol*, **58**, 4529–32.

Ulmer, J.B., Donnelly, J.J., et al. 1993. Heterologous protection against influenza by injection of DNA encoding a viral protein. *Science*, **259**, 1745–9.

Ulmer, J.B., Deck, R.R., et al. 1996. Generation of MHC class I-restricted cytotoxic T lymphocytes by expression of a viral protein in muscle cells: antigen presentation by non-muscle cells. *Immunology*, **86**, 59–67.

Verthelyi, D., Ishii, K.J., et al. 2001. Human peripheral blood cells differentially recognize and respond to two distinct CPG motifs. *J Immunol*, **166**, 2372–7.

Vinner, L., Nielsen, H.V., et al. 1999. Gene gun DNA vaccination with Rev-independent synthetic HIV-1 gp160 envelope gene using mammalian codons. *Vaccine*, **17**, 2166–75.

Wang, B., Dang, K., et al. 1997. Mucosal immunization with a DNA vaccine induces immune responses against HIV-1 at a mucosal site. *Vaccine*, **15**, 821–5.

Wang, Z., Trilo, P., et al. 2004. Detection of integration of plasmid DNA into host genomic DNA following intramuscular injection and electroporation. *Gene Ther*, **11**, 711–21.

Widera, G., Austin, M., et al. 2000. Increased DNA vaccine delivery and immunogenicity by electroporation in vivo. *J Immunol*, **164**, 4635–40.

Wolff, J.A., Malone, R.W., et al. 1990. Direct gene transfer into mouse muscle *in vivo*. *Science*, **247**, 1465–8.

Wu, Y. and Kipps, T.J. 1997. Deoxyribonucleic acid vaccines encoding antigens with rapid proteosome-dependent degradation are highly efficient inducers of cytolytic T lymphocytes. *J Immunol*, **159**, 6037–43.

Xiang, Z. and Ertl, H.C. 1995. Manipulation of the immune response to a plasmid-encoded viral antigen by coinoculation with plasmids expressing cytokines. *Immunity*, **2**, 129–35.

Xiang, Z.Q., He, Z., et al. 1997. The effect of interferon-gamma on genetic immunization. *Vaccine*, **15**, 896–8.

Yew, N.S., Przybylska, M., et al. 2001. High and sustained transgene expression *in vivo* from plasmid vectors containing a hybrid ubiquitin promoter. *Mol Ther*, **4**, 75–82.

Yi, A.K. and Krieg, A.M. 1998. Rapid induction of mitogen-activated protein kinases by immune stimulatory CpG DNA. *J Immunol*, **161**, 4493–7.

Yi, A.K., Tuetken, R., et al. 1998. CpG motifs in bacterial DNA activate leukocytes through the pH-dependent generation of reactive oxygen species. *J Immunol*, **160**, 4755–61.

Zabner, J., Fasbende, A.J., et al. 1995. Cellular and molecular barriers to gene transfer by a cationic lipid. *J Biol Chem*, **270**, 18997–9007.

Zhang, X., Collins, L. and Fabre, J.W. 2001. A powerful cooperative interaction between a fusogenic peptide and lipofectamine for the enhancement of receptor-targeted, non-viral gene delivery via integrin receptors. *J Gene Med*, **3**, 560–8.

45

Adjuvants and subunit vaccines

GIUSEPPE DEL GIUDICE AND RINO RAPPUOLI

Adjuvants are substances that, when used in combination with vaccine antigens, induce a stronger and more effective response to the vaccine compared with that induced by the vaccine alone. Most vaccines currently used, especially those consisting of inactivated (killed) microorganisms and those containing purified molecules, are given together with adjuvants. Despite the major efforts made in the past decades to develop new vaccine adjuvants (Edelman 2000), the first adjuvants ever reported in the scientific literature, i.e. aluminum salts, still remain the standard adjuvants licensed for use in human beings.

The development of aluminum salts as the first adjuvants and the development of the first subunit vaccines are strictly linked together. An ideal subunit vaccine is a vaccine that contains the microbial antigen(s) critical in the pathogenesis of the infection, against which we want to induce a protective immune response. Thus, historically bacterial toxins in their inactivated forms remain the first subunit vaccines ever developed. This was made possible by the demonstration of the anti-tetanus immunity conferred to rabbits by immunization with attenuated tetanus toxin (von Behring and Kitasato 1890), and by the demonstration that formalin treatment fully inactivated the diphtheria toxin and guinea-pigs immunized with the formalin-treated toxin were protected against a lethal challenge (Glenny and Hopkins 1923; Ramon 1923). The first attempts to enhance the immunogenicity of these toxoids in animals were reported by Ramon (1925), who observed that the highest antibody titers were obtained in animals in which local inflammatory reactions were induced by the concomitant injection of other substances, such as sterilized tapioca, aluminum salts, lanolin, tannin, kaolin, etc. The use of aluminum hydroxide as an adjuvant to increase the immunogenicity of the diphtheria toxoid was introduced the following year by Glenny et al. (1926).

The approaches toward the development of new vaccines foresee, more and more, the use of purified components of the microorganisms, as native or recombinant proteins, or as synthetic peptides, either alone or conjugated to bacterial poly- or oligosaccharides. These highly purified proteins are less immunogenic than the traditional toxoids and inactivated vaccines, which contain impurities and are much less characterized at the molecular level. Thus, for new generation vaccines adjuvants stronger than aluminum salts are required to induce appropriate effective protective immunity. The correct construction of the vaccine molecule and the use of an appropriate adjuvant system will also be crucial for the induction of the most suitable immune effector mechanisms necessary to confer protection. We had to wait until the second half of the 1990s to see new vaccine adjuvants being approved for use in human beings. Several reasons may have limited the adoption of new vaccine adjuvants (Del Giudice et al. 2001b), among which are safety issues, and the appropriateness of a given adjuvant for the particular vaccine in terms of physical interaction, quality of the effector immune response to induce, and route of immunization that one wants to use. There is, however, hope that research now in progress will result in the development of new adjuvants to be used with existing vaccines, or with newly developed subunit vaccines.

ADJUVANTS

General considerations on mechanisms of action and routes of delivery

Despite the fact that vaccine adjuvants have been in use for more than 70 years, very little is known about the exact mechanisms involved in their biological effects. The depot effect postulated for aluminum salts and other adjuvants cannot by itself explain all the immunological phenomena that are triggered by vaccine adjuvants and bring about the activation and recruitment of professional antigen-presenting cells (APC) which, in turn, induce activation and expansion of antigen-specific T- and then of B-cell populations. The depot effect of aluminum salts, resulting in a reduced rate of antigen clearance from the site of injection, was first suggested by Glenny et al. (1931). However, a large series of experimental data has clearly shown that a slow release of the vaccine over time is very unlikely to contribute to the adjuvanticity of aluminum compounds (Gupta et al. 1996). Very many adjuvants, including aluminum salts, have been postulated to exert their adjuvanticity through their ability to activate APCs and increase the expression of major histocompatibility complex (MHC) class II molecules and several co-stimulatory molecules (Ulanova et al. 2001); however, the exact mechanisms leading to these phenomena are still unclear.

Over the past few years, there have been major advances in the field of innate immunity (Janeway and Medzhitov 2002) which have led to the recognition of several molecules and their relevant ligands as important elements in first-line defense against invading microorganisms. These findings are turning out to be instrumental in understanding the mechanisms of adjuvanticity of several substances, mainly those derived from bacterial components. The family of Toll-like receptors (TLR), first described in *Drosophila*, is emerging as a key player in the delivery of initial signals not only by invading pathogens, but also by some of their components, which may eventually be used as vaccine adjuvants.

Activation of cells by bacterial lipopolysaccharide (LPS) requires the presence on APCs of an intact TLR4: this will induce the expression of inflammatory cytokines and co-stimulatory molecules (Medzhitov et al. 1997). In addition to LPS, TLR4 is also implicated in the recognition of the heat shock protein (HSP) of 60 kDa (hsp60) (Ohashi et al. 2000) and lipoteichoic acid (Takeuchi et al. 1999), which have been known for some time to have adjuvant activity (Edelman 2000).

By forming heterodimers with TLR1 and TLR6, TLR2 recognizes several microbial components, such as peptidoglycan, bacterial lipoproteins, and zymosan (Aliprantis et al. 1999; Brightbill et al. 1999). It is likely that the strong adjuvant activity of complete Freund's adjuvant, which contains mycobacteria, and of monophosphoryl lipid A (MPL), derived from the bacterial cell wall, may be at least partly explained by the interaction with TLR2.

Finally, the strong immunostimulatory effect of unmethylated CpG DNA oligodeoxynucleotides (see below and see Chapter 44, Naked DNA vaccines), which leads to strong induction of a T-helper (Th) 1)-type response, has been shown to be mediated by the specific recognition of TLR9 by these motifs (Hemmi et al. 2000). This leads to activation of macrophages and dendritic cells (DC), upregulation of MHC class I molecules and co-stimulatory molecules, and the production of proinflammatory (Th1-type) cytokines.

Several adjuvants do not, however, contain any microbial components and, thus, there is no indication that their mechanism(s) of action is mediated by interactions with TLR, e.g. it is very unlikely that aluminum salts exert their adjuvanticity through a TLR, because aluminum hydroxide behaves as a good adjuvant in genetic knock-out mice lacking MyD-88, an adaptor molecule in the TLR-signaling pathway (Schnare et al. 2001).

Another point deserves comment. It is now very well known that adjuvants can profoundly affect the polarization of the T-cell response (and thereby of the effector – and possibly protective – immune response) induced by vaccines. Just to give a few examples, it is known that aluminum adjuvants can induce, in animals and humans, the production of antigen-specific IgE antibody (Nagel et al. 1979; Gupta and Relyveld 1991). This is very probably mediated by the high propensity of aluminum salts to polarize the $CD4^+$ T-cell response toward a Th2-type response, through an increased expression of IL-4 (Ulanova et al. 2001). At the other extreme, there is the example of the unmethylated CpG DNA oligodeoxynucleotides (see below), which lead to an exquisite, strongly polarized $CD4^+$ Th1-type response. In addition, activation of antigen-specific cytolytic $CD8^+$ cells may require the use of other adjuvants and/or delivery systems, such as bacterial or viral delivery systems, immunization with naked DNA, lipidation of the antigen, etc., most of which are discussed in other chapters of this book (see Chapter 22, The role of CD8 T cells in the control of infectious disease and malignancies; 41, New vaccine technologies, and Chapter 43, Live vaccine carriers), and will not be specifically covered here.

Finally, because of their intrinsic anatomical characteristics and being the portal of entry of most pathogens, mucosal surfaces represent ideal sites for vaccine delivery. Live-attenuated vaccines (e.g. polio and salmonella vaccines) are given orally. However, nonreplicating, purified antigens are poorly immunogenic when delivered mucosally and may even induce a state of tolerance. The best mucosal immunogens are those with an inherent ability to attach to epithelial cells, e.g. the *Escherichia coli* heat-labile enterotoxin (LT), cholera toxin (CT), bacterial fimbriae, some lectins, etc. (De-Aizpurua and Russell-Jones 1988). The existing adjuvants and the vast majority of those under investigation are specifically designed for parenteral administration. It is thus clear that strong and safe adjuvants specifically designed for delivery of vaccines at the mucosal surface are strongly needed. A lot of exciting research is currently being devoted to this issue, and it is briefly summarized in this chapter.

New vaccine adjuvants

It goes without saying that vaccine adjuvants can be evaluated as such only when they are associated with a vaccine. Consequently, in the following sections, adjuvants are always discussed in the context of their use in association with specific subunit vaccines. Space limitations preclude detailed discussion of all adjuvants under experimental and clinical evaluation (Table 45.1 gives an overview). Experimental adjuvants, such as complete and incomplete Freund's adjuvants (Freund et al. 1937), are not considered because of the major safety issues linked to them, although vaccines adjuvanted with incomplete Freund's adjuvant have been developed for veterinary use (McKercher and Graves 1977), and some have even been employed in humans in the past (Salk et al. 1952). Major emphasis will be given to those innovative adjuvants that in recent years have successfully become a reality in the vaccine field and to those that are receiving more attention within the scientific community. Readers interested in more detailed, technical information on specific adjuvants not covered here are referred to the literature published in the past few years (Edelman 1997; O'Hagan 2000; O'Hagan et al. 2001; Kenney et al. 2002).

ADJUVANTS LICENSED FOR USE IN HUMANS

MF59

MF59 is an oil-in-water emulsion consisting of uniformly small (<250 nm in diameter) and stable droplets of the natural and fully metabolizable oil squalene (a natural metabolite of cholesterol and a normal component of cell membranes), which is stabilized by the addition of two emulsifiers (Ott et al. 2000). The adjuvant is very stable over several years at 4°C and exhibits high versatility because it can be successfully formulated with fully soluble antigens (e.g. viral recombinant antigens), hydrophobic proteins (e.g. the influenza virus hemagglutinin (HA)), and particulate antigens (e.g. the hepatitis B virus (HBV) surface antigen (HbsAg) containing the pre-S2 region).

The fine mechanisms of the adjuvanticity of MF59 are not fully understood yet. The depot effect does not appear to play a major role because the adjuvant does not affect the distribution of the co-injected vaccine antigen (Dupuis et al. 2000). Two days after intramuscular injection, MF59 localizes in cells with the characteristics of mature macrophages. This adjuvant clearly induces an influx of macrophages at the site of injection, which appears to depend on the presence of chemokine receptor 2 (Dupuis et al. 2001). Irrespective of the mechanism(s) of adjuvanticity, from the data available it is clear that MF59 preferentially polarizes the immune response toward a Th2-type functional phenotype, as evidenced by the preferential induction of antigen-specific IgG1 antibody and Th2-type cytokines such as interleukin 4 and 5 (IL-4 and IL-5), using a variety of model vaccines (Valensi et al. 1994; Singh et al. 1998).

The successful results obtained with this adjuvant in the preclinical setting were instrumental in the move toward clinical studies in humans which, as in the case of influenza, have led to the licensing of the MF59-adjuvanted vaccine. Indeed, MF59 strongly enhanced (from 5 to >100 times) the immunogenicity of flu vaccines in various animal species (Ott et al. 1995). It fully restored the ability of old mice to mount a strong antibody response to flu vaccine equal to that observed in young, fully immunologically competent mice (Higgins et al. 1996), and increased the protective efficacy of the vaccine, even at lower doses (Cataldo and Van Nest 1997). In addition, this enhanced response was not affected by pre-existing immunity against the influenza virus (Higgins et al. 1996). This is particularly important because flu immunization is carried out every year and pre-existing immunity can negatively influence the efficacy of subsequent immunizations. The very strong adjuvanticity of MF59 has also been demonstrated with several other viral and bacterial vaccines, not only in mice, but also in monkeys, e.g. MF59 induced up to a 127-fold increase of the immunogenicity of a Chinese hamster ovary (CHO) cell-derived HBV vaccine containing the pre-S2 region compared with conventional, alum-adjuvanted vaccine, with protective antibody titers persisting for several months (Traquina et al. 1996). Similarly, in baby baboons it dramatically enhanced the protective (bactericidal) antibody response after immunization of conjugate vaccines against *Haemophilus influenzae* type b (Hib) and *Neisseria meningitidis* group C (MenC) (Granoff et al. 1997). Finally, MF59 induced a strong and persisting antibody response against recombinant FimH from uropathogenic *E. coli* in cynomologus monkeys, which were protected against bacteriuria and pyuria induced by an infectious challenge (Langermann et al. 2000).

Conventional, nonadjuvanted influenza vaccines exhibit a 70–90 percent efficacy in young adults (Advisory Committee on Immunization Practices 2001). However, this efficacy dramatically drops in older individuals, with a prevention of the clinical illness in only 5–33 percent of the immunized patients (Strassburg et al. 1986), probably as a result of reduced immunogenicity of influenza vaccines in older individuals (Keren et al. 1988). It is thus clear that more efficacious, improved

Table 45.1 *Vaccine adjuvants under investigation: state of advancement*

Adjuvant	Clinical experience	Licensure
Mineral salts		
Aluminum hydroxide	✓	✓
Aluminum phosphate	✓	✓
Calcium phosphate	✓	✓
Bacterial products		
Cell wall skeleton of *Mycobacterium phlei* (Detox)	✓	
Muramyl dipeptides and tripeptides:		
Threonyl MDP (SAF-1)	✓	
Butyl-ester MDP (Murabutide)	✓	
Dipalmitoyl phosphatidylethanolamine MTP	✓	
Monophosphoryl lipid A (MPL)	✓	
MPL + alum (AS04)	✓	
Lipid A derivatives (e.g. OM 174)	✓	
CpG oligonucleotides	✓	
E. coli heat-labile enterotoxin (LT), LT mutants, LTB	✓	
Cholera toxin B subunit (CTB), CT mutants	✓	
Trehalose dimycolate		
Emulsions		
Water-in-oil emulsions:		
Mineral oil (Freund's incomplete)	✓	
Vegetable oil (peanut oil)	✓	
Squalene and squalane	✓	
Montanide ISA 720, ISA 51	✓	
Oil-in-water:		
MF59 (squalene + Tween80 + Span 85)	✓	✓
Surface-active agents		
Nonionic block polymer surfactants	✓	
Saponin (QS-21)	✓	
QS-21 + MPL (AS02)	✓	
Dimethyl dioctadecyl ammonium bromide (DDA)		
Microparticles		
Virosomes	✓	✓
Liposomes	✓	
Immunostimulating complexes (ISCOMs and Iscomatrix)	✓	
Meningococcal outer membrane proteins (proteosomes)	✓	
Biodegradable polymer microspheres:		
Polylactide and polyglycolide	✓	
Polyphosphazenes	✓	
Chitosan and derivatives	✓	
Polyanions		
Dextran		
Double-stranded polynucleotides		
Polyacrylics		
Polymethylmethacrylate		
Acrylic acid cross-linked with allyl sucrose (Carbopol)		
Cytokines and complement factors		
IL-2	✓	
IFN-α	✓	
IFN-γ	✓	
GM-CSF	✓	
IL-12	✓	
IL-6		
C3d		

vaccines against influenza are needed. When given to older people, the MF59 trivalent subunit vaccine against influenza exhibited a very good safety profile, with local reactions that were mild and of short duration and, importantly, did not increase after repeated immunizations in the following influenza seasons (Minutello et al. 1999; Podda 2001). A consistent finding of several clinical trials carried out was increased immunogenicity of the MF59-adjuvanted vaccine compared with the conventional vaccine, which was observed even after repeated immunizations (Minutello et al. 1999; Podda 2001). This confirmed the lack of interference by pre-existing immunity previously observed in animals (Higgins et al. 1996). Two observations are of particular interest. First, a significant increased immunogenicity of the MF59-adjuvanted vaccine was observed in older participants with chronic diseases, such as respiratory and cardiovascular diseases, and diabetes mellitus. Second, the use of MF59 increased the immunogenicity to heterovariant strains of the influenza virus (Podda 2001). More recently, MF59 was shown to enhance dramatically the immunogenicity to an A/H5N3 antigen, from a potentially pandemic strain of influenza virus (Nicholson et al. 2001). This study clearly showed that protective antibody titers were reached with reduced amounts of flu antigens per dose if the adjuvant was used. In addition, the induced antibody persisted for a much longer time and was significantly boosted by a secondary immunization 16 months after the first (Stephenson et al. 2003).

The MF59-adjuvanted subunit vaccine against influenza is now licensed and available in most European countries. The clinical experience with the MF59 adjuvant is much wider than its use with the influenza vaccine. MF59 has been tested in formulation of vaccines against HBV, hepatitis C virus (HCV), herpes simplex virus (HSV), human papillomavirus (HPV), cytomegalovirus (CMV), human immunodeficiency virus-1 (HIV-1), and is being also tested in humans with bacterial vaccines (Podda and Del Giudice 2003). Two major findings from these studies should be highlighted. First, MF59 was shown to enhance strongly the immunogenicity of an HBV vaccine containing the pre-S2 region, conferring seroprotection to 89 percent of immunized patients already after the first dose of the vaccine (Heineman et al. 1999). Second, recombinant proteins from CMV and HIV-1 formulated with MF59 and given to toddlers (second year of life) and newborns (within the first 3 days of life) were more immunogenic and safer than the same vaccines given to adults (Borkowsky et al. 2000; Cunningham et al. 2001; McFarland et al. 2001; Mitchell et al. 2002). Furthermore, as in the case of flu vaccine, the use of the MF59 adjuvant allowed the use of a significantly reduced amount of vaccine to induce high antibody and cellular immune responses, compared with the same vaccine given with alum as adjuvant (Borkowsky et al. 2000).

Virosomes

Virosomes are spherical, unilamellar vesicles with a mean diameter of 150 nm containing 70 percent egg yolk phosphatidylcholine and 20 percent synthetic phosphoethanolamine. The influenza virus hemagglutinin (HA) and trace quantities of viral neuraminidase (NA) from the H1N1 A/Singapore 6/86 virus strain are intercalated within the phospholipid bilayer. The role of the HA in the preparation of these vesicles appears to be that of binding to sialic residues on the cells to enhance endocytosis and fusion of the virosome with endosomes, with the final objective of enhancing the uptake of the associated vaccine and its resulting immunogenicity (Gluck 1999).

Several vaccines have been formulated with virosomes and tested for their safety and immunogenicity in clinical trials in humans, among which are the inactivated hepatitis A virus (HAV) vaccine (Holzer et al. 1996), the influenza subunit vaccine (Conne et al. 1997), diphtheria and tetanus toxoids (Zurbriggen and Gluck 1999), and vaccine combinations (Mengiardi et al. 1995). Virosome-adjuvanted vaccines against HAV and influenza virus have been licensed in several countries. More recently this technology has been applied to the delivery of synthetic peptides from malaria parasites (Poeltl-Frank et al. 1999; Moreno et al. 2001) and from HCV (Hunziker et al. 2002), showing the possibility of inducing priming of peptide-specific cytotoxic T lymphocytes (CTL).

ADJUVANTS AT AN ADVANCED STAGE OF DEVELOPMENT

MPL, QS-21, and their association (AS02)

Monophosphoryl lipid (MPL) A is derived from the LPS of *Salmonella minnesota*. Its adjuvant activity seems to be mediated by its interaction with the TLR2. MPL appears to enhance the migration and maturation of DCs (De Becker et al. 2000) and to promote the generation of Th1-type responses, with enhanced expression of the B7.1 co-stimulatory molecule, and the production of IL-2, IFN-γ, and IL-12 (Moore et al. 1999). The preferential activation of Th1-type cells was also demonstrated in vivo using a 3-deacylated form of MPL. Indeed, immunization of cotton rats with a recombinant respiratory syncytial virus (RSV) chimeric glycoprotein (Prince et al. 2000) or a formalin-inactivated RSV vaccine together with MPL (Prince et al. 2001) significantly reduced the degree of Th2-mediated alveolitis and interstitial pneumonitis after challenge with infectious virus.

MPL has been tested in humans using vaccines against different pathogens, cancer, and allergies. However, probably as a result of not having a very strong intrinsic adjuvanticity and/or an appropriate safety profile, MPL is now being used mainly in association with other adjuvants. One of the best associations studied is with aluminium salts (referred to as AS04, formerly SBAS4). This adjuvant combination enhanced the immunogenicity of HBV vaccine given to volunteers with different immunization schedules (Thoelen et al. 1998; Ambrosch et al. 2000). This vaccine, however, induced a higher local reactogenicity than the conventional alum-adjuvanted vaccine, and did not enhance the immune response in HLA-DQ2-positive participants, who are poor responders to the HBV vaccine (Desombere et al. 2002).

The other well-investigated association is the one with QS-21, referred to as AS02 and formerly SBAS2. QS-21 is an acylated 3,28-*o*-bisdesmodic triterpene saponin (M_r = 1990 Da) derived from the bark of the South American tree *Quillaja saponaria* Molina (Jacobsen et al. 1996). Tested in different animal models and also in several human trials with different vaccine constructs (against HIV-1, influenza, HSV, HBV, malaria, cancer, etc.), QS-21 appears to augment both Th1- and Th2-type responses (Moore et al. 1999) and to favor the in vivo priming of antigen-specific $CD8^+$ cytotoxic cells (Newman et al. 1997), although this last activity still remains controversial (Evans et al. 2001). In HIV clinical trials comparing different adjuvants, QS-21 was associated with moderate-to-severe local reactions (Keefer et al. 1997); it appears, however, that these can be reduced by decreasing the amount of adjuvant used.

The combination of MPL and QS-21 adjuvants in an oil-in-water formulation (AS02) has been clinically tested in tuberculosis, HBV, HPV, HIV-1, cancer, etc. (Kenney et al. 2002). The best experience of this adjuvant system is, however, with a malaria vaccine both in challenge trials and in efficacy trials in endemic areas. A recombinant *Plasmodium falciparum* circumsporozoite vaccine fused with HBsAg plus AS02 (referred to as RTS,S/AS02) protected six of seven immunized volunteers against a challenge with infectious sporozoites. Interestingly, in this study protection correlated well with anti-sporozoite antibody titers, and was not observed in volunteers immunized with the same vaccine formulated with the AS04 (MPL + alum) adjuvant system (Stoute et al. 1997). Six months after the last immunization specific antibody titers decreased to a half/third of the peak titers. After a new challenge with sporozoites, only two of the previously protected participants were still protected, and no correlation was observed between antibody titers and protection (Stoute et al. 1998). The immune response to the vaccine was clearly polarized toward a Th1-type functional phenotype (Stoute et al. 1998; Lalvani et al. 1999). In a subsequent challenge study in a larger number of participants receiving different immunization schedules, this vaccine exhibited an overall protective efficacy of 41 percent (Kester et al. 2001). When tested in malaria-endemic areas to evaluate its protective efficacy against natural *P. falciparum* infection, the RTS,S/AS02 vaccine showed a 34 percent efficacy (71 percent in the first week of follow-up, 0 percent in the last 6 weeks). After a fourth dose of the vaccine 1 year later, the efficacy was 41 percent (Bojang et al. 2001).

This adjuvant system is now under evaluation using other plasmodial antigens as vaccine candidates. An AS02-adjuvanted LSA-3-based vaccine conferred protection to chimpanzees against a sporozoite challenge (Daubersiers et al. 2000). However, an AS02-adjuvanted RTS,S vaccine containing the sporozoite protein TRAP was not efficacious in the human challenge model (Kenney et al. 2002).

ISCOMs and Iscomatrix

Immunostimulating complexes (ISCOM) are cage-like structures of about 40 nm diameter containing the saponin Quil A, cholesterol, and phospholipids. Antigens are incorporated within the ISCOM structure. However, not all antigens incorporate spontaneously into ISCOMs, unless extensive antigen modifications are introduced. Iscomatrix is totally identical to ISCOMs except for the fact that antigen is not incorporated, but simply mixed with the particles or chemically coupled to them (Barr et al. 1998; Sjolander et al. 1998; Sjolander et al. 2001). Interestingly, ISCOMs have been shown in different models to exert their adjuvanticity not only after parenteral, but also after mucosal, administration (Hu et al. 2001). The adjuvant effect of ISCOMs both parenterally and mucosally requires the induction of the production of IL-12. Indeed, their adjuvanticity is significantly reduced in IL-12 knock-out mice, but not in mice lacking the IL-6, IL-4, or IFN-γ receptors, or the inducible nitric oxide synthase (Grdic et al. 1999; Mowat et al. 1999; Smith et al. 1999). It has been proposed that ISCOMs act by specifically targeting adjuvant and antigen to APCs, such as macrophages and/or DCs (Mowat et al. 1999). This peculiar targeting property may allow the antigen to enter the route of antigen processing that will result in the presentation of relevant epitopes within the context of MHC-I antigens, thus leading to the priming of antigen-specific MHC-I-restricted $CD8^+$ CTLs. Indeed, this is certainly the case in mice (Sambhara et al. 1998) and priming of CTL responses has also been shown in monkeys (Sjolander et al. 2001). The induction of a strong and long-lasting CTL response has been shown in rhesus monkeys immunized with the core protein of HBV adsorbed on to Iscomatrix (Polakos et al. 2001). In this and other experiments in rhesus monkeys, ISCOM-adjuvanted vaccine induced strong proliferative responses of $CD4^+$ cells able to produce both Th1- and Th2-type cytokines (Verschoor et al. 1999).

ISCOMs have been tested in a wide variety of animal species (Barr et al. 1998; Sjolander et al. 1998). In addition, ISCOM-adjuvanted vaccines have been clearly shown to confer protection against infectious challenge in relevant animal models, e.g. against genital infection with *Chlamydia trachomatis* in mice (Igietseme and Murdin 2000) and HIV-1 in rhesus monkeys (Verschoor et al. 1999). It must also be mentioned that immunization of macaques with ISCOMs containing measles virus HA and fusion proteins induced high titers of neutralizing antibodies even in the presence of maternal antibodies, which, in monkeys receiving conventional attenuated measles vaccine, were able to abrogate the induction of protective antibodies (Van Binnendijk et al. 1997).

The results of the first trials in humans with Iscomatrix-adjuvanted influenza vaccines have been reported recently. In one study, the ISCOM-adjuvanted influenza vaccine induced $CD8^+$ CTL responses in 50–60 percent of participants compared with only 5 percent of those receiving the conventional vaccine (Ennis et al. 1999). In a subsequent study, the adjuvanted vaccine accelerated the appearance of anti-influenza virus antibody response against the three strains present in the vaccine, induced strong antigen-specific proliferative responses, and induced CTL responses in a higher proportion of vaccinees (Rimmelzwaan et al. 2001).

CpG

The immunostimulatory properties of bacterial DNA have been known for some time (see Chapter 44, Naked DNA vaccines). However, only relatively recently this property was recognized to be linked to the presence of unmethylated CpG motifs in bacterial DNA, which are absent in vertebrate DNA. CpG motifs are C-G deoxynucleotides linked by a phosphodiester bond, and flanked by appropriate bases, which can vary depending on the animal species in which they will be used (Krieg 2002). The immune modulatory effects of CpG motifs depend on their interaction with the TLR9. Mice lacking the TLR9 do not exhibit the CpG-driven effects (Hemmi et al. 2000). In addition, cells transfected with the murine or human receptor acquire the ability to respond to the more appropriate CpG motifs (Bauer et al. 2001). In humans the expression of TLR9 is highest in those cells that are more consistently directly activated by CpG motifs, such as B cells and DCs (Bauer et al. 2001; Krug et al. 2001). CpG motifs induce strong activation of B cells with production of IL-6 (Yi et al. 1996a); they also increased expression of MHC-II molecules and co-stimulatory molecules such as CD80 and CD86 (Davis et al. 1998), and an overall anti-apoptopic effect associated with increased NFκB activity and c-*myc* expression (Yi et al. 1996b). CpG motifs strongly activate plasmacytoid DCs inducing increased expression of MHC, adhesion, and co-stimulatory molecules, and enhanced ability to produce cytokines such as TNFα, IFN-α, and IL-12 (Hartmann and Weiner 1999; Kadowaki et al. 2001; Krug et al. 2001). The outcome of these activation phenomena will be the polarization of the immune response toward a strong Th1-type functional phenotype. This polarization is so prominent that it also takes place when CpG oligonucleotides are administered in association with other adjuvants, such as aluminum salts, known specifically to induce Th2-type responses, and when they are given neonatally in individuals who are prone to develop Th2-type immune responses (Brazolot Millan et al. 1998). These characteristics are now being exploited for the development of vaccines against cancer and allergies (Krieg 2002). CpG has also been shown to act as a strong mucosal adjuvant (McCluskie et al. 2001).

CpG motifs are now under investigation as vaccine adjuvants in different models, e.g. they have shown optimal adjuvanticity in rhesus monkeys immunized with a heat-killed vaccine candidate against *Leishmania* (Verthelyi et al. 2002) and in orangutans, in which they overcome hyporesponsiveness to an HBV vaccine (Davis et al. 2000). In human phase 1 studies with HBV vaccine, CpG motifs were well tolerated, except for an increased frequency of local pain and flu-like symptoms compared with the currently available vaccine, and induced protective levels of antibodies in 75 percent of vaccinees after the first dose and 100 percent after the second dose (Kenney et al. 2002).

CpG DNA is among the strongest adjuvant systems available to date for the induction of Th1-type immune responses. However, some concerns have been raised about the risk of inducing or reactivating autoimmune phenomena in susceptible individuals, because of their strong immunomodulatory activity mainly at the level of B cells and DCs (Bachmaier et al. 1999; Tsunoda et al. 1999; Miyata et al. 2000) and their ability to activate microglial cells in vitro and in vivo (Dalpke et al. 2002).

Mutants of bacterial toxins as mucosal adjuvants

The ADP-ribosylating toxins LT and CT remain the strongest mucosal adjuvants known so far. Their toxicity, however, seriously limits their use in humans because very limited amounts cause diarrhea in recipients (Levine et al. 1983). These toxins consist of two subunits: the A subunit, which contains the enzymatic activity, and the B subunit, which binds to the G_{M1} ganglioside and other glycolipids. After internalization into the cell, the A subunit of the toxin is proteolytically cleaved, binds to NAD, and transfers the ADP-ribose group to the α subunit of Gs, a GTP-binding protein that regulates the activity of adenylyl cyclase (Holmes 1997). This enzyme becomes permanently activated and causes accumulation of cAMP and secretion of electrolytes and water (Field et al. 1989).

The first approach to develop mucosal adjuvants derived from these toxins, but devoid of their toxic activity, was to use their B subunit (Holmgren et al. 1997). It is now clear, however, that the B subunit alone is a very poor adjuvant. The activity originally reported was very probably the result of traces of wild-type toxin still contaminating the preparation of the B subunit. The most successful approach to develop nontoxic derivatives of the toxins while still retaining their strong mucosal adjuvanticity has been to produce mutants by site-directed mutagenesis (Freytag and Clements 1999; Rappuoli et al. 1999; Pizza et al. 2001). Some mutations at the active enzymatic site, such as at position 63 in the A subunit (e.g. LTK63 and CTK63 (S → K substitution)), results in total loss of enzymatic activity and toxic properties in vitro and in vivo, even at doses up to 1 mg. Other mutants, such as the LTR72 (in which there is an A → R substitution), retain some residual enzymatic and toxic activity, although at levels several orders of magnitude lower that those observed with the wild-type toxin (Giuliani et al. 1998). Mutants have also been developed to make the toxin resistant to the proteolytic cleavage of the A subunit. The prototype of these mutants, referred to as LTG192 (R → G substitution), however, retains most of the toxic properties of the wild-type parent molecule both in vitro (cytotoxicity on Y1 cells) and in vivo (rabbit ileal loop) (Giannelli et al. 1997).

All these mutants (and others not reported here because of space limitation) behave as strong mucosal adjuvants in mice and other animal models, when co-administered with recombinant proteins, synthetic peptides, and other vaccine constructs, and to favor the development of protective immunity in appropriate challenge models (Pizza et al. 2001). Interestingly, LTK63 and LTR72 mutants also exhibited a strong adjuvanticity when delivered systemically (Jakobsen et al. 2002) and transdermally (Scharton-Kersten et al. 2000). The mucosal adjuvanticity of these mutants was potentiated when the vaccine and the adjuvant were delivered intranasally together with nanoparticles, favoring the uptake of the vaccine at the mucosal level (Baudner et al. 2002). Furthermore, not only did these mutants prime $CD4^+$ T cells; they also primed $CD8^+$ CTLs specific for the co-administered antigen (Simmons et al. 1999), irrespective of the route used for immunization. If CT and CT mutants appear to activate predominantly Th2-type responses (Braun et al. 1999), LT mutants induce more widespread responses, with a preferential induction of Th1-type responses (Takahashi et al. 1996), even in newborn mice that are genetically prone to mount Th2 responses.

From the data available so far, it is clear that the holotoxin structure of the mutants is important for a strong adjuvanticity; indeed, as mentioned above, the B subunit alone is a very poor adjuvant. The enzymatic activity is not necessary itself, because the LTK63 mutant exhibits an important adjuvanticity. A residual enzymatic activity (as in the case of the LTR72 mutant) enhances the adjuvanticity of the molecule in a dose-independent manner.

Clinical experience with these molecules is still limited. The LT or CT B subunits have been extensively tested and shown to be safe after oral delivery together with an inactivated cholera vaccine (Holmgren et al. 1997) and with a vaccine against enterotoxigenic *E. coli* (ETEC) (Hall et al. 2001). The safety of this subunit has also been shown in humans after intranasal immunization (Bergquist et al. 1997). The LTG192 mutant at the level of the protease-sensitive loop has been tested in humans with a whole-cell *Helicobacter pylori* candidate vaccine (Kotloff et al. 2001). In agreement with the animal studies, it caused unwanted effects, such as diarrhea, in about a third of the recipients at doses as small as 25 μg. The LTK63 mutant is now being tested as an intranasal adjuvant in a phase 1 clinical trial together with a subunit influenza vaccine.

SUBUNIT VACCINES

Subunit vaccines consist of one or more antigens, purified from the microorganism or produced by recombinant DNA technology or chemical synthesis, which are able to protect against disease. It is clear that the development of subunit vaccines requires knowledge of the protective antigen(s), the ability to produce and purify them on a large scale, and the ability to prove their protective efficacy in appropriate animal models in vivo and/or in relevant in vitro assays suited to quantify immune responses that correlate with protection. The knowledge of the effector immune response necessary to confer protection in vivo is also very important in order to construct the vaccine with the most suitable formulation (e.g. the most appropriate adjuvant system) and to deliver it via the most effective route. Subunit vaccines against a wide panoply of pathogenic microorganisms are now under development: some are still at the experimental, preclinical stage; others are being tested in clinical trials in humans (at different phase of development); others, finally, have been licensed for human use (Table 45.2).

The identification of protective antigens is a complex problem, which involves approaches that can differ for viruses, bacteria, and parasites. Viruses have generally small genomes encoding a few proteins, the selection of which for vaccine development is relatively easier than with larger microorganisms. Envelope proteins and glycoproteins are the primary candidates for the induction of neutralizing antibodies, whereas core antigens are usually good candidates for CTL responses. For bacteria and parasites, which have complex genomes, there can be several hundred potential candidate antigens. Therefore, the identification of the potential candidates for the development of subunit vaccines has to be based on a rational approach combining genetic, biochemical, and immunological studies. Until very recently, the starting point was often represented by studies on the pathogenic mechanisms of disease, with the definition of molecules critical in the induction of pathology in the host and/or in the survival of the microorganisms. This approach has been particularly

Table 45.2 *Status of development of subunit vaccines*[a]

Pathogen	Vaccine construct	Preclinical	Phase of clinical development I	II	III	Licensure
Viruses						
Cytomegalovirus	Recombinant glycoproteins			√		
Dengue virus	Recombinant envelope	√				
Ebola virus	Recombinant subunit	√				
Epstein–Barr virus	Recombinant glycoprotein			√		
Hantaan virus	Recombinant subunit	√				
Hepatitis A virus	Proteins in vectors	√				
Hepatitis B virus	Yeast-derived HBsAg					√
Hepatitis C virus	Recombinant envelope proteins		√			
Hepatitis E virus	Recombinant proteins			√		
Herpes simplex viruses 1 and 2	Recombinant glycoproteins				√	
HIV-1	Recombinant glycoproteins				√	
HIV-2	Recombinant glycoproteins	√				
Human papillomavirus	Recombinant proteins/VLPs				√	
Influenza virus	Subunit plus MF59					√
	Recombinant HA			√		
Measles virus	Recombinant HA and fusion proteins	√				
Norwalk virus	Recombinant proteins		√			
Parainfluenza virus	Purified HN and F proteins	√				
Respiratory syncytial virus	Purified proteins and fusions			√		
Rotavirus	Recombinant VPs	√				
Varicella-zoster virus	Recombinant glycoproteins	√				
West Nile Virus	Recombinant envelope protein	√				
Bacteria						
Bacillus anthracis	Recombinant subunit	√				
Bordetella pertussis	Purified/Recombinant antigens					√
Borrelia burgdorferi	Recombinant OspA					√[b]
Chlamydia pneumoniae	Purified MOMP, hsp	√				
Chlamydia trachomatis	Purified major outer membrane protein (MOMP)	√				
Clostridium botulinum	Toxoid			√		
Clostridium difficile	Toxoids			√		
Enterohemorrhagic *E. coli*	Nontoxic mutant toxins/conjugates	√				
Enterotoxigenic *E. coli*	LTB		√			
Uropathogenic *E. coli*	Recombinant FimH		√			
Group A streptococci	Conjugates/M protein			√		
Group B streptococci	Conjugates			√		
Haemophilus ducreyi	Various proteins	√				
H. influenzae nontypeable	Recombinant proteins/Conjugates			√		
H. influenzae type b	Conjugates					√
Helicobacter pylori	Recombinant antigens		√			
Legionella pneumophila	Purified proteins	√				
Leptospira spp.	Recombinant protein	√				
Listeria monocitogenes	Recombinant protein	√				
Moraxella catarrhalis	Various proteins in conjugates	√				
Mycobacterium tuberculosis	Recombinant proteins	√				
Mycoplasma pneumoniae	Purified/Recombinant proteins	√				
Neisseria gonorrheae	Recombinant proteins		√			
N. meningitidis group A	Conjugates			√		
N. meningitidis group B	Recombinant proteins		√			
N. meningitidis group C	Conjugates					√

(Continued over)

Table 45.2 *Status of development of subunit vaccines*[a] *(Continued)*

Pathogen	Vaccine construct	Preclinical	Phase of clinical development I	II	III	Licensure
N. meningitidis group W135	Conjugates		√			
N. meningitidis group Y	Conjugates		√			
Porphyromonas gingivalis	Recombinant proteins	√				
Pseudomonas aeruginosa	Purified proteins/Conjugates				√	
Rickettsia rickettsii	Recombinant surface proteins	√				
Salmonella typhi	Purified Vi					√
	Conjugated Vi				√	
Shigella dysenteriae	Conjugate			√		
Shigella flexneri	Conjugate			√		
Shigella sonnei	Conjugate				√	
Staphylococcus aureus	Conjugate				√	
Staphylococcal enterotoxin B	Recombinant toxin	√				
Streptococcus pneumoniae	Conjugate					√
	Recombinant proteins		√			
Treponema pallidum	Surface lipoproteins	√				
Vibrio cholerae	Conjugate LPS	√				
Yersinia pestis	Recombinant subunit	√				
Fungi						
Blastomyces dermatitidis	Purified/Recombinant proteins	√				
Candida albicans	Surface oligomannosyl epitope	√				
Coccidioides immitis	Purified/Recombinant proteins	√				
Cryptococcus neoformans	Conjugate		√			
Histoplasma capsulatum	Purified/Recombinant proteins	√				
Paracoccidioides brasiliensis	Purified/Recombinant proteins	√				
Pythium insidiosum	Purified proteins	√				
Parasites						
Ancylostoma duodenale	Recombinant protein	√				
Brugia malayi	Purified antigens	√				
Entamoeba histolytica	Recombinant antigens	√				
Leishmania spp.	Recombinant antigens	√				
Onchocerca volvulus	Recombinant antigens	√				
Plasmodium falciparum	Recombinant CSP				√	
	Recombinant asexual stage antigens			√		
	Recombinant sexual stage antigens	√				
Plasmodium vivax	Recombinant cirumsporozoite protein		√			
	Recombinant asexual stage antigens	√				
	Recombinant sexual stage antigens	√				
Schistosoma spp.	Purified/Recombinant larval antigens	√				
Toxoplasma gondii	Recombinant surface proteins	√				
Trichomonas vaginalis	Recombinant protein	√				
Trypanosoma cruzi	Recombinant antigen	√				

a) Only purified antigens, recombinant antigens, and conjugated constructs are included. Conventional vaccines (e.g. tetanus and diphtheria toxoids), naked DNA constructs, and synthetic peptides are not included.
b) This vaccine is not commercially available any longer.

successful for those molecules produced only by pathogenic bacteria, such as bacterial toxins and capsular polysaccharides (a few examples follow). However, in several instances the situation may be more complex and the approach to vaccine development may lead to the selection of antigens which, after being tested in animals, are discarded because they do not induce protective responses in humans. The selection then starts again. More recently another way of selecting potentially protective antigens has been applied to vaccine development. Thanks to the progress in computer science and molecular biology, it is now possible to sequence the entire bacterial genome in a short period of time. This permits the comprehensive testing of all the potentially protective antigens in appropriate animal models, and to select vaccine candidates that would not have been selected based on conventional approaches. Examples of the application of both the conventional and genomic approaches to vaccine development follow.

Past and present: from toxoids and capsular polysaccharides to conjugate vaccines

TOXOIDS AND POLYSACCHARIDES

The first subunit vaccines developed have been the diphtheria and tetanus toxoids (Rappuoli 1997a; Relyveld 1996). As already mentioned at the beginning, the seminal observation leading to the development of these vaccines was that both diseases were caused by a toxin that was produced by the bacterium, and that serum antibodies able to neutralize the toxin were sufficient to protect from disease. The semipurified toxins are inactivated essentially by chemical (formaldehyde) treatment and used as vaccines. For these two vaccines, the titers of serum antitoxin antibodies correlate well with protection. Tetanus and diphtheria toxoids are among the most used vaccines worldwide, because they are part of the pediatric immunizations, which are done within the frame of the Expanded Programme of Immunization of the WHO and Unicef.

In the case of encapsulated bacteria, the choice of the capsular polysaccharide as the antigen of choice for the development of subunit vaccines was based on the observation that mutants without the capsule are nonpathogenic because they are highly sensitive to serum complement. In the case of meningococci, group-specific immunity against disease is mediated by serum antibodies directed against the group-specific capsular polysaccharide (Goldschneider et al. 1969a), through a complement-mediated bactericidal activity (Goldschneider et al. 1969b) and opsonophagocytosis (Vioarsson et al. 1994).

Purified capsular polysaccharides have been used to develop vaccines against MenC, *N. meningitidis* group A (MenA), *N. meningitidis* group Y (MenY), and *N. meningitidis* group MenW135 (MenW135) (Jodar et al. 2002; Morley and Pollard 2002), against 23 serotypes of *S. pneumoniae* (Wuorimaa and Kayhty 2002), against Hib (Ward and Zangwill 1999), and against *Salmonella typhi* using the Vi polysaccharide (Plotkin and Bouveret-Le Cam 1995). All these vaccines have several drawbacks. Capsular polysaccharides are T-independent antigens and they induce transient antibody responses (mostly of IgM and IgG2 isotypes) mainly in individuals aged over 18 years. Their immunogenicity and efficacy are very poor or absent in infants. Furthermore, polysaccharides do not induce immunological memory and repeated immunization not only fails to induce any increase in specific antibody titers, but can also in some cases even induce tolerance in adults (Granoff et al. 1998a). In the case of meningococcal meningitis, polysaccharide vaccines have been proved efficacious in adults and in controlling a MenA epidemic in Africa (Hassan-King et al. 1988). However, the vaccine had limited effects on bacterial colonization and transmission (Hassan-King et al. 1988; Wenger et al. 1997). In the case of pneumococci, the efficacy of the 23-valent polysaccharide vaccine against pneumonia and invasive diseases still remains controversial (Wuorimaa and Kayhty 2002). There is agreement, however, on the fact that this vaccine does not have any effect on carriage rates in children and adults (Dagan et al. 1996).

CONJUGATE VACCINES

The solution to these drawbacks was found by putting together the first and the second subunit vaccines, i.e. the toxoids and the polysaccharides. During the 1920s it was formally demonstrated that the immunogenicity of saccharides was significantly increased when animals were immunized with the sugar covalently linked to a protein, which thus behaved as a carrier molecule (Avery and Goebel 1929). It is now clear that this procedure converts T-independent antigens into T-dependent antigens by providing a source of appropriate T-cell epitopes (present in the carrier protein) that are able to prime carrier-specific T cells; these will provide help to B cells for the production of sugar-specific antibodies. This technology has now been successfully applied to the development of conjugate vaccines replacing simple polysaccharide vaccines. The carrier proteins used in the development of conjugate vaccines are essentially tetanus toxoid, diphtheria toxoid, and the nontoxic mutant of diphtheria toxin, the crossreacting material (CRM) 197 (see below). The only limitation that this technology faces may relate to the overload of carrier protein that patients would receive in the situation where all conjugated vaccines used the same carrier. Indeed, carriers not only help the production of anti-oligosaccharide antibodies, they also induce specific antibodies against themselves. Anti-carrier antibodies present at the moment of immunization with a given conjugate vaccine may suppress the induction of anti-oligosaccharide antibodies. This has been well documented in animals (Barrios et al. 1992), although conflicting observations have been reported so far in humans. Nevertheless, active research is now in progress to select new carrier molecules that would avoid the potential drawbacks of epitope suppression, e.g. synthetic peptides containing selected $CD4^+$ epitopes have been used (Alexander et al. 2000). Alternately, recombinant proteins corresponding to strings of several universal $CD4^+$ T-cell epitopes have been successfully tested as carrier proteins in mice (Falugi et al. 2001).

Hib

The first conjugate vaccine developed has been the vaccine against Hib (Ward and Zangwill 1999). Conjugated Hib vaccines have been shown to be highly immunogenic and efficacious, and to induce immune memory, Ig isotype switching, and antibody affinity maturation in children aged less than 18 months. All these responses could not be induced after the use of unconjugated polysaccharide vaccine. These vaccines have now been introduced in several countries worldwide (often in association with diphtheria, tetanus, and pertussis vaccines), and their use is being implemented in less developed countries. In the countries where it is used to immunize infants, often starting at the age of 2 months, the conjugated Hib vaccine has contributed to the dramatic reduction in the incidence of invasive Hib diseases (Peltola 2000), e.g. in the USA, from its introduction to 1996, the incidence of Hib invasive disease (i.e. meningitis, sepsis) among children aged less than 5 years had declined by more than 99 percent (Anonymous 1998), a decline that has been maintained also in the following years (Anonymous 2002). It is interesting that among the same pediatric population the incidence of invasive disease caused by nontype b *H. influenzae* remained unchanged (>1 per 100 000 children) since the introduction of the Hib vaccine (Anonymous 2002), suggesting that other serotypes are not overtaking, at least up to now, the ecological niche vacated by Hib. The same dramatic drop of incidence of invasive Hib disease has been reported from several countries (Ward and Zangwill 1999), and more recently from a regional study in Italy (Gallo et al. 2002). Immunization clearly also reduces the carriage of Hib, leading to a reduced transmission of the bacteria to unimmunized patients (Murphy et al. 1993).

Meningococci

The successful approach of conjugate vaccine development against Hib prompted several groups and governmental health authorities to consider the development of a conjugate vaccine against MenC. MenC and MenA vaccines had been already developed and tested favorably in humans for their safety and immunogenicity (Lieberman et al. 1996). However, until very recently the development of a MenA vaccine was almost discontinued by major vaccine companies because of the high prevalence of this group of neisseriae in poor countries, such as those in sub-Saharan Africa (Anonymous 1997), whereas the MenC vaccine was fully developed and finally licensed in several countries. The MenC vaccine, containing as carrier protein the CRM197, was strongly immunogenic (Richmond et al. 2001), and in the UK it exhibited an efficacy of 97 percent among adolescents (15–19 year olds) and 92 percent among toddlers (2–3 year olds) (Ramsay et al. 2001). Longer follow-ups will be required to evaluate whether group C meningococci may be replaced by other strains not contained in the vaccine, as observed with the multivalent pneumococcal vaccine (Eskola et al. 2001), or may undergo C-to-B capsule switching as already documented in neisseriae (Vogel et al. 2000). For the time being, vaccine manufacturers are actively working to develop conjugated vaccines against MenA, MenY, and MenW135 to be incorporated into a tetravalent anti-neisserial vaccine. No major technical problems are foreseen for these vaccines. The real obstacle preventing the development of a definitive anti-neisserial vaccine still remains the problem in producing a vaccine against group B meningococci (MenB) (see below).

Pneumococci

Over the past 16 years, since the first report of a monovalent penumococcal conjugate vaccine (Schneerson et al. 1986), mono-, bi-, tetra-, penta-, hepta-, octa-, nona-, and undecavalent conjugated vaccines against pneumococci have been developed using various carrier proteins, and tested in a large number of clinical trials (Wuorimaa and Kayhty 2002). The conjugate vaccine that has been licensed for human use in Europe and the USA contains polysaccharides from seven serotypes (4, 6B, 9V, 14, 18C, 19F, and 23F) conjugated to the CRM197 as carrier protein. This vaccine has been shown to be safe and highly immunogenic in all age groups (Eskola 2000) and to prime memory responses in early life (Ahman et al. 1998). Importantly, it exhibited 56 percent efficacy in preventing acute otitis media caused by the *S. pneumoniae* strains covered by the vaccine (although protection varied widely among serotypes) (Eskola et al. 2001), and 73 percent efficacy in preventing clinically diagnosed and radiologically confirmed pneumonia in infants (Black et al. 2000). Experiments in mice have recently shown that these vaccines can also be delivered mucosally (intranasally) at birth with nontoxic mutants of LT as mucosal adjuvants and can protect animals against a lethal challenge with pneumococci (Jakobsen et al. 2002), suggesting the possibility of immunizing against these pathogens very early in life by alternate routes.

Other conjugate vaccines

A similar approach is now under consideration for the development of subunit vaccines against other pathogens, e.g. a conjugate vaccine consisting of the capsular polysaccharide Vi of *S. enterica* serovar Typhi conjugated to a nontoxic recombinant *Pseudomonas aeruginosa* exotoxin A, was more than 90 percent efficacious against typhoid fever after two immunizations, 6 weeks apart, in 2- to 5-year-old children in a highly endemic area (Lin et al. 2001). Other conjugate vaccines are under development against various serotypes of group B streptococci using the type-specific capsular polysaccharides (Paoletti et al. 2000; Paoletti and Kasper 2002), and against *Shigella sonnei* and *S. flexneri* 2a using the *O*-specific polysaccharide of LPS

(Cohen et al. 1997; Ashkenazi et al. 1999; Passwell et al. 2001).

Recombinant DNA approach for subunit vaccines

It is not always easy to develop subunit vaccines using molecules directly purified from a given microorganism. In several instances, for many reasons, it is necessary to produce the appropriate antigens by genetic engineering. The issue remains, both for native antigens and for recombinant proteins, of how to select the vaccine candidates. The conventional biotechnological approach to identify microbial components suitable for vaccine development generally starts with the pathogens being cultivated in the laboratory. (This implies that this approach can be very difficult or impossible to apply to microorganisms that *cannot* be grown in the laboratory.) The components of the pathogens are then identified sequentially using biochemical, immunological, and genetic methodologies. The identification of potential vaccine candidates requires the separation of each single microbial constituent. This approach takes time, allows only one protein to be taken into consideration each time, and, importantly, permits the identification of only those antigens that are expressed or can be purified in large quantities. In many cases the most abundant proteins are not the most suitable vaccine candidates, and the genetic tools to identify less abundant candidates may be inadequate or not available. It is also possible that antigens expressed during the infection in vivo are not equally well expressed in vitro during cultivation. This approach can take several years to be successful, and in some cases it can totally fail to identify the relevant vaccine candidates. Once a suitable antigen is identified, most often it is expressed in genetically engineered prokaryotic or eukaryotic vectors, and then purified as a recombinant protein. This conventional approach to vaccine development has been successful in some instances, although it took a long time to provide vaccines against pathogens for which the solution was easy. However, this approach has failed (at least up to now) for those complex pathogens, such as bacteria and parasites, for which obvious major protective antigens were not readily available. Some examples of the successes and the failures of the conventional recombinant DNA approach to the development of subunit vaccines follow.

SUCCESSES IN THE DEVELOPMENT OF SUBUNIT VACCINES

HBV vaccine

The first recombinant subunit vaccine developed was the one against HBV (Valenzuela et al. 1982). This development was particularly fortunate because it was already known that the surface antigen of the virus (the HBsAg) circulated in the bloodstream in large quantities, and that the antibody response to the HBsAg was responsible for protection (Mahoney and Kane 1999). The yeast- and mammalian cell-derived vaccine has replaced the first-generation, plasma-derived vaccine. This vaccine is highly effective: it induces seroprotective levels of antibodies (i.e. >10 mIU/ml) in >95 percent of individuals and prevents the development of chronic hepatitis in at least 75 percent of immunized infants born to hepatitis Be antigen (HBeAg)-positive mothers (Poovorawan et al. 1992). This vaccine has now been incorporated into the routine infant or adolescent immunization programs of 129 countries worldwide (Van Damme and Vorsters 2002). In addition to preventing both acute and chronic diseases, mass immunization against HBV has clearly reduced the incidence of hepatocellular carcinoma in children from Taiwan, where it dropped from 0.70/100 000 children in 1981–86 to 0.57 in 1986–90, and further to 0.36 in 1991–94 (Chang et al. 1997, 2000). The HBV vaccine can therefore be considered as the first successful anti-cancer vaccine.

Recent work is now concentrated on improving the efficacy of this vaccine by, for example, using novel adjuvants such as MF59 (Heineman et al. 1999), the AS04 (MPL + aluminum hydroxide) adjuvant system (Desombere et al. 2002), or the CpG oligonucleotides (Davis et al. 2000). The final objective of this work is to reduce the number of nonresponders to the currently available vaccine, and to attempt the development of a therapeutic vaccine for individuals with chronic hepatitis using either available recombinant vaccines or synthetic constructs containing selected HBcAg CTL epitopes (Engler et al. 2001).

Acellular vaccine against pertussis

A genetically detoxified pertussis toxin was the first bacterial recombinant subunit vaccine developed (Rappuoli 1997b; Del Giudice et al. 1998). Instead of preparing toxoids through chemical treatment, as in the case of diphtheria and tetanus toxins, the approach consisted of knocking out the enzymatic (toxic) activity of the pertussis toxin by substituting in the S1 subunit of the amino acids that were critical for enzymatic activity. The mutant at the level of amino acid positions 2 and 179 (Pizza et al. 1989) was further characterized and associated with other *Bordetella pertussis* antigens such as filamentous HA (FHA) and pertactin for the development of an acellular pertussis vaccine (Rappuoli 1997b; Del Giudice et al. 1998). The vaccine containing the genetically detoxified toxin was shown to be safe and efficacious in various trials. It is interesting that, 5–6 years after the primary immunization schedule, this vaccine still exhibited an efficacy of about 80 percent (Salmaso et al. 2001).

The genetic detoxification of ADP-ribosylating toxins was then extended to LT and CT to develop safe and effective mucosal adjuvants. These molecules have already been discussed above. The genetic detoxification will now also be possible for the anthrax toxin, after the elucidation of its fine structure (Lacy and Collier 2002), for the development of a new generation of safer and more effective anthrax vaccines.

Lyme disease

The search for antigens suitable for the development of protective vaccines against Lyme disease, a tick-borne bacterial infection caused by *Borrelia burgdorferi*, has essentially concentrated on outer surface proteins (Osp). In preclinical studies, the recombinant OspA, OspB, and OspC gave the best levels of protection against infectious challenge (Fikrig et al. 1992). The vaccine developed consisted, however, of one single recombinant – lipidated protein, OspA – which in 1999 was recommended for use in 15- to 70-year-old people living or visiting areas at risk of tick bites (ACIP 1999). In large human trials, this vaccine exhibited an overall efficacy of 80–90 percent after three doses of vaccine (Sigal et al. 1998; Steere et al. 1998). As OspA is expressed by *B. burgdorferi* when it develops in the tick, protection conferred by this vaccine is mediated by a transmission-blocking immunity, through anti-OspA antibodies that are able to destroy and eliminate the spirochetes in the midgut of the ticks (De Silva et al. 1996).

Based on observations made in mice (Feng et al. 1995), some concerns were raised on the risk that Lyme arthritis could be induced by OspA-based vaccines. Human DRB1*0401-positive synovial fluid T cells can respond to OspA; this is most probably the result of the recognition of the OspA amino acid sequence 165–173 which is homologous to a sequence present within the α_L chain of human LFA-1 (amino acids 332–340) (Gross et al. 1998). It is not clear yet whether this vaccine can really induce Lyme arthritis via antigenic mimicry, at least in susceptible individuals. A recent comprehensive post-licensure study on serious adverse events after the administration of over 1.4 million doses of the Lyme disease vaccine did not detect unexpected or unusual patterns. Importantly, the number of reported arthritis-related events were much lower than those expected by the safety data reported in the efficacy trial (Lathrop et al. 2002).

FAILURES IN THE DEVELOPMENT OF SUBUNIT VACCINES

Among the examples of failures of the conventional approach to development of subunit vaccines are three diseases, which account for a heavy burden of morbidity and mortality: AIDS, tuberculosis, and malaria. In these three cases, the complexity of the pathogens, the effector immune mechanisms to be induced, and the systems required for this induction are such that multifaceted approaches are required in order to achieve adequate protective efficacy.

In the case of AIDS, the conventional approaches to vaccine development have essentially focused onto the proteins of the HIV-1 envelope, mainly the gp120, facing the serious problem of antigen variability and, as a consequence, the poor ability of these vaccine constructs to induce antibodies that are able also to neutralize heterologous viral strains. More recent approaches are based on the selection of more conserved antigen candidates, such as regulatory proteins of HIV-1 (see below). On the other hand, observations coming from both experimentally infected animals and naturally infected individuals strongly suggest a central role for CTLs, together with antibodies, in conferring sustained immunity against HIV-1. This has implied the development of a panoply of approaches aimed at inducing both antibody and CTL responses through the use of various delivery systems for both DNA and protein constructs. Many of these constructs have been tested, or are being tested in phase 1 and 2 clinical trials. One of them is in phase 3 (efficacy) trial. All these 'trials and tribulations' in the field of HIV-1 vaccines have been extensively reviewed in the past few years in excellent reviews (Johnston and Flores 2001; Weiss 2001; Graham 2002; Letvin et al. 2002; Lifson and Martin 2002; McMichael and Hanke 2002).

A live-attenuated vaccine against tuberculosis (the so-called bacillus Calmette–Guérin (BCG)) has been available for more than 70 years. Despite the fact that it is one of the most used vaccines in the world, its efficacy remains controversial, e.g. it protects infants against disseminated tuberculosis, but not adults against the pulmonary disease (Fine 1995). In consideration of the increasing burden of this disease, the development of new efficacious vaccines against tuberculosis is highly desirable. Several factors, however, limit its development, including the intracellular location of *Mycobacterium tuberculosis*, which leads to the need for the development of Th1-type and MHC class I-restricted CTL responses for efficacious clearance of the bacteria. A further problem is the lack of ideal experimental animal models of infection. Surface antigens, such as the antigen 85, hsp60, ESAT-6, etc. have been tested in the preclinical setting, mainly in the form of DNA vaccines, but also as recombinant antigens. However, most of the approaches rely on the development of viable mycobacterial vaccines and on mixed approaches (Ridzon and Hannan 1999; Kaufmann 2000, 2001).

The situation is even more complex for malaria, the burden of which is increasing as a result of drug resistance and worsening of environmental and social conditions, mainly in Africa (Greenwood and Mutabingwa 2002). Immunity against malaria parasites is not only species specific (thus requiring specific constructs for *P. falciparum*, *P. vivax*, *P. malariae*, and *P. ovale*), but also specific for each stage of development. In addition, antigenic variability has been widely described in malaria parasites. Antigens specific for the pre-erythrocytic forms (sporozoites and liver stages), several antigens of asexual forms, and other sexual forms of the parasites have been characterized and produced under different forms by recombinant DNA technology. Furthermore, the effector mechanisms required for protection are different for pre-erythrocytic vaccines (Th1-type, CTLs) and for erythrocytic (both sexual and asexual) vaccines (mainly, but not exclusively, antibodies). Some of the recombinant antigens have also been tested in still nonideal animal models (primates) and some also in humans, as in the case of the circumsporozoite protein fused to the HBsAg particle (referred to as RTS,S) and formulated with the so-called AS02 adjuvant system (MPL + QS-21 (Stoute et al. 1997; Bojang et al. 2001; see also above)). Despite the low levels of transient protection reported, these constructs must be considered as first-generation candidates that still need optimization for their application in malaria-endemic areas (Good 2001; Richie and Saul 2002). It is likely that an ideal malaria vaccine in the future will consist of a mixture of antigens from the different stages of development of the parasite.

There is hope that the comprehensive genomic approach will provide the solution in the selection of the most appropriate antigens in the development of effective vaccines against malaria and tuberculosis.

Genomics applied to vaccine development

The possibility of access to the whole genome sequences of microorganisms, even the most complex, has entirely changed the perspectives and ways of thinking in the process toward vaccine development. By completely reverting the conventional approach (hence the definition of 'reverse vaccinology' coined by one of us (R.R.) (Rappuoli 2000)), the genomic approach does not start from microbiology, but from the comprehensive genomic sequence of the pathogen and, by strict computer analysis, it can predict those antigens that are most likely to be vaccine candidates. One of the novelties of this approach is that cultivation of the pathogen is not required. This avoids handling of dangerous pathogens and also offers the possibility to conceive the development of vaccines for pathogens that cannot be cultured. In addition, the analysis of the potential vaccine candidates takes into consideration virtually all the proteins of the microorganism, irrespective of whether they are expressed in vitro and/or in vivo, the abundance of the protein, whether it is immunogenic in vivo during natural infection, etc. In this respect, this approach is totally unbiased, because all proteins are equally screened as potential vaccine candidates. The feasibility of the genomic approach relies heavily on the availability of a high-throughput system allowing the screening for the development of protective immunity of a very large number of potential candidates reproducibly and in a relatively short period of time. The availability of good animal models of infection and protection, and the availability of immunological correlates of protection, can enormously help the identification of good vaccine candidates. Unfortunately, good correlates of protection are rarely available and this limits the effectiveness of the approach, e.g. despite the fact that the genome of *Helicobacter pylori* has been available for a few years, the development of a vaccine against *H. pylori* has been based up to now essentially on the conventional approaches detailed above (Del Giudice et al. 2001a, b). The other limit of the genomic approach is inherent to molecular biology, and refers to its inability to identify nonprotein antigens, such as polysaccharides, which are components of successful vaccines (see above), and to identify CD1-restricted antigens such as glycolipids, which represent new promising vaccine candidates, as in the case of tuberculosis (Schaible and Kaufmann 2000).

THE GENOMIC APPROACH TO BACTERIAL VACCINES

Group B meningococci. The first bacterial pathogen to be tackled using the genomic approach was the MenB, for which all the conventional approaches used so far have consistently failed. This is even more dramatic because MenB still remains the most prevalent cause of meningococcal meningitis in a very large portion of the world (Rosenstein et al. 2001).

Unlike MenC, for which a conjugate vaccine now exists and for MenA, MenW135, and MenY, for which conjugate vaccines are under development, the use of capsular polysaccharide as the basis of a vaccine against MenB is highly problematic. The MenB capsular polysaccharide is identical to a carbohydrate ($\alpha(2\rightarrow8)N$-acetyl neuraminic acid or polysialic acid), which is widely expressed by human cells, e.g. neural cells during ontogenesis (Finne et al. 1987). This renders this structure very poorly immunogenic (Zollinger et al. 1997). Moreover, the administration of this polysaccharide as a conjugate may elicit antibodies crossreacting against the self-antigen (Hayrinen et al. 1995; Granoff et al. 1998b).

Another approach to vaccine development against MenB is based on surface-exposed proteins contained in outer membrane vesicles (OMV). These vesicles contain the major porin proteins, other proteins of molecular masses between 60 and 100 kDa, and LPS. In different efficacy trials, OMV-based MenB vaccines have been shown to elicit serum bactericidal antibody responses and to protect against the development of meningococcal disease (Bjune et al. 1991; de Moraes et al. 1992; Boslego et al. 1995; Tappero et al. 1999). On the one hand, these trials demonstrated that the development of efficacious vaccines against MenB was feasible, but, on the other, they clearly showed the intrinsic limitations of the OMV-based approach, mainly as a result of the high degree of sequence and antigenic variability of the major proteins that they contain (mainly class 1 porin protein, PorA). Indeed, OMV vaccines induced protective (bactericidal) antibodies at all ages only against the homologous strain of bacteria; they failed, however, to induce protection against heterologous strains, mainly among the youngest children (Tappero et al. 1999), i.e. those more susceptible to meningococcal diseases. To enhance the number of potential strains covered by the vaccine, OMVs were prepared from two strains, each expressing three different PorA proteins. This hexavalent PorA vaccine exhibited poor activity in infants in which a fourth dose was required to induce substantial bactericidal antibody titers (Cartwright et al. 1999). Furthermore, as a result of the extremely high variability of the PorA proteins, such a vaccine would have the potential to cover less than 50 percent of the circulating MenB strains (Tondella et al. 2000), without considering the risk of antigenic drift or the emergence of pathogenic PorA-negative strains.

The attempts to develop noncapsular, non-OMV vaccines using potentially conserved proteins have also failed so far. The proteins that have mostly been investigated are either variable at the level of amino acid sequence, such as the transferrin-binding protein B (TbpB) (Rokbi et al. 2000), or expressed by only about 50 percent of the MenB strains circulating, such as the neisserial surface protein A (NspA) (Moe et al. 1999).

To identify novel potential vaccine candidates able to induce protective immunity against all MenB strains, the genomic approach was applied by sequencing and deciphering the entire genome of the virulent strain MC58 (Tettelin et al. 2000). While the work of nucleotide sequencing was still in progress, unassembled DNA fragments were investigated to identify open reading frames that potentially coded for novel surface-exposed or exported proteins. Computer analysis predicted more than 600 novel antigens, 350 of which were successfully expressed in prokaryotic cells, purified and used to immunize mice. The immune sera were then tested to confirm to surface location of the antigens by fluorescence activated cell sorter (FACS) analysis and to evaluate the presence of antibodies with bactericidal activity against a broad range of MenB strains, the titers of which are known to correlate with protective immunity against meningococci. Of the 85 novel surface-exposed antigens, 25 identified induced bactericidal antibodies at titers, for some of these antigens, similar to those induced by efficacious OMV vaccines. By analyzing in detail the nucleotide and amino acid sequences in large numbers of strains, it was evident that most of these newly described antigens were very well conserved in strains representative of the circulating meningococcal population, thus suggesting the potential of their use to induce protective immunity against a broad range of strains (Pizza et al. 2000). Some of these conserved antigens that could induce bactericidal antibodies in mice against large panel of MenB strains are now being developed for testing in phase 1 trials in humans.

The information derived from the genome is also being exploited to identify those bacterial antigens that are selectively expressed in vivo at the moment of interaction with the endothelial cells. Using DNA microarrays of MenB it has been shown that the contact of the bacterium with the cell induces upregulation of 189 genes, 40 percent of which are located at the bacterial surface. Five of these surface antigens, not originally retained by the first screening of potential candidates, induce bactericidal antibodies in mice and may represent additional promising vaccine candidates against MenB (Grifantini et al. 2002).

Other bacteria

The genomic, reverse vaccinology approach is now being exploited for the identification of vaccine candidates for the development of vaccines against tuberculosis (Cole et al. 1998), syphilis (Norris and Weinstock 2000), group B streptococci (Tettelin et al. 2002), pneumococci (Wizemann et al. 2001), *Chlamydia pneumoniae* (Montigiani et al. 2002), and others. The entire genomes of many bacteria have been published or are going to be published. The reader is referred to the website www.tigr.org for detailed and fast-growing information. Again, the availability of high-throughput screening systems will enormously help in accelerating the selection of vaccine candidates to move from experimental laboratory models to clinical testing.

THE GENOMIC APPROACH TO PARASITE VACCINES

The attempts made to develop a vaccine against malaria have already been mentioned above. Despite the preliminary results obtained in the field with a recombinant pre-erythrocytic vaccine construct given with a particular adjuvant system (see above), there is still a long way to go before the successful development of an efficacious vaccine able to combat this disease. Malaria, together with AIDS and tuberculosis, remains one of the most dangerous diseases threatening human health. The increase of resistance to anti-malarial drugs and anti-vector insecticides makes the development of an efficacious vaccine of paramount priority. A panoply of plasmodial antigens has been identified as potential vaccine candidates; some have been tested in clinical trials in humans, but none has so far provided the desired breakthrough (Richie and Saul 2002). The final solution may derive from the genomic approach. Of the 14 chromosomes of *P. falciparum*, two have been fully sequenced (Gardner et al. 1998; Bowman et al. 1999), whereas the annotation for others is in progress (website www.tigr.org). The analysis of the whole genome will show which genes are expressed by the parasite at its different developmental stages (sporozoite, live stages, and asexual and sexual erythrocytic stages). Expression of genes predicted to be immunogenic as recombinant proteins or as DNA vaccines will eventually provide the effective vaccine against malaria. The task is not easy, because malaria species that infect humans can infect only particular monkey species, thus limiting the possibilities of high-throughput screening of the candidate antigens, and requiring more and more clinical trials with new candidate vaccine constructs. However, it is encouraging that in recent years there has been an increasing involvement of governments and nonprofit foundations, which has significantly increased the amount of funds allocated for malaria vaccine research and development (Nossal 2000).

Active work is now in progress toward the sequencing of the genome of the other human malaria parasite, *P. vivax*, trypanosomes, *Schistosoma mansoni*, *Brugia malayi*, and other parasites (website www.tigr.org).

THE GENOMIC APPROACH TO VIRAL VACCINES

Despite their small size and the fact that viral genomes have been available for a long time, the information derived from the genomic approach has been poorly exploited for vaccine development. The best example, and also the first, of reverse vaccinology applied to virus discovery and the development of vaccines against viral infections is given by the HCV. The virus cannot be cultured and it has never been observed by electron microscopy. Identification of the etiological agent was only possible through cloning and sequencing of the HCV genome (Choo et al. 1989), which allowed the prediction of the envelope proteins; these were then shown to induce protective immune responses in chimpanzees (Choo et al. 1994).

Until very recently, most of the attention has been focused on proteins from the viral particle, such as those of the envelope and the core of the virus particle. The best example is provided by the long-term efforts to develop HIV-1 vaccines based on different forms of the major envelope protein gp120 and/or on the other structural proteins encoded by the *gag* gene. It is now evident that other proteins, which are expressed in too limited amounts to be purified from the virus or which are not structural proteins (e.g. Tat, Nef, Rev, and Pol), can be protective in relevant experimental animal models and may be exploited for the development of vaccines in humans (Cafaro et al. 1999, 2001; Osterhaus et al. 1999; Pauza et al. 2000; Ensoli and Cafaro 2002). The promising results obtained so far with these 'unusual' antigens strongly suggest that we have to change our way of thinking about the way of inducing protective immune responses and to consider that even nonstructural, nonexposed proteins, and even naturally poorly immunogenic antigens, can represent potential candidate vaccines when they are correctly expressed and appropriately delivered to the host, e.g. it has been shown that the HIV-1 Tat protein is able to target to DCs and to favor their maturation and function, thereby enhancing antigen-specific T-cell responses (Fanales-Belasio et al. 2002), a finding totally unexpected based on the information available from the conventional approaches to vaccine development.

ACKNOWLEDGMENTS

We thank Derek O'Hagan and Maria Lattanzi for the supervision of Tables 45.1 and 45.2, respectively, Paolo Ruggiero and Samuele Peppoloni for critical reading of the manuscript, and Catherine Mallia and Fabiola Lai for superb secretarial assistance.

REFERENCES

Advisory Committee on Immunization Practices (ACIP) 1999. Recommendations for the use of Lyme disease vaccine. *MMWR*, **48**, 1–17, 21–5.

Advisory Committee on Immunization Practices (ACIP) 2001. Prevention and control of influenza. *MMWR*, **50**, 1–46.

Ahman, H., Kayhty, H., et al. 1998. Streptococcus pneumoniae capsular polysaccharide-diphtheria toxoid conjugate vaccine is immunogenic in early infancy and able to induce immunologic memory. *Pediatr Infect Dis J*, **17**, 211–16.

Alexander, J., Del Guercio, M.F., et al. 2000. Linear PADRE T helper epitope and carbohydrate B cell epitope conjugate induce specific high titer IgG antibody responses. *J Immunol*, **164**, 1625–33.

Aliprantis, A.O., Yang, R.B., et al. 1999. Cell activation and apoptosis by bacterial lipoproteins through toll-like receptor-2. *Science*, **285**, 736–9.

Ambrosch, F., Wiedermann, G., et al. 2000. A hepatitis B vaccine formulated with a novel adjuvant system. *Vaccine*, **18**, 2095–101.

Anonymous. 1997. Response to epidemic meningitis in Africa. *Wkly Epidemiol Rec*, **42**, 313–18.

Anonymous. 1998. Progress toward eliminating *Haemophilus influenzae* type b disease among infants and children – Unites States, 1987–1997. *MMWR*, **47**, 993–8.

Anonymous. 2002. Progress toward elimination of *Haemophilus influenzae* type b invasive disease among infants and children – United States, 1998–2000. *MMWR*, **51**, 234–7.

Ashkenazi, S., Passwell, J.H., et al. 1999. Safety and immunogenicity of *Shigella sonnei* and *Shigella flexneri* 2a O-specific polysaccharide conjugates in children. *J Infect Dis*, **179**, 1565–8.

Avery, O. and Goebel, W. 1929. Chemo-immunological studies on conjugated carbohydrate-proteins. II. Immunological specificity of synthetic sugar-protein antigens. *J Exp Med*, **50**, 533–50.

Bachmaier, K., Neu, N., et al. 1999. Chlamydia infections and heart disease linked through antigenic mimicry. *Science*, **283**, 1335–9.

Barr, I.G., Sjolander, A. and Cox, J.C. 1998. ISCOMs and other saponin-based adjuvants. *Adv Drug Deliv Rev*, **32**, 247–71.

Barrios, C., Lussow, A., et al. 1992. Mycobacterial heat shock proteins as carrier molecules. II. The use of the 70-kDa mycobacterial heat shock protein as carrier for conjugated vaccines can circumvent the need for adjuvants and Bacillus Calmette–Guérin priming. *Eur J Immunol*, **22**, 1365–72.

Baudner, B.C., Balland, O., et al. 2002. Enhancement of protective efficacy following intranasal immunization with vaccine plus a nontoxic LTK63 mutant delivered with nanoparticles. *Infect Immun*, **70**, 4785–90.

Bauer, S., Kirschning, C.J., et al. 2001. Human TLR9 confers responsiveness to bacterial DNA via species-specific CpG motif recognition. *Proc Natl Acad Sci USA*, **98**, 9237–42.

Bergquist, C., Johansson, E.L., et al. 1997. Intranasal vaccination of humans with recombinant cholera toxin B subunit induces systemic and local antibody responses in the upper respiratory tract and the vagina. *Infect Immun*, **65**, 2676–84.

Bjune, G., Hoiby, E.A., et al. 1991. Effect of outer membrane vesicle vaccine against group B meningococcal disease in Norway. *Lancet*, **338**, 1093–6.

Black, S., Shinefield, H., et al. 2000. Efficacy, safety, and immunogenicity of heptavalent pneumococcal conjugate vaccine in children. Northern California Kaiser Permanente Vaccine Study Center Group. *Pediatr Infect Dis J*, **19**, 187–95.

Bojang, K.A., Milligan, P.J., et al. 2001. Efficacy of RTS,S/AS02 malaria vaccine against *Plasmodium falciparum* infection in semi-immune adult men in The Gambia: a randomised trial. *Lancet*, **358**, 1927–34.

Borkowsky, W., Wara, D., et al. 2000. Lymphoproliferative responses to recombinant HIV-1 envelope antigens in neonates and infants receiving gp120 vaccines. *J Infect Dis*, **181**, 890–6.

Boslego, J., Garcia, J., et al. 1995. Efficacy, safety and immunogenicity of a meningococcal group B (15:P1.3) outer membrane protein vaccine in Iquique, Chile. Chilean National Committee for Meningococcal Disease. *Vaccine*, **13**, 821–9.

Bowman, S., Lawson, D., et al. 1999. The complete nucleotide sequence of chromosome 3 of *Plasmodium falciparum*. *Nature*, **400**, 532–8.

Braun, M.C., He, J., et al. 1999. Cholera toxin suppresses interleukin (IL)-12 production and IL-12 receptor β1 and β2 chain expression. *J Exp Med*, **189**, 541–52.

Brazolot Millan, C.L., Weeratna, R., et al. 1998. CpG DNA can induce strong Th1 humoral and cell-mediated immune responses against hepatitis B surface antigen in young mice. *Proc Natl Acad Sci USA*, **95**, 15553–8.

Brightbill, H.D., Libraty, D.H., et al. 1999. Host defense mechanisms triggered by microbial lipoproteins through toll-like receptors. *Science*, **285**, 732–6.

Cafaro, A., Caputo, A., et al. 1999. Control of SHIV-89.6P-infection of cynomolgus monkeys by HIV-1 Tat vaccine. *Nature Med*, **5**, 643–50.

Cafaro, A., Titti, F., et al. 2001. Vaccination with DNA containing tat coding sequences and unmethylated CpG motifs protects cynomolgous monkeys upon infection with simian/human immunodeficiency virus (SHIV89.6P). *Vaccine*, **19**, 2862–77.

Cartwright, K., Morris, R., et al. 1999. Immunogenicity and reactogenicity in UK infants of a novel meningococcal vesicle vaccine containing multiple class 1 (PorA) outer membrane proteins. *Vaccine*, **17**, 2612–19.

Cataldo, D.M. and Van Nest, G. 1997. The adjuvant MF59 increases the immunogenicity and protective efficacy of subunit influenza vaccine in mice. *Vaccine*, **15**, 1710–15.

Chang, M.H., Chen, C.J., et al. 1997. Universal hepatitis B vaccination in Taiwan and the incidence of hepatocellular carcinoma in children. *N Engl J Med*, **336**, 1855–9.

Chang, M.H., Shau, W.Y., et al. 2000. Hepatitis B vaccination and hepatocellular carcinoma rates in boys and girls. *JAMA*, **284**, 3040–2.

Choo, Q.L., Kuo, G., et al. 1989. Isolation of a cDNA clone derived from a blood-borne non-A and non-B viral hepatitis genome. *Science*, **244**, 359–62.

Choo, Q.L., Kuo, G., et al. 1994. Vaccination of chimpanzees against infection by the hepatitis C virus. *Proc Natl Acad Sci USA*, **91**, 1294–8.

Cohen, D., Ashkenazi, S., et al. 1997. Double-blind vaccine-controlled randomised efficacy trial of an investigational *Shigella sonnei* conjugate vaccine in young adults. *Lancet*, **349**, 155–9.

Cole, S.T., Brosch, R., et al. 1998. Deciphering the biology of *Mycobacterium tuberculosis* from the complete genome sequence. *Nature*, **393**, 537–44.

Conne, P., Gauthey, L., et al. 1997. Immunogenicity of trivalent subunit versus virosome-formulated vaccine in geriatric patients. *Vaccine*, **15**, 1675–9.

Cunningham, C.K., Wara, D.W., et al. 2001. Safety of 2 recombinant human immunodeficiency virus type 1 (HIV-1) envelope vaccines in neonates born to HIV-1-infected women. *Clin Infect Dis*, **32**, 801–7.

Dagan, R., Melamed, R., et al. 1996. Nasopharyngeal colonization in southern Israel with antibiotic-resistant pneumococci during the first 2 years of life: relation to serotypes likely to be included in pneumococcal conjugate vaccines. *J Infect Dis*, **174**, 1352–5.

Dalpke, A.H., Schaefer, M.K.H., et al. 2002. Immunostimulatory CpG-DNA activates murine microglia. *J Immunol*, **168**, 4854–63.

Daubersiers, P., Thomas, A.W., et al. 2000. Protection against *Plasmodium falciparum* malaria in chimpanzees by immunization with the conserved pre-erythrocytic liver-stage antigen 3. *Nature Med*, **6**, 1258–63.

Davis, H.L., Weeratna, R., et al. 1998. CpG DNA is a potent enhancer of specific immunity in mice immunized with recombinant hepatitis B surface antigen. *J Immunol*, **160**, 870–6.

Davis, H.L., Suparto, I., et al. 2000. CpG DNA overcomes hyporesponsiveness to hepatitis B vaccine in orangutans. *Vaccine*, **18**, 1920–4.

De-Aizpurua, D.H. and Russell-Jones, I. 1988. Oral vaccination: identification of classes of proteins that provoke an immune response upon oral feeding. *J Exp Med*, **167**, 440–51.

De Becker, G., Moulin, V., et al. 2000. The adjuvant monophosphoryl lipid A increases the function of antigen-presenting cells. *Int Immunol*, **12**, 807–15.

De Moraes, J.C., Perkins, B.A., et al. 1992. Protective efficacy of a serogroup B meningococcal vaccine in Sao Paulo, Brazil. *Lancet*, **340**, 1074–8.

De Silva, A.M., Telford, S.R., et al. 1996. Borrelia burgdorferi OspA is an arthropod-specific transmission-blocking Lyme disease vaccine. *J Exp Med*, **183**, 271–5.

Del Giudice, G., Pizza, M. and Rappuoli, R. 1998. Molecular basis of vaccination. *Mol Aspects Med*, **19**, 1–70.

Del Giudice, G., Covacci, A., et al. 2001a. The design of vaccines against *Helicobacter pylori* and their development. *Annu Rev Immunol*, **19**, 523–63.

Del Giudice, G., Podda, A. and Rappuoli, R. 2001b. What are the limits of adjuvanticity? *Vaccine*, **20**, Suppl. 1, S38–41.

Desombere, I., Van der Wielen, M., et al. 2002. Immune response of HLA DQ2 positive subjects, vaccinated with HbsAg/AS04, a hepatitis B vaccine with a novel adjuvant. *Vaccine*, **20**, 2597–602.

Dupuis, M., McDonald, D.M. and Ott, G. 2000. Distribution of adjuvant MF59 and antigen gD2 after intramuscular injection in mice. *Vaccine*, **18**, 434–9.

Dupuis, M., Denis-Mize, K., et al. 2001. Immunization with the adjuvant MF59 induces macrophage trafficking and apoptosis. *Eur J Immunol*, **31**, 2910–18.

Edelman, R. 1997. Adjuvants for the future. In: Levine, M.M., Woodrow, G.C., et al. (eds), *New generation vaccines*, 2nd edn. New York: Marcel Dekker, 173–92.

Edelman, R. 2000. An overview of adjuvant use. In: O'Hagan, D. (ed.), *Vaccine adjuvants: Preparation methods and research protocols*. Totowa, NJ: Humana Press, 1–27.

Engler, O.B., Dai, W.J., et al. 2001. Peptide vaccines against hepatitis B virus: from animal model to human studies. *Mol Immunol*, **38**, 457–65.

Ennis, F.A., Cruz, J., et al. 1999. Augmentation of human influenza A virus-specific cytotoxic T lymphocyte memory by influenza vaccine and adjuvanted carriers (ISCOMS). *Virology*, **259**, 256–61.

Ensoli, B. and Cafaro, A. 2002. HIV-1 Tat vaccines. *Virus Res*, **82**, 91–101.

Eskola, J. 2000. Immunogenicity of pneumococcal conjugate vaccines. *Pediatr Infect Dis J*, **19**, 388–93.

Eskola, J., Kilpi, T., et al. 2001. Efficacy of a pneumococcal conjugate vaccine against acute otitis media. *N Engl J Med*, **344**, 403–9.

Evans, T.G., McElrath, M.J., et al. 2001. QS-21 promotes an adjuvant effect allowing for reduced antigen dose during HIV-1 envelope subunit immunization in humans. *Vaccine*, **19**, 2080–91.

Falugi, F., Petracca, R., et al. 2001. Rationally designed strings of promiscuous CD4+ T cell epitopes provide help to *Haemophilus influenzae* type b oligosaccharide: a model for new conjugate vaccines. *Eur J Immunol*, **31**, 3816–24.

Fanales-Belasio, E., Moretti, S., et al. 2002. Native HIV-1 Tat protein targets monocyte-derived dendritic cells and enhances their maturation, function, and antigen-specific T cell responses. *J Immunol*, **168**, 197–206.

Feng, S., Barthold, S.W., et al. 1995. Lyme disease in human DR4Dw4-transgenic mice. *J Infect Dis*, **172**, 286–9.

Field, M., Rao, M.C. and Chang, E.B. 1989. Intestinal electrolyte transport and diarrhoeal disease. 2. *N Engl J Med*, **321**, 800–6.

Fikrig, E., Barthold, S.W., et al. 1992. Role of OspA, OspB, and flagellin in protective immunity to Lyme borreliosis in laboratory mice. *Infect Immun*, **59**, 553–9.

Fine, P.E. 1995. Variation in protection by BCG: implications of and for heterologous immunity. *Lancet*, **346**, 1339–45.

Finne, J., Bitter-Suermann, D., et al. 1987. An IgG monoclonal antibody to group B meningococci cross-reacts with developmentally regulated polysialic acid units of glycoproteins in neural and extraneural tissues. *J Immunol*, **138**, 4402–7.

Freund, J., Casals, J. and Hosmer, E.P. 1937. Sensitization and antibody formation after injection of tubercle bacilli and paraffin oil. *Proc Exp Biol Med*, **37**, 509–13.

Freytag, L.C. and Clements, J.D. 1999. Bacterial toxins as mucosal adjuvants. *Curr Top Microbiol Immunol*, **236**, 215–36.

Gallo, G., Ciofi degli Atti, M.L., et al. 2002. Impact of regional Hib vaccination programme in Italy. *Vaccine*, **20**, 993–5.

Gardner, M.J., Tettelin, H., et al. 1998. Chromosome 2 sequence of the human malaria parasite *Plasmodium falciparum*. *Science*, **282**, 1126–32.

Giannelli, V., Fontana, M.R., et al. 1997. Protease susceptibility and toxicity of heat-labile enterotoxins with a mutation in the active site or in the protease-sensitive loop. *Infect Immun*, **65**, 331–4.

Giuliani, M.M., Del Giudice, G., et al. 1998. Mucosal adjuvanticity and immunogenicity of LTR72, a novel mutant of *Escherichia coli* heat-labile enterotoxin with partial knockout of ADP-ribosyltransferase activity. *J Exp Med*, **187**, 1123–32.

Glenny, A.T. and Hopkins, B.E. 1923. Diphtheria toxoid as an immunizing agent. *Br J Exp Pathol*, **4**, 283–8.

Glenny, A.T., Pope, C.G., et al. 1926. The antigenic value of toxoid precipitated by potassium alum. *J Pathol Bacteriol*, **29**, 38–9.

Glenny, A.T., Buttle, A.H. and Stevens, M.F. 1931. Rate of disappearance of diphtheria toxoid injected into rabbits and guinea pigs: toxoid precipitated with alum. *J Pathol Bacteriol*, **34**, 267–75.

Gluck, R. 1999. Adjuvant activity of immunopotentiating reconstituted influenza virosomes (IRIVs). *Vaccine*, **17**, 1782–7.

Goldschneider, I., Gotschlich, E.C. and Artenstein, M.S. 1969a. Human immunity to the meningococcus. I. The role of humoral antibodies. *J Exp Med*, **129**, 1307–26.

Goldschneider, I., Gotschlich, E.C. and Artenstein, M.S. 1969b. Human immunity to the meningococcus. II. Development of natural immunity. *J Exp Med*, **129**, 1327–48.

Good, M.F. 2001. Towards a blood-stage vaccine for malaria: are we following all the leads? *Nat Rev Immunol*, **1**, 117–25.

Graham, B.S. 2002. Clinical trials of HIV vaccines. *Annu Rev Med*, **53**, 207–21.

Granoff, D.M., McHugh, Y.E., et al. 1997. MF59 adjuvant enhances antibody response to infant baboons immunized with *Haemophilus influenzae* type b and *Neisseria meningitidis* group C oligosaccharide-CRM197 conjugate vaccine. *Infect Immun*, **65**, 1710–15.

Granoff, D.M., Gupta, R.K., et al. 1998a. Induction of immunologic refractoriness in adults by meningococcal C polysaccharide vaccination. *J Infect Dis*, **178**, 870–4.

Granoff, D.M., Bartoloni, A., et al. 1998b. Bactericidal monoclonal antibodies that define unique meningococcal B polysaccharide epitopes that do not cross-react with human polysialic acid. *J Immunol*, **160**, 5028–36.

Grdic, D., Smith, R., et al. 1999. The mucosal adjuvant effects of cholera toxin and immune-stimulating complexes differ in their requirement for IL-12, indicating different pathways of action. *Eur J Immunol*, **29**, 1774–84.

Greenwood, B. and Mutabingwa, T. 2002. Malaria in 2002. *Nature*, **415**, 670–2.

Grifantini, R., Bartolini, E., et al. 2002. Previously unrecognized vaccine candidates against group B meningococcus identified by DNA microarrays. *Nat Biotechnol*, **20**, 914–21.

Gross, D.M., Forsthuber, T., et al. 1998. Identification of LFA-1 as a candidate autoantigen in treatment-resistant Lyme arthritis. *Science*, **281**, 703–6.

Gupta, R.K. and Relyveld, E.H. 1991. Adverse reactions after injection of adsorbed diphtheria-pertussis-tetanus (DPT) vaccine are not only due to pertussis organisms or pertussis components in the vaccine. *Vaccine*, **9**, 699–702.

Gupta, R.K., Chang, A.C., et al. 1996. In vivo distribution of radioactivity in mice after injection of biodegradable polymer microspheres containing ^{14}C-labeled tetanus toxoid. *Vaccine*, **14**, 1412–16.

Hall, E.R., Wierzba, T.F., et al. 2001. Induction of antifimbria and antitoxin antibody responses in Egyptian children and adults by an oral, killed enterotoxigenic *Escherichia coli* plus cholera toxin B subunit vaccine. *Infect Immun*, **69**, 2853–7.

Hartmann, G. and Weiner, G.J. 1999. CpG DNA: a potent signal for growth, activation, and maturation of human dendritic cells. *Proc Natl Acad Sci USA*, **96**, 1119–29.

Hassan-King, M.K.A., Wall, R.A. and Greenwood, B.M. 1988. Meningococcal carriage, meningococcal disease and vaccination. *J Infect*, **16**, 55–9.

Hayrinen, J., Jennings, H., et al. 1995. Antibodies to polysialic acid and its N-propyl derivative: binding properties and interaction with human embryonal brain glycopeptides. *J Infect Dis*, **171**, 1481–90.

Heineman, T.C., Clements-Mann, M.L., et al. 1999. A randomized, controlled study in adults of the immunogenicity of a novel hepatitis B vaccine containing MF59 adjuvant. *Vaccine*, **17**, 2769–28.

Hemmi, H., Tekeuchi, O., et al. 2000. A Toll-like receptor recognizes bacterial DNA. *Nature*, **408**, 740–5.

Higgins, D.A., Carlson, J.R. and Van Nest, G. 1996. MF59 enhances the immunogenicity of influenza vaccine in both young and old mice. *Vaccine*, **14**, 478–84.

Holmes, R.K. 1997. Heat-labile enterotoxins (*Escherichia coli*). In: Rappuoli, R. and Montecucco, C. (eds), *Guidebook to protein toxins and their use in cell biology*. Oxford: Oxford University Press, 30–3.

Holmgren, J., Jertborn, M. and Svennerholm, A.M. 1997. New and improved vaccines against cholera. II. Oral B subunit killed whole-cell cholera vaccine. In: Levine, M.M., Woodrow, G.C., et al. (eds), *New generation vaccines*, 2nd edn. New York: Marcel Dekker, 459–68.

Holzer, B.R., Hatz, C., et al. 1996. Immunogenicity and adverse effects of an inactivated virosome versus alum-adsorbed hepatitis A vaccine: a randomized controlled trial. *Vaccine*, **14**, 982–6.

Hu, K.F., Lovgtren-Bengtsson, K. and Morein, B. 2001. Immunostimulating complexes (ISCOMs) for nasal vaccination. *Adv Drug Deliv Rev*, **51**, 149–59.

Hunziker, I.P., Grabscheid, B., et al. 2002. In vitro studies of core-peptides bearing immunopotentiating reconstituted influenza virosomes as a non-live prototype vaccine against hepatitis C virus. *Int Immunol*, **14**, 615–26.

Igietseme, J.U. and Murdin, A. 2000. Induction of protective immunity against *Chlamydia trachomatis* genital infection by a vaccine based on major outer membrane protein-lipophilic immune response-stimulating complexes. *Infect Immun*, **68**, 6798–806.

Jacobsen, N.E., Fairbrother, W.J., et al. 1996. Structure of the saponin adjuvant QS-21 and its base-catalyzed isomerization product by ^{1}H- and natural abundance ^{13}C NMR spectroscopy. *Carbohydr Res*, **280**, 1–14.

Jakobsen, S.T., Bjarnarson, S., et al. 2002. Intranasal immunization with penumococcal conjugate vaccines with LTK63, a non toxic mutant of heat-labile enterotoxin, as adjuvant rapidly induces protective immunity against lethal pneumococcal infections in neonatal mice. *Infect Immun*, **70**, 1443–52.

Janeway, C.A. Jr. and Medzhitov, R. 2002. Innate immune recognition. *Annu Rev Immunol*, **20**, 197–216.

Jodar, L., Feavers, I.M., et al. 2002. Development of vaccines against meningococcal disease. *Lancet*, **359**, 1499–508.

Johnston, M.I. and Flores, J. 2001. Progress in HIV vaccine development. *Curr Opin Pharmacol*, **1**, 504–10.

Kadowaki, N., Ho, S., et al. 2001. Subsets of human dendritic cell precursors express different toll-like receptors and respond to different microbial antigens. *J Exp Med*, **194**, 863–70.

Kaufmann, S.H.E. 2000. Is the development of a new tuberculosis vaccine possible? *Nat Med*, **6**, 955–60.

Kaufmann, S.H.E. 2001. How can immunology contribute to the control of tuberculosis? *Nat Rev Immunol*, **1**, 20–30.

Keefer, M.C., Wolff, M., et al. 1997. Safety profile of phase I and II preventive HIV type, 1 envelope vaccination: experience of the NIAID AIDS Vaccine Evaluation Group. *AIDS Res Hum Retroviruses*, **13**, 1163–77.

Kenney, R.T., Rabinovich, N.R., et al. 2002. Second meeting on novel adjuvants currently in/close to human clinical testing. *Vaccine*, **20**, 2155–63.

Keren, G., Segev, S., et al. 1988. Failure of influenza vaccination in the aged. *J Med Virol*, **25**, 85–9.

Kester, K.E., McKinney, D.A., et al. 2001. Efficacy of recombinant circumsporozoite protein vaccine regimens against experimental *Plasmodium falciparum* malaria. *J Infect Dis*, **183**, 640–7.

Kotloff, K.L., Sztein, M.B., et al. 2001. Safety and immunogenicity of oral inactivated whole-cell *Helicobacter pylori* vaccine with adjuvant among volunteers with or without subclinical infection. *Infect Immun*, **69**, 3581–90.

Krieg, A.M. 2002. CpG motifs in bacterial DNA and their immune effects. *Annu Rev Immunol*, **20**, 709–60.

Krug, A., Towarowski, A., et al. 2001. Toll-like receptor expression reveals CpG DNA as a unique microbial stimulus for plasmacytoid dendritic cells which synergizes with CD40 ligand to induce high amounts of IL-12. *Eur J Immunol*, **31**, 3026–37.

Lacy, D.B. and Collier, R.J. 2002. Structure and function of anthrax toxin. *Curr Top Microbiol Immunol*, **271**, 61–85.

Lalvani, A., Moris, P., et al. 1999. Potent induction of focused Th1-type cellular and humoral immune responses by RTS,S/SBAS2, a recombinant *Plasmodium falciparum* malaria vaccine. *J Infect Dis*, **180**, 1656–64.

Langermann, S., Moellby, R., et al. 2000. Vaccination with FimH adhesin protects cynomolgus monkeys from colonization and infection by uropathogenic *Escherichia coli*. *J Infect Dis*, **181**, 774–8.

Lathrop, S.L., Ball, R., et al. 2002. Adverse event reports following vaccination for Lyme disease: December 1998–July 2000. *Vaccine*, **20**, 1603–8.

Letvin, N.L., Barouch, D.H. and Montefiori, D.C. 2002. Prospects for vaccine protection against HIV-1 infection and AIDS. *Annu Rev Immunol*, **20**, 73–99.

Levine, M.M., Kaper, J.B., et al. 1983. New knowledge on pathogenesis of bacterial enteric infections as applied to vaccine development. *Microbiol Rev*, **47**, 510–50.

Lieberman, J.M., Chiu, S.S., et al. 1996. Safety and immunogenicity of a serogroup A/C *Neisseria meningitidis* oligosaccharide-protein conjugate vaccine in young children: a randomized controlled trial. *JAMA*, **275**, 1499–503.

Lifson, J.D. and Martin, M.A. 2002. AIDS vaccines. One step forwards, one step back. *Nature*, **415**, 272–3.

Lin, F.Y., Ho, V.A., et al. 2001. The efficacy of a *Salmonella typhi* Vi conjugate vaccine in two- to-five-year-old children. *N Engl J Med*, **344**, 1263–9.

McCluskie, M.J., Weeratna, R.D., et al. 2001. The potential of CpG oligodeoxynucleotides as mucosal adjuvants. *Crit Rev Immunol*, **21**, 103–20.

McFarland, E.J., Borkowsky, W., et al. 2001. Human immunodeficiency virus type, 1 (HIV-1) gp120-specific antibodies in neonates receiving an HIV-1 recombinant gp120 vaccine. *J Infect Dis*, **184**, 1331–5.

McKercher, P.D. and Graves, J.H. 1977. A review of the current status of oil adjuvants in foot-and-mouth disease vaccines. *Dev Biol Stand*, **35**, 107–12.

McMichael, A. and Hanke, T. 2002. The quest for an AIDS vaccine: is the CD8+ T-cell approach feasible? *Nat Rev Immunol*, **2**, 283–91.

Mahoney, F.J. and Kane, M. 1999. Hepatitis B vaccine. In: Plotkin, S.A. and Orenstein, W.A. (eds), *Vaccines*, 3rd edn. Philadelphia: Saunders, 158–82.

Medzhitov, R., Preston-Hurlburt, P. and Janeway, C.A. Jr. 1997. A human homologue of the *Drosophila* Toll protein signals activation of adaptive immunity. *Nature*, **388**, 394–7.

Mengiardi, B., Berger, R., et al. 1995. Virosomes as carriers for combined vaccines. *Vaccine*, **13**, 1306–15.

Minutello, M., Senatore, F., et al. 1999. Safety and immunogenicity of an inactivated subunit influenza vaccine combined with MF59 adjuvant emulsion in elderly subjects, immunized for three consecutive influenza seasons. *Vaccine*, **17**, 99–104.

Mitchell, D.K., Holmes, S.J., et al. 2002. Immunogenicity of a recombinant human cytomegalovirus gB vaccine in seronegative toddlers. *Pediatr Infect Dis J*, **21**, 133–8.

Miyata, M., Kobayashi, H., et al. 2000. Unmethylated oligo-DNA containing CpG motifs aggravates collagen-induced arthritis in mice. *Arthritis Rheum*, **43**, 2578–82.

Moe, G.R., Tan, S. and Granoff, D.M. 1999. Differences in surface expression of NspA among *Neisseria meningitidis* group B strains. *Infect Immun*, **67**, 5664–75.

Montigiani, S., Falugi, F., et al. 2002. Genomic approach for analysis of surface proteins in *Chlamydia penumoniae*. *Infect Immun*, **70**, 368–79.

Moore, A., McCarthy, L. and Mills, K.H. 1999. The adjuvant combination monophosphoryl lipid A and QS-21 switches T cell responses induced with a soluble recombinant HIV protein from Th2 to Th1. *Vaccine*, **17**, 2517–27.

Moreno, R., Jiang, L., et al. 2001. Exploiting conformationally constrained peptidomimetics and an efficient human-compatible delivery system in synthetic vaccine design. *Chembiochem*, **2**, 838–43.

Morley, S.L. and Pollard, A.J. 2002. Vaccine prevention of meningococcal disease, coming soon? *Vaccine*, **20**, 666–87.

Mowat, A.M., Smith, R.E., et al. 1999. Oral vaccination with immune stimulating complexes. *Immunol Lett*, **65**, 133–40.

Murphy, T.V., Pastor, P., et al. 1993. Decreased *Haemophilus* colonization in children vaccinated with *Haemophilus influenzae* type b conjugate vaccine. *J Pediatr*, **122**, 517–23.

Nagel, J.E., White, C., et al. 1979. IgE synthesis in man. II. Comparison of tetanus and diphtheria IgE antibody in allergic and nonallergic children. *J Allergy Clin Immunol*, **63**, 308–14.

Newman, M.J., Wu, J.Y., et al. 1997. Induction of cross-reactive cytotoxic T-lymphocyte responses specific for HIV-1 gp120 using saponin adjuvant (QS-21) supplemented subunit vaccine formulations. *Vaccine*, **15**, 1001–7.

Nicholson, K.G., Colegate, A.E., et al. 2001. Safety and antigenicity of non-adjuvanted and MF59-adjuvanted influenza A/Duck/Singapore/97 (H5N3) vaccine: a randomized trial of two potential vaccines against H5N1 influenza. *Lancet*, **357**, 1937–43.

Norris, S.J. and Weinstock, G.M. 2000. The genome sequence of *Treponema pallidum*, the syphilis spirochete: will clinicians benefit? *Curr Opin Infect Dis*, **13**, 29–36.

Nossal, G.J. 2000. The global alliance for vaccine and immunization – a millennium challenge. *Nat Immunol*, **1**, 5–8.

O'Hagan, D.T. (ed.) 2000. *Vaccine adjuvants: Preparation methods and research protocols*. Totowa, NJ: Humana Press.

O'Hagan, D.T., MacKichan, M.L. and Singh, M. 2001. Recent developments in adjuvants for vaccines against infectious diseases. *Biomol Eng*, **18**, 69–85.

Ohashi, K., Burkart, V., et al. 2000. Heat shock protein 60 is a putative endogenous ligand of the toll-like receptor-4 complex. *J Immunol*, **164**, 558–61.

Osterhaus, A.D., van Baalen, C.A., et al. 1999. Vaccination with Rev and Tat against AIDS. *Vaccine*, **17**, 2713–14.

Ott, G., Barchfeld, G.L. and Van Nest, G. 1995. Enhancement of humoral response against human influenza vaccine with the simple submicron oil/water emulsion adjuvant MF59. *Vaccine*, **13**, 1557–62.

Ott, G., Radhakrishnan, R., et al. 2000. The adjuvant MF59: a 10-year perspective. In: O'Hagan, D. (ed.), *Vaccine adjuvants: Preparation methods and research protocols*. Totowa, NJ: Humana Press, 211–28.

Paoletti, L.C. and Kasper, D.L. 2002. Conjugate vaccines against group B *Streptococcus* types IV and VII. *J Infect Dis*, **186**, 123–6.

Paoletti, L.C., Madoff, L.C. and Kasper, D.L. 2000. Surface structures of group B Streptococcus important in human immunity. In: Fischetti, V.A., Novick, R.P., et al. (eds), *Gram-positive pathogens*. Washington, DC: American Society for Microbiology, 137–53.

Passwell, J.H., Harlev, E., et al. 2001. Safety and immunogenicity of improved *Shigella* O-specific polysaccharide-protein conjugate vaccines in adults in Israel. *Infect Immun*, **69**, 1351–7.

Pauza, C.D., Trivedi, P., et al. 2000. Vaccination with Tat toxoid attenuates disease in simian/HIV-challenged macaques. *Proc Natl Acad Sci USA*, **97**, 3515–19.

Peltola, H. 2000. Worldwide *Haemophilus influenzae* type b disease at the beginning of the, 21st century: global analysis of the disease burden 25 years after the use of the polysaccharide vaccine and a decade after the advent of conjugates. *Clin Microbiol Rev*, **13**, 302–17.

Pizza, M., Covacci, A., et al. 1989. Mutants of pertussis toxin suitable for vaccine development. *Science*, **246**, 497–500.

Pizza, M., Scarlato, V., et al. 2000. Whole genome sequencing to identify vaccine candidates against serogroup B meningococcus. *Science*, **287**, 1816–20.

Pizza, M., Giuliani, M.M., et al. 2001. Mucosal vaccines: non toxic derivatives of LT and CT as mucosal adjuvants. *Vaccine*, **19**, 2534–41.

Plotkin, S.A. and Bouveret-Le Cam, N. 1995. A new typhoid vaccine composed of the Vi capsular polysaccharide. *Arch Intern Med*, **155**, 2293–9.

Podda, A. 2001. The adjuvanted influenza vaccines with novel adjuvants: experience with the MF59-adjuvanted vaccine. *Vaccine*, **19**, 2673–80.

Podda, A. and Del Giudice, G. 2003. MF59 adjuvant emulsion. In: Levine, M.M. and Kaper, J.B. (eds), *New generation vaccines*, 3rd edn. New York: Marcel Dekker, 223–35.

Poeltl-Frank, F., Zurbriggen, R., et al. 1999. Use of reconstituted influenza virus virosomes as an immunopotentiating delivery system for a peptide-based vaccine. *Clin Exp Immunol*, **117**, 496–503.

Polakos, N.K., Drane, D., et al. 2001. Characterization of hepatitis C virus core-specific immune responses primed in rhesus macaques by a nonclassical ISCOM vaccine. *J Immunol*, **166**, 3589–98.

Poovorawan, Y., Sanpavat, S., et al. 1992. Long term efficacy of hepatitis B vaccine in infants born to hepatitis B e antigen-positive mothers. *Pediatr Infect Dis J*, **11**, 816–21.

Prince, G.A., Capiau, C., et al. 2000. Efficacy and safety studies of a recombinant chimeric respiratory syncytial virus FG glycoprotein vaccine in cotton rats. *J Virol*, **74**, 10287–92.

Prince, G.A., Denamur, F., et al. 2001. Monophosphoryl lipid A adjuvant reverses a principal histologic parameter of formalin-inactivated respiratory syncytial virus-vaccine induced disease. *Vaccine*, **19**, 2048–54.

Ramon, G. 1923. Sur le pouvoir floculant et sur les propriétés immunisantes d'une toxine diphthérique rendue anatoxique (anatoxine). *CR Acad Sci (Paris)*, **177**, 1338–40.

Ramon, G. 1925. Sur la production des antitoxins. *CR Acad Sci (Paris)*, **181**, 157–9.

Ramsay, M.E., Andrews, N., et al. 2001. Efficacy of meningococcal serogroup C conjugate vaccine in teenagers and toddlers in England. *Lancet*, **357**, 195–6.

Rappuoli, R. 1997a. New and improved vaccines against diphtheria and tetanus. In: Levine, M.M., Woodrow, G.C., et al. (eds), *New generation vaccines*, 2nd edn. New York: Marcel Dekker, 417–36.

Rappuoli, R. 1997b. Rational design of vaccines. *Nat Med*, **3**, 374–6.

Rappuoli, R. 2000. Reverse vaccinology. *Curr Opin Microbiol*, **3**, 445–50.

Rappuoli, R., Pizza, M., et al. 1999. Structure and mucosal adjuvanticity of cholera and *Escherichia coli* heat-labile enterotoxins. *Immunol Today*, **20**, 493–500.

Relyveld, E.H. 1996. A history of toxoids. In: Plotkin, S. and Fantini, B. (eds), *Vaccinia, vaccination and vaccinology: Jenner, Pasteur and their successors*. Paris: Elsevier, 95–105.

Richie, T.L. and Saul, A. 2002. Progress and challenges for malaria vaccines. *Nature*, **415**, 694–701.

Richmond, P., Borrow, R., et al. 2001. Ability of three different meningococcal C conjugate vaccines to induce immunologic memory after a single dose in UK toddlers. *J Infect Dis*, **183**, 160–3.

Ridzon, R. and Hannan, M. 1999. Tuberculosis vaccines. *Science*, **286**, 1298–300.

Rimmelzwaan, G.F., Nieuwkoop, N., et al. 2001. A randomized, double blind study in young healthy adults comparing cell mediated and humoral immune responses induced by influenza ISCOM® vaccines and conventional vaccines. *Vaccine*, **19**, 1180–7.

Rokbi, B., Renauld-Mongenie, G., et al. 2000. Allelic diversity of the two transferrin binding protein B gene isotypes among a collection of *Neisseria meningitidis* strains representative of serogroup B disease: implication for the composition of a recombinant TbpB-based vaccine. *Infect Immun*, **68**, 4938–47.

Rosenstein, N.E., Perkins, B.A., et al. 2001. Meningococcal disease. *N Engl J Med*, **344**, 1378–88.

Salk, J.E., Bailey, M.L. and Laurent, A.M. 1952. The use of adjuvants in studies on influenza immunization. II. Increased antibody formation in human subjects inoculated with influenza virus vaccine in a water-in-oil emulsion. *Am J Hyg*, **55**, 439–56.

Salmaso, S., Mastrantonio, P., et al. 2001. Sustained efficacy during the first 6 years of life of 3-component acellular pertussis vaccines administered in infancy: the Italian experience. *Pediatrics*, **108**, E81.

Sambhara, S., Woods, S., et al. 1998. Heterotypic protection against influenza by immune stimulating complexes is associated with the induction of cross-reactive cytotoxic T lymphocytes. *J Infect Dis*, **177**, 1266–74.

Schaible, U.E. and Kaufmann, S.H.E. 2000. CD1 molecules and CD1-dependent T cells in bacterial infections: a link from innate to acquired immunity? *Semin Immunol*, **12**, 527–35.

Scharton-Kersten, T., Yu, J., et al. 2000. Transcutaneous immunization with bacterial ADP-ribosylating exotoxins, subunits, and unrelated adjuvants. *Infect Immun*, **68**, 5306–13.

Schnare, M., Barton, G.L., et al. 2001. Toll-like receptors control activation of adaptive immune responses. *Nature Immunol*, **2**, 947–50.

Schneerson, R., Robbins, J., et al. 1986. Quantitative and qualitative analyses of serum antibodies elicited in adults by *Haemophilus influenzae* type b and pneumococcus type 6A capsular polysaccharide-tetanus toxoid conjugates. *Infect Immun*, **52**, 519–28.

Sigal, L.H., Zahradnik, J.M., et al. 1998. A vaccine consisting of recombinant *Borrelia burgdorferi* outer-surface protein A to prevent Lyme disease. *N Engl J Med*, **339**, 216–22.

Simmons, C.P., Mastroeni, P., et al. 1999. MHC class I-restricted cytotoxic lymphocyte responses induced by enterotoxin-based mucosal adjuvants. *J Immunol*, **163**, 6502–10.

Singh, M., Carlson, J.R., et al. 1998. A comparison of biodegradable microparticles and MF59 as systemic adjuvants for recombinant gD from HSV-2. *Vaccine*, **16**, 1822–7.

Sjolander, A., Cox, J.C. and Barr, I.G. 1998. ISCOMs: an adjuvant with multiple functions. *J Leukoc Biol*, **64**, 713–23.

Sjolander, A., Drane, D., et al. 2001. Immune responses to ISCOM® formulations in animal and primate models. *Vaccine*, **19**, 2661–5.

Smith, R.E., Donachie, A.M., et al. 1999. Immune-stimulating complexes induce an IL-12-dependent cascade of innate immune responses. *J Immunol*, **162**, 5536–46.

Steere, A.C., Sikand, V.K., et al. 1998. Vaccination against Lyme disease with recombinant *Borrelia burgdorferi* outer-surface lipoprotein A with adjuvant. *N Engl J Med*, **339**, 209–15.

Stephenson, I., Nicholson, K.G., et al. 2003. Boosting immunity to influenza H5N1 with MF59-adjuvanted H5N3 A/Duck/Singapore/97 vaccine in a primed human population. *Vaccine*, **21**, 1687–93.

Stoute, J.A., Slaoui, M., et al. 1997. A preliminary evaluation of a recombinant circumsporozoite protein vaccine against *Plasmodium falciparum* malaria. *N Engl J Med*, **336**, 86–91.

Stoute, J.A., Kester, K.E., et al. 1998. Long-term protection and immune responses following immunization with the RTS,S malaria vaccine. *J Infect Dis*, **178**, 1139–44.

Strassburg, M.A., Greenland, S., et al. 1986. Influenza in the elderly: report of an outbreak and review of vaccine effectiveness reports. *Vaccine*, **4**, 38–44.

Takahashi, I., Marinaro, M., et al. 1996. Mechanisms of mucosal immunogenicity and adjuvancy of *Escherichia coli* labile enterotoxin. *J Infect Dis*, **173**, 627–35.

Takeuchi, O., Hoshino, K., et al. 1999. Differential roles of TLR2 and TLR4 in recognition of gram-negative and gram-positive bacterial cell wall components. *Immunity*, **11**, 443–51.

Tappero, J.W., Lagos, R., et al. 1999. Immunogenicity of 2 serogroup B outer-membrane protein meningococcal vaccines: a randomized controlled trial in Chile. *JAMA*, **281**, 1502–7.

Tettelin, H., Saunders, N.J., et al. 2000. Complete genome sequence of *Neisseria meningitidis* serogroup B strain MC58. *Science*, **287**, 1809–15.

Tettelin, H., Masignani, V., et al. 2002. Complete genome sequence and comparative genomic analysis of an emerging human pathogen, serotype V *Streptococcus agalactiae*. *Proc Natl Acad Sci USA*, **99**, 12391–6.

Thoelen, S., Van Damme, P., et al. 1998. Safety and immunogenicity of a hepatitis B vaccine formulated with a novel adjuvant system. *Vaccine*, **16**, 708–14.

Tondella, M.L., Popovic, T., et al. 2000. Distribution of *Neisseria meningitidis* serogroup B serosubtypes and serotypes circulating in the United States. The Active Bacterial Core Surveillance Team. *J Clin Microbiol*, **38**, 3323–38.

Traquina, P., Morandi, M., et al. 1996. MF59 adjuvant enhances the antibody response to recombinant hepatitis B surface antigen vaccine in primates. *J Infect Dis*, **174**, 1168–75.

Tsunoda, I., Tolley, N.D., et al. 1999. Exacerbation of viral and autoimmune animal models for multiple sclerosis by bacterial DNA. *Brain Pathol*, **9**, 481–93.

Ulanova, M., Tarkowski, A., et al. 2001. The common vaccine adjuvant aluminium hydroxide upregulates accessory properties of human monocytes via an-interleukin-4-dependent mechanism. *Infect Immun*, **69**, 1151–9.

Valensi, J.P.M., Carlson, J.R. and Van Nest, G.A. 1994. Systemic cytokine profiles in BALB/c mice immunized with trivalent influenza vaccine containing MF59 oil emulsion and other advanced adjuvants. *J Immunol*, **153**, 4029–39.

Valenzuela, P., Medina, A., et al. 1982. Synthesis and assembly of hepatitis B virus surface antigen particles in yeast. *Nature*, **298**, 347–50.

Van Binnendijk, R.S., Poolen, C.M., et al. 1997. Protective immunity in macaques vaccinated with live attenuated, recombinant, and subunit measles vaccines in the presence of passively acquired antibodies. *J Infect Dis*, **175**, 524–32.

Van Damme, P. and Vorsters, A. 2002. Hepatitis B control in Europe by universal vaccination programmes: the situation in 2001. *J Med Virol*, **67**, 433–9.

Verschoor, E.J., Mooij, P., et al. 1999. Comparison of immunity generated by nucleic acid-, MF59- and ISCOM-formulated human immunodeficiency virus type, 1 vaccines in rhesus macaques: evidence for viral clearance. *J Virol*, **73**, 3292–300.

Verthelyi, D., Kenney, R.T., et al. 2002. CpG oligodeoxynucleotides as vaccine adjuvants in primates. *J Immunol*, **168**, 1659–63.

Vioarsson, G., Jonsdottir, I., et al. 1994. Opsonization and antibodies to capsular and cell wall polysaccharides of *Streptococcus pneumoniae*. *J Infect Dis*, **170**, 592–9.

Vogel, U., Claus, H. and Frosch, M. 2000. Rapid serogroup switching in *Neisseria meningitidis*. *N Engl J Med*, **342**, 219–20.

von Behring, E. and Kitasato, S. 1890. Ueber das Zustandekommen der Diphtherie-Immunitaet und der Tetanus-Immunitaet die Tieren. *Deutsch Med Wochenschr*, **16**, 1113–14.

Ward, J.I. and Zangwill, K.M. 1999. Haemophilus influenzae vaccines. In: Plotkin, S.A. and Orenstein, W.A. (eds), *Vaccines*, 3rd edn. Philadelphia: Saunders, 183–221.

Weiss, R.A. 2001. Gulliver's travel in HIVland. *Nature*, **410**, 963–7.

Wenger, J., Tikhomirov, E., et al. 1997. Meningococcal vaccine in sub-saharan Africa. *Lancet*, **350**, 1709–10.

Wizemann, T.M., Heinrichs, J.H., et al. 2001. Use of a whole genome approach to identify vaccine molecules affording protection against *Streptococcus pneumoniae* infection. *Infect Immun*, **69**, 1593–8.

Wuorimaa, T. and Kayhty, H. 2002. Current state of pneumococcal vaccines. *Scand J Immunol*, **56**, 111–29.

Yi, A.K., Klinman, D.M., et al. 1996a. Rapid activation by CpG motifs in bacterial DNA. Systemic induction of IL-6 transcription through an antioxidant-sensitive pathway. *J Immunol*, **157**, 5394–402.

Yi, A.K., Hornbeck, P., et al. 1996b. CpG DNA rescue of murine B lymphoma cells from anti-IgM-induced growth arrest and programmed cell death is associated with increased expression of c-myc and bcl-xL. *J Immunol*, **157**, 4918–25.

Zollinger, W.D., Moran, E.E., et al. 1997. Bactericidal antibody responses of juvenile rhesus monkeys immunized with group B *Neisseria meningitidis* capsular polysaccharide-protein conjugate vaccines. *Infect Immun*, **65**, 1053–60.

Zurbriggen, R. and Gluck, R. 1999. Immunogenicity of IRIV- versus alum-adjuvanted diphtheria and tetanus toxoid vaccines in influenza primed mice. *Vaccine*, **17**, 1301–5.

46

Mathematical models of vaccination

GRAHAM F. MEDLEY AND D. JAMES NOKES

INTRODUCTION

The purpose of this chapter is to introduce the use of mathematical models in the design of vaccination programs. Like any other healthcare interventions, the aim is to reduce disease, and the success of the program can be measured in terms of the amount of disease prevented, i.e. a quantity. Whenever a problem can be expressed in quantitative terms (i.e. numbers), it lends itself to mathematical formulation, and a whole host of techniques can be used to help solve it. Many people have an aversion to mathematics, but this should not prevent its use when its use is clearly indicated. In this context mathematics is acting as a supporting subject. Just as the development of diagnostics often requires support and insight from chemistry, so the control of infectious disease can make use of mathematics. However, we are not attempting to produce a manual for mathematical models, or indeed convert those with an aversion to equations; rather we seek to explain the content of models and the conclusions that flow from them.

Models (mathematical or otherwise) are conceptual simplifications of complex biological problems. As such, they are always open to the criticism that some relevant and important process or factor is missing. The adage that 'all models are wrong, but some are useful' is true. The decisions taken about which processes are to be included (and which are to be omitted) are critical to determining the usefulness of a model. This is true of mathematical models of problems in other subjects, e.g. engineering. It is clear that judicious use of mathematics can make bridges safer, even when many of the potential complexities cannot be modeled. The definitive test is always when the bridge is actually built and, indeed, there are good examples of bridges failing when the models clearly missed out important processes. However, the next time you are passing over a bridge, it is of some comfort to think that somebody has performed some calculations to demonstrate that it can take your weight.

The principal reason for using mathematical models in the design of vaccination programs is that appropriate experiments are impossible, usually on logistic grounds. If somebody develops a vaccine that they believe induces a protective immune response, there is an agreed route through which they can demonstrate efficacy and safety. It might then be suggested that this vaccine, if given to 75 percent of the population, will prevent 1 500 deaths per year. The only way of demonstrating the potential impact of the vaccine at the population level without actually introducing the program is to model it, i.e. use quantitative frameworks to predict the potential outcome. Note that this is true of the majority of public health interventions – designating 'treatment' and 'control' populations is usually not possible. Clearly, to predict the impact of a vaccine even reasonably accurately requires that we can initially predict the outcome of infection without any intervention.

Just as mathematics has become a mainstay of engineering, so mathematical or quantitative descriptions of pathogen transmission dynamics are increasingly used to support decision-making in design of control programs against infectious disease. Our emphasis in this chapter is on the insights that modeling provides and in what ways these might be instructive in vaccine program design. This chapter concentrates on vaccination, and the central questions of vaccination program design is: 'Who should be vaccinated, what with, and when?'

These are nontrivial questions, and the literature addressing them is substantial and growing. An introduction is given by Anderson and May (1991), which provides a (rather technical) base for more recent advances. More accessible reviews include Nokes and Anderson (1988) and Fine (1993). Consequently, in this chapter, we concentrate on the situation for which the results are best-established: viruses with single serotypes, where immunity after infection is long lasting. The classic examples (archetypal viruses) are measles, mumps, and rubella (MMR). It is no coincidence that this is the simplest circumstance – a consensus on the population biology and epidemiology of more complicated infections is yet to be found.

BASIC CONCEPTS

In this section, we introduce the central idea of infectious disease epidemiology: it is a dynamic process driven proximately by the rate of infection and, ultimately, the availability of people to be infected.

Individual vs population

The population level patterns (epidemiology) of infectious disease are very different from noninfectious disease. An infected individual acts as a potential source of infection to others in a population – an individual with a noninfectious condition poses no such risk. With infectious disease there is a necessary relationship between the *incidence* and *prevalence*: if the prevalence of infection is zero, then there is no possibility of incidence being anything other than zero (Figure 46.1), i.e. if nobody is infected with smallpox, nobody can become infected with smallpox. This is not the case for noninfectious or noncommunicable disease, where the individual risk of developing the disease is little influenced by the amount of disease in the population.

It follows from this simple observation that infectious disease has to be studied at a population or community level if it is to be controlled. The risk of disease to an individual depends on the health (infection) status of all the other individuals with whom they come into contact. Likewise, an intervention that acts on an individual will have consequences for everybody else in the population. If you successfully vaccinate 20 percent of a population, the remaining 80 percent who were unvaccinated will still receive some protection from infection because they have fewer people from whom to acquire infection.

An important distinction must be drawn between infection and disease. Infected individuals are not guaranteed to develop disease and, for most pathogens, most infections are relatively asymptomatic. However, an individual infected with influenza but without clinical symptoms can transmit the virus to another individual who subsequently dies. It follows that control of infectious disease at the population level requires that it is infection that is considered rather than disease. Unfortunately, most data available are highly biased towards cases of clinical disease, and uncomplicated infection is usually unobserved unless special effort is made.

Transmission dynamics and susceptibility

It is also clear that incidence is dependent on susceptibility to infection: if there are no susceptible individuals to infect, the incidence is, again, necessarily zero. If it were possible to make everybody immune to measles tomorrow, nobody would become infected. This relationship between prevalence and incidence gives an inherent nonlinearity in patterns of infectious disease. Under simple assumptions of random transmission (see below), we can write the incidence of infection as the product of three numbers. Suppose that individuals in a population contact each other at some rate, c, and there are X susceptible and Y infected individuals, making a total population size of N ($=X + Y$). Then the rate at which each susceptible contacts an infected individual is:

$$c\frac{Y}{N} \qquad (46.1)$$

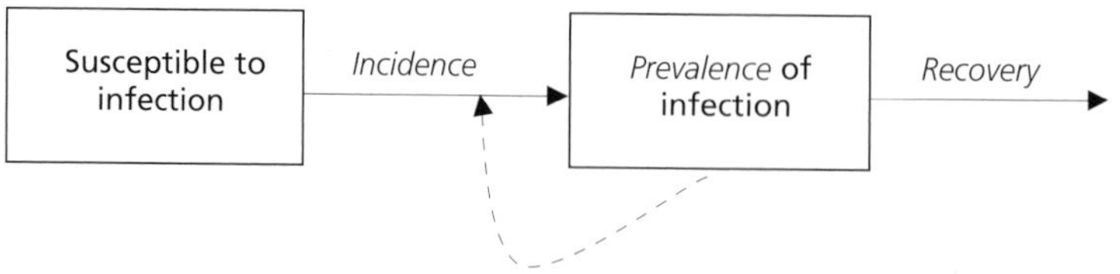

Figure 46.1 *Relationship between incidence and prevalence for an infectious disease. The boxes represent two sorts of individuals: those who might be infected (i.e. are susceptible to infection) and those who are infected. The prevalence of infection is the number of individuals currently infected, and is expressed as a proportion or percentage. The solid arrows represent time-dependent rates of movement of individuals. Incidence is a measure of the rate at which individuals become infected, and is often expressed as a proportion of the population per unit time (the attack rate). Recovery from infection can generally be the result of immunological clearance of infection or death of the infected individual. The dotted line represents the dependence of incidence on prevalence.*

For example, suppose that the contact rate is 10 individuals per week, and half of the population is infected, then the average susceptible will contact 5 infected people per week. Now suppose that on each contact between a susceptible and infected individual there is a probability, p, that transmission occurs (i.e. the susceptible becomes infected). Consequently, the rate of infection per susceptible is:

$$pc\frac{Y}{N} \tag{46.2}$$

This quantity is also known as the 'force of infection'. Continuing our numerical example, if the probability of transmission is 0.1, the rate of infection per susceptible is 0.5 per week. This can be translated into an average time before infection of 1/0.5 = 2 weeks. The unsurprising result is that the more infected individuals there are in a population, the more likely that each susceptible becomes infected, and the faster they become infected.

The total rate of infection in the population (i.e. taking into account all the susceptibles) is the incidence (e.g. the number of cases of infection per week):

$$pc\frac{Y}{N}X = \frac{pcY(N-Y)}{N} \tag{46.3}$$

This relationship is drawn in Figure 46.2. The implicit assumption for this simple example is that individuals are either susceptible or infected. Lack of either susceptible or infected individuals reduces incidence. Incidence is greatest when there is a plentiful supply of both. This nonlinear relationship between incidence and susceptibles and infecteds is what creates 'transmission dynamics'. During an epidemic, the number of infected individuals starts small, but a positive incidence means that infection increases, increasing incidence further, and so on. Eventually, the numbers of susceptibles will be depleted, and incidence will start to fall. Thus, changes in incidence at any point in time have important consequences in the future, making prediction of the dynamic (through time) changes intrinsically complicated.

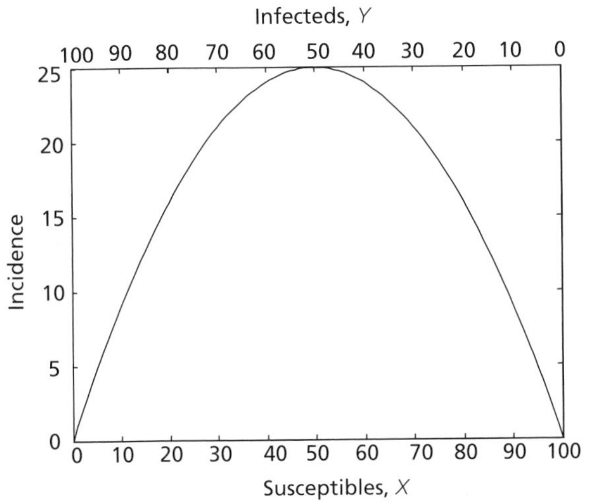

Figure 46.2 *The relationship between incidence (number of new cases per unit time), and the numbers of susceptibles in a population of 100 individuals. The incidence is zero when either there is nobody to infect (X = 0, Y = 100) or there are no infectious individuals (X = 100, Y = 0). See text (Equation 46.3).*

The simplest dynamic model

The preceding section makes it clear that there are intimate links between rates of infection, prevalence of infection, and proportion susceptible. To understand these links and the dynamic consequence of changing any of these quantities (e.g. reducing susceptibility by vaccinating), it is necessary to consider them together in a single model framework. Mathematics provides the tools to do this.

Imagine a closed population such as the passengers and crew on a cruise liner, i.e. a population in which birth, death, immigration, and emigration do not usually occur. This implies that we are thinking of a relatively short time period. Let us consider the simplest situation (i.e. the MMR paradigm). We can divide the population into three mutually exclusive groups or classes: susceptible, infected (and infectious), and recovered (and immune).

In this case, the only process occurring as far as the susceptible population is concerned is infection, which occurs at a rate given in Equation 46.3. The number of infected individuals is being increased by infection (at the same rate as susceptibles are lost), but also decreased by recovery. The immune population is increased in the same manner, i.e. as each person recovers and leaves the infected class, he or she enters the immune class. We can tie these processes together by considering the rate at which the populations are changing. Figure 46.3 sketches a 'flow diagram' indicating the three classes of individual and the rates of flow between them.

As before, we define X and Y to be the numbers susceptible and infected respectively, and introduce Z as the numbers immune. We can then say that the rate of change of X is written as dX/dt. This quantity has units of 'people per unit time': if it is zero, the susceptible population is not changing; if it is greater than zero the susceptible population is increasing; if it is less than zero (negative) the susceptible population is decreasing. Taking all the assumptions together, the equations for this simplest model are:

$$\frac{dX}{dt} = -pc\frac{Y}{N}X \tag{46.4}$$

$$\frac{dY}{dt} = +pc\frac{Y}{N}X - \frac{1}{D}Y \tag{46.5}$$

$$\frac{dZ}{dt} = \frac{1}{D}Y \tag{46.6}$$

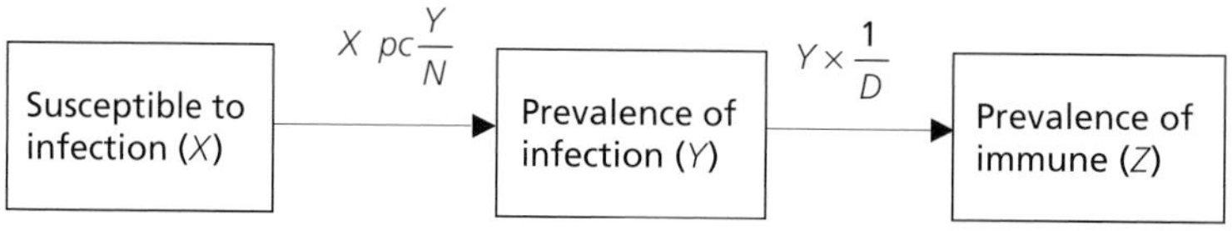

Figure 46.3 *A flow diagram for the simplest possible model of a microparasitic infection that produces a solid, life-long immunity (e.g. mumps, measles, and rubella or MMR). In comparison with Figure 46.1, we have now introduced an explicit immune class of individuals, and added variables (X, Y, and Z), which are the numbers of individuals within each class. The total population is N = X + Y + Z. Each individual in the population falls into one, and only one, class. The arrows between the classes represent the flow of individuals, and the rate of flow is given as an equation. See text (Equations 46.4–46.6).*

The incidence rates are as previously (see Equation 46.3). The recovery rate is written as $1/D$ where D is the duration of infection. Note that the parameter c is a rate and D is a duration, and must be expressed in the same time units, i.e. it is wrong to include c as five contacts per week and D as a duration of 14 days. The only other information necessary to solve these equations is the 'initial conditions', i.e. the numbers in each class at the start.

We are not going to enter into a mathematical discussion of these equations, but rather simply state that they are easily solved in many computer packages. Figure 46.4 gives an example of such a solution. The epidemic is shown as the bold line, reaching a peak prevalence of 40 people in 100 infected after 4 weeks. The susceptible population falls continuously, although note that a small proportion of people escape infection. The immune population (dashed line) rises throughout as people pass from susceptible through infected and recover.

One thing that should be clear from this model is that the shape of the epidemic is determined by both the availability of infection and the susceptibility. The reason that everybody does not become infected on the first day is that infection is rare, but the prevalence of infection increases because the rate of infection is greater than the rate of recovery. The reason that infection prevalence falls after 4 weeks is that only about 30 people are susceptible, so the rate of recovery is greater than the rate of infection.

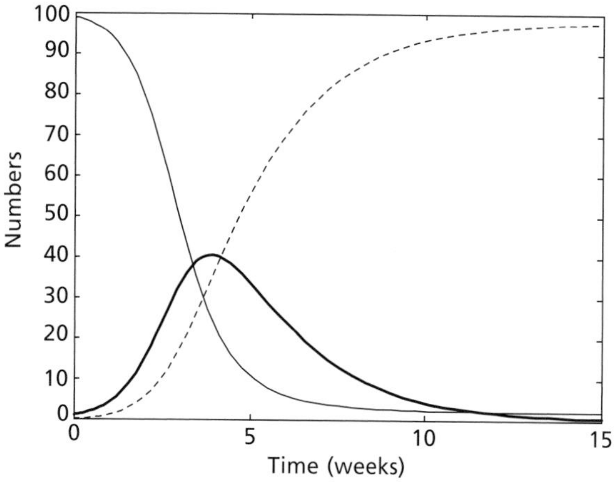

Figure 46.4 *An example outcome from the simplest model (see text, Equations 46.4–46.6). The lines show the numbers in each class: susceptible (X), infectious (Y, bold) and immune (Z, dashed). The parameters are: c = 20 per week, p = 0.1, and D = 2 weeks. The initial conditions are X = 99, Y = 1, and Z = 0.*

Statistical and political complications

Generally, for infectious disease studies, individuals cannot be considered as statistically independent observations. For infectious disease, the incidence is a (nonlinear, complex) function of the prevalence. Noninfectious disease epidemiology is essentially a statistical study of the relationship between risks and disease where individuals can be treated as heterogeneous, but independent, replicates. This makes observational research into infectious disease more difficult and, to some extent, the appropriate methods are still under development (e.g. see Becker 1989).

Infectious disease also introduces conflicts between populations and individuals, because of the interdependence. Some of these conflicts are discussed in Medley (1996), but a couple of examples will demonstrate. No vaccine is completely free from risk of adverse reactions, so each parent would like their children to avoid both infection and vaccine. This is possible only if all other parents have their children vaccinated, i.e. everybody would like everybody else to use the vaccine, because then they would not have to (see also Nokes and Anderson 1988, 1991).

Another conflict arises if chemotherapy is available to prolong the infectious life of infected individuals. Clearly, such a therapy is advantageous to the individual, but will almost certainly increase the total number of people infected, which is disadvantageous to the population (e.g. Anderson et al. 1991). These conflicts are occasionally seen when those responsible for the health of populations (e.g. government departments) enforce control measures that are apparently detrimental to individuals. A conflict arises because the best policy depends on the perspective taken: what is best for an individual might not be the best for the population, and vice versa.

PROCESSES OF INFECTIOUS DISEASE EPIDEMIOLOGY

Having introduced the basic concepts, in this section we go through the processes that drive infectious disease epidemiology, and hence form the components of mathematical descriptions of infectious disease dynamics.

Routes of transmission

Pathogens must be passed from one individual to another if they are going to survive, even if only because no host is immortal. From an evolutionary point of view, the pathogen that transmits the most is the most successful (the 'fittest'), and will out-compete the less transmissible. From an epidemiological viewpoint, if the transmission dynamics of infection, and hence the impact of vaccination, are to be predicted, a critical knowledge is how many and which individuals are infected by an infectious case.

Transmission can be classified in a number of ways. In Table 46.1 we give a classification system based on three criteria. First, infections can be considered in terms of their ultimate source: other people, other animal species (zoonotic), or the environment. Second, within each of these categories, the route of transmission essentially defines who is likely to be exposed, e.g. an infection that can use the maternal route will potentially infect children; a sexually transmitted pathogen will potentially infect sexual partners, etc. Vectors can transmit both human and zoonotic pathogens. Third, the mode of infection essentially defines the physical manner in which the pathogen transfers from one individual to another, so that children can be infected maternally via a number of modes (e.g. across the placenta or via breast milk). Thus, knowing the route of transmission helps define the at-risk contacts of an infected individual, and knowing the mode of transmission helps define control strategies to reduce the risk of those individuals. Distinction should also be made between transmission modes that are contaminative (i.e. there is no multiplication of the pathogen) and reservoir; multiplication of malaria within the vector reservoir is different from the contamination of shared drug-injecting equipment with HIV.

Quantification of transmission probability

Contact between an infectious and a susceptible individual does not guarantee transmission. To estimate a probability of transmission given a contact, the contacts have to be defined and countable. This is not straightforward, e.g. for sexually transmitted infections (STI) there is the possibility of measuring the contact rates and transmission probability in terms of both sexual partnerships and sexual acts (within a partnership) (see Blower and Boe 1993).

Suppose that we are interested in transmission of HIV from intravenous drug-using women. There are three routes through which infection can pass, and hence three groups who might be infected: children, equipment-sharing partners, and sexual partners. Suppose that these women have, on average, one child every 4 years; then the contact rate, c_1, for this route is 0.25 different children per year. Likewise we can define c_2 as the average number of different injecting partners per year,

Table 46.1 *Classification of transmission*

Source	Route	Mode	Examples (organism)
Human	Maternal	Transplacental	*Toxoplasma gondii*, rubella, CMV, *Treponema pallidum*
		Transmammary	HIV, CMV
	Environmental contamination	Food borne	HAV, *Vibrio cholerae*
		Other (fomite) ingestion	*Shigella* spp.
	'Close contact'	Respiratory (airborne)	Influenza 2, RSV, *Bordetella pertussis*, MMR
		Oral–fecal	*V. cholerae*, rotavirus
		Physical (nonsexual)	HBV, HSV1, EBV
	Sexual	Genital–genital, anogenital, etc.	HIV, HBV, HSV2 *Neisseria gonorrhoeae*, *Treponema pallidum*
	Vector-borne	Vector-borne	*Plasmodium* spp., urban YFV, dengue
	Blood-borne	Needle sharing/transfusion	HBV, HIV, HCV
Zoonotic	Physical contact	Various	Rabies, Q-fever, brucellosis, *Campylobacter* spp.
	Vector-borne	Vector-borne	*Yersinia pestis*, jungle YFV, *Borrelia burgdorferi*
Environmental	Environment	Respiratory (airborne)	*Legionella* spp.
		Oral/Mechanical	*Clostridium tetani*, *Listeria* spp., *Mycobacterium bovis*

CMV, cytomegalovirus; EBV, Epstein–Barr virus; HAV, hepatitis A virus; HBV, hepatitis B virus; HCV, hepatitis C virus; HIV, human immunodeficiency virus; HSV, herpes simplex virus; MMR, measles, mumps, and rubella; RSV, respiratory syncytial virus; YFV, yellow fever virus.

and c_3 as the average number of different sexual partners per year. If the probability of a child becoming infected from its infectious mother is p_1, and similarly for p_2 and p_3, the total average rate of people infected by each infected woman is:

$$c_1p_1 + c_2p_2 + c_3p_3 \qquad (46.7)$$

There is considerable blurring across boundaries in Table 46.1, as with any attempt to impose categories on to continuous scales, e.g. when does close contact, oral–fecal transmission become food-borne environmental contamination? One can see the difficulty in defining the nonsexual 'close contact' rates (although see Edmunds et al. 1997). This is also complicated by the fact that close contact modes and sexual modes are not mutually exclusive – if two individuals are close enough to touch, they can transmit via the respiratory mode. In this sense, the sexual route is a 'very close contact'. Figure 46.5 schematically demonstrates that, within the close contact/sexual routes, there is a relationship between the number of contacts and intimacy of contact (which is very probably correlated to probability of transmission). Thus, we speak to more people than we touch, and touch more people than we have sex with.

By defining a transmission mode as 'respiratory', we are defining the lower limit of its transmission modes, because it will also be transmitted during more intimate contacts. Figure 46.6 schematically illustrates that this lower limit will not always coincide with the maximum transmission route: how much influenza is sexually transmitted (that is, transmitted during sexual contact)?

Social and environmental setting

Having defined and quantified transmission in terms of contact rates, the next level of complexity is determining with whom the contact occurs. The simplest assumption is that all individuals within the population are equally likely to contact all other individuals. This is in fact the underlying rationale behind Equations 46.1–46.3, and the effect is that doubling the number of infectious individuals doubles the rate at which each (and every) susceptible contacts an infectious individual. In reality this is rarely the case – we do not have an equal chance of meeting everybody. Social systems effectively mean that we have a group of people we meet much more often (e.g. family, close friends, and work colleagues), and have a very low chance of meeting most other people.

There are a large number of variables that determine who our contacts are. These include age, gender, occupation, and geography. Taking age as an example, people tend to mix with individuals of the same age, although parents and teachers with children are examples of mixing across age groups. Geography is somewhat spurious, because it does determine much of the contact, but behavior tends to be overriding, so that it is possible to have more regular and closer contact with family members in North America, than with next-door neighbors in the UK.

There is also considerable heterogeneity in the amount of contact, so that some individuals have much higher contact rates than others. The individuals with the highest contact rates are simultaneously at greatest risk of becoming infected, and have the greatest opportunity for infecting others. In the context of STIs, these high-contact individuals are termed the 'core group', but all infections have a 'core group', and the same phenomenon is probably universal for infectious agents (Woolhouse et al. 1997).

In much work in the literature, there is an implicit assumption that the rate of infection is determined by the density (or size) of the population, rather than being

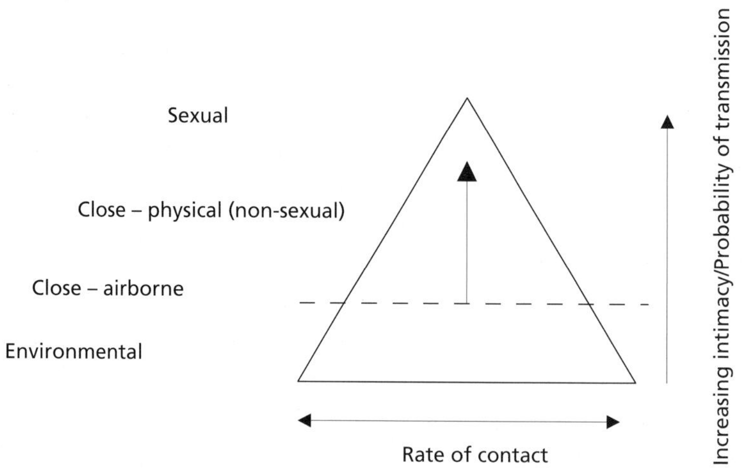

Figure 46.5 *Schematic diagram representing the relationship between the frequency and intimacy of contact. The higher up the triangle, the greater the probability of transmission, but the lower the rate of that contact. The horizontal line represents a hypothetical infection which is transmissible via direct airborne spread, but shows that it is also transmissible by other routes (see text).*

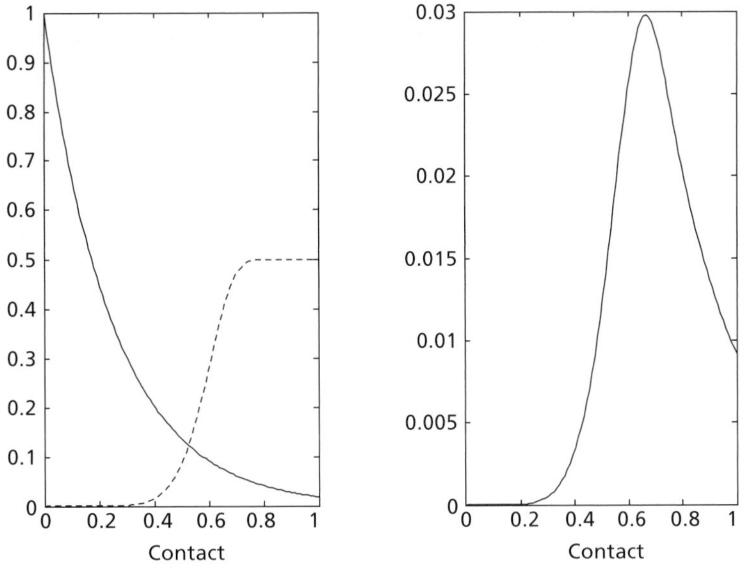

Figure 46.6 *Putative relationships between (relative) contact rate, c (solid line left panel), and probability of transmission, p (dashed line left panel), varying with increased intimacy of contact. The right-hand panel shows the product c*p over the same scale, i.e. the effective contact rate. Note that if the contact rate falls and probability of transmission reaches a plateau, this latter relationship will always have a single maximum, and the maximum will be at or before the maximum transmission probability is reached.*

determined by contact explicitly. In this case, Equation 46.2 is rewritten as:

$$\beta Y \qquad (46.8)$$

where β is a 'transmission coefficient'. This formulation is known as the 'mass action' assumption: the name derives from similar models (and assumptions) in chemical and physical processes. If the population size (N) is constant, the two assumptions (contact-driven and mass action – Equations 46.2 and 46.8, respectively) are equivalent, and the transmission coefficient subsumes the population size. If the population size is changing, the two are equivalent only if the contact rate is a linear function of the population size (i.e. if doubling the number of people doubles the average rate of contact). This might be a fair approximation for transmission via more environmental routes (such as airborne), but is unlikely to be true for more sociological routes (such as sexual contact).

It is clear that much of this discussion about social and environmental setting and its relationship to transmission rates depends on the population under consideration. For any model, defining the population is a critical step, because it effectively defines the scope of the model, which then determines what is outside the model, e.g. producing a model of pneumococcal transmission in school might be erroneous if most of the transmission occurs in households. The other important feature to come out of this discussion is that heterogeneities (i.e. differences) are critically important. The simplest model formulations have everything identical. In biology, this is very rarely the case – most hosts and most pathogens are distinct from each other. This theme is picked up continuously through the remainder of the chapter.

Natural history

For the purposes of describing transmission dynamics, the natural history of infection charts the progress of *an individual* through time, starting with exposure and successful infection. Within each infected individual, there is a dynamic duel fought between pathogen and immunity – vaccines are designed to give immunity the upper hand (Nowak and May 2000). But, at a population level, there are four characteristics of relevance: (1) the time course of infectiousness; (2) the immunity to subsequent infection (i.e. susceptibility); (3) the time course of immune markers of (past) infection; and (4) the time course of disease. Figure 46.7 shows schematic pictures of these four aspects for three diseases. Measles, mumps, and rubella are archetypal viral infections, where the infection, disease, and immune response to infection all occur over a matter of days. The infection (and infectiousness) is curtailed by the immune response that persists for life, and antibody markers of previous infection can be found in the serum and saliva of most individuals, although their concentration may fall over a period of years without re-exposure.

For bacterial infections (e.g. *N. gonorrhoea*, *Streptococcus pneumoniae*), the timescale of infection is months, there is no solid immunity, and immune markers are generally not persistent.

For hepatitis B virus (HBV), there are two possible outcomes of infection. After initial exposure, and a risk of acute hepatitis, the majority of individuals recover and become immune to re-infection, i.e. the natural history is as for measles, but with a timescale of months rather than days. However, as illustrated, some

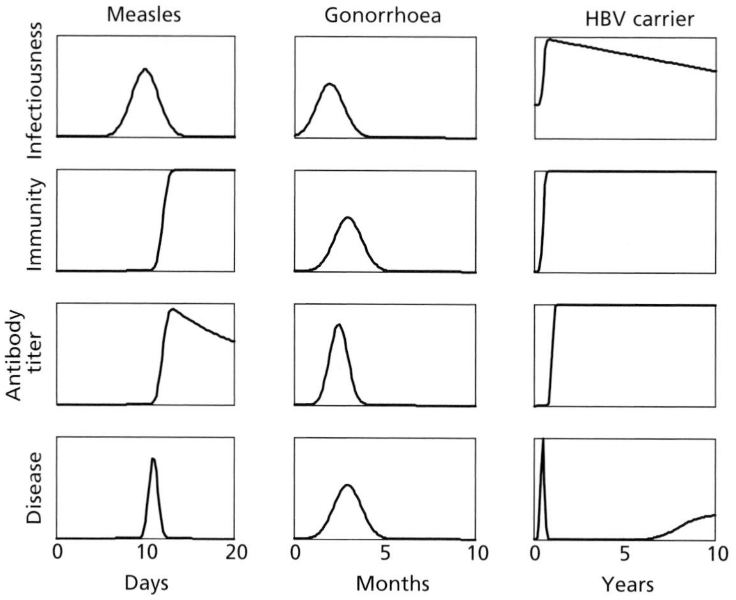

Figure 46.7 *Schematic representation of three different natural histories without intervention (treatment). The three columns show (left to right) measles, gonorrhea, and* hepatitis B virus *carriage. Note the different time scales (i.e. the time since infection). The four rows show (top to bottom) the infectiousness, the immunity to reinfection, the titer of antibodies (markers of previous infection), and the risk of disease and/or symptoms.*

individuals develop a carrier state, and remain more or less continually infectious, although they are probably immune to further infection, and maintain some antibody markers of infection. The risk of cancer and cirrhosis increases with duration of carriage.

To develop a mathematical description of the natural history, the most common (and common-sense) approach is to divide the population into a series of mutually exclusive categories or classes of individuals (as was done in Figure 46.3). Figure 46.8 illustrates such compartments for the three infections in Figure 46.7. The arrows denote the flow or movement of individuals between categories. For measles, there are only three states: susceptible, infectious, resistant (SIR), and individuals move from susceptible to infectious (when infected) and from infectious to immune as they recover. This is the classic 'SIR' model. Frequently, an exposed category is added between susceptible and infectious to include those individuals who are infected but not yet infectious: this is the SEIR model. For most bacterial infections there is no effective solid immunity, so individuals return to susceptible after resolution of infection:

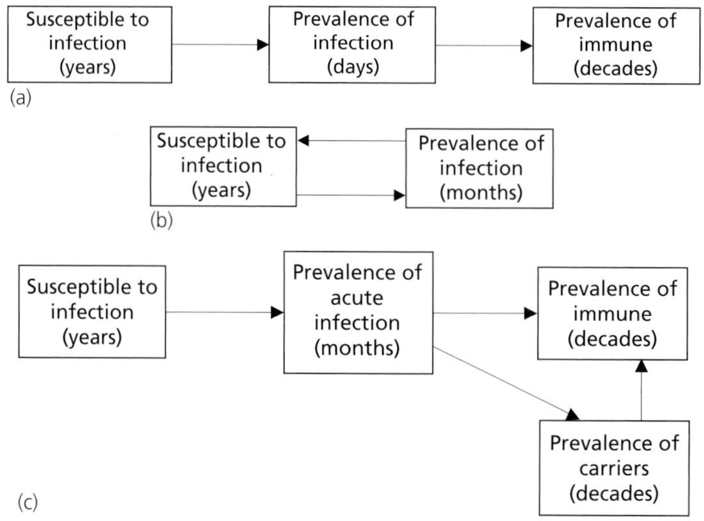

Figure 46.8 *Compartmental model structures for the natural histories of three infections illustrated in Figure 46.7.* **(a)** *Measles,* **(b)** *bacterial sexually transmitted disease, and* **(c)** hepatitis B virus. *The duration of stay within each compartment is written in braces. The first two model structures are SIR and SIS respectively.*

the SIS model. Again, if there is a period of immunity after infection, before recovery of susceptibility, an SIRS framework is possible, as seems likely for respiratory syncytial virus (RSV) and rotavirus. For HBV, the compartmental model should include both consequences of initial (acute) infection: immunity and carriage. Note that carriage can resolve, so that there is a flow from carriers to immune. Figure 46.8 is not exhaustive: indeed there are a great many possibilities for sewing together compartments representing the natural histories of different pathogens (which might be different in different host populations). But note that the compartments are based on what happens within individuals.

Figure 46.8 also shows the duration of stay within each compartment. This is important, because it largely determines the prevalence of each compartment, i.e. what percentage of individuals are in which state. A short duration stage has a lower prevalence than a long duration stage, e.g. the prevalence of people whose 40th birthday is today is much lower than the prevalence of people in their 40s: because it takes only one day to have a 40th birthday, but 10 years to move between 40 and 50.

As discussed below, for the purposes of understanding transmission, the duration of infectiousness (D) is the most important parameter of the natural history.

Pathogen heterogeneities

> Measles occupies a rather unique position in epidemiological theory, as it is largely an infection of childhood with very clear-cut immunizing characteristics, so that the susceptible population (and its new 'recruits') are fairly well defined. (Bartlett 1960, p. 73)

We can perhaps add mumps and rubella, but most other pathogens display variation, particularly with respect to immunity determinants. Agents with antigenic diversity (e.g. influenza virus, rhinoviruses, rotavirus) appear to have natural histories like the second type in Figures 46.7 and 46.8, i.e. every infection is like a new one. The typical scenario might be that of a strain of influenza, which follows a similar life history to that of, say, measles, but, unlike measles, the solid immunity generated to the specific strain is not solid across strains. Thus an individual's immunity to 'influenza' as a whole is compromised by the antigenic diversity (existing or immune selected), such that in a subsequent season previously infected individuals succumb to a new (drifted) variant. From a host viewpoint, this looks like loss of immunity to influenza. From the virus's viewpoint, all those hosts that were previously infected and immune are now susceptible and ripe for re-infection.

This picture is complicated by the concepts of partial and temporary immunity. If immunity is partial, it is effective against a proportion of the pathogen population, whereas, if it is temporary, it is effective against the whole pathogen population, but this immunity wanes. Further complication arises if the immunity is to disease rather than infection: for RSV and rotavirus disease is usually expressed or most severe on first infection.

Basic reproduction number

The processes outlined above (transmission, contact, and natural history) are the determinants of the epidemiology of an infectious disease in a given host population. That HBV has a different epidemiology in developed versus developing countries, or that STIs are different from childhood viral infections, is the result of differences in these three processes.

To understand the population dynamics of infection, we should capture the processes as they determine transmission from person to person. This can be done in terms of a single number: the basic reproduction number, R_0 (pronounced R-zero or R-nought). This turns out to be the central concept in infectious disease epidemiology.

Consider a completely susceptible population (i.e. without any immunity), with a single infected case introduced. In this situation, the transmission that derives from the infected case will be maximal – it is the ideal situation for the pathogen. The infected case will be infectious for a period determined by the natural history, and in the simplest circumstance we can represent this by the parameter D. This determines the time window or duration over which infection can occur.

During this period, the case will make contact with susceptible people at a rate c, which is determined by the transmission route and the population characteristics (environment and behavior). So, overall, the number of potential infectees (secondary cases) will be cD – the number of contacts during the infectious period. But not all will become infected, and we can write p as a transmission probability, i.e. given that a susceptible contacts an infectious person, p is the probability that transmission will occur. So the basic reproduction number can be defined as:

$$R_0 = pcD \qquad (46.9)$$

Note that this is a single number and is defined as the average number of secondary cases that are derived from one primary case in a completely susceptible population. As previous discussion on heterogeneity in transmission and natural history illustrates, the word 'average' in this definition glosses over much complexity, but the concept conveys the essential idea that the maximal expected transmission in a given setting can be quantified in terms of route of transmission, environmental/behavioral setting, and natural history.

The most important concept resulting from R_0 is that of a threshold value for an epidemic to occur. If an infection is to be able to propagate through a population, i.e. to cause an epidemic, each new infection will have to (on average) infect at least one other person. So for an epidemic to occur:

$$R_0 > 1 \tag{46.10}$$

Imagine, if $R_0 = 2$, each infectious case will create a chain of new cases, so that one case becomes 2, which beget 4 cases, which beget 8 cases, and so forth.

Effective reproduction number

Given that susceptibility is the key quantity – the food on which infection feeds – there ought to be some way of determining a sufficient supply of susceptibles required to maintain infection. This idea is captured in the *effective reproduction number*, *R*. This is defined as the average number of secondary cases from each primary case. Note the similarity with the definition of the basic reproduction number, which differs only by having the extra condition of a completely susceptible population. The effective reproduction number does not have this condition – it is more general and applies regardless of the state of the population.

There is a simple relationship between these two reproduction numbers. The assumption previously was that each contact (potential transmission) that the infectious case had was with a susceptible person. However, if only a proportion of the population is susceptible, x, then the number of contacts each infectious case has during the infectious period is xcD, and consequently:

$$R = pxcD = xR_0 \tag{46.11}$$

When everybody is susceptible, $x = 1$, and $R = R_0$. If there are no susceptibles, $x = 0$, and $R = 0$, i.e. there can be no transmission.

Host population effects

Viruses survive in host populations, so, not surprisingly, the population dynamics of hosts is an important factor in determining the epidemiology of a virus. There are two aspects that we concentrate on here: the availability of susceptible hosts and the variability of the effect of infection on different hosts. A key concept is that hosts are not identical, and we emphasize the role of host age.

In Figure 46.4 the epidemic ends and the virus that caused it will become eliminated from the host population. This is because all (but a small fraction of) hosts have been infected and are immune, and there is no susceptibility available for the virus to exploit. Pathogens need susceptibility to survive. A pathogen with a different natural history, e.g. one with sufficient antigenic diversity, might be able to re-infect hosts, thus creating susceptibility. The other principal source of susceptibles is the arrival of new hosts through birth or immigration. An alternative strategy is for the pathogen to find a site in which it can survive the longer term and wait for susceptibility to return. A carrier state and survival in the environment are both examples of such strategies; vertical transmission is also a good adaptation for a virus to survive in a small population of hosts.

We can adapt the simplest model in Equations 46.4–46.6 to include a supply of susceptibles. Imagine that, in our population, individuals leave the population after 20 weeks on average, and they are immediately replaced by susceptibles, in order to keep the population constant. This can be thought of as birth/death or immigration/emigration, and is captured in a parameter, μ. We also include partial immunity by adding a parameter, π, which we define as the proportion of recovering hosts that are immediately susceptible (so that $1 - \pi$ become immune). The equations for this system are:

$$\frac{dX}{dt} = \mu N - pc\frac{Y}{N}X + \pi\frac{1}{D}Y - \mu X \tag{46.12}$$

$$\frac{dY}{dt} = +pc\frac{Y}{N}X - \frac{1}{D}Y - \mu Y \tag{46.13}$$

$$\frac{dZ}{dt} = (1-\pi)\frac{1}{D}Y - \mu Z \tag{46.14}$$

Four examples of the results are shown in Figure 46.9. Introduction of a trickle of susceptibility that does not depend on infection (through birth/death) results in the infection being maintained in the population – the supply of susceptibles is enough to keep all the chains of transmission from going extinct. Note that this introduces 'damped oscillations', as the infection reaches its endemic, equilibrium prevalence. Decreasing partial immunity increases the prevalence of infection and reduces the amplitude of the oscillations.

This model (Equations 46.12–46.14) is an example of a 'toy model' or 'thought experiment' in which the underlying effect of explicitly stated assumptions can be investigated. Nobody would pretend that a framework such as this be used for quantitative prediction or designing control programs. More complicated models, e.g. introducing explicit host age, gender, and pathogen diversity, would be required for these purposes. However, these more complex models tend to echo the important results from the simpler models, which are consequently often more useful for developing understanding. A fuller review of the dynamics of SIR and SIS models is given by Gomes et al. (2004).

Dynamic equilibria

Implicit in Figure 46.9 is that if there are sufficient susceptibles to maintain an infection in a host population, i.e. it becomes endemic; then the prevalence of infection tends toward a constant equilibrium. This can

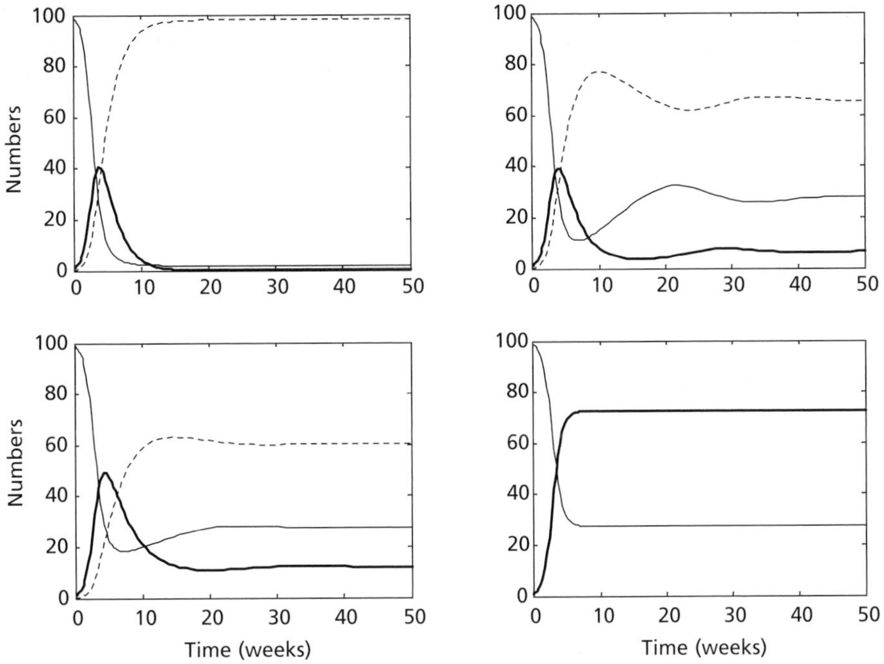

Figure 46.9 *The effect of supplying susceptibles on epidemic propagation (see text and Equations 46.12–46.14). The first panel shows the epidemic with no susceptible supply (SIR – as Figure 46.4). The second panel introduces birth/death (with μ = 0.05 so that each individual has an expectancy of staying 20 weeks in the population). The third panel introduces partial immunity (μ = 0.05, π = 0.5). The fourth panel shows the SIS situation, with no immunity (μ = 0.05, π = 1.0). The remaining parameters are as Figure 46.4.*

be related back to the effective reproduction number. At endemicity, on average, each case will give rise to one other case, i.e. $R = 1$, and prevalence is constant.

This equilibrium is also dynamically stable. Figure 46.10 shows the situation where additional susceptibles are either added or removed from a population at endemic equilibrium. The removal of susceptibles (e.g. by a one-time vaccination campaign – left column in Figure 46.10) results in a decrease in transmission ($R < 1$) and consequently the number of infectious individuals. Susceptibles entering the population are less likely to get infected than at equilibrium, so their prevalence rises, as does R. When $R = 1$ the number of infectious individuals bottoms out, and starts to rise as the numbers of susceptibles increases and $R > 1$. A small epidemic ensues. The addition of susceptibles (right column in Figure 46.10) immediately results in an epidemic ($R > 1$) during which the additional susceptibles are 'consumed'. In both cases susceptibility and infection return to equilibrium where $R = 1$.

The value $R = 1$ is a special situation, and decreasing or increasing the proportion susceptible moves R away from this value, although infection dynamics will act to increase or decrease the proportion susceptible and bring R = 1. The value $R = 1$ occurs when the proportion susceptible is at a *critical value*:

$$x^* = \frac{1}{R_0} \qquad (46.15)$$

Transmission dynamics acts to keep the proportion susceptible at this critical value.

BASIC PRINCIPLES OF VACCINATION

Having discussed some of the basic concepts and potential complexities, we turn, at last, to the effects of vaccination. For each individual host, successful vaccination is a short cut in the natural history that results in moving from susceptible to immune without the infection. For the pathogen, vaccination means removing susceptibility, i.e. potential hosts. As we have seen, susceptibility is a key quantity in determining the population level dynamics of infection, so vaccination will have dynamic consequences. In particular, because individuals are not independent, vaccinating some hosts will have consequences for those hosts who are not vaccinated.

Herd immunity and reproduction numbers

An important concept in infectious disease is that of herd immunity, which is often confused so we adopt a particular definition. A population (herd) can be said to be immune to a specific pathogen when that infection is not endemic and cannot be introduced. In particular, the in-migration of infected people will not result in continuous chains of transmission and an epidemic. A more poetic term is 'community immunity'.

For an epidemic to occur, and consequently the infection has the potential to become endemic, the effective reproduction number must be greater than one. In a

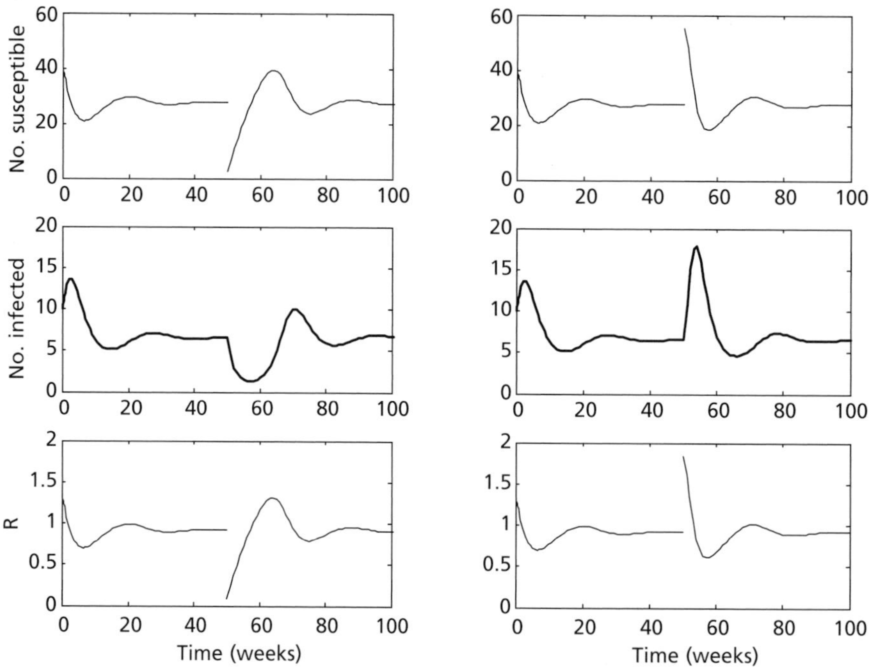

Figure 46.10 *Dynamic effect of increasing or decreasing the proportion susceptible at one point in time. The model (Equations 46.12–46.14); μ = 0.05, π = 0.0) is run for 50 weeks, then either 90 percent of susceptibles are moved to immune class (left panels) or the number of susceptibles is doubled by movement from the immune class (right panels). The rows show the effect on susceptible class (top row), infected class (middle) and effective reproduction number (bottom) (immune population not shown). Note that susceptible numbers and effective reproduction numbers are linear transformations of each other (Equation 46.11).*

completely susceptible population, the basic and effective reproduction numbers are equal, but reduction in susceptibility directly (and linearly) reduces the effective reproduction number (R_0 remains unchanged by susceptibility). Without any natural infection in the population, we can divide the population into two categories: the proportion susceptible, x, and the proportion who have been successfully made immune to infection through vaccination, p_v. Figure 46.11 shows the relationships between these quantities. If the proportion susceptible is forced below its critical value, x^*, by immunization, there are insufficient susceptibles to permit an epidemic. The proportion of the population that must be immunized to achieve this is:

$$p_v^* = 1 - x^* = 1 - \frac{1}{R_0} \tag{46.16}$$

Thus, if $R_0 = 2$ then $p_v^* = 0.5$ so that immunizing more than 50 percent of the population will mean that, if the infection is introduced, $R < 1$ and an epidemic will not occur.

The tantalizing upshot is that a population is immune to an epidemic even though a proportion of the individuals remains susceptible. The unvaccinated individuals derive their protection from the vaccinated. Vaccination of individuals not only protects them directly, but also protects the unvaccinated. Much of the theory of immunization is about working out how large the proportion susceptible can be without leaving the community vulnerable to pathogen invasion.

Vaccination and susceptibility

In the previous section, we considered the introduction of a pathogen *after* the introduction of vaccination. However, the more usual situation is introduction of the vaccine into a population in which the pathogen is already endemic.

The fundamental concept is that, while an infection remains endemic within a population, vaccination does not reduce the proportion susceptible in the population. Instead it replaces those with a previous history of infection (and now immune) with those vaccinated. This is illustrated in Figure 46.12, using the simple model of Equations 46.12–46.14, but allowing a proportion, v, of births to enter the immune class directly (i.e. they are vaccinated before any exposure). As susceptible individuals are removed by vaccination into the immune class, the proportion susceptible *temporarily* declines. The dynamic effect is very similar to that shown in Figure 46.10. Eventually, for a given vaccination rate (which does not eliminate the infection, $v < 0.7$) there is a balance achieved between input to the susceptible pool (from births) and output from the susceptible pool, which is now divided up by the processes of infection *and* vaccination. The upshot is that the proportion susceptible regains its pre-vaccine level, but not so the proportion infected, because removal of susceptibles is now a process shared between infection and immunization.

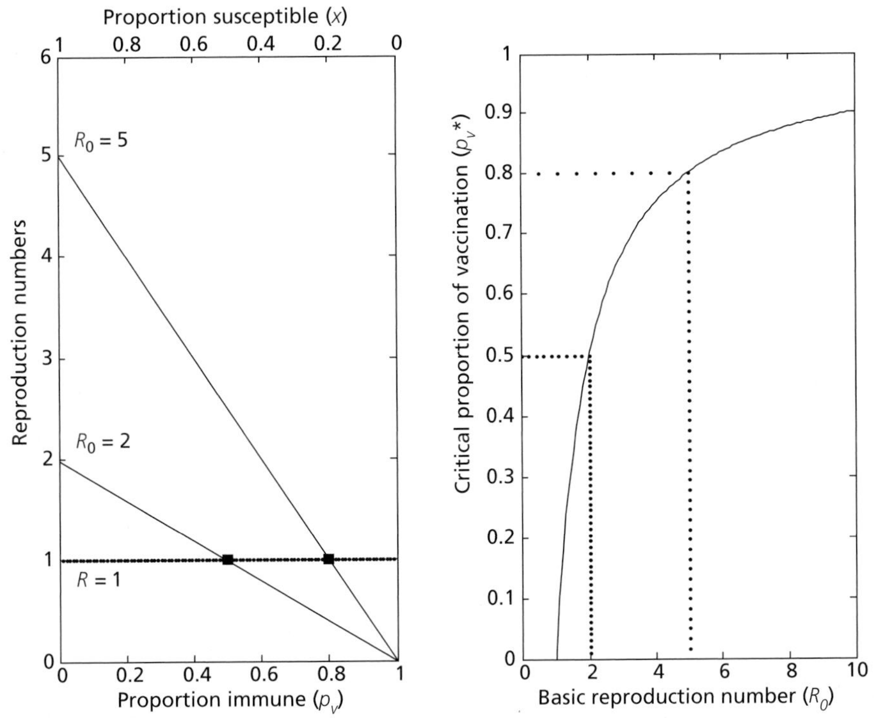

Figure 46.11 *Community immunity: the relationships between the proportion vaccinated,* p_v*, the proportion susceptible, x, and the reproduction numbers,* R_0 *and R. The left panel gives two examples, for* $R_0 = 5$ *and* $R_0 = 2$*. As the proportion immunized increases, so the effective reproduction number (solid lines) in each case decreases linearly. The critical value, i.e. R = 1, is marked. The right panel shows the relationship between the basic reproduction number and the immunization proportion required for R = 1. The two examples (*$R_0 = 5$ *and* $R_0 = 2$*) are marked as dotted lines.*

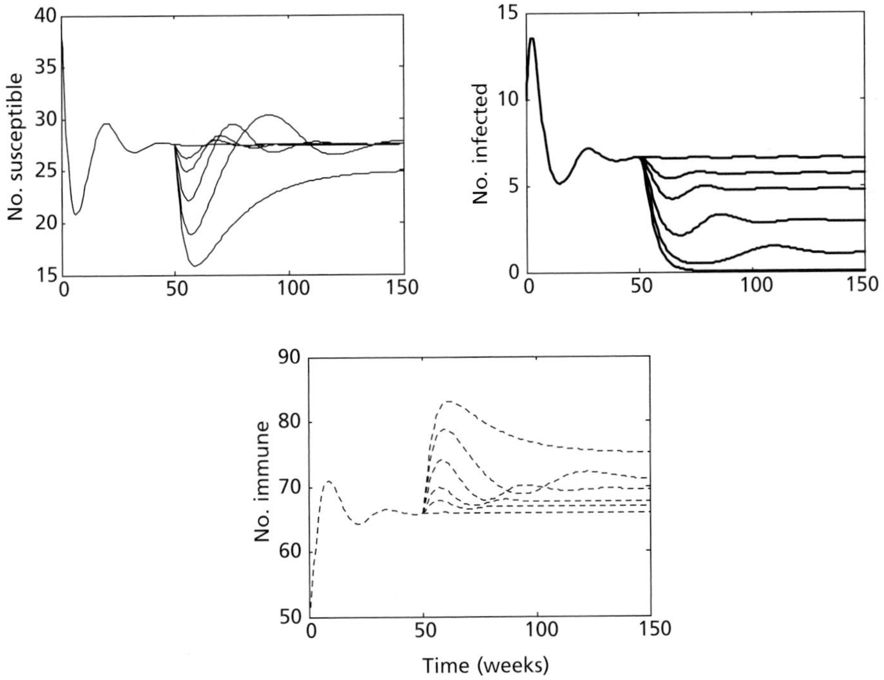

Figure 46.12 *Illustration of the dynamic effects of immunization using the model defined in Equations 46.12–46.14, modified to include vaccination at birth (see text). The panels show the numbers of susceptible, infected, and immune respectively. The model is run to equilibrium for 50 weeks, and immunization introduced at six levels (v = 0, 0.1, 0.2, 0.4, 0.6, and 0.75 where v = 0 is no vaccination). Here* $R_0 = 3.33$ *and* $p_v^* = 0.7$*.*

Only when immunization forces the proportion susceptible below the critical proportion, x^*, does the pathogen become extinct. For this example, when $v = 0.75$, which is greater than 0.7, there are not sufficient susceptibles entering the population for $R = 1$ to be maintained. In this case the infection becomes extinct, but a proportion of the population (25 percent) remains susceptible and 75 percent are immune. Note that the threshold required to eliminate infection from a population is the same as that required to protect a population from invasion (i.e. herd immunity). Again, it is not necessary to immunize all the members of a population to eliminate the infection.

Time (dynamic) effects of vaccination

Following the introduction of a vaccine, given a high enough coverage to appreciably reduce the proportion susceptible, cases of infection will decrease, often markedly so. This is particularly the case with infections that have short latent and infectious periods. A period of low incidence occurs, which is frequently ended by an alarming rebound in cases. This rebound, after what has been termed a 'honeymoon period' (McLean 1992), arises because of a rebound in the proportion susceptible well above the epidemic threshold, while incidence is low (see above and Figure 46.10). The rebound is an expected epidemiological consequence of vaccination and not a failure of vaccination policy as such, although they are frequently ascribed to a failure in vaccine or vaccine delivery. In the longer term, although vaccination coverage remains below that required for elimination, epidemics are likely to continue but less frequently than was the case before vaccination. This is because after each epidemic the rate of replenishment of the susceptible pool to epidemic proportions is reduced compared with pre-vaccination in proportion to level of vaccine coverage.

In general the impact of vaccination programs may not be immediate, because the targeting of single age classes generates only a gradually increasing proportion of the population with vaccine-induced immunity. The extreme of this would be a program of universal infant vaccination for an infection transmitted by sexual contact, such that a lag of a decade would arise before those protected by vaccination aged into the at-risk sexually active groups. In response to this it is now common to introduce routine immunization procedures with an initial one-off catch-up program of vaccination to a wide segment of the risk population.

Age effects of vaccination

Given that vaccination will tend to result in a reduction in the proportion infected, and hence lower the force of infection (see above and Figures 46.10 and 46.12), the average time for an individual, following birth, to be exposed and infected will increase. Thus the average age at infection will increase as a result of vaccination. The relationship between the transmission potential of an infection (R_0), the proportion vaccinated, v, and the long-term (equilibrium) average age at infection, A_v, is:

$$A_v = \frac{L}{R_0(1-v)} \tag{46.17}$$

where L is the life expectancy at birth. This is shown in Figure 46.13 for an archetypal virus (also assuming one survival type where all individuals born live until the average life expectancy from birth). Clearly, the effect on A_v is greater for higher levels of coverage, for less transmissible infections (lower R_0), the younger the age at delivery (i.e. where the proportion susceptible is higher), and for nonselective rather than selective vaccination.

The implications of increasing the average age at infection are various (Nokes and Anderson 1988; Anderson and May 1991), dependent, for example, on the age-related nature of disease caused by infection (see also Coleman et al. 2001). Where, like measles, the risk of mortality declines with age, a rise in age at infection in those who missed vaccination will translate into an additional indirect benefit of the vaccine program.

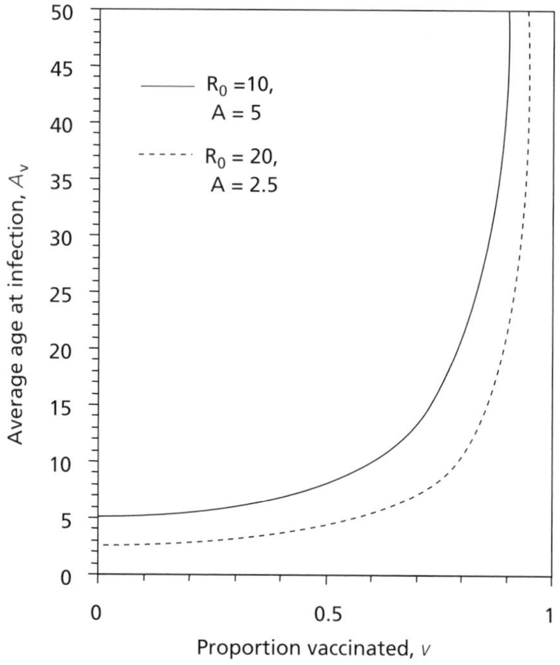

Figure 46.13 Vaccination increases the average age at infection. The relationship between the proportion vaccinated at birth, v, and the new average age at infection under such vaccination pressure, A_v, is shown for two infections with different reproductive capacities. Where the value of R_0 (20) is highest, and thus the average age at infection, A, in the absence of vaccination is lowest, the impact of a specific level of vaccine coverage on A_v is, in absolute terms, less than for the infection with lower R_0 (higher A) – although the proportional change is equal. (Adapted from McLean 1992.)

This would also apply to HBV infection and the risk of developing long-term carriage (Medley et al. 2001). In contrast, where the risk of disease increases appreciably with age, e.g. the risk of intrauterine infection from rubella which increases nonlinearly in relation to fertility, the beneficial effect of a particular vaccine program in reducing cases of infection may be severely undermined by the increased risk of severe disease arising from those cases that remain and occur at an older age (Anderson and Grenfell 1986). Observational evidence that supports this theoretical prediction was a recent epidemic of rubella among women of childbearing age in Greece (Panagiotopoulos et al. 1999).

In parallel with the increase in average age at infection resulting from vaccination, the average age of the proportion susceptible will increase (Nokes and Anderson 1988). Again, this is supported by data (Ukkonen and Von Bonsdorf 1988; Ukkonen 1996; Bahri et al. 2003). As different age groups show differing behavior, e.g. mixing patterns, changes in the age distribution of susceptibles may appreciably alter the observed epidemiology of the infection where the behavior in question is related to the route of transmission. For example, studies demonstrate that the susceptible risk of exposure to a variety of viral infections (e.g. MMR, HBV, pertussis) changes with age, presumably because of age-related changes in mixing, and other behavioral characteristics (Anderson and May 1985; Nokes et al. 1986; Edmunds et al. 1997). A general trend appears to be for a decrease in the force of infection with increasing age. Thus, vaccination tends to move susceptibles into older age groups where they are both less likely to acquire infection and less likely to transmit it. One outcome of this phenomenon is that the predicted vaccination coverage for herd immunity is diminished.

Vaccine characteristics

Vaccines are usually imperfect. The immunogenic and reactogenic characteristics of vaccines are central to predictions of their impact at a population level. Most successful vaccines have been developed against infectious agents possessing a single serotype, i.e. all variants are antigenically similar, and the host immune system sees them as the same entity with equal variant specific to variant cross-immunity. The immunogenic properties have been classified into three parameters: take, degree, and duration (Halloran et al. 1992; McLean and Blower 1993): 'take' is the proportion of vaccinated individuals who produce an immunological response to the vaccine; 'degree' is the degree of protection provided by the immunological response generated by the vaccine; and 'duration' is the time span of the immunological response.

These three attributes capture both variability between individuals (take) and the average response within those individuals that respond (degree and duration). The efficacy of a vaccine is the combined effect of a vaccine within an individual (and is a combination of all three characteristics). The effectiveness of a vaccine is a measure of the combined effect of a vaccine within a population. The effectiveness thus includes the results of herd immunity, and includes the protection given to the nonvaccinated individuals.

Delivering the vaccine

Mechanisms for delivering vaccine to the target population vary considerably. The reasons for these differences arise from (1) the need to target individuals most at risk, e.g. *Haemophilus influenzae* in infants versus hepatitis B in drug-using adults; (2) existence of mechanisms by which to deliver vaccines efficiently, e.g. maternal–child health services or general practice clinics; and (3) different transmission routes.

From the perspective of representing the delivery mechanisms accurately in models, the key characteristics are (1) age at delivery, (2) proportion receiving vaccine, (3) vaccine failure rate, and (4) selectivity of vaccination based on past disease, risk group, or vaccine history. Model structures may need to alter to reflect the particular mechanisms of delivery, e.g. universal infant vaccination might be modeled most simply as the redirection of a proportion (v) of all individuals born into the population into a vaccine-immunized class whereas the remainder ($1 - v$) enter other population classes – usually the susceptible class (see Figure 46.12). This assumes 0 percent primary vaccine failure, no influence of maternal-derived specific antibody, and random delivery of vaccine, i.e. no overt selection procedure for vaccination. However, this simple model might not adequately describe the situation if the vaccine is neutralized by the presence of maternal antibody (e.g. live attenuated vaccines), or must be delivered across a range of age classes as in campaign or catch-up programs. In these instances, it will be more appropriate to consider age classes within the model structure.

The assumption of random delivery is implicit within most models, and in the estimation of summary parameters such as the herd immunity threshold. The basic assumption is that all susceptibles are equal, insofar as prevention of infection in any individual will prevent an equal number of future infections that would have arisen had that individual not been vaccinated. However, not all individuals are equal with respect to transmission: certain age groups may have higher rates of contact within their own and with other age groups (e.g. important in transmission of aerosol-transmitted infection); core groups exist in relation to the transmission of infections by sexual contact; super-spreaders have been suspected in recent severe acute respiratory syndrome (SARS) outbreaks in east Asia (Riley et al. 2003). So, targeting such groups with vaccine has a disproportionately large, indirect, protective effect at the community level. In a different way, the control of smallpox through targeted vaccination of contacts to suspected cases illustrates a nonrandom delivery mechanism. In either case, the level of effective coverage required to develop herd immunity will be significantly less than that predicted through random delivery of vaccination, provided, of course, that the identification of 'super-spreaders' or contacts is accurate.

From an economic perspective, selectivity in delivery of vaccine may have cost–benefit implications, e.g. the benefits of selectively targeting highest risk groups (such as individuals attending STI clinics receiving HBV vaccine), with reduced numbers of vaccines delivered, may be outweighed by the costs associated with delivering the vaccine, which might involve prior screening for susceptibility and counseling (Williams et al. 1996).

Vaccination by repeated campaigns

The usual notion of a vaccination program is to vaccinate individuals as they pass some age gateway, e.g. infant vaccination schedules for diphtheria/tetanus/polio (DTP), HBV, *Haemophilus influenzae* b (Hib). However, vaccination across an age segment of a population has gained prominence in the last two decades either as one-off campaigns for the prevention of suspected epidemics or for 'catch-up' purposes, or repeated campaigns or pulses of vaccine aimed toward elimination. The idea is not new, and indeed, in the late 1950s, modeling studies of measles campaign interventions helped select the time interval between measles campaigns in west Africa, and led to temporary elimination of measles circulation for 3 years. More recently, repeated national vaccination days through social mobilization significantly contributed to the success in Latin America and the Caribbean in controlling measles and polio in the early to mid-1990s. This strategy has subsequently been extended globally for polio with remarkable success, and increasingly is part of accelerated measles control programs.

The principle underlying the idea of pulse vaccination is the targeting and removal of a large proportion of susceptible individuals in a short space of time through vaccination, thus suppressing the proportion susceptible below the threshold required to maintain chains of transmission, i.e. $R < 1$. This leads to a rapid decline in incident cases, particularly if the infectious agent in question has a short infectious period. If this process is repeated at a frequency that prevents the susceptible proportion ever rising to epidemic proportions, inevitably the infection must be eliminated.

This principle is schematically presented in the Figure 46.14. Based on this understanding it is possible to establish some simple expressions characterizing the frequency of campaigns given a particular level of campaign vaccine coverage. At its simplest, if a proportion v' of the population (i.e. of susceptibles if applied at random) is effectively vaccinated in a single pulse, then the time taken until the effective reproductive number attains unity ($R = 1$), is the pulse interval, given by:

$$T_v = \frac{v' x^*}{f} = v' A \quad (46.18)$$

where f is the proportion of the population born each unit of time (e.g. year) and A is the average age at infection (before vaccination) (Nokes and Swinton 1997). Furthermore, if routine universal immunization (at

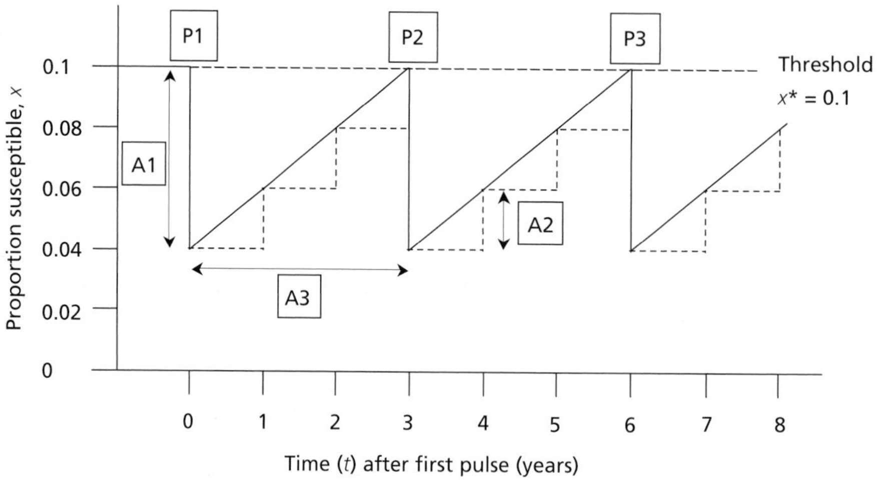

Figure 46.14 *Principle of pulse vaccination. A proportion, $v' = 0.6$ (i.e. 60 percent) of all individuals are vaccinated in pulses P1–P3 at times 0, 3, 6, . . . et seq., when the proportion of the population susceptible is at its epidemic threshold (i.e. $x = x^* = 0.1$ or 10 percent, arrow A1). Thus the proportion susceptible is reduced by 6 percent (i.e. $v'x^* = 0.06$). Subsequent to each pulse, susceptibles increase at a maximum rate of $f = 0.02$ per year (A2) as a result of births (i.e. 2 percent of the population are born – and die – each year), assuming no continued infection (which would otherwise reduce the rate of replenishment of susceptibles). Thus, in 3 years (A3) the deficit in susceptibles caused by the vaccine pulse has been recruited by births, regaining epidemic proportion ($x = x^*$) whence a further pulse is due. (Taken from Nokes and Swinton 1997.)*

around birth) is in place, at an effective coverage of v, then this slows the rate of replenishment of the susceptible pool, and extends the pulse interval:

$$T_v = \frac{v' A}{1 - v} \tag{46.19}$$

Thus we obtain some general concepts about what is important in determining the program requirements for control through pulse vaccination, namely epidemiology and demography (i.e. x^* and f, which define A) and programmatics (i.e. v' and v). So that, given two infections that differ in their transmissibility such that one has a lower average age at infection than the other, then, within the same demographic context, control of infection 1 will either require more frequent pulses, or higher level campaign coverage, than infection 2. This is of some practical value in informing policy makers. In particular, the timing of pulses should be determined by the infection.

More generally vaccination is applied to specific age groups, e.g. under 5 year olds, where it is assumed most susceptibles are, and thus vaccine (which is usually delivered irrespective of past history of disease or vaccination) will be most efficiently used. Consequently, if effective vaccine coverage is not 100 percent, susceptible individuals may accumulate in older age groups, beyond the reach of childhood vaccination, which may alter the predictions of when subsequent pulses are required. This strategy may also accumulate numbers of at-risk individuals, e.g. women of childbearing age susceptible to rubella.

Again, this model deals with the issues very simplistically. More useful models for predictive purposes require explicit descriptions of these features, i.e. age structure, age-related mixing rates, accurate demographic schedules (Nokes and Swinton 1997). Such models thus become more specific to particular locations and setting and less general, i.e. they lose the quality of general insights to be gained from the 'too simple' models.

MODEL APPLICATION

In this section, we discuss some examples where models have been used to address specific problems. There are many types of model, some of which we have referenced here: none of them is 'right' in the sense that it captures reality; many of them will be 'useful' in the sense that they provide insight, understanding, and some quantitative predictions.

The question remains, for the non-modeler, of how to judge the quality of a model. There are two aspects. First, the assumptions used to design the model should be clearly and explicitly stated. You, the reader, should decide what processes you think are important (e.g. host age and gender) and determine if they are included. To simplify, models usually have to 'average' over heterogeneities, e.g. if the modeler does not believe that host gender has any effect, the model will have 'people' as its fundamental unit, implicitly taking an average of male and female. If there are significant differences between genders, the average will not be sensible and the model results are less likely to be useful.

Second, and more difficult for the nonspecialist, is that the model defined should be analyzed and solved properly. The best advice is to treat the model as any other technical, laboratory procedure. In that case you will be looking for some demonstration that the results are reliable, and that, in defined and known circumstances, the model produces the expected results.

Design of vaccination programmes: MMR

Rubella occupies a unique position in viral infections. A solid, life-long immunity develops after either infection or vaccination, and the disease caused by infection is solely related to infection during pregnancy. The objective of a vaccination program is clear – to reduce the incidence of congenital rubella syndrome (CRS). Given the relative simplicity, there have been several models developed that address this problem (e.g. Anderson and May 1983; Anderson and Grenfell 1986; Massad et al. 1994, 1995; van der Heijden et al. 1998; Edmunds et al. 2000).

The results of these models (borne out by observation) demonstrate the dangers of vaccinating at coverages well below that required for elimination. Although those individuals vaccinated are protected, those who are not vaccinated experience an increased average age at infection and hence a greater risk of disease. The population level benefit derived from the vaccinated does not necessarily outweigh the worsened situation in the unvaccinated. This situation is complicated when vaccine is available through private purchase, because the distribution of benefit and detriment might be expected to exacerbate inequalities (Vynnycky et al. 2003).

To prevent recurrent epidemics in a vaccinated population, it has become increasingly common to recommend multiple schedules, i.e. vaccine is offered twice at different ages (Babad et al. 1995). The two-dose MMR vaccine program in the UK was supported by modeling, as was the MR 'catch-up' campaign (Gay et al. 1995).

Design of vaccination programmes: hepatitis B virus

The disease caused by HBV infection can be divided into acute and chronic. Acute disease occurs during the weeks and months after infection, and, like many other viral infections (e.g. rubella), the risk of disease probably increases with age at infection. If the immune response is able to clear the infection, the individual is left solidly immune to further infection. The alternative outcome is that a chronic infection develops and individuals become infectious carriers, and can remain so for many years. The risk of developing chronic carriage is highly age dependent: over 90 percent for infected infants and perhaps 5 percent for adults. The sequelae of chronic carriage include cirrhosis and primary hepatic cancer. There are safe, cheap, and effective vaccines to prevent acute infection. How should they be used?

The answer to this question will depend on the epidemiology of the infection, which varies dramatically across the globe. In The Gambia (west Africa) HBV is a childhood infection, with over 80 percent of children infected by the age of 10 years. The exact route of transmission is essentially unknown. As the risk of developing carriage is higher for those infected as children, the proportion of the population with chronic infection in areas of high endemicity is also high (perhaps as high as 10 percent). In complete contrast, in countries such as the UK, HBV is essentially an adult infection, with the majority of transmission associated with sexual contact or intravenous drug use. Consequently, carriage is relatively rare, and certainly less than 1 percent in the general population (Hahne et al. 2004). Between these two extremes, there is a whole range of endemicities (e.g. Coursaget et al. 1994).

There is little doubt that immunization is indicated in areas of high endemicity (e.g. Edmunds et al. 1996), but in low endemic populations the risk of infection is so low that there is some debate as to whether mass immunization is required, and is essentially a cost-effectiveness issue (see below). However, the relationship between average age at infection and probability of developing carriage provides a possible explanation for the global variation in HBV endemicity (Medley et al. 2001). If this process is important, the effect of vaccination is further enhanced.

Cost-effectiveness and health economics

Decisions concerning the implementation of any public health intervention should involve a consideration of the economic costs and expected health gains. Models of the type discussed here are capable of providing predictions of the latter, but care needs to be taken to ensure that the two frameworks are compatible in terms of scope (or perspective) and discounting. In particular, the prediction of the health impact of introducing a vaccine should include consideration of the effect on unprotected individuals (Edmunds et al. 1999).

Quantitative prediction

As mathematical models deal with numbers, for most non-modelers it would seem that the principal use of models should be to provide quantitative predictions. However, we hope that this chapter has demonstrated that accurate quantitative prediction is very difficult, and that qualitative prediction and increased understanding are the best output. Even in situations where the only value of the model is numerical prediction (e.g. Ghani et al. 2003), the predictions provide a test of our understanding; if the predictions are wrong, clearly there are processes that are not included or fully understood – the model is wrong. Note, however, that, if predictions prove correct, this is not proof of model correctness. In situations where models are intended to guide policy, testing them against data through prediction does provide some validation. When models are not validated against data, they have no such empirical support.

Evolution

Another unique feature of infectious disease (in contrast to noninfectious) is that the organisms involved (hosts and pathogens) are subject to evolutionary change. As pathogens usually have a much shorter generation time than their hosts, they are expected to evolve faster. In terms of vaccination, a pathogen strain that is able to circumvent the immunity provided by a vaccine has a large population of 'susceptibles' to infect. However, McLean (1995) argues persuasively that, even if such an escape mutant occurs, it will be less infectious and therefore easier to control than the original pathogen. Until such an event arises and is well documented, these predictions remain untested.

CONCLUSIONS

Given a reasonable understanding of the natural history of an infection within the typical individual and the key factors leading to transmission between individuals, mathematical models may be developed that capture the essence of infection dynamics within a population of hosts. Such models can be put to various uses in relation to vaccine intervention, ranging from developing our understanding of underlying principles to detailed cost-effectiveness analyses.

To date, most modeling work has been undertaken retrospectively to understand why things have or have not happened as a result of vaccine intervention. However, the understanding that arises from using quantitative methods to study the transmission dynamics of infectious disease is becoming widespread. Fine (1994) suggests that it is as much the conceptual issues that modeling has developed which has been instructive to those on the policy-making committees, rather than a targeted modeling study that has led the specific decision being made.

Our own perspective, of course, is that modeling should be a requirement for the assessment of any public health intervention, including vaccination. But that this modeling should take its place as a source of information and a vehicle for testing knowledge and understanding, rather than as a definitive prediction of outcome. To return to our bridge analogy – building a bridge without predicting its effect on traffic flow or probability of collapse is irresponsible, so why implement a vaccination program without calculating its expected effects?

REFERENCES

Anderson, R.M. and Grenfell, B.T. 1986. Quantitative investigations of different vaccination policies for the control of congenital-rubella syndrome (CRS) in the United Kingdom. *J Hygiene*, **96**, 305–33.

Anderson, R.M. and May, R.M. 1983. Vaccination against rubella and measles: quantitative investigations of different policies. *J Hygiene*, **90**, 259–325.

Anderson, R.M. and May, R.M. 1985. Vaccination and herd-immunity to infectious diseases. *Nature*, **318**, 323–9.

Anderson, R.M. and May, R.M. 1991. *Infectious diseases of humans: dynamics and control*. Oxford: Oxford University Press.

Anderson, R.M., Gupta, S. and May, R.M. 1991. Potential of community-wide chemotherapy or immunotherapy to control the spread of HIV-1. *Nature*, **350**, 356–9.

Babad, H.R., Nokes, D.J., et al. 1995. Predicting the impact of measles vaccination in England and Wales – model validation and analysis of policy options. *Epidemiol Infect*, **114**, 319–44.

Bahri, O., Ben Halima, M., et al. 2003. Measles surveillance and control in Tunisia: 1979–2000. *Vaccine*, **21**, 440–5.

Bartlett, M.S. 1960. *Stochastic population models in ecology and epidemiology*. London: Methuen & Co. Ltd.

Becker, N.G. 1989. *Analysis of infectious disease data (Monographs on Applied Probability and Statistics)*. London: Chapman & Hall/CRC.

Blower, S.M. and Boe, C. 1993. Sex acts, sex partners, and sex budgets – implications for risk factor-analysis and estimation of HIV transmission probabilities. *J AIDS Hum Retrovirol*, **6**, 1347–52.

Coleman, P.G., Perry, B.D. and Woolhouse, M.E.J. 2001. Endemic stability – a veterinary idea applied to human public health. *Lancet*, **357**, 1284–6.

Coursaget, P., Gharbi, Y., et al. 1994. Familial clustering of hepatitis B virus infections and prevention of perinatal transmission by immunization with a reduced number of doses in an area. *Vaccine*, **12**, 275–8.

Edmunds, W.J., Medley, G.F. and Nokes, D.J. 1996. The transmission dynamics and control of hepatitis B virus in the Gambia. *Statist Med*, **15**, 2215–33.

Edmunds, W.J., O'Callaghan, C.J. and Nokes, D.J. 1997. Who mixes with whom? A method to determine the contact patterns of adults that may lead to the spread of airborne infections. *Proc R Soc Lond Ser B*, **264**, 949–57.

Edmunds, W.J., Medley, G.F. and Nokes, D.J. 1999. Evaluating the cost-effectiveness of vaccination programs: A dynamic perspective. *Statist Med*, **18**, 3263–82.

Edmunds, W.J., van de Heijden, O.G., et al. 2000. Modeling rubella in Europe. *Epidemiol Infect*, **125**, 617–34.

Fine, P.E.M. 1993. Herd immunity: history, theory, practice. *Epidemiol Rev*, **15**, 265–302.

Fine, P.E.M. 1994. The contribution of modeling to vaccination policy. In: Cutts, F.T. and Smith, P.G. (eds), *Vaccination and world health*. Chichester: John Wiley & Sons Ltd, 177–94.

Gay, N.J., Hesketh, L.M., et al. 1995. Interpretation of serological surveillance data for measles using mathematical-models – implications for vaccine strategy. *Epidemiol Infect*, **115**, 139–56.

Ghani, A.C., Ferguson, N.M., et al. 2003. Short-term projections for variant Creutzfeldt-Jakob disease onsets. *Statist Methods Med Res*, **12**, 191–201.

Gomes, M.G.M., White, L.J. and Medley, G.F. 2004. Infection, reinfection, and vaccination under suboptimal immune protection: epidemiological perspectives. *J Theor Biol*, **228**, 539–49.

Hahne, S., Ramsay, M., et al. 2004. Incidence and routes of transmission of hepatitis B virus in England and Wales, 1995–2000: implications for immunization policy. *J Clin Virol*, **29**, 211–20.

Halloran, M.E., Haber, M. and Longini, I.M. 1992. Interpretation and estimation of vaccine efficacy under heterogeneity. *Am J Epidemiol*, **136**, 328–43.

McLean, A.R. 1992. Mathematical modeling of the immunization of populations. *Rev Med Virol*, **2**, 141–52.

McLean, A.R. 1995. Vaccination, evolution and changes in the efficacy of vaccines: a theoretical framework. *Proc R Soc Lond Ser B*, **261**, 389–93.

McLean, A.R. and Blower, S.M. 1993. Imperfect vaccines and herd immunity to HIV. *Proc R Soc Lond Ser B*, **253**, 9–13.

Massad, E., Burattini, M.N., et al. 1994. A model-based design of a vaccination strategy against rubella in a nonimmunized community of Sao-Paulo State, Brazil. *Epidemiol Infect*, **112**, 579–94.

Massad, E., Azevedoneto, R.S., et al. 1995. Assessing the efficacy of a mixed vaccination strategy against rubella in Sao-Paulo, Brazil. *Int J Epidemiol*, **24**, 842–50.

Medley, G.F. 1996. Conflicts between individual and communities in treatment and control. In: Isham, V.S. and Medley, G.F. (eds), *Mathematical models of human diseases*. Cambridge: Cambridge University Press.

Medley, G.F., Lindop, N.A., et al. 2001. Hepatitis-B virus endemicity: heterogeneity, catastrophic dynamics and control. *Nat Med*, **7**, 619–24.

Nokes, D.J. and Anderson, R.M. 1988. The use of mathematical models in the epidemiological study of infectious diseases and in the design of mass immunization programs. *Epidemiol Infect*, **101**, 1–20.

Nokes, D.J. and Anderson, R.M. 1991. Vaccine safety versus vaccine efficacy in mass immunization programs. *Lancet*, **338**, 1309–12.

Nokes, D.J. and Swinton, J. 1997. Vaccination in pulses: a strategy for global eradication of measles and polio? *Trends Microbiol*, **5**, 14–19.

Nokes, D.J., Anderson, R.M. and Anderson, M.J. 1986. Rubella epidemiology in South East England. *J Hygiene*, **96**, 291–304.

Nowak, M. and May, R.M. 2000. *Virus dynamics: mathematical principles of immunology and virology*. Oxford: Oxford University Press.

Panagiotopoulos, T., Antoniadou, I. and Valassi-Adam, E. 1999. Increase in congenital rubella occurrence after immunization in Greece: retrospective survey and systematic review. *BMJ*, **319**, 1462–7.

Riley, S., Fraser, C., et al. 2003. Transmission dynamics of the etiological agent of SARS in Hong Kong: Impact of public health interventions. *Science*, **300**, 1961–6.

Ukkonen, P. 1996. Rubella immunity and morbidity: Impact of different vaccination programs in Finland 1979–1992. *Scand J Infect Dis*, **28**, 31–5.

Ukkonen, P. and Von Bonsdorf, C.-H. 1988. Rubella immunity and morbidity; effects of vaccination in Finland. *Scand J Infect Dis*, **20**, 255–9.

van der Heijden, O.G., Conyn-van Spaendonck, M.A.E., et al. 1998. A model-based evaluation of the national immunization program against rubella infection and congenital rubella syndrome in The Netherlands. *Epidemiol Infect*, **121**, 653–71.

Vynnycky, E., Gay, N.J. and Cutts, F.T. 2003. The predicted impact of private sector MMR vaccination on the burden of congenital rubella syndrome. *Vaccine*, **21**, 2708–19.

Williams, J.R., Nokes, D.J., et al. 1996. The transmission dynamics of hepatitis B in the UK: A mathematical model for evaluating costs and effectiveness of immunization programs. *Epidemiol Infect*, **116**, 71–89.

Woolhouse, M.E.J., Dye, C., et al. 1997. Heterogeneities in the transmission of infectious agents: Implications for the design of control programs. *Proc Natl Acad Sci USA*, **94**, 338–42.

Index

Notes

(Fig.) and (Tab.) refer to figures and tables respectively. *vs.* indicates a comparison or differential diagnosis.

To save space in the index, the following abbreviations have been used

APCs - antigen-presenting cells
BCE - B-cell epitope
BCR - B-cell receptor
CTL - cytotoxic T cell (lymphocyte)
G-CSF - granulocyte colony stimulating factor
HLA - human leukocyte antigen
ICAM - intercellular adhesion molecule
IL - interleukin
LT - *Escherichia coli* heat labile enterotoxin
M-CSF - macrophage colony stimulating factor
MHC - major histocompatibility complex
NK cells - natural killer cells
SCF - stem cell factor
SLE - systemic lupus erythematosus
TCE- T-cell epitope
TCR - T-cell receptor
Th1 - T helper cells type 1
Th2 - T helper cells type 2

Complete table of contents for *Topley & Wilson's Microbiology and Microbial Infections*

VIROLOGY, VOLUMES 1 AND 2

BACTERIOLOGY, VOLUMES 1 AND 2

MEDICAL MYCOLOGY

PARASITOLOGY

IMMUNOLOGY